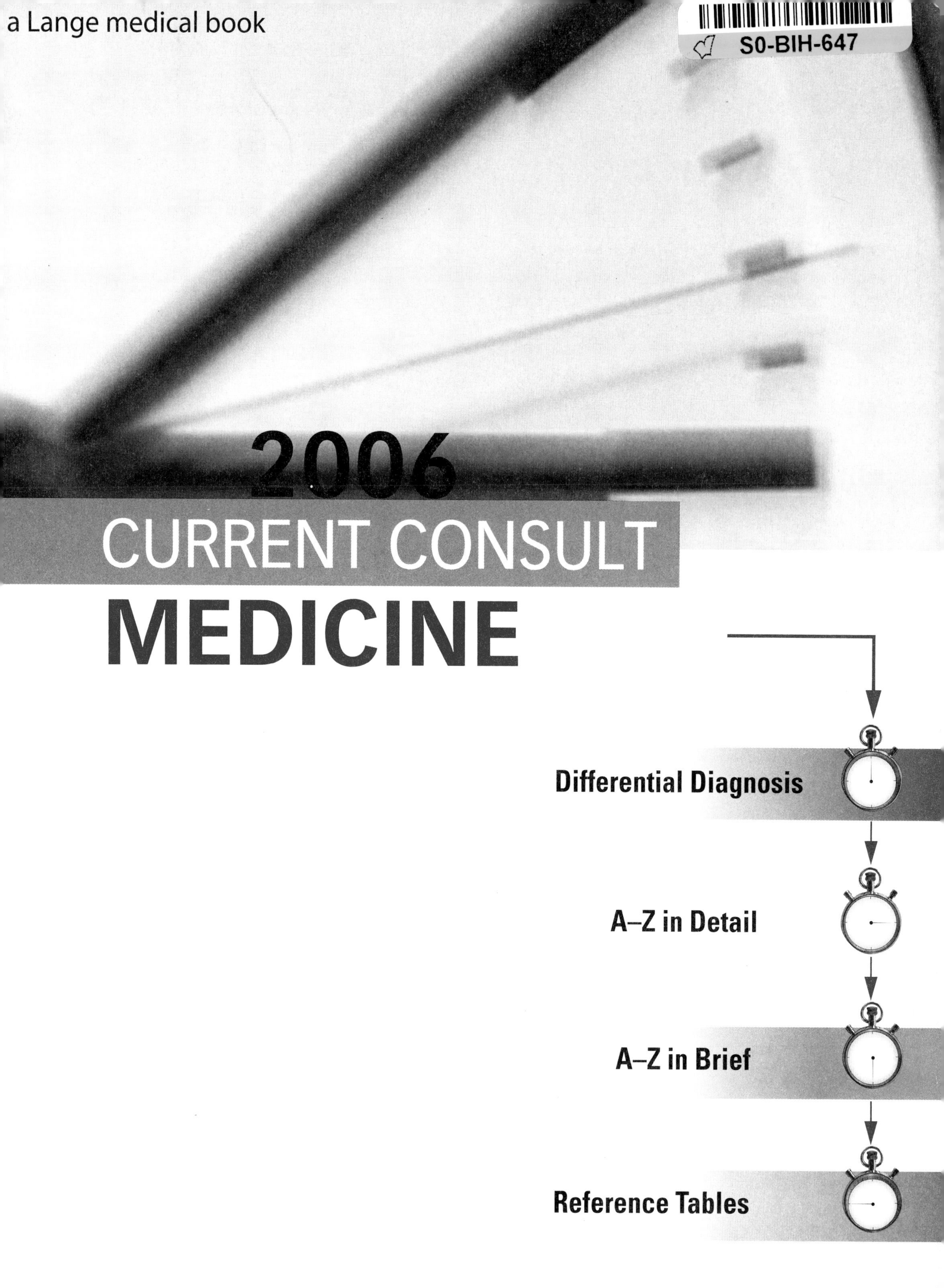
a Lange medical book
S0-BIH-647
2006
CURRENT CONSULT
MEDICINE
Differential Diagnosis
A–Z in Detail
A–Z in Brief
Reference Tables

a Lange medical book

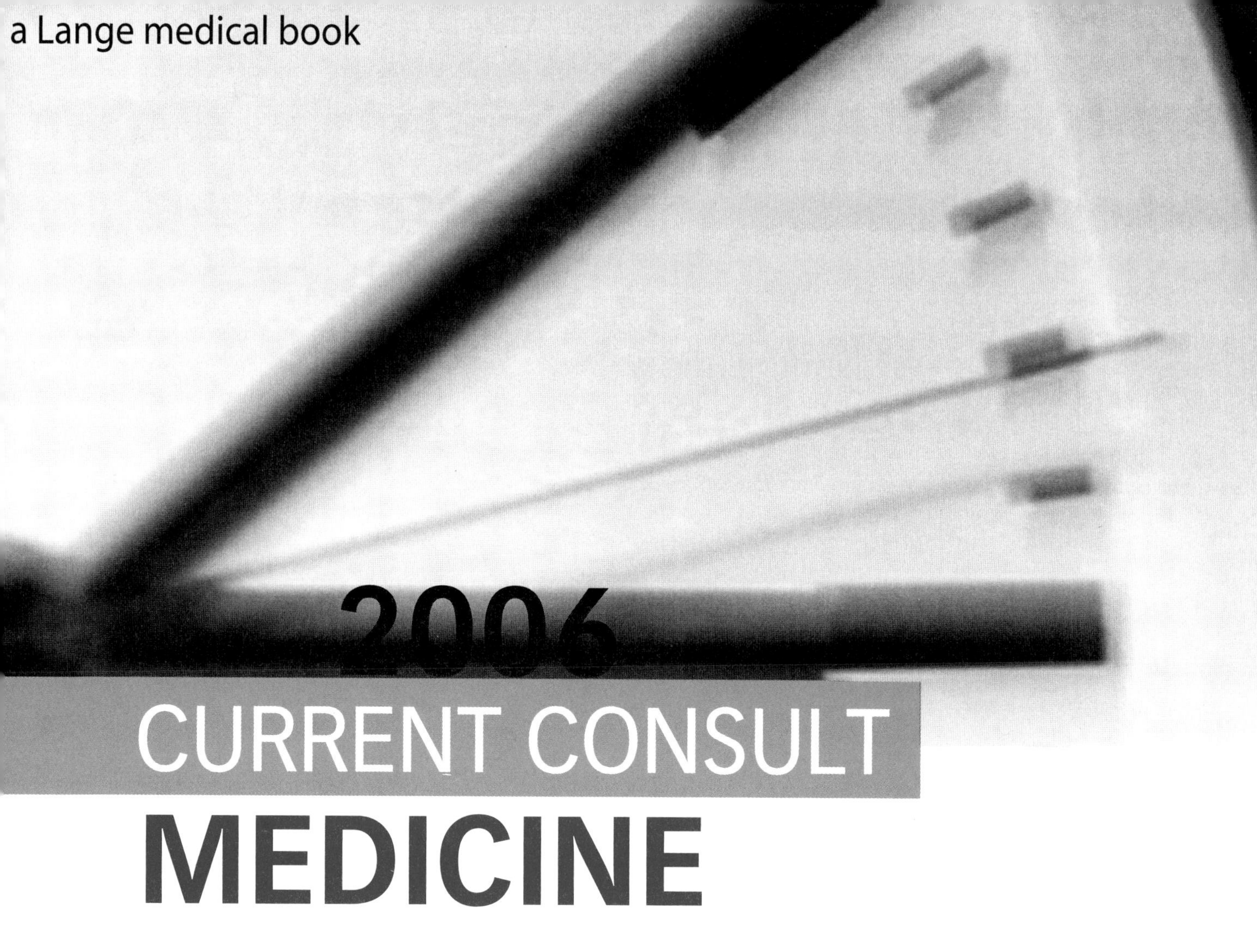

2006 CURRENT CONSULT MEDICINE

Edited by

Maxine A. Papadakis, MD
Professor of Clinical Medicine
Associate Dean for Student Affairs
School of Medicine
University of California, San Francisco

Stephen J. McPhee, MD
Professor of Medicine
Division of General Internal Medicine
Department of Medicine
University of California, San Francisco

Lange Medical Books/McGraw-Hill
Medical Publishing Division

New York Chicago San Francisco Lisbon
London Madrid Mexico City Milan New Delhi
San Juan Seoul Singapore Sydney Toronto

Current Consult: Medicine, 2006

1234567890 QPDQPD 098765

ISBN: 0-07-145892-1

Notice

Medicine is an ever-changing science. As new research and clinical experience broaden our knowledge, changes in treatment and drug therapy are required. The authors and the publisher of this work have checked with sources believed to be reliable in their efforts to provide information that is complete and generally in accord with the standards accepted at the time of publication. However, in view of the possibility of human error or changes in medical sciences, neither the authors nor the publisher nor any other party who has been involved in the preparation or publication of this work warrants that the information contained herein is in every respect accurate or complete, and they disclaim all responsibility for any errors or omissions or for the results obtained from use of the information contained in this work. Readers are encouraged to confirm the information contained herein with other sources. For example and in particular, readers are advised to check the product information sheet included in the package of each drug they plan to administer to be certain that the information contained in this work is accurate and that changes have not been made in the recommended dose or in the contraindications for administration. This recommendation is of particular importance in connection with new or infrequently used drugs.

This book was set by Silverchair Science + Communications, Inc.
The editors were Jason Malley, Harriet Lebowitz, and Barbara Holton.
The production supervisor was Philip Galea.
The art manager was Charissa Baker.
The text was designed by Eve Siegel.
The index was prepared by Kathrin Unger.
Quebecor Dubuque was printer and binder.

This book is printed on acid-free paper.

INTERNATIONAL EDITION ISBN: 0-07-110549-2

CURRENT CONSULT

Medicine: 4 Parts

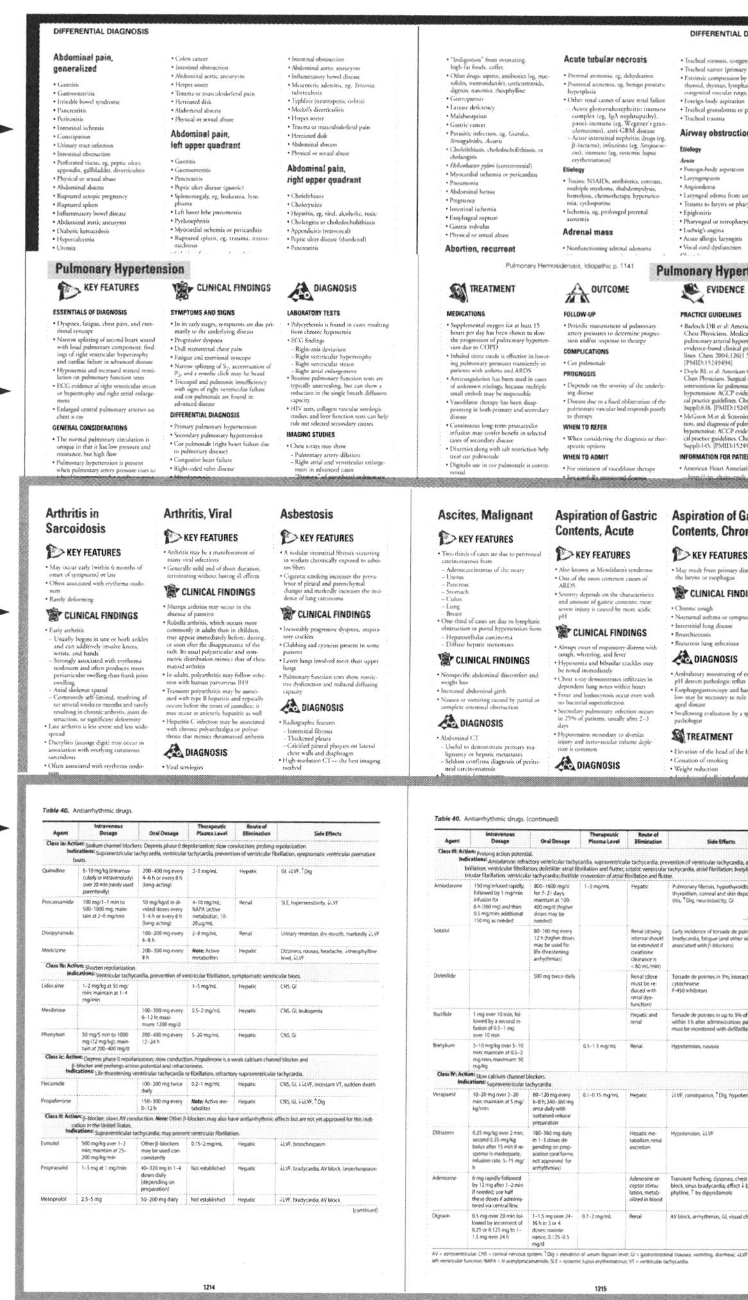

CONTENTS: Alphabetical

CONTENTS: Topical

Fluid & Electrolyte Disorders

Gastrointestinal Disorders

Genetics

Geriatrics

Gynecology

Infectious Diseases: Spirochetal

Infectious Diseases: Viral & Rickettsial

Kidney

Liver, Biliary Tract, & Pancreas

Lung

Musculoskeletal Disorders

Neurologic Disorders

Nutrition

Obstetrics

Physical Agent–Related Disorders

Poisoning & Overdose

Psychiatric Disorders

Skin, Hair, & Nails

CONTENTS: Reference Tables

Liver, Biliary Tract, and Pancreas

Gynecology

Obstetrics

Allergic Disorders

Musculoskeletal Disorders

Fluid & Electrolyte Disorders

Urology

Kidney

Neurology

Psychiatry

Endocrinology

Lipid Abnormalities

HIV Infection

Infectious Diseases

Poisoning

Genetic Disorders

Cancer

Authors & Contributors

Associate Editor

Roni F. Zeiger, MD

Fellow in Medical Informatics, VA Palo Alto Health Care System, Palo Alto, California; Clinical Instructor of Medicine, Stanford University School of Medicine, Stanford, California

Authors

Daniel C. Adelman, MD

Adjunct Professor of Medicine, Division of Allergy and Immunology, University of California, San Francisco

Michael J. Aminoff, MD, DSc, FRCP

Professor of Neurology, University of California, San Francisco; Attending Physician, University of California Medical Center, San Francisco

Robert B. Baron, MD, MS

Professor of Medicine; Associate Dean for Continuing Medical Education; Vice Chief and Director, Educational Programs, Division of General Internal Medicine; Director, Primary Care Internal Medicine Residency Program, University of California, San Francisco

Thomas Bashore, MD

Professor of Medicine; Director of Cardiology Fellowship Program, Duke University Medical Center, Durham, North Carolina

Timothy G. Berger, MD

Professor of Clinical Dermatology, Department of Dermatology, University of California, San Francisco

Peter R. Carroll, MD, FACS

Professor and Chair, Department of Urology, University of California, San Francisco

Henry F. Chambers, MD

Professor of Medicine, University of California, San Francisco; Chief, Division of Infectious Diseases, San Francisco General Hospital

Mark S. Chesnutt, MD

Associate Professor of Medicine, Pulmonary & Critical Care Medicine; Director, Medical Critical Care, Oregon Health & Science University, Portland

Richard Cohen, MD, MPH

Clinical Professor, Division of Occupational and Environmental Medicine, University of California, San Francisco

William R. Crombleholme, MD

Professor of Clinical Obstetrics & Gynecology, Columbia University College of Physicians and Surgeons, New York; Chairman, Department of Obstetrics and Gynecology, The Stamford Hospital, Stamford, Connecticut

Stuart J. Eisendrath, MD

Professor of Clinical Psychiatry, University of California, San Francisco

Paul A. Fitzgerald, MD

Clinical Professor of Medicine, Department of Medicine, Division of Endocrinology, University of California, San Francisco

Lawrence S. Friedman, MD

Professor of Medicine, Harvard Medical School, Boston, Massachusetts; Chair, Department of Medicine, Newton-Wellesley Hospital, Newton, Massachusetts; Assistant Chief of Medicine, Massachusetts General Hospital, Boston, Massachusetts

Masafumi Fukagawa, MD, PhD

Associate Professor and Director, Division of Nephrology and Dialysis Center, Kobe University School of Medicine, Japan

Armando E. Giuliano, MD

Chief of Surgical Oncology, John Wayne Cancer Institute; Director, Joyce Eisenberg Keefer Breast Center, Saint John's Health Center, Santa Monica, California

Ralph Gonzales, MD, MSPH

Associate Professor of Medicine, Epidemiology & Biostatistics, Division of General Internal Medicine, Department of Medicine, University of California, San Francisco

Christopher B. Granger, MD

Associate Professor, Department of Medicine, Division of Cardiology, Duke University Medical Center, Durham, North Carolina

Richard J. Hamill, MD

Professor, Division of Infectious Diseases, Departments of Medicine and Molecular Virology & Microbiology, Baylor College of Medicine, Houston, Texas

G. Michael Harper, MD

Associate Clinical Professor of Medicine, Geriatric Medicine, University of California School of Medicine, San Francisco; Director of Geriatrics Fellowship Training Program, San Francisco Veterans Affairs Medical Center, San Francisco, California

David B. Hellmann, MD, FACP

Mary Betty Stevens Professor of Medicine; Chairman, Department of Medicine, Johns Hopkins Bayview Medical Center, Johns Hopkins University School of Medicine, Baltimore

Harry Hollander, MD

Professor of Clinical Medicine and Director, Categorical Medicine Residency Program, University of California, San Francisco

Robert K. Jackler, MD
Sewall Professor and Chair, Department of Otolaryngology-Head and Neck Surgery, Stanford University School of Medicine, Stanford, California

Richard A. Jacobs, MD, PhD
Clinical Professor of Medicine and Clinical Pharmacy, Division of Infectious Diseases, University of California, San Francisco

C. Bree Johnston, MD
Associate Professor of Clinical Medicine, Division of Geriatrics, Department of Medicine, Veterans Affairs Medical Center, University of California, San Francisco

Michael J. Kaplan, MD
Professor, Department of Otolaryngology-Head and Neck Surgery; Professor, Neurosurgery and Surgery, Stanford University School of Medicine, Stanford, California

Mitchell H. Katz, MD
Clinical Professor of Medicine, Epidemiology & Biostatistics, University of California, San Francisco; Director of Health, San Francisco Department of Public Health

Jeffrey L. Kishiyama, MD
Assistant Clinical Professor of Medicine, University of California, San Francisco

Kiyoshi Kurokawa, MD, MACP
Adjunct Professor, Division of Health Policy, Research Center for Advanced Science, The University of Tokyo, Tokyo, Japan

Jonathan E. Lichtmacher, MD
Assistant Clinical Professor of Psychiatry, University of California, San Francisco; Associate Director, Adult Psychiatry Clinic, Langley Porter Hospitals and Clinics, University of California, San Francisco

Charles A. Linker, MD
Clinical Professor of Medicine; Director, Bone Marrow Transplant Program, Division of Hematology/Oncology, University of California, San Francisco

H. Trent MacKay, MD, MPH
Professor of Obstetrics and Gynecology, Uniformed Services, University of the Health Sciences, Bethesda, Maryland; Associate Director, Women's Health Services, National Naval Medical Center, Bethesda, Maryland

Umesh Masharani, MB, BS; MRCP(UK)
Associate Clinical Professor of Medicine, Division of Endocrinology and Metabolism, University of California, San Francisco

Barry M. Massie, MD
Professor of Medicine, University of California, San Francisco; Chief, Cardiology Division, San Francisco Veterans Affairs Medical Center

Stephen J. McPhee, MD
Professor of Medicine, Division of General Internal Medicine, Department of Medicine, University of California, San Francisco

Kenneth R. McQuaid, MD
Professor of Clinical Medicine, University of California, San Francisco; Director of Endoscopy, San Francisco Veterans Affairs Medicine Center

Louis M. Messina, MD
Professor and Chief, Division of Vascular Surgery, University of California, San Francisco

Brent R.W. Moelleken, MD, FACS
Plastic and Reconstructive Surgery; Assistant Clinical Professor, Division of Plastic Surgery, Attending Physician, University of California, Los Angeles Medical Center; Private Practice, Beverly Hills, California

Ana Moran, MD
Clinical Fellow, Department of Infectious Diseases, Baylor College of Medicine, Houston, Texas

Gail Morrison, MD
Vice Dean for Education, Director of Academic Programs, and Professor of Medicine, School of Medicine, Division of Renal-Electrolytes, University of Pennsylvania Health System, Philadelphia

Kent R. Olson, MD
Medical Director, San Francisco Division, California Poison Control System, University of California, San Francisco

Maxine A. Papadakis, MD
Professor of Clinical Medicine and Associate Dean for Student Affairs, School of Medicine, University of California, San Francisco

Thomas J. Prendergast, MD
Associate Professor of Medicine and Anesthesiology, Section of Pulmonary and Critical Care Medicine, Dartmouth-Hitchcock Medical Center, Lebanon, New Hampshire

Reed E. Pyeritz, MD, PhD
Professor of Medicine and Genetics; Chief, Division of Medical Genetics, University of Pennsylvania Health System and School of Medicine, Philadelphia

Paul Riordan-Eva, FRCS, FRCOphth
Consultant Ophthalmologist, King's College Hospital, London, United Kingdom

Hope S. Rugo, MD
Clinical Professor of Medicine and Director, Breast Oncology Clinical Trials Program, University of California, San Francisco Comprehensive Cancer Center

Wayne X. Shandera, MD

Assistant Professor of Internal Medicine, Baylor College of Medicine, Houston, Texas

Samuel A. Shelburne, MD

Assistant Professor, Department of Internal Medicine, Baylor College of Medicine, Houston, Texas

Marshall L. Stoller, MD

Professor of Urology and Vice Chairman, Department of Urology, University of California, San Francisco

John H. Stone, MD, MPH

Associate Professor of Medicine, Division of Rheumatology, Johns Hopkins University; Director, Johns Hopkins Vasculitis Center, Baltimore, Maryland

Suzanne Watnick, MD

Assistant Professor of Medicine, Division of Nephrology and Hypertension, Oregon Health & Science University, Portland; Director, Dialysis Unit, Portland VA Medical Center, Portland, Oregon

Andrew R. Zolopa, MD

Associate Professor of Medicine, Division of Infectious Diseases and Geographic Medicine, Stanford University, Stanford, California

Contributors

Erika Leemann

Medical student, University of California, San Francisco

Norna Ludeman

Medical student, University of California, San Francisco

Margaret E.M. Van Meter

Medical student, University of California, San Francisco

Guide To *Current Consult: Medicine*

To get practical, expert information on diagnosis and treatment when you just have a few minutes, rely on *Current Consult: Medicine.* It is a single-source reference designed for quick-and-easy access to the information you need in the clinical setting. The 4 parts of the book, which are color-coded, include:

Differential Diagnosis: THE DARK BLUE PAGES
A–Z in Detail: THE WHITE PAGES
A–Z in Brief: THE LIGHT BLUE PAGES
Reference Tables: THE GRAY PAGES

The **DIFFERENTIAL DIAGNOSIS** entries provide a comprehensive outline of differential diagnoses and disease etiologies for over 400 disorders and symptoms. It is derived from Diagnosaurus, the PDA program that has become an extraordinarily popular differential diagnosis tool.

The **A–Z IN DETAIL** and **A–Z IN BRIEF** present the right amount of information on each topic to give you the key diagnostic and treatment features of more than 860 diseases. To save you time, the disease entries are alphabetized. The bulleted form promotes rapid comprehension so that you can immediately apply what you learn from this quick consult on current medical practice. Each disease entry in the A–Zs IN DETAIL includes:

- Key Features: Essentials of diagnosis and general considerations
- Clinical Findings: Symptoms and signs and differential diagnosis
- Diagnosis: Laboratory tests, imaging studies, and diagnostic procedures
- Treatment: Medications, surgery, and therapeutic procedures
- Outcome: Complications, prognosis, when to refer, and when to admit sections
- Evidence: Up-to-date clinical guidelines, targeted references, and Web sites for clinicians and patients

The **REFERENCE TABLES** display specific diagnostic and treatment options to help you find the best solutions to immediate clinical problems. Using these tables, you can quickly pinpoint individual drugs and dosages.

The authors of *Current Consult: Medicine* are those you already know and trust from *Current Medical Diagnosis & Treatment,* the leading medicine textbook for both hospital and outpatient settings, now in its 45th annual edition. These authors provide the latest expert information on adult primary care topics that include gynecology, obstetrics, dermatology, otolaryngology, psychiatry, neurology, geriatrics, urology, toxicology, and ophthalmology.

HOW TO USE *CURRENT CONSULT: MEDICINE*

If you know the diagnosis for which you need an immediate consult, go directly to that disorder in the **A–Z IN DETAIL** (WHITE PAGES). In addition to the disease entries in the white pages, you will see page numbers at the top of some of the white pages that direct you to specific disorders selected for the **A–Z IN BRIEF** (LIGHT BLUE PAGES).

If, instead, you are searching for a differential diagnosis, consult the **DIFFERENTIAL DIAGNOSIS** section (DARK BLUE PAGES). After identifying the most likely disorder(s), go to **A–Z IN DETAIL** (WHITE PAGES) to get diagnosis and treatment information.

If you want to find specifics about drugs and dosages, go to the **REFERENCE TABLES** (GRAY PAGES). (See the CONTENTS: REFERENCE TABLES at the front of the book for a list of tables arranged by topics. Also, the index at the back of the book can guide you to the appropriate table for a specific drug.)

Current Consult: Medicine offers these unique features:

- Leaders in their medical specialties provide you with their expertise
- Content organized into 4 easy-to-use sections
- Bulleted clinical information and specific treatment options to give you the current medical consult you need.

PDA VERSION OF *CURRENT CONSULT: MEDICINE*

For electronic access, *Current Consult: Medicine* is also available as a PDA program (Palm and Pocket PC) on a CD, which can be purchased at your local bookstore or ordered at www.accessmedbooks.com.

Maxine A. Papadakis, MD
Stephen J. McPhee, MD
San Francisco, California
December 2005

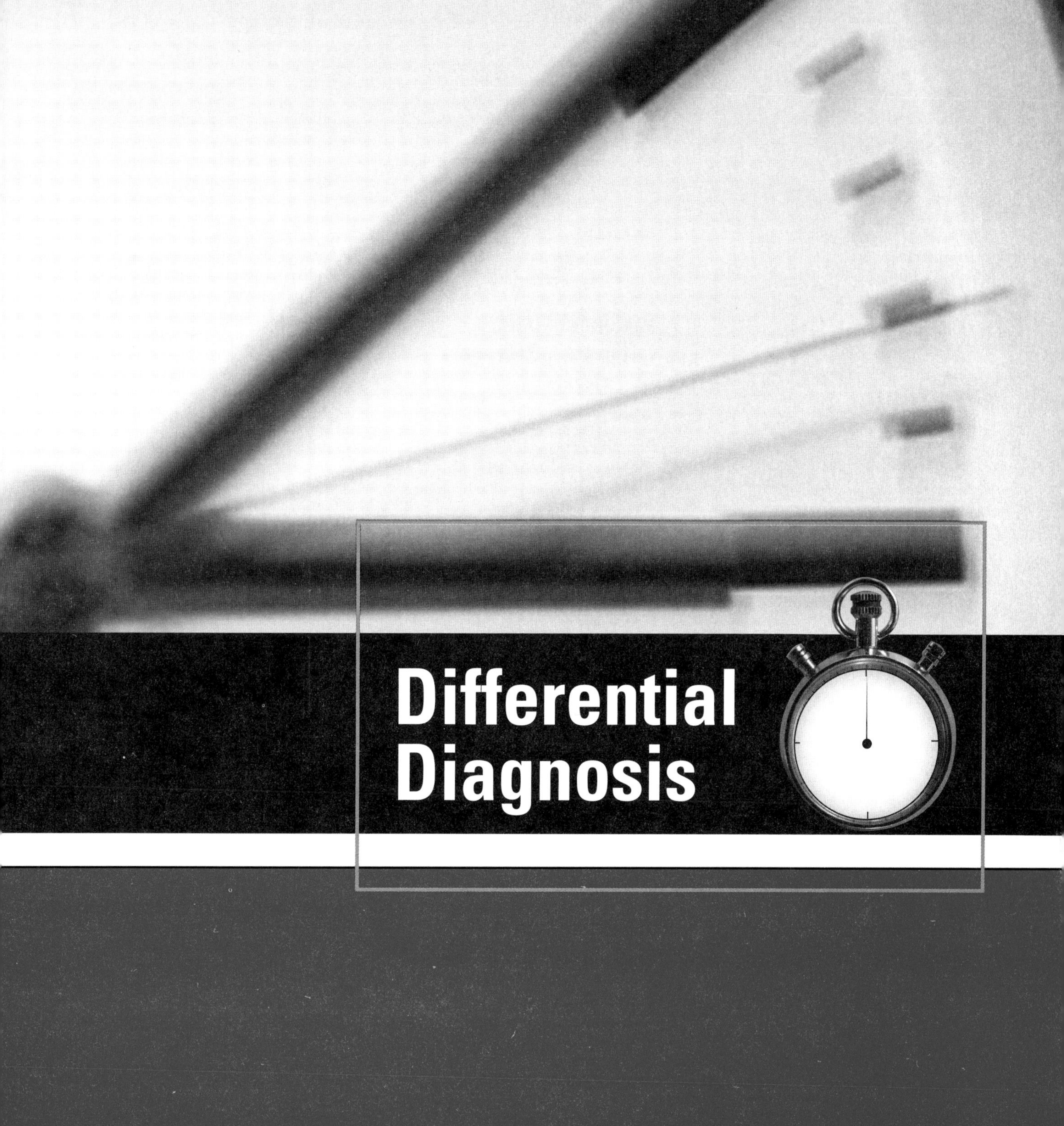

Differential Diagnosis

Abdominal pain, generalized

- Gastritis
- Gastroenteritis
- Irritable bowel syndrome
- Pancreatitis
- Peritonitis
- Intestinal ischemia
- Constipation
- Urinary tract infection
- Intestinal obstruction
- Perforated viscus, eg, peptic ulcer, appendix, gallbladder, diverticulitis
- Physical or sexual abuse
- Abdominal abscess
- Ruptured ectopic pregnancy
- Ruptured spleen
- Inflammatory bowel disease
- Abdominal aortic aneurysm
- Diabetic ketoacidosis
- Hypercalcemia
- Uremia
- Parasitic infection, eg, giardia, strongyloides, ascaris, tapeworms
- Adrenal insufficiency
- Lead poisoning
- Iron poisoning
- Polyarteritis nodosa
- Henoch-Schönlein purpura
- Porphyria, eg, acute intermittent porphyria
- Familial Mediterranean fever
- Black widow spider bite

Abdominal pain, left lower quadrant

- Diverticulitis
- Gastroenteritis or colitis
- Constipation
- Irritable bowel syndrome
- Gynecologic: pelvic inflammatory disease, ovarian torsion, ruptured ovarian cyst, tubo-ovarian abscess, endometriosis, ectopic pregnancy, mittelschmerz
- Intestinal ischemia
- Cystitis
- Hernia, eg, femoral, inguinal, umbilical
- Testicular, eg, epididymitis, testicular torsion
- Prostatitis
- Urinary calculi
- Inflammatory bowel disease
- Colon cancer
- Intestinal obstruction
- Abdominal aortic aneurysm
- Herpes zoster
- Trauma or musculoskeletal pain
- Herniated disk
- Abdominal abscess
- Physical or sexual abuse

Abdominal pain, left upper quadrant

- Gastritis
- Gastroenteritis
- Pancreatitis
- Peptic ulcer disease (gastric)
- Splenomegaly, eg, leukemia, lymphoma
- Left lower lobe pneumonia
- Pyelonephritis
- Myocardial ischemia or pericarditis
- Ruptured spleen, eg, trauma, mononucleosis
- Splenic infarct, eg, endocarditis
- Urinary calculi
- Functional or nonulcer dyspepsia
- Gastric cancer
- Diverticulitis
- Herpes zoster
- Intestinal ischemia
- Trauma or musculoskeletal pain
- Herniated disk
- Abdominal abscess
- Physical or sexual abuse

Abdominal pain, right lower quadrant

- Appendicitis
- Gastroenteritis or colitis
- Irritable bowel syndrome
- Gynecologic: pelvic inflammatory disease, ovarian torsion, ruptured ovarian cyst, tubo-ovarian abscess, endometriosis, ectopic pregnancy, mittelschmerz
- Cystitis
- Hernia, eg, femoral, inguinal, umbilical
- Testicular, eg, epididymitis, testicular torsion
- Prostatitis
- Diverticulitis
- Colon cancer
- Urinary calculi
- Intestinal ischemia
- Intestinal obstruction
- Abdominal aortic aneurysm
- Inflammatory bowel disease
- Mesenteric adenitis, eg, *Yersinia*, tuberculosis
- Typhlitis (neutropenic colitis)
- Meckel's diverticulitis
- Herpes zoster
- Trauma or musculoskeletal pain
- Herniated disk
- Abdominal abscess
- Physical or sexual abuse

Abdominal pain, right upper quadrant

- Cholelithiasis
- Cholecystitis
- Hepatitis, eg, viral, alcoholic, toxic
- Cholangitis or choledocholithiasis
- Appendicitis (retrocecal)
- Peptic ulcer disease (duodenal)
- Pancreatitis
- Functional or nonulcer dyspepsia
- Liver abscess
- Liver, pancreatic, or biliary tract cancer
- Ischemic hepatopathy (shock liver)
- Hepatic vein obstruction (Budd-Chiari syndrome)
- Right lower lobe pneumonia
- Pyelonephritis
- Urinary calculi
- Fitz-Hugh-Curtis syndrome (with pelvic inflammatory disease)
- Liver cell adenoma
- Herpes zoster
- Trauma or musculoskeletal pain
- Herniated disk
- Abdominal abscess
- Intestinal ischemia
- Physical or sexual abuse

Abdominal pain, upper or epigastric

- Functional or nonulcer dyspepsia (most common)
- Peptic ulcer disease
- Gastroesophageal reflux
- Gastritis, eg, NSAIDs, alcohol, stress, *Helicobacter pylori*, pernicious anemia
- Pancreatitis or pancreatic cancer

- "Indigestion" from overeating, high-fat foods, coffee
- Other drugs: aspirin, antibiotics (eg, macrolides, metronidazole), corticosteroids, digoxin, narcotics, theophylline
- Gastroparesis
- Lactase deficiency
- Malabsorption
- Gastric cancer
- Parasitic infection, eg, *Giardia, Strongyloides, Ascaris*
- Cholelithiasis, choledocholithiasis, or cholangitis
- *Helicobacter pylori* (controversial)
- Myocardial ischemia or pericarditis
- Pneumonia
- Abdominal hernia
- Pregnancy
- Intestinal ischemia
- Esophageal rupture
- Gastric volvulus
- Physical or sexual abuse

Abortion, recurrent

Etiology

- Luteal phase insufficiency (insufficient progesterone)
- Diabetes mellitus
- Hypothyroidism
- Congenital anatomic lesion, eg, septate uterus
- Acquired anatomic lesion, eg, incompetent cervix, intrauterine adhesions, submucous uterine leiomyoma (fibroid)
- Polycystic ovary syndrome
- Antiphospholipid antibody syndrome or other hypercoagulable state
- Balanced chromosomal translocation

Abortion, spontaneous

- Incompetent cervix
- Ectopic pregnancy
- Menses or menorrhagia
- Prolapsed uterine leiomyoma (fibroid)
- Hydatidiform mole
- Cervical neoplasm or lesion

Acanthosis nigricans

- Nevi
- Reticulated pigment anomaly (Dowling-Degos disease)
- Confluent and reticulated papillomatosis (of Gougerot and Carteaud)

Acute tubular necrosis

- Prerenal azotemia, eg, dehydration
- Postrenal azotemia, eg, benign prostatic hyperplasia
- Other renal causes of acute renal failure
  - Acute glomerulonephritis: immune complex (eg, IgA nephropathy), pauci-immune (eg, Wegener's granulomatosis), anti-GBM disease
  - Acute interstitial nephritis: drugs (eg, β-lactams), infections (eg, *Streptococcus*), immune (eg, systemic lupus erythematosus)

Etiology

- Toxins: NSAIDs, antibiotics, contrast, multiple myeloma, rhabdomyolysis, hemolysis, chemotherapy, hyperuricemia, cyclosporine
- Ischemia, eg, prolonged prerenal azotemia

Adrenal mass

- Nonfunctioning adrenal adenoma
- Metastatic cancer, eg, lung, breast, renal cell, lymphoma, melanoma
- Cortisol-producing adenoma
- Aldosterone-producing adenoma
- Adrenal carcinoma
- Pheochromocytoma
- Cyst or myelolipoma

Aggressive behavior

- Drugs, eg, PCP, alcohol, cocaine, amphetamines, anabolic steroids
- Impulse control disorder
- Psychiatric disease, eg, schizophrenia, personality disorder, mania
- Psychosis due to other causes

Airway obstruction, bronchi

Etiology

- Pulmonary secretions
- Aspiration
- Foreign body
- Bronchogenic carcinoma
- Extrinsic compression by mass
- Metastatic tumor

Airway obstruction, trachea

Etiology

- Tracheal stenosis, acquired (intubation, trauma)
- Tracheal stenosis, congenital
- Tracheal tumor (primary or metastatic)
- Extrinsic compression by tumor of lung, thyroid, thymus; lymphadenopathy; congenital vascular rings; aneurysms
- Foreign-body aspiration
- Tracheal granulomas or papillomas
- Tracheal trauma

Airway obstruction, upper

Etiology

Acute

- Foreign-body aspiration
- Laryngospasm
- Angioedema
- Laryngeal edema from airway burns
- Trauma to larynx or pharynx
- Epiglottitis
- Pharyngeal or retropharyngeal abscess
- Ludwig's angina
- Acute allergic laryngitis
- Vocal cord dysfunction

Chronic

- Carcinoma of larynx or pharynx
- Laryngeal or subglottic stenosis
- Laryngeal granulomas or webs
- Bilateral vocal cord paralysis
- Vocal cord dysfunction

Alcohol withdrawal

- Withdrawal from other sedatives, eg, benzodiazepines or opioids
- Drug intoxication, eg, cocaine, amphetamines
- Delirium due to medical illness, eg, hypoxia, hepatic encephalopathy, thiamine deficiency, bacteremia
- Anxiety disorder
- Hallucinosis due to other causes, eg, schizophrenia, amphetamine psychosis
- Seizure due to other causes, eg, hypoglycemia, epilepsy

Alkaline phosphatase increased

Etiology

- Obstructive hepatobiliary disease (GGT increased)
- Bone disease, eg, bone metastases, Paget's disease, osteomalacia, osteosarcoma, hyperparathyroidism (GGT normal)

- Pregnancy (third trimester)
- Gastrointestinal disease, eg, bowel infarction or perforated viscus
- Hepatitis, eg, viral, alcoholic, toxic
- Infiltrative liver disease, eg, tuberculosis, sarcoidosis, lymphoma, amyloidosis
- Hemochromatosis

Altered mental status

Drugs

- Opioids, alcohol, sedatives, antipsychotics, withdrawal, others

Metabolic

- Hypoxia, hypoglycemia, hyperglycemia, hypercalcemia, hypernatremia, hyponatremia, uremia, hepatic encephalopathy, hypothyroidism, hyperthyroidism, vitamin B_{12} or thiamine deficiency, carbon monoxide poisoning, Wilson's disease

Infectious

- Meningitis, encephalitis, bacteremia, urinary tract infection, pneumonia, neurosyphilis

Structural

- Space-occupying lesion, eg, brain tumor, subdural hematoma, hydrocephalus

Vascular

- Stroke, subarachnoid hemorrhage, coronary ischemia, hypertensive encephalopathy, CNS vasculitis, thrombotic thrombocytopenic purpura, disseminated intravascular coagulation, hyperviscosity

Psychiatric

- Schizophrenia, depression

Other

- Seizure, hypothermia, heat stroke, ICU psychosis, "sundowning"

Altered mental status in a diabetic

- Hypoglycemia
- Diabetic ketoacidosis
- Hyperglycemic hyperosmolar state
- Lactic acidosis, eg, severe infection, metformin use
- Stroke
- Sepsis
- Uremia

Altered mental status in HIV/AIDS

- Mass lesion: toxoplasmosis, CNS lymphoma, brain abscess, metastatic tumor, cryptococcoma
- Other infections: bacterial meningitis, cryptococcal meningitis, herpes simplex virus encephalitis, neurosyphilis, tuberculous meningitis, bacteremia
- Other: AIDS dementia, progressive multifocal leukoencephalopathy, stroke, seizure, depression, metabolic, eg, hypoxia, hypoglycemia, uremic or hepatic encephalopathy

Alveolar hemorrhage, diffuse

Etiology

Immune causes

- Goodpasture's syndrome
- Systemic lupus erythematosus
- Wegener's granulomatosis
- Systemic necrotizing vasculitis
- Pulmonary capillaritis associated with idiopathic rapidly progressive glomerulonephritis

Nonimmune causes

- Coagulopathy
- Mitral stenosis
- Necrotizing pulmonary infection (eg, aspergillosis, cytomegalovirus, herpes simplex virus)
- Idiopathic pulmonary hemosiderosis
- Recent bone marrow transplant
- Drugs (penicillamine)
- Toxins (trimellitic anhydride)

Amaurosis fugax

- Emboli from carotid
- Cardiac emboli
- Choroidal or retinal vascular spasm (especially younger patients)
- Severe occlusive carotid disease
- Aortic dissection
- Increased intracranial pressure (more transient, bilateral)
- Takayasu's arteritis
- Hyperviscosity, eg, polycythemia vera, leukemia, Waldenström's macroglobulinemia

Amenorrhea, primary

Etiology

Hypothalamic-pituitary causes (low-normal FSH)

- Idiopathic delayed puberty
- Pituitary tumor
- Hypothalamic amenorrhea, eg, stress, weight change, exercise
- Anorexia nervosa
- Hypothyroidism
- Cushing's syndrome
- GnRH or gonadotropin deficiency, eg, Kallmann syndrome
- Craniopharyngioma

Excess testosterone (low-normal FSH)

- Adrenal tumor or adrenal hyperplasia
- Polycystic ovary syndrome
- Ovarian tumor
- Androgenic steroids

Ovarian causes (high FSH)

- Gonadal dysgenesis, eg, Turner syndrome
- Autoimmune ovarian failure
- Rare ovarian enzyme deficiencies

Pseudohermaphroditism (high LH)

- Testosterone synthesis defect
- Complete androgen resistance (testicular feminization)

Anatomic defect (normal FSH)

- Vaginal agenesis, absent uterus, atrophic endometrium, imperforate hymen

Pregnancy (high hCG)

Amylase increased

Etiology

- Acute pancreatitis, pancreatic pseudocyst, or pancreatic duct obstruction (eg, cholecystitis, choledocholithiasis, pancreatic cancer)
- Intestinal obstruction or infarction
- Mumps (salivary amylase; may cause pancreatitis)
- Parotitis due to other causes, eg, sarcoidosis
- Diabetic ketoacidosis
- Penetrating duodenal ulcer
- Peritonitis
- Ruptured ectopic pregnancy
- Pelvic inflammatory disease
- Abdominal surgery
- Macroamylasemia
- Narcotic administration

Anal fissure

Etiology

- Trauma
- Crohn's disease
- Tuberculosis
- Leukemia

Anemia, general approach

Etiology

Macrocytic (MCV >100)

- Megaloblastic anemia: folic acid or vitamin B_{12} deficiency
- Liver disease (target cells)
- Alcoholism
- Reticulocytosis
- Hypothyroidism
- Myelodysplastic syndrome
- Antiretrovirals, eg, AZT

Microcytic (MCV < 80)

- Iron deficiency
- Thalassemia
- Anemia of chronic disease
- Sideroblastic anemia
- Lead poisoning

Normocytic (MCV 80–100)

- Low reticulocyte count
- Iron deficiency (especially early)
- Anemia of chronic disease
- Chronic renal disease (low erythropoietin)
- Hypothyroidism, adrenal insufficiency, or hypopituitarism
- Primary bone marrow disorder
  - Aplastic anemia
  - Malignancy, eg, multiple myeloma, leukemia, metastases
  - Myelofibrosis
  - Myelodysplastic syndrome
  - Infection, eg, parvovirus B19 (causes red cell hypoplasia or aplastic anemia)
- High reticulocyte count
- Blood loss
- Hemolysis
  - Coombs positive (immune): autoimmune, drugs, infection, lymphoproliferative disease, Rh or ABO incompatibility
  - Coombs negative: intrinsic red cell disease
    1. Abnormal hemoglobin: sickle cell disease, thalassemia, methemoglobinemia
    2. Membrane defect: hereditary spherocytosis, hereditary elliptocytosis, paroxysmal nocturnal hemoglobinuria
    3. Enzyme defect: G6PD deficiency, pyruvate kinase deficiency
  - Coombs negative: extrinsic disease
    1. Microangiopathic hemolytic anemia, eg, thrombotic thrombocytopenic purpura, disseminated intravascular coagulation, prosthetic valve hemolysis
    2. Splenic sequestration
    3. Infection: malaria, *Clostridium*, *Borrelia*
    4. Burns

Anemia, hemolytic

Etiology

Coombs positive (immune)

- Autoimmune, drugs, infection, lymphoproliferative disease, Rh or ABO incompatibility

Coombs negative

- Intrinsic red cell disease
  - Abnormal hemoglobin: sickle cell disease, thalassemia, methemoglobinemia
  - Membrane defect: hereditary spherocytosis, hereditary elliptocytosis, paroxysmal nocturnal hemoglobinuria
  - Enzyme defect: G6PD deficiency, pyruvate kinase deficiency
- Extrinsic disease
  - Microangiopathic hemolytic anemia: thrombotic thrombocytopenic purpura, hemolytic uremic syndrome, disseminated intravascular coagulation, prosthetic valve hemolysis, metastatic adenocarcinoma, vasculitis, malignant hypertension, HELLP syndrome
  - Splenic sequestration
  - Infection: malaria, *Clostridium*, *Borrelia*
  - Burns

Anemia, iron deficiency

- Microcytic anemia due to other causes: thalassemia, anemic of chronic disease, sideroblastic anemia, lead poisoning

Etiology

- Blood loss: gastrointestinal, menstrual, repeated blood donation
- Deficient diet
- Increased requirements: pregnancy, lactation
- Hemoglobinuria, eg, paroxysmal nocturnal hemoglobinuria
- Malabsorption, eg, gastric surgery, celiac disease
- Hemolysis
- Pulmonary hemosiderosis (iron sequestration)

Anemia, macrocytic

Etiology

- Megaloblastic anemia: folic acid or vitamin B_{12} deficiency
- Liver disease (target cells)
- Alcoholism
- Reticulocytosis
- Hypothyroidism
- Myelodysplastic syndrome
- Antiretrovirals, eg, AZT

Anemia, microcytic

Etiology

- Iron deficiency
- Thalassemia
- Anemic of chronic disease (low-normal MCV)
- Sideroblastic anemia
- Lead poisoning

Anemia, normocytic

Etiology

Low reticulocyte count

- Iron deficiency (especially early)
- Anemia of chronic disease (low-normal MCV)
- Chronic renal disease (low erythropoietin)
- Hypothyroidism, adrenal insufficiency, or hypopituitarism
- Primary bone marrow disorder:
  - Aplastic anemia
  - Malignancy, eg, multiple myeloma, leukemia, metastases
  - Myelofibrosis
  - Myelodysplastic syndrome
  - Infection, eg, parvovirus B19 (causes red cell hypoplasia or aplastic anemia)

High reticulocyte count

- Blood loss
- Hemolysis
  - Coombs positive (immune): autoimmune, drugs, infection, lymphoproliferative disease, Rh or ABO incompatibility
  - Coombs negative: intrinsic red cell disease
    1. Abnormal hemoglobin: sickle cell disease, thalassemia, methemoglobinemia
    2. Membrane defect: hereditary spherocytosis, hereditary elliptocytosis, paroxysmal nocturnal hemoglobinuria
    3. Enzyme defect: G6PD deficiency, pyruvate kinase deficiency
  - Coombs negative: extrinsic disease
    1. Microangiopathic hemolytic anemia, eg, thrombotic thrombocytopenic purpura, disseminated intravascular coagulation, prosthetic valve hemolysis
    2. Splenic sequestration
    3. Infection: malaria, *Clostridium*, *Borrelia*
    4. Burns

Angular cheilitis

- Candidiasis

- Iron deficiency
- Malnutrition
- Glucagonoma

Anion gap, decreased

Etiology

Decreased anion gap and metabolic acidosis

- Plasma cell dyscrasias, eg, multiple myeloma (cationic paraproteins accompanied by chloride and bicarbonate)
- Bromide or lithium intoxication

Decreased anion gap without acidosis

- Hypoalbuminemia (decreased unmeasured anion)
- Severe hyperlipidemia

Ankle pain

- Ankle sprain, eg, anterior talofibular ligament
- Fibular fracture
- Tibial avulsion fracture
- Arthritis, eg, gout, rheumatoid arthritis
- Posterior tibial tendinitis (pain posterior to medial malleolus)
- Peroneal tendonitis (pain at lateral malleolus)
- Arterial insufficiency ulcer with or without osteomyelitis
- Neuropathic arthropathy (Charcot joint)
- Avascular necrosis

Anorectal pain

- Hemorrhoids
- Perianal abscess
- Perianal fistula, eg, Crohn's disease
- Infectious proctitis, eg, gonorrhea, syphilis, chlamydia
- Rectal prolapse or intussusception
- Anal skin tag
- Anal fissure, eg, trauma, Crohn's disease, tuberculosis, leukemia
- Anorectal herpes simplex
- Anogenital warts (condyloma acuminata)
- Primary syphilis (chancre)
- Secondary syphilis (condyloma lata)
- Lymphogranuloma venereum (proctocolitis, perianal ulcer, anorectal strictures or fistulas)
- Pruritus ani
- Anal or rectal cancer
- Proctalgia fugax or levator ani syndrome
- Rectocele
- Solitary rectal ulcer syndrome

Anovulation in reproductive years

- Polycystic ovary syndrome
- Hypothalamic amenorrhea, eg, stress, weight change, exercise
- Obesity
- Hypothyroidism or hyperthyroidism
- Hyperprolactinemia
- Premature ovarian failure
- Discontinuation of oral contraceptives
- Cushing's syndrome
- Congenital adrenal hyperplasia
- Androgen-secreting tumor (adrenal, ovarian)
- Pregnancy

Anticholinergic poisoning

Etiology

- Atropine
- Scopolamine
- Tricyclic antidepressants
- Antihistamines
- Amantadine
- Phenothiazines (hypotension, small pupils)

Anxiety

- Generalized anxiety disorder
- Hyperthyroidism
- Medication or substance abuse, eg, caffeine, nicotine, cocaine, amphetamines, pseudoephedrine
- Medication or substance withdrawal, eg, alcohol, benzodiazepines
- Major depressive disorder
- Adjustment disorder
- Somatoform disorder (eg, somatization)
- Other anxiety disorder, eg, obsessive-compulsive disorder, panic disorder
- Pheochromocytoma

Aortic insufficiency

- Aortic dissection
- Graham Steell murmur (pulmonary insufficiency secondary to pulmonary hypertension)
- Mitral stenosis
- Tricuspid stenosis
- Dock's murmur of stenotic left anterior descending artery

Etiology

- Congenitally bicuspid aortic valve
- Hypertension
- Valvular calcification
- Infective endocarditis
- Rheumatic heart disease
- Aortic root (or arch) disease: Marfan syndrome, aortic dissection, temporal (giant cell) arteritis, Takayasu's arteritis, ankylosing spondylitis, syphilis, Reiter's syndrome (reactive arthritis), cystic medial necrosis, sinus of Valsalva aneurysm, relapsing polychondritis

Aortic stenosis

- Aortic sclerosis
- Mitral regurgitation
- Hypertrophic obstructive cardiomyopathy
- Supravalvular aortic stenosis
- Congenital subvalvular aortic stenosis

Etiology

- Valvular calcification, especially of congenitally bicuspid aortic valve
- Rheumatic heart disease

Arthritis

- Osteoarthritis (degenerative joint disease) or inflammatory osteoarthritis
- Connective tissue disease, eg, rheumatoid arthritis, systemic lupus erythematosus, scleroderma, Sjögren's syndrome, adult Still's disease
- Seronegative spondyloarthropathy, eg, reactive arthritis (Reiter's syndrome), psoriatic arthritis, ankylosing spondylitis, inflammatory bowel disease
- Infection, eg, *Staphylococcus aureus* septic arthritis, gonococcal arthritis, endocarditis, hepatitis B or hepatitis C, parvovirus B19, Lyme disease, rubella or post-rubella vaccination
- Crystal-induced, eg, gout, pseudogout
- Trauma
- Other joint disease, eg, Charcot (neuropathic) joint, sarcoidosis, tumor, paraneoplastic syndrome (eg, hypertrophic pulmonary osteoarthropathy, leukemia), avascular necrosis, amyloidosis, coagulopathy, sickle cell disease, Henoch-Schönlein purpura, relapsing polychondritis, Behçet's syndrome, Whipple's disease, palindromic rheumatism, ochronosis (alkaptonuria)

- Other non-joint disease, eg, tendonitis, bursitis, polymyalgia rheumatica, reflex sympathetic dystrophy

Arthritis, acute, multijoint

- Reactive arthritis (Reiter's syndrome)
- Crystal-induced, eg, gout, pseudogout
- Infection, eg, gonococcal arthritis, endocarditis, hepatitis B, parvovirus B19, rubella or post-rubella vaccination
- Connective tissue disease, eg, rheumatoid arthritis, systemic lupus erythematosus, scleroderma, Sjögren's syndrome, adult Still's disease

Arthritis, acute, one joint

Inflammatory
- Infection, eg, *Staphylococcus aureus* septic arthritis, gonococcal arthritis, endocarditis, parvovirus B19
- Crystal-induced, eg, gout, pseudogout
- Reactive arthritis (Reiter's syndrome)
- Uncommon: other seronegative spondyloarthropathy, connective tissue disease

Noninflammatory
- Trauma
- Nontraumatic bleed, eg, coagulopathy
- Sickle cell crisis

Arthritis, chronic, multijoint

Inflammatory
- Connective tissue disease, eg, rheumatoid arthritis, systemic lupus erythematosus, scleroderma, Sjögren's syndrome, adult Still's disease
- Seronegative spondyloarthropathy, eg, reactive arthritis (Reiter's syndrome), psoriatic arthritis, ankylosing spondylitis, inflammatory bowel disease
- Crystal-induced, eg, gout, pseudogout
- Inflammatory osteoarthritis
- Lyme disease
- Paraneoplastic syndrome (especially in elderly, eg, hypertrophic pulmonary osteoarthropathy)

Noninflammatory
- Osteoarthritis (degenerative joint disease)

Arthritis, chronic, one joint

Noninflammatory
- Osteoarthritis (degenerative joint disease; DJD)
- Hemarthrosis (bleed)
- Sickle cell disease
- Repeated trauma (causing DJD)
- Charcot (neuropathic) joint, eg, diabetes mellitus, syphilis

Inflammatory
- Opportunistic infection, eg, tuberculosis of bone and joints, fungal, sporotrichosis

Arthritis, migratory

- Rheumatic fever
- Palindromic rheumatism
- Gonococcal arthritis
- Lyme disease
- Viral, eg, HIV, hepatitis B, hepatitis C
- Adult Still's disease
- Sarcoidosis
- Henoch-Schönlein purpura
- Relapsing polychondritis
- Whipple's disease

Arthritis & inflammatory bowel disease

- Reactive arthritis (Reiter's syndrome)
- Ankylosing spondylitis
- Psoriatic arthritis
- Whipple's disease

Arthritis & skin nodules

- Rheumatoid arthritis
- Tophaceous gout
- Sarcoidosis
- Systemic lupus erythematosus
- Palindromic rheumatism
- Rheumatic fever
- Multicentric reticular histiocytosis
- Endocarditis
- Hepatitis B with polyarteritis nodosa
- Coccidioidomycosis

Ascites

Etiology

Normal peritoneum
- Portal hypertension (serum-ascites albumin gradient [SAAG] ≥1.1 g/dL)
  - Liver disease
    1. Cirrhosis (most common)
    2. "Mixed ascites" (portal hypertension with secondary process, eg, malignancy, infection)
    3. Alcoholic hepatitis
    4. Fulminant hepatic failure
    5. Massive hepatic metastases
    6. Hepatic fibrosis
    7. Acute fatty liver of pregnancy
  - Hepatic congestion (usually SAAG ≥1.1 g/dL and ascites total protein >2.5 g/dL)
    1. Congestive heart failure, constrictive pericarditis, tricuspid insufficiency
    2. Budd-Chiari syndrome, veno-occlusive disease
  - Portal vein occlusion
- Hypoalbuminemia (SAAG < 1.1 g/dL)
  - Nephrotic syndrome
  - Protein-losing enteropathy
  - Severe malnutrition with anasarca

Miscellaneous conditions (SAAG < 1.1 g/L)
  - Chylous ascites
  - Pancreatic ascites
  - Bile ascites
  - Nephrogenic ascites
  - Urine ascites
  - Myxedema (SAAG ≥1.1 g/dL)
  - Ovarian disease

Diseased peritoneum (SAAG < 1.1 g/dL except in "mixed ascites" with portal hypertension and secondary process, eg, infection, malignancy)
- Infections
  - Bacterial peritonitis
  - Tuberculous peritonitis
  - Fungal peritonitis
  - HIV-associated peritonitis
- Malignant conditions
  - Peritoneal carcinomatosis
  - Primary mesothelioma
  - Pseudomyxoma peritonei
  - Massive hepatic metastases
  - Hepatocellular carcinoma
- Other conditions
  - Familial Mediterranean fever
  - Vasculitis
  - Granulomatous peritonitis
  - Eosinophilic peritonitis

Ascites, chylous

Etiology

- Lymphatic obstruction, eg, lymphoma
- Postoperative trauma
- Cirrhosis
- Tuberculosis
- Pancreatitis
- Filariasis

Ascites, malignant

Etiology

- Peritoneal carcinomatosis: adenocarcinoma of ovary, uterus, pancreas, stomach, colon, lung, breast

- Hepatocellular carcinoma causing lymphatic obstruction or portal hypertension
- Diffuse hepatic metastases

Ascites (common causes)

Etiology

- Cirrhosis (80–85%)
- Malignancy (10%)
- Congestive heart failure (3%)
- Tuberculous peritonitis
- Dialysis-related
- Bile or pancreatic ascites
- Lymphatic tear (chylous ascites)
- Nephrotic syndrome

Aspirated foreign body

- Asthma with mucus plugging
- Bronchiolitis
- Ludwig's angina
- Epiglottitis
- Laryngospasm, eg, anaphylaxis
- Lung cancer
- Substernal goiter
- Tracheal cystadenoma

Aspiration of gastric contents, chronic

Etiology

- Achalasia
- Esophageal stricture
- Scleroderma
- Esophageal carcinoma
- Esophagitis
- Gastroesophageal reflux disease
- Disorders of the larynx

Asplenia & infection risk

Etiology

- Encapsulated organisms: *Streptococcus pneumoniae, Haemophilus influenzae, Neisseria meningitidis*
- *Capnocytophaga canimorsus* (dog bites)
- Intraerythrocytic parasites, eg, malaria, babesiosis
- Others: *Salmonella typhi*, *Klebsiella*, herpes zoster, group B streptococci, enterococcus, *Bacteroides*

AST/ALT increased

Etiology

- Acute viral hepatitis (ALT > AST)
- Toxic hepatitis, eg, acetaminophen
- Alcoholic hepatitis (AST < ALT)
- Cirrhosis (AST > ALT)
- Vascular: right-sided congestive heart failure, shock liver, Budd-Chiari syndrome
- Biliary tract obstruction (followed by increased alkaline phosphatase and bilirubin)
- Nonalcoholic fatty liver disease (formerly NASH)
- Metabolic, eg, hemochromatosis, Wilson's disease
- Liver abscess
- Hepatocellular or metastatic cancer
- Drugs, eg, INH, statins
- Heart or skeletal muscle injury
- Celiac sprue (ALT)

AST/ALT > 500–1000

- Acetaminophen, *Amanita* mushroom, other toxins
- Viral, especially hepatitis A
- Shock liver (ischemia)
- Budd-Chiari syndrome
- Right-sided heart failure

Ataxia

- Intoxication, eg, alcohol, phenytoin
- Cerebellar infarct, mass, or hemorrhage
- Cerebellar degeneration, eg, alcoholism
- Parkinsonism
- Vascular (multi-infarct) dementia
- Multiple sclerosis
- Wernicke's encephalopathy
- Hydrocephalus
- Metabolic: hyponatremia, hypothyroidism, vitamin B_{12} deficiency
- Paraneoplastic syndrome, eg, breast, ovarian
- Progressive multifocal leukoencephalopathy in AIDS
- Lyme disease
- Neurosyphilis
- Inherited ataxia, eg, Friedreich's

Atrial fibrillation

- Frequent premature atrial contractions
- Atrial flutter (especially if variable block)
- Multifocal atrial tachycardia
- Sinus tachycardia
- Sinus arrhythmia
- Atrial tachycardia
- Supraventricular tachycardia
- Ventricular tachycardia

Etiology

- Rheumatic heart disease
- Dilated cardiomyopathy
- Pulmonary disease, eg, chronic obstructive pulmonary disease, pulmonary embolism
- Mitral stenosis
- Mitral regurgitation
- Mitral valve prolapse
- Coronary artery disease
- Atrial septal defect
- Atrial myxoma
- Hypertension
- Hypertrophic obstructive cardiomyopathy
- Thyrotoxicosis (hyperthyroidism)
- Pericarditis
- Chest trauma or chest surgery
- Medications: theophylline, beta-agonists
- Alcohol withdrawal
- Sepsis

Atrial flutter

- Sinus tachycardia
- Supraventricular tachycardia
- Atrial tachycardia
- Junctional tachycardia
- Atrial fibrillation

Etiology

- Chronic obstructive pulmonary disease
- Rheumatic heart disease
- Coronary artery disease
- Congestive heart failure
- Atrial septal defect

Atrial myxoma

- Infective endocarditis
- Systemic lupus erythematosus (with Libman-Sacks endocarditis)
- Lymphoma
- Mitral stenosis
- Cor triatriatum (congenital atrial anomaly)

Atrioventricular block (first, second, or third degree)

Etiology

- Increased vagal tone (first degree or Mobitz type I)
- Drugs: digitalis, calcium channel blockers, beta blockers, clonidine, other sympatholytics, amiodarone, other antiarrhythmics

- Age-related conduction system fibrosis or calcification (Lev's disease)
- Cardiac infiltrative disease (eg, amyloid, sarcoidosis, hemochromatosis)
- Myocardial ischemia or myocardial infarction
- Myocarditis
- Chagas' disease

Auricle diseases

- Skin cancer
- Traumatic auricular hematoma
- Cauliflower ear (cartilage dissolution post-trauma)
- Cellulitis
- Chondritis or perichondritis
- Relapsing polychondritis
- Chondrodermatitis nodularis helicis
- Discoid lupus erythematosus
- Cutaneous leishmaniasis

Autonomic insufficiency

Etiology

- Diabetes
- Adrenal insufficiency
- Spinal cord lesion
- Guillain-Barré syndrome
- Parkinsonism
- Chronic idiopathic orthostatic hypotension
- Shy-Drager syndrome (multiple system atrophy)

Bacteremia & sepsis

- Other types of shock: cardiogenic, hypovolemic, neurogenic, anaphylactic
- Toxic shock syndrome

Etiology

- Genitourinary system
- Hepatobiliary tract
- Gastrointestinal tract
- Lungs
- Indwelling catheter
- Surgical wound
- Decubitus ulcer

Belching

- Normal belching: air ingestion from rapid eating, carbonated beverages, gum chewing, smoking
- Excessive belching: aerophagia (air swallowing, often subconscious)

Bitemporal hemianopsia

- Pituitary tumor
- Craniopharyngioma
- Meningioma
- Aneurysm of circle of Willis
- Sarcoidosis
- Metastatic carcinoma

Bleeding, general approach

Etiology

Defect in platelet number or function (gum bleeding, petechiae, bruising)

- Thrombocytopenia, eg, idiopathic and thrombotic, thrombotic thrombocytopenic purpura, leukemia
- Acquired disorder, eg, aspirin-induced platelet dysfunction, uremia, myeloproliferative disorder, autoantibody
- Hereditary disorder, eg, von Willebrand's disease, Glanzmann's thrombasthenia

Defect in coagulation (skin and deep muscle bleeding)

- Acquired disorder, eg, liver disease, vitamin K deficiency, anticoagulants, disseminated intravascular coagulation, factor VIII antibodies
- Hereditary disorder, eg, hemophilia A

Blistering diseases (bullae)

- Pemphigus
- Bullous pemphigoid
- Drug eruption
- Erythema multiforme major or toxic epidermal necrolysis
- Bullous impetigo
- Contact dermatitis
- Dermatitis herpetiformis
- Cicatricial pemphigoid
- Paraneoplastic pemphigus
- Linear IgA dermatosis
- Pemphigus foliaceus
- Porphyria cutanea tarda
- Epidermolysis bullosa
- Staphylococcal scalded skin syndrome
- Herpes gestationis
- Graft-versus-host disease
- Disseminated *Vibrio vulnificus* (cirrhosis, seafood or seawater exposure)
- Ecthyma gangrenosum (neutropenic, pseudomonal)

Bone pain & pathologic fractures

- Osteoporosis (fracture)
- Malignancy, primary or metastatic (fracture)
- Hyperparathyroidism (bone pain)
- Hyperthyroidism (osteopenia)
- Cushing's syndrome (osteopenia)
- Osteogenesis imperfecta (fracture)
- Osteomalacia or rickets (bowing and pseudofractures)
- Multiple myeloma (bone pain, fracture)
- Paget's disease (bone pain)
- Leukemia (bone pain)
- Gaucher disease (fracture)
- Beta thalassemia (fracture)

Bone tumors

- Metastatic cancer
- Osteomyelitis
- Posttraumatic lesion
- Metabolic bone disease, eg, Paget's disease, hyperparathyroidism, osteoporosis
- Arthritis

Bradycardia

- Medications (eg, calcium channel blockers, beta blockers, digitalis, clonidine, other sympatholytics, amiodarone, other antiarrhythmics)
- Normal (especially athletes)
- Sick sinus syndrome
- Vasovagal response
- Atrioventricular block
- Hypothermia
- Hypothyroidism
- Myocardial ischemia involving right coronary artery
- Increased intracranial pressure (Cushing's reflex)
- Cardiac infiltrative disease (eg, amyloid, sarcoidosis, hemochromatosis)

Bradycardia, relative

- Typhoid fever (enteric fever)
- Legionnaire's disease
- Brucellosis
- Leptospirosis
- Psittacosis
- Q fever
- Viral hemorrhagic fever, eg, yellow fever

- Infections affecting cardiac conduction: acute rheumatic fever, viral myocarditis, Lyme disease, endocarditis
- Noninfectious causes: intrinsic cardiac conduction disease, beta blockers, calcium channel blockers, drug fever, neoplasm (eg, lymphoma), factitious fever, CNS lesion

Brain mass in HIV/AIDS

- Toxoplasmosis
- CNS lymphoma
- Bacterial brain abscess
- Fungal brain abscess, eg, *Aspergillus*, *Histoplasma*
- Cryptococcoma
- *Nocardia* brain abscess
- Tuberculoma
- Other primary or metastatic tumor

Brain tumors (brain mass)

- Primary brain tumor, eg, glioblastoma multiforme, meningioma, pituitary adenoma, neurofibroma, lymphoma
- Metastases, eg, lung, breast, renal, gastrointestinal, melanoma, lymphoma
- Brain abscess
- Cerebral infarction or intracerebral hemorrhage
- Subdural hematoma
- Multiple sclerosis
- Cryptococcoma
- Neurocysticercosis
- Tuberculoma

Breast lump or mass

- Fibrocystic condition, breast or cyst
- Breast fibroadenoma
- Breast cancer
- Intraductal papilloma
- Lipoma
- Breast abscess (mastitis)
- Fat necrosis
- Phyllodes tumor

Breast pain

- Premenstrual syndrome or cyclic mastalgia
- Fibrocystic condition, breast or cyst
- Pregnancy
- Breast-feeding
- Breast abscess (mastitis)
- Onset of menopause
- Breast cancer
- Breast fibroadenoma
- Trauma
- Estrogen replacement therapy
- Breast augmentation disorder (implants)
- Shingles
- Gynecomastia (men)

Bronchiectasis

- Chronic obstructive pulmonary disease
- Asthma
- Bronchiolitis
- Allergic bronchopulmonary aspergillosis

Etiology

- Cystic fibrosis
- Infection: tuberculosis, fungal, lung abscess, pneumonia, parasites
- Localized airway obstruction: retained foreign body, tumor, mucoid impaction
- Abnormal lung defense mechanisms
  - Hypogammaglobulinemia
  - Common variable immunodeficiency
  - Selective IgA, IgM, and IgG subclass deficiency
  - Acquired immunodeficiency from cytotoxic drugs, AIDS, lymphoma, leukemia, multiple myeloma, chronic renal disease, chronic liver disease
  - Alpha-1-antiprotease deficiency with cigarette smoking
  - Mucociliary clearance disorders (immotile cilia syndrome)
  - Rheumatic disease, eg, rheumatoid arthritis

Bruit

- Carotid stenosis (cervical bruit)
- Temporal (giant cell) arteritis (near clavicle)
- Renal artery bruit (epigastric)
- Peripheral vascular disease (femoral bruit)
- Abdominal aortic aneurysm
- Thoracic aortic aneurysm
- Takayasu's arteritis or "pulseless disease" (various bruits)

Budd-Chiari syndrome (hepatic vein obstruction)

- Cholecystitis
- Shock liver
- Cirrhosis
- Hepatic congestion from right-sided congestive heart failure
- Metastatic cancer involving the liver

Etiology

- Caval webs
- Myeloproliferative disease, eg, polycythemia vera
- Right-sided congestive heart failure or constrictive pericarditis
- Neoplasm compressing hepatic vein
- Paroxysmal nocturnal hemoglobinuria
- Behçet's syndrome
- Oral contraceptives or pregnancy
- Hypercoagulable state
- Post bone-marrow transplant
- "Bush teas" (pyrrolizidine alkaloids)

BUN increased with normal GFR

Etiology

- Prerenal azotemia
- Catabolic states
- High-protein diets
- Gastrointestinal bleeding
- Glucocorticoids
- Tetracycline

Cafe au lait spots

- Idiopathic
- Neurofibromatosis
- McCune-Albright syndrome

Calf pain

- Muscular strain
- Baker's (popliteal) cyst
- Deep vein thrombosis
- Claudication (arterial insufficiency)
- Superficial thrombophlebitis
- Varicose veins
- Achilles tendon rupture
- Myositis, eg, polymyositis, dermatomyositis
- Vasculitis, eg, polyarteritis nodosa, thromboangiitis obliterans (Buerger's disease)
- Spinal stenosis (pseudoclaudication; usually back and thigh pain)

Cancer of unknown primary

- Poorly differentiated: lymphoma, germ cell tumor, melanoma, neuroendocrine, prostate
- Adenocarcinoma: breast, prostate, pancreatic, hepatobiliary, lung, colorectal, ovarian

- Squamous cell (depending on location of adenopathy): head and neck, genital, anorectal, cervical, lung
- Others: melanoma, sarcoma, thyroid

Cardiac tamponade

- Tension pneumothorax
- Restrictive cardiomyopathy
- Constrictive pericarditis
- Right ventricular infarction
- Left ventricular failure

Etiology

- Malignancy
- Hemopericardium, eg, aortic dissection, iatrogenic cardiac perforation
- Uremia
- Less common: infection (viral, bacterial, tuberculous), radiation, myxedema, Dressler's syndrome, systemic lupus erythematosus

Cardiac tumors

Metastases (most common)

- Bronchogenic carcinoma
- Breast cancer
- Melanoma
- Lymphoma
- Renal cell carcinoma
- Kaposi's sarcoma (in AIDS)

Primary cardiac tumors

- Atrial myxoma (most common primary tumor)
- Rhabdomyoma
- Fibrous histiocytoma
- Hemangioma
- Sarcoma

Cardiomyopathy, primary dilated

- Hypertrophic obstructive cardiomyopathy
- Restrictive cardiomyopathy

Etiology

- Idiopathic
- Alcoholic
- Viral myocarditis
- Postpartum
- Cocaine
- Endocrinopathies: hyperthyroidism, acromegaly, pheochromocytoma
- Amyloidosis
- Sarcoidosis
- Hemochromatosis
- Diabetes mellitus
- Doxorubicin
- Genetic

Cardiomyopathy, restrictive

- Constrictive pericarditis
- Hypertrophic obstructive cardiomyopathy
- Hypertensive heart disease
- Ischemic heart disease
- Dilated cardiomyopathy

Etiology

- Amyloidosis
- Radiation-induced
- Fibrosis after open-heart surgery
- Sarcoidosis
- Hemochromatosis
- Carcinoid
- Scleroderma
- Diabetes mellitus
- Endomyocardial fibrosis

Carotid pulse, bisferiens

- Hypertrophic obstructive cardiomyopathy
- Mixed aortic stenosis and aortic insufficiency

Cataract

- Corneal opacity, eg, scar, pterygium
- Refractive error
- Macular degeneration (atrophic)
- Diabetic retinopathy
- Glaucoma
- Anterior ischemic optic neuropathy, eg, temporal (giant cell) arteritis

Etiology

- Senile cataract
- Congenital, eg, rubella, cytomegalovirus, galactosemia
- Trauma
- Systemic disease, eg, diabetes mellitus, atopic dermatitis, myotonic dystrophy
- Corticosteroids (topical or systemic)
- Uveitis

Catatonia or stiffness

Severe stiffness or catatonia

- Catatonic schizophrenia
- Parkinson's disease
- Catatonic syndrome due to other CNS causes, eg, viral encephalitis, CNS bleed
- Neuroleptic-induced catatonia
- Seizure or status epilepticus
- Neuroleptic malignant syndrome
- Malignant hyperthermia
- Tetany, eg, hypocalcemia (usually distal muscles)
- Dystonic reaction to neuroleptics, eg, torticollis
- Huntington's disease
- Tetanus
- Strychnine poisoning
- Lethal catatonia
- Stiff-person syndrome
- Meningitis (stiff neck)

Mild stiffness

- Arthritis, eg, osteoarthritis, rheumatoid arthritis, pseudogout
- Early parkinsonism
- Fibromyalgia
- Polymyalgia rheumatica

Cervical (cervix) lesions

- Cervical polyp
- Nabothian cyst
- Cervical cancer or cervical intraepithelial neoplasia
- Cervical ectropion
- Cervical ectopy (columnar epithelium on face of os, common in adolescence)
- Cervicitis, eg, chlamydia, gonorrhea, herpes simplex virus, *Trichomonas* infection (severe)
- Genital warts (condyloma acuminata)
- Cervical ulcer: herpes simplex virus, syphilis, chancroid
- Granuloma inguinale
- Leiomyomas
- Endometriosis
- Deformity or hypoplasia due to DES exposure in utero

Cervical discharge

- Chlamydia
- Gonorrhea
- Herpes simplex virus
- *Trichomonas* infection (severe)
- Pelvic inflammatory disease
- Cervical polyp
- Cervical cancer

- Uterine cancer
- Reaction to douches, tampons, diaphragm

Cervical lymphadenopathy

- Upper respiratory tract infection
- Bacterial infection of upper extremities
- Metastasis from squamous cell carcinoma in mouth, pharynx, larynx, upper esophagus
- Lymphoma
- Tuberculous lymphadenitis (scrofula)
- Cat-scratch disease
- Sarcoidosis
- Lyme disease
- Toxoplasmosis
- Autoimmune adenopathy
- Kikuchi's disease (histiocytic necrotizing lymphadenitis)
- Tularemia
- Actinomycosis (cervicofacial)
- Drug-induced pseudolymphoma (classically phenytoin)

Cervicitis

Etiology

- Chlamydia
- Gonorrhea
- Herpes simplex virus
- *Trichomonas* infection (severe)
- Pelvic inflammatory disease
- Cervical inflammation due to vaginitis
- Cervical ectropion
- Cervical ectopy (columnar epithelium on face of os, common in adolescence)
- Cervical cancer
- Reaction to douches, tampons, diaphragm

Chest pain

Don't miss

- Myocardial ischemia, pericarditis, aortic dissection, pulmonary embolism, tension pneumothorax, esophageal rupture

Cardiovascular

- Myocardial ischemia (angina, myocardial infarction), pericarditis, aortic stenosis, aortic dissection, pulmonary embolism, cardiomyopathy, myocarditis, mitral valve prolapse, pulmonary hypertension, hypertrophic obstructive cardiomyopathy, carditis (eg, acute rheumatic fever), aortic insufficiency, right ventricular hypertrophy

Pulmonary

- Pneumonia, pleuritis, bronchitis, pneumothorax, tumor

Gastrointestinal

- Esophageal rupture, gastroesophageal reflux disease, esophageal spasm, Mallory-Weiss syndrome, peptic ulcer disease, biliary disease, pancreatitis, functional gastrointestinal pain

Musculoskeletal

- Cervical or thoracic disk disease or arthritis, shoulder arthritis, costochondritis (anterior chest wall syndrome or Tietze's syndrome), subacromial bursitis

Other

- Anxiety or panic attack, herpes zoster, breast disorders, chest wall tumors, thoracic outlet syndrome, mediastinitis

Chest pain, pleuritic

- Pneumonia
- Upper respiratory tract infection
- Rib fracture
- Pulmonary embolism
- Pneumothorax
- Pericarditis
- Aspiration pneumonia
- Myocarditis
- Mesothelioma
- Pleurodynia (coxsackievirus)

Cheyne-Stokes respiration

- Neurologic disease (coma, stroke, hemorrhage, tumor, meningitis)
- Severe congestive heart failure
- Hypoxia
- Normal at high altitude (especially during sleep)

Cholestasis

Etiology

Extrahepatic causes

- Choledocholithiasis or cholangitis
- Pancreatic tumor
- Biliary stricture
- Primary sclerosing cholangitis (intra- and extrahepatic)
- Carcinoma of the bile ducts
- Compression of common duct by metastatic cancer
- Gallbladder cancer extending to common duct
- Choledochal cyst
- Sepsis
- Parasites, eg, *Ascaris, Clonorchis, Fasciola hepatica*, hydatid disease

Intrahepatic causes

- Primary biliary cirrhosis
- Infiltrative disease, eg, tuberculosis, sarcoidosis, lymphoma, amyloidosis
- Drug-induced cholestasis, eg, chlorpromazine, estrogen
- Autoimmune cholangitis (like PBC but AMA negative)
- Idiopathic adulthood ductopenia

Cholesterol decreased

Etiology

- Malnutrition
- Malignancy or chronic infection, eg, AIDS
- Malabsorption
- Hyperthyroidism
- Cirrhosis

Cholesterol increased

Etiology

- Idiopathic
- Hypothyroidism
- Nephrotic syndrome
- Chronic renal insufficiency
- Obstructive liver disease
- Diabetes mellitus
- Anorexia nervosa
- Cushing's syndrome
- Familial, eg, familial hypercholesterolemia
- Drugs: oral contraceptives, thiazides (short-term effect), beta blockers (short-term effect), corticosteroids, cyclosporine

Cholinergic poisoning

Etiology

- Carbamate insecticide, eg, neostigmine, physostigmine
- Nicotine
- Organophosphates
- Poisonous mushrooms

Chorea

Etiology

- Huntington's disease
- Wilson's disease
- Sydenham's chorea
- Senile chorea
- Benign hereditary chorea
- Drugs, eg, antipsychotics, levodopa, anticholinergics, phenytoin, carbamazepine, lithium, amphetamines, oral contraceptives, bromocriptine

Cirrhosis

- Edema or ascites due to other causes, eg, congestive heart failure, nephrotic syndrome, myxedema
- Hepatomegaly due to other causes, eg, hepatitis, hepatocellular carcinoma
- Encephalopathy due to other causes, eg, uremia, thiamine deficiency
- Upper gastrointestinal bleeding due to other causes, eg, peptic ulcer disease, Mallory-Weiss syndrome
- Noncirrhotic causes of portal hypertension, eg, portal or splenic vein thrombosis, schistosomiasis

Etiology

- Chronic hepatitis C or hepatitis B
- Alcoholism
- Nonalcoholic fatty liver disease
- Cryptogenic
- Metabolic, eg, hemochromatosis, Wilson's disease, alpha-1 antiprotease deficiency
- Primary biliary cirrhosis
- Secondary biliary cirrhosis (chronic obstruction due to stone, stricture, neoplasm)
- Congestive heart failure or constrictive pericarditis ("cardiac cirrhosis")
- Other: Budd-Chiari syndrome, cystic fibrosis, autoimmune hepatitis, *Clonorchis sinensis* infection, glycogen storage disease

Claudication, lower extremity

- Peripheral arterial disease
- Musculoskeletal pain
- Lumbar spinal stenosis (neurogenic or pseudoclaudication)
- Deep vein thrombosis
- Lumbar disk disease
- Peripheral neuropathy
- Nocturnal leg cramps
- Arterial embolism
- Thromboangiitis obliterans (Buerger's disease)
- Polyarteritis nodosa
- Unilateral claudication in young, athletic person: popliteal artery entrapment, trauma, compression by Baker's cyst, popliteal adventitial cystic disease

Claudication, upper extremity

- Thoracic outlet syndrome
- Takayasu's arteritis ("pulseless disease")
- Thromboangiitis obliterans (Buerger's disease)
- Hand-arm vibration syndrome or hypothenar hammer (jackhammer) syndrome

Clubbed digits

Etiology

- Chronic lung infection, eg, bronchiectasis, cystic fibrosis, lung abscess, tuberculosis, empyema
- Malignancy of lung or pleura, eg, hypertrophic pulmonary osteoarthropathy with bronchogenic carcinoma
- Chronic interstitial lung disease, eg, idiopathic pulmonary fibrosis
- Pulmonary arteriovenous malformation
- Cyanotic congenital heart disease
- Infective endocarditis
- Cirrhosis
- Inflammatory bowel disease
- Congenital or idiopathic
- Thyroid acropachy associated with hyperthyroidism

Coma

Etiology

Intracranial causes

- Anoxic brain injury or head trauma
- Ischemic stroke or intracerebral hemorrhage
- Subarachnoid hemorrhage
- Meningitis or encephalitis
- Brainstem hemorrhage, infarct, or mass
- Mass lesion causing brainstem compression
- Subdural hematoma
- Seizure

Metabolic causes

- Hypoglycemia
- Diabetic ketoacidosis
- Hyperglycemic hyperosmolar state
- Drugs, eg, alcohol, opioids, sedatives, antidepressants, salicylates
- Uremic or hepatic encephalopathy
- Hypernatremia or hyponatremia
- Hypercalcemia
- Hypothermia
- Heat stroke
- Myxedema
- Carbon monoxide poisoning

Congestive heart failure

- Chronic obstructive pulmonary disease
- Pneumonia
- Cirrhosis
- Peripheral venous insufficiency
- Nephrotic syndrome
- Myxedema (hypothyroidism)

Etiology

Left ventricular failure

- Ischemic cardiomyopathy (eg, myocardial infarction)
- Hypertension
- Cardiomyopathy (eg, idiopathic, alcoholic)
- Valvular disease (eg, aortic stenosis, aortic insufficiency, mitral regurgitation)
- Volume overload including thiazolidinediones, eg, rosiglitazone
- Arrhythmia, eg, atrial fibrillation
- High-output states
- Chagas' disease

Right ventricular failure

- Usually left ventricular failure (left-sided congestive heart failure)
- Cor pulmonale (right heart failure due to pulmonary disease)
- Chronic pulmonary embolism
- Right-sided valve disease

Diastolic dysfunction

- Left ventricular hypertrophy
- Hypertension
- Hypertrophic obstructive cardiomyopathy
- Restrictive cardiomyopathy
- Diabetes

High output heart failure

- Hyperthyroidism
- Severe anemia
- Arteriovenous shunting
- Paget's disease of the bone
- Beriberi
- Hepatic hemangiomatosis
- Sepsis
- Carcinoid

Congestive heart failure, right-sided

- Congestive heart failure, left-sided
- Cirrhosis
- Peripheral venous insufficiency
- Nephrotic syndrome

Etiology

- Usually left ventricular failure (left-sided congestive heart failure)
- Cor pulmonale (right heart failure due to pulmonary disease)

- Chronic pulmonary embolism
- Right-sided valve disease

Conjunctivitis

- Uveitis
- Acute glaucoma
- Foreign body or corneal abrasion
- Keratitis (corneal ulcer or inflammation), eg, herpes simplex
- Scleritis or episcleritis
- Dacryocystitis (lacrimal sac infection)

Etiology

- Viral infection, eg, adenovirus
- Bacterial infection, eg, *Staphylococcus, Streptococcus, Haemophilus, Pseudomonas, Moraxella, Chlamydia*, gonococci
- Allergic conjunctivitis
- Reactive arthritis (Reiter's syndrome)
- Keratoconjunctivitis sicca (dry eyes)
- Chemical irritants
- Systemic disease, eg, measles, Kawasaki syndrome, epidemic or scrub typhus, trichinosis

Constipation

Most common
- Inadequate fiber or fluid intake
- Poor bowel habits

Systemic disease
- Endocrine: hypothyroidism, hyperparathyroidism, diabetes mellitus
- Metabolic: hypercalcemia, hypokalemia, uremia, porphyria
- Neurologic: Parkinson's disease, multiple sclerosis, sacral nerve damage (pelvic surgery, tumor), paraplegia, autonomic neuropathy
- Rheumatologic: scleroderma, amyloidosis
- Medications: narcotics, diuretics, calcium channel blockers, anticholinergics, psychotropics, calcium, iron, NSAIDs, clonidine, sucralfate, cholestyramine
- Infectious: typhoid fever

Structural abnormalities
- Anorectal: rectal prolapse, rectocele, rectal intussusception, anorectal stricture, anal fissure, solitary rectal ulcer syndrome
- Pelvic floor dysfunction, eg, hysterectomy
- Obstructing colonic mass, eg, cancer
- Colonic stricture: radiation, ischemia, diverticulosis
- Hirschsprung's disease
- Chagas' disease
- Idiopathic megarectum

Slow colonic transit
- Idiopathic: isolated to colon
- Psychogenic
- Eating disorders
- Chronic intestinal pseudo-obstruction

Other
- Irritable bowel syndrome

Constricted pupil

- Opioids (pinpoint)
- Other causes of sympatholytic poisoning, eg, benzodiazepines, clonidine
- Horner's syndrome
- Myotic drugs, eg, pilocarpine
- Neurosyphilis (Argyll Robertson pupils)
- Pontine infarct
- Uveitis
- Inflammatory adhesions between iris and lens (posterior synechiae)
- Cholinergic poisoning, eg, organophosphates
- Physiologic anisocoria (unequal pupils, react normally)

Cough, acute

- Viral upper respiratory infection or postviral cough (most common)
- Bacterial upper respiratory infection
- Postnasal drip (allergic rhinitis)
- Pneumonia
- Pulmonary edema, eg, congestive heart failure
- Pulmonary embolism
- Aspiration pneumonia

Cough, chronic

- Top 3 causes: postnasal drip, asthma, gastroesophageal reflux disease

Pulmonary infection
- Postviral
- Bronchitis, especially in smokers
- Bronchiectasis
- Tuberculosis
- Cystic fibrosis
- *Mycobacterium avium* complex
- Pertussis
- *Mycoplasma*
- Chlamydia
- Respiratory syncytial virus
- Parasites, eg, ascariasis, paragonimiasis

Pulmonary noninfectious
- Asthma (cough-variant asthma)
- Beta blockers causing asthma
- Chronic obstructive pulmonary disease
- ACE inhibitors
- Irritant inhalation, eg, smoking
- Endobronchial lesion, eg, tumor
- Interstitial lung disease
- Sarcoidosis
- Chronic microaspiration

Nonpulmonary
- Gastroesophageal reflux disease
- Postnasal drip (allergic rhinitis)
- Sinusitis
- Congestive heart failure
- Laryngitis
- Ear canal or tympanic membrane irritation
- Psychogenic or habit cough

Cranial nerve 3 palsy

Etiology

- Microvascular infarction, eg, diabetes mellitus, hypertension
- Sarcoidosis
- Space-occupying lesion, especially posterior inferior cerebellar artery aneurysm
- Ophthalmoplegic migraine
- Brainstem infarct or vertebrobasilar insufficiency
- Temporal (giant cell) arteritis
- Uncal herniation

Cranial nerve 6 palsy

Etiology

- Microvascular infarction, eg, diabetes mellitus, hypertension
- Wernicke's encephalopathy
- Increased intracranial pressure, eg, pseudotumor cerebri
- Tuberculous meningitis
- Sphenoid sinusitis
- Cavernous sinus thrombosis
- Brainstem infarct or vertebrobasilar insufficiency
- Multiple sclerosis
- Temporal (giant cell) arteritis

Cranial nerve palsy

Etiology

- Microvascular infarction, eg, diabetes mellitus, hypertension

- Multiple sclerosis
- Acute or chronic otitis media
- Malignant otitis externa
- Infiltrating process at skull base: meningitis, sarcoidosis, intracranial metastases, lymphoma, nasopharyngeal cancer
- Brainstem infarct or vertebrobasilar insufficiency
- Arterial dissection, eg, internal carotid, vertebral
- Compression by aneurysm or tumor
- Neurosyphilis
- Systemic lupus erythematosus
- Neurofibromatosis
- Paget's disease
- Myasthenia gravis
- Guillain-Barré syndrome
- Diphtheria
- Glomus jugulare (middle ear tumor)
- Pituitary apoplexy
- Graves' ophthalmopathy (not a palsy, but affects extraocular movements)

Cyanosis

- Hypoxia, eg, pneumonia, pulmonary embolism, congestive heart failure, valvular heart disease, hypotension, shunt, severe anemia, high altitude
- Cold exposure
- Raynaud's syndrome
- Reflex sympathetic dystrophy
- Methemoglobinemia
- Thoracic outlet syndrome
- Polyarteritis nodosa

Decubitus ulcers

- Herpes simplex
- Skin cancer
- Pyoderma gangrenosum
- Ecthyma gangrenosum (neutropenic, pseudomonal)

Dementia

- Delirium
- Depression (pseudodementia)
- Vision or hearing impairment

Etiology

Reversible causes

- Hypothyroidism or hyperthyroidism
- Depression
- Drugs, eg, anticholinergics, sedatives, antipsychotics, opioids
- Vitamin B_{12} or thiamine deficiency
- Hypercalcemia
- Uremic or hepatic encephalopathy
- Space-occupying lesion, eg, brain tumor, subdural hematoma
- Neurosyphilis
- HIV
- Normal pressure hydrocephalus
- Wilson's disease
- Sleep apnea
- Chronic meningitis

Irreversible causes

- Alzheimer's disease
- Vascular (multi-infarct) dementia
- Parkinson's disease
- Dementia with Lewy bodies
- Huntington's disease
- Frontotemporal dementia, eg, Pick's disease
- Progressive supranuclear palsy
- Creutzfeldt-Jakob disease

Depression

- Normal grief response
- Bipolar disorder
- Alcohol, sedative, or opiate abuse
- Stimulant withdrawal, eg, cocaine, amphetamines
- Anxiety disorder, eg, generalized anxiety disorder, post-traumatic stress disorder
- Domestic violence
- Hypothyroidism
- Dementia, parkinsonism, or stroke
- Other chronic medical illness, eg, anemia, chronic infection, renal failure
- Drug-induced, eg, reserpine, corticosteroids, oral contraceptives, clonidine, levodopa
- Cushing's syndrome
- Personality disorder, eg, borderline

Dermatitis, exfoliative (exfoliative erythroderma)

- Psoriasis
- Seborrheic dermatitis
- Drug eruption
- Toxic shock syndrome (staphylococcal or streptococcal)
- Scarlet fever
- Staphylococcal scalded skin syndrome
- Erythema multiforme major or toxic epidermal necrolysis

Etiology

- Idiopathic
- Drug eruption
- Seborrheic dermatitis
- Contact dermatitis
- Atopic dermatitis
- Psoriasis
- Cancer (Sézary syndrome of cutaneous T cell lymphoma, Hodgkin's disease)
- Pityriasis rubra pilaris

Desquamative erythema

- Toxic shock syndrome (staphylococcal or streptococcal)
- Scarlet fever
- Kawasaki syndrome
- Staphylococcal scalded skin syndrome
- Exfoliative erythroderma syndrome (eg, underlying psoriasis, eczema, drug eruption)
- Erythema multiforme major or toxic epidermal necrolysis

Diarrhea, acute

Infectious: noninflammatory (nonbloody)

- Viruses: Norwalk virus, rotavirus, adenoviruses, astrovirus, coronavirus
- Preformed toxin (food poisoning): *Staphylococcus aureus, Bacillus cereus, Clostridium perfringens*
- Toxin production: enterotoxigenic *Escherichia coli, Vibrio cholerae, Vibrio parahaemolyticus*
- Protozoa: *Giardia lamblia, Cryptosporidium, Cyclospora, Isospora*

Infectious: invasive or inflammatory

- *Shigella, Salmonella, Campylobacter,* enteroinvasive *E. coli, E. coli* O157:H7, *Yersinia enterocolitica, Clostridium difficile* (eg, pseudomembranous colitis), *Entamoeba histolytica, Neisseria gonorrhoeae, Listeria monocytogenes*

Associated with unprotected anal intercourse

- *Neisseria gonorrhoeae,* syphilis, lymphogranuloma venereum, herpes simplex

Noninfectious

- Drug reaction, especially antibiotics
- Ulcerative colitis, Crohn's disease (inflammatory)
- Ischemic colitis (inflammatory)
- Fecal impaction (stool may leak around impaction)
- Laxative abuse

- Radiation colitis (inflammatory)
- Emotional stress

Diarrhea, chronic

Common

- Irritable bowel syndrome, lactase deficiency, parasites, caffeine, alcohol, laxative abuse

Osmotic

- Lactase deficiency
- Medications: antacids, lactulose, sorbitol, Olestra
- Factitious: magnesium-containing antacids or laxatives

Secretory

- Hormonal: Zollinger-Ellison syndrome (gastrinoma), carcinoid, VIPoma, medullary thyroid carcinoma
- Laxative abuse: phenolphthalein, cascara, senna
- Villous adenoma
- Medications

Inflammatory conditions

- Inflammatory bowel disease
- Microscopic colitis (lymphocytic or collagenous)
- Cancer with obstruction and pseudo-diarrhea
- Radiation colitis

Malabsorption

- Small bowel: celiac sprue, Whipple's disease, tropical sprue, eosinophilic gastroenteritis, small bowel resection, Crohn's disease
- Lymphatic obstruction: lymphoma, carcinoid, tuberculosis, mycobacterium avium complex, Kaposi's sarcoma, sarcoidosis, retroperitoneal fibrosis
- Pancreatic insufficiency: chronic pancreatitis, cystic fibrosis, pancreatic cancer
- Bacterial overgrowth, eg, diabetes mellitus
- Reduced bile salts: ileal resection, Crohn's disease, postcholecystectomy

Motility disorders

- Irritable bowel syndrome
- Postsurgical: vagotomy, partial gastrectomy, blind loop with bacterial overgrowth
- Systemic disease: diabetes mellitus, hyperthyroidism, scleroderma
- Caffeine or alcohol use

Chronic infections

- Parasites: giardiasis, amebiasis, strongyloidiasis

Other

- Ischemic colitis
- Adrenal insufficiency

Diarrhea in diabetes

- Sorbitol in dietetic foods
- Celiac sprue
- Pancreatic insufficiency
- Bacterial overgrowth
- Visceral autonomic neuropathy

Diarrhea in HIV/AIDS

- Viral: cytomegalovirus, adenovirus, HIV (AIDS enteropathy)
- Bacterial: *Campylobacter, Salmonella, Shigella, Clostridium difficile, Mycobacterium avium* complex, tuberculosis
- Protozoal: *Cryptosporidium, Entamoeba histolytica, Giardia, Isospora,* microsporidia
- HIV-associated malabsorption

Dilated pupil

- Cranial nerve 3 palsy
- Iris damage due to acute glaucoma
- Mydriatic drugs, eg, atropine
- Sympathomimetic poisoning, eg, amphetamines, cocaine
- Anticholinergic poisoning, eg, atropine, tricyclic antidepressants
- Physiologic anisocoria (unequal pupils, react normally)

Diplopia or ophthalmoplegia

- Microvascular infarction, eg, diabetes mellitus, hypertension
- Wernicke's encephalopathy
- Multiple sclerosis
- Myasthenia gravis
- Graves' ophthalmopathy
- Botulism
- Internal carotid artery aneurysm or carotid dissection
- Posterior inferior cerebellar artery aneurysm
- Other mass compressing nerves to extraocular muscles
- Brainstem infarct
- Neurosyphilis
- Systemic lupus erythematosus
- Sarcoidosis
- Pseudotumor cerebri
- Muscle entrapment from orbital blow-out fracture
- Orbital cellulitis
- Sphenoid sinusitis
- Cavernous sinus thrombosis
- Ophthalmoplegic migraine
- Temporal (giant cell) arteritis
- Tuberculous meningitis
- Diphtheria
- Progressive supranuclear palsy
- Progressive external ophthalmoplegia (mitochondrial myopathy)
- Other causes of cranial nerve palsy

Monocular diplopia (with one eye closed)

- Refractive error
- Early cataract
- Lens dislocation, eg, Marfan syndrome, homocystinuria
- Corneal opacity, eg, scar, pterygium

Drug eruption, fixed

- Bullous pemphigoid
- Erythema multiforme
- Sweet's syndrome (acute febrile neutrophilic dermatosis)
- Genital lesions: psoriasis, lichen planus, syphilis

Dry eyes (keratoconjunctivitis sicca)

- Allergic conjunctivitis
- Chronic blepharitis
- Age-related
- Dry environment
- Abnormal lipid component of tears, eg, blepharitis
- Autoimmune disease, eg, Sjögren's syndrome, systemic lupus erythematosus
- Xerophthalmia (vitamin A deficiency)
- Sarcoidosis
- Pemphigoid or Stevens-Johnson syndrome
- Impaired eyelid or lacrimal gland function
- Systemic or topical drugs

Dry mouth (xerostomia)

- Sjögren's syndrome
- Mumps
- Sarcoidosis
- Drugs: psychiatric, anticholinergic, antihypertensive
- Local irradiation
- Diabetes mellitus
- Lymphoma

- Psychogenic
- Idiopathic

Dysarthria

Etiology

- Painful oral ulcers, eg, herpes simplex, aphthous ulcers
- Cerebral stroke or subarachnoid hemorrhage
- Brainstem or cerebellar infarct, mass, or hemorrhage
- Multiple sclerosis
- Pseudobulbar palsy
- Amyotrophic lateral sclerosis
- Poliomyelitis
- Guillain-Barré syndrome
- Myasthenia gravis
- Botulism
- Parkinsonism
- Huntington's disease
- Wilson's disease
- Trauma to cranial nerve V or XII
- Diphtheria
- Macroglossia, eg, amyloidosis, hypothyroidism

Dysmenorrhea

Etiology

- Primary dysmenorrhea
- Endometriosis
- Adenomyosis (uterine endometriosis)
- Pelvic inflammatory disease
- Uterine leiomyomas (fibroids)
- Intrauterine device
- Pelvic pain syndrome
- Endometrial polyp
- Cervicitis
- Retroverted uterus
- Cervical stenosis
- Cystitis
- Interstitial cystitis

Dyspareunia

- Vulvodynia or vulvar vestibulitis
- Vaginismus
- Insufficient vaginal lubrication
- Atrophic vaginitis
- Vulvovaginitis, cervicitis, or pelvic inflammatory disease
- Endometriosis
- Lichen sclerosus
- Ovarian tumor
- Pelvic adhesions
- Remnants of the hymen

Dysphagia

Etiology

Esophageal dysphagia

Mechanical obstruction (solids worse than liquids)

- Esophageal web, ring (eg, Schatzki's), or diverticulum (intermittent dysphagia, not progressive)
- Peptic stricture (chronic heartburn, progressive dysphagia)
- Esophageal cancer (progressive dysphagia, age >50)

Motility disorder (solids and liquids)

- Achalasia (progressive dysphagia)
- Diffuse esophageal spasm (intermittent, not progressive)
- Scleroderma (chronic heartburn)

Oropharyngeal dysphagia

Neurologic disorders

- Brainstem stroke, mass lesion
- Amyotrophic lateral sclerosis, multiple sclerosis, pseudobulbar palsy, postpolio syndrome, Guillain-Barré syndrome
- Parkinson's disease, Huntington's disease, dementia
- Tardive dyskinesia

Muscular and rheumatologic disorders

- Myopathy, polymyositis
- Oculopharyngeal dystrophy
- Sjögren's syndrome

Metabolic disorders

- Thyrotoxicosis, amyloidosis, Cushing's disease, Wilson's disease
- Drugs: anticholinergics, phenothiazines

Infectious disease

- Polio, diphtheria, botulism, Lyme disease, syphilis, mucositis (*Candida*, herpes)

Structural disorders

- Zenker's diverticulum
- Cervical osteophytes, cricopharyngeal bar, proximal esophageal webs
- Oropharyngeal tumors
- Postsurgical or radiation changes
- Pill-induced injury

Motility disorders

- Upper esophageal sphincter dysfunction

Dyspnea

Acute

- Asthma, pneumonia, pulmonary edema, pneumothorax, pulmonary embolism, metabolic acidosis, acute respiratory distress syndrome, panic attack

Pulmonary

- Airflow obstruction (asthma, chronic obstructive pulmonary disease, upper airway obstruction), restrictive lung disease (interstitial lung disease, pleural thickening or effusion, respiratory muscle weakness, obesity), pneumonia, pneumothorax, pulmonary embolism, aspiration, acute respiratory distress syndrome

Cardiac

- Myocardial ischemia, congestive heart failure, valvular obstruction, arrhythmia, cardiac tamponade

Metabolic

- Acidosis, hypercapnia, sepsis

Hematologic

- Anemia, methemoglobinemia

Psychiatric

- Anxiety

Dyspnea, episodic

- Congestive heart failure
- Asthma
- Acute or chronic bronchitis
- Recurrent pulmonary emboli

Dystonia

Etiology

- Dystonia, idiopathic torsion
- Focal torsion dystonia, eg, blepharospasm, torticollis, oromandibular dystonia, writer's cramp
- Perinatal anoxia or birth trauma
- Kernicterus
- Wilson's disease
- Huntington's disease
- Parkinsonism
- Encephalitis lethargica
- Drugs, eg, antipsychotics
- Tetanus

Dysuria

- Cystitis
- Urethritis, eg, gonorrhea, chlamydia
- Pyelonephritis
- Vaginitis
- Epididymitis
- Balanitis
- Prostatitis
- Interstitial cystitis

- Urethral syndrome
- Genital herpes
- Atrophic vaginitis
- Reactive arthritis (Reiter's syndrome)

Ear canal diseases

- Cerumen impaction (ear wax)
- Otitis externa (external otitis)
- Malignant otitis externa (osteomyelitis)
- Ear pruritus
- Osteoma
- Exostoses
- Squamous cell carcinoma
- Cholesteatoma
- Seborrheic dermatitis

Ear pain

- Acute otitis media
- Otitis externa
- Chronic otitis media
- Auditory (eustachian) tube dysfunction
- Mastoiditis
- Referred pain: sinusitis, tooth pain, cancer of upper aerodigestive tract
- Temporomandibular joint syndrome
- Trauma or barotrauma
- Foreign body
- Osteoma
- Cholesteatoma
- Ramsay-Hunt syndrome (herpes zoster oticus)
- Acoustic neuroma
- Bullous myringitis
- Glossopharyngeal neuralgia

Ear pruritus

- Otitis, externa (external otitis)
- Seborrheic dermatitis
- Psoriasis
- Excoriation
- Excessive ear cleaning

Eczema, nummular or discoid

- Tinea corporis
- Psoriasis
- Xerosis (dry skin)
- Impetigo
- Contact dermatitis
- Lichen simplex chronicus
- Pityriasis rosea

Edema, lower extremity

Cardiovascular

- Congestive heart failure (right-sided)
- Pericardial effusion
- Pericarditis
- Tricuspid regurgitation
- Tricuspid stenosis
- Pulmonary stenosis
- Cor pulmonale
- Venous insufficiency (most common)
- Venous obstruction

Noncardiovascular

- Cirrhosis
- Low albumin (nephrotic syndrome, malnutrition, protein-losing enteropathy)
- Cellulitis
- Premenstrual fluid retention
- Drugs (vasodilators, eg, calcium channel blockers, salt-retaining medications, eg, NSAIDs, thiazolidinediones)
- Musculoskeletal (Baker's cyst, gastrocnemius tear, compartment syndrome)
- Lymphatic obstruction
- Preeclampsia-eclampsia
- Myxedema
- Lymphatic filariasis
- Eosinophilic fasciitis

Edema, unilateral

- Deep vein thrombosis
- Venous insufficiency
- Baker's cyst (rupture or obstruction of popliteal vein)
- Cellulitis
- Trauma
- Lymphatic obstruction, eg, obstruction by pelvic tumor
- Reflex sympathetic dystrophy
- Tumor or fibrosis obstructing iliac vein
- May-Thurner syndrome (left iliac vein compressed by right common iliac artery)
- Loiasis (*Loa loa* infection)

Edema, upper extremity

- SVC syndrome
- Upper extremity deep vein thrombosis
- Lymphatic obstruction
- Reflex sympathetic dystrophy
- Eosinophilic fasciitis

EKG: electrical alternans

- Pericardial effusion
- Dilated cardiomyopathy
- Transient electrical alternans with supraventricular tachycardia

EKG: left atrial enlargement

- Left ventricular hypertrophy
- Coronary artery disease
- Mitral valve disease
- Cardiomyopathy

EKG: left axis deviation

- Left anterior fascicular block
- Inferior myocardial infarction
- Ventricular pre-excitation (Wolff-Parkinson-White pattern)
- Chronic obstructive pulmonary disease

EKG: long QT

Etiology

Electrolyte abnormalities

- Hypokalemia
- Hypomagnesemia
- Hypocalcemia

Drugs (selected examples)

- Class Ia antiarrhythmics (quinidine, procainamide)
- Class Ic antiarrhythmics (propafenone)
- Class III antiarrhythmics (amiodarone, bretylium, sotalol)
- Tricyclic antidepressants
- Astemizole, terfenadine
- Antibiotics: erythromycin, trimethoprim-sulfamethoxazole, levofloxacin, ketoconazole, itraconazole
- Phenothiazines, haloperidol
- Prednisone

Miscellaneous

- Congenital long QT syndrome
- Third-degree A-V block
- Second-degree A-V block
- Left ventricular hypertrophy
- Myocardial ischemia
- Significant bradycardia
- Stroke or subarachnoid hemorrhage
- Hypothermia

EKG: low voltage

Myocardial causes

- Multiple or massive myocardial infarctions
- Infiltrative disease (eg, amyloidosis, sarcoidosis, hemochromatosis)

Nonmyocardial causes

- Pericardial effusion
- Chronic obstructive pulmonary disease
- Pleural effusion
- Obesity
- Anasarca
- Myxedema (due to skin changes, pericardial effusion, and myocardial disease)
- Subcutaneous emphysema

EKG: right atrial enlargement

- Right ventricular hypertrophy

EKG: right axis deviation

- Right ventricular hypertrophy
- Anteroapical myocardial infarction
- Ventricular pre-excitation (Wolff-Parkinson-White pattern)
- Left posterior fascicular block

EKG: short QT

- Hypercalcemia
- Digoxin
- Thyrotoxicosis
- Increased sympathetic tone

EKG: ST depression or T wave inversion

- Subendocardial ischemia
- Right bundle branch block (V1)
- Left bundle branch block (V5-V6)
- Left ventricular hypertrophy with repolarization abnormality (V5-V6)
- Subarachnoid hemorrhage
- Right ventricular hypertrophy (V1-V3)
- Hypokalemia
- Digoxin

EKG: ST elevation

- Acute myocardial infarction
- Vasospasm (Prinzmetal's angina)
- Pericarditis
- Left bundle branch block (V1-V3)
- Left ventricular hypertrophy with repolarization abnormality (V1-V3)
- Early repolarization (normal variant)
- Ventricular pacemaker
- Cocaine
- Myocarditis

EKG: U waves

- Hypokalemia
- Bradycardia
- Digoxin
- Antiarrhythmic drugs

EKG: wide QRS

- Bundle branch block or intraventricular conduction delay
- Ventricular ectopy
- Pacemaker
- Hyperkalemia
- Wolff-Parkinson-White syndrome
- Drugs: tricyclic antidepressants, class Ia antiarrhythmics (eg, quinidine), class Ic antiarrhythmics (eg, propafenone), phenothiazines

Elbow pain

- Epicondylitis, lateral ("tennis elbow") or medial ("golf elbow")
- Olecranon bursitis
- Arthritis, eg, rheumatoid arthritis, gout, osteoarthritis, septic arthritis
- Fracture
- Tendonitis of distal insertion of biceps
- Ulnar nerve entrapment at elbow
- Avascular necrosis
- Metastatic or primary tumor

Encephalitis, viral

- Aseptic or bacterial meningitis
- Lymphocytic choriomeningitis
- Encephalitis accompanying exanthematous diseases of childhood: measles, varicella, infectious mononucleosis, rubella
- Nonparalytic poliomyelitis
- Subarachnoid hemorrhage, stroke, brain tumor, brain abscess
- Lupus cerebritis
- Behçet's syndrome
- Lyme disease or neurosyphilis
- Toxoplasmosis or cryptococcosis
- Encephalitis following vaccination (for rabies, measles, pertussis)
- Reye's syndrome
- Toxic encephalitis, eg, drugs, poisons, Shiga toxin
- Amebic meningoencephalitis (*Naegleria fowleri*) or granulomatous amebic encephalitis (*Acanthamoeba*)
- African trypanosomiasis (sleeping sickness)

Etiology

- Herpes simplex, mumps, HIV, poliovirus, rabies, cytomegalovirus
- Viral and mosquito-borne (arboviruses): St. Louis, California, Japanese B, Western equine, Eastern equine, West Nile encephalitis

Eosinophilia

Etiology

- Drug hypersensitivity
- Allergic state, eg, asthma, urticaria, atopic dermatitis
- Tissue invasion by parasites, eg, ascariasis, visceral larva migrans
- Other skin disorder, eg, pemphigoid, dermatitis herpetiformis
- Malignancy, especially lymphoma
- Connective tissue disease, eg, Churg-Strauss syndrome, polyarteritis nodosa, eosinophilic fasciitis
- Eosinophilic pulmonary syndrome
- Fungal infection, eg, coccidioidomycosis
- Idiopathic
- Other: adrenal insufficiency, cholesterol emboli, eosinophilic leukemia

Eosinophilic pulmonary syndromes

Etiology

- Chronic eosinophilic pneumonia
- Acute eosinophilic pneumonia (Loefﬂer's syndrome)
- Drugs: nitrofurantoin, phenytoin, ampicillin, penicillin, sulfonamides, acetaminophen, ranitidine, methotrexate
- Helminth infection: ascariasis, hookworm, strongyloidiasis, paragonimiasis, toxocariasis (visceral larva migrans), tropical pulmonary eosinophilia (*Wuchereria bancrofti, Brugia malayi*)
- Allergic bronchopulmonary aspergillosis
- Churg-Strauss syndrome
- Systemic hypereosinophilic syndromes
- Eosinophilic granuloma (Langerhans cell histiocytosis, histiocytosis X)

- Malignancy
- Numerous interstitial lung diseases
- Toxins: inhaled crack cocaine, heroin, Scotchguard, sulfite pesticides

Epistaxis

- Nasal trauma, eg, nose picking, forceful nose blowing, foreign body
- Allergic rhinitis or viral rhinitis
- Dry nasal mucosa
- Deviated septum
- Chronic sinusitis
- Inhaled steroids
- Cocaine use
- Alcohol use
- Antiplatelet drugs, eg, aspirin, clopidogrel
- Thrombocytopenia, eg, idiopathic thrombocytopenic purpura, thrombotic thrombocytopenic purpura
- Hemophilia
- Hereditary hemorrhagic telangiectasia (Osler-Weber-Rendu syndrome)
- Polycythemia vera
- Leukemia
- Wegener's granulomatosis
- Nasal tumor

Erectile dysfunction

- Diabetes mellitus
- Atherosclerosis (Leriche syndrome: impotence and claudication)
- Hypogonadism (primary or secondary testicular failure)
- Stroke
- Local trauma
- Hyperprolactinemia
- Hyperthyroidism
- Cushing's syndrome
- Addison's disease
- Acromegaly
- Multiple sclerosis
- Spinal cord trauma or tumor
- Psychogenic
- Drugs (selected): alcohol, tobacco, recreational drugs, SSRIs, clonidine, thiazides, spironolactone, tricyclic antidepressants, antihistamines, beta blockers (uncommon)

Erythema, figurate (shaped)

- Urticaria
- Erythema multiforme
- Erythema migrans (Lyme disease)
- Cellulitis & erysipelas
- Cellulitis
- Erysipeloid
- Arthropod bites (insect bites)

Erythromelalgia

- Raynaud's phenomenon
- Venous insufficiency
- Arterial insufficiency
- Peripheral neuropathy

Etiology

- Idiopathic
- Polycythemia vera
- Essential thrombocytosis
- Drugs: bromocriptine, nifedipine, felodipine, desmopressin
- Hypertension
- Gout

Erythroplakia

- Usually dysplasia or carcinoma

Esophageal motility disorders

- Achalasia (idiopathic)
- Chagas' disease
- Pseudoachalasia (tumor invading gastroesophageal junction)
- Diffuse esophageal spasm
- Scleroderma
- Nutcracker esophagus

Esophagitis

Etiology

- Infectious: *Candida*, herpes simplex virus, cytomegalovirus
- Reflux esophagitis
- Pill-induced esophagitis: NSAIDs, KCl, AZT, alendronate, iron, antibiotics
- Caustic esophageal injury (alkali or acid ingestion)
- Radiation esophagitis

Eyelid disorders

- Blepharitis
- Hordeolum (sty)
- Chalazion
- Entropion or ectropion
- Xanthelasma (lipid disorder or idiopathic)
- Tumor, eg, verrucae, papilloma, basal or squamous cell carcinoma, melanoma
- Dacryocystitis (lacrimal sac infection)

Eye pain

- Viral or bacterial conjunctivitis
- Foreign body or corneal abrasion
- Keratitis (corneal ulcer or inflammation), eg, herpes simplex
- Trauma
- Acute glaucoma
- Orbital or periorbital cellulitis
- Ultraviolet (actinic) keratitis
- Eyelid disorder, eg, hordeolum, chalazion, blepharitis
- Inverted eyelash (eg, entropion)
- Dacryocystitis (lacrimal sac infection)
- Decreased tearing, eg, age-related, Sjögren's syndrome, anticholinergics
- Sinusitis
- Migraine or cluster headache
- Temporal (giant cell) arteritis
- Ophthalmic zoster (pain may precede rash)
- Uveitis
- Scleritis or episcleritis
- Optic neuritis
- Intracranial mass

Facial, tooth, or jaw pain

- Dental caries or abscess
- Sinusitis
- Temporal arteritis
- Trigeminal neuralgia
- TMJ syndrome
- Migraine
- Sialadenitis (eg, parotitis)
- Sialolithiasis (salivary gland calculi)
- Otitis media
- Orbital or periorbital cellulitis
- Peritonsillar abscess
- Ludwig's angina (retropharyngeal infection)
- Carotid dissection
- Glossopharyngeal neuralgia
- Atypical facial pain
- Postherpetic neuralgia
- Bruxism (teeth grinding)
- Dental misalignment
- Acoustic neuroma
- Trauma
- Glaucoma

- Dacryocystitis (lacrimal sac infection)
- Angina pectoris
- Numb chin syndrome (mental neuropathy) due to malignancy in mandible

Facial erythema

- Erysipelas
- Cellulitis
- Impetigo
- Acne rosacea
- Contact dermatitis
- Seborrheic dermatitis
- Systemic lupus erythematosus
- Herpes zoster (shingles)
- Tinea
- Angioedema
- Necrotizing fasciitis
- Erysipeloid
- Dermatomyositis (purplish rash on upper eyelids)

Facial palsy (Bell's palsy)

Etiology

- Bell's palsy (idiopathic)
- HIV
- Lyme disease
- Sarcoidosis
- Ramsay Hunt syndrome (herpes zoster of geniculate ganglion)
- Acoustic neuroma
- Acute or chronic otitis media
- Malignant otitis externa
- Guillain-Barré syndrome
- Tumor, eg, parotid, temporal bone tumor
- Brainstem infarct

Falls & gait disorders

- Visual impairment
- Gait impairment due to:
  - Podiatric disorder, eg, ingrown nail
  - Arthritis
  - Muscular weakness, eg, myopathy
  - Cerebellar ataxia, eg, alcoholism
  - Sensory ataxia, eg, vitamin B_{12} deficiency, neurosyphilis
  - Other neurologic disorder, eg, parkinsonism, dementia in elderly, spinal stenosis, multiple sclerosis, peripheral neuropathy
- Environmental hazards, eg, poor lighting, stairs, rugs, uneven floors
- Polypharmacy, eg, benzodiazepines, opioids, phenothiazines, vasodilators, diuretics
- Alcohol use
- Orthostatic or postprandial hypotension
- Vertigo, presyncope, syncope, or dysequilibrium
- Medical illness, eg, pneumonia, myocardial infarction, anemia, hyponatremia
- Other contributing factors: urinary urgency, peripheral edema, insomnia

Fatigue

- Hypothyroidism
- Anemia
- Depression
- Sleep apnea or insufficient sleep
- Infection, eg, tuberculosis, hepatitis, endocarditis, HIV, Lyme disease
- Diabetes mellitus
- Congestive heart failure, chronic obstructive pulmonary disease, or chronic renal failure
- Cancer
- Alcoholism
- Hypercalcemia
- Drugs, eg, sedatives, beta blockers
- Chronic fatigue syndrome
- Somatoform disorder (eg, somatization)
- Fibromyalgia
- Mononucleosis
- Autoimmune disease
- Adrenal insufficiency
- Iron deficiency even in absence of anemia

Fecal incontinence

- Acute or chronic diarrhea
- Perianal fistula, eg, Crohn's disease
- Rectal prolapse

Etiology

- Hemorrhoids or anal skin tags (disrupt anal seal)
- Proctitis
- Irritable bowel syndrome
- Constipation with "overflow" incontinence
- Chronic diarrhea due to other causes
- Sphincter damage, eg, traumatic childbirth, episiotomy, rectal prolapse, surgery, cancer
- Neurologic, eg, pudendal nerve damage (obstetric trauma), diabetes mellitus, aging, dementia, multiple sclerosis, spinal cord injury, cauda equina syndrome

Fever

Common causes

- Infection
  - Bacterial, viral, rickettsial, fungal, parasitic
  - CNS, sinusitis, dental, endocarditis, pneumonia, liver, biliary system, gastrointestinal, peritonitis, abdominal abscess, urinary tract infection, prostatitis, sexually transmitted disease, cellulitis, soft tissues, bone, joints
- Autoimmune disease
- CNS disease including head trauma, mass lesion
- Malignancy, especially lymphoma, leukemia, renal cell carcinoma, primary or metastatic liver cancer

Less common causes

- Cardiovascular disease, eg, myocardial infarction, deep vein thrombosis, pulmonary embolism
- Gastrointestinal disease, eg, inflammatory bowel disease, alcoholic hepatitis, granulomatous hepatitis
- Miscellaneous, eg, drug fever, sarcoidosis, familial Mediterranean fever, tissue injury, hematoma, factitious fever

Hyperthermia

- Heat stroke, neuroleptic malignant syndrome, malignant hyperthermia

Fever, hospital-acquired

- Noninfectious: drug fever, postoperative atelectasis or tissue necrosis, hematoma, pancreatitis, pulmonary embolism, myocardial infarction, ischemic colitis
- Pneumonia
- Bacteremia, eg, indwelling catheter, wound, abscess, pneumonia, GU or gastrointestinal tract
- Wound infection, eg, decubitus ulcer
- *Clostridium difficile* colitis

Fever, postoperative

- Wind: pneumonia, atelectasis
- Water: urinary tract infection
- Wound: wound infection
- Walking: deep vein thrombosis from immobilization
- Wonderdrugs: drug fever

Fever, postpartum

- Endometritis
- Urinary tract infection
- Pneumonia
- Septic pelvic vein thrombosis or pelvic abscess
- Retained products of conception

- Deep vein thrombosis or pulmonary embolism (including amniotic embolism)
- Wound infection
- Mastitis
- Thyroiditis

Fever, relapsing or recurrent

- Malaria
- Typhoid fever (enteric fever)
- Brucellosis
- Borreliosis
- Lymphoma (especially Hodgkin's disease)
- Tuberculosis
- Rat bite fever
- Occult abscess
- Trench fever (*Bartonella quintana*)
- Familial Mediterranean fever

Fever and rash

Diffuse maculopapular rash

- Viral exanthem: measles, rubella (German measles), erythema infectiosum ("slapped-cheek" disease), exanthem subitum (roseola), primary HIV infection, infectious mononucleosis, dengue
- Other infection: typhoid fever, secondary syphilis, Lyme disease, leptospirosis, rat bite fever, relapsing fever, ehrlichiosis, epidemic typhus, endemic typhus, scrub typhus, erythema marginatum (rheumatic fever)
- Noninfectious: drug rash (with drug fever or unrelated infection), systemic lupus erythematosus, adult Still's disease

Peripheral eruption

- Meningococcemia or gonococcemia
- Secondary syphilis
- Rocky Mountain spotted fever
- Erythema multiforme
- Bacterial endocarditis
- Hand, foot, and mouth disease

Desquamative erythema

- Toxic shock syndrome (staphylococcal or streptococcal)
- Scarlet fever
- Kawasaki syndrome
- Staphylococcal scalded skin syndrome
- Exfoliative erythroderma syndrome (eg, underlying psoriasis, eczema, drug eruption)
- Erythema multiforme major or toxic epidermal necrolysis

Vesicles or bullae

- Varicella (chickenpox)
- Staphylococcal scalded skin syndrome
- Erythema multiforme major or toxic epidermal necrolysis
- Hand, foot, and mouth disease
- Rickettsialpox
- Ecthyma gangrenosum (neutropenic, pseudomonal)
- Disseminated *Vibrio vulnificus* (cirrhosis, seafood or seawater exposure)

Purpura or petechiae

- Bacterial endocarditis
- Meningococcemia or gonococcemia
- Rocky Mountain spotted fever
- Purpura fulminans (severe disseminated intravascular coagulation)
- Thrombotic thrombocytopenic purpura
- Other: epidemic typhus, rat bite fever, enteroviral petechial rash, viral hemorrhagic fever

Other

- Urticarial vasculitis (serum sickness, connective tissue disease, infection, idiopathic)
- Nodules due to disseminated infection (eg, fungal), erythema nodosum, Sweet's syndrome (acute febrile neutrophilic dermatosis)
- Pustular psoriasis

Fever in immunocompromised patient

Neutropenia

- Gram-negative enteric organisms
- *Pseudomonas*
- Gram-positive cocci, eg, *S. aureus*, *S. epidermidis*
- *Candida*
- *Aspergillus* and other fungi

Cellular immune defect (HIV, lymphoma, immunosuppressive drugs)

- Bacteria: *Listeria*, *Legionella*, *Salmonella*, *Mycobacterium*
- Viruses: herpes simplex virus, varicella, cytomegalovirus
- Fungi: *Cryptococcus*, *Coccidioides*, *Histoplasma*, *Pneumocystis*
- Protozoa: *Toxoplasma*

Humoral immune defect (congenital, multiple myeloma, chronic lymphocytic leukemia)

- Encapsulated organisms: *Streptococcus pneumoniae*, *Haemophilus influenzae*, *Neisseria meningitidis*

Asplenia (functional or anatomic)

- Encapsulated organisms: *Streptococcus pneumoniae*, *Haemophilus influenzae*, *Neisseria meningitidis*

Noninfectious causes

- Transplant rejection
- Organ ischemia or necrosis
- Thrombophlebitis
- Lymphoma

Fever in parenteral drug user

- Community-acquired pneumonia
- Endocarditis
- Complications of endocarditis, eg, pulmonary septic emboli, epidural abscess, osteomyelitis
- Skin abscess, cellulitis, myositis, necrotizing fasciitis
- Pelvic inflammatory disease
- Urinary tract infection

Fever in returning traveler

- Malaria
- Typhoid fever (enteric fever)
- Prodrome of hepatitis A, B, or E
- Dengue
- Amebiasis or amebic liver abscess
- Rickettsial spotted fever, eg, Mediterranean spotted fever, rickettsialpox, Rocky Mountain spotted fever
- Tuberculosis
- Visceral leishmaniasis
- Acute HIV infection
- Leptospirosis
- Acute schistosomiasis
- Yellow fever
- Scrub typhus
- African trypanosomiasis
- Rabies

Fever of unknown origin

Infection

- Tuberculosis, endocarditis, osteomyelitis, urinary tract infection, sinusitis, occult abscess (intra-abdominal, dental, brain), cholangitis, primary HIV, Epstein-Barr virus, cytomegalovirus, systemic mycosis, toxoplasmosis, brucellosis, Q fever, cat-scratch disease, salmonellosis, malaria

Neoplasm

- Hodgkin's or non-Hodgkin's lymphoma, leukemia, primary or metastatic liver cancer, renal cell carcinoma, atrial myxoma, others

Autoimmune

- Adult Still's disease, systemic lupus erythematosus, cryoglobulinemia, polyarteritis nodosa, temporal (giant cell) arteritis, polymyalgia rheumatica, Wegener's granulomatosis

Other

- Drug fever, sarcoidosis, granulomatous or alcoholic hepatitis, Crohn's disease, ulcerative colitis, factitious fever, thyroiditis, hematoma, recurrent pulmonary emboli, hypersensitivity pneumonitis, familial Mediterranean fever, Whipple's disease

Flatfoot

- Idiopathic
- Posterior tibial tendon rupture, eg, acute flatfoot after ankle sprain

Flatus (flatulence, gas)

- Carbohydrate-rich food
- Air swallowing
- Lactase deficiency
- Malabsorption, eg, celiac sprue
- Irritable bowel syndrome
- Parasites, eg, *Giardia*, *Strongyloides*, *Trichuris* (whipworm)
- Gas-producing foods: beans, peas, lentils, broccoli, Brussels sprouts, cauliflower, cabbage, parsnips, leeks, onions, beer, coffee

Flexor (volar) tenosynovitis

- Overuse
- Disseminated gonococcal infection
- Rheumatic fever
- Arthritis, eg, rheumatoid arthritis, psoriatic arthritis, osteoarthritis
- Sarcoidosis
- Fungal or atypical mycobacterial infection, eg, *Mycobacterium marinum*

Floaters

- Benign vitreous opacities
- Posterior vitreous detachment
- Vitreous hemorrhage
- Posterior uveitis
- Retinal detachment or tear (acute onset, especially with flashing lights)
- Cysticercosis

Focal segmental glomerulosclerosis

Etiology

- Heroin use
- Morbid obesity
- HIV
- Reflux nephropathy
- Idiopathic

Foot drop

Etiology

- Peroneal nerve compression
- L5 radiculopathy
- Diabetes mellitus
- Polyarteritis nodosa
- Charcot-Marie-Tooth disease
- Lyme disease

Foot pain

- Ingrown toenail
- Bunions, warts, calluses, corns
- Plantar fasciitis
- Morton's neuroma
- Metatarsalgia, eg, rheumatoid arthritis
- Pes planus (flatfoot)
- Bursitis of first MTP (inflamed bunion)
- Metatarsal stress fracture
- Arthritis, eg, gout, psoriatic arthritis, rheumatoid arthritis, osteoarthritis
- Poorly fitting shoes
- Lumbar disk herniation
- Achilles tendinitis
- Retrocalcaneal bursitis
- Tarsal tunnel syndrome
- Peripheral neuropathy, eg, diabetes mellitus, alcoholism
- Arterial insufficiency
- Diabetic or arterial insufficiency ulcer with or without osteomyelitis
- Polyarteritis nodosa, thromboangiitis obliterans (Buerger's disease), Raynaud's syndrome
- Erythromelalgia

FUO in HIV/AIDS

- Disseminated *mycobacterium avium* complex
- *Pneumocystis* pneumonia (PCP)
- Cytomegalovirus infection
- Disseminated histoplasmosis
- Lymphoma
- Tuberculosis
- Cryptococcal meningitis
- Drug fever
- Sinusitis
- *Salmonella* infection
- Kaposi's sarcoma
- Neurosyphilis
- Visceral leishmaniasis

Galactorrhea

- Physiologic: pregnancy, postpartum
- Idiopathic (normal prolactin level in parous woman)
- Hyperprolactinemia, eg, medications, prolactinoma, hypothyroidism
- Benign or malignant neoplasm
- Nipple stimulation
- Mastitis
- Oral contraceptives or estrogen replacement therapy

Gastric tumor

Benign

- Gastric epithelial polyp
- Adenomatous polyp
- Submucosal: benign stromal tumor (leiomyoma), pancreatic rest

Malignant

- Gastric adenocarcinoma
- Gastric lymphoma (primary, eg, MALT-oma, or secondary)
- Gastric carcinoid
- Leiomyosarcoma
- Kaposi's sarcoma

Gastritis

- Peptic ulcer disease
- Functional or nonulcer dyspepsia
- Gastroesophageal reflux disease or hiatal hernia
- Biliary disease or pancreatitis
- Gastric or pancreatic cancer
- Viral gastroenteritis
- "Indigestion" from overeating, high-fat foods, coffee
- Angina pectoris
- Severe pain: esophageal rupture, gastric volvulus, ruptured aortic aneurysm

Etiology

- Erosive gastritis: NSAIDs, alcohol, stress, caustic ingestion, radiation
- Portal gastropathy
- *Helicobacter pylori* gastritis
- Pernicious anemia gastritis
- Uncommon infections: necrotizing gastritis; cytomegalovirus or *Candida* (common in immunosuppressed); *Anisakis marina* (raw fish)

- Chronic granulomatous inflammation: tuberculosis, syphilis, fungal infection, sarcoidosis, Crohn's disease
- Eosinophilic gastritis
- Lymphocytic gastritis

Gastrointestinal bleeding, lower

Etiology

- Diverticulosis
- Vascular ectasias (angiodysplasias), eg, idiopathic arteriovenous malformation, CREST syndrome, hereditary hemorrhagic telangiectasias
- Colonic polyps
- Colorectal cancer
- Inflammatory bowel disease
- Hemorrhoids
- Anal fissure
- Ischemic colitis
- Infectious colitis
- Radiation colitis or proctitis
- Iron or bismuth subsalicylate ingestion (false melena)

Rare causes

- Aortoenteric fistula
- Vasculitis
- Solitary rectal ulcer
- NSAID-induced ulcers of small bowel or right colon
- Small bowel diverticula
- Colonic varices

Gastrointestinal bleeding, occult

Etiology

- Malignancy
- Vascular ectasias (angiodysplasias), eg, idiopathic arteriovenous malformation, CREST syndrome, hereditary hemorrhagic telangiectasias
- Portal hypertensive gastropathy
- Peptic ulcer disease
- Ulcerated polyp
- Infections, eg, hookworm, tuberculosis
- Drugs, eg, NSAIDs, aspirin
- Inflammatory bowel disease
- Malabsorption, especially celiac sprue
- Menstrual or pregnancy-associated iron loss
- Idiopathic

Gastrointestinal bleeding, upper

Etiology

- Hemoptysis
- Peptic ulcer disease
- Esophageal varices
- Gastric or duodenal varices (rare)
- Erosive gastritis, eg, NSAIDs, alcohol, stress
- Mallory-Weiss syndrome
- Portal hypertensive gastropathy
- Vascular ectasias (angiodysplasias), eg, idiopathic arteriovenous malformation, CREST syndrome, hereditary hemorrhagic telangiectasias
- Gastric cancer

Rare causes

- Erosive esophagitis
- Aortoenteric fistula
- Dieulafoy's lesion (aberrant gastric submucosal artery)
- Hemobilia (blood in biliary tree), eg, iatrogenic, malignancy
- Pancreatic cancer
- *Hemosuccus pancreaticus* (pancreatic pseudoaneurysm)

Gastroparesis

- Mechanical obstruction of stomach, small intestine, or colon

Etiology

- Endocrine: diabetes mellitus, hypothyroidism, cortisol insufficiency
- Postsurgical: vagotomy, partial gastric resection, fundoplication, gastric bypass, Whipple procedure
- Neurologic: Parkinson's disease, muscular and myotonic dystrophy, autonomic dysfunction, multiple sclerosis, postpolio syndrome, porphyria
- Rheumatologic: scleroderma
- Infection: postviral, Chagas' disease
- Other: amyloidosis, paraneoplastic, drugs, anorexia nervosa, idiopathic

Gingival hyperplasia

- Gingivitis
- Leukemia
- Scurvy (vitamin C deficiency)
- Kaposi's sarcoma
- Drugs: phenytoin, cyclosporine, calcium channel blockers, ethosuximide, atropine/diphenoxylate (Lomotil)
- Familial gingival fibromatosis

Glomerulonephritis

Etiology

Immune complex

- IgA nephropathy
- Endocarditis
- Systemic lupus erythematosus
- Cryoglobulinemia
- Postinfectious glomerulonephritis
- Membranoproliferative
- Henoch-Schönlein purpura

Pauci-immune (ANCA+)

- Wegener's granulomatosis
- Churg-Strauss syndrome
- Microscopic polyarteritis

Anti-GBM

- Goodpasture's syndrome
- Anti-GBM glomerulonephritis

Other

- Malignant hypertension
- Thrombotic thrombocytopenic purpura

Glomerulonephropathies

- Nephritic syndrome or glomerulonephritis (hematuria, proteinuria, HTN, renal insufficiency)
- Nephrotic syndrome (heavy proteinuria, hypoalbuminemia, hyperlipidemia, edema)

Glossitis

- Nutritional deficiency, eg, niacin (pellagra), riboflavin, pyridoxine, vitamin B_{12}, folic acid, iron, vitamin E
- Drug reaction
- Dehydration
- Irritants
- Pernicious anemia
- Psoriasis
- Glucagonoma
- Median rhomboid glossitis

Glossodynia

- Diabetes mellitus
- Drugs, eg, diuretics
- Tobacco
- Dry mouth (xerostomia)
- Oral candidiasis

Glucosuria

Etiology

- Hyperglycemia, eg, diabetes mellitus, gestational diabetes, Cushing's syndrome

- Nondiabetic (benign) glycosuria: genetic, Fanconi's syndrome, chronic renal failure, pregnancy
- Lead toxicity

Goiter

- Benign multinodular goiter
- Iodine-deficient goiter
- Pregnancy (in areas of iodine deficiency)
- Graves' disease
- Hashimoto's thyroiditis
- Subacute (de Quervain's) thyroiditis
- Drugs causing hypothyroidism: lithium, amiodarone, propylthiouracil, methimazole, phenylbutazone, sulfonamides, interferon α, iodide
- Infiltrating disease, eg, malignancy, sarcoidosis
- Suppurative thyroiditis
- Riedel's thyroiditis

Etiology

Causes of endemic goiter

- Iodine deficiency (most common)
- Foods: sorghum, millet, maize, cassava, turnip
- Mineral deficiency: selenium, iron
- Water pollutants

Gynecomastia

- Breast cancer
- Fatty breast enlargement of obesity
- Breast abscess (mastitis)
- Metastatic cancer, eg, prostate

Etiology

- Physiologic: neonatal, pubertal, aging, obesity
- Endocrine: hyperprolactinemia, hyperthyroidism, Klinefelter syndrome, hypogonadism
- Systemic disease: chronic liver or renal disease
- Neoplasms: adrenal, testicular, lung, liver, breast
- Drugs (selected): alcohol, amiodarone, anabolic steroids, cimetidine, diazepam, digoxin, estrogens, finasteride, flutamide, INH, ketoconazole, marijuana, omeprazole, opioids, progestins, protease inhibitors & antiretrovirals, spironolactone, testosterone, tricyclic antidepressants

Halitosis (bad breath)

- Gingivitis
- Dental caries
- Dental abscess
- Sinusitis
- Gastroesophageal reflux
- Cancer of upper aerodigestive tract
- Zenker's diverticulum

Hallucinations

- Schizophrenia
- Major depressive or manic episode with psychotic features
- Drugs or substance abuse, eg, steroids, cocaine, amphetamines, alcohol withdrawal
- Psychotic symptoms associated with dementia
- Delirium
- CNS disease, eg, complex partial seizures, brain tumor, neurosyphilis
- Nutritional deficiency, eg, thiamine, vitamin B_{12}
- Heavy metal poisoning, eg, mercury
- Endocrinopathy, eg, hypothyroidism, Cushing's syndrome
- Other psychotic disorder, eg, schizoaffective or schizophreniform disorder, delusional disorder (nonbizarre delusions, minimal impairment of daily functioning), brief psychotic disorder
- Personality disorder, eg, paranoid, schizotypal, schizoid

Hand pain

- Trauma or overuse, eg, fracture, dislocation, tendinitis
- Trigger finger
- Arthritis, eg, osteoarthritis (DIP and PIP joints), rheumatoid arthritis (MCPs, not DIPs), psoriatic arthritis, reactive arthritis (Reiter's syndrome), gout, septic arthritis
- Finger: felon (infected pad), paronychia, subungual hematoma
- Area of first CMC joint: osteoarthritis, DeQuervain's tenosynovitis, scaphoid fracture (snuffbox pain)
- Carpal tunnel syndrome
- Pronator teres syndrome (median nerve entrapment at level of pronator teres)
- Flexor tenosynovitis, eg, overuse, rheumatoid arthritis, gonococcal
- Dupuytren's contracture
- Ulnar nerve entrapment at the wrist
- Brachial plexus neuropathy
- Cervical nerve root compression, eg, herniated disk
- Superficial radial neuropathy (cheiralgia paresthetica or handcuff neuropathy)
- Reflex sympathetic dystrophy
- Thoracic outlet syndrome
- Vascular, eg, Raynaud's syndrome, thromboangiitis obliterans (Buerger's disease), erythromelalgia
- Angina pectoris (left-sided pain)

HDL decreased

Etiology

- Obesity
- "Metabolic syndrome" (insulin resistance, hypertriglyceridemia)
- Malnutrition
- Sedentary lifestyle
- Cigarette smoking
- Familial
- Beta blockers (short-term effect)

Headache

Don't miss

- Subarachnoid hemorrhage
- Meningitis
- Temporal (giant cell) arteritis
- Glaucoma
- Hypertension
- Cerebral ischemia
- Arterial dissection (carotid or vertebral)
- Brain tumor

Intracranial

- Migraine
- Cluster headache
- Subarachnoid hemorrhage
- Meningitis
- Brain abscess
- Temporal (giant cell) arteritis
- Hypertension
- Caffeine, alcohol, or drug withdrawal
- Pseudotumor cerebri
- Subdural hemorrhage
- Cerebral ischemia
- Arterial dissection (carotid or vertebral)
- Arteriovenous malformation
- Head injury
- Neurocysticercosis
- Venous sinus thrombosis (intracranial venous thrombosis)
- Post-lumbar puncture
- Carbon monoxide poisoning

Extracranial

- Tension headache
- Sinusitis

- Cervical arthritis
- Glaucoma
- Refractive error
- Dental abscess
- Otitis media
- Temporomandibular joint syndrome
- Depression
- Somatoform disorder (eg, somatization)
- Trigeminal neuralgia
- Glossopharyngeal neuralgia

Headache, cough-associated

- Idiopathic
- Intracranial lesion, usually posterior fossa, eg, Arnold-Chiari malformation

Hearing loss

Conductive (external or middle ear)

- Cerumen impaction (ear wax)
- Transient auditory tube dysfunction (upper respiratory infection, allergies)
- Acute or chronic otitis media
- Mastoiditis
- Otosclerosis
- Disruption of ossicles
- Trauma or barotrauma
- Glomus tympanicum (middle ear tumor)
- Paget's disease

Sensory

- Presbycusis (age-related)
- Excessive noise exposure
- Ménière's disease (endolymphatic hydrops)
- Labyrinthitis
- Head trauma
- Ototoxicity, eg, salicylates, aminoglycosides, loop diuretics, cisplatin
- Occlusion of ipsilateral auditory artery (acute)
- Hereditary hearing loss
- Autoimmune: systemic lupus erythematosus, Wegener's granulomatosis, Cogan's syndrome
- Other systemic causes: diabetes mellitus, hypothyroidism, hyperlipidemia, renal failure, infections (eg, measles, mumps, syphilis)

Neural

- Acoustic neuroma
- Multiple sclerosis
- Cerebrovascular disease

Heartburn

- Gastroesophageal reflux disease (most common)
- Hiatal hernia (causing gastroesophageal reflux disease)
- Gastritis
- Peptic ulcer disease
- Functional or nonulcer dyspepsia
- Esophagitis, eg, candidiasis
- Angina pectoris
- Cholelithiasis
- Esophageal motility disorder

Heart sound, fixed split S_2

- Atrial septal defect

Heart sound, loud P_2

- Pulmonary hypertension

Heart sound, loud S_1

- Mitral stenosis
- Short PR interval

Heart sound, paradoxically split S_2 (or no split)

- Aortic stenosis
- Left ventricular failure
- Left bundle branch block

Heart sound, S_3

- Normal (eg, young or pregnant)
- Congestive heart failure
- Volume overload

Heart sound, S_4

- Normal (especially athletes)
- Hypertension
- Coronary artery disease
- Aortic stenosis
- Cardiomyopathy

Heart sound, widely split S_2

- Right bundle branch block

Heel pain

- Plantar fasciitis
- Enthesopathy due to seronegative spondyloarthropathy (eg, ankylosing spondylitis)
- Achilles tendinitis
- Metatarsal stress fracture
- Retrocalcaneal bursitis
- Tarsal tunnel syndrome
- Genital herpes simplex (referred pain from sacral ganglion)

Hematochezia

- Gastrointestinal bleeding (lower)
- Gastrointestinal bleeding (massive)

Hematuria

- Cystitis
- Urinary calculi
- Benign prostatic hyperplasia (usually microscopic hematuria)
- Renal cell carcinoma
- Transitional cell carcinoma (urethra, bladder, ureter, or renal pelvis)
- Glomerulonephritis, eg, IgA nephropathy
- Polycystic kidney disease
- Anticoagulant use
- Prostate cancer
- Papillary necrosis, eg, NSAID overuse, diabetes mellitus, sickle cell trait or disease
- Renal infarction
- Interstitial nephritis
- Medullary sponge kidney
- Radiation or chemical cystitis, eg, cyclophosphamide
- Atrophic vaginitis (usually microscopic hematuria)
- Schistosomiasis
- Menses

Hemoglobinuria

Etiology

- Hemolysis, eg, thrombotic thrombocytopenic purpura, prosthetic heart valve, march hemoglobinuria
- Paroxysmal nocturnal hemoglobinuria

Hemoptysis

Airways

- Bronchitis
- Bronchiectasis
- Bronchogenic carcinoma

Pulmonary vasculature

- Left-sided congestive heart failure
- Mitral stenosis
- Pulmonary embolism

- Arteriovenous malformation

Pulmonary parenchyma
- Pneumonia
- Lung abscess
- Tuberculosis
- Aspergilloma
- Parasites, eg, paragonimiasis, ascariasis, hookworm, strongyloidiasis
- Goodpasture's syndrome
- Wegener's granulomatosis
- Systemic lupus erythematosus
- Crack cocaine inhalation
- Idiopathic pulmonary hemosiderosis
- Leukemia

Iatrogenic
- Transbronchial lung biopsy
- Anticoagulation
- Pulmonary artery rupture by PA line

Hepatic failure, acute

Etiology

- Viral: hepatitis B (common), hepatitis A, hepatitis D (in presence of B), hepatitis E (especially in pregnancy), hepatitis C (rare), herpes simplex virus, cytomegalovirus, infectious mononucleosis, parvovirus B19
- Toxins (predictable): acetaminophen (common), *Amanita* mushrooms, tetracycline, valproic acid, carbon tetrachloride
- Toxins (idiosyncratic): INH, NSAIDs, halothane, ecstasy, kava
- Vascular: right-sided congestive heart failure, shock liver, portal vein thrombosis, Budd-Chiari syndrome
- Metabolic & other: Wilson's disease, acute fatty liver of pregnancy, HELLP syndrome, Reye's syndrome, hyperthermia or hypothermia, lymphoma

Hepatitis, acute

Etiology

Causes of acute hepatitis
- Viral: hepatitis A, hepatitis B, hepatitis C, hepatitis D (in presence of B), hepatitis E, infectious mononucleosis, cytomegalovirus, herpes simplex virus, parvovirus B19
- Other infections, eg, leptospirosis, secondary syphilis, brucellosis, Q fever
- Alcoholic hepatitis
- Toxins (predictable): acetaminophen, *Amanita* mushrooms, tetracycline, valproic acid
- Toxins (idiosyncratic): INH, NSAIDs, statins, azole antifungals, halothane, ecstasy, kava
- Vascular: right-sided congestive heart failure, shock liver, portal vein thrombosis, Budd-Chiari syndrome
- Metabolic: Wilson's disease, acute fatty liver of pregnancy, Reye's syndrome
- Autoimmune hepatitis
- Lymphoma or metastatic cancer

Causes of cholestasis (selected)
- Extrahepatic: choledocholithiasis, pancreatic tumor, biliary stricture, primary sclerosing cholangitis (intra- and extrahepatic)
- Intrahepatic: primary biliary cirrhosis, autoimmune cholangitis, infiltrative disease (eg, tuberculosis, sarcoidosis, lymphoma, amyloidosis), drugs

Hepatitis, chronic

Etiology

- Viral: hepatitis B, hepatitis C, hepatitis D (in presence of B)
- Alcoholic cirrhosis
- Genetic and metabolic: hemochromatosis, Wilson's disease, alpha-1-antiprotease deficiency
- Autoimmune hepatitis
- Chronic hepatitis due to drugs, eg, nitrofurantoin, methyldopa, INH

Hepatomegaly

- Viral, eg, hepatitis A, hepatitis B, hepatitis C, hepatitis E, infectious mononucleosis, cytomegalovirus
- Bacterial, eg, leptospirosis, brucellosis
- Protozoal and helminthic, eg, malaria, leishmaniasis, amebiasis, schistosomiasis, toxoplasmosis, fascioliasis, clonorchiasis, filariasis
- Liver disease, alcoholic
- Toxic hepatitis
- Fatty liver disease, nonalcoholic
- Cirrhosis
- Congestive heart failure
- Hepatocellular carcinoma or metastatic cancer
- Leukemia or myeloproliferative disease
- Hemochromatosis
- Primary biliary cirrhosis
- Budd-Chiari syndrome
- Autoimmune hepatitis
- Infiltrative disease, eg, sarcoidosis, amyloidosis
- Carcinoma of the biliary tract
- Normal variant, eg, Riedel's lobe
- Sickle cell disease
- Polycystic disease of the liver
- Glycogen storage disease

Hiccups (singultus)

Self-limited
- Idiopathic
- Gastric distension, eg, carbonated beverage, air swallowing, overeating
- Sudden temperature changes, eg, hot then cold beverage, hot then cold shower
- Alcohol ingestion
- Excitement, stress, or laughing

Recurrent or persistent
- CNS: neoplasm, infection, stroke, trauma
- Metabolic: uremia, hypocapnia (hyperventilation)
- Vagus or phrenic nerve irritation:
  - Head & neck: ear foreign body, goiter, neoplasm
  - Thorax: pneumonia, empyema, neoplasm, myocardial infarction, pericarditis, aneurysm, esophageal obstruction, reflux esophagitis
  - Abdomen: subphrenic abscess, hepatomegaly, hepatitis, cholecystitis, gastric distension, gastric neoplasm, pancreatitis, pancreatic malignancy
- Surgical: general anesthesia, postoperative
- Psychogenic
- Idiopathic

Hip pain

- Hip joint arthritis, eg, osteoarthritis, rheumatoid arthritis, septic arthritis, gout
- Trochanteric bursitis
- Hip fracture
- Sciatica
- Sacroiliitis, eg, ankylosing spondylitis
- Lumbar facet joint degenerative arthritis
- Lumbar disk herniation
- Ischial bursitis
- Piriformis syndrome
- Iliopsoas bursitis
- Claudication (arterial insufficiency)
- Polymyalgia rheumatica
- Fibromyalgia
- Meralgia paresthetica (compression of lateral femoral cutaneous nerve; anterolateral thigh pain)

- Avascular necrosis
- Hip dislocation

Hirsutism & virilization

- Idiopathic or familial
- Polycystic ovary syndrome
- Drugs, eg, minoxidil, cyclosporine, phenytoin, anabolic steroids, diazoxide, some progestins
- Congenital adrenal hyperplasia (may be late-onset)
- Ovarian tumor or adrenal tumor
- Adrenocorticotrophic hormone-induced Cushing's syndrome

Hoarseness

- Laryngitis
- Voice overuse
- Vocal cord nodules, polyps, or papillomas
- Laryngeal cancer
- Lung cancer (with paralysis of recurrent laryngeal nerve)
- Unilateral vocal cord paralysis
- Hypothyroidism
- Substernal goiter, thyroiditis, multinodular goiter, or thyroid cancer
- Gastroesophageal reflux
- Angioedema

Horner's syndrome

Etiology

- Pancoast tumor (lung cancer)
- Neck trauma or tumor
- Lung abscess or tuberculoma
- Internal carotid dissection
- Brainstem infarct (Wallenberg or lateral medullary syndrome)
- Demyelinating disease, eg, multiple sclerosis
- Syringomyelia
- Cluster headache
- Substernal goiter

Hyperacusis

- Idiopathic
- Hearing loss (recruitment causing sensitivity to loud sounds despite reduced sensitivity to softer ones)
- Bell's palsy
- Migraine
- Adrenal insufficiency

Hypercoagulable state

Etiology

Acquired

- Immobility or postoperative state
- Cancer
- Inflammatory disorders, eg, ulcerative colitis
- Myeloproliferative disorder, eg, polycythemia vera, essential thrombocytosis
- Estrogens, pregnancy
- Heparin-induced thrombocytopenia
- Lupus anticoagulant
- Anticardiolipin antibodies
- Nephrotic syndrome
- Paroxysmal nocturnal hemoglobinuria
- Disseminated intravascular coagulation
- Congestive heart failure

Congenital

- Activated protein C resistance, eg, Factor V Leiden
- Prothrombin 20210 mutation
- Antithrombin III deficiency
- Protein C deficiency
- Protein S deficiency
- Hyperhomocysteinemia
- Dysfibrinogenemia
- Abnormal plasminogen

Hyperglycemia

Etiology

Endocrinopathies

- Diabetes mellitus, Cushing's syndrome, acromegaly, pheochromocytoma, glucagonoma, somatostatinoma

Drugs

- Glucocorticoids, thiazides, phenytoin, niacin, oral contraceptives, pentamidine

Pancreatic insufficiency

- Subtotal pancreatectomy, chronic pancreatitis, hemochromatosis ("bronze diabetes"), cystic fibrosis, hemosiderosis

Other

- Gestational diabetes, cirrhosis, Schmidt syndrome (polyglandular failure: Addison's disease, autoimmune thyroiditis, diabetes)

Hyperhidrosis

- Anxiety
- Idiopathic
- Hyperthyroidism
- Infection or malignancy
- Hypoglycemia
- Menopause
- Pheochromocytoma
- Reflex sympathetic dystrophy

Hyperpigmentation

- Pigmented nevi
- Ephelides (juvenile freckles)
- Lentigines (senile freckles, liver spots)
- Postinflammatory (eg, acne, atopic dermatitis)
- Chronic venous insufficiency
- Melasma (chloasma)
- Neurofibromatosis (café au lait spots, axillary freckling)
- Hemochromatosis
- Addison's disease
- Acanthosis nigricans
- Hyperbilirubinemia (eg, primary biliary cirrhosis)
- Ochronosis (alkaptonuria)
- Pellagra (niacin deficiency)
- Porphyria cutanea tarda
- Wilson's disease
- Whipple's disease
- Scleroderma
- Vitamin B_{12} deficiency
- Folic acid deficiency
- Medications: chloroquine, chlorpromazine, minocycline, amiodarone
- Topicals: benzoyl peroxide, tretinoin, fluorouracil
- Fixed drug eruption to laxatives (phenolphthalein), trimethoprim-sulfamethoxazole, NSAIDs, tetracyclines
- Exogenous pigment exposure: carotenemia, argyria, gold, tattooing, arsenic
- Berloque hyperpigmentation (phototoxicity form citrus or celery)
- Visceral leishmaniasis (kala azar)
- POEMS syndrome (polyneuropathy, organomegaly, endocrinopathy, monoclonal gammopathy, skin changes)

Hypersensitivity pneumonitis

- Sarcoidosis
- Asthma
- Atypical pneumonia
- Collagen vascular disease, eg, systemic lupus erythematosus
- Idiopathic pulmonary fibrosis
- Lymphoma

Etiology

- Farmer's lung (moldy hay)
- Humidifier lung (contaminated humidifier, heating, or air conditioning)
- Bird fancier's lung (pigeon breeder's disease)
- Bagassosis (moldy sugar cane fiber)
- Sequoiosis (moldy redwood sawdust)
- Maple bark stripper's disease
- Mushroom picker's disease (moldy compost)
- Suberosis (moldy cork dust)
- Detergent worker's lung (enzyme additives)

Hypersomnia

- Insomnia of any cause limiting nighttime sleep
- Inadequate sleep time (lifestyle)
- Sleep apnea
- Narcolepsy
- Primary insomnia (primary CNS hypersomnolence)
- Drugs, eg, sedatives, opiates
- Depression
- Hypothyroidism
- Kleine-Levin syndrome

Hypertension

- Essential hypertension
- "White-coat" hypertension
- Cuff too small

Secondary hypertension

- Adrenal
- Primary hyperaldosteronism, Cushing's syndrome (or steroid therapy), pheochromocytoma
- Renal
- Chronic renal disease, renal artery stenosis (atherosclerotic or fibromuscular dysplasia), polyarteritis nodosa
- Oral contraceptives, alcohol, NSAIDs, pregnancy-associated, hypercalcemia, hyperthyroidism, obstructive sleep apnea, obesity, coarctation of the aorta, acromegaly, increased intracranial pressure

Hyperthermia

Etiology

- Heat stroke
- Neuroleptic malignant syndrome
- Malignant hyperthermia (anesthetic-associated)
- Serotonin syndrome, eg, SSRI used with monoamine oxidase inhibitor
- Other drugs: anticholinergics, antihistamines, tricyclic antidepressants, monoamine oxidase inhibitors, salicylates, amphetamines, cocaine, PCP, LSD
- Thyrotoxicosis
- Prolonged seizures

Hyperuricemia, endogenous

Etiology

Primary hyperuricemia

- Increased production of purine
  - Idiopathic
  - Specific enzyme defects (eg, Lesch-Nyhan syndrome, glycogen storage diseases)
  - Decreased renal clearance of uric acid (idiopathic)

Secondary hyperuricemia

- Increased purine catabolism and turnover
  - Myeloproliferative disorders (eg, chronic myelogenous leukemia)
  - Lymphoproliferative disorders (eg, non-Hodgkin's lymphoma)
  - Carcinoma and sarcoma (disseminated)
  - Chronic hemolytic anemias
  - Cytotoxic drugs
  - Psoriasis
  - Decreased renal clearance of uric acid
  - Intrinsic kidney disease
  - Functional impairment of tubular transport
    1. Drug-induced (eg, thiazides, probenecid)
    2. Hyperlacticacidemia (eg, lactic acidosis, alcoholism)
    3. Hyperketoacidemia (eg, diabetic ketoacidosis, starvation)
    4. Diabetes insipidus (vasopressin-resistant)
    5. Bartter's syndrome

Hyperventilation

Etiology

- Anxiety
- Hypoxemia
- Acidemia
- Pregnancy
- Obstructive lung disease
- Interstitial lung disease
- Sepsis
- Hepatic failure
- Fever
- Pain
- Central neurogenic hyperventilation (in comatose)

Hypoglycemia

Etiology

- Surreptitious or excess use of insulin or sulfonylurea
- Liver failure
- Acute alcohol intoxication
- Renal failure
- Sepsis
- Hypopituitarism
- Adrenal insufficiency
- Myxedema
- Insulinoma (pancreatic B cell tumor)
- Postprandial (reactive) hypoglycemia: postgastrectomy, occult diabetes, idiopathic
- Drugs: pentamidine, sulfamethoxazole (eg, TMP-SMX), quinine
- Extrapancreatic tumors (rare): hepatocellular carcinoma, retroperitoneal sarcoma, adrenocortical carcinoma
- Anti-insulin antibodies or antibodies to insulin receptors (very rare)

Hypogonadism, male

Etiology

Hypogonadotropic (low or normal LH)

- Hypopituitarism, eg, pituitary adenoma
- Cushing's syndrome
- Hypothyroidism
- Hyperprolactinemia
- Hemochromatosis
- Estrogen-secreting tumor (testicular, adrenal)
- Idiopathic
- GnRH agonist therapy, eg, leuprolide
- Drugs: alcohol, ketoconazole, spironolactone, marijuana, prior androgens, phenytoin, cimetidine, intrathecal opioids
- Anorexia nervosa
- Cirrhosis
- Serious illness or malnutrition
- Kallmann syndrome
- Prader-Willi syndrome

Hypergonadotropic (primary testicular failure; high LH)

- Male climacteric (andropause or male menopause)

- Klinefelter syndrome
- Orchitis, eg, mumps, gonorrhea, tuberculosis, leprosy
- Radiation therapy
- Cancer chemotherapy
- Autoimmune
- Uremia
- Testicular trauma or torsion
- Lymphoma
- Myotonic dystrophy
- Androgen insensitivity
- Idiopathic

Hypopigmentation or depigmentation

- Postinflammatory (eg, acne, atopic dermatitis)
- Vitiligo
- Albinism
- Tinea versicolor (pityriasis versicolor)
- Pityriasis alba (pityriasis simplex)
- Seborrheic dermatitis
- Piebaldism (white forelock)
- Tuberous sclerosis
- Halo nevi or halo around melanoma
- Leukoderma
- Liquid nitrogen treatment
- Intralesional corticosteroids
- Morphea (localized scleroderma)
- Lichen sclerosis
- Hansen's disease (leprosy)

Hypopituitarism

- Anorexia nervosa (hypogonadotropic hypogonadism)
- Serious illness (hypogonadotropic hypogonadism, functional suppression of TSH and thyroxine)
- Severe malnutrition (hypogonadotropic hypogonadism)
- Hypothyroidism
- Addison's disease
- High-dose glucocorticoids (secondary adrenal insufficiency for months)
- Cachexia due to other causes (eg, carcinoma, tuberculosis)
- Empty sella syndrome

Etiology

Mass lesions

- Pituitary adenoma (prolactinoma, nonfunctioning, growth hormone-secreting)
- Granuloma
- Brain tumor (eg, craniopharyngioma, meningioma, germinoma, glioma, chondrosarcoma, chordoma of the clivus)
- Rathke's cleft cyst
- Intracranial aneurysm
- Pituitary apoplexy (hemorrhage in pituitary tumor)
- Metastatic carcinoma

Without mass lesion

- Idiopathic
- Trauma
- Cranial irradiation
- Hemochromatosis
- Sarcoidosis
- Surgery
- Encephalitis
- Autoimmune
- Stroke
- Status post-coronary artery bypass graft
- Postpartum pituitary necrosis (Sheehan's syndrome)
- Langerhans cell histiocytosis
- Eclampsia-preeclampsia
- Sickle cell disease
- African trypanosomiasis

Hypotension or shock

Low stroke volume

- Hypovolemia, eg, hemorrhage, vomiting, diarrhea, burns, "third spacing"
- Pneumothorax
- Pulmonary embolism
- Cardiac tamponade
- "Pump failure" due to myocardial ischemia or cardiomyopathy
- Aortic stenosis
- Aortic insufficiency
- Mitral regurgitation
- Aortic dissection
- Rupture of ventricular septum or free wall

Abnormal heart rate

- Bradycardia
- Tachycardia

Low systemic vascular resistance

- Sepsis
- Adrenal insufficiency
- Anaphylaxis
- Drugs, eg, vasodilators
- Neurogenic shock

Hypothermia

Etiology

- Cold exposure including drowning
- Infection
- Other causes of altered mental status, eg, hypoglycemia, drugs, stroke
- Hypothyroidism
- Anorexia or malnutrition (poor fat stores)
- Adrenal insufficiency
- Burns
- Spinal cord injury

Hypothermia of extremities

Etiology

- Cold exposure
- Raynaud's syndrome
- Polyarteritis nodosa
- Reflex sympathetic dystrophy
- Thoracic outlet syndrome
- Acrocyanosis (vasospastic disorder)
- Chilblain (erythema pernio)
- Chilblain lupus erythematosus

Hypoventilation, chronic

Etiology

- Obstructive or central sleep apnea
- Obesity-hypoventilation syndrome (Pickwickian syndrome)
- Central alveolar hypoventilation (brainstem disorder)
- Primary alveolar hypoventilation (Ondine's curse)
- Neuromuscular disorder, eg, myasthenia gravis, poliomyelitis, spinal cord trauma
- Chronic obstructive pulmonary disease
- Chronic hypnotic use

Hypoxia and normal CXR

- Asthma
- Pulmonary embolism
- Early pneumonia
- Early interstitial lung disease
- Early pneumocystis pneumonia
- Shunt, eg, atrial or ventricular septal defect, arteriovenous malformation, atelectasis
- Pulmonary hypertension
- Chronic alveolar hypoventilation

Immobility (especially in elderly)

- Weakness, eg, disuse, anemia, malnutrition, electrolyte abnormality, neurologic disorder, myopathy

- Stiffness, eg, arthritis, parkinsonism, polymyalgia rheumatica
- Bone pain, eg, vertebral fracture, metastases, Paget's disease
- Joint pain, eg, arthritis, hip fracture
- Bursa or muscle pain, eg, bursitis, polymyalgia rheumatica, claudication, pseudoclaudication (spinal stenosis)
- Foot pain, eg, ingrown nail, plantar warts, bunions, calluses & corns
- Imbalance (often multifactorial):
  - Neurologic disease, eg, stroke, cervical myelopathy, peripheral neuropathy, vestibular or cerebellar disorder
  - Orthostatic or postprandial hypotension
  - Drugs, eg, antihypertensives, diuretics, sedatives, neuroleptics, antidepressants
- Anxiety or depression

Infertility, female

- Male factor, eg, hypogonadism, varicocele, alcohol or drug use, immotile cilia syndrome
- Polycystic ovary syndrome
- Premature ovarian failure
- Hyperprolactinemia
- Hypothyroidism
- Inadequate luteal progesterone or short luteal phase
- Endometriosis
- Uterine leiomyomas (fibroids) or polyps
- Prior pelvic inflammatory disease
- Pelvic adhesions, eg, pelvic surgery, therapeutic abortion, ectopic pregnancy, septic abortion, intrauterine device use
- Cervical factors, eg, unfavorable mucus, antisperm antibodies

Infertility, male

- Female infertility
- Erectile dysfunction
- Hypogonadism (deficient testosterone from primary or secondary testicular failure)
- Spermicidal lubricants
- Cryptorchism
- Epididymitis
- Retrograde ejaculation, eg, diabetic neuropathy
- Varicocele
- Ejaculatory duct obstruction
- Vas deferens obstruction
- Absent seminal emission from sympathetic nerve injury, eg, pelvic or retroperitoneal surgery
- Hernia repair damaging vas deferens or testicular blood supply
- Drugs: sulfasalazine, nitrofurantoin affect sperm motility (see also drugs in Hypogonadism)

Insomnia

- Acute: emotional stress, physical discomfort, jet lag
- Alcohol abuse
- Stimulants, eg, caffeine, nicotine, cocaine, pseudoephedrine
- Depression
- Poor sleep hygiene, eg, daytime naps, TV in bed
- Mania or bipolar disorder
- Medical illness, eg, chronic obstructive pulmonary disease, uremia, hyperthyroidism, hepatic encephalopathy, gastroesophageal reflux disease
- Nocturia, eg, diuretics, benign prostatic hyperplasia, urinary incontinence, congestive heart failure
- Restless leg syndrome
- Menopause
- CNS disease, eg, complex partial seizures, brain tumor, neurosyphilis
- Medications, eg, corticosteroids, SSRIs, theophylline, benzodiazepine withdrawal
- Circadian rhythm disorder

Interstitial lung disease

Etiology

Drug-related

- Amiodarone
- Antibacterials (nitrofurantoin, sulfonamides)
- Antineoplastics (bleomycin, cyclophosphamide, methotrexate, nitrosoureas)
- Antirheumatics (gold salts, penicillamine)
- Phenytoin

Environmental & occupational

- Inorganic dust (asbestos, silica, hard metals, beryllium)
- Organic dust or hypersensitivity pneumonitis (thermophilic actinomycetes, avian antigens, *Aspergillus* spp.)
- Gases, fumes, vapors (chlorine, isocyanates, paraquat, sulfur dioxide)
- Ionizing radiation
- Talc (injection drug users)

Infections

- Disseminated fungus (coccidioidomycosis, blastomycosis, histoplasmosis)
- Disseminated mycobacteria
- *Pneumocystis jiroveci* pneumonia
- Viruses

Primary pulmonary syndromes

- Idiopathic fibrosing interstitial pneumonia [idiopathic pulmonary fibrosis (IPF)]:
  - Acute interstitial pneumonitis
  - Desquamative interstitial pneumonia
  - Nonspecific interstitial pneumonitis
  - Usual interstitial pneumonia
  - Respiratory bronchiolitis-associated interstitial lung disease
- Bronchiolitis obliterans-organizing pneumonia

Systemic disorders

- Acute respiratory distress syndrome
- Amyloidosis
- Ankylosing spondylitis
- Autoimmune disease: dermatomyositis, polymyositis, rheumatoid arthritis, systemic sclerosis (scleroderma), systemic lupus erythematosus
- Chronic eosinophilic pneumonia
- Goodpasture's syndrome
- Idiopathic pulmonary hemosiderosis
- Inflammatory bowel disease
- Eosinophilic granuloma (Langerhans cell histiocytosis, histiocytosis X)
- Lymphangitic carcinomatosis
- Lymphangioleiomyomatosis
- Pulmonary edema
- Pulmonary venous hypertension
- Sarcoidosis
- Wegener's granulomatosis

Interstitial nephritis

- Acute tubular necrosis
- Acute glomerulonephritis
- Prerenal azotemia
- Chronic glomerulopathy, eg, diabetic nephropathy
- Hypertensive nephrosclerosis
- Obstructive uropathy

Etiology

Acute

- Antibiotics: β-lactams, sulfa, ciprofloxacin, erythromycin, tetracycline, vancomycin, rifampin, ethambutol
- NSAIDs
- Diuretics: thiazides, furosemide

- Other drugs: phenytoin, allopurinol, cimetidine
- Infections: *Streptococcus*, leptospirosis, cytomegalovirus, Epstein-Barr virus, histoplasmosis, Rocky Mountain spotted fever, *Legionella*, *Mycoplasma*, *Toxoplasma*
- Immune: systemic lupus erythematosus, Sjögren's syndrome, sarcoidosis, cryoglobulinemia

Chronic

- Obstructive uropathy
- Vesicoureteral reflux (reflux nephropathy)
- Analgesic nephropathy
- Heavy metals: lead, cadmium, mercury, bismuth
- Multiple myeloma
- Gout

Intestinal ischemia, acute

- Diverticulitis
- Appendicitis
- Peptic ulcer disease or gastritis
- Acute pancreatitis or cholecystitis
- Myocardial infarction
- Vasculitis, eg, polyarteritis nodosa

Etiology

- Emboli, eg, atrial fibrillation
- Thrombosis of mesenteric vessel
- Low flow due to congestive heart failure or arterial spasm (eg, ergotamine or cocaine)
- Mesenteric vein occlusion
- Postcoarctectomy syndrome (mesenteric vasoconstriction after coarctation repair)

Intestinal ischemia, chronic

- Peptic ulcer disease
- Gastroesophageal reflux disease
- Chronic pancreatitis
- Irritable bowel syndrome
- Visceral malignancy
- Vasculitis, eg, polyarteritis nodosa

Etiology

- Atherosclerosis

Intracranial pressure, increased

Etiology

- Space-occupying lesion, eg, brain tumor, brain abscess
- Pseudotumor cerebri
- Subdural hematoma
- Meningitis
- Cerebral edema, eg, trauma, encephalitis, infarction
- Malignant hypertension
- Venous sinus thrombosis
- Dural arteriovenous malformation
- Hydrocephalus
- Neurocysticercosis

Intraocular pressure, increased

Etiology

- Acute (angle-closure) glaucoma
- Open-angle glaucoma (primary)
- Open-angle glaucoma secondary to uveitis, trauma
- Corticosteroids (topical or systemic)
- Ophthalmic zoster

Jaundice (icterus)

Hyperbilirubinemia

- Unconjugated (indirect bilirubin)
- Increased production: hemolysis, hematoma, pulmonary infarction
- Impaired uptake and storage: posthepatitis hyperbilirubinemia, Gilbert's syndrome, Crigler-Najjar syndrome, drugs
- Conjugated (direct bilirubin)
- Biliary obstruction: choledocholithiasis, pancreatic tumor, biliary stricture, primary sclerosing cholangitis, biliary duct carcinoma
- Hepatocellular damage or intrahepatic cholestasis: hepatitis (eg, alcoholic, viral), hepatic cirrhosis, biliary cirrhosis, drugs, sepsis, cholangitis, liver abscess, Budd-Chiari syndrome, infectious mononucleosis, spirochetal infection, infiltrative disease (tuberculosis, sarcoidosis, lymphoma), industrial toxins
- Hereditary bilirubin excretion defect: Dubin-Johnson syndrome, Rotor's syndrome

Other causes of yellow skin

- Carotenemia (excessive beta-carotene ingestion, especially in hypothyroidism)

Jaundice in pregnancy

- Viral hepatitis (including herpes simplex virus-related)
- Acute fatty liver of pregnancy
- Choledocholithiasis
- Idiopathic cholestasis of pregnancy
- HELLP syndrome (hemolysis, elevated liver enzymes, low platelets)
- Primary biliary cirrhosis

Joint effusion by joint fluid type

Etiology

Group I: Noninflammatory (200–300 WBC, < 25% PMNs)

- Osteoarthritis
- Trauma (may be hemorrhagic)
- Osteochondritis dissecans
- Osteochondromatosis
- Neuropathic arthropathy (may be hemorrhagic)
- Subsiding or early inflammation
- Hypertrophic osteoarthropathy (group I or II)
- Pigmented villonodular synovitis (may be hemorrhagic)

Group II: Inflammatory (3000–50,000 WBC, >50% PMNs)

- Rheumatoid arthritis
- Gout or pseudogout
- Reactive arthritis (Reiter's syndrome)
- Ankylosing spondylitis
- Psoriatic arthritis
- Arthritis accompanying inflammatory bowel disease
- Rheumatic fever (group I or II)
- Systemic lupus erythematosus (group I or II)
- Scleroderma (group I or II)
- Tuberculosis of bone & joints
- Mycotic infection

Group III: Purulent (>50,000 WBC, >75% PMNs)

- Pyogenic bacterial infection (septic arthritis)

Hemorrhagic

- Hemophilia or other bleeding disorder
- Trauma with or without fracture
- Neuropathic arthropathy
- Pigmented villonodular synovitis
- Synovioma
- Hemangioma and other benign neoplasms

Keratitis (corneal ulcer or inflammation)

- Corneal abrasion or foreign body
- Conjunctivitis
- Uveitis
- Acute glaucoma

Etiology

- Bacterial, eg, *Pseudomonas*, *Moraxella*, *Staphylococcus*, pneumococcus
- Herpes simplex keratitis
- Ophthalmic zoster
- Fungal keratitis
- *Acanthamoeba* keratitis
- Contact lenses (especially soft)
- Neurotrophic keratitis (lack of corneal sensation)
- Exposure keratitis (inadequate eyelid closure)
- Severe dry eyes
- Severe allergic eye disease
- Behçet's syndrome
- Topical steroids

Kidneys, large

- Diabetes mellitus
- Polycystic kidney disease
- HIV-associated nephropathy
- Amyloidosis
- Scleroderma
- Lymphoma
- Bilateral hydronephrosis

Knee effusion

Etiology

- Trauma, eg, fracture, ligament or meniscal injury, overuse syndrome
- Infection, eg, gonococcal arthritis, *Staphylococcus aureus* septic arthritis, Lyme disease, tuberculosis of bone & joints
- Gout or pseudogout
- Seronegative spondyloarthropathy, eg, reactive arthritis (Reiter's syndrome)
- Rheumatoid arthritis
- Osteoarthritis or inflammatory osteoarthritis
- Hemarthrosis due to bleeding disorder
- Malignant or benign tumor

Knee pain

- Patellofemoral syndrome
- Iliotibial band syndrome
- Patellar tendonitis
- Anserine bursitis
- Meniscus tear (medial > lateral)
- Medial or lateral collateral ligament strain or tear
- Cruciate ligament tear (anterior > posterior)
- Prepatellar bursitis
- Baker's (popliteal) cyst
- Arthritis, eg, osteoarthritis, rheumatoid arthritis, gout, pseudogout, septic arthritis, reactive arthritis (Reiter's syndrome)
- Medial plica syndrome
- Osgood-Schlatter disease
- Osteochondritis dissecans
- Neuropathic arthropathy (Charcot joint)
- Tumor, eg, osteosarcoma
- Referred pain from hip, eg, avascular necrosis
- Referred pain from back, eg, sciatica
- Fracture

Kussmaul's sign

- Constrictive pericarditis
- Restrictive cardiomyopathy

Laryngeal tumor

- Vocal cord nodules
- Vocal cord polyps
- Laryngeal papillomas
- Laryngeal granulomas
- Laryngeal leukoplakia
- Laryngeal squamous cell carcinoma

Leukoplakia (oral leukoplakia)

- Hyperkeratosis due to irritation, eg, dentures, tobacco, cheek biting
- Dysplasia or carcinoma
- Lichen planus
- Oral candidiasis
- Oral hairy leukoplakia
- White sponge nevus
- Secondary syphilis
- Necrotizing sialometaplasia
- Pseudoepitheliomatous hyperplasia

Lift, parasternal

- Right ventricular hypertrophy
- Cor pulmonale
- Pulmonary hypertension
- Left atrial enlargement
- Pulmonary stenosis

Limb ischemia, acute

- Lumbar spinal stenosis (neurogenic or pseudoclaudication)
- Musculoskeletal pain
- Peripheral neuropathy, eg, diabetes mellitus, alcoholism
- Osteomyelitis

Etiology

- Emboli, eg, atrial fibrillation, cholesterol emboli after aortic instrumentation
- Thrombosis
- Trauma
- Thromboangiitis obliterans (Buerger's disease)

Livedo reticularis

- Benign idiopathic
- Occult malignancy
- Polyarteritis nodosa
- Cholesterol emboli
- Antiphospholipid antibody syndrome
- Systemic lupus erythematosus
- Dermatomyositis
- Rheumatoid arthritis
- Thromboangiitis obliterans (Buerger's disease)

Liver mass

- Hepatocellular carcinoma
- Metastatic cancer
- Cavernous hemangioma
- Liver cell adenoma
- Cyst, eg, congenital, echinococcal (hydatid), associated with polycystic kidney disease
- Pyogenic liver abscess
- Amebic liver abscess
- Focal nodular hyperplasia

Low back pain

- Muscular strain
- Osteoarthritis
- Herniated disk
- Spinal stenosis
- Sciatica
- Sacroiliitis, eg, ankylosing spondylitis
- Rheumatoid arthritis
- Metastatic cancer
- Compression fracture, eg, osteoporosis, multiple myeloma
- Osteomyelitis or epidural abscess
- Cauda equina tumor
- Ischial bursitis
- Piriformis syndrome
- Fibromyalgia

- Polymyalgia rheumatica
- Aortic aneurysm
- Duodenal ulcer
- Urinary calculi or pyelonephritis
- Pancreatitis
- Prostatitis
- Hip osteoarthritis

Lung cavities, multiple

- Septic emboli
- Metastatic cancer
- Wegener's granulomatosis
- Tuberculosis
- Coccidioidomycosis

Lung cavity

- Lung abscess
- Tuberculosis
- Aspergilloma
- Mycetoma (eg, *Nocardia brasiliensis*)
- Lung cancer
- Lung infarction
- Wegener's granulomatosis
- Coccidioidomycosis
- Histoplasmosis

Lung disease, drug-induced

Etiology

- Asthma: beta blockers, aspirin, NSAIDs, histamine, methacholine, acetylcysteine, aerosolized pentamidine, any nebulized medication
- Chronic cough: ACE inhibitors
- Pulmonary infiltration:
  - with eosinophilia: amitriptyline, amiodarone
  - without eosinophilia: sulfonamides, penicillin, methotrexate, crack cocaine
- Drug-induced systemic lupus erythematosus: hydralazine, procainamide, isoniazid, chlorpromazine, phenytoin
- Interstitial pneumonitis/fibrosis: nitrofurantoin, cyclophosphamide, phenytoin
- Pulmonary edema: aspirin, chlordiazepoxide, cocaine, heroin
- Pleural effusion: bromocriptine, nitrofurantoin, any drug inducing systemic lupus erythematosus
- Mediastinal widening: phenytoin, corticosteroids, methotrexate
- Respiratory failure:
  - Neuromuscular blockade: aminoglycosides, succinylcholine
  - CNS depression: sedatives, opioids, alcohol, tricyclic antidepressants

Lung disease, lower lobe

- Alpha-1 antiprotease deficiency
- Asbestosis (parenchymal)
- Tuberculosis (primary)

Lung disease, upper lobe

- Silicosis
- Tuberculosis
- Ankylosing spondylitis
- Sarcoidosis
- Eosinophilic granuloma (Langerhans cell histiocytosis, histiocytosis X)
- Cystic fibrosis
- Hypersensitivity pneumonitis (extrinsic allergic alveolitis)
- Histoplasmosis

Lymphadenopathy, generalized

Infection
- Viral, eg, infectious mononucleosis (Epstein-Barr virus, cytomegalovirus), hepatitis, herpes simplex virus, varicella, rubella, acute HIV infection or AIDS
- Bacterial, eg, streptococci, staphylococci, cat-scratch disease, tuberculosis, syphilis, tularemia, chancroid, plague, leprosy
- Fungal, eg, histoplasmosis, coccidioidomycosis
- Chlamydial, eg, lymphogranuloma venereum
- Parasitic, eg, toxoplasmosis, leishmaniasis, trypanosomiasis, filariasis
- Rickettsial, eg, scrub typhus

Malignancy
- Hodgkin's or non-Hodgkin's lymphoma
- Leukemia
- Metastatic cancer
- Virchow's (left supraclavicular) node: gastrointestinal (classically gastric) cancer
- Sister Mary Joseph (umbilical) node: gastrointestinal cancer
- Right subclavian node: lung cancer

Immunologic disease
- Rheumatoid arthritis, systemic lupus erythematosus, dermatomyositis, Sjögren's syndrome
- Drug hypersensitivity
- Serum sickness

Other
- Sarcoidosis
- Amyloidosis
- Lipid storage disease, eg, Gaucher, Niemann-Pick
- Hyperthyroidism
- Castleman's disease (giant lymph node hyperplasia)
- Dermatopathic lymphadenitis
- Kikuchi's disease (histiocytic necrotizing lymphadenitis)
- Kawasaki syndrome
- Eosinophilic granuloma (Langerhans cell histiocytosis, histiocytosis X)
- Familial Mediterranean fever
- Drug-induced pseudolymphoma (classically phenytoin)

Lymphedema

Etiology

- Congenital
- Trauma
- Regional lymph node dissection
- Irradiation
- Bacterial or fungal infection
- Lymphoproliferative disease
- Filariasis

Lymphocytosis

Etiology

- Viral infection, eg, infectious mononucleosis
- Chronic lymphocytic leukemia
- Pertussis
- Lymphoma in leukemic phase

Macroglossia

- Amyloidosis
- Acromegaly
- Hypothyroidism
- Multiple myeloma
- Down syndrome
- Lymphoma
- Angioedema
- Hemangioma

Malabsorption

Etiology

- Small bowel: celiac sprue, Whipple's disease, tropical sprue, eosinophilic gastroenteritis, small bowel resection, Crohn's disease

- Lymphatic obstruction: lymphoma, carcinoid, tuberculosis, *Mycobacterium avium* complex, Kaposi's sarcoma, sarcoidosis, retroperitoneal fibrosis
- Pancreatic insufficiency: chronic pancreatitis, cystic fibrosis, pancreatic cancer
- Bacterial overgrowth, eg, diabetes
- Reduced bile salts: ileal resection, Crohn's disease, postcholecystectomy
- Strongyloidiasis

Malingering

- Factitious disorder (Munchausen syndrome)
- Somatoform disorder
- Organic disease producing symptoms

Mania

- Bipolar disorder (manic depression)
- Substance abuse, eg, cocaine, amphetamines
- Hypomania
- Cyclothymic disorder (depression and hypomania)
- Schizophrenia
- Hyperthyroidism
- Medications, eg, corticosteroids, thyroxine
- CNS disease, eg, complex partial seizures, brain tumor, neurosyphilis
- Personality disorder, eg, borderline, narcissistic

Mediastinal mass

Anterior
- Thymoma
- Teratoma
- Thyroid lesion
- Lymphoma
- Mesenchymal tumors (lipoma, fibroma)

Middle
- Lymphadenopathy
- Pulmonary artery enlargement
- Aneurysm of aorta or innominate artery
- Developmental cyst (bronchogenic, enteric, pleuropericardial)
- Dilated azygos or hemiazygos vein
- Foramen of Morgagni hernia

Posterior
- Hiatal hernia
- Neurogenic tumor (neurilemmoma, neurofibroma, neurosarcoma, ganglioneuroma, pheochromocytoma)
- Meningocele
- Esophageal tumor
- Foramen of Bochdalek hernia
- Thoracic spine disease
- Extramedullary hematopoiesis

Melena

- Gastrointestinal (upper or lower) bleeding
- Iron or bismuth subsalicylate ingestion (false melena)

Membranous nephropathy

Etiology

- Infections: hepatitis B, endocarditis, syphilis, malaria
- Autoimmune: systemic lupus erythematosus, mixed connective tissue disease, thyroiditis
- Non-Hodgkin's lymphoma
- Carcinomas: colorectal, renal cell, bronchogenic, thyroid cancer
- Drugs: gold, penicillamine, captopril
- Idiopathic

Meningitis

- Subarachnoid hemorrhage
- Encephalitis
- "Neighborhood reaction" causing abnormal CSF, eg, brain abscess, epidural abscess, vertebral osteomyelitis, mastoiditis, sinusitis, brain tumor
- Dural sinus thrombosis
- Noninfectious meningeal irritation: carcinomatous meningitis, sarcoidosis, systemic lupus erythematosus, drugs (eg, NSAIDs, TMP-SMX), pneumonia, shigellosis
- If fever and rash: gonococcemia, infective endocarditis, thrombotic thrombocytopenic purpura, Rocky Mountain spotted fever, viral exanthem
- Seizure due to other causes, eg, febrile seizure
- Amebic meningoencephalitis (*Naegleria fowleri*)

Etiology

Purulent meningitis
- 18–50 years: *S. pneumoniae* (pneumococcal), *N. meningitidis* (meningococcal)
- >50 years: *S. pneumoniae* (pneumococcal), *N. meningitidis* (meningococcal), *Listeria*, gram-negative bacilli
- Impaired cellular immunity: *Listeria*, gram-negative bacilli, *S. pneumoniae* (pneumococcal)
- Postsurgical or posttraumatic: *S. aureus*, *S. pneumoniae* (pneumococcal), gram-negative bacilli

Aseptic meningitis
- Mumps, coxsackievirus, echoviruses
- Infectious mononucleosis
- Leptospirosis, syphilis, Lyme disease

Chronic meningitis
- Tuberculous meningitis or atypical mycobacteria
- Fungi: *Cryptococcus*, *Coccidioides*, *Histoplasma*
- Spirochetes: syphilis, Lyme disease, leptospirosis
- Other: brucellosis, HIV infection, neurocysticercosis

Menorrhagia

- Uterine leiomyomas (fibroids)
- Endometrial polyp
- Adenomyosis (uterine endometriosis)
- Bleeding disorder, eg, von Willebrand's disease, thrombocytopenia, leukemia
- Hypothyroidism

Metastases to bone

- Lung cancer
- Breast cancer
- Prostate cancer
- Multiple myeloma (not truly metastatic)
- Renal cell carcinoma
- Others: skin, oral, esophageal, cervical, gastric, colorectal, melanoma

Metastases to brain

- Parenchymal: lung cancer, breast cancer, renal cell carcinoma, gastrointestinal, melanoma, lymphoma
- Leptomeningeal: breast cancer, lymphoma, leukemia, prostate cancer

Metastases to kidney

- Cysts (simple, acquired, polycystic kidney disease, medullary sponge kidney, medullary cystic kidney)
- Renal cell carcinoma
- Metastases, eg, lung, breast, gastric, contralateral kidney
- Renal abscess
- Transitional cell carcinoma of renal pelvis

- Adrenal tumor
- Renal oncocytoma
- Renal angiomyolipoma
- Lymphoma
- Nephrolithiasis
- Renal infarction

Metastases to liver

- Gastrointestinal tract, eg, colorectal cancer
- Lung cancer
- Breast cancer
- Malignant melanoma
- Prostate cancer
- Thyroid cancer
- Skin cancer
- Carcinoid
- Most cancers can metastasize to liver

Metastases to lung

- Renal cell carcinoma
- Breast cancer
- Colon cancer
- Cervical cancer
- Malignant melanoma
- Almost every cancer can metastasize to lung

Metastases to meninges

- Leukemia or lymphoma
- Breast cancer
- Lung cancer
- Malignant melanoma
- Prostate cancer

Metastases to skin

- Metastatic melanoma
- Breast cancer
- Others: colorectal, lung, renal cell, bladder, ovarian, cervical, prostate

Methemoglobinemia

- Hypoxia, eg, congestive heart failure
- Right-to-left shunt, eg, arteriovenous fistula
- Cold exposure
- Sulfhemoglobinemia
- Carbon monoxide poisoning

Etiology

- Dapsone
- Benzocaine
- Pyridium
- Primaquine
- Sulfonamides
- Aniline
- Nitrites
- Nitrogen oxide gases
- Nitrobenzene

Microalbuminuria

Etiology

- Early proteinuria of any cause
- Acute hyperglycemia
- Urinary tract infection
- Marked hypertension
- Congestive heart failure
- Menses (false positive)

Microangiopathic hemolytic anemia

Etiology

- Thrombotic thrombocytopenic purpura
- Hemolytic uremic syndrome
- Disseminated intravascular coagulation
- Prosthetic valve hemolysis
- Metastatic adenocarcinoma
- Vasculitis
- Malignant hypertension
- HELLP syndrome (hemolysis, elevated liver enzymes, low platelets)

Midcycle spotting

- Ovulation bleeding (normal)
- Sexually transmitted disease
- Oral contraceptive pill (OCP) with low estrogen dose, first months of OCP use, or OCP not taken at same time each day
- Depo-Provera or intrauterine device use

Mitral regurgitation

- Aortic stenosis
- Aortic sclerosis
- Tricuspid regurgitation
- Hypertrophic obstructive cardiomyopathy
- Atrial septal defect
- Ventricular septal defect

Etiology

- Myxomatous degeneration (eg, mitral valve prolapse, Marfan syndrome)
- Infective endocarditis
- Subvalvular dysfunction (papillary muscle dysfunction or ruptured chordae tendinae)
- Rheumatic heart disease
- Dilated cardiomyopathy
- Congenital cleft mitral valve
- Left atrial myxoma (rare)

Mitral stenosis

- Mitral valve prolapse
- Atrial myxoma
- Cor triatriatum (congenital atrial anomaly)

Etiology

- Usually rheumatic heart disease
- Rarely: systemic lupus erythematosus, rheumatoid arthritis, mitral annular calcification, carcinoid, congenital

Murmur, diastolic

- Aortic regurgitation
- Mitral stenosis
- Tricuspid stenosis
- Patent ductus arteriosus (continuous murmur)
- Graham Steell murmur (pulmonary insufficiency secondary to pulmonary hypertension)

Murmur, systolic

- Aortic stenosis
- Aortic sclerosis
- Mitral regurgitation
- Mitral valve prolapse
- Flow murmur (anemia, pregnancy, hyperthyroidism, sepsis)
- Tricuspid regurgitation
- Hypertrophic obstructive cardiomyopathy
- Pulmonary stenosis
- Atrial septal defect
- Ventricular septal defect
- Coarctation of the aorta

Muscle cramps or tetany

Nocturnal leg cramps

- Idiopathic
- Diabetes
- Parkinson's disease
- CNS or spinal cord disease
- Peripheral neuropathy
- Hemodialysis

- Peripheral vascular disease
- Pregnancy
- Drugs: cisplatin, vincristine

Other causes of muscle cramps

- Muscle injury, eg, sports
- Dehydration
- Hypocalcemia, hypokalemia, hyponatremia, hypoglycemia, hyperkalemia, hypermagnesemia
- Alkalosis (eg, vomiting, hyperventilation)
- Arterial insufficiency (claudication)
- Restless leg syndrome
- Dystonia
- Hyperthyroidism
- Hypothyroidism
- Celiac disease
- Amyotrophic lateral sclerosis
- Black widow spider bite
- McArdle's disease (muscle fatigue, cramping, high CK)

Myelofibrosis

- Other myeloproliferative disorder, eg, chronic myelogenous leukemia
- Bone marrow infiltrative process, eg, metastatic cancer, tuberculosis, fungal infection
- Other causes of bone marrow fibrosis: Hodgkin's disease, hairy cell leukemia

Myocarditis, acute

- Angina or myocardial infarction
- Pneumonia
- Congestive heart failure

Etiology

Infectious myocarditis

- Viral, eg, coxsackie (most common), HIV
- Rickettsial, eg, scrub typhus, Rocky-Mountain spotted fever, Q fever
- Diphtheria
- Chagas' disease
- Toxoplasmosis
- Trichinosis (*Trichinella* infection)

Drug-induced & toxic myocarditis

- Doxorubicin
- Emetine
- Catecholamines (eg, pheochromocytoma)
- Phenothiazines
- Lithium
- Chloroquine
- Disopyramide
- Antimony-containing compounds
- Arsenicals
- Hypersensitivity to sulfonamides, penicillins, aminosalicylic acid
- Radiation
- Cocaine

Myoclonus

Etiology

- Anoxic brain injury
- Epilepsy
- Uremic or hepatic encephalopathy
- Idiopathic
- Drugs, eg, levodopa, alcohol, drug withdrawal
- Lipid storage diseases
- Ramsay Hunt syndrome type II (rare degenerative disorder)
- Subacute sclerosing panencephalitis
- Creutzfeldt-Jakob disease
- Spinal cord lesion (segmental myoclonus)

Myopathy

Etiology

- Alcoholism
- Endocrine: hypothyroidism, hyperthyroidism, Cushing's syndrome
- Chronic hypokalemia
- Polymyositis
- Dermatomyositis
- HIV myopathy
- Hyperparathyroidism
- Muscular dystrophy, eg, Duchenne, Becker, limb-girdle, facioscapulohumeral
- Myotonic dystrophy
- Myotonia congenita
- Inclusion body myositis
- Mitochondrial myopathy
- Sarcoidosis
- Drugs: corticosteroids, statins, clofibrate, colchicine, chloroquine, zidovudine, emetine, aminocaproic acid, bretylium, penicillamine, drugs causing hypokalemia

Myositis

Muscle inflammation

- Polymyositis
- Dermatomyositis
- Systemic lupus erythematosus
- Scleroderma
- Sjögren's syndrome
- Inclusion body myositis
- Trichinosis (*Trichinella* infection)
- Sarcocystosis

Other causes of proximal muscle weakness

- Polymyalgia rheumatica
- Endocrine: hypothyroidism, hyperthyroidism, Cushing's syndrome
- Alcoholism
- Drugs: corticosteroids, statins, clofibrate, colchicine, chloroquine, emetine, aminocaproic acid, bretylium, penicillamine, drugs causing hypokalemia
- HIV myopathy
- Hyperparathyroidism
- Spinal stenosis
- Osteomalacia
- Mitochondrial myopathy

Nail disorders, miscellaneous

- Nail pitting: psoriasis, alopecia areata, hand eczema
- Beau's lines (transverse) after serious illness
- Longitudinal groove: genetic or trauma
- Nail atrophy: congenital, trauma, vascular or neuralgic disease
- Spoon nails: anemia
- Nail hyperpigmentation: zidovudine, doxorubicin, cyclophosphamide, bleomycin, daunorubicin, fluorouracil, hydroxyurea, melphalan, mechlorethamine, nitrosoureas

Nails, discolored or thick

- Onychomycosis (tinea unguium)
- Psoriasis
- Keratoderma blennorrhagica (with reactive arthritis or Reiter's syndrome)
- Crusted (Norwegian) scabies
- Lichen planus
- Allergy to nail polish or nail glue

Nails, distorted

- Chronic inflammation of nail matrix
- Warts, tumors, nevi, or cysts impinging on nail matrix
- Lichen planus
- Allergy to nail polish or nail glue
- Keratosis follicularis (Darier disease)

Nasal deformity or saddle nose

- Syphilis

- Wegener's granulomatosis
- Relapsing polychondritis
- Rhinophyma (rosacea)
- Trauma
- Nasopharyngeal carcinoma
- Polymorphic reticulosis (lethal midline granuloma)
- Mucocutaneous leishmaniasis
- Hansen's disease (leprosy)
- Paracoccidioidomycosis
- Sarcoidosis

Nasal polyps

- Idiopathic
- Cystic fibrosis

Nasal tumors

- Nasal polyps
- Inverted papilloma
- Juvenile angiofibroma
- Nasopharyngeal carcinoma (usually squamous cell, also adenocarcinoma, mucosal melanoma, sarcoma, non-Hodgkin's lymphoma)
- Wegener's granulomatosis
- Sarcoidosis
- Polymorphic reticulosis (lethal midline granuloma)

Nausea and vomiting

Infections
- Norwalk or rotavirus
- "Food poisoning" by toxins from *B. cereus, S. aureus, C. perfringens*
- Hepatitis A or B
- Meningitis or encephalitis
- Acute systemic infections

Hepatobiliary or pancreatic disease
- Acute pancreatitis
- Cholecystitis or cholelithiasis

Topical gastrointestinal irritants
- Alcohol, NSAIDs, oral antibiotics

Systemic drugs
- Antitumor chemotherapy
- Alcohol
- Calcium channel blockers
- Opioids

Mechanical obstruction
- Gastric outlet obstruction: peptic ulcer disease, malignancy, gastric volvulus
- Small intestine: adhesions, hernias, volvulus, Crohn's disease, carcinomatosis

Dysmotility
- Gastroparesis: diabetic, medications, postviral, postvagotomy
- Small intestine: scleroderma, amyloidosis, chronic intestinal pseudo-obstruction, familial myoneuropathies

Peritonitis
- Perforated viscus
- Appendicitis
- Spontaneous bacterial peritonitis

Vestibular disorders
- Labyrinthitis, Ménière's disease, motion sickness, migraine

Increased intracranial pressure
- CNS tumors
- Subdural or subarachnoid hemorrhage

Psychogenic
- Anticipatory vomiting
- Bulimia
- Psychiatric disorders

Other
- Myocardial infarction, hypercalcemia, kidney stones, pyelonephritis, diabetic ketoacidosis, uremia, pregnancy, radiation therapy, adrenal crisis, parathyroid disease, hypothyroidism, paraneoplastic syndrome

Neck mass

- Reactive lymphadenopathy, eg, pharyngitis, tuberculous lymphadenitis (scrofula), cat-scratch disease, Lyme disease
- Lymphoma
- Skin abscess
- Parotitis
- Goiter or thyroiditis
- Branchial cleft cyst
- Thyroglossal duct cyst
- Metastasis from squamous cell carcinoma in mouth, pharynx, larynx, upper esophagus
- Metastatic thyroid carcinoma
- Sarcoidosis
- Cervical rib
- Zenker's diverticulum
- Carotid artery aneurysm
- Carotid body tumor
- Autoimmune adenopathy
- Kikuchi's disease (histiocytic necrotizing lymphadenitis)
- Esophageal diverticulum

Neck pain

- Acute or chronic cervical strain, eg, poor sleeping posture, whiplash injury
- Osteoarthritis, eg, cervical spondylosis on x-ray
- Herniated disk (discogenic neck pain)
- Rheumatoid arthritis
- Ankylosing spondylitis
- Compression fracture
- Osteomyelitis
- Meningitis
- Metastatic cancer
- Spinal stenosis
- Fibromyalgia
- Deep neck infection, eg, Ludwig's angina
- Thyroiditis
- Shoulder disorder
- Subarachnoid hemorrhage
- Thoracic outlet syndrome
- Temporal (giant cell) arteritis
- Carotid artery aneurysm or carotid dissection
- If myelopathy (eg, bilateral upper extremity findings, lower extremity spasticity or weakness, bladder dysfunction): osteoarthritis, rheumatoid arthritis, ankylosing spondylitis, motor neuron disease, multiple sclerosis, spinal cord tumor, syringomyelia, tropical spastic paresis (HTLV-1)

Neck stiffness

- Meningitis
- Subarachnoid hemorrhage
- Cervical arthritis, eg, osteoarthritis, rheumatoid arthritis
- Cervical strain, eg, poor sleeping posture, whiplash injury
- Fibromyalgia
- Polymyalgia rheumatica
- Tetanus

Nephrotic syndrome

- Congestive heart failure
- Cirrhosis
- Venous insufficiency
- Protein-losing enteropathy
- Malnutrition
- Hypothyroidism

Etiology

- Diabetes mellitus
- Lupus nephritis
- Amyloidosis
- HIV-associated nephropathy
- Multiple myeloma

- Idiopathic
  - Membranous nephropathy
  - Minimal change disease
  - Focal segmental glomerulosclerosis
  - Membranoproliferative glomerulonephritis

Neurogenic bladder

- Stroke
- Multiple sclerosis
- Parkinson's disease
- Spinal cord lesion or injury
- Diabetes mellitus
- Pelvic surgery or trauma
- Tabes dorsalis (neurosyphilis)
- Herniated lumbar disk

Neutropenia

Etiology

Bone marrow disorders
- Aplastic anemia
- Drugs: sulfonamides, chlorpromazine, procainamide, penicillin, cephalosporins, cimetidine, methimazole, phenytoin, chlorpropamide, antiretrovirals
- Cyclic neutropenia
- Pure white cell aplasia
- "Chronic benign neutropenia" in African-American and other populations
- Congenital (rare)

Peripheral disorders
- Hypersplenism
- Sepsis
- Immune destruction, eg, systemic lupus erythematosus
- Felty's syndrome (with rheumatoid arthritis and splenomegaly)
- HIV infection
- Acute viral infection
- Large granular lymphocytosis

Neutrophilia

Etiology

- Bacterial infection
- Inflammation, eg, rheumatoid arthritis, inflammatory bowel disease
- Malignancy or myeloproliferative disorder, eg, chronic myelogenous leukemia
- Corticosteroid administration
- Physiologic stress

Nipple discharge

- Galactorrhea, eg, pregnancy, postpartum, hyperprolactinemia
- Mammary duct ectasia
- Intraductal papilloma
- Breast cancer
- Oral contraceptives or estrogen replacement
- Subareolar abscess
- Fibrocystic breast disease

Nipple or areolar lesions

- Atopic dermatitis (eczema)
- Contact or irritant dermatitis
- Trauma, eg, breast-feeding
- Breast abscess (mastitis)
- Candidiasis
- Seborrheic keratosis
- Fox-Fordyce spots (sebaceous glands)
- Breast cancer, especially Paget's disease
- Bowen's disease (squamous cell carcinoma in situ)

Nocturia

- Benign prostatic hyperplasia
- Congestive heart failure (fluid redistribution)
- Diabetes mellitus
- Diuretic use
- Cystitis
- Urinary incontinence
- Obstructive sleep apnea

Nodules, subcutaneous

- Rheumatoid nodules (rheumatoid arthritis or rheumatic fever)
- Erythema nodosum
- Gout
- Lipoma
- Coccidioidomycosis
- Endocarditis (Osler's nodes)
- Sarcoidosis
- Polyarteritis nodosa
- Foreign-body granuloma
- Sporotrichosis
- Subcutaneous granuloma annulare
- Lupus panniculitis
- Calcinosis cutis
- Parasites, eg, cysticercosis, loiasis, paragonimiasis, onchocerciasis

Nonalcoholic fatty liver disease

Etiology

- Obesity
- Diabetes mellitus
- Hypertriglyceridemia
- Corticosteroids
- Cushing's syndrome
- Starvation or rapid weight loss
- Hypobetalipoproteinemia
- Total parenteral nutrition
- Drugs: corticosteroids, amiodarone, tamoxifen
- Wilson's disease
- Jejunoileal bypass
- Poisons: carbon tetrachloride, yellow phosphorus
- Microvesicular steatosis (nonalcoholic fatty liver disease usually macrovesicular): Reye's syndrome, valproic acid toxicity, tetracycline, acute fatty liver of pregnancy

Other causes of hepatomegaly
- Alcoholic fatty liver disease
- Hepatitis, eg, viral, alcoholic, toxic
- Cirrhosis
- Congestive heart failure
- Hepatocellular carcinoma or metastatic cancer

Obesity

- Increased caloric intake
- Fluid retention: congestive heart failure, cirrhosis, nephrotic syndrome
- Cushing's syndrome, eg, exogenous corticosteroids (central obesity)
- Hypothyroidism (edema and fat accumulation)
- Alcoholism (via hypercortisolism)
- Menopause (decreased metabolic rate)
- Polycystic ovary syndrome
- Syndrome X (obesity, diabetes, and hypertension)
- Insulinoma (hypoglycemia causing overeating)
- Insulin or thiazolidinedione therapy (worsen obesity)
- Other drugs, eg, antipsychotics, antidepressants
- Pregnancy
- Growth hormone deficiency
- Hypothalamic disorders
- Congenital leptin deficiency (morbid obesity)

- Defects in α-MSH (melanocortin 4) receptor (morbid obesity)
- Genetic syndromes of obesity and mental retardation
  - Prader-Willi syndrome (hypotonia, hypogonadism)
  - Laurence-Moon-Bardet-Biedl syndrome (polydactyly, renal anomalies, retinitis pigmentosa, hypogonadism)
  - Cohen's syndrome (microcephaly, hypotonia, short stature, ocular anomalies, neutropenia)
  - Biemond syndrome (diabetes mellitus, polydactyly, coloboma, facial anomalies, hypogonadism)

Obstruction of large intestine

Etiology

- Mechanical colonic obstruction, eg, malignancy, diverticulitis, volvulus, fecal impaction
- Toxic megacolon due to inflammatory bowel disease or *Clostridium difficile* colitis
- Megacolon due to Chagas' disease, Hirschsprung's disease (aganglionic), multiple sclerosis, sacral nerve damage, myxedema (hypothyroidism)
- Chronic intestinal pseudo-obstruction
- Acute colonic pseudo-obstruction (Ogilvie's syndrome), associated with:
  - Trauma, burns, or postoperative
  - Respiratory failure
  - Malignancy
  - Myocardial infarction or congestive heart failure
  - Pancreatitis
  - Stroke or subarachnoid hemorrhage
  - Intestinal ischemia
  - Drugs, eg, opioids, anticholinergics

Obstruction of small intestine

Etiology

- Mechanical obstruction of small intestine or proximal colon, eg, adhesions, volvulus, Crohn's disease
- Acute paralytic ileus due to:
  - Gastrointestinal or abdominal surgery
  - Peritoneal irritation, eg, peritonitis, pancreatitis, ruptured viscus
  - Severe medical illness, eg, sepsis, electrolyte abnormality
  - Drugs, eg, opioids, anticholinergics
  - Myxedema (hypothyroidism)
- Chronic intestinal pseudo-obstruction

Obstructive voiding symptoms

- Benign prostatic hyperplasia (especially with anticholinergics)
- Urethral stricture
- Neurogenic bladder
- Prostate cancer
- Bladder cancer
- Extrinsic compression, eg, pelvic or gastrointestinal tumor, radiation-induced fibrosis
- Urethral carcinoma
- Meatal stenosis

Occupational pulmonary disease

Etiology

Pneumoconiosis

Obstructive airway disorders

- Occupational asthma
- Industrial bronchitis
- Byssinosis (textile workers)

Toxic lung injury

- Smoke inhalation
- Toxic gas inhalation
- Silo-filler's disease

Lung cancer

- Asbestos, others

Pleural diseases

- Asbestos exposure
- Talc inhalation

Other

- Berylliosis

Odynophagia

- Infectious esophagitis: *Candida*, herpes simplex virus, cytomegalovirus
- Pill-induced esophagitis: NSAIDs, KCl, AZT, alendronate, iron, antibiotics
- Caustic esophageal injury (alkali or acid ingestion)
- Radiation esophagitis
- Reflux esophagitis

Olfactory dysfunction

- Anatomic blockage of nares, eg, polyps, septal deformity, nasal tumor
- Viral rhinitis
- Allergic rhinitis
- Idiopathic
- CNS tumor in olfactory groove (cribriform plate) or temporal lobe
- Head trauma
- Parkinson's disease
- Alzheimer's disease

Oligomenorrhea & amenorrhea

- Pregnancy
- Menopause or perimenopause
- Polycystic ovary syndrome
- Hypothalamic amenorrhea, eg, stress, weight change, exercise
- Hyperprolactinemia
- Hypothyroidism or hyperthyroidism
- Diabetes mellitus
- Premature ovarian failure
- Other endocrine causes: Cushing's syndrome, Addison's disease, hypopituitarism (pituitary tumor), androgen-secreting tumor (adrenal, ovarian), congenital adrenal hyperplasia, acromegaly, Turner syndrome
- Anorexia nervosa
- Endometrial scarring (Asherman's syndrome)
- Anabolic steroids

Onycholysis

- Excess water, soap, detergent, alkali
- Candidiasis
- Nail hardeners
- Photosensitive drug eruption
- Hyperthyroidism
- Hypothyroidism
- Keratoderma blennorrhagica (with reactive arthritis or Reiter's syndrome)
- Lichen planus
- Allergy to nail polish or nail glue

Opioid withdrawal

- Other drug withdrawal, eg, alcohol, benzodiazepines, amphetamines, cocaine
- Nausea or vomiting due to other causes
- Influenza or other viral syndrome

Optic disc swelling

- Glaucomatous cupping

Etiology

- Increased intracranial pressure (papilledema)
- Optic neuritis, eg, multiple sclerosis
- Anterior ischemic optic neuropathy, eg, temporal (giant cell) arteritis
- Severe hypertensive retinopathy
- Central retinal vein occlusion
- Posterior uveitis
- Posterior scleritis
- Optic disc drusen (pseudopapilledema)
- Optic nerve sheath meningioma
- Optic nerve infiltration by sarcoidosis, leukemia, or lymphoma

Optic neuritis

- Anterior ischemic optic neuropathy, eg, temporal (giant cell) arteritis
- Papilledema
- Retinal detachment
- Macular degeneration (exudative)
- Retinal artery or vein occlusion
- Vitreous hemorrhage
- Compressive lesion or intrinsic optic nerve tumor

Etiology

- Multiple sclerosis
- Viral infection, eg, measles, mumps, influenza, herpes zoster
- Autoimmune, eg, systemic lupus erythematosus
- Spread of inflammation from meninges, orbital tissues, paranasal sinuses

Oral lesions in HIV/AIDS

- Oral candidiasis
- Oral hairy leukoplakia
- Kaposi's sarcoma
- Necrotizing ulcerative periodontitis
- Oral ulcers: herpes simplex, aphthous ulcers, cytomegalovirus, histoplasmosis, herpes zoster, lymphoma

Oral ulcers

- Aphthous ulcer (canker sore, ulcerative stomatitis)
- Herpes simplex virus infection
- Erythema multiforme
- Drug reaction
- Pemphigus
- Bullous pemphigoid
- Systemic lupus erythematosus
- Lichen planus
- Coxsackievirus (herpangina, hand-foot-mouth disease)
- Acute HIV infection
- Parvovirus
- Varicella zoster
- Syphilis
- Oral candidiasis
- Behçet's syndrome
- Reactive arthritis
- Inflammatory bowel disease
- Squamous cell carcinoma
- Necrotizing ulcerative gingivostomatitis (Vincent's fusospirochetal disease)

Orthopnea

- Congestive heart failure (left-sided)
- Asthma
- Gastroesophageal reflux disease
- Sleep apnea

Osmolar gap

Etiology

- Methanol
- Ethylene glycol
- Isopropyl alcohol
- Ethanol toxicity
- Acetone
- Propylene glycol
- Severe alcoholic or diabetic ketoacidosis
- Lactic acidosis

Otitis media, chronic

- Otitis externa
- Auditory (eustachian) tube dysfunction
- Mastoiditis
- Tympanosclerosis (scarred tympanic membrane)
- Referred pain: sinusitis, tooth pain
- Temporomandibular joint syndrome
- Foreign body
- Cholesteatoma
- Bullous myringitis
- Nasopharyngeal carcinoma

Ovarian tumor

- Benign ovarian tumor, eg, follicle cyst, corpus luteum cyst
- Malignant ovarian tumor
- Teratoma (usually benign)
- Tubo-ovarian abscess
- Endometriosis
- Colon cancer
- Ectopic pregnancy
- Metastases to ovary, eg, gastrointestinal, breast
- Hydatidiform mole

Pain, chronic

- Major depressive disorder
- Somatoform disorder, eg, pain disorder associated with psychological factors
- Anxiety disorder, eg, general anxiety disorder, post-traumatic stress disorder
- Factitious disorder
- Malingering
- Organic disease producing symptoms

Palpitations

Cardiac
- Arrhythmia
- Valvular regurgitation

Noncardiac
- Exercise-associated
- Thyrotoxicosis
- Anemia
- Anxiety

Pancreatitis, acute

- Acute cholecystitis or cholangitis
- Penetrating duodenal ulcer
- Pancreatic pseudocyst
- Ischemic colitis
- Small bowel obstruction
- Abdominal aortic aneurysm
- Kidney stone
- Nonpancreatic causes of increased amylase

Etiology

- Gallstone
- Alcohol
- Hypertriglyceridemia
- Hypercalcemia
- Abdominal trauma or surgery
- Post-ERCP
- Drugs, eg, azathioprine, mercaptopurine, pentamidine, didanosine (ddI), valproic acid, tetracycline, estrogen, sulfonamides, thiazides, glucocorticoids
- Viral, eg, mumps, HIV
- Vasculitis
- Pregnancy

- Pancreas divisum
- Penetrating duodenal ulcer
- Pancreatic cancer
- Parasites, eg, *Clonorchis*, *Ascaris*
- Peritoneal dialysis
- Cardiopulmonary bypass

Pancreatitis, chronic

- Cholelithiasis
- Diabetes mellitus
- Malabsorption due to other causes
- Intractable duodenal ulcer
- Pancreatic cancer
- Irritable bowel syndrome

Etiology

- Alcoholism
- Chronic pancreatic obstruction by stricture, stone, or tumor
- Hyperparathyroidism
- Hereditary pancreatitis
- Abdominal trauma
- Tropical pancreatitis (tropical Africa & Asia)
- Autoimmune chronic pancreatitis
- Idiopathic

Pancytopenia

Etiology

Bone marrow disorders
- Aplastic anemia
- Myelodysplastic syndrome
- Acute leukemia
- Myelofibrosis
- Infiltrative disease: lymphoma, myeloma, carcinoma, hairy cell leukemia
- Megaloblastic anemia
- Paroxysmal nocturnal hemoglobinuria
- Bone marrow irradiation
- Genetic, eg, Fanconi's anemia

Nonmarrow disorders
- Hypersplenism
- Systemic lupus erythematosus
- Infection: tuberculosis, AIDS, leishmaniasis, brucellosis, histoplasmosis. (Viruses causing aplastic anemia: hepatitis, Epstein-Barr virus, HIV, parvovirus B19)

Panic

- Supraventricular tachycardia or angina pectoris
- Hyperthyroidism
- Pheochromocytoma
- Medication or substance abuse, eg, caffeine, nicotine, cocaine, amphetamines, pseudoephedrine
- Other anxiety disorder, eg, obsessive-compulsive disorder, post-traumatic stress disorder
- Somatoform disorder (eg, somatization)

Papillary necrosis

- Renal tuberculosis
- Medullary sponge kidney

Etiology

- Analgesic nephropathy
- Diabetes mellitus
- Sickle cell trait or disease
- Pyelonephritis
- Urinary tract obstruction
- Renal vein thrombosis
- Tuberculosis
- Cirrhosis

Papules and nodules

Skin-colored, white, or yellow
- Skin tag (acrochordon)
- Warts
- Basal cell carcinoma
- Squamous cell carcinoma
- Sebaceous (epidermal inclusion) cyst
- Lipoma
- Xanthoma
- Molluscum contagiosum
- Nevus (intradermal)
- Sebaceous hyperplasia
- Milia
- Keratosis pilaris
- Granuloma annulare
- Rheumatoid nodules
- Gout
- Sarcoidosis
- Calcinosis cutis
- Metastases (color variable)
- Calluses or corns
- Gummas (tertiary syphilis)
- Sporotrichosis
- Foreign-body granuloma

Brown
- Seborrheic keratosis
- Nevus (compound, intradermal)
- Melanoma
- Dermatofibroma
- Neurofibroma

Red
- Insect bites
- Acne vulgaris
- Cherry angioma
- Hemangioma
- Folliculitis
- Inflamed sebaceous (epidermal inclusion) cyst
- Furuncle
- Scabies
- Erythema nodosum
- Basal cell carcinoma
- Keratoacanthoma
- Prurigo nodularis
- Miliaria (heat rash)
- Urticaria
- Sporotrichosis

Blue, violaceous, or purple
- Vasculitis (palpable purpura)
- Lichen planus
- Melanoma
- Kaposi's sarcoma
- Blue nevus
- Venous lake
- Mycosis fungoides (cutaneous T cell lymphoma)
- Endocarditis (Osler's nodes)

Parasites involving the lung

- Ascariasis
- Hookworm
- Strongyloidiasis
- Paragonimiasis
- Toxocariasis (visceral larva migrans)
- Tropical pulmonary eosinophilia (*Wuchereria bancrofti*, *Brugia malayi*)
- Echinococcosis (hydatid disease)
- Amebic abscess

Parasomnias

- Nightmares or sleep terrors
- Sleepwalking: idiopathic, dementia, drugs (marijuana, alcohol), partial complex seizures
- Enuresis (bedwetting)

Paresthesias

- Alcoholism
- Diabetes mellitus

- Entrapment neuropathy, eg, carpal tunnel syndrome, tarsal tunnel syndrome, meralgia paresthetica
- Hypocalcemia
- Multiple sclerosis
- Spinal cord lesion
- Nerve root compression
- Herpes zoster
- Transient ischemic attack
- Guillain-Barré syndrome
- Trigeminal neuralgia
- Migraine
- Partial seizure
- Reflex sympathetic dystrophy
- Thoracic outlet syndrome
- Brachial plexus neuropathy

Parkinsonism

Etiology

- Parkinson's disease (idiopathic)
- Vascular parkinsonism (due to stroke)
- Essential tremor
- Depression
- Wilson's disease
- Huntington's disease
- Normal pressure hydrocephalus
- Shy-Drager syndrome
- Progressive supranuclear palsy
- Cortical-basal ganglionic degeneration
- Creutzfeldt-Jakob disease
- Drugs causing parkinsonism: antipsychotics, reserpine, metoclopramide
- West Nile virus

Paronychia

- Bacterial
- Candidiasis
- Felon (finger pad infection)
- Associated conditions: hypoparathyroidism, celiac sprue, acrodermatitis enteropathica, reactive arthritis (Reiter's syndrome)

Pelvic pain, acute

- Pelvic inflammatory disease
- Ectopic pregnancy
- Appendicitis
- Urinary calculi
- Primary dysmenorrhea
- Septic abortion
- Ruptured ovarian cyst or tumor
- Ovarian torsion
- Tubo-ovarian abscess
- Degeneration of leiomyoma (fibroid)
- Endometriosis
- Diverticulitis
- Cystitis

Pelvic pain, chronic

Gynecologic
- Endometriosis, adenomyosis (uterine endometriosis), pelvic adhesions, prior pelvic inflammatory disease or chronic pelvic inflammatory disease, uterine leiomyomas (fibroids), ovarian tumor

Gastrointestinal
- Irritable bowel syndrome, inflammatory bowel disease, diverticulosis, constipation, colon cancer, abdominal hernia

Urologic
- Detrusor overactivity, interstitial cystitis, urinary calculi, urethral syndrome, bladder cancer

Musculoskeletal
- Myofascial pain, low back pain, disk disease, nerve entrapment, muscle strain or spasm

Psychiatric
- Somatization, depression, physical or sexual abuse, anxiety

Penile pain

- Urethritis
- Herpes simplex
- Balanitis, eg, candidiasis
- Paraphimosis (in uncircumcised)
- Peyronie's disease
- Priapism
- Prostatitis
- Passage of a urinary calculus
- Trauma

Penile papules & other lesions

- Pearly penile papules (benign)
- Genital warts (condyloma)
- Molluscum contagiosum
- Syphilis
- Scabies
- Lice
- Herpes simplex (vesicles & ulcers)
- Lichen planus (lacy white patches)
- Psoriasis (plaques)
- Neoplasm
- Bowenoid papulosis
- Vitiligo (white patches)

Penile ulcer

- Herpes simplex
- Primary syphilis (chancre)
- Chancroid
- Lymphogranuloma venereum
- Granuloma inguinale
- Trauma
- Behçet's syndrome (usually glans)
- Systemic lupus erythematosus (usually glans)
- Neoplasm (usually glans)
- Lichen planus

Perianal fistula

Etiology

- Crohn's disease
- Lymphogranuloma venereum
- Cancer
- Rectal tuberculosis

Pericardial effusion

- Cardiac tamponade
- Restrictive cardiomyopathy
- Constrictive pericarditis
- Pericarditis
- Hemopericardium
- Congestive heart failure

Etiology

- Malignancy, eg, lung, breast, leukemia
- Infection, eg, viral, bacterial, mycobacterial, *Mycoplasma*
- Iatrogenic, eg, catheterization, pacemaker placement, postcardiotomy
- Idiopathic
- Uremia
- Radiation-induced
- Collagen vascular disease, eg, systemic lupus erythematosus
- Anticoagulation
- Aortic dissection
- Myxedema (hypothyroidism)

Pericarditis

- Myocardial infarction
- Aortic dissection
- Pneumothorax
- Pneumonia
- Pleurisy

- Costochondritis (anterior chest wall syndrome or Tietze's syndrome)
- Pericardial effusion
- Cholecystitis

Etiology

Infectious
- Viral (especially coxsackie and echovirus, also influenza, Epstein-Barr, varicella, hepatitis, mumps, HIV)
- Idiopathic (many likely viral)
- Tuberculous
- Bacterial, eg, extension from pulmonary infection, Lyme disease

Noninfectious
- Malignancy, eg, lung, breast, renal cell, lymphoma
- Uremia
- Dressler's syndrome (post-MI or post-cardiotomy)
- Radiation
- Systemic lupus erythematosus (including drug-induced, eg, procainamide, hydralazine)
- Rheumatoid arthritis
- Scleroderma
- Mixed connective tissue disease
- Drugs: minoxidil, penicillins
- Myxedema

Periorbital edema or swelling

- Allergies (allergic rhinitis)
- Nephrotic syndrome
- Orbital or periorbital cellulitis
- Hypothyroidism (myxedema)
- Herniated fat (usually in elderly)
- Angioedema
- Dermatomyositis
- Cavernous sinus thrombosis
- Mononucleosis (early)
- Trichinosis (*Trichinella* infection)
- Otorhinolaryngeal tumor
- Chagas' disease
- Dacryocystitis (lacrimal sac infection)

Peripheral neuropathy (mononeuropathy)

Etiology

- Nerve entrapment or compression
- Less often systemic disease, eg, diabetes mellitus, amyloidosis, rheumatoid arthritis, lead poisoning
- Peripheral nerve tumor (rare except in neurofibromatosis)

Examples
- Carpal tunnel syndrome
- Ulnar entrapment, eg, cubital tunnel syndrome
- Radial nerve palsy (wrist drop)
- Femoral neuropathy
- Meralgia paresthetica
- Sciatica
- Common peroneal nerve palsy
- Tarsal tunnel syndrome

Peripheral neuropathy (polyneuropathy)

Etiology

Metabolic and Systemic
- Diabetes mellitus
- Alcoholism
- Uremia
- Thiamine deficiency
- Vitamin B_{12} deficiency
- Multiple myeloma
- Amyloidosis
- Cryoglobulinemia
- Hypothyroidism or hyperthyroidism
- Sarcoidosis
- Paraneoplastic syndrome, eg, lung cancer
- Neuropathy associated with critical illness

Infectious and Inflammatory
- Hansen's disease (leprosy)
- HIV/AIDS
- Lyme disease
- Diphtheritic neuropathy
- Polyarteritis nodosa
- Rheumatoid arthritis
- Temporal (giant cell) arteritis

Toxic
- Metals: lead, mercury, arsenic, thallium
- Drugs: isoniazid, phenytoin, pyridoxine, nitrofurantoin, vincristine
- Industrial agents or pesticides: acrylamide, organophosphates, hexacarbon solvents, methyl bromide, carbon disulfide

Hereditary
- Charcot-Marie-Tooth disease (hereditary motor and sensory neuropathy, HMSN type I & II)
- Porphyria
- Friedrich's ataxia
- Dejerine-Sottas disease (HMSN type III)
- Refsum disease (HMSN type IV)

Mostly motor
- Guillain-Barré syndrome
- Chronic inflammatory demyelinating polyneuropathy (CIDP)
- Porphyria
- Diphtheritic neuropathy
- Toxic neuropathy
- Poliomyelitis
- Periodic paralysis syndrome

PFTs, DLCO (diffusion capacity) decreased

- Emphysema
- Interstitial lung disease
- Pulmonary embolism
- Pneumocystis pneumonia

PFTs, DLCO (diffusion capacity) increased

- Pulmonary hemorrhage
- Asthma
- Congestive heart failure (acute)
- Pregnancy

PFTs, obstructive disease

- Asthma
- Chronic obstructive pulmonary disease
- Bronchiectasis
- Bronchiolitis
- Airway obstruction, upper

PFTs, restrictive disease

Decreased lung compliance
- Interstitial lung disease
- Pneumonia
- Sarcoidosis
- Acute respiratory distress syndrome

Decreased muscle strength
- Neuromuscular disease (eg, myasthenia gravis, Guillain-Barré)
- Diaphragm dysfunction
- Phrenic nerve injury

Extrapulmonic disease
- Pleural effusion
- Pleural thickening
- Obesity
- Kyphoscoliosis

Pharyngitis

- Viral, eg, adenovirus, herpes simplex virus

- Group A streptococci
- Infectious mononucleosis
- Gonorrhea
- *Mycoplasma*
- *Chlamydia pneumoniae*
- Influenza
- Diphtheria
- Necrotizing gingivostomatitis (Vincent's angina, trench mouth)
- *Arcanobacterium haemolyticum*

Other causes of sore throat

- Peritonsillar abscess
- Oral candidiasis
- Epiglottitis
- Acute HIV infection
- Dry mouth (xerostomia)
- Nasopharyngeal carcinoma
- Glossopharyngeal neuralgia
- With rash: meningococcemia, toxic shock syndrome, drug eruption, viral exanthem

Photophobia

- Migraine
- Corneal abrasion
- Meningitis or encephalitis
- Uveitis
- Acute glaucoma
- Viral or bacterial conjunctivitis
- Keratitis (corneal ulcer or inflammation), eg, herpes simplex
- Systemic viral infection, eg, measles
- Severe dry eyes
- Ultraviolet (actinic) keratitis
- Aphakia (absence of lens)
- Albinism
- Eyestrain from refractive error
- Optic neuritis

Pigmented lesions

- Freckles (ephelides, juvenile freckles)
- Lentigo, eg, solar lentigo (liver spots, senile freckles)
- Seborrheic keratosis
- Acquired nevus (mole), eg, junctional nevus, compound nevus
- Congenital nevus
- Dysplastic (atypical) nevus
- Blue nevus
- Halo nevus
- Malignant melanoma
- Café au lait spots
- Pigmented basal cell carcinoma (uncommon)
- Diabetic dermopathy

Platelet disorders, qualitative

Etiology

Acquired disorders

- Drugs: aspirin, NSAIDs, antibiotics
- Uremia
- Myeloproliferative disorder, eg, polycythemia vera, essential thrombocytosis
- Autoantibody
- Paraproteins, eg, multiple myeloma
- Fibrin degradation products

Hereditary disorders

- von Willebrand's disease
- Glanzmann's thrombasthenia
- Bernard-Soulier syndrome
- Storage pool disease, eg, gray platelet syndrome

Platypnea

- Arteriovenous malformation at lung bases

Pleural effusion

- Atelectasis
- Chronic pleural thickening
- Lobar consolidation
- Subdiaphragmatic process

Etiology

Transudates

- Congestive heart failure (most common)
- Cirrhosis with ascites
- Nephrotic syndrome
- Peritoneal dialysis
- Myxedema
- Acute atelectasis
- Constrictive pericarditis
- Superior vena cava obstruction
- Pulmonary embolism
- Urinothorax (due to obstructive uropathy)

Exudates

- Pneumonia (parapneumonic effusion)
- Cancer
- Pulmonary embolism
- Empyema
- Tuberculosis
- Connective tissue disease (eg, rheumatoid arthritis)
- Viral infection
- Fungal infection
- Rickettsial infection
- Parasitic infection (eg, *Paragonimus*)
- Asbestosis
- Meigs' syndrome
- Pancreatic disease
- Uremia
- Chronic atelectasis
- Trapped lung
- Chylothorax
- Sarcoidosis
- Drug reaction
- Post-myocardial infarction syndrome
- Esophageal rupture

Pleural plaques (masses or thickening)

Malignant tumors

- Metastatic cancer
- Mesothelioma
- Bronchogenic carcinoma
- Lymphoma (subpleural tumor plaque)
- Thymoma

Benign tumors

- Lipoma
- Fibrous tumor
- Neurogenic

Other

- Asbestosis plaques
- Nonspecific response to: inflammation, trauma, neoplasm, radiation
- Talc inhalation
- Extramedullary hematopoiesis

Pleuritis (pleurisy)

Etiology

- Upper respiratory tract infection
- Pneumonia
- Rib fracture
- Pneumothorax
- Pulmonary embolism
- Pneumothorax
- Pericarditis
- Aspiration pneumonia
- Mesothelioma

Pneumaturia

- Fistula between bladder & gastrointestinal tract, eg, diverticulitis, carcinoma, Crohn's disease, radiation enteritis

- Infection with gas-producing organisms (rare)

Pneumoconiosis

- Tuberculosis
- Sarcoidosis
- Histoplasmosis
- Coccidioidomycosis
- Idiopathic pulmonary fibrosis

Etiology

Metal dusts

- Siderosis (mining, welding)
- Stannosis (mining, tin-working, smelting)
- Baritosis (glass & insecticide manufacturing)

Coal dust

- Coal worker's pneumoconiosis (common)

Inorganic dusts

- Silicosis (rock mining, stonecutting; common)

Silicate dusts

- Asbestosis (mining, insulation, construction, shipbuilding; common)
- Talcosis (mining, insulation, construction, shipbuilding)
- Kaolin pneumoconiosis (pottery, cement work)
- Shaver's disease (corundum manufacture)

Pneumonia, anaerobic, & lung abscess

- Tuberculosis
- Bronchogenic carcinoma
- Fungal infection, eg, histoplasmosis
- Bronchiectasis
- Cavitary bacterial pneumonia
- Pulmonary vasculitis, eg, Wegener's granulomatosis

Etiology

- Usually polymicrobial
- *Prevotella melaninogenica*
- *Peptostreptococcus*
- *Fusobacterium nucleatum*
- *Bacteroides*

Pneumonia, community-acquired

- Bacterial pneumonia
- Viral pneumonia
- Aspiration pneumonia
- *Pneumocystis* pneumonia
- Bronchitis
- Lung abscess
- Tuberculosis
- Pulmonary embolism
- Myocardial infarction
- Sarcoidosis
- Lung cancer
- Hypersensitivity pneumonitis
- Bronchiolitis or bronchiolitis obliterans organizing pneumonia

Etiology

Bacterial

- *Streptococcus pneumoniae* (most common)
- *Haemophilus influenzae*
- *Mycoplasma pneumoniae* (young adults, summer & fall)
- *Chlamydia pneumoniae* (young adults)
- *Staphylococcus aureus* (influenza epidemics, IV drug use, bronchiectasis)
- *Neisseria meningitides*
- *Moraxella catarrhalis* (lung disease, elderly)
- *Klebsiella pneumoniae* (alcohol, diabetes)
- *Legionella* spp. (contaminated construction site, water source, or air conditioner)

Viral

- Influenza virus
- Respiratory syncytial virus
- Adenovirus
- Parainfluenza virus

Special risk factors

- *Chlamydia psittaci* (psittacosis): birds
- *Coxiella burnetii* (Q fever): cattle, sheep, goats; especially newborns or products of conception
- *Francisella tularensis* (tularemia): tick or skinning rabbit
- Endemic fungi (*Blastomyces*: Ohio & Mississippi River valleys; *Coccidioides*: Southwest United States or Latin America; *Histoplasma*: Ohio & Mississippi River valleys)
- Sin nombre virus (hantavirus pulmonary syndrome): rodent waste, Southwest United States
- Severe acute respiratory syndrome (SARS): travel to endemic area within 10 days before symptom onset, including mainland China, Hong Kong, Singapore, Taiwan, Vietnam, and Toronto

Pneumonia, hospital-acquired

- Bacterial pneumonia
- Viral pneumonia
- Aspiration pneumonia
- Pneumocystis pneumonia
- Bronchitis
- Lung abscess
- Tuberculosis
- Pulmonary embolism
- Myocardial infarction
- Sarcoidosis
- Lung cancer
- Hypersensitivity pneumonitis
- Bronchiolitis or bronchiolitis obliterans organizing pneumonia

Etiology

More common

- *Pseudomonas aeruginosa*
- *Staphylococcus aureus*
- *Enterobacter*
- *Klebsiella pneumoniae*
- *Escherichia coli*

Less common

- *Proteus*
- *Serratia marcescens*
- *H. influenzae*
- Streptococci
- *Acinetobacter*

Pneumonia, recurrent or persistent

- Lung cancer (postobstructive pneumonia)
- Hypersensitivity pneumonitis
- Eosinophilic pneumonia
- Bronchiolitis obliterans organizing pneumonia
- *Mycobacterium avium* complex
- Asplenism

Pneumonia in immunocompromised patient

- Bacterial pneumonia
- Pneumocystis pneumonia
- Tuberculosis
- Fungal pneumonia, eg, coccidioidomycosis, histoplasmosis, cryptococcosis, aspergillosis, candidiasis
- Cytomegalovirus

- Lymphoma
- Kaposi's sarcoma

Pneumothorax

- Myocardial infarction
- Pulmonary embolism
- Pneumonia
- Chronic obstructive pulmonary disease
- Asthma
- Pleural effusion
- Aortic dissection
- Pericarditis
- Aortic aneurysm rupture

Etiology

Primary pneumothorax

- Apical bleb rupture (tall, thin males age 10–30)

Secondary pneumothorax

- Chronic obstructive pulmonary disease (ruptured bleb or bulla)
- Asthma
- Cystic fibrosis
- Tuberculosis
- *Pneumocystis* pneumonia
- Menstruation (catamenial pneumothorax)
- Interstitial lung disease, eg, sarcoidosis, lymphangioleiomyomatosis (LAM), eosinophilic granuloma (Langerhans cell histiocytosis, histiocytosis X)

Tension pneumothorax

- Penetrating or blunt trauma
- Lung infection
- Cardiopulmonary resuscitation
- Positive-pressure mechanical ventilation

Traumatic or iatrogenic

- Penetrating or blunt trauma
- Thoracentesis
- Pleural biopsy
- Percutaneous or transbronchial lung
- Central line placement
- Positive-pressure mechanical ventilation

Podagra

- Gout
- Trauma
- Cellulitis
- Sarcoidosis
- Pseudogout
- Psoriatic arthritis
- Bursitis of first MTP joint (inflamed bunion)

Polycythemia

Etiology

- Relative ("spurious") polycythemia
- Polycythemia vera (primary polycythemia)
- Secondary polycythemia
  - Hypoxia: cardiac disease, pulmonary disease, high altitude
  - Carboxyhemoglobin (smoking)
  - Renal cyst or hydronephrosis
  - Erythropoietin-secreting tumors (rare): renal cell or hepatocellular carcinoma, adrenal tumor, cerebellar hemangioma, uterine leiomyoma
  - Abnormal hemoglobins (rare)

Polydipsia

- Diabetes mellitus
- Diabetes insipidus
- Hypercalcemia
- Psychogenic polydipsia (associated with schizophrenia)
- Sjögren's syndrome
- Anticholinergics
- Primary hyperaldosteronism

Polyps of colon and small intestine

Etiology

- Mucosal neoplastic: adenoma (tubular, villous, or tubulovillous)
  - Nonfamilial (sporadic) adenomatous polyps
  - Familial adenomatous polyposis
- Mucosal nonneoplastic: hyperplastic, juvenile, hamartoma, inflammatory
  - Hamartomatous polyposis syndromes, eg, Peutz-Jeghers syndrome, familial juvenile polyposis, Cowden's syndrome
- Submucosal: lipoma, lymphoid aggregates, carcinoid, pneumatosis cystoides intestinalis

Polyuria

- Osmotic diuresis: diabetes mellitus, mannitol infusion, radiocontrast media, high-protein tube feeds
- Drugs: diuretics, lithium, caffeine
- Diabetes insipidus
- Hypercalcemia, eg, hyperparathyroidism
- Psychogenic polydipsia (eg, schizophrenia)
- Excess IV fluids
- Chronic renal failure (early)
- Diuretic phase of acute tubular necrosis
- Hypokalemia
- Post-transurethral resection of the prostate
- Cushing's syndrome
- Primary hyperaldosteronism
- Inability to concentrate urine: sickle cell trait or disease, chronic pyelonephritis, amyloidosis
- Anxiety

Portal hypertension

Etiology

- Cirrhosis (most common)
- Portal vein thrombosis
- Splenic vein thrombosis
- Schistosomiasis
- Noncirrhotic intrahepatic portal sclerosis
- Arterial-portal vein fistula

Postcholecystectomy pain

- Retained common bile duct stone
- Common bile duct stricture
- Dilated cystic duct remnant
- Sphincter of Oddi spasm or stenosis
- Foreign-body granuloma
- Traction on common duct by long cystic duct
- Functional pain
- Pain due to nonbiliary disease, eg, peptic ulcer disease

Premature ovarian failure

Etiology

- Surgical bilateral oophorectomy
- Autoimmune
- X chromosome mosaicism
- Pelvic irradiation or chemotherapy
- Hysterectomy (even without oophorectomy)
- Turner syndrome
- Myotonic dystrophy
- Galactosemia
- Mumps oophoritis
- Familial or idiopathic

Proptosis (exophthalmos)

- Graves' ophthalmopathy

- Orbital cellulitis
- Orbital pseudotumor
- Tumor, eg, hemangioma, optic nerve glioma
- Trauma or orbital hemorrhage
- Retracted eyelid (normal variant)
- Inflammatory disease, eg, Wegener's granulomatosis, sarcoidosis
- Carotid cavernous fistula, dural arteriovenous malformation, or cavernous sinus thrombosis
- Posterior scleritis
- Hand-Schuller-Christian disease (eosinophilic granuloma)

Prostatodynia

- Chronic bacterial prostatitis
- Nonbacterial prostatitis
- Urethritis
- Cystitis
- Interstitial cystitis
- Prostatic abscess
- Prostate cancer
- Perirectal abscess
- Proctitis
- Diverticulitis
- Anal fissure or fistula

Proteinuria

Etiology

- Functional (benign): acute illness, exercise, "orthostatic proteinuria"
- Overload: multiple myeloma, rhabdomyolysis, leukemia
- Glomerular: diabetes, postinfectious glomerulonephritis, HIV, systemic lupus erythematosus, amyloid, IgA nephropathy, membranous nephropathy
- Tubulointerstitial: acute tubular necrosis, aminoglycosides, interstitial nephritis, Wilson's disease, Fanconi's syndrome
- Other: polycystic kidney disease, preeclampsia-eclampsia

Pruritus (itching)

Skin diseases
- Xerosis (dry skin)
- Scabies
- Urticaria
- Atopic dermatitis
- Contact dermatitis
- Arthropod bites (insect bites)
- Pediculosis (lice)
- Dermatitis herpetiformis
- Anogenital pruritus
- Lichen simplex chronicus
- Drug reaction
- Urticarial eruptions of pregnancy
- Folliculitis

Non-skin diseases
- Uremia
- Hyperbilirubinemia or cholestasis
- Hepatitis C
- Amphetamine or cocaine use
- Hypothyroidism or hyperthyroidism
- Intestinal parasites
- Lymphoma, leukemia, other malignancy
- Polycythemia vera
- Iron deficiency anemia
- Psychiatric

Pseudogout & chondrocalcinosis

- Gouty arthritis
- Septic arthritis
- Rheumatoid arthritis
- Reactive arthritis (Reiter's syndrome)
- Osteoarthritis

Etiology

Causes of chondrocalcinosis
- Pseudogout
- Hemochromatosis
- Hyperparathyroidism
- Ochronosis (alkaptonuria)
- Diabetes mellitus
- Hypothyroidism
- Wilson's disease
- Gouty arthritis

PT increased

Etiology

- Liver disease
- Warfarin therapy
- Vitamin K deficiency
- Factor VII deficiency or inhibitor
- Heparin therapy (PTT increased more than PT)
- Disseminated intravascular coagulation (PT & PTT increased)
- Rare isolated factor deficiencies (II, V, X, I)

Ptosis

- Cranial nerve 3 palsy (dilated or normal pupil), eg, diabetic neuropathy, posterior inferior cerebellar artery aneurysm
- Horner's syndrome (constricted pupil)
- Myasthenia gravis
- Botulism
- Age-related (sagging eyelid)
- Eyelid inflammation or deformity
- Congenital
- Progressive external ophthalmoplegia (mitochondrial myopathy)

PTT increased

Etiology

Congenital factor deficiencies
- Contact factors (no clinical bleeding)
- Factor XII (no clinical bleeding)
- Factor XI
- Factor IX (hemophilia B)
- Factor VIII (hemophilia A)
- Factor VIII (von Willebrand's disease)
- Factor I (afibrinogenemia)

Anticoagulants
- Factor VIII inhibitor (postpartum, idiopathic, or after factor VIII infusions)
- Lupus anticoagulant (no clinical bleeding)
- Heparin
- Warfarin (PT increased more than PTT)

Other
- Disseminated intravascular coagulation (PT & PTT increased)
- Liver disease (PT increased more than PTT)
- Vitamin K deficiency (PT increased more than PTT)

Pulmonary edema, acute

Etiology

Cardiogenic
- Congestive heart failure
- Myocardial infarction
- Myocardial ischemia
- Volume overload of left ventricle: mitral regurgitation, aortic insufficiency, ventricular septal defect
- Mitral stenosis

Noncardiogenic
- Acute respiratory distress syndrome
- Sepsis

- Disseminated intravascular coagulation
- Increased intracerebral pressure (eg, intracerebral bleed or stroke)
- Aspiration pneumonia
- High altitude
- Drug reaction
- Transfusion reaction
- Salicylate intoxication
- Radiographic contrast allergy
- Inhaled toxins, eg, smoke inhalation

Pulmonary embolism

- Myocardial infarction
- Pneumonia
- Pericarditis
- Congestive heart failure
- Pleuritis (pleurisy)
- Pneumothorax
- Pericardial tamponade

Etiology

- Thromboembolism (most common)
- Fat embolism
- Air embolism
- Amniotic fluid embolism
- Septic embolism (eg, endocarditis)
- Tumor embolism (eg, renal cell carcinoma)
- Foreign-body embolism (eg, talc in IV drug use)
- Parasite egg embolism (schistosomiasis)

Pulmonary hypertension

- Primary pulmonary hypertension
- Secondary pulmonary hypertension
- Cor pulmonale (right heart failure due to pulmonary disease)
- Congestive heart failure
- Right-sided valve disease
- Mitral stenosis

Etiology

- Primary pulmonary hypertension
- Chronic pulmonary embolism
- Chronic obstructive pulmonary disease
- Interstitial lung disease
- Sleep apnea
- Pickwickian syndrome (obesity-hypoventilation syndrome)
- Scleroderma or other connective tissue disease
- Left to right intracardiac shunt
- Drugs or toxins: fenfluramine, dexfenfluramine, phentermine, bleomycin, amiodarone, talc (via IV drug use)
- Radiation
- Pulmonary veno-occlusive disease
- Valve disease: mitral stenosis, mitral regurgitation, aortic stenosis
- Left-sided heart failure
- Atrial myxoma
- High altitude (chronic mountain sickness)
- Polycythemia vera
- Cirrhosis with portal hypertension
- HIV
- Schistosomiasis
- Sickle cell disease

Pulmonary insufficiency

Etiology

- Pulmonary hypertension (usually)
- Rare: congenital, rheumatic heart disease, endocarditis, carcinoid

Pulmonary nodule, solitary

- Bronchogenic carcinoma
- Granuloma (tuberculous, fungal)
- Lung abscess
- Hamartoma
- Metastatic cancer
- Arteriovenous malformation
- Resolving pneumonia
- Rheumatoid nodule
- Pulmonary infarction
- Carcinoid
- Pseudotumor (loculated fluid in a fissure)

Pulmonary nodules (multiple)

- Metastatic cancer
- Bronchogenic carcinoma
- Lymphoproliferative cancer
- Tuberculosis
- Lung abscess
- Granulomas (eg, tuberculous, fungal)
- Coccidioidomycosis
- Histoplasmosis
- Sarcoidosis
- Silicosis
- Coal worker's pneumoconiosis
- *Mycobacterium avium complex* (MAC)
- Arteriovenous malformations
- Rheumatoid nodules
- Hamartomas
- Wegener's granulomatosis
- Methotrexate-induced
- Eosinophilic granuloma (Langerhans cell histiocytosis, histiocytosis X)
- Congenital cysts
- Echinococcosis (hydatid disease)
- Paragonimiasis

Pulmonary-renal syndromes

- Goodpasture's syndrome
- Severe congestive heart failure (pulmonary edema and prerenal azotemia)
- Renal failure (with hypervolemia and pulmonary edema)
- Microscopic polyangiitis (polyarteritis nodosa)
- Systemic lupus erythematosus
- Henoch-Schönlein purpura
- Wegener's granulomatosis
- Churg-Strauss syndrome
- Legionnaire's disease
- Renal vein thrombosis with pulmonary embolism

Pulse, absent or decreased

- Peripheral vascular disease
- Takayasu's arteritis or "pulseless disease" (various pulses)
- Temporal (giant cell) arteritis (temporal artery)
- Thromboangiitis obliterans or Buerger's disease (distal pulses)
- Aortic dissection (decreased or unequal pulses)
- Coarctation of the aorta (femoral pulses)

Pulseless electrical activity (PEA)

- CHEAPMD (mnemonic)
  - **C**ardiac tamponade
  - **H**ypoxia, hypovolemia, hypothermia, hyperkalemia
  - **E**mbolism (massive pulmonary embolism)
  - **A**cidosis
  - **P**neumothorax (tension pneumothorax)
  - **M**yocardial infarction
  - **D**rug overdose, eg, tricyclic antidepressant, digoxin, beta blocker, calcium channel blocker

Pulse pressure, wide

High output states
- Thyrotoxicosis
- Pregnancy
- Beriberi heart disease
- Vasodilating drugs

Increased run-off of LV outflow
- Aortic regurgitation
- Patent ductus arteriosus

Other
- Old age (rigid arteries)
- Severe bradycardia

Pulsus alternans

- Low ejection fraction
- Large pericardial effusion

Pulsus paradoxus

- Asthma
- Chronic obstructive pulmonary disease
- Pericardial effusion
- Cardiac tamponade
- Constrictive pericarditis (rarely)

Purine content of foods

Etiology

Note
- The consumption of large amounts of a food containing a small concentration of purines may provide a greater purine load than consumption of a small amount of food containing a large concentration of purines.

Low-purine foods
- Refined cereals and cereal products, cornflakes, white bread, pasta, flour, arrowroot, sago, tapioca, cakes
- Milk, milk products, and eggs
- Sugar, sweets, and gelatin
- Butter, polyunsaturated margarine, and all other fats
- Fruit, nuts, and peanut butter
- Lettuce, tomatoes, and green vegetables (except those listed below)
- Cream soups made with low-purine vegetables but without meat or meat stock
- Water, fruit juice, cordials, and carbonated drinks

High-purine foods
- All meats, including organ meats, and seafood
- Meat extracts and gravies
- Yeast and yeast extracts, beer, and other alcoholic beverages
- Beans, peas, lentils, oatmeal, spinach, asparagus, cauliflower, and mushrooms

Purpura, nonpalpable

- Trauma
- Senile or solar purpura
- Corticosteroid use
- Idiopathic (autoimmune) thrombocytopenic purpura
- Thrombotic thrombocytopenic purpura
- Disseminated intravascular coagulation
- Other thrombocytopenia or platelet dysfunction
- Clotting factor defect
- Vitamin K deficiency
- Warfarin necrosis
- Amyloidosis
- Waldenström's macroglobulinemia
- Scurvy
- Ehlers-Danlos syndrome

Purpura, palpable

Vasculitis
- Polyarteritis nodosa
- Rheumatoid arthritis
- Wegener's granulomatosis
- Churg-Strauss syndrome
- Henoch-Schönlein purpura
- Systemic lupus erythematosus
- Hypersensitivity (leukocytoclastic) vasculitis

Infection or emboli
- Meningococcemia
- Gonococcemia
- Endocarditis
- Rocky Mountain spotted fever
- *Aspergillus*
- Candidiasis
- Ecthyma gangrenosum (neutropenic, pseudomonal)

Other
- Sarcoidosis
- Cryoglobulinemia
- Ulcerative colitis
- Crohn's disease
- Medications

Pustules

- Acne vulgaris
- Acne rosacea
- Folliculitis
- Candidiasis
- Tinea
- Miliaria (heat rash)
- Gonococcemia
- Vesicles (can be pustular)
- Scabies
- Keratosis pilaris
- Hidradenitis suppurativa

Pyoderma gangrenosum

- Ulcer secondary to underlying infection (eg, mycobacterial, fungal, tertiary syphilis, amebiasis)
- Ulcer secondary to underlying neoplasm
- Folliculitis
- Arthropod bites (insect bites)
- Sweet's syndrome (acute febrile neutrophilic dermatosis)
- Vasculitis (eg, Wegener's granulomatosis)
- Warfarin necrosis

Pyuria

- Cystitis
- Urethritis
- Epididymitis
- Orchitis
- Prostatitis
- Pyelonephritis
- Perinephric abscess
- Renal tuberculosis (sterile pyuria)

Rash, annular

- Tinea corporis (body ringworm)
- Psoriasis
- Secondary syphilis
- Erythema multiforme
- Pityriasis rosea
- Nummular (discoid) eczema
- Discoid lupus erythematosus
- Erythema migrans (Lyme disease)
- Granuloma annulare
- Erythema nodosum (nodular)

Rash, intertriginous

- Tinea cruris (jock itch)
- Candidiasis
- Intertrigo
- Seborrheic dermatitis

- Cellulitis
- Psoriasis of body folds ("inverse psoriasis")
- Erythrasma
- Tinea versicolor (pityriasis versicolor) (rarely)
- Scratching due to lice
- Contact dermatitis

Rash, morbilliform

- Drug eruption
- Viral exanthem
- Secondary syphilis
- Early erythema multiforme major
- Scarlet fever
- Toxic shock syndrome
- Acute HIV infection
- Acute graft-versus-host disease

Rash, palms and soles

- Tinea
- Warts
- Dyshidrotic eczema (pompholyx, dyshidrosis)
- Secondary syphilis
- Dermatophytid reaction (allergy or sensitivity to fungi)
- Erythema multiforme
- Rocky Mountain spotted fever
- Drug eruption
- Janeway lesions or Osler's nodes (bacterial endocarditis)
- Cholesterol emboli
- Contact dermatitis (palms)
- Pitted keratolysis (soles)
- Keratoderma blennorrhagica (with reactive arthritis or Reiter's syndrome)
- Psoriasis
- Gonococcemia or meningococcemia
- Hand, foot, and mouth disease
- Toxic shock syndrome
- Lichen planus (ulcerative)
- Melanoma
- Calluses or corns
- Rat bite fever
- Arsenic poisoning

Raynaud's syndrome

- Raynaud's disease (idiopathic)
- Livedo reticularis
- Acrocyanosis
- Erythromelalgia

Red eye

- Conjunctivitis (viral, bacterial, allergic)
- Uveitis
- Acute glaucoma
- Foreign body or corneal abrasion
- Keratitis (corneal ulcer or inflammation), eg, herpes simplex
- Scleritis or episcleritis
- Trauma
- Subconjunctival hemorrhage
- Eyelid disorder, eg, hordeolum, chalazion, blepharitis
- Cluster headache

Red eye, circumcorneal (ciliary injection)

- Corneal abrasion or keratitis
- Intraocular inflammation, eg, uveitis
- Acute glaucoma

Reflexes, delayed relaxation

Etiology

- Hypothyroidism
- Diabetes mellitus
- Pernicious anemia
- Hypothermia

Renal cysts

- Renal cell carcinoma
- Renal abscess
- Transitional cell carcinoma of renal pelvis
- Adrenal tumor
- Renal oncocytoma
- Renal angiomyolipoma
- Metastases, eg, lung, breast, stomach, contralateral kidney
- Lymphoma
- Nephrolithiasis
- Renal infarction

Renal failure, acute

Etiology

Prerenal azotemia

- Dehydration
- Hemorrhage, eg, gastrointestinal bleeding
- Congestive heart failure
- Renal artery stenosis including fibromuscular dysplasia
- NSAIDs, ACE inhibitors

Postrenal azotemia

- Obstruction, eg, benign prostatic hypertrophy, bladder tumor, pelvic mass

Intrinsic renal disease

- Acute tubular necrosis
- Toxins: NSAIDs, antibiotics, contrast, multiple myeloma, rhabdomyolysis, hemolysis, chemotherapy, hyperuricemia, cyclosporine
- Ischemia, eg, prolonged prerenal azotemia
- Acute glomerulonephritis
- Immune complex: IgA nephropathy, endocarditis, systemic lupus erythematosus, cryoglobulinemia, postinfectious glomerulonephritis, membranoproliferative, Henoch-Schönlein purpura
- Pauci-immune (ANCA+): Wegener's granulomatosis, Churg-Strauss syndrome, microscopic polyarteritis
- Anti-GBM: Goodpasture's syndrome, anti-GBM glomerulonephritis
- Other: malignant hypertension, thrombotic thrombocytopenic purpura, scleroderma renal crisis, preeclampsia-eclampsia
- Acute interstitial nephritis
- Drugs: beta-lactams, sulfa, diuretics, NSAIDs, rifampin, phenytoin, allopurinol
- Infections: *Streptococcus*, leptospirosis, cytomegalovirus, histoplasmosis, Rocky Mountain spotted fever
- Immune: systemic lupus erythematosus, Sjögren's syndrome, sarcoidosis, cryoglobulinemia

Renal failure, chronic

Etiology

Glomerulopathies

- Primary glomerular diseases
- IgA nephropathy
- Focal segmental glomerulosclerosis
- Membranoproliferative glomerulonephritis
- Membranous nephropathy
- Secondary glomerular diseases
- Diabetic nephropathy (very common)
- Hypertensive nephropathy
- Amyloidosis
- Postinfectious glomerulonephritis
- HIV-associated nephropathy
- Collagen vascular diseases, eg, systemic lupus erythematosus
- Sickle cell nephropathy

Tubulointerstitial nephritis
- Drug hypersensitivity
- Heavy metals
- Analgesic nephropathy
- Vesicoureteral reflux
- Idiopathic

Obstructive uropathy
- Prostatic disease
- Urinary calculi
- Retroperitoneal fibrosis or tumor

Vascular diseases
- Hypertensive nephrosclerosis (very common)
- Renal artery stenosis including fibromuscular dysplasia

Hereditary diseases
- Polycystic kidney disease
- Medullary cystic kidney disease
- Alport's syndrome

Renal failure in HIV/AIDS

Etiology

- Typical causes of acute renal failure
- HIV-associated nephropathy
- Acute tubular necrosis due to pentamidine, amphotericin, foscarnet, cidofovir, aminoglycosides, rifampin, acyclovir
- Interstitial nephritis due to TMP-SMX, sulfadiazine, acyclovir
- Nephrolithiasis due to indinavir
- Postinfectious glomerulonephritis
- Membranous nephropathy due to hepatitis B, syphilis
- Membranoproliferative glomerulonephritis due to hepatitis C, cryoglobulinemia
- Ureteral compression due to lymphoma, lymphadenopathy
- IgA immune-complex deposition
- Thrombotic thrombocytopenic purpura

Renal tubular acidosis

Other causes of normal gap metabolic acidosis
- Gastrointestinal loss of HCO_3^-, eg, diarrhea, pancreatic ileostomy or ileal loop bladder
- Renal tubular acidosis
- Recovery from diabetic ketoacidosis
- Dilutional acidosis from rapid administration of 0.9% NaCl
- Carbonic anhydrase inhibitors
- Chloride retention or administration of HCl equivalent or NH_4Cl

Etiology

- Type I (distal H^+ secretion defect): low serum K^+, urine pH >5.5, associated with autoimmune disease, hypercalcemia
- Type II (proximal HCO_3^- reabsorption defect): low serum K^+, urine pH <5.5, associated with multiple myeloma, drugs (eg, sulfa)
- Type III (rare): normal serum K^+, urine pH <5.5, associated with renal insufficiency
- Type IV (hyporeninemic hypoaldosteronism): high serum K^+, urine pH <5.5, associated with diabetes mellitus, drugs (eg, NSAIDs)

Respiratory failure, acute

Airway disorders
- Asthma
- Chronic obstructive pulmonary disease exacerbation
- Airway obstruction

Pulmonary edema
- Left ventricular dysfunction
- Mitral regurgitation or mitral stenosis
- Volume overload states
- Acute respiratory distress syndrome
- Re-expansion

Parenchymal lung disorders
- Pneumonia or aspiration pneumonitis
- Interstitial lung disease
- Lung contusion

Pulmonary vascular disorders
- Pulmonary thromboembolism

Chest wall, diaphragm, and pleural disorders
- Flail chest
- Pneumothorax
- Pleural effusion
- Massive ascites

Neuromuscular and related disorders
- Guillain-Barré syndrome
- Myasthenia gravis
- Poliomyelitis
- Botulism
- Organophosphates or aminoglycosides
- Spinal cord injury
- Phrenic nerve injury or dysfunction
- Hypokalemia, hypophosphatemia
- Myxedema

CNS disorders
- Drugs: sedative, hypnotic, opioid, anesthetics
- Brainstem disorder
- Intracranial hypertension
- CNS infections

Increased CO_2 production
- Fever, infection, seizures, drugs

Respiratory tract infections, recurrent

- Seasonal allergies (allergic rhinitis)
- Selective IgA deficiency
- Common variable immunodeficiency
- Anatomic abnormalities

Retinal artery occlusion

- Ophthalmic artery occlusion
- Ophthalmic migraine
- Retinal detachment
- Retinal vein occlusion

Etiology

- Emboli from carotid or heart
- Vasculitis, eg, temporal (giant cell) arteritis
- Internal carotid dissection
- Thrombophilia

Retinal detachment

- Retinal artery or vein occlusion
- Vitreous hemorrhage
- Macular degeneration (exudative)
- Anterior ischemic optic neuropathy, eg, temporal (giant cell) arteritis
- Amaurosis fugax (transient ischemic attack)

Retinal vein occlusion

- Retinal artery occlusion
- Retinal detachment
- Anterior ischemic optic neuropathy, eg, temporal (giant cell) arteritis
- Papilledema
- Diabetic retinopathy
- Hypertensive retinopathy

Retinopathy

Etiology

- Diabetic retinopathy
- Hypertensive retinopathy

- Radiation retinopathy
- Retinal vein occlusion
- Anterior ischemic optic neuropathy, eg, temporal (giant cell) arteritis
- Sickle cell retinopathy
- Retinopathy of severe anemia
- Retinopathy due to autoimmune disease, eg, systemic lupus erythematosus
- Emboli from IV drug use (talc retinopathy)
- Eales' disease (idiopathic retinal vasculitis)

Rhinitis (nasal congestion)

- Viral rhinitis (common cold)
- Allergic rhinitis
- Sinusitis (rhinosinusitis)
- Vasomotor rhinitis (eg, cold air- or irritant-induced)
- Nasal polyposis
- Rhinitis medicamentosa
- Foreign body
- Wegener's granulomatosis
- CSF leak

Rickettsial diseases

Etiology

- Typhus group: epidemic (louse-borne) typhus, scrub typhus, endemic typhus, California flea rickettsiosis
- Spotted fever group: Rocky Mountain spotted fever, rickettsialpox, RMSF-like, Boutonneuse fever, Kenya tick typhus, South African tick fever, Indian tick typhus, Queensland tick typhus, North Asian tick typhus
- Other: ehrlichiosis (human monocytic and human granulocytic), Q fever

Sacroiliitis

- Causes or mimics of sacroiliitis: ankylosing spondylitis, reactive arthritis (Reiter's syndrome), psoriatic arthritis, inflammatory bowel disease, osteitis condensans ilii, hyperparathyroidism, Whipple's disease
- Diffuse idiopathic skeletal hyperostosis (in elderly)
- Synovitis-acne-pustulosis-hyperostosis-osteitis syndrome
- Sciatica
- Lumbar disk herniation, spinal stenosis, or facet joint degenerative arthritis
- Ochronosis (alkaptonuria)

Salivary gland tumor

- Sialadenitis
- Sialolithiasis (salivary gland calculi)
- Lymphadenopathy (eg, from conjunctivitis, otitis media, sinusitis)
- Metastatic submandibular lymph node

Scaly lesions

- Atopic dermatitis (eczema)
- Seborrheic dermatitis
- Psoriasis
- Tinea, eg, tinea corporis, cruris, or pedis
- Contact dermatitis
- Stasis dermatitis (due to venous insufficiency)
- Xerosis (dry skin)
- Lichen simplex chronicus (circumscribed neurodermatitis)
- Tinea versicolor (pityriasis versicolor)
- Nummular eczema (discoid eczema, nummular dermatitis)
- Intertrigo
- Secondary syphilis
- Pityriasis rosea
- Discoid lupus erythematosus
- Exfoliative dermatitis (exfoliative erythroderma)
- Actinic keratoses
- Cutaneous T cell lymphoma (mycosis fungoides)
- Bowen's disease (squamous cell carcinoma in situ)
- Paget's disease

Scleritis or episcleritis

- Conjunctivitis
- Keratitis
- Uveitis
- Acute glaucoma
- Corneal abrasion

Etiology

- Autoimmune: rheumatoid arthritis, systemic lupus erythematosus, polyarteritis nodosa, Wegener's granulomatosis, relapsing polychondritis, inflammatory bowel disease, sarcoidosis
- Infectious: ophthalmic zoster, herpes simplex, Lyme disease, HIV, syphilis, tuberculosis

Seizure

- Syncope
- Cardiac arrhythmia
- Stroke or transient ischemic attack
- Pseudoseizure
- Panic attack
- Migraine
- Narcolepsy

Etiology

- Idiopathic (epilepsy)
- Hypoglycemia
- Drugs: alcohol withdrawal, cocaine, amphetamines, benzodiazepine withdrawal, heroin withdrawal, SSRIs
- Electrolyte abnormality, eg, hyponatremia, hypocalcemia
- Infection: bacterial meningitis, herpes encephalitis, neurocysticercosis, neurosyphilis
- Space-occupying lesion, eg, brain tumor, arteriovenous malformation
- Trauma
- Stroke
- CNS vasculitis, eg, systemic lupus erythematosus
- Uremia
- Febrile seizures
- Congenital abnormality or perinatal injury
- Degenerative disease, eg, Alzheimer's disease

Seizure in HIV/AIDS

Etiology

- CNS toxoplasmosis
- Cryptococcal meningitis
- Herpes encephalitis
- Bacterial meningitis
- CNS lymphoma
- Neurosyphilis

Septal perforation

- Nose picking
- Prior surgery
- Cocaine use
- Wegener's granulomatosis

Seronegative spondyloarthropathy

Etiology

- Reactive arthritis (Reiter's syndrome)
- Psoriatic arthritis
- Ankylosing spondylitis

- Arthritis associated with inflammatory bowel disease
- Ochronosis (alkaptonuria; mimics ankylosing spondylitis)

Sexual dysfunction, women

- Depression
- Dyspareunia
- Chronic pelvic pain
- Menopause
- Oral contraceptive use
- Hypothyroidism
- Hyperprolactinemia
- Diabetes mellitus
- Cushing's syndrome
- Addison's disease
- Hypopituitarism
- Drugs: alcohol, recreational drugs, SSRIs, tricyclic antidepressants
- Physical or sexual abuse
- Anorexia nervosa
- Multiple sclerosis

Shoulder pain

- Rotator cuff tendonitis ("impingement") or tear
- Subacromial bursitis
- Biceps tendonitis
- Osteoarthritis (AC joint; rare in glenohumeral joint)
- Frozen shoulder (adhesive capsulitis)
- Acromioclavicular separation
- Neck disorder, eg, osteoarthritis, herniated disk (discogenic neck pain), tumor
- Rheumatoid arthritis or septic arthritis
- Calcific tendinitis
- Shoulder dislocation or fracture
- Avascular necrosis
- Polymyalgia rheumatica
- Fibromyalgia
- Thoracic outlet syndrome
- Brachial plexus neuropathy
- Referred pain from gallbladder, heart, diaphragm, Pancoast tumor
- Metastatic or primary tumor

Shunt (right to left, anatomic shunts)

Etiology

Pulmonary

- Arteriovenous fistula (eg, idiopathic arteriovenous malformation, Osler-Weber-Rendu, hepatopulmonary)
- Atelectasis
- Pulmonary edema
- Pneumonia
- Acute respiratory distress syndrome

Cardiac

- Atrial septal defect
- Ventricular septal defect
- Patent foramen ovale
- Patent ductus arteriosus

Sialolithiasis or sialadenitis

- Sialolithiasis (salivary gland calculi)
- Bacterial sialadenitis
- Salivary gland tumor
- Facial cellulitis
- Dental abscess
- TMJ syndrome
- Trigeminal neuralgia
- Lymphadenopathy (eg, from conjunctivitis, otitis media, sinusitis)
- Parotid enlargement due to starch ingestion

Etiology

- Viral: mumps, HIV, influenza, Epstein-Barr virus, cytomegalovirus, coxsackie
- Bacterial infection, eg, *S. aureus*
- Sjögren's syndrome
- Sarcoidosis
- Amyloidosis
- Alcohol
- Bulimia
- Dehydration
- Diabetes, cirrhosis, chronic pancreatitis
- Vitamin deficiency
- Acromegaly
- Drugs: antithyroid drugs, iodine, cholinergics, eg, phenothiazines

Sick sinus syndrome

- Sinus bradycardia
- Atrioventricular block
- Tachy-brady syndrome

Etiology

- Drugs: digitalis, calcium channel blockers, beta blockers, clonidine, other sympatholytics, amiodarone, other antiarrhythmics
- Age-related conduction system fibrosis or calcification (Lev's disease)
- Cardiac infiltrative disease (eg, amyloid, sarcoidosis, hemochromatosis)
- Chagas' disease

Sinopulmonary syndromes

Infection

- HIV
- Aspergillosis

Allergic

- Asthma and allergic rhinitis
- ABPA and allergic fungal sinusitis

Idiopathic

- Wegener's granulomatosis
- Churg-Strauss syndrome

Altered defenses

- Cystic fibrosis
- Immotile cilia syndrome
- Common variable immunodeficiency
- IgA deficiency
- IgG subclass deficiency
- Complement deficiency

Sinusitis, chronic

- Wegener's granulomatosis
- Neoplasm
- Cystic fibrosis
- Immotile cilia syndrome (eg, Kartagener's)
- Aspergillosis

Small intestinal tumor

Benign

- Adenomatous polyp
- Villous adenoma
- Lipoma
- Benign stromal tumor (leiomyoma)
- Crohn's disease (may mimic tumor)

Malignant

- Adenocarcinoma, especially in ampulla of Vater
- Lymphoma (primary or secondary)
- Carcinoid
- Leiomyosarcoma
- Kaposi's sarcoma

Sneezing

- Allergic rhinitis
- Upper respiratory tract infection
- Influenza
- Nasal polyp
- Deviated septum

Spasticity

Etiology

- Stroke

- Cerebral palsy
- Anoxic brain injury, head trauma, or space-occupying lesion
- Spinal cord tumor or injury
- Multiple sclerosis

Spells (nonspecific)

- Neurologic: syncope or presyncope, vertigo, transient ischemic attack, absence seizure, temporal lobe seizure, pseudoseizure, migraine, narcolepsy, multiple sclerosis, porphyria
- Psychiatric: anxiety, panic attack, conversion disorder, domestic violence
- Cardiac: arrhythmia, mitral valve prolapse
- Pulmonary: pulmonary embolism, pulmonary hypertension
- Endocrine: hypoglycemia, hypocalcemia, pheochromocytoma, carcinoid, hyperthyroidism, hypothyroidism, hot flashes (menopausal)
- Rheumatologic: CNS vasculitis
- Drugs, eg, alcohol, cocaine, withdrawal
- Infectious: Lyme disease, neurosyphilis

Spinal cord tumor

- Primary tumor, eg, ependymoma, meningioma, neurofibroma
- Lymphoma, leukemia, multiple myeloma
- Metastases: prostate cancer, breast cancer, lung cancer, renal cell carcinoma, colon cancer, melanoma
- Epidural abscess
- Multiple sclerosis
- Tuberculosis (Pott's disease)

Splenomegaly

- Infections, eg, mononucleosis (Epstein-Barr virus), cytomegalovirus, acute HIV, endocarditis, histoplasmosis, malaria, schistosomiasis, leishmaniasis, filariasis
- Chronic hemolytic anemia
- Leukemia
- Lymphoma
- Extramedullary hematopoiesis, eg, myelofibrosis, marrow toxin
- Polycythemia vera
- Essential thrombocytosis
- Cirrhosis or noncirrhotic portal hypertension
- Congestive heart failure
- Immune thrombocytopenias
- Splenic vein thrombosis
- Rheumatoid arthritis (Felty's syndrome)
- Systemic lupus erythematosus
- Sarcoidosis
- Wilson's disease
- Amyloidosis
- Budd-Chiari syndrome
- Gaucher disease
- Niemann-Pick disease
- Splenic cysts, hemangiomas, hamartomas, fibromas
- Metastases, eg, melanoma
- Eosinophilic granuloma (Langerhans cell histiocytosis, histiocytosis X)

Splinter hemorrhages

- Trauma
- Endocarditis
- Antiphospholipid antibody syndrome
- Rheumatoid vasculitis
- Trichinosis (*Trichinella* infection)
- Scurvy

Stroke

- Transient ischemic attack
- Ischemic stroke
- Intracerebral hemorrhage
- Subdural or epidural hematoma
- Space-occupying lesion, eg, brain tumor
- Seizure (Todd's paralysis)
- Migraine
- Peripheral causes of vertigo, eg, Ménière's disease
- Hypoglycemia
- Guillain-Barré syndrome
- Multiple sclerosis
- Aortic dissection

Etiology

- Embolic: atrial fibrillation, carotid atherosclerosis, left ventricular aneurysm, dilated cardiomyopathy, acute myocardial infarction, endocarditis, mechanical valve, mitral valve prolapse, aortic arch atherosclerosis, atrial myxoma, patent foramen ovale
- Thrombotic: atherosclerosis, small vessel ischemia, vasculitis, eg, systemic lupus erythematosus, polycythemia, thrombocytosis, sickle cell disease, meningovascular syphilis, arterial dissection or aneurysm, eg, intracerebral carotid or vertebral
- Hemorrhagic: hypertension, amyloidosis, conversion of ischemic stroke, cocaine

Sudden death

Cardiac causes

- Ventricular fibrillation
- Acute myocardial infarction
- Complete heart block
- Sinus node arrest
- Hypertrophic obstructive cardiomyopathy
- Congestive heart failure
- Long QT syndrome
- Atrial myxoma
- Mitral valve prolapse
- Pre-excitation syndrome (eg, Wolff-Parkinson-White)
- Chagas' disease
- Coronary anomalies
- Brugada syndrome
- Arrhythmogenic right ventricular dysplasia

Noncardiac causes & Associated conditions

- Pulmonary embolism
- Asthma
- Aortic dissection
- Ruptured aortic aneurysm
- Intracerebral hemorrhage
- Tension pneumothorax
- Anaphylaxis
- Electrolyte abnormalities
- Cocaine or other drug use
- Primary pulmonary hypertension
- Aortic stenosis
- Pulmonary stenosis

Sympatholytic poisoning

Etiology

- Barbiturates
- Benzodiazepines, other sedatives
- Gamma-hydroxybutyrate
- Clonidine
- Ethanol
- Opioids

Sympathomimetic poisoning

Etiology

- Amphetamines
- Cocaine
- Ephedrine, pseudoephedrine
- PCP (pupils normal or small)
- Phenylpropanolamine (bradycardia common)

- Theophylline toxicity

Syncope

- Seizure
- Transient ischemic attack or stroke
- Hypoglycemia
- Narcolepsy
- Vertigo

Etiology

Cardiac

- Arrhythmia (ventricular tachycardia, supraventricular tachycardia, sick sinus syndrome, sinus bradycardia, sinus arrest, atrioventricular block)
- Aortic stenosis
- Myocardial infarction
- Hypertrophic obstructive cardiomyopathy
- Pulmonary hypertension, pulmonary embolism, pulmonary stenosis
- Atrial myxoma

Noncardiac

- Orthostatic or postural hypotension
  - Hypovolemia
  - Drugs, eg, beta blockers, calcium channel blockers, vasodilators, diuretics
  - Autonomic insufficiency, eg, diabetes, adrenal insufficiency, spinal cord lesion, Guillain-Barré syndrome, chronic idiopathic orthostatic hypotension
- Situational, eg, micturition, defecation, cough, swallow
- Carotid sinus hypersensitivity

Tachycardia

Narrow & regular

- Sinus tachycardia
- Atrial flutter
- AV node re-entry tachycardia
- Atrial ventricular re-entry tachycardia (AVRT)
- Wolff-Parkinson-White syndrome (subset of AVRT)
- Atrial tachycardia
- Junctional tachycardia

Narrow & irregular

- Atrial fibrillation
- Frequent premature atrial contractions
- Atrial flutter with variable block
- Multifocal atrial tachycardia
- Sinus arrhythmia

Wide & regular

- Ventricular tachycardia
- Supraventricular tachycardia with aberrancy (eg, pre-existing bundle branch block, rate-related bundle branch block, or WPW)

Wide & irregular

- Torsades de pointes
- Frequent PVCs

Tachycardia, multifocal atrial

- Atrial fibrillation
- Frequent premature atrial contractions
- Atrial flutter (especially if variable block)

Etiology

- Pulmonary disease, eg, chronic obstructive pulmonary disease
- Hypokalemia
- Hypomagnesemia

Tachycardia, paroxysmal supraventricular

Etiology

- Digitalis toxicity
- AV node re-entry tachycardia
- Atrial ventricular re-entry tachycardia (AVRT)
- Wolff-Parkinson-White syndrome (subset of AVRT)

Tachycardia, sinus

- Fever
- Exercise
- Emotion
- Pain
- Anemia
- Heart failure
- Shock
- Hyperthyroidism
- Drugs
- Alcohol withdrawal

Tachycardia, ventricular

- Supraventricular tachycardia with aberrancy (eg, pre-existing bundle branch block, rate-related bundle branch block, or WPW)
- Atrial flutter or atrial fibrillation with aberrancy
- Hyperkalemia (severe)
- Torsades de pointes
- Frequent PVCs

Etiology

- Myocardial infarction
- Dilated cardiomyopathy
- Coronary artery disease
- Hypertrophic obstructive cardiomyopathy
- Mitral valve prolapse
- Myocarditis
- Long QT

Telangiectasia

- Actinic (sun) damage
- Cirrhosis ("spiders")
- Acne rosacea
- Basal cell carcinoma
- Hereditary hemorrhagic telangiectasia (Osler-Weber-Rendu syndrome)
- Scleroderma or CREST syndrome
- Systemic lupus erythematosus
- Dermatomyositis
- Pregnancy
- Necrobiosis lipoidica diabeticorum

Testicular mass or swelling

- Inguinal hernia
- Hydrocele
- Testicular cancer
- Epididymitis
- Orchitis
- Testicular torsion
- Varicocele
- Testicular cyst (epidermoid cyst)
- Lymphoma
- Metastases (rare): prostate, lung, gastrointestinal, melanoma, kidney
- Lymphedema, eg, filariasis (elephantiasis)

Testicular pain (scrotal pain, groin pain)

- Trauma
- Epididymitis
- Testicular torsion
- Inguinal hernia
- Hydrocele
- Varicocele
- Orchitis
- Torsion of appendix of testis or epididymis
- Testicular tumor
- Prostatitis
- Urinary calculi

- Renal disorder
- Hip joint arthritis, eg, osteoarthritis, septic arthritis
- Iliopsoas bursitis
- Ilioinguinal, iliohypogastric, or genitofemoral neuralgia
- Lumbosacral disk or cord disease

Thalassemias

- Iron deficiency anemia
- Other hemoglobinopathy, eg, sickle thalassemia, hemoglobin C disorders
- Sideroblastic anemia
- Anemia of chronic disease

Etiology

Alpha thalassemia syndromes

- Silent carrier (3 alpha globin genes, normal hematocrit)
- Alpha thalassemia minor or trait (2 genes, hematocrit 32–40%, MCV 60–75)
- Hemoglobin H disease (3 genes, hematocrit 22–32%, MCV 60–70)
- Hydrops fetalis (0 genes)

Beta thalassemia syndromes

- Beta thalassemia minor
- Beta thalassemia intermedia
- Beta thalassemia major

Thrombocytopenia

Etiology

Decreased production (bone marrow disorder)

- Aplastic anemia
- Hematologic malignancies
- Myelodysplastic syndrome
- Megaloblastic anemia
- Chronic alcoholism
- Other infiltrative process, eg, myelofibrosis, infection

Increased destruction

- Immune disorders
  - Idiopathic (autoimmune) thrombocytopenic purpura
  - Drug-induced, eg, heparin, sulfonamides, thiazides, quinine
  - Secondary (chronic lymphocytic leukemia, systemic lupus erythematosus)
  - Posttransfusion purpura
- Disseminated intravascular coagulation
- Thrombotic thrombocytopenic purpura
- Hemolytic uremic syndrome
- Sepsis
- Viral infections, AIDS
- Liver failure
- Preeclampsia-eclampsia

Splenic sequestration

Thrombocytosis

Etiology

Reactive thrombocytosis (usually platelets < 1,000,000)

- Inflammatory disease, eg, rheumatoid arthritis, ulcerative colitis
- Chronic infection
- Iron deficiency anemia
- Postsplenectomy (transient)

Myeloproliferative disorder

- Essential thrombocytosis
- Polycythemia vera
- Chronic myelogenous leukemia
- Myelofibrosis

Thyroid nodules

- Adenoma, colloid nodule, or cyst
- Benign multinodular goiter
- Thyroid cancer
- Hashimoto's thyroiditis (may be nodular)
- Metastatic cancer

Tinnitus

- Idiopathic
- Excessive noise exposure
- Ménière's disease
- Labyrinthitis
- Acute otitis media
- Chronic otitis media
- Auditory (eustachian) tube dysfunction
- Ototoxicity, eg, salicylates, aminoglycosides, loop diuretics, cisplatin
- Glomus tumor
- Any cause of sensory hearing loss

Pulsatile tinnitus (like hearing one's heartbeat)

- Glomus tumor
- Carotid stenosis or carotid dissection
- Arteriovenous malformation
- Aneurysm
- Pseudotumor cerebri

Toxidromes (poisoning syndromes)

Etiology

- Sympathomimetic poisoning
- Sympatholytic poisoning
- Cholinergic poisoning
- Anticholinergic poisoning
- Acetaminophen poisoning
- Amphetamines or cocaine intoxication
- Beta blocker overdose
- Carbon monoxide poisoning
- Chemical warfare agents (eg, cholinergic poisoning)
- Digitalis overdose
- Iron poisoning
- Isoniazid (INH) poisoning
- Lead poisoning
- Methanol and ethylene glycol poisoning
- Methemoglobinemia
- Opioid overdose
- Salicylate poisoning
- Tricyclic antidepressant overdose

Transient ischemic attack

- Stroke
- Hypoglycemia
- Seizure (Todd's paralysis)
- Syncope
- Migraine
- Peripheral causes of vertigo, eg, Ménière's disease

Etiology

- Embolic: atrial fibrillation, carotid atherosclerosis, left ventricular aneurysm, dilated cardiomyopathy, acute myocardial infarction, endocarditis, mechanical valve, mitral valve prolapse, aortic arch atherosclerosis, atrial myxoma, patent foramen ovale
- Thrombotic: atherosclerosis, small vessel ischemia, vasculitis, eg, systemic lupus erythematosus, polycythemia, thrombocytosis, sickle cell disease, meningovascular syphilis, arterial dissection or aneurysm, eg, intracerebral carotid or vertebral
- Hemorrhagic: hypertension, amyloidosis, conversion of ischemic stroke, cocaine

Traveler's diarrhea

- Most common: Enterotoxigenic *E. coli*, *Shigella*, *Campylobacter*
- Less common: *Aeromonas*, *Salmonella*, noncholera vibrios, *Entamoeba histolytica*, *Giardia lamblia*, adenoviruses, rotavirus
- Chronic watery diarrhea: *Entamoeba histolytica*, *Giardia lamblia*, tropical sprue (rare)

- From unprotected anal intercourse: *Neisseria gonorrhoeae,* syphilis, lymphogranuloma venereum, herpes simplex virus

Tremor

Etiology

- Enhanced physiologic tremor, eg, anxiety
- Essential tremor
- Parkinson's disease
- Hyperthyroidism
- Hepatic encephalopathy
- Cerebellar tremor, eg, multiple sclerosis
- Adult-onset idiopathic dystonia
- Wilson's disease
- Drugs: caffeine, alcohol withdrawal, sympathomimetics, antipsychotics, theophylline, metoclopramide, lithium, levothyroxine, tricyclic antidepressants, valproic acid, reserpine
- Psychogenic tremor

Tricuspid regurgitation

- Mitral regurgitation
- Aortic stenosis
- Pulmonary stenosis
- Atrial septal defect
- Ventricular septal defect

Etiology

- Right ventricular overload due to left ventricular failure
- Infective endocarditis
- Pulmonary hypertension
- Right ventricular or inferior myocardial infarction
- Rheumatic heart disease
- Carcinoid syndrome
- Systemic lupus erythematosus
- Myxomatous degeneration or mitral valve prolapse
- Ebstein's anomaly

Triglycerides increased

Etiology

- Alcohol
- Obesity
- "Metabolic syndrome" (insulin resistance, low HDL)
- Diabetes mellitus
- Chronic renal insufficiency
- Lipodystrophy, eg, protease inhibitors
- Pregnancy
- Familial
- Drugs: oral contraceptives, isotretinoin, thiazides (short-term effect), beta blockers (short-term effect), corticosteroids, bile acid-binding resins

TSH decreased

Etiology

- Primary hyperthyroidism, eg, Graves' disease, toxic multinodular goiter, toxic thyroid nodule, subacute thyroiditis, early Hashimoto's disease
- Thyroid hormone administration
- Severe nonthyroidal illness
- Dopamine or dopamine agonists (levodopa, bromocriptine)
- Pregnancy
- hCG-secreting trophoblastic tumor
- Acute psychiatric illness
- Acute glucocorticoid administration
- Other drugs, eg, NSAIDs, amphetamines, octreotide, opioids, nifedipine, verapamil
- "Subclinical" hyperthyroidism: low TSH, clinically euthyroid, normal T4, common in elderly (10%), risk of atrial fibrillation and osteoporosis

TSH increased

Etiology

- Primary hypothyroidism
- "Subclinical" hypothyroidism: high TSH, clinically euthyroid, normal T4
- Autoimmune disease (assay interference)
- Recovery from nonthyroidal illness
- Acute psychiatric illness
- Drugs: dopamine antagonists (eg, metoclopramide), phenothiazines, atypical antipsychotics
- Levothyroxine malabsorption due to iron, sucralfate, aluminum hydroxide antacids, calcium supplements, soy milk
- Rare cases of hyperthyroidism due to inappropriate pituitary TSH secretion, eg, neoplasm

Ulcer, leg

- Venous stasis ulcers (due to venous insufficiency)
- Arterial insufficiency (arterial ulcer)
- Stasis dermatitis (due to venous insufficiency)
- Diabetic neuropathy
- Bacterial pyoderma (eg, infected wound or bite)
- Trauma
- Pressure ulcer
- Vasculitis, eg, thromboangiitis obliterans (Buerger's disease)
- Rheumatoid arthritis or Felty's syndrome
- Pyoderma gangrenosum
- Underlying skin cancer
- Sickle cell anemia
- Embolic disease (including cholesterol emboli)
- Cryoglobulinemia
- Erythema induratum (associated with tuberculosis)
- Other underlying infection (eg, fungal, tertiary syphilis, leishmaniasis, amebiasis, dracunculiasis)
- Calciphylaxis

Ulcer and eschar

- Cutaneous anthrax
- Warfarin necrosis
- Antiphospholipid antibody syndrome
- Aspergillosis
- Mucormycosis
- Brown recluse spider bite
- Cutaneous leishmaniasis
- Ecthyma gangrenosum (neutropenic, pseudomonal)
- Tularemia
- Rickettsialpox
- Plague

Upper respiratory tract infection (upper respiratory infection)

- Allergic rhinitis
- Sinusitis (rhinosinusitis)
- Pharyngitis
- Bronchitis
- Otitis media
- Asthma
- Influenza
- Pneumonia
- Mononucleosis
- Laryngitis
- Pertussis
- Epiglottitis

Urethral discharge, men

- Gonorrhea

- Nongonococcal urethritis, eg, chlamydia, *Ureaplasma urealyticum*, trichomoniasis
- Balanitis, eg, candidiasis
- Reactive arthritis (Reiter's syndrome)
- Urethral carcinoma

Urethral discharge, women

- Gonorrhea
- Nongonococcal urethritis, eg, chlamydia, *Ureaplasma urealyticum*
- Trichomoniasis
- Candidiasis
- Cystitis
- Reactive arthritis (Reiter's syndrome)
- Urethral carcinoma

Urinary frequency

- Cystitis
- Urethritis
- Pyelonephritis
- Diabetes mellitus
- Diabetes insipidus
- Excess fluid intake
- Diuretics
- Caffeine, alcohol
- Chronic urinary retention
- Neurogenic bladder
- Interstitial cystitis
- Urethral syndrome
- Extrinsic bladder compression, eg, pelvic tumor, radiation-induced fibrosis
- Urinary calculi
- Anxiety

Urinary incontinence

- Cystitis
- Prostatitis
- Interstitial cystitis
- Medications, eg, diuretics, alcohol, caffeine, hypnotics
- Polyuria, eg, diabetes mellitus, diabetes insipidus, hypercalcemia
- Vesicovaginal or ureterovaginal fistula
- Dementia
- Normal pressure hydrocephalus

Etiology

Transient incontinence: DIAPPERS

- Delirium
- Infection
- Atrophic vaginitis or urethritis
- Pharmacology, eg, anticholinergics, diuretics, hypnotics
- Psychiatric disorders, eg, psychosis, depression
- Excess urine, eg, edema, hyperglycemia, hypercalcemia
- Restricted mobility
- Stool impaction

Established incontinence

- Detrusor overactivity (urge incontinence or "overactive" bladder)
- Urethral incompetence (stress incontinence, eg, multiparity, pelvic surgery)
- Urethral obstruction (eg, benign prostatic hyperplasia; can also present as urge or overflow)
- Detrusor underactivity (overflow incontinence, eg, neurogenic bladder, anticholinergics)
- Mixed incontinence (urge and stress)

Urinary tract infection

- Acute cystitis
- Pyelonephritis
- Acute bacterial prostatitis
- Chronic bacterial prostatitis

Urinary tract obstruction

- Benign prostatic hyperplasia (especially with anticholinergics or over-the-counter sympathomimetics)
- Bilateral ureteral calculi
- Urethral stricture
- Neurogenic bladder
- Prostate cancer
- Bladder cancer
- Extrinsic compression, eg, pelvic or gastrointestinal tumor, radiation-induced fibrosis
- Urethral carcinoma
- Meatal stenosis

Urinary urgency

- Cystitis
- Urethritis
- Pyelonephritis
- Neurogenic bladder
- Interstitial cystitis
- Urethral syndrome
- Urinary calculi

Urine, cloudy

- Urinary tract infection
- Alkaline urinary pH
- Chyluria (lymph in urine) due to fistula with lymphatics, eg, filariasis, tuberculosis, retroperitoneal tumor

Urine, dark

- Hematuria
- Biliary tract obstruction
- Hepatitis
- Dehydration (concentrated urine)
- Hemolytic anemia
- Rhabdomyolysis
- Ingestion of beets
- Phenazopyridine (Pyridium) use
- Alkaptonuria (ochronosis)
- Acute intermittent porphyria

Urticaria & angioedema

- Vasculitis
- Erythema multiforme
- Contact dermatitis (eg, poison oak or ivy)
- Pityriasis rosea
- Erythema migrans (Lyme disease)

Etiology

- Arthropod-related skin lesions (insect bites)
- Drugs (nonallergic), eg, codeine, morphine
- Physical factors: heat, cold urticaria, solar, pressure, water, vibratory
- Cholinergic urticaria: exercise, excitement, hot showers
- Drugs (allergic): penicillin, aspirin
- Other allergic causes: feathers, dander, shellfish, tomatoes, strawberries, vaccines, chemicals, cosmetics
- Infection, eg, otitis media, sinusitis, hepatitis
- Serum sickness
- Angioedema: complement-mediated (hereditary or acquired), ACE inhibitors

Uveitis (iritis, cyclitis, choroiditis, retinitis)

- Acute glaucoma
- Keratitis (corneal ulcer or inflammation), eg, herpes simplex
- Conjunctivitis
- Scleritis or episcleritis
- Retinal detachment
- Intraocular tumor, eg, retinoblastoma, leukemia, melanoma

- CNS lymphoma
- Retained intraocular foreign body

Etiology

- HLA-B27-related conditions: ankylosing spondylitis, reactive arthritis (Reiter's syndrome), psoriasis, inflammatory bowel disease
- Behçet's syndrome
- Herpes simplex or zoster infection
- Sarcoidosis
- Tuberculosis, syphilis, toxoplasmosis
- AIDS: cytomegalovirus, herpes simplex virus, herpes zoster, mycobacteria, *Cryptococcus*, *Toxoplasma*, *Candida*
- Vogt-Koyanagi-Harada syndrome (uveitis, alopecia, poliosis, vitiligo, hearing loss)
- Autoimmune retinal vasculitis

Vaginal bleeding, abnormal premenopausal (increased or irregular)

- Ovulation bleeding (spotting episode between menses)
- Anovulatory cycle (dysfunctional uterine bleeding)
- Polycystic ovary syndrome (type of anovulatory cycle)
- Pregnancy
- Ectopic pregnancy
- Spontaneous abortion
- Uterine leiomyomas (fibroids)
- Endometrial polyp
- Cervicitis or pelvic inflammatory disease
- Adenomyosis (uterine endometriosis)
- Cervical cancer
- Cervical polyp
- Endometrial hyperplasia
- Endometrial cancer
- Hypothyroidism
- Hyperprolactinemia
- Diabetes mellitus
- Bleeding disorder, eg, von Willebrand's disease
- Hydatidiform mole

Vaginal bleeding, postmenopausal

- Atrophic endometrium
- Endometrial hyperplasia or proliferation
- Endometrial cancer
- Atrophic vaginitis
- Perimenopausal bleeding
- Endometrial polyp
- Unopposed exogenous estrogen
- Cervical cancer
- Uterine leiomyomas (fibroids)
- Trauma
- Bleeding disorder
- Cervical polyp
- Cervical ulcer
- Vaginal cancer
- Vulvar cancer

Vaginal bleeding, third-trimester

- Placental causes: placenta previa, placental abruption, vasa previa
- Infection, eg, vaginitis, cervicitis
- Labor (blood or mucus plug)
- Ruptured cervical blood vessel (eg, by intercourse)
- Bleeding disorder
- Cervical cancer

Vaginal discharge

- Normal vaginal discharge
- Bacterial vaginosis
- *Trichomonas* vaginitis
- *Candida* vulvovaginitis
- Cervicitis
- Pelvic inflammatory disease
- Reaction to douches, tampons, condoms, soap
- Cervical cancer
- Uterine cancer

Vaginitis

Etiology

- Normal vaginal discharge
- Bacterial vaginosis
- *Trichomonas* vaginitis
- *Candida* vulvovaginitis
- Atrophic vaginitis
- Genital warts (condyloma acuminata)
- Friction from intercourse
- Reaction to douches, tampons, condoms, soap

Varicocele

Etiology

- Usually due to elevated hydrostatic pressure or incompetent valves in the internal spermatic vein
- Left-sided (more common): may also be due to left renal vein obstruction, eg, renal cell carcinoma
- Right-sided: may also be due to retroperitoneal malignancy obstructing right spermatic vein

Vasculitis, hypersensitivity (leukocytoclastic)

- Polyarteritis nodosa
- Henoch-Schönlein purpura
- Meningococcemia
- Disseminated gonococcal infection
- Cryoglobulinemia

Vasculitis syndromes

- Polyarteritis nodosa: fever, hypertension, abdominal pain, often hepatitis B or C
- Microscopic polyangiitis: overlaps with PAN, glomerulonephritis, pulmonary hemorrhage
- Churg-Strauss syndrome: asthma, transient pulmonary infiltrates
- Wegener's granulomatosis: respiratory disease and glomerulonephritis
- Temporal (giant cell) arteritis: headache, jaw claudication, blindness, associated with polymyalgia rheumatica
- Takayasu's arteritis: young Asian women, aortic arch vasculitis
- Henoch-Schönlein purpura: children, palpable purpura, abdominal pain
- Hypersensitivity (leukocytoclastic) vasculitis: lower extremity palpable purpura; associated with drugs, neoplasms, connective tissue disease, viral or bacterial infection, cryoglobulinemia, serum sickness
- Thromboangiitis obliterans (Buerger's disease): smokers, extremity ischemia
- Behçet's syndrome: oral and genital ulcers, ocular lesions
- Kawasaki syndrome: children, fever, rash, conjunctivitis, cardiac disease

Vertigo

By episode duration

- Auditory symptoms present
  - Seconds: perilymphatic fistula
  - Hours: endolymphatic hydrops (Ménière's disease, syphilis)
  - Days: labyrinthitis, labyrinthine concussion (head trauma)
  - Months: acoustic neuroma, ototoxicity

- Auditory symptoms absent
  - Seconds: positioning vertigo (cupulolithiasis), vertebrobasilar insufficiency, cervical vertigo (head-extension vertigo), diplopia
  - Hours: recurrent vestibulopathy (Ménière's disease without auditory symptoms), vestibular migraine
  - Days: vestibular neuronitis, head trauma
  - Months: vertebrobasilar insufficiency, arteriovenous malformation, brainstem or cerebellar tumor, cerebellar degeneration, multiple sclerosis, vertebrobasilar migraine

Drugs

- Anticonvulsants (eg, phenytoin), antibiotics (eg, aminoglycosides, doxycycline, metronidazole), hypnotics (eg, diazepam), analgesics (eg, aspirin), alcohol

Vesicles

- Herpes simplex virus infection (cold sore, genital herpes)
- Varicella (chicken pox)
- Herpes zoster (shingles)
- Contact dermatitis
- Scabies
- Dyshidrotic eczema (pompholyx, dyshidrosis)
- Vesicular tinea
- Dermatitis herpetiformis
- Atopic dermatitis (eczema) (acute)
- Dermatophytid reaction (allergy or sensitivity to fungi)
- Miliaria (heat rash)
- Porphyria cutanea tarda
- Photodermatitis
- Smallpox
- Rickettsialpox
- Hand, foot, and mouth disease

Visual loss, acute

Inflamed (red) eye

- Acute glaucoma
- Uveitis
- Keratitis (corneal ulcer or inflammation), eg, herpes simplex
- Conjunctivitis (blurry)

Uninflamed eye

- Retinal detachment
- Central retinal vein occlusion
- Central retinal artery occlusion
- Vitreous hemorrhage
- Macular degeneration (exudative)
- Anterior ischemic optic neuropathy, eg, temporal (giant cell) arteritis
- Optic neuritis, eg, multiple sclerosis
- Papilledema
- Hyperglycemia (blurry; subacute)
- Polycythemia vera (blurry; subacute)
- Trauma
- Conversion disorder
- Episodic: amaurosis fugax (transient ischemic attack), ophthalmic migraine
- Diplopia

Visual loss, chronic

- Refractive error
- Cataract
- Macular degeneration (atrophic)
- Diabetic retinopathy
- Glaucoma
- Corneal opacity, eg, scar, pterygium
- Chronic uveitis
- Pituitary tumor (bitemporal)
- Other types of retinopathy, eg, hypertensive, sickle cell, severe anemia, radiation, systemic lupus erythematosus, talc (emboli from IV drug use)
- Cerebrovascular disease or brain tumor affecting visual pathways
- Intraorbital tumor
- Toxic optic neuropathy, eg, methanol
- Lens dislocation, eg, Marfan syndrome, homocystinuria
- Other worldwide causes: trachoma, Hansen's disease (leprosy), onchocerciasis, xerophthalmia (vitamin A deficiency)

Vitreous hemorrhage

Etiology

- Diabetic retinopathy
- Retinal tear (with or without retinal detachment)
- Retinal vein occlusion
- Macular degeneration (exudative)
- Blood dyscrasias
- Trauma
- Subarachnoid hemorrhage

Vocal cord paralysis

Etiology

- Recurrent laryngeal nerve damage: thyroid or other neck surgery, lung cancer, thyroid cancer
- Laryngeal cancer
- Esophageal cancer
- Intubation injury
- Cricoarytenoid arthritis (in rheumatoid arthritis)
- Glottic or subglottic stenosis
- Skull base tumor involving cranial nerves IX, X, and XI
- Idiopathic

Vulvar lesions

- Genital warts (condyloma acuminata)
- Contact dermatitis
- Vulvovaginal candidiasis
- Ulcer: herpes simplex virus, chancroid, syphilis, granuloma inguinale, lymphogranuloma venereum, Behçet's syndrome
- Vulvar cancer
- Vulvar intraepithelial neoplasia
- Vulvar vestibulitis
- Bartholin's cyst or abscess
- Epidermal cyst
- Epithelial polyp
- Lichen sclerosus
- Hypertrophic vulvar dystrophy
- Lichen planus
- Psoriasis
- Cicatricial pemphigoid
- Hidradenitis suppurativa
- Lichen simplex chronicus
- Papillary hidradenoma
- Paget's disease
- Melanoma
- Vitiligo
- Molluscum contagiosum
- Pediculosis (lice)

Weakness

General

- Disuse of muscles
- Anemia
- Malnutrition
- Electrolyte abnormality, eg, hypercalcemia, hypokalemia, hyponatremia
- Endocrine disease, eg, hypothyroidism, diabetes mellitus, Cushing's syndrome, Addison's disease, hyperaldosteronism
- Chronic lung or heart disease
- Malingering

Upper motor neuron disease

- Stroke
- Space-occupying lesion, eg, brain tumor
- Spinal cord lesion

- Multiple sclerosis

Lower motor neuron disease

- Anterior horn cell, eg, poliomyelitis, amyotrophic lateral sclerosis, West Nile virus
- Motor nerve root, eg, disk protrusion
- Nerve plexus, eg, brachial plexus neuropathy
- Peripheral nerve, eg, diabetes mellitus, alcoholism, heavy metals, Guillain-Barré syndrome
- Neuromuscular junction, eg, myasthenia gravis, Eaton-Lambert syndrome, botulism, organophosphate poisoning, tick paralysis, drug-induced, eg, aminoglycoside
- Myopathy, eg, polymyositis, corticosteroids, hypothyroidism, alcohol
- Other: aortic dissection, periodic paralysis, eg, hypokalemic, hyperkalemic, thyrotoxic

Weakness, proximal muscle

Muscle inflammation

- Polymyositis
- Dermatomyositis
- Systemic lupus erythematosus
- Scleroderma
- Sjögren's syndrome
- Inclusion body myositis
- Trichinosis (*Trichinella* infection)
- Sarcocystosis

Other causes of proximal muscle weakness

- Polymyalgia rheumatica
- Endocrine: hypothyroidism, hyperthyroidism, Cushing's syndrome
- Alcoholism
- Drugs: corticosteroids, statins, clofibrate, colchicine, chloroquine, emetine, aminocaproic acid, bretylium, penicillamine, drugs causing hypokalemia
- HIV myopathy
- Hyperparathyroidism
- Spinal stenosis
- Osteomalacia
- Mitochondrial myopathy
- Diabetic lumbosacral plexopathy

Weeping or encrusted lesions

Etiology

- Impetigo
- Contact dermatitis (acute)
- Any vesicular dermatitis can become crusted

Weight loss, involuntary

Medical

- Malignancy
- Gastrointestinal disorders, eg, malabsorption, pancreatic insufficiency, peptic ulcer
- Hyperthyroidism
- Chronic heart, lung, or renal disease
- Uncontrolled diabetes mellitus
- Intestinal ischemia
- Dysphagia
- Anorexia due to azotemia
- Hypercalcemia
- Tuberculosis
- Subacute bacterial endocarditis

Psychosocial

- Depression
- Dementia
- Alcoholism
- Anorexia nervosa
- Loss of teeth, poor denture fit
- Social isolation
- Poverty
- Inability to buy or prepare food

Drug related

- NSAIDs
- Antiepileptics
- Digoxin
- SSRIs

Wheezing

- Asthma
- Chronic obstructive pulmonary disease
- Congestive heart failure (cardiac asthma)
- Acute bronchitis
- Pneumonia
- Gastroesophageal reflux disease
- Airway obstruction (eg, tumor, goiter)
- Foreign-body aspiration
- Aspiration pneumonia
- Interstitial lung disease
- Pulmonary embolism
- Angioedema or anaphylaxis
- Carcinoid syndrome
- Vocal cord dysfunction
- Ascariasis

Wrist drop (radial nerve palsy)

Etiology

- Radial nerve compression
- Diabetes mellitus
- Lead poisoning

Wrist pain

- Sprain
- Area of first CMC joint: osteoarthritis, DeQuervain's tenosynovitis, scaphoid fracture (snuffbox pain)
- Carpal tunnel syndrome
- Pronator teres syndrome (median nerve entrapment at level of pronator teres)
- Lunate fracture or dislocation
- Colles (distal radius) fracture
- Triangular fibrocartilage complex injury
- Arthritis, eg, rheumatoid arthritis, osteoarthritis, reactive arthritis (Reiter's syndrome), psoriatic arthritis, gout or pseudogout, septic arthritis
- Dorsal ganglion (may be ventral)
- Superficial radial neuropathy (cheiralgia paresthetica or handcuff neuropathy)

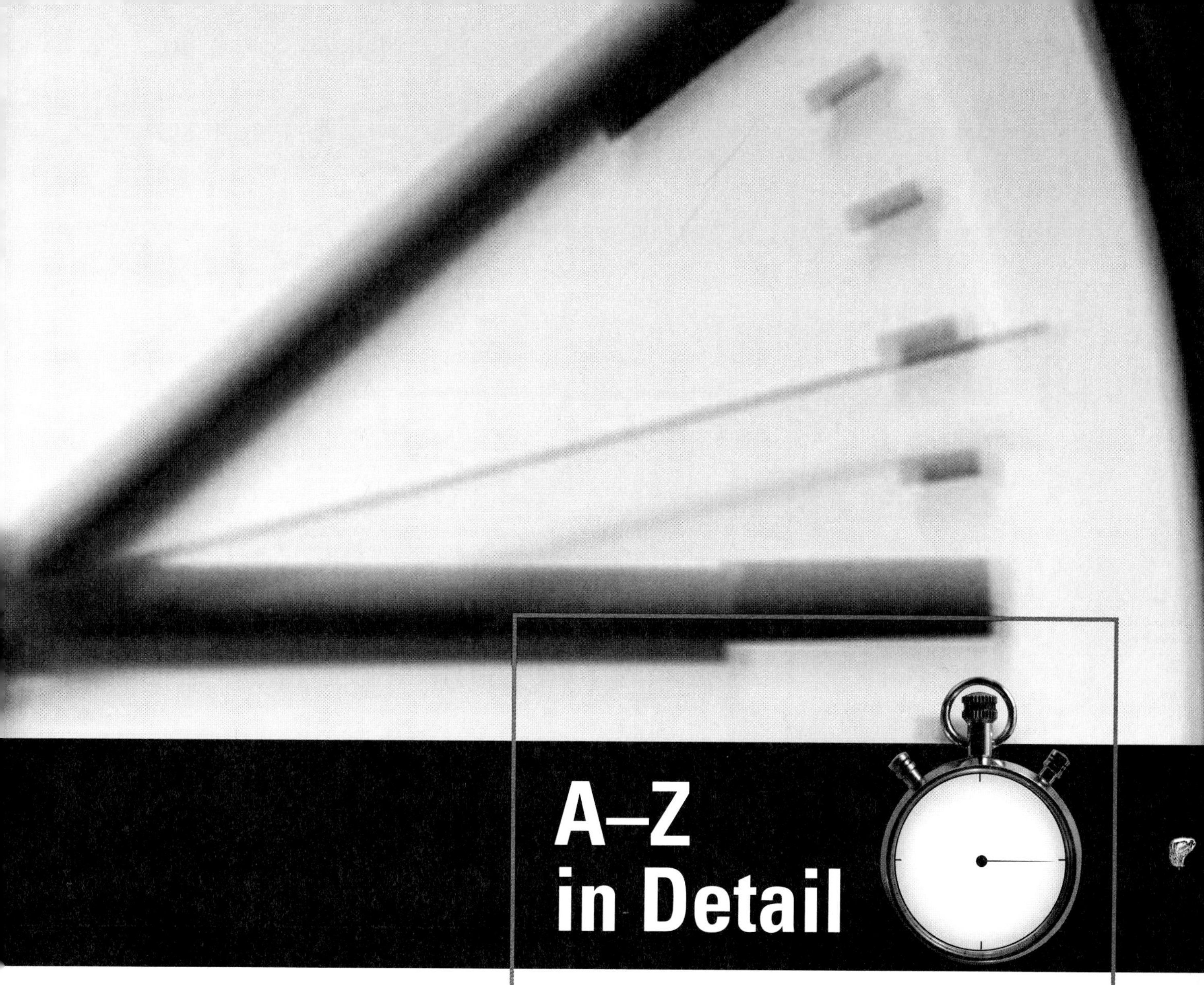

A–Z in Detail

Abdominal Aortic Aneurysm

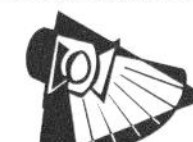

KEY FEATURES

ESSENTIALS OF DIAGNOSIS

- Defined as an aortic diameter > 3 cm
- Most are asymptomatic, detected during a routine physical examination or imaging performed for another reason
- Severe back or abdominal pain and hypotension indicate rupture
- Concomitant atherosclerotic occlusive disease of lower extremities in 25%

GENERAL CONSIDERATIONS

- More than 90% of abdominal aneurysms originate below the renal arteries, many extend into the common iliac arteries
- Half are < 5 cm in diameter
- On routine ultrasound surveillance, two thirds will increase in size to require repair
- Yearly rupture risk is 2% for 4- to 5.4-cm aneurysms, 7% for 6- to 6.9-cm aneurysms, and 25% for 7-cm aneurysms
- Patients with chronic obstructive pulmonary disease are more likely to experience rupture of smaller aneurysms
- More than one third of patients with popliteal aneurysms have abdominal aortic aneurysms

DEMOGRAPHICS

- Aortic aneurysm is present in 5–8% of the population older than 65
- Incidence has tripled over the last 30 years

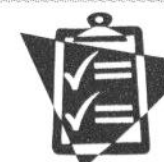

CLINICAL FINDINGS

SYMPTOMS AND SIGNS

- Asymptomatic aneurysms: prominent aortic pulsation on routine physical examination and incidental finding on abdominal ultrasonogram or CT scan: coexisting renal or lower extremity arterial occlusive disease present in 25%, popliteal artery aneurysms in 15%
- Symptomatic aneurysms: midabdominal or lower back pain (or both)
- Inflammatory aortic aneurysms: low-grade fever, elevated sedimentation rate, and recent upper respiratory tract infection
- Infected aneurysms (rare): fever of unknown origin, peripheral emboli, positive blood cultures, caused by septic emboli to a normal aorta or bacterial colonization of an existing aneurysm
- Ruptured aneurysms: severe back, abdominal, or flank pain and hypotension; 90% of patients die before reaching the hospital or in the perioperative period

DIFFERENTIAL DIAGNOSIS

- Asymptomatic abdominal aortic aneurysms: intraabdominal tumor, iliac aneurysm, or mesenteric artery aneurysm
- Symptomatic/ruptured abdominal aortic aneurysms: acute myocardial infarction, aortic dissection, renal stones, gastroenteritis, bowel obstruction, and bowel infarction

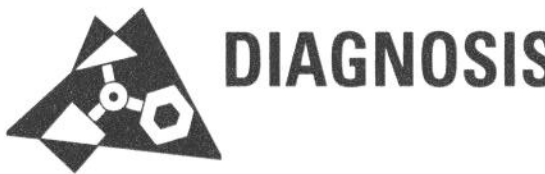

DIAGNOSIS

LABORATORY TESTS

- Preoperative evaluation: electrocardiogram, serum creatinine, hematocrit and hemoglobin, and type and cross-match

IMAGING STUDIES

- Abdominal ultrasonography: indicated for screening and for monitoring aneurysm growth (annually for aneurysms > 3.5 cm in diameter)
- Abdominal radiograph: curvilinear calcifications are much less accurate
- Contrast-enhanced CT scanning: precisely sizes the aneurysm, defines its relationship to the renal arteries
- MRI: as sensitive and specific as CT and useful if renal insufficiency precludes contrast-enhanced CT
- Aortography/CT angiogram: indicated before elective aneurysm repair when arterial occlusive disease of the visceral or lower extremity arteries is suspected or when endograft repair is being considered
- Preoperative evaluation: assessment of cardiac risk and ultrasound examination of the carotid arteries

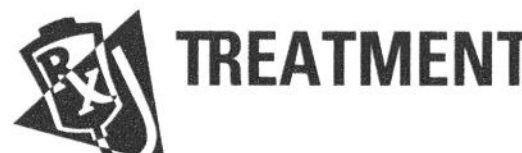

TREATMENT

MEDICATIONS

- β-Blockers and oral roxithromycin, 300 mg daily for 30 days, decrease the expansion rate of small aneurysms

SURGERY

- In asymptomatic good-risk patients, surgery advised when aneurysm diameter > 5 cm
- In poor-risk patients, surgery advised when aneurysm diameter > 6 cm
- Urgent repair advised for symptomatic aneurysms irrespective of diameter
- Ruptured aneurysms require emergent surgery
- Open repair: surgical resection and synthetic graft replacement for most thoracic, abdominal, juxtarenal, and infrarenal aortic aneurysms with diameter > 5 cm
- Endovascular repair: uniiliac or bifurcated endovascular stent grafts, deployed via the common femoral arteries, can be considered for infrarenal aneurysms with favorable anatomy
- Endovascular repair can be done by a percutaneous route or by bilateral inguinal incisions under epidural anesthesia, and thus has made repair of aortic aneurysms feasible in elderly high-risk patients
- Long-term durability of endovascular grafts needs to be established

THERAPEUTIC PROCEDURES

- Physical examination
- Ultrasonogram of abdominal aorta every 6 months

OUTCOME

FOLLOW-UP

- Open repair: yearly physical examination
- Endovascular repair: routine surveillance, CT abdomen, and physical examination

COMPLICATIONS

- Open repair: acute myocardial infarction, arrhythmia, bleeding, respiratory failure, limb ischemia, renal failure, stroke, ischemic colitis, bowel infarction, liver dysfunction, acalculous cholecystitis, graft infection, graft-enteric fistula
- Endovascular repair: persistent filling of the aneurysm (endoleak), graft migration, graft thrombosis, graft infection (rare), renal failure, conversion to open repair

PROGNOSIS

- Mortality following elective open or endovascular repair is 1–5%
- A patient with > 5-cm aortic aneurysm and life expectancy of > 1 year has a 3-fold greater chance of dying of rupture than of dying from surgical resection
- 5-year survival after surgical repair is 60–80%
- 5–10% will develop another aortic aneurysm adjacent to the graft or in the thoracic aorta

WHEN TO REFER

- Any patient with an aneurysm ≥ 4.0 cm
- Any patient with a symptomatic or suspected ruptured abdominal aortic aneurysm

WHEN TO ADMIT

- All patients with symptomatic or suspected ruptured abdominal aortic aneurysms or suspected infected aneurysms

PREVENTION

- Blood pressure control
- Cardiovascular risk assessment and treatment
- Smoking cessation
- Screening of family members older than 65

EVIDENCE

PRACTICE GUIDELINES

- Brewster DC et al: Guidelines for the treatment of abdominal aortic aneurysms. Report of a subcommittee of the Joint Council of the American Association for Vascular Surgery and Society for Vascular Surgery. J Vasc Surg 2003;37:1106. [PMID: 12756363]

INFORMATION FOR PATIENTS

- Cleveland Clinic: Abdominal Aortic Aneurysm
  - http://www.clevelandclinic.org/health/health-info/docs/2400/2455.asp?index=9513
- MedlinePlus: Abdominal Aortic Aneurysm
  - http://www.nlm.nih.gov/medlineplus/ency/article/000162.htm
- MedlinePlus: Abdominal Aortic Aneurysm interactive tutorial
  - http://www.nlm.nih.gov/medlineplus/tutorials/abdominalaorticaneurysm.html

REFERENCES

- Ashton HA et al: The Multicentre Aneurysm Screening Study (MASS) into the effect of abdominal aortic aneurysm screening on mortality in men: a randomized controlled trial. Lancet 2002;360:1531. [PMID: 12443589]
- Ohki T et al: Increasing incidence of midterm and long-term complications after endovascular graft repair of abdominal aortic aneurysms: a note of caution based on a 9-year experience. Ann Surg 2001;234:323. [PMID: 11524585]
- Vammen S et al: Randomized double-blind controlled trial of roxithromycin for prevention of abdominal aortic aneurysm expansion. Br J Surg 2001;88:1066. [PMID: 11488791]

Author(s)

Louis M. Messina, MD

Lawrence M. Tierney, Jr., MD

Abortion

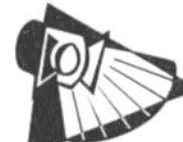

KEY FEATURES

ESSENTIALS OF DIAGNOSIS

- In the United States, 87% of abortions are performed before 11 weeks' gestation and only 1.4% after 20 weeks
- If abortion is chosen, every effort should be made to encourage an early procedure

GENERAL CONSIDERATIONS

- The abortion-related maternal mortality rate has fallen markedly since the legalization of abortion in the United States in 1973
- While numerous state laws limiting access to abortion and a federal law banning a rarely-used variation of dilation and evacuation have been enacted, abortion remains legal and available until fetal viability under Roe v. Wade
- The long-term sequelae of repeated induced abortions are uncertain regarding increased rates of fetal loss or premature labor
- Adverse sequelae can be minimized by performing early abortion with minimal cervical dilation or by the use of osmotic dilators to induce gradual cervical dilation

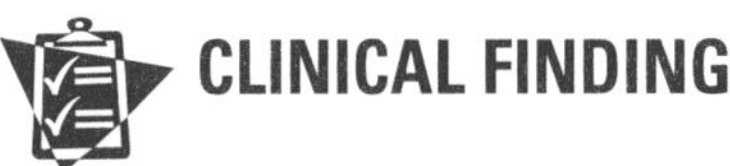

CLINICAL FINDINGS

SYMPTOMS AND SIGNS

- Pregnancy at less than the gestational age of viability

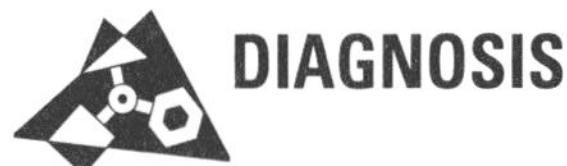

DIAGNOSIS

LABORATORY TESTS

- Determine if patient is Rh positive or negative
- Pregnancy test

DIAGNOSTIC PROCEDURES

- Establish date of last menstrual period (LMP) by pelvic exam or ultrasound

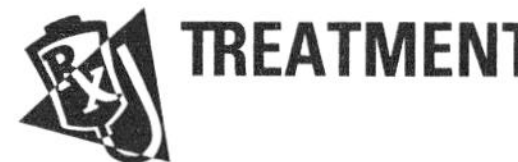

TREATMENT

MEDICATIONS

- Mifepristone (RU 486) 600 mg as a single dose
  - FDA-approved oral abortifacient
  - Followed by a prostaglandin vaginally or orally in 36–48 h
  - Combination 95% successful in terminating pregnancies of up to 9 weeks' duration with minimum complications
- Although not approved by the FDA for this indication, a combination of intramuscular methotrexate, 50 mg/m^2 of body surface area, followed 7 days later by vaginal misoprostol, 800 µg, is 98% successful in terminating pregnancy at 8 weeks or less; minor side effects of nausea, vomiting, and diarrhea are common. There is a 5–10% incidence of hemorrhage or incomplete abortion requiring curettage, but there are no known long-term complications

THERAPEUTIC PROCEDURES

- Abortion in the first trimester is performed by vacuum aspiration under local anesthesia
- A similar technique, dilation and evacuation, is generally used in the second trimester, with general or local anesthesia
- Techniques using intra-amniotic instillation of hypertonic saline solution or various prostaglandin regimens, along with osmotic dilators, are also occasionally used after 18 weeks from the LMP but are more difficult for the patient

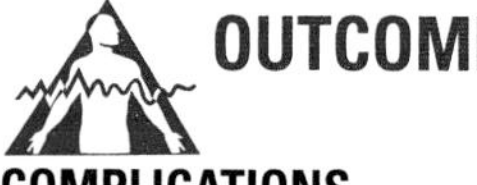

OUTCOME

COMPLICATIONS

- Retained products of conception (often associated with infection and heavy bleeding) and unrecognized ectopic pregnancy
- Immediate analysis of the removed tissue for placenta can exclude or corroborate the diagnosis of ectopic pregnancy
- Women presenting with fever, bleeding, or abdominal pain after abortion should be examined; use of broad-spectrum antibiotics and reaspiration of the uterus are frequently necessary

PROGNOSIS

- Legal abortion has a mortality rate of < 1:100,000. Rates of morbidity and mortality rise with length of gestation

WHEN TO ADMIT

- Hospitalization is advisable if acute salpingitis requires IV administration of antibiotics
- Complications following illegal abortion often need emergency care for hemorrhage, septic shock, or uterine perforation

PREVENTION

- Contraception should be thoroughly discussed and provided at the time of abortion
- Prophylactic antibiotics are indicated: for instance, a one-dose regimen is doxycycline, 200 mg PO 1 h before the procedure. Many prescribe tetracycline, 500 mg four times daily, for 5 days after the procedure for all patients as presumptive treatment for chlamydia
- Rh immune globulin should be given to all Rh-negative women following abortion

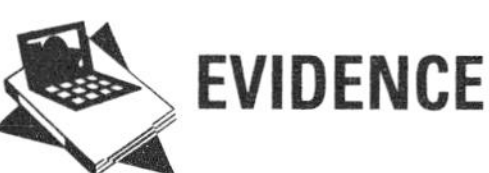

EVIDENCE

PRACTICE GUIDELINES

- National Abortion Federation Clinical Policy Guidelines, 2004.
  - http://www.guideline.gov/summary/summary.aspx?doc_id=5092&nbr=3559
- American College of Obstetricians and Gynecologists (ACOG) Practice Bulletin. Clinical management guidelines for obstetrician-gynecologists. Medical management of abortion. Obstet Gynecol 2001;97:suppl 1. [PMID: 11501565]

WEB SITES

- National Abortion Federation: Professional Education Resources
  - http://www.prochoice.org/education/resources/med_educational_resources.html#curriculum
- Kaiser Family Foundation Fact Sheet: Abortion in the U.S.
  - http://www.kff.org/womenshealth/loader.cfm?url=/commonspot/security/getfile.cfm&PageID=14273
- Kaiser Family Foundation Update: Abortion Policy and Politics
  - http://www.kff.org/womenshealth/loader.cfm?url=/commonspot/security/getfile.cfm&PageID=14091

INFORMATION FOR PATIENTS

- American College of Obstetricians and Gynecologists
  - http://www.medem.com/medlb/article_detaillb.cfm?article_ID=ZZZ2K98T77C&sub_cat=2006
  - http://www.medem.com/search/article_display.cfm?path=TANQUERAYM_ContentItem&mstr=/M_ContentItem/ZZZHSWHG97C.html&soc=ACOG&srch_typ=NAV_SERCH
- ACOG: Pregnancy Choices
  - http://www.medem.com/medlb/article_detaillb.cfm?article_ID=ZZZHSWHG97C&sub_cat=2005
- ACOG: Induced Abortion
  - http://www.medem.com/medlb/article_detaillb.cfm?article_ID=ZZZ2K98T77C&sub_cat=2006
- MedlinePlus: Abortion
  - http://www.nlm.nih.gov/medlineplus/ency/article/002912.htm

REFERENCES

- Grimes DA et al: Induced abortion: an overview for internists. Ann Intern Med 2004;140:620. [PMID: 15096333]
- Stubblefield PG et al: Methods for induced abortion: Obstet Gynecol 2004;104:174. [PMID: 15229018]

Author(s)

H. Trent MacKay, MD, MPH

Abortion, Spontaneous

KEY FEATURES

ESSENTIALS OF DIAGNOSIS

- Intrauterine pregnancy at less than 20 weeks
- Low or falling levels of human chorionic gonadotropin (hCG)
- Bleeding or midline cramping pain, or both
- Open cervical os
- Complete or partial expulsion of products of conception

GENERAL CONSIDERATIONS

- Defined as termination of gestation prior to the 20th week of pregnancy
- 75% of cases occur before the 16th week, with 75% of these before the 8th week
- Almost 20% of clinically recognized pregnancies terminate in spontaneous abortion
- More than 60% of cases result from chromosomal defects
- About 15% of cases are associated with maternal trauma, infection, dietary deficiency, diabetes mellitus, hypothyroidism, or anatomic malformations
- There is no evidence that psychic stimuli such as severe fright, grief, anger, or anxiety can induce termination
- There is no evidence that electromagnetic fields are associated with an increased risk of termination
- It is important to distinguish women with incompetent cervix from more typical early abortion, premature labor, or rupture of the membranes

DEMOGRAPHICS

- Predisposing factors
  - History of incompetent cervix
  - Cervical conization or surgery
  - Cervical injury
  - Diethylstilbestrol exposure
  - Anatomic abnormalities of the cervix

CLINICAL FINDINGS

SYMPTOMS AND SIGNS

- **Incompetent cervix**
  - Classically presents as "silent" cervical dilation (without contractions) between weeks 16 and 28
- **Threatened abortion**
  - Bleeding or cramping without termination
  - The cervix is not dilated
- **Inevitable abortion**
  - The cervix is dilated and membranes may be ruptured
  - Passage of products of conception has not occurred, but is considered inevitable
- **Complete abortion**
  - The fetus and placenta are completely expelled
  - Pain ceases, but spotting may persist
- **Incomplete abortion**
  - Some portion of the products of conception remain in the uterus
  - Cramps are usually mild; bleeding is persistent and often excessive
- **Missed abortion**
  - The pregnancy has ceased to develop, but the conception has not been expelled
  - There is brownish vaginal discharge but no free bleeding
  - Symptoms of pregnancy disappear

DIFFERENTIAL DIAGNOSIS

- Ectopic pregnancy
- Hydatidiform mole
- Incompetent cervix
- Anovular bleeding in a nonpregnant women
- Menses or menorrhagia
- Cervical neoplasm or lesion

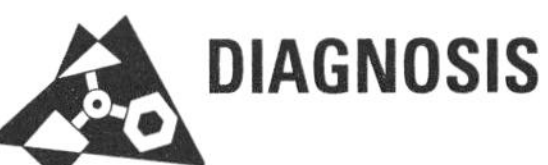

DIAGNOSIS

LABORATORY TESTS

- Falling levels of hCG
- Complete blood count should be obtained if bleeding is heavy
- Rh type should be determined and Rho(D) Ig given if the type is Rh negative
- All recovered tissue should be preserved and assessed by a pathologist

IMAGING STUDIES

- Ultrasound can identify the gestational sac 5–6 weeks from the last menstrual period, a fetal pole at 6 weeks, and fetal cardiac activity at 6–7 weeks
- With accurate dating, a small, irregular sac without a fetal pole is diagnostic of an abnormal pregnancy

Abortion, Recurrent p. 1018

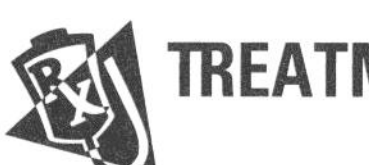

TREATMENT

MEDICATIONS

- Antibiotics should be used only if there is evidence of infection
- Hormonal treatment is contraindicated in **threatened abortion**
- Prostaglandin vaginal suppositories may be used in termination for **missed** or **inevitable abortion**

SURGERY

- **Incomplete abortion** is treated with prompt removal of any remaining products of conception to stop bleeding and prevent infection

THERAPEUTIC PROCEDURES

- **Threatened abortion**
  - Can be treated with bed rest for 24–48 h with gradual resumption of activities
  - Abstinence from coitus and douching
- **Missed** or **inevitable abortion**
  - Requires evacuation
  - Dilation with laminaria insertion and aspiration is preferred for missed abortion, though prostaglandin suppositories are an alternative
- **Incompetent cervix**
  - Treated with cerclage and restriction of activities
  - Cervical cultures for *Neisseria gonorrhoeae, Chlamydia*, and group B *Streptococcus* should be obtained before the procedure

OUTCOME

FOLLOW-UP

- With recurrent first-trimester losses (3 or more) chromosomal analysis of tissue may be informative

COMPLICATIONS

- Retained tissue and prolonged bleeding can occur with prostaglandin use

WHEN TO REFER

- Missed abortion
- Inevitable or incomplete abortion

WHEN TO ADMIT

- Vital signs unstable from excessive bleeding
- When evacuation of uterine contents cannot be done as an outpatient

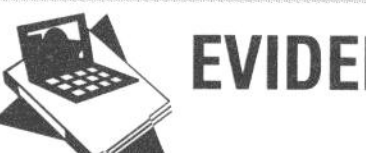

EVIDENCE

PRACTICE GUIDELINES

- ACOG practice bulletin. American College of Obstetricians and Gynecologists. Management of recurrent pregnancy loss. Number 24, February 2001. (Replaces Technical Bulletin Number 212, September 1995.) American College of Obstetricians and Gynecologists. Int J Gynaecol Obstet 2002;78:179. [PMID: 12360906]

WEB SITE

- Guidelines, Recommendations, and Evidence-Based Medicine in Obstetrics
  - http://matweb.hcuge.ch/matweb/endo/cours_4e_MREG/obstetrics_gynecology_guidelines.htm

INFORMATION FOR PATIENTS

- American College of Obstetricians and Gynecologists: Early Pregnancy Loss: Miscarriage and Molar Pregnancy
  - http://www.medem.com/medlb/article_detaillb.cfm?article_ID=ZZZJESDP97C&sub_cat=2005
- March of Dimes: Miscarriage
  - http://www.marchofdimes.com/professionals/681_1192.asp
- MedlinePlus: Miscarriage
  - http://www.nlm.nih.gov/medlineplus/ency/article/001488.htm
- Torpy JM: JAMA patient page. Miscarriage. JAMA 2002;288:1936. [PMID: 12377095]
  - http://www.medem.com/MedLB/article_detaillb.cfm?article_ID=ZZZZIS5Y47D&sub_cat=2005

REFERENCES

- Bukulmez O et al: Luteal phase defect: myth or reality. Obstet Gynecol Clin North Am 2004;31:727. [PMID: 15550332]
- George L et al: Plasma folate levels and risk of spontaneous abortion. JAMA 2002;288:1867. [PMID: 12377085]
- Hurd WW et al: Expectant management versus elective curettage for the treatment of spontaneous abortion. Fertil Steril 1997;68:601. [PMID: 9341597]

Author(s)

William R. Crombleholme, MD

Acanthamoeba Infections

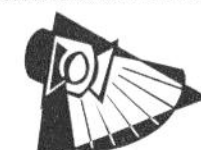

KEY FEATURES

ESSENTIALS OF DIAGNOSIS

Syndromes

- Encephalitis
- Skin lesions
- Keratitis
- Granulomatous dissemination to many tissues

GENERAL CONSIDERATIONS

Granulomatous lesions

- Free-living amebas of the genus *Acanthamoeba*
- Found in soil and in fresh, brackish, and thermal water as trophozoites (15–45 μm) or cysts (10–25 μm)
- Several species, including *A castellanii* and *A culbertsoni*, cause a number of poorly defined syndromes, especially in debilitated or immunosuppressed patients
  - Subacute and chronic multifocal granulomatous necrotizing encephalitis
  - Skin lesions (ulcers or hard nodules in which ameba may be detected)
  - Granulomatous dissemination to many tissues
- Portals of entry may include the skin, eyes, or respiratory tract
- A commensal nasal carrier state is established

Keratitis

- *Acanthamoeba* keratitis and uveitis occur
- Most cases are associated with wearing contact lenses
- Others are associated with penetrating corneal trauma or exposure to contaminated water

CLINICAL FINDINGS

SYMPTOMS AND SIGNS

Encephalitis

- Mental status abnormalities
- Meningismus
- Neurological features of a space-occupying lesion

Keratitis

- Waxing and waning clinical course over several months
- Severe ocular pain, photophobia, tearing, blurred vision, and conjunctival injection
- Partial or 360-degree paracentral stromal ring infiltrate on ophthalmological examination
- Recurrent corneal epithelial breakdown
- A corneal lesion refractory to the usual medications

DIFFERENTIAL DIAGNOSIS

- Many cases of *Acanthamoeba* keratitis are misdiagnosed as viral keratitis

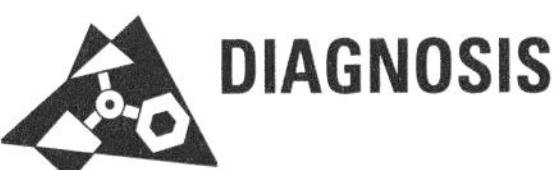

DIAGNOSIS

LABORATORY TESTS

Encephalitis

- Cerebrospinal fluid lymphocytosis may be present
- Brain biopsy, culture, or cerebrospinal fluid wet mounts using specific fluorescent stains

Keratitis

- The diagnosis can be confirmed by vigorously scraping the cornea with a swab or platinum-tipped scapula
- The material is microscopically examined as a wet preparation for cysts and motile trophozoites, after staining by immunofluorescent techniques and after being cultured using various media
- Isolates can be identified by isoenzyme analysis and DNA profiles
- Because of variable drug sensitivities, each isolate should be tested for drug susceptibility

IMAGING STUDIES

- Focal consolidation on chest films may be present in patients with encephalitis

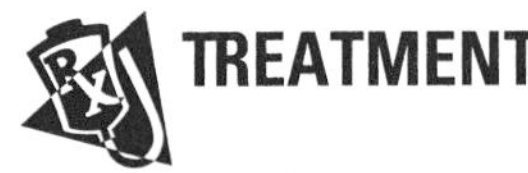

TREATMENT

MEDICATIONS

Granulomatous lesions

- Ketoconazole, miconazole, itraconazole, sulfonamides, clotrimazole, pentamidine, paromomycin, propamidine, neomycin, amphotericin B, cotrimoxazole, or flucytosine can be tried
- No treatment has been proved effective

Keratitis

- Treat with topical propamidine isothionate (0.1%) with either chlorhexidine digluconate (0.02%), polyhexamethylene biguanide, or neomycin-polymyxin B-gramicidin
- Topical miconazole has also been used
- Oral itraconazole or ketoconazole can be added for deep keratitis
- Use of corticosteroid therapy is controversial

THERAPEUTIC PROCEDURES

- In spite of medical treatment of keratitis, penetrating keratoplasty is often necessary to excise diseased tissue
- Corneal grafting can be done after the amebic infection has been eradicated

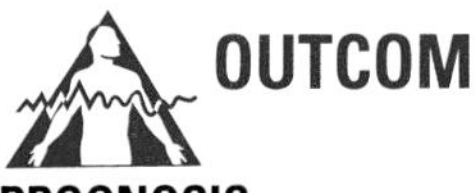

OUTCOME

PROGNOSIS

- With early treatment, many patients can expect cure and a good visual result
- Untreated encephalitis can lead to death in weeks to months
- Untreated keratitis can progress slowly over months and can lead to blindness

WHEN TO REFER

- All patients with keratitis should be referred to an ophthalmologist

WHEN TO ADMIT

- All cases of encephalitis

PREVENTION

- Prevention of keratitis requires immersion of contact lenses in disinfectant solutions or heat sterilization
  - Lenses should not be cleaned in homemade saline solutions
  - Lenses should not be worn while swimming

EVIDENCE

PRACTICE GUIDELINES

- National Guideline Clearinghouse
  - http://www.guideline.gov/summary/summary.aspx?doc_id=2603

WEB SITE

- Centers for Disease Control and Prevention—Division of Parasitic Diseases
  - http://www.cdc.gov/ncidod/dpd/parasites/acanthomoeba/default.htm

INFORMATION FOR PATIENTS

- Centers for Disease Control and Prevention
  - http://www.cdc.gov/ncidod/dpd/parasites/acanthomoeba/factsht_acanthamoeba.htm

REFERENCES

- Kumar R et al: Recent advances in the treatment of *Acanthamoeba* keratitis. Clin Infect Dis 2002;35:434. [PMID: 12145728]
- McCulley JP et al: The diagnosis and management of *Acanthamoeba* keratitis. CLAO J 2000;26:47. [PMID: 10656311]
- Moshari A et al: Chorioretinitis after keratitis caused by *Acanthamoeba*: case report and review of the literature. Ophthalmology 2001;108:2232. [PMID: 11733264]

Achalasia

KEY FEATURES

ESSENTIALS OF DIAGNOSIS

- Gradual, progressive dysphagia for solids and liquids
- Regurgitation of undigested food
- Barium esophagogram shows "bird's beak" distal esophagus
- Esophageal manometry confirms diagnosis

GENERAL CONSIDERATIONS

- Idiopathic motility disorder characterized by loss of peristalsis in the distal two-thirds (smooth muscle) of the esophagus and impaired relaxation of the lower esophageal sphincter
- Cause unknown

DEMOGRAPHICS

- Increased incidence with advancing age

CLINICAL FINDINGS

SYMPTOMS AND SIGNS

- Gradual onset of dysphagia for solid foods and, in the majority, liquids also
- Symptoms persist for months to years
- Substernal chest pain, discomfort, or fullness
- Regurgitation of undigested food
- Nocturnal regurgitation
- Coughing or aspiration
- Weight loss is common
- Physical examination unhelpful

DIFFERENTIAL DIAGNOSIS

- Chagas' disease
- Primary or metastatic tumors at the gastroesophageal junction
- Diffuse esophageal spasm
- Scleroderma esophagus
- Peptic stricture

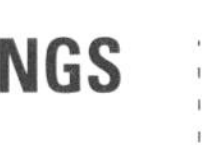

DIAGNOSIS

IMAGING STUDIES

- Chest x-ray: air-fluid level in an enlarged, fluid-filled esophagus
- Barium esophagography
  - Esophageal dilation
  - Loss of esophageal peristalsis
  - Poor esophageal emptying
  - A smooth, symmetric "bird's beak" tapering of the distal esophagus

DIAGNOSTIC PROCEDURES

- Endoscopy to exclude a distal stricture or carcinoma
- Esophageal manometry confirms the diagnosis; characteristic features include:
  - Complete absence of peristalsis
  - Elevated lower esophageal sphincter pressure with incomplete relaxation during swallowing

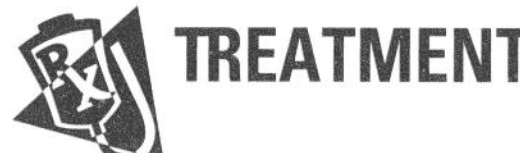

TREATMENT

MEDICATIONS

- Calcium channel blockers (nifedipine) may provide temporary symptomatic improvement

SURGERY

- Surgical myotomy
  - Modified Heller cardiomyotomy of the lower esophageal sphincter and cardia plus an antireflux procedure (fundoplication) results in improvement in >85%; now routinely performed laparoscopically

THERAPEUTIC PROCEDURES

- Botulinum toxin injection
  - Endoscopically guided injection of botulinum toxin directly into the lower esophageal sphincter results in improvement in 85%
  - Symptom relapse occurs in >50% within 6–9 months
- 75% of initial responders to botulinum toxin injection who relapse improve with repeated injections
- Pneumatic dilation; goal is to disrupt lower esophageal sphincter
  - Over 75–85% of patients experience good to excellent relief of dysphagia after 1–3 sessions
  - >50–70% achieve long-term relief

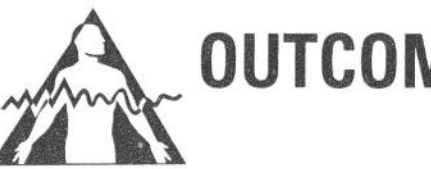

OUTCOME

FOLLOW-UP

- No follow-up necessary unless symptoms recur

COMPLICATIONS

- Perforations occur in <3% of pneumatic dilations, may require operative repair
- Increased risk of squamous cell esophageal cancer

PROGNOSIS

- After successful dilation or myotomy, patients have near-normal swallowing, although esophageal peristalsis is absent

WHEN TO REFER

- Patients with achalasia should be evaluated by a gastrointestinal specialist

EVIDENCE

PRACTICE GUIDELINES

- Patient Care Committee, Society for Surgery of the Alimentary Tract. Esophageal achalasia. SSAT patient care guidelines. J Gastrointest Surg 2004;8(3):367
- National Guideline Clearinghouse
  - http://www.guideline.gov/summary/summary.aspx?doc_id=3259&nbr=2485&string=achalasia
- The Society for Surgery of the Alimentary Tract
  - http://www.ssat.com//cgi-bin/achalasia.cgi?affiliation=student&referer=

INFORMATION FOR PATIENTS

- MEDLINEplus
  - http://www.nlm.nih.gov/medlineplus/ency/article/000267.htm
- Society of Thoracic Surgeons
  - http://www.sts.org/doc/4120

REFERENCES

- Mikaeli J et al: Pneumatic balloon dilation in achalasia: a prospective comparison of safety and efficacy with different balloon diameters. Aliment Pharmacol Ther 2004;20:431. [PMID: 15298637]
- Vela M et al: Complexities of managing achalasia at a tertiary referral center: use of pneumatic dilation, Heller myotomy, and botulinum toxin injection. Am J Gastroenterol 2004;99:1029. [PMID: 15180721]

Author(s)

Kenneth R. McQuaid, MD

Acidosis, Lactic

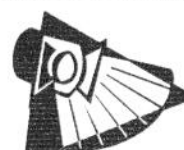

KEY FEATURES

ESSENTIALS OF DIAGNOSIS

- Severe acidosis with hyperventilation
- Blood pH below 7.30
- Serum bicarbonate < 15 mEq/L
- Anion gap > 15 mEq/L
- Absent serum ketones
- Serum lactate > 5 mmol/L

GENERAL CONSIDERATIONS

- Characterized by overproduction of lactic acid (tissue hypoxia), deficient removal (hepatic failure), or both (circulatory collapse)
- Occurs often in severely ill patients suffering from cardiac decompensation, respiratory or hepatic failure, septicemia, or infarction of bowel or extremities
- With the discontinuance of phenformin therapy in the United States, lactic acidosis in diabetics is uncommon but occasionally occurs with use of metformin. It must be considered in the acidotic diabetic, especially if the patient is seriously ill

Etiology

- Tissue hypoxia, eg, cardiogenic, septic, or hemorrhagic shock; seizure; carbon monoxide or cyanide poisoning
- Hepatic failure
- Ischemic bowel
- Infarction of extremities
- Diabetes, especially with metformin use
- Ketoacidosis
- Renal failure
- Infection
- Leukemia or lymphoma
- Drugs: ethanol, methanol, salicylates, isoniazid
- AIDS
- Idiopathic

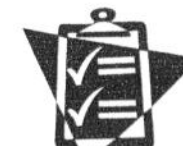

CLINICAL FINDINGS

SYMPTOMS AND SIGNS

- Main clinical feature is marked hyperventilation
- When lactic acidosis is secondary to tissue hypoxia or vascular collapse, the clinical presentation is variable, being that of the prevailing catastrophic illness
- In idiopathic, or spontaneous, lactic acidosis, onset is rapid (usually over a few hours), blood pressure is normal, peripheral circulation is good, and there is no cyanosis

DIFFERENTIAL DIAGNOSIS

Other causes of metabolic acidosis

- Diabetic ketoacidosis
- Starvation ketoacidosis
- Alcoholic ketoacidosis
- Renal failure (acute or chronic)
- Ethylene glycol toxicity
- Methanol toxicity
- Salicylate toxicity
- Other: paraldehyde, metformin, isoniazid, iron, rhabdomyolysis

DIAGNOSIS

LABORATORY TESTS

- High anion gap [serum sodium minus the sum of chloride and bicarbonate anions (in mEq/L) should be no greater than 15]. A higher value indicates the existence of an abnormal compartment of anions
- Plasma bicarbonate and blood pH are quite low, indicating the presence of severe metabolic acidosis
- Ketones are usually absent from plasma and urine or at least not prominent
- In the absence of azotemia, hyperphosphatemia may be clue to the presence of lactic acidosis for reasons that are not clear
- The diagnosis is confirmed by demonstrating, in a sample of blood that is promptly chilled and separated, a plasma lactic acid concentration of 5 mmol/L or higher (values as high as 30 mmol/L have been reported)
- Normal plasma values average 1 mmol/L, with a normal lactate–pyruvate ratio of 10:1. This ratio is greatly exceeded in lactic acidosis

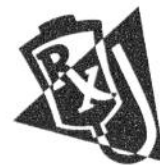

TREATMENT

- Empirical antibiotic coverage for sepsis should be given after culture samples are obtained if the cause of lactic acidosis is unknown
- Alkalinization with IV sodium bicarbonate to keep the pH above 7.2 in the emergency treatment of lactic acidosis is controversial; as much as 2000 mEq in 24 h has been used. However, there is no evidence that the mortality rate is favorably affected by administering bicarbonate

THERAPEUTIC PROCEDURES

- Aggressive treatment of the precipitating cause is the main component of therapy, such as ensuring adequate oxygenation and vascular perfusion of tissues
- Hemodialysis may be useful when large sodium loads are poorly tolerated

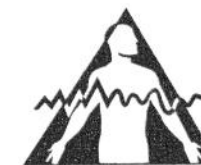

OUTCOME

PROGNOSIS

- Mortality rate of spontaneous lactic acidosis is high
- Prognosis in most cases is that of the primary disorder that produced the lactic acidosis

WHEN TO ADMIT

- All patients because of the high mortality rate

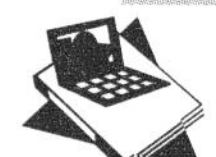

EVIDENCE

PRACTICE GUIDELINES

- National Guideline Clearinghouse: Surviving Sepsis Campaign Guidelines for Management of Severe Sepsis and Septic Shock
  - http://www.guideline.gov/summary/summary.aspx?doc_id=4911
- Canadian Diabetes Association: Gestational Diabetes Mellitus
  - http://www.diabetes.ca/cpg2003/downloads/gdm.pdf

REFERENCES

- Salpeter S et al: Risk of fatal and nonfatal lactic acidosis with metformin use in type 2 diabetes mellitus. Cochrane Database Syst Rev 2003:CD002967. [PMID: 12804446]
- Forsythe SM et al: Sodium bicarbonate for the treatment of lactic acidosis. Chest 2000;117:260. [PMID: 10631227]

Author(s)

Umesh Masharani, MB, BS, MRCP (UK)

Acidosis, Metabolic, Decreased or Normal Anion Gap

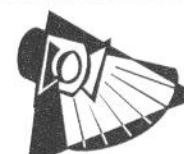

KEY FEATURES

ESSENTIALS OF DIAGNOSIS

- The hallmark of this disorder is that the low HCO_3^- of metabolic acidosis is associated with hyperchloremia, so that the anion gap remains normal
- The anion gap helps determine the cause of the metabolic acidosis
- Decreased HCO_3^-, seen also in respiratory alkalosis, but the pH distinguishes between the two disorders

GENERAL CONSIDERATIONS

- The most common causes are gastrointestinal HCO_3^- loss and defects in renal acidification (renal tubular acidoses). The urinary anion gap can differentiate between these two common causes

HCO_3^- loss

- **Normal anion gap (6–12 mEq)**
- Gastrointestinal loss of HCO_3^-, eg, diarrhea, pancreatic ileostomy, or ileal loop bladder
- Renal tubular acidosis
- Recovery from diabetic ketoacidosis
- Dilutional acidosis from rapid administration of 0.9% NaCl
- Carbonic anhydrase inhibitors
- Chloride retention or administration of HCl equivalent or NH_4Cl
- **Decreased anion gap (< 6 mEq)**
- Plasma cell dyscrasias, eg, multiple myeloma (cationic paraproteins accompanied by chloride and bicarbonate)
- Bromide or lithium intoxication
- **Decreased anion gap without acidosis**
- Hypoalbuminemia (decreased unmeasured anion)
- Severe hyperlipidemia

Renal tubular acidoses (RTA)

- **Type I (distal H^+ secretion defect)**
- Due to selective deficiency in H^+ secretion in the distal nephron
- Low serum K^+
- Despite acidosis, urinary pH cannot be acidified (urine pH > 5.5)
- Associated with autoimmune disease, hypercalcemia
- **Type II (proximal HCO_3^- reabsorption defect)**
- Due to a selective defect in the proximal tubule's ability to adequately reabsorb filtered HCO_3^-
- Low serum K^+
- Urine pH < 5.5
- Associated with multiple myeloma and drugs, eg, sulfa, carbonic anhydrase inhibitors (acetazolamide)
- **Type III (rare)**
- Associated with glomerular insufficiency (glomerular filtration rate [GFR] 20–30 mL/min
  - Further reduction in GFR results in increased anion gap acidosis of uremia
- Ability to generate adequate NH_3 is impaired, with subsequent decreased $NH_4^+Cl^-$ excretion
- Normal serum K^+
- Urine pH < 5.5
- **Type IV (hyporeninemic hypoaldosteronism)**
- Only RTA characterized by hyperkalemic, hyperchloremic acidosis
- Defect is aldosterone deficiency or antagonism, which impairs distal nephron Na^+ reabsorption and K^+ and H^+ excretion
- Urine pH < 5.5
- Renal salt wasting is frequently present
- Most common in diabetic nephropathy, tubulointerstitial renal diseases, AIDS, and hypertensive nephrosclerosis

CLINICAL FINDINGS

SYMPTOMS AND SIGNS

- Symptoms are mainly those of the underlying disorder
- Compensatory hyperventilation may be misinterpreted as a primary respiratory disorder
- When acidosis is severe, Kussmaul respirations (deep, regular, sighing respirations) occur and are indicative of intense stimulation of the respiratory center

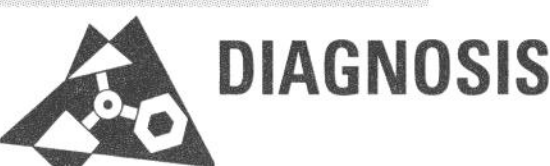

DIAGNOSIS

LABORATORY TESTS

- See Table 86
- Blood pH, serum HCO_3^-, and P_{CO_2} are decreased
- Anion gap is normal (hyperchloremic) or decreased
- Hyperkalemia may be seen
- Urinary anion gap from a random urine sample $[(Na^+ + K^+] - Cl^-]$ reflects the ability of the kidney to excrete NH_4Cl as in the following equation: $Na^+ + K^+ + NH_3^+ = Cl^- + 80$ where 80 is the average value for the difference in the urinary anions and cations other than Na^+, K^+, NH_3^+, and Cl^-
- Therefore, urinary anion gap is equal to $80 - NH_3^+$; this gap aids in the distinction between gastrointestinal and renal causes of hyperchloremic acidosis:
  - If the cause of the metabolic acidosis is gastrointestinal HCO_3^- loss (diarrhea), renal acidification ability remains normal and NH_4Cl excretion increases in response to the acidosis. The urinary anion gap is negative (eg, –30 mEq/L)
  - If the cause is distal RTA, the urinary anion gap is positive (eg, +25 mEq/L), since the basic lesion in the disorder is the inability of the kidney to excrete H^+ and thus the inability to increase NH_4Cl excretion
  - In Type II (proximal) RTA, the kidney has defective HCO_3^- reabsorption, leading to increased HCO_3^- excretion rather than decreased NH_4Cl excretion. Thus, the urinary anion gap is often negative
- Urinary pH may not as readily differentiate between renal and gastrointestinal etiologies

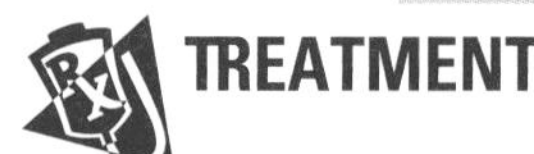

TREATMENT

MEDICATIONS

- See Table 86
- Treatment of RTA is mainly achieved by administration of alkali (either as bicarbonate or citrate) to correct metabolic abnormalities and prevent nephrocalcinosis and renal failure
- Type I distal RTA: supplementation of bicarbonate is necessary since acid accumulates systemically
- Proximal RTA: correction of low serum bicarbonate is not indicated except in severe cases
  - Large amounts of alkali (10–15 mEq/kg/day) may be required because much of the alkali is secreted into the urine, which exacerbates hypokalemia
  - A mixture of sodium and potassium salts, such as K-Shohl, is preferred

OUTCOME

COMPLICATIONS

- The hyperkalemia can be exacerbated by drugs, including angiotensin-converting enzyme inhibitors, aldosterone receptor blockers such as spironolactone, and nonsteroidal anti-inflammatory drugs

WHEN TO REFER

- If expertise is needed in determining the etiology of the metabolic acidosis
- If consultation is needed on whether bicarbonate should be administered

WHEN TO ADMIT

- Respiratory muscle weakness from severe hypokalemia

EVIDENCE

WEB SITE

- National Kidney Foundation
  - http://www.kidney.org/

INFORMATION FOR PATIENTS

- National Kidney and Urologic Diseases Information Clearinghouse: Renal Tubular Acidosis
  - http://kidney.niddk.nih.gov/kudiseases/pubs/tubularacidosis/index.htm
- MedlinePlus: Metabolic Acidosis
  - http://www.nlm.nih.gov/medlineplus/ency/article/000335.htm
- MedlinePlus: Distal Renal Tubular Acidosis
  - http://www.nlm.nih.gov/medlineplus/ency/article/000493.htm
- MedlinePlus: Proximal Renal Tubular Acidosis
  - http://www.nlm.nih.gov/medlineplus/ency/article/000497.htm

REFERENCES

- Fall PJ: A stepwise approach to acid-base disorders. Practical patient evaluation for metabolic acidosis and other conditions. Postgrad Med 2000;107:249. [PMID: 10728149]
- Smulders YM et al: Renal tubular acidosis: pathophysiology and diagnosis. Arch Intern Med 1996;156:1629. [PMID: 8694660]

Author(s)

Masafumi Fukagawa, MD, PhD
Kiyoshi Kurokawa, MD, MACP
Maxine A. Papadakis, MD

Acidosis, Metabolic, Increased Anion Gap

KEY FEATURES

ESSENTIALS OF DIAGNOSIS

- Decreased HCO_3^-, seen also in respiratory alkalosis, but pH distinguishes between the two disorders
- Calculation of the anion gap useful in determining the cause of the metabolic acidosis
- Hallmark of this disorder is that metabolic acidosis (thus low HCO_3^-) is associated with normal serum Cl^-, so that the anion gap increases

GENERAL CONSIDERATIONS

- Normochloremic (increased anion gap) metabolic acidosis generally results from addition to the blood of nonchloride acids such as lactate, acetoacetate, β-hydroxybutyrate, and exogenous toxins (exception: uremia, with underexcretion of organic acids and anions)

Etiology

- Lactic acidosis
  - Type A (tissue hypoxia): cardiogenic, septic, or hemorrhagic shock; seizure; carbon monoxide or cyanide poisoning
  - Type B (nonhypoxic): hepatic or renal failure, ischemic bowel, diabetes especially with metformin use, ketoacidosis, infection, leukemia or lymphoma, drugs (ethanol, methanol, salicylates, isoniazid), AIDS, idiopathic (usually in debilitated patients)
- Diabetic ketoacidosis
- Starvation ketoacidosis
- Alcoholic ketoacidosis
  - Frequently mixed disorders (10% have triple acid-base disorder)
  - Acid-base disorders in alcoholism include metabolic acidosis of three types (ketoacidosis, lactic acidosis, and hyperchloremic acidosis from bicarbonate loss in urine from ketonuria); metabolic alkalosis from volume contraction and vomiting; respiratory alkalosis from alcohol withdrawal, pain, sepsis, or liver disease
- Uremic acidosis (usually at glomerular filtration rate < 20 mL/min)
- Ethylene glycol toxicity
- Methanol toxicity
- Salicylate toxicity (mixed metabolic acidosis with respiratory alkalosis)
- Other: paraldehyde, isoniazid, iron, rhabdomyolysis

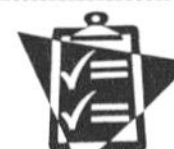

CLINICAL FINDINGS

SYMPTOMS AND SIGNS

- Symptoms are mainly those of the underlying disorder
- Compensatory hyperventilation may be misinterpreted as a primary respiratory disorder
- When severe, Kussmaul respirations (deep, regular, sighing respirations indicating intense stimulation of the respiratory center) occur

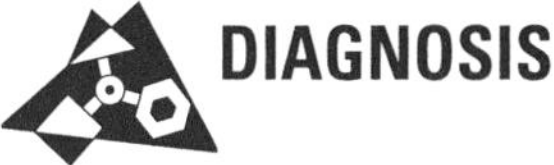

DIAGNOSIS

LABORATORY TESTS

- See Table 85
- Blood pH, serum HCO_3^-, and PCO_2 are decreased
- Anion gap is increased (normochloremic)
- Hyperkalemia may be seen
- In lactic acidosis, lactate levels are at least 4–5 mEq/L but commonly 10–30 mEq/L
- The diagnosis of alcoholic ketoacidosis is supported by the absence of a diabetic history and no evidence of glucose intolerance after initial therapy

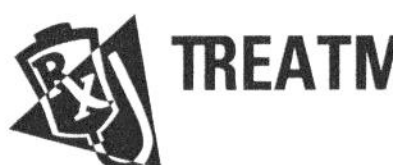

TREATMENT

MEDICATIONS

- Supplemental HCO_3^- is indicated for treatment of hyperkalemia but is controversial for treatment of increased anion gap metabolic acidosis
- Administration of large amounts of HCO_3^- may have deleterious effects, including hypernatremia, hyperosmolality, and worsening of intracellular acidosis
- In salicylate intoxication, alkali therapy must be started unless blood pH is already alkalinized by respiratory alkalosis, because the increment in pH converts salicylate to more impermeable salicylic acid and thus prevents central nervous system damage
- The amount of HCO_3^- deficit can be calculated as follows: Amount of HCO_3^- deficit = 0.5 × bodyweight × (24 – HCO_3^-)
- Half of the calculated deficit should be administered within the first 3–4 h to avoid overcorrection and volume overload
- In methanol intoxication, ethanol is administered as a competitive substrate for alcohol dehydrogenase, the enzyme that metabolizes methanol to formaldehyde

THERAPEUTIC PROCEDURES

- Treatment is aimed at the underlying disorder, such as insulin and volume resuscitation to restore tissue perfusion
- Lactate will later be metabolized to produce HCO_3^- and increase pH

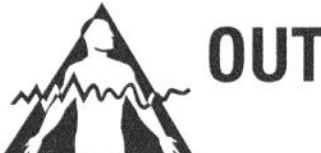

OUTCOME

PROGNOSIS

- The mortality rate of lactic acidosis exceeds 50%

WHEN TO ADMIT

- Because of the high mortality rate, all patients with lactic acidosis should be admitted
- Most other patients with significant metabolic acidosis are admitted as well

PREVENTION

- Avoid metformin use if there is tissue hypoxia or renal insufficiency
- Acute renal failure can occur rarely with the use of radiocontrast agents in patients on metformin therapy. Metformin should be temporarily halted on the day of the test and for 2 days after injection of radiocontrast agents to avoid potential lactic acidosis if renal failure occurs

EVIDENCE

PRACTICE GUIDELINES

- American Diabetes Association: Hyperglycemic Crises in Diabetes, 2004
  - http://www.guideline.gov/summary/summary.aspx?doc_id=4694&nbr=3428

INFORMATION FOR PATIENTS

- MedlinePlus: Metabolic Acidosis
  - http://www.nlm.nih.gov/medlineplus/ency/article/000335.htm
- American Diabetes Association: Ketoacidosis
  - http://www.diabetes.org/type-1-diabetes/ketoacidosis.jsp
- MedlinePlus: Alcoholic Ketoacidosis
  - http://www.nlm.nih.gov/medlineplus/ency/article/000323.htm

REFERENCES

- Adrogue HJ et al: Management of life threatening acid base disorders. First of two parts. N Engl J Med 1998;338:26. [PMID: 9414329]
- Adrogue HJ et al: Management of life-threatening acid-base disorders. Second of two parts. N Engl J Med 1998;338:107. [PMID: 9420343]
- John M et al: Hyperlactatemia syndromes in people with HIV infection. Curr Opin Infect Dis 2002;15:23. [PMID: 119649029]
- Kraut JA et al: Use of base in the treatment of severe acidemic states. Am J Kidney Dis 2001;38:703. [PMID: 11576874]

Author(s)

Masafumi Fukagawa, MD, PhD
Kiyoshi Kurokawa, MD, MACP
Maxine A. Papadakis, MD

Acne Vulgaris

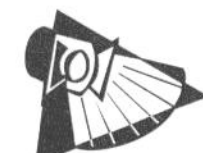

KEY FEATURES

ESSENTIALS OF DIAGNOSIS

- Occurs at puberty, though onset may be delayed into the third or fourth decade
- Open and closed comedones are the hallmark of acne vulgaris
- The most common of all skin conditions
- Severity varies from purely comedonal to papular or pustular inflammatory acne to cysts or nodules
- Face and trunk may be affected
- Scarring may be a sequela of the disease or picking and manipulating by the patient

GENERAL CONSIDERATIONS

- The disease is activated by androgens in those who are genetically predisposed
- The skin lesions parallel sebaceous activity
- Pathogenic events include plugging of the infundibulum of the follicles, retention of sebum, overgrowth of the acne bacillus *(Propionibacterium acnes)* with resultant release of and irritation by accumulated fatty acids, and foreign body reaction to extrafollicular sebum
- When a resistant case of acne is encountered in a woman, hyperandrogenism may be suspected

DEMOGRAPHICS

- Acne vulgaris is more common and more severe in males
- 12% of women and 3% of men over age 25 have acne vulgaris

CLINICAL FINDINGS

SYMPTOMS AND SIGNS

- See Table 7
- Mild soreness, pain, or itching
- Lesions occur mainly over the face, neck, upper chest, back, and shoulders
- Comedones are the hallmark
- Closed comedones are tiny, flesh-colored, noninflamed bumps that give the skin a rough texture or appearance
- Open comedones typically are a bit larger and have black material in them
- Inflammatory papules, pustules, ectatic pores, acne cysts, and scarring are also seen
- Acne may have different presentations at different ages

DIFFERENTIAL DIAGNOSIS

- Acne rosacea (face)
- Bacterial folliculitis (face or trunk)
- Tinea (face or trunk)
- Topical corticosteroid use (face)
- Perioral dermatitis (face)
- Pseudofolliculitis barbae (ingrown beard hairs)
- Miliaria (heat rash) (trunk)
- Eosinophilic folliculitis (trunk)
- Hyperandrogenic states in women
- Pustules on the face can also be caused by tinea infections

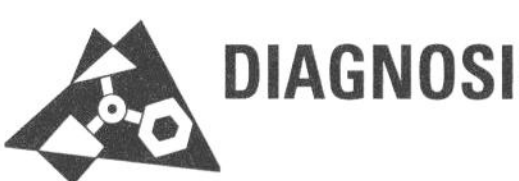

DIAGNOSIS

LABORATORY TESTS

- Culture in refractory cases

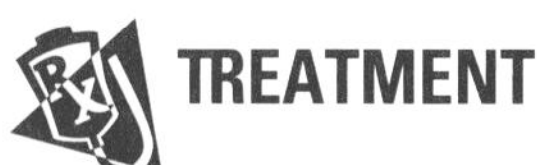

TREATMENT

MEDICATIONS

- See Table 6

Comedonal acne

- Soaps play little part and, if any are used, they should be mild
- Topical retinoids
  - Tretinoin is very effective: start with 0.025% cream (not gel) twice weekly at night, then build up to as often as nightly; a pea-sized amount is sufficient to cover half the entire face; wait 20 min after washing to apply
  - Adapalene gel 0.1% and reformulated tretinoin (Renova, Retin A Micro, Avita), and tazarotene gel 0.05% or 0.1% are other options if standard tretinoin preparations cause irritation
  - Lesions may flare in the first 4 weeks of treatment; the drug is contraindicated in pregnancy
- Benzoyl peroxide is available in many concentrations but 2.5% is as effective as 10% and less irritating

Papular inflammatory acne

- Antibiotics are the mainstay, used topically or orally
- **Mild acne**
  - The first choice of topical antibiotics is the combination of erythromycin or clindamycin with benzoyl peroxide topical gel; clindamycin (Cleocin T) lotion (least irritating), gel, or solution, or topical erythromycin gel or solution may be used twice daily and benzoyl peroxide in the morning (a combination of erythromycin or clindamycin with benzoyl peroxide is available as a prescription item)
  - The addition of tretinoin 0.025% cream or 0.01% gel at night enhances efficacy
- **Moderate acne**
  - Tetracycline, 500 mg twice daily, erythromycin, 500 mg twice daily, doxycycline, 100 mg twice daily, and minocycline, 50–100 mg twice daily, are all effective; tetracycline, minocycline, and doxycycline are contraindicated in pregnancy
  - If the skin is clear, taper the dose by 250 mg for tetracycline and erythro-

mycin, by 100 mg for doxycycline, every 6–8 weeks—while treating with topicals—to arrive at the lowest systemic dose needed; lowering the dose to zero without other therapy usually results in recurrence of the acne
- Oral contraceptives or spironolactone (50–100 mg daily) may be added as an antiandrogen in women with antibiotic-resistant acne or in women in whom relapse occurs after isotretinoin therapy

- **Severe cystic acne**
  - Isotretinoin (Accutane) should be used before significant scarring occurs or if symptoms are not promptly controlled by antibiotics
  - Informed consent must be obtained before its use in all patients
  - Dosage of 0.5–1 mg/kg/day for 20 weeks for a cumulative dose of at least 120 mg/kg is usually adequate
  - The drug is teratogenic and must not be used in pregnancy; obtain two serum pregnancy tests before starting the drug in a female and every month thereafter; sufficient medication for only 1 month should be dispensed; two forms of effective contraception must be used
  - Side effects of dry skin and mucous membranes occur in most patients; if headache occurs, consider pseudotumor cerebri; at higher dosages, elevation of cholesterol and triglycerides and a lowering of high-density lipoproteins can occur; minor elevations of liver function tests and fasting blood sugar can occur; moderate to severe myalgias necessitate decreasing the dosage or stopping the drug
- Monitor baseline and Q week cholesterol, triglycerides, and liver function studies when using isotretinoin

THERAPEUTIC PROCEDURES

- Comedones may be removed with a comedo extractor but will recur if not prevented by treatment
- In otherwise moderate acne, injection of triamcinolone acetonide (2.5 mg/mL, 0.05 mL per lesion) may hasten resolution of deeper papules and cysts
- Cosmetic improvement may be achieved by excision and punch-grafting of deep scars and by dermabrasion of inactive acne lesions, particularly flat, superficial scars

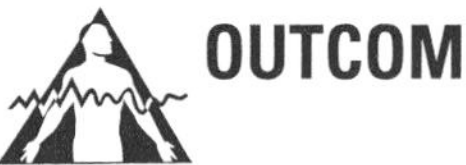

OUTCOME

COMPLICATIONS

- Cyst formation
- Pigmentary changes in pigmented patients
- Severe scarring
- Psychological problems may result

PROGNOSIS

- The disease flares intermittently in spite of treatment
- The condition may persist through adulthood and may lead to severe scarring if left untreated
- Antibiotics continue to improve skin for the first 36 months of use
- Relapse during treatment may suggest the emergence of resistant *P acnes*
- Remissions following systemic treatment with isotretinoin may be lasting in up to 60% of cases
- Relapses after isotretinoin usually occur within 3 years and require a second course in up to 20% of patients

WHEN TO REFER

- Failure to respond to standard regimens
- When the diagnosis is in question
- Fulminant scarring disease (acne fulmincans)

PREVENTION

- Foods do not cause or exacerbate acne
- Educate patients not to manipulate lesions
- Avoid topical exposure to oils, cocoa butter, and greases

EVIDENCE

PRACTICE GUIDELINES

- Institute for Clinical Systems Improvement. Acne management. 2003
  - http://www.guideline.gov/summary/summary.aspx?doc_id=4164&nbr=3189
- Madden WS et al: Treatment of acne vulgaris and prevention of acne scarring: Canadian consensus guidelines. J Cutan Med Surg 2000;4(Suppl 1):S2. [PMID: 11749902]

WEB SITE

- American Academy of Dermatology
  - http://www.aad.org

INFORMATION FOR PATIENTS

- National Institute of Arthritis, and Musculoskeletal and Skin Diseases: Acne
  - http://www.niams.nih.gov/hi/topics/acne/acne.htm
- MedlinePlus: Acne Interactive Tutorial
  - http://www.nlm.nih.gov/medlineplus/tutorials/acne.html
- American Academy of Dermatology: What is Acne?
  - http://www.skincarephysicians.com/acnenet/acne.html
- Torpy JM et al: JAMA patient page: Acne. JAMA 2004;292:764. [PMID: 15304474]

REFERENCES

- Johnson BA: Use of systemic agents in the treatment of acne vulgaris. Am Fam Physician 2000;62:1823. [PMID: 11057839]
- Thiboutot D: New treatments and therapeutic strategies for acne. Arch Fam Med 2000;9:179. [PMID: 10693736]

Author(s)

Timothy G. Berger, MD

Acromegaly & Gigantism

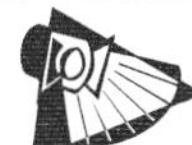

KEY FEATURES

ESSENTIALS OF DIAGNOSIS

- Excessive growth of hands (increased glove and ring size), feet (increased shoe width), jaw (prognathism, protrusion of lower jaw), and internal organs
- Gigantism if growth hormone (GH) excess before closure of epiphyses; acromegaly if after closure
- Coarsening of facial features; deeper voice
- Amenorrhea, headaches, visual field loss, sweating, weakness
- Soft, doughy, sweaty handshake
- Serum GH not suppressed following oral glucose
- Elevated insulin-like growth factor 1 (IGF-1)
- Radiographs: terminal phalangeal "tufting." CT or MRI: pituitary tumor in 90%

GENERAL CONSIDERATIONS

- GH exerts much of its effects through release of IGF-1 from liver and other tissues
- Nearly always caused by pituitary adenoma, usually macroadenomas (>1 cm). May be locally invasive but < 1% are malignant
- GH-secreting pituitary tumors usually cause hypogonadism by cosecretion of prolactin or direct pressure on pituitary
- Usually sporadic, rarely familial
- May be associated with endocrine tumors of parathyroids or pancreas (multiple endocrine neoplasia type 1 [MEN-1])
- Acromegaly may be seen in McCune-Albright syndrome and as part of Carney's complex (atrial myxoma, acoustic neuroma, and spotty skin pigmentation)
- Rarely caused by ectopic growth hormone-releasing hormone or GH secreted by lymphoma, hypothalamic tumor, bronchial carcinoid, or pancreatic tumor

CLINICAL FINDINGS

SYMPTOMS AND SIGNS

- Tall stature
- Enlarged hands and soft, doughy, sweaty handshake
- Fingers widen and rings no longer fit
- Carpal tunnel syndrome is common
- Feet grow, particularly in width
- Facial features coarsen
- Hat size increases, tooth spacing widens
- Mandible becomes more prominent
- Macroglossia and hypertrophy of pharyngeal and laryngeal tissue cause deep, coarse voice and may cause obstructive sleep apnea
- Goiter may be noted
- Hypertension (50%) and cardiomegaly
- Weight gain
- Arthralgias, degenerative arthritis, and spinal stenosis may occur
- Colon polyps common
- Skin: hyperhidrosis, thickening, cystic acne, and acanthosis nigricans
- Symptoms of hypopituitarism
  - Hypogonadism: decreased libido, impotence, irregular menses or amenorrhea common
  - Secondary hypothyroidism sometimes occurs, hypoadrenalism is unusual
  - Headaches and temporal hemianopia

DIFFERENTIAL DIAGNOSIS

- Familial tall stature, coarse features, or large hands and feet
- Physiological growth spurt
- Pseudoacromegaly (acromegaly features, insulin resistance)
- Inactive ("burned-out") acromegaly (spontaneous remission due to pituitary adenoma infarction)
- Myxedema
- Isolated prognathism (jaw protrusion)
- Aromatase deficiency or estrogen receptor deficiency causing tall stature
- Other causes of increased growth hormone level: exercise or eating prior to test, acute illness or agitation, hepatic or renal failure, malnourishment, diabetes mellitus, drugs: estrogens, β-blockers, clonidine

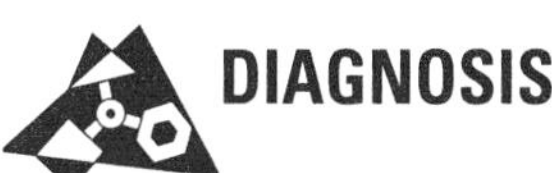

DIAGNOSIS

LABORATORY TESTS

- IGF-1 levels >5 times normal in most acromegalics
- Glucose tolerance test: glucose syrup 75 g PO, GH measured 60 min later; acromegaly excluded if GH < 1 μg/L (IRMA or chemiluminescent assays) or < 2 μg/L (older radioimmunoassays) and if IGF-1 is normal
- Prolactin may be elevated (cosecreted by many GH-secreting tumors)
- Insulin resistance usually present, often causing hyperglycemia (common) and diabetes mellitus (30%)
- Thyroid-stimulating hormone and free thyroxine may show secondary hypothyroidism
- Serum phosphorus frequently elevated
- Serum calcium elevated if hyperparathyroidism as in MEN-1

IMAGING STUDIES

- MRI shows pituitary tumor in 90%
- MRI superior to CT, especially postoperatively
- Skull x-rays may show enlarged sella and thickened skull
- Radiographs may show tufting of terminal phalanges of fingers and toes
- Lateral view of foot shows increased thickness of heel pad

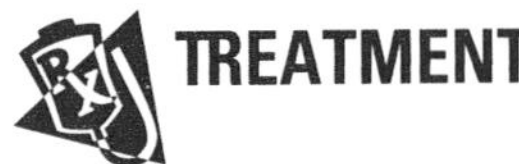

TREATMENT

MEDICATIONS

- Dopamine agonists are used if surgery does not produce clinical remission or normalization of GH. Most successful if tumor secretes both prolactin and GH—with cabergoline 0.25–1.0 mg PO twice weekly, one-third of such tumors shrink by >50%
- Octreotide or lanreotide (somatostatin analogs) used if acromegaly persists despite pituitary surgery; suppress GH to < 5 ng/mL in 60% of patients within 3–6 months
- Responders who tolerate short-acting octreotide 50 μg SQ TID are switched to long-acting octreotide 20 mg IM Q month
- Octreotide dose adjusted up to 40 mg IM Q month to maintain serum GH between 1 ng/mL and 2.5 ng/mL, keeping IGF-1 levels normal
- Lanreotide SR 30 mg SQ Q 7–14 days (not available in the United States)
- Lanreotide Autogel 60–120 mg SQ Q 28 days, better tolerated than lanreotide SR (not available in the United States)
- Pegvisomant, a GH receptor antagonist, 10–30 mg/day SQ, following IGF-1 levels

SURGERY

- Endoscopic transnasal, transsphenoidal resection is treatment of choice for acromegaly caused by pituitary adenoma; the normal pituitary is often preserved
- GH levels fall immediately
- About 10% get infection, cerebrospinal fluid leak, or hypopituitarism
- Hyponatremia can occur 4–13 days postoperatively. Serum sodium must be monitered closely

THERAPEUTIC PROCEDURES

- Pituitary irradiation suggested if not cured by surgical and medical therapy. Stereotactic radiosurgery (cyber knife or gamma knife) preferred
- Heavy particle radiation available in certain centers

OUTCOME

FOLLOW-UP

- Postoperatively, normal pituitary function usually preserved
- Postoperative GH levels >5 ng/mL and rising IGF-1 levels usually indicate recurrent tumor
- Soft tissue swelling regresses but bone enlargement is permanent
- Hypertension frequently persists
- Carpal tunnel syndrome and diaphoresis often improve within a day of surgery

COMPLICATIONS

- Hypopituitarism
- Hypertension
- Glucose intolerance or frank diabetes mellitus
- Cardiac enlargement and cardiac failure
- Carpal tunnel syndrome
- Arthritis of hips, knees, and spine
- Spinal cord compression may be seen
- Visual field defects may be severe and progressive
- Tumor may be locally invasive, particularly into the cavernous sinus
- Acute loss of vision or cranial nerve palsy if tumor undergoes spontaneous hemorrhage and necrosis (pituitary apoplexy)
- Intubation may be difficult due to macroglossia and hypertrophy of pharyngeal and laryngeal tissue

PROGNOSIS

- Untreated or persistent acromegaly usually causes premature cardiovascular disease and progressive acromegalic symptoms
- Transsphenoidal pituitary surgery successful in 80–90% if tumor < 2 cm and GH < 50 ng/mL
- Conventional radiation therapy (alone) produces remission in 40% by 2 years and 75% by 5 years
- Gamma knife radiation reduces GH levels an average of 77%, with 20% in remission at 12 months
- Heavy particle pituitary radiation produces remission in 70% by 2 years and 80% by 5 years
- Radiation therapy usually produces some degree of hypopituitarism
- Conventional radiation therapy may cause some degree of organic brain syndrome and predisposes to small strokes

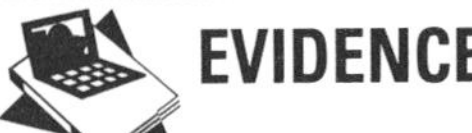

EVIDENCE

PRACTICE GUIDELINES

- AACE Practice Guidelines:
  - http://www.aace.com/clin/guidelines/AcromegalyGuidelines2004.pdf
- Melmed S et al: Guidelines for acromegaly management. J Clin Endocrinol Metab 2002;87:4054. [PMID:12213843]
- Scandinavian Workshop on the Treatment of Acromegaly. Treatment guidelines for acromegaly. Report from a Scandinavian workshop: first Scandinavian Workshop on the Treatment of Acromegaly. Growth Horm IGF Res 2001;11:72. [PMID:11472072]

WEB SITE

- National Institute of Diabetes and Digestive and Kidney Diseases (NIDDK)—Endocrine and metabolic diseases
  - http://www.niddk.nih.gov/health/endo/pubs/acro/acro.htm

INFORMATION FOR PATIENTS

- Acromegaly.org
  - www.acromegaly.org
- Mayo Clinic—Acromegaly
  - http://www.mayoclinic.com/invoke.cfm?id=IEC8F4CO-4627-4349-A3C7F1DE85AE7702

REFERENCES

- Bourrdelot A et al: Clinical, hormonal and magnetic resonance imaging (MRI) predictors of transsphenoidal surgery outcome in acromegaly. Eur J Endocrinol 2004;150:763. [PMID: 15191345]
- Cozzi R et al: Cabergoline addition to depot somatostatin analogues in resistant acromegalic patients: efficacy and lack of predictive value of prolactin status. Clin Endocrinol (Oxf) 2004;61:209. [PMID: 15272916]
- Paisley AN et al: Pegvisomant: a novel pharmacotherapy for the treatment of acromegaly. Expert Opin Biol Ther 2004;4:421. [PMID: 15006735]
- Pham CJ et al: Preliminary visual field preservation after staged CyberKnife radiosurgery for perioptic lesions. Neurosurgery 2004;54:799. [PMID: 15046645]

Author(s)

Paul A. Fitzgerald, MD

Actinomycosis

KEY FEATURES

ESSENTIALS OF DIAGNOSIS

- History of recent dental infection or abdominal trauma
- Chronic pneumonia or indolent intra-abdominal or cervicofacial abscess
- Sinus tract formation

GENERAL CONSIDERATIONS

- Organisms are anaerobic, gram-positive, branching filamentous bacteria (1 μm in diameter) that may fragment into bacillary forms
- Occur in the normal flora of the mouth and tonsillar crypts
- When introduced into traumatized tissue and associated with other anaerobic bacteria, actinomycetes become pathogens
- The most common site of infection is the cervicofacial area (about 60% of cases)
- Infection typically follows extraction of a tooth or other trauma
- Lesions may develop in the gastrointestinal tract or lungs following ingestion or aspiration of the organism from its endogenous source in the mouth

CLINICAL FINDINGS

SYMPTOMS AND SIGNS

Cervicofacial actinomycosis

- Develops slowly, becomes markedly indurated, and the overlying skin becomes reddish or cyanotic
- Abscesses eventually drain to the surface
- Persist for long periods
- Sulfur granules—masses of filamentous organisms—may be found in the pus
- There is usually little pain unless there is secondary infection

Thoracic actinomycosis

- Fever, cough, sputum production
- Night sweats, weight loss
- Pleuritic pain
- Multiple sinuses may extend through the chest wall to the heart or abdomen

Abdominal actinomycosis

- Pain in the ileocecal region
- Spiking fever and chills
- Vomiting
- Weight loss
- Irregular abdominal masses may be palpated
- Pelvic inflammatory disease caused by actinomycetes has been associated with prolonged use of an intrauterine contraceptive device
- Sinuses draining to the exterior may develop

DIFFERENTIAL DIAGNOSIS

- Lung cancer
- Tuberculous lymphadenitis (scrofula)
- Other cause of cervical lymphadenopathy
- Nocardiosis
- Crohn's disease
- Pelvic inflammatory disease from another cause

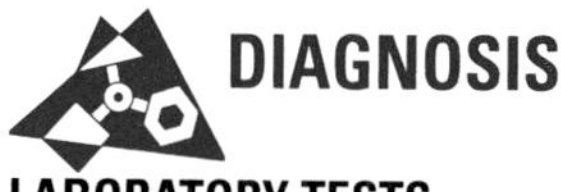

DIAGNOSIS

LABORATORY TESTS

- Organisms may be demonstrated as a granule or as scattered branching gram-positive filaments in the pus
- Anaerobic culture is necessary to distinguish from *Nocardia*

IMAGING STUDIES

- Chest x-ray shows areas of consolidation and, in many cases, pleural effusion
- Abdominal pelvic CT scanning reveals an inflammatory mass that may extend to involve bone

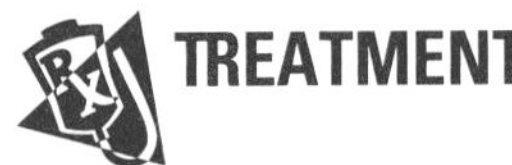

TREATMENT

MEDICATIONS

- Penicillin G is the drug of choice, 10 to 20 million units IV for 24 weeks, followed by penicillin V, 500 mg PO four times daily
- Sulfonamides such as sulfamethoxazole may be an alternative regimen at a total daily dosage of 2–4 g

SURGERY

- Drainage and resection may be beneficial

THERAPEUTIC PROCEDURES

- Therapy should be continued for weeks to months after clinical manifestations have disappeared in order to ensure cure
- Response to therapy is slow

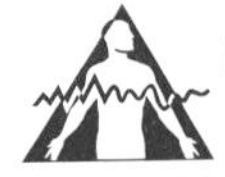

OUTCOME

PROGNOSIS

- With penicillin and surgery, the prognosis is good
- The difficulties of diagnosis may result in extensive destruction of tissue before therapy is started

WHEN TO REFER

- Refer early to an infectious disease specialist for diagnosis and management

WHEN TO ADMIT

- All patients with thoracic or abdominal actinomycosis
- Patients with cervicofacial actinomycosis if the diagnosis is in question, to control symptoms, or initiate IV antibiotics

EVIDENCE

PRACTICE GUIDELINES

- Cayley J et al: Recommendations for clinical practice: actinomyces like organisms and intrauterine contraceptives. The Clinical and Scientific Committee. Br J Fam Plann 1998;23:137. [PMID: 9882769]

WEB SITE

- Karolinska Institute: Diseases and Disorders—Links Pertaining to Bacterial Infections and Mycoses
  - http://www.mic.ki.se/Diseases/C01.html

INFORMATION FOR PATIENTS

- National Institutes of Health: Actinomycosis
  - http://www.nlm.nih.gov/medlineplus/ency/article/000599.htm
- National Institutes of Health: Pulmonary Actinomycosis
  - http://www.nlm.nih.gov/medlineplus/ency/article/000074.htm

REFERENCES

- Sudhakar SS et al: Short-term treatment of actinomycosis: two cases and a review. Clin Infect Dis 2004;38:444. [PMID: 14727221]
- Wagenlehner FM et al: Abdominal actinomycosis. Clin Microbiol Infect 2003;9:881. [PMID: 14616714]

Author(s)

Henry F. Chambers, MD

Acute Respiratory Distress Syndrome (ARDS)

KEY FEATURES

ESSENTIALS OF DIAGNOSIS

- Acute onset of respiratory failure
- Bilateral radiographic pulmonary infiltrates
- Absence of elevated left atrial pressure
- Ratio of $PAO_2/FIO_2 < 200$, regardless of the level of peak end-expiratory pressure (PEEP)

GENERAL CONSIDERATIONS

- Acute hypoxemic respiratory failure following a systemic or pulmonary insult without evidence of heart failure
- Common risk factors
  - Sepsis, aspiration of gastric contents
  - Shock, infection
  - Lung contusion
  - Trauma
  - Toxic inhalation
  - Near-drowning
  - Multiple blood transfusion (see Table 38)
- Damage to capillary endothelial and alveolar epithelial cells is found, regardless of the cause of ARDS

Systemic causes

- Trauma, sepsis, shock, burns
- Pancreatitis
- Multiple transfusions
- Disseminated intravascular coagulation (DIC) and thrombotic thrombocytopenia purpura (TTP)
- Drugs
  - Opioids
  - Aspirin
  - Phenothiazines
  - Tricyclic antidepressants
  - Amiodarone
  - Chemotherapeutics
  - Nitrofurantoin
  - Protamine
- Cardiopulmonary bypass
- Head injury
- Paraquat

Pulmonary causes

- Aspiration of gastric contents
- Embolism of thrombus, fat, air, or amniotic fluid
- Miliary tuberculosis
- Diffuse pneumonia
- Acute eosinophilic pneumonia
- Bronchiolitis obliterans with organizing pneumonia (BOOP)
- Upper airway obstruction
- Free-base cocaine smoking
- Near-drowning
- Toxic gas inhalation
  - Nitrogen dioxide
  - Chlorine
  - Sulfur dioxide
  - Ammonia
  - Smoke inhalation
- Oxygen toxicity
- Lung contusion
- Radiation
- High-altitude exposure
- Lung reexpansion or reperfusion

CLINICAL FINDINGS

SYMPTOMS AND SIGNS

- Rapid onset of profound dyspnea, usually 12–48 hours after the initiating event
- Labored breathing and tachypnea, with crackles on examination
- Marked hypoxemia refractory to supplemental oxygen
- Multiple-organ failure is seen in many patients

DIFFERENTIAL DIAGNOSIS

- Because ARDS is a syndrome, the concept of differential diagnosis applies only in considering the precipitating illness or injury
- Cardiogenic (hydrostatic) pulmonary edema
- Pneumonia
- Diffuse alveolar hemorrhage
- BOOP

DIAGNOSIS

LABORATORY TESTS

- Tests to identify the systemic or pulmonary causes of ARDS are indicated

IMAGING STUDIES

- Chest x-ray shows diffuse or patchy bilateral infiltrates that rapidly become confluent
- Air bronchograms are seen in 80% of cases
- Features of congestive heart failure (pleural effusions, cardiomegaly, venous engorgement in upper lung zones) are absent

DIAGNOSTIC PROCEDURES

- When indicated to rule out cardiogenic pulmonary edema, Swan-Ganz catheterization will demonstrate pulmonary capillary wedge pressures < 18 mm Hg

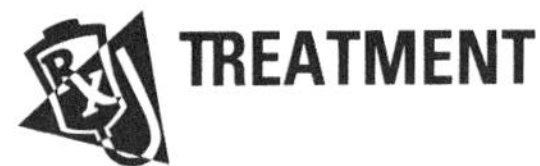

TREATMENT

MEDICATIONS

- Medications directed at the underlying cause of ARDS are indicated
- Intravascular volume should be maintained at the lowest level required to maintain adequate cardiac output
- Diuretics may be needed to reduce pulmonary capillary wedge pressure and improve oxygenation
- Judicious use of inotropes to maintain cardiac output at higher levels of PEEP may be necessary
- Achieving supranormal oxygen delivery through the use of inotropes and blood transfusion is not clinically useful and may be harmful
- Sedatives, analgesics, and antipyretics may be used to decrease oxygen consumption
- Systemic corticosteroids have not been shown to reliably improve outcomes

THERAPEUTIC PROCEDURES

- Intubation and mechanical ventilation are usually required to treat hypoxemia
- The lowest levels of PEEP and FIO_2 needed to maintain a PAO_2 >60 mm Hg
- The use of small tidal volume ventilation (6 mL/kg of ideal body weight) has been shown to reduce mortality by 10% in a large multicenter trial
- PEEP may be increased as long as cardiac output and O_2 delivery are not impaired and pulmonary pressures are not excessive
- Prone positioning may improve oxygenation in selected patients

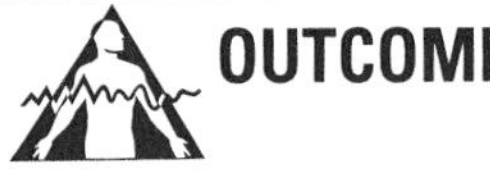

OUTCOME

FOLLOW-UP

- Efforts should be made to decrease FIO_2 below 60% as early as possible
- For patients who recover, no specific follow-up is required

COMPLICATIONS

- Complications are those associated with ICU level care and mechanical ventilation

PROGNOSIS

- Mortality is 30–40% in ARDS, 90% when associated with sepsis
- Median survival is 2 weeks
- Many patients with ARDS die when support is withdrawn
- Survivors of ARDS are left with some pulmonary symptoms, which tend to improve over time
- Mild abnormalities of oxygenation, diffusion capacity, and lung mechanics may persist in some survivors

WHEN TO REFER

- Care of patients with ARDS should involve a clinician who is familiar with the syndrome, typically an intensivist or pulmonologist

WHEN TO ADMIT

- Because of the profound hypoxemia that defines ARDS, all patients need admission and intensive care

PREVENTION

- No measures have been identified to effectively prevent ARDS
- Prophylactic PEEP and methylprednisolone are not helpful in patients at risk

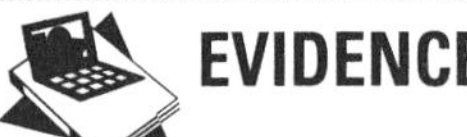

EVIDENCE

INFORMATION FOR PATIENTS

- National Institutes of Health
  - http://www.nlm.nih.gov/medlineplus/ency/article/000103.htm

REFERENCES

- Adhikari N et al: Pharmacologic therapies for adults with acute lung injury and acute respiratory distress syndrome. Cochrane Database Syst Rev 2004;(4):CD004477. [PMID:15495113]
- Kallet RH. Evidence-based management of acute lung injury and acute respiratory distress syndrome. Respir Care 2004;49:793. [PMID:15222911]
- Matthay MA et al: Future research directions in acute lung injury: summary of a National Heart, Lung, and Blood Institute Working Group. Am J Respir Crit Care Med 2003;167:1027. [PMID:12663342]
- Richard C et al: Early use of the pulmonary artery catheter and outcomes in patients with shock and acute respiratory distress syndrome: a randomized controlled trial. JAMA 2003;290:2713. [PMID:14645314]
- Schwarz MI et al: "Imitators" of the ARDS: implications for diagnosis and treatment. Chest 2004;125:1530. [PMID: 15078770]
- Ventilation with lower tidal volumes as compared with traditional tidal volumes for acute lung injury and the acute respiratory distress syndrome. The Acute Respiratory Distress Syndrome Network. N Engl J Med 2000;342:1301. [PMID 10793162]

Author(s)

Mark S. Chesnutt, MD
Thomas J. Prendergast, MD

Adrenocortical Insufficiency, Acute (Adrenal Crisis)

Adenovirus Infections p. 1019

KEY FEATURES

ESSENTIALS OF DIAGNOSIS

- Weakness, abdominal pain, fever, confusion, nausea, vomiting, and diarrhea
- Low blood pressure, dehydration; skin pigmentation may be increased
- Serum potassium high, sodium low, blood urea nitrogen high
- Cosyntropin ($ACTH_{1\text{-}24}$) unable to stimulate a normal increase in serum cortisol

GENERAL CONSIDERATIONS

- Acute adrenal insufficiency is an emergency caused by insufficient cortisol
- May occur in course of chronic, treated adrenal insufficiency, or as its presenting manifestation
- Acute adrenal crisis is more common in primary adrenal insufficiency (adrenal gland disorder; Addison's disease) than secondary adrenocortical hypofunction (pituitary gland disorder)
- May occur following stress, eg, trauma, surgery, infection, or prolonged fasting in patient with latent insufficiency
- May result from withdrawal of adrenocortical hormone replacement in patient with chronic adrenal insufficiency or temporary insufficiency related to withdrawal of exogenous glucocorticoids
- May occur following bilateral adrenalectomy or removal of a functioning adrenal tumor that had suppressed the other adrenal
- May result from injury to both adrenals by trauma, hemorrhage, anticoagulant therapy, thrombosis, infection, or, rarely, metastatic carcinoma
- May occur after pituitary necrosis, or when thyroid hormone replacement is given to a patient with adrenal insufficiency
- Adrenal crisis may occur in infancy or childhood in congenital adrenal hyperplasia, congenital adrenal hypoplasia, Allgrove syndrome, adrenoleukodystrophy

CLINICAL FINDINGS

SYMPTOMS AND SIGNS

- Headache, lassitude, nausea and vomiting, abdominal pain, and diarrhea
- Confusion or coma
- Fever, as high as 40.6°C or more
- Low blood pressure
- Recurrent hypoglycemia and reduced insulin requirements in patients with preexisting type 1 diabetes mellitus
- Cyanosis, dehydration, skin hyperpigmentation, and sparse axillary hair (if hypogonadism also present)
- Meningococcemia may cause purpura and adrenal insufficiency secondary to adrenal infarction (Waterhouse-Friderichsen syndrome)

DIFFERENTIAL DIAGNOSIS

- Other cause of shock, eg, sepsis, cardiogenic, hypovolemic, anaphylaxis
- Hyperkalemia due to other cause, eg, renal failure, rhabdomyolysis, angiotensin-converting enzyme inhibitors, angiotensin receptor blockers, spironolactone
- Hyponatremia due to other cause, eg, syndrome of inappropriate antidiuretic hormone, cirrhosis, vomiting
- Abdominal pain due to other cause
- Low serum cortisol-binding globulin in critical illness, causing low total serum cortisol; serum free cortisol levels normal

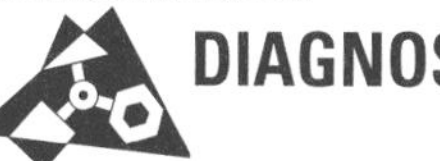

DIAGNOSIS

LABORATORY TESTS

- Eosinophil count may be high
- Hyponatremia or hyperkalemia (or both) usually present
- Hypoglycemia common
- Hypercalcemia may be present
- Blood, sputum, or urine culture may be positive if bacterial infection is precipitating cause
- Cosyntropin stimulation test: synthetic $ACTH_{1\text{-}24}$ (cosyntropin), 0.25 mg, given SQ, IM, or IV, and serum cortisol obtained 45 min later. Normally, cortisol rises to ≥20 μg/dL. For patients on glucocorticoids, hydrocortisone must not be given for at least 8 h before test. Other glucocorticoids (eg, prednisone, dexamethasone) do not interfere with specific assays for cortisol
- Plasma ACTH markedly elevated if patient has primary adrenal disease (generally >200 pg/mL)

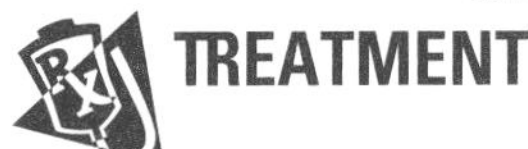

TREATMENT

MEDICATIONS

- If diagnosis is suspected, draw blood sample for cortisol determination and treat with hydrocortisone 100–300 mg IV and saline *immediately*, without waiting for results
- Then continue hydrocortisone 50–100 mg IV Q 6 h for first day, Q 8 h the second day, and taper as clinically appropriate
- Broad-spectrum antibiotics given empirically while waiting for initial culture results
- $D_{50}W$ to treat hypoglycemia with careful monitoring of serum electrolytes, blood urea nitrogen, and creatinine
- When patient is able to take oral medication, give hydrocortisone 10–20 mg PO Q 6 h, and taper to maintenance levels. Most require hydrocortisone twice daily: 10–20 mg Q AM, 5–10 mg Q PM
- Mineralocorticoid therapy is not needed when large amounts of hydrocortisone are being given, but as the dose is reduced, may need to add fludrocortisone 0.05–0.2 mg PO QD. Some never require fludrocortisone or become edematous at doses >0.05 mg once or twice weekly

THERAPEUTIC PROCEDURES

- Once the crisis is over, must assess degree of permanent adrenal insufficiency and establish cause if possible

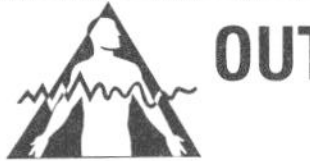

OUTCOME

FOLLOW-UP

- Repeat cosyntropin stimulation test

COMPLICATIONS

- Shock and death if untreated
- Sequelae of infection that commonly precipitate adrenal crisis

PROGNOSIS

- Rapid treatment usually life-saving
- Frequently unrecognized and untreated since manifestations mimic more common conditions; lack of treatment leads to shock that is unresponsive to volume replacement and vasopressors, resulting in death

EVIDENCE

PRACTICE GUIDELINES

- Arlt W et al: Adrenal insufficiency. Lancet 2003;361:1881. [PMID: 12788587]
- Clinical practice parameters for hemodynamic support of pediatric and neonatal patients in septic shock. American College of Critical Care Medicine, 2002
  - http://www.sccm.org/pdf/hemodynamic%20peds%20guidelines.pdf
- Cooper MS et al: Corticosteroid insufficiency in acutely ill patients. N Engl J Med 2003;348:727. [PMID: 12594318]
- Oelkers W et al: Therapeutic strategies in adrenal insufficiency. Ann Endocrinol (Paris) 2001;62:212. [PMID: 11353897]

WEB SITE

- National Adrenal Disease Foundation
  - http://medhelp.org/www/nadf.htm

INFORMATION FOR PATIENTS

- MEDLINEplus–Acute adrenal crisis
  - http://www.nlm.nih.gov/medlineplus/ency/article/000357.htm

REFERENCES

- Hamrahian AH et al: Measurements of serum free cortisol in critically ill patients. N Engl J Med 2004;350:1629. [PMID: 15084695]
- Marik PE et al: Adrenal insufficiency in the critically ill: a new look at an old problem. Chest 2002;122:1784. [PMID: 12426284]
- Vella A et al: Adrenal hemorrhage: a 25-year experience at the Mayo Clinic. Mayo Clin Proc 2001;76:161. [PMID: 11213304]

Author(s)

Paul A. Fitzgerald, MD

Adrenocortical Insufficiency, Chronic (Addison's Disease)

KEY FEATURES

ESSENTIALS OF DIAGNOSIS

- Weakness, easy fatigability, anorexia, weight loss; nausea and vomiting, diarrhea; abdominal pain, muscle and joint pains; amenorrhea
- Sparse axillary hair; increased skin pigmentation, especially of creases, pressure areas, and nipples
- Hypotension, small heart
- Serum sodium may be low; potassium, calcium, and urea nitrogen may be elevated; neutropenia, mild anemia, eosinophilia, and relative lymphocytosis may be present
- Plasma cortisol levels low or fail to rise after administration of cosyntropin
- Plasma ACTH level elevated

GENERAL CONSIDERATIONS

- Autoimmune destruction of adrenals is most common cause in the United States. May occur alone or as part of an autoimmune polyglandular failure syndrome
- May be associated with autoimmune thyroid disease, hypoparathyroidism, diabetes mellitus type 1, vitiligo, alopecia areata, celiac sprue, primary ovarian failure, testicular failure, and pernicious anemia
- Combination of Addison's disease and hypothyroidism is Schmidt's syndrome
- Tuberculosis is common cause in areas of high prevalence; now rare
- Bilateral adrenal hemorrhage may occur with sepsis, heparin-associated thrombocytopenia or anticoagulation, antiphospholipid antibody syndrome, surgery (postoperatively) or trauma, or spontaneously
- Adrenoleukodystrophy is an X-linked disorder accounting for one-third of Addison's disease in boys. May cause hypogonadism, psychiatric symptoms, and neurologic deterioration
- Rare causes of adrenal insufficiency: lymphoma, metastatic carcinoma, coccidioidomycosis, histoplasmosis, cytomegalovirus (more frequent in AIDS), syphilitic gummas, scleroderma, amyloid disease, hemochromatosis, familial glucocorticoid deficiency, Allgrove syndrome (associated with achalasia, alacrima, and neurologic disease), X-linked adrenal leukodystrophy, and congenital adrenal hypoplasia (associated with hypogonadotropic hypogonadism)
- Congenital adrenal hyperplasia results from hereditary defects in adrenal enzymes for cortisol synthesis, eg, P-450c21 (21-hydroxylase). Severe cases manifest mineralocorticoid deficiency (salt wasting) in addition to deficient cortisol and excessive androgens
- May occur in polyglandular autoimmunity (PGA1 and PGA2)

CLINICAL FINDINGS

SYMPTOMS AND SIGNS

- Weakness and fatigability, weight loss, myalgias, arthralgias, fever
- Anorexia, nausea and vomiting
- Anxiety, mental irritability, and emotional changes common
- Diffuse tanning over nonexposed and exposed skin or multiple freckles; hyperpigmentation, especially knuckles, elbows, knees, posterior neck, palmar creases, nail beds, pressure areas, and new scars
- Vitiligo (10%)
- Hypoglycemia, when present, may worsen weakness and mental functioning, rarely leading to coma
- Other autoimmune disease manifestations
- In diabetics, increased insulin sensitivity and hypoglycemic reactions
- Hypotension and orthostasis usual; 90% have SBP < 110 mm Hg; SBP >130 mm Hg is rare
- Small heart
- Scant axillary and pubic hair (especially in women)
- Neuropsychiatric symptoms, sometimes without adrenal insufficiency, in adult-onset adrenoleukodystrophy

DIFFERENTIAL DIAGNOSIS

- Hypotension due to other cause, eg, medications
- Hyperkalemia due to other cause, eg, renal failure
- Gastroenteritis
- Occult cancer
- Anorexia nervosa
- Hyperpigmentation due to other cause, eg, hemochromatosis
- Isolated hypoaldosteronism

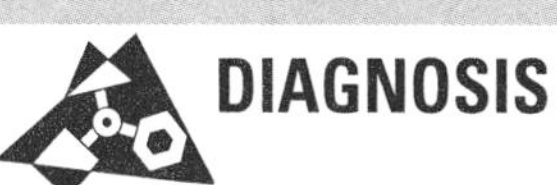

DIAGNOSIS

LABORATORY TESTS

- Moderate neutropenia, lymphocytosis, and total eosinophil count >300/μL
- In *chronic* Addison's disease, serum sodium is usually low (90%) while potassium is elevated (65%). Patients with diarrhea may not be hyperkalemic
- Fasting blood glucose may be low
- Hypercalcemia may be present
- Plasma very-long-chain fatty acid levels to screen for adrenoleukodystrophy in young men with idiopathic Addison's disease
- Plasma cortisol level low (< 5 mg/dL) at 8 am is diagnostic, especially if accompanied by simultaneous elevated ACTH (usually >200 pg/mL)
- Cosyntropin stimulation test: synthetic $ACTH_{1-24}$ (cosyntropin), 0.25 mg, given parenterally, and serum cortisol obtained 45 min later. Normally, cortisol rises to ≥20 μg/dL. For patients on glucocorticoids, hydrocortisone must not be given for at least 8 h before the test. Other glucocorticoids do not interfere with specific assays for cortisol
- Plasma ACTH markedly elevated (generally > 200 pg/mL) if patient has primary adrenal disease
- Serum DHEA > 1000 ng/mL excludes the diagnosis
- Antiadrenal antibodies detected in 50% of autoimmune Addison's disease
- Antithyroid antibodies (45%) and other autoantibodies may be present
- Elevated plasma renin activity indicates depleted intravascular volume and need for higher doses of fludrocortisone replacement
- Plasma epinephrine levels low

IMAGING STUDIES

- Chest x-ray for tuberculosis, fungal infection, or cancer
- Abdominal CT shows small noncalcified adrenals in autoimmune Addison's disease. Adrenals enlarged in about 85% of cases of metastatic or granulomatous disease. Calcification noted in cases of tuberculosis (~50%), hemorrhage, fungal infection, and melanoma

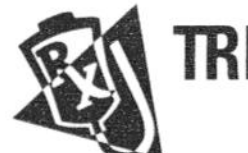

TREATMENT

MEDICATIONS

- Glucocorticoid and mineralocorticoid replacement required in most cases; hydrocortisone alone may be adequate in mild cases
- Hydrocortisone is drug of choice, usually 15–25 mg in two divided doses, two-thirds in AM and one-third in late PM or early evening
- Prednisone 2–3 mg PO Q AM and 1–2 mg PO Q PM or evening is an alternative
- Dose adjusted according to clinical response; proper dose usually results in normal WBC differential
- Glucocorticoid dose raised in case of infection, trauma, surgery, diagnostic procedures, or other stress. Maximum hydrocortisone dose for severe stress is 50 mg IV or IM Q 6 h. Lower doses, oral or parenteral, for lesser stress. Dose tapered to normal as stress subsides
- Fludrocortisone, 0.05–0.3 mg PO QD or QOD required by many patients. Dose increased for postural hypotension, hyponatremia, hyperkalemia, fatigue, or elevated plasma renin activity. Dosage decreased for edema, hypokalemia, or hypertension
- Treat all infections immediately
- In some women with adrenal insufficiency, dehydroepiandrosterone (DHEA), 50 mg PO Q AM, improves sense of well-being, mood, and sexual performance

THERAPEUTIC PROCEDURES

- "Lorenzo's oil" for adrenoleukodystrophy normalizes serum very-long-chain fatty acid concentrations but is ineffective clinically. Hematopoietic stem cell transplantation from normal donors may improve neurological manifestations

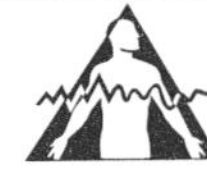

OUTCOME

FOLLOW-UP

- Follow clinically and adjust glucocorticoid and (if required) mineralocorticoid doses as needed
- Fatigue in treated patients may indicate suboptimal dosing of medication, electrolyte imbalance, or concurrent problems such as hypothyroidism or diabetes mellitus
- Glucocorticoid dose must be increased in case of physiologic stress (see above)

COMPLICATIONS

- Complications of underlying disease (eg, tuberculosis) are more likely in chronic adrenal insufficiency
- Adrenal crisis may be precipitated by intercurrent infections
- Associated autoimmune diseases are common (see above)
- Fatigue often persists despite treatment of Addison's disease
- Excessive glucocorticoid replacement can cause Cushing's syndrome

PROGNOSIS

- Normal life expectancy if adrenal insufficiency is diagnosed and treated with appropriate doses of glucocorticoids and (if required) mineralocorticoids. Most able to live fully active lives
- However, associated conditions can pose additional health risks, eg, adrenoleukodystrophy or Allgrove syndrome may result in neurological disease; patients with adrenal tuberculosis may have serious systemic infection
- Glucocorticoid and mineralocorticoid replacement must not be stopped
- Patients should wear medical alert bracelet or medal reading "Adrenal insufficiency—takes hydrocortisone"
- Higher doses of glucocorticoids must be administered to patients with infection, trauma, or surgery to prevent adrenal crisis

EVIDENCE

PRACTICE GUIDELINES

- Arlt W et al: Adrenal insufficiency. Lancet 2003;361:1881. [PMID:12788587]
- Don-Wauchope AC et al: Diagnosis and management of Addison's disease. Practitioner 2000;244:794. [PMID:11048377]

WEB SITES

- Australian Addison's Disease Association
  - http://www.addisons.org.au/
- National Adrenal Disease Foundation
  - http://medhelp.org/www/nadf.htm

INFORMATION FOR PATIENTS

- Cleveland Clinic—Addison's disease
  - http://www.clevelandclinic.org/health/health-info/docs/0800/0853.asp?index=5484

REFERENCES

- Betterle C et al: Autoimmune adrenal insufficiency and autoimmune polyendocrine syndromes: autoantibodies, autoantigens, and their applicability in diagnosis and disease prediction. Endocr Rev 2002;23:327. [PMID:12050123]
- Dorin RI et al: Diagnosis of adrenal insufficiency. Ann Intern Med 2003;139:194. [PMID: 12899587]

Author(s)

Paul A. Fitzgerald, MD

Alcoholism

KEY FEATURES

ESSENTIALS OF DIAGNOSIS

Major criteria

- Physiologic dependence as evidenced by withdrawal when intake is interrupted
- Tolerance to the effects of alcohol
- Evidence of alcohol-associated illnesses, such as alcoholic liver disease
- Continued drinking despite strong medical and social contraindications
- Impairment in social and occupational functioning
- Depression
- Blackouts

Other signs

- Alcohol stigmas: alcohol odor on breath, alcoholic facies, flushed face, scleral injection, tremor, ecchymoses, peripheral neuropathy
- Surreptitious drinking
- Unexplained work absences
- Frequent accidents, falls, or injuries
- In smokers, cigarette burns on hands or chest

GENERAL CONSIDERATIONS

- The two-phase syndrome includes problem drinking and alcohol addiction
- Problem drinking is the repetitive use of alcohol, often to alleviate anxiety or solve other emotional problems
- Alcohol addiction is a true addiction
- Alcoholism is associated with a high prevalence of lifetime psychiatric disorders, especially depression

DEMOGRAPHICS

- Most suicides and intrafamily homicides involve alcohol
- Major factor in rapes and other assaults
- Male-to-female ratios of 4:1 are converging
- Adoption and twin studies indicate some genetic influence
- Forty percent of Japanese have aldehyde dehydrogenase deficiency, which increases susceptibility to the effects of alcohol

CLINICAL FINDINGS

SYMPTOMS AND SIGNS

Acute intoxication

- Drowsiness, errors of commission, psychomotor dysfunction, disinhibition, dysarthria, ataxia, and nystagmus
- Presence of ataxia, dysarthria, and nausea and vomiting indicates a blood level above 150 mg/dL
- Lethal blood levels: 350–900 mg/dL
- Severe cases are marked by respiratory depression, stupor, seizures, shock syndrome, coma, and death
- Serious overdoses often include other sedatives combined with alcohol

Withdrawal

- Onset of withdrawal symptoms is usually 8–12 hours, with peak intensity 48–72 hours after alcohol consumption is stopped
- Anxiety, decreased cognition, tremulousness, increasing irritability, and hyperreactivity to full-blown delirium tremens
- Symptoms of mild withdrawal, including tremor, elevated vital signs, and anxiety, begin about 8 hours after the last drink and end by day 3
- Generalized seizures occur within the first 24–38 hours and are more prevalent in patients with previous withdrawal syndromes
- Delirium tremens is an acute organic psychosis
  - Usually manifest within 24–72 hours after the last drink but may occur up to 7–10 days later
  - Mental confusion, tremor, sensory hyperacuity, visual hallucinations, autonomic hyperactivity, cardiac abnormalities, diaphoresis, dehydration, electrolyte disturbances (hypokalemia, hypomagnesemia), and seizures
- The acute withdrawal syndrome often unexpectedly occurs in patients hospitalized for some unrelated reason and presents as a diagnostic problem
- Possible persistence of sleep disturbances, anxiety, depression, excitability, fatigue, and emotional volatility for 3–12 months, becoming chronic in some cases

Alcoholic hallucinosis

- Paranoid psychosis without the tremulousness, confusion, and clouded sensorium seen in withdrawal syndromes
- Occurs during heavy drinking or during withdrawal
- The patient appears normal except for the auditory hallucinations, which are frequently persecutory and may cause the patient to behave aggressively and in a paranoid fashion

Chronic alcoholic brain syndromes

- Encephalopathies characterized by
  - Increasing erratic behavior
  - Memory and recall problems
  - Emotional lability
- Wernicke's encephalopathy characterized by
  - Confusion
  - Ataxia
  - Ophthalmoplegia (typically sixth nerve)
- Korsakoff's psychosis is a sequela, characterized by
  - Both anterograde and retrograde amnesia
  - Confabulation early in the course

DIFFERENTIAL DIAGNOSIS

Alcohol dependence

- Alcoholism secondary to psychiatric disease, eg, depression, bipolar disorder, schizophrenia, borderline personality disorder
- Other sedative dependence, eg, benzodiazepines
- Other drug abuse, eg, opioids

Alcohol withdrawal

- Withdrawal from other sedatives, eg, benzodiazepines or opioids
- Drug intoxication, eg, cocaine
- Delirium due to medical illness, eg, hypoxia, hepatic encephalopathy, thiamine deficiency, bacteremia
- Anxiety disorder
- Hallucinosis due to other cause, eg, schizophrenia, amphetamine psychosis
- Seizure due to other cause, eg, hypoglycemia, epilepsy

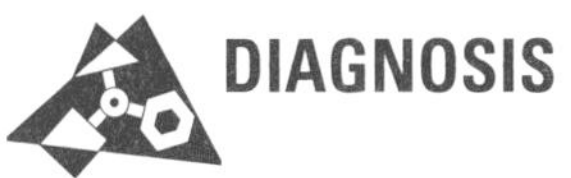

DIAGNOSIS

LABORATORY TESTS

- Blood alcohol levels < 50 mg/dL rarely cause much motor dysfunction
- Carbohydrate-deficient transferrin (CDT) can detect heavy use over a 2-week period with high specificity
- Elevations of both γ-glutamyl transpeptidase (levels >30 units/L suggest heavy drinking) and mean corpuscular volume (>95 fL in men and >100 fL in women) make a serious drinking problem likely

DIAGNOSTIC PROCEDURES

- Suspect the problem early
- CAGE questionnaire (Table 103)
- Before treating for withdrawal or hallucinosis, meticulous examination for other medical problems is necessary

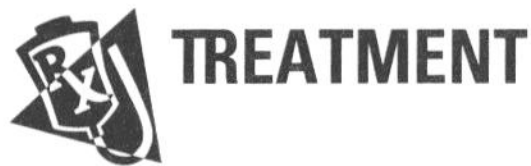

TREATMENT

MEDICATIONS

Alcoholic addiction

- Disulfiram (250–500 mg/day PO); compliance depends on motivation
- Naltrexone (50 mg/day PO) lowers relapse rates over the 3–6 months after drinking cessation, apparently by lessening the pleasurable effects of alcohol
- Haloperidol, 5 mg PO BID for the first day or so; taper drug over several days as the patient improves
- Use adequate doses of sedative to cause moderate sedation
- Antipsychotic drugs should not be used
- For some outpatients, a short course of oral tapering benzodiazepines, eg, 20 mg of diazepam initially, decreasing by 5 mg daily, may be a useful adjunct
  - In moderate to severe withdrawal, use diazepam (5–10 mg PO hourly depending on severity of withdrawal symptoms)
  - In very severe withdrawal, IV diazepam
  - After stabilization, diazepam (enough to maintain a sedated state) may be given orally every 8–12 hours
  - If withdrawal signs persist (eg, tremulousness), the dosage is increased until moderate sedation occurs
  - The dosage is then gradually reduced by 20% every 24 hours until withdrawal is complete, which usually requires a week or more of treatment
- Clonidine, 5 μg/kg PO Q 2 h, or the patch formulation, suppresses cardiovascular signs of withdrawal
- Carbamazepine, 400–800 mg/day PO, compares favorably with benzodiazepines for alcohol withdrawal
- Atenolol, as an adjunct to benzodiazepines, can reduce symptoms of alcohol withdrawal but should not be used when bradycardia is present
  - 100 mg/day PO when the heart rate is above 80 beats per minute
  - 50 mg/day for a heart rate between 50 and 80 beats per minute
- Phenytoin is not useful for alcohol withdrawal seizures unless there is a preexisting seizure disorder
- A general diet should be accompanied by vitamins in high doses
  - Thiamine, 50 mg IV initially (IV glucose given prior to thiamine may precipitate Wernicke's syndrome; concurrent administration is satisfactory)
  - Pyridoxine, 100 mg/day
  - Folic acid, 1 mg/day
  - Ascorbic acid, 100 mg BID

THERAPEUTIC PROCEDURES

- Maintain a nonjudgmental attitude
- Denial is best faced at the first meeting, preferably with family members
- Aversion behavioral therapy has been successful in some patients

OUTCOME

FOLLOW-UP

- Monitoring of vital signs and fluid and electrolyte levels is essential for the severely ill patient with withdrawal
- Alcoholic chronic brain syndrome patients require careful attention to their social and environmental care

COMPLICATIONS

- Nervous system complications
  - Chronic brain syndromes
  - Cerebellar degeneration
  - Cardiomyopathy
  - Peripheral neuropathies
- Direct liver effects
  - Cirrhosis
  - Eventual hepatic failure
- Indirect effects
  - Protein abnormalities
  - Coagulation defects
  - Hormone deficiencies
  - Increased incidence of liver neoplasms
- Alcoholic hypoglycemia can occur even with low blood alcohol levels
- Traumatic subdural hematoma with liver-induced hypocoagulability
- Fetal alcohol syndrome

PROGNOSIS

- The mortality rate from delirium tremens has steadily decreased with early diagnosis and improved treatment

WHEN TO REFER

- Alcoholics Anonymous (AA)
- Al-Anon for the spouse

WHEN TO ADMIT

- Hallucinosis or severe withdrawal symptoms
- Comorbid conditions (eg, advanced liver disease) that may decompensate during alcohol withdrawal
- Hospitalization is usually not necessary

EVIDENCE

PRACTICE GUIDELINES

- National Guideline Clearinghouse: Screening and counseling. U.S. Preventive Services Task Force, 2004
  - http://www.guideline.gov/summary/summary.aspx?doc_id=4618

WEB SITE

- National Institutes of Health: National Institute on Alcohol Abuse and Alcoholism
  - http://www.niaaa.nih.gov/

INFORMATION FOR PATIENTS

- JAMA patient page. Alcohol abuse and alcoholism.JAMA 2005;293:1694. [PMID:15811988]
- JAMA patient page: Alcohol use and heart disease. JAMA 2001;285:2040. [PMID:11336048]
- JAMA Patient Page: alcohol and driving. JAMA 2000;283:2340. [PMID: 10807396]
- National Institute on Alcohol Abuse and Alcoholism
  - http://www.niaaa.nih.gov/publications/brochures.htm

REFERENCES

- Adams WL et al: Screening for problem drinking in older primary care patients. JAMA 1996;276:1964. [PMID:897110650]
- Helping patients with alcohol problems. A health practitioner's guide. NIH Publication No. 03-3769, 2003.

Author(s)

Stuart J. Eisendrath, MD

Jonathan E. Lichtmacher, MD

Alkalosis, Metabolic

KEY FEATURES

ESSENTIALS OF DIAGNOSIS

- Characterized by high HCO_3^-, which is also seen in chronic respiratory acidosis but pH differentiates the two disorders
- Compensatory increase in Pco_2 rarely 55 mm Hg. A higher value implies a superimposed respiratory acidosis
- Effective circulating volume status and urinary chloride concentration help distinguish between saline-responsive and saline-unresponsive metabolic alkalosis

GENERAL CONSIDERATIONS

- Etiology can be classified into saline responsive or saline unresponsive (Table 87)
- **Saline responsive**
  - By far the more common disorder
  - Characterized by normotensive extracellular volume contraction
  - Less frequently, hypotension or orthostatic hypotension are seen
  - Generally associated with hypokalemia, due partly to the direct effect of alkalosis per se on renal potassium excretion and partly to secondary hyperaldosteronism from volume contraction
- **Saline unresponsive**
  - Implies a volume-expanded state as from hyperaldosteronism with accompanying hypokalemia from the renal mineralocorticoid effect

Etiology

- **Saline responsive (UCl < 10 mEq/day)**
- Excessive body bicarbonate content
  - *Renal alkalosis*
    - Diuretic therapy
    - Poorly reabsorbable anion therapy (carbenicillin, penicillin, sulfate, phosphate)
    - Posthypercapnia
  - Gastrointestinal alkalosis
    - Loss of HCl from vomiting or nasogastric suction
    - Intestinal alkalosis: chloride diarrhea
  - Exogenous alkali
    - $NaHCO_3$ (baking soda)
    - Sodium citrate, lactate, gluconate, acetate
    - Transfusions
    - Antacids
- Normal body bicarbonate content
  - Contraction alkalosis
- **Saline unresponsive (UCl > 10 mEq/day)**
- Excessive body bicarbonate content
  - Renal alkalosis, normotensive
    - Bartter's syndrome (renal salt wasting and secondary hyperaldosteronism)
    - Severe potassium depletion
    - Refeeding alkalosis
    - Hypercalcemia and hypoparathyroidism
  - Renal alkalosis, hypertensive
    - Endogenous mineralocorticoids (primary hyperaldosteronism, hyperreninism, adrenal enzyme deficiency: 11- and 17-hydroxylase, Liddle's syndrome)
    - Exogenous mineralocorticoids (licorice)

CLINICAL FINDINGS

SYMPTOMS AND SIGNS

- No characteristic symptoms or signs
- Orthostatic hypotension may occur
- Weakness and hyporeflexia occur if serum K^+ is markedly low
- Tetany and neuromuscular irritability occur rarely

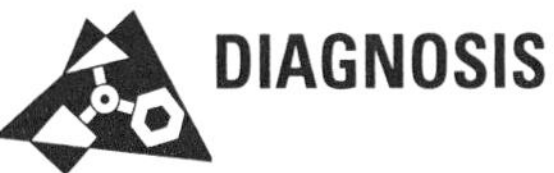

DIAGNOSIS

LABORATORY TESTS

- Elevated arterial blood pH and bicarbonate
- Arterial Pco_2 is increased
- Serum potassium and chloride are decreased
- There may be an increased anion gap
- Urinary chloride is low (< 10 mEq/day) in saline-responsive disorders
- Urinary chloride is higher (> 10 mEq/day) in saline-unresponsive disorders

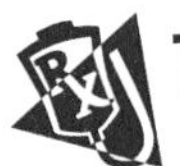

TREATMENT

MEDICATIONS

Saline-responsive metabolic alkalosis

- Correct the extracellular volume deficit with adequate amounts of 0.9% NaCl and KCl
- For alkalosis due to nasogastric suction, discontinuation of diuretics and administration of H_2-blockers can be useful
- Acetazolamide, 250–500 mg intravenously every 4–6 h, can be used if cardiovascular status prohibits adequate volume repletion
  - Watch for the development of hypokalemia
- Administration of acid can be used as emergency therapy
  - HCl, 0.1 mol/L, is infused via a central vein (the solution is sclerosing)
  - Dosage is calculated to decrease the HCO_3^- level by one-half over 24 h, assuming a HCO_3^- volume of distribution (L) of 0.5 × body weight (kg)

Saline-unresponsive metabolic alkalosis

- Block aldosterone effect with an angiotensin-converting enzyme inhibitor or with spironolactone
- Metabolic alkalosis in primary hyperaldosteronism can be treated only with potassium repletion

THERAPEUTIC PROCEDURES

- Mild alkalosis is generally well tolerated
- Severe or symptomatic alkalosis (pH > 7.60) requires urgent treatment
- Patients with marked renal insufficiency may require dialysis

SURGERY

- Therapy for saline-unresponsive metabolic alkalosis includes surgical removal of a mineralocorticoid-producing tumor

OUTCOME

WHEN TO REFER

- If expertise is needed for the work-up
- Treatment of saline-unresponsive metabolic alkalosis

WHEN TO ADMIT

- Persistent metabolic alkalosis in the absence of hypovolemia or associated with severe hypokalemia
- If administration of acid is needed for emergency therapy

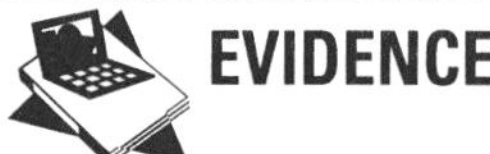

EVIDENCE

WEB SITE

- National Kidney Foundation
  - http://www.kidney.org/

INFORMATION FOR PATIENTS

- MedlinePlus: Alkalosis
  - http://www.nlm.nih.gov/medlineplus/ency/article/001183.htm
- MedlinePlus: Bartter's Syndrome
  - http://www.nlm.nih.gov/medlineplus/ency/article/000308.htm
- MedlinePlus: Milk-Alkali Syndrome
  - http://www.nlm.nih.gov/medlineplus/ency/article/000332.htm

REFERENCES

- Adrogue HJ et al: Management of life threatening acid base disorders. (Part 2.) N Engl J Med 1998;338:107. [PMID: 98069970]
- Galla JH: Metabolic alkalosis. J Am Soc Nephrol 2000;11:369. [PMID: 10665945]
- Khanna A: Metabolic alkalosis. Respir Care 2001;46:354. [PMID: 11262555]

Author(s)

Masafumi Fukagawa, MD, PhD
Kiyoshi Kurokawa, MD, MACP
Maxine A. Papadakis, MD

Allergy, Drug & Food

KEY FEATURES

ESSENTIALS OF DIAGNOSIS

- An IgE-mediated reaction to a drug
- Many drugs have toxicities or idiosyncratic reactions that are not immune mediated and therefore are not drug allergies
- 90% of food allergies are caused by peanuts, tree nuts, fish, and shellfish

GENERAL CONSIDERATIONS

- Immediate hypersensitivity
  - Previously sensitized individuals
  - Rapid development of urticaria, angioedema, or anaphylaxis
- Immune complex-mediated disorder
  - Delayed onset of urticaria accompanied by fever, arthralgias, and nephritis
- Immune hypersensitivity mechanisms
  - Drug fever
  - Stevens-Johnson syndrome
- Some drugs are clearly more immunogenic than others, and this can be reflected in the incidence of drug hypersensitivity
- Partial list of drugs frequently implicated in drug reactions
  - β-Lactam antibiotics, sulfonamides
  - Phenytoin, carbamazepine
  - Allopurinol
  - Muscle relaxants used for general anesthesia
  - Nonsteroidal antiinflammatory drugs
  - Antisera
  - Antiarrhythmic agents
- Drug toxicities, drug interactions, or idiosyncratic reactions must be distinguished from true hypersensitivity reactions because the prognosis and management differ
- Food hypersensitivity must be distinguished from more common food intolerance (eg, lactose intolerance).

DEMOGRAPHICS

- Some estimate that 10% or less of adverse reactions to drugs are true hypersensitivity reactions

CLINICAL FINDINGS

SYMPTOMS AND SIGNS

- Urticaria
- Angioedema
- Anaphylaxis
- Fever, arthralgias, nephritis
- Stevens-Johnson syndrome
- Morbilliform eruptions, lupus-like skin syndromes, cutaneous vasculitides
- Atopic dermatitis
- Oral allergy syndrome (pruritis of lips, tongue, palate without systemic anaphylaxis)

DIFFERENTIAL DIAGNOSIS

- Vasculitis
- Erythema multiforme
- Contact dermatitis (eg, poison oak or ivy)
- Erythema migrans (Lyme disease)
- Arthropod bites (insect bites)
- Physical factors: heat, cold, solar, pressure, water, vibratory
- Cholinergic urticaria: exercise, excitement, hot showers
- Other allergic causes: feathers, dander, shellfish, tomatoes, strawberries, vaccines, chemicals, cosmetics
- Infection (eg, otitis media, sinusitis, hepatitis)
- Serum sickness
- Angioedema: hereditary or acquired complement-mediated, angiotensin-converting enzyme inhibitors
- Food intolerance

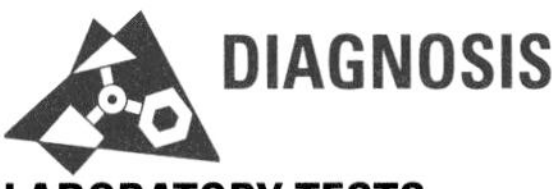

DIAGNOSIS

LABORATORY TESTS

Allergy testing

- Observed allergic reaction in the setting of a new or old drug
- Skin testing (available for very few drugs, eg, penicillin)
- A negative penicillin skin test makes penicillin allergy unlikely
- If the likelihood of immunological reaction is low—based on the history and the assessment of likely offending agents—and if no allergy testing is available, judicious test dose challenges may be considered in a monitored setting (performed only by a practitioner skilled and experienced with these procedures)
- If the likelihood of an IgE-mediated reaction is significant, these challenges are risky and rapid drug desensitization is indicated
- The gold standard for allergy food testing is skin-prick testing with actual food items, but due to the potential risk for systemic reactions, testing is usually preceded by IgE RAST testing and/or skin-prick testing with commercially available extracts.

Provocation tests

- Bronchoprovocation testing
  - Obtain serial determinations of peak expiratory flow rate (PEFR) using a portable peak flowmeter during periods of natural exposure to a suspected airborne allergen
  - May be helpful in some cases of occupational asthma
- Oral provocation
  - In most cases of suspected allergy to a food or drug, placebo-controlled oral challenge is the definitive test
  - Freeze-dried foods in large opaque capsules provide a sufficient dose of allergen for testing
  - This test should be conducted in a monitored setting and should not be administered to patients with suspected food-induced anaphylaxis

Alkalosis, Respiratory p. 1020. Alkaptonuria p. 1020.
Allergic Bronchopulmonary Aspergillosis (ABPA) p. 1020.

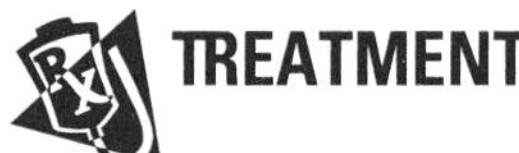

TREATMENT

MEDICATIONS

- Same as other allergic reactions (antihistamines, steroids, or subcutaneous epinephrine)
- Acute rapid desensitization can be done if the drug (eg, penicillin or insulin) must be administered
- Rapid escalation of miniscule doses of the drug is followed by full-dose administration
- This is accomplished by a course of oral or parenteral doses starting with extremely low doses (dilutions of 1×10^{-6} or 1×10^{-5} units) and increasing to the full dose over a period of hours
- Slow desensitization protocols are available for patients with late-appearing morbilliform eruptions (sulfamethoxazole-induced dermatitis in AIDS patients, aspirin, NSAIDs, allopurinol). Any history of toxic epidermal necrolysis or Stevens-Johnson syndrome is an absolute contraindication to drug readministration
- Epi-Pen, as indicated

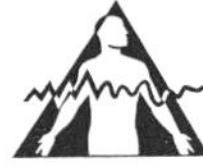

OUTCOME

WHEN TO REFER

- Refer to an allergist for specialized diagnostic or therapeutic interventions, such as oral provocation or rapid desensitization

WHEN TO ADMIT

- For rapid desensitization procedures, especially when there is a history of possible or probable anaphylaxis. This procedure carries significant risk and should be undertaken in an intensively monitored setting

PREVENTION

- The drug and all chemically related compounds should be avoided in the future
- Many antigens involved in oral allergy syndrome denature during cooking

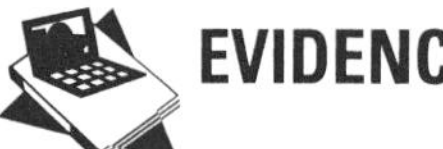

EVIDENCE

PRACTICE GUIDELINES

- Joint Task Force on Practice Parameters, the American Academy of Allergy, Asthma and Immunology, and the Joint Council of Allergy, Asthma and Immunology. Executive summary of disease management of drug hypersensitivity: a practice parameter. Ann Allergy Asthma Immunol 1999;83(6 Pt 3):665. [PMID: 10616910]

WEB SITES

- American Academy of Allergy, Asthma, and Immunology
  - http://www.aaaai.org
- MedlinePlus: Allergy
  - http://www.nlm.nih.gov/medlineplus/allergy.html

INFORMATION FOR PATIENTS

- JAMA patient page: Understanding allergies. JAMA 2000;283:424. [PMID: 10647806]
- Medem and American College of Allergy, Asthma and Immunology: Drug Reactions
  - http://www.medem.com/search/article_display.cfm?path=TANQUERAYM_ContentItem&mstr=/M_ContentItem/ZZZEA5MS2BC.html&soc=Medem-ACAAI&srch_typ=NAV_SERCH
- MedlinePlus: Drug Allergies
  - http://www.nlm.nih.gov/medlineplus/allergy.html

REFERENCES

- Drain KL: Preventing and managing drug-induced anaphylaxis. Drug Safety 2001;24:843. [PMID: 11665871]
- Fogg MI et al: Management of food allergies. Expert Opin Pharmacother 2003;4:1025. [PMID: 12831331]
- Grammer LC et al: Drug allergy and protocols for management of drug allergies, 3rd ed. Part II. General principles of prevention of allergic drug reactions. Allergy Asthma Proc 2004;25:267.
- Nigen S et al: Drug eruptions: approaching the diagnosis of drug-induced skin diseases. J Drugs Dermatol 2003;2:278. [PMID: 12848112]
- Tang AW: A practical guide to anaphylaxis. Am Fam Physician 2003;68:1325. Erratum in Am Fam Physician 2004;69:1049. [PMID: 14567487]

Author(s)

Jeffrey L. Kishiyama, MD
Daniel C. Adelman, MD

Amebiasis

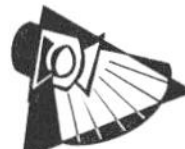

KEY FEATURES

ESSENTIALS OF DIAGNOSIS

- Mild to severe colitis
- Amebas or antigen in stools; serological tests positive with severe colitis

GENERAL CONSIDERATIONS

- The *Entamoeba* complex contains two morphologically identical species
  - *E dispar* (about 90% of the complex), which remains in the colon in a stable asymptomatic carrier state
  - *E histolytica*, whose virulence can range from asymptomatic to fulminant colitis and to extraintestinal infections
- Humans are the only established host
- The organisms exist in two forms: only cysts are infectious, since after ingestion they survive gastric acidity, which destroys trophozoites
- Transmission occurs through ingestion of cysts from fecally contaminated food or water; transmission can result from contamination of food by the hands of food handlers
- Because infection can be transmitted person-to-person, all household members and sexual partners should have their stools examined
- Flies and other arthropods also serve as mechanical vectors
- Corticosteroids and other immunosupressive drugs may convert a commensal infection into an invasive one

DEMOGRAPHICS

- The infections are worldwide but are most prevalent in tropical areas with crowded conditions
- Urban outbreaks have occurred because of common-source water contamination
- Of 500 million persons worldwide infected with *Entamoeba*, an estimated 10% (50 million) are infected with *E histolytica*
- Mortality is about 100,000 per year

CLINICAL FINDINGS

SYMPTOMS AND SIGNS

- Acute onset of severe diarrhea can occur as early as 8 days after infection
- Some patients may be asymptomatic or have mild recurrent symptoms for months to years before severe colitis or liver abscess appears
- Transition may occur from one type of intestinal infection to another, and each may give rise to hepatic abscess
- **Mild to moderate colitis (nondysenteric colitis)**
  - Few semiformed stools a day; no blood
  - Abdominal cramps, flatulence, fatigue, weight loss, abdominal distention and tenderness; fever is uncommon
  - Periods of remission and recurrence may last days to weeks; during remissions, there may be constipation
  - In some patients with chronic infection, the colon is thick and palpable, particularly over the cecum and descending colon
  - Mild hepatomegaly and tenderness
- **Severe colitis (dysenteric colitis)**
  - Several liquid stools with blood streaking
  - With larger numbers of stools, 10–20 or more, little fecal material is present, but blood (fresh or dark) and bits of necrotic tissue may be evident
  - The patient may become prostrate and toxic, with fever up to 40.5°C, colic, vomiting, diffuse abdominal tenderness, hepatic tenderness
- **Localized ulcerative lesions of the colon**
  - Rectal ulcerations may result in passage of formed stools with bloody exudate
  - Cecal ulcerations may induce mild diarrhea and simulate appendicitis
  - Amebic appendicitis is rare
- **Localized granulomatous lesions of the colon (ameboma)**
  - The masses may present as an irregular tumor(s) projecting into the bowel or as an annular constricting mass up to several centimeters in length
  - May mimic colonic carcinoma, tuberculosis, or lymphogranuloma venereum
- **Extraintestinal amebiasis**
  - See Amebic liver disease
  - Perianal skin infections
  - Lungs, brain, genitalia, and elsewhere

DIFFERENTIAL DIAGNOSIS

- Inflammatory bowel disease
- Giardiasis
- *Shigella, Salmonella, Campylobacter*
- Irritable bowel syndrome
- Lactase deficiency
- Cryptosporidiosis, cyclosporiasis
- Annular carcinoma of the bowel

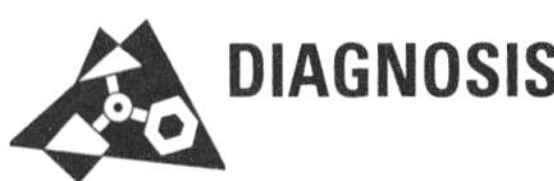

DIAGNOSIS

LABORATORY TESTS

Intestinal amebiasis

- Diagnosis is made by finding *E histolytica* or its antigen in stool or by serology
- **Microscopic stool examination**
  - Testing three specimens obtained under optimal conditions will generally detect 80% of *Entamoeba* complex infections (but does not distinguish between *E histolytica* and *E dispar*); three additional tests will raise the diagnostic rate to 90%
  - Collect three specimens at 2-day intervals or longer, with one of the three obtained after a laxative such as sodium sulfate or phosphate (Fleet's Phospho-Soda), 30–60 g in a glass of water; or bisacodyl 5–15 mL
  - If the patient has received specific therapy, antibiotics, barium, antimalarials, antidiarrheal agents (containing bismuth, kaolin, or magnesium hydroxide), or mineral oil, specimen collection should be delayed
  - *E histolytica* and *E dispar* can be differentiated by methods that are sensitive and specific and do not require culture
    - Polymerase chain reaction-based assays
    - The detection of *E histolytica*-specific galactose/N-acetyl-d-galactosamine
    - The coproantigen TechLab *Entamoeba* test (sensitivity 93%, specificity 97%) requires fresh or frozen stool specimens; preserved stool cannot be used
- **Serology**
  - The ELISA and enzyme immunoassays are positive only in the case of *E histolytica* infection
    - About 70% of patients with active intestinal disease (the frequency is lower in mild colitis, higher in dysentery) and about 10% of asymptomatic *E histolytica* cyst passers will have positive serologic tests
    - False-positive results are rare
    - The tests remain positive up to 10 years after successful treatment

- The agar gel immunodiffusion test becomes negative 36 months after eradication of the organism
- **Other tests**
  - Detection of trophozoites that contain ingested red blood cells is nearly diagnostic for invasive *E histolytica*
  - Fecal occult blood is frequently positive in amebic colitis, whereas findings for fecal leukocytes are noncontributory
  - The white blood cell count can reach 20,000/μL or higher in amebic dysentery but is not elevated in mild colitis
  - A low-grade eosinophilia is occasionally present

DIAGNOSTIC PROCEDURES

- Colonoscopy is preferred over sigmoidoscopy. The bowel should not be cleansed by laxative or enema as this washes exudate from the ulcers and destroys trophozoites
- Rectal biopsy (from the edge of the ulcer) may enhance diagnosis

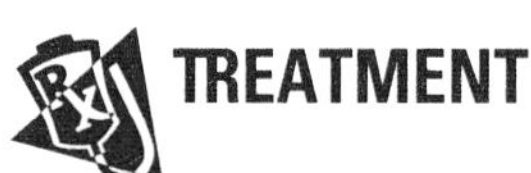

TREATMENT

MEDICATIONS

- See Table 143
- The decision to treat is based on finding *Entamoeba* cysts or trophozoites and, when feasible (rarely), differentiating *E histolytica* from *E dispar*; testing for *E histolytica* antigen in stool; and testing for serum antibody
- The **tissue amebicides** dehydroemetine and emetine act on organisms in the bowel wall but not on amebas in the bowel lumen; dehydroemetine may be the safer drug
- Chloroquine is principally active against amebas in the liver
- The **luminal amebicides** diloxanide furoate (not available in the United States), iodoquinol, and paromomycin act on organisms in the bowel lumen but are ineffective against amebas in the bowel wall or other tissues
- Tinidazole and metronidazole are effective both in the bowel lumen and bowel and in extraintestinal tissues
  - Tinidazole or metronidazole plus a luminal amebicide is the treatment of choice
  - Tinidazole has a shorter course and may be better tolerated but is more expensive than metronidazole
- Proceed with anti-*E histolytica* treatment in patients with intestinal symptoms who have *Entamoeba* organisms in the stool in whom *E dispar* and *E histolytica* cannot be differentiated because the results of the stool antigen and serum antibody tests may be falsely negative and *E histolytica* infection may be present

Severe intestinal disease

- Fluid and electrolyte therapy and opioids to control bowel motility are necessary adjuncts. Use opioids cautiously because of the risk of toxic megacolon

THERAPEUTIC PROCEDURES

- In asymptomatic cyst-passers, if stool antigen and serum antibody tests are negative, the infection is presumed to be *E dispar*, and should not be treated
- Within endemic areas, asymptomatic carriers generally are not treated because of the frequency of reinfection

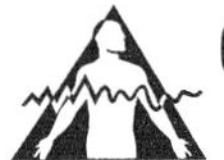

OUTCOME

FOLLOW-UP

- Examine at least three stools at 2- to 3-day intervals, starting 2–4 weeks after the end of treatment
- Colonoscopy and reexamination of stools within 3 months may be indicated

COMPLICATIONS

- See Amebic liver disease
- Rare complications include appendicitis, bowel perforation, massive mucosal sloughing, and hemorrhage; death may follow

PROGNOSIS

- The mortality rate from untreated amebic dysentery or ameboma may be high
- With chemotherapy instituted early in the course of the disease, the prognosis is good

WHEN TO REFER

- Progressive colitis despite therapy

WHEN TO ADMIT

- Severe colitis or hepatic abscess

PREVENTION

- Hand washing
- Water supplies can be boiled (briefly) or treated with iodine (0.5 mL tincture of iodine per liter for 20 min, or longer if the water is cold)
  - Cysts are resistant to standard concentrations of chlorine
  - Filters are also available to purify drinking water
- Disinfection dips for fruits and vegetables are not advised
- No drug is effective in prophylaxis

EVIDENCE

PRACTICE GUIDELINES

- National Guideline Clearinghouse
  - http://www.guideline.gov/summary/summary.aspx?doc_id=2791

WEB SITE

- Centers for Disease Control and Prevention—Division of Parasitic Diseases
  - http://www.cdc.gov/ncidod/dpd/parasites/amebiasis/default.htm

INFORMATION FOR PATIENTS

- Centers for Disease Control and Prevention
  - http://www.cdc.gov/ncidod/dpd/parasites/amebiasis/factsht_amebiasis.htm
- Nemours Foundation
  - http://kidshealth.org/parent/infections/parasitic/amebiasis.html
- National Institutes of Health
  - http://www.nlm.nih.gov/medlineplus/ency/article/000298.htm

REFERENCES

- http://www.nlm.nih.gov/medlineplus/ency/article/000298.htm
- Blessmann J et al: Treatment of asymptomatic intestinal *Entamoeba histolytica* infection. N Engl J Med 2002;347:1384. [PMID: 12397207]
- Petri WA: *Entamoeba histolytica*: clinical update and vaccine prospects. Curr Infect Dis Rep 2002;4:124. [PMID: 11927043]

Amebic Liver Disease

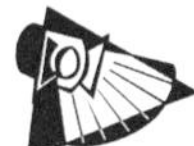

KEY FEATURES

ESSENTIALS OF DIAGNOSIS

- Fever, hepatomegaly, pain, localized tenderness
- Amebas or antigen in stool or abscess aspirate; positive serologic tests
- Abscess by ultrasound or CT scan

GENERAL CONSIDERATIONS

- *Entamoeba histolytica* is hematogenously spread from the colon to the liver
- Hepatic abscesses range from a few millimeters to 15 cm or larger, usually are single, occur more often in the right lobe (particularly the upper portion), and are more common in men

DEMOGRAPHICS

- Of 500 million persons worldwide infected with *Entamoeba*, most are infected with nonpathogenic *E dispar* and an estimated 10% (50 million) with potentially pathogenic *E histolytica*. Invasive *E histolytica* may constitute 5 million cases, with mortality in the range of 100,000 per year
- Amebic liver abscess, although a relatively infrequent (3–9%) consequence of *E histolytica* intestinal amebiasis, is not uncommon given the large number of intestinal infections

CLINICAL FINDINGS

SYMPTOMS AND SIGNS

- Many patients do not have current or a past history of intestinal symptoms
- The onset of symptoms can be sudden or gradual, ranging from a few days to many months
- Cardinal manifestations are
  - Fever (often high)
  - Pain (continuous, stabbing, or pleuritic, and sometimes severe)
  - An enlarged and tender liver
- There may be malaise or prostration, sweating, chills, anorexia, and weight loss
- The liver enlargement may present subcostally, in the epigastrium, as a localized bulging of the rib cage, or, as a result of enlargement against the dome of the diaphragm, it may produce coughing and findings of consolidation at the right lung base
- Intercostal tenderness is common
- Localizing signs on the skin over the liver may be an area of edema or a point of maximum tenderness

DIFFERENTIAL DIAGNOSIS

- Pyogenic liver abscess
- Echinococcosis (hydatid disease)
- Cholecystitis or cholangitis
- Right lower lobe pneumonia
- Pancreatitis
- Hepatocellular carcinoma

DIAGNOSIS

LABORATORY TESTS

- The white blood cell count ranges from 15,000 to 25,000/μL without eosinophilia
- Liver function test abnormalities, when present, are usually minimal
- Examination of stools for antigen and the organism is frequently negative
- Serologic tests (ELISA and enzyme immunoassay) are almost always positive by 1 week after onset of hepatic symptoms or earlier as a result of chronic intestinal infection
- The indirect hemagglutination test (a positive titer is 1:128 or a higher dilution) stays positive for as long as 10 years after successful treatment and does not distinguish between past and new infections
- The agar gel test, though less sensitive, is rapidly conducted and may detect current infection because it becomes negative 3–6 months after eradication of the organism
- Detection of trophozoites in stool that contain ingested red blood cells is nearly diagnostic for invasive *E histolytica* but may be confused with the occasional *E dispar* or macrophage that also contains the red blood cells

IMAGING STUDIES

- Elevation of the right dome of the diaphragm and the size and location of the abscess can be determined by
  - Ultrasonography (usually round or oval nonhomogeneous lesions, abrupt transition from normal liver to the lesion, hypoechoic center with diffuse echoes throughout the abscess)
  - CT scan (well-defined, round, low-density lesions with an internal, nonhomogeneous structure)
  - MRI
  - Radioisotope scanning
- After IV injection of contrast material, CT scan may show a hyperdense halo around the periphery of the abscess
- Gallium scans, infrequently useful, show a cold spot as opposed to the increased gallium uptake in the center of pyogenic abscesses

DIAGNOSTIC PROCEDURES

- As CT, MRI, and sonography do not distinguish amebic and pyogenic abscesses, percutaneous aspiration may be indicated; this is best done by an image-guided needle (risks described below)
- The aspirate is divided into serial 30- to 50-mL aliquots, but only the last sample is examined for amebas, since the organisms are found at the edge of the cyst
- Detection of amebic antigen in aspirate appears to be very sensitive

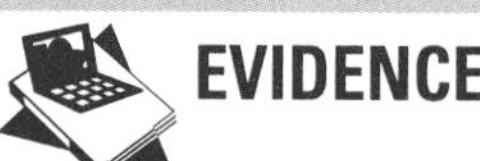

TREATMENT

MEDICATIONS

- See Table 143
- Treatment is metronidazole or tinidazole plus diloxanide furoate or iodoquinol followed by chloroquine
- There is no clinical evidence of tinidazole- or metronidazole-resistant *E histolytica*
- Chloroquine has been included in treatment to avoid rare long-term failures
- Treatment also requires a luminal amebicide (diloxanide furoate or iodoquinol), whether or not the organism is found in the stool
- If a satisfactory clinical response does not occur in 3 days, the abscess should be drained for therapeutic purposes and to exclude pyogenic abscess
- Continued failure to achieve an adequate clinical response requires changing to the potentially toxic alternative drug dehydroemetine (or emetine) plus chloroquine
- Antibiotics are added for concomitant bacterial liver abscess, although metronidazole itself is highly effective against anaerobic bacteria

THERAPEUTIC PROCEDURES

- Most treatments with tinidazole or metronidazole do not require therapeutic percutaneous drainage. When needed, the catheter method is preferred. Indications are a large abscess (> 5–10 cm), threatening rupture; the presence of a left lobe abscess (due to the risk of perforation into the peritoneum); and the absence of medical response after 3 days of metronidazole therapy to exclude pyogenic abscess
- The risks of aspiration or catheter drainage are
  - Bacterial superinfection
  - Bleeding
  - Peritoneal spillage
  - Inadvertent puncture of an infected hydatid cyst

OUTCOME

FOLLOW-UP

- Imaging defects in the liver disappear slowly (range: 3–13 months) after treatment; some calcify

COMPLICATIONS

- Without prompt treatment, the abscess may rupture into the pleural, peritoneal, or pericardial space or other contiguous organs, and death may follow

PROGNOSIS

- With chemotherapy instituted early in the course of the disease, most patients are successfully treated

WHEN TO ADMIT

- All patients should be admitted

PREVENTION

- Hand washing
- Water supplies can be boiled (briefly) or treated with iodine (0.5 mL tincture of iodine per liter for 20 min, or longer if the water is cold); cysts are resistant to standard concentrations of chlorine
- Filters are available to purify drinking water
- Disinfection dips for fruits and vegetables are not advised
- No drug is effective in prophylaxis

EVIDENCE

INFORMATION FOR PATIENTS

- National Institutes of Health
  - http://www.nlm.nih.gov/medlineplus/ency/article/000211.htm
- Centers for Disease Control and Prevention
  - http://www.cdc.gov/ncidod/dpd/parasites/amebiasis/factsht_amebiasis.htm

REFERENCE

- Weinke T et al: Amebic liver abscess—rare need for percutaneous treatment modalities. Eur J Med Res 2002;7:25. [PMID: 11827837]

Amebic Meningoencephalitis, Primary

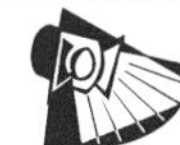

KEY FEATURES

ESSENTIALS OF DIAGNOSIS

- A fulminating, hemorrhagic, necrotizing meningoencephalitis
- It occurs in healthy children and young adults and is rapidly fatal

GENERAL CONSIDERATIONS

- It is caused by free-living amebas, most commonly by *Naegleria fowleri*
- Other causes are *Balamuthia mandrillaris* and the *Acanthamoeba* species, both of which may have a predilection for immunocompromised patients
- Nasal and throat swabs have shown a carrier state, and serologic surveys suggest that inapparent infections occur
- The organism apparently invades along the olfactory nerve to enter the central nervous system
- The incubation period varies from 2 to 15 days

DEMOGRAPHICS

- *N fowleri* is a thermophilic organism found in fresh and polluted warm lake water, domestic water supplies, swimming pools, thermal water, and sewers
- Most patients give a history of exposure to fresh water; dust is also a possible source

CLINICAL FINDINGS

SYMPTOMS AND SIGNS

- Early symptoms include headache, fever, and lethargy, often associated with rhinitis and pharyngitis
- Vomiting, disorientation, and other signs of meningoencephalitis develop within 1 or 2 days, followed by coma and then death within 7–10 days
- There may also be nonspecific myocarditis
- *B mandrillaris* meningoencephalitis runs a subacute course that can last months to 2 years

DIFFERENTIAL DIAGNOSIS

- No distinctive clinical features distinguish the infection from acute bacterial meningoencephalitis

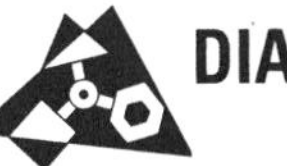

DIAGNOSIS

LABORATORY TESTS

- Lumbar or ventricular cerebrospinal fluid (CSF) contains several hundred to 25,000 leukocytes/μL (50–100% neutrophils) and erythrocytes (up to several thousand/μL)
- Protein is usually somewhat elevated, and glucose is normal or moderately reduced in CSF
- If conventional examinations for bacteria and fungi are negative, the fluid is examined for free-living amebas; phase contrast is preferred
  - A wet mount examined by an ordinary optical microscope with the aperture restricted or condenser down will enhance contrast and refractility; a warm stage is not needed
  - The fluid should not be centrifuged at speeds over 150 × *g* or refrigerated because this tends to immobilize the amebas (7–14 μm)
  - Their brisk motility distinguishes them from leukocytes of various types, which they closely resemble
  - Staining, culture, and mouse inoculation should be performed
- Precise species identification is based on morphology, demonstration of flagellate transformation (*Naegleria* only), and various immunologic methods
- Serologic testing is only useful epidemiologically; patients die before antibodies are detectable
- Diagnosis of *B mandrillaris* is based on brain biopsy; culture is not effective

IMAGING STUDIES

- With *B mandrillaris*, multiple hypodense lesions are seen with imaging studies

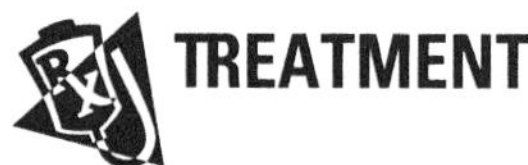

TREATMENT

MEDICATIONS

- A few well-documented survivors of *N fowleri* infection have been reported. One was treated with intravenous and intrathecal amphotericin B and another with a combination of amphotericin B, miconazole, and oral rifampin
- Several cases of *B mandrillaris* have been successfully treated with combination therapy using flucytosine, pentamidine, fluconazole, sulfadiazine, and azithromycin

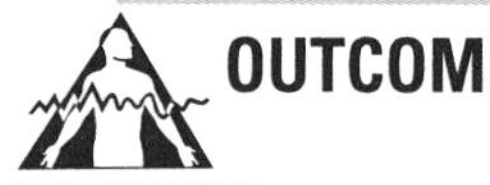

OUTCOME

PROGNOSIS

- In *B mandrillaris* infections, the usual course is subacute, with death occurring within 1 week to several months. No treatment is available

WHEN TO ADMIT

- All patients with confirmed or suspected disease

EVIDENCE

PRACTICE GUIDELINES

- National Guideline Clearinghouse
  - http://www.guideline.gov/summary/summary.aspx?doc_id=2446&nbr=1672&string=meningoencephalitis

WEB SITE

- Centers for Disease Control and Prevention—Division of Parasitic Diseases
  - http://www.cdc.gov/ncidod/dpd/parasites/naegleria/default.htm

INFORMATION FOR PATIENTS

- Centers for Disease Control and Prevention
  - http://www.cdc.gov/ncidod/dpd/parasites/naegleria/factsht_naegleria.htm

REFERENCE

- Doel I et al: Encephalitis due to a free-living amoeba (*Balamuthia mandrillaris*): case report with literature review. Surg Neurol 2000;53:611. [PMID: 10940434]

Amenorrhea, Primary p. 1021

Amenorrhea, Secondary & Menopause

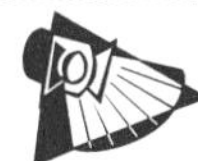

KEY FEATURES

ESSENTIALS OF DIAGNOSIS

- Secondary amenorrhea: absence of menses for 3 consecutive months in women who have passed menarche
- Menopause: termination of naturally occurring menses; usually diagnosed after 6 months of amenorrhea

GENERAL CONSIDERATIONS

Causes of secondary amenorrhea

- Pregnancy (high human chorionic gonadotropin [hCG]): most common cause. Rare: ectopic secretion of hCG by choriocarcinoma or bronchogenic carcinoma
- Hypothalamic-pituitary causes (low-normal follicle-stimulating hormone [FSH])
- "Hypothalamic amenorrhea": idiopathic, stress, strict dieting, vigorous exercise, organic illness, or anorexia nervosa
- Hyperprolactinemia, pituitary tumors, and glucocorticoid excess can suppress gonadotropins
- Hyperandrogenism (low-normal FSH): polycystic ovarian syndrome; anabolic steroids. Rare: adrenal P-450c21 deficiency, ovarian or adrenal malignancy, ectopic ACTH from malignancy, Cushing's disease
- Endometritis (normal FSH): scarring (Asherman's syndrome) occurring spontaneously, following delivery or D&C, or with tuberculosis or schistosomiasis in endemic areas
- Premature ovarian failure (high FSH) (primary hypogonadism before age 40): autoimmune, XO/XX chromosome mosaicism, bilateral oophorectomy, pelvic radiation therapy, and chemotherapy. Rare: myotonic dystrophy, galactosemia, mumps oophoritis, familial or idiopathic
- Menopause (high FSH)

DEMOGRAPHICS

- Normal age of menopause in the United States is 48–55 years (average 51.5 years)

CLINICAL FINDINGS

SYMPTOMS AND SIGNS

- Nausea and breast engorgement suggest pregnancy
- Hot flushes suggest ovarian failure
- Headache or visual field abnormalities suggest pituitary tumor. Thirst and polyuria with diabetes insipidus indicate hypothalamic or pituitary lesion. Acromegaly or gigantism indicate pituitary tumor
- Goiter suggests hyperthyroidism
- Weight loss, diarrhea, or skin darkening suggests adrenal insufficiency
- Weight loss with distorted body image suggests anorexia nervosa
- Galactorrhea suggests hyperprolactinemia due to pituitary tumor or various drugs
- Hirsutism or virilization occurs with hyperandrogenism
- Weakness, psychiatric changes, hypertension, central obesity, hirsutism, thin skin, ecchymoses suggest Cushing's syndrome or alcoholism
- Perform pelvic examination to check for uterine or adnexal enlargement
- Vasomotor instability (hot flushes), depression, irritability, fatigue, insomnia, headache, diminished libido, or rheumatological symptoms suggest menopause. Vasomotor instability in 80%, lasts seconds to many minutes; may be most severe at night or triggered by emotional stress, may persist for >5 years in 35%
- Urogenital atrophy, vaginal dryness, and dyspareunia; dysuria, frequency, and incontinence; osteoporotic fractures are late manifestations of estrogen deficiency

DIFFERENTIAL DIAGNOSIS

- Pregnancy
- Menopause or perimenopause
- Polycystic ovary syndrome
- Hypothalamic amenorrhea, eg, stress, weight change, exercise
- Hyperprolactinemia
- Hypothyroidism or hyperthyroidism
- Diabetes mellitus
- Premature ovarian failure
- Anorexia nervosa

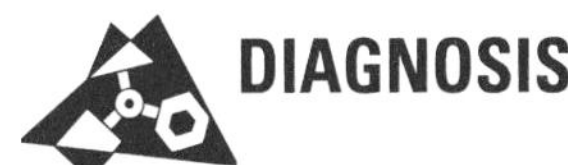

DIAGNOSIS

LABORATORY TESTS

- Serum pregnancy test for all women of childbearing age. False-positive tests may occur rarely with ectopic hCG secretion (eg, choriocarcinoma or bronchogenic carcinoma)
- Check serum prolactin, FSH, luteinizing hormone, thyroid-stimulating hormone, potassium, creatinine, and liver enzymes if not pregnant
- Check serum testosterone in hirsute or virilized women
- Perform 1-mg overnight dexamethasone suppression test (see *Cushing's syndrome*) if signs of hypercortisolism
- Perform Pap smear and vaginal smear to assess estrogen effect

IMAGING STUDIES

- Hyperprolactinemia or hypopituitarism without obvious cause should prompt pituitary MRI (see Hypopituitarism)

DIAGNOSTIC PROCEDURES

- Progestin withdrawal test: nonpregnant women with normal pelvic examination and laboratory tests are given a 10-day course of progestin (eg, medroxyprogesterone acetate 10 mg PO QD)
  - Absence of withdrawal menses indicates possible pregnancy, uterine abnormality, or estrogen deficiency
  - Occurrence of withdrawal bleeding indicates anovulation likely due to noncyclic gonadotropin secretion (eg, polycystic ovaries, idiopathic anovulation)

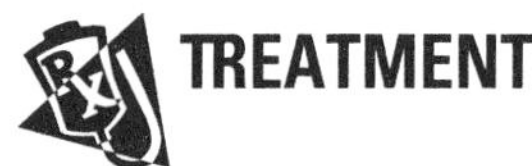

TREATMENT

MEDICATIONS

- Hormone replacement therapy (HRT) recommended for all women with premature ovarian failure (< 40 years of age) and for older women with ovarian failure on a case-by-case basis
- Lower-dose estrogen replacement is favored. Transdermal estradiol and vaginal estrogen are favored over oral estrogen. Progestins are added to conventional-dose estrogen, for women with a uterus, to avoid endometrial hyperplasia; exposure can be minimized or eliminated by using lower-dose estrogen or progestin-eluting IUDs
- Transdermal estradiol: do not apply to the breasts
- Vaginal estrogen creams, tablets, and rings: relieve vaginal dryness and discomfort, dyspareunia, urinary urgency, and dysuria; can cause endometrial proliferation with prolonged use
- Oral preparations include estrogen, estrogen plus progestin, and progestin
  - Progestin-eluting intrauterine devices (IUDs): available as levonorgestrel (eg, Norplant); replaced every 5 years. Best tolerated by parous women
- Hormone replacement therapy (HRT)
  - Benefits include improvement in hot flushes, vaginal moisture, sleep, rheumatic complaints; improved bone density and fewer fractures; protection of verbal memory (when initiated at menopause); improved skin moisture and thickness
  - Risks are dose-dependent; conventional doses carry higher risks than lower doses. Oral estrogens increase hepatic production of clotting factors (thereby increasing risks of deep vein thrombosis and stroke); increase the risk of deep vein thrombosis; can cause hypertriglyceridemia, particularly in women with preexistent hyperlipidemia, rarely resulting in pancreatitis; reduce the effectiveness of growth hormone replacement. These can be reduced or avoided by using nonoral estrogen replacement
- Estrogen replacement without progestin
  - Benefits: improvement in menopause-related depression; better control of type 2 diabetes mellitus; slightly reduced risk of breast cancer
  - Risks: increased risk of stroke among women taking conjugated equine estrogens; endometrial hyperplasia and dysfunctional uterine bleeding (DUB), endometrial carcinoma, although the absolute risk is low, and mortality from ovarian cancer, although the absolute risk is small
- Estrogen replacement with progestin
  - Benefits: women have a 0.7% lower risk for developing diabetes, reduced risk for dysfunctional uterine bleeding and endometrial carcinoma
  - Risks: conventional-dose oral combined HRT results in an increased risk for myocardial infarction (6 additional heart attacks per 10,000 women), mostly in preexistent corronary disease in the first year of therapy
- Selective estrogen receptor modulators (SERMs) (eg, raloxifene; Evista): an alternative to estrogen replacement for hypogonadal women at risk for osteoporosis who prefer not to take estrogens because of their contraindications (eg, breast or uterine cancer) or side effects

THERAPEUTIC PROCEDURES

- Treatment directed at underlying cause
- Postmenopausal women should be evaluated for osteoporosis and treated if appropriate (see Osteoporosis)

OUTCOME

FOLLOW-UP

- Hypothalamic amenorrhea: patients typically recover spontaneously but should have regular evaluations and a progestin withdrawal test about every 3 months to detect loss of estrogen effect

PROGNOSIS

- Ovarian failure (premature or menopausal): usually irreversible
- Menopause: increased bone osteoclastic activity increases risk for osteoporosis and fractures
- Menopause: increased LDL/HDL cholesterol ratio causes increased risk for atherosclerosis
- Diet adequate in protein, calories, calcium, and vitamins; calcium and vitamin D supplements and exercise for those at risk for osteoporosis
- Consider bisphosphonate if osteoporosis on bone densitometry
- Mammography recommended yearly for menopausal women receiving hormone replacement therapy
- Tamoxifen and raloxifene offer protection against osteoporosis but aggravate hot flushes

EVIDENCE

PRACTICE GUIDELINES

- Practice Committee of the American Society for Reproductive Medicine. Current evaluation of amenorrhea. Fertil Steril 2004;82:266. [PMID: 15237040]

INFORMATION FOR PATIENTS

- Mayo Clinic: Amenorrhea: When menstruation goes away
  - http://www.mayoclinic.com/invoke.cfm?id=HQ00224
- MedlinePlus: Secondary Amenorrhea
  - http://www.nlm.nih.gov/medlineplus/ency/article/001219.htm
- National Women's Health Information Center: Menopause
  - http://www.4woman.gov/faq/menopaus.htm

REFERENCES

- Anderson GL et al: Effects of conjugated equine estrogen in postmenopausal women with hysterectomy: the Women's Health Initiative randomized controlled trial. JAMA 2004;291:701. [PMID: 15082697]
- Lethaby A et al: Hormone replacement therapy in postmenopausal women: endometrial hyperplasia and irregular bleeding. Cochrane Database Syst Rev 2004;(3)CD000402. [PMID: 15266429]
- Sherwin BB: Estrogen and memory in women: how can we reconcile the findings? Horm Behav 2005;47:371. [PMID: 15708768]

Author(s)

Paul A. Fitzgerald, MD

Amphetamine & Cocaine Overdose

KEY FEATURES

ESSENTIALS OF DIAGNOSIS

- Agitation, paranoia, psychosis
- Seizures, hyperthermia
- Hypertension, tachycardia
- Hyponatremia may occur with methylenedioxymethamphetamine (MDMA, "ecstasy")

GENERAL CONSIDERATIONS

- Amphetamines and cocaine are widely abused for their euphorigenic and stimulant properties
- Both drugs may be smoked, snorted, ingested, or injected
- The toxic dose of each drug is highly variable and depends on the route of administration and individual tolerance
- Amphetamine derivatives and related drugs include methamphetamine ("crystal meth," "crank"), MDMA, and methcathinone ("cat")
- Nonprescription medications and nutritional supplements may contain stimulant or sympathomimetic drugs such as ephedrine or caffeine

CLINICAL FINDINGS

SYMPTOMS AND SIGNS

- Amphetamines and cocaine produce central nervous system stimulation and a generalized increase in central and peripheral sympathetic activity
- The onset of effects is most rapid after IV injection or smoking
- There may be anxiety, tremulousness, tachycardia, hypertension, diaphoresis, dilated pupils, agitation, muscular hyperactivity, and psychosis
- In severe intoxication, seizures and hyperthermia may occur

DIFFERENTIAL DIAGNOSIS

- Ephedrine
- Pseudoephedrine
- Anticholinergic poisoning
- Psychosis
- Heat stroke
- Alcohol or opiate withdrawal symptom

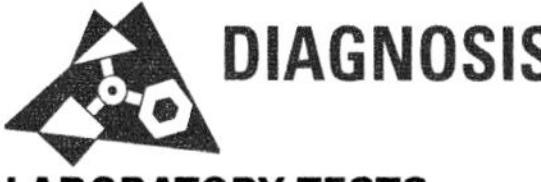

DIAGNOSIS

LABORATORY TESTS

- Amphetamines, cocaine, or the cocaine metabolite benzoylecgonine is found in the urine
- Blood screening is generally not sensitive enough to detect these drugs
- Metabolic acidosis may occur
- Hyponatremia has been reported after MDMA use
- Massive cocaine intoxication can cause QRS interval prolongation similar to tricyclic antidepressant overdose

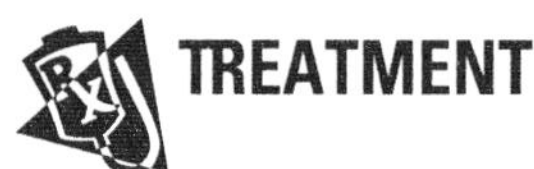

TREATMENT

MEDICATIONS

Emergency and supportive measures

- Rapidly lower the body temperature (see Hyperthermia) in patients who are hyperthermic (40°C)
- Treat agitation or psychosis with a benzodiazepine: lorazepam, 2–3 mg IV repeated PRN up to 8–10 mg, or midazolam, 0.1–0.2 mg/kg IM
- For poisoning by ingestion, administer activated charcoal 60–100 g orally or via gastric tube, mixed in aqueous slurry. Do not use for comatose or convulsing patients unless the activated charcoal can be given by gastric tube and the airway is protected by a cuffed endoctracheal tube
- Do *not* induce emesis because of the risk of seizures

Specific treatment

- Treat agitation with a sedative such as lorazepam, 2–3 mg IV
- Treat seizures with lorazepam or phenobarbital
- Treat hypertension with a vasodilator drug such as phentolamine, 1–5 mg IV, or nifedipine, 10–20 mg PO, or a combined α- and β-adrenergic blocker such as labetalol, 10–20 mg IV; do *not* administer a pure β-blocker such as propranolol alone because this may result in paradoxic worsening of the hypertension as a result of unopposed β-adrenergic effects
- Treat tachycardia or tachyarrhythmias with a short-acting β-blocker such as esmolol, 25–100 μg/kg/min by IV infusion
- Treat hyponatremia (see Hyponatremia)

OUTCOME

COMPLICATIONS

- Sustained or severe hypertension may result in intracranial hemorrhage, aortic dissection, or myocardial infarction
- Hyperthermia may cause multiorgan failure or permanent brain damage

PROGNOSIS

- Good if only a single brief seizure or mild-moderate agitation or cardiovascular effects
- Poor after severe hyperthermia (eg, temperature > 40°C) or intracranial hemorrhage

WHEN TO ADMIT

- Persistent hypertension, tachycardia
- Hyperthermia
- Multiple or prolonged seizures

EVIDENCE

PRACTICE GUIDELINES

- National Guideline Clearinghouse: VHA/DoD Clinical Practice Guideline for the Management of Substance Abuse Disorders
  - http://www.guideline.gov/summary/summary.aspx?doc_id=3169&nbr=2395&string=amphetamine

WEB SITES

- National Institute on Drug Abuse: InfoFacts: Crack and Cocaine
  - http://www.nida.nih.gov/Infofacts/cocaine.html
- eMedicine: Toxicology Articles
  - http://www.emedicine.com/emerg/TOXICOLOGY.htm

INFORMATION FOR PATIENTS

- JAMA patient page: Cocaine addiction. JAMA 2002;287:146. [PMID: 11797622]
- JAMA patient page: Drug abuse. JAMA 2000;283:1378. [PMID: 10714739]

REFERENCES

- Greene SL et al: Multiple toxicity from 3,4-methylenedioxymethamphetamine (ecstasy). Am J Emerg Med 2003; 21:121. [PMID: 12671812]
- Kashani J et al: Methamphetamine toxicity secondary to intravaginal body stuffing. J Toxicol Clin Toxicol 2004;42:987. [PMID: 15641645]

Author(s)

Kent R. Olson, MD

Amyloidosis

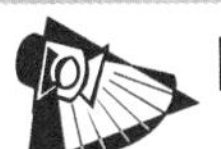

KEY FEATURES

ESSENTIALS OF DIAGNOSIS

- The diagnosis is based on clinical suspicion, family history, and preexisting long-standing infection or debilitating illness
- Microscopic examination of biopsy (eg, gingival, renal, rectal) or surgical specimens is diagnostic
- Fine-needle biopsy of subcutaneous abdominal fat is a simple and reliable method for diagnosing secondary systemic amyloidosis

GENERAL CONSIDERATIONS

- A group of disorders characterized by impaired organ function due to infiltration with insoluble protein fibrils
- Different fibrils are correlated with the clinical syndromes
- In **primary amyloidosis** (AL), the protein fibrils are monoclonal immunoglobulin light chains
- **Secondary amyloid** (AA) proteins are derived from acute-phase reactant apolipoprotein precursors
- Familial syndromes commonly cause infiltrative neuropathies
- Other types of amyloidosis may also be hereditary
- Over 20 types of fibrils have been identified in amyloid deposits
- Amyloidosis due to deposition of β_2-microglobulin in carpal ligaments occurs in chronic hemodialysis patients

CLINICAL FINDINGS

SYMPTOMS AND SIGNS

- Related to malfunction of the infiltrated organ
- The hereditary amyloidoses usually cause neuropathies

Primary amyloidosis

- Causes widespread disease
- Nephrotic syndrome and renal failure
- Cardiomyopathy and cardiac conduction defects
- Intestinal malabsorption and pseudo-obstruction
- Alzheimer's disease
- Carpal tunnel syndrome
- Macroglossia
- Peripheral neuropathy
- End-organ insufficiency of endocrine glands
- Respiratory failure
- Capillary damage with ecchymosis

Secondary amyloidosis

- Usually limited to the liver, spleen, and adrenals

DIFFERENTIAL DIAGNOSIS

- Multiple myeloma
- Hemochromatosis
- Sarcoidosis
- Waldenström's macroglobulinemia
- Metastatic cancer
- Other causes of nephrotic syndrome, eg, lupus nephritis

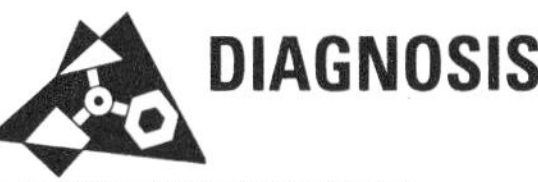

DIAGNOSIS

LABORATORY TESTS

- Monoclonal gammopathy on serum protein electrophoresis (in primary amyloidosis)

DIAGNOSTIC PROCEDURES

- Abdominal fat pad, rectal, or gingival biopsy with microscopic examination revealing amyloid protein (green birefringence under polarizing microscope after Congo red staining)
- In systemic disease, rectal or gingival biopsies show a sensitivity of about 80%, bone marrow biopsy about 50%, and abdominal fat aspiration between 70% and 80%

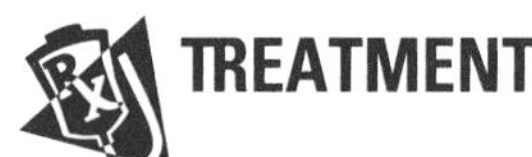

TREATMENT

MEDICATIONS

- Myeloma- or AL-associated amyloid can be treated with melphalan and prednisone

SURGERY

- Treatment of localized amyloid tumors is by surgical excision
- Some hereditary forms of amyloid are being treated with liver transplantation

THERAPEUTIC PROCEDURES

Systemic amyloidosis

- There is no effective treatment
- Supportive care/specific care pertinent to involved organs
- Hemodialysis and immunosuppressive therapy may be useful
- See *Alzheimer's disease*

Secondary disease

- Usually approached by aggressively treating the predisposing disease, but remission of fibril deposition does not occur
- Bone marrow transplant after chemotherapy has been employed in selected patients

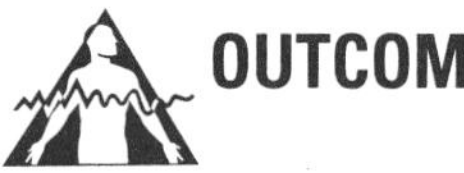

OUTCOME

PROGNOSIS

- Death usually occurs within 1–3 years of diagnosis with systemic amyloidosis

WHEN TO REFER

- Refer to a hematologist to confirm the diagnosis and for management
- Refer to a specialist on the organ(s) involved (eg, cardiologist, nephrologist)

EVIDENCE

PRACTICE GUIDELINES

- Guidelines Working Group of UK Myeloma Forum; British Committee for Standards in Haematology, British Society for Haematology: guidelines on the diagnosis and management of AL amyloidosis. Br J Haematol 2004;125:681. [PMID: 15180858]

WEB SITE

- Amyloidosis Support Network
  - http://www.amyloidosis.org

INFORMATION FOR PATIENTS

- Mayo Clinic: Amyloidosis
  - http://www.mayoclinic.com/invoke.cfm?id=DS00431

REFERENCES

- Ando Y et al: A novel tool for detecting amyloid deposits in systemic amyloidosis in vitro and in vivo. Lab Invest 2003;83:1751. [PMID: 14691293]
- Merlini G et al: Molecular mechanisms of amyloidosis. N Engl J Med. 2003;349:583. [PMID: 12904524]
- Skinner M et al: High-dose melphalan and autologous stem-cell transplantation in patients with AL amyloidosis: an 8-year study. Ann Intern Med 2004;140:85. [PMID: 14734330]

Author(s)

Jeffrey L. Kishiyama, MD
Daniel C. Adelman, MD

Anaphylaxis

Anaerobic Infections, Intra-Abdominal p. 1022. Anaerobic Infections, Skin & Soft Tissue p. 1023. Anaerobic Infections, Upper Respiratory Tract p. 1023.

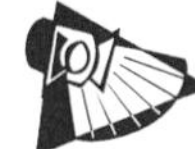

KEY FEATURES

ESSENTIALS OF DIAGNOSIS

- **Anaphylaxis**
  - Systemic reaction with cutaneous symptoms
  - Dyspnea, visceral edema, and hypotension
- **Urticaria**
  - Large, irregularly shaped, pruritic, erythematous wheals
- **Angioedema**
  - Painless subcutaneous swelling, often involving periorbital, circumoral, and facial regions
- These disorders may be diagnosed clinically, especially in the context of allergen exposure; detection of specific IgE or elevated serum tryptase can confirm diagnosis

GENERAL CONSIDERATIONS

- The most common allergens that induce this IgE antibody-mediated response are drugs, insect venoms, and foods
- A generalized release of mediators from mast cells can result in systemic anaphylaxis
- Can affect both nonatopic and atopic persons
- Isolated urticaria and angioedema are more common cutaneous forms of anaphylaxis with a better prognosis
- In about 10% of cases, chronic relapsing urticaria, angioedema, and anaphylaxis are not due to IgE-mediated hypersensitivity; consider underlying systemic disorders such as systemic mastocytosis or subclinical infection or inflammatory disorders
- Idiopathic autoimmune processes include the production of histamine-liberating autoantibodies directed against Fcε mast cell membrane receptors

DEMOGRAPHICS

In the United States

- The estimated prevalence of idiopathic anaphylaxis is 34,000 patients
- Food allergies cause an estimated 150 fatalities per year
- Most food allergy fatalities are due to peanuts, tree nuts, shellfish, and fish
- β-Lactam antibiotics may be involved in 400–800 fatalities per year
- Stinging insect venom causes about 50 fatalities per year
- 20% of the population will experience urticaria or angioedema during their lifetime

CLINICAL FINDINGS

SYMPTOMS AND SIGNS

- Hypotension/shock from widespread vasodilation
- Respiratory distress from bronchospasm or laryngeal edema
- Gastrointestinal or uterine smooth muscle contraction
- Flushing, pruritus, urticaria, and angioedema

DIFFERENTIAL DIAGNOSIS

- Other causes of shock
  - Sepsis
  - Cardiogenic
  - Hypovolemic
  - Neurogenic
- Asthma
- Adrenal insufficiency
- Vasovagal reaction

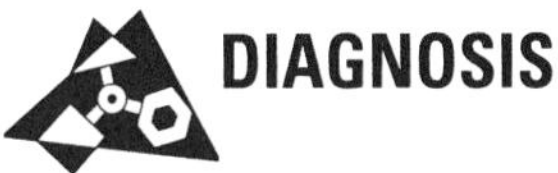

DIAGNOSIS

LABORATORY TESTS

- Based on the clinical presentation and a history of allergen exposure
- An elevated serum tryptase (a mast cell protease) measured during the episode can confirm the diagnosis
- Detection of a specific IgE, skin testing, or radioallergosorbent test (RAST) against the suspected antigen can confirm the allergic diathesis
- A serum C4 level is an adequate screening test in CI-esterase inhibitor deficiency/hereditary angioedema in patients with recurrent angioedema. The serum C4 level will usually be low when there is CI-esterase inhibitor deficiency

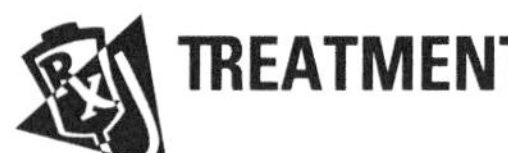

TREATMENT

MEDICATIONS

Anaphylaxis

- Epinephrine 1:1000 in a dose of 0.2–0.5 mL (0.2–0.5 mg) injected IM in the anterolateral thigh (more predictable and rapidly absorbed than injecting in the arm); repeated injections can be given every 5–15 min if necessary
- Rapid infusions of normal saline
- Inhaled β_2-adrenergic agonists, or IV aminophylline (0.5 mg/kg/h with 6-mg/kg loading dose over 30 min) for bronchospasm
- Antihistamines (H_1 and H_2 receptor antagonists) such as diphenhydramine (25–50 mg orally, intramuscularly, or intravenously every 4–6 h) and ranitidine (150 mg orally every 12 h or 50 mg intramuscularly or intravenously every 6–8 h)
- Anaphylaxis from β-adrenergic blocker drugs can be particularly problematic because of refractoriness to epinephrine and selective β-adrenergic agonists. Higher-dose adrenergic drugs are required: glucagon (0.5–1.0 mg intravenously, intramuscularly, or subcutaneously; may be repeated after 30 min) may be beneficial
- Intravenous corticosteroids (which may mitigate the late-phase response that occurs 24 h after onset)
- 12–24 h of observation
- See *Urticaria & angioedema*

THERAPEUTIC PROCEDURES

- Endotracheal intubation for laryngeal edema or severe bronchospasm

OUTCOME

FOLLOW-UP

- Follow up with an allergist and receive a subcutaneous epinephrine self-injection kit; further management may involve antihistamines or immunotherapy

WHEN TO REFER

- Early referral to an allergist may help with management
- Refer for desensitization and immunotherapy

WHEN TO ADMIT

- Patients with anaphylaxis should be admitted for 12–24 h of observation for recurrence of symptoms

PREVENTION

- Long-term combined oral antihistamine and prednisone therapy reduces the number and severity of attacks of life-threatening idiopathic anaphylaxis
- Medical therapy does not reliably prevent true IgE-mediated hypersensitivity reactions

Venom immunotherapy

- Patients with immediate hypersensitivity reactions to stinging insects and documented venom-specific IgE on allergy testing should receive a 5-year course of venom immunotherapy for prevention of anaphylaxis. Large, isolated, local reactions to insect stings are not a predisposing factor for systemic anaphylaxis
- Untreated individuals have a 50–60% risk of anaphylactic response to subsequent stings
- Venom immunotherapy provides 98% protection from life-threatening reactions on rechallenge

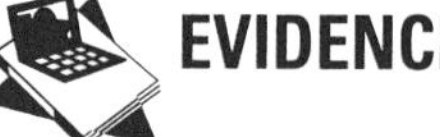

EVIDENCE

PRACTICE GUIDELINES

- Chamberlain D: Emergency medical treatment of anaphylactic reactions. Project Team of the Resuscitation Council (UK). J Accid Emerg Med 1999;16(4):243. [PMID: 10417927]
- The diagnosis and management of anaphylaxis. Joint Task Force on Practice Parameters, Work Group on Diagnosis and Management of Anaphylaxis. J Allergy Clin Immunol 1998;101:S465.
  - http://www.jcaai.org/Param/Anaphylax.htm

WEB SITES

- American Academy of Allergy, Asthma, and Immunology
  - http://www.aaaai.org
- Food Allergy & Anaphylaxis Network
  - http://www.foodallergy.org/anaphylaxis.html

INFORMATION FOR PATIENTS

- American Academy of Allergy, Asthma & Immunology: Anaphylaxis
  - http://www.aaaai.org/patients/resources/easy_reader/anaphylaxis.pdf
- American Academy of Allergy, Asthma & Immunology: What Is Anaphylaxis?
  - http://www.aaaai.org/patients/publicedmat/tips/whatisanaphylaxis.stm
- FamilyDoctor.org: Anaphylaxis
  - http://familydoctor.org/809.xml
- MedlinePlus: Anaphylaxis
  - http://www.nlm.nih.gov/medlineplus/ency/article/000844.htm

REFERENCES

- Charous BL: Natural rubber latex allergy after 12 years: recommendations and perspectives. J Allergy Clin Immunol 2002;109:31. [PMID: 11799362]
- Kaplan AP: Diagnostic tests for urticaria and angioedema. Clin Allergy Immunol 2000;15:111. [PMID: 10943290]
- Kemp SF: Anaphylaxis: a review of causes and mechanisms. J Allergy Clin Immunol 2002:110:341. [PMID: 12209078]

Author(s)

Jeffrey L. Kishiyama, MD
Daniel C. Adelman, MD

Anemia, Aplastic

Anal Cancer p. 1023. Anal Fissures p. 1024.

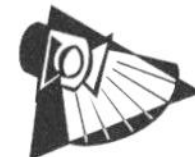

KEY FEATURES

ESSENTIALS OF DIAGNOSIS

- Pancytopenia
- No abnormal cells seen
- Hypocellular bone marrow

GENERAL CONSIDERATIONS

- In aplastic anemia, bone marrow failure and pancytopenia arise from injury to or abnormal expression of the hematopoietic stem cell

Causes of aplastic anemia

- "Idiopathic" (probably autoimmune)
- Drugs: chloramphenicol, phenylbutazone, gold salts, sulfonamides, phenytoin, carbamazepine, quinacrine, tolbutamide
- Viruses: hepatitis, Epstein-Barr virus, HIV, parvovirus B19
- Systemic lupus erythematosus
- Chemotherapy
- Radiation therapy
- Toxins: benzene, toluene, insecticides
- Posthepatitis
- Pregnancy
- Paroxysmal nocturnal hemoglobinuria
- Congenital (rare)

CLINICAL FINDINGS

SYMPTOMS AND SIGNS

- Weakness and fatigue from anemia
- Vulnerability to bacterial infections from neutropenia
- Mucosal and skin bleeding from thrombocytopenia
- Pallor, purpura, and petechiae
- Hepatosplenomegaly, lymphadenopathy, or bone tenderness should *not* be present

DIFFERENTIAL DIAGNOSIS

- Acute leukemia
- Myelodysplastic syndrome
- Bone marrow infiltrative process (eg, tumor, infection, granulomatous disease)
- Hypersplenism
- Viral infection (eg, parvovirus B19, hepatitis, HIV)
- Systemic lupus erythematosus

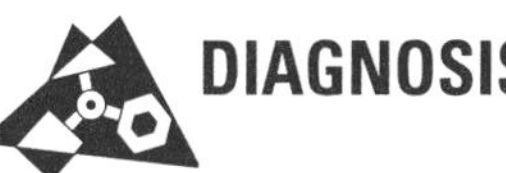

DIAGNOSIS

LABORATORY TESTS

- Pancytopenia, although in early disease only one or two cell lines may be reduced
- Anemia may be severe
- Reticulocytes always decreased
- Red blood cell morphology unremarkable
- Neutrophils and platelets reduced in number, no immature or abnormal forms seen
- Severe aplastic anemia defined by neutrophils $< 500/\mu L$, platelets $< 20,000/\mu L$, reticulocytes $< 1\%$, and bone marrow cellularity $< 20\%$

DIAGNOSTIC PROCEDURES

- Bone marrow aspirate and bone marrow biopsy appear hypocellular, with scant amounts of normal hematopoietic progenitors; no abnormal cells are seen

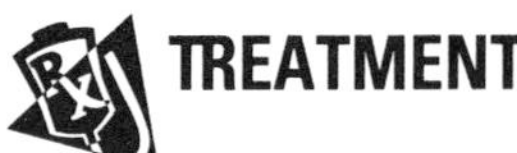

TREATMENT

MEDICATIONS

- Antibiotics to treat infections
- Immunosuppression with antithymocyte globulin (ATG) plus cyclosporine for severe aplastic anemia in adults aged > 50 or those without HLA-matched siblings
- Useful regimen is ATG, 40 mg/kg/day IV for 4 days, in combination with cyclosporine, 6 mg/kg PO BID, given in hospital in conjunction with corticosteroids, and transfusion and antibiotic support
- Corticosteroids are given with ATG (prednisone 1–2 mg/kg/day initially followed by rapid taper) to avoid complications of serum sickness
- High-dose cyclophosphamide (200 mg/kg) immunosuppression for refractory cases and in patients without suitable bone marrow donors
- Antibiotics and transfusion often required for prolonged pancytopenia (median 7 weeks of neutropenia)
- Androgens (eg, oxymetholone, 2–3 mg/kg PO QD) used commonly in past
- Despite low response rate, some patients can be maintained successfully with androgens

THERAPEUTIC PROCEDURES

- Supportive measures only for mild cases
- Allogeneic bone marrow transplantation for severe aplastic anemia in adults aged < 50 with HLA-matched siblings
- Allogeneic transplantation using unrelated donor for severe aplastic anemia in children or adults aged < 30
- Red blood cell and platelet transfusions as necessary

OUTCOME

COMPLICATIONS

- Infections
- Bleeding

PROGNOSIS

- Median survival in severe aplastic anemia without treatment is ~3 months, and 1-year survival is only 20%
- Allogeneic bone marrow transplantation is highly successful in children and young adults with HLA-matched siblings, with durable complete response rate > 80%
- ATG treatment produces partial response in ~60% of adults, usually in 4–12 weeks; long-term prognosis of responders is good
- Paroxysmal nocturnal hemoglobinuria or myelodysplasia or other clonal hematological disorders develop in < 25% of nontransplanted patients after many years of follow-up

EVIDENCE

PRACTICE GUIDELINES

- Marsh JC et al: Guidelines for the diagnosis and management of acquired aplastic anaemia. Br J Haematol 2003;123:782. Erratum in: Br J Haematol 2004;126:625. [PMID: 14632769]

INFORMATION FOR PATIENTS

- American Cancer Society: Detailed Guide: Aplastic Anemia
  - http://www.cancer.org/docroot/CRI/CRI_2_3x.asp?rnav=cridg&dt=77
- Aplastic Anemia & MDS International Foundation
  - http://www.aplastic.org/
- MedlinePlus: Idiopathic Aplastic Anemia
  - http://www.nlm.nih.gov/medlineplus/ency/article/000554.htm
- MedlinePlus: Secondary Aplastic Anemia
  - http://www.nlm.nih.gov/medlineplus/ency/article/000529.htm

REFERENCES

- Ades L et al: Long-term outcome after bone marrow transplantation for severe aplastic anemia. Blood 2004;103:2490. [PMID: 14656884]
- Frickhofen N et al: Antithymocyte globulin with or without cyclosporin A: 11-year follow-up of a randomized trial comparing treatments of aplastic anemia. Blood 2003;101:1236. [PMID: 12393680]
- Rosenfeld S et al: Antithymocyte globulin and cyclosporine for severe aplastic anemia: association between hematologic response and long-term outcome. JAMA 2003;289:1130. [PMID: 12622583]
- Young NS: Acquired aplastic anemia. Ann Intern Med 2002;136:534. [PMID: 11926789]

Author(s)

Charles A. Linker, MD

Anemia, Autoimmune Hemolytic

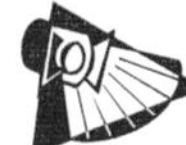

KEY FEATURES

ESSENTIALS OF DIAGNOSIS

- Acquired anemia caused by immunoglobulin G (IgG) autoantibody
- Spherocytes and reticulocytosis on peripheral blood smear
- Positive Coombs test

GENERAL CONSIDERATIONS

- Acquired disorder in which IgG autoantibody binds to red blood cell (RBC) membrane
  - Macrophages in spleen and other portions of reticuloendothelial system then remove portion of RBC membrane, forming a spherocyte because of decreased surface-to-volume ratio of RBC
  - Spherocytes less deformable and become trapped in spleen
- Causes include idiopathic (~50% of cases), systemic lupus erythematosus, chronic lymphocytic leukemia, and lymphomas
- Must be distinguished from drug-induced hemolytic anemia (eg, penicillin and other drugs), which coats RBC membrane; antibody is directed against membrane–drug complex
- Typically produces anemia of rapid onset that may be life threatening

CLINICAL FINDINGS

SYMPTOMS AND SIGNS

- Fatigue, angina pectoris, symptoms of congestive heart failure
- Jaundice and splenomegaly may be present

DIFFERENTIAL DIAGNOSIS

- Coombs positive (immune) hemolytic anemia: autoimmune, drugs, infection, lymphoproliferative disease, Rh or ABO incompatibility
- Coombs negative hemolytic anemia
- Hereditary spherocytosis
- Glucose-6-phosphate dehydrogenase deficiency
- Pyruvate kinase deficiency
- Microangiopathic hemolytic anemia: thrombotic thrombocytopenic purpura, hemolytic uremic syndrome, disseminated intravascular coagulation
- Splenic sequestration

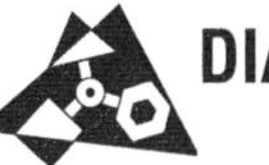

DIAGNOSIS

LABORATORY TESTS

- Anemia of variable severity, although hematocrit may be < 10%
- Reticulocytosis usually present
- Spherocytes on peripheral blood smear
- Indirect bilirubin increased
- Coincident immune thrombocytopenia (Evans syndrome) in ~10%
- Coombs antiglobulin test is basis for diagnosis; reagent is rabbit IgM antibody against human IgG or human complement
- Direct Coombs test positive: patient's RBCs mixed with Coombs reagent; agglutination indicates antibody on RBC surface
- Indirect Coombs test may or may not be positive: patient's serum mixed with panel of type O RBCs, then Coombs reagent added; agglutination indicates presence of large amount of autoantibody that has saturated binding sites on RBC and consequently appears in serum
- Micro-Coombs test is more sensitive and is necessary to make diagnosis in ~10% of cases; test indicated in patient with acquired spherocytic hemolytic anemia that may be autoimmune who has a negative direct Coombs test

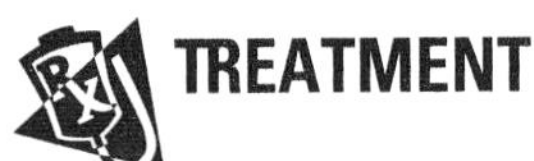

TREATMENT

MEDICATIONS

- Prednisone, 1–2 mg/kg/day in divided doses, is initial therapy
- Splenectomy if prednisone ineffective or if disease recurs on tapering dose
- Immunosuppressive agents (eg, cyclophosphamide, azathioprine, or cyclosporine in refractory cases)
- Danazol, 600–800 mg/day, is less effective than in immune thrombocytopenia
- High-dose IVIG, 1 g daily for 1 or 2 days, may be highly effective in controlling hemolysis; benefit is short lived (1–3 weeks) and it is expensive
- Rituximab, 375 mg/m^2 IV every week for 4 weeks, is effective in some cases

SURGERY

- Splenectomy is often successful

THERAPEUTIC PROCEDURES

- Transfusion may be problematic because of difficulty in performing cross-match; thus, incompatible blood may be given
- If compatible, most transfused blood survives similarly to patient's own RBCs

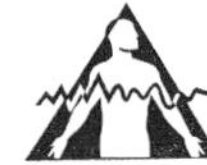

OUTCOME

COMPLICATIONS

- Possible transfusion reactions

PROGNOSIS

- Long-term prognosis is good, especially if there is no underlying autoimmune disorder or lymphoma

WHEN TO REFER

- Decisions regarding transfusions should be made in consultation with a hematologist

EVIDENCE

WEB SITES

- American Academy of Family Physicians: Hemolytic Anemia
  - http://www.aafp.org/afp/20040601/2599.html

INFORMATION FOR PATIENTS

- The Regional Cancer Center: Autoimmune Hemolytic Anemia
  - http://www.trcc.org/blood/10b_autoimmune.pdf
- MedlinePlus: Idiopathic Autoimmune Hemolytic Anemia
  - http://www.nlm.nih.gov/medlineplus/ency/article/000579.htm
- National Institutes of Health: Questions and Answers About Autoimmunity
  - http://www.niams.nih.gov/hi/topics/autoimmune/autoimmunity.htm#autoim_j

REFERENCES

- Petz LD: A physician's guide to transfusion in autoimmune hemolytic anemia. Br J Haematol 2004;124:712. [PMID: 15009058]
- Robak T: Monoclonal antibodies in the treatment of autoimmune cytopenias. Eur J Haematol 2004;72:79. [PMID: 14962245]

Author(s)

Charles A. Linker, MD

Anemia, Iron Deficiency

Anemia, Hemolytic p. 1024

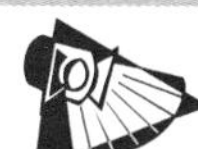

KEY FEATURES

ESSENTIALS OF DIAGNOSIS

- Absent bone marrow iron stores or serum ferritin < 12 μg/L are both pathognomonic
- Caused by bleeding in adults unless proved otherwise
- Response to iron therapy

GENERAL CONSIDERATIONS

- Most common cause of anemia worldwide
- Causes: blood loss [gastrointestinal (GI), menstrual, repeated blood donation]; deficient diet; increased requirements (pregnancy, lactation); hemoglobinuria (eg, paroxysmal nocturnal hemoglobinuria); malabsorption (eg, gastric surgery, celiac disease); hemolysis; pulmonary hemosiderosis (iron sequestration)
- Blood loss, especially GI bleeding, is by far the most important cause of iron deficiency anemia
- Women with heavy menstrual losses may require more iron than can reasonably be absorbed; thus, they often become iron deficient
- Pregnancy and lactation also increase requirement for iron, necessitating medicinal iron supplementation
- Chronic aspirin use may cause blood loss even without documented structural lesion
- In iron deficiency, search for source of GI bleeding if other sites of blood loss (menorrhagia, other uterine bleeding, and repeated blood donations) are excluded
- Diagnosis of iron deficiency anemia can involve demonstrating iron-deficient state or evaluating response to a therapeutic trial of iron replacement

DEMOGRAPHICS

- More common in women as a result of menstrual losses

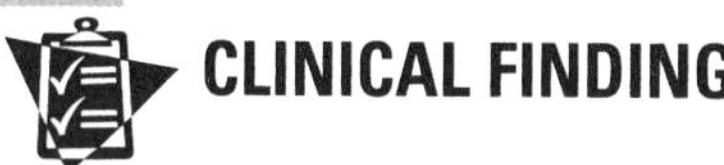

CLINICAL FINDINGS

SYMPTOMS AND SIGNS

- Symptoms of anemia (eg, easy fatigability, tachycardia, palpitations and tachypnea on exertion)
- Skin and mucosal changes (eg, smooth tongue, brittle nails, and cheilosis) in severe iron deficiency
- Dysphagia resulting from esophageal webs (Plummer-Vinson syndrome)
- Pica (ie, craving for specific foods [eg, ice chips, lettuce] often not rich in iron) is frequent

DIFFERENTIAL DIAGNOSIS

- Microcytic anemia resulting from other causes: thalassemia, anemia of chronic disease, sideroblastic anemia, or lead poisoning

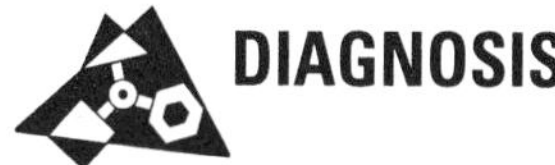

DIAGNOSIS

LABORATORY TESTS

- Hematocrit low, but mean corpuscular hemoglobin (MCV) initially normal, later MCV low
- Platelet count often increased
- Serum ferritin low; value < 30 μg/L highly reliable indicator of iron deficiency
- Serum total iron-binding capacity (TIBC) rises, serum iron < 30 μg/dL, and transferrin saturation < 15% after iron stores depleted
- Blood smear shows hypochromic microcytic cells, anisocytosis (variation in red blood cell [RBC] size), and poikilocytosis (variation in RBC shape)
- Severely hypochromic cells, target cells, hypochromic pencil-shaped cells, and occasionally small numbers of nucleated RBCs in severe iron deficiency
- Fecal occult blood testing often positive with GI bleeding

DIAGNOSTIC PROCEDURES

- Colonoscopy or flexible sigmoidoscopy may be required in evaluation of suspected GI bleeding

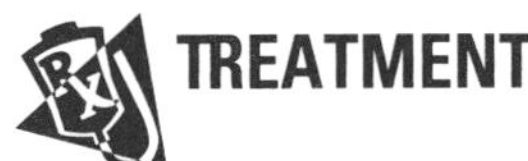

TREATMENT

MEDICATIONS

- Ferrous sulfate, 325 mg PO TID, is treatment of choice; may cause GI side effects
- Compliance improved by starting 325 mg PO QD with food, then gradually escalating dose
- Preferable to prescribe a lower dose of iron or to allow ingestion concurrent with food rather than insist on a regimen that will not be followed
- Continue iron therapy for 3–6 months after restoration of normal hematological values to replenish iron stores
- Failure of response to iron therapy is usually due to noncompliance; occasional patients absorb iron poorly; other reasons include incorrect diagnosis (anemia of chronic disease, thalassemia) and ongoing GI blood loss
- Parenteral iron indicated in intolerance of oral iron, refractoriness to oral iron, GI disease (usually inflammatory bowel disease) precluding use of oral iron, and continued blood loss that cannot be corrected
- Because of risk of anaphylaxis, parenteral iron used only for persistent anemia after reasonable trial of oral therapy
- Dose of IV iron (total 1.5–2 g) is calculated by estimating decrease in volume of RBC mass and supplying 1 mg of iron for each milliliter of volume below normal
  - Then add approximately 1 g for storage iron
  - Entire dose may be given as IV infusion over 4–6 h
  - Test dose of dilute solution given first; observe patient during entire infusion for anaphylaxis

THERAPEUTIC PROCEDURES

- Treat underlying cause such as source of GI bleeding

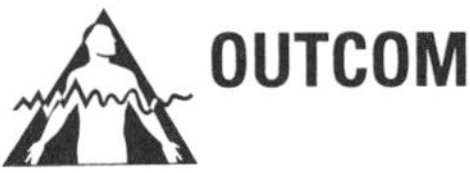

OUTCOME

FOLLOW-UP

- Recheck complete blood cell count to observe for response to iron replacement by return of hematocrit to halfway toward normal within 3 weeks and fully to baseline after 2 months
- Iron supplementation during pregnancy and lactation: included in prenatal vitamins

EVIDENCE

PRACTICE GUIDELINES

- Goddard AF et al: Guidelines for the management of iron deficiency anaemia. British Society of Gastroenterology. Gut 2000;46(Suppl 3–4):IV1. [PMID: 10862605]
- CDC Recommendations to Prevent and Control Iron Deficiency in the United States. MMWR Recomm Rep 1998;47:1
  - http://www.cdc.gov/epo/mmwr/preview/mmwrhtml/00051880.htm

WEB SITES

- NIH Office of Dietary Supplements: Iron Fact Sheet
  - http://ods.od.nih.gov/factsheets/iron.asp
- National Heart, Lung, and Blood Institute
  - http://www.nhlbi.nih.gov

INFORMATION FOR PATIENTS

- American Academy of Family Physicians: Anemia: When Low Iron Is the Cause
  - http://familydoctor.org/009.xml
- National Women's Health Information Center: Anemia
  - http://www.4woman.gov/faq/anemia.htm
- Mayo Clinic: Iron Deficiency Anemia
  - http://www.mayoclinic.com/invoke.cfm?objectid=072ADD99-C40D-4E6A-82DAA8347C662BDD

REFERENCES

- Capurso G et al: Can patient characteristics predict the outcome of endoscopic evaluation of iron deficiency anemia: a multiple logistic regression analysis. Gastrointest Endosc 2004;59:766. [PMID: 15173787]
- Yates JM et al: Iron deficiency anaemia in general practice: clinical outcomes over three years and factors influencing diagnostic evaluations. Postgrad Med J 2004;80:405. [PMID: 15254305]

Author(s)

Charles A. Linker, MD

Aneurysm, Intracranial

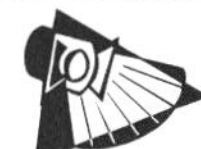

KEY FEATURES

ESSENTIALS OF DIAGNOSIS

- Subarachnoid hemorrhage or focal deficit
- "Warning leak" may precede the major hemorrhage
- Abnormal imaging studies

GENERAL CONSIDERATIONS

- Most aneurysms are located on the anterior part of the circle of Willis—particularly on the anterior or posterior communicating arteries, at the bifurcation of the middle cerebral artery, and at the bifurcation of the internal carotid artery
- Saccular aneurysms ("berry" aneurysms) occur at arterial bifurcations, are more common in adults than in children, are frequently multiple (20% of cases), and are usually asymptomatic
- May be associated with polycystic kidney disease and coarctation of the aorta

DEMOGRAPHICS

- Risk factors for aneurysm formation include smoking, hypertension, and hypercholesterolemia

CLINICAL FINDINGS

SYMPTOMS AND SIGNS

- May cause a focal neurologic deficit by compressing adjacent structures
- Most are asymptomatic or produce only nonspecific symptoms until they rupture, causing a subarachnoid hemorrhage
- Focal neurologic signs may be absent in subarachnoid hemorrhage and secondary to a focal hematoma or ischemia in the territory of the vessel with the ruptured aneurysm
- Focal arterial spasm in the area of the ruptured aneurysm may occur after 1–14 days, causing hemiplegia or other focal deficits
- Cause of vasospasm is unknown and likely multifactorial
- Vasospasm may lead to significant cerebral ischemia or infarction and increase in intracranial pressure
- Subacute hydrocephalus due to interference with the flow of cerebrospinal fluid may occur after 2 or more weeks; leads to delayed clinical deterioration and is relieved by shunting
- "Warning leaks" of a small amount of blood from the aneurysm sometimes precede the major hemorrhage by a few hours or days, leading to headaches, nausea, and neck stiffness

DIFFERENTIAL DIAGNOSIS

- Meningitis or meningoencephalitis
- Ischemic stroke
- Space-occupying lesion, eg, brain tumor
- Subdural hemorrhage
- Epidural hemorrhage
- Migraine

DIAGNOSIS

LABORATORY TESTS

- Cerebrospinal fluid is bloodstained if subarachnoid hemorrhage has occurred
- ECG evidence of arrhythmias or myocardial ischemia may occur and probably relates to excessive sympathetic activity
- Peripheral leukocytosis and transient glycosuria also common

IMAGING STUDIES

- CT scan generally confirms that subarachnoid hemorrhage has occurred, but may be normal
- Angiography (bilateral carotid and vertebral studies) indicates the size and site of the lesion, sometimes reveals multiple aneurysms, and may show arterial spasm
- If subarachnoid hemorrhage is confirmed by lumbar puncture or CT scanning but arteriogram is normal, the examination should be repeated after 2 weeks, because vasospasm may prevent detection of an aneurysm during the initial study

Anemia of Chronic Disease p. 1025. Anemia, Sideroblastic p. 1025.

TREATMENT

MEDICATIONS

- Phenytoin to prevent seizures
- Calcium channel blockers reduce or reverse experimental vasospasm, and nimodipine reduces ischemic deficits from arterial spasm without any side effects (60 mg Q4h for 21 days)

SURGERY

- Definitive treatment requires surgery and clipping of the aneurysm base, or endovascular treatment by interventional radiology

THERAPEUTIC PROCEDURES

- Major aim is to prevent further hemorrhages
- Conscious patients are confined to bed, advised against exertion or straining, treated symptomatically for headache and anxiety, and given laxatives or stool softeners
- Lower blood pressure gradually for severe hypertension, but not below a diastolic level of 90 mm Hg
- Medical management as outlined for subarachnoid hemorrhage is continued for about 6 weeks and followed by gradual mobilization

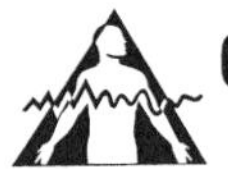

OUTCOME

FOLLOW-UP

- After surgical obliteration of aneurysms, symptomatic vasospasm may be treated by intravascular volume expansion, induced hypertension, or transluminal balloon angioplasty of involved intracranial vessels

PROGNOSIS

- Unruptured aneurysms that are symptomatic merit prompt treatment, whereas small asymptomatic ones discovered incidentally are often followed arteriographically and corrected surgically only if > 10 mm
- Greatest risk of further hemorrhage is within a few days of initial bleed; thus, early obliteration (within 2 days) is preferred
- Approximately 20% of patients will have further bleeding within 2 weeks and 40% within 6 months

WHEN TO ADMIT

- All patients need admission and referral to specialized care

EVIDENCE

PRACTICE GUIDELINES

- National Guideline Clearinghouse
  - http://www.guideline.gov/summary/summary.aspx?doc_id=5355&nbr=3658&string=intracranial+AND+aneurysm
- American Society of Interventional and Therapeutic Neuroradiology. Aneurysm endovascular therapy. AJNR Am J Neuroradiol 2001;22(8 Suppl):S4. [PMID: 11686074]

WEB SITES

- 3-D Visualization of brain aneurysms
  - http://dpi.radiology.uiowa.edu/nlm/app/aneur/brain/aneur.html
- CNS Pathology Index
  - http://medstat.med.utah.edu/WebPath/CNSHTML/CNSIDX.html

INFORMATION FOR PATIENTS

- UCSF Neurocritical Care and Stroke Patient Information
  - http://www.ucsf.edu/stroke/patinfo.htm
- National Institute of Neurological Disorders and Stroke
  - http://www.ninds.nih.gov/disorders/ceraneur/ceraneur.htm

REFERENCES

- Molyneux A et al: International Subarachnoid Aneurysm Trial (ISAT) of neurosurgical clipping versus endovascular coiling in 2143 patients with ruptured intracranial aneurysms: a randomised trial. Lancet 2002;360:1267. [PMID: 12414200]
- Roos Y et al: Antifibrinolytic therapy for aneurysmal subarachnoid hemorrhage: a major update of a Cochrane review. Stroke 2003;34:2308. [PMID: 12933970]
- Wiebers DO et al: Unruptured intracranial aneurysms: natural history, clinical outcome, and risks of surgical and endovascular treatment. Lancet 2003;362:103. [PMID: 12867109]

Author(s)

Michael J. Aminoff, MD, DSc, FRCP

Angina Pectoris

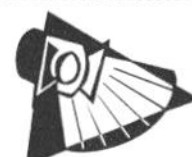

KEY FEATURES

ESSENTIALS OF DIAGNOSIS

- Precordial chest pain, usually precipitated by stress or exertion, and rapidly relieved by resting or nitrates
- Electrocardiographic, echocardiographic, or scintigraphic evidence of ischemia during pain or stress testing
- Angiographic evidence of significant obstruction of major coronary arteries

GENERAL CONSIDERATIONS

- Usually due to atherosclerotic coronary artery disease
- Less common causes: coronary vasospasm, congenital anomalies, emboli, arteritis, dissection, severe ventricular hypertrophy, severe aortic stenosis or regurgitation
- Commonly exacerbated by increased metabolic demands (eg, hyperthyroidism, anemia, tachycardias)
- Coronary vasospasm may occur spontaneously, or by exposure to cold, emotional stress, vasoconstricting medications, or cocaine

DEMOGRAPHICS

- Underdiagnosed in postmenopausal women

CLINICAL FINDINGS

SYMPTOMS AND SIGNS

- Diagnosis depends primarily on the history
- Angina most commonly arises during activity and is relieved by rest
- Patient often prefers to remain upright rather than lie down
- Rather than "pain," patient may describe tightness, squeezing, burning, pressure, choking, aching
- Discomfort behind or slightly to the left of the mid-sternum (in 80–90%)
- May radiate to left shoulder and upper arm; medial aspect of arm, elbow, forearm, wrist, and fourth and fifth fingers; or to lower jaw, nape of neck, or interscapular area
- Diagnosis strongly supported if sublingual nitroglycerin aborts or attenuates length of attack
- Physical examination during an attack often reveals a significant elevation in systolic and diastolic blood pressure
- Hypotension is a more ominous sign
- An S_3 or arrhythmia may occur (bradycardia more common with involvement of the right coronary artery)

DIFFERENTIAL DIAGNOSIS

- *Cardiovascular:* Myocardial infarction (MI), pericarditis, aortic stenosis, aortic dissection, cardiomyopathy, myocarditis, mitral valve prolapse, pulmonary hypertension, hypertrophic cardiomyopathy, carditis in acute rheumatic fever, aortic insufficiency, right ventricular hypertrophy
- *Pulmonary:* pneumonia, pleuritis, bronchitis, pneumothorax, tumor, mediastinitis
- *Gastrointestinal:* esophageal rupture, gastroesophageal reflux disease, esophageal spasm, Mallory-Weiss tear, peptic ulcer disease, biliary disease, pancreatitis, functional gastrointestinal pain
- *Musculoskeletal:* cervical or thoracic disk disease or arthritis, shoulder arthritis, costochondritis or Tietze's syndrome, subacromial bursitis
- *Other:* anxiety, herpes zoster, breast disorders, chest wall tumors, thoracic outlet syndrome

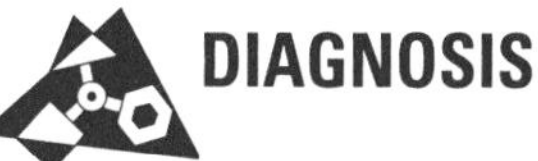

DIAGNOSIS

LABORATORY TESTS

- Obtain a fasting lipid profile
- Rule out diabetes mellitus and anemia
- Exercise testing (treadmill or bicycle) is the least expensive and most useful noninvasive procedure to confirm the diagnosis of angina, determine the severity of limitation of activity, assess prognosis, and evaluate responses to therapy

IMAGING STUDIES

- Stress scintigraphy (thallium or technetium) is indicated when patients are physically unable to exercise, the ECG is difficult to interpret (eg, LBBB), the results of exercise testing contradict the clinical impression, to more precisely localize the ischemia, to assess the completeness of revascularization, or as a prognostic indicator
- Scintigraphy can provide more information about the presence, location, and extent of coronary artery disease than exercise testing
- Scintigraphy is performed both at rest and during stressing (exercise or pharmacological stimulation)

DIAGNOSTIC PROCEDURES

- Obtain an ECG in all patients and, if possible, compare ECGs when pain is and is not present
- During anginal episodes, the ECG may reveal horizontal or downsloping ST-segment depression, or T wave flattening or inversion that reverses after ischemia disappears or, less commonly, ST-segment elevation
- ECG is normal in ~25% of patients with angina
- Coronary arteriography is the definitive diagnostic procedure
- Arteriography has a mortality rate of ~0.1% and morbidity of ~1–5%, but it is expensive
- Left ventricular angiography performed at the same time assesses left ventricular function and mitral regurgitation

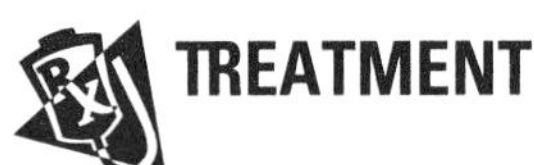

TREATMENT

MEDICATIONS

- Nitroglycerin, 0.3–0.6 mg sublingual or 0.4–0.8 mg by spray, with onset of symptoms or prophylactically 5 min before activity
- Long-acting nitrates (isosorbide dinitrate or mononitrate) for symptom management: avoid use for 8–10 h each day to avoid tolerance
- Nitrates relieve symptoms but do not benefit mortality
- β-Blockers reduce myocardial oxygen demand and benefit mortality
- Calcium channel blockers are generally not indicated except to treat coronary vasospasm
- Platelet inhibitors reduce the risk of coronary thromboembolism: aspirin (81–325 mg/day), or clopidogrel (75 mg/day) in aspirin-intolerant patients, benefits mortality

SURGERY

- Revascularization (coronary bypass grafting or angioplasty) is indicated when
  - Symptoms are unacceptable despite maximal medical therapy
  - There is > 50% stenosis of the left main coronary artery with or without symptoms
  - Triple-vessel disease coexists with either an ejection fraction < 50% or a prior MI
  - Unstable angina is present
  - Angina or severe ischemia persists on noninvasive testing after MI
- Coronary bypass grafting is generally reserved for left main and triple-vessel disease

THERAPEUTIC PROCEDURES

- Angioplasty or stenting performed during angiography
  - The procedure of choice for single-vessel disease in the setting of refractory symptoms
  - Superior to medical therapy for symptom relief, but not in preventing infarction or death
  - A high rate (~40%) of restenosis may be reduced with newer stents

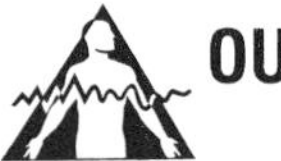

OUTCOME

WHEN TO ADMIT

- Admit patients with unremitting or unstable angina (see Angina pectoris, unstable) for cardiac evaluation, to rule out MI, and to maximize therapy, including possible emergent revascularization

PREVENTION

- Smoking cessation
- β-Blockers, nitrates, and aspirin
- Vigorous treatment of hyperlipidemia (goal LDL < 100 mg/dL, HDL > 45 mg/dL)
- Tight control of diabetes mellitus
- Goal blood pressure (< 140/90 mm Hg)
- Avoiding aggravating factors: strenuous activity, cold temperatures, strong emotion

EVIDENCE

PRACTICE GUIDELINES

- Snow V et al; American College of Physicians; American College of Cardiology Chronic Stable Angina Panel. Primary care management of chronic stable angina and asymptomatic suspected or known coronary artery disease: a clinical practice guideline from the American College of Physicians. Ann Intern Med 2004;141:562. [PMID: 15466774]
- ACC/AHA 2002 guideline update for the management of patients with unstable angina and non-ST-segment elevation myocardial infarction. A report of the American College of Cardiology/American Heart Association Task Force on Practice Guidelines
  - http://www.acc.org/clinical/guidelines/unstable/unstable.pdf

WEB SITES

- National Heart, Lung, and Blood Institute
  - http://www.nhlbi.nih.gov/
- American College of Cardiology
  - http://www.acc.org/

INFORMATION FOR PATIENTS

- National Heart, Lung, and Blood Institute: Angina
  - http://www.nhlbi.nih.gov/health/dci/Diseases/Angina/Angina_WhatIs.html
- American Heart Association: Angina Pectoris
  - http://www.americanheart.org/presenter.jhtml?identifier=4472
- MedlinePlus: Angina Interactive Tutorial
  - http://www.nlm.nih.gov/medlineplus/tutorials/angina/htm/index.htm
- American Academy of Family Physicians: Angina and Heart Disease
  - http://familydoctor.org/233.xml

REFERENCES

- Paetsch I et al: Comparison of dobutamine stress magnetic resonance, and adenosine stress magnetic resonance perfusion. Circulation 2004;110:835. [PMID: 15289384]

Author(s)

Thomas M. Bashore, MD
Christopher B. Granger, MD

Angiostrongyliasis Cantonensis

Angina Pectoris, Unstable p. 1026

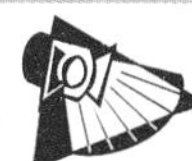

KEY FEATURES

ESSENTIALS OF DIAGNOSIS

- Meningoencephalitis
- Transient cranial neuropathies

GENERAL CONSIDERATIONS

- A nematode of rats, *Angiostrongylus cantonensis*, is the causative agent of a form of eosinophilic meningoencephalitis
- Human infection results from the ingestion of infective larvae contained in uncooked food—either the intermediate mollusk hosts (snails, slugs, planarians) or transport hosts that have ingested mollusks (crabs, shrimp, fish)
- Leafy vegetables contaminated by small mollusks or by mollusk slime may also be the source of infection, as can fingers during collection and preparation of snails for cooking
- The mollusks become infected by ingesting larvae excreted in feces of infected rodents, the definitive host
- The incubation period in humans is 1–3 weeks. Ingested larvae (0.5 × 0.025 mm) invade the central nervous system, where, during migration, they may cause extensive tissue damage; at their death, a local inflammatory reaction ensues

DEMOGRAPHICS

- The disease has been reported from Hawaii and other Pacific islands, Southeast Asia, Japan, China, Taiwan, Hong Kong, Australia, Egypt, Madagascar, Nigeria, Bombay, Cuba, Puerto Rico, Bahamas, Brazil, and New Orleans

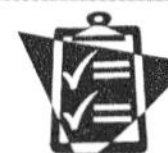

CLINICAL FINDINGS

SYMPTOMS AND SIGNS

- Meningoencephalitis, including severe headache, fever, neck stiffness, nausea and vomiting
- Multiple neurologic findings, particularly asymmetric transient cranial neuropathies
- Worms in the spinal cord may result in sensory abnormalities in the trunk or extremities
- Worms can occur in the eye

DIFFERENTIAL DIAGNOSIS

- Tuberculous, coccidioidal, or aseptic meningitis
- Neurocysticercosis
- Neurosyphilis
- Lymphoma
- Paragonimiasis
- Echinococcosis
- Gnathostomiasis

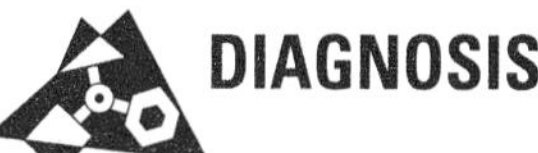

DIAGNOSIS

LABORATORY TESTS

- The spinal fluid characteristically shows elevated protein, eosinophilic pleocytosis, and normal glucose. Occasionally, the parasite can be recovered from spinal fluid
- Peripheral eosinophilia with a low-grade leukocytosis is common
- A serologic test is available from the Centers for Disease Control and Prevention

IMAGING STUDIES

- CT and MRI scans may show a central nervous system lesion

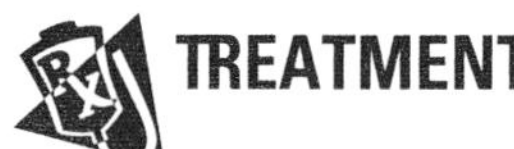

TREATMENT

MEDICATIONS

- No specific treatment is available; however, the following can be tried:
  - Albendazole (400 mg twice daily for 7 days)
  - Thiabendazole (25 mg/kg three times daily for 3 days); this dose may be toxic and need to be reduced
  - Mebendazole (100 mg twice daily for 5 days)
  - Ivermectin

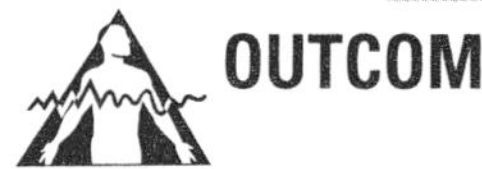

OUTCOME

COMPLICATIONS

- Parasite deaths may exacerbate central nervous system inflammatory lesions. Symptomatic treatment with analgesics or corticosteroids may be necessary

PROGNOSIS

- The illness usually persists for weeks to months, the parasite dies, and the patient then recovers spontaneously, usually without sequelae. However, fatalities have been recorded

WHEN TO ADMIT

- All patients

PREVENTION

- Controlling rat population
- Cooking snails, prawns, fish, and crabs for 3–5 min or by freezing them (–15°C for 24 h)
- Examining vegetables for mollusks before eating
- Washing contaminated vegetables to eliminate larvae contained in mollusk mucus is not always successful

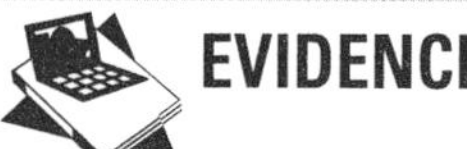

EVIDENCE

PRACTICE GUIDELINES

- National Guideline Clearinghouse
  - http://www.guideline.gov/summary/summary.aspx?doc_id=2446&nbr=1672&string=meningoencephalitis

WEB SITE

- Centers for Disease Control and Prevention—Division of Parasitic Diseases
  - http://www.cdc.gov/ncidod/dpd/parasites/angiostrongylus/default.htm

INFORMATION FOR PATIENTS

- Centers for Disease Control and Prevention
  - http://www.dpd.cdc.gov/dpdx/HTML/Angiostrongyliasis.htm
- Centers for Disease Control and Prevention—Division of Parasitic Diseases
  - http://www.cdc.gov/ncidod/dpd/parasites/angiostrongylus/factsht_angiostrongylus.htm

REFERENCE

- Wang X et al: A clinical study of eosinophilic meningoencephalitis caused by angiostrongyliasis. Chin Med J (Engl) 2002;115:1312. [PMID: 12411101]

Anisakiasis

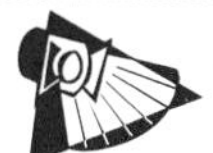

KEY FEATURES

ESSENTIALS OF DIAGNOSIS

- The majority of acute cases present as gastric anisakiasis with symptoms of nausea, vomiting, and progressive epigastric pain
- Occasionally, acute infection is followed by a chronic course
- Infection is by larval invasion of the stomach or intestinal wall by anisakid nematodes

GENERAL CONSIDERATIONS

- Humans are infected when they ingest larvae in marine fish or squid eaten raw, undercooked, salted, or lightly pickled
- Larvae liberated in the stomach attach to or partially penetrate the gastric or intestinal mucosa (small bowel is more common; colon is rare), resulting in localized ulceration, edema, and eosinophilic granuloma formation; eventually, the parasite dies
- In the **acute form**, the infection may mimic surgical abdomen
- In the **chronic form**, mild symptoms may persist for weeks to years
- Rarely, worms are coughed up and expectorated or penetrate the gut wall, enter the peritoneal cavity, and migrate
- Most larvae, however, probably fail to cause infection and are passed in feces

DEMOGRAPHICS

- The infection occurs worldwide, but most cases have been reported in Japan and The Netherlands, with a few in the United States, Scandinavia, Chile, and other countries with high fish consumption
- Raw sashimi in Japan, pickled herring in The Netherlands, and ceviche (seviche) in Latin America are sources of infection

CLINICAL FINDINGS

SYMPTOMS AND SIGNS

- Within hours after larval ingestion, there is nausea, vomiting, and epigastric pain that progressively becomes more severe
- Allergic reactions, including rare anaphylaxis, can occur
- Chest pain and hematemesis are rare
- Acute intestinal anisakiasis
  - Within 1–7 days, colicky pain appears in the lower abdomen
  - The pain is often localized at the ileocecal region, accompanied by diarrhea, nausea, vomiting, diffuse abdominal tenderness, and mild fever
- Chronic intestinal anisakiasis
  - Symptoms that mimic gastric ulcer, gastritis, gastric tumor, bowel obstruction, or inflammatory bowel disease may continue for weeks to several years

DIFFERENTIAL DIAGNOSIS

- Norwalk virus or rotavirus
- "Food poisoning" by toxins from *Bacillus cereus, Staphylococcus aureus, Clostridium perfringens*
- Appendicitis
- Peptic ulcer disease or gastritis
- Inflammatory bowel disease

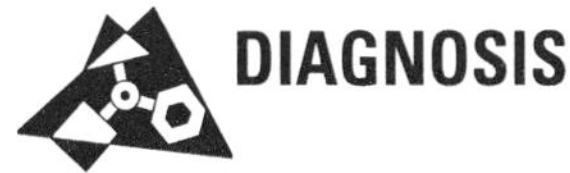

DIAGNOSIS

LABORATORY TESTS

- Stools may show occult blood, but eggs are not produced
- Mild leukocytosis and eosinophilia may be present
- ELISA and RAST serologic tests may be helpful but are not reliable in chronic disease

IMAGING STUDIES

- In acute infections, x-rays of the stomach may show a localized edematous, ulcerated area with an irregularly thickened wall, decreased peristalsis, and rigidity
  - Double-contrast technique may show the threadlike larvae
  - Small bowel x-rays may show thickened mucosa and segments of stenosis with proximal dilation
- Ultrasound examination of gastric and intestinal lesions may also be useful
- In the chronic stage, x-rays of the stomach—but not of the bowel—may be helpful

DIAGNOSTIC PROCEDURES

- In acute infection, gastroscopy is preferred because the larvae sometimes can be seen and removed from the stomach
- In the chronic stage, stomach endoscopy—but not of the bowel—may be helpful
- The diagnosis is often made only at laparotomy with surgical removal of the parasite

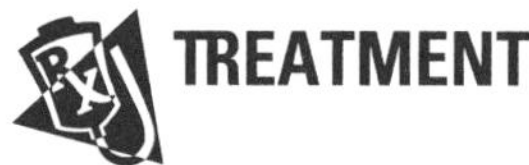

TREATMENT

MEDICATIONS

- There is no drug treatment, although one report suggests efficacy for albendazole

SURGERY

- Surgical excision of the worm may be necessary in severe cases

THERAPEUTIC PROCEDURES

- Treatment of acute and chronic lesions is limited to symptomatic measures; symptoms generally improve in 1–2 weeks
- At times, larvae can be removed by fiberoptic gastroscopy or colonoscopy

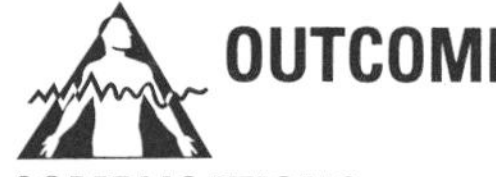

OUTCOME

COMPLICATIONS

- Chronic intestinal anisakiasis

WHEN TO REFER

- Refer for consideration of mechanical removal of the worm

PREVENTION

- Avoidance of ingestion of raw or incompletely cooked squid or marine fish, especially salmon, rockfish, herring, and mackerel; early evisceration of fish is recommended
- Larvae within fish may, with difficulty, be seen as colorless, tightly coiled or spiraled worms in 3-mm whorls or as reddish or pigmented larvae lying open in muscles or viscera
- The larvae are killed by temperatures above 60°C or by freezing at –20°C for 24 h (7 days is advised by some clinicians)
- Smoking procedures that do not bring the temperature to 60°C, marinating in vinegar, and salt-curing are not reliable

EVIDENCE

PRACTICE GUIDELINES

- National Guideline Clearinghouse
  - http://www.guideline.gov/summary/summary.aspx?doc_id=2791

INFORMATION FOR PATIENTS

- Centers for Disease Control and Prevention
  - http://www.dpd.cdc.gov/dpdx/HTML/Anisakiasis.htm

REFERENCES

- Audicana MT et al: Anisakis simplex: dangerous—dead and alive? Trends Parasitol 2002;18:20. [PMID: 11850010]
- Moore DA et al: Treatment of anisakiasis with albendazole. Lancet 2002;360:54. [PMID: 12114042]

Ankylosing Spondylitis

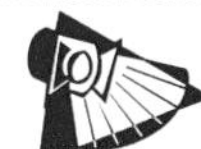

KEY FEATURES

ESSENTIALS OF DIAGNOSIS

- Chronic low backache in young adults
- Hallmark of the disease is enthesopathy, inflammation of tendons and ligaments
- Diagnostic x-ray changes in sacroiliac joints
- Accelerated erythrocyte sedimentation rate and negative serologic tests for rheumatoid factor
- HLA-B27 usually positive

GENERAL CONSIDERATIONS

- Chronic inflammatory disease of the joints of the axial skeleton, manifested clinically by pain and progressive stiffening of the spine

DEMOGRAPHICS

- The age at onset is usually in the late teens or early 20s
- The incidence is greater in males than in females

CLINICAL FINDINGS

SYMPTOMS AND SIGNS

- Gradual onset, with intermittent bouts of back pain that may radiate down the thighs
- Symptoms progress in a cephalad direction
- Motion becomes limited, with the normal lumbar curve flattened and the thoracic curvature exaggerated
- Chest expansion is often limited as a consequence of costovertebral joint involvement
- In advanced cases, the entire spine becomes fused, allowing no motion in any direction
- Transient acute arthritis of the peripheral joints occurs in about 50% of cases, and permanent changes—most commonly the hips, shoulders, and knees—are seen in about 25%
- Anterior uveitis in up to 25% of cases
- Constitutional symptoms similar to those of rheumatoid arthritis are absent in most patients

DIFFERENTIAL DIAGNOSIS

- Rheumatoid arthritis
  - Predominantly affects multiple, small, peripheral joints of the hands and feet
  - Usually spares the sacroiliac joints with little effect on the rest of the spine except for C1–C2
- Ankylosing hyperostosis (diffuse idiopathic skeletal hyperostosis [DISH], Forestier's disease)
  - Exuberant osteophyte formation
  - The osteophytes are thicker and more anterior than the syndesmophytes of ankylosing spondylitis
  - Sacroiliac joints are not affected
- Reactive arthritis (Reiter's syndrome)
- Psoriatic arthritis
- Inflammatory bowel disease
- Osteitis condensans ilii
- Hyperparathyroidism
- Whipple's disease
- Synovitis-acne-pustulosis-hyperostosis-osteitis (SAPHO) syndrome
- Sciatica
- Lumbar disk herniation, spinal stenosis, or facet joint degenerative arthritis

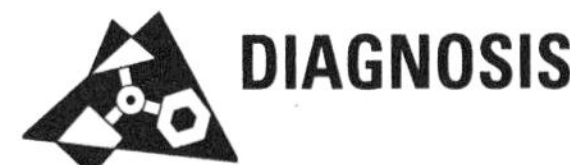

DIAGNOSIS

LABORATORY TESTS

- The erythrocyte sedimentation rate is elevated in 85% of cases
- Serologic tests for rheumatoid factor are characteristically negative
- HLA-B27 is found in 90% of patients with ankylosing spondylitis (occurs in 8% of the normal population)

IMAGING STUDIES

- The earliest radiographic changes of sclerosis and erosion are usually in the sacroiliac joints (early on may be detectable only by CT)
- Involvement of the apophysial joints of the spine, ossification of the annulus fibrosus, calcification of the anterior and lateral spinal ligaments, and squaring and generalized demineralization of the vertebral bodies may occur in more advanced stages
- "Bamboo spine" describes the late radiographic appearance of the spinal column

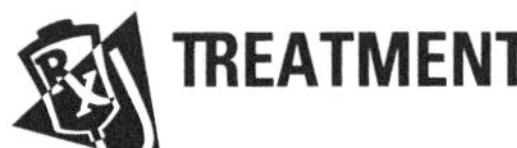

TREATMENT

MEDICATIONS

- Postural and breathing exercises
- Nonsteroidal anti-inflammatory drugs (NSAIDs)
- Sulfasalazine (1000 mg twice daily) is sometimes useful for the peripheral arthritis but has little symptomatic effect on spinal and sacroiliac joint disease
- Tumor necrosis factor inhibitors are highly effective in both the spinal and peripheral arthritis. Either etanercept (25 mg SC twice a week) or infliximab (5 mg/kg every other month) is reasonable for patients whose symptoms are refractory to physical therapy and other interventions

SURGERY

- Total hip replacement benefits those with severe hip involvement

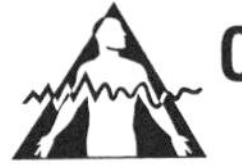

OUTCOME

COMPLICATIONS

- Spondylitic heart disease, characterized chiefly by atrioventricular conduction defects and aortic insufficiency, occurs in 3–5% of patients with longstanding severe disease
- Pulmonary fibrosis of the upper lobes, with progression to cavitation and bronchiectasis mimicking tuberculosis, may occur

PROGNOSIS

- Almost all patients have persistent symptoms over decades
- The severity of disease varies greatly, with about 10% of patients having work disability after 10 years
- Absence of severe hip disease after the first 5 years is an excellent prognostic sign

WHEN TO REFER

- Refer to a rheumatologist when diagnosis is in doubt or when the patient fails to improve while taking NSAIDs
- Refer to an ophthalmologist for symptoms of uveitis
- Refer for hip replacement

PREVENTION

- Avoid cigarette smoking, since patients are already at risk for restrictive lung disease
- Use a small pillow at night to avoid accelerating flexion deformities of the spine

EVIDENCE

WEB SITES

- Spondylitis Association of America
  - http://www.spondylitis.org/
- National Institutes of Health
  - http://medlineplus.nlm.nih.gov/medlineplus/ankylosingspondylitis.html

INFORMATION FOR PATIENTS

- Arthritis Foundation
  - http://www.arthritis.org/conditions/DiseaseCenter/ankylosing_spondylitis.asp
- Mayo Clinic
  - http://www.mayoclinic.com/invoke.cfm?id=DS00483
- Ankylosing Spondylitis International Federation
  - http://www.asif.rheumanet.org

REFERENCES

- Braun J et al: Long-term efficacy and safety of infliximab in the treatment of ankylosing spondylitis. Arthritis Rheum 2003;48:2224. [PMID: 12905476]
- Calin A et al: Outcomes of a multicentre randomised clinical trial of etanercept to treat ankylosing spondylitis. Ann Rheum Dis 2004;63:1594. [PMID: 15345498]
- Khan MA: Update on spondyloarthropathies. Ann Intern Med 2002;136:896. [PMID: 12069564]

Author(s)

David B. Hellmann, MD, FACP
John H. Stone, MD, MPH

Anorectal Infections p. 1027

Anorexia Nervosa

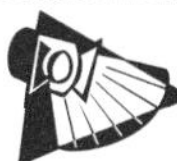

KEY FEATURES

ESSENTIALS OF DIAGNOSIS

- Disturbance of body image and intense fear of becoming fat
- Weight loss, leading to body weight 15% below expected
- In females, absence of three consecutive menstrual cycles
- Fear of weight gain and of loss of control over food intake

GENERAL CONSIDERATIONS

- Begins in the years between adolescence and young adulthood
- Occurs most commonly in females (90%), predominantly middle and upper income
- Estimated prevalence: 270 cases per 100,000 population for females and 22 per 100,000 for males
- Cause not known, probably of primary psychiatric origin
- Medical or psychiatric illnesses that can account for anorexia and weight loss must be excluded

CLINICAL FINDINGS

SYMPTOMS AND SIGNS

- Loss of body fat with severe emaciation
- Dry and scaly skin
- Increased lanugo body hair
- Parotid enlargement and edema
- In severe cases, bradycardia, hypotension, and hypothermia
- Cold intolerance
- Constipation
- Amenorrhea

DIFFERENTIAL DIAGNOSIS

- Endocrine and metabolic disorders
  - Panhypopituitarism
  - Addison's disease
  - Hyperthyroidism
  - Diabetes mellitus
- Gastrointestinal disorders
  - Malabsorption
  - Pancreatic insufficiency
  - Crohn's disease
  - Celiac sprue
- Chronic infections, eg, tuberculosis
- Cancer, eg, lymphoma
- Rare central nervous system disorders such as hypothalamic tumors
- Severe malnutrition
- Depression
- Obsessive-compulsive disorder
- Body dysmorphic disorder
- Malignancy
- AIDS
- Substance abuse

DIAGNOSIS

LABORATORY TESTS

- Check for anemia, leukopenia, electrolyte abnormalities, and elevations of blood urea nitrogen and serum creatinine
- Serum cholesterol level often increased
- Luteinizing hormone level depressed and impaired response to luteinizing hormone-releasing hormone

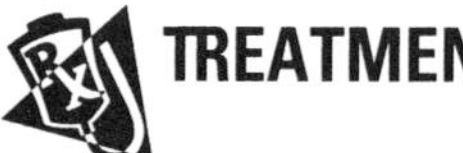

TREATMENT

MEDICATIONS

- Tricyclic antidepressants, selective serotonin reuptake inhibitors, and lithium carbonate are effective in some cases

THERAPEUTIC PROCEDURES

- Treatment goal: restoration of normal body weight and resolution of psychological difficulties
- Supportive care
- Structured behavioral therapy
- Intensive psychotherapy
- Family therapy
- Hospitalization may be necessary
- Treatment by experienced teams successful in about two-thirds of cases

OUTCOME

COMPLICATIONS

- Poor dentition
- Pharyngitis
- Esophagitis
- Aspiration
- Gastric dilatation
- Pancreatitis
- Constipation
- Hemorrhoids
- Dehydration
- Electrolyte abnormalities

PROGNOSIS

- 50% of patients continue to experience difficulties with eating behavior and psychiatric problems
- 2% to 6% of patients die of the complications of the disorder or from suicide

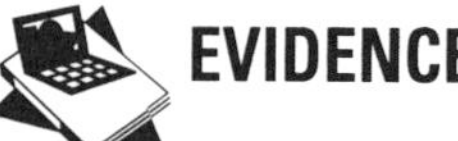

EVIDENCE

PRACTICE GUIDELINES

- Position of the American Dietetic Association: Nutrition intervention in the treatment of anorexia nervosa, bulimia nervosa, and binge eating. J Am Diet Assoc 2001;101:810. [PMID: 11478482]
- American Dietetic Association http://www.eatright.org/aanorexiainter.html.
- Ebeling H et al: A practice guideline for treatment of eating disorders in children and adolescents. Ann Med 2003;35:488. [PMID: 14649331]

INFORMATION FOR PATIENTS

- MedlinePlus—Anorexia nervosa
  - http://www.nlm.nih.gov/medlineplus/ency/article/000362.htm
- American Academy of Family Physicians
  - http://familydoctor.org/063.xml
- National Association of Anorexia Nervosa and Associated Disorders
  - http://www.altrue.net/site/anadweb/content.php?type=1&id=6982
- National Eating Disorders Association
  - http://www.nationaleatingdisorders.org/p.asp?WebPage_ID=286&Profile_ID=41142

REFERENCES

- Fairburn CG et al: Eating disorders. Lancet 2003;361:407. [PMID: 12573387]
- Fisher M: The course and outcome of eating disorders in adults and in adolescents: a review. Adolesc Med 2003;14:149. [PMID: 12529198]
- Gottero C et al: Ghrelin: a link between eating disorders, obesity and reproduction. Nutr Neurosci 2004;7:255. [PMID: 15682922]
- Kaplan AS: Psychological treatments for anorexia nervosa: a review of published studies and promising new directions. Can J Psychiatry 2002;47:235. [PMID: 11987474]
- Pompili M et al: Suicide in anorexia nervosa: a meta-analysis. Int J Eat Disord 2004;36:99. [PMID: 15185278]
- Wilson GT et al: Eating disorders guidelines from NICE. Lancet 2005;365:79. [PMID: 15639682]
- Zhu AJ et al: Pharmacologic treatment of eating disorders. Can J Psychiatry 2002;47:227. [PMID: 11987473]

Author(s)

Robert B. Baron, MD, MS

Anthrax

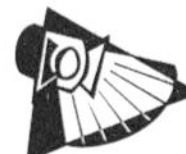

KEY FEATURES

ESSENTIALS OF DIAGNOSIS

- Appropriate epidemiological setting (eg, exposure to animals or animal hides) or potential exposure resulting from an act of bioterrorism
- A cutaneous black eschar, typically painless and on exposed areas of the skin, with marked surrounding edema and vesicles
- Nonspecific flu-like symptoms that rapidly progress to extreme dyspnea and shock in association with mediastinal widening and pleural effusions on chest x-ray

GENERAL CONSIDERATIONS

- Naturally occurring anthrax is a disease of sheep, cattle, horses, goats, and swine
- *Bacillus anthracis* is a gram-positive spore-forming aerobic rod.
  - Spores—not vegetative bacteria—are the infectious form of the organism
- Transmitted to humans from contaminated animals, animal products, or soil by inoculation of broken skin or mucous membranes, by inhalation of aerosolized spores, or, rarely, by ingestion resulting in cutaneous, inhalational, or gastrointestinal forms of anthrax, respectively
- Spores entering the lungs are ingested by macrophages and carried via lymphatics to regional lymph nodes, where they germinate
  - The bacteria rapidly multiply within the lymphatics, causing a hemorrhagic lymphadenitis
  - Invasion of the bloodstream leads to overwhelming sepsis, killing the host

CLINICAL FINDINGS

SYMPTOMS AND SIGNS

Cutaneous anthrax

- Onset occurs within 2 weeks of exposure to spores
- Initial lesion is erythematous papule, often on exposed area of skin, that vesiculates, ulcerates, and undergoes necrosis, ultimately progressing to a purple-to-black eschar
- Surrounding area is edematous and vesicular but not purulent
- Infection is usually self-limited

Inhalational anthrax

- Nonspecific viral-like symptoms
- Anterior chest pain is an early symptom of mediastinitis
- Within hours to days, the patient progresses to the fulminant stage of infection, in which signs and symptoms of overwhelming sepsis predominate
- Dissemination may occur, resulting in meningitis

Gastrointestinal anthrax

- Symptoms begin 2–5 days after ingestion of meat contaminated with anthrax spores
- Fever, diffuse abdominal pain, rebound abdominal tenderness, vomiting, constipation, and diarrhea occur
- Because the primary lesion is ulcerative, emesis is blood tinged or has coffee-ground appearance; stool may be blood tinged or melenic
- Bowel perforation can occur

DIFFERENTIAL DIAGNOSIS

Cutaneous anthrax

- Ecthyma gangrenosum (neutropenic, *Pseudomonas*)
- Tularemia
- Plague
- Brown recluse spider bite
- Aspergillosis or mucormycosis
- Antiphospholipid antibody syndrome
- Warfarin necrosis
- Rat-bite fever
- Rickettsialpox
- Orf (parapoxvirus infection)
- Cutaneous mycobacterial infection
- Cutaneous leishmaniasis

Inhalational anthrax

- Influenza
- Bacterial mediastinitis
- Fibrous mediastinitis from histoplasmosis, coccidioidomycosis, atypical or viral pneumonia, silicosis, sarcoidosis
- Other causes of mediastinal widening (eg, ruptured aortic aneurysm, lymphoma, superior vena cava syndrome)
- Tuberculosis

Gastrointestinal anthrax

- Bowel obstruction
- Perforated viscus
- Peritonitis
- Gastroenteritis
- Peptic ulcer disease

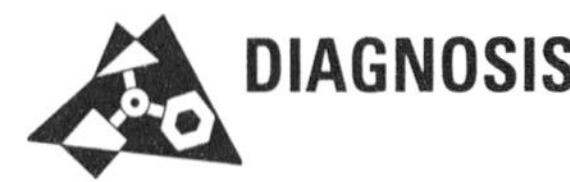

DIAGNOSIS

LABORATORY TESTS

- Pleural fluid in inhalational anthrax is hemorrhagic with few white blood cells; cerebrospinal fluid from meningitis cases is hemorrhagic
- Gram stain of fluid from a cutaneous lesion, pleural fluid, cerebrospinal fluid, unspun blood, or blood culture may show the characteristic boxcar-shaped encapsulated rods in chains
- The diagnosis is established by isolation of the organism from culture of the skin lesion (or fluid expressed from it), blood, or pleural fluid or cerebrospinal fluid in cases of meningitis
- In the absence of prior antimicrobial therapy, cultures are invariably positive

IMAGING STUDIES

- The chest x-ray is the most sensitive test for inhalational disease, being abnormal initially in every case of bioterrorism-associated disease
- Mediastinal widening from hemorrhagic lymphadenitis in 70% of the bioterrorism-related cases
- Pleural effusions were present initially or occurred over the course of illness in all cases, and approximately three fourths had pulmonary infiltrates or signs of consolidation

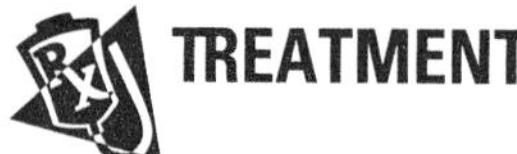

TREATMENT

MEDICATIONS

- Ciprofloxacin is considered the drug of choice (Table 135); other fluoroquinolones are probably as effective
- Doxycycline is an alternative first-line agent
- *B anthracis* may express β-lactamases that confer resistance to cephalosporins and penicillins
  - For this reason, penicillin and amoxicillin are no longer recommended for use as single agents in the treatment of disseminated disease

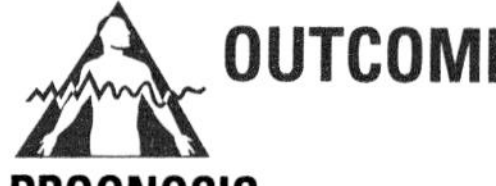

OUTCOME

PROGNOSIS

- The prognosis in cutaneous infection is excellent; death is unlikely if the infection has remained localized and lesions heal without complications in most cases
- The reported mortality rate for gastrointestinal and inhalational infections is up to 85%

WHEN TO REFER

- Any suspected case of anthrax should be immediately reported to the Centers for Disease Control and Prevention so that a complete investigation can be conducted

PREVENTION

- Ciprofloxacin is considered the drug of choice (Table 135) for treatment and for prophylaxis following exposure to anthrax spores
- There is an FDA-approved vaccine for persons at high risk of exposure to anthrax spores

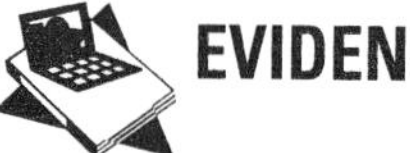

EVIDENCE

PRACTICE GUIDELINES

- National Guideline Clearinghouse
  - http://www.guideline.gov/summary/summary.aspx?doc_id=3220&nbr=2446&string=anthrax
  - http://www.guideline.gov/summary/summary.aspx?doc_id=2652&nbr=1878&string=anthrax

WEB SITES

- Centers for Disease Control and Prevention: Anthrax and Other Bioterrorism-Related Issues
  - http://www.bt.cdc.gov/
- Karolinska Institute: Directory of Bacterial Infections and Mycoses
  - http://www.mic.ki.se/Diseases/C01.html
- MedlinePlus: Anthrax
  - http://www.nlm.nih.gov/medlineplus/anthrax.html

INFORMATION FOR PATIENTS

- JAMA patient page: Anthrax. JAMA 2001;286:2626. [PMID: 11763849]
- Centers for Disease Control: Anthrax
  - http://www.cdc.gov/ncidod/dbmd/diseaseinfo/anthrax_g.htm

REFERENCES

- Borio L et al: Death due to bioterrorism-related inhalational anthrax: report of 2 patients. JAMA 2001;286:2554. [PMID: 11722269]
- Fennelly KP et al: Airborne infection with *Bacillus anthracis*—from mills to mail. Emerg Infect Dis 2004;10:996. [PMID: 15207048]
- Ferguson NE et al: Bioterrorism web site resources for infectious disease clinicians and epidemiologists. Clin Infect Dis 2003;36:1458. [PMID: 12766842]
- Reissman DB et al: One-year health assessment of adult survivors of *Bacillus anthracis* infection. JAMA 2004;291:1994. [PMID: 15113818]
- Kuehnert MJ et al: Clinical features that discriminate inhalational anthrax from other acute respiratory illnesses. Clin Infect Dis 2003;36:328. [PMID: 12539075]
- Roche KJ et al: Images in clinical medicine. Cutaneous anthrax infection. N Engl J Med 2001;345:1611. [PMID: 11704684]

Author(s)

Henry F. Chambers, MD

Antiarrhythmic Agent Overdose p. 1028

Anticoagulant Overdose

KEY FEATURES

ESSENTIALS OF DIAGNOSIS

- Prolonged prothrombin time (PT)

GENERAL CONSIDERATIONS

- Warfarin and related compounds (including ingredients of many commercial rodenticides) inhibit the clotting mechanism by blocking hepatic synthesis of vitamin K–dependent clotting factors
- Half-life of the "superwarfarins" used as rodenticides can be weeks or longer

CLINICAL FINDINGS

SYMPTOMS AND SIGNS

- Initially asymptomatic, as evidence of anticoagulant effect usually delayed for 12–24 h
- Hemoptysis
- Gross hematuria
- Bloody stools
- Hemorrhages into organs
- Widespread bruising
- Bleeding into joint spaces

DIFFERENTIAL DIAGNOSIS

- Liver disease
- Hemophilia
- Aspirin overdose

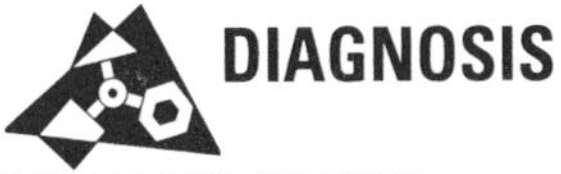

DIAGNOSIS

LABORATORY TESTS

- The PT is increased within 12–24 h (peak 36–48 h) after a single overdose
- After ingestion of brodifacoum and indanedione rodenticides (so-called superwarfarins), inhibition of clotting factor synthesis may persist for several weeks or even months after a single dose

DIAGNOSTIC PROCEDURES

- Obtain daily PT/INR for at least 2 days after acute ingestion to rule out excessive anticoagulation

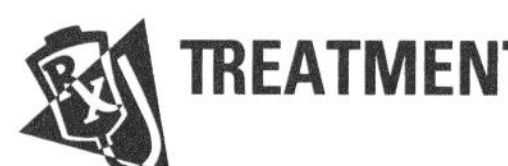

TREATMENT

MEDICATIONS

Emergency and supportive measures

- Discontinue the drug at the first sign of gross bleeding, and determine the PT

Activated charcoal

- If the patient has ingested an acute overdose, administer activated charcoal, 60–100 g PO or via gastric tube, mixed in aqueous slurry

Specific treatment

- If the PT is elevated, give phytonadione (vitamin K_1), 10–25 mg PO, and additional doses as needed to restore the PT to normal
- Do not treat prophylactically—wait for the evidence of anticoagulation (elevated PT)
- Give fresh-frozen plasma as needed to rapidly correct the coagulation factor deficit if there is serious bleeding
- If the patient is chronically anticoagulated and has strong medical indications for being maintained in that status (eg, prosthetic heart valve), give much smaller doses of vitamin K (1 mg) and fresh-frozen plasma (or both) to titrate to the desired PT
- If the patient has ingested brodifacoum or a related superwarfarin, prolonged observation (over weeks) and repeated administration of large doses of vitamin K may be required

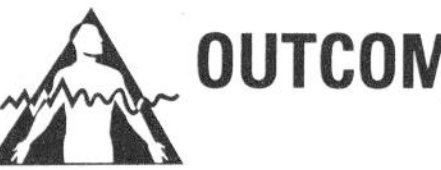

OUTCOME

FOLLOW-UP

- Serial evaluation of PT

COMPLICATIONS

- Bleeding

WHEN TO ADMIT

- Admit all patients with a history of superwarfarin ingestion for 2-day observation of the PT
- Admit all patients with active bleeding

PROGNOSIS

- Very good if no active bleeding and if close outpatient follow-up (and vitamin K treatment, if needed) is maintained (for several weeks or longer after brodifacoum overdose)

EVIDENCE

WEB SITES

- National Pesticide Information Center: Pesticide Poisonings
  - http://npic.orst.edu/rmpp.htm
- eMedicine: Toxicology Articles
  - http://www.emedicine.com/emerg/toxicology.htm

INFORMATION FOR PATIENTS

- National Institutes of Health: Anticoagulants (Systemic)
  - http://www.nlm.nih.gov/medlineplus/druginfo/uspdi/202050.html

REFERENCE

- Ingels M et al: A prospective study of acute, unintentional, pediatric superwarfarin ingestions managed without decontamination. Ann Emerg Med 2002;40:73. [PMID: 12085076]

Author(s)

Kent R. Olson, MD

Anticonvulsant Overdose

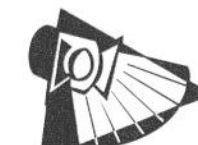

KEY FEATURES

ESSENTIALS OF DIAGNOSIS

- Ataxia, slurred speech, somnolence
- Valproic acid can cause hypernatremia, metabolic acidosis, hyperammonemia

GENERAL CONSIDERATIONS

- Rapid IV injection of phenytoin can cause acute myocardial depression and cardiac arrest owing to the solvent propylene glycol (does not occur with fosphenytoin injection)
- Phenytoin intoxication can occur with only slightly increased doses because of the small toxic-therapeutic window and zero-order kinetics

CLINICAL FINDINGS

SYMPTOMS AND SIGNS

Phenytoin

- The overdose syndrome is usually mild even with high serum levels
- The most common manifestations are ataxia, nystagmus, and drowsiness
- Choreoathetoid movements have been described

Carbamazepine

- Drowsiness, stupor, and, with high levels, coma and seizures
- Dilated pupils and tachycardia are common

Valproic acid

- Encephalopathy, which may be associated with hyperammonemia, metabolic acidosis, cerebral edema
- Produces a unique syndrome consisting of hypernatremia (from the sodium component of the salt), metabolic acidosis, hypocalcemia, elevated serum ammonia, and mild liver aminotransferase elevation
- Hypoglycemia may occur as a result of hepatic metabolic dysfunction
- Coma with small pupils, which can mimic opioid poisoning

DIFFERENTIAL DIAGNOSIS

- Opioid intoxication
- Sedative-hypnotic overdose

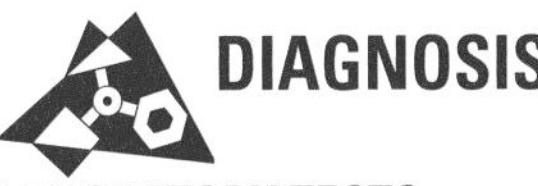

DIAGNOSIS

LABORATORY TESTS

- Carbamazepine toxicity
  - May be seen with serum levels > 20 mg/L, though severe poisoning is usually associated with concentrations > 30–40 mg/L
  - Because of erratic and slow absorption, intoxication may progress over several hours to days
- Phenytoin toxicity
  - Levels > 20 mg/L associated with ataxia, nystagmus, drowsiness
- Valproic acid
  - Obtain frequent repeated levels to rule out delayed absorption from sustained-release formulations (eg, Depakote, Depakote ER)

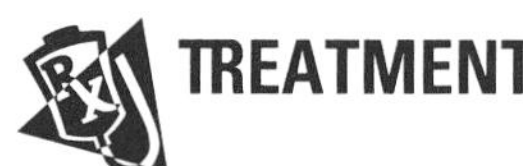

TREATMENT

MEDICATIONS

Repeat-dose charcoal

- Repeated doses of activated charcoal, 20–30 g Q3–4h, are indicated for massive ingestions of valproic acid or carbamazepine
- Sorbitol or other cathartics should *not* be used with each dose, or resulting large stool volumes may lead to dehydration or hypernatremia

Whole-bowel irrigation

- For large ingestions of carbamazepine or valproic acid, especially of sustained-release formulations, consider whole-bowel irrigation
- Administer the balanced polyethylene glycol-electrolyte solution (CoLyte, GoLYTELY) into the stomach via gastric tube at a rate of 1–2 L/h until the rectal effluent is clear

Specific treatment

- There are no specific antidotes
- Naloxone has been reported to reverse valproic acid overdose in a few anecdotal case reports

THERAPEUTIC PROCEDURES

- Consider hemodialysis for massive intoxication (eg, carbamazepine levels > 100 mg/L or valproic acid levels > 1000 mg/L)

OUTCOME

WHEN TO ADMIT

- For phenytoin-induced ataxia if adequate home care is not available
- After overdose of any drug with symptoms

EVIDENCE

PRACTICE GUIDELINES

- Guidelines from the Royal Children's Hospital, Melbourne, Australia: Anticonvulsant Poisoning
  - http://www.rch.org.au/clinicalguide/cpg.cfm?doc_id=5427

WEB SITE

- eMedicine: Toxicology Articles
  - http://www.emedicine.com/emerg/toxicology.htm

INFORMATION FOR PATIENTS

- Epilepsy Foundation: Special Concerns About Seizure Medications
  - http://www.epilepsyfoundation.org/answerplace/Life/adults/women/weimeds.cfm
- National Institutes of Health: Anticonvulsants: Hydantoin (Systemic)
  - http://www.nlm.nih.gov/medlineplus/druginfo/uspdi/202052.html
- National Institutes of Health: Anticonvulsants: Succinimide (Systemic)
  - http://www.nlm.nih.gov/medlineplus/druginfo/uspdi/202053.html
- National Institutes of Health: Anticonvulsants: Dione (Systemic)
  - http://www.nlm.nih.gov/medlineplus/druginfo/uspdi/202051.html

REFERENCES

- Cameron RJ et al: Efficacy of charcoal hemoperfusion in massive carbamazepine poisoning. J Toxicol Clin Toxicol 2002;40:507. [PMID: 12217004]
- Glick TH et al: Preventing phenytoin intoxication: safer use of a familiar anticonvulsant. J Fam Pract 2004;53:197. [PMID: 15000924]
- Singh SM et al: Extracorporeal management of valproic acid overdose: a large regional experience. J Nephrol 2004;17:43. [PMID: 15151258]

Author(s)

Kent R. Olson, MD

Antipsychotic Agent Overdose p. 1028

Anxiety & Dissociative Disorders

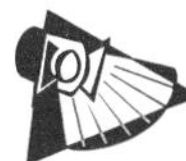

KEY FEATURES

ESSENTIALS OF DIAGNOSIS

- Overt anxiety or an overt manifestation of a defense mechanism (eg, a phobia), or both
- Not limited to an adjustment disorder
- Somatic symptoms referable to the autonomic nervous system or to a specific organ system (eg, dyspnea, palpitations, paresthesias)
- Not a result of physical disorders, psychiatric conditions (eg, schizophrenia), or drug abuse

GENERAL CONSIDERATIONS

- Group of disorders
  - Generalized anxiety disorder (GAD 300.02)
  - Panic disorder (300.01)
  - Obsessive-compulsive disorder (OCD 300.3)
  - Phobic disorder (300.2)
  - Dissociative disorder
- *GAD*
  - Symptoms are brought on by everyday activities
  - Are present on most days for at least 6 months
- *Panic disorder*
  - Symptoms occur in recurrent, short-lived episodes with unpredictable triggers
  - Somatic symptoms are often marked
- *OCD*
  - Patients experience recurrent intrusive thoughts or obsessions
  - They engage in compulsive actions or rituals to maintain control
- *Phobic disorder*
  - Symptoms occur predictably
  - Follow exposure to certain objects or situations
- *Dissociative disorder*
  - The reaction is precipitated by emotional crisis
  - The symptom produces anxiety reduction and a temporary solution of the crisis
  - Mechanisms include repression and isolation, as well as particularly limited concentration, as seen in hypnotic states

DEMOGRAPHICS

- Incidence
  - OCD: 2–5%
- Prevalence
  - Panic disorder: 3–5%, 25% with coincident OCD
- Age
  - Panic disorder: onset < 25 years
  - OCD: onset 20–35 years
- Risk factors
  - OCD: divorce or separation, unemployment

CLINICAL FINDINGS

SYMPTOMS AND SIGNS

- Anxiety or fear
- Apprehension or worry
- Difficulty concentrating
- Insomnia and fatigue
- Irritability
- Feelings of impending doom
- Recurrent thoughts or fears
- Repetitive actions and rituals
- Avoidant behaviors
- Sympathomimetic symptoms
  - Tachycardia
  - Hyperventilation
  - Tremor
  - Sweating
- Somatic symptoms
  - Headache
  - Paresthesias
  - Dizziness
  - Nausea
  - Bloating
  - Chest pain
  - Palpitations
- Examples of dissociative states
  - Fugue (the sudden, unexpected travel away from one's home with inability to recall one's past)
  - Amnesia
  - Somnambulism
  - Dissociative identity disorder (multiple personality disorder)
  - Depersonalization

DIFFERENTIAL DIAGNOSIS

- Hyperthyroidism
- Pheochromocytoma
- Sympathomimetic drug use
- Myocardial infarction
- Hypoglycemia
- Adjustment disorders
- Dissociative symptoms are similar to symptoms of temporal lobe dysfunction

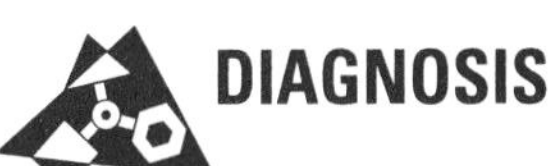

DIAGNOSIS

LABORATORY TESTS

- Thyroid-stimulating hormone
- Complete blood cell count
- Toxicology screen (if suspected)
- Glucose (as appropriate to rule out medical disorders)

IMAGING STUDIES

- Chest x-ray may be indicated
- Head CT may be useful in dissociative symptoms to rule out temporal lobe dysfunction

DIAGNOSTIC PROCEDURES

- ECG
- EEG may be useful in dissociative symptoms to rule out temporal lobe dysfunction

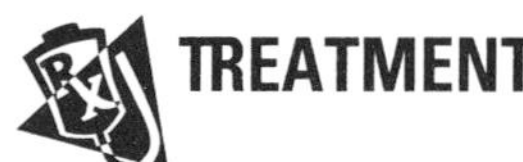

TREATMENT

MEDICATIONS

- See Table 105
- GAD
  - Benzodiazepines initially [diazepam 5–10 mg PO TID (or equivalent)]
  - Buspirone (start 15–60 mg PO divided TID)
  - Venlafaxine (start 37.5–75 mg PO QD)
  - Possibly selective serotonin reuptake inhibitors (SSRIs), paroxetine
- Panic disorder
  - Lorazepam (0.5–2 mg PO) or alprazolam SL (0.5–1 mg) as acute treatment
  - SSRIs (eg, sertraline 25 mg PO QD, titrate upward after 1 week) for ongoing treatment
- OCD
  - SSRIs, usually in doses higher than for depression (eg, fluoxetine, up to 60–80 mg PO QD)
  - Clomipramine
- Phobic disorder
  - SSRIs (paroxetine, sertraline, fluvoxamine)
  - Monoamine oxidase inhibitors
  - Gabapentin (900–3600 mg PO divided TID) for global social phobia
  - Propranolol 20–40 mg PO 1 hour before exposure for specific phobias (eg, performance)

SURGERY

- Stereotactic modified cingulotomy of limited use in severe, unremitting OCD

THERAPEUTIC PROCEDURES

- Behavioral/cognitive
  - Frequently used in conjunction with medical therapies
  - Relaxation techniques (particularly effective for physiologic symptoms in *Panic disorder*)
  - Desensitization, via graded exposure to a phobic object
  - Emotive imagery (imagining anxiety-provoking situation while using relaxation techniques)
  - Cognitive therapy
- Social
  - Support groups
  - Family counseling
  - School, vocational counseling

OUTCOME

FOLLOW-UP

- Every 1–2 weeks until stabilized, then as agreed upon with patient

COMPLICATIONS

- Alcohol and substance abuse

WHEN TO REFER

- Refer to a psychiatrist
  - If the diagnosis is in question
  - To receive recommendations on therapy
  - If first-line therapy has failed
  - If patient presents with management problems

PROGNOSIS

- Usually longstanding and difficult to treat
- All disorders relieved to varying degrees by medication and behavioral techniques (eg, 60% response rate to SSRIs for OCD)

EVIDENCE

PRACTICE GUIDELINES

- National Guideline Clearinghouse: Anxiety Disorders. Singapore Ministry of Health, 2003
  - http://www.guideline.gov/summary/summary.aspx?doc_id=5293
- Bandelow B et al: World Federation of Societies of Biological Psychiatry (WFSBP) guidelines for the pharmacological treatment of anxiety, obsessive-compulsive and posttraumatic stress disorders. World J Biol Psychiatry 2002;3:171. [PMID: 12516310]

WEB SITES

- American Psychiatric Association
  - http://www.psych.org/
- Anxiety Disorders Association of America
  - http://www.adaa.org
- Internet Mental Health
  - http://www.mentalhealth.com/t30.html

INFORMATION FOR PATIENTS

- American Psychiatric Association
  - http://www.psych.org/public_info/anxiety.cfm
- JAMA patient page: Obsessive-compulsive disorder. JAMA 1998;280:1806. [PMID:9842960]
- National Institute of Mental Health
  - http://www.nimh.nih.gov/publicat/anxiety.cfm
  - http://www.nimh.nih.gov/publicat/NIMHocd.cfm

REFERENCES

- Kaplan A et al: A review of pharmacologic treatments for obsessive compulsive disorder. Psychiatr Serv 2003;54:1111. [PMID: 12883138]
- Pohl RB et al: Sertraline in the treatment of panic disorder: a double-blind multicenter trial. Am J Psychiatry 1998;155:1189. [PMID: 9734541]
- Stein DJ et al: Efficacy of paroxetine for relapse prevention in social anxiety disorder: a 24-week study. Arch Gen Psychiatry 2002;59:1111. [PMID: 12470127]

Author(s)

Stuart J. Eisendrath, MD

Jonathan E. Lichtmacher, MD

Aortic Dissection

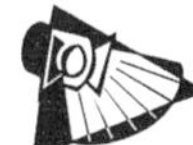

KEY FEATURES

ESSENTIALS OF DIAGNOSIS

- A history of hypertension or Marfan's syndrome is often present
- Sudden severe chest pain with radiation to the back, occasionally migrating to the abdomen and hips or groin
- Patient appears to be in shock, but blood pressure is normal or elevated; pulse discrepancy in many patients
- Acute aortic regurgitation

GENERAL CONSIDERATIONS

- Aortic dissection caused by an intimal tear allows creation of a false lumen between the media and adventitia
- More than 95% of intimal tears occur either in the ascending aorta just distal to the aortic valve (Stanford type A) or just distal to the left subclavian artery (Stanford type B)
- A false lumen can rupture into the left pleural space, retroperitoneum, pericardium, or abdominal cavity, but more commonly propagates distally to involve aortic branch vessels, producing acute ischemia of the spinal cord (3%), viscera (9%), kidney (12%), or lower extremity (9%)
- Anterograde extension can produce acute aortic regurgitation, myocardial infarction, and intrapericardial rupture with tamponade
- Risk factors include hypertension (80% of patients), Marfan's syndrome, pregnancy, bicuspid aortic valve, and coarctation of the aorta

CLINICAL FINDINGS

SYMPTOMS AND SIGNS

- Sudden excruciating ("ripping") pain in the chest or upper back, radiating into the abdomen, neck, or groin in 85%
- Hypertension in most patients
- Syncope, hemiplegia, lower extremity paralysis, or abdominal pain
- Physical examination: diminished or unequal peripheral pulses and blood pressures
- Diastolic murmur of aortic regurgitation

DIFFERENTIAL DIAGNOSIS

- Acute myocardial infarction
- Pulmonary embolus
- Esophageal rupture
- Strangulated paraesophageal hernia
- Mesenteric ischemia
- Symptomatic aortic aneurysm
- Pneumothorax/pneumonia
- Extremity arterial embolus

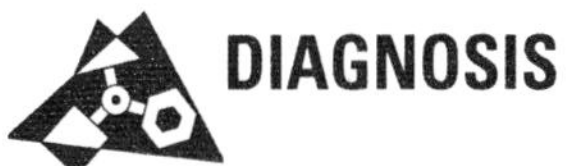

DIAGNOSIS

LABORATORY TESTS

- Electrocardiogram may be normal but often reveals left ventricular hypertrophy
- Acute ischemia suggests coronary artery involvement
- Because dissections preferentially extend into the right coronary ostium, inferior wall ischemic changes predominate

IMAGING STUDIES

- Chest x-ray film: abnormal aortic contour or a widened superior mediastinum, pleural or pericardial effusion
- Dynamic CT scanning, angiography, MRI, and transesophageal echocardiography (TEE) are all useful in diagnosis
- TEE has high sensitivity (98%) and specificity (99%)
- CT or MRI useful for serial follow-up

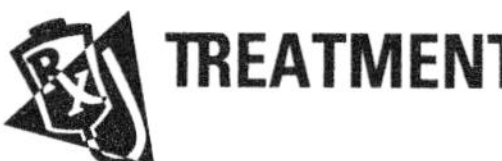

TREATMENT

MEDICATIONS

Acute management

- Vasodilator: nitroprusside (0.3–10 μg/kg/min) or fenoldopam (0.1–1.6 μg/kg/min) by continuous IV infusion to maintain systolic blood pressure of 100–120 mm Hg (Table 51)
- β-Blocker: esmolol (50–300 μg/kg/min IV), metoprolol (5–10 mg IV Q15 min), or labetalol (20–80 mg IV Q10 min or 1–2 mg/min) to decrease heart rate (Table 51)

Chronic management

- β-Blocker (eg, metoprolol 25–100 mg PO BID, atenolol 50–100 mg PO QD), often in combination with
  - Clonidine, 0.1–0.3 mg PO BID (0.1–0.3 mg TTS patch topically Q24 h), or
  - Hydralazine, 10–50 mg PO QID, or
  - Amlodipine, 2.5–10 mg PO QD, or
  - Enalapril, 2.5–20 mg PO QD

SURGERY

- Type A dissection: warrants emergent surgical repair
- Replace ascending aorta and, if necessary, the aortic valve and arch with reimplantation of the coronary and brachiocephalic vessels
- Type B dissection: manage aggressively with medications initially
- Indications for surgical treatment of type B dissections: aortic rupture; severe intractable pain; mesenteric, renal, or limb ischemia; progression of dissection
- Surgery involves obliteration of the false lumen and secondary arterial bypass if this fails to restore blood flow
- Obliteration of the false lumen involves resection of the entry point of the dissection and prosthetic tube graft interposition, open or endovascular fenestration of the dissection flap, or stent graft deployment to cover the entry point
- Chronic type B dissections: repair if patients are symptomatic or aneurysm diameter > 6 cm

THERAPEUTIC PROCEDURES

- Bed rest
- Opioids for pain relief
- Arterial line for continuous blood pressure monitoring
- Reduce aortic pressure and pulsatile flow (*dP/dt*) by lowering systemic vascular resistance and cardiac output (heart rate)

OUTCOME

FOLLOW-UP

- Acute: if nitroprusside is administered for ≥ 48 h, check serum thiocyanate level and stop the infusion if level is > 10 mg/dL to avoid toxicity
- Chronic: monitor unoperated patients with annual CT scan or MRI

PROGNOSIS

- Mortality in untreated type A dissection is 50% at 48 h and 90% at 1 month
- Mortality in untreated type B dissection is 10–20%
- Operative mortality of type A dissection approaches 20%
- Operative mortality of type B dissection is twice that of type A dissection
- 5-year survival is 70–80% for repaired type A dissections and 50–70% for repaired type B dissections

WHEN TO REFER

- Any acute aortic dissection
- Chronic dissection with diameter > 4 cm or evidence of progression

WHEN TO ADMIT

- Any acute aortic dissection
- Any symptomatic dissection

PREVENTION

- Control of hypertension
- Control of hyperlipidemia

EVIDENCE

PRACTICE GUIDELINES

- National Guideline Clearinghouse: Diagnosis and Management of Aortic Dissection
  - http://www.guideline.gov/summary/summary.aspx?ss=15&doc_id=2975&nbr=2201
- National Guideline Clearinghouse: ACR Appropriateness Criteria for Acute Chest Pain—No ECG Evidence of Myocardial Ischemia/Infarction
  - http://www.guideline.gov/summary/summary.aspx?ss=15&doc_id=3254&nbr=2480

INFORMATION FOR PATIENTS

- MedlinePlus: Aortic Dissection
  - http://www.nlm.nih.gov/medlineplus/ency/article/000181.htm
  - http://www.americanheart.org/presenter.jhtml?identifier=3005390
- Mayo Clinic: Aortic Dissection
  - http://www.mayoclinic.com/invoke.cfm?id=AN00678

REFERENCES

- Beregi J-P et al: Endovascular treatment for dissection of the descending aorta. Lancet 2000;356:482. [PMID: 10981895]
- Buffolo E et al: Revolutionary treatment of aneurysms and dissections of descending aorta: the endovascular approach. Ann Thorac Surg 2002;74:S1815. [PMID: 12440672]
- Genoni M et al: Chronic beta blocker therapy improves outcome and reduces treatment costs in chronic type B aortic dissection. Eur J Cardiothorac Surg 2001;19:606. [PMID: 11343940]
- Hagan P et al: The International Registry of Acute Aortic Dissection (IRAD): new insights into an old disease. JAMA 2000;283:897. [PMID: 10685714]

Author(s)

Louis M. Messina, MD

Appendicitis

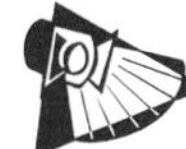

KEY FEATURES

ESSENTIALS OF DIAGNOSIS

- Early: periumbilical pain
- Later: right lower quadrant pain and tenderness
- Anorexia, nausea and vomiting, obstipation
- Tenderness or localized rigidity at McBurney's point
- Low-grade fever and leukocytosis

GENERAL CONSIDERATIONS

- The most common abdominal surgical emergency, affecting ~10% of the population
- Occurs most commonly between the ages of 10 and 30 years
- Caused by obstruction of the appendix by a fecalith, inflammation, foreign body, or neoplasm
- If untreated, gangrene and perforation develop within 36 hours

CLINICAL FINDINGS

SYMPTOMS AND SIGNS

- Vague, often colicky, periumbilical or epigastric pain
- Within 12 hours, pain shifts to right lower quadrant, with steady ache worsened by walking or coughing
- Nausea and one or two episodes of vomiting in almost all
- Constipation
- Low-grade fever (< 38°C)
- Localized tenderness with guarding in the right lower quadrant
- Rebound tenderness
- Psoas sign (pain on passive extension of the right hip)
- Obturator sign (pain with passive flexion and internal rotation of the right hip)
- Atypical presentations include
  - Pain less intense and poorly localized; tenderness minimal in the right flank
  - Pain in the lower abdomen, often on the left; urge to urinate or defecate
  - Abdominal tenderness absent, but tenderness on pelvic or rectal examination

DIFFERENTIAL DIAGNOSIS

- Gastroenteritis or colitis
- Gynecologic: pelvic inflammatory disease, tuboovarian abscess, ovarian torsion, ruptured ectopic pregnancy or ovarian cyst, mittelschmerz, endometriosis
- Urologic: testicular torsion, acute epididymitis
- Urinary calculus
- Pyelonephritis
- Diverticulitis
- Meckel's diverticulitis
- Carcinoid of the appendix
- Perforated colon cancer
- Crohn's ileitis
- Perforated peptic ulcer
- Cholecystitis
- Mesenteric adenitis
- Typhlitis (neutropenic colitis)
- Mesenteric ischemia

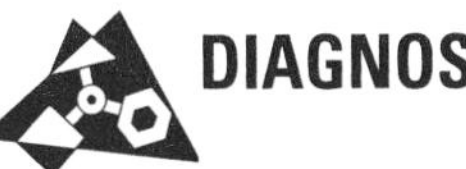

DIAGNOSIS

LABORATORY TESTS

- Moderate leukocytosis (10,000–20,000/μL) with neutrophilia
- Microscopic hematuria and pyuria in 25%

IMAGING STUDIES

- No imaging necessary in typical appendicitis
  - Imaging may be useful in patients in whom the diagnosis is uncertain
  - Imaging studies (US or CT) suggest alternative diagnosis in up to 15%
- Abdominal or transvaginal ultrasound
  - Diagnostic accuracy of >85%
  - Useful in the exclusion of adnexal disease in younger women
- Abdominal CT
  - Most accurate test for diagnosis (sensitivity and specific ≈95%)
  - Useful in suspected appendiceal perforation to diagnose a periappendiceal abscess

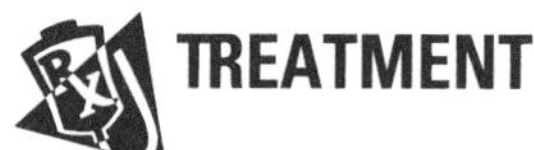

TREATMENT

MEDICATIONS

- Systemic antibiotics reduce the incidence of postoperative wound infections

SURGERY

- Surgical appendectomy by laparotomy or by laparoscopy in patients with uncomplicated appendicitis
- Emergency appendectomy in patients with perforated appendicitis with generalized peritonitis

THERAPEUTIC PROCEDURES

- Percutaneous CT-guided drainage of periappendiceal abscess, intravenous fluids and antibiotics, and interval appendectomy after 6 weeks in stable patients with perforated appendicitis

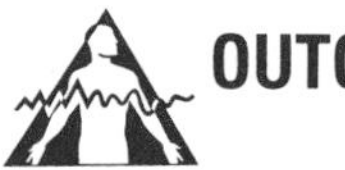

OUTCOME

COMPLICATIONS

- Perforation in 20%
- Periappendiceal abscess
- Suppurative peritonitis
- Septic thrombophlebitis (pylephlebitis) of the portal venous system

PROGNOSIS

- Mortality rate of uncomplicated appendicitis is extremely low
- Mortality rate of perforated appendicitis is 0.2%, but 15% in the elderly

EVIDENCE

PRACTICE GUIDELINES

- National Guideline Clearinghouse
  - http://www.guideline.gov/summary/summary.aspx?doc_id=4132&nbr=3168&string=appendicitishttp://www.guideline.gov/summary/summary.aspx?doc_id=4222&nbr=3227&string=appendicitis

WEB SITE

- Gastrointestinal Pathology Index
  - http://medstat.med.utah.edu/WebPath/GIHTML/GIIDX.html

INFORMATION FOR PATIENTS

- Mayo Clinic
  - http://www.mayoclinic.com/invoke.cfm?id=DS00274
- NDDIC–NIH
  - http://digestive.niddk.nih.gov/ddiseases/pubs/appendicitis/index.htm

REFERENCES

- Sauerland S et al: Laparascopic versus open surgery for suspected appendicitis. Cochrane Database Syst Rev 2004;(11)CD001546. [PMID: 15495014]
- Terasawa T et al: Systematic review: computed tomography and ultrasonography to detect acute appendicitis in adults and adolescents. Ann Intern Med 2004;141:357. [PMID: 15466771]

Author(s)

Kenneth R. McQuaid, MD

Arteriovenous Malformations, Intracranial

Arbovirus Encephalitides p. 1031.
Arsenic Poisoning p. 1031.

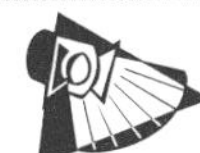

KEY FEATURES

ESSENTIALS OF DIAGNOSIS

- Sudden onsest of subarachnoid or intracerebral hemorrhage
- Distinctive neurologic signs reflect the region of the brain involved
- Signs of meningeal irritation in patients presenting with subarachnoid hemorrhage
- Seizures or focal deficits may occur

GENERAL CONSIDERATIONS

- See Table 96
- Congenital vascular malformations
  - Result from a localized maldevelopment of part of the primitive vascular plexus
  - Vary in size, ranging from massive lesions fed by multiple vessels to small lesions that are hard to identify at arteriography, surgery, or autopsy
- Symptoms may relate to hemorrhage or to cerebral ischemia due to diversion of blood by the anomalous arteriovenous shunt or venous stagnation
- Most cerebral arteriovenous malformations are **supratentorial** and in the middle cerebral artery territory
- **Infratentorial** lesions: brainstem or cerebellar arteriovenous malformations
- Small arteriovenous malformations are more likely to bleed than large ones
- Arteriovenous malformations that have bled once are more likely to bleed again
- Bleeding unrelated to sex or lesion site
- Hemorrhage is intracerebral and subarachnoid (with 10% of cases fatal)

DEMOGRAPHICS

- Up to 70% of arteriovenous malformations bleed, most commonly before the age of 40
- Approximately 10% of cases are associated with arterial aneurysm, while 1–2% of patients with aneurysms have arteriovenous malformations

CLINICAL FINDINGS

SYMPTOMS AND SIGNS

Supratentorial lesions

- Initial symptoms
  - Hemorrhage in 30–60% of cases
  - Recurrent seizures in 20–40%
  - Headache in 5–25%
  - Miscellaneous complaints (including focal deficits) in 10–15%
- Focal or generalized seizures may accompany or follow hemorrhage, or may be the initial presentation, especially with frontal or parietal arteriovenous malformations
- Headaches, especially when the external carotid arteries are involved (sometimes simulate migraine but usually are nonspecific in character)
- In patients with subarachnoid hemorrhage, examination may reveal an abnormal mental status and signs of meningeal irritation
- Symptoms of increased intracranial pressure may be present—headache, visual obscurations, obtundation
- A cranial bruit may be present but may also be found with aneurysms, meningiomas, acquired arteriovenous fistulas, and arteriovenous malformations involving the scalp, calvarium, or orbit
- Bruits are best heard over the ipsilateral eye or mastoid region and help in lateralization but not localization
- Absence of a bruit does not exclude an arteriovenous malformation

Infratentorial lesions

- Brainstem arteriovenous malformations are often clinically silent but may hemorrhage, cause obstructive hydrocephalus, or lead to progressive or relapsing brainstem deficits
- Cerebellar arteriovenous malformations may also be clinically inconspicuous but sometimes lead to cerebellar hemorrhage

DIFFERENTIAL DIAGNOSIS

- Aneurysmal hemorrhage
- Intracerebral hemorrhage from other causes
- Space-occupying lesion, eg, brain tumor

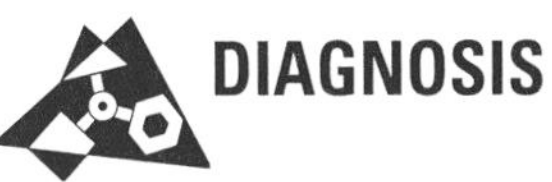

DIAGNOSIS

IMAGING STUDIES

- CT scanning
  - Indicates whether subarachnoid or intracerebral bleeding has recently occurred
  - Helps localize its source, and may reveal the arteriovenous malformation
- Arteriography
  - If the source of hemorrhage is not evident on the CT scan, arteriography is necessary to exclude aneurysm or arteriovenous malformation. MR angiography is not always sensitive enough for this purpose
  - Even if the findings on CT scan suggest arteriovenous malformation, bilateral arteriography of the internal and external carotid and vertebral arteries is required to establish the nature of the lesion
  - Arteriovenous malformations typically appear as a tangled vascular mass with distended tortuous afferent and efferent vessels, a rapid circulation time, and arteriovenous shunting
- MRI typically reveals the lesion but does not define its blood supply
- Plain radiographs of the skull are often normal unless an intracerebral hematoma is present, in which case there may be changes suggestive of raised intracranial pressure and displacement of a calcified pineal gland

DIAGNOSTIC PROCEDURES

- If the CT scan shows no evidence of bleeding but subarachnoid hemorrhage is diagnosed clinically, the cerebrospinal fluid should be examined
- Electroencephalography is usually indicated in patients presenting with seizures and may show consistently focal or lateralized abnormalities resulting from the underlying cerebral arteriovenous malformation

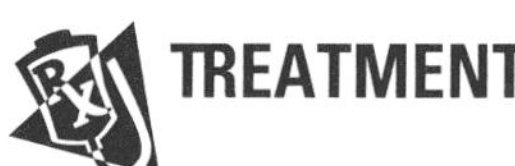

TREATMENT

MEDICATIONS

- In patients presenting solely with seizures, anticonvulsant drug treatment is usually sufficient, and surgery is unnecessary

SURGERY

- Surgical treatment to prevent further hemorrhage is justified with arteriovenous malformations that have bled, provided that the lesion is accessible and the patient has a reasonable life expectancy
- Surgical treatment is appropriate if intracranial pressure is increased and to prevent further progression of a focal neurologic deficit
- Definitive operative treatment consists of excision of the arteriovenous malformation if it is surgically accessible

THERAPEUTIC PROCEDURES

- Inoperable arteriovenous malformations are sometimes treated solely by embolization; although the risk of hemorrhage is not reduced, neurologic deficits may be stabilized or even reversed by this procedure
- Other techniques are injection of a vascular occlusive polymer through a flow-guided microcatheter and permanent occlusion of feeding vessels by positioning detachable balloon catheters in the desired sites and then inflating them with quickly solidifying contrast material
- Stereotactic radiosurgery with the gamma knife is also useful in the management of inoperable cerebral arteriovenous malformations

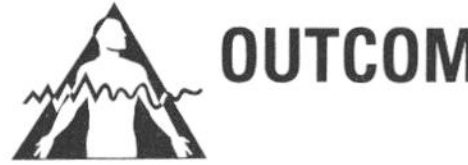

OUTCOME

FOLLOW-UP

- Serial MRIs help monitor malformations that are not treated surgically

COMPLICATIONS

- Communicating or obstructive hydrocephalus may occur and lead to symptoms

PROGNOSIS

- Depends on site of malformation and whether it has bled

WHEN TO REFER

- All patients

EVIDENCE

PRACTICE GUIDELINES

- Ogilvy CS et al: AHA Scientific Statement: recommendations for the management of intracranial arteriovenous malformations. Stroke 2001;32:1458. [PMID: 11387517]
- National Guideline Clearinghouse
  - http://www.guideline.gov/summary/summary.aspx?doc_id=4360&nbr=3285&string=arteriovenous+AND+malformations
- American Society of Interventional and Therapeutic Neuroradiology. Embolization of spinal arteriovenous fistulae, spinal arteriovenous malformations, and tumors of the spinal axis. AJNR Am J Neuroradiol 2001;22(8 Suppl):S28. [PMID: 11686072]

WEB SITE

- The Whole Brain Atlas
  - http://www.med.harvard.edu/AANLIB/home.html

INFORMATION FOR PATIENTS

- Columbia University College of Physicians and Surgeons Cerebrovascular Center
  - http://cpmcnet.columbia.edu/dept/cerebro/AVM.html
- National Institute of Neurological Disorders and Stroke
  - http://www.ninds.nih.gov/disorders/avms/detail_avms.htm
- UCSF Neurocritical Care and Stroke Patient Information
  - http://www.ucsf.edu/stroke/patinfo.htm#avm

REFERENCES

- Al-Shahi R et al: A systematic review of the frequency and prognosis of arteriovenous malformations of the brain in adults. Brain 2001;124:1900. [PMID: 11571210]
- Fleetwood IG et al: Arteriovenous malformations. Lancet 2002;359:863. [PMID: 11897302]

Author(s)

Michael J. Aminoff, MD, DSc, FRCP

Arthritis, Gonococcal

Arthritis & Inflammatory Bowel Diseases p. 1031.
Arthritis in Sarcoidosis p. 1032.

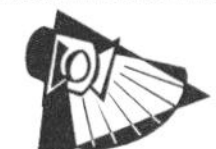

KEY FEATURES

ESSENTIALS OF DIAGNOSIS

- Prodromal migratory polyarthralgias
- Tenosynovitis most common sign
- Purulent monarthritis in 50%
- Characteristic skin rash
- Most common in young women during menses or pregnancy
- Symptoms of urethritis frequently absent
- Dramatic response to antibiotics

GENERAL CONSIDERATIONS

- Usually occurs in otherwise healthy individuals
- Most common cause of infectious arthritis in large urban areas
- Recurrent disseminated gonococcal infection occurs when there is a congenital deficiency of complement components, especially C7 and C8

DEMOGRAPHICS

- Two to three times more common in women than in men and is especially common during menses and pregnancy
- Gonococcal arthritis is also common in male homosexuals
- Rare after age 40

CLINICAL FINDINGS

SYMPTOMS AND SIGNS

- One to 4 days of migratory polyarthralgias involving the wrist, knee, ankle, or elbow
- Thereafter, two patterns emerge, one (60%) characterized by tenosynovitis and the other (40%) by purulent monarthritis, most frequently involving the knee
- Less than half of patients have fever
- Less than one-fourth have genitourinary symptoms
- Most patients will have asymptomatic but highly characteristic skin lesions: two to ten small necrotic pustules distributed over the extremities, especially the palms and soles

DIFFERENTIAL DIAGNOSIS

- Reactive arthritis (Reiter's syndrome)
  - Can produce acute monarthritis in a young person but is distinguished by negative cultures, sacroiliitis, and failure to respond to antibiotics
- Lyme disease involving the knee
  - Less acute
  - Does not show positive cultures
  - May be preceded by known tick exposure and characteristic rash
- Infective endocarditis with septic arthritis
- Nongonococcal septic arthritis
- Gout or pseudogout
- Rheumatic fever
- Sarcoidosis
- Meningococcemia

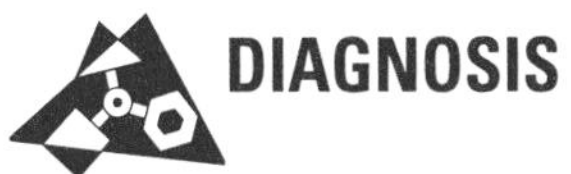

DIAGNOSIS

LABORATORY TESTS

- The synovial fluid white blood cell count is typically over 50,000 cells/μL
- The synovial fluid Gram stain is positive in one-fourth of cases and culture in less than half
- Positive blood cultures are seen in 40% of patients with tenosynovitis and virtually never in patients with suppurative arthritis
- Urethral, throat, and rectal cultures should be done in all patients, since they are often positive in the absence of local symptoms
- The peripheral blood leukocyte count averages 10,000 cells/μL and is elevated in < one-third of patients

IMAGING STUDIES

- Radiographs are usually normal or show only soft tissue swelling

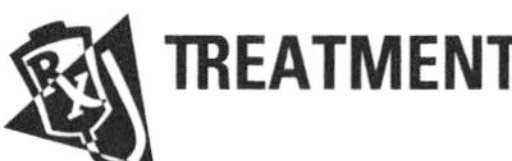

TREATMENT

MEDICATIONS

- Approximately 25% of patients have absolute or relative resistance to penicillin. Therefore, give ceftriaxone, 1 g IV daily (or cefotaxime, 1 g IV Q8 h; or ceftizoxime, 1 g IV Q8 h; or spectinomycin, 2 g IM Q12 h, for patients with β-lactam allergy)
- Once improvement from parenteral antibiotics has been achieved for 24–48 h, patients can be switched to cefixime, 400 mg PO twice daily, or ciprofloxacin, 500 mg PO twice daily, to complete a 7- to 10-day course

THERAPEUTIC PROCEDURES

- Generally responds dramatically in 24–48 h after initiation of antibiotics so that daily joint aspirations are rarely needed

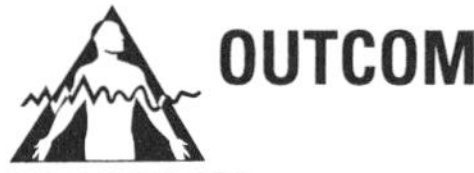

OUTCOME

PROGNOSIS

- Complete recovery is the rule

WHEN TO REFER

- When diagnosis is in doubt
- Report to the public health department for tracing contacts

WHEN TO ADMIT

- While outpatient treatment has been recommended in the past, the rapid rise in gonococci resistant to penicillin makes initial inpatient treatment advisable
- Patients in whom gonococcal arthritis is suspected should be admitted to the hospital to confirm the diagnosis, to exclude endocarditis, and to start treatment

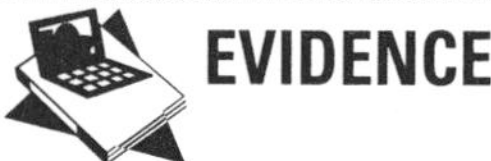

EVIDENCE

PRACTICE GUIDELINES

- National Guideline Clearinghouse
  - http://www.guideline.gov/summary/summary.aspx?doc_id=3045

INFORMATION FOR PATIENTS

- National Institutes of Health
  - http://www.nlm.nih.gov/medlineplus/ency/article/000453.htm

REFERENCES

- Bardin T: Gonococcal arthritis. Best Pract Res Clin Rheumatol 2003;17:201. [PMID: 12787521]
- Sieper J et al: Diagnosing reactive arthritis: role of clinical setting in the value of serologic and microbiologic assays. Arthritis Rheum 2002;46:319. [PMID: 11840434]

Author(s)

David B. Hellmann, MD, FACP
John H. Stone, MD, MPH

Arthritis, Nongonococcal Acute Bacterial (Septic)

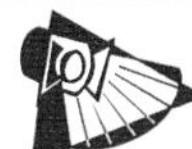

KEY FEATURES

ESSENTIALS OF DIAGNOSIS

- Sudden onset of acute arthritis, usually monarticular, most often in large weight-bearing joints and wrists
- Previous joint damage or injection drug use are common risk factors
- Infection with causative organisms commonly found elsewhere in body
- Joint effusions are usually large, with white blood cell counts commonly > 50,000/μL

GENERAL CONSIDERATIONS

- A disease of an abnormal host
- Key risk factors are persistent bacteremia (eg, injection drug use, endocarditis) and damaged joints (eg, rheumatoid arthritis)
- *Staphylococcus aureus* is the most common cause of nongonococcal septic arthritis, followed by group A and group B streptococci
- Gram-negative septic arthritis is seen in injection drug users and in other immunocompromised patients
- *Staphylococcus epidermidis* is the usual organism in prosthetic joint arthritis

CLINICAL FINDINGS

SYMPTOMS AND SIGNS

- Sudden onset, with pain, swelling, and heat of one joint—most frequently the knee
- Unusual sites, such as the sternoclavicular or sacroiliac joint, can be involved in injection drug users
- Chills and fever are common but are absent in up to 20% of patients
- Infection of the hip usually does not produce apparent swelling but results in groin pain greatly aggravated by walking

DIFFERENTIAL DIAGNOSIS

- Gout and pseudogout are excluded by the failure to find crystals on synovial fluid analysis
- Acute rheumatic fever and rheumatoid arthritis commonly involve many joints
- Still's disease may mimic septic arthritis, but laboratory evidence of infection is absent

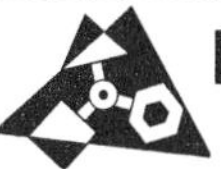

DIAGNOSIS

LABORATORY TESTS

- Blood cultures are positive in approximately 50% of patients
- The leukocyte count of the synovial fluid exceeds 50,000/μL and often 100,000/μL, with 90% or more polymorphonuclear cells
- Gram stain of the synovial fluid is positive in 75% of staphylococcal infections and in 50% of gram-negative infections

IMAGING STUDIES

- Radiographs are usually normal early in the disease, but evidence of demineralization may be present within days of onset
- Bony erosions and narrowing of the joint space followed by osteomyelitis and periostitis may be seen within 2 weeks

DIAGNOSTIC PROCEDURES

- Joint aspiration is required to establish the diagnosis

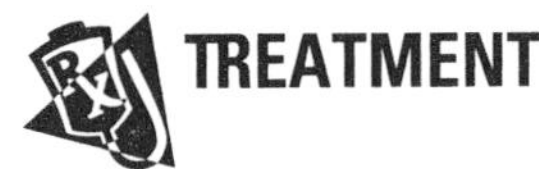

TREATMENT

MEDICATIONS

- Prompt systemic antibiotic therapy of any septic arthritis should be based on the best clinical judgment of the causative organism
- If the organism cannot be determined clinically, treatment should be started with bactericidal antibiotics effective against staphylococci, pneumococci, and gram-negative organisms

SURGERY

- Immediate surgical drainage is reserved for septic arthritis of the hip, because that site is inaccessible to repeated aspiration
- For most other joints, surgical drainage is used only if medical therapy fails over 2–4 days to improve the fever and the synovial fluid volume, white blood cell count, and culture results

THERAPEUTIC PROCEDURES

- Rest, immobilization, and elevation are used at the onset of treatment. Early active motion exercises within the limits of tolerance will hasten recovery
- Frequent (even daily) local aspiration is indicated to complement antibiotic therapy when synovial fluid rapidly reaccumulates and causes symptoms

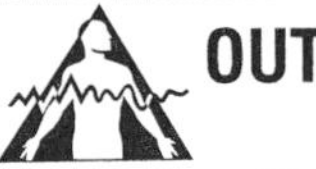

OUTCOME

COMPLICATIONS

- Bony ankylosis and articular destruction occur if treatment is delayed or inadequate

PROGNOSIS

- With prompt antibiotic therapy and no serious underlying disease, functional recovery is usually good
- Five to 10% of patients with an infected joint die, chiefly from respiratory complications of sepsis
- The mortality rate is 30% for patients with polyarticular sepsis

WHEN TO REFER

- Refer to an orthopedist if the infected joint is not easy to aspirate repeatedly (eg, hip)

WHEN TO ADMIT

- Admit for presumed or confirmed septic arthritis

EVIDENCE

INFORMATION FOR PATIENTS

- American Association for Clinical Chemistry
  - http://www.labtestsonline.org/understanding/conditions/septic.html
- National Institutes of Health
  - http://www.nlm.nih.gov/medlineplus/ency/article/000430.htm

REFERENCES

- Ross JJ: Pneumococcal septic arthritis. Clin Infect Dis 2003;36:319. [PMID: 12539074]
- Ross JJ et al: Sternoclavicular septic arthritis: review of 180 cases. Medicine (Baltimore) 2004;83:139. [PMID: 15118542]
- Zimmerli W et al: Prosthetic-joint infections. N Engl J Med 2004;351:1645. [PMID: 15483283]

Author(s)

David B. Hellmann, MD, FACP
John H. Stone, MD, MPH

Arthritis, Reactive (Reiter's Syndrome)

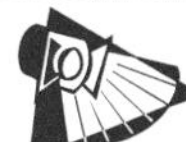

KEY FEATURES

ESSENTIALS OF DIAGNOSIS

- Oligoarthritis, conjunctivitis, urethritis, and mouth ulcers most common features
- Usually follows dysentery or a sexually transmitted infection
- Fifty to 80% of patients are HLA-B27 positive

GENERAL CONSIDERATIONS

- Reiter's syndrome (also called reactive arthritis) is a clinical tetrad
  - Urethritis
  - Conjunctivitis (or, less commonly, uveitis)
  - Mucocutaneous lesions
  - Aseptic arthritis
- Most cases develop within days or weeks after definite or implicated triggers
  - Dysentery: *Shigella, Salmonella, Yersinia, Campylobacter*
  - Sexually transmitted disease: *Chlamydia trachomatis, Ureaplasma urealyticum*, gonorrhea
  - Other: *Chlamydia pneumoniae, Clostridium difficile*
- Gonococcal arthritis can initially mimic Reiter's syndrome, but the marked improvement after 24–48 h of antibiotic administration and the culture results distinguish the two disorders

DEMOGRAPHICS

- Most commonly in young men
- The gender ratio: 1:1 after enteric infections but 9:1 with male predominance after sexually transmitted infections
- Associated with HLA-B27 in 80% of white patients and 50–60% of blacks

CLINICAL FINDINGS

SYMPTOMS AND SIGNS

- The arthritis is most commonly asymmetric and frequently involves the large weight-bearing joints (chiefly the knee and ankle)
- Sacroiliitis or ankylosing spondylitis is observed in at least 20% of patients
- Systemic symptoms including fever and weight loss are common at the onset of disease
- The mucocutaneous lesions may include circinate balanitis, stomatitis, and keratoderma blenorrhagicum, indistinguishable from pustular psoriasis
- Carditis and aortic regurgitation may occur

DIFFERENTIAL DIAGNOSIS

- Gonococcal arthritis
- Psoriatic arthritis
- Ankylosing spondylitis
- Rheumatoid arthritis
- Arthritis associated with inflammatory bowel disease

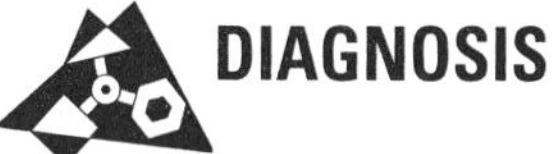

DIAGNOSIS

LABORATORY TESTS

- HLA B-27 test is useful in the diagnosis

IMAGING STUDIES

- X-ray signs of permanent or progressive joint disease may be seen in the sacroiliac as well as the peripheral joints

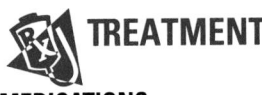

TREATMENT

MEDICATIONS

- Nonsteroidal anti-inflammatory drugs (NSAIDs) have been the mainstay of therapy
- Corticosteroids are typically not helpful
- Tetracycline (250 mg four times daily) given for 3 months to patients with Reiter's syndrome associated with *C trachomatis* reduces the duration of symptoms
- Patients who do not respond to NSAIDs and tetracycline may respond to sulfasalazine, 1000 mg twice daily
- Antitumor necrosing factor agents (etanercept, infliximab) are reasonable therapies for patients with refractory disease

OUTCOME

PROGNOSIS

- While most signs of the disease disappear within days or weeks, the arthritis may persist for several months or even years
- Recurrences involving any combination of the clinical manifestations are common and are sometimes followed by permanent sequelae, especially in the joints

WHEN TO REFER

- Refer to a rheumatologist for progressive symptoms despite therapy

PREVENTION

- Antibiotics given at the time of a nongonococcal sexually transmitted infection reduce the chance that Reiter's syndrome will develop

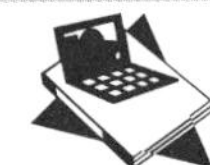

EVIDENCE

PRACTICE GUIDELINES

- National Guideline Clearinghouse
  - http://www.guideline.gov/summary/summary.aspx?doc_id=3045

INFORMATION FOR PATIENTS

- American Academy of Family Physicians
  - http://familydoctor.org/handouts/448.html
- National Institute of Arthritis and Musculoskeletal and Skin Diseases
  - http://www.niams.nih.gov/hi/topics/reactive/reactive.htm

REFERENCES

- Kvien TK et al: Three month treatment of reactive arthritis with azithromycin: a EULAR double blind, placebo controlled study. Ann Rheum Dis 2004;63:1113. [PMID: 15308521]
- Sieper J et al: Diagnosing reactive arthritis: role of clinical setting in the value of serologic and microbiologic assays. Arthritis Rheum 2002;46:319. [PMID: 11840434]

Author(s)

David B. Hellmann, MD, FACP
John H. Stone, MD, MPH

Ascariasis

Arthritis, Viral p. 1032. Asbestosis p. 1032.

KEY FEATURES

ESSENTIALS OF DIAGNOSIS

- Pulmonary phase
  - Transient cough
  - Dyspnea
  - Wheezing
  - Urticaria
  - Eosinophilia
  - Transient pulmonary infiltrates
- Intestinal phase
  - Vague upper abdominal discomfort
  - Occasional vomiting
  - Abdominal distention
- Eggs in stools
- Worms passed per rectum, nose, or mouth

GENERAL CONSIDERATIONS

- *Ascaris lumbricoides* is the most common intestinal helminth
- Adult worms live in the upper small intestine
- After fertilization, the female produces enormous numbers of eggs that pass in feces
- Direct transmission between humans does not occur, as the eggs must remain on the soil for 2–3 weeks before they become infective; thereafter, they can survive for years
- Infection occurs through ingestion of mature eggs in fecally contaminated food and drink
- Egg production begins 60–75 days after ingestion of infective eggs. Adult worms (20–40 cm × 3–6 mm) live for 1 year or more
- As a result of their migration and induction of hypersensitivity, larvae in the lung cause capillary and alveolar damage and symptoms of the pulmonary phase

DEMOGRAPHICS

- An estimated 1 billion people are infected worldwide
- It is cosmopolitan in distribution and is found in high prevalence wherever there are low standards of hygiene and sanitation (including focally in the southeastern United States) or where human feces are used as fertilizer

CLINICAL FINDINGS

SYMPTOMS AND SIGNS

- Pulmonary phase
  - Low-grade fever
  - Nonproductive cough
  - Blood-tinged sputum
  - Wheezing
  - Dyspnea
  - Substernal pain
- There may be urticaria and localized rales
- Rarely, larvae lodge ectopically in the brain, kidney, eye, spinal cord, etc, and may be symptomatic
- Small numbers of adult worms in the intestine usually produce no symptoms
- With heavy infection, peptic ulcer-like symptoms or vague preprandial or postprandial abdominal discomfort may be seen
- Adult worms may be coughed up, vomited, or emerge through the nose or anus
- Adult worms may migrate into the common bile duct, pancreatic duct, appendix, diverticula, and other sites, which may lead to cholangitis, cholecystitis, cholelithiasis, pyogenic liver abscess, pancreatitis, or obstructive jaundice
- With very heavy infestations, masses of worms may cause intestinal obstruction, volvulus, intussusception, or death

DIFFERENTIAL DIAGNOSIS

- Asthma
- Allergic bronchopulmonary aspergillosis (ABPA)
- Acute eosinophilic pneumonia (Löffler's syndrome)
- Paragonimiasis
- Tropical pulmonary eosinophilia (*Wuchereria bancrofti*, *Brugia malayi*)
- Hookworm disease
- Strongyloidiasis
- Toxocariasis (visceral larva migrans)
- Peptic ulcer disease
- Other causes of cholangitis, cholecystitis, pancreatitis, appendicitis, diverticulitis

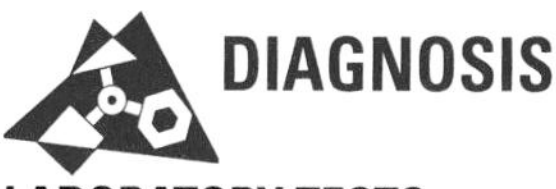

DIAGNOSIS

LABORATORY TESTS

- During the pulmonary phase, eosinophils may reach 30–50% and remain high for about a month; larvae are occasionally found in sputum
- During the intestinal phase, diagnosis usually depends on finding the characteristic eggs in feces
- Occasionally, an adult worm spontaneously passed per rectum or orally reveals an unsuspected infection
- Serologic tests are not useful, and there is no eosinophilia in the intestinal phase

IMAGING STUDIES

- During the larval migratory phase, chest radiographs may show transitory, patchy, ill-defined asymmetric infiltrations (Löffler's syndrome)
- Radiologic examination of the abdomen (with or without barium) may show the presence of worms
- In intestinal obstruction, plain abdominal films show air-filled levels and multiple linear images of ascarides in dilated bowel loops; ultrasonography can also demonstrate the dilated bowel and worm mass

DIAGNOSTIC PROCEDURES

- The diagnosis of biliary ascariasis can be made by endoscopic retrograde cholangiopancreatography, which has the therapeutic potential of removing the worms

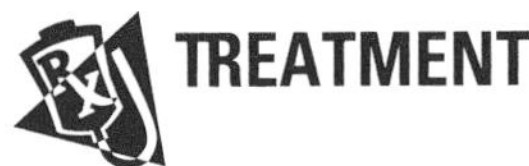

TREATMENT

MEDICATIONS

- Albendazole and pyrantel pamoate are the treatments of choice
- Ascariasis, hookworm, and trichuriasis infections, which often occur together, may be treated simultaneously by albendazole, mebendazole, or oxantel-pyrantel pamoate
- In pregnancy, ascariasis should be treated after the first trimester
- Drug treatment should not be used in the migratory phase
- **Albendazole**
  - In light infections, a single dose (400 mg) results in cure rates over 95%; in heavy infections, a 2- to 3-day course is indicated
  - Side effects, including migration of ascaris through the nose or mouth, are rare
  - The drug is contraindicated in pregnancy
- **Pyrantel pamoate**
  - A single oral dose of 10 mg base/kg (maximum, 1 g) results in 85–100% cure rates; it may be given before or after meals
  - Infrequent and mild side effects include vomiting, diarrhea, headache, dizziness, and drowsiness
- **Mebendazole**
  - Although highly effective when given in a dosage of 100 mg twice daily before or after meals for 3 days, a single 500-mg dose is often sufficient
  - Gastrointestinal side effects are infrequent
  - The drug is contraindicated in pregnancy
- **Piperazine**
  - The dosage for piperazine (as the hexahydrate) is 75 mg/kg body weight (maximum, 3.5 g) for 2 days in succession, giving the drug orally before or after breakfast
  - For heavy infestations, treatment should be continued for 4 days in succession or the 2-day course should be repeated after 1 week
  - Gastrointestinal symptoms and headache occur occasionally; central nervous system symptoms (temporary ataxia and exacerbation of seizures) are rare
  - Allergic symptoms have been attributed to piperazine
  - The drug should not be used for patients with hepatic or renal insufficiency or in those with a history of seizures or chronic neurological disease
- **Levamisole**
  - Not approved in the US for ascariasis
  - A single oral dose of 150 mg is highly effective
  - Occasional mild and transient side effects are nausea, vomiting, abdominal pain, headache, and dizziness
- **Ivermectin**
  - One dose (200 µg/kg) had a cure rate of 78%; with two doses given at a 10-day interval the cure rate increased to 99%
  - This drug is under evaluation for mass treatment of intestinal helminth infections and ectoparasites

THERAPEUTIC PROCEDURES

- In intestinal obstruction or biliary ascariasis, surgery may be avoided by nasogastric suction followed by a standard dose of an anthelmintic given via the tube
- In biliary ascariasis, endoscopic removal of the worm under ultrasonographic guidance is often successful; treatment by injection of a solution of albendazole or piperazine into the common duct followed by systemic treatment has also been effective

OUTCOME

FOLLOW-UP

- Stools should be rechecked at 2 weeks after treatment and patients retreated until all ascarids are removed
- Because anesthesia stimulates worms to hypermotility, they should be removed in advance in infected patients undergoing elective surgery
- The complications caused by wandering adult worms require that all *Ascaris* infections be treated and eradicated

WHEN TO REFER

- If there is difficulty in making the diagnosis or progressive symptoms despite therapy

WHEN TO ADMIT

- Intestinal obstruction or biliary ascariasis

EVIDENCE

WEB SITE

- Centers for Disease Control and Prevention—Division of Parasitic Diseases
  - http://www.cdc.gov/ncidod/dpd/parasites/ascaris/default.htm

INFORMATION FOR PATIENTS

- Centers for Disease Control and PreventionDivision of Parasitic Diseases
  - http://www.cdc.gov/ncidod/dpd/parasites/ascaris/factsht_ascaris.htm
- National Institute of Allergy and Infectious Disease
  - http://www.niaid.nih.gov/factsheets/roundwor.htm
- Nemours Foundation
  - http://kidshealth.org/parent/infections/stomach/ascariasis.html

REFERENCES

- Crompton DW: Ascaris and ascariasis. Adv Parasitol 2001;48:285. [PMID: 11013758]
- Dib J et al: Hepato-biliary ascariasis. Gastrointest Endosc 2000;51:594. [PMID: 10805849]
- Misra SP et al: Clinical features and management of biliary ascariasis in non-endemic areas. Postgrad Med J 2000;76:29. [PMID: 10622777]
- Ogata H et al: Multilocular pyogenic hepatic abscess complicating *Ascaris lumbricoides* infestation. Intern Med 2000;39:228. [PMID: 10772125]

Ascites

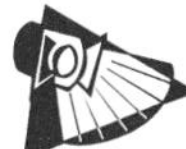

KEY FEATURES

ESSENTIALS OF DIAGNOSIS

- Pathologic accumulation of fluid in the peritoneal cavity

GENERAL CONSIDERATIONS

- Two broad categories of ascites
  - Ascites associated with a normal peritoneum
  - Ascites due to a diseased peritoneum (Table 54)
- Most common cause is portal hypertension secondary to chronic liver disease (>80% of cases)
- Other causes
  - Infections (tuberculous peritonitis)
  - Intra-abdominal malignancy
  - Inflammatory disorders of the peritoneum
  - Ductal disruptions (chylous, pancreatic, biliary)
- Risk factors for ascites include causes of liver disease
  - Ethanol consumption
  - Transfusions
  - Tattoos
  - Intravenous drug use
  - History of viral hepatitis or jaundice
  - Birth in an area endemic for hepatitis
- History of cancer or marked weight loss suggests malignancy
- Fevers suggest infected peritoneal fluid, including bacterial peritonitis (spontaneous or secondary)

DEMOGRAPHICS

- Tuberculous peritonitis occurs in
  - Immigrants
  - Immunocompromised hosts
  - Severely malnourished alcoholics
- Cirrhosis with portal hypertensive ascites most commonly caused by chronic alcoholism or chronic viral infection (hepatitis B or C)

CLINICAL FINDINGS

SYMPTOMS AND SIGNS

- Increasing abdominal girth
- Abdominal pain
- In portal hypertension: large abdominal wall veins with cephalad flow; inferiorly directed flow implies hepatic vein obstruction
- In portal hypertension and chronic liver disease
  - Palmar erythema
  - Cutaneous spider angiomas
  - Gynecomastia
  - Dupuytren's contracture
  - Asterixis
- In right-sided congestive heart failure or constrictive pericarditis: elevated jugular venous pressure
- In acute alcoholic hepatitis or Budd-Chiari syndrome: large tender liver
- In congestive heart failure or nephrotic syndrome: anasarca
- In malignancy: firm lymph nodes in the left supraclavicular region or umbilicus

DIFFERENTIAL DIAGNOSIS

- See Table 54
- Cirrhosis (80–85%)
- Malignancy (10%)
- Congestive heart failure (3%)
- Tuberculous peritonitis
- Dialysis-related
- Bile or pancreatic ascites
- Lymphatic tear (chylous ascites)
- Nephrotic syndrome

DIAGNOSIS

LABORATORY TESTS

- Ascitic fluid cell count: normal cell count is < 500 leukocytes/μL and < 250 polymorphonuclear neutrophils (PMNs)/μL
- PMN count of >250/μL (neutrocytic ascites), with >75% of all white blood cells (WBCs) being PMNs usually indicates bacterial peritonitis
- Ascitic fluid culture and Gram's stain in suspected peritonitis
- Elevated WBCs with a predominance of lymphocytes occur in tuberculosis or peritoneal carcinomatosis
- Cloudy ascitic fluid suggests infection
- Milky fluid occurs in chylous ascites
- Bloody fluid suggests traumatic paracentesis, malignant ascites
- Serum-ascites albumin gradient (SAAG) classifies ascites into portal hypertensive and nonportal hypertensive causes (Table 54)
- SAAG is calculated by subtracting the ascitic fluid albumin from the serum albumin
  - SAAG >1.1 g/dL suggests underlying portal hypertension
  - SAAG < 1.1 g/dL implicates nonportal hypertensive causes
- ~4% of patients have "mixed ascites," due to underlying cirrhosis with portal hypertension complicated by a second cause for ascites (such as malignancy or tuberculosis)
- An elevated SAAG and a high ascitic fluid total protein level (>2.5 g/dL)
  - In hepatic congestion secondary to cardiac disease or Budd-Chiari syndrome
  - In up to 20% of cases of uncomplicated cirrhosis
- Ascitic fluid glucose is low in tuberculous peritonitis
- Ascitic fluid amylase is elevated in pancreatic ascites or a perforation of the gastrointestinal tract
- Ascitic fluid bilirubin concentration is greater than the serum bilirubin in perforation of the biliary tree
- Ascitic fluid creatinine is elevated in leakage of urine from the bladder or ureters

IMAGING STUDIES

- Ultrasound and CT imaging is useful in
  - Distinguishing between causes of portal and nonportal hypertensive ascites, such as thrombosis of the hepatic veins (Budd-Chiari syndrome) or portal veins
  - Detecting lymphadenopathy and masses

– Permiting directed percutaneous needle biopsies of abnormal lymph nodes or solid organic masses

DIAGNOSTIC PROCEDURES

- Physical examination is insensitive for detecting ascites until >1500 mL of fluid
- Cytologic examination if peritoneal carcinomatosis is suspected
- Abdominal paracentesis is indicated
  - In all patients with new-onset ascites to diagnose bacterial peritonitis
  - In all patients admitted to the hospital with cirrhosis and ascites
  - In patients with known ascites who develop clinical deterioration (fever, abdominal pain, rapid worsening of renal function, or worsened hepatic encephalopathy)
- When fluid volume is small or fluid is loculated, abdominal ultrasound confirms presence of ascites and facilitates paracentesis
- Laparoscopy permits direct visualization and biopsy of the peritoneum, liver, and some intra-abdominal lymph nodes in suspected peritoneal tuberculosis or malignancy

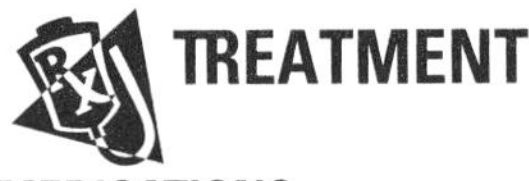

TREATMENT

MEDICATIONS

- Portal hypertensive ascites: diuretics. such as spironolactone, 100 mg/day, and furosemide, 40 mg/day
- Dose increased every 5–7 days until diuresis achieved, to maximum of 400 mg/day aldactone and 160 mg/day furosemide
- Goal is to lose 0.5 kg/day
- Careful monitoring of serum sodium, potassium, and creatinine required

SURGERY

- Peritovenous shunt in patients with refractory ascites due to portal hypertension

THERAPEUTIC PROCEDURES

- In ascites caused by portal hypertension, dietary sodium restriction to 1–2 g/day; fluid intake restriction if serum Na < 125 mEq/L
- TIPS (transjugular intrahepatic portosystemic shunt) effectively controls 75% of carefully selected patients with portal hypertension and refractory ascites
- Large-volume paracentesis (4–6 L) is indicated for patients with massive ascites or ascites refractory to diuretics
- Intravenous albumin should be administered with large-volume paracentesis to reduce acute and long-term complications: 10 g albumin/L of ascites removed

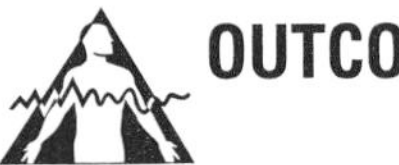

OUTCOME

COMPLICATIONS

- Portal hypertensive ascites: spontaneous bacterial peritonitis occurs in 20–30%; patients with ascites total protein < 1 g/dL are at higher risk (40%)
- Massive ascites
  - Ruptured umbilical hernia
  - Hepatic hydrothorax
  - Respiratory compromise
  - Poor nutritional intake
- Peritoneovenous shunts
  - Shunt occlusion
  - Disseminated intravascular coagulation
  - Bacterial infection
  - Variceal hemorrhage
- TIPS: encephalopathy in 30% and shunt stenosis or occlusion in 30–60% within 1 year, requiring periodic revisions

PROGNOSIS

- In patients with cirrhosis, ascites is a poor prognostic indicator, with 50% survival at 2 years

WHEN TO ADMIT

- Suspected peritonitis

EVIDENCE

PRACTICE GUIDELINES

- Runyon BA; Practice Guidelines Committee, American Association for the Study of Liver Diseases (AASLD). Management of adult patients with ascites due to cirrhosis.Hepatology 2004;39(3):841
- National Guideline Clearinghouse
  - http://www.guideline.gov/summary/summary.aspx?doc_id=4116&nbr=3161&string=Ascites

WEB SITE

- American Association for the Study of Liver Diseases
  - http://www.aasld.org

INFORMATION FOR PATIENTS

- Cancerbacup
  - http://www.cancerbacup.org.uk/info/ascites.htm
- MEDLINEplus
  - http://www.nlm.nih.gov/medlineplus/ency/article/000286.htm
- Merck Manual
  - http://www.merck.com/pubs/mmanual/section4/chapter38/38e.htm

REFERENCES

- Jeffrey J et al: Ascitic fluid analysis: the role of biochemistry and haematology. Hosp Med 2001;62:282. [PMID:11885888]
- Krige JE et al: ABC of diseases of the liver, pancreas, and biliary system: portal hypertension 2. Ascites, encephalopathy, and other conditions. BMJ 2001;322:416. [PMID:11179165]
- Runyon BA: Ascites. Clin Liver Dis 2000;4:151. [PMID:11232182]

Author(s)

Kenneth R. McQuaid, MD

Aspergillosis

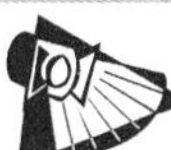

KEY FEATURES

- *Aspergillus fumigatus* is the usual cause of aspergillosis, although many species of *Aspergillus* can cause disease
- These fungi often colonize burn eschar and debris in the external ear canal
- Clinical illness results from abnormal immune response or tissue invasion, which can occur rarely in immunocompetent adults
- Life-threatening invasive aspergillosis usually occurs in profound immunodeficiency, particularly prolonged severe neutropenia
- Allergic bronchopulmonary aspergillosis (ABPA) occurs in asthmatics and sometimes in cystic fibrosis

CLINICAL FINDINGS

ABPA
  - Worsening bronchospasm develops in patients with asthma or cystic fibrosis
  - Waxing and waning course with gradual improvement but may cause saccular bronchiectasis and end-stage fibrotic lung disease
- In immunocompetent patients, aspergillosis causes
  - Chronic sinusitis
  - Aspergillomas, colonization of preexisting pulmonary cavities, found incidentally by chest x-ray film or in symptomatic patients who present with hemoptysis
- In immunocompromised patients, invasive aspergillosis causes
  - Pulmonary disease, leading to severe necrotizing pneumonia
  - Pleuritic chest pain, reflecting tissue infarction
  - Ulcerative tracheobronchitis that coexists with parenchymal pulmonary disease in AIDS patients
  - Hematogenous dissemination to CNS, skin, and other organs

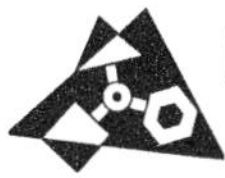

DIAGNOSIS

- ABPA
  - Fleeting pulmonary infiltrates, eosinophilia, high IgE levels, and *Aspergillus* precipitins in the blood
  - Aspergillomas of the lung appear on chest x-ray film or CT scan as "fungus ball" within a cavity
- Invasive aspergillosis
  - Chest x-ray film initially shows patchy infiltration, then severe necrotizing pneumonia
  - Elevated serum lactate dehydrogenase (resulting from tissue infarction)
  - Blood cultures of very low yield
  - Unlike in ABPA, serologic tests have low sensitivity
  - Detection of galactomannan by ELISA has sensitivity of 89% and specificity of 98% for invasive disease, although multiple determinations should be obtained
  - Isolation of *Aspergillus* from pulmonary secretions does not necessarily imply invasive disease
  - Mainstay of diagnosis is biopsy demonstration of *Aspergillus* in tissue as branched septate hyphae, although specimens do not invariably grow the organism

TREATMENT

- **ABPA:** for acute exacerbations, prednisone, 1 mg/kg/day PO tapered slowly over several months; itraconazole, 200 mg PO QD for 16 weeks appears to improve pulmonary function and decrease steroid requirements
- **Sinus disease:** long-term antifungal therapy (eg, itraconazole or voriconazole, 200 mg PO BID for weeks to months) and surgical débridement
- **Aspergillomas:** if symptomatic, surgical resection; itraconazole may yield some benefit; intracavitary amphotericin B and bronchoscopic removal have little success
- **Invasive aspergillosis**
  - Reversal of any correctable immunosuppression
  - Early diagnosis and high-dose amphotericin B when diagnosis likely or proven
  - Increase amphotericin dose rapidly to 0.8–1.5 mg/kg/day IV as tolerated for several weeks, then use doses of 0.6 mg/kg/day until clinical resolution
  - Lipid formulations of amphotericin B have less nephrotoxicity, allowing administration of higher doses (eg, 5–10 mg/kg/day), but are more costly
  - Voriconazole (6 mg/kg IV twice on first day, followed by 4 mg/kg IV BID) is a recently developed triazole with potent anti-*Aspergillus* activity and excellent oral absorption that has been demonstrated to be more effective than conventional amphotericin B with fewer adverse effects
  - Caspofungin acetate, 70 mg IV load, then 50 mg QD IV, is approved for invasive aspergillosis in patients refractory to or intolerant of other treatments. Caspofungin may be added to amphotericin B in critically ill patients not responding to amphotericin B
  - Surgical resection of invasive pulmonary aspergillosis warrants further study after promising results in neutropenic patients

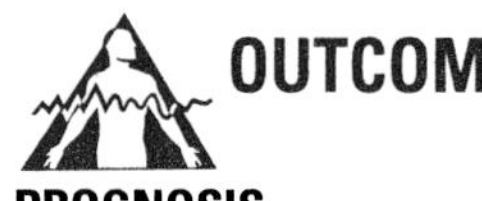

OUTCOME

PROGNOSIS

- Invasive aspergillosis
  - Can be life-threatening, particularly in profound immunodeficiency and prolonged severe neutropenia
  - In such patients, mortality rate of pulmonary or disseminated disease is > 50%

EVIDENCE

PRACTICE GUIDELINES

- Infectious Diseases Society of America: Practice guidelines for diseases caused by *Aspergillus*
  - http://www.journals.uchicago.edu/CID/journal/issues/v30n4/99126/991226.html
- Infectious Diseases Society of America: Guidelines for the use of antimicrobial agents in neutropenic patients with unexplained fever
  - http://www.journals.uchicago.edu/CID/journal/issues/v25n3/se34_551/se34_551.web.pdf
- Infectious Diseases Society of America: Summary of the guidelines for preventing opportunistic infections among hematopoietic stem cell transplant recipients
  - http://www.journals.uchicago.edu/CID/journal/issues/v33n2/001547/001547.html

REFERENCES

- Maertens J et al: Efficacy and safety of caspofungin for treatment of invasive aspergillosis in patients refractory to or intolerant of conventional antifungal therapy. Clin Infect Dis 2004;39:1563. [PMID: 15578352]
- Klont RR: Utility of *Aspergillus* antigen detection in specimens other than serum specimens.Clin Infect Dis 2004;39:1467. [PMID: 15546083]

Author(s)

Samuel A. Shelburne, MD

Richard J. Hamill, MD

Asthma

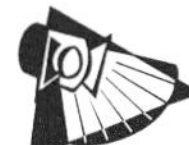

KEY FEATURES

ESSENTIALS OF DIAGNOSIS

- Episodic or chronic symptoms of airflow obstruction
  - Breathlessness
  - Cough
  - Wheezing
  - Chest tightness
- Symptoms frequently worse at night or in the early morning
- Prolonged expiration and diffuse wheezes on physical examination
- Limitation of airflow on pulmonary function testing or positive bronchoprovocation challenge
- Complete or partial reversibility of airflow obstruction, either spontaneously or after bronchodilator therapy

GENERAL CONSIDERATIONS

- Affects 5% of the population
- Accounts for 470,000 hospital admissions and 5000 deaths annually in the United States
- Prevalence, hospitalizations, and fatal asthma have all increased in the United States over the past 20 years

DEMOGRAPHICS

- Men and women are affected equally
- Hospitalization rates have been highest among blacks and children
- Death rates for asthma are consistently highest among blacks aged 15–24 years

CLINICAL FINDINGS

SYMPTOMS AND SIGNS

- See Tables 12 and 13
- Episodic wheezing and difficulty breathing, chest tightness, and cough
- Symptoms are frequently worse at night
- Common aeroallergens
  - Dust mites
  - Cockroaches
  - Cats
  - Pollen
- Nonspecific precipitants
  - Exercise
  - Respiratory tract infections
  - Postnasal drip
  - Aspiration
  - Gastroesophageal reflux
  - Changes in weather
  - Stress
- Tobacco smoke increases symptoms and decreases lung function
- Certain medications (including aspirin and nonsteroidal anti-inflammatory drugs) may be triggers
- Nasal findings consistent with allergy and evidence of allergic skin disorders
- Wheezing with normal breathing or a prolonged forced expiratory phase

DIFFERENTIAL DIAGNOSIS

Upper airway disorders

- Vocal cord paralysis
- Vocal cord dysfunction syndrome
- Foreign body aspiration
- Laryngotracheal mass
- Tracheal stenosis
- Tracheomalacia
- Angioedema
- Airway edema from inhalation injury

Lower airway disorders

- Chronic obstructive pulmonary disease
- Bronchiectasis
- Allergic bronchopulmonary aspergillosis
- Cystic fibrosis
- Eosinophilic pneumonia
- Bronchiolitis obliterans

Other

- Congestive heart failure (cardiac asthma)
- Gastroesophageal reflux disease
- Pulmonary embolism
- Churg-Strauss syndrome

Psychiatric

- Conversion disorder

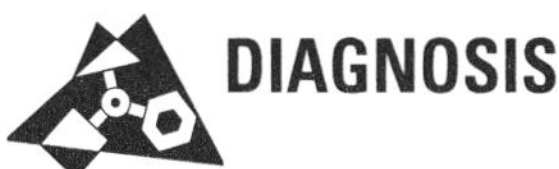

DIAGNOSIS

LABORATORY TESTS

- See Tables 12 and 13
- Spirometry (FEV_1, FVC, FEV_1/FVC) before and after the administration of a short-acting bronchodilator
- Significant reversibility of obstruction is demonstrated by an increase of >12% and 200 mL in FEV_1 or >15% and 200 mL in FVC after inhaling a bronchodilator
- Arterial blood gases may show a respiratory alkalosis and an increase in the alveolar–arterial oxygen difference; in severe exacerbations, hypoxemia develops and the $PaCO_2$ normalizes
- An increased $PaCO_2$ and respiratory acidosis may portend respiratory failure

IMAGING STUDIES

- Chest x-rays show only hyperinflation, but may include bronchial wall thickening and diminished peripheral lung vascular shadows
- Chest x-rays if pneumonia or complications of asthma are suspected

DIAGNOSTIC PROCEDURES

- Bronchial provocation testing with histamine, methacholine, or exercise is useful when asthma is expected and spirometry is nondiagnostic
- Skin testing for sensitivity to environmental allergens may be useful in persistent asthma

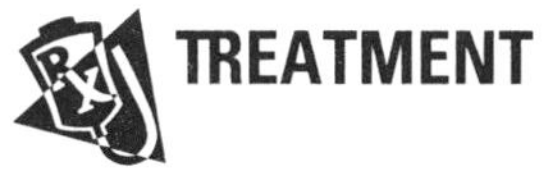

TREATMENT

MEDICATIONS

- See Tables 14 and 15

Long-term control therapy

- Inhaled corticosteroids
- Systemic corticosteroids
- Long-acting β_2-agonists
- Combination inhaled corticosteroid and long-acting β_2-agonist
- Leukotriene modifiers
- Mediator inhibitors
- Phosphodiesterase inhibitors

Quick-relief therapy

- See Table 16
- Short-acting inhaled β_2-agonists
- Anticholinergics
- Glucocorticoids

- Antimicrobials
  - No role in routine asthma exacerbations
  - Fever and purulent sputum and evidence of pneumonia or bacterial sinusitis may suggest a benefit

Acute exacerbations

- Repetitive or continuous use of inhaled short-acting β_2-agonist
- Early administration of systemic corticosteroids
- Treatment or removal of any identified trigger to the exacerbation
- **Mild exacerbations** [peak expiratory flow (PEF) >80%]
  - Double the usual dose of inhaled steroids after acute treatment
- **Moderate exacerbations** (PEF 50–80%)
  - A course of oral corticosteroids
- **Severe exacerbations** (PEF < 50%)
  - Rapid inititiation of high-dose bronchodilators and systemic corticosteroids and careful observation

Chronic asthma

- Treatment is guided by an assessment of asthma severity (see Table 12)
- Mild intermittent asthma
  - Short-acting β_2-agonists
  - Control therapy added if >2 uses/week
- Mild persistent asthma
  - Daily use of either low-dose inhaled steroid OR cromolyn or neodocromil
  - Sustained-release theophylline or leukotriene modifier is less desirable
  - Short-acting β_2-agonists
- Moderate persistent asthma
  - Daily use of medium-dose OR low–medium-dose inhaled steroid with long-acting inhaled β_2-agonist
  - Daily use of long-acting inhaled β_2-agonist OR sustained-release theophylline or long-acting β_2-agonist tablets
  - Short-acting β_2-agonists
- Severe persistent asthma
  - Daily use of high-dose inhaled corticosteroid AND long-acting bronchodilator or sustained-release theophylline or long-acting β_2-agonist tablets
  - Daily use of systemic corticosteroids
  - Short-acting β_2-agonists

THERAPEUTIC PROCEDURES

- Desensitization to specific allergens
- Intubation and mechanical ventilation for patients with impending respiratory failure; permissive hypercapnia to limit airway pressures

OUTCOME

FOLLOW-UP

- Patient self-assesment is a primary method of monitoring
- PEF monitoring can provide objective measurement to guide treatment
  - A 20% change in PEF from day to day or AM to PM suggests inadequate control
  - PEF < 200 L/min indicates severe obstruction
- Follow-up visits should be at least biannual to maintain control and evaluate medication adjustments
- Repeat spirometry at least every 1–2 years after symptoms have stabilized

COMPLICATIONS

- Exhaustion, dehydration, and tussive syncope
- Cor pulmonale
- Airway infection
- Acute hypercapnic and hypoxic respiratory failure in severe disease

PROGNOSIS

- Good with regular follow-up and care

WHEN TO REFER

- Lack of response to therapy or progressive disease

WHEN TO ADMIT

- Patients with acute exacerbations who have an inadequate response to initial therapy
- Admission should be considered for patients with a PEF or FEV_1 < 70% of predicted; admission is likely for PEF < 50%
- The duration and severity of symptoms, as well as severity of prior exacerbations and psychosocial issues, should be taken into account

PREVENTION

- Patients should be taught to recognize early symptoms of an exacerbation and initiate a predetermined action plan
- Pneumococcal and annual influenza vaccination
- Environmental measures to reduce exposure to allergens should occur

EVIDENCE

PRACTICE GUIDELINES

- National Institutes of Health
  - http://www.nhlbi.nih.gov/guidelines/asthma/index.htm
- National Guideline Clearinghouse
  - http://www.guideline.gov/summary/summary.aspx?ss=15&doc_id=3444&nbr=2670&string=asthma
  - http://www.guideline.gov/summary/summary.aspx?doc_id=3734&nbr=2960&string=asthma

INFORMATION FOR PATIENTS

- JAMA patient page: Adult asthma. JAMA 2004;292:402
- National Institute of Allergy and Infectious Disease
  - http://www2.niaid.nih.gov/newsroom/focuson/asthma01/basics.htm

REFERENCES

- Barnes PJ et al: How do corticosteroids work in asthma? Ann Intern Med 2003;139:359. [PMID:12965945]
- Busse WW et al: Asthma. N Engl J Med 2001;344:350. [PMID:11172168]
- Guidelines for the diagnosis and management of asthma. National Asthma Education and Prevention Program: Expert Panel Report 2. National Institutes of Health, Publication No. 97-4051, Bethesda, MD, 1997.
- Rodrigo GJ et al: Acute asthma in adults: a review. Chest 2004;125:1081. [PMID:15006973]
- Sin DD et al: Pharmacological management to reduce exacerbations in adults with asthma: a systemic review and meta-analysis. JAMA 2004;292:367. [PMID:15265853]
- Walker S et al: Anti-IgE for chronic asthma in adults and children. Cochrane Database Syst Rev 2004;3:CD003559. [PMID 15266491]

Author(s)

Mark S. Chesnutt, MD

Thomas J. Prendergast, MD

Atrial Fibrillation

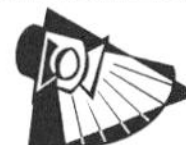

KEY FEATURES

ESSENTIALS OF DIAGNOSIS

- Irregularly irregular heart rhythm
- Untreated, the atrial rate is 400–600 bpm; the ventricular response is irregular, ranging from 80 bpm to 180 bpm

GENERAL CONSIDERATIONS

- The most common chronic arrhythmia, affecting nearly 10% of individuals older than 80
- Rarely life-threatening
- If the ventricular rate is rapid enough, it can precipitate hypotension, myocardial ischemia, or myocardial dysfunction

CLINICAL FINDINGS

SYMPTOMS AND SIGNS

- Irregularly irregular pulse
- Often occurs paroxysmally before becoming the established rhythm
- Older or inactive individuals may have relatively few symptoms; however, some patients are made uncomfortable by the irregular rhythm
- In patients with heart disease, rheumatic disease, and other valvular heart disease, dilated cardiomyopathy, atrial septal defect, hypertension, coronary heart disease, and thyrotoxicosis can cause attacks
- In patients with normal hearts, pericarditis, chest trauma, thoracic or cardiac surgery, pulmonary disease, electrolyte disturbances, acute alcohol excess or withdrawal, and medications such as theophylline and β-adrenergic agonists can cause attacks

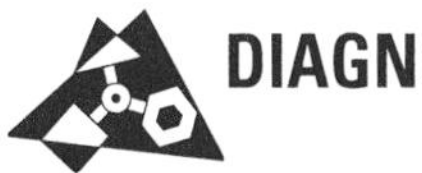

DIAGNOSIS

LABORATORY TESTS

- ECG
  - Lack of normal P waves and an irregular, rapidly fluctuating baseline
  - Irregular ventricular rhythm, with heart rate usually 80–180 bpm
- Echocardiography
  - Visualization of fibrillating atria with irregular ventricular contractions
  - Recommended in patients with newly diagnosed atrial fibrillation to exclude occult valvular or myocardial disease
- Ambulatory ECG monitoring or event recorders are indicated when paroxysmal atrial fibrillation is suspected
- Obtain thyroid-stimulating hormone level to exclude thyrotoxicosis

TREATMENT

MEDICATIONS

- Up to two-thirds of patients with a first episode will spontaneously revert to sinus rhythm within 24 h
- If atrial fibrillation persists for > 1 week, spontaneous conversion is unlikely, and management consists of rate control and anticoagulation
- Rate control is defined as ventricular rate of 50–100 bpm with usual daily activities and not exceeding 120 bpm except with moderate to strenuous activity
- Conventional rate-control agents used singly or, in younger adults, often in combination, include β-blockers, digoxin, and calcium channel blockers (Table 40)
- In patients with heart failure, coronary artery disease, or ongoing ischemia, β-blockers (metoprolol or esmolol) are preferred
- If hypertension is present or β-blockers are contraindicated, calcium channel blockers (diltiazem or verapamil) are effective
- Amiodarone is useful when rate control with other agents is incomplete or contraindicated or when cardioversion is anticipated
- Do not use digoxin, verapamil, or β-blockers if atrial fibrillation is associated with a known or suspected accessory pathway

THERAPEUTIC PROCEDURES

- Urgent electrical cardioversion is indicated in patients with shock or severe hypotension, pulmonary edema, or ongoing myocardial infarction or ischemia, even if atrial fibrillation has been present for > 48 h
- Elective electrical or pharmacologic cardioversion is recommended in patients with an initial episode of recent onset when there is an identifiable precipitating factor and in those who remain symptomatic despite aggressive efforts at rate control
- If cardioversion is planned and the duration of atrial fibrillation exceeds 2–3 days or is unknown, perform a transesophageal echocardiography to exclude an atrial thrombus and attempt electrical cardioversion while the patient remains sedated
- If thrombus is present, delay cardioversion until after 3–4 weeks of therapeutic warfarin anticoagulation (goal INR of 2–3)
- Use heparin while awaiting therapeutic warfarin anticoagulation in atrial fibrillation with mitral stenosis, a history of embolic events, or demonstrated thrombus on transesophageal echocardiography
- After cardioversion, maintain therapeutic anticoagulation for at least 1–6 mo
- Patients with paroxysmal or persistent atrial fibrillation who fail to convert should be anticoagulated indefinitely, except for "lone atrial fibrillation" (age < 60 and no associated heart disease, hypertension, atherosclerotic vascular disease, or diabetes)
- For refractory atrial fibrillation (causing persistent symptoms or limiting activity despite vigorous efforts at rate control and cardioversion), consider radiofrequency atrioventricular node ablation and permanent pacing

OUTCOME

COMPLICATIONS

- Propensity for stroke from embolization of an atrial thrombus

WHEN TO REFER

- For elective cardioversion or radiofrequency atrioventricular node ablation and permanent pacing

WHEN TO ADMIT

- When the patient is hemodynamically unstable and immediate treatment is required

EVIDENCE

PRACTICE GUIDELINES

- Fuster V et al: America College of Cardiology/American Heart Association Task Force on Practice Guidelines; European Society of Cardiology Committee for Practice Guidelines and Policy Conferences (Committee to Develop Guidelines for the Management of Patients With Atrial Fibrillation); North American Society of Pacing and Electrophysiology: ACC/AHA/ESC Guidelines for the Management of Patients With Atrial Fibrillation: Executive Summary. Circulation 2001;104:2118. [PMID: 11673357]
- Rockson SG et al: Comparing the guidelines: anticoagulation therapy to optimize stroke prevention in patients with atrial fibrillation. J Am Coll Cardiol 2004;43:929. [PMID: 15028346]
- Snow V et al: Management of newly detected atrial fibrillation: a clinical practice guideline from the American Academy of Family Physicians and the American College of Physicians. Ann Intern Med 2003;139:1009. [PMID: 14678921]

WEB SITE

- American College of Cardiology Foundation
  - Management of Patients with Atrial Fibrillation - Executive Summary http://www.acc.org/clinical/guidelines/atrial%5Ffib/exec%5Fsumm/exec%5Ffigures.htm.

INFORMATION FOR PATIENTS

- Parmet S et al: JAMA patient page. Atrial fibrillation. JAMA 2003;290:1118. [PMID: 12941685]
- American Heart Association
  - http://www.americanheart.org/presenter.jhtml?identifier=4451

REFERENCES

- Fang MC et al: Anticoagulation for atrial fibrillation. Cardiol Clin 2004;22:47. [PMID: 14994847]
- Finta B et al: Catheter ablation therapy for atrial fibrillation. Cardiol Clin 2004;22:127. [PMID: 14994853]
- Gillinov AM et al: Advances in the surgical treatment of atrial fibrillation. Cardiol Clin 2004;22:147. [PMID: 14994854]
- Joglar JA et al: Electrical cardioversion of atrial fibrillation. Cardiol Clin 2004;22:101. [PMID: 14994851]
- McNamara RL et al: Management of atrial fibrillation: review of the evidence for the role of pharmacologic therapy, electrical cardioversion, and echocardiography. Ann Intern Med 2003;139:1018. [PMID: 14678922]
- Mead GE et al: Electrical cardioversion for atrial fibrillation and flutter. Cochrane Database Syst Rev 2002;(1):CD002903. [PMID: 11869642]
- Tamariz LJ et al: Pharmacological rate control of atrial fibrillation. Cardiol Clin 2004;22:35. [PMID: 14994846]
- Wijffels MC et al: Rate versus rhythm control in atrial fibrillation. Cardiol Clin 2004;22:63. [PMID: 14994848]

Author(s)

Thomas M. Bashore, MD

Christopher B. Granger, MD

Auditory Tube Dysfunction

Atrial Flutter p. 1034. Atrial Septal Defect p. 1035. Atropine and Anticholinergic Poisoning p. 1035.

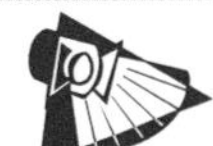

KEY FEATURES

ESSENTIALS OF DIAGNOSIS

- Aural fullness
- Fluctuating hearing
- Discomfort with barometric pressure change

GENERAL CONSIDERATIONS

- The tube that connects the middle ear to the nasopharynx—the auditory tube, or eustachian tube—provides ventilation and drainage for the middle ear cleft
- The auditory tube is normally closed, opening only during the act of swallowing or yawning

Hypofunctioning (narrowed) auditory tube

- When auditory tube function is compromised, air trapped within the middle ear becomes absorbed and negative pressure results
- The most common causes are diseases associated with edema of the tubal lining, such as viral upper respiratory tract infections and allergy

Overly patent auditory tube

- A relatively uncommon problem that may be quite distressing
- May develop during rapid weight loss, or may be idiopathic

CLINICAL FINDINGS

SYMPTOMS AND SIGNS

Hypofunctioning auditory tube

- Usually there is a sense of fullness in the ear and mild to moderate impairment of hearing
- When the tube is only partially blocked, swallowing or yawning may elicit a popping or crackling sound
- Examination reveals retraction of the tympanic membrane and decreased mobility on pneumatic otoscopy

Overly patent auditory tube

- Fullness in the ear
- Autophony, an exaggerated ability to hear oneself breathe and speak
- In contrast to a hypofunctioning auditory tube, the aural pressure is often made worse by exertion and may diminish during an upper respiratory tract infection.
- Although physical examination is usually normal, respiratory excursions of the tympanic membrane may occasionally be detected during vigorous breathing

DIFFERENTIAL DIAGNOSIS

- Cerumen impaction (ear wax)
- Acute or chronic otitis media
- Temporomandibular joint disfunction
- Paget's disease
- Head trauma

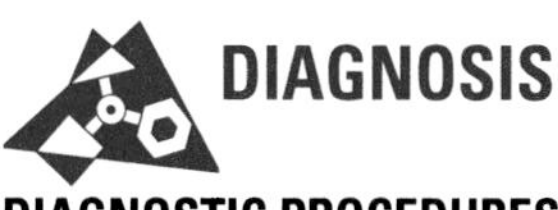

DIAGNOSIS

DIAGNOSTIC PROCEDURES

- Clinical diagnosis

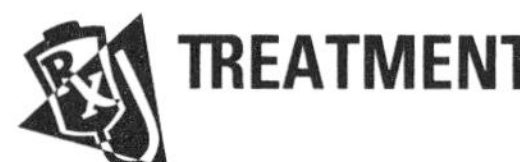

TREATMENT

MEDICATIONS

Hypofunctioning auditory tube

- Systemic and intranasal decongestants (eg, pseudoephedrine, 60 mg PO Q4 h; oxymetazoline, 0.05% spray Q8–12 h) combined with autoinflation by forced exhalation against closed nostrils may hasten relief
- Allergic patients may also benefit from desensitization or intranasal corticosteroids (eg, beclomethasone dipropionate, two sprays in each nostril twice daily for 2–6 weeks)

Overly patent auditory tube

- Avoidance of decongestant products

SURGERY

Hypofunctioning auditory tube

- In medically refractory tube hypofunction, insertion of a tympanostomy tube is often helpful

Overly patent auditory tube

- Rarely, surgical narrowing of the auditory tube is indicated, and the same is true of insertion of a ventilating tube to reduce the outward stretch of the ear drum during phonation

THERAPEUTIC PROCEDURES

- Autoinflation should not be recommended to patients with active intranasal infection, because this maneuver may precipitate middle ear infection

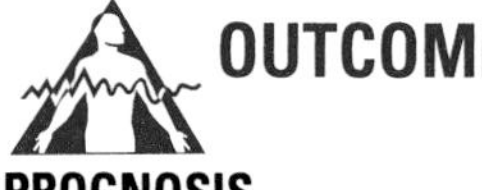

OUTCOME

PROGNOSIS

- Following a viral illness, this disorder is usually transient, lasting days to weeks

WHEN TO REFER

- Refer to an otolaryngologist if symptoms persist despite medical therapy or if there is persistent hearing loss

PREVENTION

- Avoid chronic decongestant use
- Avoid exacerbants of air travel, rapid altitudinal change, and underwater diving
- Control associated sinonasal disease

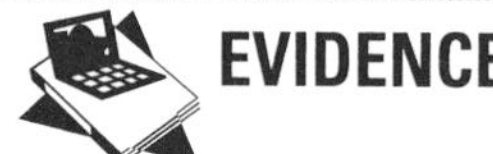

EVIDENCE

WEB SITES

- Baylor College of Medicine: Otolaryngology Resources
  - http://www.bcm.tmc.edu/oto/othersa.html

INFORMATION FOR PATIENTS

- McKinley Health Center, University of Illinois: Eustachian Tube Dysfunction
  - http://www.mckinley.uiuc.edu/handouts/eusttube/eusttube.html
- Vestibular Disorders Association: Inner Ear Anatomy
  - http://www.vestibular.org/gallery.html
- MedlinePlus: Eustachian Tube Patency
  - http://www.nlm.nih.gov/medlineplus/ency/article/001630.htm

REFERENCES

- Kujawski OB et al: Laser eustachian tuboplasty. Otol Neurotol 2004;25:1. [PMID: 14724483]
- Licameli GR: The eustachian tube. Update on anatomy, development, and function. Otolaryngol Clin North Am 2002;35:803. [PMID: 12487082]
- van Heerbeek N: Therapeutic improvement of eustachian tube function: a review. Clin Otolaryngol 2002;27:50. [PMID:11903373]

Author(s)

Robert K. Jackler, MD

Michael J. Kaplan, MD

Babesiosis

Avascular Necrosis of Bone p. 1036

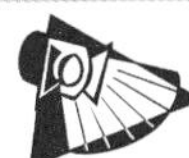 KEY FEATURES

ESSENTIALS OF DIAGNOSIS

- Fever, chills, headache, myalgia, fatigue
- Nausea, vomiting
- Hemolytic anemia, moderate
- Intraerythrocytic parasites on staining of thick and thin blood smears; no gametocytes
- Specific IgM antibody in 1–4 weeks

GENERAL CONSIDERATIONS

- Babesiae are tick-borne protozoal parasites of wild and domestic animals
- In Europe, the infection is caused by *Babesia divergens*
- In the United States, Taiwan, China, Japan, Egypt, South Africa, Mexico, Switzerland, and South America, the infection is caused by *Babesia microti*
- New *Babesia* species or strains (WA1 and others) have been described in California, Washington, Georgia, and Kentucky
- Natural hosts for *B microti* are wild and domestic animals, particularly the white-footed mouse and white-tailed deer. The extension of the deer's habitat is increasing human infection
- Humans are infected as a result of *Ixodes scapularis* (*I dammini*) tick bites (mainly nymphal) but also by blood transfusion and perinatally
- Coinfections with Lyme disease and ehrlichiosis occur
- Without passing through an exoerythrocytic stage, *B microti* enters the red blood cell and multiplies, resulting in cell rupture followed by infection of other cells
- The incubation period is 1 week to several months; parasitemia is evident in 2–4 weeks
- All *B divergens* infections (transmitted by *I ricinus*) have been in splenectomized patients

DEMOGRAPHICS

- In the United States, *B microti* infections have occurred in the coastal and island areas of northeastern and mid-Atlantic states as well as Wisconsin, Minnesota, Missouri, Washington, and California

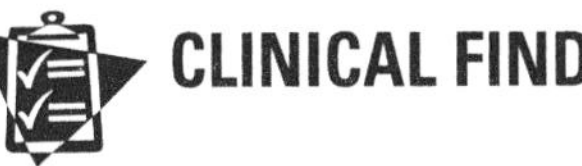

CLINICAL FINDINGS

SYMPTOMS AND SIGNS

- Irregular fever, chills, headache, diaphoresis, myalgia, and fatigue but without malaria-like periodicity of symptoms
- Nausea, vomiting, jaundice, arthralgia, and emotional lability
- Some patients have hemoglobinuria, hepatosplenomegaly, or thrombocytopenia
- *B divergens* infections in splenectomized patients present with rapidly progressive high fever, severe hemolytic anemia, jaundice, hemoglobinuria, and renal failure

DIFFERENTIAL DIAGNOSIS

- Malaria
- Infectious mononucleosis
- Viral hepatitis
- Ehrlichiosis
- Lyme disease

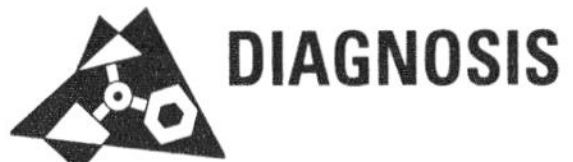

DIAGNOSIS

LABORATORY TESTS

- The intraerythrocytic parasite (2–3 μm) can be identified on Giemsa-stained thick and thin blood smears; no gametocytes and no intracellular pigment are seen
- A single red cell may contain different stages of the parasite, and parasitemia can exceed 10%. Repeated smears may be necessary
- The organism must be differentiated from malarial parasites, particularly *Plasmodium falciparum*
- Isolation can be attempted by inoculating patient blood into hamsters or gerbils
- Antibody is detectable within 1–4 weeks after onset of symptoms and persists for 6–12 months
- Testing with specific antigens in the immunofluorescent test is relatively species specific, with a titer of 1:1024 or greater considered diagnostic; antibody titers against *Plasmodium* are generally low or absent
- Detection of specific IgM antibody confirms the diagnosis
- The polymerase chain reaction method, where available, is more sensitive for low parasitemias but of equal specificity
- Other findings include hemolytic anemia, thrombocytopenia, low-grade leukocytosis or leukopenia, and abnormal liver and renal function tests

IMAGING STUDIES

- Imaging studies may detect morphologic changes in the spleen

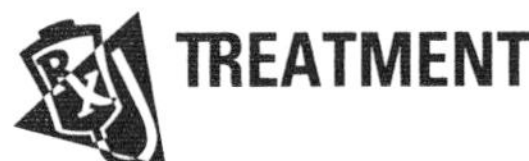

TREATMENT

MEDICATIONS

- No drug treatment is fully satisfactory
- Everyone, even those mildly ill, should be treated with a 7–10 day course of atovaquone (750 mg every 12 hours) plus azithromycin (600 mg once daily)
- The alternative treatment is a 7-day course of quinine (650 mg three times daily) plus clindamycin (600 mg three times daily orally or 1200 mg twice daily IV)
- Exchange transfusion with antibiotics has been successful in several severely ill asplenic patients and patients with parasitemia greater than 10%
- Management of *B divergens* infection can be attempted with exchange transfusion and clindamycin-quinine plus atovaquone or trimethoprim-sulfamethoxazole plus pentamidine

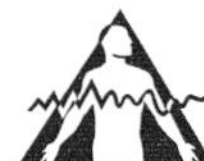

OUTCOME

COMPLICATIONS

- Severe complications include acute respiratory, cardiac, and renal failure

PROGNOSIS

- Although parasitemia may continue for months, with or without symptoms, the disease is self-limited and, after several weeks or months, most patients recover without sequelae
- Splenectomized, older, or immunosuppressed persons are most likely to have severe manifestations; case fatality rates in the United States may reach 5%
- The death rate among splenectomized patients with *B divergens* infection is over 40%

WHEN TO REFER

- Patients not responding to therapy

WHEN TO ADMIT

- All splenectomized, older, or immunosuppressed patients

EVIDENCE

WEB SITE

- Centers for Disease Control and Prevention—Division of Parasitic Diseases
  - http://www.cdc.gov/ncidod/dpd/parasites/babesia/default.htm

INFORMATION FOR PATIENTS

- American Academy of Family Physicians
  - http://familydoctor.org/handouts/689.html
- American College of Emergency Physicians
  - http://www.acep.org/1.2737.0.html

REFERENCES

- Krause PJ: Babesiosis. Med Clin North Am 2002;86:361. [PMID: 11982307]
- Krause PJ et al: Disease-specific diagnosis of coinfecting tickborne zoonoses: babesiosis, human granulocytic ehrlichiosis, and Lyme disease. Clin Infect Dis 2002;34:1184. [PMID: 11941544]
- Ranque S: The treatment of babesiosis. N Engl J Med 2000;343:1454. [PMID: 11236790]

Baldness

KEY FEATURES

ESSENTIALS OF DIAGNOSIS

Forms of hair loss

- Baldness due to scarring (cicatricial baldness)
- Baldness not due to scarring
- Androgenetic (male pattern) baldness
- Telogen effluvium
- Alopecia areata
- Drug-induced alopecia
- Trichotillomania (the pulling out of one's own hair)

GENERAL CONSIDERATIONS

Baldness due to scarring

- Irreversible and permanent, thus it is important to treat the scarring process as early as possible
- May occur following chemical or physical trauma, lichen planopilaris, severe bacterial or fungal infections, severe herpes zoster, chronic discoid lupus erythematosus, scleroderma, and excessive ionizing radiation
- The specific cause is often suggested by the history, the distribution of hair loss, and the appearance of the skin, as in lupus erythematosus

Baldness not due to scarring

- Nonscarring alopecia may occur in association with various systemic diseases such as systemic lupus erythematosus, secondary syphilis, hyperthyroidism or hypothyroidism, iron deficiency anemia, and pituitary insufficiency

Androgenetic baldness

- The most common form of alopecia is of genetic predetermination

Telogen effluvium

- A transitory increase in the number of hairs in the telogen (resting) phase of the hair growth cycle
- May occur spontaneously, may appear at the termination of pregnancy, may be precipitated by "crash dieting," high fever, stress from surgery or shock, or malnutrition, or may be provoked by hormonal contraceptives
- Latent period of 2–4 months
- The prognosis is generally good
- A major important cause is iron deficiency

Alopecia areata

- Unknown cause but is believed to be an immunologic process
- Occasionally associated with Hashimoto's thyroiditis, pernicious anemia, Addison's disease, and vitiligo

Drug-induced alopecia

- Becoming increasingly important
- Incriminated drugs include
  - Thallium
  - Excessive and prolonged use of vitamin A
  - Retinoids
  - Antimitotic agents
  - Anticoagulants
  - Antithyroid drugs
  - Oral contraceptives
  - Trimethadione
  - Allopurinol
  - Propranolol
  - Indomethacin
  - Amphetamines
  - Salicylates
  - Gentamicin
  - Levodopa
- While chemotherapy-induced alopecia is very distressing, it must be emphasized to the patient before treatment that it is invariably reversible

CLINICAL FINDINGS

SYMPTOMS AND SIGNS

Androgenetic baldness

- The earliest changes occur at the anterior portions of the calvarium on either side of the "widow's peak" and on the crown (vertex) of the skull
- The extent of hair loss is variable and unpredictable
- Occurs in both women and men

Alopecia areata

- Typically, there are patches that are perfectly smooth and without scarring
- Tiny hairs 2–3 mm in length, called "exclamation hairs," may be seen
- Telogen hairs are easily dislodged from the periphery of active lesions
- The beard, brows, and lashes may be involved
- Involvement may extend to all of the scalp hair (alopecia totalis) or to all scalp and body hair (alopecia universalis)
- The patches of hair loss are irregular and growing hairs are always present, since they cannot be pulled out until they are long enough

DIFFERENTIAL DIAGNOSIS

- Scarring (cicatricial)
  - Chemical or physical trauma
  - Lichen planopilaris
  - Bacterial or fungal infection (severe)
  - Herpes zoster (shingles) (severe)
  - Discoid lupus erythematosus
  - Scleroderma
  - Excessive ionizing radiation
- Nonscarring
  - Androgenic (male pattern) baldness
  - Telogen effluvium
  - Alopecia areata
  - Trichotillomania
  - Drug-induced alopecia
  - Systemic lupus erythematosus
  - Secondary syphilis
  - Hyperthyroidism
  - Hypothyroidism
  - Iron deficiency anemia
  - Pituitary insufficiency

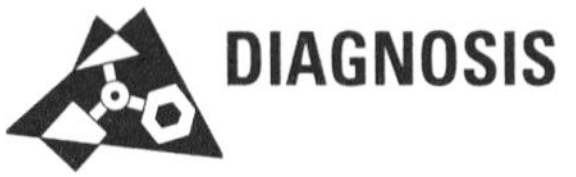

DIAGNOSIS

LABORATORY TESTS

- Hair loss in women
- Serum testosterone, DHEAS, iron, total iron-binding capacity, and thyroid function tests and a complete blood cell count will identify most other causes of hair thinning in premenopausal women

Telogen effluvium

- Diagnosed by the presence of large numbers of hairs with white bulbs coming out upon gentle tugging
- Counts of hairs lost on combing or shampooing often exceed 150 per day, compared with an average of 70–100

DIAGNOSTIC PROCEDURES

- Biopsy is useful in the diagnosis of scarring alopecia, but specimens must be taken from the active border and not from the scarred central zone

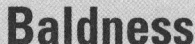

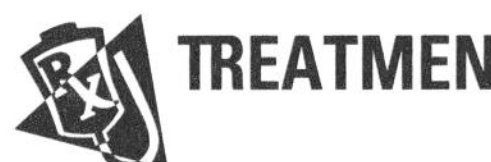

TREATMENT

MEDICATIONS

Androgenetic baldness

- Rogaine extra strength
  - Solution containing 50 mg/mL of minoxidil; available over the counter; best results achieved in persons with recent onset (< 5 years) and smaller areas of alopecia
  - Approximately 40% of patients treated twice daily for 1 year will have moderate to dense growth
- Finasteride (Propecia): 1 mg PO daily, has similar efficacy to Rogaine and may be additive to minoxidil; used only in males

Hair loss or thinning in women

- May be treated with minoxidil

Alopecia areata

- Intralesional corticosteroids are frequently effective
- Triamcinolone acetonide in a concentration of 2.5–10 mg/mL is injected in aliquots of 0.1 mL at approximately 1- to 2-cm intervals, not exceeding a total dose of 30 mg per month for adults
- Alternatively, anthralin 0.5% ointment used daily, may help some patients

THERAPEUTIC PROCEDURES

Baldness not due to scarring

- The only treatment necessary is prompt and adequate control of the underlying disorder, in which case hair loss may be reversible

Alopecia areata

- Alopecia areata is usually self-limiting, with complete regrowth of hair in 80% of patients, but some mild cases are resistant
- Support groups for patients with extensive alopecia areata are very beneficial

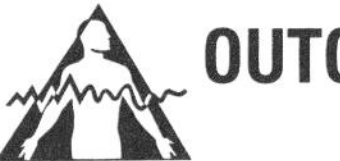

OUTCOME

FOLLOW-UP

- Women who complain of thin hair but show little evidence of alopecia need follow-up, because more than 50% of the scalp hair can be lost before the clinician can perceive it

COMPLICATIONS

- Scarring alopecia can be very disfiguring

WHEN TO REFER

- All scarring alopecias except clearly diagnosed discoid lupus erythematosis and posttraumatic
- Diagnosis and management questions

EVIDENCE

PRACTICE GUIDELINES

- MacDonald Hull SP et al; British Association of Dermatologists: Guidelines for the management of alopecia areata. Br J Dermatol 2003;149:692. [PMID: 14616359]
- Recommendations to diagnose and treat adult hair loss disorders or alopecia in primary care settings (nonpregnant female and male adults). University of Texas at Austin, 2004
  - http://www.guideline.gov/summary/summary.aspx?

WEB SITES

- American Academy of Dermatology
  - http://www.aad.org
- National Alopecia Areata Foundation
  - http://www.naaf.org/

INFORMATION FOR PATIENTS

- American Academy of Family Physicians: Hair Loss and Its Causes
  - http://familydoctor.org/081.xml
- Mayo Clinic: Baldness
  - http://www.mayoclinic.com/invoke.cfm
- MedlinePlus: Alopecia Interactive Tutorial
  - http://www.nlm.nih.gov/medlineplus/tutorials/alopecia.html
- National Institute of Arthritis and Musculoskeletal and Skin Diseases: Alopecia Areata
  - http://www.niams.nih.gov/hi/topics/alopecia/alopecia.htm
- American Medical Association: Male Pattern Baldness
  - http://www.medem.com/MedLB/article_detaillb.cfm?

REFERENCES

- Bertolino AP: Alopecia areata. A clinical overview. Postgrad Med 2000;107:81. [PMID: 10887448]
- Madani S et al: Alopecia areata update. J Am Acad Dermatol 2000;42:549. [PMID: 10727299]
- Price VH: Treatment of hair loss. N Engl J Med 1999;341:964. [PMID: 10498493]

Author(s)

Timothy G. Berger, MD

Basal Cell Carcinoma

Bartholin's Duct Cyst & Abscess p. 1038

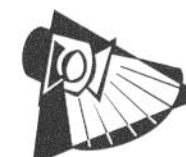

KEY FEATURES

ESSENTIALS OF DIAGNOSIS

- Slow-growing lesions
- Pearly or translucent appearance
- Telangiectatic vessels easily visible

GENERAL CONSIDERATIONS

- Most common form of cancer
- They occur on sun-exposed skin in otherwise normal fair-skinned individuals
- Clinicians should examine the skin routinely, looking for bumps, patches, and scabbed lesions

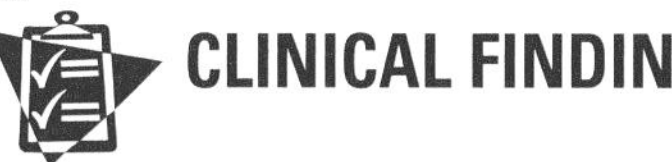

CLINICAL FINDINGS

SYMPTOMS AND SIGNS

- The most common presentation is a papule or nodule that may have a scab or erosion
- Occasionally the nodules have a brown-gray color or have stippled pigment (pigmented basal cell carcinoma)
- Grow slowly, attaining a size of 1–2 cm or more in diameter, often after years of growth
- There is a waxy, "pearly" appearance, with telangiectatic vessels easily visible
- Pearly or translucent quality of the lesions is most diagnostic, a feature best appreciated if the skin is stretched
- Less common types include morpheaform or scar-like lesions; these are hypopigmented, somewhat thickened plaques
- On the back and chest, basal cell carcinomas appear as reddish, somewhat shiny, scaly plaques
- When examining the face, look at the eyelid margins and medial canthi, the nose and alar folds, the lips, and then around and behind the ears
- Basal cell carcinomas of the medial canthi are particularly dangerous

DIFFERENTIAL DIAGNOSIS

- Squamous cell carcinoma
- Actinic keratosis
- Intradermal nevi
- Fibrous papule of the nose
- Seborrheic keratosis (unpigmented type)
- Sebaceous (epidermal inclusion) cyst
- Sebaceous hyperplasia
- Keratoacanthoma
- Molluscum contagiosum
- Melanoma
- Paget's disease

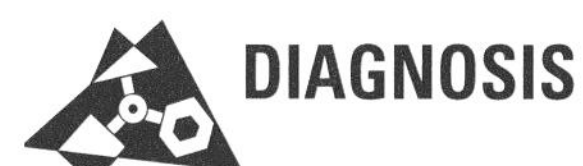

DIAGNOSIS

DIAGNOSTIC PROCEDURES

- Lesions suspected to be basal cell carcinomas should be biopsied, by shave or punch biopsy
- Biopsy confirms the diagnosis

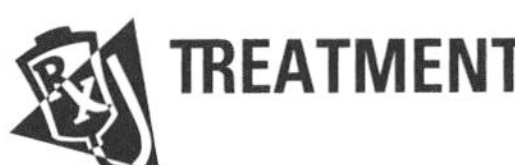

TREATMENT

MEDICATIONS

- Imiquimod cream 5% three times a week for 10 weeks may be effective for nonfacial, superficial (by biopsy) basal cell cancers

SURGERY

- Therapy is aimed at eradication with minimal cosmetic deformity, often by excision and suturing with recurrence rates of 5% or less
- The technique of three cycles of curettage and electrodesiccation depends on the skill of the operator and is not recommended for head and neck lesions
- After 4–6 weeks of healing, it leaves a broad, hypopigmented, at times hypertrophic scar
- Mohs surgery—removal of the tumor followed by immediate frozen section histopathologic examination of margins with subsequent reexcision of tumor-positive areas and final closure of the defect—gives the highest cure rates (98%) and results in least tissue loss

THERAPEUTIC PROCEDURES

- Radiotherapy is effective and sometimes appropriate for older individuals (over 65), but recurrent tumors after radiation therapy are more difficult to treat and may be more aggressive

OUTCOME

FOLLOW-UP

- Patients must be monitored for the first 1 to 2 years to detect new or recurrent lesions

COMPLICATIONS

- Neglected lesions may ulcerate and produce great destruction

PROGNOSIS

- Metastases almost never occur
- Most recurrences appear in the first 1 to 2 years
- Recurrent lesions around the nose and ears may track along cartilage underneath the skin, requiring treatment of much more extensive areas than are apparent from inspection

WHEN TO REFER

- If confirmation of the need for biopsy is required or to perform biopsy

PREVENTION

- Sun avoidance, particularly in children, is essential to lower the incidence of new basal cell cancers

EVIDENCE

PRACTICE GUIDELINES

- Miller SJ et al; NCCN Basal Cell and Squamous Cell Skin Cancer Practice Guidelines Panel. National Comprehensive Cancer Network: Basal Cell and Squamous Cell Skin Cancers v.1.2004
  - http://www.nccn.org/professionals/physician_gls/PDF/nmsc.pdf
- US Preventive Services Task Force: Counseling to prevent skin cancer, 2003
  - http://www.ahrq.gov/clinic/uspstf/uspsskco.htm

WEB SITES

- National Cancer Institute: Skin Cancer Information for Patients and Health Professionals
  - http://www.cancer.gov/cancertopics/types/skin
- American Academy of Dermatology
  - http://www.aad.org

INFORMATION FOR PATIENTS

- Skin Cancer Foundation: Basal Cell Carcinoma
  - http://www.skincancer.org/basal/index.php
- American Cancer Society: Nonmelanoma Skin Cancer
  - http://www.cancer.org/docroot/CRI/CRI_2_3x.asp?rnav=cridg&dt=51
- MedlinePlus: Skin Cancer Interactive Tutorial
  - http://www.nlm.nih.gov/medlineplus/tutorials/skincancer.html
- American Academy of Family Physicians: Skin Cancer: Saving Your Skin from Sun Damage
  - http://familydoctor.org/159.xml

REFERENCES

- Garner KL et al: Basal and squamous cell carcinoma. Prim Care 2000;27:447. [PMID: 10815054]
- Jerant AF et al: Early detection and treatment of skin cancer. Am Fam Physician 2000;62:357. [PMID: 10929700]

Author(s)

Timothy G. Berger, MD

Bell's Palsy

Behçet's Syndrome p. 1038

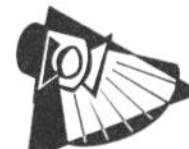

KEY FEATURES

ESSENTIALS OF DIAGNOSIS

- Sudden onset of lower motor neuron facial palsy
- May have hyperacusis or impaired taste
- No other neurologic abnormalities

GENERAL CONSIDERATIONS

- Idiopathic lower motor neuron facial paresis
- Attributed to an inflammatory reaction of the facial nerve near the stylomastoid foramen or in the bony facial canal
- Reactivation of herpes simplex virus has been postulated

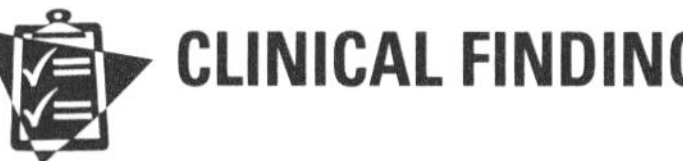

CLINICAL FINDINGS

SYMPTOMS AND SIGNS

- Generally comes on abruptly, but it may worsen over 1 or 2 days
- Pain about the ear often precedes or accompanies the weakness but usually lasts for only a few days
- There may be ipsilateral restriction of eye closure and difficulty with eating and fine facial movements
- A disturbance of taste is common, owing to involvement of chorda tympani fibers, and hyperacusis due to involvement of fibers to the stapedius occurs occasionally

DIFFERENTIAL DIAGNOSIS

- HIV-related facial neuropathies
- Lyme disease
- Sarcoidosis
- Ramsay Hunt syndrome (herpes zoster of geniculate ganglion)
- Acoustic neuroma
- Acute or chronic otitis media
- Malignant otitis externa
- Guillain-Barré syndrome
- Tumor, eg, parotid, temporal bone tumor
- Brainstem infarct

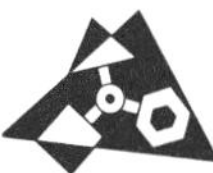

DIAGNOSIS

- The clinical features are characteristic
- Electromyography and nerve excitability or conduction studies provide a guide to prognosis

LABORATORY TESTS

- To exclude other causes of facial neuropathy (see Differential Diagnosis)

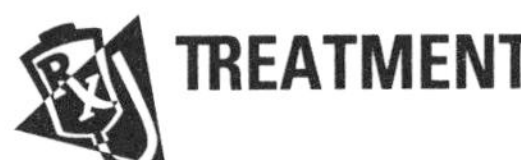

TREATMENT

MEDICATIONS

- The only medical treatment that may influence the outcome is administration of corticosteroids, but studies supporting this approach have been criticized
- Many clinicians nevertheless routinely prescribe corticosteroids for patients seen within 5 days of onset. Others prescribe them only when the palsy is clinically complete or there is severe pain
- Treatment with prednisone, 60 or 80 mg PO QD in divided doses for 4 or 5 days, followed by tapering of the dose over the next 7–10 days, is a satisfactory regimen
- It is helpful to protect the eye with lubricating drops (or lubricating ointment at night) and a patch if eye closure is not possible
- The role of acyclovir or other antiviral agents is unclear

SURGERY

- There is no evidence that surgical procedures to decompress the facial nerve are of benefit

THERAPEUTIC PROCEDURES

- The management is controversial
- Approximately 60% recover completely without treatment. Considerable improvement occurs in most other cases, and only about 10% of all patients have permanent disfigurement or other long-term sequelae
- Treatment is unnecessary in most cases but is indicated when an unsatisfactory outcome can be predicted. The best clinical guide to progress is the severity of the palsy during the first few days after presentation

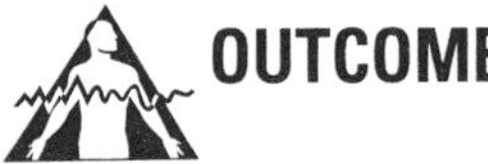

OUTCOME

PROGNOSIS

- Patients with clinically complete palsy when first seen are less likely to make a full recovery than those with an incomplete one
- A poor prognosis for recovery is also associated with advanced age, hyperacusis, and severe initial pain

EVIDENCE

PRACTICE GUIDELINES

- Grogan PM et al: Practice parameter: steroids, acyclovir, and surgery for Bell's palsy (an evidenced-based review): report of the Quality Standards Subcommittee of the American Academy of Neurology. Neurology 2001;56:830. [PMID: 11294918]

INFORMATION FOR PATIENTS

- American Academy of Otolaryngology—Head and Neck Surgery
  - http://www.entnet.org/healthinfo/topics/bells.cfm
- National Institute of Neurological Disorders and Stroke
  - http://www.ninds.nih.gov/disorders/bells/bells.htm

REFERENCES

- Gilden DH: Clinical practice. Bell's palsy. N Engl J Med 2004;351:1323. [PMID: 15385659]
- Holland NJ et al: Recent developments in Bell's palsy. BMJ 2004;329:553. [PMID: 15345630]

Author(s)

Michael J. Aminoff, MD, DSc, FRCP

Benign Prostatic Hyperplasia

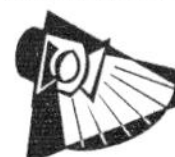

KEY FEATURES

ESSENTIALS OF DIAGNOSIS

- Obstructive or irritative voiding symptoms
- May have enlarged prostate on rectal examination
- Absence of urinary tract infection, neurological disorder, urethral stricture disease, prostatic or bladder malignancy

GENERAL CONSIDERATIONS

- Smooth, firm, elastic enlargement of the prostate

Etiology

- Multifactorial
- Endocrine: dihydrotestosterone (DHT)
- Aging

DEMOGRAPHICS

- The most common benign tumor in men
- Incidence is age related
- Prevalence
  - ~20% in men aged 41–50
  - ~50% in men aged 51–60
  - > 90% in men aged 80 and older
- Symptoms are also age related: at age 55, ~25% of men report obstructive voiding symptoms

CLINICAL FINDINGS

SYMPTOMS AND SIGNS

- Can be divided into obstructive and irritative complaints
- Obstructive symptoms
  - Hesitancy
  - Decreased force and caliber of stream
  - Sensation of incomplete bladder emptying
  - Double voiding (urinating a second time within 2 h)
  - Straining to urinate
  - Postvoid dribbling
- Irritative symptoms
  - Urgency
  - Frequency
  - Nocturia
- American Urological Association (AUA) Symptom Index (Table 90) should be calculated for all patients starting therapy
- Seven questions quantitate the severity of obstructive or irritative complaints on a scale of 0–5. Thus, the score can range from 0 to 35

DIFFERENTIAL DIAGNOSIS

- Prostate cancer
- Urinary tract infection
- Neurogenic bladder
- Urethral stricture

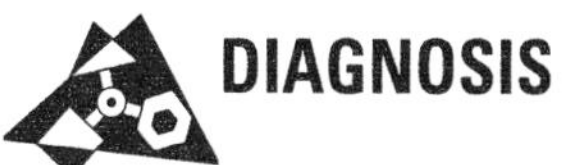

DIAGNOSIS

DIAGNOSTIC PROCEDURES

- History to exclude other possible causes of symptoms
- Physical examination, digital rectal examination (DRE), and a focused neurological examination
- DRE: note size and consistency of the prostate
- Examine lower abdomen for a distended bladder
- If possibility of cancer, further evaluation is needed by serum prostate-specific antigen (PSA), transrectal ultrasound, and biopsy

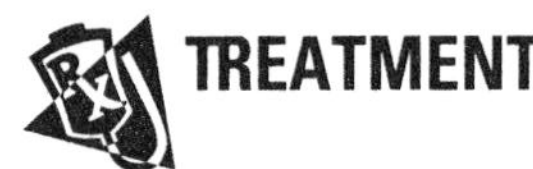

TREATMENT

MEDICATIONS

- α-Blockers
  - Prazosin 1 mg PO QHS for 3 nights, increasing to 1 mg PO BID and then titrating up to 2 mg PO BID if necessary
  - Terazosin 1 mg PO QD for 3 days, increasing to 2 mg PO QD for 11 days, then 5–10 mg PO QD if necessary
  - Doxazosin 1 mg PO QD for 7 days, increasing to 2 mg PO QD for 7 days, then 4–8 mg PO QD if necessary
  - Tamsulosin 0.4 mg PO QD, increased to 0.8 mg PO QD if necessary
- 5α-Reductase inhibitors
  - Finasteride 5 mg PO QD—6 months of therapy required for maximum effects on prostate size (20% reduction) and symptomatic improvement
- Combination therapy
  - α-Blocker and 5α-reductase inhibitor

SURGERY

- Indications
  - Refractory urinary retention (failing at least one attempt at catheter removal)
  - Large bladder diverticula
  - Recurrent urinary tract infection
  - Recurrent gross hematuria
  - Bladder stones
  - Renal insufficiency
- Transurethral resection of the prostate (TURP): operative complications
  - Bleeding
  - Urethral stricture or bladder neck contracture
  - Perforation of the prostate capsule with extravasation
  - Transurethral resection syndrome
  - A hypervolemic, hyponatremic state resulting from the absorption of the hypotonic irrigating solution
- TURP: postoperative complications
  - Retrograde ejaculation (75%)
  - Impotence (5–10%)
  - Urinary incontinence (< 1%)
- Transurethral incision of the prostate (TUIP): lower rate of retrograde ejaculation reported (25%)
- Open simple prostatectomy: when prostate is too large to remove endoscopically (> 100 g), concomitant bladder diverticulum, bladder stone, when dorsal lithotomy positioning is not possible
- Minimally invasive approaches
  - Laser therapy—(Nd:YAG) and holmium-YAG lasers used
  - TULIP (transurethral laser-induced prostatectomy) under transrectal ultrasound guidance
  - Visually directed laser techniques under cystoscopic control
  - Interstitial laser therapy usually under cystoscopic control
  - Advantages of laser surgery include outpatient surgery, minimal blood loss, rare occurrence of transurethral resection syndrome, and ability to treat patients while receiving anticoagulation therapy.
  - Disadvantages of laser surgery include lack of tissue for pathological examination, longer postoperative catheterization time, more frequent irritative voiding complaints, and expense of laser fibers and generators
  - Transurethral needle ablation of the prostate (TUNA)
  - Transurethral electrovaporization of the prostate
  - Hyperthermia—microwave thermotherapy
  - High-intensity focused ultrasound (HIFU)
  - Intraurethral stents

THERAPEUTIC PROCEDURES

- Watchful waiting: only for patients with mild symptoms (AUA scores 0–7)
- With watchful waiting, ~10% progress to urinary retention, and half demonstrate marked improvement or resolution of symptoms

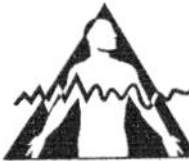

OUTCOME

FOLLOW-UP

- Follow American Urological Association Symptom Index for benign prostatic hyperplasia (Table 90)

EVIDENCE

PRACTICE GUIDELINES

- AUA Practice Guidelines Committee. AUA guideline on management of benign prostatic hyperplasia (2003). Chapter 1: Diagnosis and treatment recommendations. J Urol 2003;170(2 Pt 1):530. [PMID: 12853821]

WEB SITE

- Male Genital Pathology Index
  - http://medstat.med.utah.edu/WebPath/MALEHTML/MALEIDX.html

INFORMATION FOR PATIENTS

- MedlinePlus—Benign prostatic hyperplasia
  - http://www.nlm.nih.gov/medlineplus/ency/article/000381.htm
- Mayo Clinic
  - http://www.mayoclinic.com/invoke.cfm?id=DS00027

REFERENCES

- Andersson SO et al: Prevalence of lower urinary tract symptoms in men aged 45-79 years: a population-based study of 40 000 Swedish men. BJU Int 2004;94:327. [PMID: 15291861]
- Kaplan SA: Use of alpha-adrenergic inhibitors in treatment of benign prostatic hyperplasia and implications on sexual function. Urology 2004;63:428. [PMID: 15028431]
- Lee KL et al: Molecular and cellular pathogenesis of benign prostatic hyperplasia. J Urol 2004;172(5 Pt 1):1784. [PMID: 15540721]
- O'Sullivan M et al: Effects of transurethral resection of prostate on the quality of life of patients with benign prostatic hyperplasia. J Am Coll Surg 2004;198:394. [PMID: 14992742]
- Poulakis V et al: Transurethral electrovaporization vs transurethral resection for symptomatic prostatic obstruction: a meta-analysis. BJU Int 2004;94:89. [PMID: 15217438]

Author(s)

Marshall L. Stoller, MD

Peter R. Carroll, MD

Biliary Tract Carcinoma

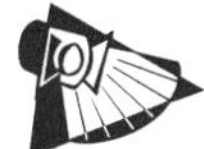

KEY FEATURES

ESSENTIALS OF DIAGNOSIS

- Obstructive jaundice, usually painless, often with dilated biliary tree
- Pain is more common in gallbladder carcinoma than cholangiocarcinoma
- A Courvoisier (dilated) gallbladder may be detected

GENERAL CONSIDERATIONS

Gallbladder carcinoma

- The diagnosis is often made unexpectedly at surgery
- Cholelithiasis (often large, symptomatic stones) is usually present
- **Risk factors**
  - Chronic infection of the gallbladder with *Salmonella typhi*
  - Gallbladder polyps over 1 cm in diameter
  - Mucosal calcification of the gallbladder (porcelain gallbladder)
  - Anomalous pancreaticobiliary ductal junction
  - Genetic factors include k-*ras* and *p53* mutations
- **TNM classification**
  - Tis, carcinoma in situ
  - T1, invasion of the subepithelial fibro-(muscular) connective tissue
  - T2, invasion beyond the wall of the bile duct
  - T3, invasion of branches of the portal vein (right or left), hepatic artery, or liver
  - T4, invasion of the main portal vein, common hepatic artery, and/or regional organs

Carcinoma of the bile ducts (cholangiocarcinoma)

- Two-thirds arise at the confluence of the hepatic ducts (Klatskin tumors), and one-fourth arise in the distal extrahepatic bile duct; the remainder are intrahepatic
- Staging is similar to that for carcinoma of the gallbladder
- There is an increased frequency with ulcerative colitis, especially with primary sclerosing cholangitis
- In southeast Asia, infection of the bile ducts with helminths (*Clonorchis sinensis, Opisthorchis viverrini, Fasciola hepatica*) is associated with chronic cholangitis and an increased risk of cholangiocarcinoma

DEMOGRAPHICS

Carcinoma of the bile ducts

- Accounts for 3% of all cancer deaths in the United States, and the incidence and mortality rates have increased dramatically in the past 2 decades
- Affects both sexes equally but is more prevalent in individuals aged 50–70
- Found in approximately 2% of people operated on for biliary tract disease

CLINICAL FINDINGS

SYMPTOMS AND SIGNS

- Progressive jaundice is the most common symptom
- Pain in the right upper abdomen with radiation into the back is usually present early in the course of gallbladder carcinoma, but this occurs later in the course of bile duct carcinoma
- Anorexia and weight loss are common and often associated with fever and chills due to cholangitis
- Rarely, hematemesis or melena results from erosion of the tumor into a blood vessel (hemobilia). Fistula formation between the biliary system and adjacent organs may also occur
- The course is usually one of rapid deterioration, with death occurring within a few months
- A palpable gallbladder with obstructive jaundice usually is said to signify malignant disease (Courvoisier's law); however, this clinical generalization has proved to be only 50% accurate
- Hepatomegaly is usually present and is associated with liver tenderness
- Ascites may occur with peritoneal implants
- Pruritus and skin excoriations

DIFFERENTIAL DIAGNOSIS

- Biliary stricture
- Hepatocellular or pancreatic carcinoma
- Primary sclerosing cholangitis
- Primary biliary cirrhosis
- Choledocholithiasis

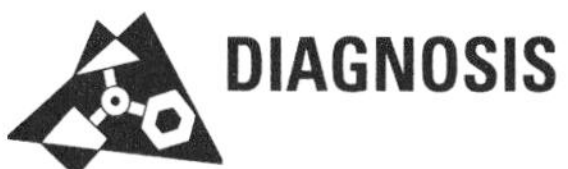

DIAGNOSIS

LABORATORY TESTS

- Predominantly conjugated hyperbilirubinemia, with total serum bilirubin values ranging from 5 to 30 mg/dL
- There is usually concomitant elevation of the alkaline phosphatase and serum cholesterol. Aspartate aminotransferase is normal or minimally elevated
- An elevated CA 19-9 level may help distinguish cholangiocarcinoma from a benign biliary stricture (in the absence of cholangitis)

IMAGING STUDIES

- Ultrasonography and CT may show a gallbladder mass in gallbladder carcinoma and an intrahepatic mass or biliary dilation in carcinoma of the bile ducts. CT may also show involved regional lymph nodes
- MRI with magnetic resonance cholangiopancreatography permits visualization of the biliary tree and detection of vascular invasion and obviates the need for angiography
- Positron emission tomography (PET) may detect cholangiocarcinomas as small as 1 cm

DIAGNOSTIC PROCEDURES

- The most helpful diagnostic studies before surgery are either percutaneous transhepatic or endoscopic retrograde cholangiography with biopsy and cytological specimens, though false-negative biopsy and cytology results are common
- Fine-needle aspiration of tumors under endoscopic ultrasonographic guidance, choledochoscopy, and intraductal ultrasonography have potential roles in the diagnosis of cholangiocarcinoma

Bernard-Soulier Syndrome p. 1038. Berylliosis p. 1039.
β-Blocker Overdose p. 1039. Biliary Stricture p. 1039.

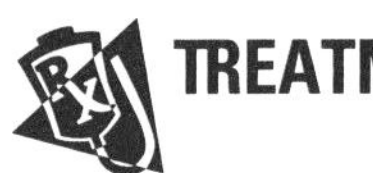

TREATMENT

MEDICATIONS

- There is limited response to chemotherapy such as with gemcitabine

SURGERY

- In young and fit patients, curative surgery may be attempted if the tumor is well localized
- If the tumor is unresectable at laparotomy, biliary-enteric bypass can be performed
- Although cholangiocarcinoma is generally considered a contraindication to liver transplantation because of rapid tumor recurrence, a 60% 5-year survival rate has been reported in patients with a single peripheral cholangiocarcinoma undergoing either transplantation or resection, with clear resection margins and no lymph node involvement

THERAPEUTIC PROCEDURES

- When disease progresses despite treatment, meticulous efforts at palliative care are essential
- Palliation can be achieved by placement of a self-expandable metal stent via the endoscopic or percutaneous transhepatic route. Plastic stents are less expensive but more prone to occlude than metal ones; they are suitable for patients expected to survive only a few months
- There may be a role for palliative photodynamic therapy. Radiotherapy may relieve pain and contribute to biliary decompression

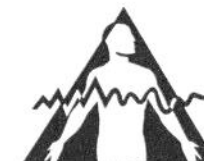

OUTCOME

PROGNOSIS

- The 5-year survival rate for localized carcinoma of the gallbladder (stage 1, T1a, N0, M0) is as high as 80% with laparoscopic cholecystectomy but drops to 15%, even with a more extended open resection, if there is muscular invasion (T1b)
- Carcinoma of the bile ducts is curable by surgery in less than 10% of cases
  - Few patients survive more than 12 months after surgery

PREVENTION

- The frequency of carcinoma with choledochal cysts is over 14% at 20 years, and surgical excision is recommended

EVIDENCE

PRACTICE GUIDELINES

- Khan SA et al: British Society of Gastroenterology. Guidelines for the diagnosis and treatment of cholangiocarcinoma: consensus document. Gut 2002;51(Suppl 6):VI1. [PMID: 12376491]
- National Guideline Clearinghouse
  - http://www.guideline.gov/summary/summary.aspx?doc_id=5689&nbr=3827&string=cholangiocarcinoma

WEB SITE

- Carcinoma of the Ampulla of Vater Demonstration Case
  - http://www.brighamrad.harvard.edu/Cases/bwh/hcache/43/full.html

INFORMATION FOR PATIENTS

- Mayo Clinic
  - http://www.mayoclinic.com/invoke.cfm?id=DS00425
- National Institutes of Health
  - http://www.nlm.nih.gov/medlineplus/ency/article/000291.htm
  - http://www.cancer.gov/cancerinfo/pdq/treatment/gallbladder/patient

REFERENCES

- Gores GJ (guest ed.): Cholangiocarcinoma: pathogenesis, diagnosis, and management. Semin Liver Dis 2004;24:113.
- Rajagopalan V et al: Gallbladder and biliary tract carcinoma: a comprehensive review, Parts I and II. Oncology (Huntingt) 2004;18:889 and 2004;18:1049. [PMID: 11573044; 15328897]
- Shaib YH et al: Rising incidence of intrahepatic cholangiocarcinoma in the United States: a true increase? J Hepatol 2004;40:472. [PMID: 15123362]

Author(s)

Lawrence S. Friedman, MD

Bipolar Disorder

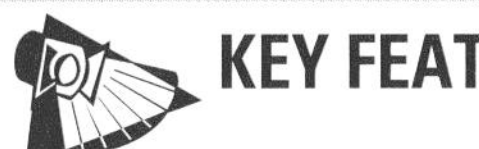

KEY FEATURES

ESSENTIALS OF DIAGNOSIS

- Episodic mood shifts into mania, major depression, hypomania, and mixed states

GENERAL CONSIDERATIONS

- Manic episodes
  - Begin abruptly and may be triggered by life stresses
  - Last days to months—generally shorter than depressive episodes
  - Most common in spring and summer months
- Cyclothymia
  - Chronic mood disturbances with episodes of depression and hypomania
  - Symptoms are milder than those in a manic or depressive episode, but have at least a 2-year duration
  - Symptoms occasionally escalate to a full-blown manic or depressive episode, warranting a diagnosis of bipolar I or bipolar II disorder

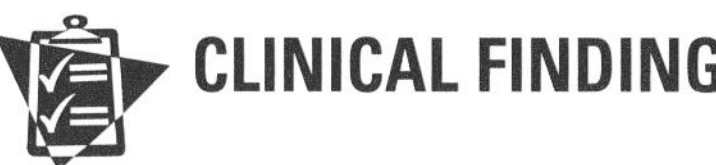

CLINICAL FINDINGS

SYMPTOMS AND SIGNS

- Manic episodes
  - Mood ranging from euphoria to irritability
  - Overinvolvement in life activities
  - Flight of ideas with distractibility
  - Sleep disruption, little need for sleep
  - Racing thoughts
  - Behaviors may initially attract others
  - Irritability, mood lability, aggression, and grandiosity usually lead to problems in relationships
  - Excessive spending, resignation from a job, a hasty marriage or divorce, sexual acting out, or exhibitionism may occur
  - Atypical episodes involve gross delusions, paranoid ideations, and auditory hallucinations
  - "Rapid cyclers" experience four or more discrete episodes of mood disturbance per year
- Most depressions
  - Lowered mood, varying from mild sadness to intense feelings of guilt, worthlessness, and hopelessness
  - Difficulty in thinking, including inability to concentrate, ruminations, and lack of decisiveness
  - Loss of interest, with diminished involvement in work and recreation
  - Somatic complaints such as
    - Headache
    - Disrupted, lessened, or excessive sleep
    - Loss of energy
    - Change in appetite
    - Decreased sexual drive
  - Anxiety
- Some severe depressions
  - Psychomotor retardation or agitation
  - Delusions of a hypochondriacal or persecutory nature
  - Withdrawal from activities
  - Physical symptoms of major severity, eg,
    - Anorexia
    - Insomnia
    - Reduced sexual drive
    - Weight loss
    - Various somatic complaints
  - Suicidal ideation

DIFFERENTIAL DIAGNOSIS

- Schizophrenia and other psychotic disorders
- Intoxication with stimulants
- Major depressive episode
- Hypothryoidism
- Dysthymia

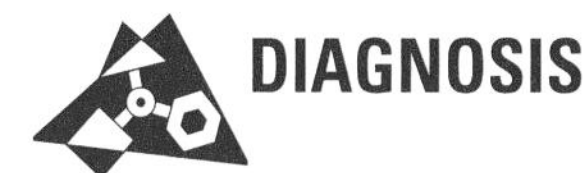

DIAGNOSIS

LABORATORY TESTS

- Consider thyroid-stimulating hormone
- Consider toxicology screen

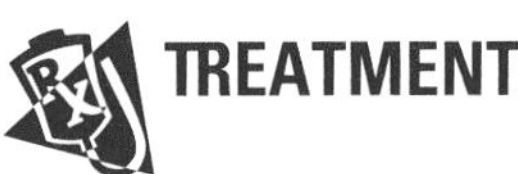

TREATMENT

MEDICATIONS

- Mania
  - Haloperidol (5–10 mg PO or IM Q 2–3 h)
  - Alternatively, atypical neuroleptics (olanzapine 5–20 mg QD) may be used initially to treat agitation and psychosis
  - Clonazepam (1–2 mg PO Q 4–6 h) may be used instead of or in conjunction with a neuroleptic to control acute behavioral symptoms
  - Lithium (1200–1800 mg PO QD targeted to therapeutic serum level)
    - Effective in acute mania or hypomania, but takes several days to take effect
    - As prophylaxis, can limit the frequency and severity of mood swings in 70% of patients
  - Valproic acid (750 mg/day divided and titrated to therapeutic levels) can be loaded to therapeutic levels in 2–3 days
  - Carbamazepine (800–1600 mg/day)
    - Used in patients intolerant or unresponsive to lithium
    - Also more effective than lithium in rapid cyclers
  - Calcium channel blockers (verapamil) have been used in refractory patients
  - Lamotrigine (25–50 mg/day titrated slowly upward) has good efficacy for bipolar depression
- Depression
  - See Depression

THERAPEUTIC PROCEDURES

- Electroconvulsive therapy is effective in treatment of manic disorders in pregnant women, in whom medications are contraindicated

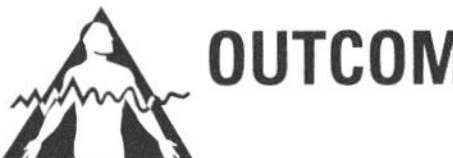

OUTCOME

FOLLOW-UP

- Lithium levels should be measured 5–7 days after initiation and dose changes, monthly to bimonthly early in treatment, and every 6–12 months in stable patients
- Thyroid and kidney function should be monitored every 3–4 months in patients on lithium
- Liver function and blood counts must be monitored in patients taking valproic acid or carbamazepine
- Weight, fasting blood sugar, and lipids must be monitored in patients taking most atypical antipsychotics

COMPLICATIONS

- Suicide (see Depression)
- Drug–drug interactions complicate therapy with all agents—careful review of concomitant medications is needed
- Lithium toxicity occurs at serum levels >2 mEq/L (see Lithium Toxicity)
- Long-term lithium use can cause cogwheel rigidity and other extrapyramidal signs

PROGNOSIS

- Good prognosis with adequate treatment
- Compliance with lithium is adversely affected by the loss of some hypomanic experiences valued by the patient

WHEN TO REFER

- When diagnosis is in question or when standard management strategies are ineffective
- Any question of suicidiality or irrational behavior

WHEN TO ADMIT

- In a depressive episode, patients who are at risk of suicide or self-harm
- Manic patients whose judgment is sufficiently impaired to make them a risk to themselves or others

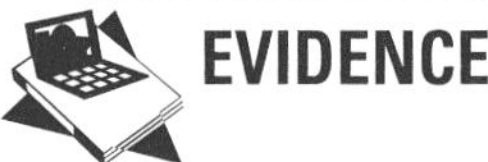

EVIDENCE

PRACTICE GUIDELINES

- National Guideline Clearinghouse: American Psychiatric Association
  - http://www.guideline.gov/summary/summary.aspx?doc_id=3302

WEB SITES

- American Psychiatric Association
  - http://www.psych.org/
- Internet Mental Health
  - http://www.mentalhealth.com/t30.html
- National Institute of Mental Health
  - http://www.nimh.nih.gov

INFORMATION FOR PATIENTS

- American Psychiatric Association
  - http://www.psych.org/public_info/bipolar.cfm
- National Institute of Mental Health
  - http://www.nimh.nih.gov/publicat/bipolar.cfm

REFERENCES

- Krishnan KR: Psychiatric and medical comorbidities of bipolar disorder. Psychosom Med 2005;67:1. [PMID: 15673617]
- Viguera AC et al: Reproductive decisions by women with bipolar disorder after prepregnancy psychiatric consultation. Am J Psychiatry 2002;159:2102. [PMID: 12450965]

Author(s)

Stuart J. Eisendrath, MD

Jonathan E. Lichtmacher, MD

Bites, Animal & Human

KEY FEATURES

ESSENTIALS OF DIAGNOSIS

- Cat and human bites are more likely to become infected than dog bites
- Bites to the hand are of special concern because of the possiblity of closed-space infection
- Antibiotic prophylaxis indicated for noninfected bites of the hand and hospitalization required for infected hand bites
- All infected wounds need to be cultured to direct therapy

GENERAL CONSIDERATIONS

- Biting animals are usually known by their victims, and most biting incidents are provoked (ie, bites occur while playing with the animal or after surprising the animal or waking it abruptly from sleep)
- The animal inflicting the bite, the location of the bite, and the type of injury inflicted are all important determinants of whether they become infected
- Bites of the head, face, and neck are less likely to become infected than bites on the extremities
- Failure to elicit a history of provocation is important, because an unprovoked attack raises the possibility of rabies
- **Human bites** are usually inflicted by children while playing or fighting; in adults, bites are associated with alcohol use and closed-fist injuries that occur during fights
- Infections following human bites are variable
  - Bites inflicted by children rarely become infected, because they are superficial
  - Bites by adults become infected in 15–30% of cases, with a particularly high rate of infection in closed-fist injuries
- **Cat bites** are more likely to become infected than human bites—between 30% and 50% of all cat bites become infected
- **Dog bites,** for unclear reasons, become infected only 5% of the time
- **Puncture wounds** become infected more frequently than lacerations, probably because the latter are easier to irrigate and debride
- The bacteriology of dog and cat bites is polymicrobial with over 50% of infections caused by aerobes and anaerobes and 36% caused by aerobes alone. Pure anaerobic infections are rare
- *Pasteurella* species are the single most common pathogen—75% of cat bites and 50% of dog bites
- Other common aerobes include streptococci, staphylococci, *Moraxella*, and *Neisseria*
- Common anaerobes include *Fusobacterium, Bacteroides, Porphyromonas,* and *Prevotella*
- Human bites, like dog and cat bites, are a mixture of aerobes and anaerobes in over 50% and aerobes alone in 44%
- Staphylococci, streptococci, and *Eikenella corrodens* (isolated in 30% of infections) are the most common anaerobes
- *Prevotella* and *Fusobacterium* are the most common anaerobes
- Although the above named organisms are the most common, numerous others have been isolated such as *Capnocytophaga* (dogs and cats), *Pseudomonas,* and *Haemophilus,* emphasizing the need to culture all infected wounds to define bacteriology
- HIV transmission following a bite has been rarely reported; saliva not contaminated with blood is very low risk

DEMOGRAPHICS

- About 900 dog bite injuries require emergency department attention each day, most often in urban areas
- Dog bites occur most commonly in the summer months

CLINICAL FINDINGS

SYMPTOMS AND SIGNS

Dog and cat bites

- Early infections (within 24 h after the bite) are characterized by rapid onset and progression, fever, chills, cellulitis, and local adenopathy

Human bites

- **Early infections** can produce a rapidly progressive necrotizing infection
- **Late infections** (longer than 24 h after the bite) present with local swelling and erythema. Drainage and systemic symptoms may or may not be present

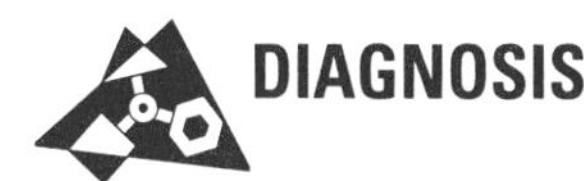

DIAGNOSIS

LABORATORY TESTS

- Because the bacteriology of the infections is so variable, always culture infected wounds and adjust therapy appropriately, especially if the patient is not responding to initial empiric treatment

IMAGING STUDIES

- X-ray films should be obtained to look for fractures and the presence of foreign bodies

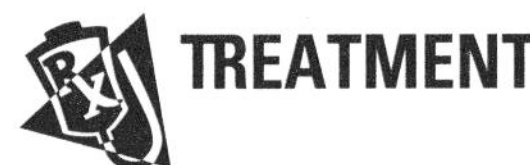

TREATMENT

MEDICATIONS

Prophylactic antibiotics

- Prophylaxis is indicated in high-risk bites, eg, cat bites in any location and hand bites by any animal or by humans
- The most commonly used antibiotic for prophylaxis is amoxicillin-clavulanate (Augmentin) 500 mg three times a day for 3–5 days
- In the penicillin-allergic patient, clindamycin plus a fluoroquinolone is given
- Immunocompromised and asplenic patients are at risk for developing overwhelming bacteremia and sepsis following animal bites and should also receive prophylaxis, even for low-risk bites

Antibiotics

- Infected wounds require antibiotics, administered either orally or intravenously, depending on individualized clinical decisions
- *Pasteurella multocida* is best treated with penicillin or a tetracycline
  - Other active agents include second- and third-generation cephalosporins, fluoroquinolones, or azithromycin and clarithromycin
  - Response to therapy is slow, and therapy should be continued for at least 2–3 weeks
- Human bites frequently require IV therapy with a β-lactam plus a β-lactamase inhibitor combination (Unasyn, Timentin, Zosyn), a second-generation cephalosporin with anaerobic activity (cefoxitin, cefotetan, cefmetazole) or, in the penicillin-allergic patient, clindamycin plus a fluoroquinolone

THERAPEUTIC PROCEDURES

- Careful examination to assess the extent of the injury (tendon laceration, joint space penetration) is critical to appropriate care
- Vigorous cleansing and irrigation of the wound as well as debridement of necrotic material are the most important factors in decreasing the incidence of infections
- If wounds require closure for cosmetic or mechanical reasons, suturing can be done
- Never suture an infected wound, and wounds of the hand should generally not be sutured since a closed-space infection of the hand can result in loss of function

OUTCOME

FOLLOW-UP

- Careful follow-up is required every 1–2 days to assess improvement

COMPLICATIONS

- Osteomyelitis
- Tendon rupture
- Abscess

PROGNOSIS

- Generally good, but resolution may be slow, especially with *Pasteurella* infections

WHEN TO REFER

- Bites to the hand
- Failure to improve within 2–3 days

WHEN TO ADMIT

- Human bites to the hand are usually admitted to the hospital

PREVENTION

- All patients must be evaluated for the need for tetanus (Tables 132 and 133) and rabies prophylaxis (see Rabies)

EVIDENCE

PRACTICE GUIDELINES

- Update on emerging infections from the Centers for Disease Control and Prevention. Update rabies postexposure prophylaxis guidelines. Ann Emerg Med 1999;33:590. [PMID: 10216339]

INFORMATION FOR PATIENTS

- National Institutes of Health
  - http://www.nlm.nih.gov/medlineplus/ency/article/000034.htm
- The Mayo Clinic
  - http://www.mayoclinic.com/invoke.cfm?id=FA00044
  - http://www.mayoclinic.com/invoke.cfm?id=FA00057

REFERENCES

- Brook I: Microbiology and management of human and animal bite wound infections. Prim Care 2003;30:25. [PMID: 12825249]
- Medeiros I et al: Antibiotic prophylaxis for mammalian bites. Cochrane Database Syst Rev 2001;(2)CD001738. [PMID: 11406003]
- Talan DA et al: Clinical presentation and bacteriologic analyses of infected human bites in patients presenting to emergency departments. Clin Infect Dis 2003;37:1481. [PMID: 14614671]

Author(s)

Richard A. Jacobs, MD, PhD

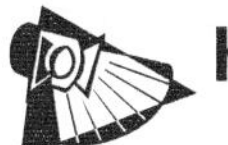

KEY FEATURES

ESSENTIALS OF DIAGNOSIS

- Localized rash with pruritus
- Furuncle-like lesions containing live arthropods
- Tender erythematous patches that migrate ("larva migrans")
- Generalized urticaria or erythema multiforme in some patients

GENERAL CONSIDERATIONS

- Body lice, fleas, bedbugs, and mosquitoes should be considered
- Some arthropods (eg, most pest mosquitoes and biting flies) are readily detected as they bite, whereas in others reactions may be delayed for many hours; many are allergic
- Spiders are often incorrectly believed to be the source of bites; they rarely attack humans, though the brown spider (*Loxosceles laeta, Loxosceles reclusa*) may cause severe necrotic reactions and death due to intravascular hemolysis, and the black widow spider (*Latrodectus mactans*) may cause severe systemic symptoms and death
- In addition to arthropod bites, the most common lesions are venomous stings (wasps, hornets, bees, ants, scorpions) or bites (centipedes), furuncle-like lesions due to fly maggots or sand fleas in the skin, and a linear creeping eruption due to a migrating larva
- Fleas: *Ctenocephalides felis* and *Ctenocephalides canis* are the most common species found on cats and dogs, and both species attack humans; the human flea is *Pulex irritans*
- Bedbugs: found in crevices of beds or furniture
- Ticks: usually picked up by brushing against low vegetation; ticks may transmit Rocky Mountain Spotted Fever, Lyme Disease, Relapsing Fever, and Ehrlichiosis (see separate diagnoses)
- Chiggers or red bugs are larvae of trombiculid mites
- Bird and rodent mites: larger than chiggers, bird mites infest pigeon lofts or nests of birds in eaves; bites are multiple anywhere on the body
- Mites in stored products
  - White and almost invisible; infest products such as vanilla pods, sugar, straw, cottonseeds, cereals
  - Persons who handle these products may be attacked on the hands and forearms and sometimes on the feet
- Caterpillars of moths with urticating hairs: hairs are blown from cocoons or carried by emergent moths, causing severe and often seasonally recurrent outbreaks after mass emergence; the gypsy moth is a cause in eastern United States
- Tungiasis
  - Due to the burrowing flea known as *Tunga penetrans* and found in Africa, the West Indies, and South and Central America
  - The female burrows under the skin, sucks blood, swells to 0.5 cm, and then ejects her eggs onto the ground

CLINICAL FINDINGS

SYMPTOMS AND SIGNS

- Individual bites are often in clusters and tend to occur either on exposed parts (eg, midges and gnats) or under clothing, especially around the waist or at flexures (eg, small mites or insects in bedding or clothing)
- The reaction is often delayed for 1–24 h or more
- Pruritus is almost always present and may be all but intolerable once the patient starts to scratch
- Secondary infection may follow scratching
- Urticarial wheals are common; papules may become vesicular
- Flea saliva and bedbugs produce papular urticaria in sensitized individuals
- Chiggers or red bugs
  - A few species attack humans, often around the waist, on the ankles, or in flexures, raising intensely itching erythematous papules after a delay of many hours
  - The red chiggers may sometimes be seen in the center of papules that have not yet been scratched
- Tungiasis: ulceration, lymphangitis, gangrene, and septicemia may result, in some cases with lethal effect

DIFFERENTIAL DIAGNOSIS

- Scabies
- Lice
- Fleas
- Bedbugs
- Ticks
- Chiggers or red bugs
- Bird or rodent mites
- Tungiasis (burrowing flea)

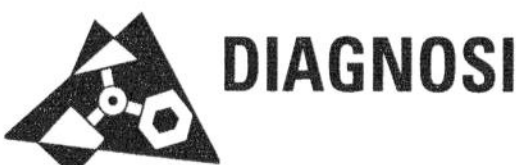

DIAGNOSIS

- Diagnosis is based on the clinical features, but may be aided by searching for exposure to arthropods and by considering the patient's occupation and recent activities

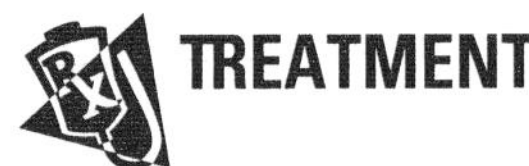

TREATMENT

MEDICATIONS

- Corticosteroid lotions or creams are helpful
- Calamine lotion or a cool wet dressing is always appropriate
- Topical antibiotics may be applied if secondary infection is suspected
- Localized persistent lesions may be treated with intralesional corticosteroids
- Stings produced by many arthropods may be alleviated by applying papain powder (Adolph's Meat Tenderizer) mixed with water, or aluminum chloride hexahydrate (Xerac AC)
- To break the life cycle of the flea, one must repeatedly treat the home and pets, using quick-kill insecticides, residual insecticides, and a growth regulator
- Tungiasis: ethyl chloride spray will kill the insect when applied to the lesion, and disinfestation may be accomplished with insecticide applied to the terrain; simple surgical excision is usually performed

THERAPEUTIC PROCEDURES

- Living arthropods should be removed carefully with tweezers after application of alcohol and preserved in alcohol for identification

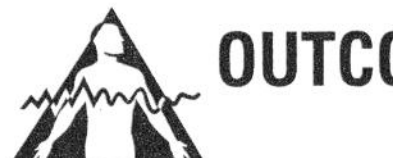

OUTCOME

WHEN TO REFER

- If there is a question about the diagnosis, if recommended therapy is ineffective, or specialized treatment is necessary

PREVENTION

- Avoidance of contaminated areas
- Personal cleanliness
- Disinfection of clothing, bedclothes, and furniture as indicated
- Benzyl benzoate and dimethylphthalate are excellent acaricides
  - Clothing should be impregnated by spray or by dipping in a soapy emulsion

EVIDENCE

PRACTICE GUIDELINES

- The diagnosis and management of urticaria: a practice parameter Part I: acute urticaria/angioedema Part II: chronic urticaria/angioedema. Joint Task Force on Practice Parameters for Allergy and Immunology, 2000
  - http://www.guideline.gov/summary/summary.aspx?doc_id=3622&nbr=2848

WEB SITE

- Centers for Disease Control and Prevention
  - http://www.cdc.gov/

INFORMATION FOR PATIENTS

- American College of Allergy, Asthma & Immunology: Insect Stings
  - http://www.medem.com/medlb/article_detaillb.cfm?article_ID=ZZZMO0FIA9C&sub_cat=530
- Mayo Clinic: Insect Bites and Stings
  - http://www.mayoclinic.com/invoke.cfm?id=fa00046
- Centers for Disease Control and Prevention: Protection against Mosquitoes and Other Arthropods
  - http://www.cdc.gov/travel/bugs.htm
- Nemours Foundation: Bug Bites and Stings (Bedbug, Bee, Black Widow Spider, Brown Recluse Spider, Chigger, Fire Ant, Flea, Gnat, Louse, Mosquito, Scorpion, Tarantula, Tick)
  - http://kidshealth.org/kid/ill_injure/

REFERENCE

- Elston DM et al: What's eating you? Bedbugs. Cutis 2000;65:262. [PMID: 10826083]

Author(s)

Timothy G. Berger, MD

Bladder Cancer

Bites, Snake p. 1040. Bites, Spider & Scorpion p. 1040.

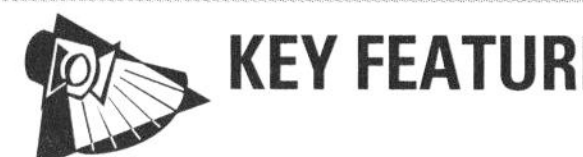

KEY FEATURES

ESSENTIALS OF DIAGNOSIS

- Irritative voiding symptoms
- Gross or microscopic hematuria
- Positive urinary cytology in most patients
- Filling defect within bladder noted on imaging

GENERAL CONSIDERATIONS

- Second most common urological cancer
- More common in men than women (2.7:1)
- Mean age at diagnosis is 65 years
- Risk factors: cigarette smoking, exposure to industrial dyes and solvents

Pathology

- Transitional cell carcinomas ~90%
- Squamous cell cancers ~7%
- Adenocarcinomas ~2%
- Bladder cancer staging is based on the extent of bladder wall penetration and the presence of either regional or distant metastases
- Natural history is based on tumor recurrence and progression to higher stage disease. Both are related to tumor grade and stage

CLINICAL FINDINGS

SYMPTOMS AND SIGNS

- Hematuria is the presenting symptom in 85–90%
- Irritative voiding symptoms in a small percent
- Masses detected on bimanual examination with large-volume or deeply infiltrating cancers
- Lymphedema of the lower extremities with locally advanced cancers or metastases to pelvic lymph nodes
- Hepatomegaly or supraclavicular lymphadenopathy with metastatic disease

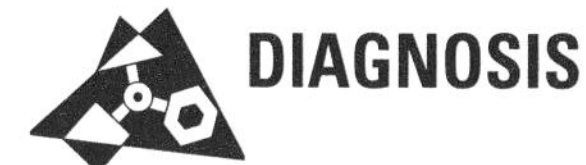

DIAGNOSIS

LABORATORY TESTS

- Urinalysis—hematuria; on occasion, pyuria
- Azotemia
- Anemia

IMAGING STUDIES

- Intravenous urography, ultrasound, CT, MRI show filling defects within the bladder

DIAGNOSTIC PROCEDURES

- Cytology useful in detecting disease at initial presentation or recurrence
- Cytology very sensitive (80–90%) in detecting cancers of higher grade and stage. Sensitivity enhanced by flow cytometry
- Imaging done primarily for evaluating the upper urinary tract and staging
- Cystourethroscopy and biopsy
- Diagnosis and staging are by cystoscopy and transurethral resection of bladder tumor (TURBT)
- TURBT can be done under general or regional anesthesia
- Resection down to muscular elements of the bladder
- Random bladder and, on occasion, prostatic urethral biopsies

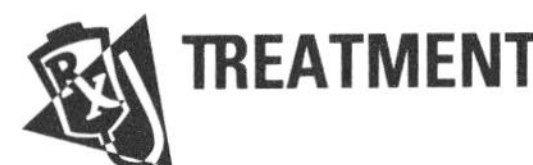

TREATMENT

MEDICATIONS

- Patients with superficial cancers (Ta, T1) are treated with complete TURBT and selective use of intravesical chemotherapy
- Patients with large, high-grade, recurrent Ta lesions, T1 cancers, and carcinoma in situ are treated with intravesical chemotherapy after TURBT
- Patients with more invasive (T2, T3) but still localized cancers require more aggressive surgery (radical cystectomy), or the combination of chemotherapy and selective surgery
- Patients with evidence of lymph node or distant metastases should undergo systemic chemotherapy
- Intravesical chemotherapy
  - Immunotherapeutic or chemotherapeutic agents administered weekly for 6 weeks
  - Maintenance therapy after the initial induction regimen includes Bacillus Calmette-Guérin, thiotepa, mitomycin, or doxorubicin

SURGERY

- Transurethral resection is diagnostic, allows for proper staging, and controls superficial cancers
- Partial cystectomy is indicated in patients with cancers in a bladder diverticulum
- Radical cystectomy with urinary diversion—a conduit of small or large bowel—or continent forms of diversion available

THERAPEUTIC PROCEDURES

- Radiotherapy: external beam therapy over a 6- to 8-week period
- Chemotherapy (systemic)
  - Cisplatin-based combination chemotherapy
  - Adjuvant chemotherapy when the primary tumor invades perivesical fat or adjacent organs or when lymph node metastases are found—used for patients being treated with radical cystectomy
  - Combination radiotherapy and systemic chemotherapy or surgery, radiotherapy, and systemic chemotherapy

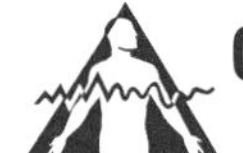

OUTCOME

COMPLICATIONS

- Intravesical chemotherapy: side effects include irritative voiding symptoms and hemorrhagic cystitis
- Radiotherapy: approximately 10–15% of patients develop bladder, bowel, or rectal complications; local recurrence is common (30–70%)

PROGNOSIS

- Chemotherapy (systemic)
  - Partial response in 15–35%
  - Complete response in 15–45%

EVIDENCE

PRACTICE GUIDELINES

- Oosterlinck W et al: Guidelines on bladder cancer. Eur Urol 2002;41:105. [PMID: 12074395]
- Segal R et al; Cancer Care Ontario Practice Guidelines Initiative Genitourinary Cancer Disease Site Group: Adjuvant chemotherapy for deep muscle-invasive transitional cell bladder carcinoma—a practice guideline. Can J Urol 2002;9:1625. [PMID: 12431323]

INFORMATION FOR PATIENTS

- American Urological Association
  - http://www.urologyhealth.org/adult/index.cfm?cat=03&topic=37
- Cleveland Clinic — Bladder cancer
  - http://www.clevelandclinic.org/health/health-info/docs/1300/1379.asp?index=6150
- Mayo Clinic
  - http://www.mayoclinic.com/invoke.cfm?id=DS00177

REFERENCES

- Donat SM: Evaluation and follow-up strategies for superficial bladder cancer. Urol Clin North Am 2003;30:765. [PMID: 14680313]
- Golka K et al: Occupational exposure and urological cancer. World J Urol 2004;21:382. [PMID: 14648102]
- Madeb R et al: Gender, racial and age differences in bladder cancer incidence and mortality. Urol Oncol 2004;22:86. [PMID: 15082003]

Author(s)

Marshall L. Stoller, MD
Peter R. Carroll, MD

Botulism

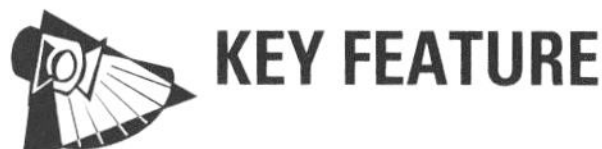

KEY FEATURES

ESSENTIALS OF DIAGNOSIS

- History of recent ingestion of home-canned or smoked foods or of injection drug use and demonstration of toxin in serum or food
- Sudden onset of diplopia, dry mouth, dysphagia, dysphonia, and muscle weakness progressing to respiratory paralysis
- Pupils are usually fixed and dilated

GENERAL CONSIDERATIONS

- A paralytic disease caused by botulinum neurotoxin, which is produced by *Clostridium botulinum*, a ubiquitous, strictly anaerobic, spore-forming bacillus found in soil
- Four toxin types—A, B, E, and F—cause human disease
- Botulinum toxin inhibits release of acetylcholine at the neuromuscular junction
- Naturally occurring botulism occurs in one of three forms
  - Food-borne botulism
  - Infant botulism
  - Wound botulism
- **Food-borne botulism** is caused by ingestion of preformed toxin present in canned, smoked, or vacuum-packed foods such as home-canned vegetables, smoked meats, and vacuum-packed fish
- **Infant botulism** is associated with ingestion of honey. Honey consumption is safe for children 1 year of age or older
- **Wound botulism** typically occurs in association with injection drug use. It results from organisms present in the gut or wound that elaborate toxin in vivo
- Botulinum toxin is extremely potent and is classified by the Centers for Disease Control and Prevention (CDC) as a high-priority agent because of its potential for use as an agent of bioterrorism

DEMOGRAPHICS

- Approximately 170 cases of botulism have been reported to the CDC over a year. Of these, 20% were food-borne and wound botulism and the remainder were infant botulism

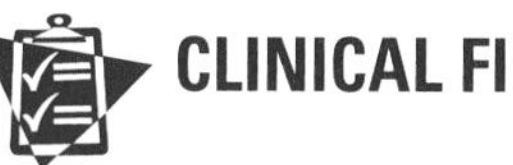

CLINICAL FINDINGS

SYMPTOMS AND SIGNS

- Twelve to 36 h after ingestion of the toxin, visual disturbances appear, particularly diplopia and loss of accommodation
- Ptosis, cranial nerve palsies with impairment of extraocular muscles, and fixed dilated pupils are characteristic signs
- Other symptoms are dry mouth, dysphagia, and dysphonia
- The sensory examination is normal
- The sensorium remains clear and the temperature normal
- Respiratory paralysis may lead to death unless mechanical assistance is provided

DIFFERENTIAL DIAGNOSIS

- Poliomyelitis
- Guillain-Barré syndrome
- Myasthenia gravis
- Brainstem infarct or vertebrobasilar insufficiency
- Tick paralysis
- Organophosphate poisoning

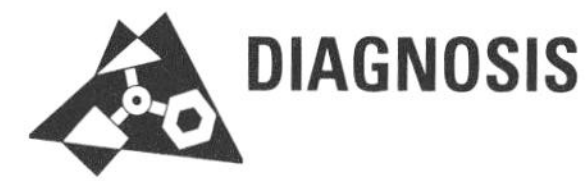

DIAGNOSIS

LABORATORY TESTS

- Toxin in patients' serum and in suspected foods may be shown by mouse inoculation and identified with specific antiserum

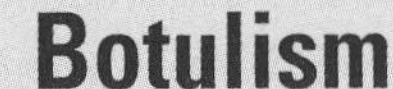

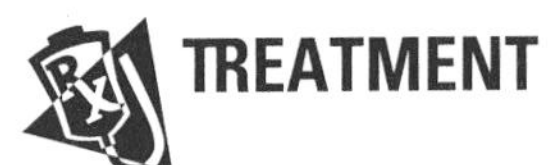

TREATMENT

MEDICATIONS

- If botulism is suspected, the CDC should be contacted for advice and help with procurement of botulinus antitoxin and for assistance in obtaining assays for toxin. During off hours, the CDC provides assistance via a recorded message at 404-639-2206

THERAPEUTIC PROCEDURES

- Respiratory failure is managed with intubation and mechanical ventilation

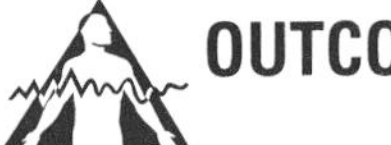

OUTCOME

PROGNOSIS

- Early nervous system involvement leads to respiratory paralysis and death in untreated cases

WHEN TO REFER

- All cases should be reported to the public health authorities
- Obtain immediate expert infectious and neurological consultation

WHEN TO ADMIT

- All suspected and proven cases because of the high fatality rate

PREVENTION

- Botulism toxin is destroyed by high temperatures; persons who eat home-canned foods should consider boiling the food for 10 min before eating it

EVIDENCE

PRACTICE GUIDELINES

- National Guideline Clearinghouse
  - http://www.guideline.gov/summary/summary.aspx?doc_id=3619

WEB SITES

- CDC
  - http://www.bt.cdc.gov/agent/botulism/index.asp
- CDC—Division of Bacterial and Mycotic Diseases
  - http://www.cdc.gov/ncidod/dbmd/diseaseinfo/botulism_a.htm
- Karolinska Institute—Directory of Bacterial Infections and Mycoses
  - http://www.mic.ki.se/Diseases/C01.html

INFORMATION FOR PATIENTS

- Centers for Disease Control—Bioterrorism
  - http://www.bt.cdc.gov/agent/botulism/factsheet.asp
- JAMA patient page: Food-borne illnesses. JAMA 1999;281:1866. [PMID: 10340376]

REFERENCES

- Merrison AF et al: Wound botulism associated with subcutaneous drug use. BMJ 2002;326:1020. [PMID: 12411365]
- Shapiro RL et al: Botulism in the United States: a clinical and epidemiologic review. Ann Intern Med 1998;129:221. [PMID: 9696731]

Author(s)

Henry F. Chambers, MD

Brain Abscess

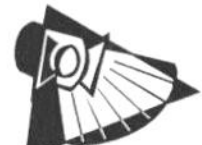

KEY FEATURES

ESSENTIALS OF DIAGNOSIS

- Symptoms and signs of expanding intracranial mass
- May be signs of primary infection or congenital heart disease
- Fever may be absent

GENERAL CONSIDERATIONS

- Presents as an intracranial space-occupying lesion
- May be a sequela of ear or nose disease, a complication of infection elsewhere in the body, or an infection introduced intracranially by trauma or surgical procedures
- Most common infective organisms are streptococci, staphylococci, and anaerobes; mixed infections are not uncommon

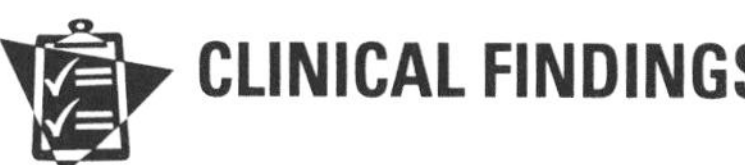

CLINICAL FINDINGS

SYMPTOMS AND SIGNS

- Headache, drowsiness, inattention, confusion, and seizures are early symptoms
- Increasing intracranial pressure and focal neurologic deficits are later signs
- There may be little or no systemic evidence of infection

DIFFERENTIAL DIAGNOSIS

- Other rapidly expanding intracranial space-occupying lesions

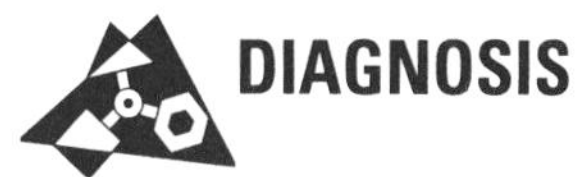

DIAGNOSIS

LABORATORY TESTS

- Examination of the cerebrospinal fluid does not help in diagnosis and may precipitate a herniation syndrome

IMAGING STUDIES

- CT scan of the head characteristically shows an area of contrast enhancement surrounding a low-density core (similar to metastatic neoplasms)
- MRI permits earlier recognition of focal cerebritis or an abscess
- Arteriography indicates the presence of a space-occupying lesion (avascular mass with displacement of normal cerebral vessels) but provides no clue to the nature of the lesion

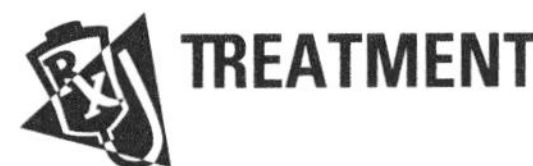

TREATMENT

MEDICATIONS

- IV antibiotics, combined with surgical drainage (aspiration or excision) if necessary to reduce the mass effect, or to establish the diagnosis
- Broad-spectrum antibiotics are used if the infecting organism is unknown (Table 128); a common regimen is penicillin G (2 million units Q2 h IV) plus either chloramphenicol (1–2 g IV Q6 h), metronidazole (750 mg IV Q6 h), or both; nafcillin is added if *Staphylococcus aureus* is suspected
- Antimicrobial treatment is usually continued parenterally for 6–8 weeks, then orally for another 2–3 weeks
- Dexamethasone (4–25 mg four times daily, depending on severity, followed by tapering of dose, depending on response) may reduce any associated edema; IV mannitol is sometimes required

THERAPEUTIC PROCEDURES

- Aspiration or excision if necessary to reduce mass effect or to establish the diagnosis

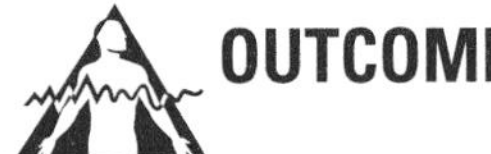

OUTCOME

FOLLOW-UP

- Monitor patient by serial CT scans or MRI every 2 weeks and at deterioration

COMPLICATIONS

- Seizures
- Focal neurologic deficits

PROGNOSIS

- Abscesses smaller than 2 cm can often be cured medically

WHEN TO ADMIT

- When the diagnosis is suspected

EVIDENCE

PRACTICE GUIDELINES

- Evaluation and management of intracranial mass lesions in AIDS. Report of the Quality Standards Subcommittee of the American Academy of Neurology. Neurology 1998;50:21. [PMID: 9443452]
- National Guideline Clearinghouse
  - http://www.guideline.gov/summary/summary.aspx?doc_id=3821&nbr=3047&string=brain+AND+abscess
  - http://www.guideline.gov/summary/summary.aspx?doc_id=2446&nbr=1672&string=brain+abscess

WEB SITES

- The Whole Brain Atlas
  - http://www.med.harvard.edu:80/AANLIB/home.html
- CNS Pathology Index
  - http://medstat.med.utah.edu/WebPath/CNSHTML/CNSIDX.html

INFORMATION FOR PATIENTS

- National Institutes of Health
  - http://www.nlm.nih.gov/medlineplus/ency/article/000783.htm

REFERENCE

- Roos KL: Acute bacterial infections of the central nervous system. In: *Neurology and General Medicine*, ed 3. Aminoff MJ (editor). Churchill Livingstone, 2001.

Author(s)

Michael J. Aminoff, MD, DSc, FRCP

Brain Tumor, Primary

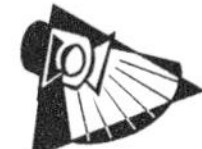

KEY FEATURES

ESSENTIALS OF DIAGNOSIS

- Personality changes, intellectual decline, emotional lability, seizures, headaches, nausea
- Increased intracranial pressure in some patients
- Neuroradiologic evidence of space-occupying lesion

GENERAL CONSIDERATIONS

- Half of all primary intracranial neoplasms (Table 99) are gliomas and the remainder meningiomas, pituitary adenomas, neurofibromas, and other tumors
- Certain tumors (eg, neurofibromas, hemangioblastomas, and retinoblastomas) have a familial basis
- May lead to a generalized disturbance of cerebral function and symptoms of increased intracranial pressure

DEMOGRAPHICS

- Tumors may occur at any age, but some gliomas are age-specific (Table 99)

CLINICAL FINDINGS

SYMPTOMS AND SIGNS

Herniation symptoms

- Temporal lobe uncus herniation with compression of the third cranial nerve, midbrain, and posterior cerebral artery
  - Ipsilateral pupillary dilation
  - Followed by stupor, coma, decerebrate posturing, and respiratory arrest
- Cerebellar tonsillar displacement causing medullary compression; apnea, circulatory collapse, and death

Focal deficits

- **Frontal lobe lesions**
  - Progressive intellectual decline, slowing of mental activity, personality changes, and contralateral grasp reflexes
  - Expressive aphasia if the posterior part of the left inferior frontal gyrus is involved
  - Anosmia secondary to pressure on the olfactory nerve
  - Precentral lesions may cause focal motor seizures or contralateral pyramidal deficits
- **Temporal lobe lesions**
  - Seizures with olfactory or gustatory hallucinations, motor automatisms, and impairment of external awareness without actual loss of consciousness
  - Depersonalization, emotional changes, behavioral disturbances, sensations of déjà vu or jamais vu
  - Micropsia or macropsia (objects appear smaller or larger than they are), visual field defects (crossed upper quadrantanopia), and auditory illusions or hallucinations
  - Left-sided lesions may lead to dysnomia and receptive aphasia, while right-sided involvement may disturb the perception of musical notes and melodies
- **Parietal lobe lesions**
  - May cause sensory seizures
  - Contralateral disturbances of sensation, sensory loss or inattention (cortical in type and involves postural sensibility and tactile discrimination, so that the appreciation of shape, size, weight, and texture is impaired)
  - Objects placed in the hand may not be recognized (astereognosis)
  - Extensive lesions may produce contralateral hyperpathia and spontaneous pain (thalamic syndrome)
  - Optic radiation involvement leads to a contralateral homonymous field defect that sometimes consists solely of lower quadrantanopia
  - Left angular gyrus lesions cause Gerstmann's syndrome (alexia, agraphia, acalculia, right-left confusion, and finger agnosia), whereas involvement of the left submarginal gyrus causes ideational apraxia
  - Anosognosia (denial, neglect, or rejection of a paralyzed limb) is seen in patients with lesions of the nondominant (right) hemisphere
  - Constructional apraxia and dressing apraxia may also occur with right-sided lesions
- **Occipital lobe lesions**
  - Crossed homonymous hemianopia or a partial field defect
  - Left-sided or bilateral lesions may cause visual agnosia; irritative lesions on either side can cause unformed visual hallucinations
  - Bilateral occipital lobe involvement causes cortical blindness with preservation of pupillary responses to light and lack of awareness of the defect by the patient
  - Loss of color perception, prosopagnosia (inability to identify a familiar face), simultagnosia (inability to integrate and interpret a composite scene as opposed to its individual elements), and Balint's syndrome (failure to turn the eyes to a particular point in space, despite preservation of spontaneous and reflex eye movements), denial of blindness or a field defect (Anton's syndrome)
- **Brainstem and cerebellar lesions**
  - Brainstem lesions lead to cranial nerve palsies, ataxia, incoordination, nystagmus, and pyramidal and sensory deficits in the limbs
  - Intrinsic brainstem tumors, such as gliomas, cause an increase in intracranial pressure, usually late
  - Marked ataxia of the trunk if the vermis cerebelli is involved
  - Ipsilateral appendicular deficits (ataxia, incoordination and hypotonia of the limbs) if the cerebellar hemispheres are affected
- **False localizing signs**
  - Neurologic signs other than by direct compression or infiltration, leading to errors of clinical localization
  - Include third or sixth nerve palsy and bilateral extensor plantar responses produced by herniation syndromes, and an extensor plantar response occurring ipsilateral to a hemispheric tumor because the opposite cerebral peduncle is compressed against the tentorium

DIFFERENTIAL DIAGNOSIS

- Metastatic intracranial tumors
  - Cerebral metastases
  - Leptomeningeal metastases (carcinomatous meningitis)
- Intracranial mass lesions in AIDS patients

Brain Death p. 1042. Brain Mass, AIDS p. 1043.
Brain Metastases p. 1043.

Brain Tumor, Primary

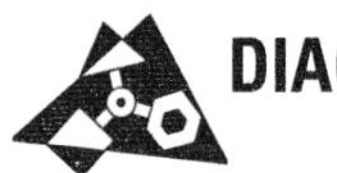

DIAGNOSIS

IMAGING STUDIES

- MRI with gadolinium
  - Best for tumors in the posterior fossa
- CT scanning
  - Characteristic appearance of meningiomas on CT scanning is virtually diagnostic
  - Noncontrast CT shows a lesion in the parasagittal and sylvian regions, olfactory groove, sphenoidal ridge, or tuberculum sellae with a homogeneous area of increased density, which enhances uniformly with contrast
- Arteriography
  - May show stretching or displacement of normal cerebral vessels by the tumor and tumor vascularity
  - An avascular mass may be due to tumor, hematoma, abscess, or any space-occupying lesion
  - In patients with normal hormone levels and an intrasellar mass, angiography used to distinguish between a pituitary adenoma and an arterial aneurysm

DIAGNOSTIC PROCEDURES

- Lumbar puncture is rarely necessary; the findings are seldom diagnostic, herniation syndrome is a risk

TREATMENT

MEDICATIONS

- Corticosteroids help reduce cerebral edema and are usually started before surgery
- Herniation is treated with IV dexamethasone (10–20 mg as a bolus, followed by 4 mg Q6 h) and IV mannitol (20% solution given in a dose of 1.5 g/kg over about 30 min)
- Anticonvulsants in standard doses (Table 98): controversial whether to start these prophylactically or only after a first seizure

SURGERY

- Complete surgical removal if the tumor is extra-axial (eg, meningioma, acoustic neuroma) or is not in a critical or inaccessible region of the brain (eg, cerebellar hemangioblastoma)
- Surgery may be diagnostic and may relieve intracranial pressure symptoms even if the neoplasm cannot be completely removed
- Simple surgical shunting procedures help in cases with obstructive hydrocephalus

THERAPEUTIC PROCEDURES

- Treatment depends on the type and site of the tumor (Table 99) and the condition of the patient
- For those patients whose disease deteriorates despite treatment, palliative care is important
- With malignant gliomas, radiation therapy increases median survival rates regardless of preceding surgery; chemotherapy provides additional benefit
- Indications for irradiation for other primary intracranial neoplasms depend on tumor type and accessibility and the feasibility of complete surgical removal

WHEN TO REFER

- All patients should be referred to specialized care

WHEN TO ADMIT

- Altered sensorium
- Specialized treatment or surgery

EVIDENCE

PRACTICE GUIDELINES

- National Guideline Clearinghouse
  - http://www.guideline.gov/summary/summary.aspx?doc_id=2438&nbr=1664&string=primary+intracerebral+neoplasm

WEB SITES

- Anaplastic Astrocytoma Demonstration Case
  - http://www.brighamrad.harvard.edu/Cases/bwh/hcache/49/full.html
- The Whole Brain Atlas
  - http://www.med.harvard.edu/AANLIB/home.html
- University of Utah CNS Pathology Index
  - http://medstat.med.utah.edu/WebPath/CNSHTML/CNSIDX.html

INFORMATION FOR PATIENTS

- National Cancer Institute
  - http://www.cancer.gov/cancerinfo/wyntk/brain
- Patient Education Institute
  - http://www.nlm.nih.gov/medlineplus/tutorials/braincancer.html

REFERENCES

- Behin A et al: Primary brain tumours in adults. Lancet 2003;361:323. [PMID: 12559880]
- Sarin R et al: Medical decompressive therapy for primary and metastatic intracranial tumours. Lancet Neurol 2003;2:357. [PMID: 12849152]
- Wen PY et al: Malignant gliomas. Curr Neurol Neurosci Rep 2004;4:218. [PMID: 15102348]
- Whittle IR: Surgery for gliomas. Curr Opin Neurol 2002;15:663. [PMID: 12447103]
- Wrensch M et al: Epidemiology of primary brain tumors: current concepts and review of the literature. Neurooncology 2002;4:278. [PMID: 12356358]

Author(s)

Michael J. Aminoff, MD, DSc, FRCP

Breast Cancer, Female

Breast Abscess p. 1043. Breast Augmentation Disorders p. 1044.

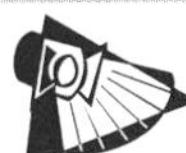

KEY FEATURES

ESSENTIALS OF DIAGNOSIS

- Early findings: single, nontender, firm to hard mass with ill-defined margins; mammographic abnormalities and no palpable mass
- Later findings: skin or nipple retraction; axillary lymphadenopathy; breast enlargement, redness, edema, pain; fixation of mass to skin or chest wall

GENERAL CONSIDERATIONS

- Second most common cancer in women
- Second most common cause of cancer death in women
- Develops in 1 of every 8–9 American women in her lifetime
- ~213,000 new cases and ~41,000 deaths from breast cancer in US women estimated for 2005

DEMOGRAPHICS

- Mean and median age: 60–61 years
- More common in whites
- 3–4 times increased risk in those whose mother or sister had breast cancer, risk is further increased if family member had premenopausal or bilateral disease
- 1.5 times increased incidence if nulliparous or first full-term pregnancy at age > 35
- Slight increased risk if menarche at age < 12 or natural menopause at age >50
- Increased incidence in fibrocystic disease with proliferative changes, papillomatosis, or atypical ductal epithelial hyperplasia
- Women with prior breast cancer develop contralateral cancer at a rate of 1–2% per year
- Increased risk with long-term use of hormone replacement therapy
- Increased risk if history of uterine cancer
- 85% lifetime risk in women with *BRCA1* gene mutations
- Increased risk with *BRCA2*, ataxia-telangiectasia, and *P53* gene mutations

CLINICAL FINDINGS

SYMPTOMS AND SIGNS

- Presenting complaint is a lump (usually painless) in 70%
- Less frequently
  - Breast pain
  - Nipple discharge
  - Erosion, retraction, enlargement, or itching of the nipple
  - Redness, generalized hardness, enlargement, or shrinking of the breast
  - Axillary mass or swelling of the arm (rare)
- With metastatic disease, back or bone pain, jaundice, or weight loss
- Physical examination is done with patient sitting arms at sides and then overhead, and supine with arm abducted
- Findings include
  - Nontender, firm or hard mass with poorly delineated margins
  - Skin or nipple retraction
  - Breast asymmetry
  - Erosions of nipple epithelium
  - Watery, serous or bloody discharge
- Metastatic disease suggested by
  - Firm or hard axillary nodes > 1 cm
  - Axillary nodes that are matted or fixed to skin or deep structures indicate advanced disease (at least stage III)
- Advanced stage (stage IV) cancer suggested by ipsilateral supraclavicular or infraclavicular nodes

DIFFERENTIAL DIAGNOSIS

- Fibrocystic disease or cyst
- Fibroadenoma
- Intraductal papilloma
- Lipoma
- Fat necrosis
- Breast abscess
- Phyllodes tumor

DIAGNOSIS

LABORATORY TESTS

- Alkaline phosphatase increased in liver or bone metastases
- Serum calcium elevated in advanced disease
- Carcinoembryonic antigen (CEA) and CA 15-3 or CA 27-29 are tumor markers for recurrent breast cancer
- Cytological examination of breast nipple discharge occasionally helpful

IMAGING STUDIES

- Mammography
- Breast ultrasound may differentiate cystic from solid masses
- MRI and positron emission tomography (PET) may play a role in imaging atypical lesions but only after diagnostic mammography
- CT scan of chest, abdomen, pelvis, and brain may demonstrate metastases
- Bone scan may show bony metastases in symptomatic patients
- PET scan is under investigation as single test for evaluation of breast, lymphatics, and metastases

DIAGNOSTIC PROCEDURES

- Fine-needle aspiration (FNA) or core biopsy
- Open biopsy under local anesthesia if needle biopsy inconclusive
- Computerized stereotactic or ultrasound guided core needle biopsies for nonpalpable lesions found on mammogram
- TNM staging (I–IV)

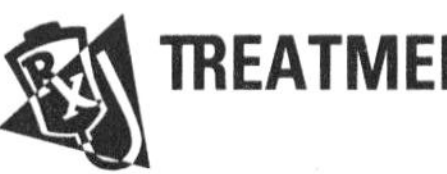

TREATMENT

MEDICATIONS

Potentially curable disease

- Adjuvant chemotherapy improves survival
- Tamoxifen or aromatase inhibitors in hormone receptor-positive patients
- CMF (cyclophosphamide, methotrexate, fluorouracil)
- AC (Adriamycin [doxorubicin], cyclophosphamide) with taxanes (docetaxel or paclitaxel)
- Tamoxifen plus chemotherapy with AC or PAF (prednisone, adriamycin, fluorouracil) lowers recurrence rates more than tamoxifen alone in postmeno-

pausal women with estrogen receptor-positive tumors

Metastatic disease

- For hormone receptor-positive postmenopausal patients, palliative tamoxifen (20 mg PO QD) or aromatase inhibitors
- For patients who initially respond to tamoxifen, but then relapse, consider aromatase inhibitors
- For metastatic disease, chemotherapy should be considered if visceral metastases (especially brain or lung lymphangitic); if hormonal treatment is unsuccessful or disease progresses after initial response to hormonal manipulation; or tumor is estrogen receptor-negative
- AC achieves response rate of ~85%
- Combinations of cyclophosphamide, vincristine, methotrexate, fluorouracil, and taxanes achieve response rates of up to 60–70%
- Paclitaxel achieves response rate of 30–40%
- Trastuzumab, a monoclonal antibody that binds to HER-2/*neu* receptors on the cancer cell, is highly effective in HER-2/*neu*-expressive cancers
- High-dose chemotherapy and autologous bone marrow or stem cell transplantation produce no improvement in survival over conventional chemotherapy

SURGERY

- Surgery indicated for stage I and II cancers
- Disease-free survival rates are similar with partial mastectomy plus axillary dissection followed by radiation therapy and with modified radical mastectomy (total mastectomy plus axillary dissection)
- Large size and multifocal tumors, fixation to the chest wall, or involvement of the nipple or overlying skin are relative contraindications to breast-conserving therapy
- Axillary dissection generally indicated in women with invasive cancer
- Sentinel node biopsy is an alternative to axillary dissection in selected patients

THERAPEUTIC PROCEDURES

- Radiotherapy after partial mastectomy improves local control: 5–6 weeks of 5 daily fractions to a total dose of 5000–6000 cGy; may also improve survival after total mastectomy

OUTCOME

FOLLOW-UP

- Examine patient every 6 months for the first 2 years after diagnosis; thereafter, annually

COMPLICATIONS

- Pleural effusion occurs in almost half of patients with metastatic breast cancer
- Local recurrence occurs in 8%
- Significant edema of the arm occurs in about 10–30%; more commonly if radiotherapy to axilla after surgery

PROGNOSIS

- Stage of breast cancer is the most reliable indicator of prognosis
- Increasing number of involved axillary nodes correlates directly with lower survival rates
- Estrogen and progesterone receptor-positive primary tumors have a more favorable course
- Tumors with marked aneuploidy or high grade have a poor prognosis
- HER-2/*neu* oncogene amplification, epidermal growth factor receptors, and cathepsin D have some prognostic value
- Clinical cure rate of localized invasive breast cancer treated with most accepted methods of therapy is 75–90%
- When axillary lymph nodes are involved, the survival rate drops to 50–60% at 5 years and 30–40% at 10 years

WHEN TO REFER

- Women with exceptional family histories should be referred for genetic counseling and testing

WHEN TO ADMIT

- For definitive therapy by lumpectomy, axillary node dissection or sentinel node biopsy, or mastectomy after diagnosis by FNA or core needle biopsy
- For complications of metastatic disease

PREVENTION

- Screening by combination of clinical examination and mammography: 80–85% detectable only by mammogram; 50% detectable only by examination
- Monthly breast self-examination controversial
- Clinical examination every 2–3 years in women age 20–40, annually in women age > 40
- Mammography every 1–2 years in women 50–79
- For women at high risk for developing breast cancer, tamoxifen yields a 50% reduction in breast cancer if taken for 5 years; raloxifene studies are ongoing

EVIDENCE

PRACTICE GUIDELINES

- Carlson RW et al: NCCN Breast Cancer Practice Guidelines Panel. National Comprehensive Cancer Network: Breast Cancer v.1.2004.
  - http://www.nccn.org/professionals/physician_gls/PDF/breast.pdf

WEB SITE

- National Cancer Institute: Breast Cancer Information for Patients and Health Professionals
  - http://www.cancer.gov/cancertopics/types/breast

INFORMATION FOR PATIENTS

- MedlinePlus: Breast Cancer Interactive Tutorial
  - http://www.nlm.nih.gov/medlineplus/tutorials/breastcancer.html

REFERENCES

- Albain KS: Adjuvant chemotherapy for lymph node-negative, estrogen receptor-negative breast cancer: a tale of three trials. J Natl Cancer Inst 2004;96:1801. [PMID: 15601631]
- Citron ML: Dose density in adjuvant chemotherapy for breast cancer. Cancer Invest 2004;22:555. [PMID: 15565814]
- Giordano SH et al: Breast cancer treatment guidelines in older women. J Clin Oncol 2005;23:783. [PMID: 15681522]
- Grube BJ et al: The current role of sentinel node biopsy in the treatment of breast cancer. Adv Surg 2004;38:121. [PMID: 15515617]
- Narod SA et al: Prevention and management of hereditary breast cancer. J Clin Oncol 2005;23:1656. [PMID: 15755973]
- Rossouw JE et al: Risks and benefits of estrogen plus progestin in healthy postmenopausal women: principal results from the Women's Health Initiative randomized controlled trial. JAMA 2002;288:321. [PMID: 12117397]

Author(s)

Armando E. Giuliano, MD

Bronchiectasis

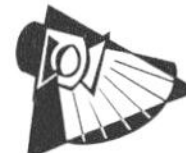

KEY FEATURES

ESSENTIALS OF DIAGNOSIS

- Chronic productive cough with dyspnea and wheezing
- Recurrent pulmonary infections requiring antibiotics
- A history of recurrent pulmonary infection or inflammation or a predisposing condition
- Radiographic findings of dilated, thickened airways and scattered, irregular opacities

GENERAL CONSIDERATIONS

- A congenital or acquired disorder of large bronchi characterized by abnormal dilation and destruction of bronchial walls
- May be localized or diffuse
- May be caused by recurrent inflammation or infection
- Cystic fibrosis causes 50% of all cases
- Can result from abnormal lung defenses (immunodeficiency states, α_1-antiprotease deficiency, mucociliary clearance disorders, rheumatic disease)
- Airways are often colonized with gram-negative bacilli (especially *Pseudomonas*), *Staphylococcus aureus*, and *Aspergillus* species
- Causes
  - Cystic fibrosis
  - Infection
    - Tuberculosis
    - Fungal
    - Abscess
    - Pneumonia
  - Abnormal lung defense mechanisms
    - Hypogammaglobulinemia
    - Common variable immunodeficiency
    - Selective IgA, IgM, and IgG subclass deficiency
    - Acquired immunodeficiency from cytotoxic drugs, AIDS, lymphoma, leukemia, multiple myeloma, chronic renal disease, chronic liver disease
    - α_1-Antiprotease deficiency with cigarette smoking
    - Mucociliary clearance disorders (immotile cilia syndrome)
    - Rheumatic disease, eg, rheumatoid arthritis
  - Localized airway obstruction

CLINICAL FINDINGS

SYMPTOMS AND SIGNS

- Chronic cough with production of copious, purulent sputum
- Recurrent pneumonia
- Hemoptysis
- Weight loss and anemia common
- Persistent basilar crackles commonly found on examination
- Clubbing infrequent in mild cases, but present in severe disease
- Obstructive pulmonary dysfunction with hypoxemia seen in moderate or severe disease

DIFFERENTIAL DIAGNOSIS

- Chronic obstructive pulmonary disease
- Asthma
- Bronchiolitis
- Allergic bronchopulmonary aspergillosis

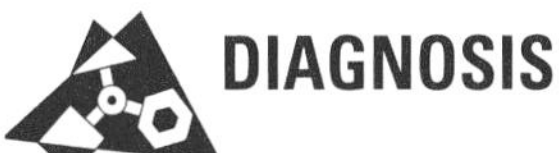

DIAGNOSIS

LABORATORY TESTS

- Sputum smear and culture for bacterial, mycobacterial, and fungal organisms
- Sweat chloride testing
- Quantitative immunoglobulins
- α_1-Antitrypsin level
- Excluding patients with humoral immunodeficiencies, most patients have panhypergammaglobulinemia, reflecting an immune response to chronic airway infection

IMAGING STUDIES

- Chest x-ray shows dilated, thickened central airways and scattered, irregular opacities
- High-resolution CT scanning is the diagnostic test of choice

Breast Cancer, Male p. 1044. Breast Fat Necrosis p. 1045.
Breast Fibroadenoma p. 1045. Bronchial Obstruction p. 1045.

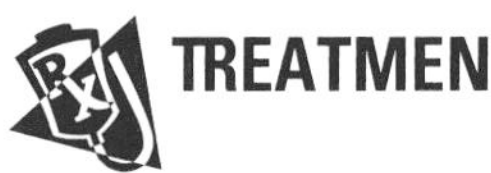

TREATMENT

MEDICATIONS

- Antibiotics should be used in acute exacerbations
- Empiric therapy for 10–14 days with amoxicillin or amoxicillin clavulanate, ampicillin or tetracycline, or trimethoprim-sulfamethoxazole
- Sputum smears and cultures should guide therapy where possible
- Preventive or suppressive antibiotics are frequently given to patients with increased purulent sputum, although this practice is not guided by clinical trial data
- Inhaled aerosolized aminoglycosides reduce *Pseudomonas* colonization, but improve FEV_1 and reduce hospitalizations only in cystic fibrosis patients
- Inhaled bronchodilators are commonly used as maintenance therapy and in acute exacerbations

SURGERY

- Resection is reserved for the few patients with localized bronchiectasis and adequate pulmonary function who fail to respond to conservative treatment
- Surgical treatment may be necessary to stop bleeding in some cases of massive hemoptysis

THERAPEUTIC PROCEDURES

- Daily chest physiotherapy with postural drainage and chest percussion
- Bronchoscopy may be needed to evaluate hemoptysis, remove retained secretions, and rule out obstructing lesions
- Pulmonary angiography with embolization may be required to control massive hemoptysis

OUTCOME

FOLLOW-UP

- Monitor serial pulmonary function tests and sputum cultures

COMPLICATIONS

- Hemoptysis
- Hypoxemia
- Cor pulmonale
- Amyloidosis
- Secondary visceral abscesses at distal sites

PROGNOSIS

- Depends on cause and severity

WHEN TO REFER

- Most cases should be referred to a pulmonary, allergy, clinical immunology, or infectious disease specialist to assist in the evaluation and treatment

WHEN TO ADMIT

- Hypoxia
- Moderate-to-severe acute airflow obstruction
- Severe infection

PREVENTION

- Influenza vaccine
- Pneumococcal vaccine
- Regular chest physiotherapy

EVIDENCE

INFORMATION FOR PATIENTS

- American Lung Association
  - http://www.lungusa.org/site/apps/s/content.asp?c=dvLUK9O0E&b=34706&ct=67356
- National Institutes of Health
  - http://www.nlm.nih.gov/medlineplus/ency/article/000144.htm

REFERENCES

- Barker AF: Bronchiectasis. N Engl J Med 2002;346:1383. [PMID:11986413]
- Silverman E et al: Current management of bronchiestasis: review and 3 case studies. Heart Lung 2003;32:59. [PMID: 12571549]

Author(s)

Mark S. Chesnutt, MD
Thomas J. Prendergast, MD

Bronchiolitis Obliterans & Organizing Pneumonia

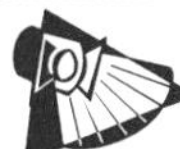

KEY FEATURES

ESSENTIALS OF DIAGNOSIS

- Dry cough, dyspnea, and a flu-like illness of abrupt onset, but lasting from days to several months
- Patchy, bilateral ground glass or alveolar infiltrates on chest x-ray
- Pulmonary function tests (PFTs) demonstrate restrictive pattern and hypoxemia
- Lung biopsy may be necessary to confirm diagnosis

GENERAL CONSIDERATIONS

- Diagnosis is difficult on clinical grounds alone

DEMOGRAPHICS

- Affects men and women equally
- Most patients between ages 50 and 70

CLINICAL FINDINGS

SYMPTOMS AND SIGNS

- Abrupt onset, frequently weeks to a few months after a flu-like illness
- Dyspnea and dry cough are common
- Constitutional symptoms such as fatigue, fever, and weight loss are common
- Crackles are heard in most patients
- Wheezing in approximately one-third of patients
- Clubbing is uncommon

DIFFERENTIAL DIAGNOSIS

- Idiopathic interstitial pneumonias
- Idiopathic pulmonary fibrosis
- Interstitial lung disease due to infection (eg, fungal, tuberculosis, *Pneumocystis jiroveci* pneumonia, viral)
- Drug-induced fibrosis, eg, amiodarone, bleomycin
- Sarcoidosis
- Pneumoconiosis
- Hypersensitivity pneumonitis
- Asbestosis

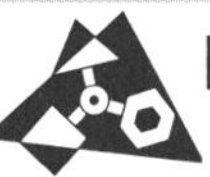

DIAGNOSIS

LABORATORY TESTS

- PFTs typically show a restrictive pattern with hypoxemia, but obstruction is seen in 25%
- High-resolution CT scan shows subpleural consolidation and bronchial wall thickening and dilation

IMAGING STUDIES

- Chest x-ray typically shows bilateral ground-glass or alveolar infiltrates
- Solitary pneumonia-like infiltrates or a diffuse interstitial pattern may be seen

DIAGNOSTIC PROCEDURES

- Lung biopsy shows buds of loose connective tissue and inflammatory cells filling alveoli and distal bronchioles

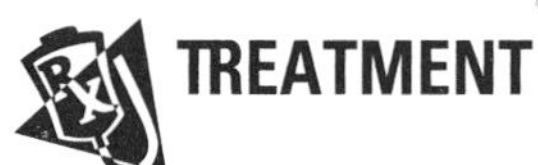

TREATMENT

MEDICATIONS

- Prednisone, 1 mg/kg/day for 2–3 months, tapered slowly to 20–40 mg/day and usually continued for at least 6 months

OUTCOME

FOLLOW-UP

- Monitor serial chest x-rays and PFTs

COMPLICATIONS

- Irreversible scarring or fibrosis of the lung
- Respiratory failure
- Complications of chronic steroid use

PROGNOSIS

- Two-thirds of patients respond rapidly to corticosteroids
- Long-term prognosis is generally good for steroid-responsive patients
- Relapses are common

WHEN TO REFER

- The majority of patients with suspected or confirmed disease should be seen by a pulmonologist

WHEN TO ADMIT

- Respiratory failure
- Signs of acute infection

PREVENTION

- Measures to prevent steroid-induced bone mineral loss

EVIDENCE

REFERENCES

- Cordier JF: Cryptogenic organizing pneumonia. Clin Chest Med 2004;25:727. [PMID:15564018]
- Epler GR: Bronchiolitis obliterans organizing pneumonia. Arch Intern Med 2001;161:158. [PMID:11176728]
- Ryu JH et al: Bronchiolar disorders. Am J Respir Crit Care Med 2003;168:1277. [PMID:14644923]
- Wright JL: Diseases of the small airways. Lung 2001;179:375. [PMID:12040427]

Author(s)

Mark S. Chesnutt, MD

Thomas J. Prendergast, MD

Bronchogenic Carcinoma

KEY FEATURES

ESSENTIALS OF DIAGNOSIS

- New cough or change in chronic cough
- Dyspnea, hemoptysis, anorexia
- New or enlarging mass; persistent infiltrate, atelectasis, or pleural effusion on chest radiograph or CT scan
- Cytologic or histologic findings of lung cancer in sputum, pleural fluid, or biopsy specimen

GENERAL CONSIDERATIONS

- Leading cause of cancer deaths
- 90% of lung cancer in men and 79% in women are attributable to smoking
- **Small cell lung cancer** (SCLC)
  - Prone to early hematogenous spread
  - Is rarely amenable to resection
  - Has a very aggressive course
- **Non–small cell lung cancer** (NSCLC)
  - Spreads more slowly
  - Early disease may be cured with resection
- Histologic types
  - **Squamous cell carcinoma** (25–35%) arises from bronchial epithelium; it is usually centrally located and intraluminal
  - **Adenocarcinoma** (35–40%) arises from mucous glands as a peripheral nodule or mass
  - **Small cell carcinoma** (15–20%) is of bronchial origin, begins centrally, and infiltrates submucosally
  - **Large cell carcinoma** (5–10%) is a heterogeneous group and presents as a central or peripheral mass
  - **Bronchioloalveolar cell carcinoma** (2%) arises from epithelial cells distal to the terminal bronchiole and spreads intraalveolarly

DEMOGRAPHICS

- Mean age at diagnosis is 60 years
- Environmental risk factors include tobacco smoke, radon gas, asbestos, metals, and industrial carcinogens
- A familial predisposition is recognized
- Chronic obstructive pulmonary disease, pulmonary fibrosis, and sarcoidosis are associated with an increased risk of lung cancer

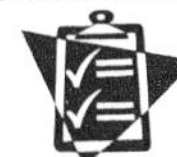

CLINICAL FINDINGS

SYMPTOMS AND SIGNS

- 75–90% are symptomatic at diagnosis
- The presentation depends on
  - Type and location of tumor
  - Extent of spread
  - Presence of paraneoplastic syndromes
- Anorexia, weight loss, and asthenia in 55–90%
- New or changed cough in up to 60%
- Hemoptysis in 5–30%
- Pain, often from bony metastases, in 25–40%
- Local spread may result in endobronchial obstruction and postobstructive pneumonia, effusions, or a change in voice due to recurrent laryngeal nerve involvement
- Superior vena cava (SVC) syndrome and Horner's syndrome
- Liver metastases are associated with asthenia and weight loss
- Possible presentation of brain metastases
  - Headache
  - Nausea and vomiting
  - Seizures
  - Altered mental status
- **Paraneoplastic syndromes** (Table 156) are not necessarily indicative of metastasis
  - Syndrome of inappropriate antidiuretic hormone secretion occurs in 15% of SCLC patients
  - Hypercalcemia occurs in 10% of SCLC patients

DIFFERENTIAL DIAGNOSIS

- Pneumonia
- Tuberculosis
- Metastatic cancer to lung
- Benign pulmonary nodule or nodules
- Lymphoma
- *Mycobacterium avium* complex
- Sarcoidosis
- Fungal pneumonia
- Bronchial carcinoid tumor
- Foreign body aspiration (retained)

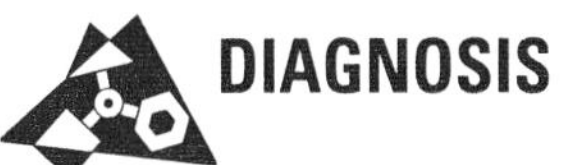

DIAGNOSIS

LABORATORY TESTS

- See Tables 25 and 26
- Tissue or cytology specimen is needed for diagnosis
- Sputum cytology is highly specific, but insensitive; yield is best with lesions in central airways
- Serum tumor markers are neither sensitive nor specific
- Complete blood cell count, renal panel, calcium, liver function tests, and lactate dehydrogenase are a routine part of staging
- Pulmonary function tests are required in all NSLC patients prior to surgery
  - Preop FEV_1 >2 L is adequate to undergo surgery
  - Estimate of postresection FEV_1 is needed if < 2 L preresection
  - Postresection FEV_1 >800 mL or >40% predicted is associated with a low incidence of perioperative complications

IMAGING STUDIES

- Nearly all patients have abnormal findings on chest x-ray or CT
  - Hilar adenopathy and mediastinal thickening (squamous cell)
  - Infiltrates, single or multiple nodules (bronchioloalveolar cell)
  - Central or peripheral masses (large cell)
  - Hilar and mediastinal abnormalities (small cell)
- Chest CT is the most important modality in staging to determine resectability
- For staging, brain MRI, abdominal CT, or radionuclide bone scanning should be targeted to symptoms or signs
- PET imaging can help confirm no metastates in NSCLC patients who are candidates for surgical resection

DIAGNOSTIC PROCEDURES

- Thoracentesis can be diagnostic in the setting of malignant effusions (50–65%)
- If pleural fluid cytology is nondiagnostic after two thoracenteses, thoracoscopy is preferred to blind pleural biopsy
- Fine-needle aspiration of palpable supraclavicular or cervical lymph nodes is frequently diagnostic
- Tissue diagnostic yield from bronchoscopy is 10–90%
- Transthoracic needle biopsy has a sensitivity of 50–90%

- Mediastinoscopy, VATS, or thoracotomy is necessary where less invasive techniques are not diagnostic

Staging

- See Table 25
- NSCLC is staged with the TNM international staging system:
  - Stages I and II disease may be cured surgically
  - Stage IIIA disease may benefit from surgery
  - Stage IIIB and IV disease does not benefit from surgery

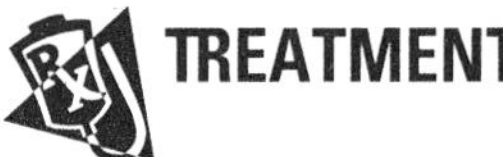

TREATMENT

MEDICATIONS

- See Table 154

Neoadjuvant chemotherapy in NSCLC

- Administration in advance of surgery or radiation therapy
- There is no consensus on the survival impact in stages I and II disease but it is widely used in stage IIIA and IIIB disease

Adjuvant chemotherapy in NSCLC

- Administration of drugs after surgery or radiation therapy
- Multidrug platinum-based therapy shows a trend toward improved survival in stage I and N0 stage II disease (on the order of 3 months at 5 years)
- Data are conflicting for stage IIIA or node-positive stage II disease
- Stage IIIA and IIIB disease, which cannot be treated surgically, has improved survival when treated with combination chemo- and radiation therapy
- Performance status and symptom control in stage IIIB and stage IV disease may be improved by chemotherapy

Chemotherapy in SCLC

- 80–100% response to cisplatin/etoposide in limited stage disease (50–70% complete response)
- 60–80% response to cisplatin/etoposide in extensive disease (15–40% complete response)
- Remissions last a median of 6–8 months
- Median survival is 3–4 months after recurrence

SURGERY

- Resection of solitary brain metastases
  - Does not improve survival
  - May improve quality of life in combination with radiation therapy

NSCLC

- Stages I and II are treated with surgical resection where possible
- Stage IIIA disease should be treated with multimodal protocols
- Selected stage IIIB patients who undergo resection after multimodal therapy have shown long-term survival
- Stage IV patients are treated palliatively

THERAPEUTIC PROCEDURES

- Radiation therapy is used as part of multimodal regimens in NSCLC
- Intraluminal radiation is an alternative palliative approach to intraluminal disease
- Palliative care
  - Pain control at the end of life is essential
  - External-beam radiation therapy is useful to control
    - Dyspnea
    - Hemoptysis
    - Pain from bony metastases
    - Obstruction from SVC syndrome
    - Solitary brain metastases

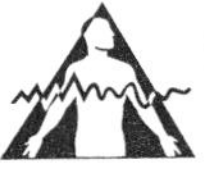

OUTCOME

FOLLOW-UP

- Depends on type and stage of cancer as well as the patient's functional status and comorbid conditions

COMPLICATIONS

- SVC syndrome
- Paraneoplastic syndromes
- Venous thrombosis
- Postobstructive pneumonia

PROGNOSIS

- See Table 27
- The overall 5-year survival rate is 15%
- Squamous cell carcinoma may have a better prognosis than adenocarcinoma or large cell carcinoma

WHEN TO REFER

- All patients deserve an evaluation by a multidisciplinary lung cancer evaluation and treatment program
- A palliative care specialist should be involved in advanced disease care

WHEN TO ADMIT

- Respiratory distress, altered mental status, pain control

PREVENTION

- Smoking cessation
- Screening in high-risk, asymptomatic patients has no proven benefit

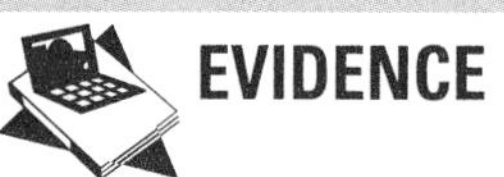

EVIDENCE

PRACTICE GUIDELINES

- Back PB: Screening for lung cancer: The guidelines. Chest 2003;123:83S
- Rivera MP et al: Diagnosis of lung cancer: the guidelines. Chest 2003;123(1 Suppl):129S.

INFORMATION FOR PATIENTS

- American Lung Association
  - http://www.lungusa.org/site/apps/s/content.asp?c=dvLUK9O0E&b=34706&ct=67325
- JAMA patient page: Lung cancer. JAMA 2003;289:380. [PMID: 12532974]
- Mayo Clinic
  - http://www.mayoclinic.com/invoke.cfm?ed=DS00038

REFERENCES

- American College of Chest Physicians; Health and Science Policy Committee: Diagnosis and management of lung cancer: ACCP evidence-based guidelines. Chest 2003;123(1 Suppl): 1S. [PMID: 12527560]
- Barnes DJ. The changing face of lung cancer. Chest 2004;126:1718. [PMID: 15596660]
- Bilello KS et al: Epidemiology, etiology, and prevention of lung cancer. Clin Chest Med 2002;23:1. [PMID: 11901905]
- Gerber RB et al: Paraneoplastic syndromes associated with bronchogenic carcinoma. Clin Chest Med 2002;23:257. [PMID: 11901915]
- Lardinois D et al: Staging of non-small cell lung cancer with integrated positron-emission tomography and computed tomography. N Engl J Med 2003;348:2500. [PMID: 12815135]
- Macbeth F et al: Palliative treatment for advanced non-small cell lung cancer. Hematol Onc Clin North Am 2004;18:115. [PMID: 15005285]
- Patel JD. Bach PB. Kris MG. Lung cancer in US women: a contemporary epidemic. JAMA 2004;291:1763. [PMID: 15082704]
- Spira A et al: Multidisciplinary management of lung cancer. N Engl J Med 2004;350:379. [PMID: 14736930]

Author(s)

Mark S. Chesnutt, MD

Thomas J. Prendergast, MD

Brucellosis

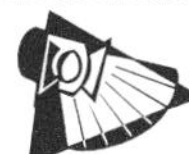

KEY FEATURES

ESSENTIALS OF DIAGNOSIS

- History of animal exposure, ingestion of unpasteurized milk or cheese
- Insidious onset: easy fatigability, headache, arthralgia, anorexia, sweating, irritability
- Intermittent fever, especially at night, which may become chronic and undulant
- Cervical and axillary lymphadenopathy; hepatosplenomegaly
- Lymphocytosis, positive blood culture, elevated agglutination titer

GENERAL CONSIDERATIONS

- The infection is transmitted from animals to humans. *Brucella abortus* (cattle), *Brucella suis* (hogs), and *Brucella melitensis* (goats) are the main agents
- Transmission to humans occurs by
  - Contact with infected meat (slaughterhouse workers)
  - Placentas of infected animals (farmers, veterinarians)
  - Ingestion of infected unpasteurized milk or cheese
- The incubation period varies from a few days to several weeks
- The disorder may become chronic

DEMOGRAPHICS

- In the United States, brucellosis is very rare except in the midwestern states (*B suis*) and in visitors or immigrants from countries where brucellosis is endemic (eg, Mexico, Spain, South American countries)

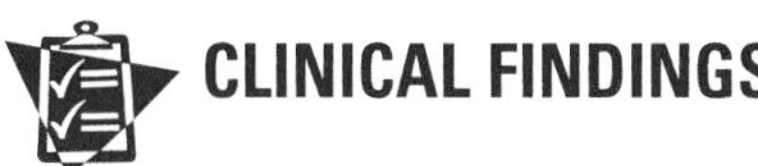

CLINICAL FINDINGS

SYMPTOMS AND SIGNS

- Insidious onset of weakness, weight loss, low-grade fevers, sweats, and exhaustion with minimal activity
- Headache, abdominal or back pains with anorexia and constipation, and arthralgia
- Epididymitis occurs in 10% of cases in men
- 50% of cases have peripheral lymph node enlargement and splenomegaly; hepatomegaly is less common
- The **chronic form** may assume an undulant nature, with periods of normal temperature between acute attacks; symptoms may persist for years, either continuously or intermittently

DIFFERENTIAL DIAGNOSIS

- Lymphoma
- Tuberculosis
- Infective endocarditis
- Q fever
- Typhoid fever
- Tularemia
- Malaria
- Infectious mononucleosis
- Influenza
- HIV infection
- Disseminated fungal infection, eg, histoplasmosis, coccidioidomycosis

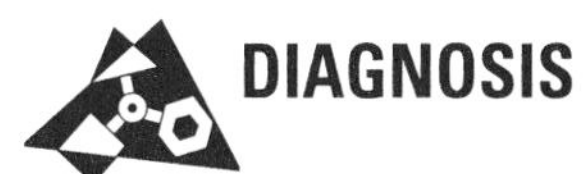

DIAGNOSIS

LABORATORY TESTS

- Early in the course of infection, the organism can be recovered from the blood, cerebrospinal fluid, urine, and bone marrow
- Most modern culture systems can detect growth of the organism in blood by 7 days; cultures are more likely to be negative in chronic cases
- The diagnosis often is made by serological testing
- Rising serological titers or an absolute agglutination titer of greater than 1:100 supports the diagnosis

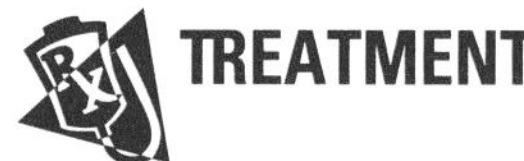

TREATMENT

MEDICATIONS

- Combination regimens of two or three drugs are more effective
- Either doxycycline plus rifampin or streptomycin (or both) *or* trimethoprim-sulfamethoxazole plus rifampin or streptomycin (or both) is effective in doses as follows for 21 days
  - Doxycycline, 100–200 mg/day in divided doses
  - Trimethoprim, 320 mg/day, plus sulfamethoxazole, 1600 mg/day in divided doses
  - Rifampin, 600–1200 mg/day
  - Streptomycin, 500 mg intramuscularly twice a day
- Longer courses of therapy (eg, several months) may be required to cure relapses, osteomyelitis, or meningitis

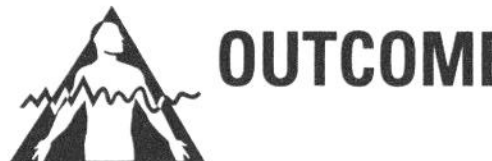

OUTCOME

COMPLICATIONS

Most frequent

- Bone and joint lesions such as spondylitis and suppurative arthritis (usually of a single joint)
- Endocarditis
- Meningoencephalitis

Less common

- Pneumonitis with pleural effusion
- Hepatitis
- Cholecystitis

WHEN TO REFER

- Refer to an infectious disease specialist to confirm the diagnosis or for management of proven cases

WHEN TO ADMIT

- Suspected or known complications such as endocarditis or meningoencephalitis

EVIDENCE

WEB SITES

- CDC—Division of Bacterial and Mycotic Diseases
  - http://www.cdc.gov/ncidod/dbmd/
- CDC—Emerging Infectious Diseases
  - http://www.cdc.gov/ncidod/EID/vol3no2/corbel.htm
- Karolinska Institute—Directory of bacterial infections and mycoses
  - http://www.mic.ki.se/Diseases/C01.html

INFORMATION FOR PATIENTS

- Centers for Disease Control
  - http://www.cdc.gov/ncidod/dbmd/diseaseinfo/brucellosis_g.htm
- National Institutes of Health
  - http://www.nlm.nih.gov/medlineplus/ency/article/000597.htm

REFERENCE

- Yagupsky P: Detection of brucellae in blood cultures. J Clin Microbiol 1999;37:3437. [PMID: 10523530]

Author(s)

Henry F. Chambers, MD

Bullous Pemphigoid

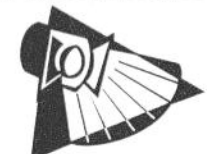

KEY FEATURES

ESSENTIALS OF DIAGNOSIS

- Large, tense blisters that rupture, leaving denuded areas that heal without scarring
- Caused by autoantibodies to two specific components of the hemidesmosome

GENERAL CONSIDERATIONS

- Relatively benign pruritic disease characterized by tense blisters in flexural areas, usually remitting in 5 or 6 years, with a course characterized by exacerbations and remissions
- Oral lesions are present in about one-third of affected persons
- The disease may occur in various forms, including localized and urticarial
- There is no statistical association with internal malignant disease

DEMOGRAPHICS

- Most patients are over the age of 60 (often in their 70s and 80s)
- Men are affected twice as frequently as women

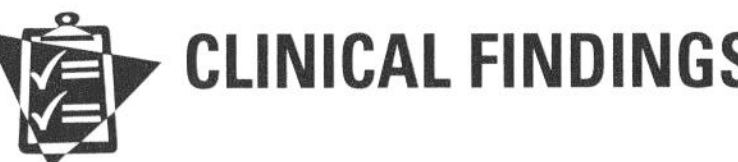

CLINICAL FINDINGS

SYMPTOMS AND SIGNS

- See Table 7
- Characterized by tense blisters in flexural areas
- Predilection for groin, axillae, flexor forearms, thighs and shins, though may occur anywhere; some have oral involvement
- Appearance of blisters may be preceded by urticarial or edematous lesions for months
- May occur in various forms, including localized, vesicular, vegatating, erythematous, erythrodermic, and nodular
- Course characterized by exacerbations and remissions

DIFFERENTIAL DIAGNOSIS

- Pemphigus
- Drug eruptions
- Erythema multiforme major or toxic epidermal necrolysis
- Bullous impetigo
- Contact dermatitis
- Dermatitis herpetiformis
- Cicatricial pemphigoid
- Paraneoplastic pemphigus
- Linear IgA dermatosis
- Pemphigus foliaceus
- Porphyria cutanea tarda
- Epidermolysis bullosa
- Staphylococcal scalded skin syndrome
- Herpes gestationis
- Graft-versus-host disease

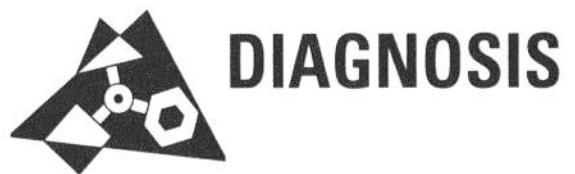

DIAGNOSIS

LABORATORY TESTS

- Circulating anti-basement membrane antibodies can be found in the sera of patients in about 70% of cases

DIAGNOSTIC PROCEDURES

- The diagnosis is made by biopsy and direct immunofluorescence examination
- Light microscopy shows a subepidermal blister
- With direct immunofluorescence, IgG and C3 are found at the dermal–epidermal junction

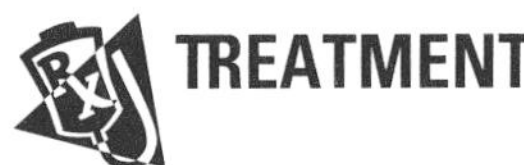

TREATMENT

MEDICATIONS

- If the patient has only a few blisters, ultrapotent topical corticosteroids may be adequate (Table 6)
- Prednisone at dosages of 60–80 mg/day is often used to achieve rapid control of more widespread disease
- Although slower in onset of action, tetracycline or erythromycin, 1–1.5 g/day, alone or combined with nicotinamide—not nicotinic acid or niacin!—(up to 1.5 g/day), if tolerated, may control the disease in patients who cannot use corticosteroids or may allow decreasing or eliminating corticosteroids after control is achieved
- Dapsone is particularly effective in mucous membrane pemphigoid
- If these drugs are not effective, methotrexate, 5–25 mg weekly, or azathioprine, 50 mg one to three times daily, may be used as steroid-sparing agents
- Mycophenolate mofetil (1 g twice daily) or IV immunoglobulin as used for pemphigus vulgaris may be used in refractory cases

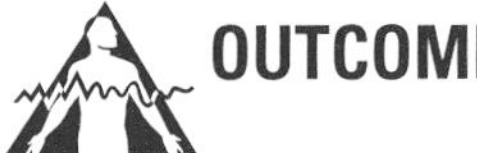

OUTCOME

PROGNOSIS

- Usually remitting in 5–6 years

WHEN TO REFER

- If there is a question about the diagnosis, if recommended therapy is ineffective, or specialized treatment is necessary

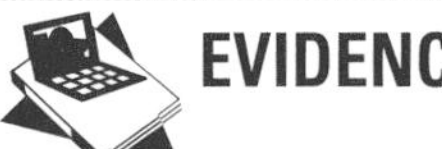

EVIDENCE

PRACTICE GUIDELINES

- British Association of Dermatologists. Wojnarowska F et al: Guidelines for the management of bullous pemphigoid. Br J Dermatol 2002;147:214. [PMID: 12174090]

WEB SITE

- American Academy of Dermatology
  - http://www.aad.org

INFORMATION FOR PATIENTS

- American Osteopathic College of Dermatology: Bullous Pemphigoid
  - http://www.aocd.org/skin/dermatologic_diseases/bullous_pemphigoid.html
- MedlinePlus: Bullous Pemphigoid
  - http://www.nlm.nih.gov/medlineplus/ency/article/000883.htm
- International Pemphigus Foundation: About Pemphigoid
  - http://www.pemphigus.org/typesofgoid.html

REFERENCES

- Ahmed AR: Intravenous immunoglobulin therapy for patients with bullous pemphigoid unresponsive to conventional immunosuppressive treatment. J Am Acad Dermatol 2001;45:825. [PMID: 11756944]
- Heilborn JD et al: Low-dose oral pulse methotrexate as monotherapy in elderly patients with bullous pemphigoid. J Am Acad Dermatol 1999;40(5 Part 1):741. [PMID: 10321603]
- Nousari HC et al: Pemphigus and bullous pemphigoid. Lancet 1999;354:667. [PMID: 10466686]

Author(s)

Timothy G. Berger, MD

Burns

KEY FEATURES

ESSENTIALS OF DIAGNOSIS

- Assess body surface area affected by burns
- Evaluate depth of burn to categorize as first- or second-degree burn
- Consider patient age and associated illness or injury

GENERAL CONSIDERATIONS

- Only second- and third-degree burns are included in calculating the total burn surface area (TBSA)
- Distinguishing between second- and third-degree burns is not necessary because both are generally treated as full-thickness (third-degree) burns with early excision and grafting

DEMOGRAHICS

- About 1.25 million burn injuries occur yearly in the United States
- About 51,000 victims of acute burns are hospitalized each year in the United States

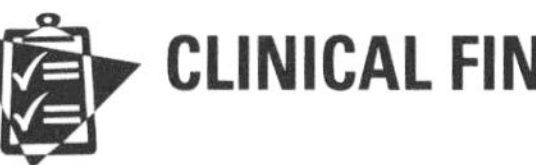

CLINICAL FINDINGS

SYMPTOMS AND SIGNS

- First-degree burns do not blister initially
- Second-degree burns blister. Hairs are absent or easily extracted, sweat glands become less visible, and the skin appears smoother

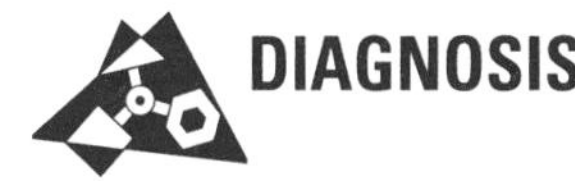

DIAGNOSIS

IMAGING STUDIES

- Chest radiographs, usually normal initially, may show acute respiratory distress syndrome in 24–48 h with severe inhalation injury

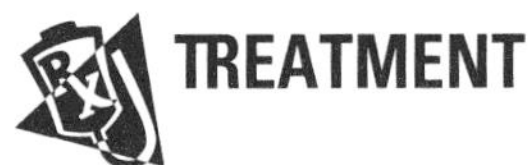

TREATMENT

MEDICATIONS

- **Crystalloids:** fluid resuscitation may be instituted simultaneously with initial resuscitation
  - Parkland formula for fluid requirement in first 24 h: lactated Ringer's injection (4 mL/kg body weight per percent TBSA)
  - Deep electrical burns and inhalation injury increase fluid requirement
  - Adequacy of resuscitation determined clinically: urine output and specific gravity, blood pressure, central venous catheter, or Swan-Ganz catheter readings
  - Half of calculated fluid given in first 8-h period (measured from hour of injury); remaining fluid, split in half, delivered over next 16 h
  - Very large volume of fluid may be needed
- **β-Blockade:** routine β-blockade (propranolol, adjusting dose to decrease resting heart rate by 20%, for up to 4 weeks) may reverse some of catecholamine-mediated hypermetabolic response after severe burns
- **Colloids:** avoid in routine burn resuscitation because of risk of glomerular filtration decline and association with pulmonary edema

SURGERY

- Because full-thickness circumferential burn may develop ischemia under constricting eschar, escharotomy incisions through anesthetic eschar can save life/limb
- Early excision/grafting of burned areas critical, as soon as 24 h after injury or when patient will hemodynamically tolerate procedure
- Wounds that do not heal in 7–10 days (ie, third-degree burns) best treated by excision and autograft

THERAPEUTIC PROCEDURES

- Establish airway; evaluate cervical spine, head injuries; stabilize fractures
- Supplemental oxygen
- Intubate if inhalation injury suspected
- **Vascular access:** remove clothing and establish venous access, preferably with percutaneous large-bore (14- or 16-gauge) IV line through nonburned skin (eg, femoral lines) (hypovolemic shock may develop with major burns)
  - Avoid emergent subclavian lines in volume-depleted patient because of pneumothorax and subclavian vein laceration risk
  - *All lines should be changed within 24 h because of high risk of nonsterile placement*
- Protect wound with topical antibiotic (eg, silver sulfadiazine)
- Clean burned areas thoroughly daily

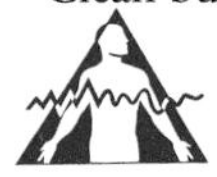

OUTCOME

FOLLOW-UP

- A Foley catheter is essential for monitoring urinary output
- Monitor inhalation injuries with serial blood gas determination and bronchoscopy

COMPLICATIONS

- Consider comorbid conditions
- Suspect smoke inhalation injury when nasal hairs are singed, mechanism of burn involves closed spaces, sputum is carbonaceous, or carboxyhemoglobin level > 5% in nonsmokers
- Electrical injury that causes burns may also produce cardiac arrhythmias, which require immediate attention and muscle necrosis. Test for elevated creatine kinase levels when rhabdomyolysis suspected
- Pancreatitis occurs in severe burns along with multiorgan failure
- Nearly all burn patients have one or more septicemic episodes during hospital course; gram positives initially, *Pseudomonas* later

PROGNOSIS

- The Baux Score (age + percent burn) predicts mortality after major burn
- Female sex, concomitant nonburn injury, electrical cause of burn, and pediatric age presage poorer outcome
- Physical therapy and psychosocial support are essential

WHEN TO REFER

- Burn units offer the extensive support needed for patients with burns

PREVENTION

- Prophylactic antibiotics in burn patients are increasingly being used
- Maintain normal core body temperature with burns > 20% of TBSA; keep room temperature at 30°C
- If tube feedings are not tolerated, begin total parenteral nutrition (TPN) because of markedly increased metabolic rate
- As much as 4000–6000 kcal/day TPN may be required in postburn period. Start enteric feedings as soon as patient tolerates

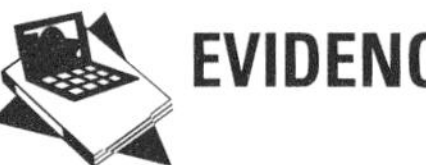

EVIDENCE

PRACTICE GUIDELINES

- American Burn Association: Inhalation injury: diagnosis. J Am Coll Surg 2003;196:307. [PMID: 12632576]

INFORMATION FOR PATIENTS

- American Academy of Family Physicians: Taking Care of Burns
  - http://familydoctor.org/638.xml
- MedlinePlus: Burns interactive tutorial
  - http://www.nlm.nih.gov/medlineplus/tutorials/burns/htm/index.htm
- Shriners Hospital: Burn Prevention Tips
  - http://www.shrinershq.org/prevention/burntips/index.html
- Mayo Clinic: Burns
  - http://www.mayoclinic.com/invoke.cfm?id=FA00022

REFERENCES

- Atiyeh BS et al: State of the art in burn treatment. World J Surg 2005;29:131. [PMID: 15654666]
- Herndon DN et al: Support of the metabolic response to burn injury. Lancet 2004;363:1895. [PMID: 15183630]

Author(s)

Brent R. W. Moelleken, MD, FACS

Cancer, Overview

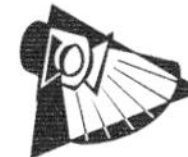

KEY FEATURES

ESSENTIALS OF DIAGNOSIS

- In the United States, second most common cause of death after cardiovascular disease
- In 2004, ~1.4 million new cases of invasive cancer and > 560,000 cancer deaths
- One of every 2 men and 1 of every 3 women will develop invasive cancer in their lifetime

GENERAL CONSIDERATIONS

- Cause of most cancers unknown
- DNA mutations in protooncogenes or deletion of tumor suppressor genes (eg, *P53*), or both, cause abnormal cellular proliferation
- Overexpression of *Bcl-2* in breast, colon, prostate, head and neck, and ovarian cancer is one mechanism of resistance to chemotherapy and radiation therapy
- Certain chromosomal abnormalities are associated with specific malignancies and can be used to assess prognosis and determine treatment
- Autoimmune suppression may contribute to development of cancer
- Hereditary predisposition to some cancers, linked to gene mutations, is a relatively rare cause of cancer
- Somatic genetic mutations can be caused by environmental exposure, genetic susceptibility to environmental toxins, infectious agents, physical agents, and drugs, including chemotherapeutic agents such as alkylating agents and topoisomerase II inhibitors

DEMOGRAPHICS

- U.S. incidence and mortality data for common cancers: Table 151
- Lifetime risk of diagnosis or death for 5 leading cancers in the United States: Table 152
- Median age at diagnosis of cancer is 68
- Risk factors for cancer: tobacco use, diet, alcohol consumption, obesity, parity, length of lactation, and certain occupations

CLINICAL FINDINGS

SYMPTOMS AND SIGNS

- Anorexia
- Malaise
- Weight loss
- Fever
- Local effects of tumor growth
- Paraneoplastic syndromes (Table 156)

DIFFERENTIAL DIAGNOSIS

- Depression
- Thyroid disease
- Metabolic disorders (renal, liver disease)
- Chronic infection
- Rheumatologic disease

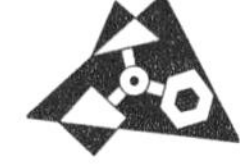

DIAGNOSIS

LABORATORY TESTS

- Tumor markers primarily used for assessing response to therapy in advanced disease
- Tumor markers should only be used for screening in special circumstances

IMAGING STUDIES

- Plain x-rays occasionally helpful
- CT, MRI
- PET or PET/CT scan may be more sensitive for certain cancers
- Bone scan to assess for skeletal metastases

DIAGNOSTIC PROCEDURES

- Surgical staging for early-stage disease
- Sentinel lymph node biopsy reduces complications of axillary node dissection in breast cancer
- **Staging**
  - TNM system: used to indicate the extension of cancer before definitive therapy begins: extent of untreated primary tumor (T); regional lymph node involvement (N); distant metastases (M)
  - Staging of certain tumors (lymphomas, Hodgkin's disease) differs to reflect their natural history and to better direct treatment decisions
  - Pathological characteristics of certain tumors add prognostic information (eg, estrogen receptors, tumor grade)
  - Overexpression or underproduction of oncogene products (Her-2/*neu* in breast cancer), infection of cancer cells with specific viral genomes (HPV subtypes in cervical cancer), and certain chromosomal translocations or deletions (alteration of the retinoic acid receptor gene in acute promyelocytic leukemia) have prognostic significance and may direct therapy

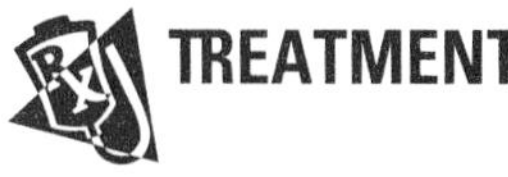

TREATMENT

MEDICATIONS

- Systemic chemotherapy
  - As curative therapy for certain malignancies
  - Preoperatively as "neoadjuvant" therapy to reduce size and extent of primary tumor, allowing complete excision at surgery
  - As adjuvant therapy to decrease rate of relapse, improve disease-free interval, and improve cure rate
  - As palliative therapy for symptoms and to prolong survival in some patients with incurable malignancies
  - As intensive therapy in combination with bone marrow transplant to improve cure rate in certain cancers, with targeted biological therapy to enhance response
- Regional administration of active chemotherapeutic agents into tumor site can result in palliation and prolonged survival
- Types of cancer responsive to chemotherapy and current treatments of choice: Table 153
- Dosage schedules and toxicities of common chemotherapeutic agents: Table 154
- Hormonal therapy (or ablation) used in treatment and palliation of breast, prostate, endometrial cancers
- Bisphosphonates used to reduce bone pain and fractures in bone metastases
- Other supportive care medications include white and red cell growth factors, pain medications

SURGERY

- Resection is treatment of choice for GI, genitourinary, CNS, breast, thyroid, and skin cancers and sarcomas
- Cryosurgical ablation being evaluated for localized breast and prostate cancer
- Resection of isolated metastases and limited recurrences may result in long-term disease-free survival

THERAPEUTIC PROCEDURES

- Radiation therapy used primarily or in combination with surgery and/or chemotherapy for cancers of the larynx, oral cavity, pharynx, esophagus, breast, lung, colorectum, uterine cervix, vagina, prostate, skin, brain, and spinal cord and Hodgkin's and non-Hodgkin's lymphomas

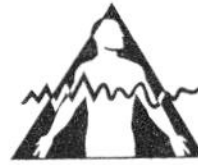

OUTCOME

FOLLOW-UP

- Monitor for toxicities and need for supportive care (Table 155)
- Evaluate tumor response by examination, radiographic imaging, and tumor markers
  - Partial: ≥ 50% reduction in sum of diameters of original tumor masses
  - Complete: disappearance of detectable tumor
  - Progression: increase in tumor size by ≥ 20% or any new lesions

COMPLICATIONS

- **Cancer**
  - Spinal cord compression
  - Hypercalcemia
  - Hyperuricemia and acute urate nephropathy
  - Malignant carcinoid syndrome
  - Malignant effusions
  - Infection
  - Mucositis/esophagitis
  - GI symptoms
  - Pain
  - Anorexia/weight loss
  - Paraneoplastic syndromes (Table 156)
- **Therapy**
  - Toxicities of commonly chemotherapeutic agents: Table 154
  - Acute radiation toxicity: fatigue, malaise, anorexia, nausea, vomiting, local skin changes, diarrhea, mucosal ulceration of irradiated area, bone marrow suppression, pneumonitis, congestive heart failure, gastroenteritis
  - Long-term radiation toxicity: increased cardiac mortality with chest radiation, secondary leukemias and solid tumors, decreased function of the radiated organ, myelopathy, osteonecrosis, and hyperpigmentation and basal cell carcinoma of involved skin

PROGNOSIS

- Functional status at diagnosis (or start of treatment) is major prognostic factor and determinant of outcome with or without tumor-directed therapy
- Depends on stage and tumor biology

WHEN TO REFER

- Patients with strong family histories need referral for genetic screening, counseling

WHEN TO ADMIT

- Oncological emergencies
- Fever and neutropenia after chemotherapy
- Intractable pain

PREVENTION

Primary

- Smoking cessation
- Diets rich in vegetables and fruit and low in saturated fats
- Reduced exposure to UV light; regular use of sunscreen
- Aspirin and NSAIDs for colon cancer, polyps
- Vitamin E for prostate cancer
- Calcium for colon polyps and selenium for prostate cancer
- Tamoxifen for breast cancer
- Oral contraceptives for ovarian cancer
- Bilateral prophylactic oophorectomy or mastectomy

Secondary

- Mammography
- Pap smear and human papillomavirus testing
- Fecal occult blood testing, sigmoidoscopy, and colonoscopy
- Prostate-specific antigen in combination with digital rectal examination controversial for prostate cancer screening
- Adjuvant chemo-, hormone, and/or radiation therapy to prevent recurrence

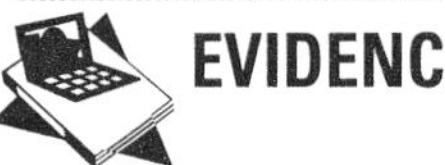

EVIDENCE

PRACTICE GUIDELINES

- National Comprehensive Cancer Network: Clinical Practice Guidelines in Oncology
  - http://www.nccn.org/professionals/physician_gls/f_guidelines.asp

WEB SITES

- National Cancer Institute: Statistics, Clinical Trials, Information for Professionals and Patients
  - http://www.cancer.gov/
- American Cancer Society: Cancer Reference Information
  - http://www.cancer.org/docroot/CRI/CRI_0.asp

INFORMATION FOR PATIENTS

- National Cancer Institute: Cancer: Questions and Answers
  - http://cis.nci.nih.gov/fact/6_7.htm
- National Cancer Institute: Cancer Information Sources
  - http://cis.nci.nih.gov/fact/2_1.htm

REFERENCES

- *AJCC Cancer Staging Manual/American Joint Committee on Cancer*, ed 6. Springer, 2002. (The bible of TNM staging)
- Chlebowski RT et al: Reducing the risk of breast cancer. N Engl J Med 2000;343:191. [PMID: 10900280]
- Janne PA et al: Chemoprevention of colorectal cancer. N Engl J Med 2000;342:1960. [PMID: 10874065]
- Lieberman DA et al: Use of colonoscopy to screen asymptomatic adults for colorectal cancer. Veterans Affairs Cooperative Study Group 380. N Engl J Med 2000;343:162. [PMID: 10900274]
- Mandel JS et al: The effect of fecal occult-blood screening on the incidence of colorectal cancer. N Engl J Med 2000;343:1603. [PMID: 11096167]
- Sawaya GF et al: Clinical practice. Current approaches to cervical cancer screening. N Engl J Med 2001;344:1603. [PMID: 11372013]
- Smith TJ et al: American Society of Clinical Oncology 1998 Update of Recommended Breast Cancer Surveillance Guidelines. J Clin Oncol 1999;17:1080. [PMID: 10071303]

Author(s)

Hope Rugo, MD

Candidiasis

KEY FEATURES

ESSENTIALS OF DIAGNOSIS

- Common normal flora and opportunistic pathogen
- Mucosal diseases are most common symptomatic infections and include vaginitis, oral thrush, and esophagitis
- Catheter-associated fungemia in hospitalized patients
- Diagnosis of invasive systemic disease requires biopsy or evidence of retinal disease

GENERAL CONSIDERATIONS

- Cutaneous and oral lesions
- Persistent oral or vaginal candidiasis should arouse suspicion of HIV infection
- Fungemia in immunocompromised patients on fluconazole prophylaxis is increasingly due to imidazole-resistant *Candida albicans* or non-*albicans* species

DEMOGRAPHICS

- Mucocutaneous disease occurs with cellular immunodeficiency
- Vulvovaginal candidiasis occurs with pregnancy, uncontrolled diabetes mellitus, broad-spectrum antibiotics, corticosteroids, HIV
- Invasive candidiasis occurs with prolonged neutropenia, recent surgery, broad-spectrum antibiotics, IV catheters (especially for total parenteral nutrition), IV drug use, and renal failure
- Candidal endocarditis occurs with repeated inoculation with injection drug use and direct inoculation during valvular heart surgery causing infection of prosthetic valves in first few months following surgery

CLINICAL FINDINGS

SYMPTOMS AND SIGNS

- Esophageal candidiasis
  - Substernal odynophagia, gastroesophageal reflux, or nausea without substernal pain
  - Oral candidiasis may not be present
- Vulvovaginal candidiasis
  - Acute vulvar pruritus
  - Burning vaginal discharge
  - Dyspareunia
- Disseminated candidiasis
  - Fluffy white retinal infiltrates (in < 50%)
  - Raised, erythematous skin lesions that may be painful (in < 50%)
  - Brain, meninges, and myocardial involvement
- Hepatosplenic candidiasis: fever and variable abdominal pain weeks after chemotherapy for hematological cancers, when neutrophil counts have recovered
- Candidal endocarditis
  - Splenomegaly
  - Petechiae
  - Large-vessel embolization

DIFFERENTIAL DIAGNOSIS

- Esophageal
  - Herpes simplex virus (HSV) esophagitis
  - Cytomegalovirus (CMV) esophagitis
  - Varicella-zoster virus esophagitis
  - Pill esophagitis, eg, nonsteroidal anti-inflammatory drugs, bisphosphonates, KCl
  - Gastroesophageal reflux disease
- Vulvovaginal
  - Bacterial vaginosis
  - *Trichomonas* vaginitis
  - Normal vaginal discharge
- Disseminated
  - Histoplasmosis
  - Coccidioidomycosis
  - Tuberculosis
  - Bacterial endocarditis
  - Aspergillosis

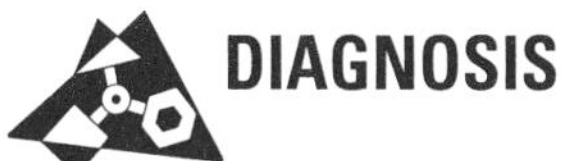

DIAGNOSIS

LABORATORY TESTS

- Disseminated candidiasis
  - Blood cultures are positive in only about 50% of cases
  - While candidemia can be benign, positive blood cultures are sufficient to initiate treatment for disseminated disease
  - Positive mucosal cultures (sputum, urine) may be clue to underlying disseminated candidiasis
  - However, isolated sputum or urine cultures generally represent colonization rather than true infection
  - No current antigens have acceptable sensitivity or specificity for distinguishing colonization from true infection
- Hepatosplenic candidiasis: blood cultures are generally negative, alkaline phosphatase elevated, definitive diagnosis established by tissue biopsy and culture
- Candidal endocarditis requires either positive culture from blood, emboli, or from vegetations found at time of valve replacement

IMAGING STUDIES

- Usually normal in disseminated disease
- For esophageal candidiasis, barium swallow does not allow clear distinction from HSV or CMV esophagitis
- Hepatosplenic candidiasis: abdominal CT scan shows hepatosplenomegaly with multiple low-density defects in the liver and spleen

DIAGNOSTIC PROCEDURES

- Esophageal candidiasis is best confirmed by endoscopy with biopsy and culture
- For mucosal disease KOH prep will demonstrate yeast and pseudohyphae
- Definitive proof of invasive disease requires sterile site histologic tests or culture or both
- Fundoscopic evaluation may be helpful in suspected fungemia

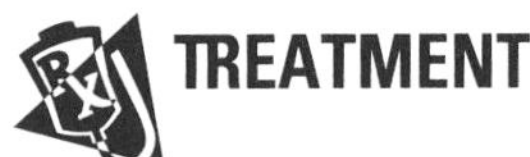

TREATMENT

MEDICATIONS

- Esophageal candidiasis
  - Fluconazole, 100–200 mg PO QD, or itraconazole solution, 100 mg PO QD for 10–14 days
  - Voriconazole 200 mg PO BID for refractory cases or cases that develop while on other azoles
  - Caspofungin acetate, 50 mg/day IV, has FDA approval for esophageal candidiasis with low toxicity
  - Amphotericin B, 0.3 mg/kg/IV for 10–14 days is reserved for patients who have not responded to other therapies
- Vulvovaginal candidiasis
  - Topical azoles, eg, clotrimazole 100 mg vaginally QD for 7 days, or miconazole 200 mg vaginally QD for 3 days
  - Fluconazole 150 mg PO once has equivalent efficacy with better patient acceptance
  - Weekly fluconazole therapy, 150 mg PO, helps prevent relapses in patients prone to multiple recurrences
- Candidal funguria
  - Benefit from treatment of asymptomatic candiduria has not been demonstrated
  - Frequently resolves without therapy following discontinuation of antibiotics or removal of bladder catheter
  - Fluconazole, 200 mg PO QD for 7–14 days, if symptoms persist
- Candidal fungemia
  - Fluconazole 400–800 mg IV QD with switch to PO therapy when stable; has equivalent efficacy to amphotericin B
  - Amphotericin B, 0.3–0.5 mg/kg/day IV, has excellent efficacy
  - Caspofungin acetate, 70 mg IV for first day then 50 mg/day IV, has equal efficacy to amphotericin B and likely better results versus fluconazole for azole resistant strains
  - Voriconazole, 6 mg/kg IV BID × 2 doses then 4 mg/kg IV BID, has increased in vitro activity versus many strains compared with fluconazole
  - Lipid formulations to amphotericin B reduce toxicity allowing for higher doses but are more costly

OUTCOME

COMPLICATIONS

- Candidal funguria: rare ureteral obstruction and dissemination
- Candidal fungemia: endophthalmitis; often no complications if fungemia resolves with removal of IV catheters
- Candidal endocarditis: valve destruction (usually aortic or mitral) is common

PROGNOSIS

- Esophageal candidiasis: relapse common in HIV infection

PREVENTION

- Fluconazole prophylaxis for high-risk patients undergoing induction chemotherapy
- Minimize unnecessary broad-spectrum antibiotics and IV catheters

EVIDENCE

PRACTICE GUIDELINES

- Infectious Diseases Society of America—Practice guidelines for the treatment of candidiasis.
  - http://www.journals.uchicago.edu/CID/journal/issues/v38n2/32301/32301.web.pdf

WEB SITE

- Project Inform
  - http://www.ProjectInform.org

INFORMATION FOR PATIENTS

- CDC Disease Information
  - http://www.cdc.gov/ncidod/dbmd/diseaseinfo/candidiasis_g.htm
- JAMA patient page: HIV infection: the basics. JAMA 2002;288:268. [PMID: 12123237]
- Mayo Clinic
  - http://www.mayoclinic.com/invoke.cfm?id=DS00408
- MedlinePlus
  - http://www.nlm.nih.gov/medlineplus/ency/article/000626.htm

REFERENCES

- Mora-Durate J et al: Comparison of caspofungin and amphotericin B for invasive candidiasis. N Engl J Med 2002;347:2020. [PMID: 12490683]
- Raad I et al: Management of central venous catheters in patients with cancer and candidemia. Clin Infect Dis 2004;38:1119. [PMID: 15095217]
- Sobel JD et al: Maintenance fluconazole therapy for recurrent vulvovaginal candidiasis. N Engl J Med 2004;351:876. [PMID: 15329425]

Author(s)

Samuel A. Shelburne, MD
Richard J. Hamill, MD

Candidiasis, Mucocutaneous

Candidiasis, Oral p. 1048. Carbon Monoxide Poisoning p. 1049. Carcinoid Syndrome, Malignant p. 1049.

KEY FEATURES

ESSENTIALS OF DIAGNOSIS

- Candidal intertrigo
- Oral candidiasis
- Angular cheilitis
- Perianal candidiasis
- Candidal paronychia
- Severe pruritus of vulva, anus, or body folds
- Superficial denuded, beefy-red areas with or without satellite vesicopustules
- Whitish curd-like concretions on the oral and vaginal mucous membranes
- Yeast on microscopic examination of scales or curd

GENERAL CONSIDERATIONS

- Superficial fungal infection that may involve almost any cutaneous or mucous surface of the body
- Particularly likely to occur in diabetics, during pregnancy, and in obese persons who perspire freely
- Antibiotics and oral contraceptive agents may be contributory

DEMOGRAPHICS

- Oral candidiasis more common in elderly, debilitated, malnourished, diabetic, or HIV-infected patients as well as those taking antibiotics, systemic corticosteroids, or chemotherapy

CLINICAL FINDINGS

SYMPTOMS AND SIGNS

- See Table 7
- Itching may be intense
- Burning is reported, particularly around the vulva and anus
- Lesions consist of superficially denuded, beefy-red areas in the depths of the body folds
  - Groin and the intergluteal cleft
  - Beneath the breasts
  - Angles of the mouth
  - Umbilicus
- The peripheries of the denuded lesions are superficially undermined, and there may be satellite vesicopustules
- Whitish, curd-like concretions may be present on the surface of the mucosal lesions
- Paronychia and interdigital erosions may occur

DIFFERENTIAL DIAGNOSIS

- **Cutaneous candidiasis**
  - Intertrigo
  - Seborrheic dermatitis
  - Tinea cruris (jock itch)
  - Psoriasis of body folds ("inverse psoriasis")
  - Erythrasma
  - Contact dermatitis
  - Tinea versicolor (pityriasis versicolor) (rarely)
- **Oral candidiasis**
  - Leukoplakia
  - Lichen planus
  - Dysplasia or carcinoma
  - Geographic tongue
  - Herpes simplex
  - Erythema multiforme
  - Pemphigus
  - Oral hairy leukoplakia

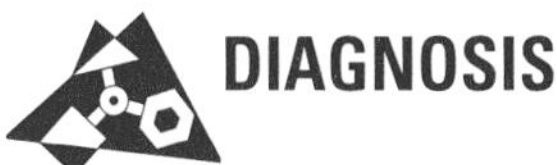

DIAGNOSIS

LABORATORY TESTS

- Clusters of budding cells and hyphae can be seen under high power when skin scales or curd-like lesions have been cleared in 10% KOH

Carcinoid Tumors, Bronchial p. 1049. Carcinoid Tumors, Gastric p. 1050.

Candidiasis, Mucocutaneous

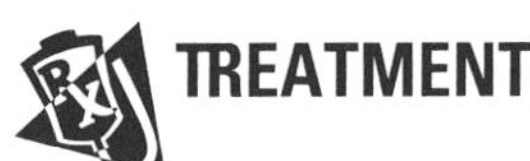

TREATMENT

MEDICATIONS

- See Table 6
- Apply ciclopirox cream, nystatin cream, 100,000 units/g, or miconazole, econazole, ketoconazole, or clotrimazole cream three or four times daily
- Gentian violet, 1%, or carbolfuchsin paint (Castellani's paint) may be applied once or twice weekly as an alternative, but these preparations are messy

Vaginal candidiasis

- Single-dose fluconazole (150 mg) is effective; intravaginal clotrimazole, miconazole, terconazole, or nystatin may also be used
- Chronic suppressive therapy may be required for recurrent or "intractable" cases
- Non-albicans candidal species may be identified by culture in some refractory cases and may respond to oral itraconazole, 200 mg twice daily for 2–4 weeks

Balanitis

- Most frequent in uncircumcised men
- Topical imidazole cream or nystatin ointment is the initial treatment if the lesions are mildly erythematous or superficially erosive
- Soaking with dilute aluminum acetate for 15 min twice daily may quickly relieve burning or itching
- Chronicity and relapses, especially after sexual contact, suggest reinfection from a sexual partner who should be treated
- Severe purulent balanitis is usually due to bacteria
  - If it is so severe that phimosis occurs, oral antibiotics—some with activity against anaerobes—are required
  - If rapid improvement does not occur, urologic consultation is indicated

THERAPEUTIC PROCEDURES

- Affected parts should be kept dry and exposed to air as much as possible
- If possible, discontinue systemic antibiotics

OUTCOME

PROGNOSIS

- Cases of cutaneous candidiasis range from the easily cured to the intractable and prolonged

WHEN TO REFER

- If there is a question about the diagnosis, if recommended therapy is ineffective, or if specialized treatment is necessary

PREVENTION

- Keep skin dry and cool
- Keep good glucose control in diabetics

EVIDENCE

PRACTICE GUIDELINES

- Pappas PG et al; Infectious Diseases Society of America: Guidelines for treatment of candidiasis. Clin Infect Dis 2004;38:161. [PMID: 14699449]
  - http://www.guideline.gov/summary/summary.aspx?doc_id=4545&nbr=3359
- Association for Genitourinary Medicine, Medical Society for the Study of Venereal Disease (London). 2002 national guideline on the management of vulvovaginal candidiasis
  - http://www.guideline.gov/summary/summary.aspx?doc_id=3033&nbr=2259
- Roberts DT et al; British Association of Dermatologists: Guidelines for treatment of onychomycosis. Br J Dermatol 2003;148:402. [PMID: 12653730]

WEB SITES

- American Academy of Dermatology
  - http://www.aad.org
- Centers for Disease Control and Prevention
  - http://www.cdc.gov/ncidod/dbmd/diseaseinfo/

INFORMATION FOR PATIENTS

- American Academy of Family Physicians: Vaginal Yeast Infections
  - http://familydoctor.org/206.xml
- Mayo Clinic: Oral Thrush
  - http://www.mayoclinic.com/invoke.cfm?id=DS00408
- MedlinePlus: Cutaneous Candidiasis
  - http://www.nlm.nih.gov/medlineplus/ency/article/000880.htm
- MedlinePlus: Paronychia
  - http://www.nlm.nih.gov/medlineplus/ency/article/001444.htm

REFERENCE

- Ringdahl EN: Treatment of recurrent vulvovaginal candidiasis. Am Fam Physician 2000;61:3306. [PMID: 10865926]

Author(s)

Timothy G. Berger, MD

Celiac Disease

Cardiomyopathy, Hypertrophic p. 1050. Cardiomyopathy, Peripartum p. 1051. Cardiomyopathy, Primary Dilated p. 1051. Carotid Artery Aneurysm p. 1052.

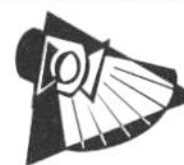

KEY FEATURES

ESSENTIALS OF DIAGNOSIS

- Typical symptoms
  - Weight loss
  - Chronic diarrhea
  - Abdominal distention
  - Growth retardation
- Atypical symptoms
  - Dermatitis herpetiformis
  - Iron deficiency anemia
  - Osteoporosis
- Abnormal serologic test results
- Abnormal small bowel biopsy
- Clinical improvement on gluten-free diet

GENERAL CONSIDERATIONS

- Also known as gluten enteropathy or celiac sprue
- Diffuse damage to the proximal small intestinal mucosa results in malabsorption of most nutrients
- Typical symptoms commonly manifest between 6 months and 24 months of age
- Up to 50% of cases present with atypical symptoms in childhood or adulthood
- More than 10% of adults with iron deficiency have undiagnosed celiac disease
- Removal of gluten from the diet results in resolution of symptoms and intestinal healing in most patients
- Celiac disease may be associated with other autoimmune disorders

DEMOGRAPHICS

- Occurs in 1:250 whites of northern European ancestry but is rare in Africans and Asians
- Clinical diagnosis made in only 1:5000 persons in the United States, so most cases are undiagnosed

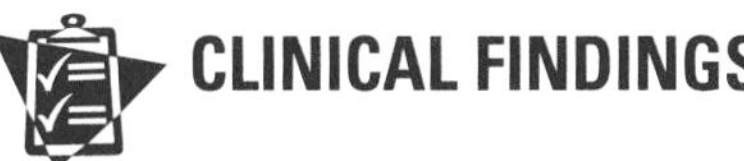

CLINICAL FINDINGS

SYMPTOMS AND SIGNS

- Infants (< 2 years)
  - Diarrhea, weight loss, abdominal distention, weakness, muscle wasting, or growth retardation
  - Stools characteristically loose to soft, large, floating, oily or greasy, and foul-smelling; may also be watery and frequent (up to 10–12 daily)
- Children and adults
  - Chronic diarrhea or flatulence
  - Weight loss (variable)
  - Fatigue
  - Short stature
  - Osteoporosis
  - Dental enamel hypoplasia
  - Anemia
- Physical examination
  - In mild cases: may be normal
  - In more severe cases: may reveal signs of malabsorption, loss of muscle mass or subcutaneous fat, pallor, easy bruising, hyperkeratosis, or bone pain
- Abdominal examination may reveal distention with hyperactive bowel sounds
- Dermatitis herpetiformis in < 10%

DIFFERENTIAL DIAGNOSIS

- Irritable bowel syndrome
- Malabsorption due to other cause, eg, pancreatic insufficiency, reduced bile salts, lymphatic obstruction, bacterial overgrowth, tropical sprue
- Lactase deficiency
- Viral gastroenteritis, eosinophilic gastroenteritis
- Whipple's disease
- Giardiasis
- Mucosal damage caused by acid hypersecretion associated with gastrinoma

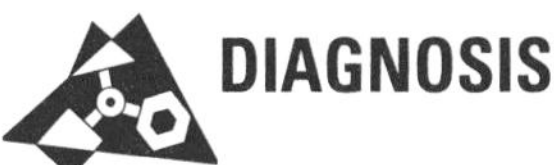

DIAGNOSIS

LABORATORY TESTS

- Complete blood cell count, prothrombin time, albumin, and serum iron or ferritin, red cell folate, vitamin B_{12} level, vitamin A and D levels, serum calcium, and alkaline phosphatase
- Iron deficiency or megaloblastic anemia occurs because of iron or folate or vitamin B_{12} malabsorption
- Elevations of prothrombin time
- Nonanion gap acidosis and hypokalemia in severe diarrhea
- Steatorrhea
  - Detected by a qualitative (Sudan stain) or quantitative 72-hour stool assessment for fecal fat while patients are consuming a 100-g fat diet
  - Excretion of more than 10 g/day of fat is abnormal
- d-Xylose test for malabsorption
- Serologic tests
  - IgA endomysial antibody or IgA tissue transglutaminase antibody have >90% sensitivity and >95% specificity for diagnosis
  - Either is excellent screening test in patients in whom there is a low to moderate suspicion for diagnosis
  - A negative test result reliably excludes diagnosis whereas a positive test is virutally diagnostic
  - IgG or IgA antigliandin antibodies present in >85%; however, low specificity (85–90%) limits usefulness as screening test
- Serologic test results become undetectable 8–12 months after dietary gluten withdrawal

IMAGING

- Dual-energy x-ray densitometry scanning for osteoporosis

DIAGNOSTIC PROCEDURES

- Mucosal biopsy: endoscopic mucosal biopsy of the distal duodenum or proximal jejunum confirms diagnosis

Carotid Body Tumor p. 1052. Carotid Dissection p. 1053.

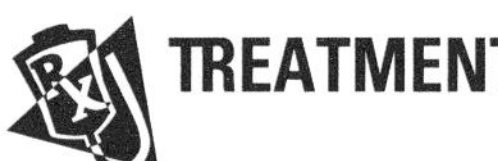

TREATMENT

- Removal of all gluten from the diet
- Most patients with celiac disease also have lactose intolerance either temporarily or permanently and should avoid dairy products until the intestinal symptoms have improved on the gluten-free diet

MEDICATIONS

- Nutrient supplements (folate, iron, vitamin B_{12}, calcium, vitamins A and D) in initial stages of therapy, as necessary
- Calcium, vitamin D, and bisphosphonate therapy for osteoporosis

OUTCOME

FOLLOW-UP

- Improvement in symptoms within a few weeks on the gluten-free diet

PROGNOSIS

- Excellent prognosis with appropriate diagnosis and treatment
- Celiac disease that is truly refractory to gluten withdrawal carries a poor prognosis
  - May be caused by ulcerative jejunitis or enteropathy or by associated T-cell lymphoma, which occurs in up to 10% of patients

EVIDENCE

PRACTICE GUIDELINES

- American Gastroenterological Association medical position statement: celiac sprue. Gastroenterology 2001;120:1522. [PMID: 11313323]
- Ciclitira PJ et al: AGA technical review on celiac sprue. American Gastroenterological Association. Gastroenterology 2001;120:1526. [PMID:11313324]
- National Guideline Clearinghouse
  - http://www.guideline.gov/summary/summary.aspx?doc_id=3697&nbr=2923&string=celiac+AND+sprue

WEB SITES

- Celiac and gluten free support page
  - http://www.celiac.com
- National Institute of Diabetes and Digestive and Kidney Diseases (NIDDK), NIH
  - http://www.niddk.nih.gov
- WebPath: Gastrointestinal Pathology Index
  - http://medstat.med.utah.edu/WebPath/GIHTML/GIIDX.html

INFORMATION FOR PATIENTS

- JAMA patient page: Celiac disease. JAMA 2002;287:1484
- Mayo Clinic
  - http://www.mayoclinic.com/invoke.cfm?id=DS00319
- National Institute of Diabetes and Digestive and Kidney Diseases (NIDDK), NIH
  - http://digestive.niddk.nih.gov/ddiseases/pubs/celiac/index.htm

REFERENCES

- Farrell RJ et al: Celiac sprue. N Engl J Med 2002;346:180. [PMID:11796853]
- Green PH et al: Coeliac disease. Lancet 2003;362:383. [PMID: 12907013]
- Shan L et al: Structural basis for gluten intolerance in celiac sprue. Science 2002;297:2275. [PMID:12351792]

Author(s)

Kenneth R. McQuaid, MD

Cellulitis & Erysipelas

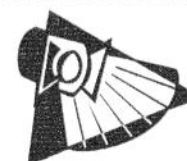

KEY FEATURES

ESSENTIALS OF DIAGNOSIS

- Diffuse, spreading infection of the skin

GENERAL CONSIDERATIONS

Cellulitis

- Usually due to gram-positive cocci, though gram-negative rods such as *Escherichia coli* may be responsible
- The major portal of entry for lower leg cellulitis is toe web tinea pedis with fissuring of the skin at this site

Erysipelas

- A superficial form of cellulitis that occurs classically on the cheek, caused by β-hemolytic streptococci
- Edematous, spreading, circumscribed, hot, erythematous area, with or without vesicles or bullae
- Pain, chills, fever, and systemic toxicity may be striking
- Erysipeloid, unlike erysipelas, is a benign bacillary infection producing redness of the skin of the fingers or the backs of the hands in fishermen and meat handlers

CLINICAL FINDINGS

SYMPTOMS AND SIGNS

- See Table 7

Cellulitis

- The lesion is hot and red
- Pain at the lesion, malaise, chills, and moderate fever
- Usually on the lower leg
- In case of venous stasis, the only clue to cellulitis may be a new localized area of tenderness
- Recurrent attacks may sometimes affect lymphatic vessels, producing a permanent swelling called "solid edema"

Erysipelas

- Central face frequently involved
  - A bright red spot appears first, very often near a fissure at the angle of the nose
  - This spreads to form a tense, sharply demarcated, glistening, smooth, hot area
  - The margin characteristically makes noticeable advances in days or even hours
- The lesion is somewhat edematous and can be pitted slightly with the finger
- Vesicles or bullae occasionally develop on the surface
- The lesion does not usually become pustular or gangrenous and heals without scar formation

DIFFERENTIAL DIAGNOSIS

- Deep venous thrombosis
- Venous stasis
- Candidiasis
- Anthrax
- Erysipeloid
- Contact dermatitis
- Herpes zoster (shingles)
- Scarlet fever
- Angioedema
- Necrotizing fasciitis
- Sclerosing panniculitis
- Underlying osteomyelitis
- Systemic lupus erythematosus

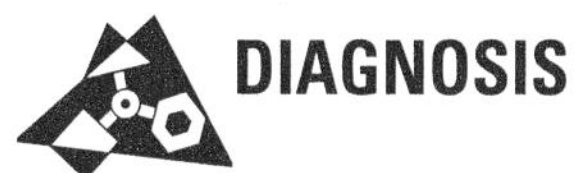

DIAGNOSIS

LABORATORY TESTS

- Attempts to isolate the responsible organism by injecting and then aspirating saline are successful in 20% of cases
- Leukocytosis and an increased sedimentation rate are almost invariably present but are not specific
- Blood cultures may be positive

Cellulitis & Erysipelas

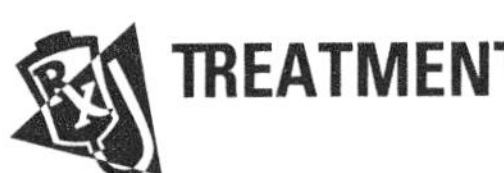

TREATMENT

MEDICATIONS

- Intravenous or parenteral antibiotics effective against group A β-hemolytic streptococci and staphylococci may be required for the first 24–48 h
- In mild cases or following the initial parenteral therapy, dicloxacillin or cephalexin, 250–500 mg PO QID for 7–10 days, is usually adequate
- In patients in whom intravenous treatment is not instituted, the first dose of oral antibiotic can be increased to 750–1000 mg to achieve rapid high blood levels

Erysipelas

- Place the patient at bed rest with the head of the bed elevated
- Intravenous antibiotics as above are indicated for the first 48 hours in all but the mildest cases
- A 7-day course is completed with penicillin VK, 250 mg, dicloxacillin, 250 mg, or a first-generation cephalosporin, 250 mg, PO QID
- Either erythromycin, 250 mg PO QID for 7–14 days, or clarithromycin, 250 mg PO BID for 7–14 days, is a good alternative in penicillin-allergic patients

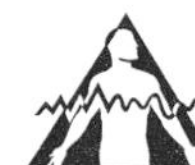

OUTCOME

COMPLICATIONS

- Unless erysipelas is promptly treated, death may result from extension of the process and systemic toxicity, particularly in the very young and in the aged

PROGNOSIS

- Erysipelas was at one time a life-threatening infection. It can now usually be quickly controlled with systemic penicillin or erythromycin therapy

WHEN TO REFER

- If there is a question about the diagnosis, if recommended therapy is ineffective, or specialized treatment is necessary

WHEN TO ADMIT

- All but the mildest cases of erysipelas
- Cellulitis with systemic toxicity or in need of IV antibiotics

EVIDENCE

WEB SITES

- National Institute of Allergy and Infectious Disease
  - http://www.niaid.nih.gov
- American Academy of Dermatology
  - http://www.aad.org

INFORMATION FOR PATIENTS

- National Institute of Allergy and Infectious Disease: Group A Streptococcal Infections
  - http://www.niaid.nih.gov/factsheets/strep.htm
- MedlinePlus: Erysipelas
  - http://www.nlm.nih.gov/medlineplus/ency/article/000618.htm

REFERENCES

- Baddour LM: Cellulitis syndromes: an update. Int J Antimicrob Agents 2000;14:113. [PMID: 2018804]
- Roldan YB et al: Erysipelas and tinea pedis. Mycoses 2000;43:181. [PMID: 10948816]

Author(s)

Timothy G. Berger, MD

Cerebrovascular Disease, Occlusive

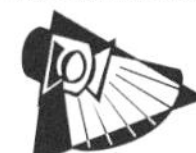

KEY FEATURES

ESSENTIALS OF DIAGNOSIS

- A stroke is defined as a sudden onset of a neurological deficit that persists beyond 24 h
- A transient ischemic attack (TIA) is defined as the sudden onset of a neurological deficit that resolves completely within 24 h

GENERAL CONSIDERATIONS

- Most strokes are caused by emboli occluding small cerebral arteries
- Emboli consist of platelet aggregates that form on irregular or ulcerated surfaces or plaque debris liberated by turbulent flow and intraplaque hemorrhage from the carotid bifurcation, from the heart (eg, mural thrombus or atrial myxoma), or from the aortic arch
- Stroke is also caused by intracerebral hemorrhage (from trauma, hypertension, or a ruptured cerebral aneurysm) or by small-vessel occlusive disease in the pons, basal ganglia, and internal capsule (lacunar infarcts)
- Risk of stroke for carotid artery stenosis < 60% is 1.6% per year; risk for > 60% stenosis is 3.2% per year; risk for > 80% stenosis is 5–10% per year
- Increased stroke risk is also associated with rapid progression of carotid disease and with plaque heterogeneity or ulceration
- Risk factors for carotid disease include hypertension, diabetes mellitus, hypercholesterolemia, advanced age, smoking, and coronary artery disease
- A single TIA is associated with a 26% risk of subsequent stroke

DEMOGRAPHICS

- Every year, half a million people in the United States suffer a stroke
- 15–30% of strokes are fatal

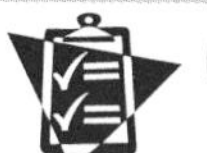

CLINICAL FINDINGS

SYMPTOMS AND SIGNS

- Carotid artery occlusive disease: contralateral weakness or sensory loss, expressive aphasia, and amaurosis fugax (transient partial or complete loss of vision in the ipsilateral eye)
- Vertebrobasilar occlusive disease: brainstem and cerebellar symptoms, including dysarthria, diplopia, vertigo, ataxia, and hemiparesis or quadriparesis
- Cervical bruits
- Diminished or absent pulses in the neck or arms
- Hollenhorst plaques (bright, refractile cholesterol emboli) in the retinal arteries
- Blood pressure difference between the two arms of > 10 mm Hg

DIFFERENTIAL DIAGNOSIS

- Acute myocardial infarction
- Carotid dissection
- Syncope
- Intracranial hemorrhage

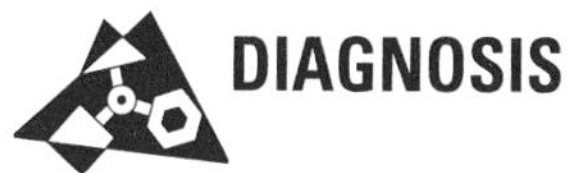

DIAGNOSIS

IMAGING STUDIES

- Duplex carotid ultrasonography provides both physiological (flow) and anatomic (plaque characterization) information; percent stenosis is derived from measurement of blood flow velocities, with sensitivity and specificity > 90%
- Gadolinium-enhanced magnetic resonance angiography (MRA) or CT angiography (CTA) provides anatomic information and cross-sectional imaging for measurement of degree of stenosis and characterizes the arch intracranial circulation and vertebral arteries
  - MRA can provide more detailed information about plaque composition, but is time consuming and can overestimate degree of stenosis
  - CTA is fast but requires contrast and can be limited in cases with severe arterial calcification
- Ultrasonography plus MRA or CTA estimates percent stenosis better than conventional angiography
- Conventional or CT angiography is used in cases of suspected carotid occlusion before nonoperative management is elected because a small percentage will have internal carotid artery "string sign" lesions that require urgent revascularization
- Because catheter angiography has a 1% risk of procedure-related stroke, it is reserved for patients with greatly disparate ultrasound and CTA or MRA findings, those suspected of vertebrobasilar insufficiency or intracranial lesions, those unable to undergo MRA or CTA, and those potentially requiring endovascular intervention
- Noncontrast CT head for any patients with TIA/CVA

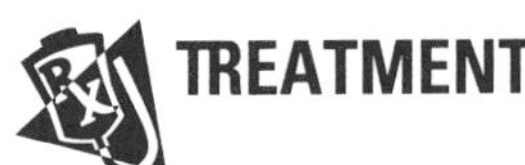

TREATMENT

MEDICATIONS

- Asymptomatic diagnosis: antiplatelet medication (eg, aspirin, 81 mg PO QD, ticlopidine, 250 mg PO BID, or clopidogrel, 75 mg PO BID) to reduce the likelihood of thrombosis and microemboli
- Acute TIA: aspirin, 81 mg PO QD, or clopidogrel, 75 mg PO QD, for urgent surgery
- Acute stroke: aspirin, 81 mg PO QD, or clopidogrel, 75 mg PO QD, in preparation for surgery in 5–8 weeks
- Clopidogrel for patients with neurological symptoms secondary to intracerebral disease not amenable to surgical reconstruction

SURGERY

Acute stroke

- Delay surgery until neurological examination stabilizes (5–8 weeks)
- Carotid endarterectomy, antiplatelet therapy, and risk factor modification

Transient ischemic attacks

- Carotid endarterectomy plus antiplatelet, and risk factor modification
  - Highly effective in preventing stroke and death in symptomatic patients with > 70% carotid stenosis
  - More modest benefit–risk ratio in symptomatic patients with 50–69% carotid stenosis

Asymptomatic carotid stenosis

- Risk of stroke is ~5% per year in asymptomatic patients with > 80% carotid stenosis
- Carotid endarterectomy in good-risk asymptomatic patients with > 60% stenosis affords an overall risk reduction of 53% compared with aspirin alone

THERAPEUTIC PROCEDURES

- Percutaneous techniques: carotid angioplasty and stenting indicated in patients who are not good candidates for surgery

OUTCOME

COMPLICATIONS

- Carotid endarterectomy morbidity–mortality rate is < 5%; endarterectomy has a ~1–2% mortality rate and ~1–4% risk of neurological complications
- Carotid stenting has a 5–18% risk of periprocedural stroke or TIA and 8–14% per year incidence of recurrent stenosis (compared with < 4% per year with surgery)

PROGNOSIS

- In symptomatic patients, endarterectomy reduces stroke risk 5- to 10-fold at 5 years; there is a 5–15% incidence of late stroke after uncomplicated endarterectomy often related to contralateral carotid or intracranial disease
- Restenosis occurring < 2 years after endarterectomy is due to intimal hyperplasia, which responds well to angioplasty and stenting
- Restenosis > 2 years after endarterectomy is more often related to progression of atherosclerotic disease
- Repeat surgery or stenting is advised for symptomatic restenoses or > 80% stenoses

WHEN TO REFER

- Asymptomatic carotid stenosis > 60%
- Symptomatic carotid disease

WHEN TO ADMIT

- Patients with acute or crescendo TIAs for heparin anticoagulation and evaluation for surgery

PREVENTION

- Risk factor modification: control of hypertension, hyperlipidemia, and diabetes

EVIDENCE

PRACTICE GUIDELINES

- Albers GW et al: Antithrombotic and thrombolytic therapy for ischemic stroke: the Seventh ACCP Conference on Antithrombotic and Thrombolytic Therapy. Chest 2004;126(Suppl):483S. [PMID: 15383482]
- Coull BM et al: Anticoagulants and antiplatelet agents in acute ischemic stroke: report of the Joint Stroke Guideline Development Committee of the American Academy of Neurology and the American Stroke Association (a division of the American Heart Association). Stroke 2002;33:1934. [PMID: 12105379]
- Streefkerk HJ et al: Cerebral revascularization. Adv Tech Stand Neurosurg 2003;28:145. [PMID: 12627810]

WEB SITE

- National Institute of Neurological Disorders and Stroke
  - http://www.ninds.nih.gov/

INFORMATION FOR PATIENTS

- Cleveland Clinic: Stroke
  - http://www.clevelandclinic.org/health/health-info/docs/2100/2179.asp?index=9074
- Mayo Clinic: Stroke
  - http://www.mayoclinic.com/invoke.cfm?objectid=487C37FA-C927-45BF-84821670F1635148
- MedlinePlus: Stroke Secondary to Atherosclerosis
  - http://www.nlm.nih.gov/medlineplus/ency/article/000738.htm
- National Institute of Neurological Disorders and Stroke: Stroke Information Page
  - http://www.ninds.nih.gov/disorders/stroke/stroke.htm

REFERENCES

- Barnett HJM et al: Causes and severity of ischemic stroke in patients with internal carotid artery stenosis. JAMA 2000;283:1429. [PMID: 10732932]
- Endovascular versus surgical treatment in patients with carotid stenosis in the Carotid and Vertebral Artery Transluminal Angioplasty Study (CAVATAS): a randomised trial. Lancet 2001;357:1729. [PMID: 11403808]

Author(s)

Louis M. Messina, MD

Cervical Cancer

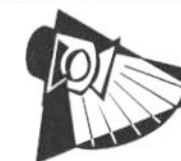

KEY FEATURES

ESSENTIALS OF DIAGNOSIS

- Abnormal uterine bleeding and vaginal discharge
- Cervical lesion may be visible on inspection as a tumor or ulceration
- Vaginal cytology usually positive; must be confirmed by biopsy

GENERAL CONSIDERATIONS

- Cancer appears first in the intraepithelial layers (the preinvasive stage, or carcinoma in situ)
- Preinvasive cancer (CIN III) is a common diagnosis in women 25–40 years of age and is etiologically related to infection with the human papillomavirus

DEMOGRAPHICS

- Multiparity
- Smoker
- Early initiation of intercourse
- Multiple sex partners

CLINICAL FINDINGS

SYMPTOMS AND SIGNS

- The most common signs are metrorrhagia, postcoital spotting, and cervical ulceration
- Bloody or purulent, odorous, nonpruritic discharge may appear after invasion
- Bladder and rectal dysfunction or fistulas and pain are late symptoms

DIFFERENTIAL DIAGNOSIS

- Cervical intraepithelial neoplasia
- Cervical ectropion
- Cervical ectopy (columnar epithelium on face of os, common in adolescence)
- Genital warts (condyloma acuminata)
- Cervical polyp
- Cervicitis
- Nabothian cyst
- Granuloma inguinale

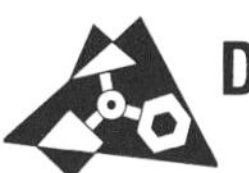

DIAGNOSIS

LABORATORY TESTS

- Positive Papanicolaou smear

IMAGING STUDIES

- Further staging assessment beyond biopsy may be carried out by abdominal and pelvic CT scanning or MRI

DIAGNOSTIC PROCEDURES

- **Cervical biopsy and endocervical curettage, or conization**
  - These procedures are necessary steps after a positive Papanicolaou smear to determine the extent and depth of invasion of the cancer
  - Even if the smear is positive, treatment is never justified until definitive diagnosis has been established through biopsy
- **"Staging," or estimate of gross spread of cancer of the cervix**
  - The depth of penetration of the malignant cells beyond the basement membrane is a reliable clinical guide to the extent of primary cancer within the cervix and the likelihood of metastases
  - It is customary to stage cancers of the cervix under anesthesia as shown in Table 66

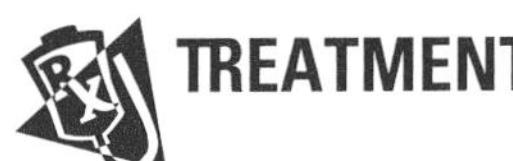

TREATMENT

- **Carcinoma in situ (stage 0)**
  - In women who have completed childbearing, total hysterectomy is the treatment of choice
  - In women who wish to retain the uterus, acceptable alternatives include cervical conization or ablation of the lesion with cryotherapy or laser
- **Invasive carcinoma**
  - Microinvasive carcinoma (stage IA) is treated with simple, extrafascial hysterectomy
  - Stage IB and stage IIA cancers may be treated with either radical hysterectomy or radiation therapy
  - Stage IIB and stage III and IV cancers must be treated with radiation therapy
  - Because radical surgery results in fewer long-term complications than irradiation and may allow preservation of ovarian function, it may be the preferred mode of therapy in younger women without contraindications to major surgery
- **Emergency measures**
  - Vaginal hemorrhage originates from gross ulceration and cavitation in stage II–IV cervical carcinoma
  - Ligation and suturing of the cervix are usually not feasible, but ligation of the uterine or hypogastric arteries may be lifesaving when other measures fail
  - Styptics such as Monsel's solution or acetone are effective, although delayed sloughing may result in further bleeding
  - Wet vaginal packing is helpful
  - Emergency irradiation usually controls bleeding

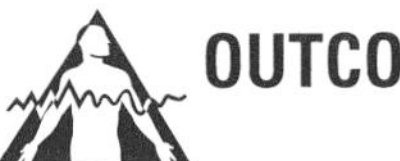

OUTCOME

FOLLOW-UP

- Carcinoma in situ
- Close follow-up with Papanicolaou smears every 3 months for 1 year and every 6 months for another year is necessary after cryotherapy or laser

COMPLICATIONS

- Metastases to regional lymph nodes occur with increasing frequency from stage I to stage IV
- The ureters are often obstructed lateral to the cervix, causing hydroureter, hydronephrosis, and renal insufficiency
- Almost two-thirds of untreated patients die of uremia when ureteral obstruction is bilateral
- Pain in the back, in the distribution of the lumbosacral plexus, is often indicative of neurologic involvement
- Gross edema of the legs may be indicative of vascular and lymphatic stasis due to tumor
- Vaginal fistulas to the rectum and urinary tract
- 10–20% of patients with extensive invasive carcinoma die of hemorrhage

PROGNOSIS

- Two to 10 years are required for carcinoma to penetrate the basement membrane and invade the tissues; death usually occurs in 3–5 years in untreated or unresponsive patients
- The overall 5-year relative survival rate is 68% in white women and 55% in black women in the United States
- Survival rates are inversely proportional to the stage of cancer: stage 0, 99–100%; stage IA, > 95%; stage IB-IIA, 80–90%; stage IIB, 65%; stage III, 40%; stage IV, < 20%

WHEN TO REFER

- All patients with invasive cervical cancer should be referred to a gynecologic oncologist

PREVENTION

- Regular Papanicolaou smears (Table 150)
- Smoking cessation

EVIDENCE

PRACTICE GUIDELINES

- Teng N et al; NCCN Cervical Cancer Practice Guidelines Panel. National Comprehensive Cancer Network: Cervical Cancer v.1.2004.
  - http://www.nccn.org/professionals/physician_gls/PDF/cervical.pdf
- American College of Obstetricians and Gynecologists. Diagnosis and treatment of cervical carcinomas. ACOG Practice Bulletin 35, 2002.
  - http://www.guideline.gov/summary/summary.aspx?ss=15&doc_id=3983&nbr=3122

WEB SITES

- National Cancer Institute: Cervical Cancer Information for Patients and Health Professionals
  - http://www.cancer.gov/cancerinfo/types/cervical
- Cervical Cancer Screening: Collection of articles
  - http://bmj.com/cgi/collection/cervical_screening

INFORMATION FOR PATIENTS

- American Cancer Society: Cervical Cancer
  - http://www.cancer.org/docroot/CRI/CRI_2_3x.asp?dt=8
- CDC: Basic Facts on Cervical Cancer Screening and the Pap Test
  - http://www.cdc.gov/cancer/nbccedp/bccpdfs/cc_basic.pdf
- MedlinePlus: Cervical Cancer
  - http://www.nlm.nih.gov/medlineplus/ency/article/000893.htm
- National Cancer Institute
  - http://www.cancer.gov/cancerinfo/wyntk/cervix

REFERENCES

- ACOG Practice Bulletin. Diagnosis and treatment of cervical carcinomas, number 35, May 2002. Obstet Gynecol 2002;99:855. [PMID: 11978302]
- Lonky NM: Reducing death from cervical cancer: examining the prevention paradigms. Obstet Gynecol Clin North Am 2002;29:599. [PMID: 12509087]

Author(s)

H. Trent MacKay, MD, MPH

Cervical Intraepithelial Neoplasia

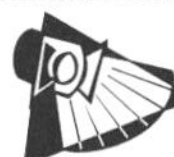

KEY FEATURES

ESSENTIALS OF DIAGNOSIS

- The presumptive diagnosis is made by an abnormal Pap smear of an asymptomatic woman with no grossly visible cervical changes
- Diagnose by colposcopically directed biopsy
- Increased in women with HIV

GENERAL CONSIDERATIONS

- Cervical infection with the human papillomavirus (HPV) is associated with a high percentage of all cervical dysplasias and cancers
  - There are over 70 recognized HPV subtypes, of which types 6 and 11 tend to cause mild dysplasia, while types 16, 18, 31, and others cause higher-grade cellular changes
- The varying degrees of dysplasia are defined by the degree of cellular atypia (Table 65)
- The cervical intraepithelial neoplasia (CIN) classification is used along with a description of abnormal cells, including evidence of HPV. The term "squamous intraepithelial lesions (SIL)," low-grade or high-grade, is increasingly used
- HPV testing of cytologic smears may be useful for triage of atypia (atypical squamous cells of unknown significance; ASCUS)

DEMOGRAPHICS

- Cervical cancer almost never occurs in virginal women
  - It is epidemiologically related to the number of sexual partners a woman has had and the number of other female partners a male partner has had
- Long-term oral contraceptive users, smokers, and women exposed to second-hand smoke are at increased risk
- Women with HIV infection appear to be at increased risk for the disease and of recurrent disease after treatment

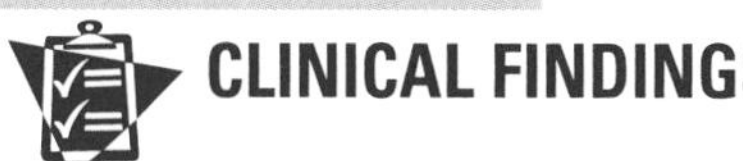

CLINICAL FINDINGS

SYMPTOMS AND SIGNS

- There are no specific symptoms or signs of cervical intraepithelial neoplasia

DIFFERENTIAL DIAGNOSIS

- Cervical cancer
- Cervical ectropion
- Cervical ectopy (columnar epithelium on face of os, common in adolescence)
- Genital warts (condyloma acuminata)
- Cervical polyp
- Cervicitis
- Nabothian cyst
- Granuloma inguinale

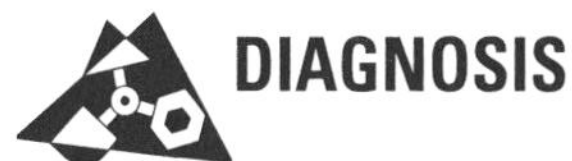

DIAGNOSIS

LABORATORY TESTS

Cytologic examination (Papanicolaou smear)

- Specimens should be taken from a nonmenstruating patient, spread on a single slide, and fixed or rinsed directly into preservative solution if a thin-layer slide system (ThinPrep) is to be used
- A specimen should be obtained from the squamocolumnar junction with a wooden or plastic spatula and from the endocervix with a cotton swab or nylon brush

DIAGNOSTIC PROCEDURES

Colposcopy

- Viewing the cervix with 10–20× magnification allows for assessment of the size and margins of an abnormal transformation zone and determination of extension into the endocervical canal
- The application of 3–5% acetic acid (vinegar) dissolves mucus, and the acid's desiccating action sharpens the contrast between normal and actively proliferating squamous epithelium
- Abnormal changes include white patches and vascular atypia, which indicate areas of greatest cellular activity
- Paint the cervix with Lugol's solution [strong iodine solution (Schiller's test)]. Normal squamous epithelium will take the stain; nonstaining squamous epithelium should be biopsied. (The single-layered, mucus-secreting endocervical tissue will not stain either but can readily be distinguished by its darker pink, shinier appearance.)

Biopsy

- Colposcopically directed punch biopsy and endocervical curettage are office procedures
- If colposcopic examination is not available, the normal-appearing cervix shedding atypical cells can be evaluated by endocervical curettage and multiple punch biopsies of nonstaining squamous epithelium or biopsies from each quadrant of the cervix
- All visibly abnormal cervical lesions should be biopsied

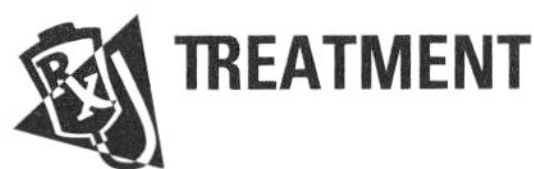

TREATMENT

SURGERY

Conization of the cervix

- Conization is surgical removal of the entire transformation zone and endocervical canal
- It should be reserved for cases of severe dysplasia or cancer in situ (CIN III), particularly those with endocervical extension
- The procedure can be performed with the scalpel, the CO_2 laser, the needle electrode, or by large-loop excision

THERAPEUTIC PROCEDURES

- Treatment varies depending on the degree and extent of cervical intraepithelial neoplasia
- Biopsies should always precede treatment

Cauterization or cryosurgery

- The use of either hot cauterization or freezing (cryosurgery) is effective for noninvasive small lesions visible on the cervix without endocervical extension

CO_2 laser

- This well-controlled method minimizes tissue destruction
- It is colposcopically directed and requires special training
- May be used with large visible lesions
- Involves the vaporization of the transformation zone on the cervix and the distal 5–7 mm of the endocervical canal

Loop resection

- When the CIN is clearly visible in its entirety, a wire loop can be used for excisional biopsy
- Cutting and hemostasis are effected with a low-voltage electrosurgical machine (Bovie)
- This office procedure with local anesthesia is quick and uncomplicated

OUTCOME

FOLLOW-UP

- All types of dysplasia must be observed and treated if they persist or become more severe
- Because recurrence is possible—especially in the first 2 years after treatment—and because the false-negative rate of a single cervical cytologic test is 20%, close follow-up is imperative
- Cytologic examination should be repeated at 3-month intervals for at least 1 year

PROGNOSIS

- At present, the malignant potential of a specific lesion cannot be predicted. Some lesions remain stable for long periods of time; some regress; and others advance
- Adequately treated CIN very rarely progresses to invasive disease

WHEN TO REFER

- Patients with abnormal Papanicolaou smears or visible cervical lesions should be referred for colposcopy

PREVENTION

- Preventive measures include the following
  - Regular cytologic screening to detect abnormalities
  - Limiting the number of sexual partners
  - Using a diaphragm or condom for coitus
  - Stopping smoking
  - Avoiding exposure to second-hand smoke
- Women with HIV infection should receive regular cytologic screening and should be monitored closely after treatment for cervical intraepithelial neoplasia
- A prophylactic vaccine against HPV-16 has been shown to be effective and additional clinical trials are underway. A therapeutic vaccine to treat existing HPV infections is in early stages of development.
- Because of the very low rate of abnormal Papanicolaou smears in women who have undergone hysterectomy for benign disease, routine screening is not justified in this population

EVIDENCE

PRACTICE GUIDELINES

- Wright TC et al; American Society for Colposcopy and Cervical Pathology. 2001 consensus guidelines for the management of women with cervical intraepithelial neoplasia
  - http://www.guideline.gov/summary/summary.aspx?doc_id=3868&nbr=3078

WEB SITE

- Colposcopy Atlas
  - http://lib-sh.lsuhsc.edu/fammed/atlases/colpo.html

INFORMATION FOR PATIENTS

- National Cancer Institute
  - http://www.cancer.gov/cancerinfo/wyntk/cervix
- JAMA Patient Page: Papillomavirus. JAMA 2002;287:2452. [PMID: 12004891]
- American Cancer Society: Pap Test
  - http://www.cancer.org/docroot/PED/content/PED_2_3X_Pap_Test.asp?sitearea=PED
- National Cancer Institute: HPV and Cancer
  - http://cis.nci.nih.gov/fact/3_20.htm
- American Academy of Family Physicians: Pap Smears: When Yours is Slightly Abnormal
  - http://familydoctor.org/223.xml
- American Medical Association: Cervical Dysplasia
  - http://www.medem.com/MedLB/article_detaillb.cfm?article_ID=ZZZIY13X59C&sub_cat=9
- National Library of Medicine: Colposcopy Interactive Tutorial
  - http://www.nlm.nih.gov/medlineplus/tutorials/colposcopy.html

REFERENCES

- Schreckenberger C et al: Vaccination strategies for the treatment and prevention of cervical cancer. Curr Opin Oncol 2004;16:485. [PMID: 15314520]
- Stoler MH: New Bethesda terminology and evidence-based management guidelines for cervical cytology findings. JAMA 2002;287:2140. [PMID: 11966390]
- Wright TC Jr et al: 2001 Consensus guidelines for the management of women with cervical cytological abnormalities. JAMA 2002;287:2120. [PMID: 11966387]

Author(s)

H. Trent MacKay, MD, MPH

Cholangitis & Choledocholithiasis

Cervical Polyps p. 1054. Cervicitis p. 1055.
Chancroid p. 1055.

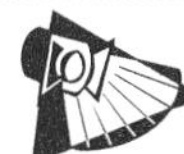

KEY FEATURES

ESSENTIALS OF DIAGNOSIS

- Often a history of biliary colic or jaundice
- Sudden onset of severe right upper quadrant or epigastric pain, which may radiate to the right scapula or shoulder
- Occasional patients present with painless jaundice
- Nausea and vomiting
- Fever, which may be followed by hypothermia and gram-negative shock, jaundice, and leukocytosis
- Abdominal films may reveal gallstones

GENERAL CONSIDERATIONS

- Common duct stones usually originate in the gallbladder but may also form spontaneously in the common duct after cholecystectomy
- The stones are frequently "silent" unless there is obstruction
- Biliary colic results from rapid increases in common bile duct pressure due to obstructed bile flow

DEMOGRAPHICS

- About 15% of patients with gallstones have choledocholithiasis (common bile duct stones). The percentage rises with age, and the frequency in elderly people with gallstones may be as high as 50%

CLINICAL FINDINGS

SYMPTOMS AND SIGNS

- See Table 63
- Biliary pain with jaundice
- Frequently recurring attacks of right upper abdominal pain that is severe and persists for hours
- Chills and fever associated with severe colic
- **Charcot's triad** [pain, fever (and chills), and jaundice] is characteristic of cholangitis
- Altered sensorium, lethargy, and septic shock connote acute suppurative cholangitis and constitute an endoscopic or surgical emergency
- Hepatomegaly may be present in calculous biliary obstruction, and tenderness is usually present in the right upper quadrant and epigastrium

DIFFERENTIAL DIAGNOSIS

- Cancer of the pancreas, ampulla of Vater, or common duct
- Acute hepatitis
- Biliary stricture
- Chronic cholestatic liver disease, eg, primary biliary cirrhosis, primary sclerosing cholangitis, drug toxicity
- Pancreatitis
- Sepsis due to other causes
- Underlying *Ascaris* or *Clonorchis*, or hydatid disease

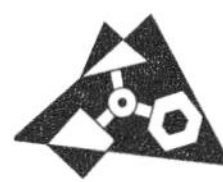

DIAGNOSIS

LABORATORY TESTS

- Bilirubinuria and elevation of serum bilirubin are present if the common duct is obstructed; levels commonly fluctuate
- Serum alkaline phosphatase elevation is suggestive of obstructive jaundice
- Serum amylase elevations may be present in secondary pancreatitis
- Acute obstruction of the bile duct rarely produces a transient striking increase in serum aminotransferase levels (> 1000 units/L)
- Hypoprothrombinemia can result from obstructed flow of bile to the intestine
- When extrahepatic obstruction persists for more than a few weeks, differentiation of obstruction from chronic cholestatic liver disease becomes progressively more difficult

IMAGING STUDIES

- Ultrasonography, CT scan, and radionuclide imaging may demonstrate dilated bile ducts and impaired bile flow
- Endoscopic ultrasonography, helical CT, and MR cholangiography can accurately demonstrate common duct stones and, if available, may be used when there is low or intermediate risk for choledocholithiasis

DIAGNOSTIC PROCEDURES

- Endoscopic retrograde cholangiopancreatography (ERCP) or percutaneous transhepatic cholangiography is the best means to determine the cause, location, and extent of obstruction
- If the likelihood that obstruction is caused by a stone is high, ERCP is the procedure of choice because it permits papillotomy or balloon dilation of the papilla with stone extraction or stent placement; balloon dilation is associated with a higher rate of pancreatitis than is sphincterotomy

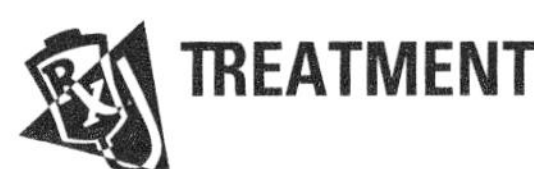

TREATMENT

MEDICATIONS

Hypoprothrombinemia

- Treat with 10 mg of parenteral vitamin K or water-soluble oral vitamin K (phytonadione, 5 mg) in 24–36 h

Cholangitis

- Ciprofloxacin, 250 mg IV Q 12 h
- Alternatively, in severely ill patients, give mezlocillin, 3 g IV Q 4 h, plus either metronidazole, 500 mg IV Q 6 h (if there has been no prior manipulation of the duct) or gentamicin (2 mg/kg IV as loading dose, plus 1.5 mg/kg every 8 h adjusted for renal function) (or both)
- Aminoglycosides should not be given for more than a few days because the risk of aminoglycoside nephrotoxicity is increased in patients with cholestasis

SURGERY

- At cholecystectomy, operative cholangiography via the cystic duct should be considered. If stones in the common duct are found, common duct exploration can be performed or a postoperative ERCP and sphincterotomy can be planned
- Following operative choledochostomy, a simple catheter or T tube is placed in the common duct for decompression. A properly placed tube should drain bile at the operating table and continuously thereafter; otherwise, it should be considered blocked or dislocated. The volume of bile drainage varies from 100 to 1000 mL daily (average, 200–400 mL). Above-average drainage may be due to obstruction at the ampulla (usually by edema)
- Choledocholithiasis discovered at laparoscopic cholecystectomy may be managed via laparoscopic removal or, if necessary, conversion to open surgery or by postoperative endoscopic sphincterotomy

THERAPEUTIC PROCEDURES

- Nutrition should be restored by a high-carbohydrate, high-protein diet and vitamin supplementation
- Common duct stone with cholelithiasis and cholecystitis is usually treated by endoscopic papillotomy and stone extraction followed by laparoscopic cholecystectomy. For the poor-risk patient, cholecystectomy may be deferred because the risk of subsequent cholecystitis is low
- ERCP should be performed before cholecystectomy in patients with gallstones and jaundice (serum total bilirubin >5 mg/dL), a dilated common bile duct (>7 mm), or stones in the bile duct seen on ultrasound or CT
- When biliary pancreatitis resolves rapidly, the stone usually passes into the intestine, and ERCP prior to cholecystectomy is not necessary if an intraoperative cholangiogram is done
- In the postcholecystectomy patient with choledocholithiasis, endoscopic papillotomy with stone extraction is preferable to transabdominal surgery
- Lithotripsy (endoscopic or external), direct cholangioscopy, or biliary stenting may be therapeutic for large stones. For the patient with a T tube and common duct stone, the stone may be extracted via the T tube
- Urgent ERCP, sphincterotomy, and stone extraction are generally indicated for choledocholithiasis complicated by ascending cholangitis
- Emergent decompression of the bile duct, generally by ERCP, for patients who are septic or fail to improve on antibiotics within 12–24 h
- If sphincterotomy cannot be performed, decompression by a biliary stent or nasobiliary catheter can be done. Once decompressed, antibiotics are generally continued for another 3 days

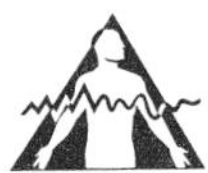

OUTCOME

FOLLOW-UP

- Postoperative antibiotics are not given routinely after biliary tract surgery; intraoperative bile cultures are taken
- If biliary tract infection was present preoperatively or is apparent at operation, ampicillin (500 mg IV Q 6 h) with gentamicin (1.5 mg/kg Q 8 h) and metronidazole (500 mg Q 6 h) or ciprofloxacin (250 mg IV Q 12 h) or a third-generation cephalosporin (eg, cefoperazone, 1–2 g IV Q 12 h) is administered postoperatively until the sensitivity tests on culture specimens are available
- A T-tube cholangiogram should be done before the tube is removed, usually about 3 weeks after surgery. A small amount of bile frequently leaks from the tube site for a few days

COMPLICATIONS

- Common duct obstruction lasting longer than 30 days results in liver damage leading to cirrhosis
- Hepatic failure with portal hypertension occurs in untreated cases

PROGNOSIS

- Medical therapy alone is most likely to fail in patients with tachycardia, serum albumin < 3 g/dL, serum bilirubin >50 μmol/L, and prothombin time >14 s on admission

EVIDENCE

PRACTICE GUIDELINES

- Eisen et al: American Society for Gastrointestinal Endoscopy. Standards of Practice Committee. An annotated algorithm for the evaluation of choledocholithiasis.Gastrointest Endosc 2001;53(7):864.
- National Guideline Clearinghouse
  - http://www.guideline.gov/summary/summary.aspx?doc_id=5513&nbr=3756&string=choledocholithiasis

WEB SITE

- Choledocholithiasis Demonstration Case
  - http://www.brighamrad.harvard.edu/Cases/bwh/hcache/99/full.html

INFORMATION FOR PATIENTS

- Mayo Clinic
  - http://www.mayoclinic.com/invoke.cfm?id=DS00165
- National Institutues of Health
  - http://www.nlm.nih.gov/medlineplus/ency/article/000290.htm
  - http://www.nlm.nih.gov/medlineplus/ency/article/000274.htm

REFERENCE

- Tse F et al: The elective evaluation of patients with suspected choledocholithiasis undergoing laparoscopic cholecystectomy. Gastrointest Endosc 2004;60:437. [PMID: 15332044]

Author(s)

Lawrence S. Friedman, MD

Cholecystitis, Acute

Cholecystectomy, Pre- & Post-Syndrome p. 1055

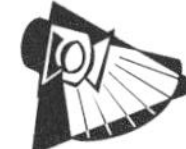

KEY FEATURES

ESSENTIALS OF DIAGNOSIS

- Steady, severe pain and tenderness in the right hypochondrium or epigastrium
- Nausea and vomiting
- Fever and leukocytosis

GENERAL CONSIDERATIONS

- Associated with gallstones in over 90% of cases
- Occurs when a stone becomes impacted in the cystic duct and inflammation develops behind the obstruction
- Acalculous cholecystitis should be considered when unexplained fever or right upper quadrant pain occurs within 2–4 weeks of major surgery or in a critically ill patient who has had no oral intake for a prolonged period
- Primarily as a result of ischemic changes secondary to distention, gangrene may develop, resulting in perforation. Although generalized peritonitis is possible, the leak usually remains localized and forms a chronic, well-circumscribed abscess cavity
- Acute cholecystitis caused by infectious agents (eg, cytomegalovirus, cryptosporidiosis, or microsporidiosis) may occur in patients with AIDS

CLINICAL FINDINGS

SYMPTOMS AND SIGNS

- The acute attack is often precipitated by a large or fatty meal
- Relatively sudden, severe, steady pain that is localized to the epigastrium or right hypochondrium and may gradually subside over a period of 12–18 h
- Vomiting occurs in about 75% of patients and in 50% affords variable relief
- Right upper quadrant abdominal tenderness is almost always present and is usually associated with muscle guarding and rebound pain
- A palpable gallbladder is present in about 15% of cases
- Jaundice
  - Present in about 25% of cases
  - When persistent or severe, suggests the possibility of choledocholithiasis
  - May also result from compression of the common bile or hepatic duct by a cystic duct that is inflamed because of an impacted stone (Mirizzi's syndrome)
- Fever is usually present

DIFFERENTIAL DIAGNOSIS

- Perforated viscus, eg, peptic ulcer, diverticulitis
- Acute pancreatitis
- Appendicitis
- Acute hepatitis or liver abscess
- Right lower lobe pneumonia
- Myocardial infarction
- Radicular pain in T6–T10 dermatome, eg, preeruptive zoster

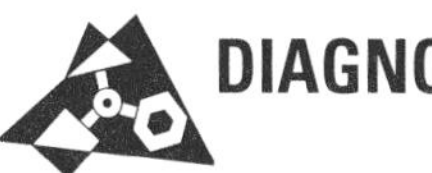

DIAGNOSIS

LABORATORY TESTS

- The white blood cell count is usually high (12,000–15,000/μL)
- Total serum bilirubin values of 1–4 mg/dL may be seen even in the absence of common duct obstruction
- Serum aminotransferase and alkaline phosphatase are often elevated—the former as high as 300 units/mL, or even higher when associated with ascending cholangitis
- Serum amylase may also be moderately elevated

IMAGING STUDIES

- Plain films of the abdomen may show radiopaque gallstones in 15% of cases
- ^{99m}Tc hepatobiliary imaging (using iminodiacetic acid compounds) (HIDA scan) is useful in demonstrating an obstructed cystic duct, which is the cause of acute cholecystitis in most patients. This test is reliable if the bilirubin is under 5 mg/dL (98% sensitivity and 81% specificity for acute cholecystitis)
- Right upper quadrant abdominal ultrasound may show the presence of gallstones but is not sensitive for acute cholecystitis (67% sensitivity, 82% specificity)

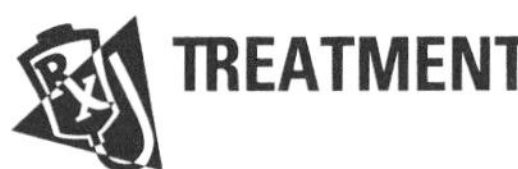

TREATMENT

MEDICATIONS

- Will usually subside on a conservative regimen (withholding of oral feedings, intravenous alimentation, analgesics, and antibiotics)
- Meperidine may be preferable to morphine for pain because of less spasm of the sphincter of Oddi

SURGERY

- Because of the high risk of recurrent attacks (up to 10% by 1 month and over 30% by 1 year), cholecystectomy—generally laparoscopically—should generally be performed within 2–3 days after hospitalization
- Surgical treatment of chronic cholecystitis is the same as for acute cholecystitis. If indicated, cholangiography can be performed during laparoscopic cholecystectomy. Choledocholithiasis can also be excluded by either pre- or postoperative endoscopic retrograde or magnetic resonance cholangiopancreatography

THERAPEUTIC PROCEDURES

- In high-risk patients, ultrasound-guided aspiration of the gallbladder or percutaneous cholecystostomy may postpone or even avoid the need for surgery. Cholecystectomy is mandatory when there is evidence of gangrene or perforation

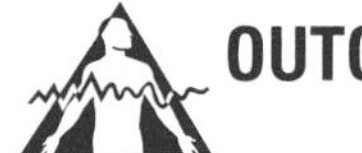

OUTCOME

FOLLOW-UP

- If nonsurgical treatment has been elected, watch the patient (especially if diabetic or elderly) for recurrent symptoms, evidence of gangrene of the gallbladder, or cholangitis

COMPLICATIONS

Gangrene of the gallbladder

- Continuation or progression of right upper quadrant abdominal pain, tenderness, muscle guarding, fever, and leukocytosis after 24–48 h suggests severe inflammation and possible gangrene of the gallbladder
- Necrosis may develop without definite signs in the obese, diabetic, elderly, or immunosuppressed patient
- See *Cholangitis & choledocholithiasis*

Chronic cholecystitis and other complications

- Results from repeated episodes of acute cholecystitis or chronic irritation of the gallbladder wall by stones
- Calculi are usually present
- In about 5% of cases, the villi of the gallbladder undergo polypoid enlargement due to deposition of cholesterol ("strawberry gallbladder," cholesterolosis). In other instances, adenomatous hyperplasia of the gallbladder wall may be so marked as to give the appearance of a myoma (pseudotumor)
- Hydrops of the gallbladder results when acute cholecystitis subsides but cystic duct obstruction persists, producing distention of the gallbladder with a clear mucoid fluid
- A stone in the neck of the gallbladder may compress the bile duct and cause jaundice (Mirizzi's syndrome)
- Cholelithiasis with chronic cholecystitis may be associated with acute exacerbations of gallbladder inflammation, common duct stone, fistulization to the bowel, pancreatitis, and, rarely, carcinoma of the gallbladder
- Calcified (porcelain) gallbladder may have a high association with gallbladder carcinoma (particularly when the calcification is mucosal rather than intramural) and appears to be an indication for cholecystectomy

PROGNOSIS

- The mortality rate of cholecystectomy is less than 1%, but hepatobiliary tract surgery in the elderly has a mortality rate of 5–10%
- A successful surgical procedure is generally followed by complete resolution of symptoms

EVIDENCE

PRACTICE GUIDELINES

- National Guideline Clearinghouse
  - http://www.guideline.gov/summary/summary.aspx?doc_id=5513&nbr=3756&string=cholecystitis
  - http://www.guideline.gov/summary/summary.aspx?doc_id=3258&nbr=2484&string=cholecystitis

WEB SITES

- Acute Acalculous Cholecystitis Demonstration Case
  - http://www.brighamrad.harvard.edu/Cases/bwh/hcache/55/full.html
- Acute Cholecystitis Demonstration Case
  - http://www.brighamrad.harvard.edu/Cases/bwh/hcache/96/full.html

INFORMATION FOR PATIENTS

- JAMA patient page: Acute cholecystitis. JAMA 2003;289:124.
- Mayo Clinic
  - http://www.mayoclinic.com/invoke.cfm?objectid=7E7F8A87-F164-441E-BB6E7731D06D9B47
- National Institutes of Health
  - http://www.nlm.nih.gov/medlineplus/ency/article/000264.htm

REFERENCES

- Alobaidi M et al: Current trends in imaging evaluation of acute cholecystitis. Emerg Radiol 2004;10:256. [PMID: 15290472]
- Trowbridge RL et al: Does this patient have acute cholecystitis? JAMA 2003;289:80. [PMID: 12503981]

Author(s)

Lawrence S. Friedman, MD

Cholelithiasis (Gallstones)

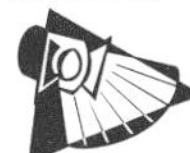

KEY FEATURES

ESSENTIALS OF DIAGNOSIS

- Biliary pain
- Gallstones in gallbladder on ultrasound
- Patients may be asymptomatic

GENERAL CONSIDERATIONS

- Gallstones are classified according to their predominant chemical composition as cholesterol or calcium bilirubinate stones. The latter comprise less than 20% of the stones found in Europe or the United States but 30–40% of the stones found in Japan

DEMOGRAPHICS

- Gallstones are more common in women than in men and increase in incidence in both sexes and all races with aging
- In the United States, over 10% of men and 20% of women have gallstones by age 65; the total exceeds 20 million people. Although cholesterol gallstones are less common in black people, cholelithiasis attributable to hemolysis occurs in over a third of individuals with sickle cell anemia
- Native Americans of both the Northern and Southern Hemispheres have a high rate of cholesterol cholelithiasis, probably because of a predisposition resulting from "thrifty" (*LITH*) genes that promote efficient calorie utilization and fat storage
- As many as 75% of Pima and other American Indian women over the age of 25 years have cholelithiasis
- Obesity is a risk factor for gallstones, especially in women, while rapid weight loss increases the risk of symptomatic gallstone formation
- Diabetes and elevated serum insulin levels (insulin resistance syndrome) are risk factors for gallstones
- Prolonged fasting (over 5–10 days) can lead to formation of biliary "sludge" (microlithiasis), which usually resolves with refeeding but can lead to gallstones or biliary symptoms
- Pregnancy is associated with an increased risk of gallstones and of symptomatic gallbladder disease
- Hormone replacement therapy conveys a slight risk for biliary tract surgery

CLINICAL FINDINGS

SYMPTOMS AND SIGNS

- See Table 63
- Cholelithiasis is frequently asymptomatic and is discovered incidentally
- "Symptomatic" cholelithiasis usually means characteristic right upper quadrant or epigastric discomfort or pain (biliary pain)
- Occasional patients present with small intestinal obstruction due to "gallstone ileus" as the initial manifestation of cholelithiasis

DIFFERENTIAL DIAGNOSIS

- Acute cholecystitis
- Acute pancreatitis
- Peptic ulcer disease
- Appendicitis
- Acute hepatitis
- Myocardial infarction
- Radicular pain in T6–T10 dermatome, eg, preeruptive zoster

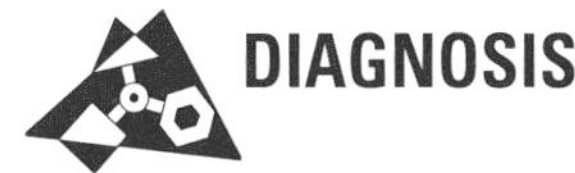

DIAGNOSIS

LABORATORY TESTS

- Table 63
- Laboratory tests are normal in persons with asymptomatic gallstones

IMAGING STUDIES

- Ultrasound is the most sensitive imaging modality
- CT is an alternative but usually not necessary

DIAGNOSTIC PROCEDURES

- See *Cholecystitis, acute* or *Cholangitis & choledocholithiasis*

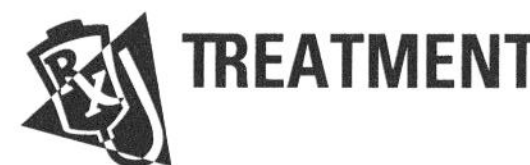

TREATMENT

MEDICATIONS

- Cheno- and ursodeoxycholic acids
  - When given orally for up to 2 years dissolve some cholesterol stones
  - May be considered in selected patients who refuse cholecystectomy
  - Dose is 7 mg/kg/day of each or 8–13 mg/kg of ursodeoxycholic acid in divided doses daily
  - They are most effective in patients with a functioning gallbladder, as determined by gallbladder visualization on oral cholecystography, and multiple small "floating" gallstones (representing not more than 15% of patients with gallstones)
  - In 50% of patients, gallstones recur within 5 years after treatment is stopped

SURGERY

- There is generally no need for prophylactic cholecystectomy in an asymptomatic person unless the gallbladder is calcified or gallstones are over 3 cm in diameter
- Laparoscopic cholecystectomy is the treatment of choice for symptomatic gallbladder disease. The minimal trauma to the abdominal wall makes it possible for patients to go home within 2 days after the procedure and to return to work within 7 days (instead of weeks for those undergoing standard open cholecystectomy). If problems are encountered, the surgery can be converted to a conventional open cholecystectomy. See *Cholangitis & choledocholithiasis*
- A conservative approach to biliary pain is advised in pregnant patients, but for patients with repeated attacks of biliary pain or acute cholecystitis, cholecystectomy can be performed—even by the laparoscopic route—preferably in the second trimester

THERAPEUTIC PROCEDURES

- Enterolithotomy alone is considered adequate treatment in most patients with gallstone ileus
- Lithotripsy in combination with bile salt therapy for single radiolucent stones less than 20 mm in diameter is no longer generally employed in the United States

OUTCOME

COMPLICATIONS

- Cholecystectomy may increase the risk of esophageal and proximal small intestinal adenocarcinoma because of increased duodenogastric reflux and changes in intestinal exposure to bile, respectively
- There may be persistence of symptoms after removal of the gallbladder (see *Cholecystectomy, pre- and post-syndrome* in Diseases in Brief section)

PROGNOSIS

- Symptoms (biliary pain) develop in 10–25% of patients with gallstones by 10 years

PREVENTION

- Low-carbohydrate, low-fat, and high-fiber diets and physical activity may help prevent gallstones, and consumption of caffeinated coffee appears to protect against gallstones in women

EVIDENCE

PRACTICE GUIDELINES

- National Guideline Clearinghouse
  - http://www.guideline.gov/summary/summary.aspx?doc_id=5513&nbr=3756&string=gallstones
- Patient Care Committee, Society for Surgery of the Alimentary Tract. Treatment of gallstone and gallbladder disease. SSAT patient care guidelines. J Gastrointest Surg 2004;8:363. [PMID: 15115004]

WEB SITE

- Choledocholithiasis Demonstration Case
  - http://www.brighamrad.harvard.edu/Cases/bwh/hcache/99/full.html

INFORMATION FOR PATIENTS

- Mayo Clinic
  - http://www.mayoclinic.com/invoke.cfm?objectid=7E7F8A87-F164-441E-BB6E7731D06D9B47
- National Digestive Diseases Information Clearinghouse
  - http://win.niddk.nih.gov/publications/gallstones.htm
- National Institutes of Health
  - http://www.nlm.nih.gov/medlineplus/ency/article/000273.htm

REFERENCES

- Lublin M et al: Symptoms before and after laparoscopic cholecystectomy for gallstones. Am Surg 2004;70:836. [PMID: 15529838]
- Tsai CJ et al: Long-term intake of dietary fiber and decreased risk of cholecystectomy in women. Am J Gastroenterol 2004;99:1364. [PMID: 15233680]
- Tsai CJ et al: The effect of long-term intake of cis unsaturated fats on the risk for gallstone disease in men: a prospective cohort study. Ann Intern Med 2004;141:514. [PMID: 15466768]

Author(s)

Lawrence S. Friedman, MD

Cholera

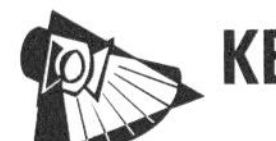

KEY FEATURES

ESSENTIALS OF DIAGNOSIS

- History of travel in endemic area or contact with infected person
- Voluminous diarrhea
- Stool is liquid, gray, turbid, and without fecal odor, blood, or pus ("rice water stool")
- Rapid development of marked dehydration
- Positive stool cultures and agglutination of vibrios with specific contaminated food or water

GENERAL CONSIDERATIONS

- An acute diarrheal illness caused by certain serotypes of *Vibrio cholerae*
- The toxin activates adenylyl cyclase in intestinal epithelial cells of the small intestines, producing hypersecretion of water and chloride ion and a massive diarrhea of up to 15 L/day
- Occurs in epidemics under conditions of crowding, war, and famine (eg, in refugee camps) and where sanitation is inadequate
- Infection is acquired by ingestion of contaminated food or water

DEMOGRAPHICS

- Rarely seen in the United States until 1991, when epidemic cholera returned to the Western Hemisphere, originating as an outbreak in coastal cities of Peru. The epidemic spread to involve several countries in South and Central America as well as Mexico, and cases have been imported into the United States
- A major cause of epidemic diarrhea throughout the developing world

CLINICAL FINDINGS

SYMPTOMS AND SIGNS

- See Table 131
- A sudden onset of severe, frequent watery diarrhea (up to 1 L/h)
- The liquid stool is gray, turbid, and without fecal odor, blood, or pus ("rice water stool")
- Dehydration and hypotension develop rapidly
- The disease is toxin mediated, and fever is unusual

DIFFERENTIAL DIAGNOSIS

- Viral gastroenteritis
- Other small intestinal diarrhea, eg, salmonellosis, enterotoxigenic *Escherichia coli*
- Vasoactive intestinal polypeptide-producing pancreatic tumor (pancreatic cholera)
- Food poisoning, eg, *Staphylococcus aureus*

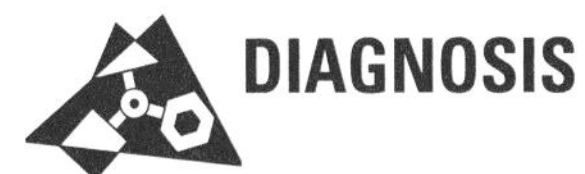

DIAGNOSIS

LABORATORY TESTS

- Stool culture

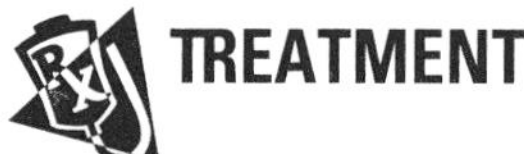

TREATMENT

MEDICATIONS

- Antimicrobial therapy will shorten the course of illness
- Several antimicrobials are active against *V cholerae*, including tetracycline, ampicillin, chloramphenicol, trimethoprim-sulfamethoxazole, and fluoroquinolones

THERAPEUTIC PROCEDURES

- Fluid replacement
- In mild or moderate illness, oral rehydration is usually adequate

OUTCOME

COMPLICATIONS

- Death results from profound hypovolemia

PROGNOSIS

- 25–50% fatality if untreated

WHEN TO ADMIT

- Severe diarrhea
- Moderate to severe dehydration in need of parenteral fluid replacement
- Inability to maintain fluid replacement because there can be rapid development of dehydration

PREVENTION

- A vaccine is available that confers short-lived, limited protection
- Vaccine may be required for entry into or reentry after travel to some countries
- Vaccine is administered in two doses 1–4 weeks apart. A booster dose every 6 months is recommended for persons remaining in areas where cholera is a hazard
- Vaccination programs are expensive and not particularly effective in managing outbreaks of cholera. When outbreaks occur, efforts should be directed toward establishing clean water and food sources and proper waste disposal

EVIDENCE

PRACTICE GUIDELINES

- National Guideline Clearinghouse
  - http://www.guideline.gov/summary/summary.aspx?doc_id=2791

WEB SITES

- CDC—Division of Bacterial and Mycotic Diseases
  - http://www.cdc.gov/ncidod/dbmd/
- Karolinska Institute—Directory of bacterial infections and mycoses
  - http://www.mic.ki.se/Diseases/C01.html

INFORMATION FOR PATIENTS

- Centers for Disease Control
  - http://www.cdc.gov/ncidod/dbmd/diseaseinfo/cholera_g.htm
- JAMA patient page: Preventing dehydration from diarrhea. JAMA 2001;185:362.

REFERENCE

- Guerrant RL et al: How intestinal bacteria cause disease. J Infect Dis 1999;179(Suppl 2):S331. [PMID: 10081504]

Author(s)

Henry F. Chambers, MD

Chronic Fatigue Syndrome

Chromoblastomycosis p. 1056

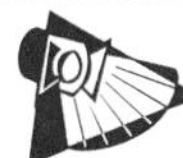

KEY FEATURES

ESSENTIALS OF DIAGNOSIS

- Weight loss
- Fever
- Sleep-disordered breathing
- Substance use
- Depression

GENERAL CONSIDERATIONS

- Fatigue often attributable to overexertion, poor physical conditioning, sleep disturbance, obesity, undernutrition, and emotional problems
- The lifetime prevalence of significant fatigue (present for at least 2 weeks) is about 25%

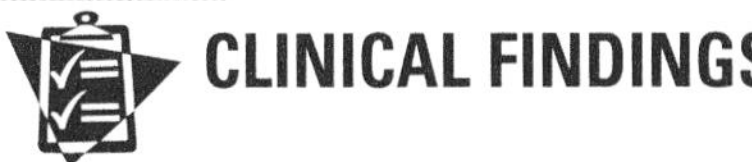

CLINICAL FINDINGS

SYMPTOMS AND SIGNS

- Screen for psychiatric disorders
- Evaluation and classification of unexplained chronic fatigue involves history and physical examination, mental status examination (abnormalities require appropriate psychiatric, psychological, or neurological examination), and screening laboratory tests
- Fatigue is classified as chronic fatigue syndrome if criteria for severity of fatigue are met and four or more of the following symptoms are concurrently present for 6 or more months
  - Impaired memory or concentration
  - Sore throat
  - Tender cervical or axillary lymph nodes
  - Muscle pain
  - Multijoint pain
  - New headaches
  - Unrefreshing sleep
  - Postexertion malaise
- Fatigue is classified as idiopathic chronic fatigue if criteria for fatigue severity or the symptoms are not met

DIFFERENTIAL DIAGNOSIS

- Hypothyroidism
- Anemia
- Depression
- Obstructive sleep apnea or insufficient sleep
- Infection, eg, tuberculosis, hepatitis, endocarditis, HIV, Lyme disease
- Diabetes mellitus
- Congestive heart failure, chronic obstructive pulmonary disease, or chronic renal failure
- Cancer
- Alcoholism
- Hypercalcemia
- Drugs, eg, sedatives, β-blockers
- Somatoform disorder (somatization)
- Fibromyalgia
- Mononucleosis
- Autoimmune disease

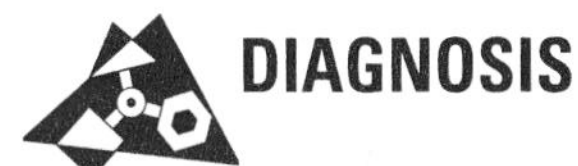

DIAGNOSIS

LABORATORY TESTS

- Obtain complete blood count, erythrocyte sedimentation rate, serum electrolytes, glucose, blood urea nitrogen, creatinine, calcium, liver and thyroid function tests, antinuclear antibody, urinalysis, and tuberculin skin test
- Consider, as indicated, serum cortisol, rheumatoid factor, immunoglobulin levels, Lyme serology in endemic areas, and HIV antibody test

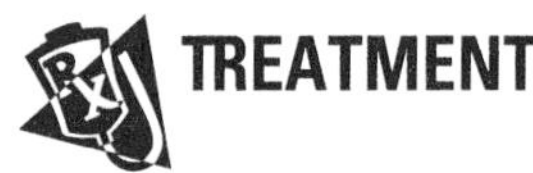

TREATMENT

MEDICATIONS

- Treat affective or anxiety disorder only if present
- Treat postural hypotension with fludrocortisone, 0.1 mg/day, and increased dietary sodium

THERAPEUTIC PROCEDURES

- For chronic fatigue syndrome, treatment involves a comprehensive multidisciplinary intervention
  - Optimal medical management of coexisting disorders, eg, depression
  - Cognitive-behavioral therapy
  - Graded exercise program

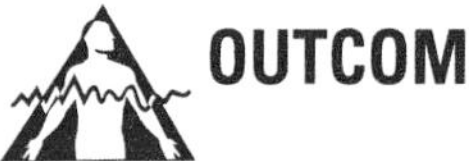

OUTCOME

PROGNOSIS

- Although few patients are cured, the treatment effect can be substantial
- Full recovery is eventually possible in many cases

EVIDENCE

PRACTICE GUIDELINES

- Veterans Health Administration, Department of Defense: VHA/DoD clinical practice guideline for the management of medically unexplained symptoms: chronic pain and fatigue. 2001.
  - http://www.oqp.med.va.gov/cpg/cpgn/mus/mus_base.htm
- Working Group of the Royal Australasian College of Physicians: Chronic fatigue syndrome. Clinical practice guidelines—2002. Med J Aust 2002;176(Supp l):S23.
  - http://www.mja.com.au/public/guides/cfs/cfs2.html

WEB SITE

- Agency for Healthcare Research and Quality: Defining and Managing Chronic Fatigue Syndrome
  - http://www.ahrq.gov/clinic/epcsums/cfssum.htm

INFORMATION FOR PATIENTS

- American Academy of Family Physicians: Chronic Fatigue Syndrome
  - http://familydoctor.org/x1598.xml
- Mayo Clinic: Chronic Fatigue Syndrome
  - http://www.mayoclinic.com/invoke.cfm?id=DS00395
- National Center for Infectious Diseases: Chronic Fatigue Syndrome
  - http://www.cdc.gov/ncidod/diseases/cfs/info.htm
- National Institute of Allergy and Infectious Diseases: Chronic Fatigue Syndrome
  - http://www.niaid.nih.gov/factsheets/cfs.htm

REFERENCES

- Powell P et al: Randomised controlled trial of patient education to encourage graded exercise in chronic fatigue syndrome. BMJ 2001;322:1. [PMID: 11179154]
- Whiting P et al: Interventions for the treatment and management of chronic fatigue syndrome: a systematic review. JAMA 2001;286:1360. [PMID: 11560542]

Author(s)

Ralph Gonzales, MD

Chronic Obstructive Pulmonary Disease (COPD)

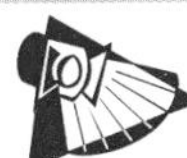

KEY FEATURES

ESSENTIALS OF DIAGNOSIS

- History of cigarette smoking
- Chronic cough and sputum production (bronchitis) and dyspnea (emphysema)
- Rhonchi, decreased intensity of breath sounds, and prolonged expiration on physical examination
- Airflow limitation on pulmonary function testing

GENERAL CONSIDERATIONS

- Airflow obstruction due to chronic bronchitis or emphysema; most patients have features of both
- Obstruction
  - Is progressive
  - May be accompanied by airway hyperreactivity
  - May be partially reversible
- Chronic bronchitis is characterized by excessive mucous secretions with productive cough for 3 months or more in at least 2 consecutive years
- Emphysema is abnormal enlargement of distal air spaces and destruction of bronchial walls without fibrosis
- Cigarette smoking is the most important cause
  - About 80% of patients have had a significant exposure to tobacco smoke
- Air pollution, airway infection, familial factors, and allergy have been implicated in chronic bronchitis
- α_1-Antitrypsin deficiency has been implicated in emphysema

CLINICAL FINDINGS

SYMPTOMS AND SIGNS

- Presentation
  - Usually at 40–50 years of age
  - Cough
  - Sputum production
  - Shortness of breath
- Dyspnea initially occurs only with heavy exertion, progressing to symptoms at rest in severe disease
- Frequent exacerbations lead to eventual disability
- Viral infections precede exacerbations in the majority of patients
- Late-stage COPD characterized by
  - Pneumonia
  - Pulmonary hypertension
  - Cor pulmonale
  - Respiratory failure
- Death usually occurs during an exacerbation of COPD in association with respiratory failure
- Clinical findings may be absent early
- Patients are often dichotomized as "pink puffers" or "blue bloaters" depending on whether emphysema or bronchitis predominates (Table 17)

DIFFERENTIAL DIAGNOSIS

- Bronchial asthma
- Bronchiectasis, which features recurrent pneumonia and hemoptysis, with distinct radiographic findings
- Severe α_1-antitrypsin deficiency
- Cystic fibrosis, which is seen in children and young adults

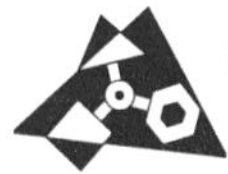

DIAGNOSIS

LABORATORY TESTS

- Sputum examination may reveal
  - *Streptococcus pneumoniae*
  - *Haemophilus influenzae*
  - *Moraxella catarrhalis*
  - Cultures correlate poorly with exacerbations
- ECG shows sinus tachycardia, abnormalities consistent with cor pulmonale in severe disease, and/or supraventricular tachycardias and ventricular irritability
- Arterial blood gas values
  - May show only an increased A–a Do_2 in early disease
  - Unnecessary unless hypoxemia or hypercapnia is suspected
  - Show hypoxemia in advanced disease
  - Compensated respiratory acidosis with worsening acidemia during exacerbations
- Spirometry
  - Objectively measures pulmonary function and assesses severity
  - Early changes are reductions in mid-expiratory flow and abnormal closing volumes
  - FEV_1 and FEV_1/FVC are reduced later in disease
  - FVC is reduced in severe disease
  - Lung volume measurements show an increase in total lung capacity (TLC), residual volume (RV), and an elevation of RV/TLC indicating air trapping
- α_1-Antitrypsin level in young patients with emphysema

IMAGING STUDIES

- Chest x-ray may show hyperinflation, especially when emphysema predominates
- Parenchymal bullae or subpleural blebs are pathognomonic of emphysema
- Nonspecific peribronchial and perivascular markings with chronic bronchitis
- Enlargement of central pulmonary arteries in advanced disease

TREATMENT

MEDICATIONS

- Supplemental oxygen
  - In hospitalized patients, O_2 should not be withheld for fear of worsening acidemia
  - Longer survival, reduced hospitalizations, and better quality of life in advanced disease
  - Unless therapy is intended only for night-time or exercise use, 15 hours of nasal oxygen per day is required
  - For most patients, a flow rate of 1–3 L achieves a Pao_2 >55 mm Hg
  - Medicare covers 80% of costs for patients who meet requirements (Table 18)
- Bronchodilators are the most important pharmacologic agents (Tables 15 and 16)
  - **Ipratropium bromide** (2–4 puffs via MDI Q 6 h) is first-line therapy, because it is longer-acting and without sympathomimetic side effects
  - Short-acting β-agonists (**albuterol, metaproterenol**) have a shorter onset of action and are less expensive
  - At maximal doses, bronchodilation of β-agonists is equivalent to ipratropium, but with side effects of tremor, tachycardia, and hypokalemia
  - Ipratropium and β-agonists together are more effective than either alone
  - Oral **theophylline** is a third-line agent for patients who fail ipratropium or β-agonists
- Corticosteroids
  - COPD is generally not steroid responsive; 10% of stable outpatients have more than a 20% increase in FEV_1 compared with placebo
- Antibiotics improve outcomes slightly when used to treat acute exacerbations
  - Regimens include tremethoprim-sulfamethoxaxole, 160/800 mg BID, amoxicillin or amoxicillin-clavulanate 500 mg TID, or doxycycline, 100 mg BID
- Opioids: severe dyspnea in spite of optimal management may warrant a trial of an opioid
- Sedative-hypnotic drugs (diazepam 5 mg TID) may benefit very anxious patients with intractable dyspnea

SURGERY

- The 1-year survival with lung transplantation is 75%, which offers substantial improvement in pulmonary function and exercise performance
- Lung volume reduction surgery in highly selected patients results in modest improvements in pulmonary function, exercise performance, and dyspnea; surgical mortality rates at experienced centers are 4–10%

THERAPEUTIC PROCEDURES

- Noninvasive positive-pressure ventilation
  - Reduces the need for intubation
  - Shortens ICU lengths of stay
  - May reduce the risk of nosocomial infection and antibiotic use
- Smoking cessation is the single most important goal
- Cough suppressants and sedatives should be avoided as routine measures
- Graded physical exercise programs
- Measure theophylline levels in hospitalized patients

OUTCOME

COMPLICATIONS

- Pulmonary hypertension, cor pulmonale, and chronic respiratory failure are common in advanced disease
- Spontaneous pneumothorax occurs in a small fraction of emphysematous patients
- Hemoptysis may result from chronic bronchitis or bronchogenic carcinoma

PROGNOSIS

- Median survival for severe disease (FEV_1 < 1 L) is 4 years
- Degree of dysfunction at presentation is the most important predictor of survival

WHEN TO REFER

- Progressive and/or severe airflow obstruction and/or symptoms
- α_1-Antitrypsin deficiency
- Large bullae

WHEN TO ADMIT

- Acute exacerbations that fail to respond to measures for ambulatory patients
- Acute respiratory failure
- Cor pulmonale or pneumothorax

PREVENTION

- Largely preventable by eliminating chronic exposure to tobacco smoke
- Smoking cessation slows the decline in FEV_1 in middle-aged smokers with mild obstructive disease
- Vaccination against influenza and pneumococcal infection

EVIDENCE

PRACTICE GUIDELINES

- National Collaborating Centre for Chronic Conditions: Chronic obstructive pulmonary disease. National clinical guideline on management of chronic obstructive pulmonary disease in adults in primary and secondary care. Thorax 2004;59(Suppl 1):1
- Sinuff T, Keenan SP: Clinical practice guideline for the use of noninvasive positive pressure ventilation in COPD patients with acute respiratory failure. J Crit Care 2004;19:82
- Pauwels RA et al: Global strategy for the diagnosis, management, and prevention of chronic obstructive pulmonary disease: National Heart, Lung, and Blood Institute and World Health Organization Global Initiative for Chronic Obstructive Lung Disease (GOLD): executive summary. Respir Care 2001;46:798

INFORMATION FOR PATIENTS

- JAMA patient page: Chronic obstructive pulmonary disease. JAMA 2003;290:2362. [PMID:14600198]
- Mayo Clinic
  - http://www.mayoclinic.com/invoke.cfm?id=DS00296

REFERENCES

- Alsaeedi A et al: The effects of inhaled corticosteriods in chronic obstructive pulmonary disease: a systemic review of randomized placebo-controlled trials. Am J Med 2002;113:59. [PMID: 12106623]
- Bach PB et al: Management of acute exacerbations of chronic obstructive pulmonary disease: a summary and appraisal of published evidence. Ann Intern Med 2001;134:600. [PMID: 11296189]
- Fishman A et al: A randomized trial comparing lung-volume reduction surgery with medical therapy for severe emphysema. N Engl J Med 2003;348:2059. [PMID: 12759479]
- Gluck O et al: Recognizing and treating glucocorticoid-induced osteoporosis in patients with pulmonary diseases. Chest 2004;125:1859. [PMID: 15136401]
- Hersh CP et al: Predictors of survival in severe, early onset COPD. Chest 2004;126:1443. [PMID: 15539711]
- Hogg JC et al: The nature of small-airway obstruction in chronic obstructive pulmonary disease. N Engl J Med 2004;350:2645. [PMID: 15215480]
- Pauwels RA et al: Global strategy for the diagnosis, management, and prevention of chronic obstructive pulmonary disease. NHLBI/WHO Global Initiative for Chronic Obstructive Lung Disease (GOLD) Workshop summary. Am J Respir Crit Care Med 2001;163:1256. [PMID: 11316667]
- Sin DD et al: Contemporary management of chronic obstructive pulmonary disease: scientific review. JAMA 2003;290:2301. [PMID: 14600189]
- Wouters EF. Management of severe COPD. Lancet 2004;364:883. [PMID: 15351196]

Author(s)

Mark S. Chesnutt, MD

Thomas J. Prendergast, MD

Churg-Strauss Syndrome p. 1056

Cirrhosis

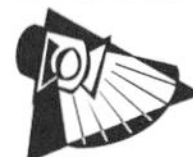

KEY FEATURES

ESSENTIALS OF DIAGNOSIS

- End result of injury that leads to both fibrosis and nodular regeneration
- Generally irreversible
- The clinical features result from hepatic cell dysfunction, portosystemic shunting, and portal hypertension

GENERAL CONSIDERATIONS

- The most common histological classification is micronodular, macronodular, and mixed forms cirrhosis. Each form may be seen at different stages of the disease

Micronodular cirrhosis

- Regenerating nodules are ≤1 mm
- Typical of alcoholic liver disease (Laennec's cirrhosis)

Macronodular cirrhosis

- Characterized by larger nodules, up to several centimeters in diameter, and may contain central veins
- Corresponds to postnecrotic (posthepatic) cirrhosis; but may not follow episodes of massive necrosis

Etiology of cirrhosis

- Chronic hepatitis C or B
- Alcoholism
- Nonalcoholic fatty liver disease
- Cryptogenic
- Metabolic, eg, hemochromatosis, α_1-antiprotease deficiency, Wilson's disease
- Primary biliary cirrhosis
- Secondary biliary cirrhosis (chronic obstruction due to stone, stricture, neoplasm)
- Congestive heart failure or constrictive pericarditis
- Other: Budd-Chiari syndrome, cystic fibrosis, autoimmune hepatitis, *Clonorchis sinensis* infection, glycogen storage disease

DEMOGRAPHICS

- Eighth leading cause of death in the United States

CLINICAL FINDINGS

SYMPTOMS AND SIGNS

- Can be asymptomatic for long periods
- Symptoms may be insidious or, less often, abrupt
- Weakness, fatigability, disturbed sleep, muscle cramps, anorexia, and weight loss are common
- Nausea and occasional vomiting
- Jaundice—usually not an initial sign—is mild at first, increasing in severity
- Abdominal pain from hepatic enlargement and stretching of Glisson's capsule or from ascites
- Hematemesis is the presenting symptom in 15–25%
- In women
  - Amenorrhea
- In men
  - Impotence, loss of libido, sterility, and gynecomastia
- In 70% of cases, the liver is enlarged and firm with a sharp or nodular edge; the left lobe may predominate
- Splenomegaly occurs in 35–50%
- Ascites, pleural effusions, peripheral edema, and ecchymoses are late findings
- Fever
  - May be a presenting symptom in up to 35%
  - Usually reflects associated alcoholic hepatitis, spontaneous bacterial peritonitis, or intercurrent infection

Encephalopathy

- Day-night reversal, asterixis, tremor, dysarthria, delirium, drowsiness
- Coma occurs late except when precipitated by an acute hepatocellular insult or gastrointestinal bleeding

Skin

- Spider nevi on the upper half of the body
- Palmar erythema, Dupuytren's contractures
- Glossitis and cheilosis from vitamin deficiencies are common
- Dilated superficial veins of the abdomen and thorax that fill from below when compressed

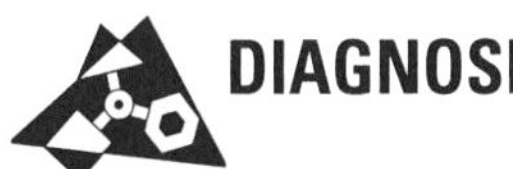

DIAGNOSIS

LABORATORY TESTS

- Laboratory abnormalities are either absent or minimal in quiescent cirrhosis
- Anemia
  - Usually macrocytic, from suppression of erythropoiesis by alcohol, folate deficiency, hypersplenism, hemolysis, and blood loss from the gastrointestinal tract
- White blood cell count
  - May be low, reflecting hypersplenism, or high, suggesting infection
- Thrombocytopenia is secondary to alcoholic marrow suppression, sepsis, folate deficiency, or splenic sequestration
- Prolongation of the prothrombin time from failure of hepatic synthesis of clotting factors
- Modest elevations of aspartate aminotransferase and alkaline phosphatase and progressive elevation of the bilirubin. Serum albumin is low; γ-globulin is increased and may be as high as in autoimmune hepatitis
- Patients with alcoholic cirrhosis may have elevated serum cardiac troponin I levels of uncertain significance
- See *Ascites* or *Peritonitis, spontaneous bacterial*

IMAGING STUDIES

- Upper gastrointestinal barium studies may show esophageal or gastric varices
- Ultrasound can assess liver size and detect ascites or hepatic nodules, including small hepatocellular carcinomas. Together with Doppler studies, it may establish patency of the splenic, portal, and hepatic veins
- Hepatic nodules can be characterized by contrast-enhanced CT scan or MRI. Nodules suspicious for malignancy may be biopsied under ultrasound or CT guidance

DIAGNOSTIC PROCEDURES

- Perform diagnostic paracentesis for new ascites
- Esophagogastroduodenoscopy confirms the presence of varices and detects specific causes of bleeding
- Liver biopsy

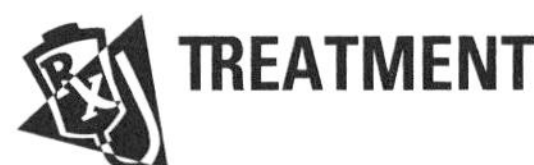

TREATMENT

MEDICATIONS

Ascites and edema

- Restrict sodium intake to 400–800 mg/day
- Restrict fluid intake (800–1000 mL/day) for hyponatremia (sodium < 125 mEq/L)
- Ascites may rapidly decrease on bed rest and dietary sodium restriction alone
- **Diuretics**
  - Use spironolactone if there is no response to salt restriction. The initial dose is 100 mg daily and may be increased by 100 mg every 3–5 days (up to a maximal conventional daily dose of 400 mg/day, though higher doses have been used) until diuresis is achieved, typically preceded by a rise in the urinary sodium concentration. Monitor for hyperkalemia
  - Substitute amiloride, 5–10 mg orally daily, if painful gynecomastia develops from spironolactone
  - Diuresis can be augmented with the addition of furosemide, 40–160 mg/day. Monitor for prerenal azotemia, blood pressure, urine output, mental status, and serum electrolytes, especially potassium

Anemia

- For iron deficiency anemia, give ferrous sulfate, 0.3 g enteric-coated tablets, PO TID after meals
- Treat macrocytic anemia associated with alcoholism with folic acid, 1 mg/day PO QD
- Packed red blood cell transfusions may be necessary to replace blood loss

Hemorrhagic tendency

- Treat severe hypoprothrombinemia with vitamin K (eg, phytonadione, 5 mg PO or SQ QD)
- When this treatment is ineffective, use large volumes of fresh frozen plasma. Because the effect is transient, plasma infusions are indicated only for active bleeding or before an invasive procedure
- Use of recombinant factor VII may be an alternative

SURGERY

- Liver transplantation is indicated in selected cases of irreversible, progressive liver disease
  - Absolute contraindications include malignancy (except small hepatocellular carcinomas in a cirrhotic liver), sepsis, and advanced cardiopulmonary disease (except pulmonary arteriovenous shunting due to portal hypertension and cirrhosis)

THERAPEUTIC PROCEDURES

- The most important principle is abstinence from alcohol
- Diet
  - Should have adequate calories (25–35 kcal/kg/day) in compensated cirrhosis and 35–40 kcal/kg/day in those with malnutrition
  - Protein should include 1.0–1.2 g/kg/day in compensated cirrhosis and 1.5 g/kg/day in those with malnutrition
  - For hepatic encephalopathy, protein intake should be reduced to 60–80 g/day
- Vitamin supplementation is desirable
- The goal of weight loss with ascites without associated peripheral edema should not exceed 0.5–0.7 kg/day
- Transjugular intrahepatic portosystemic shunt (TIPS)
  - In refractory ascites, reduces ascites recurrence and the risk of hepatorenal syndrome. Preferred to peritoneovenous shunts because of the high rate of complications from the latter
  - Increases the rate of hepatic encephalopathy compared with repeated large-volume paracentesis
  - Survival benefit has not been shown

OUTCOME

COMPLICATIONS

- Upper gastrointestinal tract bleeding from varices, portal hypertensive gastropathy, or gastroduodenal ulcer
- Hepataocellular carcinoma
- Spontaneous bacterial peritonitis
- Hepatorenal or hepatopulmonary syndrome
- Increased risk of systemic infection
- Increased risk of diabetes mellitus

PROGNOSIS

- Factors determining survival include ability to stop alcohol intake and the Child-Turcotte-Pugh class (Table 62)
- The Model for End-Stage Liver Disease (MELD) is used to determine priorities for donor livers. Hematemesis, jaundice, and ascites are unfavorable signs
- In patients with a low MELD score (< 21), a low serum sodium concentration (< 135 mEq/L) and persistent ascites predict a high mortality rate
- In established cases with severe hepatic dysfunction (serum albumin < 3 g/dL, bilirubin >3 mg/dL, ascites, encephalopathy, cachexia, and upper gastrointestinal bleeding), only 50% survive 6 months. The risk of death is associated with renal insufficiency, cognitive dysfunction, ventilatory insufficiency, age ≥65 years, and prothrombin time ≥16 s
- Liver transplantation has markedly improved survival, particularly for patients referred for evaluation early

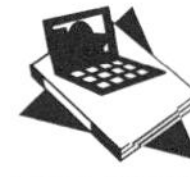

EVIDENCE

PRACTICE GUIDELINES

- Agence Nationale d'Accreditation et d'Evaluation en Sante (ANAES). Consensus conference. Treatment of hepatitis C. Gastroenterol Clin Biol 2002;26. [PMID: 12180305]
- Runyon BA: Practice Guidelines Committee, American Association for the Study of Liver Diseases (AASLD). Management of adult patients with ascites due to cirrhosis. Hepatology 2004;39:841. [PMID: 14999706]

WEB SITES

- Diseases of the Liver
  - http://cpmcnet.columbia.edu/dept/gi/cirrhosis.html
- Hepatic Pathology Index
  - http://medstat.med.utah.edu/WebPath/LIVEHTML/LIVERIDX.html

INFORMATION FOR PATIENTS

- JAMA Patient Page. Torpy JM et al: Hepatitis C. JAMA 2003;289:2450.
- Mayo Clinic
  - http://www.mayoclinic.com/invoke.cfm?objectid=810D975F-9E56-4C4C-820C7E031BC945C6

REFERENCES

- Ginés P et al: Management of cirrhosis and ascites. N Engl J Med 2004;350:1646. [PMID: 15084697]
- Hoeper MM et al: Portopulmonary hypertension and hepatopulmonary syndrome. Lancet 2004;363:1461. [PMID: 15121411]
- Runyon BA: Management of adult patients with ascites due to cirrhosis. Hepatology 2004;39:841. [PMID: 14999706]

Author(s)

Lawrence S. Friedman, MD

Cirrhosis, Primary Biliary

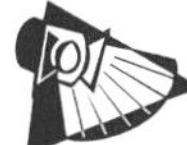

KEY FEATURES

ESSENTIALS OF DIAGNOSIS

- Middle-aged women
- Often asymptomatic
- Elevation of alkaline phosphatase, antimitochondrial antibodies (+AMA), elevated IgM, increased cholesterol
- Characteristic liver biopsy
- In later stages, can present with fatigue, jaundice, features of cirrhosis, xanthelasma, xanthomata, steatorrhea

GENERAL CONSIDERATIONS

- Chronic disease of the liver characterized by autoimmune destruction of intrahepatic bile ducts and cholestasis
- Insidious in onset, occurs usually in women aged 40–60, and is often detected by the chance finding of elevated alkaline phosphatase levels
- Infection with *Chlamydia pneumoniae* and *Novospingobium aromaticivorans* may be triggering or causative agents; viral triggers are also suspected
- Patients with a clinical and histological picture of primary biliary cirrhosis but no AMAs are said to have "autoimmune cholangitis," which has been associated with lower serum IgM levels and a greater frequency of smooth muscle and antinuclear antibodies

DEMOGRAPHICS

- Estimated incidence and prevalence rates in the United States are 4.5 and 65.4 per 100,000, respectively, in women, and 0.7 and 12.1 per 100,000, respectively, in men

CLINICAL FINDINGS

SYMPTOMS AND SIGNS

- Many are asymptomatic for years
- The onset of clinical illness is insidious and is heralded by fatigue and pruritus. With progression, physical examination reveals hepatosplenomegaly
- Xanthomatous lesions may occur in the skin and tendons and around the eyelids
- Jaundice and signs of portal hypertension are late findings
- The risk of osteoporosis is increased, as in patients with other forms of chronic liver disease

DIFFERENTIAL DIAGNOSIS

- Chronic biliary tract obstruction (stone or stricture)
- Carcinoma of the bile ducts
- Primary sclerosing cholangitis
- Sarcoidosis
- Cholestatic drug toxicity (eg, chlorpromazine)
- Chronic hepatitis
- Fascioliasis (sheep liver fluke)
- Some patients have overlapping features of primary biliary cirrhosis and autoimmune hepatitis

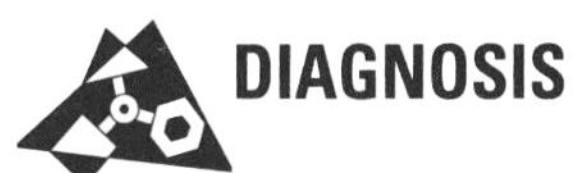

DIAGNOSIS

LABORATORY TESTS

- Blood cell counts are normal early in the disease
- Liver biochemical tests reflect cholestasis with elevation of alkaline phosphatase, cholesterol (especially high-density lipoproteins), and, in later stages, bilirubin
- AMAs (directed against pyruvate dehydrogenase or other 2-oxo-acid enzymes in mitochondria) are present in 95% of patients, and serum IgM levels are elevated

DIAGNOSTIC PROCEDURES

- Liver biopsy permits histological staging: I, portal inflammation with granulomas; II, bile duct proliferation, periportal inflammation; III, interlobular fibrous septa; and IV, cirrhosis

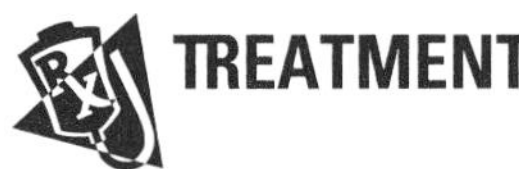

TREATMENT

MEDICATIONS

- Treatment is primarily symptomatic
- Because of its lack of toxicity, ursodeoxycholic acid (10–15 mg/kg/day in one or two doses) is the preferred medical treatment
- Colchicine (0.6 mg twice daily) and methotrexate (15 mg/week) may improve symptoms and serum levels of alkaline phosphatase and bilirubin
- Methotrexate may also improve liver histology
- Penicillamine, corticosteroids, and azathioprine are not beneficial
- Mycophenolate mofetil is under study
- For pruritis
  - Cholestyramine (4 g) or colestipol (5 g) in water or juice three times daily may be beneficial
  - Rifampin, 150–300 mg orally twice daily, is inconsistently beneficial
  - Opioid antagonists (eg, naloxone, 0.2 µg/kg/min by intravenous infusion, or naltrexone, 50 mg/day by mouth) may help
  - The 5-HT_3 serotonin receptor antagonist ondansetron may also provide some benefit
  - Plasmapheresis may be needed for refractory pruritus
- Deficiencies of vitamins A, K, and D may occur if steatorrhea is present and is aggravated when cholestyramine or colestipol is administered
- Calcium supplementation (500 mg three times daily) may help prevent osteomalacia but is of uncertain benefit in osteoporosis

SURGERY

- For patients with advanced disease, liver transplantation is the treatment of choice

OUTCOME

COMPLICATIONS

- Steatorrhea, xanthomas, xanthelasma, osteoporosis, osteomalacia, and portal hypertension
- It may be associated with Sjögren's syndrome, autoimmune thyroid disease, Raynaud's syndrome, scleroderma, hypothyroidism, and celiac disease

PROGNOSIS

- The disease is progressive
- Among asymptomatic patients, at least one-third will become symptomatic within 15 years
- Ursodeoxycholic acid treatment
  - Slows progression of the disease (particularly in early-stage disease)
  - Reduces risk of developing esophageal varices
  - Delays need for liver transplantation
  - Improves long-term survival
- Without liver transplantation, survival averages 7–10 years once symptoms develop
- In advanced disease, adverse prognostic markers are older age, high serum bilirubin, edema, low albumin, prolonged prothrombin time, and variceal hemorrhage
- The risk of hepatobiliary malignancies appears to be increased
- Liver transplantation is associated with a 1-year survival rate of 85–90%. The disease recurs in the graft in 20% of patients by 3 years, but this does not seem to affect survival

EVIDENCE

WEB SITES

- Diseases of the Liver
  - http://cpmcnet.columbia.edu/dept/gi/disliv.html
- Pathology Index
  - http://www-medlib.med.utah.edu/WebPath/LIVEHTML/LIVER-IDX.html

INFORMATION FOR PATIENTS

- National Digestive Diseases Information Clearinghouse
  - http://digestive.niddk.nih.gov/ddiseases/pubs/primarybiliarycirrhosis/index.htm
- National Institutes of Health
  - http://www.nlm.nih.gov/medlineplus/ency/article/000282.htm

REFERENCES

- Bergasa NV et al: Primary biliary cirrhosis: report of a focus study group. Hepatology 2004;40:1013. [PMID: 15382160]
- Talwalkar JA et al: Primary biliary cirrhosis. Lancet 2003;362:53. [PMID: 12853201]

Author(s)

Lawrence S. Friedman, MD

Clonorchiasis & Opisthorchiasis

Clonidine Overdose p. 1056

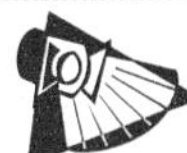

KEY FEATURES

ESSENTIALS OF DIAGNOSIS

- Clinically and epidemiologically, clonorchiasis and opisthorchiasis are identical
- Acute symptoms are fever, tender liver, urticaria, and arthralgias
- Cholangiocarcinoma has been causally linked with prolonged *Clonorchis* and *Opisthorchis* infection

GENERAL CONSIDERATIONS

- Snails become infected when they ingest clonorchiasis and opisthorchiasis eggs shed into water in human or animal feces
  - Larval forms escape from the snails, penetrate the flesh of various freshwater fish, and encyst as metacercariae
  - Fish-eating mammals—including dogs, cats, and pigs—and humans maintain the life cycle
- Human infection results from eating either raw or undercooked fish
- In humans, the ingested parasites excyst in the duodenum and ascend the bile ducts, where they mature and remain throughout their lives (15–25 years), shedding eggs in the bile
- In size, the worms are 7–20 × 1.5–3 mm
- In chronic infection, bile duct thickening, periductal fibrosis, dilation, biliary stasis, and secondary infection occcur; little fibrosis occurs in the portal tracts

DEMOGRAPHICS

- Infection by *Clonorchissinensis*, the Chinese liver fluke, is endemic in areas of Japan, Korea, China, Taiwan, Southeast Asia, and the far eastern part of Russia
- Over 20 million people are affected and in some communities prevalence is over 80%
- Opisthorchiasis is caused by worms of the genus *Opisthorchis*, generally either *O felineus* (central, eastern, and southern Europe, eastern Asia, Southeast Asia, India) or *O viverrini* (Thailand, Laos, Vietnam)

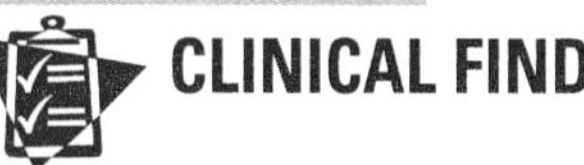

CLINICAL FINDINGS

SYMPTOMS AND SIGNS

- Most patients are asymptomatic
- Acute symptoms follow entry of immature worms into the biliary ducts and may persist for several weeks
- In acute infections, findings include
  - Malaise
  - Low-grade fever
  - An enlarged, tender liver
  - Pain in the hepatic area or epigastrium
  - Urticaria, arthralgia
  - Jaundice
- In chronic infections, findings include
  - Weakness
  - Anorexia
  - Epigastric pain
  - Diarrhea
  - Prolonged low-grade fever
  - Intermittent episodes of right upper quadrant pain
  - Localized hepatic area tenderness
  - Progressive hepatomegaly

DIFFERENTIAL DIAGNOSIS

- Opisthorchiasis (clinically identical)
- Fascioliasis (sheep liver fluke)
- Ascariasis
- Toxocariasis (visceral larva migrans)
- Echinococcosis (hydatid disease)
- Whipple's disease
- Celiac sprue or tropical sprue

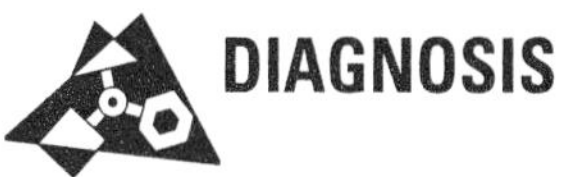

DIAGNOSIS

LABORATORY TESTS

Acute infection

- Difficult to diagnose, since ova may not appear in the feces until 3–4 weeks after onset of symptoms
- There may be leukocytosis, eosinophilia, elevated serum alanine aminotransferase, and elevated bilirubin
- Diagnosis is made by finding characteristic eggs in stools (repeated tests may be necessary) or duodenal aspirate (sensitivity approaches 100%)
- In severe infection, the number of eggs per gram of feces may not reflect the heavy worm burden; and in complete biliary obstruction, eggs can be detected in bile only by needle aspiration or at surgery

Chronic infection

- Liver function tests are normal except in severe cases
- Leukocytosis varies according to the intensity of infection; eosinophilia may be present
- In advanced chronic disease, liver function tests will indicate parenchymal damage
- The ELISA is the preferred serologic test (sensitivity, 77%); however, unless a specific monoclonal antibody is used, cross-reactions are common with other trematode and cestode infections, tuberculosis, and liver cancer

IMAGING STUDIES

- In advanced chronic disease, CT and sonography may show diffuse dilation of small intrahepatic bile ducts with no or minimal dilation of the large intrahepatic and extrahepatic ducts

DIAGNOSTIC PROCEDURES

- In advanced chronic disease, transhepatic cholangiograms may show alternating stricture and dilation of the biliary tree, with worms visualized as filling defects

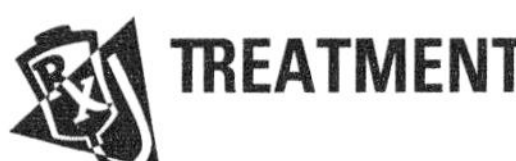

TREATMENT

MEDICATIONS

- The drug of choice is praziquantel. The dosage is 25 mg/kg three times daily for 2 days (with a 4- to 6-h interval between doses) for *Clonorchis* infections and 1 day of treatment may be sufficient for *Opisthorchis* infections
- Albendazole, at a dosage of 400 mg twice daily for 7 days, appears to be less effective (cures, 40–65%)
- In relapsing cholangitis, antibiotics are indicated to cover biliary pathogens
- In severe disease, treatment may be facilitated by endoscopic nasobiliary drainage plus antiparasitic medication

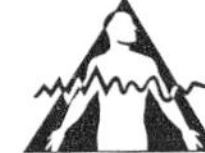

OUTCOME

COMPLICATIONS

- Intrahepatic bile duct calculi may occur that may lead to recurrent pyogenic cholangitis, biliary abscess, or endophlebitis of the portal-venous branches. This may gradually result in destruction of the liver parenchyma, fibrosis, and, rarely, cirrhosis with jaundice and ascites
- Chronic cholecystitis, cholelithiasis, and a nonfunctional, enlarged gallbladder may occur
- Flukes may enter the pancreatic duct, causing acute pancreatitis or cholelithiasis
- Cholangiocarcinoma has been causally linked with prolonged *Clonorchis* and *Opisthorchis* infection

PROGNOSIS

- Treatment cure rates over 95% can be anticipated for *Clonorchis* infections treated with praziquantel
- The disease is rarely fatal, but patients with advanced infections and impaired liver function may succumb more readily to other diseases

PREVENTION

- Pickling, smoking, or drying may not suffice to kill the metacercariae

EVIDENCE

WEB SITES

- Centers for Disease Control and Prevention—Division of Parasitic Diseases
  - http://www.cdc.gov/ncidod/dpd/parasites/clonorchis/default.htm
  - http://www.cdc.gov/ncidod/dpd/parasites/opisthorcis/default.htm

INFORMATION FOR PATIENTS

- Centers for Disease Control and Prevention
  - http://www.dpd.cdc.gov/dpdx/HTML/Clonorchiasis.htm
  - http://www.dpd.cdc.gov/dpdx/HTML/opisthorchiasis.htm

REFERENCES

- Chan HH et al: The clinical and cholangiographic picture of hepatic clonorchiasis. J Clin Gastroenterol 2002;34:183. [PMID: 11782616]
- Watanapa P et al: Liver fluke-associated cholangiocarcinoma. Br J Surg 2002;89:962. [PMID: 12153620]

Coccidioidomycosis

Clostridial Myonecrosis p. 1057. Coagulopathy of Liver Disease p. 1057.
Coal Worker's Pneumoconiosis p. 1058. Coarctation of the Aorta p. 1058.

KEY FEATURES

ESSENTIALS OF DIAGNOSIS

- Primary infection is an influenza-like illness with malaise, fever, backache, headache, and cough
- Arthralgia and periarticular swelling of knees and ankles
- Erythema nodosum common
- Dissemination may result in meningitis, bone lesions, or skin and soft tissue abscesses
- Chest x-ray varies widely from pneumonitis to cavitation
- Serologic tests useful for diagnosis
- Spherules containing endospores demonstrable in sputum or tissues

GENERAL CONSIDERATIONS

- Consider this diagnosis in any obscure illness in a patient who has been in an endemic area
- Infection results from inhalation of *Coccidioides immitis*, a mold that grows in soil of southwestern United States, Mexico, and Central and South America
- Dissemination occurs in < 1% of immunocompetent hosts, but mortality of disseminated disease is high

DEMOGRAPHICS

- Disseminated coccidioidomycosis occurs in about 0.1% of white and 1% of nonwhite patients. Filipinos and blacks and pregnant women of all races especially susceptible
- In HIV-infected people in endemic areas, coccidioidomycosis is a common opportunistic infection

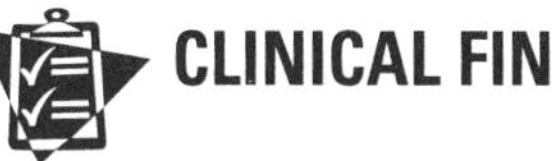

CLINICAL FINDINGS

SYMPTOMS AND SIGNS

Primary coccidioidomycosis

- Incubation period is 10–30 days
- Symptoms, usually respiratory, in 40%
- Nasopharyngitis with fever and chills; bronchitis with dry or slightly productive cough; pleuritic chest pain
- Arthralgias with periarticular swelling of knees and ankles
- Erythema nodosum 2–20 days after symptom onset
- Persistent pulmonary lesions in 5%

Disseminated coccidioidomycosis

- Can involve any organ
- Productive cough
- Enlarged mediastinal lymph nodes
- Lung abscesses, empyema
- Fungemia with diffuse miliary infiltrates on chest x-ray and early death in immunocompromised patients
- Meningitis in 30–50%
- Bone lesions at bony prominences
- Subcutaneous abscesses and verrucous skin lesions
- Lymphadenitis may progress to suppuration
- Mediastinal and retroperitoneal abscesses
- Disseminated in HIV-infected patients more often shows miliary infiltrates, lymphadenopathy, multiple organ involvement and meningitis, but skin lesions are uncommon

DIFFERENTIAL DIAGNOSIS

- Histoplasmosis, cryptococcosis, nocardiosis, blastomycosis
- Sarcoidosis
- Pneumoconiosis, eg, silicosis
- Tuberculosis
- Upper respiratory tract infection
- Atypical pneumonia
- Lymphoma (including lymphocytic interstitial pneumonitis)

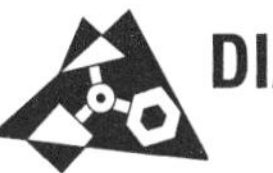

DIAGNOSIS

LABORATORY TESTS

- In primary coccidioidomycosis, moderate leukocytosis and eosinophilia
- IgM antibodies are positive in early disease
- In disseminated coccidioidomycosis, persistent or rising serum complement fixation titer (≥ 1:16); titers can be used to assess treatment adequacy
  - Complement fixation titer may be low in meningitis without other disseminated disease
  - In HIV-infected patients, complement fixation false-negative rate is as high as 30%
- In coccidioidal meningitis, cerebrospinal fluid (CSF) complement-fixing antibodies in > 90%. CSF shows increased cell count, lymphocytosis, and reduced glucose; positive culture in 30%
- Spherules filled with endospores in biopsy specimens, can be cultured
- Blood cultures rarely positive in disseminated disease

IMAGING STUDIES

- Chest x-ray film findings vary
  - Nodular infiltrates and thin-walled cavities most common
  - Hilar lymphadenopathy suggests localized disease
  - Mediastinal adenopathy suggests dissemination
  - Pleural effusions
  - Abscesses
  - Bronchiectasis
  - Lytic bone lesions

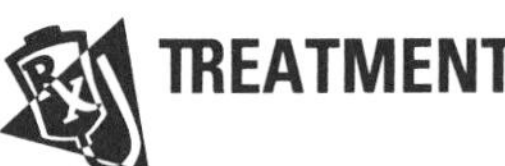

TREATMENT

MEDICATIONS

- For disease limited to the chest with no evidence of progression, symptomatic therapy
- For progressive pulmonary or extrapulmonary disease, IV amphotericin B until favorable clinical response and declining complement fixation titer
- For severe meningitis, lumbar intrathecal amphotericin B daily in increasing doses up to 1–5 mg/day, usually given with IV amphotericin B 0.6 mg/kg/day, until clinically stable. Then, taper intrathecal amphotericin to once every 6 weeks, or give oral azole therapy indefinitely
- For mild meningitis, fluconazole, 400 mg PO QD, suppresses manifestations in about 75% of patients but must be continued indefinitely, probably lifelong
- For chest, bone, and soft tissue disease, fluconazole, 200–400 mg PO QD, or itraconazole, 400 mg PO QD, continued for ≥ 6 months after disease inactive to prevent relapse

SURGERY

- Thoracic surgery is occasionally indicated for giant, infected, or ruptured cavities
- Surgical drainage useful for soft tissue abscesses and bone disease
- Following extensive surgical manipulation of infected tissue, give amphotericin B, 1 mg/kg/day IV, until disease is inactive, then change to oral azole therapy

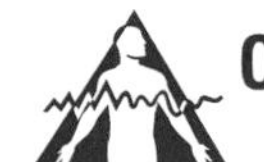

OUTCOME

FOLLOW-UP

- Follow the decrease in serum complement fixation titers
- Perform serial complement fixation titers after therapy; rising titers indicate relapse and warrant reinstitution of therapy

COMPLICATIONS

- Lung abscesses may rupture into pleural space, producing empyema, and may extend to bones, skin, and occasionally pericardium and myocardium
- Hydrocephalus may complicate chronic meningitis necessitating CSF shunting

PROGNOSIS

- Good for patients with limited disease
- Nodules, cavities, and fibrosis may rarely progress after long periods of stability or regression
- Disseminated and meningeal forms have mortality rates exceeding 50% in the absence of therapy

EVIDENCE

PRACTICE GUIDELINES

- 2001 USPHS/IDSA Guidelines for the Prevention of Opportunistic Infections in Persons Infected with Human Immunodeficiency Virus. US Department of Health and Human Services, Public Health Service
  - http://aidsinfo.nih.gov/guidelines/op_infectionsOI_112801.pdf
- Infectious Diseases Society of America—Practice guidelines for the treatment of coccidioidomycosis
  - http://www.journals.uchicago.edu/CID/journal/issues/v30n4/990665/990665.web.pdf

WEB SITE

- AIDS Info by the USDHHS
  - http://aidsinfo.nih.gov/

INFORMATION FOR PATIENTS

- Centers for Disease Control and Prevention—Coccidioidomycosis
  - http://www.cdc.gov/ncidod/dbmd/diseaseinfo/coccidioidomycosis_t.htm
- MedlinePlus
  - http://www.nlm.nih.gov/medlineplus/ency/article/001322.htm

REFERENCES

- Crum NF et al: Coccidioidomycosis: a descriptive survey of a reemerging disease. Clinical characteristics and current controversies. Medicine 2004;83:149. [PMID: 15118543]
- Galgiani JN et al: Practice guidelines for the treatment of coccidioidomycosis. Clin Infect Dis 2000;30:658. [PMID: 10770727]
- Stevens DA et al: Intrathecal amphotericin in the management of coccidioidal meningitis. Semin Respir Infect 2001;16:263. [PMID: 11739548]

Author(s)

Samuel A. Shelburne, MD

Richard J. Hamill, MD

Colitis, Antibiotic-Associated

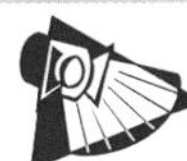

KEY FEATURES

ESSENTIALS OF DIAGNOSIS

- Most cases of antibiotic-associated diarrhea are attributable to *Clostridium difficile* and are usually mild and self-limited
- Symptoms vary from mild to fulminant
- Diagnosis in mild-to-moderate colitis is established by stool toxin assay
- Flexible sigmoidoscopy provides most rapid diagnosis in severe colitis

GENERAL CONSIDERATIONS

- Antibiotic-associated diarrhea is common
- Characteristically occurs during antibiotic exposure, is dose related, and resolves spontaneously after discontinuation
- Most cases of diarrhea are mild and self-limited and do not require evaluation or treatment
- Antibiotic-associated colitis is usually caused by *C difficile,* which colonizes 5% of healthy adults and >20% of hospitalized patients
- *C difficile*-induced colitis most often occurs in hospitalized patients who are severely ill or malnourished or receiving chemotherapy or enteral tube feedings
- *C difficile* is the major cause of diarrhea in patients hospitalized for >3 days, affecting 7 of 1000 patients
- *C difficile*-induced colitis most commonly develops after use of ampicillin, clindamycin, and third-generation cephalosporins
- Symptoms begin during or shortly after antibiotic therapy but may be delayed for up to 8 weeks

DEMOGRAPHICS

- Hospitalized or recently hospitalized patients
- Elderly or debilitated patients
- Recent antibiotic exposure
- External tube feeding
- Recent abdominal surgery

CLINICAL FINDINGS

SYMPTOMS AND SIGNS

- Mild-to-moderate greenish, foul-smelling watery diarrhea with lower abdominal cramps in most patients
- Physical examination normal, or mild left lower quadrant tenderness
- With more serious illness, abdominal pain, profuse watery diarrhea with up to 30 stools per day
- Usually low-grade fever
- Abdominal tenderness mild unless severe disease

DIFFERENTIAL DIAGNOSIS

- Antibiotic-associated diarrhea (not related to *C difficile*)
- Other drug reaction
- Diarrhea due to enteral feedings
- Ischemic colitis
- Other bacterial diarrhea
- Inflammatory bowel disease
- Rarely, other organisms (staphylococci, *Clostridium perfringens*) are associated with pseudomembranous colitis

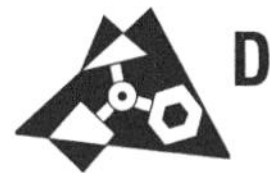

DIAGNOSIS

LABORATORY TESTS

- Mild disease: no or minimal leukocytosis
- Severe disease: leukocytosis as high as 50,000/μL
- Fecal leukocytes in only 50%
- Stool toxin cytotoxicity assay (toxin B) has sensitivity of 95% and specificity of 90%
- Rapid enzyme immunoassays (EIA) (2–4 hours) for toxins A and B have a 70–85% sensitivity with 1 stool specimen, 90% sensitivity with 2 specimens
- Culture for *C difficile* is the most sensitive test, but it is slower (2–3 days), more costly, and less specific, so is not used in most clinical settings

IMAGING STUDIES

- Abdominal radiographs: useful in detecting toxic dilation or megacolon, mucosal edema, or "thumbprinting"
- Abdominal CT: useful in detecting colonic edema

DIAGNOSTIC PROCEDURES

- Flexible sigmoidoscopy
  - May show no abnormalities or only patchy or diffuse, nonspecific colitis in mild to moderate symptoms
  - True pseudomembranous colitis (yellow adherent plaques scattered over hyperemic mucosa) evident in patients with severe illness
- Pseudomembranous colitis limited to proximal colon in 10% and therefore missed by sigmoidoscopy

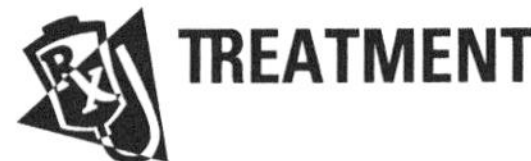

TREATMENT

MEDICATIONS

- Acute therapy
  - Metronidazole, 500 mg PO TID for 10–14 days
  - Vancomycin, 125 mg PO QID is equally effective, but more expensive, so reserved for
    - Patients who are intolerant of metronidazole
    - Pregnant women and children
    - Patients with severe disease who do not respond rapidly to metronidazole
    - Patients who fail to respond to metronidazole
- Relapse therapy
  - Vancomycin, 125 mg PO QID for 7 days; BID for 7 days; QD for 7 days; QOD for 7 days; and Q3D for 2 weeks
  - *Saccharomyces boulardii* (nonpathogenic yeast) 1 g/day for 4 weeks in combination with antibiotic reduces recurrences

SURGERY

- Total abdominal colectomy may be required in patients with toxic megacolon, perforation, sepsis, or hemorrhage

THERAPEUTIC PROCEDURES

- Discontinue offending antibiotic, if possible

OUTCOME

COMPLICATIONS

- In chronic untreated colitis
  - Weight loss
  - Protein-losing enteropathy
- In fulminant disease
  - Dehydration
  - Electrolyte imbalance
  - Toxic megacolon
  - Perforation
  - Death

PROGNOSIS

- Relapse occurs in 10–25%
- Fulminant colitis with progression to toxic megacolon:
  - High fever
  - Profound leukocytosis (>20,000/μL)
  - Diarrhea
  - Paradoxical ileus with decreased bowel movement, dilation, and thickening of colon on CT

WHEN TO REFER

- Lack of improvement after 3–5 days of therapy
- Fulminant colitis or toxic megacolon
- Multiple relapses

WHEN TO ADMIT

- Severe colitis: pain, diarrhea, dehydration, temperature >38.5°C, abdominal tenderness, leukocytosis

PREVENTION

- Fastidious hand washing and use of disposable gloves minimize transmission of *C difficile*

EVIDENCE

PRACTICE GUIDELINES

- Jabbar A et al: Gastroenteritis and antibiotic-associated diarrhea. Prim Care 2003;30:63. [PMID:12825250]

INFORMATION FOR PATIENTS

- Mayo Clinic
  - http://www.mayoclinic.com/invoke.cfm?id=DS00454
- Merck Manual
  - http://www.merck.com/mmhe/sec09/ch127/ch127a.html?alt=pf?qt=antibiotic%20associated%20colitis&alt=sh

REFERENCES

- Antibiotic-associated diarrhea. N Engl J Med 2002;346:334. [PMID: 11821511]
- Brickes E et al: Antibiotic treatment for *Clostridium difficile*-associated diarrhea in adults. Cochrane Database Syst Rev 2005;(1) CD004610. [PMID: 15674956]

Author(s)

Kenneth R. McQuaid, MD

Colonic Pseudoobstruction, Acute (Ogilvie's Syndrome)

Colitis, Microscopic p. 1059

KEY FEATURES

ESSENTIALS OF DIAGNOSIS

- Severe abdominal distention
- Massive dilation of cecum or right colon
- Arises in postoperative state or with severe medical illness
- May be precipitated by electrolyte imbalances, medications
- Absent to mild abdominal pain; minimal tenderness

GENERAL CONSIDERATIONS

- Spontaneous massive dilation of the cecum and proximal colon in hospitalized patients
- Progressive cecal dilation may lead to spontaneous perforation
- Etiology unknown
- Associated conditions
  - Trauma, burns
  - Respiratory failure
  - Malignancy
  - Myocardial infarction or CHF
  - Pancreatitis
  - Stroke or subarachnoid hemorrhage
  - Ischemic colitis
  - Use of drugs, eg, opioids, anticholinergics

DEMOGRAPHICS

- Occurs mainly in hospitalized patients with recent trauma, surgery (especially cardiothoracic), or severe medical illness
- May be precipitated by electrolyte imbalance or narcotics

CLINICAL FINDINGS

SYMPTOMS AND SIGNS

- Sometimes asymptomatic
- Constant but mild abdominal pain
- Nausea and vomiting
- Abdominal distention
- Bowel movements may be absent in up to 40%. Flatus or stool continues to pass
- Abdominal tenderness with some degree of guarding or rebound tenderness; however, signs of peritonitis absent unless perforation has occurred
- Fever suggests colonic perforation

DIFFERENTIAL DIAGNOSIS

- Mechanical colonic obstruction, eg, malignancy, diverticulitis, volvulus, fecal impaction
- Toxic megacolon due to inflammatory bowel disease or *Clostridium difficile* colitis, cytomegalovirus

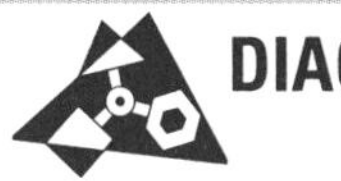

DIAGNOSIS

LABORATORY TESTS

- Obtain complete blood cell count, serum sodium, potassium, magnesium, phosphorus, and calcium
- Leukocytosis suggests colonic perforation

IMAGING STUDIES

- Plain film radiographs demonstrate colonic dilation, usually cecum and proximal colon
- Varying amounts of small intestinal dilation and air-fluid levels
- Cecal diameter >10–12 cm associated with increased risk of colonic perforation

DIAGNOSTIC PROCEDURES

- Hypaque (diatrizoate meglumine) enema to exclude colonic obstruction and to decompress the colon and evacuate distal fecal material

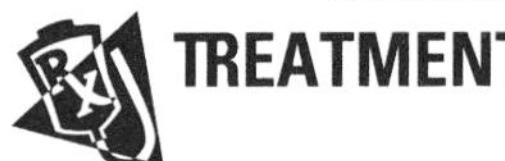

TREATMENT

MEDICATIONS

- Discontinue opioids, anticholinergics, and calcium channel blockers, if possible
- Correct electrolyte abnormalities
- Oral laxatives are not helpful and may cause perforation
- In patients with sustained or progressive cecal dilation to ≥10–12 cm and in those with signs of clinical deterioration, administering neostigmine, 2 mg IV as a single dose, results in rapid (within 30 minutes) colonic decompression in 75–90%

THERAPEUTIC PROCEDURES

- Treat underlying illness
- Conservative treatment is recommended if no or minimal abdominal tenderness, no fever, no leukocytosis, and a cecal diameter < 12 cm
- Place a nasogastric tube and a rectal tube
- Roll patients periodically from side to side
- Enemas if large amounts of stool on radiography
- Conservative treatment successful in >80%
- Colonoscopic decompression in patients who fail to respond to neostigmine, successful in up to 90%; dilation recurs in up to 50%

SURGERY

- In patients in whom colonoscopy is unsuccessful, a tube cecostomy placed through a small laparotomy or percutaneously with radiologic guidance can decompress the colon

OUTCOME

FOLLOW-UP

- Watch for signs of worsening distention or abdominal tenderness
- Assess cecal size by abdominal radiographs every 12 hours
- Cardiac monitoring after neostigmine for possible bradycardia that may require atropine administration

COMPLICATIONS

- Colonic perforation

PROGNOSIS

- Prognosis related to the underlying illness
- With aggressive therapy, perforation unusual

WHEN TO REFER

- Failure to improve within 24 hours of conservative therapy
- Signs of perforation

WHEN TO ADMIT

- Usually occurs in hospitalized patients

EVIDENCE

PRACTICE GUIDELINES

- Cappell MS et al: The role of sigmoidoscopy and colonoscopy in the diagnosis and management of lower gastrointestinal disorders: endoscopic findings, therapy, and complications. Med Clin North Am 2002;86:1253. [PMID: 12510454]
- Eisen GM et al: Standards of Practice Committee of the American Society for Gastrointestinal Endoscopy. Acute colonic pseudo-obstruction. Gastrointest Endosc 2002;56:789. [PMID:12447286]

INFORMATION FOR PATIENTS

- MEDLINEplus—Primary or idiopathic intestinal pseudo-obstruction
  - http://www.nlm.nih.gov/medlineplus/ency/article/000253.htm
- NIDDK/NIH—Intestinal pseudo-obstruction
  - http://digestive.niddk.nih.gov/ddiseases/pubs/intestinalpo/index.htm

REFERENCES

- Eisen GM et al: Acute colonic pseudo-obstruction. Gastrointest Endosc 2002;56:789. [PMID:12447286]
- Kahi CJ et al: Bowel obstruction and pseudo-obstruction. Gastroenterol Clin North Am 2003; 32:1229. [PMID: 14696305]
- Loftus C et al: Assessment of predictors of response to neostigmine for acute colonic pseudo-obstruction. Am J Gastroenterol 2002;97:3118. [PMID:12492198]

Author(s)

Kenneth R. McQuaid, MD

Colorectal Cancer

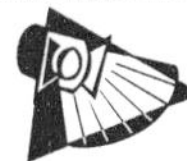

KEY FEATURES

ESSENTIALS OF DIAGNOSIS

- Symptoms or signs depend on tumor location
- Proximal colon: fecal occult blood, anemia
- Distal colon: change in bowel habits, hematochezia
- Characteristic findings on barium enema or CT colonography
- Diagnosis established with colonoscopy and biopsy

GENERAL CONSIDERATIONS

- Almost all colon cancers are adenocarcinomas
- ~50% occur distal to the splenic flexure (descending rectosigmoid) within reach of detection by flexible sigmoidoscopy
- Most colorectal cancers arise from malignant transformation of an adenomatous polyp
- Up to 5% of colorectal cancers are caused by inherited autosomal dominant germline mutations resulting in polyposis syndromes or hereditary nonpolyposis colorectal cancer
- Risk factors
  - Age
  - History of colorectal cancer or adenomatous polyps, breast, uterine, or ovarian cancer
  - Family history of colorectal cancer
  - Inflammatory bowel disease (ulcerative colitis and Crohn's colitis)
  - Diets rich in fats and red meat
  - Race (higher risk in blacks than in whites)

DEMOGRAPHICS

- Second leading cause of death due to malignancy in the United States
- ~ 6% of Americans will develop colorectal cancer and 40% of those will die of the disease
- ~134,000 new cases and 55,000 deaths occur annually in the United States

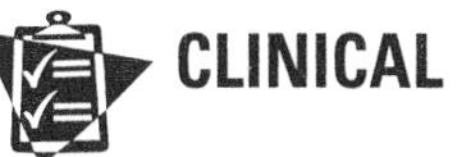

CLINICAL FINDINGS

SYMPTOMS AND SIGNS

- Adenocarcinomas grow slowly and may be asymptomatic
- Symptoms depend on the location of the cancer
- Right-sided colon cancers cause
  - Iron deficiency anemia
  - Fatigue
  - Weakness from chronic blood loss
- Left-sided colon cancers cause
  - Obstructive symptoms
  - Colicky abdominal pain
  - Change in bowel habits
  - Constipation alternating with loose stools
  - Stool streaked with blood
- Rectal cancers cause
  - Rectal tenesmus
  - Urgency
  - Recurrent hematochezia
- Physical examination usually normal, except in advanced disease: mass may be palpable in the abdomen
- Hepatomegaly suggests metastatic spread

DIFFERENTIAL DIAGNOSIS

- Diverticulosis or diverticulitis
- Hemorrhoids
- Adenomatous polyps
- Ischemic colitis
- Inflammatory bowel disease
- Irritable bowel syndrome
- Infectious colitis
- Iron deficiency due to other cause

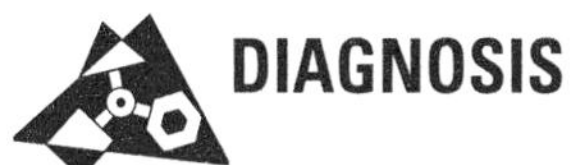

DIAGNOSIS

LABORATORY TESTS

- Complete blood cell count may reveal iron deficiency anemia
- Liver function tests elevated in metastatic disease
- Fecal occult blood tests positive
- Carcinoembryonic antigen (CEA) level elevated in 70%, should normalize after complete surgical resection

IMAGING STUDIES

- Barium enema or CT colonography ("virtual colonoscopy") for initial diagnosis, if colonoscopy not available
- Abdominal and chest CT scan for preoperative staging
- Pelvic MRI and endorectal ultrasonography may guide operative management of rectal cancer

DIAGNOSTIC PROCEDURES

- Colonoscopy is the diagnostic procedure of choice because it visualizes the whole colon and permits biopsy of lesions
- Staging by TNM system correlates with the patient's long-term survival, used to determine which patients should receive adjuvant therapy (Table 56)

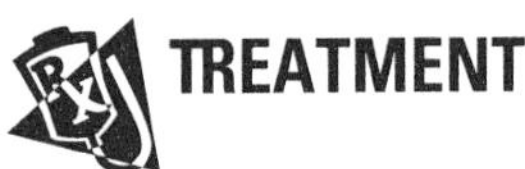

TREATMENT

MEDICATIONS

- Postoperative adjuvant chemotherapy with fluorouracil and leucovorin (± oxaliplatin) for 6 months for stage III disease improves 5-year disease-free survival rate to 65%
- Combination therapy with fluorouracil, leucovorin, and either oxaliplatin or irinotecan for stage IV disease yields tumor response rate of 40% and increases overall survival (mean 17–20 months)
- Monoclonal antibodies to endothelial growth factor (bevacizumab) and epidermal growth factor receptor (cetuximab) demonstrate further improvement in tumor response rates for stage IV disease

SURGERY

- Resection of the primary colonic or rectal cancer
- Regional lymph node removal to determine staging
- For rectal carcinoma, in selected patients, transanal excision
- For all other patients with rectal cancer, low anterior resection with a colorectal anastomosis or an abdominoperineal resection with a colostomy
- For unresectable rectal cancer, diverting colostomy, laser fulguration, or placement of an expandable wire stent
- For metastatic disease, resection of isolated (1 to 3) liver or lung metastases

THERAPEUTIC PROCEDURES

- Radiation therapy used for selected patients with locally advanced (T3 or T4) colon cancer
- Combined preoperative or postoperative adjuvant pelvic radiation and chemotherapy with fluorouracil for both stage II and stage III rectal cancers
- Local ablative techniques (cryosurgery, embolization) for unresectable hepatic metastases

OUTCOME

FOLLOW-UP

- After resection surgery, patients should be evaluated every 3–6 months for 3–5 years with history, physical examination, fecal occult blood testing, liver function tests, and CEA determinations
- A rise in CEA level that had normalized initially after surgery is suggestive of cancer recurrence
- Colonoscopy within 6–12 months and then every 3–5 years
- Change in the patient's clinical picture, abnormal liver function tests, or a rising CEA level warrant chest radiography and abdominal CT

PROGNOSIS

- 5-year survival rates:
  - Stage I: 80–100%, even with no adjuvant therapy
  - Stage II (node-negative disease), 50–75%, with no adjuvant therapy, although patients with advanced local stage II disease (T3–T4) should be considered for study protocols of adjuvant chemotherapy or radiotherapy
  - Stage III (node-positive disease), 30–50%, improved by postoperative adjuvant chemotherapy
- Long-term survival rates:
  - Stage I, >90%
  - Stage II, >70%
  - Stage III with fewer than four positive lymph nodes, 67%
  - Stage III with more than four positive lymph nodes, 33%
  - Stage IV, < 5%
- For each stage, rectal cancers have a worse prognosis
- Tumors that have microsatellite instability have a more favorable prognosis
- Tumors that have chromosomal instability (detection or loss of heterozygosity of one or more tumor suppressor genes [eg, *APC, p 53, DC2*]) have better response to adjuvant chemotherapy

PREVENTION

- Screening for colorectal neoplasms should be offered to every patient age >50 (Table 57)
- Chemoprevention: prolonged regular use of aspirin and other nonsteroidal antiinflammatory drugs may decrease the risk of colorectal neoplasia; however, routine use as chemotherapeutic agent not recommended currently

EVIDENCE

PRACTICE GUIDELINES

- National Guideline Clearinghouse
  - http://www.guideline.gov/summary/summary.aspx?doc_id=3057&nbr=2283&string=colorectal+AND+cancer
  - http://www.guideline.gov/summary/summary.aspx?doc_id=4006&nbr=3135&string=colorectal+AND+cancer
  - http://www.guideline.gov/summary/summary.aspx?doc_id=5655&nbr=3798&string=colorectal+AND+cancer
- Practice parameters for colon cancer. Dis Colon Rectum 2004;47:1269. [PMID: 15484340]
  - http://www.fascrs.org/
- Screening for colorectal cancer: recommendations and rationale. United States Preventive Services Task Force, 2002
  - http://www.ahrq.gov/clinic/3rduspstf/colorectal/
- Winawer S et al: American Gastroenterological Association. Colorectal cancer screening and surveillance: clinical guideline and rationale—update based on new evidence. Gastroenterology 2003;124:544. [PMID: 12557158]

WEB SITES

- WebPath Gastrointestinal Pathology Index
  - http://medstat.med.utah.edu/WebPath/GIHTML/GIIDX.html

INFORMATION FOR PATIENTS

- JAMA patient page: Colon cancer screening. JAMA 2003;289:1334
- Medline Plus
  - http://www.nlm.nih.gov/medlineplus/colorectalcancer.html
- National Cancer Institute
  - http://cancernet.nci.nih.gov/cancertopics/types/colon-and-rectal

REFERENCES

- Andre T et al: Oxaliplatin, fluorouracil, and leucovorin as adjuvant treatment for colon cancer. N Engl J Med 2004;350:2343. [PMID: 15175436]
- Pfister DG et al: Clinical practice. Surveillance strategies after curative treatment of colorectal cancer. N Engl J Med 2004;350:2375. [PMID: 15175439]
- Screening for colorectal cancer: recommendations and rationale. Ann Intern Med 2002;137:129. [PMID:11821507]
- Walsh JM et al: Colorectal cancer screening. Scientific review. JAMA 2003;289:1288. [PMID: 12633191]
- Walsh JM et al: Colorectal cancer screening. Clinical applications. JAMA 2003;289:1297. [PMID: 12633192]
- Weitz J et al: Colorectal cancer. Lancet 2005;365:153. [PMID 15639298]

Author(s)

Kenneth R. McQuaid, MD

Common Variable Immunodeficiency

Colorectal Cancer, Hereditary Nonpolyposis p. 1059

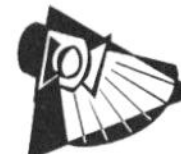

KEY FEATURES

ESSENTIALS OF DIAGNOSIS

- Defect in terminal differentiation of B cells, with absent plasma cells and deficient synthesis of secreted antibody
- Increased susceptibility to pyogenic infections—frequent sinopulmonary infections
- Confirmation by evaluation of serum immunoglobulin levels and deficient functional antibody responses

GENERAL CONSIDERATIONS

- A heterogeneous immunodeficiency disorder clinically characterized by an increased incidence of recurrent infections, autoimmune phenomena, and neoplastic diseases
- The most common cause of panhypogammaglobulinemia in adults
- The onset is usually during adolescence or early adulthood but can occur at any age
- Paradoxically, there is an increased incidence of autoimmune disease (20%), though patients may not display the usual serological markers
- Gastrointestinal disorders are commonly associated

DEMOGRAPHICS

- The prevalence is about 1:80,000 in the United States

CLINICAL FINDINGS

SYMPTOMS AND SIGNS

- Increased susceptibility to pyogenic infections
- Most patients suffer from recurrent sinusitis
- Bronchitis, otitis, pharyngitis, and pneumonia are also common
- Autoimmune disease
- Sprue-like syndrome, with diarrhea, steatorrhea, malabsorption, protein-losing enteropathy, and hepatosplenomegaly
- Lymphadenopathy
- Increased incidence of cancers—lymphoma, gastric, and skin

DIFFERENTIAL DIAGNOSIS

- Secondary immunodeficiency, eg, AIDS, corticosteroid use, leukemia
- Selective IgA deficiency
- Multiple myeloma
- Cystic fibrosis
- Asplenism
- Celiac sprue
- Systemic lupus erythematosus
- X-linked agammaglobulinemia
- Immunodeficiency with thymoma
- Wegener's granulomatosis

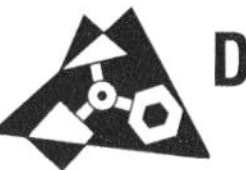

DIAGNOSIS

LABORATORY TESTS

- The pattern of immunoglobulin isotype deficiency is variable
- Typically present with significantly depressed IgG levels (usually less than 250 mg/dL), but over time all antibody classes (IgG, IgA, and IgM) may decrease
- Decreased to absent functional antibody responses to protein antigen immunizations establish the diagnosis
- Autoimmune cytopenias are common

DIAGNOSTIC PROCEDURES

- Biopsies of enlarged lymph nodes show marked reduction in plasma cells
- Noncaseating granulomas are frequently found in the spleen, liver, lungs, or skin

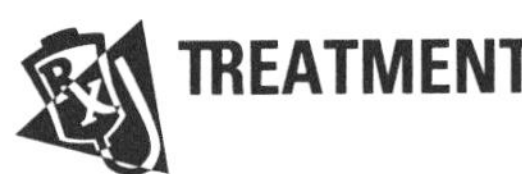

TREATMENT

MEDICATIONS

- Antibiotics at the first sign of infection; since antibody deficiency predisposes to high-risk pyogenic infections, antibiotic should cover encapsulated bacteria
- Monthly intravenous immune globulin (IGIV) is effective in decreasing the incidence of potentially life-threatening infections and increasing quality of life

OUTCOME

FOLLOW-UP

- Quarterly until "trough" immunoglobulin levels stabilize within age-adjusted "normal range"; semiannually thereafter for assessment of quantitative immunoglobulin levels and clinical assessment

COMPLICATIONS

- Infections may be of prolonged duration or associated with unusual complications such as meningitis or sepsis
- There is an increased propensity for the development of B cell neoplasms (50- to 400-fold increased risk of lymphoma), gastric carcinomas, and skin cancers

PROGNOSIS

- Good to excellent with monthly replacement immunoglobulin therapy

WHEN TO REFER

- Refer to confirm the need for intravenous immune globulin
- May need early referral to an infectious disease specialist for severe or prolonged infections
- May need referral to a medical oncologist for staging and treatment of cancer

WHEN TO ADMIT

- For severe or rapidly progressive infections

EVIDENCE

WEB SITES

- American Academy of Allergy, Asthma, and Immunology
  - http://www.aaaai.org
- Immune Deficiency Foundation
  - http://www.primaryimmune.org

INFORMATION FOR PATIENTS

- National Institutes of Health: Primary Immune Deficiency
  - http://www.niaid.nih.gov/factsheets/pid.htm#common
- National Primary Immunodeficiency Resource Center: Common Variable Immunodeficiency
  - http://www.info4pi.org/patienttopatient/index.cfm?section=patienttopatient&content=syndromes&area=4&CFID=3169571&CFTOKEN=2854607
- National Primary Immunodeficiency Resource Center: FAQ's
  - http://npi.jmfworld.org/faq/index.cfm?section=faq&CFID=3169571&CFTOKEN=2854607

REFERENCES

- Giannouli S et al: Autoimmune manifestations in common variable immunodeficiency. Clin Rheumatol 2004;23:449. [PMID: 15278751]
- Sneller MC: Common variable immunodeficiency. Am J Med Sci 2001;321:42. [PMID: 11202479]
- Tcheurekdjian H et al: Quality of life in common variable immunodeficiency requiring intravenous immunoglobulin therapy. Ann Allergy Asthma Immunol 2004;93:160. [PMID: 15328676]

Author(s)

Jeffrey L. Kishiyama, MD
Daniel C. Adelman, MD

Congestive Heart Failure

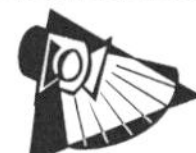

KEY FEATURES

ESSENTIALS OF DIAGNOSIS

- Left ventricular (LV) congestive heart failure (CHF): exertional dyspnea, cough, fatigue, orthopnea, paroxysmal nocturnal dyspnea, cardiac enlargement, rales, gallop rhythm, and pulmonary venous congestion
- Right ventricular (RV) CHF: elevated venous pressure, hepatomegaly, dependent edema; usually due to LV failure

GENERAL CONSIDERATIONS

- CHF occurs as a result of depressed contractility with fluid retention and/or impaired cardiac output, or diastolic dysfunction with fluid retention
- Acute exacerbations of chronic CHF are caused by patient nonadherence to or alterations in therapy, excessive salt and fluid intake, arrhythmias, excessive activity, pulmonary emboli, intercurrent infection, or progression of the underlying disease
- High-output CHF is caused by thyrotoxicosis, beriberi, severe anemia, arteriovenous shunting, and Paget's disease
- Systolic dysfunction is caused by myocardial infarction (MI), ethanol abuse, long-standing hypertension, viral myocarditis (including HIV), Chagas' disease, and idiopathic dilated cardiomyopathy
- Diastolic dysfunction is associated with abnormal filling of a ("stiff") left ventricle; it is caused by chronic hypertension, LV hypertrophy, and diabetes

CLINICAL FINDINGS

SYMPTOMS AND SIGNS

- Symptoms of diastolic dysfunction are often difficult to distinguish clinically from those of systolic dysfunction
- LV CHF: exertional dyspnea progressing to orthopnea and then dyspnea at rest
- Paroxysmal nocturnal dyspnea
- Chronic nonproductive cough (often worse in recumbency)
- Nocturia
- Fatigue and exercise intolerance
- RV CHF: anorexia, nausea, and right upper quadrant pain due to chronic passive congestion of the liver and gut
- Tachycardia, hypotension, reduced pulse pressure, cold extremities, and diaphoresis
- Long-standing severe CHF: cachexia or cyanosis
- Physical examination in LV CHF: crackles at lung bases, pleural effusions and basilar dullness to percussion, expiratory wheezing, and rhonchi; parasternal lift, an enlarged and sustained LV impulse, a diminished first heart sound; S_3 gallop; S_4 gallop in diastolic dysfunction
- RV CHF: elevated jugular venous pressure, abnormal pulsations, such as regurgitant *v* waves; tender or nontender hepatic enlargement, heptojugular reflux, and ascites; peripheral pitting edema sometimes extending to the thighs and abdominal wall

DIFFERENTIAL DIAGNOSIS

- Chronic obstructive pulmonary disease (COPD)
- Pneumonia
- Cirrhosis
- Peripheral venous insufficiency
- Nephrotic syndrome

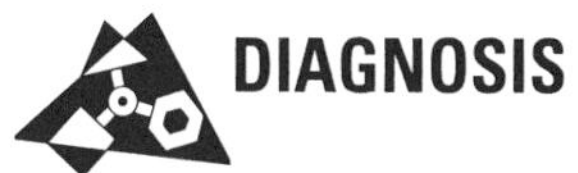

DIAGNOSIS

LABORATORY TESTS

- Obtain complete blood cell count, blood urea nitrogen, serum electrolytes, creatinine, thyroid-stimulating hormone
- ECG: arrhythmia, MI, or nonspecific changes including low-voltage, intraventricular conduction delay, LV hypertrophy, and repolarization changes
- "B-type" natriuretic peptide (BNP) elevation is a sensitive indicator of symptomatic (diastolic or systolic) CHF but may be less specific, especially in older patients, women, and patients with COPD

IMAGING STUDIES

- Chest x-ray: cardiomegaly, dilation of the upper lobe veins, perivascular or interstitial edema, alveolar fluid, and bilateral or right-sided pleural effusions
- Echocardiography: to assess ventricular size and function, valvular abnormalities, pericardial effusions, intracardiac shunts, and segmental wall motion abnormalities
- Radionuclide angiography: measures LV ejection fraction and assesses regional wall motion
- Stress imaging: ECG abnormalities or suspected myocardial ischemia

DIAGNOSTIC PROCEDURES

- ECG: rule out valvular lesions, myocardial ischemia, arrhythmias, alcohol- or drug-induced myocardial depression, intracardiac shunts, high-output states, hyperthyroidism and hypothyroidism, medications, hemochromatosis, sarcoidosis, and amyloidosis
- Left heart catheterization: to exclude significant valvular disease and to delineate presence and extent of coronary artery disease
- Right heart catheterization: to select and monitor therapy in patients not responding to standard therapy

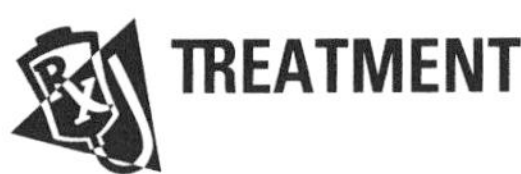

TREATMENT

MEDICATIONS

- Systolic dysfunction: a diuretic and an angiotensin-converting enzyme (ACE) inhibitor (or angiotensin receptor blocker in ACE-intolerant patients) with subsequent addition of a β-blocker
- Diuretics (Table 46): thiazide, loop, thiazide and loop, or thiazide and spironolactone
- Aldosterone blockers: spironolactone 25 mg QD; may decrease to 12.5 mg or increase to 50 mg depending on renal function, K^+, and symptoms
- ACE inhibitors (Table 48), started at low doses and titrated to dosages proved effective in clinical trials (eg, captopril 50 mg PO TID, enalapril 10 mg PO BID, lisinopril 10 mg PO QD) over 1–3 months
- Angiotensin receptor blockers (Table 48) for ACE-intolerant patients
- β-Blockers (Table 47): in stable patients, started at low doses and titrated gradually and with great care, eg, carvedilol started at 3.125 mg PO BID, increased to 6.25, 12.5, and 25 mg BID at intervals of ~2 weeks, or extended-release metoprolol, starting at 12.5 or 25 mg once daily and increasing to 50, 75, 100, 150, and 200 mg at 2-week or longer intervals
- Digoxin
- Positive inotropic agents (eg, dobutamine and milrinone): use limited to patients with hypoperfusion, rapidly deteriorating renal function, failed response to intravenous diuretics, and awaiting cardiac transplantation
- Anticoagulation: for patients with LV CHF associated with atrial fibrillation or large recent (within 3–6 months) MI
- Diastolic dysfunction: diuretics, rigorous blood pressure control

SURGERY

- Coronary revascularization may improve symptoms and prevent progression
- Bypass surgery provides more complete revascularization than angioplasty
- Cardiac transplantation for advanced heart failure
- Implantable defibrillators for chronic heart failure and ischemic or nonischemic cardiomyopathy with ejection fraction < 35%
- Biventricular pacing (resynchronization) for patients with moderate to severe systolic CHF and LV dyssynchrony

THERAPEUTIC PROCEDURES

- Moderate salt restriction (2–2.5 g sodium or 5–6 g salt per day)
- Temporary restriction of activity

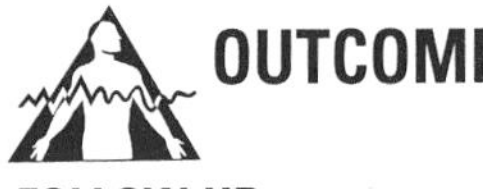

OUTCOME

FOLLOW-UP

- Monitor patients taking diuretics and ACE inhibitors for hypokalemia, renal failure
- Case management, home monitoring of weight and clinical status, and patient adjustment of diuretics can prevent rehospitalizations

COMPLICATIONS

- Myocardial ischemia in patients with underlying coronary artery disease
- Asymptomatic and symptomatic arrhythmias, especially nonsustained ventricular tachycardia
- Sudden death and unexplained syncope

PROGNOSIS

- Poor prognosis, with annual mortality rates ~5% in stable patients with mild symptoms to ~30–50% in patients with advanced, progressive symptoms
- Poorer prognosis with severe LV dysfunction (ejection fractions < 20%), nonsustained ventricular tachycardia, major limitation of exercise capacity, secondary renal insufficiency, hyponatremia, and elevated plasma catecholamine levels
- 30–50% of hospitalized patients will be readmitted within 3–6 months
- Posttransplant 1-year survival rate ≥ 80–90%, and 5-year survival rate ≥ 70%

PREVENTION

- Antihypertensive therapy
- Antihyperlipidemic therapy
- Treat valvular lesions early (aortic stenosis and mitral and aortic regurgitation)

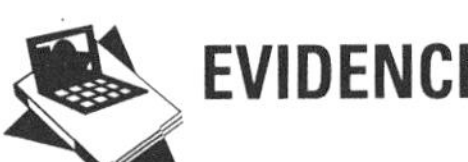

EVIDENCE

PRACTICE GUIDELINES

- ACC/AHA guidelines for the evaluation and management of chronic heart failure in the adult, 2001.
  - http://www.acc.org/clinical/guidelines/failure/pdfs/hf_fulltext.pdf
- Liu P et al: Canadian Cardiovascular Society. The 2002/3 Canadian Cardiovascular Society consensus guideline update for the diagnosis and management of heart failure. Can J Cardiol 2003;19:347. [PMID: 12704478]

WEB SITES

- National Heart, Lung, and Blood Institute
  - http://www.nhlbi.nih.gov/
- American College of Cardiology
  - http://www.acc.org/

INFORMATION FOR PATIENTS

- National Heart, Lung, and Blood Institute: Heart Failure
  - http://www.nhlbi.nih.gov/health/dci/Diseases/Hf/HF_WhatIs.html
- American Heart Association: Heart Failure
  - http://www.americanheart.org/presenter.jhtml?identifier=1486
- MedlinePlus: Congestive Heart Failure Interactive Tutorial
  - http://www.nlm.nih.gov/medlineplus/tutorials/congestiveheartfailure/htm/index.htm
- American Academy of Family Physicians: Heart Failure
  - http://familydoctor.org/119.xml

REFERENCES

- Angeja BG et al: Evaluation and management of diastolic heart failure. Circulation 2003;107:659. [PMID: 12578862]
- Bardy GH: Sudden Cardiac Death in Heart Failure (SCD-Heft) Investigators: Amiodarone or an implantable cardioverter-defibrillator for congestive heart failure. N Engl J Med 2005;352:225. [PMID: 15659722]
- Bristow MR et al: Comparison of Medical Therapy, Pacing, and Defibrillation in Heart Failure (COMPANION) Investigators: Cardiac-resynchronization therapy with or without an implantable defibrillator in advanced congestive heart failure. N Engl J Med 2004;350:2140. [PMID: 15152059]
- Brozena SC et al: The new staging system for heart failure. What every primary care physician should know. Geriatrics 2003;58:31. [PMID: 12813870]
- Cleland JG et al: The effect of cardiac resynchronization on morbidity and mortality in heart failure. N Engl J Med 2005;352:1539. [PMID: 15753115]
- Maisel AS et al: Rapid measurement of B-type natriuretic peptide in the emergency diagnosis of heart failure. N Engl J Med 2002;347:161. [PMID: 12124404]

Author(s)

Thomas M. Bashore, MD

Christopher B. Granger, MD

Conjunctivitis

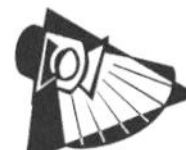

KEY FEATURES

ESSENTIALS OF DIAGNOSIS

- The most common eye disease, also known as "pink eye"
- Diffuse redness of the bulbar and tarsal conjunctiva
- Usually mild to moderate ocular irritation and discharge, clear cornea, and normal visual acuity

GENERAL CONSIDERATIONS

- Usually due to bacterial (including gonococcal or chlamydial) or viral infections
- Other common causes include atopy, chemical irritants, and keratoconjunctivitis sicca (dry eyes)
- Mode of transmission of infectious conjunctivitis is usually direct contact via fingers, towels, etc to the other eye, or to other persons
- Clinically important to differentiate conjunctivitis from acute uveitis, acute glaucoma, and corneal disorders

DEMOGRAPHICS

- Precise incidence is unknown, but very common
- Men and women affected equally
- Age group affected depends on the underlying cause
- Trachoma (*Chlamydia trachomatis*) is a major cause of blindness worldwide
- Gonococcal conjunctivitis and inclusion conjunctivitis (*C trachomatis*) are caused by the agents involved in the respective genital tract diseases and typically occur in sexually active adults
- Viral conjunctivitis is more common in children than adults, with contaminated swimming pools or ophthalmologists' offices often being the source of epidemics
- Keratoconjunctivitis sicca is common in elderly women and sometimes associated with systemic diseases (Sjögren's syndrome)
- Allergic eye disease typically begins in late childhood or young adulthood and usually in people with atopy

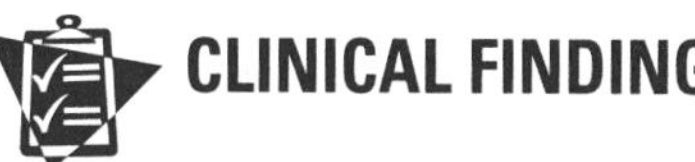

CLINICAL FINDINGS

SYMPTOMS AND SIGNS

Bacterial conjunctivitis

- Staphylococci, streptococci, *Haemophilus, Pseudomonas,* and *Moraxella* are the most common organisms isolated
- Purulent discharge
- Usually self-limited, lasting 10–14 days if untreated

Gonococcal conjunctivitis

- Exposure to infected genital secretions is the usual mode of transmission
- Copious purulent discharge
- An ophthalmologic emergency because corneal involvement may rapidly lead to perforation and blindness

Chlamydial conjunctivitis

- Trachoma usually causes recurrent conjunctivitis and epithelial keratitis during childhood leading to corneal scarring in adulthood
- Inclusion conjunctivitis produces follicular conjunctivitis with redness, discharge, and irritation, and nontender preauricular lymphadenopathy

Viral conjunctivitis

- Adenoviruses are the most common causative agents
- Copious watery discharge with severe ocular irritation and possibly visual loss due to keratitis
- Subconjunctival hemorrhages occasionally occur
- There may be pharyngitis, fever, malaise, and preauricular lymphadenopathy

Keratoconjunctivitis sicca

- Due to hypofunction of the lacrimal glands, excessive evaporation of tears, abnormalities of the lipid component of tears, or mucin deficiency
- Ocular dryness, redness, or foreign body sensation
- Marked discomfort, photophobia, and excessive mucus in severe cases
- Corneal ulceration may develop

Allergic eye disease

- Itching is strongly suggestive of allergic eye disease
- Allergic conjunctivitis is a benign disease characterized by conjunctival hyperemia and edema, often of sudden onset, that may be seasonal (hay fever conjunctivitis) or perennial
- Vernal keratoconjunctivitis, characterized by large "cobblestone" papillae on the upper tarsal conjunctiva, and atopic keratoconjunctivitis, characterized by chronic papillary conjunctivitis with fibrosis, are potentially blinding diseases

DIFFERENTIAL DIAGNOSIS

- See Table 9
- Acute anterior uveitis (iritis)
- Acute (angle-closure) glaucoma
- Corneal trauma (eg, foreign body or abrasion)
- Corneal infection or inflammation (eg, corneal ulcer or herpes simplex keratitis)
- Scleritis or episcleritis

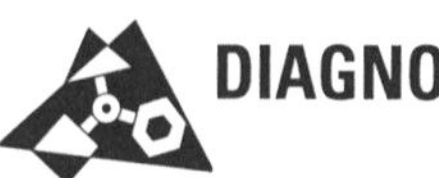

DIAGNOSIS

- Diagnosis is usually clinical
- If there is copious purulent discharge, conjunctival swab for Gram stain and bacterial culture to identify gonoccocal infection
- For suspected inclusion conjunctivitis or trachoma, immunologic tests or polymerase chain reaction on conjunctival samples
- For suspected keratoconjunctivitis sicca, Schirmer's test to measure tear production

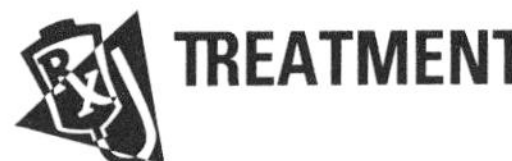

TREATMENT

MEDICATIONS

- See Table 10
- Choice of therapeutic agent should be dictated by underlying cause
- Mild bacterial conjunctivitis: sulfonamide or erythromycin ophthalmic solution or ointment
- Gonococcal conjunctivitis: ceftriaxone 1 g IM but admit to hospital if corneal involvement
- Chlamydial conjunctivitis: single dose therapy with azithromycin or oral tetracycline, erythromycin, doxycyline for 3–4 weeks
- Viral conjunctivitis: if corneal involvement, weak topical corticosteroids under the supervision of an ophthalmologist
- Keratoconjunctivitis sicca: artificial tears (preparations with methylcellulose or polyvinyl alcohol are longer lasting)
- Allergic keratoconjunctivitis: topical antihistamine, nonsteroidal anti-inflammatory or mast cell stabilizing agents, or if severe, topical corticosteroids under the supervision of an ophthalmologist

SURGERY

- Correction of eyelid deformities and corneal transplantation in the later stages of trachoma

THERAPEUTIC PROCEDURES

- Warm compresses and rest can be helpful and are often the only therapy necessary for mild bacterial or viral conjunctivitis

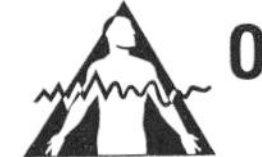

OUTCOME

FOLLOW-UP

- Most cases of bacterial or viral conjunctivitis do not require follow-up
- Recurrent bacterial conjunctivitis requires ophthalmologic assessment for predisposing factors such as blepharitis
- Gonococcal and inclusion conjunctivitis require follow-up for other sexually transmitted diseases
- Chronic moderate or severe allergic eye disease or keratoconjunctivitis sicca should be managed by an ophthalmologist

COMPLICATIONS

- Corneal ulceration, perforation or scarring, resulting in visual loss, may complicate gonococcal conjunctivitis, trachoma, keratoconjunctivitis sicca, or severe allergic eye disease

PROGNOSIS

- Most cases of conjunctivitis have an excellent prognosis, although long-term treatment may be required in keratoconjunctivitis sicca and chronic allergic eye disease

WHEN TO REFER

- Refer patients with copious purulent discharge, corneal involvement, loss of visual acuity, severe pain, or lack of response to treatment to an ophthalmologist
- Refer patients (or their mothers in the case of neonates) with inclusion conjunctivitis or gonococcal conjunctivitis for identification of genital tract infection and other sexually transmitted diseases to an internist or gynecologist

WHEN TO ADMIT

- Admit patients with gonococcal conjunctivitis involving the cornea

EVIDENCE

PRACTICE GUIDELINES

- American Academy of Ophthalmology
  - http://www.aao.org/aao/education/library/ppp/upload/Conjunctivitis_.pdf
- American Family Physician (Cochrane Interpretation)
  - http://www.aafp.org/afp/20021101/cochrane.html
- American Academy of Ophthalmology Cornea/External Disease Panel, Preferred Practice Patterns Committee. Conjunctivitis, 2003
  - http://www.guideline.gov/summary/summary.aspx?doc_id-4354&nbr=3280

WEB SITES

- American Academy of Ophthalmology
  - http://www.aao.org
- National Eye Institute
  - http://www.nei.nih.gov

INFORMATION FOR PATIENTS

- American Academy of Family Physicians: Allergic Conjunctivitis
  - http://familydoctor.org/678.xml
- Cleveland Clinic Foundation: Conjunctivitis
  - http://www.clevelandclinic.org/health/health-info/docs/1900/1951.asp?index=8614
- Keratoconjunctivitis sicca
  - http://www.medem.com/medlb/article_detaillb.cfm?article_ID=ZZZXQXXV1ED&sub_cat=37
- MD Consult
  - http://home.mdconsult.com/das/patient/view/29760586/10055/6553.html/top?sid=192484919

REFERENCES

- Lee JS et al: Gonococcal keratoconjunctivitis in adults. Eye 2002;16:646. [PMID: 12194086]
- Owen CG et al: Topical treatments for seasonal allergic conjunctivitis: systematic review and meta-analysis of efficacy and effectiveness. Br J Gen Pract 2004;54:451. [PMID: 15186569]
- Solomon AW et al: Mass treatment with single-dose azithromycin for trachoma. N Engl J Med 2004;351:1962. [PMID: 15525721]

Author(s)

Paul Riordan-Eva, FRCOphth
Richard A. Jacobs, MD, PhD

Constipation

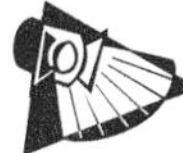

KEY FEATURES

ESSENTIALS OF DIAGNOSIS

- Defined as two or fewer bowel movements per week or excessive difficulty and straining at defecation

GENERAL CONSIDERATIONS

- Common complaint
- May be intermittent or chronic
- Most commonly caused by diet, medications, or immobility
- May be caused by systemic diseases, structural abnormalities, or abnormal motility
- Fecal impaction: predisposing factors
  - Severe psychiatric disease
  - Prolonged bed rest and debility
  - Neurogenic disorders of the colon
  - Spinal cord disorders

DEMOGRAPHICS

- Increased incidence with advancing age

CLINICAL FINDINGS

SYMPTOMS AND SIGNS

- Decreased appetite
- Nausea and vomiting
- Abdominal pain and distention
- Paradoxical "diarrhea"
- Firm feces palpable on digital rectal examination

DIFFERENTIAL DIAGNOSIS

- Inadequate fiber or fluid intake
- Poor bowel habits
- Irritable bowel syndrome

Systemic disease

- Endocrine
  - Hypothyroidism
  - Hyperparathyroidism
  - Diabetes mellitus
- Metabolic
  - Hypercalcemia
  - Hypokalemia
  - Uremia
  - Porphyria
- Neurologic
  - Parkinson's disease
  - Multiple sclerosis
  - Sacral nerve damage (pelvic surgery, tumor)
  - Paraplegia
  - Autonomic neuropathy
- Rheumatologic
  - Scleroderma
  - Amyloidosis
- Medications
  - Narcotics
  - Diuretics
  - Calcium channel blockers
  - Anticholinergics
  - Psychotropics
  - Calcium, iron
  - Nonsteroidal anti-inflammatory drugs
  - Clonidine
  - Sucralfate
  - Cholestyramine
- Infectious: Chagas' disease

Structural abnormalities

- Anorectal
  - Rectal prolapse
  - Rectocele
  - Rectal intussusception
  - Anorectal stricture
  - Anal fissure
  - Solitary rectal ulcer syndrome
- Pelvic floor dysfunction (hysterectomy)
- Obstructing colonic mass (cancer)
- Colonic stricture
  - Radiation
  - Ischemia
  - Diverticulosis
- Hirschsprung's disease
- Chagas' disease

Slow colonic transit

- Idiopathic: isolated to colon
- Psychogenic
- Eating disorders
- Chronic intestinal pseudoobstruction

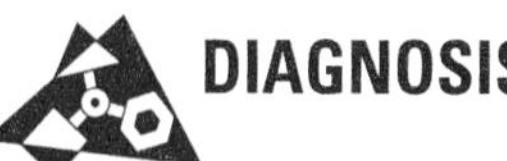

DIAGNOSIS

LABORATORY TESTS

- Complete blood cell count
- Serum electrolytes
- Serum calcium
- Serum thyroid-stimulating hormone
- Fecal occult blood test

IMAGING STUDIES

- Colonoscopy or flexible sigmoidoscopy and barium enema

DIAGNOSTIC PROCEDURES

- Diet, fluid, and medication history
- Physical examination
- Colonic transit and pelvic floor function studies for severe constipation unresponsive to life-style changes and laxatives

Constipation

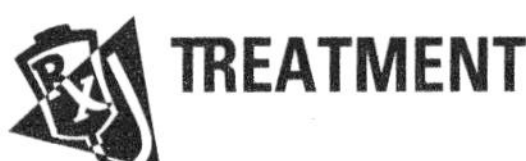

TREATMENT

MEDICATIONS

- Fiber supplements
  - Psyllium
  - Methylcellulose
  - Polycarbophil
- Stool surfactant agents
  - Docusate sodium, 50–200 mg/day or
  - Mineral oil, 14–45 mL/day, orally or rectally
- Saline laxatives
  - Magnesium-containing saline laxatives (milk of magnesia, magnesium sulfate)
  - Sodium phosphate or magnesium citrate
- Nonabsorbable carbohydrate laxatives: sorbitol (70%) or lactulose, 15–30 mL PO QD or BID
- Polyethylene glycol 3350 powder (Miralax), 17 g once or twice daily
- Stimulant agents
  - Bisacodyl
  - Senna
  - Cascara
  - Castor oil
- Tegaserod 6 mg twice daily
- Fecal impaction
  - Initial treatment: enemas (saline, mineral oil, or diatrizoate) or digital disruption
  - Long-term treatment: maintaining soft stools and regular bowel movements

SURGERY

- Subtotal colectomy with ileorectal anastomosis rarely required for severe intractable colonic inertia
- Disimpaction under anesthesia sometimes required for severe impaction

THERAPEUTIC PROCEDURES

- Biofeedback therapy for pelvic floor dysfunction

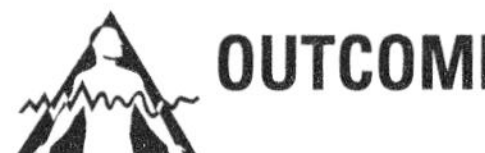

OUTCOME

COMPLICATIONS

- Fecal impaction
- Large bowel obstruction with pain, distention, nausea and vomiting

PROGNOSIS

- Most patients successfully treated with lifestyle changes and intermittent or chronic laxatives

WHEN TO REFER

- Severe constipation unresponsive to laxatives
- Suspected pelvic floor dysfunction (prolonged straining, difficulty with evacuation)

WHEN TO ADMIT

- Severe fecal impaction

EVIDENCE

PRACTICE GUIDELINES

- American Gastroenterological Association medical position statement: guidelines on constipation. American Gastroenterological Association, 2001
  - http://www2.gastrojournal.org/scripts/om.dll/serve?action=get-media&id=a0060001761&trueID=pdf_0060001761&location=jgast0011906&type=pdf&name=x.pdf
- Jones MP et al: Lack of objective evidence of efficacy of laxatives in chronic constipation. Dig Dis Sci 2002;47:2222. [PMID:12395895]
- Petticrew M et al: Effectiveness of laxatives in adults. Qual Health Care 2001;10:268. [PMID:11743157]

INFORMATION FOR PATIENTS

- Cleveland Clinic
  - http://www.clevelandclinic.org/health/health-info/docs/0000/0062.asp?index=4059
- Mayo Clinic
  - http://www.mayoclinic.com/invoke.cfm?objectid=2D434692-F005-495C-A5EB2AFBD98CA2A5
- National Digestive Diseases Information Clearinghouse—Constipation
  - http://digestive.niddk.nih.gov/ddiseases/pubs/constipation/index.htm

REFERENCES

- Lembo A et al: Chronic constipation. N Engl J Med 2003;349:1360. [PMID: 14523145]
- Prather CM: Subtypes of constipation: sorting out the confusion. Rev Gastroenterol Disord 2004;4(Suppl 2):S11. [PMID: 15184810]

Author(s)

Kenneth R. McQuaid, MD

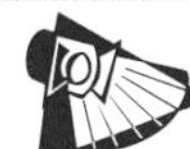

KEY FEATURES

GENERAL CONSIDERATIONS

- Contraception should be available to all women and men of reproductive ages
- Education about and access to contraception are especially important for sexually active teenagers and for women following childbirth or abortion
- Intrauterine devices (IUDs) are not abortifacients

Intrauterine devices

- IUDs include the Mirena (which releases levonorgestrel) and the copper-bearing TCu380A
- The hormone-containing IUDs have the advantage of reducing cramping and menstrual flow
- Nulliparity is not a contraindication to IUD use
- The Mirena may have a protective effect against upper tract infection similar to that of oral contraceptives
- Contraindications to use of IUDs are outlined in Table 70
- A copper-containing IUD can be inserted within 5 days following a single episode of unprotected mid-cycle coitus as a postcoital contraceptive
- An IUD should not be inserted into a pregnant uterus
- If pregnancy occurs as an IUD failure, there is a greater chance of spontaneous abortion if the IUD is left in situ (50%) than if it is removed (25%)
- Spontaneous abortion with an IUD in place is associated with a high risk of severe sepsis, and death can occur rapidly
- Women using an IUD who become pregnant should have the IUD removed if the string is visible
- It can be removed at the time of abortion if this is desired
- If the string is not visible and the patient wants to continue the pregnancy, she should be informed of the serious risk of sepsis and, occasionally, death with such pregnancies
- She should be informed that any flu-like symptoms such as fever, myalgia, headache, or nausea warrant immediate medical attention for possible septic abortion
- Since the ratio of ectopic to intrauterine pregnancies is increased among IUD wearers, clinicians should search for adnexal masses in early pregnancy and should always check the products of conception for placental tissue following abortion

Diaphragm and cervical cap

- The diaphragm (with contraceptive jelly) is a safe and effective contraceptive method with features that make it acceptable to some women and not others
- Failure rates range from 6% to 16%, depending on the motivation of the woman and the care with which the diaphragm is used
- The advantages of this method are that it has no systemic side effects and gives significant protection against pelvic infection and cervical dysplasia as well as pregnancy
- The disadvantages are that it must be inserted near the time of coitus and that pressure from the rim predisposes some women to cystitis after intercourse
- The cervical cap (with contraceptive jelly) is similar to the diaphragm but fits snugly over the cervix only (the diaphragm stretches from behind the cervix to behind the pubic symphysis)
- The cervical cap is more difficult to insert and remove than the diaphragm
- Failure rates are 16% (typical use) and 9% (perfect use) in nulliparous women and 32% and 26%, respectively, in parous women
- The main advantages are that it can be used by women who cannot be fitted for a diaphragm because of a relaxed anterior vaginal wall or by women who have discomfort or develop repeated bladder infections with the diaphragm
- Because of the small risk of toxic shock syndrome, a cervical cap or diaphragm should not be left in the vagina for over 12–18 h, nor should these devices be used during the menstrual period (see above)

Contraceptive foam, cream, film, sponge, jelly, and suppository

- Available without prescription, easy to use, and fairly effective, with reported failure rates of 2–30%
- All contain the spermicide nonoxynol-9, which also has some virucidal and bactericidal activity
  - Nonoxynol-9 does not appear to adversely affect the vaginal colonization of hydrogen peroxide-producing lactobacilli
  - A 2002 study suggests that nonoxynol-9 is not protective against HIV infection, particularly in women who have frequent intercourse
- Advantages include being simple to use and easily available
- Disadvantage is a slightly higher failure rate than the diaphragm or condom

Condom

- The **male** sheath of latex or animal membrane affords good protection against pregnancy
  - Equivalent to that of a diaphragm and spermicidal jelly
  - Latex (but not animal membrane) condoms also offer protection against sexually transmitted disease (STD) and cervical dysplasia
  - For protection against HIV transmission, a latex condom along with spermicide during vaginal or rectal intercourse is advised
  - A spermicide, such as vaginal foam, used with a condom, has a failure rate approaching that of oral contraceptives
  - Condoms coated with spermicide are available in the United States
  - The disadvantages of condoms are dulling of sensation and spillage of semen due to tearing, slipping, or leakage with detumescence of the penis
- The polyurethane **female** condom has failure rates from 5% to 21%
  - Efficacy is comparable to that of the diaphragm
  - The only female-controlled method that offers significant protection from both pregnancy and STDs

Contraception, IUD & Barrier Methods

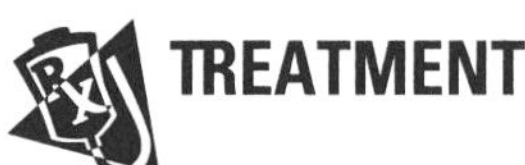

TREATMENT

THERAPEUTIC PROCEDURES

Intrauterine devices

- IUD insertion can be performed during or after the menses, at midcycle to prevent implantation, or later in the cycle if the patient is not pregnant
- Wait for 6–8 weeks postpartum before inserting an IUD
- When insertion is performed during lactation, there is greater risk of uterine perforation or embedding of the IUD
- Insertion immediately following abortion is acceptable if there is no sepsis and if follow-up insertion a month later will not be possible; otherwise, it is wise to wait until 4 weeks postabortion
- IUDs can be tried in these cases, as they often cause decreased bleeding and cramping with menses. Nonsteroidal anti-inflammatory drugs are also helpful in decreasing bleeding and pain

OUTCOME

COMPLICATIONS

- **Pelvic infection**
  - There is an increased risk of pelvic infection during the first month following insertion
  - The subsequent risk of pelvic infection appears to be primarily related to the risk of acquiring STDs
  - Infertility rates do not appear to be increased among women who have previously used the currently available IUDs
  - At the time of insertion, women with an increased risk of STDs should be screened for gonorrhea and chlamydiosis
  - Women with a history of recent or recurrent pelvic infection are not good candidates for IUD use
- **Menorrhagia or severe dysmenorrhea**
  - The copper IUD can cause heavier menstrual periods, bleeding between periods, and more cramping, so it is generally not suitable for women who already suffer from these problems. However, hormone-releasing IUDs can be tried in these cases, as they often cause decreased bleeding and cramping with menses. Nonsteroidal anti-inflammatory drugs are also helpful in decreasing bleeding and pain
- **Complete or partial expulsion**
  - Spontaneous expulsion of the IUD occurs in 10–20% of cases during the first year of use. Any IUD should be removed if the body of the device can be seen or felt in the cervical os
- **Missing IUD strings**
  - If the transcervical tail cannot be seen, this may signify unnoticed expulsion, perforation of the uterus with abdominal migration of the IUD, or simply retraction of the string into the cervical canal or uterus owing to movement of the IUD or uterine growth with pregnancy
  - Once pregnancy is ruled out, probe for the IUD with a sterile sound or forceps designed for IUD removal, after administering a paracervical block
  - If the IUD cannot be detected, pelvic ultrasound will demonstrate the IUD if it is in the uterus, or anteroposterior and lateral x-rays of the pelvis with another IUD or a sound in the uterus as a marker can confirm an extrauterine IUD
  - If the IUD is in the abdominal cavity, remove by laparoscopy or laparotomy
  - Open-looped all-plastic IUDs such as the Lippes Loop can be left in the pelvis without danger, but ring-shaped IUDs may strangulate a loop of bowel and copper-bearing IUDs may cause tissue reaction and adhesions

PROGNOSIS

- The IUD is highly effective, with failure rates similar to those achieved with surgical sterilization
- Women who are not in mutually monogamous relationships should use condoms for protection from STDs
- The Mirena is approved for 5 years use and the Tcu380A for 10 years

PREVENTION

- Perforations of the uterus are less likely if insertion is performed slowly, with care taken to follow directions applicable to each type of IUD

EVIDENCE

PRACTICE GUIDELINES

- Black A et al; Contraception Guidelines Committee. Canadian Contraception Consensus, 2004.
  - http://sogc.medical.org/sogcnet/sogc_docs/common/guide/pdfs/ps143_3.pdf (Barrier)
  - http://sogc.medical.org/sogcnet/sogc_docs/common/guide/pdfs/ps143_2.pdf (IUD)

WEB SITES

- Gynecology Handbook
  - http://www.vh.org/Providers/ClinRef/FPHandbook/13.html

INFORMATION FOR PATIENTS

- American College of Obstetricians and Gynecologists: Birth Control
  - http://www.medem.com/MedLB/article_detaillb.cfm?article_ID=ZZZ48OI527C&sub_cat=5
- Mayo Clinic: IUDs
  - http://www.mayoclinic.com/invoke.cfm?id=WO00087

REFERENCES

- ACOG Committee on Practice Bulletins-Gynecology: ACOG practice bulletin. Clinical Management Guidelines for Obstetrician-Gynecologists. Number 59, January 2005. Intrauterine device. Obstet Gynecol 2005;105:223. [PMID: 15625179]
- Holmes KK et al: Effectiveness of condoms in preventing sexually transmitted infections. Bull World Health Organ 2004;82:454. [PMID: 15356939]
- Raymond EG et al: Contraceptive effectiveness and safety of five nonoxynol-9 spermicides: a randomized trial. Obstet Gynecol 2004;103:430. [PMID: 14990402]
- Van Damme L et al: Effectiveness of COL-1492, a nonoxynol-9 vaginal gel, on HIV-1 transmission in female sex workers: a randomised controlled trial. Lancet 2002;360:971. [PMID: 12383665]

Author(s)

H. Trent MacKay, MD, MPH

Contraception, Oral, Injections, & Implants

KEY FEATURES

GENERAL CONSIDERATIONS

- Contraception should be available to all women and men of reproductive ages
- Education about contraception and access to contraceptive pills or devices are especially important for sexually active teenagers and for women following childbirth or abortion

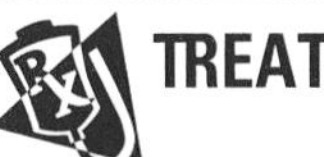

TREATMENT

MEDICATIONS

Oral contraceptives

- **Combined oral contraceptives**
  - Oral contraceptives have a theoretical failure rate of < 0.3% if taken absolutely on schedule and a typical failure rate of 8%
  - The primary mode of action is suppression of ovulation
  - The pills can be started on the first day of the menstrual cycle, on the first Sunday after the onset of the cycle, or on any day of the cycle. If started on any day other than the first day of the cycle, a backup method should be used. A pill is taken daily for 21 days, followed by 7 days of placebos or no medication, and this schedule is continued for each cycle
  - There are also pills packaged to be taken continuously for 84 days, followed by 7 days of placebos. If an active pill is missed at any time, and no intercourse occurred in the past 5 days, two pills should be taken immediately and a backup method should be used for 7 days. If intercourse occurred in the previous 5 days, emergency contraception should be used immediately, and the pills restarted the following day. A backup method should be used for 5 days
- **Benefits of oral contraceptives**
  - There are many noncontraceptive advantages to oral contraceptives. Menstrual flow is lighter, resultant anemia is less common, and dysmenorrhea is relieved for most women
  - Functional ovarian cysts generally disappear with oral contraceptive use, and new cysts do not occur
  - Pain with ovulation and postovulatory aching are relieved
  - The risk of ovarian and endometrial cancer is decreased, and the risks of salpingitis and ectopic pregnancy may be diminished
  - Acne is usually improved
  - The frequency of developing myomas is lower in long-term users (> 4 years). There is a beneficial effect on bone mass
- **Selection of an oral contraceptive**
  - Any of the combination oral contraceptives containing 35 μg or less of estrogen are suitable for most women
  - There is some variation in potency of the various progestins in the pills, but there are essentially no clinically significant differences for most women among the progestins in the low-dose pills
  - Women who have acne or hirsutism may benefit from use of one of the pills containing the third-generation progestins, desogestrel or norgestimate, as they are the least androgenic
  - The low-dose oral contraceptives commonly used in the United States are listed in Table 68
- **Drug interactions**
  - Drugs that interact with oral contraceptives to decrease their efficacy include phenytoin, phenobarbital (and other barbiturates), primidone, carbamazepine, and rifampin. Women taking these drugs should use another means of contraception for maximum safety
- **Contraindications and adverse effects**
  - Oral contraceptives have been associated with many adverse effects (Table 69)
- **Minor side effects**
  - Nausea and dizziness may occur in the first few months of pill use
  - A weight gain of 2–5 lb commonly occurs
  - Spotting or breakthrough bleeding between menstrual periods may occur, especially if a pill is skipped or taken late; this may be helped by switching to a pill of slightly greater potency
  - Missed menstrual periods may occur, especially with low-dose pills. A pregnancy test should be performed if pills have been skipped or if two or more menstrual periods are missed
  - Depression, fatigue, and decreased libido can occur
  - Chloasma may occur, as in pregnancy, and is increased by exposure to sunlight

Progestin minipill

- **Efficacy and methods of use**
  - Formulations containing 0.35 mg of norethindrone or 0.075 mg of norgestrel are available in the United States
  - Efficacy is similar to that of combined oral contraceptives, with failure rates of 1–4% being reported
  - The minipill is begun on the first day of a menstrual cycle and then taken continuously for as long as contraception is desired
- **Advantages**
  - The low dose and absence of estrogen make the minipill safe during lactation; it may increase the flow of milk
  - It is often tried by women who want

minimal doses of hormones and by patients who are over age 35
  - It can be used by women with uterine myomas or sickle cell disease (S/S or S/C)
- **Complications and contraindications**
  - Minipill users often have bleeding irregularities (eg, prolonged flow, spotting, or amenorrhea); such patients may need monthly pregnancy tests
  - Ectopic pregnancies are more frequent, and complaints of abdominal pain should be investigated with this in mind
  - The contraindications listed in Table 69 apply to the minipill
  - Minor side effects of combination oral contraceptives such as weight gain and mild headache may also occur with the minipill

Contraceptive injections and implants

- **Long-acting progestins**
  - Progestin medroxyprogesterone acetate IM, 150 mg every 3 months
  - A new subcutaneous preparation, containing 104 mg of DMPA, is available in the United States
  - It has a contraceptive efficacy of 99.7%
  - Common side effects include irregular bleeding, amenorrhea, weight gain, and headache. It is associated with bone mineral loss
  - Users commonly have irregular bleeding initially and subsequently develop amenorrhea
  - Ovulation may be delayed after the last injection
  - Contraindications are similar to those for the minipill
  - A monthly injectable containing both depot medroxyprogesterone acetate and an estrogen, estradiol cypionate (Lunelle), is highly effective, with a first-year pregnancy rate of 0.2% and a side effect profile similar to that of oral contraceptives, although it is not being marketed currently
  - The other long-acting progestin is the Norplant system, a contraceptive implant containing levonorgestrel, which is no longer marketed in the United States

Other hormonal methods

- A transdermal contraceptive patch containing 150 µg norelgestromin and 20 µg ethinyl estradiol and measuring 20 cm^2 is available. The patch is applied to the lower abdomen, upper torso, or buttock once a week for 3 consecutive weeks, followed by 1 week without the patch. The mechanism of action, side effects, and efficacy are similar to those associated with oral contraceptives, though compliance may be better
- A contraceptive vaginal ring that releases 120 µg of etonogestrel and 15 µg of ethinyl estradiol daily is available. The ring is soft and flexible and is placed in the upper vagina for 3 weeks, removed, and replaced 1 week later. The efficacy, mechanism of action, and systemic side effects are similar to those associated with oral contraceptives. In addition, users may experience an increased incidence of vaginal discharge

OUTCOME

FOLLOW-UP

- Patients using hormonal contraception are usually seen annually for a review of pertinent history, breast and pelvic examination with Pap smear

COMPLICATIONS

- Serious complications of combined hormonal contraception include
  - Venous thromboembolism: 10–30/100,000 annually
  - Myocardial infarction: 40/100,000 annually in smokers over age 35
  - Hypertension: 1% incidence

EVIDENCE

PRACTICE GUIDELINES

- Black A et al; Contraception Guidelines Committee. Canadian Contraception Consenus, 2004.
  - http://sogc.medical.org/sogcnet/sogc_docs/common/guide/pdfs/ps143_2.pdf
- FFPRHC Guidance: emergency contraception (April 2003). J Fam Plan Reprod Health Care. 2003;29:9. [PMID: 12681030]

WEB SITES

- Gynecology Handbook for Family Practitioners
  - http://www.vh.org/Providers/ClinRef/FPHandbook/13.html
- US Food and Drug Administration: Birth Control Guide
  - http://www.fda.gov/fdac/features/1997/babytabl.html

INFORMATION FOR PATIENTS

- American College of Obstetricians and Gynecologists
  - http://www.medem.com/MedLB/article_detaillb.cfm?article_ID=ZZZ48OI527C&sub_cat=5
- National Women's Health Information Center: Birth Control Methods
  - http://www.4woman.gov/faq/birthcont.htm
- National Women's Health Information Center: Emergency Contraception
  - http://www.4woman.gov/faq/econtracep.htm
- US Food and Drug Administration: What Kind of Birth Control Is Best for You?
  - http://www.fda.gov/opacom/lowlit/brthcon.html

REFERENCES

- Hatcher RA et al: *Contraceptive Technology*, 18th edition. New York, Ardent Media, 2004.
- Kaunitz AM: Injectable long-acting contraceptives. Clin Obstet Gynecol 2001;44:73. [PMID: 11219248]
- Reproductive Health and Research; World Health Organization: Medical Eligibilty Criteria for Contraceptive Use. WHO/RHR 2004, Geneva.
  - http://www.who.int/reproductive-health/publications/RHR_00_2_medical_eligibility_criteria_3rd/index.htm
- Reproductive Health and Research; World Health Organization: Selected Practice Recommendations for Contraceptive Use. WHO/RHR 2004, Geneva.
  - http://www.who.int/reproductive-health/publications/rhr_02_7/index.htm
- Seibert C et al: Prescribing oral contraceptives for women older than 35 years of age. Ann Intern Med 2003;138:54. [PMID: 12513046]
- Veres S et al: A comparison between the vaginal ring and oral contraceptives. Obstet Gynecol 2004;104:555. [PMID: 15339769]

Author(s)

H. Trent MacKay, MD, MPH

Cough

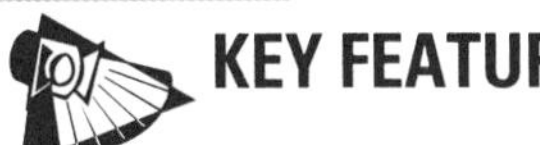

KEY FEATURES

ESSENTIALS OF DIAGNOSIS

- Duration of cough
- Dyspnea (at rest or with exertion)
- Constitutional symptoms
- Tobacco use history
- Vital signs (temperature, respiratory rate, heart rate)
- Chest examination

GENERAL CONSIDERATIONS

- Cough results from stimulation of mechanical or chemical afferent nerve receptors in the bronchial tree
- Cough illness syndromes are defined as acute (< 3 weeks) or persistent (> 3 weeks)
- In about 25% of cases, persistent cough has multiple contributors

CLINICAL FINDINGS

SYMPTOMS AND SIGNS

- Timing and character of cough are usually not useful in establishing cause
- Acute cough syndromes: most due to viral respiratory tract infections; less common causes include congestive heart failure (CHF), hay fever (allergic rhinitis), and environmental factors
- Search for additional features of infection such as fever, nasal congestion, and sore throat
- Dyspnea (at rest or with exertion) may reflect a more serious condition
- Persistent cough is usually due to
  - Angiotensin-converting enzyme (ACE) inhibitor therapy
  - Postnasal drip
  - Asthma
  - Gastroesophageal reflux disease (GERD)
- Less common causes of persistent cough
  - Bronchogenic carcinoma
  - Chronic bronchitis
  - Bronchiectasis
  - Other chronic lung disease
  - CHF
- Signs of pneumonia
  - Tachycardia
  - Tachypnea
  - Fever
  - Rales
  - Decreased breath sounds
  - Fremitus
  - Egophony
- Signs of acute bronchitis: wheezing and rhonchi
- Signs of chronic sinusitis: postnasal drip
- Signs of chronic obstructive pulmonary disease (COPD)
  - Abnormal match test (inability to blow out a match from 10 inches away)
  - Maximum laryngeal height < 4 cm (measured from the sternal notch to the cricoid cartilage at end expiration)
- Signs of CHF
  - Abnormal jugular venous pressure
  - Positive hepatojugular reflux

DIFFERENTIAL DIAGNOSIS

Acute cough

- Viral upper respiratory infection or postviral cough (most common)
- Postnasal drip (allergic rhinitis)
- Pneumonia
- Pulmonary edema
- Pulmonary embolism
- Aspiration pneumonia

Persistent cough

- Top three causes: postnasal drip, asthma, GERD
- Pulmonary infection
  - Postviral
  - Chronic bronchitis, especially in smokers
  - Bronchiectasis
  - Tuberculosis
  - Cystic fibrosis
  - *Mycobacterium avium* complex
  - Pertussis
  - *Mycoplasma, Chlamydia,* respiratory syncytial virus (underrecognized in adults)
- Pulmonary noninfectious
  - Asthma (cough-variant asthma)
  - β-blockers causing asthma
  - COPD
  - ACE inhibitors
  - Irritant inhalation (eg, smoking), endobronchial lesion, (eg, tumor), interstitial lung disease, sarcoidosis, chronic microaspiration
- Nonpulmonary
  - GERD
  - Postnasal drip (allergic rhinitis)
  - Sinusitis
  - CHF
  - Laryngitis
  - Ear canal or tympanic membrane irritation
  - Psychogenic or habit cough

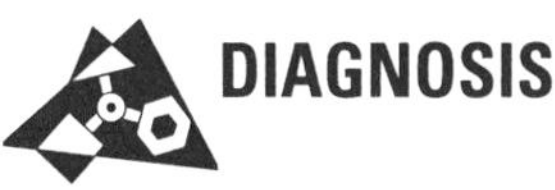

DIAGNOSIS

LABORATORY TESTS

- Pulse oximetry or arterial blood gas measurement
- Peak expiratory flow rate or spirometry

IMAGING STUDIES

- Acute cough: obtain chest radiograph if abnormal vital signs or chest examination; higher index of suspicion in elderly and/or immunocompromised
- Persistent cough: obtain chest radiograph if unexplained cough lasts more than 3–6 weeks

DIAGNOSTIC PROCEDURES

- Reserve procedures for patients who do not respond to therapeutic trials
- Sinus CT scan for cough with postnasal drip
- Spirometry (if normal, possible methacholine challenge) for cough with wheezing or possible asthma, though pulmonary function tests are often normal in cough variant asthma
- Esophageal pH monitoring for cough with GERD symptoms

Contraception, Periodic Abstinence p. 1061. Contraception, Sterilization p. 1061.
Cor Pulmonale p. 1061.

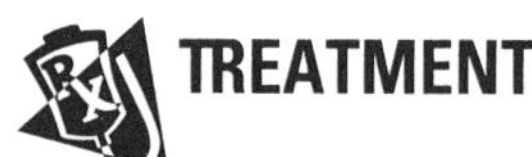

TREATMENT

MEDICATIONS

- If symptoms of postnasal drip, asthma, or GERD, begin with treatment for that condition, otherwise, undertake empiric trials with a maximum strength regimen for one condition for 2–4 weeks, followed by the next if no response
- For postnasal drip: decongestants, nasal steroids, with or without antibiotics
- For asthma: inhaled albuterol
- For GERD: proton pump inhibitors

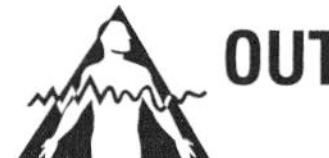

OUTCOME

WHEN TO REFER

- Refer patients with cough due to chronic sinusitis unresponsive to medications to otolaryngologist
- Refer patients with cough due to GERD unresponsive to medications to gastroenterologist or surgeon

WHEN TO ADMIT

- Pneumonia, if moderate to severe
- Bronchiectasis exacerbation, if moderate to severe
- COPD exacerbation, if moderate to severe

EVIDENCE

PRACTICE GUIDELINES

- Gonzales R et al: Principles of appropriate antibiotic use for treatment of uncomplicated acute bronchitis in adults: background. Ann Intern Med 2001;134:521. [PMID: 11255532]
- Irwin RS et al: Managing cough as a defense mechanism and symptom. A consensus panel report of the American College of Chest Physicians. Chest 1998;114(2 Suppl):133S.
  - http://www.chestjournal.org/cgi/reprint/114/2/133S
- Institute for Clinical Systems Improvement (ICSI): Chronic obstructive pulmonary disease, 2004.
  - http://www.icsi.org/knowledge/detail.asp?catID=29&itemID=157
- Institute for Clinical Systems Improvement (ICSI): Viral upper respiratory infection (VURI) in adults and children, 2004.
  - http://www.icsi.org/knowledge/detail.asp?catID=29&item=203

INFORMATION FOR PATIENTS

- American Academy of Family Physicians: Chronic Cough: Causes and Cures
  - http://familydoctor.org/237.xml
- American College of Chest Physicians: Managing Cough as Defense Mechanism and as a Symptom
  - http://www.chestnet.org/education/patient/guides/cough/
- MedlinePlus: Cough
  - http://www.nlm.nih.gov/medlineplus/ency/article/003072.htm

REFERENCE

- Metlay JP et al: Testing strategies in the initial management of patients with community-acquired pneumonia. Ann Intern Med 2003;138:109. [PMID: 12529093]

Author(s)

Ralph Gonzales, MD

Coxsackievirus Infections p. 1062

Crohn's Disease

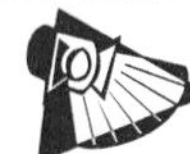

KEY FEATURES

ESSENTIALS OF DIAGNOSIS

- Insidious onset
- Intermittent bouts of low-grade fever, diarrhea, and right lower quadrant pain
- Right lower quadrant mass and tenderness
- Perianal disease with abscess, fistulas
- Radiographic evidence of ulceration, stricturing, or fistulas of the small intestine or colon

GENERAL CONSIDERATIONS

- Crohn's disease is a transmural process
- Crohn's may involve
  - Small bowel only, most commonly the terminal ileum (ileitis) in ~33% of cases
  - Small bowel and colon, most often the terminal ileum and adjacent proximal ascending colon (ileocolitis) in ~50%
  - Colon alone in 20%
- Chronic illness with exacerbations and remissions
- Treatment is directed both toward symptomatic improvement and controlling the disease process

DEMOGRAPHICS

- Increased in Europeans, North Americans, and Ashkenazi Jews
- Increased risk among first-degree relatives
- Increased risk in smokers

CLINICAL FINDINGS

SYMPTOMS AND SIGNS

- Fevers
- Abdominal pain
- Liquid bowel movements
- Abdominal tenderness or abdominal mass

Chronic inflammatory disease

- Malaise, loss of energy
- Diarrhea, nonbloody, intermittent
- Cramping or steady right lower quadrant or periumbilical pain
- Focal tenderness, right lower quadrant
- Palpable, tender mass in the lower abdomen

Intestinal obstruction

- Postprandial bloating, cramping pains, and loud borborygmi

Fistulization with or without infection

- Sinus tracts and fistulas can result in intra-abdominal or retroperitoneal abscesses manifested by fevers, chills, and a tender abdominal mass
- Bacterial overgrowth with diarrhea, weight loss, and malnutrition
- Bladder or vagina recurrent infections
- Cutaneous fistulas
- Perianal disease
  - Anal fissures
  - Perianal abscesses
  - Fistulas

Extraintestinal manifestations

- Oral aphthous lesions
- Gallstones
- Nephrolithiasis with stones

DIFFERENTIAL DIAGNOSIS

- Ulcerative colitis
- Irritable bowel syndrome
- Appendicitis
- *Yersinia enterocolitica* enteritis
- Mesenteric adenitis
- Intestinal lymphoma
- Segmental colitis due to ischemic colitis, tuberculosis, amebiasis, chlamydia
- Diverticulitis with abscess
- Nonsteroidal anti-inflammatory drug–induced colitis
- Perianal fistula due to other cause

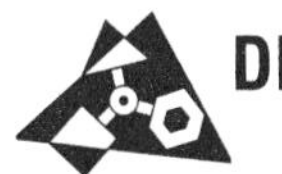

DIAGNOSIS

LABORATORY TESTS

- Obtain complete blood cell count, erythrocyte sedimentation rate or C-reactive protein, serum albumin
- Anemia of chronic inflammation, blood loss, iron deficiency, or vitamin B_{12} malabsorption
- Leukocytosis with abscesses
- Sedimentation rate or C-reactive protein elevated
- Stool for routine pathogens, ova and parasites, and *Clostridium difficile* toxin
- Antibodies to the yeast *Saccharomyces cerevisiae* (ASCA) are found in 60–70%

IMAGING STUDIES

- Upper gastrointestinal series with small bowel follow-through
- Barium enema
- Capsuled (video) imaging of small intestine

DIAGNOSTIC PROCEDURES

- Colonoscopy
- Biopsy of intestine reveals granulomas in 25%

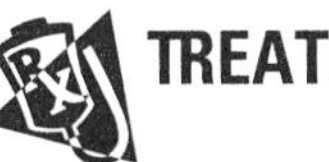

TREATMENT

MEDICATIONS

Treatment of diarrhea

- Cholestyramine (2–4 g) or colestipol (5 g) PO BID–TID before meals in terminal ileal Crohn's
- Broad-spectrum antibiotics if bacterial overgrowth
- Antidiarrheal agents
  - Loperamide (2–4 mg), diphenoxylate with atropine (one tablet), or tincture of opium (5–15 drops) QID PRN
  - Not used in patients with active severe colitis

Treatment of exacerbations

- 5-Aminosalicylic acid agents: sulfasalazine, 1.5–2 g PO BID; mesalamine (Asacol), 0.8–1.2 g PO QID, or its slow-release form (Pentasa), 1 g PO QID, for mild to moderate small bowel and ileocecal disease
- Antibiotics: metronidazole, 10 mg/kg/day for ileocolitis, colitis, or perianal disease, ciprofloxacin, 500 mg PO BID for ileitis or perianal disease
- Broad-spectrum antibiotics, and, if malnourished, total parenteral nutrition (TPN), for abscess

- Corticosteroids: prednisone, 40–60 mg/day for 2–3 weeks, tapering by 5 mg/week until dosage is 20 mg/day, then by 2.5 mg/week or every other week
- Ileal-release preparation of topically active compound budesonide, 9 mg PO QD for 8 weeks for terminal ileal disease
- Immunomodulatory drugs
  - Azathioprine (2–2.5 mg/kg) and mercaptopurine (1–1.5 mg/kg) useful for fistulas and in long-term treatment
  - Methotrexate (25 mg IM weekly for 12 weeks, followed by 12.5–15 mg IM once weekly) for patients who fail to respond to azathioprine
  - Infliximab, 5 mg/kg given at 0, 2, and 6 weeks is useful in moderate to severe Crohn's; results in closure of fistulas in ~50% and improvement in ~75%

Maintenance of remission

- Mesalamine (Asacol), 800 mg PO TID or Pentasa, 500–750 mg PO QID
- Corticosteroids should not be used
- Azathioprine, mercaptopurine, and methotrexate help maintain remission
- Chronic infliximab (every 8 weeks) appropriate for some patients with moderate to severe disease

SURGERY

- At least one surgical procedure required by >50% of patients
- Indications for surgery are intractability to medical therapy, intra-abdominal abscess, massive bleeding, and obstruction with fibrous stricture
- Incision and drainage for abscess
- Surgical resection of the stenotic area or stricturoplasty in small bowel obstruction
- Surgical fistulotomy; avoid in active Crohn's disease

THERAPEUTIC PROCEDURES

- Percutaneous drainage for abscess
- Nasogastric suction and intravenous fluids for small bowel obstruction
- Well-balanced diet
- Avoid lactose-containing foods since lactose intolerance is common
- Fiber supplementation for patients with colonic involvement
- Low-roughage diet for patients with obstructive symptoms
- Low-fat diet for patients with fat malabsorption
- Iron supplement if documented deficiency
- Vitamin B_{12} 100 μg IM every month if prior terminal ileal resection
- TPN used short term in patients with active disease and progressive weight loss or in malnourished patients awaiting surgery
- TPN used long term in subset of patients with extensive intestinal resections resulting in short bowel syndrome with malnutrition

OUTCOME

COMPLICATIONS

- Abscess
- Small bowel obstruction
- Fistulas
- Perianal disease
- Hemorrhage (unusual)
- Malabsorption

PROGNOSIS

- With proper medical and surgical treatment, most patients are able to cope with this chronic disease and its complications
- Few patients die of Crohn's disease

WHEN TO ADMIT

- Hospitalize patients with persisting symptoms despite oral steroids or those with high fever, persistent vomiting, evidence of intestinal obstruction, severe weight loss, severe abdominal tenderness, or suspicion of an abscess

PREVENTION

- Colonoscopy screening to detect dysplasia or cancer recommended for patients with a history of 8 or more years of Crohn's colitis

EVIDENCE

PRACTICE GUIDELINES

- ACR Appropriateness criteria for imaging recommendations for patients with Crohn's disease. American College of Radiology, 2001
  - http://www.acr.org/cgi-bin/fr?tmpl:appcrit,pdf:0181-192_crohns_disease_ac.pdf
- American Gastroenterological Associates Medical Position Statement: Perianal Crohn's disease. Gastroenterology 2003;125:1503 [PMID: 14598267]
- Management of Crohn's disease in adults. American College of Gastroenterology, 2001
  - http://www-east.elsevier.com/ajg/issues/9603/ajg3671fla.htm
- National Guideline Clearinghouse
  - http://www.guideline.gov/summary/summary.aspx?doc_id=4582&nbr=3372&string=Crohns

WEB SITES

- WebPath Gastrointestinal Pathology Index
  - http://medstat.med.utah.edu/WebPath/GIHTML/GIIDX.html

INFORMATION FOR PATIENTS

- Cleveland Clinic—Crohn's disease
  - http://www.clevelandclinic.org/health/health-info/docs/2300/2371.asp?index=9357
- NIH—Patient Education Institute—Crohn's
  - http://www.nlm.nih.gov/medlineplus/tutorials/crohnsdiseas.html

REFERENCES

- Colombel JF et al: The safety profile of infliximab in patients with Crohn's disease: the Mayo Clinic experience of 500 patients. Gastroenterology 2004;126:19. [PMID: 14699483]
- Regueiro M: Update in medical treatment of Crohn's disease. J Clin Gastroenterol 2000;31:282. [PMID: 11129268]
- Sands B et al: Infliximab maintenance therapy for fistulizing Crohn's disease. N Engl J Med 2004;350:876. [PMID: 14985485]

Author(s)

Kenneth R. McQuaid, MD

Cryptococcosis

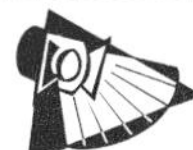

KEY FEATURES

ESSENTIALS OF DIAGNOSIS

- Infection is due to *Cryptococcus neoformans*, an encapsulated budding yeast that is found worldwide in soil and in dried bird droppings
- *C neoformans* variety *neoformans* accounts for majority of disease worldwide and is especially problematic is immunocompromised patients
- *C neoformans* var *gattii* causes localized infections (cryptococcomas) in tropical climates and has close association with eucalyptus plants
- *C neoformans* has a special predilection for the central nervous system and is the most common fungal cause of meningitis
- The polysaccharide capsule is a major virulence factor and provides the basis for antigen testing that is widely available and quite useful in establishing the diagnosis

GENERAL CONSIDERATIONS

- Infection is acquired through inhalation of the organisms into the lungs where infection may remain localized or disseminate
- Progressive pulmonary disease can occur in either HIV infected or noninfected patients in the absence of dissemination
- Predisposing factors for dissemination include HIV, underlying malignancy, and receipt of corticosteroids
- Widespread pulmonary disease common in HIV patients with meningitis
- Disseminated disease in immunocompetent patients can be especially recalcitrant to therapy

DEMOGRAPHICS

- Symptomatic cryptococcal pneumonia rarely develops in immunocompetent patients but can occur
- Progressive lung disease and dissemination usually occur in immunocompromised patients, eg, those with HIV infection, corticosteroid therapy, or hematologic malignancy

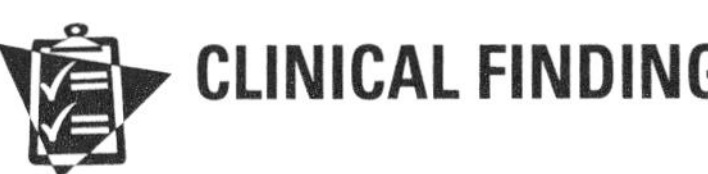

CLINICAL FINDINGS

SYMPTOMS AND SIGNS

- Disseminated cryptococcosis most commonly manifests as meningitis, which usually begins with headache, then confusion; cranial nerve abnormalities, nausea, and vomiting may occur
- Nuchal rigidity and meningeal signs in about 50%, but uncommon in HIV-infected patients
- Intracerebral mass lesions (cryptococcomas) are rare
- Obstructive hydrocephalus may occur
- In AIDS, extrameningeal disease (lungs, blood, urinary tract) is common
- Immune reconstitution following highly active antiretroviral therapy (HAART) therapy in HIV-infected patients may lead to "paradoxical exacerbations" of meningitis likely representing immune reaction to residual cryptococcal antigen

DIFFERENTIAL DIAGNOSIS

- Histoplasmosis
- Coccidioidomycosis
- Tuberculous meningitis
- Neurosyphilis
- *Acanthamoeba* (amebic encephalitis)
- Toxoplasmosis
- Lyme meningitis

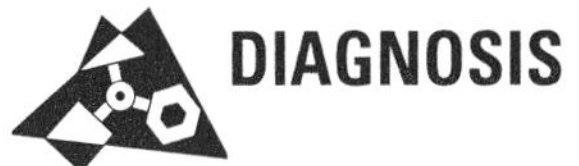

DIAGNOSIS

LABORATORY TESTS

- In HIV-infected patients with cryptococcosis, serum cryptococcal antigen positive in 95%
- In patients with crypotococcal meningitis, cerebrospinal fluid (CSF) shows increased opening pressure, variable pleocytosis, increased protein, decreased glucose, and budding encapsulated fungus cells
- Up to 50% of AIDS patients have no CSF pleocytosis
- CSF positive for cryptococcal capsular antigen in > 90%
- CSF positive culture in > 90%
- Blood cultures also have good yield, especially in HIV-infected patients

IMAGING STUDIES

- Chest x-ray may show bilateral interstitial infiltrates, which are nonspecific
- MRI or CT scan of brain may show meningeal enhancement but this is generally mild, especially in HIV-infected patients where immune response is minimal
- For immune reconstitution disease in HIV-infected patients treated with HAART, may see marked enhancement of meninges on CT or MRI indicative of enhanced immune response

DIAGNOSTIC PROCEDURES

- Given the high propensity of the organism for the CSF, lumbar puncture is mandatory for any patient with disseminated disease
- Examination of CSF via fungal stain, culture, and antigen tests usually sufficient to establish diagnosis

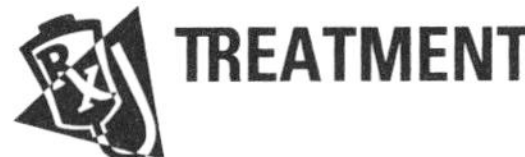

TREATMENT

MEDICATIONS

Acute therapy

- Mild AIDS-related cryptococcal meningitis
  - Fluconazole, 400 mg PO QD, for minimum of 10 weeks for patients with intact level of consciousness and CSF cryptococcal antigen titer < 1:128. Fluconazole plus flucytosine may also be efficacious
- Higher-risk patients: amphotericin B, 0.7–1 mg/kg/day IV for 14 days, followed by 8 weeks of fluconazole, 400 mg PO QD, achieves clinical response and CSF sterilization in about 70%. Switch from amphotericin B to fluconazole after clinical improvement and conversion of CSF culture to negative
- Early addition of flucytosine, 100 mg/kg/day PO divided QID, prevents late relapses but does not substantially improve cure rates
- Non–AIDS-related cryptococcal meningitis: similar treatment, though mortality is higher
  - High dose amphotericin B not tolerated because of underlying illnesses and older age
  - Lipid formulations of amphotericin B have equivalent efficacy with reduced nephrotoxicity
  - Continue therapy until CSF culture is negative and CSF antigen titers are < 1:8

Maintenance therapy

- AIDS-related cryptococcal meningitis: fluconazole, 200 mg PO QD chronically, after acute therapy to prevent > 50% relapse rate
- Secondary prophylaxis can be discontinued after minimum of 6 months in patients responding to HAART with CD4 > 200/μL on two determinations
- Non–AIDS-related cryptococcal meningitis: fluconazole, 200 mg PO QD for 3 months, is recommended by some experts

THERAPEUTIC PROCEDURES

- Repeated lumbar punctures or ventricular shunting is done to relieve high CSF pressures or hydrocephalus
- Corticosteroids may be helpful in patients with immune reconstitution "paradoxical exacerbations" of meningitis but are of no benefit in typical disease

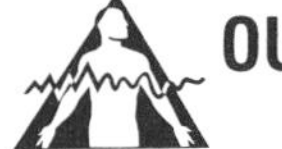

OUTCOME

COMPLICATIONS

- Obstructive hydrocephalus

PROGNOSIS

- Poor prognosis indicated by
  - Activity of predisposing conditions
  - Older age
  - Organ failure
  - Lack of CSF pleocytosis
  - High initial antigen titer in serum or CSF
  - Decreased mental status
  - Disease outside central nervous system
- Fluconazole maintenance therapy after HIV-related meningitis in patients whose CSF has been sterilized by induction therapy
  - Decreases relapse rate 10-fold compared with placebo
  - Decreases relapse rate 3-fold compared with weekly amphotericin B

EVIDENCE

PRACTICE GUIDELINES

- Practice Guidelines from the Infectious Diseases Society of America
  - http://www.journals.uchicago.edu/CID/journal/issues/v30n4/991230.web.pdf2001
- USPHS/IDSA Guidelines for the Prevention of Opportunistic Infections in Persons Infected with Human Immunodeficiency Virus. US Department of Health and Human Services, Public Health Service
  - http://aidsinfo.nih.gov/guidelines/op_infectionsOI_112801.pdf

WEB SITE

- Centers for Disease Control and Prevention
  - http://www.cdc.gov/ncidod/dbmd/diseaseinfo/cryptococcosis_t.htm

INFORMATION FOR PATIENTS

- Centers for Disease Control and Prevention—Cryptococcosis
  - http://www.cdc.gov/ncidod/dbmd/diseaseinfo/cryptococcosis_t.htm
- JAMA Patient Page: HIV infection: the basics. JAMA 2002;288:268. [PMID: 12123237]
- MedlinePlus—Cryptococcosis
  - http://www.nlm.nih.gov/medlineplus/ency/article/001328.htm

REFERENCES

- Brouwer AE et al: Combination antifungal therapies for HIV-associated cryptococcal meningitis: a randomised trial. Lancet 2004;363:1764. [PMID: 15172774]
- Mussini C et al: Discontinuation of maintenance therapy for cryptococcal meningitis in patients with AIDS treated with highly active antiretroviral therapy: an international observational study. Clin Infect Dis 2004;38:565. [PMID: 14765351]
- Saag MS et al: Practice guidelines for the management of cryptococcal disease. Clin Infect Dis 2000;30:710. [PMID: 10770733]

Author(s)

Samuel A. Shelburne, MD
Richard J. Hamill, MD

Cryptosporidiosis

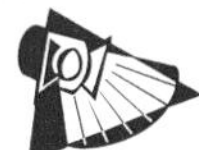

KEY FEATURES

ESSENTIALS OF DIAGNOSIS

In immunocompetent patients

- Diarrhea, mild to severe with flatulence and bloating. Mucus but no blood
- Low-grade fever, malasie, weight loss
- Generally self-limited in days to weeks

In immunocompromised patients

- Severe watery diarrhea
- Malabsorption, weight loss
- Blood and leukocytes seldom present

GENERAL CONSIDERATIONS

- Coccidiosis is an intracellular infection of intestinal epithelial cells by spore-forming protozoa
- The causes of coccidiosis are *Cryptosporidium* spp, particularly *C parvum* and *C hominis; Isospora belli; Cyclospora cayetanensis; Sarcocystis bovihominis* and *S suihominis;* all but the *Sarcocystis* species complete their life cycle in a single host. Diarrhea caused by any of these organisms is usually clinically similar
- Cryptosporidiosis is a zoonosis in which infections in farm animals (cattle, goats, turkeys, and others) can be transmitted to humans; however, most human infections are acquired from humans
- The organism is highly infectious (few parasites can induce infection) and readily transmitted fecal-orally in health and day care settings and in households
- The incubation period appears to be 1–12 days

DEMOGRAPHICS

- These infections occur worldwide, particularly in the tropics and in regions where hygiene is poor
- Clustering occurs in households, day care centers, and among sexual partners
- The prevalence of asymptomatic human carriers in the United States is estimated to be about 1.5%
- Outbreaks are of particular concern, as exemplified by the 1993 epidemic in Milwaukee in which 400,000 persons became ill

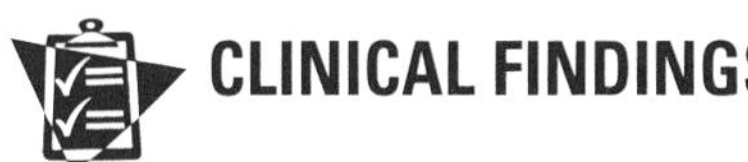

CLINICAL FINDINGS

SYMPTOMS AND SIGNS

In immunocompetent patients

- Infection varies from no symptoms to a mild diarrhea with flatulence and bloating to severe and frequent watery diarrhea in which the onset may be explosive
- Mucus may be present in stools, but no microscopic or gross blood
- May also have low-grade fever, malaise, anorexia, abdominal cramps, vomiting, dehydration, and myalgia
- Symptoms are generally self-limited, lasting under 30 days
- Weight loss can be marked

In immunodeficient patients

- The diarrhea can be profuse (up to 15 L daily has been reported), with cholera-like watery movements, accompanied by severe malabsorption, electrolyte imbalance, and marked weight loss
- Mucus is seen in the stools, but blood and leukocytes are seldom present
- The diarrhea may recur or persist
- Fever is uncommon
- In AIDS, 10–20% of patients develop cryptosporidiosis at some time during their illness; infection may involve any part of the gastrointestinal tract including the biliary tract (sclerosing cholangitis), respiratory tract infection, hepatitis, pancreatitis, lymphadenopathy, and hepatosplenomegaly may occur, as well as multisystem involvement

DIFFERENTIAL DIAGNOSIS

- *I belli, C cayetanensis,* and *S bovihominis*
- Giardiasis
- Viral gastroenteritis, eg, rotavirus
- Other traveler's diarrhea, eg, *Escherichia coli*
- Cholera
- Other cause of diarrhea in AIDS, eg, cytomegalovirus colitis

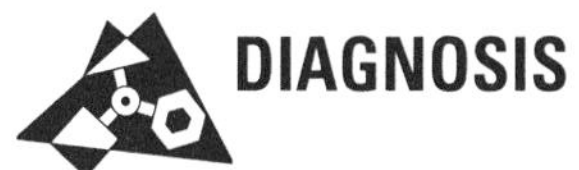

DIAGNOSIS

LABORATORY TESTS

- Three stool specimens should be obtained fresh and in preservative over 5–7 days
- Diagnosis is by detecting the organism by the modified acid-fast staining method; a minimum of two concentrated specimens should be tested
- Commercially available antigen detection kits improve on the diagnosis
  - Direct fluorescent antibody methods have sensitivities and specificities of 99–100%
  - Enzyme immunoassays have sensitivities and specificities of 93–100%
  - Some of the kits can be used with both fresh and frozen specimens
  - Other kits, however, can be used only if the specimen is fresh
- The polymerase chain reaction offers an alternative mode of diagnosis
- Tests for serum antibody are useful epidemiologically but not for patient diagnosis
- Stools rarely show white or red blood cells
- Blood leukocytosis and eosinophilia are uncommon

IMAGING STUDIES

- Radiologic changes have been reported in the stomach, intestines, and bile ducts in severe disease

DIAGNOSTIC PROCEDURES

- The organisms can also be detected by duodenal aspiration or biopsy
- In AIDS patients with unexplained diarrhea, the organism should also be looked for in sputum and bronchoalveolar lavage fluid; specimens obtained from lung tissue have sometimes been positive in patients with negative stool specimens

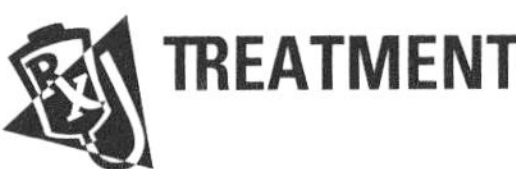

TREATMENT

MEDICATIONS

- Most acute infections in immunocompetent persons are self-limited and do not require treatment
- No treatment has been successful
- Nitazoxamide has recently been approved in the US for use in children; evaluation in adults (500 mg twice daily for 3 days) continues
- Other drugs that have been tried are
  - Roxithromycin (300 mg twice daily for 4 weeks)
  - Spiramycin (1 g three times daily for 2 weeks or longer)
  - Paromomycin (25–35 mg/kg/day in three or four divided doses; duration uncertain)
  - Zidovudine (AZT), azithromycin (600 mg daily), octreotide, eflornithine, letrazuril, nitazoxamide, hyperimmune bovine colostrum, and lactobacillus

THERAPEUTIC PROCEDURES

- Supportive treatment for severe or chronic diarrhea includes fluid and electrolyte replacement and, in chronic cases, parenteral nutrition

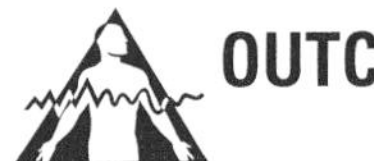

OUTCOME

FOLLOW-UP

- Symptoms are generally self-limited in **immunocompetent patients**
- Parasitologic clearance, however, may take several months
- The diarrhea may recur or persist in **immunodeficient patients,** and passage of organisms continues for months to indefinitely
- Oocysts passed in stools are fully sporulated and infectious; therefore, hospitalized patients should be isolated and stool precautions strictly observed

WHEN TO REFER

- Persistent diarrhea, particularly in the immunocompromised patient
- Malabsoption, progressive weight loss

WHEN TO ADMIT

- Profuse diarrhea causing hypotension or electrolyte imbalance

PREVENTION

- Measures to reduce exposure to the organisms are recommended for immunodeficient patients. These include reduced exposure to swimming in fresh water
- Since chlorine disinfection of water is not effective, adequate filtration is required. However, because of the oocysts' small size (2–5 μm), filtration is difficult and unreliable (the < 1-μm filters used frequently become obstructed)

EVIDENCE

PRACTICE GUIDELINES

- National Guideline Clearinghouse
  - http://www.guideline.gov/summary/summary.aspx?doc_id=3080
  - http://www.guideline.gov/summary/summary.aspx?doc_id=2573

WEB SITE

- Centers for Disease Control and Prevention—Division of Parasitic Diseases
  - http://www.cdc.gov/ncidod/dpd/parasites/cryptosporidiosis/default.htm

INFORMATION FOR PATIENTS

- Centers for Disease Control and Prevention
  - http://www.cdc.gov/ncidod/dpd/parasites/cryptosporidiosis/factsht_cryptosporidiosis.htm
  - http://www.cdc.gov/ncidod/dpd/parasites/cryptosporidiosis/factsht_crypto_prevent_water.htm

REFERENCES

- Chappell CL et al: Cryptosporidiosis. Curr Opin Infect Dis 2002;15:523. [PMID: 12686887]
- Chen XM et al: Cryptosporidiosis. N Engl J Med 2002;346:1723. [PMID: 12037153]

Cushing's Syndrome (Hypercortisolism)

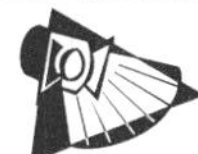

KEY FEATURES

ESSENTIALS OF DIAGNOSIS

- Central obesity, muscle wasting, thin skin, easy bruisability, psychological changes, hirsutism, purple striae
- Osteoporosis, hypertension, poor wound healing
- Hyperglycemia, glycosuria, leukocytosis, lymphocytopenia, hypokalemia
- Elevated serum cortisol and urinary free cortisol. Lack of normal suppression by dexamethasone

GENERAL CONSIDERATIONS

- Cushing's "syndrome" refers to manifestations of excessive corticosteroids
- Commonly due to supraphysiologic doses of glucocorticoid drugs; rarely due to excessive corticosteroid production
- Excessive corticosteroid production is often due to Cushing's "disease" (~43% of cases), ie, hypercortisolism due to ACTH hypersecretion by the pituitary. Usually caused by benign pituitary adenoma
- ~10% due to nonpituitary neoplasms (eg, small-cell lung carcinoma) that produce excessive ectopic ACTH
- ~15% due to ACTH from a source that cannot be initially located
- ~32% due to excessive autonomous secretion of cortisol by the adrenals independent of ACTH (serum ACTH usually low). Usually due to unilateral adrenal tumor of three types
  - Benign adrenal adenomas are generally small tumors that produce mostly cortisol
  - Adrenal carcinomas usually large and can produce excessive androgens as well as cortisol
  - ACTH-independent bilateral adrenal hyperplasia can also produce hypercortisolism

DEMOGRAPHICS

- Spontaneous Cushing's syndrome is rare: 2.6 new cases yearly per million population
- ACTH-secreting pituitary adenoma (Cushing's "disease") >3 times more common in women than men

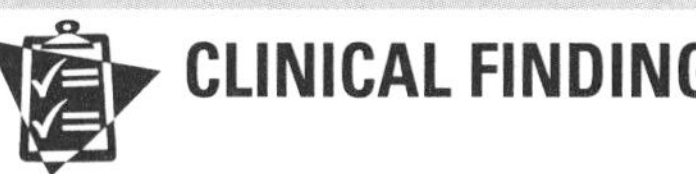

CLINICAL FINDINGS

SYMPTOMS AND SIGNS

- Central obesity with plethoric "moon face," "buffalo hump," supraclavicular fat pads, protuberant abdomen, and thin extremities
- Oligomenorrhea or amenorrhea (or impotence in males)
- Weakness, backache, headache
- Hypertension
- Osteoporosis or avascular bone necrosis
- Acne, superficial skin infections, purple striae (especially around the thighs, breasts, and abdomen), easy bruising, and impaired wound healing
- Thirst and polyuria (with or without glycosuria); renal calculi
- Glaucoma
- Mental symptoms range from diminished concentration to increased mood lability to psychosis
- Increased susceptibility to opportunistic infections
- Hirsutism and virilization may occur with adrenal carcinomas

DIFFERENTIAL DIAGNOSIS

- Chronic alcoholism (alcoholic pseudo-Cushing's syndrome)
- Diabetes mellitus
- Depression (may have hypercortisolism)
- Osteoporosis due to other cause
- Obesity due to other cause
- Primary hyperaldosteronism
- Anorexia nervosa (high urine free cortisol)
- Striae distensae ("stress marks") seen in adolescence and in pregnancy
- Lipodystrophy from antiretroviral agents

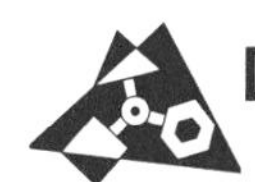

DIAGNOSIS

LABORATORY TESTS

- Glucose tolerance impaired due to insulin resistance
- Polyuria and glycosuria
- Leukocytosis; relative granulocytosis and lymphopenia
- Hypokalemia (not hypernatremia), particularly with ectopic ACTH secretion
- Dexamethasone suppression test is the easiest screening test for hypercortisolism
  - Give dexamethasone, 1 mg PO, at 11 PM and measure serum cortisol at about 8 AM next morning
  - Plasma cortisol < 5 μg/dL (fluorometric assay) or < 2 μg/dL (HPLC assay) excludes Cushing's syndrome with 98% certainty
  - Antiseizure drugs (eg, phenytoin, phenobarbital, primidone) and rifampin accelerate the metabolism of dexamethasone, causing a false-positive dexamethasone suppression test
- If not excluded, measure 24-hour urine for free cortisol and creatinine
  - High 24-hour urine free cortisol (or free cortisol to creatinine ratio of >95 μg cortisol/g creatinine) helps confirm hypercortisolism
  - Misleadingly high urine free cortisol occurs with high fluid intake
- Midnight serum cortisol level >7.5 μg/dL is indicative of Cushing's syndrome; must be NPO for 3 hours and have IV established in advance for blood draw
- Because of the inconvenience of obtaining a midnight blood specimen for serum cortisol, salivary cortisol assays have proved useful
  - The saliva must be collected in special tubes and analyzed in reference laboratories
  - Using an enzyme-linked immunosorbent assay, midnight salivary cortisol levels are normally < 0.15 mg/dL (4.0 nmol/L)
  - If consistently > 0.25 mg/dL (7.0 nmol/L) they are nearly diagnostic of endogenous Cushing's syndrome
- If hypercortisolism is confirmed
  - Plasma ACTH below normal indicates probable adrenal tumor
  - High or normal ACTH indicates pituitary or ectopic tumors
  - Blood for ACTH assay must be collected in a plastic tube, placed on ice, and processed quickly to avoid falsely low results
- In patients with ACTH-dependent Cushing's syndrome, chest masses may be the source of ACTH, but opportunistic infections are common, so it is prudent to biopsy a chest mass to confirm the pathologic diagnosis prior to resection

IMAGING STUDIES

- Pituitary MRI shows adenoma in ~50% of cases of ACTH-dependent Cushing's syndrome
- CT of chest and abdomen can help locate source of ectopic ACTH, in lungs (carcinoid or small-cell carcinomas), thymus, pancreas, or adrenals
- CT of adrenals can localize adrenal tumor in most cases of non-ACTH-dependent Cushing's syndrome

- CT scanning fails to detect the source of ACTH in about 40% of patients with ectopic ACTH secretion
- ^{111}In-octreotide scanning is also useful in detecting occult tumors, but ^{18}FDG-PET scanning is not usually helpful. Some ectopic ACTH-secreting tumors elude discovery, necessitating bilateral adrenalectomy

DIAGNOSTIC PROCEDURES

- If pituitary MRI is normal or shows incidental irregularity, selective inferior petrosal venous sampling for ACTH is performed (with corticotropin-releasing hormone stimulation) where available to confirm pituitary ACTH source, distinguishing it from an occult nonpituitary tumor secreting ACTH

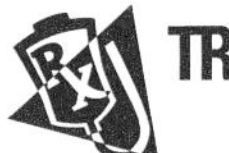

TREATMENT

MEDICATIONS

- Hydrocortisone replacement required temporarily after resection of pituitary adenoma or adrenal adenoma (see above)
- Ketoconazole, 200 mg PO Q6 h, for patients with Cushing's disease who are not surgical candidates; must monitor liver enzymes
- Mitotane for metastatic adrenal carcinomas; ketoconazole or metyrapone may suppress hypercortisolism in unresectable adrenal carcinoma; however, metyrapone may exacerbate female virilization
- Bisphosphonates for patients with osteoporosis

SURGERY

- Selective transsphenoidal resection of pituitary adenoma indicated in Cushing's disease, after which remainder of pituitary usually returns to normal function. However, corticotrophs require 6–36 months to recover normal function; thus, hydrocortisone replacement is required temporarily
- Bilateral laparoscopic adrenalectomy if no remission (or recurrence) after pituitary surgery
- Laparoscopic resection for adrenal neoplasms secreting cortisol. Because contralateral adrenal is suppressed, postoperative hydrocortisone replacement is required until recovery
- Surgical resection of ectopic ACTH-secreting tumors

THERAPEUTIC PROCEDURES

- Stereotactic pituitary radiosurgery (gamma knife) normalizes urine free cortisol in two-thirds of patients within 12 months
- Conventional radiation therapy cures 23%

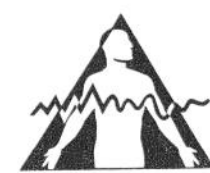

OUTCOME

COMPLICATIONS

- If untreated, produces serious morbidity and even death
- Complications of hypertension or diabetes mellitus
- Increased susceptibility to infections
- Compression fractures of osteoporotic spine, aseptic necrosis of femoral head
- Nephrolithiasis
- Depression, dementia, psychosis
- Following bilateral adrenalectomy for Cushing's disease, progressive enlargement of pituitary adenoma may cause local effects (eg, visual field impairment) and hyperpigmentation (Nelson's syndrome)

PROGNOSIS

- Cushing's syndrome due to benign adrenal adenoma has 5-year survival rate of 95% and 10-year survival rate of 90% following successful adrenalectomy
- Patients with Cushing's disease from pituitary adenoma have similar survival if pituitary surgery is successful
- Transsphenoidal surgery fails in ~10–20%
- Despite complete remission after transsphenoidal surgery, ~15–20% recur over 10 years
- Bilateral laparoscopic adrenalectomy may be required, but is often complicated by infection
  - Recurrence of hypercortisolism may occur owing to growth of adrenal remnant stimulated by high ACTH levels
- Prognosis with ectopic ACTH-producing tumors depends on aggressiveness and stage of tumor
- Patients with ACTH of unknown source have 5-year survival rate of 65% and 10-year survival rate of 55%
- Patients with adrenal carcinoma have median survival of 7 months

WHEN TO REFER

- If abnormal dexamethasone suppression test

WHEN TO ADMIT

- For transsphenoidal hypophysectomy, adrenalectomy, resection of ectopic ACTH-secreting tumor

EVIDENCE

PRACTICE GUIDELINES

- Morris D et al: The medical management of Cushing's syndrome. Ann NY Acad Sci 2002;970:119. [PMID: 12381547]
- Nieman LK: Diagnostic tests for Cushing's syndrome. Ann NY Acad Sci 2002;970:112. [PMID: 12381546]

INFORMATION FOR PATIENTS

- American Academy of Family Physicians—Cushing's syndrome and Cushing's disease
  - http://familydoctor.org/623.html
- NIDDK/NIH—Cushing's Syndrome
  - http://www.niddk.nih.gov/health/endo/pubs/cushings/cushings.htm
  - http://www.medhelp.org/www/nadf4.htm
  - http://pituitary.mgh.harvard.edu/cushings.htm

REFERENCES

- Allolio B et al: Management of adrenocortical carcinoma. Clin Endocrinol (Oxf) 2004;60:273. [PMID: 15008991]
- Hammer GD et al: Transsphenoidal microsurgery for Cushing's disease: initial outcome and longterm results. J Clin Endocrinol Metab 2004;89:6348. [PMID: 15579802]
- Hoybye C et al: Transsphenoidal surgery in Cushing's disease: 10 years of experience in 34 consecutive cases. J Neurosurg 2004;100:634. [PMID: 15070117]
- Liu C et al: Cavernous and inferior petrosal sinus sampling in the evaluation of ACTH-dependent Cushing's syndrome. Clin Endocrinol 2004:61:478. [PMID: 15473881]
- Swearingen B et al: Diagnostic errors after inferior petrosal sinus sampling. J Clin Endocrinol Metab 2004;89:3752. [PMID: 15292301]
- Yaneva M et al: Midnight salivary cortisol for the initial diagnosis of Cushing's syndrome of various causes. J Clin Endocrinol Metab 2004;89:3345. [PMID: 15240613]

Author(s)

Paul A. Fitzgerald, MD

Cyclosporiasis

Cyanide Poisoning p. 1062

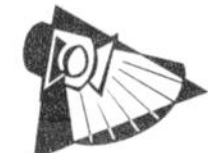

KEY FEATURES

ESSENTIALS OF DIAGNOSIS

In immunocompetent patients

- Mild to severe diarrhea; mucus may be present in the stool but blood is absent
- Low-grade fever, vomiting, malaise

In immunodeficient patients

- Diarrhea may be profuse
- Occasionally, severe malabsorption and weight loss
- Blood and leukocytes are seldom present

GENERAL CONSIDERATIONS

- The causes of coccidiosis are *Cryptosporidium* spp, particularly *C parvum* and *C hominis*; *Isospora belli*; *Cyclospora cayetanensis*; *Sarcocystis bovihominis* and *Sarcocystis suihominis*; all but the *Sarcocystis* species complete their life cycle in a single host. Diarrhea caused by any of these organisms is usually clinically similar
- The *Cyclospora* species in humans appear to be distinct to humans only
- The infectious agents are oocysts (spores) transmitted directly from person to person or by contaminated water or food
- *Cyclospora* require time outside the host to sporulate and become infectious
- Outbreaks in the United States have been attributed to imported fresh fruit and vegetables
- Is a cause of traveler's diarrhea; institutional and community outbreaks of diarrhea; and acute and chronic diarrhea in immunodeficient patients, including those with AIDS, in whom the infection can be life-threatening
- The pathogenesis of the diarrhea is not well understood; no enterotoxin has been identified

DEMOGRAPHICS

- Occurs worldwide, particularly in the tropics and in regions where hygiene is poor

CLINICAL FINDINGS

SYMPTOMS AND SIGNS

- The diarrhea caused by the coccidial and microsporidial agents is clinically indistinguishable
- The incubation period is 2–11 days
- Rarely, the organisms invade the biliary tree. Voluminous secretory or malabsorption diarrhea (including vitamin B_{12}, d-xylose, and fat absorption dysfunction) can result

In immunocompetent patients

- Infection varies from no symptoms to a mild diarrhea with flatulence and bloating to severe and frequent watery diarrhea in which the onset may be explosive
- Mucus may be present in stools, but no microscopic or gross blood is found
- There may be low-grade fever, malaise, anorexia, abdominal cramps, vomiting, and myalgia. These symptoms are generally self-limited, lasting a few days to several weeks
- Illness can be self-limited or persist with weight loss

In immunodeficient patients

- The diarrhea can be profuse (up to 15 L daily has been reported), with cholera-like watery movements, accompanied by severe malabsorption, electrolyte imbalance, and marked weight loss
- Fever is uncommon
- Mucus is seen in the stools, but blood and leukocytes are seldom present
- The diarrhea may recur or persist

DIFFERENTIAL DIAGNOSIS

- *C parvum*, *I belli*, *S bovihominis*, and *S suihominis*
- Giardiasis
- Viral gastroenteritis, eg, rotavirus
- Other traveler's diarrhea, eg, *Escherichia coli*
- Cholera
- Other causes of diarrhea in AIDS, eg, cytomegalovirus colitis

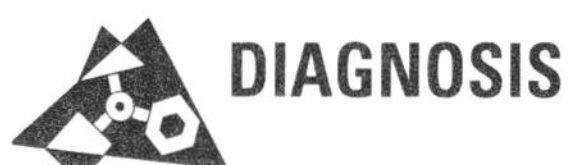

DIAGNOSIS

LABORATORY TESTS

- Three stool specimens collected over 5–7 days should be stored both as fresh specimens and in preservative and processed by flotation or concentration methods to detect the distinctive oocysts (8–10 μm)
- The laboratory should be notified that *Cyclospora* are being investigated because specific fecal examinations are needed
- Antibodies have been detected and titers increase during convalescence

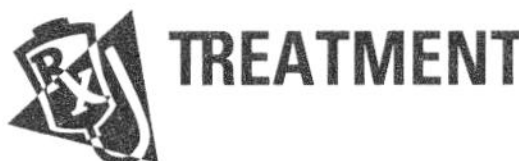

TREATMENT

MEDICATIONS

- Trimethoprim (TMP, 160 mg)-sulfamethoxazole (SMZ, 800 mg) twice daily for 7 days is effective; in HIV infections, higher doses (four times daily for 10 days) and long-term maintenance (three times weekly) are needed
- For patients intolerant of TMP-SMZ, ciprofloxacin (500 mg twice daily for 7 days) can be tried

THERAPEUTIC PROCEDURES

- Most acute infections in immunocompetent persons are self-limited and do not require treatment
- Supportive treatment for severe or chronic diarrhea includes fluid and electrolyte replacement and, in chronic cases, parenteral nutrition

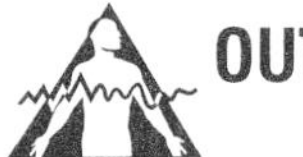

OUTCOME

FOLLOW-UP

- Parasitological clearance may take several months even in immunocompetent patients
- Passage of organisms continues for months to indefinitely in immunodeficient persons

WHEN TO REFER

- Refer to an infectious disease specialist or gastroenterologist if diarrhea persists despite antibiotic therapy, particularly in immunocompromised patients
- Refer for secretory or malabsorption diarrhea
- Refer for progressive weight loss

WHEN TO ADMIT

- Profuse diarrhea causing hypotension or electrolyte imbalance

PREVENTION

- Measures to reduce exposure to the organism are recommended for immunocompromised patients. These include reduced exposure to swimming in fresh water and boiling of drinking water (1 min) or use of a filter that removes particles over 1 μm in size

EVIDENCE

WEB SITE

- Centers for Disease Control and Prevention—Division of Parasitic Diseases
  - http://www.cdc.gov/ncidod/dpd/parasites/cyclospora/default.htm

INFORMATION FOR PATIENTS

- Centers for Disease Control and Prevention
  - http://www.cdc.gov/ncidod/dpd/parasites/cyclospora/factsht_cyclospora.htm
  - http://www.cdc.gov/ncidod/dbmd/diseaseinfo/travelersdiarrhea_g.htm
- Directors of Health Promotion and Education
  - http://www.astdhpphe.org/infect/cyclospora.html

REFERENCES

- Eberhand ML et al: *Cyclospora* spp. Curr Opin Infect Dis 2002;15:519. [PMID: 12686886]
- Herwaldt BL: *Cyclospora cayetanensis:* a review, focusing on the outbreaks of cyclosporiasis in the 1990s. Clin Infect Dis 2000;31:1040. [PMID: 11049789]

Cystic Fibrosis

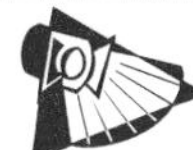

KEY FEATURES

ESSENTIALS OF DIAGNOSIS

- Chronic or recurrent cough, sputum production, dyspnea, and wheezing
- Recurrent infections or chronic colonization of the airways with *Haemophilus influenzae, Pseudomonas aeruginosa, Staphylococcus aureus*, or *Burkholderia cepacia*
- Pancreatic insufficiency, recurrent pancreatitis, distal intestinal obstruction syndrome, chronic hepatic disease, nutritional deficiencies, or male urogenital abnormalities
- Bronchiectasis and scarring on chest radiographs
- Airflow obstruction on spirometry
- Sweat chloride concentration above 60 mEq/L on two occasions or mutations in genes known to cause cystic fibrosis

GENERAL CONSIDERATIONS

- Most common fatal hereditary disorder of whites in the United States
- Autosomal recessive disorder due to mutations affecting a membrane chloride channel (the cystic fibrosis transmembrane conductance regulator, or CFTR)
- At least 1000 mutations to the CFTR gene are described, with "ΔF508" accounting for 60% of cases
- Pathophysiology results from production of an abnormal mucous in exocrine glands, which leads to tissue destruction and, in the respiratory tract, impairs mucociliary clearance
- Variety of mutations is reflected in wide range of pulmonary and nonpulmonary manifestations

DEMOGRAPHICS

- Affects 1 in 3200 whites; 1 in 25 is a carrier

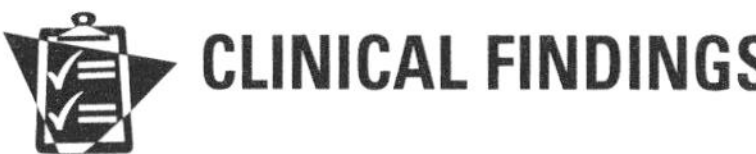

CLINICAL FINDINGS

SYMPTOMS AND SIGNS

- Disease should be suspected in young adults with a history of chronic lung disease, pancreatitis, or infertility
- Productive cough, decreased exercise tolerance, and recurrent hemoptysis are typical
- Sinus pain or pressure with purulent nasal discharge is common
- Pulmonary manifestations
  - Bronchitis
  - Bronchiectasis
  - Pneumonia
  - Atelectasis
  - Peribronchial and parenchymal scarring
- Common extrapulmonary manifestations
  - Steatorrhea
  - Diarrhea
  - Adominal pain
- Advanced disease manifestations
  - Hypoxemia
  - Hypercapnia
  - Cor pulmonale
- Nearly all male patients have congenital absence of the vas deferens with azoospermia
- Findings include
  - Digital clubbing
  - Increased anterioposterior chest diameter
  - Apical crackles

DIFFERENTIAL DIAGNOSIS

- Chronic obstructive pulmonary disease
- Asthma
- α_1-Antitrypsin deficiency
- Bronchiolitis
- Celiac disease (celiac sprue)
- Chronic sinusitis

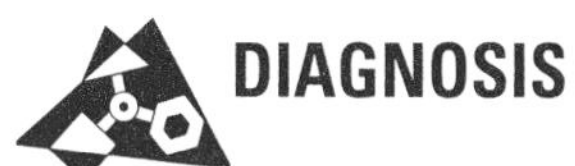

DIAGNOSIS

LABORATORY TESTS

- Arterial blood gases reveal hypoxemia, with compensated respiratory acidosis in advanced disease
- Pulmonary function tests
  - A mixed obstructive and restrictive pattern
  - Reduced FVC, airflow rates, and total lung capacity
  - Air trapping and reduced diffusion capacity are common
- Genotyping, measurement of nasal membrane potential difference, semen analysis, or assessment of pancreatic function can play a role in diagnosis
- Sputum cultures
  - Frequently show *S aureus* and *P aeruginosa*
  - Occasionally show *H influenzae, Stenotrophomonas maltophilia,* and *B cepacia*

IMAGING STUDIES

- Hyperinflation is seen early in chest x-rays
- Peribronchial cuffing, mucus plugging, bronchiectasis, atelectasis, and increased interstitial markings are sometimes seen
- High-resolution CT is the test of choice to confirm bronchiectasis

DIAGNOSTIC PROCEDURES

- Chloride sweat test reveals elevated sodium and chloride levels; two tests on different days are required for accurate diagnosis
- A normal sweat chloride test does not exclude the diagnosis

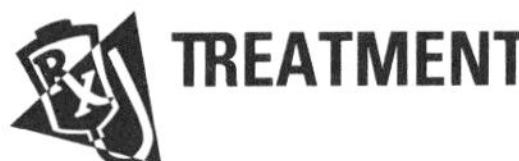

TREATMENT

MEDICATIONS

- Inhaled bronchodilators should be considered in patients who demonstrate an increase in FEV_1 of 12% in response to treatment
- rhDNase, 2.5 mg nebulized daily, thins sputum by cleaving extracellular DNA from neutrophils that accumulate in sputum and increase viscosity
- Antibiotics are used to treat airway infection based on results of sputum culture and sensitivity testing
- Aerosolized antibiotics (tobramycin and others) are sometimes helpful, but there is concern regarding development of resistant *B cepacia* and side effects such as bronchospasm

SURGERY

- Lung transplantation is the only definitive therapy for advanced disease; double-lung or heart-lung transplantation is required
- 3-year survival rates after transplantation are about 55%

THERAPEUTIC PROCEDURES

- Mechanical interventions to clear lower airway secretions
  - Postural drainage
  - Chest percussion or vibration
  - Positive expiratory pressure
  - Flutter valve breathing devices
  - Directed cough

OUTCOME

FOLLOW-UP

- Regular assessment of FEV_1
- Nutritional status

COMPLICATIONS

- Pneumothorax and hemoptysis are common
- Cor pulmonale is seen in late disease
- Patients have increased risk of gastrointestinal malignancies, osteopenia, and arthropathies
- Biliary cirrhosis, gallstones, and pancreatitis are seen
- Resistant infections, including methicillin-resistant *Staphylococcus aureus* and *B cepacia*

PROGNOSIS

- Median survival is at 31 years, but is increasing
- Death results from pulmonary infections or as a result of chronic respiratory failure and cor pulmonale

WHEN TO REFER

- All patients with suspected or confirmed cystic fibrosis should be referred to a Cystic Fibrosis Center of Excellence for evaluation and treatment recommendations

WHEN TO ADMIT

- Increased cough, sputum production, shortness of breath, decline in FEV_1, weight loss, constitutional symptoms, hemoptysis

PREVENTION

- Vaccination against pneumococcal infection and annual influenza vaccination are recommended
- Screening of family members and genetic counseling are suggested

EVIDENCE

PRACTICE GUIDELINES

- National Guideline Clearinghouse
  - http://www.guideline.gov/summary/summary.aspx?doc_id=3273&nbr=2499&string=cystic+fibrosis

INFORMATION FOR PATIENTS

- Cystic Fibrosis Foundation website
  - http://www.cff.org
- Mayo Clinic
  - http://www.mayoclinic.com/invoke.cfm?id=DS00287
- National Institutes of Health
  - http://www.nlm.nih.gov/medlineplus/cysticfibrosis.html

REFERENCES

- Boucher RC. New concepts of the pathogenesis of cystic fibrosis lung disease. Eur Respir J 2004;23:146. [PMID: 14738247]
- Ellaffi M et al: One-year outcome after severe pulmonary exacerbation in adults with cystic fibrosis. Am J Respir Crit Care Med 2005;171:158. [PMID: 15502116]
- Gibson RL et al: Pathophysiology and management of pulmonary infections in cystic fibrosis. Am J Respir Crit Care Med 2003;168:918. [PMID: 14555458]
- Yankaskas JR et al: Cystic fibrosis adult care: concensus conference report. Chest 2004;125(1 Suppl):1S. [PMID: 14734689]

Author(s)

Mark S. Chesnutt, MD

Thomas J. Prendergast, MD

Cysticercosis

KEY FEATURES

ESSENTIALS OF DIAGNOSIS

- History of exposure to *Taenia solium* in an endemic region; concomitant or past intestinal tapeworm infection
- Seizures, headache, and other findings of a focal space-occupying central nervous system (CNS) lesion
- Subcutaneous or muscular nodules (5–10 mm); calcified lesions on x-rays of soft tissues
- Calcified or uncalcified cysts by CT scan or MRI; positive serological tests

GENERAL CONSIDERATIONS

- Human cysticercosis is infection by the larval (cysticercus) stage of the tapeworm *T solium*
- Cysticerci complete their development within 2–4 months after larval entry and live for months to years
- Initially, the live larva within a thin-walled cyst (vesicular cyst) is minimally antigenic. When the host immune response or chemotherapy results in gradual death of the cyst, there may be cyst enlargement (colloidal cyst) with mechanical compression, inflammation with pericyst edema, and vasculitis that can result in small cerebral infarcts; increased intracranial pressure and cerebrospinal fluid changes may follow. As the cyst degenerates over 2–7 years, it may disappear or be replaced by a granuloma, calcification, or residual fibrosis. Cysts at different life cycle stages—active (live), transitional, and inactive (dead)—may be in the same organ
- Locations of cysts in order of frequency are the CNS, subcutaneous tissues and striated muscle, globe of the eye, and, rarely, other tissues. Cysts reach 5–10 mm in soft tissues but may be larger (up to 5 cm) in the CNS

DEMOGRAPHICS

- Worldwide, an estimated 20 million persons are infected
- Yearly, about 400,000 persons have neurological symptoms and 50,000 die from the disease
- Antibody prevalence rates to 10% are recognized in some endemic areas

CLINICAL FINDINGS

SYMPTOMS AND SIGNS

Neurocysticercosis

- May be asymptomatic
- When symptomatic, the incubation period is highly variable (usually from 1 to 5 years but sometimes shorter)
- Acute invasive stage results from extensive acute spread of cysticerci to the brain parenchyma. Rarely, fever, headache, myalgia, marked eosinophilia, and coma may occur
- Parenchymal cysts can present singly or multiply and may be scattered or in clumps. Findings include epilepsy (focal or generalized), focal neurological deficits, intracranial hypertension, and altered mental status
- Subarachnoid space and meningeal cysts may result in obstructive hydrocephalus, intracranial hypertension, arterial thrombosis, and cranial nerve palsy (most often of the optic nerve)
- Ventricular cysts may float freely (usually singly) or may be attached to the ventricular wall. They are usually asymptomatic but can cause increased intracranial pressure
- Racemose cysts are rare grape-like irregular clusters and may reach over 10 cm in diameter. They can cause marked adhesive arachnoiditis and obstructive hydrocephalus
- Spinal cord cysts can cause arachnoiditis (meningitis, radiculopathy) or pressure symptoms

Ophthalmocysticercosis

- Usually there is a single cyst, free-floating in the vitreous or under the retina
- Presenting symptoms include periorbital pain, scotomas, and progressive deterioration of visual acuity
- Findings may include disk hemorrhage, retinal detachment, iridocyclitis, and chorioretinitis

Subcutaneous and striated muscle cysticercosis

- Usually asymptomatic
- May present as nodules that tend to appear and disappear, or they may die and calcify and be detected on radiographs

DIFFERENTIAL DIAGNOSIS

- Seizure due to other cause, eg, epilepsy, bacterial meningitis
- Primary or metastatic cancer
- Tuberculoma
- Echinococcosis (hydatid disease)
- Bacterial or fungal brain abscess
- Toxoplasmosis
- Neurosyphilis

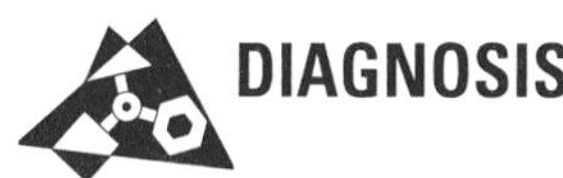

DIAGNOSIS

LABORATORY TESTS

- The serum enzyme-linked immunoelectrotransfer blot (EITB) assay has nearly 100% specificity and 94–98% sensitivity; when used with cerebrospinal fluid, however, both parameters are lower. The EITB sensitivity drops about 50% if only one or two cysts are present and is also low in patients with only calcified cysts
- The older ELISA has a 63% specificity and 65% sensitivity with serum; paradoxically, the ELISA with cerebrospinal fluid has a high specificity (95%) and sensitivity (87%) for both IgM and IgG antibody. False-positives can occur with previous exposure
- Cerebrospinal fluid typically shows increased protein, decreased glucose, and a cellular reaction of mainly lymphocytes and eosinophils; eosinophilia may be over 20% and is diagnostically important. Lumbar puncture is contraindicated in case of increased intracerebral pressure

IMAGING STUDIES

- Initially, use nonenhanced CT and then MRI and enhanced CT. Brain or spinal cord cystic lesions can show the scolex ("hole-with-dot")
- Spinal cysticercosis is evaluated by CT myelography or MRI
- Plain radiographs of muscle may detect oval or linear calcified lesions (4–10 × 2–5 mm). Plain skull films may demonstrate one or more cerebral calcifications (generally 5–10 mm; sometimes 1–2 mm when only the scolex is calcified)

DIAGNOSTIC PROCEDURES

- The diagnosis of neurocysticercosis is by demonstration of characteristic lesions on CT or MRI scan; by visualization of the parasite by ophthalmoscopic examination (subretinal or in the anterior chamber); or by finding the parasite in histological sections of brain or spinal cord tissue (not usually recommended)
- A probable diagnosis is based on the presence of various combinations of other major and minor criteria
- Highly suggestive of the diagnosis is finding the organism in excisional biopsies of skin or subcutaneous pea-sized nodules or a varied radiological appearance on brain scans

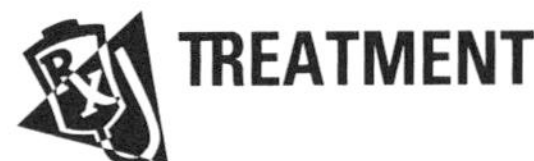

TREATMENT

MEDICATIONS

- Single enhancing lesions may be treated only with anticonvulsants; some experts do add albendazole or praziquantel treatment; however, patients with only calcified cysts do not need these drugs
- During the acute phase of encephalitis, if intracranial hypertension is present, mannitol (2 g/kg/day) and corticosteroids are used but drug treatment is withheld

Albendazole

- The dosage is 400 mg PO BID with a fatty meal
- Seven to 14 days of treatment may be sufficient, but a longer course (up to 28 days) is advisable; it can be repeated as necessary
- Up to 3 months of treatment may be needed for ventricular and subarachnoid cysts

Praziquantel

- Give 50–100 mg/kg/day PO in three divided doses for 15–30 days
- For both drugs, ingestion with a fatty meal enhances absorption

Other measures

- Phenytoin, phenobarbital, carbamazepine, cimetidine, and corticosteroids, when administered with praziquantel, reduce serum levels of the latter
- For patients with seizures, anticonvulsants should be given during drug treatment and probably for an indefinite time afterward
- Give corticosteroids at time of treatment to prevent the marked inflammatory reactions around dying parasites. Prednisone, 1 mg/kg/day in two or three divided doses, starting 1–2 days before use of the drug and continuing at diminishing doses for about 14 days afterward, is used. The reaction usually subsides in 48–72 h, but continuing severity may require steroids in higher dosage and mannitol
- Subarachnoiditis and vasculitis are treated with albendazole or praziquantel plus a corticosteroid
- An ophthalmological examination should be done; if cysticercocidal drugs are given in the presence of ocular or spinal cysts, irreparable damage can occur

SURGERY

- Surgery can remove accessible orbital, cisternal, ventricular, cerebral, meningeal, and spinal cord cysts. Obstructive hydrocephalus requires cerebrospinal fluid diversion plus a corticosteroid

THERAPEUTIC PROCEDURES

- Medical treatment, which is usually preferable to surgery, is most effective for parenchymal cysts; less effective for intraventricular, subarachnoid, or racemose cysts
- When only one or a few live parenchymal cysts are present, it is unclear whether medical treatment is preferable to symptomatic management followed by normal death of the parasites. Some clinicians wait 3 months with selected patients to see if cysts will spontaneously disappear

OUTCOME

PROGNOSIS

- The fatality rate for untreated neurocysticercosis is about 50%. Drug treatment has reduced the mortality rate to about 5–15%
- Surgical procedures to relieve intracranial hypertension along with use of steroids to reduce edema improve the prognosis for those not effectively treated with the drugs

WHEN TO REFER

- All patients should be referred to a clinician with expertise in these disorders

WHEN TO ADMIT

- Treatment should be conducted in a hospital

PREVENTION

- All family members should examine their stools over several days for passage of proglottids, and stool specimens should be sent to the laboratory to be examined for proglottids and eggs

EVIDENCE

PRACTICE GUIDELINES

- Garcia HH et al: Current consensus guidelines for treatment of neurocysticercosis. Clin Microbiol Rev 2002;15:747. [PMID: 12364377]

WEB SITE

- CDC—Division of Parasitic Diseases
  - http://www.cdc.gov/ncidod/dpd/parasites/cysticercosis/default.htm

INFORMATION FOR PATIENTS

- Centers for Disease Control
  - http://www.cdc.gov/ncidod/dpd/parasites/cysticercosis/factsht_cysticercosis.htm
- National Institutes of Health
  - http://www.nlm.nih.gov/medlineplus/ency/article/000627.htm

REFERENCES

- Katti MK: Proposed diagnostic criteria for neurocysticercosis. Neurology 2002;58:1315. [PMID: 11973827]
- Thaler DE, Frosch MP: Case records of the Massachusetts General Hospital. Weekly clinicopathological exercises. Case 16-2002. A 41-year-old woman with global headache and an intracranial mass. N Engl J Med 2002;346:1651. [PMID: 12023999]
- Verma L et al: Optic nerve cysticercosis. Arch Ophthalmol 2002;120:1408. [PMID: 12365933]

Cystitis, Acute

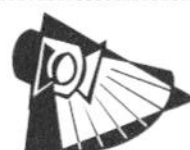

KEY FEATURES

ESSENTIALS OF DIAGNOSIS

- Irritative voiding symptoms
- Patient usually afebrile
- Positive urine culture; blood cultures may also be positive

CLINICAL FINDINGS

SYMPTOMS AND SIGNS

- Frequency, urgency, dysuria, suprapubic discomfort, gross hematuria
- Suprapubic tenderness, no systemic toxicity

DIFFERENTIAL DIAGNOSIS

- **In women**
  - Vulvovaginitis
  - Pelvic inflammatory disease
- **In men**
  - Urethritis
  - Prostatitis
- **In both**
  - Pelvic irradiation
  - Chemotherapy (cyclophosphamide)
  - Bladder carcinoma
  - Interstitial cystitis
  - Voiding dysfunction disorders
  - Psychosomatic disorders

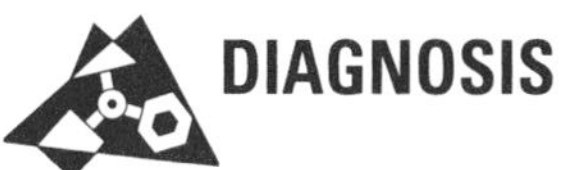

DIAGNOSIS

LABORATORY TESTS

- Urinalysis: pyuria, hematuria, bacteriuria
- Urine culture: positive, though colony counts > 10^5/mL not essential
- Urine culture and sensitivity

IMAGING STUDIES

- Imaging warranted only if pyelonephritis, recurrent infections, or anatomic abnormalities are suspected

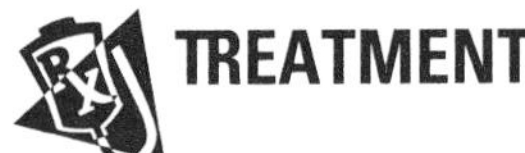

TREATMENT

MEDICATIONS

- Uncomplicated cystitis: cephalexin, nitrofurantoin, or fluoroquinolone single-dose or for 1–3 days (see regimens below)
- Avoid trimethoprim-sulfamethoxazole due to resistant organisms
- Cephalexin, 250–500 mg PO Q6 h for 1–3 days
- Ciprofloxacin, 250–500 mg PO Q12 h for 1–3 days
- Nitrofurantoin (macrocrystals), 100 mg PO Q12 h for 7 days
- Norfloxacin, 400 mg PO Q12 h for 1–3 days
- Ofloxacin, 200 mg PO Q12 h for 1–3 days
- Trimethoprim-sulfamethoxazole, 160/800 mg, 2 tablets PO once if organism is sensitive; increasing resistance noted (≥ 20%)

THERAPEUTIC PROCEDURES

- Symptomatic relief: hot sitz baths or urinary analgesics (phenazopyridine, 200 mg PO TID)
- Uncomplicated cystitis in men warrants elucidation of underlying problem

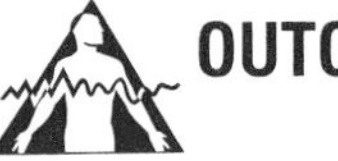

OUTCOME

PROGNOSIS

- Infections typically respond rapidly to treatment
- Failure to respond suggests resistance to the selected drug or anatomic abnormalities requiring further investigation

EVIDENCE

PRACTICE GUIDELINES

- National Guideline Clearinghouse
  - http://www.guideline.gov/summary/summary.aspx?doc_id=3264&nbr=2490&string=acute+AND+cystitis

INFORMATION FOR PATIENTS

- American College of Obstetricians and Gynecologists
  - http://www.medem.com/MedLB/article_detaillb.cfm?article_ID=ZZZ1LJ5770D&sub_cat=2008
- National Kidney and Urologic Diseases Information Clearinghouse
  - http://kidney.niddk.nih.gov/kudiseases/pubs/utiadult/index.htm
- Mayo Clinic
  - http://www.mayoclinic.com/invoke.cfm?id=DS00286

REFERENCES

- Fihn SD: Clinical practice. Acute uncomplicated urinary tract infection in women. N Engl J Med 2003;349:259. [PMID: 12867610]
- Naber KG: Treatment options for acute uncomplicated cystitis in adults. J Antimicrob Chemother 2000;46 Suppl 1:23. [PMID: 11051620]
- Nicolle LE: Empirical treatment of acute cystitis in women. Int J Antimicrob Agents 2003;22:1. [PMID: 12842322]

Author(s)

Marshall L. Stoller, MD
Peter R. Carroll, MD

Cystitis, Interstitial

KEY FEATURES

ESSENTIALS OF DIAGNOSIS

- Pain with bladder filling that is relieved by emptying
- Often associated with urgency and frequency
- Submucosal petechiae on cystoscopic examination
- Diagnosis of exclusion

GENERAL CONSIDERATIONS

- Etiology unknown
- Most likely several diseases with similar symptoms
- Associated diseases include severe allergies, irritable bowel syndrome, or inflammatory bowel disease

DEMOGRAPHICS

- Prevalence of between 18 and 40 per 100,000 people
- Both sexes, but majority of patients are women
- Mean age at onset of 40 years

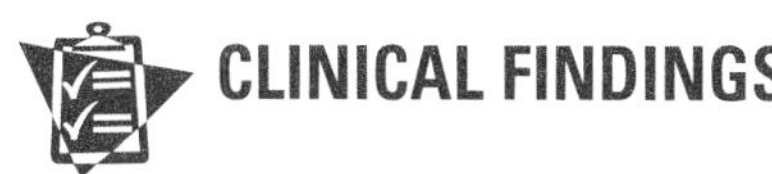

CLINICAL FINDINGS

SYMPTOMS AND SIGNS

- History: pain with bladder filling that is relieved with urination, or urgency, frequency, and nocturia
- Physical examination: should exclude genital herpes, vaginitis, or a urethral diverticulum

DIFFERENTIAL DIAGNOSIS

- Exposure to radiation (radiation cystitis) or cyclophosphamide (chemical cystitis)
- Bacterial vaginitis
- Genital herpes
- Urethral diverticulum
- Urethral carcinoma
- Bladder carcinoma
- Eosinophilic cystitis
- Tuberculous cystitis

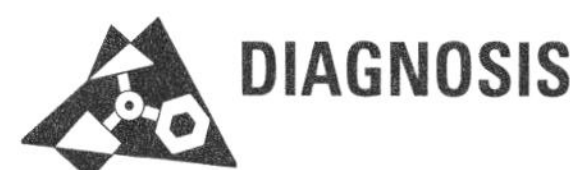

DIAGNOSIS

LABORATORY TESTS

- Negative urine culture and cytology
- Urinalysis and urine culture to exclude infectious causes
- Urinary cytology to exclude bladder malignancy

DIAGNOSTIC PROCEDURES

- Urodynamic testing assesses bladder sensation and compliance and excludes detrusor instability or neurogenic bladder
- The bladder is distended with fluid (hydrodistention) to detect glomerulations (submucosal hemorrhage), which typically are present in at least three quadrants of the bladder
- Bladder biopsy to exclude other causes

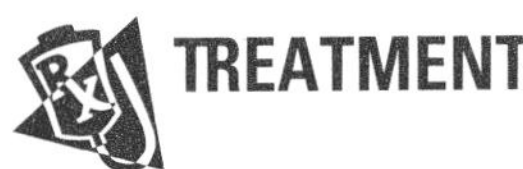

TREATMENT

DIET

- Avoid foods that exacerbate symptoms (eg, tomatoes)

MEDICATIONS

- Amitriptyline
- Nifedipine and other calcium channel blockers
- Pentosan polysulfate sodium (Elmiron)—an oral synthetic sulfated polysaccharide—helps restore integrity to the epithelium of the bladder
- Intravesical instillation of dimethyl sulfoxide (DMSO)
- Intravesical instillation of heparin and Bacillus Calmette-Guérin

SURGERY

- Cystourethrectomy with urinary diversion in extreme cases

PROCEDURES

- Symptomatic relief from hydrodistention

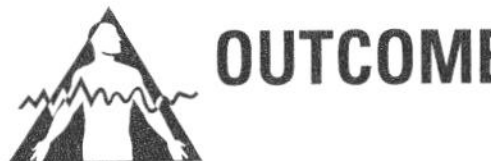

OUTCOME

PROGNOSIS

- No cure, but most patients achieve symptomatic relief

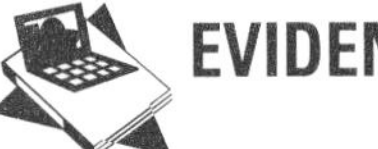

EVIDENCE

PRACTICE GUIDELINES

- Lukban JC et al: Current management of interstitial cystitis. Urol Clin North Am 2002;29:649. [PMID: 12476528]
- MaLossi J et al: Interstitial cystitis: diagnosis and treatment options. Curr Womens Health Rep 2002;2:298. [PMID: 12150758]

INFORMATION FOR PATIENTS

- Mayo Clinic
  - http://www.mayoclinic.com/invoke.cfm?id=DS00497
- National Kidney and Urologic Diseases and Kidney Diseases
  - http://kidney.niddk.nih.gov/kudiseases/pubs/interstitialcystitis/index.htm
- The National Women's Health Information Center
  - http://www.4woman.gov/faq/intcyst.htm

REFERENCES

- Buffington CA: Comorbidity of interstitial cystitis with other unexplained clinical conditions. J Urol 2004;172(4 Pt 1):1242. [PMID: 15371816]
- Chancellor MB et al: Treatment of interstitial cystitis. Urology 2004;63(3 Suppl 1):85. [PMID: 15013658]
- Nickel JC: Interstitial cystitis: a chronic pelvic pain syndrome. Med Clin North Am 2004;88:467. [PMID: 15049588]
- Parsons CL: Diagnosing chronic pelvic pain of bladder origin. J Reprod Med 2004;49(3 Suppl):235. [PMID: 15088862]

Author(s)

Marshall L. Stoller, MD
Peter R. Carroll, MD

Decompression Sickness

Cytomegalovirus (CMV) Infection p. 1063

KEY FEATURES

ESSENTIALS OF DIAGNOSIS

- Respiratory gases are compressed into the blood and other tissues by the greatly increased pressures at low depths
- Gases dissolved in the blood and other tissues escape as the external pressure decreases during ascent from depths > 9 m (30 ft)

GENERAL CONSIDERATIONS

- The appearance of symptoms depends on:
  - depth and duration of submersion
  - degree of physical exertion
  - age, weight, and physical condition of the diver
  - rate of ascent
- The release of gas bubbles and (particularly) the location of their release determine the symptoms
  - The size and number of gas bubbles (notably nitrogen) escaping from the tissues depend on the difference between the atmospheric pressure and the partial pressure of the gas dissolved in the tissues
- Predisposing factors include exercise, injury, patent foramen ovale, obesity, dehydration, alcoholic excess, hypoxia, some medications (eg, narcotics, antihistamines), and cold
- Asthma, pneumothorax, reduced pulmonary function, lung cysts, and thoracic trauma may be contraindications to diving

CLINICAL FINDINGS

SYMPTOMS AND SIGNS

- The onset of acute symptoms occurs within 30 min in 50% of cases and almost invariably within 6 h
- Symptoms are highly variable
  - Pain (largely in the joints) from gas bubble formation (bends)
  - Headache
  - Fatigue
  - Numbness
  - Confusion
  - Pruritic rash
  - Visual disturbances
  - Nausea, vomiting
  - Loss of hearing
  - Weakness, paralysis
  - Dizziness, vertigo
  - Dyspnea
  - Paresthesias
  - Aphasia
  - Coma
- Pulmonary decompression sickness (chokes) presents with burning, pleuritic substernal pain, cough, and dyspnea

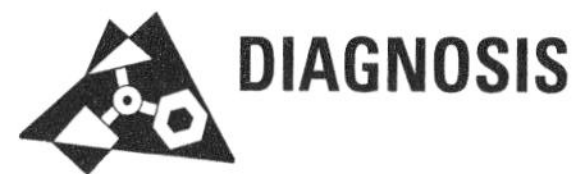

DIAGNOSIS

DIAGNOSTIC PROCEDURES

- Early recognition and prompt treatment are very important

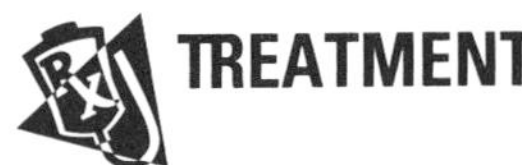

TREATMENT

MEDICATIONS

- Aspirin may be given for pain
- Narcotics should be used cautiously to avoid obscuring the patient's response to recompression

THERAPEUTIC PROCEDURES

- Complete alleviation of decompression symptoms is possible with treatment given up to 2 weeks postinjury
- Administer continuous 100% oxygen as a first aid measure whether or not cyanosis is present

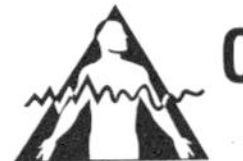

OUTCOME

COMPLICATIONS

Sequelae

- Hemiparesis
- Neurological dysfunction
- Bone damage

WHEN TO REFER

- Rapid transportation to a treatment facility for recompression, hyperbaric oxygen, hydration treatment of plasma deficits, and supportive measures are necessary to relieve symptoms and prevent permanent impairment
- Call the local public health department or nearest naval facility for information on the nearest compression center
- The National Divers Alert Network at Duke University (919-684-8111) provides assistance in the management of underwater diving accidents

EVIDENCE

PRACTICE GUIDELINES

- Bove AA et al: *Diving Medicine,* 4th ed, WB Saunders, 2003.
- British Thoracic Society Fitness to Dive Group, Subgroup of the British Thoracic Society Standards of Care Committee: British Thoracic Society guidelines on respiratory aspects of fitness for diving. Thorax 2003;58:3.
  - http://thorax.bmjjournals.com/cgi/content/full/58/1/3

INFORMATION FOR PATIENTS

- American Academy of Family Physicians: Scuba Diving Safety
  - http://familydoctor.org/156.xml
- Divers Alert Network: Diving Medicine: Frequently Asked Questions
  - http://www.diversalertnetwork.org/medical/faq/index.asp
- Aetna: InteliHealth: Decompression Sickness
  - http://www.intelihealth.com/IH/ihtIH/WSIHW000/35263/35269/322059.html?d=dmtHealthAZ

REFERENCES

- De Gorordo A et al: Diving emergencies. Resuscitation 2003;59:171. [PMID: 14625107]
- Hamilton-Farrell M et al: Barotrauma. Injury 2004;35:359. [PMID: 15037370]

Author(s)

Richard Cohen, MD, MPH

Decubitous Ulcers

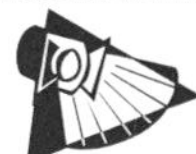

KEY FEATURES

ESSENTIALS OF DIAGNOSIS

- A special type of ulcer caused by impaired blood supply and tissue nutrition
- Results from prolonged pressure over bony or cartilaginous prominences

GENERAL CONSIDERATIONS

- Occur most readily in the elderly, paralyzed, debilitated, and unconscious patients

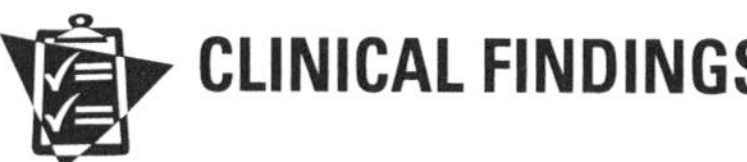

CLINICAL FINDINGS

SYMPTOMS AND SIGNS

- The skin overlying the sacrum and hips is most commonly involved, but bedsores may also be seen over the occiput, ears, elbows, heels, and ankles

DIFFERENTIAL DIAGNOSIS

- Herpes simplex virus
  - In immunocompromised patients, particularly if there is a scalloped border, representing the erosions of herpetic vesicles
- Skin cancer
  - In the perianal area, a nonhealing ulcer may be cancer
- Pyoderma gangrenosum
  - Rapidly expanding ulcers associated with inflammatory bowel disease
- Ecthyma gangrenosum
  - Ucerating lesion, commonly due to *Pseudomonas*, observed in neutropenic patients

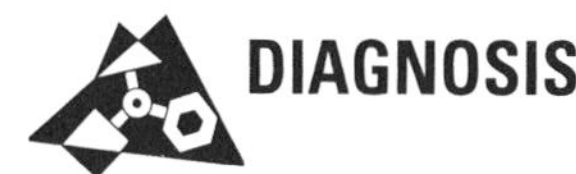

DIAGNOSIS

LABORATORY TESTS

- Based on clinical appearance
- Suspect an alternative diagnosis if ulcers not healing properly

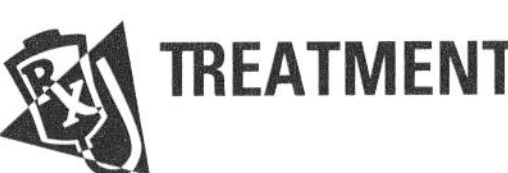

TREATMENT

MEDICATIONS

- See Table 6
- **Early lesions**
  - Treat with topical antibiotic powders and adhesive absorbent bandage (Gelfoam)
  - Once clean, they may be treated with hydrocolloid dressings such as Duo-Derm
- **Established lesions**
  - Topical antiseptics are not recommended
  - Systemic antibiotics may be required for deep infections if the patient is systemically ill, but should otherwise be avoided because they will promote antibiotic resistance

SURGERY

- Established lesions require surgery for débridement, cleansing, and dressing

THERAPEUTIC PROCEDURES

- For established lesions a spongy foam pad placed under the patient may work best in some cases

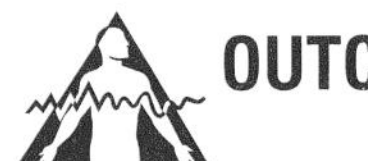

OUTCOME

COMPLICATIONS

- Low-grade infection may occur

WHEN TO REFER

- If there is a question about the diagnosis, if recommended therapy is ineffective, or if specialized treatment is necessary

PREVENTION

- Good nursing care, good nutrition, and maintenance of skin hygiene are important preventive measures
- The skin and the bed linens should be kept clean and dry
- Bedfast, paralyzed, moribund, listless, or incontinent patients who are candidates for the development of decubiti must be turned frequently (at least every hour) and must be examined at pressure points for the appearance of small areas of redness and tenderness
- Water-filled mattresses, rubber pillows, alternating-pressure mattresses, and thick papillated foam pads are useful in prevention and in the treatment of lesions
- "Donut" devices should not be used

EVIDENCE

PRACTICE GUIDELINES

- Agency for Health Care Policy and Research. Pressure ulcers in adults: prediction and prevention. 1992 (review 2000)
  - http://www.guideline.gov/summary/summary.aspx?doc_id=2601&nbr=1827
- Agency for Health Care Policy and Research. Treatment of pressure ulcers. 1994 (review 2000)
  - http://www.guideline.gov/summary/summary.aspx?doc_id=810&nbr=8

WEB SITE

- University of Alabama at Birmingham: Prevention of Pressure Sores Slideshow
  - http://www.spinalcord.uab.edu/show.asp?durki=34911

INFORMATION FOR PATIENTS

- American Academy of Family Physicians: Pressure Sores
  - http://familydoctor.org/039.xml
- MedlinePlus: Pressure Ulcer
  - http://www.nlm.nih.gov/medlineplus/ency/article/007071.htm
- Torpy JM et al: JAMA patient page. Pressure ulcers. JAMA 2003;289:254. [PMID: 12517212]
- University of Alabama at Birmingham: Prevention of Pressure Sores Through Skin Care
  - http://www.spinalcord.uab.edu/show.asp?durki=21486

REFERENCE

- Theaker C: Risk factors for pressure sores in the critically ill. Anaesthesia 2000;55:221. [PMID: 10671839]

Author(s)

Timothy G. Berger, MD

Deep Vein Thrombosis

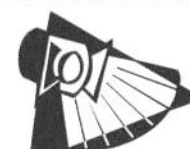

KEY FEATURES

ESSENTIALS OF DIAGNOSIS

- Pain in the calf or thigh, new leg edema
- History of congestive heart failure, recent surgery, trauma, neoplasia, oral contraceptive use, or prolonged inactivity
- Physical signs unreliable
- Duplex ultrasonogram is diagnostic

GENERAL CONSIDERATIONS

- Cause often multifactorial
- Virchow's triad: stasis, vascular injury, and hypercoagulability
- Chronic venous insufficiency with venous stasis disease occurs in ~35% of patients
- In 80% of patients thrombosis begins in the deep veins of the calf
- Propagation into the popliteal and femoral veins then occurs in ~25% of patients
- About 3% of patients undergoing major general surgical procedures develop symptomatic deep vein thrombosis
- Major risk factors: certain operations, particularly total hip replacement; prolonged bed rest or immobility; hypercoagulable state; occult or known malignancy
- Other risk factors: advanced age, type A blood group, obesity, previous thrombosis, multiparity, use of oral contraceptives, inflammatory bowel disease, and systemic lupus erythematosus

DEMOGRAPHICS

- 800,000 new cases per year

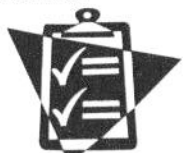

CLINICAL FINDINGS

SYMPTOMS AND SIGNS

- Half of patients have no symptoms or signs
- Dull ache, tightness, or pain in the calf or leg, especially when walking
- Edema of the involved calf, distension of the superficial venous collaterals, low-grade fever, and tachycardia
- Homans' sign positive in 50% of patients
- Cyanosis of the skin (phlegmasia cerulea dolens) in iliofemoral venous thrombosis
- A pale, cool extremity (phlegmasia alba dolens) if reflex arterial spasm is superimposed

DIFFERENTIAL DIAGNOSIS

- Localized muscle strain or contusion
- Baker's cyst (rupture or obstruction of popliteal vein)
- Achilles tendon rupture
- Cellulitis
- Superficial thrombophlebitis
- Lymphedema from lymphatic obstruction (eg, by pelvic tumor)
- Reflex sympathetic dystrophy
- Tumor or retroperitoneal fibrosis obstructing iliac vein or inferior vena cava
- May-Thurner syndrome (external compression of the left iliac vein by the right common iliac artery)
- Edema secondary to heart, liver, or kidney failure or pregnancy

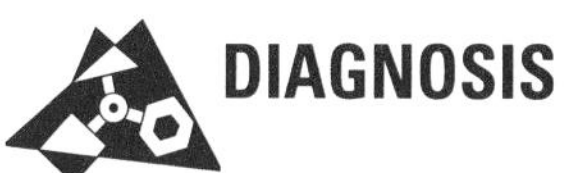

DIAGNOSIS

LABORATORY TESTS

- Obtain complete blood cell count, prothrombin time/International Normalized Ratio (INR), partial thromboplastin time (PTT)
- Consider hypercoagulable workup in cases of recurrent or spontaneous deep vein thrombosis or with family history of hypercoagulable state

IMAGING STUDIES

- Duplex ultrasonography has high sensitivity and specificity
- Ascending contrast venography has 100% sensitivity and 96% specificity but is invasive and rarely indicated to make the diagnosis
- MRA is considered in cases in which there is high clinical suspicion of deep venous thrombosis but ultrasonogram is negative

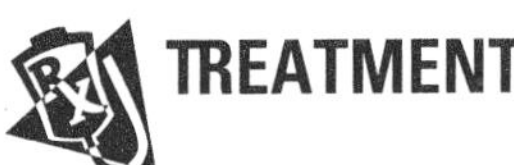

TREATMENT

MEDICATIONS

- Patients with thrombus in the deep veins or with symptomatic calf vein thrombosis should be anticoagulated
- Unfractionated heparin (initial bolus 100 U/kg followed by 10 U/kg/h, dosed to a goal PTT = 1.5–2 times normal) or therapeutic dose low-molecular-weight heparin (eg, enoxaparin, 1 mg/kg SC BID)
- Warfarin is started after therapeutic heparinization to maintain a goal INR = 2.0–3.0 for 3–6 months
- Lifelong anticoagulation is recommended after a second episode of deep venous thrombosis (DVT), and in factor V Leiden mutations, homozygous activated protein C resistance, antiphospholipid antibody, and deficiencies of antithrombin III, protein C or protein S
- Fibrinolytic agents (eg, alteplase) indicated for acute iliofemoral venous thrombosis complicated by phlegmasia within 1 week after clot formation

OUTCOME

FOLLOW-UP

- Patients with asymptomatic calf vein thrombosis may be monitored expectantly (without anticoagulation) with serial ultrasound examination

COMPLICATIONS

- Pulmonary embolism
- Varicose veins
- Chronic venous insufficiency
- Bleeding complications (more common with alteplase than anticoagulants)

PROGNOSIS

- Mortality is related to pulmonary embolism, which occurs in 60% of patients with inadequately treated proximal lower extremity DVT

PREVENTION

- Elevation of the foot of the bed
- Footboard
- Early ambulation
- Graduated compression stockings
- Sequential compression devices
- Unfractionated heparin, 5000 U SC BID, or low-molecular-weight heparin (LMWH) (eg, enoxaparin, 30 mg SC BID)
- LMWH is more effective and has lower risk of bleeding complications in orthopedic surgery patients
- Avoidance of dehydration and femoral catheters or blood draws

EVIDENCE

PRACTICE GUIDELINES

- Abdel-Razeq H et al: Guidelines for diagnosis and treatment of deep venous thrombosis and pulmonary embolism. Methods Mol Med 2004;93:267. [PMID: 14733339]
- American College of Emergency Physicians (ACEP) Clinical Policies Committee; ACEP Clinical Policies Subcommittee on Suspected Lower-Extremity Deep Venous Thrombosis: Clinical policy: critical issues in the evaluation and management of adult patients presenting with suspected lower-extremity deep venous thrombosis. Ann Emerg Med 2003;42:124. [PMID: 12827132]
- Buller HR et al: Antithrombotic therapy for venous thromboembolic disease: the Seventh ACCP Conference on Antithrombotic and Thrombolytic Therapy. Chest 2004;126(3 Suppl):401S. [PMID: 15383479]

INFORMATION FOR PATIENTS

- American Academy of Orthopaedic Surgeons: Deep Vein Thrombosis
  - http://orthoinfo.aaos.org/fact/thr_report.cfm?Thread_ID=264&topcategory=Hip&all=all
- Mayo Clinic: Thrombophlebitis
  - http://www.mayoclinic.com/invoke.cfm?id=DS00223
- MedlinePlus: Deep Venous Thrombosis
  - http://www.nlm.nih.gov/medlineplus/ency/article/000156.htm

REFERENCES

- Breddin HK et al: Effects of a low-molecular weight heparin on thrombus regression and recurrent thromboembolism in patients with deep-vein thrombosis. N Engl J Med 2001;344:626. [PMID: 11228276]
- Forster A et al: Tissue plasminogen activator for the treatment of deep venous thrombosis of the lower extremity: a systematic review. Chest 2001;119:572. [PMID: 11171740]
- Lopez-Beret P et al: Systematic study of occult pulmonary thromboembolism in patients with deep venous thrombosis. J Vasc Surg 2001;33:515. [PMID: 11241121]

Author(s)

Louis M. Messina, MD

Delirium

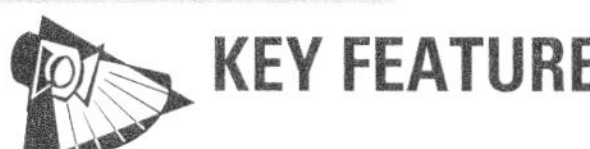

KEY FEATURES

ESSENTIALS OF DIAGNOSIS

- Acute confusional state
- Transient global disorder of attention, with clouding of consciousness
- Usually a result of systemic problems (eg, drugs, hypoxemia)

GENERAL CONSIDERATIONS

- The organic problem may be a primary brain disease or a secondary manifestation of some general disorder
- The causes of cognitive disorders are listed in Table 109
- Should be considered a syndrome of acute brain dysfunction analogous to acute renal failure
- Delirium can coexist with dementia

DEMOGRAPHICS

- Alcohol or substance withdrawal is the most common cause of delirium in the general hospital

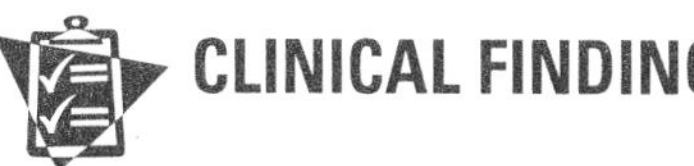

CLINICAL FINDINGS

SYMPTOMS AND SIGNS

- Onset is usually rapid
- The mental status fluctuates (impairment is usually least in the morning), with varying inability to concentrate, maintain attention, and sustain purposeful behavior
- "Sundowning"—mild to moderate delirium at night
  - More common in patients with preexisting dementia
  - May be precipitated by hospitalization, drugs, and sensory deprivation
- There is a marked deficit of memory and recall
- Anxiety and irritability are common
- Amnesia is retrograde (impaired recall of past memories) and anterograde (inability to recall events after the onset of the delirium)
- Orientation problems follow the inability to retain information
- Perceptual disturbances (often visual hallucinations) and psychomotor restlessness with insomnia are common
- Autonomic changes include tachycardia, dilated pupils, and sweating
- Physical findings vary according to the cause

DIFFERENTIAL DIAGNOSIS

- *Drugs:* opioids, alcohol, sedatives, antipsychotics
- *Metabolic:* hypoxia, hypoglycemia, hyperglycemia, hypercalcemia, hypernatremia, hyponatremia, uremia, hepatic encephalopathy, hypothyroidism, hyperthyroidism, vitamin B_{12} or thiamine deficiency, carbon monoxide poisoning, Wilson's disease
- *Infectious:* meningitis, encephalitis, bacteremia, urinary tract infections, pneumonia, neurosyphilis
- *Structural:* space-occupying lesion, eg, brain tumor, subdural hematoma, hydrocephalus
- *Vascular:* stroke, subarachnoid hemorrhage, hypertensive encephalopathy, CNS vasculitis, thrombotic thrombocytopenic purpura, disseminated intravascular coagulation, hyperviscosity
- *Psychiatric:* schizophrenia, depression
- *Other:* seizure, hypothermia, heat stroke, ICU psychosis

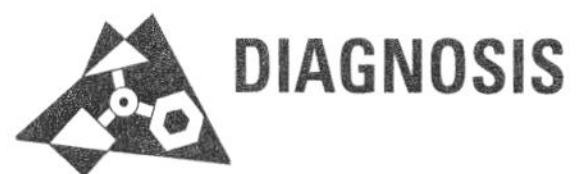

DIAGNOSIS

LABORATORY TESTS

- Comprehensive physical examination including a search for neurologic abnormalities, infection, or hypoxia
- Routine laboratory tests may include
  - Serum electrolytes
  - Serum glucose
  - Blood urea nitrogen
  - Serum creatinine
  - Liver function tests
  - Thyroid function tests
  - Arterial blood gases
  - Complete blood count
  - Serum calcium, phosphorus, magnesium, vitamin B_{12}, folate
  - Blood cultures
  - Urinalysis
  - Cerebrospinal fluid analysis
- See Table 109

IMAGING STUDIES

- Electroencephalography, CT, MRI, positron emission tomography, and single-photon emission computed tomography evaluations may be helpful in diagnosis

DIAGNOSTIC PROCEDURES

- The EEG usually shows generalized slowing

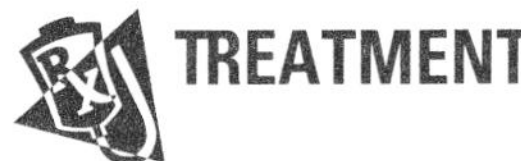

TREATMENT

MEDICATIONS

- The first aim of treatment is to identify and correct the etiologic medical problem
- Discontinue drugs that may be contributing to the problem (eg, analgesics, corticosteroids, cimetidine, lidocaine, anticholinergic drugs, central nervous system depressants, mefloquine)
- Ideally, the patient should be monitored without further medications while the evaluation is carried out
- Two indications for medication in delirious states
  - Behavioral control (eg, pulling out lines)
  - Subjective distress (eg, pronounced fear due to hallucinations)
  - If these indications are present, medications may be given
- If there is any hint of alcohol or substance withdrawal, a benzodiazepine such as lorazepam (1–2 mg every hour) can be given parenterally
- If there is little likelihood of withdrawal syndrome, haloperidol is often used in doses of 1–10 mg every hour
- Once the underlying condition has been identified and treated, adjunctive medications can be tapered

THERAPEUTIC PROCEDURES

- In addition to the medication, a pleasant, comfortable, nonthreatening, and physically safe environment with adequate nursing or attendant services should be provided

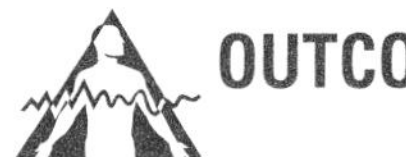

OUTCOME

PROGNOSIS

- The prognosis is good for recovery of mental functioning in delirium when the underlying condition is reversible
- The average duration is about 1 week, with full recovery in most cases

EVIDENCE

PRACTICE GUIDELINES

- National Guideline Clearinghouse: American Psychiatric Association, 1999
  - http://www.guideline.gov/summary/summary.aspx?doc_id=2180

WEB SITES

- American Academy of Family Physicians
  - http://www.aafp.org/afp/20030301/1027.html
- American Psychiatric Association
  - http://www.psych.org/
- Internet Mental Health
  - http://www.mentalhealth.com/t30.html

INFORMATION FOR PATIENTS

- Torpy JM et al: JAMA patient page: Delirium. JAMA 2004;291:1794. [PMID: 15082707]
- National Cancer Institute
  - http://www.cancer.gov/cancerinfo/pdq/supportivecare/delirium/patient
- National Institutes of Health
  - http://www.nlm.nih.gov/medlineplus/ency/article/000740.htm

REFERENCES

- Gleason OC: Delirium. Am Fam Physician 2003;67:1027 [PMID: 12643363]
- Sirois F: Steroid psychosis: a review. Gen Hosp Psychiatry 2003;25:27 [PMID: 12583925]

Author(s)

Stuart J. Eisendrath, MD
Jonathan E. Lichtmacher, MD

Delirium in Elderly

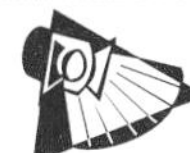

KEY FEATURES

ESSENTIALS OF DIAGNOSIS

- Rapid onset of acute confusional state
- Fluctuates during the day
- Inability to concentrate, maintain attention, or sustain purposeful behavior
- Altered level of consciousness ranging from hyperalert to drowsy or stuporous
- Increased anxiety and irritability
- The majority of delirium is initiated by problems outside the central nervous system

GENERAL CONSIDERATIONS

- Delirium is the pathophysiologic consequence of an underlying general medical condition such as infection, coronary ischemia, hypoxemia, or metabolic derangement
- Although the acutely agitated, "sundowning" elderly patient often comes to mind when considering delirium, many episodes are more subtle
- A key component is review of medications, as a large number of drugs, the addition of a new agent, or the discontinuation of an agent known to cause withdrawal symptoms is associated with the development of delirium

DEMOGRAPHICS

- Approximately 25% of delirious patients are demented, and 40% of demented hospitalized patients are delirious
- Cognitive impairment is an important risk factor
- Other risk factors
  - Male sex
  - Severe illness
  - Hip fracture
  - Fever or hypothermia
  - Hypotension
  - Malnutrition
  - Polypharmacy and use of psychoactive medications
  - Sensory impairment
  - Use of restraints
  - Use of IV lines or urinary catheters
  - Metabolic disorders
  - Depression
  - Alcoholism

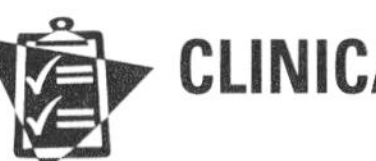

CLINICAL FINDINGS

SYMPTOMS AND SIGNS

- An acute, fluctuating disturbance of consciousness
- Change in cognition or the development of perceptual disturbances
- Inattention, inability to focus on tasks
- Disorientation, confusion
- Irritability
- Mental status may fluctuate throughout the day
- Agitation or may be subdued
- Mental slowing
- Hallucinations are common

DIFFERENTIAL DIAGNOSIS

- Depression
- Mania
- Once the diagnosis of delirium has been made, an underlying cause should be sought. The underlying causes are wide-ranging
- Dementia, especially Lewy body dementia
- Psychotic disorders
- Seizures

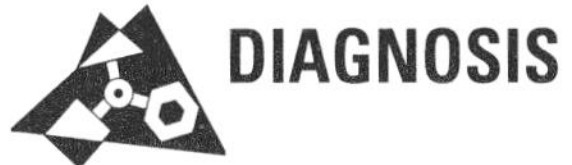

DIAGNOSIS

LABORATORY TESTS

- Laboratory evaluation is aimed at finding an underlying medical condition
- Routine studies include
  - Complete blood cell count
  - Electrolytes
  - Blood urea nitrogen and serum creatinine
  - Glucose, calcium, albumin, liver function studies
  - Urinalysis
  - ECG
- In selected cases, serum magnesium, serum drug levels, arterial blood gas measurements, blood cultures, chest x-ray films, and urinary toxin screens may be helpful

IMAGING STUDIES

- CT scanning may be indicated if there is a history of falls or if the patient does not respond to other measures

DIAGNOSTIC PROCEDURES

- Most cases of delirium do not require lumbar puncture. Consider lumbar puncture if sign of infection (fever, high white blood cell count), if no other obvious cause, or no clinical response to other measures
- Electroencephalogram may sometimes be helpful if seizures are in the differential diagnosis

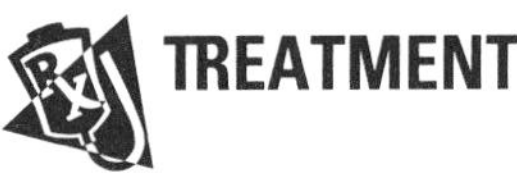

TREATMENT

MEDICATIONS

- Management entails treating the underlying cause, eliminating unnecessary medications, and avoidance of restraints
- For refractory cases in which the patient's or others' welfare is at risk, an oral antipsychotic such as risperidone 0.25–0.5 mg or haloperidol 0.5–1.0 mg at bedtime or twice a day may be necessary
- In emergency situations, starting haloperidol at 0.5 mg PO or IM and repeating every 30 min until the agitation is controlled may be necessary but is often followed by prolonged sedation or other complications
- In general, benzodiazepines should be avoided unless specifically used to treat alcohol withdrawal

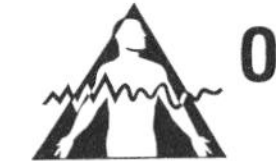

OUTCOME

FOLLOW-UP

- Patients who suffer prolonged episodes of delirium merit closer follow-up for the development of dementia if not already diagnosed

COMPLICATIONS

- May lead to increased number of iatrogenic events

PROGNOSIS

- Delirium is associated with worse clinical outcomes (higher in-hospital and postdischarge mortality, longer lengths of stay, greater probability of placement in a nursing facility), though it is unclear if delirium causes worse outcomes or is simply an ominous marker
- Most episodes clear in a matter of days after correction of the precipitant

WHEN TO REFER

- Patients in whom restraints are being considered should be referred to a geriatrician or geropsychiatrist
- Refer to a neurologist, geriatrician, or psychiatrist when the etiology is not clear or the patient is not responding to therapy

WHEN TO ADMIT

- Delirium generally signifies an underlying serious medical issue in need of treatment
- Most patients with delirium should be admitted, unless the cause is obvious, treatment is expected to result in rapid response, and they have good social support
- Uncontrollable patients should be admitted

PREVENTION

- Preventive measures include improving cognition (frequent reorientation, activities), sleep (massage, noise reduction), mobility, vision (visual aids and adaptive equipment), hearing (portable amplifiers, cerumen disimpaction), and hydration status (volume repletion)

EVIDENCE

PRACTICE GUIDELINES

- American Psychiatric Association
  - http://www.psych.org/psych_pract/treatg/pg/pg_delirium.cfm

INFORMATION FOR PATIENTS

- Torpy JM et al: JAMA patient page: Delirium. JAMA 2004;291:1794. [PMID: 15082707]
- American Psychiatric Association
  - http://www.psych.org/clin_res/Delirium.pdf
- National Institutes of Health
  - http://www.nlm.nih.gov/medlineplus/ency/article/000740.htm

REFERENCES

- Elie M: Delirium risk factors in elderly hospitalized patients. J Gen Intern Med 1998;13:204. [PMID: 9541379]
- Inouye SK: A multicomponent intervention to prevent delirium in hospitalized older patients. N Engl J Med 1999;340:669. [PMID: 10053175]
- Marcantonio ER: Reducing delirium after hip fracture: a randomized trial. J Am Geriatr Soc 2001;49:516. [PMID: 11380742]

Author(s)

G. Michael Harper, MD

C. Bree Johnston, MD

Dementia in Elderly

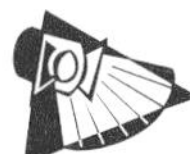

KEY FEATURES

ESSENTIALS OF DIAGNOSIS

- Persistent and progressive impairment in intellectual function
- Not due to delirium—diagnosis should not be made during an acute illness
- Primary deficit of short-term memory
- Must have other deficits (executive function, visuospatial function, language) as well

GENERAL CONSIDERATIONS

- A progressive, acquired impairment in multiple cognitive domains, at least one of which is memory
- The deficits must represent a decline in function significant enough to interfere with work or social life
- Frequently coexists with depression and delirium
- Patients have little cognitive reserve and can have acute cognitive or functional decline with a new medical illness

DEMOGRAPHICS

- Alzheimer's disease is the eighth leading cause of death in the United States with a prevalence that doubles every 5 years in the older population, reaching 30–50% at age 85
- Women suffer disproportionately, as patients (even after age adjustment) and as caregivers
- Alzheimer's disease accounts for two-thirds of cases of dementia in the United States, with vascular dementia (either alone or combined with Alzheimer's disease) and dementia with Lewy bodies accounting for much of the rest
- Risk factors are older age, family history, lower education level, and female gender

CLINICAL FINDINGS

SYMPTOMS AND SIGNS

- Memory impairment with at least one or more of the following:
  - Language impairment (initially just word finding; later, difficulty following a conversation)
  - Apraxia (inability to perform previously learned tasks)
  - Agnosia (inability to recognize objects)
  - Impaired executive function (poor abstraction and judgment)
- Alzheimer's disease
  - Typical earliest deficits are in memory and visuospatial abilities
  - Social graces may be retained despite advanced cognitive decline
  - Personality changes and behavioral difficulties (wandering, inappropriate sexual behavior, agitation) may develop as the disease progresses
  - Hallucinations typically observed only in moderate to severe dementia
  - End-stage disease characterized by near-mutism, inability to sit up, hold up the head, or track objects with the eyes, difficulty with eating and swallowing, weight loss, bowel or bladder incontinence, and recurrent respiratory or urinary infections
- "Subcortical" dementias: psychomotor slowing, reduced attention, early loss of executive function, personality changes, and benefit from cuing in tests of memory
- Dementia with Lewy bodies
  - May be confused with delirium, as fluctuating cognitive impairment is frequently observed
  - Rigidity and bradykinesia are primarily noted; tremor is rare
  - Hallucinations—classically visual and bizarre—may occur
- Frontotemporal dementias
  - Personality change (euphoria, disinhibition, apathy) and compulsive behaviors often predate memory changes
  - In contrast to Alzheimer's disease, visuospatial function is relatively preserved
- Dementia with motor findings: extrapyramidal features or ataxia

DIFFERENTIAL DIAGNOSIS

- Depression
- Delirium
- Medication effect

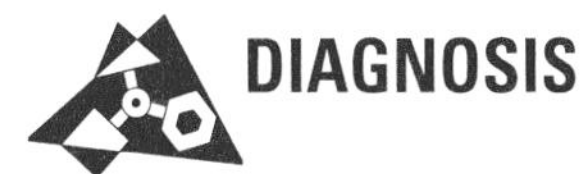

DIAGNOSIS

LABORATORY TESTS

- Recommended tests include TSH, vitamin B_{12}, complete blood count, electrolytes, blood urea nitrogen, creatinine, glucose, calcium
- Testing for HIV, neurosyphilis, and heavy metals should not be performed routinely

IMAGING STUDIES

- Obtain a head CT or MRI scan
  - In younger patients
  - If other etiologies of dementia need to be excluded, with symptoms suggestive of other etiologies including:
    - Focal neurologic signs
    - Seizures, gait abnormalities
    - Acute or subacute onset (symptoms of 6 months or less)

DIAGNOSTIC PROCEDURES

- Assess mental status
- Evaluate for deficits related to cardiovascular accidents, parkinsonism, or peripheral neuropathy
- The combination of the "clock draw" (in which the patient is asked to sketch a clock face, with all the numerals placed properly, the two clock hands positioned at a specified time) and the "three-item recall" is a fairly quick and good test; an abnormally drawn clock markedly increases the probability of dementia
- When patients fail either of these screening tests, further testing with the Mini-Mental State questionnaire, neuropsychological testing, or other instruments is warranted
- Examine for comorbid conditions that may aggravate the disability

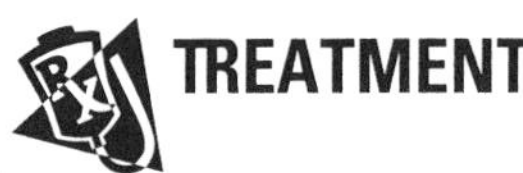

TREATMENT

MEDICATIONS

- Acetylcholinesterase inhibitors (donepezil, galantamine, rivastigmine)
  - Modest improvements in cognitive function in mild to moderate dementia
  - Do not appear to prevent progression of disability or institutionalization
  - Starting dosages: donepezil, 5 mg PO daily (maximum 10 mg daily); galantamine, 4 mg PO twice daily (maximum 12 mg twice daily); rivastigmine, 1.5 mg PO twice daily (maximum 6 mg twice daily)
  - Increase doses gradually as tolerated
  - Side effects include nausea, diarrhea, anorexia, and weight loss
  - May be modestly beneficial in improving neuropsychiatric symptoms
- Choose medications based on symptoms—depression, anxiety, psychosis
- Haloperidol may modestly reduce aggression, but not agitation; it is associated with significant adverse effects
- Risperidone, olanzapine, and quetiapine may be better tolerated than older agents but are more expensive
- Starting and target neuroleptic dosages are low (eg, haloperidol 0.5–2.0 mg; risperidone 0.25–2 mg)
- Risperidone may be associated with increased strokes
- Behavioral symptoms in dementia with Lewy bodies may improve with rivastigmine

THERAPEUTIC PROCEDURES

- Discontinue all nonessential drugs and correct, if possible, sensory deficits
- Exclude unrecognized delirium, pain, urinary obstruction, or fecal impaction
- Caregivers should speak simply to the patient, break down activities into simple component tasks, and use a "distract, not confront" approach

OUTCOME

FOLLOW-UP

- Federal regulations require drug reduction efforts at least every 6 months if antipsychotic agents are used in a nursing home patient

COMPLICATIONS

- Clinicians should be alert for signs of elder abuse when working with stressed caregivers

PROGNOSIS

- The prevalence of fully reversible dementias is under 5%
- Life expectancy with Alzheimer's disease is typically 3–15 years
- Caregiver support, counseling, and respite care can prevent or delay nursing home placement

WHEN TO REFER

- Referral for neuropsychological testing may be helpful to distinguish dementia from depression, to diagnose dementia in persons of poor education or very high premorbid intellect, and to aid diagnosis when impairment is mild
- Referral to a geriatrician or neurologist is useful if the dementia does not have the classic features of Alzheimer's disease

WHEN TO ADMIT

- Dementia complicates other medical problems, and the threshold for admission should be lower

EVIDENCE

PRACTICE GUIDELINES

- American Academy of Family Physicians. Pharmacologic Treatment of Alzheimer's
  - http://www.aafp.org/afp/20031001/1365.html
- American Geriatrics Society: Dementia
  - http://www.americangeriatrics.org/products/positionpapers/aan_dementia.shtml
- National Guideline Clearinghouse: Alzheimer's Management California Working Group for Alzheimer's Disease Management, 2002
  - http://www.guideline.gov/summary/summary.aspx?doc_id=3157
- National Guideline Clearinghouse: American Academy of Neurology. Dementia
  - http://www.guideline.gov/summary/summary.aspx?doc_id=2817

WEB SITES

- American Geriatrics Society
  - http://www.americangeriatrics.org/
- Alzheimer's Association
  - http://www.alz.org
- National Institute on Aging — Alzheimer's Disease Education and Referral Center
  - http://www.alzheimers.org/

INFORMATION FOR PATIENTS

- Alzheimer's Association
  - http://www.alz.org/AboutAD/WhatIsAD.asp
- Alzheimer's Disease Education and Referral Center
  - http://www.alzheimers.org/generalinfo.htm
- Alzheimer's Family Relief Program
  - http://www.ahaf.org
- American Academy of Neurology
  - http://www.aan.com/professionals/practice/pdfs/dem_pat.pdf
- JAMA patient page: Alzheimer disease. JAMA 2001;286:2194 [PMID: 1175749]

REFERENCES

- Courtney C et al: Long-term donepezil treatment in 565 patients with Alzheimer's disease (AD 2000): randomized double-blind trial. Lancet 2004;363:2105 [PMID: 15520051]
- Trinh NH: Efficacy of cholinesterase inhibitors in the treatment of neuropsychiatric symptoms and functional impairment in Alzheimer disease: a meta-analysis. JAMA 2003;289:210. [PMID: 12517232]

Author(s)

G. Michael Harper, MD

C. Bree Johnston, MD

Depression

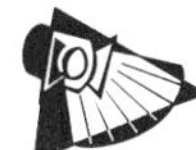

KEY FEATURES

ESSENTIALS OF DIAGNOSIS

- In most depressions
  - Lowered mood, from mild sadness to intense guilt, worthlessness, and hopelessness
  - Difficulty in thinking and concentration, with rumination and indecision
  - Loss of interest, with diminished involvement in activities
  - Somatic complaints
  - Disrupted, reduced, or excessive sleep
  - Loss of energy, appetite, and sex drive
  - Anxiety
- In some severe depressions
  - Psychomotor disturbance: retardation or agitation
  - Delusions of a hypochondriacal or persecutory nature
  - Withdrawal from activities
  - Suicidal ideation

GENERAL CONSIDERATIONS

- Sadness and grief are normal responses to loss; depression is not
- Unlike grief, depression is marked by a disturbance of self-esteem, with a sense of guilt and worthlessness
- Dysthymia is a chronic depressive disturbance with symptoms generally milder than in a major depressive episode

DEMOGRAPHICS

- Up to 30% of primary care patients have depressive symptoms

CLINICAL FINDINGS

SYMPTOMS AND SIGNS

- Anhedonia
- Withdrawal from activities
- Feelings of guilt
- Poor concentration and cognitive dysfunction
- Anxiety
- Chronic fatigue and somatic complaints
- Diurnal variation with improvement as the day progresses
- Vegetative signs
  - Insomnia
  - Anorexia
  - Constipation
- Occasionally, severe agitation and psychotic ideation
- Atypical features
  - Hypersomnia
  - Overeating
  - Lethargy
  - Rejection sensitivity
- Unlike normal sadness and grief, depression often produces frustration and irritation in the clinician

DIFFERENTIAL DIAGNOSIS

- Bipolar disorder or cyclothymia
- Adjustment disorder with depressed mood
- Dysthymia
- Premenstrual dysphoric disorder
- Major depression with postpartum onset: usually 2 weeks to 6 months postpartum
- Seasonal affective disorder
  - Carbohydrate craving
  - Lethargy
  - Hyperphagia
  - Hypersomnia

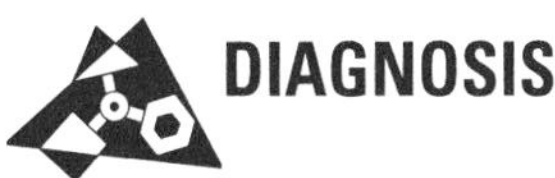

DIAGNOSIS

LABORATORY TESTS

- Complete blood cell count
- Thyroid-stimulating hormone
- Folate
- Toxicology screen may be indicated

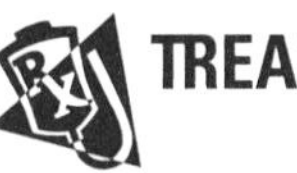

TREATMENT

MEDICATIONS

- See Table 108
- Selective serotonin reuptake inhibitors (SSRIs) and atypical antidepressants
  - Generally lack anticholinergic or cardiovascular side effects
  - Most are activating and should be given in the morning
  - Some patients may experience sedation with paroxetine, fluvoxamine, and mirtazapine
  - Clinical response varies from 2 to 6 weeks
  - Common side effects are headache, nausea, tinnitus, insomnia, nervousness
  - Sexual side effects are very common and may respond to sildenafil
  - "Serotonin syndrome" may occur when taken in conjunction with monoamine oxidase inhibitors or selegeline
  - With the exception of paroxetine, this class should be tapered over weeks to months to avoid a withdrawal syndrome
  - Fluoxetine, fluvoxamine, paroxetine, sertraline, and venlafaxine appear to be safe in pregnancy
    - Their use should be weighed against the risks of an untreated depression in the mother
- Tricyclic antidepressants (TCAs)
  - Mainstay of treatment before SSRIs
  - Clinical response lags several weeks
  - With all TCAs, start at low dose and increase by 25 mg weekly to avoid sedation and anticholinergic side effects
  - Overdose can be serious
- Monoamine oxidase inhibitors (MAOIs)
  - Third-line agents due to dietary restrictions and drug-drug interactions
  - Commonly cause orthostatic hypotension and sympathomimetic effects
  - Potential for withdrawal syndromes requires gradual tapering
- Drug selection influenced by any history of prior responses
- If response is inadequate to first agent at 6 weeks, a second agent from a different group should be substituted

- Lithium should be added when a second drug fails to produce a response
- Thyroid drug (liothyronine 25 μg/day) may be added as augmentative therapy if a second agent fails
- Stimulants such as dextroamphetamine (5–30 mg/day) and methylphenidate (10–45 mg/day) can be used for short-term treatment of medically ill and geriatric patients or in refractory cases

THERAPEUTIC PROCEDURES

- Electroconvulsive therapy (ECT) is the most effective (70–85%) treatment for severe depression
  - Indications are contraindications to medications or depression refractory to medications
  - Most common side effects are headache and memory disturbances, which are usually short-lived
- Psychological
  - Medication and psychotherapy are more effective than either modality alone
  - Psychotherapy is seldom possible in the acute phase of severe depression
- Social
  - In depressions involving alcohol abuse, early involvement in recovery programs is important to future success
  - Family, employers, and friends can help to mobilize a recently depressed patient

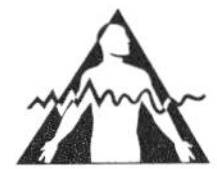

OUTCOME

FOLLOW-UP

- Medication trials should be monitored every 1–2 weeks until 6 weeks, when the effectiveness of the medication can be assessed
- If successful, medications should be continued for 6–12 months before tapering is considered
- Medications should be continued indefinitely in patients with their first episode before age 20, more than two episodes after age 40, or a single episode after age 50
- Tapering of medications should occur gradually over several months

COMPLICATIONS

- A lifetime risk of 10–15% of suicide among patients with depression
- Four major groups who attempt suicide
  - Those who are overwhelmed by problems in living
  - Those who are clearly attempting to control others
  - Those with severe depressions
  - Those with psychotic illness

PROGNOSIS

- Patients frequently respond well to a full trial of drug treatment

WHEN TO REFER

- When depression is refractory to antidepressant therapy
- When depression is moderate to severe
- When suicidality or significant loss of function is present
- With active psychosis or history of mania

WHEN TO ADMIT

- Patients at risk for suicide
- Complex treatment modalities are required

PREVENTION

- Patients at risk for suicide should receive medications in small amounts
- Guns and drugs should be removed from the patient's house
- High-risk patients should be asked not to drive

EVIDENCE

PRACTICE GUIDELINES

- Brigham and Young's Women's Hospital, 2001
  - http://www.guideline.gov/summary/summary.aspx?doc_id=3432
- Institute for Clinical Systems Improvement, 2004
  - http://www.guideline.gov/summary/summary.aspx?doc_id=5301
- National Guideline Clearinghouse

WEB SITES

- American Psychiatric Association
  - http://www.psych.org/
- National Institute of Mental Health
  - http://www.nimh.nih.gov/healthinformation/depressionmenu.cfm

INFORMATION FOR PATIENTS

- National Institute of Mental Health
  - http://www.nimh.nih.gov/publicat/depression.cfm
- JAMA patient page: Depression. JAMA 2003;289:3198. [PMID:12813126]
- JAMA patient page: Postpartum depression. JAMA 2002;287:802. [PMID: 11862958]
- JAMA patient page: Treating depression with electroconvulsive therapy. JAMA 2001;285:1390. [PMID:11280331]
- National Institutes of Health
  - http://www.nlm.nih.gov/medlineplus/ency/article/003213.htm
- American Academy of Family Physicians: Depression in Women
  - http://familydoctor.org/443.xml

REFERENCES

- Glass RM: Treating depression as a recurrent or chronic disease. JAMA 1999;281:83. [PMID:9892456]
- Glassman AH et al: Sertraline treatment of major depression in patients with acute MI or unstable angina. JAMA 2002;288:701. Erratum in JAMA 2002;288:1720. [PMID:12169073]
- Nurnberg HG et al: Treatment of antidepressant-associated sexual dysfunction with sildenafil: a randomized controlled trial. JAMA 2003;289:56. [PMID: 12503977]
- Reynolds CF et al: Nortriptyline and interpersonal psychotherapy as maintenance therapies for recurrent major depression: a randomized controlled trial in patients older than 59 years. JAMA 1999;281:39. [PMID:9892449]

Author(s)

Stuart J. Eisendrath, MD

Jonathan E. Lichtmacher, MD

Depression in Elderly

KEY FEATURES

ESSENTIALS OF DIAGNOSIS

- Older patients often present without complaining of depressed mood
- Somatization is a frequent presentation
- Older people not meeting diagnostic criteria for major depression may still have clinically significant depressive symptoms

GENERAL CONSIDERATIONS

- Compared with younger patients, geriatric patients with depression are more likely to have somatic complaints, less likely to report depressed mood or feelings of guilt, and are more likely to experience delusions
- Depression should be evaluated in any geriatric patient with unexplained functional decline
- Depression and dementia frequently coexist and should be considered as a potential exacerbating comorbidity

DEMOGRAPHICS

- Medical illness and disability—more common in older adults—are risk factors for depression
- Stroke and Parkinson's disease appear to predispose to depression
- Depression in older adults is associated with disability, increased rates of hospitalization and nursing home admission, and higher mortality
- Major depressive disorder has a slightly lower prevalence in older adults than in younger populations

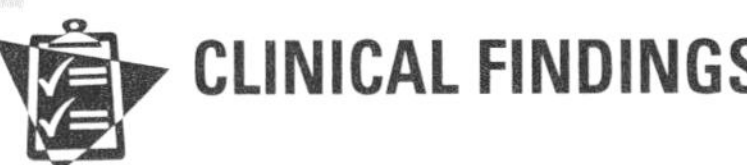

CLINICAL FINDINGS

SYMPTOMS AND SIGNS

- *DSM-IV* diagnosis requires at least five of the following symptoms for a diagnosis of major depression
  - Low mood (must be one of the symptoms)
  - Diminished interest or pleasure in most activities (must be one of the symptoms)
  - Significant weight loss or weight gain
  - Insomnia or hypersomnia
  - Fatigue
  - Feelings of worthlessness or guilt
  - Diminished ability to think or concentrate
  - Recurrent thoughts of death

DIFFERENTIAL DIAGNOSIS

- Substance-induced mood disorder (alcoholism)
- Bipolar disorder
- Grief reaction

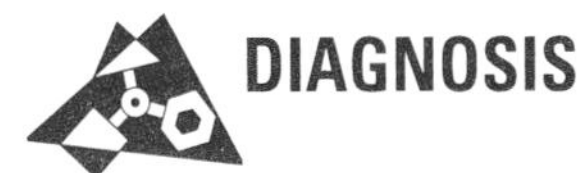

DIAGNOSIS

LABORATORY TESTS

- A simple two-question screen, "Over the last month, have you often been bothered by feeling sad, depressed or hopeless?" and "During the last month, have you often been bothered by little interest or pleasure in doing things?" is at least 96% sensitive for detecting major depression
- Positive responses can be followed up with more comprehensive interviews such as the Yesavage's Geriatric Depression Scale (Table 4)
- Ask patients and their family members about medication use (including corticosteroids, benzodiazepines, cimetidine, β-blockers, and clonidine)
- Laboratory determination of complete blood cell count; liver, thyroid, and renal function; and calcium may be helpful to rule out medical problems presenting as or contributing to depression

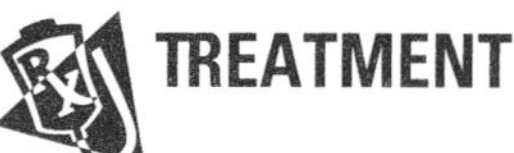

TREATMENT

MEDICATIONS

- Longer trials of antidepressants (at least 9 weeks) may be needed in elderly patients than in younger ones
- The major classes of antidepressants (tricyclics, selective serotonin reuptake inhibitors, monoamine oxidase inhibitors) have comparable efficacy in older adults
- Choice of an antidepressant should be based on side effect profile, pharmacokinetics, previous response and cost
- Cognitive behavioral therapy can improve outcomes alone or in combination with pharmacologic therapy
- Electroconvulsive therapy should be considered in case of severe or refractory depression
- See Depression for more detailed description of individual classes of antidepressants

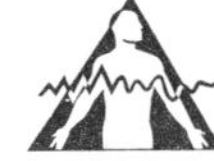

OUTCOME

FOLLOW-UP

- A significant number of older patients in whom depression develops may represent individuals with neurodegenerative disorders (eg, dementia)
- Close follow-up of a patient with a recent diagnosis of depression, with frequent assessment of mental status and neurologic examination, may disclose an additional or alternative diagnosis

COMPLICATIONS

- Risk of suicide, the most dreaded complication of depression, is highest in the geriatric age group

PROGNOSIS

- Chances for recovery are good, but it often takes over 4 weeks to respond to an antidepressant
- Patients not responding to one antidepressant will often respond to another agent
- Relapse can occur when therapy is discontinued and some patients may require long-term maintenance therapy

WHEN TO REFER

- Suicidal ideation
- Possibility of bipolar disorder
- Unresponsive to treatment
- Coexisting substance use disorder

WHEN TO ADMIT

- Suicidal ideation, especially if active plan and/or patient will not contract to seek assistance if thoughts worsen
- Patient unable to care for self
- Psychotic symptoms

PREVENTION

- Some evidence suggests increasing social activity may be helpful
- Rates of recurrence are high; a high index of suspicion is required in a patient with a previous episode

EVIDENCE

PRACTICE GUIDELINES

- American Psychiatric Association
  - http://www.psych.org/psych_pract/treatg/pg/Depression2e.book-9.cfm
- National Guideline Clearinghouse: The John A. Hartford Foundation, 2003
  - http://www.guideline.gov/summary/summary.aspx?doc_id=3512

WEB SITES

- American Psychiatric Association
  - http://www.psych.org/
- ECT On-Line
  - http://www.priory.co.uk/psych/ecctol.htm
- Psychopharmacology Tips
  - http://www.dr-bob.org/tips/
- The American Geriatrics Society
  - http://www.americangeriatrics.org

INFORMATION FOR PATIENTS

- JAMA patient page: Depression. JAMA 2000;284:1606. [PMID: 11032513]
- JAMA patient page: Psychiatric illness in older adults. JAMA 2000;283:2886. [PMID: 10896524]
- American Academy of Family Physicians
  - http://familydoctor.org/handouts/588.xml

REFERENCES

- Covinsky KE: Depressive symptoms and 3-year mortality in older hospitalized medical patients. Ann Intern Med 1999;130:563. [PMID: 10189325]
- Schulz R: Association between depression and mortality in older adults: the Cardiovascular Health Study. Arch Intern Med 2000;160:1761. [PMID: 10871968]

Author(s)

G. Michael Harper, MD
C. Bree Johnston, MD

Dermatitis, Atopic

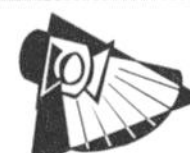

KEY FEATURES

ESSENTIALS OF DIAGNOSIS

- Pruritic, exudative, or lichenified eruption on face, neck, upper trunk, wrists, hands, antecubital and popliteal folds
- Personal or family history of allergies or asthma
- Peripheral eosinophilia, increased IgE—not needed for the diagnosis

GENERAL CONSIDERATIONS

- A chronic or intermittent pruritic, exudative, or lichenified eruption with typical distribution
- Poor prognostic factors for persistence: onset early in childhood, early generalized disease, asthma
- Personal or family history of allergic manifestations (eg, asthma, allergic rhinitis, atopic dermatitis)

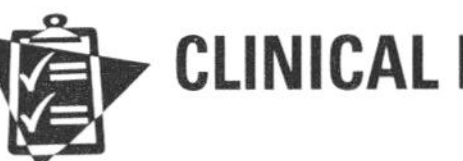

CLINICAL FINDINGS

SYMPTOMS AND SIGNS

- See Table 7
- Distribution of lesions is characteristic: face, neck, and upper trunk ("monk's cowl"), bends of elbows and knee
- Looks different at different ages and in different races, but most patients have scaly dry skin at some point
- Acute flares may present with red patches that are weepy, shiny, or lichenified and plaques and papules
- Fissures, crusts, erosions, or pustules indicate staphylococcal infection so dicloxacillin or first-generation cephalosporins may help in flares
- Pigmented persons tend to present with a papular eruption, and hypopigmented patches (pityriasis alba) are commonly seen on the cheeks and extremities

DIFFERENTIAL DIAGNOSIS

- Seborrheic dermatitis
- Contact dermatitis
- Impetigo
- Psoriasis
- Lichen simplex chronicus (circumscribed neurodermatitis)

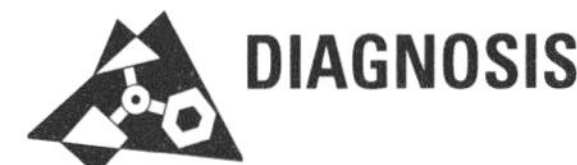

DIAGNOSIS

LABORATORY TESTS

- Clinical diagnostic criteria
  - Pruritus
  - Typical morphology and distribution (flexural lichenification)
  - Tendency toward chronicity
- Also helpful
  - Personal or family history of atopic disease
  - Xerosis-ichthyosis
  - Facial pallor with infraorbital darkening
  - Fissures under the ear lobes
  - Tendency toward hand dermatitis
  - Tendency toward repeated skin infections
  - Nipple eczema
  - Elevated serum IgE

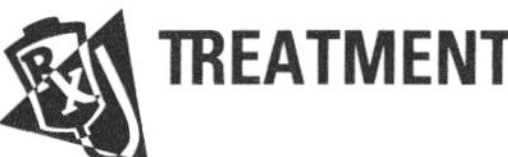

TREATMENT

MEDICATIONS

Local treatments

- Corticosteroids
  - Apply sparingly 2–4 times daily
  - Begin with hydrocortisone, Aclovate, or Desonide and use triamcinolone 0.1% for short periods
  - Taper when the dermatitis clears to avoid both tachyphylaxis, steroid side effects, and to prevent rebounds
- Doxepin cream 5%: may use up to 4 times daily; is best applied simultaneously with the topical corticosteroid; stinging and drowsiness occur in 25%
- Tacrolimus ointment (Protopic): effective as a first-line steroid-sparing agent, available in 0.03% and 0.1% and applied twice daily. Burning on application occurs in about half but may resolve with continued treatment; does not appear to cause steroid side effects and is safe on the face and eyelids
- Pimecrolimus (Elidel) cream 1% is similar, but burns less
- Use tacrolimus and pimecrolimus sparingly (limit the area) and for as brief a time as possible

Systemic and adjuvant therapies

- Immunosuppressives, oral antipruritic agents, and phototherapy

Treatment by stage of dermatitis

- Acute weeping lesions: use saline or aluminum subacetate solution (Domeboro tablets) or colloidal oatmeal (Aveeno; dispense one box) as soothing or astringent soaks or wet dressings for 10–30 min 2–4 times a day
- Lesions on extremities may be bandaged for protection at night
- Corticosteroid lotions or creams are preferred to ointments
- Tacrolimus may not be tolerated; systemic corticosteroids are last resort

Subacute or scaly lesions (lesions are dry but still red and pruritic)

- Mid- to high-potency corticosteroids in ointment form if tolerated—creams if not—should be continued until scaling and elevated skin lesions are cleared and itching is decreased; then begin a 2- to 4-week taper with topical corticosteroids

OUTCOME

COMPLICATIONS

- Treatment complications
  - Monitor for skin atrophy
  - Eczema herpeticum, a generalized herpes simplex infection manifested by monomorphic vesicles, crusts, or erosions superimposed on atopic dermatitis or other extensive eczematous processes
- Smallpox vaccination is absolutely contraindicated in patients with atopic dermatitis or a history thereof because of the risk of eczema vaccinatum
- Atopic dermatitis patients may develop generalized vaccinia by contact with recent vaccine recipients who still have pustular or crusted vaccination sites

PROGNOSIS

- Runs a chronic or intermittent course
- Affected adults may have only hand dermatitis
- Poor prognostic factors for persistence into adulthood: onset early in childhood, early generalized disease, and asthma; only 40–60% of these patients have lasting remissions

WHEN TO REFER

- If there is a question about the diagnosis, if recommended therapy is ineffective, or if specialized treatment is necessary

PREVENTION

- Avoid things that dry or irritate the skin: low humidity and dry air
- Other triggers: sweating, overbathing, animal danders, scratchy fabrics
- Do not bathe more than once daily and use soap only on armpits, groin, and feet; preferred: Dove, Eucerin, Aveeno, Basis, Alpha Keri, Purpose
- After rinsing, pat the skin dry (not rub) and then, before it dries completely, cover with a thin film of emollient such as Aquaphor, Eucerin, Vaseline
  - Triceram cream is a less greasy moisturizer and anti-inflammatory, but is much more expensive

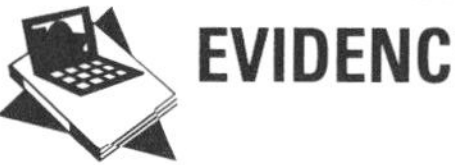

EVIDENCE

PRACTICE GUIDELINES

- Leung DY et al: Disease management of atopic dermatitis: an updated practice parameter. Joint Task Force on Practice Parameters. Ann Allergy Asthma Immunol 2004;93(3 Suppl 2):S1. [PMID: 15478395]
- Hanifin JM et al: Guidelines of care for atopic dermatitis, developed in accordance with the American Academy of Dermatology (AAD)/American Academy of Dermatology Association "Administrative Regulations for Evidence-Based Clinical Practice Guidelines." J Am Acad Dermatol 2004;50:391. [PMID: 14988682]
  - http://www.aad.org/professionals/pracmanage/guidelines/AtopicDermatitis.htm

WEB SITE

- American Academy of Dermatology
  - http://www.aad.org

INFORMATION FOR PATIENTS

- National Institute of Arthritis and Musculoskeletal and Skin Diseases: Atopic Dermatitis
  - http://www.niams.nih.gov/hi/topics/dermatitis/index.html
- National Eczema Association for Science and Education: All About Atopic Dermatitis
  - http://www.nationaleczema.org/lwe/aboutad.html
- American Academy of Dermatology: What is Eczema?
  - http://www.skincarephysicians.com/eczemanet/whatis.html

REFERENCES

- Jaffe R: Atopic dermatitis. Prim Care 2000;27:503. [PMID: 10815058]
- Leung DY et al: Atopic dermatitis. Lancet 2003:361:151. [PMID: 12531593]

Author(s)

Timothy G. Berger, MD

Dermatitis, Contact

KEY FEATURES

ESSENTIALS OF DIAGNOSIS

- Erythema and edema, with pruritus, often followed by vesicles and bullae in an area of contact with a suspected agent
- Later, weeping, crusting, or secondary infection
- A history of previous reaction to suspected contactant
- Patch test with agent positive

GENERAL CONSIDERATIONS

- An acute or chronic dermatitis that results from direct skin contact with chemicals or allergens
- **Irritant contact dermatitis**
  - Eighty percent of cases are due to excessive exposure to or additive effects of primary or universal irritants such as soaps, detergents, or organic solvents
  - The minority are due to actual contact allergy such as poison ivy or poison oak
- **Allergic contact dermatitis**
  - Occupational exposure is an important cause
  - The most common topicals causing allergic rashes include antimicrobials (especially neomycin), antihistamines, anesthetics (benzocaine), hair dyes, preservatives (eg, parabens), latex, and adhesive tape
- Weeping and crusting are typically due to allergic and not irritant dermatitis, which often appears red and scaly
- Contact dermatitis due to latex rubber in gloves is of special concern in health care workers

CLINICAL FINDINGS

SYMPTOMS AND SIGNS

- See Table 7
- The acute phase is characterized by tiny vesicles and weepy and crusted lesions
- Resolving or chronic contact dermatitis presents with scaling, erythema, and possibly thickened skin; itching, burning, and stinging may be severe
- The lesions, distributed on exposed parts or in bizarre asymmetric patterns, consist of erythematous macules, papules, and vesicles
- The affected area is often hot and swollen, with exudation and crusting, simulating and at times complicated by infection
- The pattern of the eruption may be diagnostic (eg, typical linear streaked vesicles on the extremities in poison oak or ivy dermatitis)
- The location will often suggest the cause: scalp involvement suggests hair tints, sprays, or tonics; face involvement, creams, cosmetics, soaps, shaving materials, nail polish; neck involvement, jewelry, hair dyes, etc

DIFFERENTIAL DIAGNOSIS

- Impetigo
- Scabies
- Dermatophytid reaction (allergy or sensitivity to fungi)
- Atopic dermatitis
- Pompholyx
- Asymmetric distribution, blotchy erythema around the face, linear lesions, and a history of exposure help distinguish contact dermatitis from other skin lesions
- The most commonly confused diagnosis is impetigo, in which case Gram stain and culture will rule out impetigo or secondary infection (impetiginization)

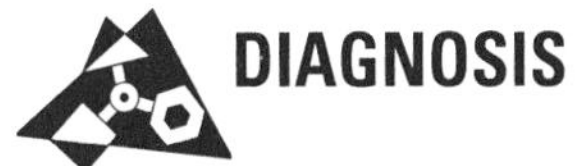

DIAGNOSIS

LABORATORY TESTS

- During the acute episode, patch testing cannot be performed; after the episode has cleared, the patch test may be useful, but not all potential allergens are available for testing; in the event of a positive reaction, the clinical relevance of the chemical agent to the dermatitis must be determined

DIAGNOSTIC PROCEDURES

- If itching is generalized and impetiginized scabies is considered, a scraping for mites should be done

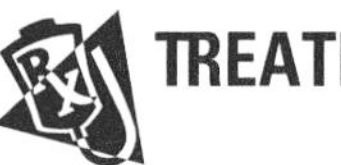

TREATMENT

- See Table 6
- Vesicular and weepy lesions often require systemic corticosteroid therapy
- Localized involvement (except on the face) can often be managed solely with topical agents
- Irritant contact dermatitis is treated by protection from the irritant and use of topical corticosteroids as for atopic dermatitis

Local measures

- Acute weeping dermatitis
  - Compresses are most often used
  - Calamine or starch shake lotions can be used between wet dressings, especially for intertriginous areas or when oozing is not marked
  - Lesions on the extremities may be bandaged with wet dressings for 30–60 min several times a day
  - Potent topical corticosteroids in gel or cream form may help suppress acute contact dermatitis and relieve itching
  - In cases where weeping is marked or in intertriginous areas, ointments will make the skin even more macerated and should be avoided
  - Topical corticosteroid preparations are fluocinonide gel, 0.05%, used BID or TID with compresses, or clobetasol or halobetasol cream, used BID for a maximum of 2 weeks—not in body folds or on the face; this should be followed by tapering of the number of applications per day or use of a mid-potency corticosteroid such as triamcinolone 0.1% cream to prevent rebound of the dermatitis
  - A soothing formulation is 0.1% triamcinolone acetonide in Sarna lotion (0.5% camphor, 0.5% menthol, 0.5% phenol)
- Subacute dermatitis (subsiding)
  - Mid-potency (triamcinolone 0.1%) to high-potency corticosteroids (amcinonide, fluocinonide, desoximetasone) are the mainstays of therapy
- Chronic dermatitis (dry and lichenified)
  - High- to highest-potency corticosteroids are used in ointment form

Systemic therapy

- For acute severe cases, give prednisone orally for 12–21 days
- Prednisone, 60 mg for 4–7 days, 40 mg for 4–7 days, and 20 mg for 4–7 days without a further taper is one useful regimen or dispense 78 5-mg pills to be taken 12 the first day, 11 the second day, and so on
- The key is to use enough corticosteroid (and as early as possible) to achieve a clinical effect and to taper slowly enough to avoid rebound
- A Medrol Dosepak (methylprednisolone) with 5 days of medication is inappropriate on both counts

OUTCOME

PROGNOSIS

- Self-limited if reexposure is prevented but often takes 2–3 weeks for full resolution

WHEN TO REFER

- Occupational allergic contact dermatitis should be referred to a dermatologist

PREVENTION

- Prompt and thorough removal of allergens by washing with water or solvents or other chemical agents may be effective if done very shortly after exposure to poison oak or ivy
- Several barrier creams (eg, Stokogard, Ivy Shield) offer some protection to patients at high risk for poison oak and ivy dermatitis if applied before exposure
- Iodoquinol cream (Vioform) may benefit nickel allergic patients
- Ingestion of rhus antigen is of limited clinical value for the induction of tolerance
- The mainstay of prevention is identification of agents causing the dermatitis and avoidance of exposure or use of protective clothing and gloves

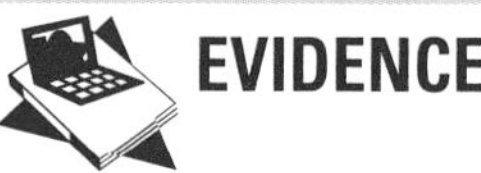

EVIDENCE

PRACTICE GUIDELINES

- Bourke J et al: Guidelines for care of contact dermatitis. Br J Dermatol 2001;145:877. [PMID: 11899139]

WEB SITE

- American Academy of Dermatology
  - http://www.aad.org

INFORMATION FOR PATIENTS

- MedlinePlus: Contact Dermatitis
  - http://www.nlm.nih.gov/medlineplus/ency/article/000869.htm
- Mayo Clinic: Dermatitis
  - http://www.mayoclinic.com/invoke.cfm?id=DS00339

REFERENCES

- Belsito DV: The diagnostic evaluation, treatment, and prevention of allergic contact dermatitis in the new millennium. J Allergy Clin Immunol 2000;105:409. [PMID: 10719287]
- Tanner TL: Rhus (Toxicodendron) dermatitis. Prim Care 2000;27:493. [PMID: 10815057]

Author(s)

Timothy G. Berger, MD

Dermatitis, Exfoliative

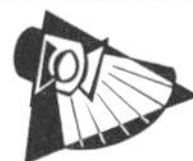

KEY FEATURES

ESSENTIALS OF DIAGNOSIS

- Scaling and erythema over most of the body
- Itching, malaise, fever, chills, weight loss

GENERAL CONSIDERATIONS

- A preexisting dermatosis is the cause in up to 65% of cases, including psoriasis, atopic dermatitis, contact dermatitis, pityriasis rubra pilaris, and seborrheic dermatitis
- Reactions to topical or systemic drugs (eg, sulfonamides) account for perhaps 20–40% of cases and cancer (cutaneous T cell lymphoma, Sézary syndrome) for 10–20%
- Causation of the remainder is indeterminable
- At the time of acute presentation, without a clear-cut prior history of skin disease or drug exposure, it may be impossible to make a specific diagnosis of the underlying condition, and diagnosis may require observation
- Generalized lymphadenopathy may be due to lymphoma or leukemia or may be part of the clinical picture of the skin disease (dermatopathic lymphadenitis)

Etiology

- Idiopathic
- Drug eruption
- Seborrheic dermatitis
- Contact dermatitis
- Atopic dermatitis
- Psoriasis
- Cancer (Sézary syndrome of cutaneous T cell lymphoma, Hodgkin's disease)
- Pityriasis rubra pilaris

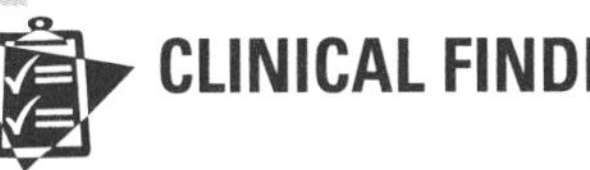

CLINICAL FINDINGS

SYMPTOMS AND SIGNS

- See Table 7
- Symptoms may include itching, weakness, malaise, fever, and weight loss
- Chills are prominent
- Redness and scaling may be generalized and sometimes includes loss of hair and nails
- Generalized lymphadenopathy
- The mucosa is spared

DIFFERENTIAL DIAGNOSIS

- Psoriasis
- Seborrheic dermatitis
- Drug eruption

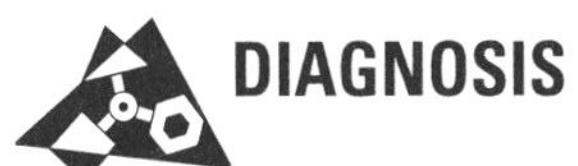

DIAGNOSIS

LABORATORY TESTS

- Peripheral leukocytes may show clonal rearrangements of the T cell receptor in Sézary syndrome

DIAGNOSTIC PROCEDURES

- A skin biopsy is required and may show changes of a specific inflammatory dermatitis or cutaneous T cell lymphoma or leukemia

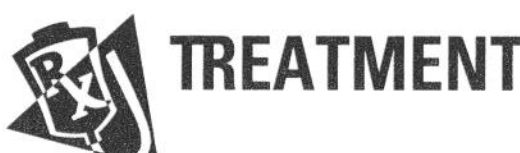

TREATMENT

MEDICATIONS

- See Table 6
- Stop all drugs, if possible
- Systemic corticosteroids may provide remarkable improvement in severe or fulminant exfoliative dermatitis, but long-term therapy should be avoided
- For cases of psoriatic erythroderma and pityriasis rubra pilaris, either acitretin or methotrexate may be indicated
- Erythroderma secondary to lymphoma or leukemia requires specific topical or systemic chemotherapy
- Suitable antibiotic drugs with coverage for *Staphylococcus* should be given when there is evidence of bacterial infection

THERAPEUTIC PROCEDURES

- Home treatment is with cool to tepid baths and application of mid-potency corticosteroids under wet dressings or with the use of an occlusive plastic suit

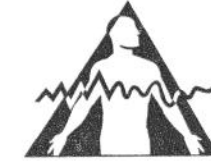

OUTCOME

FOLLOW-UP

- It may be impossible to identify the cause of exfoliative dermatitis early in the course of the disease, so careful follow-up is necessary
- Psoriasis, severe seborrheic dermatitis, and drug eruptions may have an erythrodermic phase

COMPLICATIONS

- Debility (protein loss) and dehydration may develop in patients with generalized inflammatory exfoliative erythroderma
- Sepsis
- Systemic corticosteroids must be used with caution because some patients with erythroderma have psoriasis and could develop pustular psoriasis

PROGNOSIS

- Most patients recover completely or improve greatly over time but may require chronic therapy
- Deaths are rare in the absence of cutaneous T cell lymphoma
- A minority of patients will suffer from undiminished erythroderma for indefinite periods

WHEN TO REFER

- Early referral is frequently helpful

WHEN TO ADMIT

- If the exfoliative erythroderma becomes chronic and is not manageable in an outpatient setting, hospitalize the patient
- Keep the room at a constant warm temperature and provide the same topical treatment as for an outpatient

EVIDENCE

WEB SITES

- American Academy of Dermatology
  - http://www.aad.org
- Karakayli G et al: Exfoliative Dermatitis. Am Fam Physician 1999;59:625. [PMID: 10029788]
  - http://www.aafp.org/afp/990201ap/625.html

INFORMATION FOR PATIENTS

- MedlinePlus: Exfoliative Dermatitis
  - http://www.nlm.nih.gov/medlineplus/ency/article/001610.htm
- Mayo Clinic: Dermatitis
  - http://www.mayoclinic.com/invoke.cfm?id=DS00339
- University of Virginia Health System: Generalized Exfoliative Dermatitis
  - http://www.healthsystem.virginia.edu/uvahealth/adult_derm/general.cfm

REFERENCES

- Balasubramaniam P et al: Erythroderma: 90% skin failure. Hosp Med 2004;65:100. [PMID: 14997777]
- Gallelli L et al: Generalized exfoliative dermatitis induced by interferon alfa. Ann Pharmacother 2004;38:2173. [PMID: 15522975]
- Jaffer AN et al: Exfoliative dermatitis. Erythroderma can be a sign of a significant underlying disorder. Postgrad Med 2005;117:49. [PMID: 15672891]
- Shegal VN et al: Erythroderma/exfoliative dermatitis: a synopsis. Int J Dermatol 2004;43:39. [PMID: 14693020]

Author(s)

Timothy G. Berger, MD

Diabetes Insipidus

Dermatitis Herpetiformis p. 1064. Dermatitis Seborrheic p. 1064.

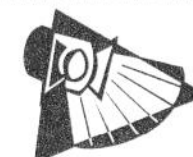

KEY FEATURES

ESSENTIALS OF DIAGNOSIS

- Polyuria (2–20 L/day); polydipsia
- Urine specific gravity usually < 1.006 during ad libitum fluid intake
- Urine is otherwise normal
- Vasopressin reduces urine output except in nephrogenic diabetes insipidus (DI)

GENERAL CONSIDERATIONS

- Uncommon disease caused by a deficiency of or resistance to vasopressin

Deficiency of vasopressin

- Primary DI (no lesion on MRI of pituitary and hypothalamus) may be familial or idiopathic
- Secondary DI is due to damage to hypothalamus or pituitary stalk by tumor, anoxic encephalopathy, surgical or accidental trauma, infection (eg, encephalitis, tuberculosis, syphilis), sarcoidosis, or multifocal Langerhans cell (eosinophilic) granulomatosis ("histiocytosis X")
- Metastases to pituitary cause DI more than pituitary adenomas (33% vs. 1%)
- Vasopressinase-induced DI may occur in last trimester of pregnancy and postpartum, often associated with oligohydramnios, preeclampsia, or hepatic dysfunction

"Nephrogenic" diabetes insipidus

- Due to defect in kidney tubules that interferes with water reabsorption
- Polyuria is unresponsive to vasopressin and patients have normal vasopressin secretion
- Congenital nephrogenic DI is X-linked, present from birth, and due to defective expression of renal vasopressin V2 receptors or vasopressin-sensitive water channels
- Acquired form less severe, seen in pyelonephritis, amyloidosis, multiple myeloma, hypokalemia, Sjögren's syndrome, sickle cell anemia, hypercalcemia, recovery from acute tubular necrosis
- May be caused by drugs, eg, glucocorticoids, diuretics, demeclocycline, tetracycline, lithium, foscarnet, methicillin

DEMOGRAPHICS

- In familial autosomal dominant central DI, symptoms begin at about age 2 years

CLINICAL FINDINGS

SYMPTOMS AND SIGNS

- Intense thirst, especially for ice water
- Polyuria
- 2 L to 20 L of fluid ingested daily, with corresponding urine volumes
- Although most patients with DI maintain fluid balance, dehydration and hypernatremia occur if patients are unable to drink or if hypothalamic thirst center is damaged by shock, anoxia, or tumor
- Partial DI presents with less intense symptoms and should be suspected in unremitting enuresis
- Diabetes insipidus also occurs in Wolfram syndrome, a rare autosomal-recessive disorder, also known by the acronym DIDMOAD (diabetes insipidus, type 1 diabetes mellitus, optic atrophy, and deafness). DIDMOAD manifestations usually present in childhood, but may not occur until adulthood, along with depression and cognitive problems

DIFFERENTIAL DIAGNOSIS

- Central versus nephrogenic DI
- Osmotic diuresis, eg, diabetes mellitus
- Polyuria from Cushing's syndrome, glucocorticoids, or lithium
- Excessive fluid intake: psychogenic polydipsia, IV fluids, CNS sarcoidosis

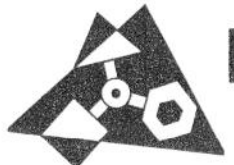

DIAGNOSIS

LABORATORY TESTS

- 24 h urine collection for volume (< 2 L/day rules out DI in adults), glucose (to screen for diabetes mellitus), creatinine (to ensure accurate collection and assess creatinine clearance)
- Serum for osmolality, glucose, potassium (hypokalemia causes polyuria), sodium, uric acid
- Urinalysis: low specific gravity but is otherwise normal, no glucosuria
- Serum osmolality greater than urine osmolality
- Hypernatremia
- In nephrogenic DI, serum vasopressin is high during modest fluid restriction
- Hyperuricemia implicates central DI
- "Vasopressin challenge test" if suspect central DI
  - Desmopressin acetate, 0.05–0.1 mL (5–10 μg) intranasally or 1 μg SQ or IV, measuring urine volume for 12 h prior to and 12 h after administration
  - Obtain serum sodium immediately if symptoms of hyponatremia
  - Patients with central DI notice reduction in thirst and polyuria
  - Serum sodium remains normal except in some salt-losing conditions
  - If marginal response, desmopressin dosage is doubled

IMAGING STUDIES

- In nonfamilial central DI, MRI of pituitary and hypothalamus to exclude mass lesions
- Absence of a posterior pituitary "bright spot" on T1-weighted MRI suggests central DI

DIAGNOSTIC PROCEDURES

- Diagnosis of DI as cause of polyuria or hypernatremia mostly requires clinical judgment

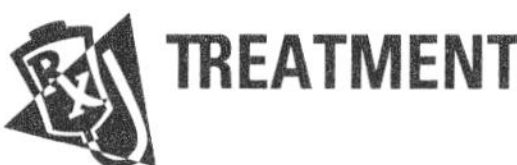

TREATMENT

MEDICATIONS

- Mild cases require only adequate fluid intake
- Reduction of aggravating factors (eg, glucocorticoids) improves polyuria
- Central DI or DI of pregancy or postpartum: desmopressin is treatment of choice
  - Intranasal: start at 0.05–0.1 mL (100 μg/mL solution) intranasally Q 12–24 h, then individualize according to thirst and polyuria. May cause sinusitis
  - Parenteral: dose is 1–4 μg IV, IM, or SC Q 12–24 h PRN thirst or hypernatremia
  - Oral: available as 0.1- and 0.2-mg tablets given in a starting dose of 0.05 mg twice daily and increased to a maximum of 0.4 mg every 8 h, if required. Particularly useful for patients with sinusitis from the nasal preparation. Mild increases in hepatic enzymes, gastrointestinal symptoms and asthenia may occur
- Hyponatremia is uncommon if minimum effective doses are used and occasional thirst is allowed
- Central and nephrogenic DI: hydrochlorothiazide 50–100 mg/day (with potassium supplement or amiloride) produces partial response
- Nephrogenic DI: indomethacin, 50 mg PO Q 8 h, or combined indomethacin-hydrochlorothiazide, indomethacin-desmopressin, or indomethacin-amiloride
- Psychotherapy for patients with compulsive water drinking. Thioridazine and lithium are best avoided if drug therapy is needed, since they cause polyuria

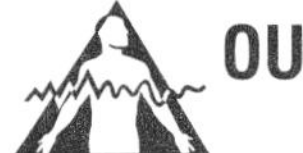

OUTCOME

COMPLICATIONS

- Without water, excessive urine output leads to severe dehydration
- Patients with impaired thirst mechanism are prone to hypernatremia, particularly when impaired mentation causes them to forget to take desmopressin
- With desmopressin acetate therapy, there is risk of water intoxication
- Desmopressin may cause nasal irritation, sinusitis, agitation, erythromelalgia

PROGNOSIS

- Chronic central DI is more an inconvenience than a dire medical condition. Desmopressin treatment allows normal sleep and activity
- Central DI appearing after pituitary surgery usually remits after days to weeks but may be permanent if upper pituitary stalk is cut
- Central DI is made transiently worse by glucocorticoids in high doses frequently given perioperatively
- Hypernatremia can occur, especially when thirst center is damaged
- Central DI itself does not reduce life expectancy if hypothalamic thirst center is intact. Prognosis is that of underlying disorder

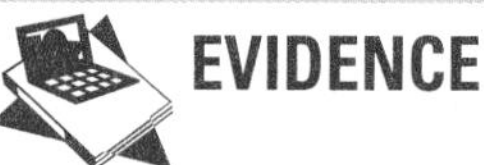

EVIDENCE

PRACTICE GUIDELINES

- Singer PA et al: Postoperative endocrine management of pituitary tumors. Neurosurg Clin North Am 2003;14:123. [PMID: 12690984]

WEB SITES

- Diabetes Insipidus Foundation
  - http://www.diabetesinsipidus.org/
- MEDLINEplus—Diabetes insipidus
  - http://www.nlm.nih.gov/medlineplus/diabetesinsipidus.html
- Nephrogenic Diabetes Insipidus Foundation
  - http://www.ndif.org/

INFORMATION FOR PATIENTS

- Mayo Clinic—Diabetes insipidus
  - http://www.mayoclinic.com/invoke.cfm?id=AN00126
- MEDLINEplus—Diabetes insipidus
  - http://www.nlm.nih.gov/medlineplus/diabetesinsipidus.html
- NIDDK/NIH—Diabetes insipidus
  - http://kidney.niddk.nih.gov/kudiseases/pubs/insipidus/index.htm

REFERENCES

- Smith CJA et al: Phenotype-genotype correlations in a series of Wolfram syndrome families. Diabetes Care 2004;27:2003. [PMID: 15277431]
- Verbalis JG: Disorders of body water homeostasis. Best Pract Res Clin Endocrinol Metab 2003;17:471. [PMID: 14687585]

Author(s)

Paul A. Fitzgerald, MD

Diabetes Mellitus, Gestational

KEY FEATURES

ESSENTIALS OF DIAGNOSIS

- Euglycemia should be established before pregnancy
- Fasting and preprandial glucose values are lower during pregnancy in both diabetic and nondiabetic women
- During pregnancy, euglycemia is 60–80 mg/dL while fasting and 30–45 min before meals and < 120 mg/dL 2 h after meals
- At least two abnormal values on a 3-h glucose tolerance test (GTT)

GENERAL CONSIDERATIONS

- Pregnancy is a natural state of insulin resistance from placental lactogen and elevated circulating estrogens and progesterone
- Depending on the population screened, a significant proportion may evidence glucose intolerance, which can have implications for adverse fetal outcome
- Type 1 diabetics express particular HLA haplotypes with anti-islet cell antibodies
- Type 2 diabetics have minimal risk of ketoacidosis

DEMOGRAPHICS

- Women at higher risk include those of Hispanic, African-American, Native American, Asian, Pacific Island, or Indigenous Australian ancestry
- Prior history of gestational diabetes
- Prior history of adverse pregnancy outcome
- First-degree relative with diabetes mellitus
- Body mass index ≥ 30

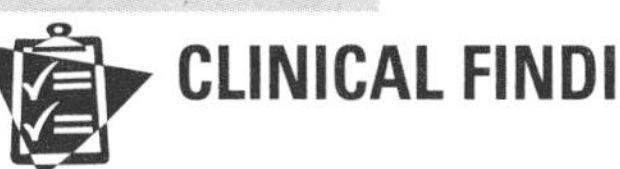

CLINICAL FINDINGS

SYMPTOMS AND SIGNS

- Polyuria and thirst
- Weakness or fatigue
- Recurrent blurred vision
- Macrosomia
- Polyhydramnios
- Often asymptomatic

DIFFERENTIAL DIAGNOSIS

- Drugs: corticosteriods, thiazides, tacrolimus
- Diabetes insipidus
- Psychogenic polydipsia
- Nondiabetic glycosuria (benign)

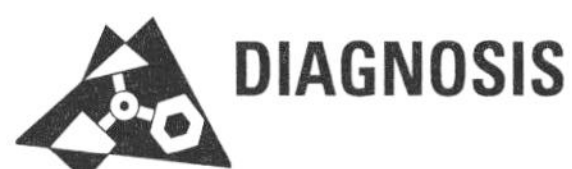

DIAGNOSIS

LABORATORY TESTS

- See Table 73
- The target for glycemic control during pregnancy is euglycemia of 60–80 mg/dL while fasting and 30–45 min before meals and < 120 mg/dL 2 h after meals
- Glycated hemoglobin levels help determine the quality of glucose control both before and during pregnancy
- Glucose challenge test at 24–28 weeks with 50 g oral glucose load and venous sample 1 h later
- Cut-off value of 130 mg/dL or higher requires follow-up with 3-h GTT
- Normal values for glucose challenge test and fasting blood sugar are ≤95 mg/dL; 1 h ≤180 mg/dL; 2 h ≤155 mg/dL; 3 h ≤140 mg/dL
- Two or more abnormal values required for diagnosis of gestational diabetes

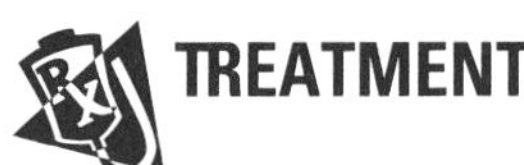

TREATMENT

MEDICATIONS

Before pregnancy

- Subcutaneous insulin in a split-dose regimen with frequent dosage adjustments
- Patients taking oral agents prior to pregnancy should be switched to insulin but glyburide may be safe and effective in pregnancy

During pregnancy

- 15% of patients with gestational diabetes require insulin during pregnancy
- Dietary therapy with 1800–2200 kcal/day
- Insulin therapy for persistent fasting blood sugar at ≥ 90 mg/dL or 2 h postprandial values of ≥ 120 mg/dL
- Glyburide may be safe and effective in pregnancy
- Continuous insulin pump therapy is very useful in type 1 diabetes mellitus

SURGERY

- Cesarean sections are performed for obstetric indications

THERAPEUTIC PROCEDURES

- The risk of fetal demise in the third trimester (stillbirth) and neonatal death increases with the level of hyperglycemia. Consequently, pregnant women with diabetes must receive regular antepartum fetal testing (nonstress testing, contraction stress testing, biophysical profile) during the third trimester
- **Timing of delivery**
  - Dictated by the quality of diabetic control, the presence or absence of medical complications, and fetal status
  - The goal is to reach 39 weeks (38 completed weeks) and then proceed with delivery
  - Confirmation of lung maturity is necessary only for delivery prior to 39 weeks

OUTCOME

FOLLOW-UP

- Patients should be evaluated 6–8 weeks postpartum by a 2-h oral glucose tolerance test (75 g glucose load)
- Following delivery, insulin dosage needs to be adjusted down to prepregnancy levels

COMPLICATIONS

- Infants of diabetic mothers are at risk for macrosomia
- Congenital anomalies result from hyperglycemia during the first 4–8 weeks of pregnancy. They occur in 4–10% of diabetic pregnancies (two to three times the rate in nondiabetic pregnancies)
- Euglycemia in the early weeks of pregnancy, when organogenesis is occurring, reduces the rate of anomalies to near-normal levels. Even so, because euglycemia is not consistently achieved, congenital anomalies are the principal cause of perinatal fetal deaths in diabetic pregnancies
- Hydramnios, preeclampsia-eclampsia, infections, and prematurity are increased even in carefully managed diabetic pregnancies

PROGNOSIS

- Pregnancy does not appear to alter the long-term consequences of diabetes, but retinopathy and nephropathy may first appear or become worse during pregnancy

WHEN TO REFER

- All women with diabetes should receive prepregnancy management by physicians experienced in diabetic pregnancies

WHEN TO ADMIT

- Failed intensive outpatient management of hypoglycemia or hyperglycemia
- Diagnosis of ketoacidosis
- Major complication of pregnancy

PREVENTION

- Prepregnancy HbA_{1c} levels of < 8% should be achieved to reduce the incidence of congenital anomalies

EVIDENCE

PRACTICE GUIDELINES

- American Academy of Family Physicians
  - http://www.aafp.org/afp/20031101/1767.html
- National Guideline Clearinghouse
  - American Diabetes Association, 2004
  - US Preventive Services Task Force, 2003
  - http://www.guideline.gov/summary/summary.aspx?doc_id=3493

WEB SITES

- American Academy of Family Physicians
  - http://www.aafp.org/afp/20031101/1775ph.html
- American Diabetes Association
  - http://www.diabetes.org
  - http://www.diabetes.org/gestational-diabetes.jsp
- Clinical Guidelines in Obstetrics and Gynecology
  - http://www.rcog.org.uk/guidelines.asp?PageID=105
- Guidelines, Recommendations, and Evidence-Based Medicine in Obstetrics
  - http://matweb.hcuge.ch/matweb/endo/cours_4e_MREG/obstetrics_gynecology_guidelines.htm

INFORMATION FOR PATIENTS

- American Academy of Family Physicians
  - http://www.aafp.org/afp/20031101/1775ph.html
- American Diabetes Association
  - http://www.diabetes.org/gestational-diabetes.jsp
- Patient Information for Obstetrics and Gynecology
  - http://www.vh.org/Patients/IHB/ObGyn.html
- National Institute of Child Health and Human Development
  - http://www.nichd.nih.gov/about/womenhealth/disorders_of_pregnancy.cfm

REFERENCES

- ACOG Practice Bulletin. Clinical management guidelines for obstetrician-gynecologists. Number 30, September 2001. Gestational diabetes. Obstet Gynecol 2001;98:525. [PMID: 11547793]
- Langer O et al: A comparison of glyburide and insulin in women with gestational diabetes mellitus. N Engl J Med 2000;343:1134. [PMID: 11036118]
- Temple R et al: Association between outcome of pregnancy and glycemic control in early pregnancy in type I diabetics: population based study. BMJ 2002;325:1275. [PMID: 12458245]

Author(s)

William R. Crombleholme, MD

Diabetes Mellitus, Type 1

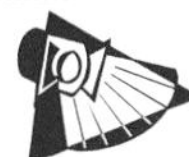

KEY FEATURES

ESSENTIALS OF DIAGNOSIS

- Polyuria, polydipsia, and weight loss associated with random plasma glucose ≥ 200 mg/dL
- Plasma glucose ≥126 mg/dL after an overnight fast, documented on more than one occasion
- Ketonemia, ketonuria, or both

GENERAL CONSIDERATIONS

- Caused by pancreatic islet B-cell destruction
- Destruction immune mediated in > 90% of cases and idiopathic in the remainder
- About 95% of type 1 patients possess either HLA-DR3 or HLA-DR4 compared with 50% of White controls. HLA-DQB1*0302 is an even more specific marker for susceptibility
- As many as 85% are positive for islet cell antibodies, antiglutamic acid decarboxylase (GAD), antiinsulin, and anti-ICA 512 (tyrosine phosphatase) antibodies at diagnosis
- The rate of pancreatic B-cell destruction ranges from rapid to slow
- Prone to ketoacidosis
- C-peptide negative 1 to 5 years after diagnosis; plasma glucagon is elevated

DEMOGRAPHICS

- Occurs mainly in 10- to 14-year olds but may occur in adults, especially when hyperglycemia first appears in the non-obese or elderly
- The highest incidence is in Scandinavia; in Finland the yearly incidence per 100,000 10- to 14-year-olds is 37. The United States averages 15 per 100,000; incidences are higher in states densely populated with persons of Scandinavian descent such as Minnesota. The lowest incidence is < 1 per 100,000 per year in China and parts of South America
- An estimated 18.2 million Americans have diabetes, of whom approximately 1 million have type 1 diabetes

CLINICAL FINDINGS

SYMPTOMS AND SIGNS

- Increased thirst and urination
- Polyphagia with weight loss
- Ketoacidosis
- Paresthesias
- Recurrent blurred vision
- Vulvovaginitis or pruritus
- Nocturnal enuresis
- Postural hypotension from lowered plasma volume

DIFFERENTIAL DIAGNOSIS

- Type 2 diabetes
- Hyperglycemia resulting from other causes (glucocorticoids, Cushing's syndrome, glucagonoma, acromegaly, pheochromocytoma, pentamidine)
- Metabolic acidosis of other causes (alcoholic ketoacidosis)
- Nondiabetic glycosuria (renal glycosuria)

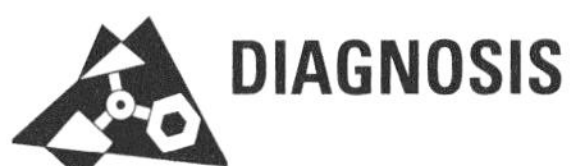

DIAGNOSIS

LABORATORY TESTS

- Fasting plasma glucose > 126 mg/dL or > 200 mg/dL 2 h after glucose load (Table 111)
- Ketonemia, ketonuria, or both
- Glucosuria (Clinistix, Diastix)
- Ketonuria (Acetest, Ketostix)
- Glycosylated hemoglobin (hemoglobin A_{1c}): reflects glycemic control over preceding 8–12 weeks
- Serum fructosamine: reflects glycemic control over preceding 2 weeks. Helpful in presence of abnormal hemoglobins or ascertaining glycemic control at time of conception among diabetic woman
- Lipoprotein abnormalities; unlike type 2 diabetes, moderately deficient control of hyperglycemia in type 1 diabetes is associated with only slight elevation of low-density lipoprotein (LDL) cholesterol and serum triglycerides and minimal change in high-density lipoprotein (HDL) cholesterol

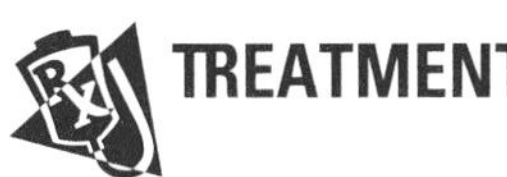

TREATMENT

MEDICATIONS

Use of insulin

- Tables 115 and 116
- Preprandial rapid-acting insulin plus basal insulin replacement with intermediate- or long-acting insulin
- Rapid-acting insulin analogs: insulin lispro, insulin aspart, insulin glulisine
- Short-acting insulins purified: regular, regular Humulin, regular Iletin II
- Intermediate-acting insulins purified: Lente Humulin, Lente Iletin II, Lente Novolin, neutral protamine Hagedorn (NPH) Humulin, NPH Iletin II, NPH Novolin
- Premixed insulins (% NPH/% regular): Novolin 70/30, Humulin 70/30 (% NPH, % insulin lispro: humalog mix 75/25), NovoLog mix 70/30
- Long-acting insulins purified: ultralente Humulin, insulin glargine

SURGERY

- Infuse intraoperatively and in immediate postoperative period: D5 0.9% saline with 20 mEq KCl IV at 100–200 mL/h. Infuse regular human insulin (25 U/250 mL 0.9% saline) into IV tubing at 1–3 U/h

- Monitor blood glucose hourly and adjust infusion for target glucose levels 100–190 mg/dL
- Patients receiving simultaneous pancreas and kidney transplants have 85% chance of pancreatic graft survival and 92% chance of renal graft survival after 1 year. Solitary pancreas transplant only for recurrent life-threatening metabolic instability
- Islet transplantation is minimally invasive (data on long-term efficacy are lacking); application is limited by need for multiple donors and potent long-term immunotherapy

THERAPEUTIC PROCEDURES

- Eucaloric healthy diet. Limit cholesterol to 300 mg QD, protein to 10–20% of total calories; keep saturated fats < 8–9% of total calories; remainder of diet made up of monounsaturated fats and carbohydrates with 20–35 g of dietary fiber
- Treat microalbuminuria with angiotensin-converting enzyme (ACE)-I inhibitor to retard diabetic nephropathy
- Treat hypertension and hyperlipidemia (reduce LDL < 100 mg/dL)
- Attempts have been made to prolong the partial clinical remission ("honeymoon") using drugs that may induce immune tolerance

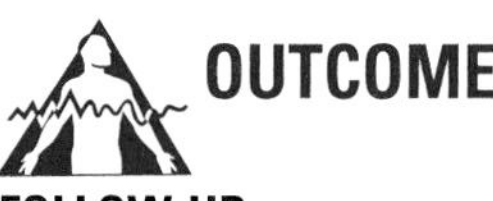

OUTCOME

FOLLOW-UP

- Glycemic control of HbA_{1c} no higher than 2% above upper limits of normal has 60% reduction in risk of diabetic retinopathy, nephropathy, and neuropathy

COMPLICATIONS

- Diabetic ketoacidosis
- Hypoglycemia and altered awareness of hypoglycemia
- Diabetic retinopathy, cataracts
- Nephropathy
- Neuropathy
- Diabetic atherothrombosis (coronary artery disease, peripheral vascular disease)
- Lipodystrophy at injection sites

PROGNOSIS

- The Diabetes Control and Complications Trial (DCCT) showed that the poor prognosis for 40% of patients with type 1 diabetes is markedly improved by optimal care
- Patients can have a full life
- Tight control (mean HbA_{1c} 7.2% normal: < 6%) in the DCCT was associated with a threefold greater risk of serious hypoglycemia as well as greater weight gain. However, no deaths occurred because of hypoglycemia, and no evidence of posthypoglycemic cognitive damage was detected
- Subsequent renal failure predicted by microalbuminuria > 30 μg/min. Risk decreased by treatment with ACE-I

WHEN TO REFER

- Team educational approach is critical. Enlist nutritionist
- Poorly controlled diabetes

WHEN TO ADMIT

- Altered mental status
- Diabetic ketoacidosis
- Marked volume disorders
- Marked electrolyte disorders
- Unstable comorbid conditions

PREVENTION

- Acetylsalicylic acid (aspirin) 81–325 mg (enteric coated) a day to reduce risk of diabetic atherothrombosis without increasing risk of vitreous bleeding
- Instruction in personal hygiene, in particular, care of feet, skin, and teeth
- Yearly diabetic eye examination
- Patient self-management training
- Self-monitoring of blood glucose
- Exercise

EVIDENCE

PRACTICE GUIDELINES

- American Diabetes Association: Clinical practice recommendations. Diabetes Care 2002;25(Suppl 1):S1.
- National Guideline Clearinghouse/ American Diabetes Association
  - http://www.guideline.gov/summary/summary.aspx?doc_id=6575&nbr=4135&string=Diabetes+AND+Mellitus
  - http://www.guideline.gov/summary/summary.aspx?doc_id=4677
- American Association of Clinical Endocrinologists
  - http://www.aace.com/clin/guidelines/diabetes_2002.pdf

WEB SITES

- CDC Diabetes Public Health Resource
  - http://www.cdc.gov/diabetes/
- American Diabetes Association
  - http://www.diabetes.org
- Joslin Diabetes Center
  - http://www.joslin.harvard.edu

INFORMATION FOR PATIENTS

- American Diabetes Association: Type 1 Diabetes
  - http://www.diabetes.org/type-1-diabetes.jsp
- American Academy of Family Physicians: Diabetes: Type 1
  - http://familydoctor.org/480.xml
- NIH—National Diabetes Education Program
  - http://www.ndep.nih.gov/diabetes/pubs/catalog.htm
- Torpy JM et al: JAMA patient page: Type 1 diabetes. JAMA 2003;290:2216. [PMID:14570956]

REFERENCE

- Atkinson MA: Type 1 diabetes: new perspectives on disease pathogenesis and treatment. Lancet 2001;358:766. [PMID:11476858]

Author(s)

Umesh Masharani, MB, BS, MRCH (UK)

Diabetes Mellitus, Type 2

KEY FEATURES

ESSENTIALS OF DIAGNOSIS

- Typically > 40 years of age
- Obesity
- Polyuria and polydipsia
- Candidal vaginitis sometimes an initial manifestation
- Often few or no symptoms
- After an overnight fast, plasma glucose ≥126 mg/dL more than once
- After 75 g oral glucose, diagnostic values are 200 mg/dL or more 2 h after the oral glucose
- Often associated with hypertension, dyslipidemia, and atherosclerosis

GENERAL CONSIDERATIONS

- Circulating endogenous insulin is sufficient to prevent ketoacidosis but inadequate to prevent hyperglycemia from tissue insensitivity
- Strong genetic influences
- Prevalence of obesity in type 2 diabetes mellitus is 30% in Chinese and Japanese, 60–70% in North Americans, Europeans, and Africans, and nearly 100% in Pima Indians and Pacific Islanders from Nauru or Samoa
- Enhancers of insulin resistance are aging, sedentary lifestyle, and abdominal-visceral obesity
- Abdominal fat, with an abnormally high waist–hip ratio, is generally associated with obesity in type 2 diabetes. This visceral obesity correlates with insulin resistance, whereas subcutaneous fat seems to have less of an association
- Both the tissue resistance to insulin and the impaired B-cell response to glucose are further aggravated by increased hyperglycemia, and both defects improve with decreased hyperglycemia

DEMOGRAPHICS

- 18.2 million Americans, or > 90% of all diabetics in the United States, have type 2 diabetes
- Middle-aged adults but occasionally juveniles
- No gender predominance

CLINICAL FINDINGS

SYMPTOMS AND SIGNS

- Polyuria and thirst
- Weakness or fatigue
- Recurrent blurred vision
- Vulvovaginitis or pruritus
- Peripheral neuropathy
- Often asymptomatic

DIFFERENTIAL DIAGNOSIS

Hyperglycemia

- Endocrinopathies: type 1 diabetes mellitus, Cushing's syndrome, acromegaly, pheochromocytoma, glucagonoma, somatostatinoma
- Drugs: glucocorticoids, thiazides, phenytoin, niacin, oral contraceptives, pentamidine
- Pancreatic insufficiency: subtotal pancreatectomy, chronic pancreatitis, hemochromatosis ("bronze diabetes"), cystic fibrosis, hemosiderosis
- Other: gestational diabetes, cirrhosis, Schmidt's syndrome (polyglandular failure: Addison's disease, autoimmune thyroiditis, diabetes)

Polyuria

- Diabetes insipidus

Hypercalcemia

- Psychogenic polydipsia

Nondiabetic glycosuria (benign)

- Genetic
- Fanconi's syndrome
- Chronic renal failure
- Pregnancy

DIAGNOSIS

LABORATORY TESTS

- Fasting plasma glucose ≥ 126 mg/dL or ≥ 200 mg/dL 2 h after glucose load (Table 111)
- Glucosuria (Clinistix, Diastix)
- Ketonuria on occasion without ketonemia (Acetest, Ketostix)
- Glycosylated hemoglobin (HbA_{1c}) reflects glycemic control over preceding 8–12 weeks
- Serum fructosamine reflects glycemic control over preceding 2 weeks. Helpful in the presence of abnormal hemoglobins and in ascertaining glycemic control at time of conception among diabetic women
- Lipoprotein abnormalities in obese type 2 diabetics include high serum triglyceride (300–400 mg/dL), low high-density lipoprotein (HDL) cholesterol (< 30 mg/dL), and a qualitative change in low-density lipoprotein (LDL) particles, differing from type 1 diabetes, which is associated with only slight elevation of LDL cholesterol and serum triglycerides and minimal change in HDL cholesterol

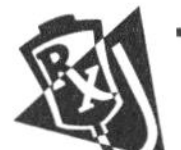

TREATMENT

MEDICATIONS

- Oral agents that stimulate insulin secretion: sulfonylureas, meglitinide analogs, d-phenylalanine derivative (Table 112)
- Insulin-sparing oral agents: biguanides, thiazolidinediones, α-glucosidase inhibitors (Table 113)
- Combination oral agents: glyburide-metformin available but limits optimal dose adjustment of individual drugs (Table 114)
- Insulin: indicated for type 2 diabetics with insulinopenia and hyperglycemia unresponsive to diet and oral hypoglycemic agents
- Preprandial rapid-acting insulin plus basal insulin replacement with an intermediate- or long-acting insulin used to attain acceptable control of blood glucose (Tables 115 and 116)

SURGERY

Major surgery

- Insulin during major surgery necessary for most type 2 diabetics, even if not previously taking insulin

- Infuse IV intraoperatively and in the immediate postoperative period: 1 L D_5W with 20 mEq KCl and 10 U regular insulin at rate of ~100 mL/h
- Monitor blood glucose hourly and adjust infusion for target glucose levels 100–250 mg/dL. If blood glucose remains > 250 mg/dL after 1–2 h, increase insulin infusion to 15 U/L

Minor surgery

- Regular human insulin or insulin lispro SC PRN to maintain glucose < 250 mg/dL
- Avoid glucose-containing solutions

THERAPEUTIC PROCEDURES

- *Diet:* Limit cholesterol to 300 mg QD, protein intake 10–20% of total calories, saturated fats < 8–9% of total calories, with remainder of diet monounsaturated fats and carbohydrates with 20–35 g of dietary fiber

OUTCOME

FOLLOW-UP

- Self-monitoring
- HbA_{1c} quarterly
- Annual screen for microalbuminuria
- Serum lipids
- Feet examination annually
- Yearly diabetic eye examination
- Treatment goals: self-monitored blood glucose, 80–120 mg/dL before meals; 100–140 mg/dL at bedtime; < 180 mg/dL 1.5–2.0 h postprandially. HbA_{1c} < 7.0%

COMPLICATIONS

- Hypoglycemia
- Ocular (diabetic cataracts and retinopathy)
- Diabetic nephropathy (microalbuminuria, progressive diabetic nephropathy)
- Gangrene of the feet
- Diabetic neuropathy (peripheral neuropathy, distal symmetric polyneuropathy, isolated peripheral neuropathy, painful diabetic neuropathy, autonomic neuropathy)
- Skin and mucous membranes (pyogenic infections, eruptive xanthomas from hypertriglyceridemia associated with poor glucose control, necrobiosis lipoidica diabeticorum, shin spots, intertriginous candida, vulvovaginitis)

WHEN TO REFER

- Team-oriented educational approach, including a nutritionist, is critical
- Poorly controlled diabetes

WHEN TO ADMIT

- Altered mental status
- Diabetic ketoacidosis
- Marked volume disorders
- Marked electrolyte disorders
- Unstable comorbid conditions

PROGNOSIS

- Antihypertensive control to a mean of 144/82 mm Hg had beneficial effects on all microvascular and all diabetes-related end points in the United Kingdom Prospective Diabetes Study

PREVENTION

- Goal of therapy is to prevent acute illness and reduce risk of long-term complications
- Lifestyle modifications can prevent or slow the development of diabetes
- Daily vigorous exercise prevents accumulation of visceral fat, which can prevent the development of diabetes
- Screen with fasting glucose at 3-year intervals beginning at age 45; screen earlier and more frequently if risk factors present

EVIDENCE

PRACTICE GUIDELINES

- National Guideline Clearinghouse: Standards of Medical Care in Diabetes
  - http://www.guideline.gov/summary/summary.aspx?doc_id=4679&nbr=3413&string=American+AND+DiabetesStandards%20of%20medical%20care%20in%20diabetes
- American Association of Clinical Endocrinologists: Medical Guidelines for the Management of Diabetes Mellitus
  - http://www.aace.com/clin/guidelines/diabetes_2002.pdf
- National Guideline Clearinghouse: Adult Diabetes Clinical Practice Guidelines
  - http://www.guideline.gov/summary/summary.aspx?doc_id=5270&nbr=3597&string=diabetes

WEB SITES

- Centers for Disease Control: Diabetes Public Health Resource
  - http://www.cdc.gov/diabetes/
- Joslin Diabetes Center
  - http://www.joslin.harvard.edu/
- American Diabetes Association
  - http://www.diabetes.org

INFORMATION FOR PATIENTS

- American Diabetes Association: Type 2 Diabetes
  - http://www.diabetes.org/type-2-diabetes.jsp
- Joslin Diabetes Center: Joslin's Online Diabetes Library
  - http://www.joslin.org/education/library/index.shtml#general
- Stevens LM: JAMA patient page: The ABCs of diabetes. JAMA 2002;287:2608. [PMID: 12025825]
- JAMA patient page: Managing type 2 diabetes. JAMA 2000;283:288.
- NIH: National Diabetes Education Program
  - http://www.ndep.nih.gov/diabetes/pubs/catalog.htm

REFERENCES

- American Diabetes Association: Clinical practice recommendations. Diabetes Care 2002;25(Suppl 1):S1
- UK Prospective Diabetes Study Group: Effect of intensive blood-glucose control with metformin on complications in overweight patients with type 2 diabetes. Lancet 1998;352:854. [PMID: 9742977]

Author(s)

Umesh Masharani, MB, BS, MRCH (UK)

Diabetic Ketoacidosis

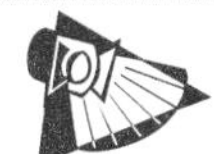

KEY FEATURES

ESSENTIALS OF DIAGNOSIS

- Hyperglycemia > 250 mg/dL
- Acidosis with blood pH < 7.3
- Serum bicarbonate < 15 mEq/L
- Serum positive for ketones

GENERAL CONSIDERATIONS

- May be the initial manifestation of type 1 diabetes
- Commonly occurs with poor compliance in type 1 diabetics, particularly when episodes are recurrent
- Develops in type 1 diabetics with increased insulin requirements during infection, trauma, myocardial infarction, or surgery
- May develop in type 2 diabetics under severe stress such as sepsis or trauma
- Common serious complication of insulin pump therapy

DEMOGRAPHICS

- Incidence is five to eight episodes per 1000 diabetic subjects annually
- Incidence in insulin pump therapy is one per 80 patient-months of treatment

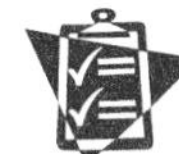

CLINICAL FINDINGS

SYMPTOMS AND SIGNS

- May begin with a day or more of polyuria, polydipsia, marked fatigue, nausea and vomiting, and, finally, mental stupor that can progress to coma
- Dehydration, possible stupor
- Rapid deep breathing and a "fruity" breath odor of acetone
- Hypotension with tachycardia indicates profound fluid and electrolyte depletion
- Mild hypothermia usually present; elevated or even a normal temperature may suggest infection
- Abdominal pain and tenderness in the absence of abdominal disease; conversely, cholecystitis or pancreatitis may occur with minimal symptoms and signs

DIFFERENTIAL DIAGNOSIS

- Lactic acidosis in type 1 diabetics, including the use of metformin
- Alcoholic ketoacidosis
- Hypoglycemia
- Hyperglycemic hyperosmolar state
- Uremia
- Starvation ketoacidosis
- Salicylate poisoning

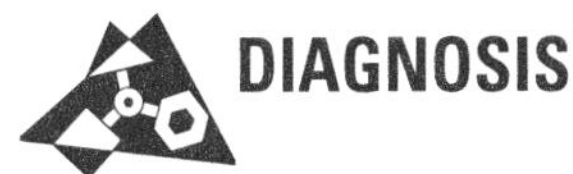

DIAGNOSIS

LABORATORY TESTS

- 4+ glycosuria, hyperglycemia
- Strong ketonuria and ketonemia [acetoacetic acid measured by nitroprusside reagents (Acetest and Ketostix)]. The more prevalent β-hydroxybutyric acid has no ketone group and is therefore not detected by conventional nitroprusside tests
- Anion-gap ketoacidosis
- Serum potassium often elevated despite total body potassium depletion
- Elevated serum amylase from salivary as well as pancreatic amylase. An elevated serum amylase is not specific for acute pancreatitis
- Serum lipase may be useful if the diagnosis of pancreatitis is being seriously considered
- Leukocytosis up to 25,000/μL with a left shift may occur with or without associated infection
- Hyperchloremic metabolic acidosis can develop during initial therapy, as keto acids are lost in the urine and a portion of the bicarbonate deficit is replaced with chloride ions from the saline therapy. This relatively benign condition reverses over a day once intravenous saline is stopped

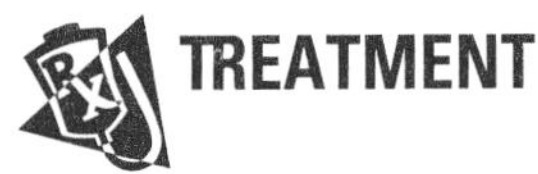

TREATMENT

MEDICATIONS

Regular insulin

- Initially in severe ketoacidosis, use only regular insulin
- Begin with loading dose of 0.1 unit/kg as IV bolus, followed by 0.1 unit/kg/h, continuously infused or given hourly as an IM injection
- "Piggy-back" insulin into the fluid line so the rate of fluid replacement can be changed without altering the insulin delivery rate
- If plasma glucose level fails to fall at least 10% in the first hour, give repeat loading dose

Fluids

- Fluid deficit is usually 4–5 L. In the first hour, give at least 1 L of 0.9% saline to reexpand contracted vascular volume
- One can then switch to 0.45% saline at a rate of 300–500 mL/h, depending on the severity of the dehydration and the cardiac and renal status
- Failure to give enough volume replacement (at least 3–4 L in 8 h) to restore normal perfusion affects satisfactory recovery
- Excessive fluid replacement (more than 5 L in 8 h) may contribute to acute respiratory distress syndrome or cerebral edema

Electrolytes

- Use **NaHCO3** only for pH < 7.1. For arterial pH 6.9–7.0, add one ampule of 7.5% NaHCO3 (44 mEq/L) to 200 mL of sterile water intravenously at a rate of 200 mL/h
  - If the pH is below 6.9, use two ampules of NaHCO3 (88 mEq) in 400 mL of sterile water at the same rate of 200 mL/h
  - For each ampule of NaHCO3, add 15 mEq/L of KCl as long as the serum potassium does not exceed 5.5 mEq/L.
  - Stop bicarbonate when pH reaches 7.1
- When blood glucose falls to 250 mg/dL or less, use 5% **glucose** solutions to maintain blood glucose 200–300 mg/dL while continuing insulin to clear ketonemia
- Total body **potassium** loss from polyuria and vomiting may be several hundred milliequivalents
  - However, initial serum potassium is usually normal or high because of extracellular shifts from acidosis
  - Potassium infusion 20–30 mEq/h should begin 2–3 h after beginning therapy, or sooner if initial serum potassium is low
  - Defer potassium replacement if serum potassium remains above 5 mEq/L, as in renal insufficiency
- **Phosphate** replacement is seldom required. However, if severe hypophosphatemia of < 0.35 mmol/L (< 1 mg/dL) develops during insulin therapy, a small amount of phosphate can be replaced as the potassium salt
  - To minimize the risk of tetany from an overload of phosphate replacement, an average deficit of 40–50 mmol phosphate should be replaced by intravenous infusion at a rate not to exceed 3 mmol/h
  - A stock solution (Abbott Laboratories) provides a mixture of 1.12 g KH_2PO_4 and 1.18 g K_2HPO_4 in a 5-mL single-dose vial representing 22 mEq potassium and 15 mmol phosphate (27 mEq); 5 mL of this stock solution in 2 L of 0.45% saline or 5% dextrose in water, infused at 400 mL/h, will replace the phosphate at the optimal rate of 3 mmol/h and provide 4.4 mEq potassium per hour
  - If serum phosphate remains below 0.35 mmol/L (1 mg/dL), repeat a 5-h infusion of potassium phosphate at a rate of 3 mmol/h

THERAPEUTIC PROCEDURES

- Use a flow sheet listing vital signs, time sequence of laboratory values (arterial pH, plasma glucose, acetone, bicarbonate, serum urea nitrogen, electrolytes, serum osmolality) in relation to therapy
- Careful monitoring of serum potassium during fluid replacement

OUTCOME

COMPLICATIONS

- Acute myocardial infarction and infarction of the bowel following prolonged hypotension
- Renal failure, especially with prior kidney dysfunction
- Cerebral edema occurs rarely
  - This is best prevented by avoiding sudden reversal of marked hyperglycemia
  - Maintaining glycemic levels of 200–300 mg/dL for the initial 24 h after correction of severe hyperglycemia reduces this risk

PROGNOSIS

- Life-threatening medical emergency with a mortality rate just under 5% in individuals younger than 40 years, but with a more serious prognosis in the elderly, who have mortality rates over 20%

WHEN TO REFER

- Recurrent diabetic ketoacidosis
- Poor compliance

WHEN TO ADMIT

- Severe ketosis, hyperosmolality
- An intensive care unit or step-down unit is preferable for more severe cases

PREVENTION

- The patient should contact a provider for persistent ketonuria
- Compliance is particularly important for juvenile-onset diabetics, particularly in the teen years. Intensive family counseling may be needed
- Urine ketones should be measured with signs of infection or in insulin pump-treated patients when capillary blood glucose is persistently high

EVIDENCE

PRACTICE GUIDELINES

- National Guideline Clearinghouse: American Diabetes Association, 2004
  - http://www.guideline.gov/summary/summary.aspx?doc_id=4694

WEB SITES

- American Diabetes Association
  - http://www.diabetes.org
- Centers for Disease Control: Diabetes
  - http://www.cdc.gov/diabetes
- Joslin Diabetes Center
  - http://www.joslin.harvard.edu

INFORMATION FOR PATIENTS

- JAMA patient page: The ABCs of diabetes. JAMA 2002;287:2608. [PMID: 12025825]
- American Diabetes Association
  - http://www.diabetes.org/type-1-diabetes/ketoacidosis.jsp
- National Institutes of Health
  - http://www.nlm.nih.gov/medlineplus/ency/article/000320.htm
- NIH: National Diabetes Education Program (multiple languages available)
  - http://www.ndep.nih.gov/diabetes/pubs/catalog.htm

REFERENCE

- Kitabchi AE et al: Management of hyperglycemic crises in patients with diabetes. Diabetes Care 2001;24:131. [PMID: 11194218]

Author(s)

Umesh Masharani, MB, BS, MRCH (UK)

Diarrhea, Acute

KEY FEATURES

ESSENTIALS OF DIAGNOSIS

- Defined as a stool weight of >250 g/24 hours, although quantification of stool weight is necessary only in some patients with chronic diarrhea
- Increased stool frequency (>2–3 bowel movements per day) or increased liquidity of feces

GENERAL CONSIDERATIONS

- Acute diarrhea (< 3 weeks) is most commonly caused by infectious agents, bacterial toxins, or drugs (Table 131)
- Recent illnesses in family members suggests infectious diarrhea
- Ingestion of improperly stored or prepared food implicates poisoning
- Exposure to unpurified water suggests *Giardia, Cryptosporidium*, or *Cyclospora*
- Recent travel abroad suggests "traveler's diarrhea"
- Antibiotic administration suggests *Clostridium difficile* colitis
- HIV infection or sexually transmitted diseases suggest AIDS-associated diarrhea
- Proctitis and rectal discharge suggest gonorrhea, syphilis, lymphogranuloma venereum, and herpes simplex

Noninflammatory diarrhea

- Watery, nonbloody diarrhea, usually small bowel source caused by either a toxin-producing bacterium or other agents (viruses, *Giardia*)
- Prominent vomiting suggests viral enteritis or *Staphylococcus aureus* food poisoning
- Diarrhea is voluminous, causing dehydration with hypokalemia and metabolic acidosis
- Fecal leukocytes are not present

Inflammatory diarrhea

- Fever and bloody diarrhea (dysentery) caused by invasion (shigellosis, salmonellosis, *Campylobacter*, or *Yersinia* infection, amebiasis, cytomegalovirus) or a toxin (*C difficile, E coli* O157:H7)
- Diarrhea small volume (< 1 L/day) with left lower quadrant cramps, urgency, and tenesmus
- Fecal leukocytes usually present

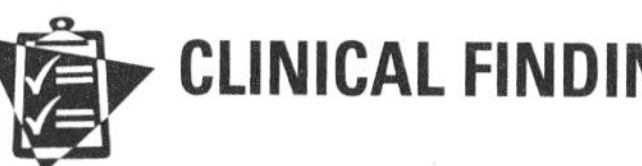

CLINICAL FINDINGS

SYMPTOMS AND SIGNS

- Increased stool frequency or liquidity
- Rectal discharge suggests proctitis
- Periumbilical cramps, bloating, nausea, or vomiting suggest noninflammatory diarrhea
- Fever, left lower quadrant cramps, urgency, and tenesmus suggest inflammatory diarrhea
- Physical examination may reveal abdominal tenderness, peritonitis

DIFFERENTIAL DIAGNOSIS

- Infectious: noninflammatory (nonbloody)
  - Viruses: Norwalk virus, rotavirus, adenoviruses, astrovirus, coronavirus
  - Preformed toxin (food poisoning): *S aureus, Bacillus cereus, Clostridium perfringens*
  - Toxin production: enterotoxigenic *E coli, Vibrio cholerae, Vibrio parahaemolyticus*
  - Protozoa: *Giardia lamblia, Cryptosporidium, Cyclospora, Isospora*
- Infectious: invasive or inflammatory
  - *Shigella, Salmonella, Campylobacter*, enteroinvasive *E coli, E coli* O157:H7, *Yersinia enterocolitica, C difficile* (eg, pseudomembranous colitis), *Entamoeba histolytica, Neisseria gonorrhoeae, Listeria monocytogenes*
- Associated with unprotected anal intercourse: *Neisseria gonorrhoeae*, syphilis, lymphogranuloma venereum, herpes simplex
- Noninfectious
  - Drug reaction, especially antibiotics
  - Ulcerative colitis, Crohn's disease (inflammatory)
  - Ischemic colitis (inflammatory)
  - Fecal impaction (stool may leak around impaction)
  - Laxative abuse
  - Radiation colitis (inflammatory)
  - Emotional stress

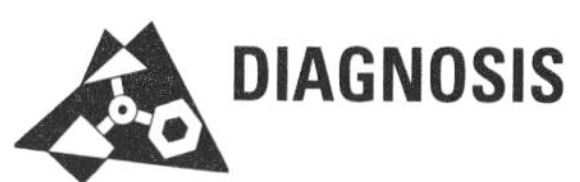

DIAGNOSIS

LABORATORY TESTS

- If diarrhea worsens or persists for >7–10 days, stool should be sent for fecal leukocyte determination, stool ovum and parasite evaluation, and stool bacterial culture
- Prompt medical evaluation when
  - Signs of inflammatory diarrhea: fever (>38.5°C), bloody diarrhea, or abdominal pain
  - Passage of six or more unformed stools in 24 hours
  - Profuse watery diarrhea and dehydration
  - Frail older patients
  - Immunocompromised patients (AIDS, post transplantation)
- Stool wet mount for amebiasis in sexually active homosexuals, those with recent travel, and those whose bacterial cultures are negative
- Stool *C difficile* toxin assay if recent history of antibiotic exposure
- Stool culture with serotyping if *E coli* O157:H7 is suspected
- Three stool examinations for ova and parasites if diarrhea persists for more than 10 days
- Stool *Giardia* antigen assay if recent camping
- Rectal swab cultures for *Chlamydia, Neisseria gonorrhoeae*, and herpes simplex virus in sexually active patients with suspected proctitis

DIAGNOSTIC PROCEDURES

- In >90% of cases, acute diarrhea is mild and self-limited, and diagnostic investigation is unnecessary
- Prompt sigmoidoscopy for severe proctitis (tenesmus, discharge, rectal pain) or for suspected *C difficile* colitis, ulcerative colitis, or ischemic colitis

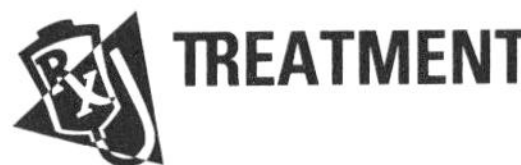

TREATMENT

MEDICATIONS

- Antidiarrheal agents may be used safely in mild to moderate diarrhea but should not be used in bloody diarrhea, high fever, or systemic toxicity
- Loperamide, 4 mg PO initially, followed by 2 mg after each loose stool (maximum: 16 mg/24 hours)
- Bismuth subsalicylate (Pepto-Bismol), 2 tablets or 30 mL PO QID
- Anticholinergic diphenoxylate with atropine contraindicated in acute diarrhea because of the rare precipitation of toxic megacolon
- Empirical antibiotic treatment recommended with moderate to severe fever, tenesmus, or bloody stools or the presence of fecal leukocytes while the stool bacterial culture is incubating
- Fluoroquinolones (eg, ciprofloxacin 500 mg, ofloxacin 400 mg, or norfloxacin 400 mg, PO BID) for 5–7 days
- Trimethoprim-sulfamethoxazole, 160/800 mg PO BID, or erythromycin, 250–500 mg PO QID
- Metronidazole (250 mg PO TID for 7 days) when *Giardia* infection is suspected
- Specific antimicrobial treatment is recommended in shigellosis, cholera, extraintestinal salmonellosis, traveler's diarrhea, *C difficile* infection, giardiasis, amebiasis, and gonorrhea, syphilis, chlamydiosis, and herpes simplex infection
- Antibiotics not recommended in nontyphoid *Salmonella, Campylobacter, Aeromonas, Yersinia*, or *E coli* O157:H7 infection except in severe disease

THERAPEUTIC PROCEDURES

- Diet
  - Adequate oral fluids containing carbohydrates and electrolytes
  - Avoidance of high-fiber foods, fats, milk products, caffeine, and alcohol
- Rehydration: oral electrolyte solutions (eg, Pedialyte, Gatorade), or intravenous fluids (lactated Ringer's injection) with severe dehydration

OUTCOME

WHEN TO ADMIT

- Hospitalization is required in patients with severe dehydration, toxicity, or marked abdominal pain, rebound tenderness

PREVENTION

- When traveling, eat only "peeled, packaged, and piping hot" foods

EVIDENCE

PRACTICE GUIDELINES

- National Guideline Clearinghouse
  - http://www.guideline.gov/summary/summary.aspx?doc_id=2791&nbr=2017&string=diarrhea
- Manatsathit S et al; Guideline for the management of acute diarrhea in adults. J Gastroenterol Hepatol 2002;Feb 17(Suppl):S54.
- Practice guidelines for the management of infectious diarrhea. Infectious Diseases Society of America, 2001
  - http://www.journals.uchicago.edu/CID/journal/issues/v32n3/001387/001387.html

INFORMATION FOR PATIENTS

- Centers for Disease Control and Prevention
  - http://www.cdc.gov/ncidod/dbmd/diseaseinfo/travelersdiarrhea_g.htm
- Mayo Clinic
  - http://www.mayoclinic.com/invoke.cfm?id=DS00292

REFERENCES

- Musher DM et al: Contagious acute gastrointestinal infections. N Engl J Med 2004;350:2417. [PMID:15575058]
- Thielman NM et al: Clinical practice: acute infectious diarrhea. N Engl J Med 2004;350:38. [PMID:14702426]
- Wingate D et al: Guidelines for adults on self-medication for the treatment of acute diarrhoea. Aliment Pharmacol Ther 2001;15:773. [PMID:11380315]

Author(s)

Kenneth R. McQuaid, MD

Diarrhea, Chronic

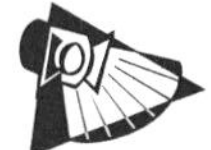

KEY FEATURES

ESSENTIALS OF DIAGNOSIS

- Defined as increased stool frequency or liquidity persisting for >3 weeks
- Classified as osmotic diarrhea, secretory diarrhea, inflammatory conditions, malabsorption syndromes, motility disorders, chronic infections, and miscellaneous

GENERAL CONSIDERATIONS

- Osmotic diarrheas resolve during fasting
- Secretory diarrhea is caused by increased intestinal secretion or decreased absorption with little change in stool output during fasting
- Motility disorders are secondary to systemic disorders or surgery due to rapid transit or to stasis of intestinal contents with bacterial overgrowth, malabsorption
- Immunocompromised patients are susceptible to *Microsporidia, Cryptosporidium*, cytomegalovirus, *Isospora belli, Cyclospora*, and *Mycobacterium avium-intracellulare* infection
- Factitious diarrhea is caused by surreptitious laxative abuse or dilution of stool

DEMOGRAPHICS

- Lactase deficiency
  - Occurs in 75% of nonwhite adults and 25% of whites
  - May be acquired with viral gastroenteritis, medical illness, or gastrointestinal surgery

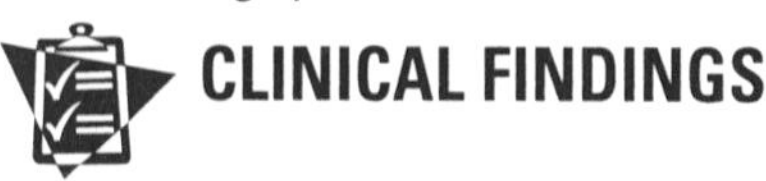

CLINICAL FINDINGS

SYMPTOMS AND SIGNS

- Osmotic diarrheas
  - Abdominal distention
  - Bloating
  - Flatulence due to increased colonic gas production
- Secretory diarrhea
  - High-volume (>1 L/day) watery diarrhea
  - Dehydration
  - Electrolyte imbalance
- Inflammatory conditions
  - Abdominal pain
  - Fever
  - Weight loss
  - Hematochezia
- Malabsorption syndromes: weight loss, osmotic diarrhea, and nutritional deficiencies

DIFFERENTIAL DIAGNOSIS

- Common
  - Irritable bowel syndrome
  - Lactase deficiency
  - Parasites
  - Caffeine
  - Alcohol
  - Laxative abuse
- Osmotic
  - Lactase deficiency
  - Medications: antacids, lactulose, sorbitol, olestra
  - Factitious: magnesium-containing antacids or laxatives
- Secretory
  - Hormonal: Zollinger-Ellison syndrome (gastrinoma), carcinoid, VIPoma, medullary thyroid carcinoma
  - Laxative abuse: phenolphthalein, cascara, senna
  - Villous adenoma
  - Medications
- Inflammatory conditions
  - Inflammatory bowel disease
  - Microscopic colitis (lymphocytic or collagenous)
  - Cancer with obstruction and pseudodiarrhea
  - Radiation colitis
- Malabsorption
  - Small bowel: celiac sprue, Whipple's disease, tropical sprue, eosinophilic gastroenteritis, small bowel resection, Crohn's disease
  - Lymphatic obstruction: lymphoma, carcinoid, tuberculosis, *M avium-intracellulare* infection, Kaposi's sarcoma, sarcoidosis, retroperitoneal fibrosis
  - Pancreatic insufficiency: chronic pancreatitis, cystic fibrosis, pancreatic cancer
  - Bacterial overgrowth, eg, diabetes
  - Reduced bile salts: ileal resection, Crohn's disease, postcholecystectomy
- Motility disorders
  - Irritable bowel syndrome
  - Postsurgical: vagotomy, partial gastrectomy, blind loop with bacterial overgrowth
  - Systemic disease: diabetes mellitus, hyperthyroidism, scleroderma
  - Caffeine or alcohol use
- Chronic infections
  - Parasites: giardiasis, amebiasis, strongyloidiasis
- Other
  - Ischemic colitis (intestinal ischemia)
  - Adrenal insufficiency

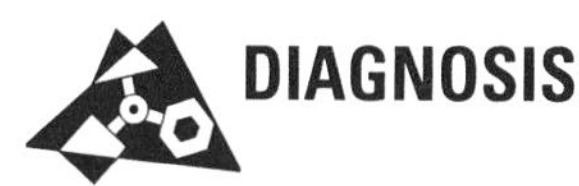

DIAGNOSIS

LABORATORY TESTS

- Obtain complete blood cell count, serum electrolytes, liver enzymes, calcium, phosphorus, albumin, thyroid-stimulating hormone, β-carotene, and prothrombin time
- Stool osmotic gap increased in osmotic diarrheas, normal in secretory diarrhea
- Fecal fat >10 g/24 hours in malabsorption syndromes
- Serologic tests for celiac sprue: serum IgG and IgA antigliadin, antiendomysial antibodies, or tissue transglutaminase antibody
- Serum VIP (VIPoma), calcitonin (medullary thyroid carcinoma), gastrin (Zollinger-Ellison syndrome), and glucagon
- Urine 5-hydroxyindoleacetic acid (carcinoid), vanillmandelic acid, metanephrines (pheochromocytoma), and histamine determinations
- Fecal leukocytes implies inflammatory diarrhea
- Stools for ova and parasites (three)
- Fecal ELISA for *Giardia*-specific antigen more sensitive and specific than ova and parasite examination

IMAGING STUDIES

- Sigmoidoscopy or colonoscopy with mucosal biopsy helpful in inflammatory bowel disease and melanosis coli
- Upper endoscopy with small bowel biopsy indicated for suspected celiac sprue, Whipple's disease, and AIDS-related *Cryptosporidium, Microsporidia*, and *M avium-intracellulare* infection
- Plain abdominal radiograph
- Abdominal CT for suspected chronic pancreatitis, pancreatic cancer
- Small intestinal barium radiography in suspected Crohn's disease, small bowel lymphoma, carcinoid, and jejunal diverticula
- Somatostatin receptor scintigraphy in suspected neuroendocrine tumors

DIAGNOSTIC PROCEDURES

- Stool analysis: 24-hour stool collection for weight and quantitative fecal fat
  - Stool weight >300 g/24 hours confirms diarrhea
  - Stool weight >1000–1500 g/24 hours suggests secretory diarrhea
  - Fecal fat >10 g/24 hours indicates a malabsorption syndrome

- Stool pH < 5.6 indicates carbohydrate malabsorption
- Stool osmolality less than serum osmolality indicates factitious diarrhea
- Stool laxative screen positive in laxative abuse
- Colonic biopsy modified acid-fast staining indicated for *Cryptosporidium* and *Cyclospora*

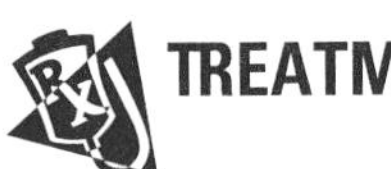

TREATMENT

MEDICATIONS

- Loperamide: 4 mg initially, then 2 mg after each loose stool (maximum: 16 mg/day)
- Diphenoxylate with atropine: 1 tablet PO TID–QID PRN
- Codeine 15–60 mg Q 4 h; deodorized tincture of opium, 10–25 drops Q 6 h PRN, safe in most patients with chronic, intractable diarrhea
- Clonidine, 0.1–0.6 mg PO BID, or a clonidine patch, 0.1–0.2 mg/day, helpful in secretory diarrheas, diabetic diarrhea, and cryptosporidiosis
- Octreotide, 50 μg to 250 μg SC TID, for secretory diarrheas due to neuroendocrine tumors (VIPomas, carcinoid) and in some cases of AIDS-related diarrhea
- Cholestyramine resin, 4 g PO QD–TID, in patients with bile salt–induced diarrhea secondary to intestinal resection or ileal disease

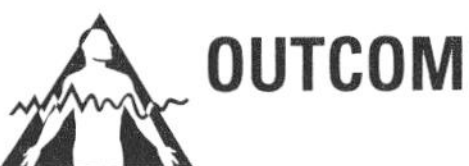

OUTCOME

COMPLICATIONS

- Dehydration
- Electrolyte abnormalities
- Malabsorption: weight loss, vitamin deficiencies

PROGNOSIS

- Cause is identifiable and treatable in almost all patients

WHEN TO ADMIT

- Secretory diarrhea with dehydration

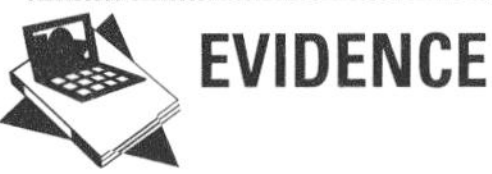

EVIDENCE

PRACTICE GUIDELINES

- Thomas PD et al: Guidelines for the investigation of chronic diarrhoea, 2nd ed. Gut 2003;52(Suppl 5):v1. [PMID:12801941]

INFORMATION FOR PATIENTS

- Cleveland Clinic—Diarrhea
  - http://www.clevelandclinic.org/health/health-info/docs/0100/0100.asp?index=4108
- Mayo Clinic
  - http://www.mayoclinic.com/invoke.cfm?id=DS00292
- JAMA patient page: Preventing dehydration from diarrhea. JAMA 2001;285:362

REFERENCES

- Camilleri M: Chronic diarrhea; a review on pathophysiology and management for the clinical gastroenterologist. Clin Gastorenterol Hepatol 2004;2:198. [PMID: 15017602]
- Schiller L: Chronic diarrhea. Gastroenterology 2004;127:287. [PMID: 15236193]

Author(s)

Kenneth R. McQuaid, MD

Diarrhea, Traveler's

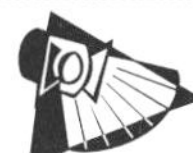

KEY FEATURES

ESSENTIALS OF DIAGNOSIS

- Usually a benign, self-limited disease occurring about a week into travel
- Prophylaxis not recommended unless there is a comorbid disease (inflammatory bowel syndrome, HIV, immunosuppressive medication)
- Single-dose therapy of a fluoroquinolone usually effective if symptoms develop

GENERAL CONSIDERATIONS

- Whenever a person travels from one country to another—particularly if the change involves a marked difference in climate, social conditions, or sanitation standards and facilities—diarrhea is likely to develop within 2–10 days
- Bacteria cause 80% of cases, with enterotoxigenic *Escherichia coli*, *Shigella* species, and *Campylobacter jejuni* being the most common pathogens
- Less common pathogens are *Aeromonas*, *Salmonella*, noncholera vibrios, *Entamoeba histolytica*, and *Giardia lamblia*
- Chronic watery diarrhea may be due to amebiasis or giardiasis or, rarely, tropical sprue
- Contributory causes include unusual food and drink, change in living habits, occasional viral infections (adenoviruses or rotaviruses), and change in bowel flora

Etiology

- Most common: enterotoxigenic *E coli*, *Shigella*, *Campylobacter*
- Less common: *Aeromonas*, *Salmonella*, noncholera vibrios, *E histolytica*, *G lamblia*, adenoviruses, rotavirus
- Chronic watery diarrhea: *E histolytica*, *G lamblia*, tropical sprue (rare)
- Associated with unprotected anal intercourse: *Neisseria gonorrhoeae*, syphilis, lymphogranuloma venereum, herpes simplex

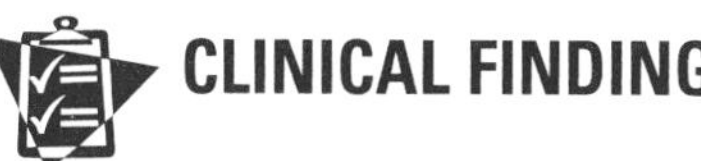

CLINICAL FINDINGS

SYMPTOMS AND SIGNS

- There may be up to 10 or even more loose stools per day, usually without mucus or blood
- Abdominal cramps, nausea, occasionally vomiting
- Fever is rare
- Aside from weakness and dehydration there are no systemic manifestations of infection
- The illness usually subsides spontaneously within 1–5 days, although 10% remain symptomatic for a week or longer, and in 2% symptoms persist for longer than a month

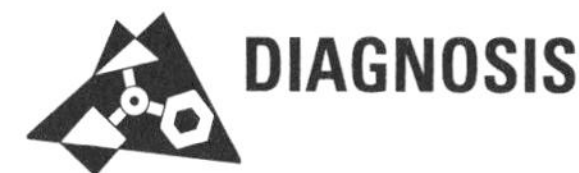

DIAGNOSIS

LABORATORY TESTS

- In patients with fever and bloody diarrhea, stool culture may be indicated, but in most cases cultures are reserved for those who do not respond to antibiotics

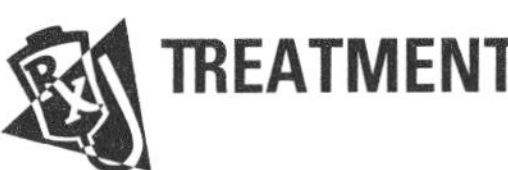

TREATMENT

MEDICATIONS

- For most patients, symptomatic therapy with opioids or loperamide is all that is required provided there is no systemic illness (fever ≥ 39°C) or dysentery (bloody stools), in which case antimotility agents should be avoided
- Packages of oral rehydration salts to treat dehydration are available over the counter in the United States (Infalyte, Pedialyte, others) and in many foreign countries
- Loperamide (4 mg loading dose, then 2 mg after each loose stool to a maximum of 16 mg/day) with a single dose of ciprofloxacin (750 mg), levofloxacin (500 mg), or ofloxacin (300 mg) cures most cases
- If diarrhea is severe, associated with fever or bloody stools, or persists despite single-dose ciprofloxacin treatment, then 3–5 days of ciprofloxacin, 500 mg twice daily, levofloxacin, 500 mg once daily, norfloxacin, 400 mg twice daily, or ofloxacin, 300 mg twice daily, can be given
- Trimethoprim-sulfamethoxazole, 160/800 mg twice daily, can be used as an alternative, but resistance is common in many areas
- Rifaximin, a nonabsorbable rifampin-like drug, is effective at 200 mg three times a day or 400 mg twice a day for 3 days. Because the drug is not systemically absorbed, it should not be used in situations where there is a high likelihood of invasive disease (eg, fever, systemic toxicity, bloody stools)

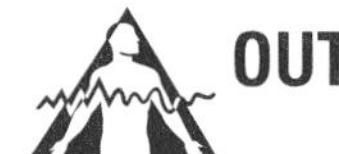

OUTCOME

PROGNOSIS

- Most illnesses are short-lived and resolve without specific therapy

WHEN TO REFER

- Persistent diarrhea despite therapy

WHEN TO ADMIT

- Dehydration
- Systemic toxicity

PREVENTION

- Recommend avoidance of fresh foods and water sources in developing countries, where infectious diarrheal illnesses are endemic
- Prophylaxis is recommended for:
  - Patients with significant underlying disease (inflammatory bowel disease, AIDS, diabetes, heart disease in the elderly, conditions requiring immunosuppressive medications)
  - Patients whose full activity status during the trip is so essential that even short periods of diarrhea would be unacceptable
- Prophylaxis is started upon entry into the destination country and is continued for 1 or 2 days after leaving
- For stays of more than 3 weeks, prophylaxis is not recommended because of the cost and increased toxicity
- Numerous antimicrobial regimens for once-daily prophylaxis are effective, such as norfloxacin, 400 mg; ciprofloxacin, 500 mg; ofloxacin, 300 mg; or trimethoprim-sulfamethoxazole, 160/800 mg
- Bismuth subsalicylate is effective but turns the tongue and the stools black and can interfere with doxycycline absorption, which may be needed for malaria prophylaxis; it is rarely used
- Because not all travelers will have diarrhea and because most episodes are brief and self-limited, an alternative approach currently recommended is to provide the traveler with a supply of antimicrobials to be taken if significant diarrhea occurs during the trip

EVIDENCE

PRACTICE GUIDELINES

- National Guideline Clearinghouse: Infectious Diarrhea. Infectious Diseases Society of America, 2001.
  - http://www.guideline.gov/summary/summary.aspx?doc_id=2791

INFORMATION FOR PATIENTS

- American Academy of Family Physicians
  - http://familydoctor.org/182.xml
- Centers for Disease Control and Prevention
  - http://www.cdc.gov/ncidod/dbmd/diseaseinfo/travelersdiarrhea_g.htm
- Centers for Disease Control and Prevention—National Center for Infectious Disease—Travelers' Health
  - http://www.cdc.gov/travel/diarrhea.htm
- National Digestive Diseases Information Clearinghouse
  - http://digestive.niddk.nih.gov/ddiseases/pubs/diarrhea/index.htm

REFERENCES

- Guerrant RL et al: Practice guidelines for the management of infectious diarrhea. Clin Infect Dis 2001;32:331. [PMID: 11170940]
- Ramzan N: Traveler's diarrhea. Gastroenterol Clin North Am 2001;30:665. [PMID: 11586551]
- Rendi-Wagner P et al: Drug prophylaxis for travelers' diarrhea. Clin Infect Dis 2002;34:628. [PMID: 11803509]
- Thielman NM et al: Clinical practice. Acute infectious diarrhea. N Engl J Med 2004;350:38. [PMID: 14702426]

Author(s)

Richard A. Jacobs, MD, PhD

Digitalis Toxicity

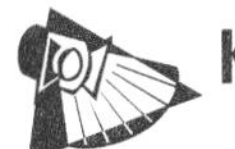

KEY FEATURES

ESSENTIALS OF DIAGNOSIS

- Intoxication may result from acute single exposure or chronic accumulation from accidental overmedication or renal insufficiency
- Hyperkalemia common after acute overdose
- Many different arrhythmias can occur

GENERAL CONSIDERATIONS

- Cardiac glycosides paralyze the Na^+-K^+-ATPase pump and have potent vagotonic effects
- Intracellular effects include enhancement of calcium-dependent contractility and shortening of the action potential duration
- Digoxin and ouabain are highly tissue bound, but digitoxin has a volume of distribution of just 0.6 L/kg, making it the only cardiac glycoside accessible to enhanced removal procedures such as hemoperfusion or repeated doses of activated charcoal

DEMOGRAPHICS

- Older age and renal impairment are associated with greater risk of chronic digoxin toxicity

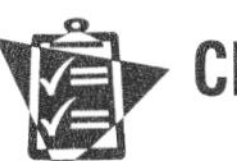

CLINICAL FINDINGS

SYMPTOMS AND SIGNS

Acute overdose

- Nausea and vomiting
- Bradycardia, atrioventricular (AV) block; junctional rhythm common in patients with underlying atrial fibrillation
- Hyperkalemia

Chronic overingestion

- Hypokalemia and hypomagnesia are more likely owing to concurrent diuretic treatment
- Ventricular arrhythmias (eg, ectopy, bidirectional ventricular tachycardia, or ventricular fibrillation)

DIFFERENTIAL DIAGNOSIS

- β-Blocker overdose
- Calcium channel blocker overdose
- Cardiotoxic plant or animal ingestion: oleander, foxglove, lily of the valley, rhododendron, toad venom

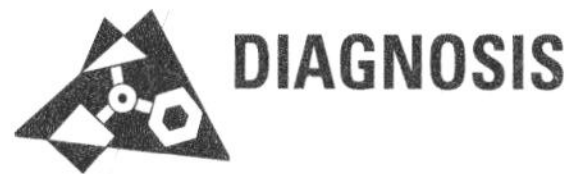

DIAGNOSIS

LABORATORY TESTS

- Serum digoxin level (**note:** levels drawn within 6 h of ingestion may be falsely elevated before complete tissue distribution)
- Serum potassium (frequent measures useful because they correlate with tissue effects)

IMAGING STUDIES

- Continuous ECG monitoring

DIAGNOSTIC PROCEDURES

- Pacemaker may be needed

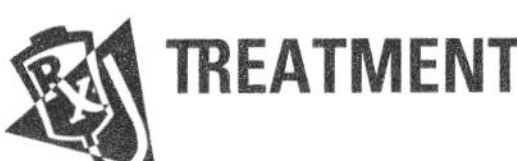

TREATMENT

MEDICATIONS

Emergency measures

- Ventricular arrhythmias: initially lidocaine, 2–3 mg/kg IV, or phenytoin, 10–15 mg/kg IV slowly over 30 min
- Bradycardia: initially atropine, 0.5–2 mg IV, or transcutaneous external cardiac pacemaker

Gut decontamination

- After acute overdose, administer activated charcoal, 60–100 g PO or via gastric tube, mixed in aqueous slurry
- Emesis not recommended because it may enhance vagotonic effects (eg, bradycardia, AV block)

Repeat-dose charcoal

- Repeated doses of activated charcoal, 20–30 g Q3–4 h, may speed elimination of digitoxin (but not digoxin) by adsorbing drug excreted into gut lumen (gut dialysis)
- Sorbitol or other cathartics should *not* be used with each dose; resulting large stool volumes may lead to dehydration or hypernatremia

Specific treatment

- Severe intoxication: administer digoxin-specific antibodies [digoxin immune Fab (ovine); Digibind]
- Digibind dose is estimated based on body burden of digoxin calculated from ingested dose or steady-state serum digoxin concentration
  - Ingested dose
    - Number of vials = ~1.5 × ingested dose (mg)
  - Serum concentration
    - Number of vials = serum digoxin (ng/mL) × body weight (kg) × 10^{-2}
    - **Note:** This is based on equilibrium digoxin level; after acute overdose, serum levels are falsely high before tissue distribution is complete, and overestimation of Digibind dose is likely
- Empirical dosing of Digibind may be used if patient's condition is relatively stable and an underlying condition (eg, atrial fibrillation) suggests residual level of digitalis activity
- Start with one or two vials and reassess clinical condition after 20–30 min
- **Note:** After administration of Digibind, serum digoxin levels may be falsely elevated depending on assay technique

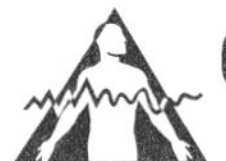

OUTCOME

FOLLOW-UP

- Monitor potassium levels and cardiac rhythm closely

COMPLICATIONS

- Cardiac arrest

WHEN TO ADMIT

- Symptomatic patients
- Asymptomatic patients after acute overdose, for monitoring at least several hours

PREVENTION

- Monitor renal function in elderly patients and obtain serum digoxin levels if symptoms of digoxin toxicity

EVIDENCE

WEB SITE

- eMedicine: Toxicology Articles
  - http://www.emedicine.com/emerg/toxicology.htm

INFORMATION FOR PATIENTS

- National Institutes of Health: Digitalis Toxicity
  - http://www.nlm.nih.gov/medlineplus/ency/article/000165.htm
- MedlinePlus: Digitalis Medicines (Systemic)
  - http://www.nlm.nih.gov/medlineplus/druginfo/uspdi/202194.html

REFERENCES

- Barrueto F Jr et al: Cardioactive steroid poisoning from an herbal cleansing preparation. Ann Emerg Med 2003;41:396. [PMID: 12605208]
- Husby P et al: Immediate control of life-threatening digoxin intoxication in a child by use of digoxin-specific antibody fragments (Fab). Paediatr Anaesth 2003;13:541. [PMID: 12846714]
- Van Deusen SK et al: Treatment of hyperkalemia in a patient with unrecognized digitalis toxicity. J Toxicol Clin Toxicol 2003;41:373. [PMID: 12870880]

Author(s)

Kent R. Olson, MD

Diphtheria

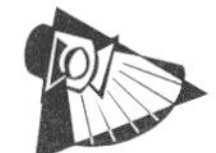

KEY FEATURES

ESSENTIALS OF DIAGNOSIS

- Tenacious gray membrane at portal of entry in pharynx
- Sore throat, nasal discharge, hoarseness, malaise, fever
- Myocarditis, neuropathy
- Culture confirms the diagnosis

GENERAL CONSIDERATIONS

- An acute infection with a toxin-producing strain of *Corynebacterium diphtheriae*
- Usually attacks the respiratory tract but may involve any mucous membrane or skin wound
- The organism is spread primarily by respiratory secretions
- Exotoxin produced by the organism is responsible for myocarditis and neuropathy. This exotoxin inhibits elongation factor, which is required for protein synthesis

DEMOGRAPHICS

- Rare in the United States and Western Europe, more likely to be encountered in persons from developing countries and those from the former Soviet Union, where vaccine programs are lacking or inadequate

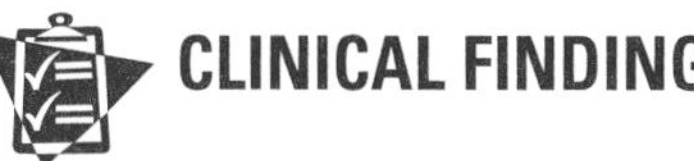

CLINICAL FINDINGS

SYMPTOMS AND SIGNS

- Nasal, laryngeal, pharyngeal, and cutaneous forms of diphtheria occur
- Nasal infection produces few symptoms other than a nasal discharge
- Laryngeal infection may lead to upper airway and bronchial obstruction
- In pharyngeal diphtheria, the most common form, a tenacious gray membrane covers the tonsils and pharynx
- Mild sore throat, fever, and malaise are followed by toxemia and prostration

DIFFERENTIAL DIAGNOSIS

- Streptococcal pharyngitis
- Oral candidiasis
- Infectious mononucleosis
- Viral pharyngitis, eg, adenovirus, herpes simplex virus
- Necrotizing gingivostomatitis (Vincent's angina, trench mouth)
- *Arcanobacterium haemolyticum* pharyngitis
- Other causes of cranial nerve or motor neuropathy, eg, myasthenia gravis, botulism, Guillain-Barré syndrome
- Myocarditis due to other causes

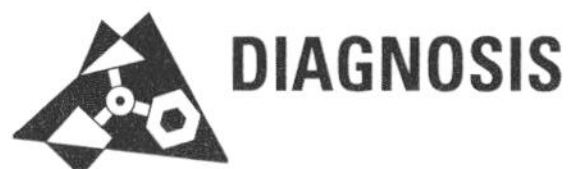

DIAGNOSIS

LABORATORY TESTS

- The diagnosis is made clinically but can be confirmed by culture of the organism

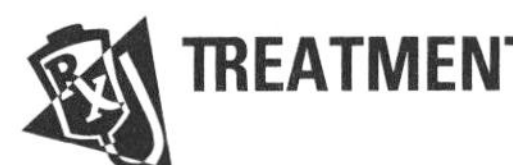

TREATMENT

MEDICATIONS

- Susceptible persons exposed to diphtheria should receive a booster dose of diphtheria toxoid plus active immunization if not previously immunized, as well as a course of penicillin or erythromycin

Antitoxin

- Prepared from horse serum
- Must be given in all cases when diphtheria is suspected
- For mild early pharyngeal or laryngeal disease, the dose is 20,000–40,000 units; for moderate nasopharyngeal disease, 40,000–60,000 units; for severe, extensive, or late (3 days or more) disease, 80,000–100,000 units

Antibiotics

- Either penicillin, 250 mg PO QID, or erythromycin, 500 mg PO QID, for 14 days is effective, though erythromycin is slightly more effective in eliminating the carrier state
- Azithromycin or clarithromycin may be as effective as erythromycin

THERAPEUTIC PROCEDURES

- Removal of membrane by direct laryngoscopy or bronchoscopy may be necessary to prevent or alleviate airway obstruction

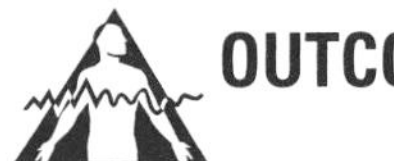

OUTCOME

FOLLOW-UP

- The patient should be isolated until three consecutive cultures at the completion of therapy have documented elimination of the organism from the oropharynx

COMPLICATIONS

- Myocarditis and neuropathy are the most common and most serious complications
- Myocarditis causes cardiac arrhythmias, heart block, and heart failure
- The neuropathy usually involves the cranial nerves first, producing diplopia, slurred speech, and difficulty in swallowing

PROGNOSIS

- Death occurs in 5–10% of respiratory cases
- Complications and deaths are much less frequent in cutaneous diphtheria

WHEN TO REFER

- This disease must be reported to the public health authorities
- Diphtheria equine antitoxin can be obtained from the Centers for Disease Control and Prevention

WHEN TO ADMIT

- All suspected or proven cases

PREVENTION

- See Table 132
- Active immunization with diphtheria toxoid is part of routine childhood immunization (usually as diphtheria-tetanus-pertussis) with appropriate booster injections
- The immunization schedule for adults is the same as for tetanus. To avoid major allergic reactions, only the "adult type" toxoid (Td) should be used
- Contacts to a case should receive erythromycin, 500 mg four times daily for 7 days, to eradicate carriage

EVIDENCE

WEB SITES

- CDC—Division of Bacterial and Mycotic Diseases
  - http://www.cdc.gov/ncidod/dbmd/diseaseinfo/diptheria_t.htm
- Karolinska Institute—Directory of Bacterial Infections and Mycoses
  - http://www.mic.ki.se/Diseases/C01.html

INFORMATION FOR PATIENTS

- JAMA patient page: Immunizations. JAMA 1999;282:102. [PMID: 10404918]
- Mayo Clinic
  - http://www.mayoclinic.com/invoke.cfm?id=DS00495
- National Coalition for Adult Immunization
  - http://www.nfid.org/factsheets/diphtadult.html
- National Institutes of Health
  - http://www.nlm.nih.gov/medlineplus/ency/article/001608.htm

REFERENCE

- Centers for Disease Control and Prevention (CDC): Fatal respiratory diphtheria in a U.S. traveler to Haiti—Pennsylvania, 2003. MMWR Morb Mortal Wkly Rep 2004;52:1285. [PMID: 14712177]

Author(s)

Henry F. Chambers, MD

Discoid Lupus Erythematosus

KEY FEATURES

ESSENTIALS OF DIAGNOSIS

- Localized red plaques, usually on the face
- Scaling, follicular plugging, atrophy, dyspigmentation, and telangiectasia of involved areas
- Histology distinctive
- Photosensitive

GENERAL CONSIDERATIONS

- Ten percent of patients with systemic lupus erythematosus (SLE) have discoid skin lesions, and 5% of patients with discoid lesions have SLE
- The disease is persistent but not life endangering unless systemic lupus intervenes, which is uncommon
- Treatment with antimalarials is effective in perhaps 60% of cases

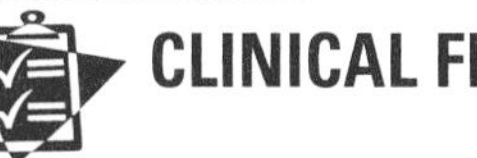

CLINICAL FINDINGS

SYMPTOMS AND SIGNS

- See Table 7
- The lesions consist of dusky red, well-localized, single or multiple plaques, 5–20 mm in diameter, usually on the face; the scalp, external ears, and oral mucous membranes may be involved
- There is atrophy, telangiectasia, depigmentation, and follicular plugging
- The lesion may be covered by dry, horny, adherent scales
- On the scalp, permanent hair loss may occur

DIFFERENTIAL DIAGNOSIS

- Psoriasis
- Seborrheic dermatitis
- Acne rosacea
- Lupus vulgaris (cutaneous tuberculosis)
- Sarcoidosis
- Bowen's disease (squamous cell carcinoma in situ)
- Polymorphous light eruption
- Lichen planopilaris

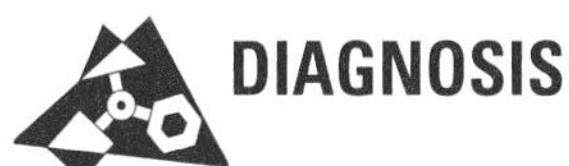

DIAGNOSIS

LABORATORY TESTS

- Diagnosis is based on the clinical appearance confirmed by skin biopsy in all cases

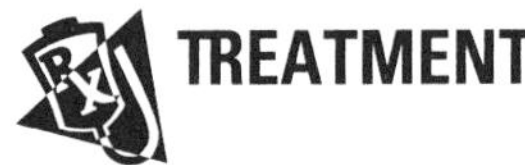

TREATMENT

MEDICATIONS

- See Table 6

General measures

- Protect from sunlight; use high-SPF (> 30) sunblock with UVB and UVA coverage daily
- **Caution:** Do not use any form of radiation therapy
- Avoid using drugs that are potentially photosensitizing (eg, thiazides, piroxicam) when possible

Local treatment

- High-potency corticosteroid creams applied each night and covered with airtight plastic film (eg, Saran Wrap); or Cordran tape; or ultra-high-potency corticosteroid cream or ointment applied twice daily without occlusion
- Local infiltration: triamcinolone acetonide suspension, 2.5–10 mg/mL, may be injected into the lesions once a month; this should be tried before systemic therapy

Systemic treatment

- Antimalarials—**Caution:** these drugs should be used only when the diagnosis is secure, because they have been associated with flares of psoriasis, which may be in the differential diagnosis; they may also cause ocular changes, and ophthalmologic evaluation is required every 6 months
- Hydroxychloroquine sulfate, 0.2–0.4 g PO daily for several months, may be effective and is often used prior to chloroquine; a 3-month trial is recommended
- Chloroquine sulfate, 250 mg daily, may be effective in some cases where hydroxychloroquine is not
- Quinacrine (Atabrine), 100 mg daily, may be the safest of the antimalarials, since eye damage has not been reported; it colors the skin yellow and is therefore not acceptable to some patients; it may be added to the above antimalarials for incomplete responses
- Isotretinoin, 1 mg/kg/day, is effective in chronic or subacute cutaneous lupus erythematosus; recurrences are prompt and predictable on discontinuation of therapy
- Thalidomide is a potent teratogen but very effective in refractory cases in doses of 50–100 mg daily

THERAPEUTIC PROCEDURES

- Monitor for neuropathy if using thalidomide
- Because of the teratogenicity of isotretinoin and thalidomide, the drugs are used with caution in women of childbearing age using effective contraception with negative pregnancy tests before and during therapy

OUTCOME

COMPLICATIONS

- Although the only morbidity may be cosmetic, this can be of overwhelming significance in more darkly pigmented patients with widespread disease
- Scarring alopecia can be prevented or lessened with close attention and aggressive therapy

PROGNOSIS

- The disease is persistent but not life endangering unless systemic lupus intervenes, which is uncommon
- Treatment with antimalarials is effective in perhaps 60% of cases

WHEN TO REFER

- If there is a question about the diagnosis, if recommended therapy is ineffective, or specialized treatment is necessary

EVIDENCE

WEB SITES

- University of Pennsylvania Dermatology Online Journal: Current Treatment of Cutaneous Lupus Erythematosus
  - http://dermatology.cdlib.org/DOJvol7num1/transactions/lupus/werth.html
- American Academy of Dermatology
  - http://www.aad.org
- National Institute of Arthritis and Musculoskeletal and Skin Diseases
  - http://www.niams.nih.gov

INFORMATION FOR PATIENTS

- Lupus Foundation of America: Skin Disease In Lupus
  - http://www.lupus.org/education/brochures/skindisease.html
- MedlinePlus: Lupus Interactive Tutorial
  - http://www.nlm.nih.gov/medlineplus/tutorials/lupus.html
- National Institute of Arthritis and Musculoskeletal and Skin Diseases: Skin Care and Lupus
  - http://www.niams.nih.gov/hi/topics/lupus/lupusguide/luppdf/skincare.pdf

REFERENCE

- Patel P et al: Cutaneous lupus erythematosus: a review. Dermatol Clin 2002;20:373. [PMID: 12170873]

Author(s)

Timothy G. Berger, MD

Disseminated Intravascular Coagulation (DIC)

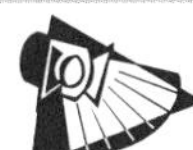

KEY FEATURES

ESSENTIALS OF DIAGNOSIS

- Underlying serious illness
- Microangiopathic hemolytic anemia may be present
- Low fibrinogen, thrombocytopenia, fibrin degradation products, and prolonged prothrombin time (PT)

GENERAL CONSIDERATIONS

- If stimulus to coagulation is too great, control mechanisms are overwhelmed, leading to DIC
- Can be thought of as a consequence of circulating thrombin (normally confined to localized area)
  - Thrombin cleaves fibrinogen to fibrin, stimulates platelet aggregation, activates factors V and VIII, and releases plasminogen activator, which generates plasmin
  - Plasmin cleaves fibrin, generating fibrin degradation products, and further inactivates factors V and VIII
- Thus, excess thrombin activity produces hypofibrinogenemia, thrombocytopenia, depletion of coagulation factors, and fibrinolysis
- Caused by a number of serious illnesses: sepsis (especially with gram-negative bacteria), severe tissue injury (especially burns and head injury), obstetric complications (amniotic fluid embolus, septic abortion, retained fetus), cancer (acute promyelocytic leukemia, mucinous adenocarcinomas), and major hemolytic transfusion reactions

CLINICAL FINDINGS

SYMPTOMS AND SIGNS

- DIC leads to both bleeding and thrombosis; bleeding is far more common, but thrombosis may dominate
- Bleeding may occur at any site; spontaneous bleeding and oozing at venipuncture sites or wounds are important clues to diagnosis
- Thrombosis most commonly manifested by digital ischemia and gangrene, but catastrophic events such as renal cortical necrosis and hemorrhagic adrenal infarction may occur
- DIC may secondarily produce microangiopathic hemolytic anemia
- Subacute DIC occurs primarily in cancer; manifested primarily as recurrent superficial and deep venous thromboses (Trousseau's syndrome)

DIFFERENTIAL DIAGNOSIS

- Severe liver disease
- Thrombotic thrombocytopenic purpura
- Sepsis-induced thrombocytopenia or anemia
- Heparin-induced thrombocytopenia
- Other microangiopathic hemolytic anemia (eg, prosthetic valve hemolysis)

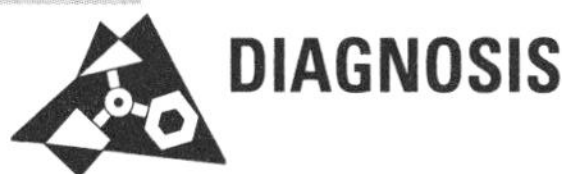

DIAGNOSIS

LABORATORY TESTS

- Serum fibrinogen low (may also occur in congenital hypofibrinogenemia, severe liver disease)
- Fibrin degradation products (eg, D-dimers) elevated (may also occur in hepatic dysfunction)
- Thrombocytopenia
- PT prolonged
- When baseline fibrinogen level is markedly elevated, initial level may be normal; because half-life is ~4 days, declining fibrinogen level confirms DIC
- Partial thromboplastin time (PTT) may or may not be prolonged
- Microangiopathic hemolytic anemia present in ~25% of cases, and peripheral blood smear shows fragmented red blood cells
- Antithrombin III levels may be markedly depleted
- When fibrinolysis is activated, levels of plasminogen and α_2-antiplasmin may be low
- Thrombocytopenia and D-dimer elevation are usually the only abnormalities in subacute DIC
- Fibrinogen level is normal, and PTT may be normal

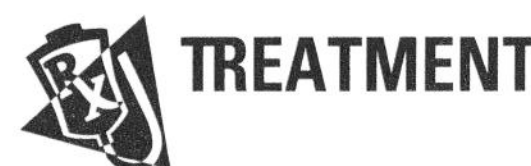

TREATMENT

MEDICATIONS

- Replacement therapy alone if underlying cause is rapidly reversible
- Platelet transfusion to maintain platelet count > 30,000/μL
- Cryoprecipitate to replace fibrinogen, aiming for plasma fibrinogen level of 150 mg/dL
- Fresh-frozen plasma may be required for coagulation factor deficiency
- Heparin is contraindicated when any increase in bleeding is unacceptable (neurosurgical procedures)
- When DIC is producing serious clinical consequences and underlying cause not rapidly reversible, heparin may be necessary
- Heparin must be used in combination with replacement therapy to prevent an unacceptable increase in bleeding
- Heparin dose is 500–750 U/h
- Heparin cannot be effective if antithrombin III is markedly depleted; measure antithrombin III level and if low, give fresh-frozen plasma to raise levels to > 50%
- Successful heparin therapy is indicated by rising fibrinogen level; it is not necessary to prolong PTT
- Fibrin degradation products decline over 1–2 days
- Improvement in platelet count may lag by 1 week behind control of coagulopathy
- If heparin and replacement therapy does not control bleeding, ε-aminocaproic acid, 1 g IV every hour, is added to decrease rate of fibrinolysis, raise fibrinogen level, and control bleeding
- Aminocaproic acid can *never* be used without heparin in DIC because of risk of thrombosis

THERAPEUTIC PROCEDURES

- Treatment of underlying disorder
- Mild DIC requires no specific therapy

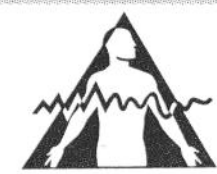

OUTCOME

PROGNOSIS

- Prognosis is that of the underlying disease

EVIDENCE

PRACTICE GUIDELINES

- Taylor FB et al: Towards definition, clinical and laboratory criteria, and a scoring system for disseminated intravascular coagulation. Thromb Haemost 2001;86:1327. [PMID: 11816725]

WEB SITE

- Postgraduate Medicine Online: Disseminated Intravascular Coagulation
  - http://www.postgradmed.com/issues/2002/03_02/messmore.htm

INFORMATION FOR PATIENTS

- MedlinePlus: Disseminated Intravascular Coagulation
  - http://www.nlm.nih.gov/medlineplus/ency/article/000573.htm

REFERENCES

- Franchini M et al: Update on the treatment of disseminated intravascular coagulation. Hematology 2004;9:81. [PMID: 15203862]
- Hoffman JN et al: Effect of long-term and high-dose antithrombin supplementation on coagulation and fibrinolysis in patients with severe sepsis. Crit Care Med 2004;32:1851. [PMID: 15343012]

Author(s)

Charles A. Linker, MD

Diverticulitis

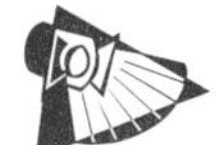

KEY FEATURES

ESSENTIALS OF DIAGNOSIS

- Intra-abdominal infection varies from microperforation (most common) with localized paracolic inflammation to macroperforation with either abscess or generalized peritonitis
- Acute abdominal pain and fever
- Left lower abdominal tenderness and mass
- Leukocytosis

GENERAL CONSIDERATIONS

- Diverticulosis is present in 25% of adults over age 40; increases with age; most asymptomatic
- Diverticulitis occurs in 10–20% of patients with diverticulosis

DEMOGRAPHICS

- Higher prevalence in societies with low fiber intake

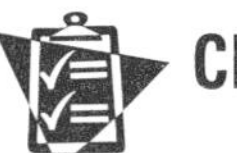

CLINICAL FINDINGS

SYMPTOMS AND SIGNS

- Abdominal pain, mild to moderate, aching, usually in the left lower quadrant
- Constipation or loose stools
- Nausea and vomiting
- Low-grade fever
- Left lower quadrant tenderness
- Palpable left lower quadrant mass
- Generalized abdominal pain and peritoneal signs in patients with free perforation

DIFFERENTIAL DIAGNOSIS

- Perforated colorectal cancer
- Infectious colitis, eg, *Campylobacter, Clostridium difficile*
- Inflammatory bowel disease
- Ischemic colitis
- Appendicitis
- Gynecologic: pelvic inflammatory disease, tuboovarian abscess, ovarian torsion, ruptured ectopic pregnancy or ovarian cyst, mittelschmerz, endometriosis
- Urinary calculus
- Ascariasis
- Gastroenteritis

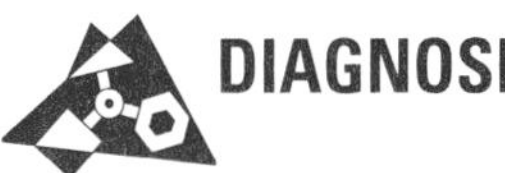

DIAGNOSIS

LABORATORY TESTS

- Leukocytosis, mild to moderate
- Stool occult blood test positive

IMAGING STUDIES

- Plain abdominal films
- Barium enema, contraindicated during acute attack; perform only after resolution of clinical symptoms to document extent of diverticulosis or presence of fistula
- CT scan
  - Scan of the abdomen in patients who do not improve rapidly after 2–4 days of empirical therapy and to confirm diagnosis
  - CT indicated in severe disease to diagnose abscess

DIAGNOSTIC PROCEDURES

- Colonoscopy
  - Contraindicated during acute attack
  - Perform only after resolution of clinical symptoms to document extent of diverticulitis and to exclude other clinical disorders
- Sigmoidoscopy with minimal air insufflation is sometimes required in acute disease to exclude other diagnoses

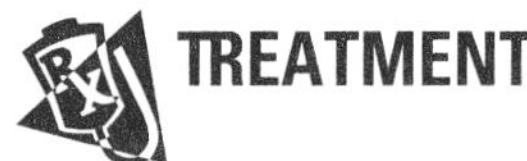

TREATMENT

MEDICATIONS

- Most patients can be managed with conservative measures
- Mild diverticulitis (mild symptoms and no peritoneal signs)
  - Clear liquid diet
  - Oral antibiotics targeting both anaerobic and gram-negative bacteria, such as amoxicillin and clavulanate potassium, 875 mg/125 mg PO BID; or metronidazole, 500 mg PO TID; plus either ciprofloxacin, 500 mg PO BID, or trimethoprim-sulfamethoxazole, 160/800 mg PO BID, for 7–10 days
- Severe diverticulitis (high fevers, leukocytosis, or peritoneal signs)
  - Nothing by mouth
  - Intravenous fluids
  - Nasogastric tube suction if ileus is present
  - Intravenous antibiotics targeting both anaerobic and gram-negative bacteria, such as either single-agent therapy with a second-generation cephalosporin (eg, cefoxitin), or piperacillin-tazobactam, or ticarcillin clavulanate; or combination therapy (eg, metronidazole or clindamycin plus an aminoglycoside) or third-generation cephalosporin (eg, ceftazidime, cefotaxime) for 7–10 days

SURGERY

- Surgical management is required in ~20–30% of cases
- Indications for surgery include
  - Free peritonitis and large abscesses
  - Fistulas
  - Colonic obstruction
- Surgery in two stages for abscesses for which catheter drainage is not possible or helpful
  - Diseased colon is resected, temporary colostomy of proximal colon is created, and distal colonic stump is either closed (forming a Hartmann pouch) or exteriorized as a mucous fistula
  - Weeks later, colon is reconnected electively

THERAPEUTIC PROCEDURES

- Percutaneous catheter drainage of localized abdominal abscess, with subsequent single-stage elective surgical resection of diseased segment of colon

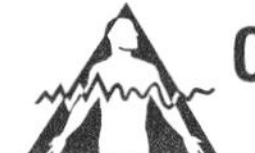

OUTCOME

FOLLOW-UP

- Colonoscopy or barium enema 4–6 weeks after recovery from diverticulitis to diagnose extent of diverticulosis and to exclude colonic malignancy

COMPLICATIONS

- Fistula formation may involve the bladder, ureter, vagina, uterus, bowel, and abdominal wall
- Stricturing of the colon with partial or complete obstruction

PROGNOSIS

- Diverticulitis recurs in one-third
- Recurrent attacks warrant elective surgical resection

WHEN TO ADMIT

- Increasing pain, fever, or inability to tolerate oral fluids
- Severe diverticulitis and patients who are elderly or immunosuppressed or who have serious comorbid disease

PREVENTION

- High-fiber diet

EVIDENCE

PRACTICE GUIDELINES

- National Guideline Clearinghouse
  - http://www.guideline.gov/summary/summary.aspx?doc_id=3258&nbr=2484&string=diverticulitis

WEB SITES

- WebPath GI Pathology Index
  - http://medstat.med.utah.edu/WebPath/GIHTML/GIIDX.html

INFORMATION FOR PATIENTS

- Cleveland Clinic—Diverticular disease
  - http://www.clevelandclinic.org/health/health-info/docs/2800/2824.asp?index=10352
- Mayo Clinic—Diverticulitis
  - http://www.mayoclinic.com/invoke.cfm?id=DS00070
- National Digestive Diseases Information Clearinghouse—Colonoscopy
  - http://digestive.niddk.nih.gov/ddiseases/pubs/colonoscopy/index.htm

REFERENCE

- Biondo S et al: Acute colonic diverticulitis in patients under 50 years of age. Br J Surg 2002;89:1137. [PMID: 12190679]
- Buckley O et al: Computed tomography in the imaging of diverticulitis. Clin Radiol 2004;59:977. [PMID:15488845]
- Whetsome D et al: Current management of diverticulitis. Curr Surg 2004;61:361. [PMID:15276340]

Author(s)

Kenneth R. McQuaid, MD

Dracunculiasis

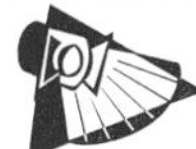

KEY FEATURES

ESSENTIALS OF DIAGNOSIS

- Worm can reach the skin and a blister develops, which can then ulcerate
- Most lesions are on the leg or foot
- Can be accompanied by a systemic allergic reaction

GENERAL CONSIDERATIONS

- This is an infection of connective and subcutaneous tissues by the nematode *Dracunculus medinensis*
- It occurs only in humans and is a major cause of disability
- Infection occurs by swallowing water containing the infected intermediate host, the crustacean cyclops (copepods, water fleas)
- In the human stomach, larvae escape from the crustacean and mature in subcutaneous connective tissue
  - After mating, the male worm dies and the gravid female (60–80 cm × 1.7–2.0 mm) moves to the surface of the body, where its head reaches the dermis and provokes a blister that ruptures on contact with water
  - Intermittently over 2–3 weeks, whenever the ulcer comes in contact with water, the uterus discharges great numbers of larvae, which are ingested by copepods
  - Most adult worms are gradually extruded; some worms retract and reemerge; and others die in the tissues, disintegrate, and may provoke a severe inflammatory reaction
- Infection does not induce protective immunity

DEMOGRAPHICS

- Since the start of the WHO eradication program, the number of infected persons has declined about 99% from over 3 million to 30,000. Endemic areas have been the Indian subcontinent; West and Central Africa north of the equator; and Saudi Arabia, Iran, and Yemen. Almost all remaining cases are reported from Sudan
- Disease occurs almost exclusively in isolated rural areas
- All ages are affected, and prevalence may reach 60%

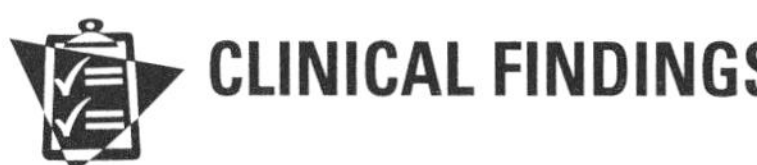

CLINICAL FINDINGS

SYMPTOMS AND SIGNS

- Infection may be at several sites
- Patients are asymptomatic during the 9- to 14-month incubation period except in the last 1–2 weeks, when the worm reaches and becomes palpable in the skin and a blister develops around its anterior end. Several hours before the head appears at the skin surface, local erythema, burning, pruritus, and tenderness often develop at the site of emergence
- There may also be a 24-h systemic allergic reaction (pruritus, fever, nausea and vomiting, dyspnea, periorbital edema, and urticaria)
- After rupture, the tissues surrounding the ulceration frequently become indurated, reddened, and tender
- Because most lesions appear on the leg or foot, patients often must give up walking and working for days to several months
- Uninfected ulcers heal in 4–6 weeks
- The worm rarely reaches ectopic sites
- Secondary infections, including tetanus, are common. Deep "cold" abscesses may result at the sites of dying, nonemergent worms

DIFFERENTIAL DIAGNOSIS

- Cutaneous larva migrans
- Loiasis (*Loa loa* infection)
- Rat bite fever
- Gnathostomiasis
- Myiasis
- Other causes of leg ulcer, eg, venous or arterial insufficiency, bacterial pyoderma, vasculitis, pyoderma gangrenosum

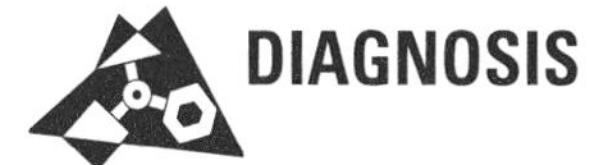

DIAGNOSIS

LABORATORY TESTS

- When an emerging adult worm is not visible in the ulcer or under the skin, the diagnosis may be made by detection of larvae in smears from discharging sinuses. Immersion of an ulcer in cold water stimulates larval expulsion
- Eosinophilia is usually present
- Skin and serological tests are not useful

IMAGING STUDIES

- Calcified worms can be recognized on radiographs

Diverticulosis p. 1065. Down Syndrome p. 1065.

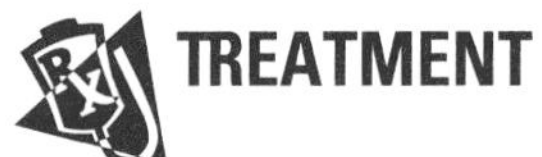

TREATMENT

MEDICATIONS

- The following drugs have an antiinflammatory effect but do not kill the adults or the larvae. This effect may alleviate symptoms, reduce duration of infection, facilitate worm removal, or expedite their spontaneous extrusion
- Metronidazole, 250 mg PO three times daily for 10 days, causes only minimal toxicity
- Mebendazole, 400–800 mg PO daily for 6 days, can be tried
- Thiabendazole, 25 mg/kg PO twice daily for 2–3 days after meals, frequently causes side effects, sometimes severe

SURGERY

- Preemergent female worms can sometimes be surgically removed intact under local anesthesia if not firmly embedded in deep fascia or around tendons

THERAPEUTIC PROCEDURES

- The patient should be at bed rest with the affected part elevated
- Cleanse the lesion, control secondary infection with topical antibiotics, and change dressings twice daily
- **Manual extraction**
  - Traditional extraction of emerging worms by gradually rolling them out a few centimeters each day on a small stick is still useful, especially when done along with chemotherapy and use of aseptic dressings
  - The process appears to be facilitated by placing the affected part in water several times a day
  - If the worm is broken during removal, however, secondary infection almost always results, leading to cellulitis, abscess formation, or septicemia

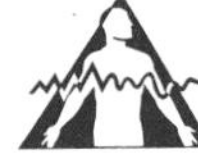

OUTCOME

COMPLICATIONS

- Ankle and knee joint infections with resultant deformity are common complications

WHEN TO REFER

- For manual or surgical extraction

PREVENTION

- The disease is prevented by use of only noncontaminated drinking water. This can be accomplished either by preventing contamination of community water supplies through use of tube wells, hand pumps, or cisterns or treating water sources with temephos; or filtering water through nets (eg, nylon nets of 100-μm pore size); or boiling water
- All persons in an endemic area should be actively immunized against tetanus

EVIDENCE

WEB SITE

- CDC—Division of Parasitic Diseases
  - http://www.cdc.gov/ncidod/dpd/parasites/dracunculiasis/default.htm

INFORMATION FOR PATIENTS

- Centers for Disease Control
  - http://www.cdc.gov/ncidod/dpd/parasites/guineaworm/factsht_guineaworm.htm

REFERENCES

- Cairncross S et al: Dracunculiasis (Guinea worm disease) and the eradication initiative. Clin Microbiol Rev 2002;15:223. [PMID: 11932231]
- Centers for Disease Control and Prevention: Progress toward global dracunculiasis eradication, June 2002. MMWR Morb Mortal Wkly Rep 2002;51:810. [PMID: 12269470]

Drowning

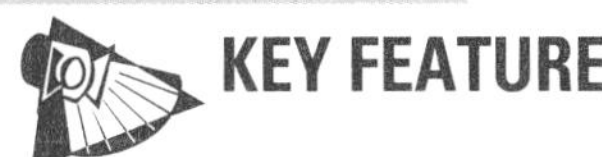

KEY FEATURES

ESSENTIALS OF DIAGNOSIS

- The asphyxia of drowning is usually due to aspiration of fluid
- May also result from airway obstruction caused by laryngeal spasm while the victim is gasping under water

GENERAL CONSIDERATIONS

- About 10% of victims develop laryngospasm after the first gulp and never aspirate water ("dry drowning")
- The rapid sequence of events after submersion—hypoxemia, laryngospasm, fluid aspiration, ineffective circulation, brain injury, and brain death—may take place within 5–10 min
- This sequence may be delayed for longer periods if the victim, especially a child, has been submerged in very cold water or if the victim has ingested significant amounts of barbiturates
- Immersion in cold water can also cause a rapid fall in the victim's core temperature, so that systemic hypothermia and death may occur before actual drowning

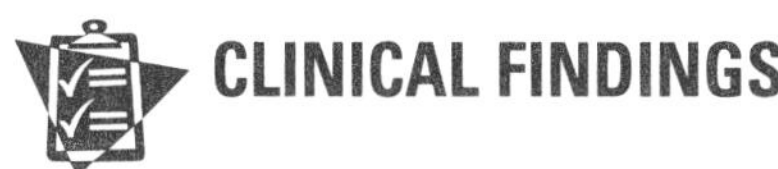

CLINICAL FINDINGS

SYMPTOMS AND SIGNS

- Unconscious, semiconscious, or awake
- Apprehensive, restless
- Complaining of headaches or chest pain
- Vomiting is common
- Cyanosis, trismus, apnea, tachypnea, and wheezing
- A pink froth from the mouth and nose indicates pulmonary edema
- Tachycardia, arrhythmias, hypotension, cardiac arrest, and circulatory shock
- With prolonged or cold-water immersion, hypothermia is likely

DIFFERENTIAL DIAGNOSIS

- Alcohol or drug intoxication
- Myocardial infarction
- Seizure
- Suicide attempt
- Head or spinal cord injury from diving
- Decompression sickness

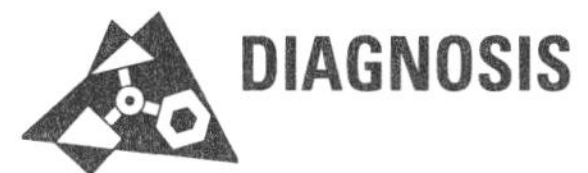

DIAGNOSIS

LABORATORY TESTS

- Urinalysis shows proteinuria, hemoglobinuria, and acetonuria
- Leukocytosis is usually present
- Pao_2 is usually decreased and $Paco_2$ increased or decreased
- The blood pH is decreased as a result of metabolic acidosis

IMAGING STUDIES

- Chest x-ray films may show pneumonitis or pulmonary edema

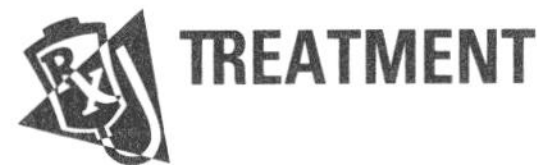

TREATMENT

MEDICATIONS

- Bronchospasm from aspirated material may require use of bronchodilators
- Antibiotics given only with clinical evidence of infection, not prophylactically
- Central venous pressure (or, better, pulmonary artery wedge pressure) guides use of vascular fluid replacement, pressors, diuretics
- Metabolic acidosis in 70% of near-drowning victims; usually corrects with adequate ventilation and oxygenation
  - Bicarbonate use (1 mEq/kg) recommended for comatose patients but is controversial

THERAPEUTIC PROCEDURES

First aid

- Immediate CPR
- Always suspect hypothermia and cervical spine injury
- Do *not* attempt to drain water from lungs
- Heimlich maneuver used only if foreign body airway obstruction suspected. Immobilize cervical spine if neck injury possible
- Do *not* stop basic life support for "hopeless" patients until core temperature = 32°C
  - Complete recovery reported after prolonged resuscitation

Hospital care

- Admit all patients
- Continuous monitoring of cardiorespiratory function; serial determination of ABGs, pH, renal function (serum creatinine), and electrolytes; and measurement of urinary output. Pulmonary edema may not appear for 24 h
- Administer O_2 immediately at highest concentration and maintain O_2 saturation at ≥ 90%
- CPAP and PEEP effectively reverse hypoxia in patients with spontaneous respirations and patent airways
- Endotracheal intubation and mechanical ventilation for patients unable to maintain open airway or normal blood gases and pH
- NG intubation to remove swallowed water and prevent aspiration
- Continuous monitoring of cardiorespiratory function; serial determination of ABGs, pH, serum creatinine, electrolytes; measurement of urinary output
- Perform serial physical examinations, chest x-rays to detect possible pneumonitis, atelectasis, pulmonary edema
- Some cases progress to irreversible CNS damage despite adequate treatment of hypoxia and shock; hyperventilation to achieve $Paco_2$ of ~30 mm Hg recommended to lower ICP
- Hypothermia: measure and manage core temperature as appropriate (see Hypothermia)

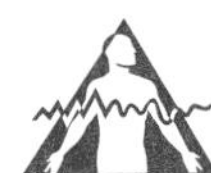

OUTCOME

FOLLOW-UP

- Keep victims of prolonged hypoxemia under close hospital observation for 2–3 days after all supportive measures have been withdrawn and clinical and laboratory findings have been stable
- Residual complications of near-drowning may include intellectual impairment, convulsive disorders, and pulmonary or cardiac disease

PROGNOSIS

- Spontaneous return of consciousness often occurs in otherwise healthy individuals when submersion is very brief
- Many other patients respond promptly to immediate ventilation
- Other patients, with more severe degrees of near-drowning, may have frank respiratory failure, pulmonary edema, shock, anoxic encephalopathy, cerebral edema, and cardiac arrest
- A few patients may be deceptively asymptomatic during the recovery period, only to deteriorate or die as a result of acute respiratory failure within the following 12–24 h

PREVENTION

- Avoidance of alcohol during recreational swimming or boating
- Swimming lessons early in life
- Use of personal flotation devices when boating

EVIDENCE

PRACTICE GUIDELINES

- European Resuscitation Council: Part 8: Advanced challenges in resuscitation. Section 3: Special challenges in ECC. 3B: Submersion or near-drowning. Resuscitation 2000;46:273. [PMID: 10978807]

INFORMATION FOR PATIENTS

- American Red Cross: Water Safety Tips
  - http://www.redcross.org/services/hss/tips/healthtips/safetywater.html
- Centers for Disease Control and Prevention: Water-Related Injuries: Fact Sheet
  - http://www.cdc.gov/ncipc/factsheets/drown.htm
- MedlinePlus: Near Drowning
  - http://www.nlm.nih.gov/medlineplus/ency/article/000046.htm
- American College of Emergency Physicians: Beach and Surf Safety
  - http://www.acep.org/webportal/PatientsConsumers/HealthSubjectsByTopic/SafetyIssues/FeatureColumnBeachAndSurfSafety.htm

REFERENCE

- Olshaker JS: Submersion. Emerg Med Clin N Am 2004;22:357. [PMID: 15163572]

Author(s)

Richard Cohen, MD, MPH

Drug Use–Related Infections

KEY FEATURES

ESSENTIALS OF DIAGNOSIS

- Common infections that occur with greater frequency in drug users
  - Skin infections
  - Hepatitis A, B, C, D
  - Aspiration pneumonia
  - Tuberculosis
  - Pulmonary septic emboli
  - Sexually transmitted diseases
  - AIDS
  - Infective endocarditis
  - Osteomyelitis
  - Septic arthritis
- Rare infections in the United States include: tetanus, malaria, and melioidosis

GENERAL CONSIDERATIONS

Skin infections

- Associated with poor hygiene and use of nonsterile technique when injecting drugs
- *Staphylococcus aureus* (including methicillin-resistant strains) and oral flora (streptococci, *Eikenella*, *Fusobacterium*, *Peptostreptococcus*) are the most common organisms, with enteric gram-negatives less common and seen in those who inject into the groin
- Cellulitis and subcutaneous abscesses occur most commonly, particularly in association with subcutaneous ("skin-popping") or intramuscular injections and the use of cocaine and heroin mixtures (probably due to ischemia)
- Myositis, clostridial myonecrosis, and necrotizing fasciitis occur infrequently but are life-threatening
- Wound botulism in association with black tar heroin occurs sporadically but often in clusters

Hepatitis

- Very common among habitual drug users
- Transmissible both by the parenteral (hepatitis B, C, and D) and by the fecal–oral route (hepatitis A)
- Multiple episodes of hepatitis with different agents can occur

Aspiration pneumonia

- Result from altered consciousness associated with drug use
- Mixed aerobic and anaerobic mouth flora are usually involved
- Complications include lung abscess, empyema, and brain abscess

Tuberculosis

- Infection with HIV has fostered the spread of tuberculosis in this population

Pulmonary septic emboli

- From venous thrombi or right-sided endocarditis

Sexually transmitted diseases

- Related to the practice of exchanging sex for drugs
- Syphilis, gonorrhea, and chancroid are the most common

AIDS

- High incidence among injection drug users and their sexual contacts and among the offspring of infected women

Infective endocarditis

- The organisms are most commonly *S aureus*, *Candida* (especially *Candida parapsilosis*), *Enterococcus faecalis*, other streptococci, and gram-negative bacteria (especially *Pseudomonas* and *Serratia marcescens*)
- Right-sided heart involvement
  - Common, and infection of more than one valve is not infrequent
  - Septic pulmonary emboli suppport diagnosis, especially in the absence of murmurs

Other vascular infections

- Septic thrombophlebitis
- Mycotic aneurysms resulting from direct trauma to a vessel with secondary infection most commonly occur in femoral arteries and less commonly in arteries of the neck. Aneurysms resulting from hematogenous spread of organisms frequently involve intracerebral vessels and thus are seen in association with endocarditis

Osteomyelitis and septic arthritis

- Osteomyelitis involving vertebral bodies, sternoclavicular joints, the pubic symphysis, the sacroiliac joints, and other sites usually results from hematogenous distribution of injected organisms or septic venous thrombi
- While staphylococci—often methicillin-resistant—are common organisms, *Serratia*, *Pseudomonas*, *Candida* (usually not *C albicans*), and other pathogens rarely encountered in spontaneous bone or joint disease are found

Tetanus

- Increased tetanus immunization has resulted in a decline in this disease
- Reported cases are generally when drugs are injected subcutaneously ("skin-popping")

Malaria

- Needle transmission occurs from injection drug users who acquired the infection in malaria-endemic areas outside the United States

Melioidosis

- This chronic pulmonary infection caused by *Burkholderia pseudomallei* is occasionally seen in debilitated drug users; most cases are reported in Asia and Australia

DEMOGRAPHICS

- There are an estimated 300,000 or more injection drug users in the United States

CLINICAL FINDINGS

SYMPTOMS AND SIGNS

- Those of the underlying infection

DIFFERENTIAL DIAGNOSIS

- Community-acquired pneumonia
- Endocarditis
- Complications of endocarditis, eg, pulmonary septic emboli, epidural abscess, osteomyelitis
- Skin abscess, cellulitis, myositis, necrotizing fasciitis
- Pelvic inflammatory disease
- Urinary tract infection

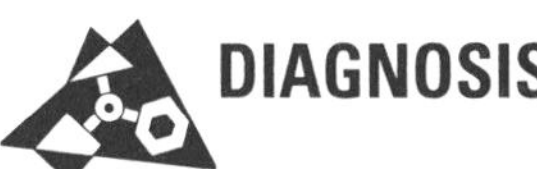

DIAGNOSIS

LABORATORY TESTS

- Appropriate cultures (blood, urine, and sputum)
- Complete blood cell count, liver function tests, urinalysis

IMAGING STUDIES

- Chest x-ray
- Classic radiographic findings are often absent in HIV patients with tuberculosis; any patient with infiltrates who does not respond to antibiotics is suspect
- Pain and fever precede radiographic changes of osteomyelitis and septic arthritis, sometimes by several weeks

DIAGNOSTIC PROCEDURES

- If blood cultures are positive for an organism that is an unusual cause of endocarditis, a transesophageal echocardiogram may be helpful. It is 90% sensitive in detecting vegetations and a negative study is strong evidence against endocarditis

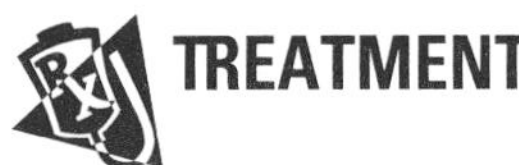

TREATMENT

MEDICATIONS

- A common and difficult clinical problem is management of the parenteral drug user who presents with fever. In general, after obtaining appropriate cultures (blood, urine, and sputum if the chest x-ray is abnormal), empiric therapy is begun (Table 28)
- If the chest x-ray suggests a community-acquired pneumonia (consolidation), therapy for outpatient pneumonia is begun with a second- or third-generation cephalosporin (many would add azithromycin or doxycycline to this regimen)
- If the chest x-ray suggests septic emboli (nodular infiltrates), therapy for presumed endocarditis is initiated, usually with a combination of nafcillin (or vancomycin if there is a high prevalence of methicillin-resistant *S aureus* or if enterococcus is a consideration) and gentamicin
- If the chest x-ray is normal and no focal site of infection can be found, endocarditis is presumed. While awaiting the results of blood cultures, empiric treatment with nafcillin (or vancomycin) and gentamicin is started
- If blood cultures are positive for organisms that frequently cause endocarditis in drug users (see above), endocarditis is presumed to be present and treated accordingly
- If blood cultures are positive for an organism that is an unusual cause of endocarditis, evaluation for an occult source of infection should go forward
- If blood cultures are negative and the patient responds to antibiotics, therapy should be continued for 7–14 days (oral therapy can be given once an initial response has occurred)
- In every patient, careful examination for an occult source of infection (genitourinary, dental, sinus, gallbladder, etc) should be done

OUTCOME

COMPLICATIONS

- See the specific diagnoses

WHEN TO REFER

- For complicated infections such as endocarditis, osteomyelitis, or septic arthritis

WHEN TO ADMIT

- Complicated infections as above
- Marked systemic toxcity

PREVENTION

- Immunizations against hepatitis A and B
- Clean needle use will decrease transmission of blood-borne pathogens

EVIDENCE

WEB SITE

- Centers for Disease Control and Prevention—National Center for HIV, STD, and TB Prevention
  - http://www.cdc.gov/idu/

INFORMATION FOR PATIENTS

- American Heart Association: Endocarditis
  - http://www.americanheart.org/presenter.jhtml?identifier=4436
- The Mayo Clinic: Cellulitis
  - http://www.mayoclinic.com/invoke.cfm?id=DS00450

REFERENCES

- Brown PD et al: Infective endocarditis in the injection drug user. Infect Dis Clin North Am 2002;16:645. [PMID: 12371120]
- Levine DP et al: Infections in injection drug users. In: *Principles and Practice of Infectious Diseases,* ed 6. Mandell GL, Bennett JR, Dolin R (editors). Elsevier, Churchill Livingstone, 2005.
- Murphy EL et al: Risk factors for skin and soft-tissue abscesses among injection drug users: a case-control study. Clin Infect Dis 2001;33:35. [PMID: 11389492]

Author(s)

Richard A. Jacobs, MD, PhD

Dysautonomia

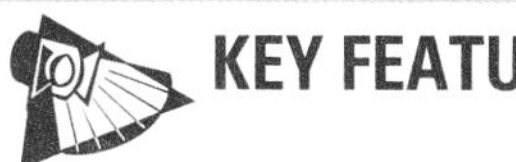

KEY FEATURES

ESSENTIALS OF DIAGNOSIS

- Features may occur in isolation or combinations and include abnormalities of blood pressure, heart rate, thermoregulatory sweating, intestinal motility, sphincter control, sexual function, respiration, and ocular function

GENERAL CONSIDERATIONS

- **Primary neurodegenerative disorders with dysautonomia**
  - Primary autonomic failure
  - Multisystem atrophy: constellation of parkinsonism, pyramidal signs, and cerebellar deficits; called Shy-Drager syndrome) when autonomic signs predominate
  - Parkinson's disease
- **CNS lesions that may exhibit features of dysautonomias (usually postural hypotension)**
  - Spinal cord transection, other myelopathies above the T6 level (eg, due to tumor or syringomyelia), or brainstem lesions such as syringobulbia and posterior fossa tumors
- **Peripheral causes**
  - Guillain-Barré syndrome may have features of marked hypotension or hypertension or cardiac arrhythmias
  - Diabetes
  - Uremia
  - Amyloidosis
  - Leprosy
  - Chagas' disease
  - Hepatic porphyria
  - Botulism
  - Lambert-Eaton myasthenic syndrome
  - Botulism and the Lambert-Eaton myasthenic syndrome may have constipation, urinary retention, and a sicca syndrome as a result of impaired cholinergic function

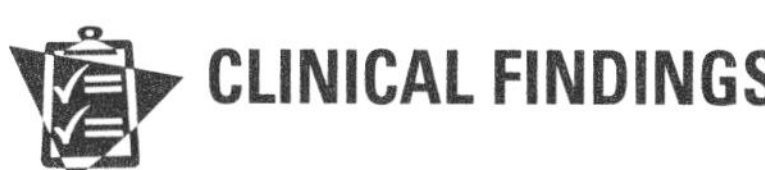

CLINICAL FINDINGS

SYMPTOMS AND SIGNS

- Syncope
- Postural hypotension
- Persistent tachycardia without other cause
- Facial flushing, hypohidrosis or hyperhidrosis
- Vomiting, constipation, diarrhea, dysphagia, abdominal distention
- Disturbances of micturition or defecation
- Apneic episodes
- Declining night vision

DIFFERENTIAL DIAGNOSIS

- Hypovolemia
- Drugs, eg, β-blockers, calcium-channel blockers, vasodilators, diuretics
- Situational syncope, eg, micturition, defecation, cough, swallow
- Postural hypotension
  - Reduced cardiac output from volume depletion, aortic stenosis or cardiomyopathy, cardiac dysrhythmias, various medications
  - Endocrine disorders such as diabetes, Addison's disease, hypothyroidism or hyperthyroidism, pheochromocytoma, and carcinoid syndrome

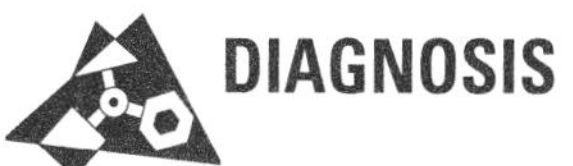

DIAGNOSIS

LABORATORY TESTS

- Serum glucose, electrolytes, renal function
- Thyroid function tests, serum serotonin, 24-h urinary metanephrines, and 5-hydroxyindoleacetic acid
- Autonomic function tests

IMAGING STUDIES

- For those with evidence of a central lesion, imaging studies will exclude a treatable structural cause

DIAGNOSTIC PROCEDURES

- Clinical evaluation focuses on excluding reversible, nonneurologic causes of symptoms
- Evaluate the Valsalva maneuver, cardiovascular response to startle, mental stress, postural change, and deep respiration, and the sudomotor (sweating) responses to warming or a deep inspiratory gasp
- Tilt-table testing may point to a neurocardiogenic cause of syncope
- Pharmacologic studies to evaluate the pupillary responses, radiologic studies of the bladder or gastrointestinal tract, uroflowmetry and urethral pressure profiles, and recording of nocturnal penile tumescence may also be necessary in selected cases

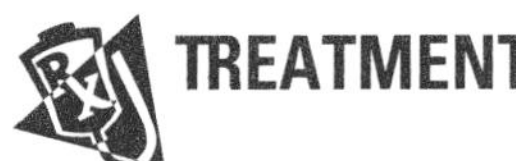

TREATMENT

MEDICATIONS

- Treatment may include wearing waist-high elastic hosiery, salt supplementation, sleeping in a semierect position (which minimizes the natriuresis and diuresis that occur during recumbency), and fludrocortisone (0.1–0.3 mg PO QD)
- Vasoconstrictor agents may be helpful and include midodrine (2.5–10 mg PO TID) and ephedrine (15–30 mg PO TID)
- Less commonly used agents are dihydroergotamine, yohimbine, and clonidine
- Refractory cases may respond to erythropoietin (epoetin alfa) or desmopressin

THERAPEUTIC PROCEDURES

- Avoid abrupt postural change, prolonged recumbency, and other precipitants (eg, straining with bowel movements)
- Medications associated with postural hypotension should be discontinued or reduced in dose
- There is no satisfactory treatment for disturbances of sweating, but an air-conditioned environment is helpful in avoiding extreme swings in body temperature
- Postprandial hypotension is helped by caffeine

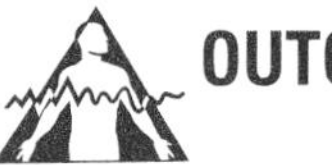

OUTCOME

WHEN TO REFER

- When the diagnosis is in question
- When symptoms do not respond to conventional therapy

EVIDENCE

PRACTICE GUIDELINES

- Gilman S et al: Consensus statement on the diagnosis of multiple system atrophy. American Autonomic Society and American Academy of Neurology. Clin Auton Res 1998;8:359. [PMID: 9869555]

WEB SITE

- Northwestern University Medical School
  - http://www.neuro.nwu.edu/meded/MOVEMENT/msa.html

INFORMATION FOR PATIENTS

- National Institute of Neurological Diseases and Stroke
  - http://www.ninds.nih.gov/disorders/dysauto/dysauto.htm
- Worldwide Education and Awareness for Movement Disorders
  - http://www.wemove.org/msa/

REFERENCES

- Chen-Scarabelli C et al: Neurocardiogenic syncope. BMJ 2004;329:336. [PMID: 15297344]
- Goldstein DS et al: Dysautonomias: clinical disorders of the autonomic nervous system. Ann Intern Med 2002;137:753. [PMID: 12416949]
- Kaufmann H et al: Why do we faint? Muscle Nerve 2001;24:981. [PMID: 11439373]

Author(s)

Michael J. Aminoff, MD, DSc, FRCP

Dysmenorrhea

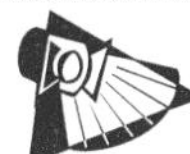

KEY FEATURES

ESSENTIALS OF DIAGNOSIS

- **Primary dysmenorrhea** is menstrual pain associated with ovular cycles in the absence of pathologic findings
- **Secondary dysmenorrhea** is menstrual pain for which an organic cause exists, such as endometriosis

GENERAL CONSIDERATIONS

Primary dysmenorrhea

- The pain usually begins within 1–2 years after the menarche and may become more severe with time
- The pain is produced by uterine vasoconstriction, anoxia, and sustained contractions mediated by prostaglandins

DEMOGRAPHICS

Primary dysmenorrhea

- The frequency of cases increases up to age 20 and then decreases with age and markedly with parity
- Fifty to 75% of women are affected at some time, and 5–6% have incapacitating pain

Secondary dysmenorrhea

- It usually begins well after menarche, sometimes even as late as the third or fourth decade of life

CLINICAL FINDINGS

SYMPTOMS AND SIGNS

Primary dysmenorrhea

- Pain is low, midline, wave-like, cramping pelvic pain often radiating to the back or inner thighs
- Cramps may last for 1 or more days and may be associated with nausea, diarrhea, headache, and flushing
- No pathologic findings on pelvic examination

Secondary dysmenorrhea

- The history and physical examination commonly suggest endometriosis or pelvic inflammatory disease

DIFFERENTIAL DIAGNOSIS

- Endometriosis
- Adenomyosis (uterine endometriosis)
- Pelvic inflammatory disease
- Uterine leiomyomas (fibroids)
- Intrauterine device
- Pelvic pain syndrome
- Endometrial polyp
- Cervicitis
- Retroverted uterus
- Cervical stenosis
- Cystitis
- Interstitial cystitis

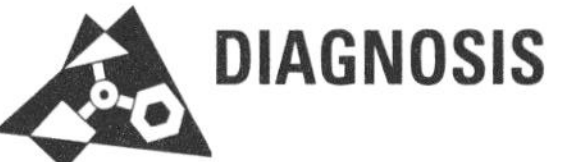

DIAGNOSIS

IMAGING STUDIES

- MRI is the most reliable method to detect submucous myomas

DIAGNOSTIC PROCEDURES

Secondary dysmenorrhea

- Laparoscopy is often needed to differentiate endometriosis from pelvic inflammatory disease
- Submucous myomas can be detected by hysterogram, by hysteroscopy, or by passing a sound or curette over the uterine cavity during D&C

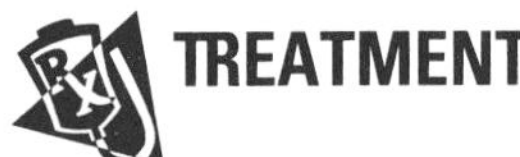

TREATMENT

MEDICATIONS

Primary dysmenorrhea

- Nonsteroidal anti-inflammatory drugs (ibuprofen, ketoprofen, mefenamic acid, naproxen) are generally helpful
- Drugs should be started at the onset of bleeding to avoid inadvertent drug use during early pregnancy
- Medication should be continued on a regular basis for 2–3 days
- Ovulation can be suppressed and dysmenorrhea usually prevented by oral contraceptives

Secondary dysmenorrhea

- Periodic use of analgesics, including the nonsteroidal anti-inflammatory drugs given for primary dysmenorrhea, may be beneficial
- Oral contraceptives may give relief, particularly in endometriosis
- Danazol and gonadotropin-releasing hormone agonists are effective in the treatment of endometriosis

SURGERY

- If disability is marked or prolonged, laparoscopy or exploratory laparotomy is usually warranted
- Definitive surgery depends upon the degree of disability and the findings at operation

THERAPEUTIC PROCEDURES

- Cervical stenosis may result from induced abortion, creating crampy pain at the time of expected menses with no blood flow; this is easily cured by passing a sound into the uterine cavity after administering a paracervical block

OUTCOME

- The expertise of a gynecologist is frequently useful in the diagnosis and treatment of secondary dysmenorrhea

EVIDENCE

PRACTICE GUIDELINES

- University of Texas at Austin: Recommendations for the treatment of dysmenorrhea
  - http://www.guideline.gov/summary/summary.aspx?doc_id=2737&nbr=1963

INFORMATION FOR PATIENTS

- American College of Obstetricians and Gynecologists: Dysmenorrhea
  - http://www.medem.com/medlb/article_detaillb.cfm?article_ID=ZZZH7MGV77C&sub_cat=2003
- Mayo Clinic: Dysmenorrhea
  - http://www.mayoclinic.com/invoke.cfm?id=DS00506
- National Women's Health Information Center: Menstruation and the Menstrual Cycle
  - http://www.4woman.org/faq/menstru.htm
- University of Utah: Dysmenorrhea
  - http://www.med.utah.edu/healthinfo/adult/gynonc/dysmen.htm

REFERENCE

- Marjoribanks J et al: Nonsteroidal anti-inflammatory drugs for primary dysmenorrhoea. Cochrane Database Syst Rev 2003;(4):CD001751. [PMID: 14583938]

Author(s)

H. Trent MacKay, MD, MPH

Dyspareunia (Painful Intercourse)

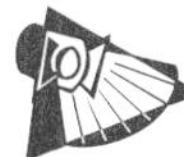

KEY FEATURES

GENERAL CONSIDERATIONS

Etiology

- Vulvovaginitis: inflammation or infection of the vagina
- Vaginismus
  - Voluntary or involuntary contraction of muscles around the introitus
  - Results from fear, pain, sexual trauma, or having learned negative attitudes toward sex during childhood
- Remnants of the hymen: a rim of hymen may remain after initial episodes of intercourse, causing pain
- Insufficient lubrication of the vagina is a frequent cause of dyspareunia in postmenopausal women
- Infection, endometriosis, tumors, or other pathologic conditions: pain occurring with deep thrusting during coitus is usually due to acute or chronic infection of the cervix, uterus, or adnexa; endometriosis; adnexal tumors; or adhesions resulting from prior pelvic disease or operation
- Vulvodynia is the most frequent cause of dyspareunia in premenopausal women

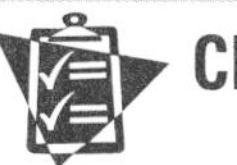

CLINICAL FINDINGS

SYMPTOMS AND SIGNS

- Questions related to sexual functioning should be asked as part of the reproductive history. Two helpful questions are, "Are you sexually active?" and "Are you having any sexual difficulties at this time?"
- During the pelvic examination, the patient should be placed in a half-sitting position and given a hand-held mirror and then asked to point out the site of pain and describe the type of pain
- Vulvovaginitis: areas of marked tenderness in the vulvar vestibule without visible inflammation
- Vulvodynia
  - A sensation of burning along with other symptoms including pain, itching, stinging, irritation, and rawness
  - Discomfort may be constant or intermittent, focal or diffuse, and experienced as either deep or superficial
  - Generally no physical findings except minimal erythema that may be associated with a subset of vulvodynia, vulvar vestibulitis

DIFFERENTIAL DIAGNOSIS

- Vulvodynia or vulvar vestibulitis
- Vaginismus
- Insufficient vaginal lubrication
- Atrophic vaginitis
- Vulvovaginitis, cervicitis, or pelvic inflammatory disease
- Endometriosis
- Lichen sclerosus
- Ovarian tumor
- Pelvic adhesions
- Remnants of the hymen

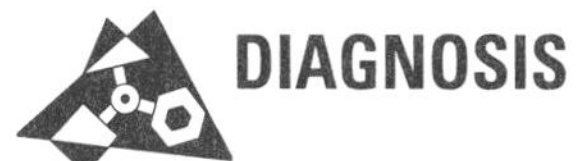

DIAGNOSIS

DIAGNOSTIC PROCEDURES

- Colposcopy to evaluate vulvovaginitis: areas of marked tenderness in the vulvar vestibule without visible inflammation occasionally show lesions resembling small condylomas

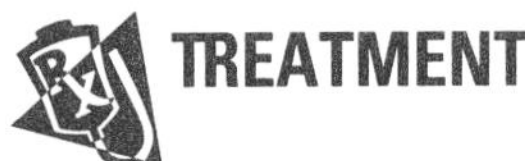

TREATMENT

THERAPEUTIC PROCEDURES

Vulvovaginitis

- Warty lesions on colposcopy or biopsy should be treated appropriately (see Vaginitis)

Vaginismus

- Sexual counseling and education may be useful
- Self-dilation, using a lubricated finger or test tubes of graduated sizes, may help. Before coitus (with adequate lubrication) is attempted, the patient and then partner should be able to painlessly introduce two fingers into the vagina

Remnants of the hymen

- Rarely, may need manual dilation of a remaining hymen under general anesthesia
- Avoid surgery

Insufficient lubrication of the vagina

- See Menopausal Syndrome
- For inadequate sexual arousal, sexual counseling is helpful
- Lubricants during sexual foreplay may be of use
- If lubrication remains inadequate, use estradiol vaginal ring worn continuously and replaced every 3 months. Concomitant progestin therapy is not needed with the ring
- Estrogen vaginal cream

Infection, endometriosis, tumors, or other pathologic conditions

- Temporarily abstain from coitus during treatment
- Consider hormonal or surgical treatment of endometriosis
- Dyspareunia from chronic pelvic inflammatory disease or extensive adhesions is difficult to treat without extirpative surgery. Couples can be advised to try coital positions that limit deep thrusting and to use manual and oral sexual techniques

Vulvodynia

- Difficult management since etiology unclear
- Surgical vestibulectomy has had success
- Antiviral, antifungal, corticosteroid, or anesthetic agents have varied success
- Pain control through behavioral therapy, biofeedback, or acupuncture has varied success
- Continuous genital burning or pain may be relieved with amitriptyline in gradually increasing doses from 10 mg PO QD to 75–100 mg PO QD

OUTCOME

WHEN TO REFER

- When symptoms persist despite first-line therapy
- For expertise in procedures

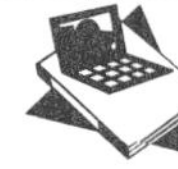

EVIDENCE

INFORMATION FOR PATIENTS

- American Academy of Family Physicians: Dyspareunia
  - http://familydoctor.org/669.xml
- American College of Obstetricians and Gynecologists: Pain During Intercourse
  - http://www.medem.com/MedLB/article_detaillb.cfm?article_ID=ZZZCYQ7I27C&sub_cat=9
- American Academy of Family Physicians: Vulvodynia
  - http://familydoctor.org/367.xml
- Mayo Clinic: Vaginal Dryness
  - http://www.mayoclinic.com/invoke.cfm?id=DS00550
- MedlinePlus: Vaginismus
  - http://www.nlm.nih.gov/medlineplus/ency/article/001487.htm
- MedlinePlus: Vulvovaginitis
  - http://www.nlm.nih.gov/medlineplus/ency/article/000897.htm

REFERENCE

- Mariani L: Vulvar vestibulitis syndrome: an overview of non-surgical treatment. Eur J Obstet Gynecol Reprod Biol 2002;101:109. [PMID: 11858882]

Author(s)

H. Trent MacKay, MD, MPH

Dyspepsia

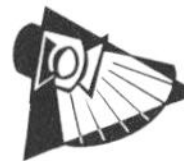

KEY FEATURES

ESSENTIALS OF DIAGNOSIS

- Pain or discomfort centered in the upper abdomen
- Upper abdominal fullness, early satiety, burning, bloating, belching, nausea, retching, or vomiting
- Heartburn (retrosternal burning) may also be present

GENERAL CONSIDERATIONS

- Functional or "nonulcer" dyspepsia is the most common cause

DEMOGRAPHICS

- Occurs in 25% of the adult population
- Accounts for 3% of office visits

CLINICAL FINDINGS

SYMPTOMS AND SIGNS

- Weight loss, persistent vomiting, and dysphagia warrant endoscopy or abdominal imaging
- Signs of serious disease: weight loss, organomegaly, abdominal mass, or fecal occult blood

DIFFERENTIAL DIAGNOSIS

- Peptic ulcer disease (in 5–15% of cases)
- Gastroesophageal reflux (in 20%)
- Gastritis, eg, nonsteroidal anti-inflammatory drugs, alcohol, stress, *Helicobacter pylori*
- Chronic pancreatitis or pancreatic cancer
- "Indigestion" from overeating, high-fat foods, coffee
- Other drugs: aspirin, antibiotics (eg, macrolides, metronidazole), corticosteroids, digoxin, iron, theophylline, and opioids
- Gastroparesis
- Lactase deficiency
- Malabsorption
- Gastric cancer (in 1%)
- Parasitic infection, eg, *Giardia, Strongyloides, Ascaris*
- Cholelithiasis, choledocholithiasis, or cholangitis
- *H pylori* (controversial)
- Myocardial ischemia or pericarditis
- Abdominal or paraesophageal hernia
- Pregnancy
- Chronic mesenteric ischemia
- Metabolic conditions: diabetes, thyroid disease, renal insufficiency
- Intra-abdominal malignancy
- Physical or sexual abuse

DIAGNOSIS

- History entails chronicity, location, and quality of the discomfort, but has limited diagnostic utility
- Under age 50 without signs of serious organic disease [dysphagia, weight loss, severe pain, vomiting, anemia, gastrointestinal (GI) bleeding]: noninvasive testing for *H pylori* (urea breath test, fecal antigen test, or serology); treat if positive
- Consider trial of proton pump inhibitors for 4–8 weeks
- If symptoms persist or recur after empirical treatment, perform esophagogastroduodenoscopy (EGD)
- Over age 50 or any age with signs of serious organic disease: upper endoscopy

LABORATORY TESTS

- Obtain complete blood cell count, serum electrolytes, liver enzymes, calcium, and thyroid-stimulating hormone

IMAGING STUDIES

- Abdominal ultrasonography indicated if pancreatic or biliary tract disease is suspected
- Upper gastrointestinal barium radiography is inferior to endoscopy

DIAGNOSTIC PROCEDURES

- Upper endoscopy indicated in all patients age >50 years with new-onset dyspepsia and in all patients with weight loss, dysphagia, recurrent vomiting, hematemesis, melena, or anemia
- Upper endoscopy helpful in reassuring patients concerned about serious underlying disease
- Noninvasive test for *H pylori*: IgG serology, fecal antigen test, or urea breath test
- Gastric emptying studies indicated for recurrent vomiting
- Ambulatory esophageal pH testing if atypical gastroesophageal reflux is suspected

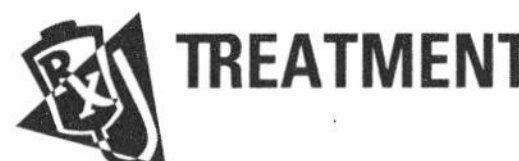

TREATMENT

MEDICATIONS

- H_2-receptor antagonists or proton pump inhibitors benefit 10–20%
- H_2-receptor antagonists (ranitidine or nizatidine, 150 mg PO BID; famotidine, 20 mg PO BID; or cimetidine, 400–800 mg PO BID)
- Proton pump inhibitors (omeprazole or rabeprazole, 20 mg, lansoprazole, 30 mg, esomeprazole or pantoprazole, 40 mg PO QD)
- Antidepressants (eg, desipramine or nortriptyline, 10–50 mg PO QHS)
- Prokinetic agent, metoclopramide 10 mg PO TID, improves symptoms in up to 60%
- *H pylori* eradication therapy benefits 5–15% (see *Helicobacter pylori* Gastritis)

THERAPEUTIC PROCEDURES

- Discontinue potentially offending medications if possible
- Reduce or discontinue alcohol and caffeine intake

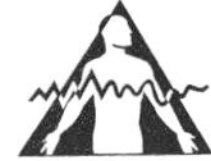

OUTCOME

FOLLOW-UP

- Reevaluate symptoms after 4–6 weeks of empirical management; if they persist or recur, further testing with EGD, possible imaging studies

PROGNOSIS

- Half to two-thirds of people affected have functional dyspepsia, ie, no demonstrable organic cause; symptoms may be chronic

WHEN TO REFER

- Dyspepsia with signs of serious organic disease
- Chronic dyspepsia unresponsive to routine therapies

WHEN TO ADMIT

- Signs of GI bleeding
- Protracted vomiting with dehydration

EVIDENCE

PRACTICE GUIDELINES

- Dyspepsia. Institute for Clinical Systems Improvement—Private Nonprofit Organization, 2003
  - http://www.icsi.org/knowledge/detail.asp?catID=29&itemID=171
- Eisen GM et al: The role of endoscopy in dyspepsia. Gastrointest Endosc 2001;54:815. [PMID:11726874]
- National Guideline Clearinghouse
  - http://www.guideline.gov/summary/summary.aspx?doc_id=3723&nbr=2949&string=dyspepsia

INFORMATION FOR PATIENTS

- Cleveland Clinic—What is indigestion?
  - http://www.clevelandclinic.org/health/health-info/docs/1700/1779.asp?index=7316
- Mayo Clinic—Nonulcer Dyspepsia
  - http://www.mayoclinic.com/invoke.cfm?id=DS00524
  - http://patients.uptodate.com/frames.asp?page=topic.asp&file=digestiv/7283&title=Dyspepsia

REFERENCES

- Moayyedi P et al: Pharmacological interventions for non-ulcer dyspepsia. Cochrane Database Syst Rev 2004;(4):CD001960. [PMID:15495023]
- Talley NJ: Dyspepsia. Gastroenterology 2003;125:1219. [PMID:14517803]
- Timmons S et al: Functional dyspepsia: motor abnormalities, sensory dysfunction, and therapeutic options. Am J Gastroenterol 2004;99:739. [PMID:15089910]

Author(s)

Kenneth R. McQuaid, MD

Dystonia, Idiopathic Torsion

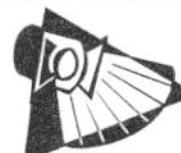

KEY FEATURES

ESSENTIALS OF DIAGNOSIS

- Dystonic movements and postures
- Normal birth and developmental history. No other neurologic signs
- Investigations (including CT scan or MRI) reveal no cause of dystonia

GENERAL CONSIDERATIONS

- May occur sporadically or on a hereditary basis, with autosomal dominant, autosomal recessive, and X-linked recessive modes of transmission
- One responsible gene is located at 9q34 (and has been named *DYT1*) and involves a unique mutation consisting of a GAG deletion in the dominantly inherited disorder and maps to the long arm of the X chromosome in the X-linked recessive form; the responsible gene in the autosomal recessive disorder is unknown
- Other autosomal dominant forms have also been recognized, with different or unidentified genetic loci
- Symptoms may begin in childhood or later and persist throughout life

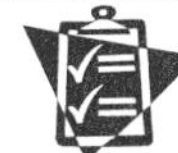

CLINICAL FINDINGS

SYMPTOMS AND SIGNS

- Onset of abnormal movements and postures in a patient with a normal birth and developmental history, no relevant past medical illness, and no other neurologic signs
- Dystonic movements of the head and neck
  - Torticollis
  - Blepharospasm
  - Facial grimacing
  - Forced opening or closing of the mouth
- The limbs may also adopt abnormal but characteristic postures
- The age at onset influences both the clinical findings and the prognosis. With onset in childhood, there is usually a family history of the disorder, symptoms commonly commence in the legs, and progression is likely until there is severe disability from generalized dystonia
- In contrast, when onset is later, a positive family history is unlikely, initial symptoms are often in the arms or axial structures, and severe disability does not usually occur, although generalized dystonia may ultimately develop in some patients

DIFFERENTIAL DIAGNOSIS

- Perinatal anoxia
- Birth trauma
- Neonatal kernicterus
- Wilson's disease
- Huntington's disease
- Parkinsonism
- Sequela of encephalitis lethargica
- Neuroleptic drug therapy
- Dopa-responsive dystonia

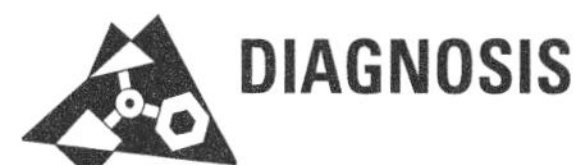

DIAGNOSIS

IMAGING STUDIES

- Investigations (including MRI or CT imaging) reveal no cause for the abnormal movements

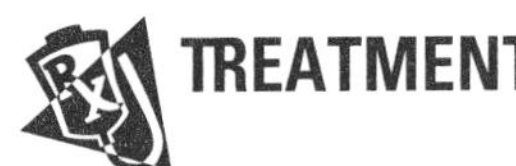

TREATMENT

MEDICATIONS

- Idiopathic torsion dystonia usually responds poorly to drugs
- Levodopa, diazepam, baclofen, carbamazepine, amantadine, or anticholinergic medication (in high dosage) is occasionally helpful
- If not, a trial of treatment with phenothiazines or haloperidol may be worthwhile
- In each case, the dose has to be individualized, depending on response and tolerance. However, the doses of these latter drugs that are required for benefit usually lead to mild parkinsonism

THERAPEUTIC PROCEDURES

- Stereotactic thalamotomy is sometimes helpful with predominantly unilateral dystonia, especially when this involves the limbs
- The utility of deep brain stimulation is under study

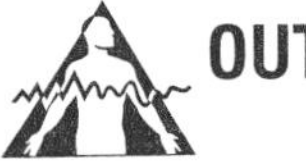

OUTCOME

PROGNOSIS

- A distinct variety of dominantly inherited dystonia, mapping to a genetic locus on chromosome 14q, is remarkably responsive to levodopa
- About one-third of patients eventually become so severely disabled that they are confined to chair or bed, while another one-third are affected only mildly

EVIDENCE

PRACTICE GUIDELINES

- Sanger TD et al: Task Force on Childhood Motor Disorders. Classification and definition of disorders causing hypertonia in childhood. Pediatrics 2003;111:e89. [PMID: 12509602]

INFORMATION FOR PATIENTS

- National Institute of Neurological Disorders and Stroke
  - http://www.ninds.nih.gov/disorders/the_dystonias/detail_the_dystonias.htm
- Worldwide Education and Awareness for Movement Disorders
  - http://www.mdvu.org/library/pediatric/dystonia/

REFERENCES

- Bressman SB et al: Diagnostic criteria for dystonia in DYT1 families. Neurology 2002;59:1780. [PMID: 12473770]
- Defazio G et al: Epidemiology of primary dystonia. Lancet Neurol 2004;3:673. [PMID: 15488460]
- Kanovsky P: Dystonia: a disorder of motor programming or motor execution? Mov Disord 2002;17:1143. [PMID: 12465050]
- Nemeth AH: The genetics of primary dystonias and related disorders. Brain 2002;125:695. [PMID: 11912106]

Author(s)

Michael J. Aminoff, MD, DSc, FRCP

Echinococcosis

KEY FEATURES

ESSENTIALS OF DIAGNOSIS

Cystic hydatid disease

- History of exposure to dogs associated with livestock in a hydatid-endemic region
- A liver cyst that may remain silent for 10–20 or more years until it becomes large enough to be palpable, to be visible as an abdominal swelling, or (rarely) to produce symptoms due to leakage or rupture
- Positive serological tests

GENERAL CONSIDERATIONS

- Parasitism by the larval stage of four *Echinococcus* species. *E granulosus* (cystic hydatid disease) and *E multilocularis* (alveolar hydatid disease) are the most important

Cystic hydatid disease (unilocular hydatid disease)

- There are two major strains, the pastoral and the sylvatic
- The **pastoral** strain—which is more pathogenic to humans—has a transmission cycle in which dogs are the definitive host, and sheep (usually) and cattle and other domestic livestock are intermediate hosts
- The **sylvatic**, or northern, strain is maintained in wolves and wild moose and reindeer
- Human infection occurs when eggs passed in dog feces are swallowed, penetrate the intestinal mucosa, enter the portal bloodstream, and are carried to the liver where they become hydatid cysts (65% of all cysts)
- Some larvae reach the lung (25%) and develop into pulmonary hydatids
- Infrequently, cysts form in the brain, bones, skeletal muscles, kidneys, spleen, or other tissues
- Cysts of the sylvatic strain tend to localize in the lungs
- In the liver, cysts may increase in size 1–30 mm in diameter per year and become enormous, but symptoms generally do not develop until they reach about 10 cm
- Some cysts die spontaneously; others may persist unchanged for years
- Part or all of the inner layer of hepatic and splenic cysts may calcify, which does not necessarily mean cyst death

Alveolar hydatid disease (multilocular hydatid disease)

- The life cycle involves foxes (sometimes wolves) as definitive hosts and microtine rodents as intermediate hosts. Domestic dogs and cats can also become infected with the adult tapeworm when they eat infected wild rodents
- Human infection is by accidental ingestion of tapeworm eggs passed in fox or dog feces

DEMOGRAPHICS

- Endemic foci of *E granulosus* are in eastern Europe, Russia, Australia, New Zealand, India, and the United Kingdom; in North America, foci are in the western United States, the lower Mississippi valley, Alaska, and northwestern Canada
- *E multilocularis* occurs only in the northern hemisphere. The highest prevalence (15%) has been reported from villages in China

CLINICAL FINDINGS

SYMPTOMS AND SIGNS

Cystic hydatid disease (liver)

- Cyst may remain asymtomatic for 20 or more years until it becomes large enough to produce symptoms
- Right upper quadrant mass that may be palpable and even visible
- Right upper quadrant pain, nausea, and vomiting
- Pressure effects by the cyst may result in biliary obstruction, with secondary bacterial cholangitis, cirrhosis, and portal hypertension
- A characteristic allergic clinical syndrome may follow intrabiliary extrusion of cyst contents—jaundice, biliary colic, urticaria, and a rise in the eosinophil count
- Rupture can occur into the pleural, pericardial, or peritoneal space or into the duodenum, colon, or renal pelvis
- If a cyst ruptures suddenly, anaphylaxis and death may occur

Alveolar hydatid disease

- Alveolar cysts primarily localize in the liver, where they may extend locally or metastasize to other tissues
- The larval mass has poorly defined borders and behaves like a neoplasm
- Lung involvement is rare, usually occurring by direct hepatic extension

DIFFERENTIAL DIAGNOSIS

- Amebic or pyogenic liver abscess
- Malignant or benign tumor of liver or other involved organ
- Fascioliasis (sheep liver fluke)
- Clonorchiasis (Chinese liver fluke)
- Choledocholithiasis
- Congenital liver cyst or liver cyst associated with polycystic kidney disease
- Cavitary pulmonary tuberculosis
- Cysticercosis

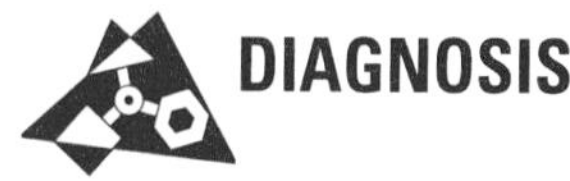

DIAGNOSIS

LABORATORY TESTS

- The immunoblot test is the test of choice (95% specific and 91% sensitive for liver cysts); the arc 5 test is also diagnostic. In both tests, cross-reactions can occur with *Taenia solium* cysticercosis infections
- The serological tests (ELISA and Western blot) are usually positive and differentiate *E granulosa* from *E multilocularis*
- In solitary lung cysts, false-negative serology results occur in up to 50% of infections
- Persons from whom cysts have been completely removed and carriers of dead cysts may become seronegative
- Eosinophilia is uncommon except after cyst rupture
- Liver function tests are usually normal

IMAGING STUDIES

Cystic hydatid disease

- The method of choice for liver and splenic cysts is sonography (specificity 90%) followed by CT and MRI; nearly pathognomonic is the presence within a hydatid cyst of daughter cysts; they must be distinguished, however, from blood clots within the cavity of simple cysts
- Chest films may show an elevated diaphragm when liver cysts are present
- Pulmonary cysts are best detected by chest films (calcification of the wall is rare); CT and MRI can also be done
- An intravenous urogram or bone scan may detect cysts at other sites

Alveolar hydatid disease

- X-rays show hepatomegaly and characteristic scattered areas of radiolucency, often outlined by 2- to 4-mm calcific rings

DIAGNOSTIC PROCEDURES

- Although the procedure was contraindicated, ultrasonic-guided percutaneous aspiration of hydatid cysts followed by injection of a scolicidal agent and use of oral albendazole is now used for diagnosis

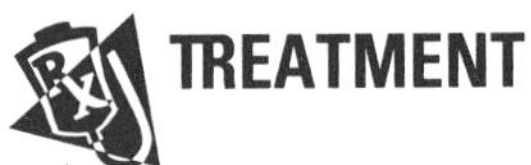

TREATMENT

MEDICATIONS

Cystic hydatid disease

- Surgical resection is now partially supplanted by antihelmintic treatment
- One approach is to give albendazole to asymptomatic patients whose cysts are small and not in danger of rupture. If, after 6–9 months, the cyst has not disappeared or clearly died, it can be removed surgically
- **Albendazole,** four tablets (800 mg) PO daily in divided doses with meals for 3 months, is the drug of choice; continue for up to 6 months if there is a response
- Relapses occur and should be retreated
- Bone cysts are more refractory and may require a year of treatment
- Drug side effects include reversible low-grade aminotransferase elevations (15%), leukopenia to 2900/μL (2%), rare gastrointestinal symptoms (including pain at cyst sites), dizziness or headache, alopecia, rash, and pruritus. The drug is contraindicated in pregnancy
- **Praziquantel** kills protoscoleces within hydatid cysts but does not affect the germinal membrane. The drug is being evaluated as adjunctive therapy with albendazole

Alveolar hydatid disease

- Long-term drug therapy (5 years to life) for patients with nonresectable masses is with oral albendazole (preferred) (800 mg day in divided doses) or with oral mebendazole (40 mg/kg/day in divided doses with fatty meals); the drugs inhibit growth of the parasite and have extended patient survival, but larval tissue is not completely destroyed

SURGERY

- The main surgical options available for liver cysts are partial hepatic resection, pericystectomy, and cystectomy
- Pulmonary cysts are treated by surgery plus chemotherapy
- Preoperatively, to reduce the risk of recurrence due to spillage, two drugs (taken with meals) are used for 1 month: albendazole, 10 mg/kg/day in two divided doses, and praziquantel, 25 mg/kg/day. Postoperatively, albendazole should be continued for 1 month; the additional use of praziquantel is under evaluation
- For alveolar hydatid disease, treatment is by surgical removal of the entire larval mass when possible, accompanied by drug treatment

THERAPEUTIC PROCEDURES

- Under ultrasonic guidance, percutaneous aspiration and injection of a scolicidal agent can be used to treat accessible cysts in patients who are inoperable or refuse surgery and are not candidates for a chemotherapeutic trial. The patient should be covered with oral albendazole
- The procedure is contraindicated for cysts that communicate with the biliary tree, those that are superficially loculated, or those that have thick internal septal divisions

OUTCOME

FOLLOW-UP

- Liver function tests and complete blood cell counts should be monitored weekly when using albendazole

PROGNOSIS

- About 15% of untreated patients eventually die because of the disease or its complications
- Ninety percent of patients with nonresectable masses die within 10 years
- 25% recurrence rates after surgery

WHEN TO REFER

- All patients should be referred to a specialist with expertise in this problem

WHEN TO ADMIT

- Patients with symptomatic cysts
- Patients who will have percutaneous aspiration of cysts or surgery

PREVENTION

- In endemic areas, prevention is by prophylactic treatment of pet dogs with 5 mg/kg of praziquantel at monthly intervals to remove adult tapeworms and by health education to prevent feeding of offal to dogs

EVIDENCE

PRACTICE GUIDELINES

- Heath DD et al: Progress in control of hydatidosis using vaccination—a review of formulation and delivery of the vaccine and recommendations for practical use in control programmes. Acta Trop 2003;85:133. [PMID: 12606090]

WEB SITE

- CDC—Division of Parasitic Diseases
  - http://www.cdc.gov/ncidod/dpd/parasites/alveolarechinococcosis/default.htm

INFORMATION FOR PATIENTS

- Centers for Disease Control
  - http://www.cdc.gov/ncidod/dpd/parasites/alveolarhydatid/factsht_alveolar_hydatid.htm
- National Institutes of Health
  - http://www.nlm.nih.gov/medlineplus/ency/article/000676.htm

REFERENCES

- Chrieki M: Echinococcosis—an emerging parasite in the immigrant population. Am Fam Physician 2002;66:817. [PMID: 12322773]
- Ozaslan E et al: Endoscopic therapy in the management of hepatobiliary hydatid disease. J Clin Gastroenterol 2002;35:160. [PMID: 12172363]
- Yorganci K et al: Surgical treatment of hydatid cysts of the liver in the era of percutaneous treatment. Am J Surg 2002;184:63. [PMID: 12135724]

Ectopic Pregnancy

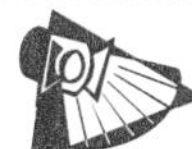

KEY FEATURES

ESSENTIALS OF DIAGNOSIS

- Amenorrhea or irregular bleeding and spotting
  - Pelvic pain, usually adnexal
  - Adnexal mass by clinical examination or ultrasound
  - Failure of serum level of human chorionic gonadotropin (hCG) to double every 48 h
- No intrauterine pregnancy on transvaginal ultrasound with serum hCG of ≥ 2000 mU/mL

GENERAL CONSIDERATIONS

- Occurs in about 1 of 150 live births, with 98% of cases being tubal pregnancies
- Implantation may also occur in the peritoneum or abdominal viscera, the ovary, and the cervix
- Undiagnosed or undetected ectopic pregnancy is the most common cause of first-trimester maternal death in the United States

DEMOGRAPHICS

- Conditions that prevent or retard migration of the fertilized ovum can predispose to ectopic implantation
- Specific risk factors are a history of infertility, pelvic inflammatory disease, ruptured appendix, and prior tubal surgery

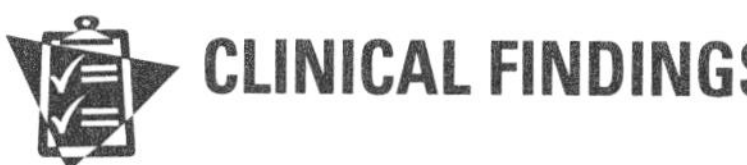

CLINICAL FINDINGS

SYMPTOMS AND SIGNS

- 40% of cases are acute
  - Sudden onset of severe, nonradiating, intermittent lancinating lower quadrant pain
  - Backache present during attacks
  - Shock in about 10%, often after pelvic examination
  - At least two-thirds of patients give a history of abnormal menstruation
- 60% of cases are chronic
  - Blood leaks from the tubal ampulla over days
  - Persistent vaginal spotting is reported
  - A pelvic mass is palpable
  - Abdominal distention and mild paralytic ileus are often present

DIFFERENTIAL DIAGNOSIS

- Acute appendicitis
- Intrauterine pregnancy (threatened abortion)
- Pelvic inflammatory disease
- Ruptured corpus luteum cyst or ovarian follicle
- Urinary calculi
- Tuboovarian abscess
- Gestational trophoblastic neoplasia, eg, hydatidiform mole
- Shock or sepsis due to other causes

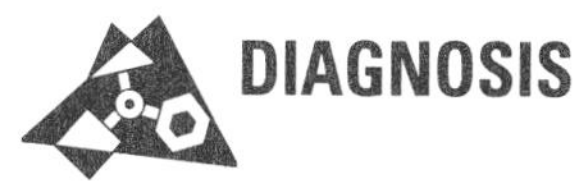

DIAGNOSIS

LABORATORY TESTS

- Complete blood cell count may show anemia and slight leukocytosis
- Serum hCG levels are lower than expected for a normal pregnancy of the same gestational age
- Serum hCG levels may rise slowly or plateau rather than double every 48 h as in viable early pregnancy or fall as in spontaneous abortion

IMAGING STUDIES

- Endovaginal ultrasound may identify the ectopic pregnancy
- An empty uterine cavity demonstrated by abdominal utrasound with an hCG of 6500 mU/mL is virtually diagnostic of an ectopic pregnancy

DIAGNOSTIC PROCEDURES

- Culdocentesis is rarely used in evaluation

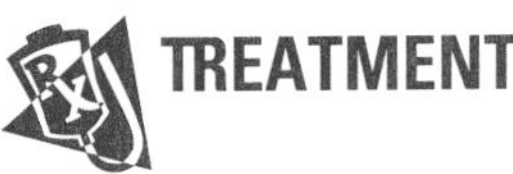

TREATMENT

MEDICATIONS

- Methotrexate (50 mg/m^2) is acceptable medical therapy for early ectopic pregnancies less than 3.5 cm and unruptured, without active bleeding
- Iron supplementation may be necessary for anemia during convalescence
- All Rh-negative paitents should receive Rho(D) Ig (300 µg)

SURGERY

- Laparoscopy is the surgical procedure of choice to both confirm and permit removal of an ectopic pregnancy without need for an exploratory laparotomy
- Salpingostomy with removal of the ectopic or partial salpingectomy can usually be performed laparoscopically
- Injection of indigo carmine into the uterine cavity with flow through the contralateral tube can demonstrate its patency

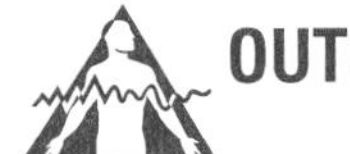

OUTCOME

COMPLICATIONS

- Tubal infertility

PROGNOSIS

- Repeat tubal pregnancy occurs in 12%
- Early ultrasound confirmation of intrauterine gestation with next pregnancy

WHEN TO REFER

- For suggestive symptoms, laboratory tests, and especially ultrasound findings that support the diagnosis

WHEN TO ADMIT

- All suspected cases of ruptured ectopic pregnancy

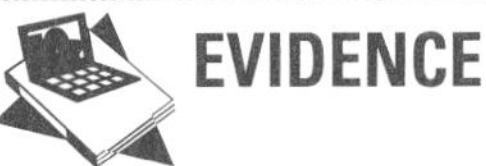

EVIDENCE

PRACTICE GUIDELINES

- ACOG Practice Bulletin. Medical management of tubal pregnancy Number 3, December 1998. Clinical management guidelines for obstetrician-gynecologists. American College of Obstetricians and Gynecologists. Int J Gynaecol Obstet 1999;65:97. [PMID: 10390113]

WEB SITES

- Ectopic Pregnancy Demonstration Case
  - http://www.brighamrad.harvard.edu/Cases/bwh/hcache/94/full.html
- Guidelines, Recommendations, and Evidence-Based Medicine in Obstetrics
  - http://matweb.hcuge.ch/matweb/endo/cours_4e_MREG/obstetrics_gynecology_guidelines.htm

INFORMATION FOR PATIENTS

- March of Dimes: Ectopic and Molar Pregnancy
  - http://www.marchofdimes.com/professionals/681_1189.asp
- MedlinePlus: Ectopic Pregnancy
  - http://www.nlm.nih.gov/medlineplus/ency/article/000895.htm
- Nemours Foundation
  - http://kidshealth.org/parent/pregnancy_newborn/pregnancy/ectopic.html

REFERENCES

- Bickell NA et al: Time and risk of ruptured tubal pregnancy. Obstet Gynecol 2004;104:789. [PMID: 15458903]
- Hajenius PJ et al: Interventions for tubal ectopic pregnancy. Cochrane Database Syst Rev 2000;(2):CD000324. [PMID: 10796710]
- Lipscomb GH et al: Methotrexate for treatment of ectopic pregnancy. Am J Obstet Gynecol 2002;186:1192. [PMID: 12066097]

Author(s)

William R. Crombleholme, MD

Edema, Lower Extremity

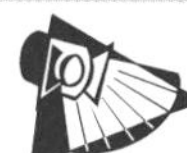

KEY FEATURES

ESSENTIALS OF DIAGNOSIS

- History of venous thromboembolism
- Lower extremity asymmetry
- Lower extremity pain
- Lower extremity dependence
- Time course: acute or chronic edema

GENERAL CONSIDERATIONS

- Lower extremities can swell in response to
  - Increased venous or lymphatic pressures
  - Decreased intravascular oncotic pressure
  - Increased capillary leak
  - Local injury or infection
- Acute lower extremity edema: deep venous thrombosis (DVT)
- Other causes of acute edema
  - Ruptured popliteal cyst
  - Calf strain or trauma
  - Cellulitis
  - Drug therapy with calcium channel blockers (particularly felodipine and amlodipine), thioglitazones, and minoxidil
- Chronic venous insufficiency is the most common cause of chronic lower extremity edema, affecting up to 2% of the population
- Other causes of chronic edema
  - Postphlebitic syndrome with valvular incompetence
  - Congestive heart failure (CHF)
  - Cirrhosis
  - Drug therapy (as above)

CLINICAL FINDINGS

SYMPTOMS AND SIGNS

- Assess heart, lungs, and abdomen for evidence of pulmonary hypertension (primary, or secondary to chronic lung disease), CHF, or cirrhosis
- Size of both calves should be measured 10 cm below the tibial tuberosity
- Swelling of the entire leg or swelling of one leg > 3 cm more than the other suggests deep venous obstruction
- Elicit pitting and tenderness
- Chronic venous insufficiency skin findings range from hyperpigmentation and stasis dermatitis to lipodermatosclerosis and atrophie blanche to skin ulceration
- Stasis dermatitis: brawny, fibrotic skin changes
- Skin ulceration can occur, particularly in the medial malleolar area, when due to chronic venous insufficiency
- Other causes of medial malleolar skin ulceration
  - Arterial insufficiency
  - Vasculitis
  - Infections (including cutaneous diphtheria)
  - Cancer

DIFFERENTIAL DIAGNOSIS

- Cardiovascular
  - CHF (right-sided)
  - Pericardial effusion
  - Pericarditis
  - Tricuspid regurgitation
  - Tricuspid stenosis
  - Pulmonic stenosis
  - Cor pulmonale
  - Venous insufficiency (most common)
  - Venous obstruction
- Noncardiovascular
  - Cirrhosis
  - Low albumin (nephrotic syndrome, malnutrition, protein-losing enteropathy)
  - Cellulitis
  - Premenstrual fluid retention
  - Drugs (vasodilators, eg, calcium channel blockers, salt-retaining medications, eg, nonsteroidal anti-inflammatory drugs, thiazolidinediones)
  - Musculoskeletal (Baker's cyst, gastrocnemius tear, compartment syndrome)
  - Lymphatic obstruction
  - Eclampsia
  - Hypothyroidism with myxedema
  - Filariasis
- Unilateral
  - DVT
  - Venous insufficiency
  - Baker's cyst
  - Cellulitis
  - Trauma
  - Lymphatic obstruction, eg, obstruction by pelvic tumor
  - Reflex sympathetic dystrophy

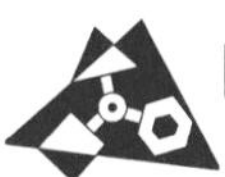

DIAGNOSIS

LABORATORY TESTS

- Serum creatinine, blood urea nitrogen
- Urinalysis
- Liver tests: alkaline phosphatase, aspartate aminotransferase, gamma glutamyltranspeptidase, total bilirubin, albumin
- Thyroid-stimulating hormone

IMAGING STUDIES

- Color duplex ultrasonography of lower extremity
- Ankle-brachial pressure index (ABPI)

DIAGNOSTIC PROCEDURES

- Consider echocardiogram

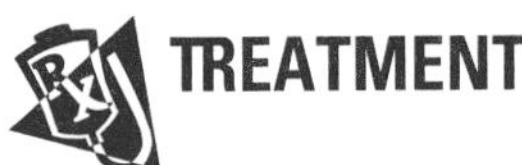

TREATMENT

THERAPEUTIC PROCEDURES

- Avoid diuretic therapy in patients with chronic venous insufficiency unless comorbid CHF or other fluid-retaining comorbid condition
- Mechanical measures effective in chronic venous insufficiency
  - Leg elevation, above the level of the heart, for 30 min three to four times daily and during sleep; and
  - Compression therapy with stockings and devices
- Refrain from using compression therapy if there are risk factors for or signs of peripheral arterial occlusive disease

OUTCOME

WHEN TO REFER

- Refer to vascular surgeon
  - Patients with chronic venous insufficiency in combination with peripheral arterial occlusive disease
  - Patients with nonhealing ulcers from chronic venous insufficiency or other causes

WHEN TO ADMIT

- Cellulitis requiring IV antibiotics
- Skin ulcers requiring grafting

EVIDENCE

WEB SITES

- Vacek JL: Chronic Edema Curbside Consult. Postgraduate Medicine Online 2000;108.
  - http://www.postgradmed.com/issues/2000/08_00/cc_aug00.htm

INFORMATION FOR PATIENTS

- Harvard Medical School, InteliHealth: Edema
  - http://www.intelihealth.com/IH/ihtIH/WSIHW000/9339/9883.html
- Mayo Clinic: Foot Swelling During Air Travel
  - http://www.mayoclinic.com/invoke.cfm?objectid=0CEA2283-31A5-4223-A11C64BC1ED3227A
- National Lymphedema Network: Lymphedema Overview
  - http://www.lymphnet.org/whatis.html

REFERENCES

- Heit JA et al: Trends in the incidence of venous stasis syndrome and venous ulcer: a 25-year population-based study. J Vasc Surg 2001;33:1022. [PMID: 11331844]
- Valencia IC et al: Chronic venous insufficiency and venous leg ulceration. J Am Acad Dermatol 2001;44:401. [PMID: 11209109]

Author(s)

Ralph Gonzales, MD

Electric Shock

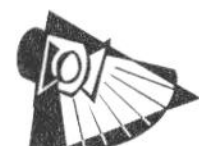

KEY FEATURES

ESSENTIALS OF DIAGNOSIS

- The extent of injury is determined by:
  - Amount and type of current
  - Duration and area of exposure
  - Pathway of the current through the body

GENERAL CONSIDERATIONS

- With alternating currents (AC) of 25–300 Hz, low voltages (< 220 Hz) tend to produce ventricular fibrillation; high voltages (> 1000 Hz), respiratory failure; intermediate voltages (220–1000 Hz), both
- More than 100 mA of domestic house current (AC) of 110 V at 60 Hz can cause ventricular fibrillation; DC current contact is more likely to cause asystole
- Lightning injuries differ from high-voltage electric shock injuries; lightning usually involves higher voltage, briefer duration of contact, asystole, nervous system injury, and multisystem pathological involvement
- Electrical burns are of three distinct types: flash (arcing) burns, flame (clothing) burns, and direct heating effect of tissues by the electric current

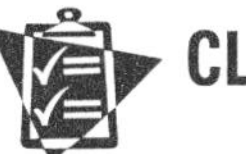

CLINICAL FINDINGS

SYMPTOMS AND SIGNS

- The lesions are usually sharply demarcated, round or oval, painless yellow-brown areas (joule burn) with inflammatory reaction
- Significant subcutaneous damage can be accompanied by little skin injury, particularly with larger skin surface area electrical contact
- Loss of consciousness
- With recovery there may be muscular pain, fatigue, headache, and nervous irritability
- The physical signs vary according to the action of the current
  - If the current passes through the heart or brainstem, death may occur immediately owing to ventricular fibrillation or apnea
  - Current passing through skeletal muscle can cause muscle necrosis and contractions severe enough to result in bone fracture
  - Current traversing peripheral nerves can cause acute or delayed neuropathy
  - Delayed effects can include damage to the spinal cord, peripheral nerves, bone, kidneys, and gastrointestinal tract and development of cataracts

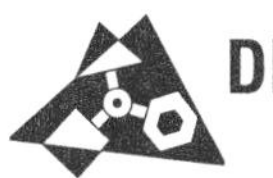

DIAGNOSIS

LABORATORY TESTS

- A urinalysis, urine myoglobin, serum creatine kinase (CK) and CK-MB, and an electrocardiogram should be obtained immediately

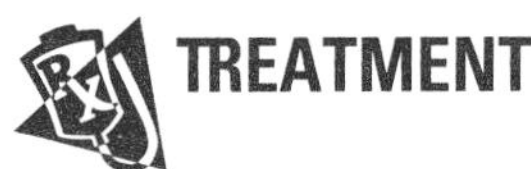

TREATMENT

THERAPEUTIC PROCEDURES

Emergency measures

- Separate victim from the electric current before initiation of CPR or other treatment; the rescuer must be protected
- Turn off the power, sever the wire with a dry wooden-handled ax, make a proper ground to divert the current, or separate the victim using nonconductive implements such as dry clothing

Hospital measures

- Evaluate for blunt trauma, dehydration, skin burns, hypertension, posttraumatic stress, acid-base disturbances, and neurological damage
- To counteract fluid losses and myoglobinuria resulting from electric shock (not lightning) burns, aggressive hydration with Ringer's lactate should seek to achieve a urine output of 50–100 mL/h

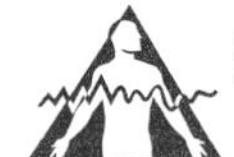

OUTCOME

COMPLICATIONS

- Complications may occur in almost any part of the body
- Most commonly include sepsis, gangrene requiring limb amputation, or neurological, cardiac, cognitive, or psychiatric dysfunction

WHEN TO ADMIT

- Lightning or unstable electric shock victims should be hospitalized
  - Observe for shock, arrhythmia, thrombosis, infarction, sudden cardiac dilation, hemorrhage, and myoglobinuria
- Indications for hospitalization include:
  - Significant arrhythmia or electrocardiographic changes
  - Large burn
  - Loss of consciousness
  - Pulmonary or cardiac symptoms
  - Evidence of significant deep tissue or organ damage
- Extra caution is indicated when the electroshock current has followed a transthoracic route (hand to hand or hand to foot) and in patients with a cardiac history

EVIDENCE

PRACTICE GUIDELINES

- European Resuscitation Council. Part 8: Advanced challenges in resuscitation. Section 3: Special challenges in ECC. 3G: Electric shock and lightning strikes. Resuscitation 2000;46:297. [PMID: 10978812]

INFORMATION FOR PATIENTS

- American College of Emergency Physicians: Safety Tips for Being Handy in the Home
  - http://www.acep.org/webportal/PatientsConsumers/HealthSubjectsByTopic/SafetyIssues/FeatureColumnSafetyTipsforBeingHan.htm
- Mayo Clinic: Electrical Shock
  - http://www.mayoclinic.com/invoke.cfm?objectid=E6844A81-4709-4E52-B0BB805D8C56E239
- Medline Plus: Electrical Injury
  - http://www.nlm.nih.gov/medlineplus/ency/article/000053.htm
- National AG Safety Database: First Aid for Electrical Accidents
  - http://www.cdc.gov/nasd/docs/d000801-d000900/d000813/d000813.html

REFERENCES

- Koumbourlis AC: Electrical injuries. Crit Care Med 2002;30(Suppl):S424. [PMID: 12528784]
- O'Keefe Gatewood M et al: Lightning injuries. Emerg Med Clin North Am 2004;22:369. [PMID: 15163573]

Author(s)

Richard Cohen, MD, MPH

Endocarditis, Infective

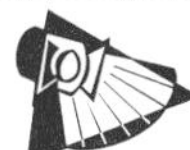

KEY FEATURES

ESSENTIALS OF DIAGNOSIS

- Preexisting organic heart lesion
- Fever
- New or changing heart murmur
- Evidence of systemic emboli
- Positive blood culture
- Evidence of vegetation on echocardiography

GENERAL CONSIDERATIONS

- Important factors that determine the clinical presentation are the nature of the infecting organism; which valve is infected; and the route of infection
- More virulent organisms, particularly *Staphylococcus aureus*
  - Rapidly progressive and destructive infection
  - Generally, acute febrile illnesses, early embolization, and acute valvular regurgitation and myocardial abscess
- Subacute presentation
  - Viridans strains of streptococci, enterococci, and a variety of other gram-positive and gram-negative bacilli, yeasts, and fungi
  - Systemic and peripheral manifestations may predominate
- Many patients have underlying cardiac disease, which is decreasing in prevalence as a risk factor
- The initiating event is colonization of the valve by bacteria during a transient or persistent bacteremia

Native valve endocarditis

- Due to viridans streptococci (60%), *S aureus* (20%), or enterococci (5–10%). Gram-negative organisms and fungi account for a small percentage
- Intravenous drug users: *S aureus* in at least 60% of cases and 80–90% of tricuspid valve infections. Enterococci and streptococci comprise the balance in about equal proportions

Prosthetic valve endocarditis

- **Early** infections (within 2 months of valve implantation) are commonly caused by staphylococci—both coagulase-positive and coagulase-negative—gram-negative organisms, and fungi
- **Late** prosthetic valve endocarditis resembles native valve endocarditis; the majority are caused by streptococci, though coagulase-negative staphylococci cause a significant proportion of cases

DEMOGRAPHICS

- Injection drug use
- Underlying valvular disease

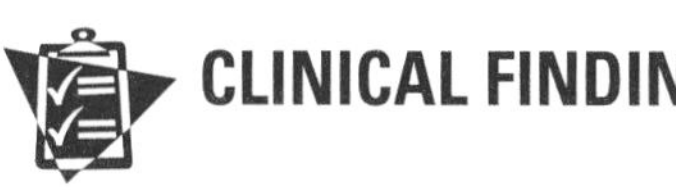

CLINICAL FINDINGS

SYMPTOMS AND SIGNS

- Most present with a febrile illness that has lasted several days to 2 weeks
- Heart murmurs
  - In the majority of cases, heart murmurs are stable
  - Changing murmur is significant diagnostically, but it is the exception rather than the rule
- Characteristic peripheral lesions occur in up to 20–25% of patients
  - Petechiae (on the palate or conjunctiva or beneath the fingernails)
  - Subungual ("splinter") hemorrhages
  - Osler nodes (painful, violaceous raised lesions of the fingers, toes, or feet)
  - Janeway lesions (painless erythematous lesions of the palms or soles)
  - Roth spots (exudative lesions in the retina)

DIFFERENTIAL DIAGNOSIS

- Valvular abnormality without endocarditis, eg, rheumatic heart disease, mitral valve prolapse, bicuspid or calcific aortic valve
- Flow murmur (anemia, pregnancy, hyperthyroidism, sepsis)
- Atrial myxoma
- Noninfective endocarditis, eg, systemic lupus erythematosus (Libman-Saks endocarditis), marantic endocarditis (nonbacterial thrombotic endocarditis)
- Hematuria due to other causes, eg, glomerulonephritis, renal cell carcinoma
- Acute rheumatic fever
- Vasculitis

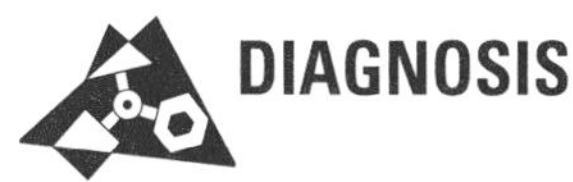

DIAGNOSIS

LABORATORY TESTS

- Blood culture is the most important diagnostic tool; to maximize the yield, obtain three sets of blood cultures at least 1 h apart before starting antibiotics
- In acute endocarditis, leukocytosis is common; in subacute cases, anemia of chronic disease and a normal white blood cell count are the rule
- Hematuria and proteinuria as well as renal dysfunction may result from emboli or immunologically mediated glomerulonephritis
- **Duke criteria** for the diagnosis
  - Major criteria of (1) two positive blood cultures for a typical microorganism of infective endocarditis; and (2) positive echocardiography (vegetation, myocardial abscess, or new partial dehiscence of a prosthetic valve) or a new regurgitant murmur
  - Minor criteria include (1) the presence of a predisposing condition; (2) fever >38°C; (3) embolic disease; (4) immunological phenomena (Osler nodes, Roth spots, glomerulonephritis, rheumatoid factor); (5) positive blood cultures not meeting the major criteria; and (6) a positive echocardiogram not meeting the major criteria
  - A definite diagnosis is made with 80% accuracy if two major criteria, one major criterion and three minor criteria, or five minor criteria are fulfilled. If none of these criteria is met and either an alternative explanation for illness is identified or the patient has defervesced within 4 days, endocarditis is highly unlikely

IMAGING STUDIES

- The chest x-ray may show the underlying cardiac abnormality and, in right-sided endocarditis, pulmonary infiltrates
- Echocardiography
  - Transthoracic echocardiography is 55–65% sensitive; therefore, it cannot rule out endocarditis but may confirm a clinical suspicion
  - Transesophageal echocardiography is 90% sensitive in detecting vegetations and is particularly useful for identifying valve ring abscesses, and pulmonary and prosthetic valve endocarditis

DIAGNOSTIC PROCEDURES

- The ECG is nondiagnostic. Changing conduction abnormalities suggest myocardial abscess formation

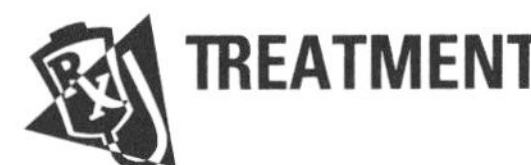

TREATMENT

MEDICATIONS

- See Table 139

SURGERY

- Valvular regurgitation resulting in acute heart failure that does not resolve promptly after institution of medical therapy is an indication for valve replacement even if active infection is present, especially if the aortic valve is involved
- Infections that do not respond to appropriate antimicrobial therapy after 7–10 days (ie, persistent fevers, positive blood cultures despite therapy) are more likely to be eradicated if the valve is replaced
- Nearly always required for fungal endocarditis and is more often necessary with gram-negative bacilli
- Infection involving the sinus of Valsalva or produces septal abscesses
- Recurrent infection with the same organism often indicates that surgery is necessary, especially with infected prosthetic valves
- Continuing embolization when the infection is otherwise responding may be an indication for surgery

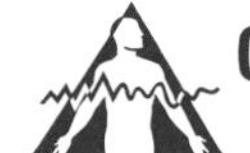

OUTCOME

FOLLOW-UP

- If infection is caused by viridans streptococci, enterococci, or coagulase-negative staphylococci, defervescence occurs in 3–4 days on average, whereas if infection is caused by *Staphylococcus aureus* or *Pseudomonas aeruginosa*, patients may remain febrile for a week or more

COMPLICATIONS

- Destruction of infected heart valves
- Myocardial abscesses leading to conduction disturbances
- Peripheral embolization
- Mycotic aneurysms
- Right-sided endocarditis, which usually involves the tricuspid valve, often leads to septic pulmonary emboli, causing infarction and lung abscesses

PROGNOSIS

- Higher morbidity and mortality associated with nonstreptococcal etiology, aortic or prosthetic valvular infection

WHEN TO REFER

- Infectious diseases consultation recommended
- Patients with signs of heart failure should be referred for surgical evaluation

WHEN TO ADMIT

- Patients with evidence of heart failure
- Patients with a nonstreptococcal etiology
- For initiation of antimicrobial therapy

PREVENTION

- Prophylactic antibiotics are given to patients with predisposing congenital or valvular anomalies who are to have any of a number of procedures (Tables 137 and 138). Current recommendations are given in Table 136

EVIDENCE

PRACTICE GUIDELINES

- Flachskampf FA et al: Working Group on Echocardiography of the European Society of Cardiology. Guidelines from the Working Group. Recommendations for performing transesophageal echocardiography. Eur J Echocardiogr 2001;2:8. [PMID: 11913372]
- National Guideline Clearinghouse
  - http://www.guideline.gov/summary/summary.aspx?doc_id=5216
- Olaison L et al: Current best practices and guidelines indications for surgical intervention in infective endocarditis. Infect Dis Clin North Am 2002;16:453. [PMID: 12092482]

WEB SITES

- CDC—Emerging Infectious Diseases
  - http://www.cdc.gov/ncidod/EID/vol10no6/03-0848.htm
- Infective Endocarditis
  - http://edcenter.med.cornell.edu/Pathology_Cases/Vascular_Infections/VI_Summary.html

INFORMATION FOR PATIENTS

- American Heart Association
  - http://www.americanheart.org/presenter.jhtml?identifier=4436
  - http://www.americanheart.org/presenter.jhtml?identifier=11086
- JAMA patient page: Endocarditis. JAMA 2002;288:128.

REFERENCES

- Cabell CH et al: Changing patient characteristics and the effect on mortality in endocarditis. Arch Intern Med 2002;162:90. [PMID: 11784225]
- Chirouze C et al; International Collaboration on Endocarditis Study Group: Prognostic factors in 61 cases of *Staphylococcus aureus* prosthetic valve infective endocarditis from the International Collaboration on Endocarditis merged database. Clin Infect Dis 2004;38:1323. [PMID: 15127349]
- Le T et al: Combination antibiotic therapy for infective endocarditis. Clin Infect Dis 2003;36:615. [PMID: 12594643]
- Olaison L et al: Enterococcal endocarditis in Sweden, 1995–1999: can shorter therapy with aminoglycosides be used? Clin Infect Dis 2002;34:159. [PMID: 11740702]

Author(s)

Henry F. Chambers, MD

Endometrial Cancer

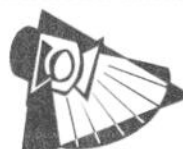

KEY FEATURES

ESSENTIALS OF DIAGNOSIS

- Abnormal bleeding is the presenting sign in 80% of cases
- Papanicolaou smear frequently negative
- After a negative pregnancy test, endometrial tissue is required to confirm the diagnosis

GENERAL CONSIDERATIONS

- Adenocarcinoma of the endometrium is the second most common cancer of the female genital tract

DEMOGRAPHICS

- Occurs most often in women 50–70 years of age
- History of unopposed estrogen in the past; this increased risk persists for 10 or more years after stopping the drug
- Obesity, nulliparity, diabetes, and polycystic ovaries with prolonged anovulation and the extended use of tamoxifen for the treatment of breast cancer are also risk factors

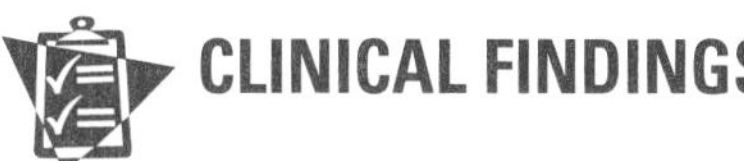

CLINICAL FINDINGS

SYMPTOMS AND SIGNS

- Vaginal bleeding
- Obstruction of the cervix with collection of pus (pyometra) or blood (hematometra) causing lower abdominal pain may occur
- However, pain generally occurs late in the disease, with metastases or infection

DIFFERENTIAL DIAGNOSIS

- Endometrial hyperplasia or proliferation
- Uterine leiomyomas (fibroids)
- Endometrial polyp
- Cervical cancer
- Atrophic endometrium
- Adenomyosis (uterine endometriosis)
- Atrophic vaginitis
- Ovarian tumor
- Leiomyosarcoma

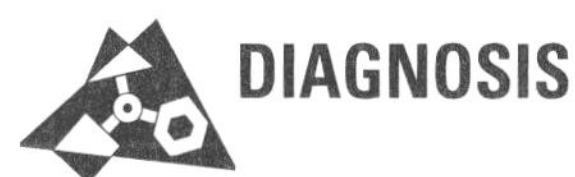

DIAGNOSIS

LABORATORY TESTS

- Papanicolaou smears of the cervix occasionally show atypical endometrial cells but are an insensitive diagnostic tool

IMAGING STUDIES

- Vaginal ultrasonography may show thickness of the endometrium indicating hypertrophy and possible neoplastic change

DIAGNOSTIC PROCEDURES

- Endocervical and endometrial sampling is the only reliable means of diagnosis. Adequate specimens of each can usually be obtained during an office procedure with local anesthesia (paracervical block)
- Simultaneous hysteroscopy can localize polyps or other lesions within the uterine cavity
- Examination under anesthesia, endometrial and endocervical sampling, chest x-ray, intravenous urography, cystoscopy, sigmoidoscopy, transvaginal sonography, and MRI for extent of disease
- The staging is based on the surgical and pathologic evaluation

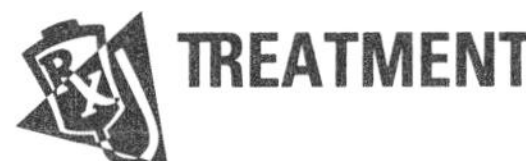

TREATMENT

MEDICATIONS

- Advanced or metastatic endometrial adenocarcinoma may be palliated with large doses of progestins, eg, medroxyprogesterone, 400 mg IM weekly, or megestrol acetate, 80–160 mg daily PO
- The role of chemotherapy alone or with irradiation is currently under investigation

SURGERY

- Treatment consists of total hysterectomy and bilateral salpingo-oophorectomy. Peritoneal material for cytologic examination is routinely taken

THERAPEUTIC PROCEDURES

- Preliminary external irradiation or intracavitary radium therapy is indicated if the cancer is poorly differentiated or if the uterus is definitely enlarged in the absence of myomas

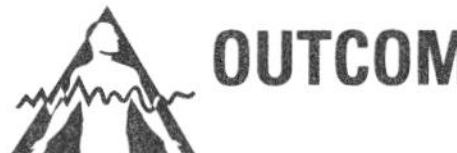

OUTCOME

FOLLOW-UP

- Examination every 3–4 months for 2 years, then every 6 months

COMPLICATIONS

- Related to therapy, radiation vs surgery

PROGNOSIS

- With early diagnosis and treatment, the 5-year survival is 80–85%

WHEN TO REFER

- All patients with carcinoma of the endometrium should be referred to a gynecologist
- If invasion deep into the myometrium has occurred or if sampled preaortic lymph nodes are positive for tumor, postoperative irradiation is indicated

PREVENTION

- Prompt endometrial sampling for patients who report abnormal menstrual bleeding or postmenopausal uterine bleeding will reveal many incipient as well as clinical cases of endometrial cancer
- Younger women with chronic anovulation are at risk for endometrial hyperplasia and subsequent endometrial cancer. They can reduce the risk of hyperplasia almost completely with the use of oral contraceptives or cyclic progestin therapy

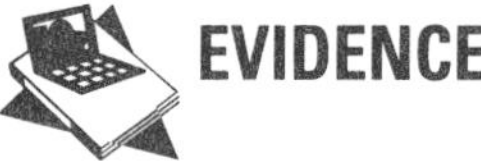

EVIDENCE

PRACTICE GUIDELINES

- American Cancer Society guidelines on testing for early endometrial cancer detection—update 2001
  - http://www.guideline.gov/summary/summary.aspx?doc_id=2749&nbr=1975
- Teng N et al; NCCN Endometrial Cancer and Uterine Sarcoma Practice Guidelines Panel. National Comprehensive Cancer Network: Uterine Cancers v.1.2004
  - http://www.nccn.org/professionals/physician_gls/PDF/uterine.pdf

WEB SITE

- National Cancer Institute: Endometrial Cancer Information for Patients and Health Professionals
  - http://www.cancer.gov/cancertopics/types/endometrial/

INFORMATION FOR PATIENTS

- American Academy of Family Physicians: Endometrial Cancer
  - http://familydoctor.org/021.xml
- American Cancer Society: Endometrial Cancer
  - http://www.cancer.org/docroot/CRI/CRI_2_3x.asp?rnav=cridg&dt=11
- JAMA patient page: Endometrial cancer. JAMA 2002;288:1678. [PMID: 12362917]
- MedlinePlus: Endometrial Cancer
  - http://www.nlm.nih.gov/medlineplus/ency/article/000910.htm
- National Institutes of Health
  - http://www.nci.nih.gov/cancerinfo/pdq/prevention/endometrial/patient/
  - http://www.nci.nih.gov/cancerinfo/pdq/treatment/endometrial/patient/#Section_92

REFERENCES

- Hernandez E: Endometrial carcinoma: a primer for the generalist. Obstet Gynecol North Am 2001;28:743. [PMID: 11766149]
- Mariani A et al: Surgical stage I endometrial cancer: predictors of distant failure and death. Gynecol Oncol 2002;87:274. [PMID: 12468325]

Author(s)

H. Trent MacKay, MD, MPH

Endometriosis

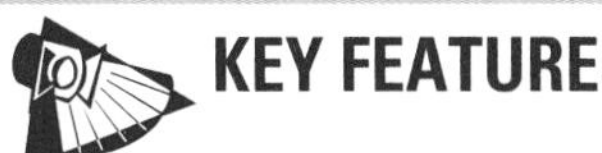

KEY FEATURES

ESSENTIALS OF DIAGNOSIS

- Pelvic pain related to menstrual cycle
- Dysmenorrhea
- Dyspareunia
- Increased frequency among infertile women

GENERAL CONSIDERATIONS

- An aberrant growth of endometrium outside the uterus, particularly in the dependent parts of the pelvis and in the ovaries
- Common cause of abnormal bleeding and secondary dysmenorrhea
- Its causes, pathogenesis, and natural course are poorly understood

DEMOGRAPHICS

- The prevalence in the United States is 6–10% among fertile women and four- to five-fold greater than that in infertile women

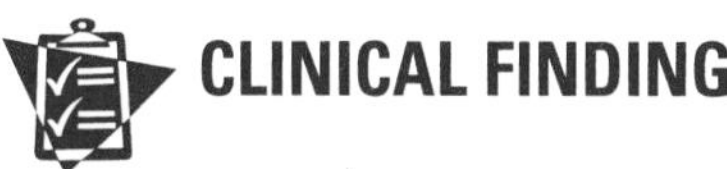

CLINICAL FINDINGS

SYMPTOMS AND SIGNS

- Aching pain tends to be constant, beginning 2–7 days before the onset of menses, and becomes increasingly severe until flow slackens
- Depending on the location and extent of the endometrial implants, infertility, dyspareunia, or rectal pain with bleeding may result
- Pelvic examination may disclose tender indurated nodules in the cul-de-sac

DIFFERENTIAL DIAGNOSIS

- Adenomyosis (uterine endometriosis)
- Pelvic inflammatory disease
- Uterine leiomyomas (fibroids)
- Primary dysmenorrhea
- Ovarian tumor
- Endometrial cancer
- Pelvic adhesions
- Irritable bowel syndrome
- Interstitial cystitis

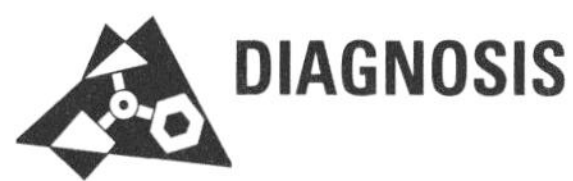

DIAGNOSIS

IMAGING STUDIES

- Ultrasound examination will often reveal complex fluid-filled masses that cannot be distinguished from neoplasms
- MRI is more sensitive and specific than ultrasound, particularly in the diagnosis of adnexal masses

DIAGNOSTIC PROCEDURES

- The clinical diagnosis of endometriosis is presumptive and is usually confirmed by laparoscopy or laparotomy

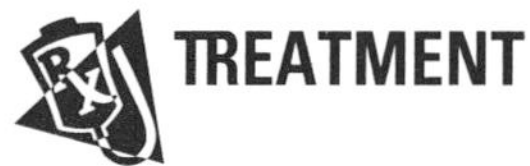

TREATMENT

MEDICATIONS

- Medications are designed to inhibit ovulation over 4–9 months to prevent cyclic stimulation of endometrial implants
- The optimum duration of therapy is not known
- The gonadotropin-releasing hormone analogs such as nafarelin nasal spray, 0.2–0.4 mg twice daily, or long-acting injectable leuprolide acetate, 3.75 mg IM monthly, used for 6 months, suppress ovulation. Side effects consisting of vasomotor symptoms and bone demineralization may be relieved by "add-back" therapy with norethindrone, 5–10 mg daily
- Danazol is used for 4–6 months in the lowest dose necessary to suppress menstruation, usually 200–400 mg twice daily. Danazol has a high incidence of androgenic side effects, including decreased breast size, weight gain, acne, and hirsutism
- Any of the combination oral contraceptives, the contraceptive patch or vaginal ring, may be used continuously for 6–12 months. Breakthrough bleeding can be treated with conjugated estrogens, 1.25 mg daily for 1 week, or estradiol, 2 mg daily for 1 week
- Medroxyprogesterone acetate, 100 mg IM every 2 weeks for four doses; then 100 mg every 4 weeks; add oral estrogen or estradiol valerate, 30 mg IM, for breakthrough bleeding. Use for 6–9 months
- Low-dose oral contraceptives can also be given cyclically; prolonged suppression of ovulation will often inhibit further stimulation of residual endometriosis, especially if taken after one of the therapies mentioned above
- Analgesics, with or without codeine, may be needed during menses. Nonsteroidal anti-inflammatory drugs may be helpful

SURGERY

- Surgical treatment of endometriosis—particularly extensive disease—is effective both in reducing pain and in promoting fertility
  - Laparoscopic ablation of endometrial implants along with uterine nerve ablation significantly reduces pain
  - Ablation of implants and, if necessary, removal of ovarian endometriomas enhance fertility, although subsequent pregnancy rates are related to the severity of disease
  - Women with disabling pain who no longer desire childbearing can be treated definitively with total abdominal hysterectomy and bilateral salpingo-oophorectomy (TAH-BSO)

THERAPEUTIC PROCEDURES

- The goal of medical treatment is to preserve the fertility of women wanting future pregnancies, ameliorate symptoms, and simplify future surgery or make it unnecessary

OUTCOME

PROGNOSIS

- The prognosis for reproductive function in early or moderately advanced endometriosis is good with conservative therapy
- Bilateral ovariectomy is curative for patients with severe and extensive endometriosis with pain. Following hysterectomy and oophorectomy, estrogen replacement therapy is indicated

WHEN TO REFER

- Refer to gynecologist for laparoscopic diagnosis and treatment

WHEN TO ADMIT

- Rarely necessary except in case of acute abdomen associated with a ruptured or bleeding endometrioma

EVIDENCE

PRACTICE GUIDELINES

- ACOG Committee on Practice Bulletins. Medical management of endometriosis. Int J Gynaecol Obstet 2000;71:183. [PMID: 11186465]
  - http://www.aafp.org/afp/20000915/practice.html

INFORMATION FOR PATIENTS

- American Association of Family Physicians: Endometriosis
  - http://familydoctor.org/x2082.xml
- MedlinePlus: Endometriosis Interactive Tutorial
  - http://www.nlm.nih.gov/medlineplus/tutorials/endometriosis.html
- MedlinePlus: Laparoscopy Interactive Tutorial
  - http://www.nlm.nih.gov/medlineplus/tutorials/diagnosticlaparoscopygeneral.html
- National Institute of Child Health & Human Development: Endometriosis
  - http://www.nichd.nih.gov/publications/pubs/endometriosis/index.htm

REFERENCES

- Giudice LC et al: Endometriosis. Lancet 2004;364:1789. [PMID: 15541453]
- Winkel CA: Evaluation and management of women with endometriosis. Obstet Gynecol 2003;102:397. [PMID: 12907119]

Author(s)

H. Trent MacKay, MD, MPH

Enterobiasis

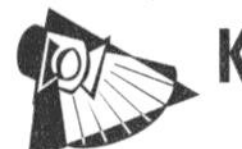

KEY FEATURES

ESSENTIALS OF DIAGNOSIS

- Nocturnal perianal and vulvar pruritus, insomnia, irritability, restlessness
- Vague gastrointestinal symptoms
- Eggs demonstrable by cellulose tape test; worms visible on perianal skin or in stool

GENERAL CONSIDERATIONS

- Humans, the only host, can harbor a few to hundreds of worms
- Adult *Enterobius vermicularis* (8–13 × 0.5 mm) inhabit the cecum and adjacent bowel areas, lying loosely attached to the mucosa. Gravid females migrate through the anus to the perianal skin and deposit eggs in large numbers. The eggs become infective in a few hours and may then infect others or be autoinfective if transferred to the mouth by contaminated food, drink, fomites, or hands. After being swallowed, the eggs hatch in the duodenum, and the larvae migrate down to the cecum
- Retroinfection occasionally occurs when the eggs hatch on the perianal skin and the larvae migrate through the anus into the large intestine
- The development of a mature ovipositing female from an ingested egg requires about 3–4 weeks. Eggs remain viable for 2–3 weeks outside the host
- The life span of the worm is 30–45 days

DEMOGRAPHICS

- More than 30% of children are infected with *E vermicularis* worldwide and this is the most prevalent nematode infection in the United States
- A second species, *E gregorii*, has been described in England

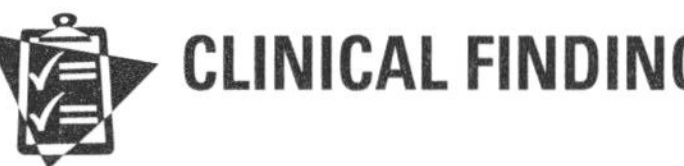

CLINICAL FINDINGS

SYMPTOMS AND SIGNS

- Many patients are asymptomatic
- The most common and important symptom is perianal pruritus (particularly at night), due to the presence of the female worms or deposited eggs
- At night, worms may occasionally be seen near the anus. Perianal scratching may result in excoriation and impetigo. Patients sometimes report a "crawling" sensation in the anal area

DIFFERENTIAL DIAGNOSIS

- Tinea or candidiasis of the anogenital region
- Hemorrhoids
- Proctitis
- Contact dermatitis
- Strongyloidiasis
- Anal fissure
- Idiopathic anogenital pruritus

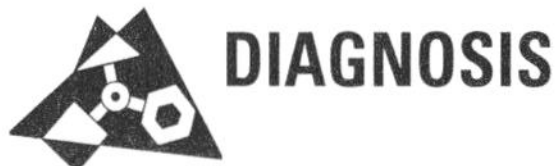

DIAGNOSIS

LABORATORY TESTS

- Diagnosis is made by finding eggs on the perianal skin (eggs are seldom found on stool examination)
  - The most reliable method is by applying a short strip of sealing cellulose pressure-sensitive tape (eg, Scotch Tape) to the perianal skin and then spreading the tape on a slide for low-power microscopic study; toluene is used to clear the preparation
  - Three such preparations made on consecutive mornings before bathing or defecation will establish the diagnosis in about 90% of cases
  - Before the diagnosis can be ruled out, five to seven such examinations are necessary
- Nocturnal examination of the perianal area or gross examination of stools may reveal adult worms, which should be placed in preservative, alcohol, or saline for laboratory examination
- The worms can sometimes be seen on anoscopy
- Eosinophilia is rare

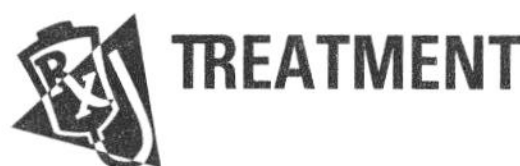

TREATMENT

MEDICATIONS

- Treatment with the following drugs should be repeated at 2 and 4 weeks: albendazole, mebendazole, and pyrantel pamoate are the drugs of choice and can be given with or without food. Albendazole and mebendazole should not be used in pregnancy. Piperazine, although effective, is not recommended because treatment requires 1 week
- **Albendazole** may reach a 100% cure rate when given as a single oral 400-mg dose. Abdominal pain and diarrhea are rare
- **Mebendazole** as a single oral 100-mg dose is also highly effective. It should be chewed for best effect. Gastrointestinal side effects are infrequent
- **Pyrantel pamoate** is highly effective, with cure rates of over 95%. It is administered as a 10-mg (base)/kg (maximum, 1 g) dose. Infrequent side effects include vomiting, diarrhea, headache, dizziness, and drowsiness. In the United States, pyrantel is available as self-medication for pinworm infection

THERAPEUTIC PROCEDURES

- Symptomatic patients should be treated, and in some situations all members of the patient's household should be treated concurrently, since for each overt case there are usually several inapparent cases. Generally, however, treatment of all nonsymptomatic cases is not necessary
- Careful washing of hands with soap and water after defecation and again before meals is important. Fingernails should be kept trimmed close and clean and scratching of the perianal area avoided. Ordinary washing of bedding will usually kill pinworm eggs; some workers recommend daily washing

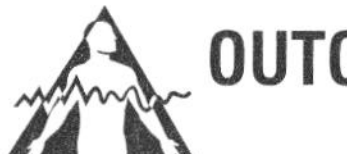

OUTCOME

COMPLICATIONS

- Rarely, worm migration—including migration through the female genital tract or into the urethra—results in ectopic inflammation (vulvovaginitis, diverticulitis, appendicitis, cystitis) or granulomatous reactions (colon, genital tract, peritoneum, and elsewhere)
- Colonic ulceration and eosinophilic colitis have been reported

PROGNOSIS

- Although annoying, the infection is benign
- Cure is readily attainable with one of several effective drugs
- Reinfection is common because of continued exposure outside the home

WHEN TO REFER

- Inability to cure the infection
- No response or progression of symptoms despite therapy

EVIDENCE

PRACTICE GUIDELINES

- Kabani A et al: Practice guidelines for ordering stool ova and parasite testing in a pediatric population. The Alberta Children's Hospital. Am J Clin Pathol 1995;104:272. [PMID: 7677114]

WEB SITE

- CDC—Division of Parasitic Diseases
  - http://www.cdc.gov/ncidod/dpd/parasites/pinworm/default.htm

INFORMATION FOR PATIENTS

- Centers for Disease Control
  - http://www.cdc.gov/ncidod/dpd/parasites/pinworm/factsht_pinworm.htm
- National Institute of Allergy and Infectious Diseases
  - http://www.niaid.nih.gov/factsheets/roundwor.htm
- National Institutes of Health
  - http://www.nlm.nih.gov/medlineplus/ency/article/001152.htm

REFERENCES

- Lohiya GS et al: Epidemiology and control of enterobiasis in a developmental center. West J Med 2000;172:305. [PMID: 10832422]
- St Georgiev V: Chemotherapy of enterobiasis (oxyuriasis). Expert Opin Pharmacother 2001;2:267. [PMID: 11336585]
- Tandan T et al: Pelvic inflammatory disease associated with *Enterobius vermicularis.* Arch Dis Child 2002;86:439. [PMID: 12023182]
- Wu ML et al: *Enterobius vermicularis.* Arch Pathol Lab Med 2000;124:647. [PMID: 10747336]

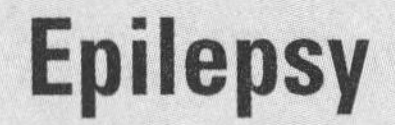

Epilepsy

Enterococcal Infections p. 1067. Enteropathy, Protein-Losing p. 1067. Eosinophilia-Myalgia Syndrome p. 1067. Epicondylitis, Lateral & Medial p. 1068.

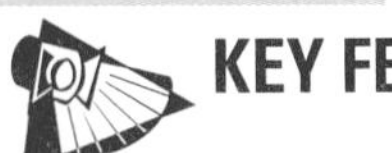

KEY FEATURES

ESSENTIALS OF DIAGNOSIS

- Recurrent seizures
- Epilepsy should not be diagnosed on the basis of a solitary seizure
- Characteristic electroencephalographic (EEG) changes may occur
- Postictal confusion or focal neurologic deficits may follow and last hours

GENERAL CONSIDERATIONS

- The most likely cause relates to the age of onset
- Idiopathic epilepsy onset is usually between the ages of 5 and 20 years
- Metabolic disorders may cause seizures
- Trauma is an important cause of seizures
  - Seizures in the first week after head injury do not imply that they will persist
  - Prophylactic anticonvulsant drugs have not been proven to reduce the incidence of posttraumatic epilepsy
- Tumors and other space-occupying lesions result in seizures that are often partial (focal), and most likely with frontal, parietal, or temporal lesions
- Vascular disease is the leading cause in patients aged 60 or older
- Alzheimer's disease and other degenerative disorders can cause seizures in later life
- Infections of the CNS (meningitis, encephalitis, or brain abscess) must be considered in all age groups as potentially reversible causes of seizures
- Causes of secondary seizures
  - CNS vasculitis, eg, systemic lupus erythematosus
  - Febrile seizures in children younger than 5 years
  - Metabolic disorders, including withdrawal from alcohol or other CNS depressant drugs, hypoglycemia, hyperglycemia, uremia, and hyponatremia
  - Trauma
  - CNS infection
  - Degenerative disease, eg, Alzheimer's disease

DEMOGRAPHICS

- Epilepsy affects approximately 0.5% of the US population

CLINICAL FINDINGS

SYMPTOMS AND SIGNS

- See Table 97
- Nonspecific prodrome in some (headache, lethargy)
- The type of aura depends on the cerebral site of origin of the seizure, eg, gustatory or olfactory hallucinations or visual hallucinations with temporal or occipital lesions
- In most patients, seizures occur unpredictably
- Fever, sleep loss, alcohol, stress, or flashing lights may precipitate seizures in some
- Clinical examination may be normal interictally unless there is a structural cause for the seizures
- Immediately postictally there may be a focal deficit (Todd's paresis) or bilateral Babinski signs
- Focal signs postictally suggest focal CNS abnormality

DIFFERENTIAL DIAGNOSIS

- Syncope
- Cardiac arrhythmia
- Stroke or transient ischemic attack
- Pseudoseizure
- Panic attack
- Migraine
- Narcolepsy

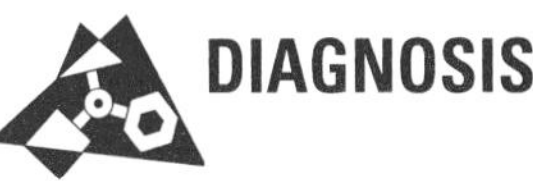

DIAGNOSIS

LABORATORY TESTS

- Complete blood count, serum glucose, liver and renal function tests, and serologic tests for syphilis

IMAGING STUDIES

- Image all patients with progressive disorder and those with new onset of seizures
- Obtain an MRI if there are focal neurologic symptoms or signs, focal seizures, or a focal EEG disturbance

DIAGNOSTIC PROCEDURES

- History is key, including eyewitness accounts
- The EEG is abnormal in only about 60% but may support clinical diagnosis of epilepsy (paroxysmal spikes or sharp waves), may guide prognosis, may help classify the seizure disorder, and is important in evaluating candidates for surgical treatment
- Repeated Holter monitoring may be necessary to establish the diagnosis of cardiac arrhythmia

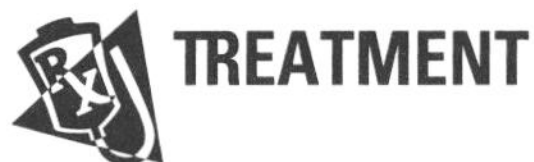

TREATMENT

MEDICATIONS

- Anticonvulsant drug treatment is generally not required for a single seizure unless further attacks occur or investigations reveal some underlying untreatable pathology
- Treatment with anticonvulsant drugs is generally not required for alcohol withdrawal seizures, which are self-limited
- See Table 98
- The drug dose is gradually increased until seizures are controlled or side effects occur
- If seizures continue despite treatment at the maximal tolerated dose, a second drug is added and the first drug is then gradually withdrawn
- In most patients, control can be achieved with a single anticonvulsant drug
- Discontinue the medication only when the patient is seizure free for at least 3 years. Dose reduction should be gradual over a period of weeks or months. If seizures recur, treatment is reinstituted with previous drugs
- A seizure recurrence after the medication is discontinued is more likely if the patient initially failed to respond to therapy, if focal or multiple types of seizures, or if EEG abnormalities persist

SURGERY

- Operative treatment or vagal nerve stimulations are best undertaken in specialized centers

THERAPEUTIC PROCEDURES

- Advise patients to avoid situations that may be dangerous or life-threatening if they have a seizure
- State laws may require clinicians to report to the public health department any patients with seizures or other episodic lapses of consciousness

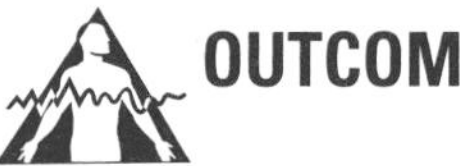

OUTCOME

FOLLOW-UP

- Dosing should not be based simply on serum levels because some patients require levels that exceed the therapeutic range ("toxic levels") but tolerate these without ill effect
- In general, the dose of an antiepileptic agent is increased depending on clinical response, not serum drug level. The trough drug level is then measured to provide a reference point for the maximum tolerated dose
- Measure serum drug levels when another drug is added to the therapeutic regimen and to assess compliance in poorly controlled patients
- Certain antiepileptic drugs may be teratogenic. Epileptic women of childbearing potential require special care

COMPLICATIONS

- See Status Epilepticus
- Residual encephalopathy after prolonged seizures or poor control of seizures

PROGNOSIS

- The risk of seizure recurrence varies in different series between about 30% and 70%

WHEN TO ADMIT

- Status epilepticus
- To video monitoring unit to distinguish pseudoseizures
- If surgery is contemplated

EVIDENCE

PRACTICE GUIDELINES

- National Guideline Clearinghouse
  - http://www.guideline.gov/summary/summary.aspx?doc_id=2439&nbr=1665&string=epilepsy
  - http://www.guideline.gov/summary/summary.aspx?doc_id=2823&nbr=2049&string=epilepsy
  - http://www.guideline.gov/summary/summary.aspx?doc_id=3526&nbr=2752&string=epilepsy
  - http://www.guideline.gov/summary/summary.aspx?doc_id=2829&nbr=2055&string=epilepsy
  - http://www.guideline.gov/summary/summary.aspx?doc_id=5091&nbr=3558&string=epilepsy
- American College of Emergency Physicians: Clinical policy: Critical issues in the evaluation and management of adult patients presenting to the emergency department with seizures. Ann Emerg Med 2004;43:605. [PMID: 15111920]
- Hirtz D et al; American Academy of Neurology: Practice parameter: treatment of the child with a first unprovoked seizure: Report of the Quality Standards Subcommittee of the American Academy of Neurology and the Practice Committee of the Child Neurology Society. Neurology 2003;60:166. [PMID: 12552027]

INFORMATION FOR PATIENTS

- Epilepsy Foundation
  - http://www.epilepsyfoundation.org/answerplace/faq.cfm
  - http://www.epilepsyfoundation.org/answerplace/index.cfm
- Epilepsy.com
  - http://www.epilepsy.com/

REFERENCES

- Alldredge BK et al: A comparison of lorazepam, diazepam, and placebo for the treatment of out-of-hospital status epilepticus. N Engl J Med 2001;345:631. [PMID: 11547716]
- Chang BS et al: Epilepsy. N Engl J Med 2003;349:1257. [PMID: 14507951]
- Schachter SC: Epilepsy: major advances in treatment. Lancet Neurol 2004;3:11. [PMID: 14693100]
- Vazquez B: Monotherapy in epilepsy: role of the newer antiepileptic drugs. Arch Neurol 2004;61:1361. [PMID: 15364680]
- Wiebe S et al: A randomized, controlled trial of surgery for temporal-lobe epilepsy. N Engl J Med 2001;345:311. [PMID: 11484687]

Author(s)

Michael J. Aminoff, MD, DSc, FRCP

Epistaxis

Epididymitis, Acute p. 1068. Epiglottitis p. 1069.

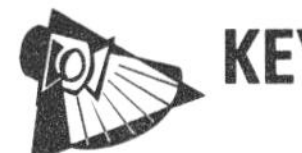

KEY FEATURES

ESSENTIALS OF DIAGNOSIS

- Bleeding from the anterior nasal cavity is by far the most common type of epistaxis encountered
- Most cases can be successfully treated by direct pressure on the bleeding site

GENERAL CONSIDERATIONS

- Bleeding from the anterior nasal cavity originates from Kiesselbach's plexus, a vascular plexus on the anterior nasal septum
- Bleeding from the posterior nasal cavity originates from the posterior half of the inferior turbinate or the top of the nasal cavity
- Predisposing factors include nasal trauma (nose picking, foreign bodies, forceful nose blowing), rhinitis, drying of the nasal mucosa from low humidity, deviation of the nasal septum, alcohol use, and antiplatelet medications

DEMOGRAPHICS

- Anterior nasal cavity bleeding is by far the most common type of epistaxis
- Only 5% of nasal bleeding originates in the posterior nasal cavity
- Less than 10% of nasal bleeding is caused by coagulopathy or tumor

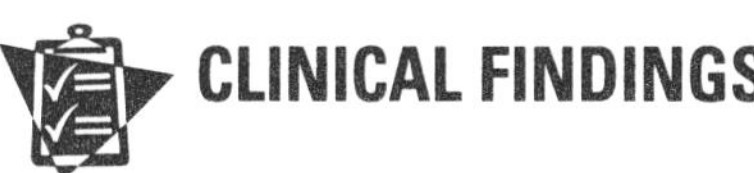

CLINICAL FINDINGS

SYMPTOMS AND SIGNS

- Bleeding from nostril or nasopharynx
- Posterior bleeding may present with hemoptysis or hematemesis

DIFFERENTIAL DIAGNOSIS

- Nasal trauma (eg, nose picking, forceful nose blowing, foreign body)
- Allergic rhinitis or viral rhinitis
- Dry nasal mucosa
- Deviated septum
- Chronic sinusitis
- Inhaled steroids
- Cocaine use
- Alcohol use
- Antiplatelet drugs (eg, aspirin, clopidogrel)
- Thrombocytopenia
- Idiopathic thrombocytopenic purpura
- Thrombotic thrombocytopenic purpura
- Hemophilia
- Hereditary hemorrhagic telangiectasia (Osler-Weber-Rendu syndrome)
- Polycythemia vera
- Leukemia
- Wegener's granulomatosis
- Nasal tumor

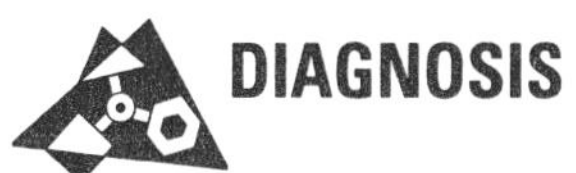

DIAGNOSIS

LABORATORY TESTS

- Laboratory assessment of bleeding parameters (platelet count, coagulation studies) may be indicated, especially in recurrent cases

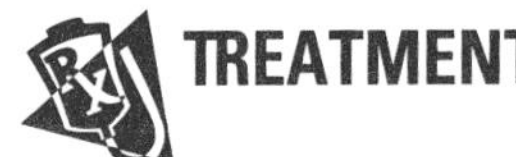

TREATMENT

- Most cases of anterior epistaxis may be successfully treated by direct pressure on the bleeding site

MEDICATIONS

- Short-acting topical nasal decongestants (eg, phenylephrine, 0.125–1% solution, one or two sprays), which act as vasoconstrictors, may be helpful
- When the bleeding does not readily subside, the nose should be examined to locate the bleeding site: topical 4% cocaine [or a topical decongestant (eg, oxymetazoline) and a topical anesthetic (eg, tetracaine)] applied either as a spray or on a cotton strip serves as an anesthetic and as a vasoconstricting agent

SURGERY

Posterior nasal bleeding

- Ligation of the nasal arterial supply (internal maxillary artery and ethmoid arteries) is a possible alternative to posterior nasal packing
- Ligation of the external carotid artery may be necessary

THERAPEUTIC PROCEDURES

Anterior nasal bleeding

- Compress the nasal alae firmly for at least 10 min
- Venous pressure is reduced in the sitting position, and leaning forward lessens the swallowing of blood
- Cauterize the bleeding site with silver nitrate, diathermy, or electrocautery
- Usually anterior packing will suffice if the bleeding has not stopped

Posterior nasal bleeding

- Placement of a pack to occlude the choana before placement of a pack anteriorly
- Narcotic analgesics reduce the discomfort and elevated blood pressure caused by a posterior pack
- Endovascular embolization of the internal maxillary artery is an alternative to surgical ligation in life-threatening hemorrhage

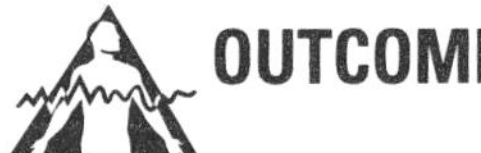

OUTCOME

FOLLOW-UP

- After control of the epistaxis, avoid vigorous exercise for several days
- Avoid hot or spicy foods and tobacco because they may cause vasodilation
- Once the acute episode has passed, carefully examine the nose and paranasal sinuses to rule out neoplasia
- Follow-up investigation of possible hypertension

COMPLICATIONS

- Sinusitis
- Aspiration or asphyxiation by blood

PROGNOSIS

- Generally self-limited with a good prognosis

WHEN TO REFER

- Refer to an otolaryngologist for persistent or recurrent bleeding
- If expertise in cauterization or localization of the bleeding site is needed
- For posterior nasal packing

WHEN TO ADMIT

- Because placing a nasal pack for posterior nasal bleeding is uncomfortable and requires oxygen supplementation to prevent hypoxia, hospitalization for several days is indicated

PREVENTION

- Avoiding nasal trauma, including nose picking
- Lubrication with petroleum jelly or bacitracin ointment
- Increased home humidity

EVIDENCE

WEB SITES

- American Academy of Otolaryngology—Head and Neck Surgery: Management of Posterior Epistaxis Interactive Module
  - http://www.entnet.org/education/COOL/epistaxisintro2.cfm
- Baylor College of Medicine Otolaryngology Resources
  - http://www.bcm.tmc.edu/oto/othersa.html

INFORMATION FOR PATIENTS

- American Academy of Family Physicians: Nosebleeds: What to Do When Your Nose Bleeds
  - http://familydoctor.org/132.xml
- American Academy of Otolaryngology—Head and Neck Surgery: Nosebleeds
  - http://www.entnet.org/healthinfo/nose/nosebleeds.cfm
- MedlinePlus: Nosebleeds
  - http://www.nlm.nih.gov/medlineplus/ency/article/003106.htm
  - http://www.nlm.nih.gov/medlineplus/ency/article/003106.htm
- MedlinePlus: Nosebleed Treatment
  - http://www.nlm.nih.gov/medlineplus/ency/article/002120.htm

REFERENCES

- Jones GL et al: The value of coagulation profiles in epistaxis management. Int J Clin Pract 2003;57:577. [PMID: 14529056]
- Middleton PM: Epistaxis. Emerg Med Australas 2004;16:428. [PMID: 15537406]
- Pond F et al: Epistaxis.Strategies for management. Aust Fam Physician 2000; 29:933. [PMID: 11059081]
- Singer AJ et al: Comparison of nasal tampons for the treatment of epistaxis in the emergency department: a randomized controlled trial. Ann Emerg Med 2005;45:134. [PMID: 15671968]

Author(s)

Robert K. Jackler, MD

Michael J. Kaplan, MD

Erectile Dysfunction

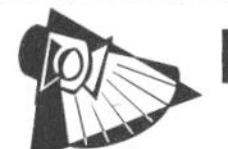

KEY FEATURES

ESSENTIALS OF DIAGNOSIS

- Consistent inability to maintain an erect penis with sufficient rigidity to allow sexual intercourse
- Affects 10 million American men
- Incidence is age related
- Affects ~25% of men aged > 65
- Most have an organic rather than psychogenic cause

GENERAL CONSIDERATIONS

Etiology

- Loss of erections: occurs from arterial, venous, neurogenic, or psychogenic causes
- Associated with concurrent medical problems (eg, diabetes mellitus), or radical pelvic or retroperitoneal surgery
- Antihypertensive medications: centrally acting sympatholytics (methyldopa, clonidine, reserpine) can cause loss of erection, while vasodilators, α-blockers, and diuretics rarely do so
- Androgen deficiency causes both loss of libido and erections and lack of emission by decreasing prostatic and seminal vesicle secretions
- Loss of orgasm: if libido and erections are intact, usually of psychological origin
- Premature ejaculation: anxiety related, due to a new partner, unreasonable expectations about performance, or emotional disorders
- Lack of emission (lack of antegrade seminal fluid during ejaculation): due to retrograde ejaculation or mechanical disruption of the bladder neck (eg, after transurethral resection of the prostate), or androgen deficiency

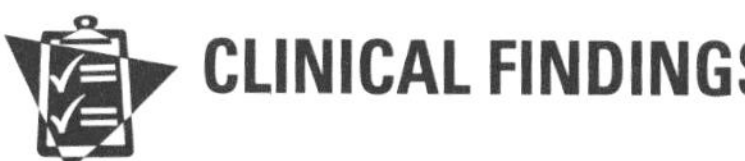

CLINICAL FINDINGS

SYMPTOMS AND SIGNS

- History: erectile dysfunction should be distinguished from problems with ejaculation, libido, and orgasm
- Degree of the dysfunction—chronic, occasional, or situational
- Timing of dysfunction
- Determine whether the patient ever has any normal erections, such as in early morning or during sleep
- Inquire about hyperlipidemia, hypertension, neurological disease, diabetes mellitus, renal failure, adrenal and thyroid disorders, and depression
- Trauma to the pelvis, pelvic surgery, or peripheral vascular surgery
- Use of drugs, alcohol, tobacco, and recreational drugs
- Physical examination: secondary sexual characteristics
- Neurological motor and sensory examination
- Peripheral vascular examination: palpation and quantification of lower extremity pulses
- Examination of genitalia, testicles, and prostate
- Evaluate for penile scarring, plaque formation (Peyronie's disease)

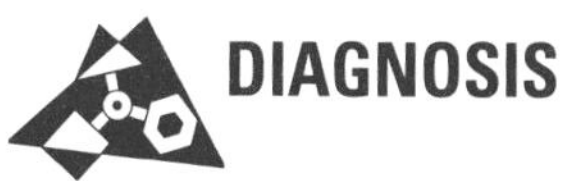

DIAGNOSIS

LABORATORY TESTS

- Complete blood count
- Urinalysis
- Lipid profile
- Serum glucose, testosterone, luteinizing hormone/follicle-stimulating hormone (LH/FSH), and prolactin
- Serum testosterone and gonadotropin (LH/FSH) levels may help localize the site of disease

IMAGING STUDIES

- Cavernous arteries duplex ultrasound
  - If poor arterial inflow, perform pelvic arteriography before arterial reconstruction
  - If normal arterial inflow, probably venous leak
- Cavernosometry (measurement of flow required to maintain erection)
- Cavernosography (contrast study of the penis to determine site and extent of venous leak)

DIAGNOSTIC PROCEDURES

- Direct injection of vasoactive substances into the penis (prostaglandin E, papaverine, or a combination of drugs). Patients who respond with a rigid erection typically require no further vascular evaluation
- Nocturnal penile tumescence testing for frequency and rigidity in patients who fail to achieve an erection with injection of vasoactive substances

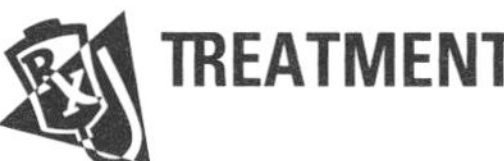

TREATMENT

MEDICATIONS

- Hormone replacement for documented androgen deficiency on endocrinological evaluation, using testosterone injections (200 mg IM Q 3 weeks) or topical patches (2.5–10 mg/day), after prostate-specific antigen and digital rectal examination screening
- Alprostadil urethral suppository pellets (125, 250, 500, and 1000 μg)
- Sildenafil, 50 mg, vardenafil 5 mg, or tadalafil, 10 mg 1 h prior to anticipated sexual activity. Contraindicated in patients receiving nitrates

SURGERY

- Penile prosthesis: rigid, malleable, hinged, or inflatable
- Surgery for disorders of the arterial system:
  - Vascular reconstruction
  - Endarterectomy and balloon dilation for proximal arterial occlusion
  - Arterial bypass procedures utilizing arterial (epigastric) or venous (deep dorsal vein) segments for distal occlusion
- Surgery for disorders of venous occlusion: ligation of certain veins (deep dorsal or emissary veins) or the crura of the corpora cavernosa

THERAPEUTIC PROCEDURES

- Vacuum constriction device: for patients with venous disorders of the penis and those who fail to achieve adequate erection with injection of vasoactive substances, use a vacuum device and rubber constriction band around proximal penis; complications are rare
- Behaviorally oriented sex therapy for men with no organic dysfunction

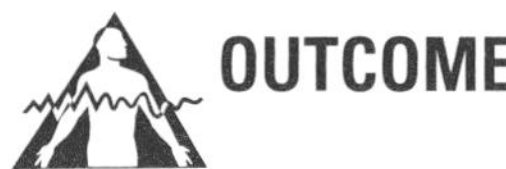

OUTCOME

PROGNOSIS

- The majority of men suffering from erectile dysfunction can be managed successfully

EVIDENCE

PRACTICE GUIDELINES

- American Association of Clinical Endocrinologists medical guidelines for clinical practice for the evaluation and treatment of male sexual dysfunction: a couple's problem—2003 update. American Association of Clinical Endocrinologists, American College of Endocrinology, 2003
- http://www.aace.com/clin/guidelines/sexdysguid.pdf
- Canadian Urological Association Guidelines Committee. Erectile dysfunction practice guidelines. Can J Urol 2002;9:1583. [PMID: 12243654]
- Wespes E et al; European Association of Urology. Guidelines on erectile dysfunction. Eur Urol 2002;41:1. [PMID: 11999460]

INFORMATION FOR PATIENTS

- Cleveland Clinic—Erectile dysfunction basics
  - http://www.clevelandclinic.org/health/health-info/docs/2900/2904.asp?index=10035
- Mayo Clinic—Erectile dysfunction
  - http://www.mayoclinic.com/invoke.cfm?objectid=F52ADDE0-FE7E-4F9D-9ACB4F34354E023C
- National Kidney and Urologic Diseases Information Clearinghouse
  - http://kidney.niddk.nih.gov/kudiseases/pubs/impotence/index.htm

REFERENCES

- Christ GJ et al: Physiology and biochemistry of erections. Endocrine 2004;23:93. [PMID: 15146085]
- Gonzalez-Cadavid NF et al: Therapy of erectile dysfunction: potential future treatments. Endocrine 2004;23:167. [PMID: 15146097]
- McVary KT: The relationship between erectile dysfunction and lower urinary tract symptoms: epidemiological, clinical, and basic science evidence. Curr Urol Rep 2004;5:251. [PMID: 15260924]

Author(s)

Marshall L. Stoller, MD
Peter R. Carroll, MD

Erythema Multiforme

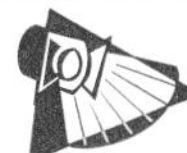

KEY FEATURES

ESSENTIALS OF DIAGNOSIS

- Sudden onset of symmetric erythematous skin lesions with history of recurrence
- May be macular, papular, urticarial, bullous, or purpuric
- "Target" lesions with clear centers and concentric erythematous rings or "iris" lesions may be noted in erythema multiforme (EM) minor; these are rare in drug-associated EM major (Stevens-Johnson syndrome)

GENERAL CONSIDERATIONS

- An acute inflammatory skin disease due to multiple causes
- EM is divided clinically into minor and major types based on the clinical findings
- ~90% of cases of EM minor follow outbreaks of herpes simplex
- **EM major** (Stevens-Johnson syndrome)
  - Toxicity and involvement of two or more mucosal surfaces (often oral and conjunctival)
  - Most often caused by drugs (sulfonamides, nonsteroidal anti-inflammatory drugs, and anticonvulsants)
  - Visceral involvement may occur, may be serious or even fatal
  - Main differential diagnosis is toxic epidermal necrolysis, and some regard this as a variant of the same disease
- EM may also present as recurring oral ulceration, with skin lesions present in only half of the cases, and is diagnosed by oral biopsy

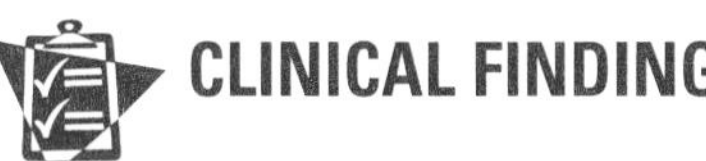

CLINICAL FINDINGS

SYMPTOMS AND SIGNS

- See Table 7
- EM major favors the trunk; EM minor on extensor surfaces, palms, soles, or mucous membranes
- Classic target lesion, most commonly seen in herpes-associated EM, consists of three concentric zones of color change, most often found acrally on the hands and feet
- Drug-associated EM is manifested by raised target-like lesions, with only two zones of color change and a central blister, or nondescript reddish or purpuric macules
- In EM major, mucous membrane ulcerations are present at two or more sites, causing pain on eating, swallowing, and urination
- Blisters are always worrisome and dictate the need for consultation

DIFFERENTIAL DIAGNOSIS

- EM minor: urticaria, drug eruption
  - Individual lesions of true urticaria itch, should come and go within 24 h, are usually responsive to antihistamines, and do not affect the mucosa
- EM major in evolution
- Sweet's syndrome (acute febrile neutrophilic dermatosis)
- EM major
  - Pemphigus
  - Bullous pemphigoid
  - Drug eruptions
  - Bullous impetigo
  - Contact dermatitis
  - Dermatitis herpetiformis
  - Cicatricial pemphigoid
  - Paraneoplastic pemphigus
  - Linear IgA dermatosis
  - Pemphigus foliaceus
  - Porphyria cutanea tarda
  - Epidermolysis bullosa
  - Staphylococcus scalded skin syndrome
  - Herpes gestationis
  - Graft-versus-host disease

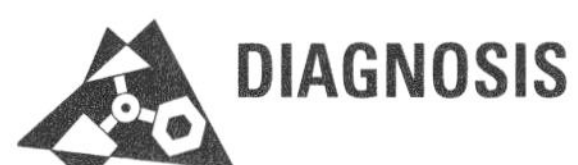

DIAGNOSIS

LABORATORY TESTS

- Blood tests are unhelpful

PROCEDURES

- Skin biopsy is diagnostic (direct immunofluorescence studies are negative)

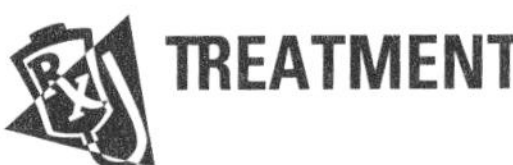

TREATMENT

MEDICATIONS

- See Table 6

EM major (Stevens-Johnson)

- No good data to support the use of corticosteroids, but they are still often prescribed
- If corticosteroids are to be tried in more severe cases, they should be used early, before blistering occurs, and in moderate to high doses (prednisone, 100–250 mg) and stopped within days if there is no dramatic response; in one trial, IGIV (0.75 g/kg/day for 4 days) yielded dramatic benefit in severe cases
- Oral and topical corticosteroids are useful in the oral variant of EM
- Antistaphylococcal antibiotics are used for secondary infection, which is uncommon
- Topical therapy is not very effective in this disease
- For oral lesions, 1% diphenhydramine elixir mixed with Kaopectate or with 1% dyclonine may be used as a mouth rinse several times daily

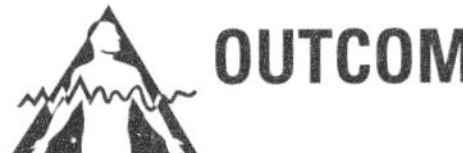

OUTCOME

FOLLOW-UP

- Patients who begin to blister with EM major should be seen daily

COMPLICATIONS

- EM major—extensive denudation, similar to an extensive burn

PROGNOSIS

- EM major—visceral involvement may occur, may be serious or even fatal
- EM minor usually lasts 2–6 weeks and may recur
- Immediate discontinuation of the inciting medication (before blistering) improves prognosis and reduces risk of death

WHEN TO REFER

- Diagnosis or suspicion of EM major

WHEN TO ADMIT

- Patients need not be admitted unless mucosal involvement interferes with hydration and nutrition; extensive denudation of skin best treated in a burn unit

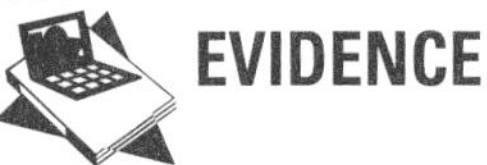

EVIDENCE

WEB SITES

- American Academy of Dermatology: Cutaneous Adverse Drug Reactions
  - http://www.aad.org/professionals/pracmanage/guidelines/CutaneousAdverseReactions.htm
- Dermatlas, Johns Hopkins University School of Medicine: Erythema Multiforme Images
  - http://dermatlas.med.jhmi.edu/derm/result.cfm?Diagnosis=98

INFORMATION FOR PATIENTS

- Mayo Clinic: Stevens-Johnson Syndrome
  - http://www.mayoclinic.com/invoke.cfm?id=AN00691
- MedlinePlus: Erythema Multiforme
  - http://www.nlm.nih.gov/medlineplus/ency/article/000851.htm
- University of Maryland Medical Center: Erythema Multiforme
  - http://www.umm.edu/dermatology-info/emulit.htm

REFERENCES

- Bachot N et al: Intravenous immunoglobulin treatment for Stevens-Johnson syndrome and toxic epidermal necrolysis: a prospective noncomparative study showing no benefit on mortality or progression. Arch Dermatol 2003;139:33. [PMID: 12533161]
- Chopra A et al: Stevens-Johnson syndrome after immunization with smallpox, anthrax, and tetanus vaccines. Mayo Clin Proc 2004;79:1193. [PMID: 15357044]
- Schechner AJ et al: Acute human immunodeficiency virus infection presenting with erythema multiforme. Am J Emerg Med 2004;22:330. [PMID: 15258890]

Author(s)

Timothy G. Berger, MD

Erythema Nodosum

KEY FEATURES

ESSENTIALS OF DIAGNOSIS

- Painful red nodules without ulceration on anterior aspects of legs
- Slow regression over several weeks to resemble contusions
- Women are predominantly affected by a ratio of 4–8:1 over men
- Some cases associated with infection or drug sensitivity

GENERAL CONSIDERATIONS

- The disease may be associated with various infectious and noninfectious conditions
  - Infection: streptococcal, coccidioidomycosis, other fungal (eg, histoplasmosis, blastomycosis), tuberculosis, syphilis, *Yersinia enterocolitica*
  - Other: sarcoidosis, medications (eg, oral contraceptives), inflammatory bowel disease, pregnancy, lymphoma, or leukemia

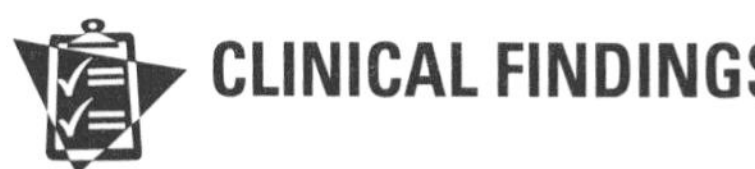

CLINICAL FINDINGS

SYMPTOMS AND SIGNS

- See Table 7
- The swellings are exquisitely tender and may be preceded by fever, malaise, and arthralgia
- They are most often located on the anterior surfaces of the legs below the knees but may occur (rarely) on the arms, trunk, and face
- The lesions, 1–10 cm in diameter, are at first pink to red; with regression, all the various hues seen in a contusion can be observed

DIFFERENTIAL DIAGNOSIS

- Erythema induratum (associated with tuberculosis)
- Nodular vasculitis
- Erythema multiforme
- Lupus panniculitis
- Poststeroid panniculitis
- Contusions or bruises
- Sweet's syndrome (acute febrile neutrophilic dermatosis)
- Subcutaneous fat necrosis (associated with pancreatitis)

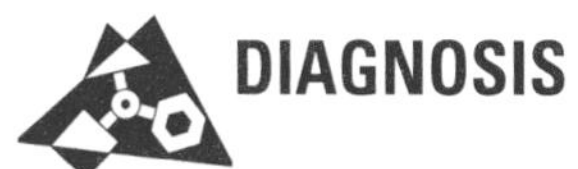

DIAGNOSIS

LABORATORY TESTS

- The histologic finding of septal panniculitis is characteristic of erythema nodosum
- Evaluation of patients presenting should include a careful history and physical examination for prior upper respiratory infection or diarrheal illness, symptoms of any deep fungal infection endemic to the area, a chest x-ray, a partial protein derivative (PPD), and two consecutive ASO titers at 2- to 4-week intervals

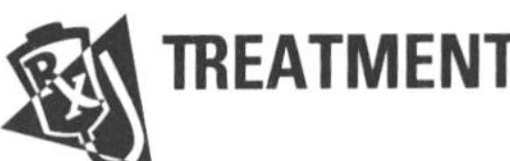

TREATMENT

MEDICATIONS

- See Table 6
- First identify and treat the underlying cause
- Primary therapy is with nonsteroidal anti-inflammatory drugs
- Saturated solution of potassium iodide, 5–15 drops three times daily, may result in prompt involution in many cases
- Side effects of potassium iodide include salivation, swelling of salivary glands, and headache
- Systemic therapy directed against the lesions themselves may include use of corticosteroids unless contraindicated by associated infection

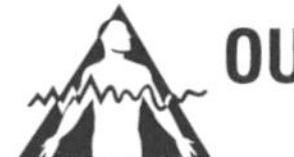

OUTCOME

PROGNOSIS

- It usually lasts about 6 weeks and may recur
- If no underlying cause is found, only a small percentage of patients will go on to develop a significant underlying illness (usually sarcoidosis) over the next year

WHEN TO REFER

- If there is a question about the diagnosis, if recommended therapy is ineffective, or specialized treatment is necessary

EVIDENCE

WEB SITES

- American Academy of Dermatology
  - http://www.aad.org
- Dermatlas, Johns Hopkins University School of Medicine: Erythema Nodosum Images
  - http://dermatlas.med.jhmi.edu/derm/result.cfm?Diagnosis=31
- Requena L et al: Erythema Nodosum. Dermatology Online Journal
  - http://dermatology.cdlib.org/DOJvol8num1/reviews/enodosum/requena.html

INFORMATION FOR PATIENTS

- American Osteopathic College of Dermatology: Erythema Nodosum
  - http://www.aocd.org/skin/dermatologic_diseases/erythema_nodosum.html
- MedlinePlus: Erythema Nodosum
  - http://www.nlm.nih.gov/medlineplus/ency/article/000881.htm
- University of Maryland Medical Center: Erythema Nodosum
  - http://www.umm.edu/dermatology-info/enodo.htm

REFERENCES

- Katugampola RP et al: Intestinal bypass syndrome presenting as erythema nodosum. Clin Exp Dermatol 2004;29:261. [PMID: 15115506]
- Mert A et al: Erythema nodosum: an experience of 10 years. Scand J Infect Dis 2004;36:424. [PMID: 15307561]

Author(s)

Timothy G. Berger, MD

Esophageal Cancer

KEY FEATURES

ESSENTIALS OF DIAGNOSIS

- Progressive solid food dysphagia
- Weight loss
- Endoscopy with biopsy establishes diagnosis

GENERAL CONSIDERATIONS

- Two histologic types
  - Squamous cell carcinoma
  - Adenocarcinoma
- Squamous cell cancer risk factors
  - Chronic alcohol and tobacco use
  - Tylosis
  - Achalasia
  - Caustic-induced esophageal stricture
  - Other head and neck cancers; in some underdeveloped countries, related to HIV infection
- Half of squamous cell cancers arise in the distal third of the esophagus
- Adenocarcinoma risk factor: Barrett's metaplasia due to chronic gastroesophageal reflux
- Most adenocarcinomas arise in the distal third of the esophagus

DEMOGRAPHICS

- Occurs usually in persons between 50 and 70 years of age
- Ratio of men to women is 3:1

CLINICAL FINDINGS

SYMPTOMS AND SIGNS

- Solid food dysphagia (>90%)
- Odynophagia
- Significant weight loss
- Coughing on swallowing or recurrent pneumonia suggests tracheoesophageal fistula from local tumor extension
- Chest or back pain mediastinal extension
- Hoarseness suggests recurrent laryngeal nerve involvement
- Physical examination often unrevealing
- Supraclavicular or cervical lymphadenopathy hepatomegaly suggests metastatic disease

DIFFERENTIAL DIAGNOSIS

- Peptic stricture
- Achalasia
- Adenocarcinoma of gastric cardia with esophageal involvement
- Esophageal web, ring (eg, Schatzki's), or diverticulum

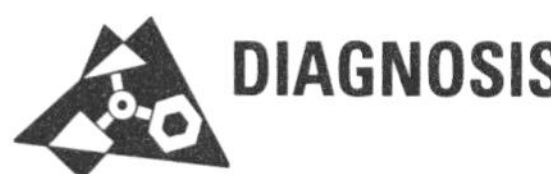

DIAGNOSIS

LABORATORY TESTS

- Anemia related to chronic disease or occult blood loss
- Elevated aminotransferase or alkaline phosphatase if hepatic metastases
- Hypoalbuminemia

IMAGING STUDIES

- Chest x-rays may show adenopathy
- Barium esophagogram
- Upper endoscopy with biopsy

DIAGNOSTIC PROCEDURES

- CT of the chest and liver for evaluation of metastases, lymphadenopathy
- Endoscopic ultrasonography with guided FNA of lymph nodes is superior to CT for evaluating local extension and lymph node involvement
- TNM classification

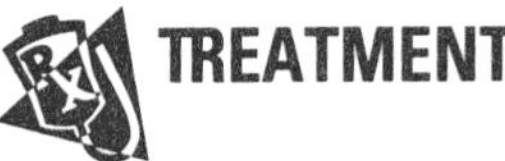

TREATMENT

MEDICATIONS

- Chemotherapy (cisplatin and fluorouracil) plus radiation therapy for patients with "curable" disease who are poor surgical candidates

SURGERY

- Surgery alone for stage I and stage IIA cancer
- Transhiatal esophagectomy with anastomosis of the stomach to the cervical esophagus
- Transthoracic excision of the esophagus with nodal resection
- Surgery with neoadjuvant chemotherapy (cisplatin and fluorouracil) and radiation therapy for patients with stage IIB and stage III cancer is used in some centers

THERAPEUTIC PROCEDURES

- Palliative therapy for patients with extensive local tumor spread (T4) or distant metastases (M1), ie, most patients with stage IIIB and stage IV tumors
  - Resection
  - Radiation therapy
  - Peroral placement of expandable permanent wire stents
  - Application of endoscopic laser therapy
  - Photodynamic therapy
- Complications of stents, perforation, migration, and tumor ingrowth occur in 20–40%
- Photodynamic therapy employs a photosensitizing agent (porfimer sodium) in combination with low-power 630-nm laser irradiation delivered endoscopically
  - Side effects include skin photosensitivity for 4–6 weeks and esophageal stricture

OUTCOME

COMPLICATIONS

- Invasion of mediastinal structures
- Tracheoesophageal fistula

PROGNOSIS

- Overall 5-year survival rate is < 15%
- Most patients present with advanced disease

WHEN TO REFER

- Dehydration due to dysphagea
- Palliative care

PREVENTION

- Adenocarcinoma: treatment of Barrett's esophagus
- Squamous cell carcinoma: eliminate cigarettes

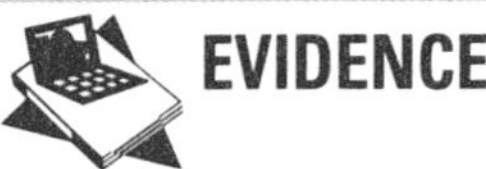

EVIDENCE

PRACTICE GUIDELINES

- Allum WH et al: Guidelines for the management of oesophageal and gastric cancer. Gut 2002;50(9Suppl 5):v1. [PMID:12049068]
- Seitz JF et al: Carcinoma of the oesophagus. Br J Cancer 2001;84(Suppl 2):61. [PMID:11355972]
- Wong RK et al: Combined modality radiotherapy and chemotherapy in nonsurgical management of localized carcinoma of the esophagus: a practice guideline. Int J Radiat Oncol Biol Phys 2003;55:930. [PMID:12605971]

INFORMATION FOR PATIENTS

- Cleveland Clinic—Esophageal cancer
  - http://www.clevelandclinic.org/health/health-info/docs/1300/1390.asp?index=6137
- National Cancer Institute
  - http://www.cancer.gov/cancerinfo/wyntk/esophagus

REFERENCES

- Enzinger PC et al: Esophageal cancer. N Engl J Med 2003;349:224. [PMID:14657432]
- Fiorica F et al: Preoperative chemoradiotherapy for esophageal cancer: a systematic review and meta-analysis. Gut 2004;53:925. [PMID:15194636]
- Weber WA et al: Imaging of esophageal and gastric cancer. Semin Oncol 2004;31:530. [PMID:15297944]

Author(s)

Kenneth R. McQuaid, MD

Esophageal Varices

Esophageal Diverticula p. 1069. Esophageal Injury, Caustic p. 1070.

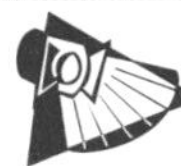

KEY FEATURES

ESSENTIALS OF DIAGNOSIS

- Dilated submucosal veins in patients with portal hypertension
- Develop in 50% of patients with cirrhosis
- One-third develop upper gastrointestinal bleeding

GENERAL CONSIDERATIONS

- Bleeding most commonly occurs in the distal 5 cm of the esophagus
- Approximately 50% of patients with cirrhosis have esophageal varices
- One-third of patients with varices develop serious bleeding

DEMOGRAPHICS

- Portal hypertension of any cause; most commonly due to cirrhosis

CLINICAL FINDINGS

SYMPTOMS AND SIGNS

- Acute gastrointestinal hemorrhage, usually severe, resulting in hypovolemia, postural vital signs, or shock

DIFFERENTIAL DIAGNOSIS

- Alcoholic gastritis
- Mallory-Weiss syndrome
- Portal hypertensive gastropathy
- Peptic ulcer disease
- Gastric or duodenal varices (rare)
- Vascular ectasias (angiodysplasias), eg, idiopathic arteriovenous malformation, CREST syndrome, hereditary hemorrhagic telangiectasia

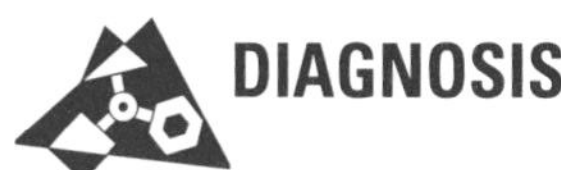

DIAGNOSIS

LABORATORY TESTS

- Complete blood cell count, platelet count, prothrombin time, INR, type and cross-match, serum liver enzymes, creatinine, blood urea nitrogen

DIAGNOSTIC PROCEDURES

- Emergent upper endoscopy after the patient's hemodynamic status has been stabilized is diagnostic

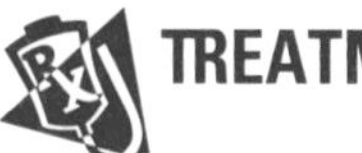

TREATMENT

MEDICATIONS

- Octreotide infusion (50-μg intravenous bolus followed by 50 μg/hour) reduces splanchnic and hepatic blood flow and portal pressures
- Combined octreotide and endoscopic therapy (band ligation or sclerotherapy) is superior to either modality alone in controlling acute bleeding and early rebleeding, and it may improve survival
- Vitamin K subcutaneously
- Lactulose 30–45 mL/hour PO until evacuation occurs, then reduced to 15–45 mL/hour Q 8–12 hours as needed to promote two or three bowel movements daily for hepatic encephalopathy
- After bleeding stops, β-blockers to reduce portal pressure: propranolol, 20 mg twice daily, or nadolol, 40 mg once daily, gradually increasing the dosage until the heart rate falls by 25% or reaches 55 beats/minute
- Combination therapy with isosorbide mononitrate (10 mg PO QD, gradually increased to 20–40 mg PO BID as tolerated) and β-blockers may be superior and reduces side effects

SURGERY

- Transvenous intrahepatic portosystemic shunts (TIPS) are indicated in the 5–10% of patients with acute variceal bleeding that cannot be controlled with pharmacologic and endoscopic therapy
- TIPS can control acute hemorrhage in >90%; however, mortality approaches 40%, especially in an actively bleeding patient with renal insufficiency, bilirubin >3.0 mg/dL, or requirement for ventilatory or blood pressure support
- TIPS reserved for patients who
  - Have recurrent (two or more) episodes of variceal bleeding who have failed endoscopic or pharmacologic

therapies, gastric varices, or portal hypertensive gastropathy
  - Are noncompliant with other therapies
  - Live in remote locations (without access to emergency care)
- Emergency portosystemic shunt, eg, selective distal splenorenal shunt, surgery can decompress portal hypertension, but is associated with a 40–60% mortality rate, seldom performed
- Liver transplantation

THERAPEUTIC PROCEDURES

- Initial management involves rapid assessment and acute resuscitation with fluids or blood products
- Transfusion of fresh frozen plasma or platelets to patients with INRs >1.8–2.0 or with platelet counts < 50,000/μL in the presence of active bleeding
- Mechanical tamponade with nasogastric tubes containing large gastric and esophageal balloons (Minnesota or Sengstaken-Blakemore tubes) provides initial control of active variceal hemorrhage in 60–90% of patients, but rebleeding occurs in 50%
- Acute endoscopic treatment with either banding or sclerotherapy
  - Arrests active bleeding in 90% of patients
  - Reduces by half (from 70%) the chance of early recurrent bleeding
- Repeat banding at intervals of 1–2 weeks until the varices are obliterated or reduced to a small size
- Banding achieves lower rates of rebleeding, complications, and death than sclerotherapy
- Sclerotherapy
  - Involves injecting the variceal trunks with ethanolamine, tetradecyl sulfate, repeating at 3–7 days, then at 1- to 3-week intervals until the varices are obliterated
  - Preferred by some endoscopists for the actively bleeding patient (in whom visualization for banding may be difficult)

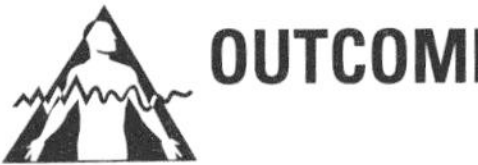

OUTCOME

FOLLOW-UP

- Stenosis and thrombosis of the TIPS stents occur in the majority over time with a consequent risk of rebleeding; periodic monitoring with Doppler ultrasonography or hepatic venography
- After obliteration of varices by endoscopic banding or sclerotherapy, repeat endoscopy every 6–12 months

COMPLICATIONS

- Encephalopathy occurs in 35% after TIPS
- Hepatic failure may occur after TIPS
- Sclerotherapy complications, including chest pain, fever, bacteremia, esophageal ulceration, stricture, and perforation, occur in 20–30%
- Complications of mechanical tamponade include esophageal and oral ulcerations, perforation, aspiration, and airway obstruction

PROGNOSIS

- Mortality rate within 2 weeks after an acute bleeding episode is 30%
- Recurrent hemorrhage occurs in 70% within 1 year (half within 6 weeks)
- Mortality rate is 60% at 2 years

WHEN TO ADMIT

- All patients with variceal hemorrhage

PREVENTION

- Prophylaxis of spontaneous bacterial peritonitis and systemic infections: norfloxacin, 400 mg (or another quinolone) PO or per nasogastric tube BID for at least 7 days
- Risk of rebleeding is 50–70% without further therapy
- Long-term treatment with sclerotherapy or band ligation reduces rebleeding to 20–50%
- Nonselective β-adrenergic blockers (propranolol, nadolol) reduce the incidence of rebleeding comparable to that of sclerotherapy or band ligation

EVIDENCE

PRACTICE GUIDELINES

- Eisen GM et al: The role of endoscopic therapy in the management of variceal hemorrhage. Gastrointest Endosc 2002;56:618. [PMID:12397264]
- National Guideline Clearinghouse
  - http://www.guideline.gov/summary/summary.aspx?doc_id=3557&nbr=2783&string=varices

WEB SITE

- WebPath Gastrointestinal Pathology Index
  - http://medstat.med.utah.edu/WebPath/GIHTML/GIIDX.html
  - http://www.guideline.gov/summary/summary.aspx?doc_id=3557&nbr=2783&string=varices

INFORMATION FOR PATIENTS

- American Academy of Family Physicians
  - http://familydoctor.org/188.xml
- Cleveland Clinic—Variceal bleeding management procedures
  - http://www.clevelandclinic.org/health/health-info/docs/1900/1930.asp?index=4721

REFERENCES

- D'Amico G et al: Emergency sclerotherapy versus vasoactive drugs for variceal bleeding in cirrhosis: a Cochrane analysis. Gastroenterology 2003;124:1277. [PMID:12730868]
- Ferguson JW et al: Review article: the management of acute variceal bleeding. Aliment Pharmacol Ther 2003;18:253. [PMID:12895210]
- Mihas AA et al: Recurrent variceal bleeding despite endoscopic and medical therapy. Gastroenterology 2004;127:621. [PMID:15300593]
- Nevens F: Review article. A critical comparison of drug therapies in currently used therapeutic strategies for variceal hemorrhage. Aliment Pharmacol Ther 2004;20(Suppl 3):18. [PMID:15335394]

Author(s)

Kenneth R. McQuaid, MD

Esophagitis, Infectious

Esophageal Webs & Rings p. 1070

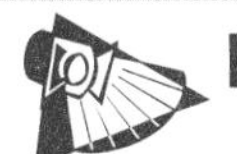

KEY FEATURES

ESSENTIALS OF DIAGNOSIS

- Odynophagia, dysphagia, and chest pain
- Occurs in immunosuppressed patients

GENERAL CONSIDERATIONS

- Occurs most commonly in immunosuppressed patients with AIDS, solid organ transplants, leukemia, and lymphoma, and in those receiving immunosuppressive drugs
- Most common pathogens: *Candida albicans*, herpes simplex, and cytomegalovirus
- *Candida* also occurs in patients who have uncontrolled diabetes mellitus and those receiving systemic corticosteroids, radiation therapy, or systemic antibiotics

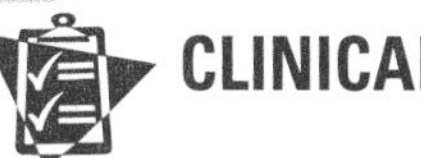

CLINICAL FINDINGS

SYMPTOMS AND SIGNS

- Odynophagia
- Dysphagia
- Substernal chest pain
- Sometimes asymptomatic (*Candida*)
- Oral thrush in 75% of patients with candidal esophagitis and 25–50% of patients with viral esophagitis
- Cytomegalovirus infection at other sites (colon and retina)
- Oral ulcers (herpes labialis) often associated with herpes simplex esophagitis

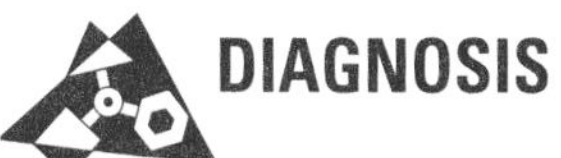

DIAGNOSIS

DIAGNOSTIC PROCEDURES

- Endoscopy with biopsy and brushings (for microbiologic and histopathologic analysis)

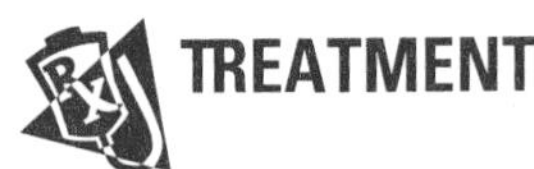

TREATMENT

MEDICATIONS

- Treatment may be empirical

Candidal esophagitis

- For patients with a normal immune system: topical nystatin, 500,000 units "swish and swallow" 5 times daily; clotrimazole troches, 10 mg dissolved in mouth 5 times daily for 7–14 days
- For immunocompromised patients (including AIDS): fluconazole, 100 mg PO QD (for 14–21 days)
- For patients not responding to oral therapy: itraconazole suspension (not capsules), 200 mg PO QD, voriconazole 200 mg PO BID, low-dose amphotericin B, 0.3–0.5 mg/kg/day, duration not standardized

Cytomegalovirus esophagitis

- For initial therapy: ganciclovir, 5 mg/kg IV Q 12 h for 3–6 weeks; after symptoms resolve, convert to oral valganciclovir, 900 mg once daily
- For patients with AIDS: immune restoration with active antiretroviral therapy (HAART) is most effective means of treating
- For patients who do not respond or cannot tolerate ganciclovir: foscarnet, 90 mg/kg IV Q 12 h for 3–6 weeks

Herpetic esophagitis

- For patients with a normal immune system: symptomatic treatment
- For immunocompromised patients: acyclovir, 200 mg PO 5 times daily, or 250 mg/m^2 IV Q 8–12, usually for 7–10 days; famciclovir, 250 mg PO TID; or valacyclovir, 1 g PO BID
- For nonresponders: foscarnet, 40 mg/kg IV Q 8 h for 21 days

OUTCOME

PROGNOSIS

- Most patients can be effectively treated with complete symptom resolution
- Chronic suppressive therapy is sometimes required for immunocompromised patients

WHEN TO REFER

- Refer patients who do not respond to empirical therapy to a gastroenterologist for upper endoscopy, brushings, and biopsy

WHEN TO ADMIT

- Severe odynophagia with inability to take adequate oral liquids

PREVENTION

- For patients with HIV infection: immune restoration with highly active antiretroviral therapy (HAART)

EVIDENCE

PRACTICE GUIDELINES

- National Guideline Clearinghouse
  - http://www.guideline.gov/summary/summary.aspx?doc_id=3259&nbr=2485&string=infectious+AND+esophagitis
  - http://www.guideline.gov/summary/summary.aspx?doc_id=3080&nbr=2306&string=esophageal+AND+candidiasis
- Pappas PG et al; Infectious Diseases Society of America: Guidelines for the treatment of candidiasis. Clin Infect Dis 2004;38:161. [PMID:14699449]
  - http://www.journals.uchicago.edu/IDSA/gidelines

INFORMATION FOR PATIENTS

- Cleveland Clinic—Esophagitis
  - http://www.clevelandclinic.org/health/health-info/docs/2800/2896.asp?index=10138
- MEDLINEplus—Candida esophagitis
  - http://www.nlm.nih.gov/medlineplus/ency/article/000643.htm
- MEDLINEplus—Herpes esophagitis
  - http://www.nlm.nih.gov/medlineplus/ency/article/000646.htm

REFERENCES

- Bobak, DA: Gastrointestinal infections caused by cytomegalovirus. Current Infect Dis Rep 2003;5:101. [PMID:12641994]
- Pappas PG et al: Guidelines for the treatment of candidiasis. Clin Infect Dis 2004;38:161. [PMID:14699449]
- Wilcox CM et al: Prospective comparison of brush cytology, viral culture, and histology for the diagnosis of ulcerative esophagitis in AIDS. Clin Gastroenterol Hepatol 2004;2:564. [PMID:15224280]

Author(s)

Kenneth R. McQuaid, MD

Falls in Elderly

Esophagitis, Pill-Induced p. 1071. Factitious Disorder p. 1071.

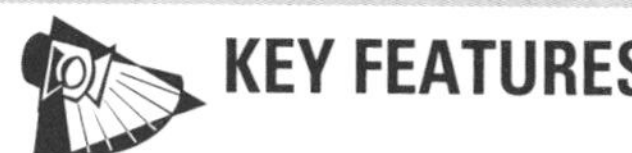

KEY FEATURES

ESSENTIALS OF DIAGNOSIS

- Falls in older people are rarely due to a single cause
- Medications and alcohol use are among the most common, significant, and reversible causes of falling

GENERAL CONSIDERATIONS

Causes of falls

- Visual impairment
- Gait impairment due to
  - Podiatric disorder (ingrown nail, ulcer)
  - Arthritis
  - Muscular weakness (myopathy, deconditioning)
  - Cerebellar ataxia (alcoholism)
  - Sensory ataxia (vitamin B_{12} deficiency, neurosyphilis)
  - Other neurologic disorders (parkinsonism, Alzheimer's disease, spinal stenosis, multiple sclerosis, peripheral neuropathy)
- Environmental hazards (poor lighting, stairs, rugs, uneven floors)
- Polypharmacy (benzodiazepines, opioids, phenothiazines, vasodilators, diuretics)
- Alcohol and illicit drug use
- Orthostatic or postprandial hypotension
- Vertigo, presyncope, syncope, or dysequilibrium
- Medical illness (pneumonia, myocardial infarction, anemia, hyponatremia)
- Other contributing factors
  - Urinary urgency
  - Peripheral edema
  - Insomnia
  - Footwear

DEMOGRAPHICS

- 30% of community-dwelling elderly fall each year, including 50% of people over age 80; of those who fall 25% have serious injuries
- About 5% of falls result in fracture
- 50% of those who fall are unable to get up without assistance
- Falls are the sixth leading cause of death for older people

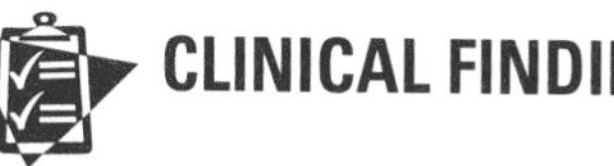

CLINICAL FINDINGS

SYMPTOMS AND SIGNS

Gait and balance tests

- Romberg test
  - Is there steadiness when patient stands with eyes closed?
- A nudge, 360-degree turn
  - Is balance maintained when the patient is pushed lightly on the sternum?
  - When turning are steps continuous or discontinuous?
- "Up and Go Test"
  - Patient is asked to stand from a sitting position without using the hands, walk 10 feet, turn around, walk back, and sit down
  - Test performance is qualitative: normal vs abnormal
  - Patient should be timed during the test: 10–15 seconds is considered normal
  - Times longer than 20 seconds are often associated with other functional impairments
- Tinetti Gait and Balance Assessment
  - Includes aspects of the above tests
  - Is most often used for formal testing
  - Evaluates step length, height, width, symmetry, and continuity
  - Evaluates steadiness with eyes closed and with gentle sternal nudge
  - Evaluates posture, sway, and use of mobility aids

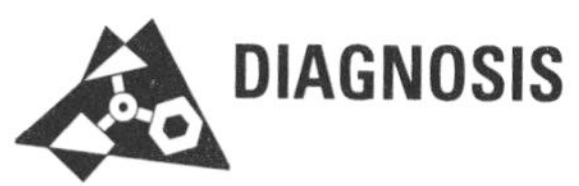

DIAGNOSIS

DIAGNOSTIC PROCEDURES

- Every older person should be asked about falls; many will not volunteer such information
- Review medications, including over-the-counter sleeping aids
- Review substance use history
- Examine for postural hypotension
- Examine for peripheral edema
- Ask about urinary symptoms

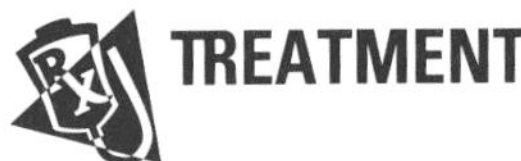

TREATMENT

MEDICATIONS

- Eliminate all nonessential medications that can interfere with gait, cause somnolence or urinary urgency

THERAPEUTIC PROCEDURES

- Home safety check: generally reimbursed by third-party payers, including Medicare
- For patients with repeated falls, make available phones at floor level, a portable phone, or a lightweight radio call system
- Exercise programs
  - Resistance training and balance retraining reduced risk 20%
  - Tai Chi programs have also shown modest benefits
- Use of an anatomically designed external hip protector reduces hip fracture risk in frail elders, but is often poorly tolerated

OUTCOME

COMPLICATIONS

- Fractures, commonly of the wrist, hip, and vertebrae
- Loss of confidence and independence and self-restricted activity because of fear of repeated falls
- Chronic subdural hematoma
  - Consider in an elderly patient who presents with new neurologic symptoms or signs, particularly obtundation
  - Headache is uncommon
- Dehydration, electrolyte imbalance, pressure sores, hypothermia, and rhabdomyolysis in patients who are unable to get up from a fall

PROGNOSIS

- Patients who fall are at high risk for subsequent falls
- Falls are associated with a higher risk of nursing home placement
- There is a high mortality rate (approximately 20% in 1 year) in elderly women with hip fractures

WHEN TO REFER

- Refer for a home safety check any elderly individual with a history of falls or balance or gait abnormalities
- Consider referral to a physical therapist for gait assessment and training (how to get up from a fall and training with special devices)
- An interdisciplinary geriatrics assessment can be useful

PREVENTION

- Remedy home hazards
- Perform a thorough gait assessment
- An abnormal gait may suggest remediable risk factor for falls, such as proximal muscle weakness, balance problems, or pain
- Modify factors outlined under General Considerations
- Determine bone density and improve if needed

EVIDENCE

PRACTICE GUIDELINES

- American Geriatrics Society
  - http://www.americangeriatrics.org/products/positionpapers/Falls.pdf
- National Guideline Clearinghouse
  - Guidelines Development Group (UK), 2000
  - University of Iowa Gerontologic Nursing Research Center, 2004

WEB SITES

- AARP Guide to Internet Resources on Aging
  - http://www.aarp.org/cyber/sd1_3.htm
- Administration on Aging
  - http://www.aoa.dhhs.gov

INFORMATION FOR PATIENTS

- JAMA patient page: Fall-induced injuries. JAMA 1999;281:1962. [PMID: 10349902]
- American Academy of Family Physicians
  - http://familydoctor.org/handouts/245.xml
- JAMA patient page: Hip fractures. JAMA 2001;285:2814. [PMID: 11419423]

REFERENCES

- Mahoney JE: Temporal association between hospitalization and rate of falls after discharge. Arch Intern Med 2000;160:2788. [PMID: 11025789]
- Ooi WL: The association between orthostatic hypotension and recurrent falls in nursing home residents. Am J Med 2000;108:106. [PMID: 11126303]
- Tinetti ME: Clinical practice. Preventing falls in elderly persons. N Engl J Med 2003;348:42. [PMID: 12510042]

Author(s)

Helen Chen, MD

C. Bree Johnston, MD

Familial Adenomatous Polyposis

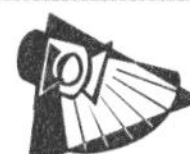

KEY FEATURES

ESSENTIALS OF DIAGNOSIS

- Hundreds to thousands of colorectal polyps evident on sigmoidoscopy or colonoscopy
- Mutation of adenomatous polyposis coli (*APC*) gene on 5q21 in 90% of affected patients; mutation in *MYH* present in some remaining patients

GENERAL CONSIDERATIONS

- Classic form of familial adenomatous polyposis (FAP) characterized by development of hundreds to thousands of colorectal polyps
- Other gastrointestinal tumors include
  - Benign gastric fundic gland polyps
  - Duodenal (especially periampullary) adenomas
  - Adenocarcinomas
- Extraintestinal manifestations include
  - Skin soft tissue tumors
  - Desmoid tumors
  - Osteomas
  - Congenital hypertrophy of retinal pigment
- Caused by autosomal dominant inheritance of mutation in *APC* gene (encodes protein involved with cell adhesion and apoptosis); location of mutation affects number of polyps formed and extracolonic features
- Attenuated variant of FAP results in fewer polyps (25–100); mutations found at 3' or 5' end of *APC* gene

DEMOGRAPHICS

- Affects 1:10,000 people
- Accounts for 1% of colorectal cancers
- Colorectal polyps develop at mean age of 15 and cancers by age 40
- 25% of patients have no family history; believed to have de novo *APC* mutation
- Colorectal cancer inevitable by age 50 unless prophylactic colectomy performed

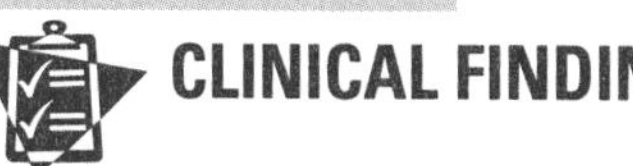

CLINICAL FINDINGS

SYMPTOMS AND SIGNS

- Iron deficiency anemia
- Hematochezia
- Obstipation due to obstructing colonic carcinoma
- Jaundice due to ampullary neoplasm or metastases to liver
- Weight loss if metastatic disease

DIFFERENTIAL DIAGNOSIS

- Sporadic colorectal cancer
- Inflammatory bowel disease with multiple inflammatory polyps
- Other nonadenomatous polyposis syndromes: Peutz-Jeghers syndrome, juvenile polyposis
- Hereditary nonpolyposis colorectal cancer also is an inherited autosomal dominant condition associated with early-onset colorectal cancer but few adenomatous polyps

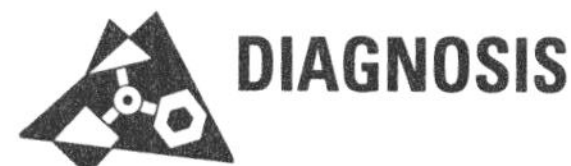

DIAGNOSIS

IMAGING STUDIES

- No imaging necessary in most cases
- Abdominal CT for evaluation of colorectal cancer or periampullary neoplasms
- Endoscopic ultrasonography and endoscopic retrograde cholangiopancreatography (ERCP) for evaluation of periampullary neoplasms

DIAGNOSTIC PROCEDURES

- Genetic counseling followed by testing (*APC* and possibly *MYH*) of first-degree relatives of patients with FAP, preferably at age 10–12; a negative result is considered true negative only if one affected member has a positive result
- Genetic counseling followed by testing in patients with > 20–100 polyps (without family history) to detect de novo classic or attenuated FAP
- Endoscopic screening beginning at age 12 for family members with *APC* mutation or for all family members, when known mutation not identified
- Classic FAP: sigmoidoscopy every year
- Attenuated FAP: colonoscopy every 2 years
- Upper endoscopy to look for periampullary tumors every 1–3 years, beginning at age 25

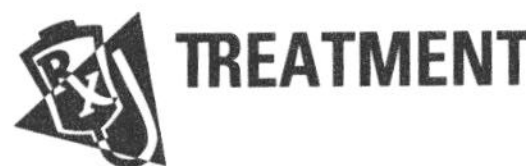

TREATMENT

MEDICATIONS

- Nonsteroidal anti-inflammatory drugs (NSAIDs), including sulindac 150 mg PO BID and celecoxib 400 mg PO BID, prevent or induce regression of duodenal polyps and rectum (after subtotal colectomy)

SURGERY

- Complete proctocolectomy with ileoanal pouch anastamosis or subtotal colectomy with ileorectal anastamosis is recommended after the development of polyposis, usually before age 20
- Ileorectal anastamosis affords superior bowel function but has 10% risk of rectal cancer
- Duodenal resection for patients with multiple or large periampullary adenomas, especially with dysplasia

THERAPEUTIC PROCEDURES

- For patients with retained rectum, sigmoidoscopy for surveillance and fulguration of polyps recommended every 6 months
- Endoscopic biopsy, removal, or fulguration of duodenal polyps and selected ampullary adenomas

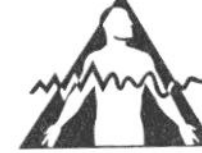

OUTCOME

FOLLOW-UP

- For patients with subtotal colectomy, surveillance sigmoidoscopy every 6 months

COMPLICATIONS

- Desmoid tumors (mesenteric fibrosis) develop in some kindreds (especially after surgery) causing obstruction and constriction of the intestines, mesenteric circulation, and ureters; these tumors cause death in > 10%

PROGNOSIS

- For patients with ileorectal anastamosis, completion proctectomy is required in 10–20% due to development of rectal cancer
- Duodenal cancer occurs in 5–10%

WHEN TO REFER

- Genetic counseling and testing should be performed by trained counselor or geneticist
- Ileoanal pouch should be performed by colorectal surgeon
- Surveillance of rectal pouch and duodenum should be performed by therapeutic gastroenterologist
- Patients with desmoid tumors

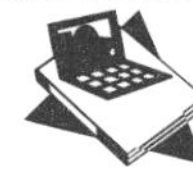

EVIDENCE

PRACTICE GUIDELINES

- American Gastroenterological Association Technical Review. Hereditary colorectal cancer and genetic testing. Gastroenterology 2001;121:198. [PMID: 11438509]

WEB SITES

- Johns Hopkins Medical Institution Gastroenterology & Hepatology Resource Center
  - http://hopkins-gi.nts.jhu.edu/pages/latin/templates/index.cfm?pg=hcc1&hccIntro_id=1&lang_id=1
- Cleveland Clinic Inherited Colorectal Cancer Registries
  - http://www.clevelandclinic.org/registries/inherited/fap.htm

INFORMATION FOR PATIENTS

- Johns Hopkins Guide for Patients and Families: Familial Adenomatous Polyposis
  - http://hopkins-gi.nts.jhu.edu/multimedia/database/hccIntro_82_FAP-Book.pdf
- National Library of Medicine Genetics Home Reference: Familial adenomatous polyposis
  - http://ghr.nlm.nih.gov/condition=familialadenomatouspolyposis

REFERENCES

- Cruz-Correa M et al: Familial adenomatous polyposis. Gastrointest Endosc 2003;58:885. [PMID: 14652558]
- Lindor NM: Recognition of genetic syndromes in families with suspected hereditary colon cancer syndromes. Clin Gastroenterol Hepatol 2004;2:366. [PMID: 15118973]
- Lynch H et al: Hereditary colorectal cancer. N Engl J Med 2003;348:919. [PMID: 12621137]

Author(s)

Kenneth R. McQuaid, MD

Fatty Liver Disease, Nonalcoholic

Familial Mediterranean Fever p. 1071. Fascioliasis p. 1072. Fasciolopsiasis p. 1072.

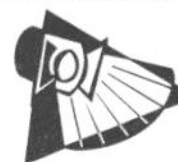

KEY FEATURES

ESSENTIALS OF DIAGNOSIS

- Often asymptomatic
- Elevated aminotransferase levels and/or hepatomegaly
- Macrovesicular and/or microvesicular steatosis on liver biopsy

GENERAL CONSIDERATIONS

Nonalcoholic fatty liver

- Besides ethanol, hepatic steatosis can be caused by obesity, diabetes mellitus, and hypertriglyceridemia
- These features are a hallmark of the insulin resistance syndrome

Nonalcoholic steatohepatitis (NASH)

- Results from "second hit" (in addition to steatosis) that leads to lipid peroxidation and oxidative stress
- Characterized histologically by macrovesicular steatosis, focal infiltration by polymorphonuclear neutrophils, and Mallory's hyalin, a picture indistinguishable from alcoholic hepatitis

Other causes of fatty liver

- Cushing's syndrome
- Starvation or rapid weight loss
- Hypobetalipoproteinemia
- Total parenteral nutrition
- Corticosteroids, amiodarone, tamoxifen
- Wilson's disease
- Jejunoileal bypass
- Poisons: carbon tetrachloride, yellow phosphorus

Causes of microvesicular steatosis

- Reye's syndrome, valproic acid toxicity, tetracycline, acute fatty liver of pregnancy
- Women in whom fatty liver of pregnancy develops often have a defect in fatty acid oxidation due to reduced long-chain 3-hydroxyacyl-CoA dehydrogenase activity

CLINICAL FINDINGS

SYMPTOMS AND SIGNS

- Hepatomegaly is present in 75% of patients with NASH, but the stigmata of chronic liver disease are uncommon

DIFFERENTIAL DIAGNOSIS

- Alcoholic fatty liver disease
- Hepatitis, eg, viral, alcoholic, toxic
- Cirrhosis
- Congestive heart failure
- Hepatocellular carcinoma or metastatic cancer

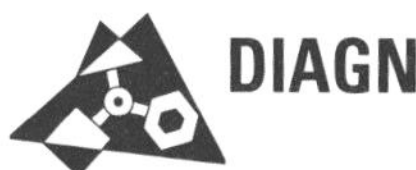

DIAGNOSIS

LABORATORY TESTS

- There may be mildly elevated aminotransferase and alkaline phosphatase levels
- In contrast to alcoholic liver disease, the ratio of alanine aminotransferase (ALT) to aspartate aminotransferase (AST) is almost always greater than 1 in NASH, but it decreases to less than 1 as advanced fibrosis and cirrhosis develop. An AST/ALT ratio >2 is highly suggestive of alcoholic liver disease

IMAGING STUDIES

- Fat in liver may be demonstrated on ultrasound, CT, or MRI; these imaging methods are insensitive for detecting inflammation and fibrosis

DIAGNOSTIC PROCEDURES

- Percutaneous liver biopsy is diagnostic and is the only way to assess the degree of inflammation and fibrosis. The risks of the procedure must be balanced against the impact of the added information on management decisions and assessment of prognosis

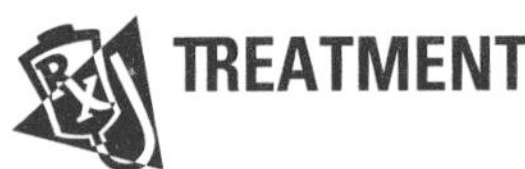

TREATMENT

MEDICATIONS

- Metformin, thiazolidinediones, vitamin E, orlistat, and betaine may reverse fatty liver and are under study
- Supplemental choline may reverse fatty liver associated with total parenteral nutrition
- Ursodeoxycholic acid, 13–15 mg/kg/day, did not improve liver function tests and liver histology in a large trial

SURGERY

- Gastric bypass may be considered in patients with a body mass index >35 kg/m^2

THERAPEUTIC PROCEDURES

- Fatty liver is readily reversible with discontinuation of alcohol or treatment of other underlying conditions
- Weight loss, dietary fat restriction, and exercise can often improve liver tests and steatosis in obese patients with fatty liver, but the benefit of such measures is less clear in patients with steatohepatitis

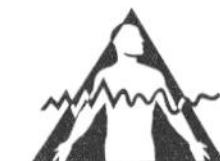

OUTCOME

COMPLICATIONS

- In patients with nonalcoholic fatty liver disease, older age, obesity, and diabetes are risk factors for advanced hepatic fibrosis and cirrhosis

PROGNOSIS

- NASH may be associated with hepatic fibrosis in 40% of cases; cirrhosis develops in 10–15%; and decompensated cirrhosis occurs in 2–5% of patients
- Hepatocellular carcinoma in cirrhosis caused by NASH can occur
- NASH may account for many cases of cryptogenic cirrhosis and can recur following liver transplantation

WHEN TO REFER

- For progressive liver diasease
- For liver biopsy

PREVENTION

- Avoid alcohol
- Maintain ideal weight
- Exercise
- Avoid hypertriglyceridemia

EVIDENCE

PRACTICE GUIDELINES

- National Guideline Clearinghouse
  - http://www.guideline.gov/summary/summary.aspx?doc_id=3491&nbr=2717&string=fatty+liver

WEB SITES

- Diseases of the Liver
  - http://cpmcnet.columbia.edu/dept/gi/fatty.html
- Pathology Index
  - http://www-medlib.med.utah.edu/WebPath/LIVEHTML/LIVER-IDX.html

INFORMATION FOR PATIENTS

- American Liver Foundation
  - http://www.liverfoundation.org/cgi-bin/dbs/articles.cgi?db=articles&uid=default&ID=1027&view_records=1
- Mayo Clinic
  - http://www.mayoclinic.com/invoke.cfm?objectid=B99683EA-2331-420F-9D023DE553EC136D
- Patient Information
  - http://patients.uptodate.com/topic.asp?file=livr_dis/5305&title=Nonalcoholic+Fatty+liver+disease

REFERENCES

- Browning JD et al: Prevalence of hepatic steatosis in an urban population in the United States: impact on ethnicity. Hepatology 2004;40:1387. [PMID: 15565570]
- Kaplan LM (ed): Obesity and the liver. Semin Liver Dis 2004;25:333.
- Sanyal AJ (guest ed): Nonalcoholic fatty liver disease. Clin Liver Dis 2004;8:481.
- Tolman KG et al: Narrative review: hepatobiliary disease in type 2 diabetes mellitus. Ann Intern Med 2004;141:946. [PMID: 15611492]

Author(s)

Lawrence S. Friedman, MD

Fever

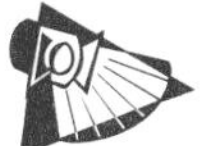

KEY FEATURES

ESSENTIALS OF DIAGNOSIS

- Localizing symptoms
- Weight loss
- Joint pain
- Intravenous substance use
- Immunosuppression or neutropenia
- History of cancer
- Travel

GENERAL CONSIDERATIONS

- Fever is a regulated rise to a new "set point" of body temperature mediated by pyrogenic cytokines
- The fever pattern is of marginal value, except for the relapsing fever of malaria, borreliosis, and lymphoma, especially Hodgkin's disease
- Most febrile illnesses are due to common infections, are short lived, and are relatively easy to diagnose
- The term FUO ("fever of undetermined origin") refers to cases of unexplained fever exceeding 38.3°C on several occasions for at least 3 weeks in patients without neutropenia or immunosuppression
- In HIV-infected individuals, prolonged unexplained fever is usually due to infections with disseminated *Mycobacterium avium*, *Pneumocystis jiroveci*, cytomegalovirus, or disseminated histoplasmosis, or to lymphoma
- In the returned traveler, consider malaria, dysentery, hepatitis, and dengue fever

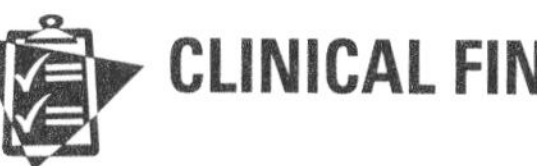

CLINICAL FINDINGS

SYMPTOMS AND SIGNS

- Fever is defined as an elevated body temperature exceeding 38.3°C
- The average normal oral body temperature taken in mid morning is 36.7°C (range 36–37.4°C)
- The normal rectal or vaginal temperature is 0.5°C higher; the axillary temperature is 0.5°C lower
- Rectal is more reliable than oral temperature, particularly in mouth breathers or in tachypneic states
- The normal diurnal temperature variation is 0.5–1°C—lowest in the early morning and highest in the evening
- There is a slight sustained temperature rise following ovulation, during the menstrual cycle, and in the first trimester of pregnancy

DIFFERENTIAL DIAGNOSIS

Common causes

- Infections
  - Bacterial
  - Viral
  - Rickettsial
  - Fungal
  - Parasitic
- Autoimmune diseases
- Central nervous system diseases
  - Head trauma
  - Mass lesions
- Malignant disease
  - Renal cell carcinoma
  - Primary or metastatic liver cancer
  - Leukemia
  - Lymphoma
- Cardiovascular diseases
  - Myocardial infarction
  - Thrombophlebitis
  - Pulmonary embolism
- Gastrointestinal diseases
  - Inflammatory bowel disease
  - Alcoholic hepatitis
  - Granulomatous hepatitis
- Miscellaneous diseases
  - Drug fever
  - Sarcoidosis
  - Familial Mediterranean fever
  - Tissue injury
  - Hematoma
  - Factitious fever

Hyperthermia

- Peripheral thermoregulatory disorders
  - Heat stroke
  - Malignant hyperthermia of anesthesia
  - Malignant neuroleptic syndrome

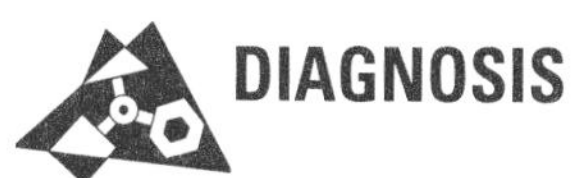

DIAGNOSIS

LABORATORY TESTS

- Obtain complete blood cell count with differential, urinalysis, erythrocyte sedimentation rate (ESR) or C-reactive protein level, liver tests (alkaline phosphatase, aspartate aminotransferase, gamma-glutamyl transpeptidase, total bilirubin)
- Obtain cultures of blood and urine

IMAGING STUDIES

- Chest x-ray film
- Abdominal ultrasound and CT scan
- Radionuclide-labeled leukocyte, gallium-67, and radiolabeled human immunoglobulin tests

DIAGNOSTIC PROCEDURES

- Temporal artery biopsy in patients aged ≥ 60 with elevated ESR

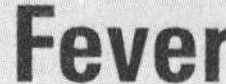

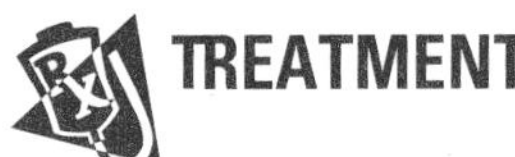

TREATMENT

MEDICATIONS

- Antipyretic therapy with aspirin or acetaminophen, 325–650 mg q4 h
- After obtaining blood and urine cultures, empiric broad-spectrum antibiotic therapy is indicated in patients
  - Who are likely to have a clinically significant infection
  - Who are clinically unstable
  - Who have hemodynamic instability
  - Who have neutropenia (neutrophils < 500/μL)
  - Who are asplenic (from surgery or sickle cell disease)
  - Who are immunosuppressed (including individuals taking systemic corticosteroids, azathioprine, cyclosporine, or other immunosuppressive medications, and those who are HIV infected)
- If a fungal infection is suspected, add fluconazole or amphotericin B

THERAPEUTIC PROCEDURES

- Most fever is well tolerated
- When temperature is < 40°C, symptomatic treatment
- When temperature is > 41°C, emergent management of hyperthermia is indicated
  - Alcohol sponges, cold sponges, ice bags, ice-water enemas, and ice baths

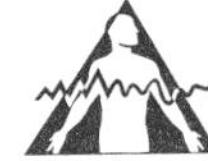

OUTCOME

PROGNOSIS

- After extensive evaluation, 25% of patients with FUO have chronic or indolent infection, 25% have autoimmune disease, 10% have malignancy; the remainder have miscellaneous other disorders or no definitive diagnosis
- Long-term follow-up of patients with initially undiagnosed FUO demonstrates that 50% become symptom-free during evaluation, 20% reach a definitive diagnosis (usually within 2 months), and 30% have persistent or recurring fever for months or years

WHEN TO REFER

- Refer patients with prolonged unexplained fever, including FUO, to infectious disease expert

WHEN TO ADMIT

- Admit for empiric broad-spectrum antibiotic therapy patients who are likely to have a clinically significant infection, who are clinically unstable, who have hemodynamic instability, who have neutropenia, who are asplenic, or who are immunosuppressed

EVIDENCE

PRACTICE GUIDELINES

- Wade JC et al: NCCN Fever and Neutropenia Practice Guidelines Panel. NCCN: Fever and neutropenia. Cancer Control 2001;8(6 Suppl 2):16. [PMID: 11760554]

WEB SITES

- World Health Organization
  - http://www.who.int/en/
- Centers for Disease Control and Prevention
  - http://www.cdc.gov
- National Institute of Allergy and Infectious Diseases/National Institutes of Health
  - http://www.niaid.nih.gov/default.htm

INFORMATION FOR PATIENTS

- American Academy of Family Physicians: Fever Flowchart
  - http://familydoctor.org/503.xml
- Mayo Clinic: Fever
  - http://www.mayoclinic.com/invoke.cfm?id=DS00077
- MedlinePlus: Fever
  - http://www.nlm.nih.gov/medlineplus/ency/article/003090.htm

REFERENCES

- Armstrong WS et al: Human immunodeficiency virus-associated fever of unknown origin: a study of 70 patients in the United States and review. Clin Infect Dis 1999;28:341. [PMID: 10064253]
- Hopkins PM: Malignant hyperthermia: advances in clinical management and diagnosis. Br J Anaesth 2000;85:118. [PMID: 10928000]
- Mackowiak PA: Concepts of fever. Arch Intern Med 1998;158:1871. [PMID: 9759682]
- Magill AJ: Fever in the returned traveler. Infect Dis Clin North Am 1998;12:445. [PMID: 9658253]
- Pizzo PA: Fever in immunocompromised patients. N Engl J Med 1999;341:893. [PMID: 10486422]

Author(s)

Ralph Gonzales, MD

Fever of Unknown Origin (FUO)

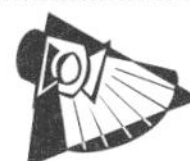

KEY FEATURES

ESSENTIALS OF DIAGNOSIS

- At least 3 weeks of fever over 38.3°C on several occasions, and no diagnosis after 3 outpatient visits or 3 days of hospitalization
- **Nosocomial FUO** occurs in a hospitalized patient with fever of 38.3°C or higher on several occasions, due to a process not present or incubating at admission, in whom initial cultures are negative and the diagnosis remains unknown after 3 days of investigation
- **Neutropenic FUO** includes fever of 38.3°C or higher in a patient on several occasions with < 500 neutrophils per microliter in whom initial cultures are negative and the diagnosis remains uncertain after 3 days
- **HIV-associated FUO** occurs in HIV-positive patients with fever of 38.3°C or higher who have been febrile for 4 weeks or more as an outpatient or 3 days as an inpatient, in whom the diagnosis remains uncertain after 3 days of investigation with at least 2 days for cultures to incubate
- Although not usually considered separately, **FUO in solid organ transplant** recipients is a common scenario with a unique differential diagnosis (see below)

GENERAL CONSIDERATIONS

Common causes

- Most cases represent unusual manifestations of common diseases and not rare or exotic diseases—eg, tuberculosis and HIV (primary infection or opportunistic infection) are more common causes than Whipple's disease
- A thorough history—including family, occupational, social (sexual practices, use of injection drugs), dietary (unpasteurized products, raw meat), exposures (animals, chemicals), and travel—may give clues to the diagnosis

Age of patient

- Infections (25–40% of cases) and cancer (25–40% of cases) account for the majority of FUOs
- In the elderly (over 65 years of age), multisystem immune-mediated diseases such as temporal arteritis, polymyalgia rheumatica, sarcoidosis, rheumatoid arthritis, and Wegener's granulomatosis account for 25–30% of all FUOs

Duration of fever

- Granulomatous diseases (granulomatous hepatitis, Crohn's disease, ulcerative colitis) and factitious fever are more likely if fever has been present for 6 months or longer
- One-fourth of patients who report being febrile for 6 months or longer have no true fever. Instead, the usual normal circadian variation in temperature (temperature 0.5–1°C higher in the afternoon than in the morning) is interpreted as abnormal
- Episodic or recurrent fever patients who meet the criteria for FUO but have fever-free periods of 2 weeks or longer are similar to those with prolonged fever
  - Infection, malignancy, and autoimmune disorders account for only 20–25% of such fevers, whereas various miscellaneous diseases (Crohn's disease, familial Mediterranean fever, allergic alveolitis) account for another 25%
  - Approximately 50% remain undiagnosed but have a benign course with eventual resolution of symptoms

Immunologic status

- In neutropenia, fungal infections and occult bacterial infection are important causes of FUO
- In the patient taking immunosuppressive medications (particularly organ transplant patients), cytomegalovirus (CMV) infections are a frequent cause of fever, as are fungal infections, nocardiosis, *Pneumocystis jiroveci* pneumonia, and mycobacterial infections

Posttransplant

- Infections immediately after transplant often involve the transplanted organ
- Following lung transplantation, pneumonia and mediastinitis are particularly common; following liver transplantation, intra-abdominal abscess, cholangitis, and peritonitis; after renal transplantation, urinary tract infections, perinephric abscesses, and infected lymphoceles
- In contrast to solid organ transplants, in bone marrow transplant patients the source of fever cannot be found in 60–70% of patients
- Most infections that occur in the first 2–4 weeks are related to the operative procedure and to hospitalization itself (wound infection, IV catheter infection, urinary tract infection from a Foley catheter) or are related to the transplanted organ
- Infections that occur between the first and sixth months are often related to immunosuppression. Reactivated herpes simplex, varicella-zoster, and CMV infections are quite common. Opportunistic infections with fungi (*Candida*, *Aspergillus*, *Cryptococcus*, *Pneumocystis*, and others), *Listeria monocytogenes*, *Nocardia*, and *Toxoplasma* are also common
- After 6 months, when immunosuppression has been reduced to maintenance levels, infections that are found in any population occur

Classification of causes of FUO

- Most patients with FUO will fit into one of five categories
  - Infection
  - Neoplasms
  - Autoimmune disorders
  - Miscellaneous causes
  - Undiagnosed FUO
- Despite extensive evaluation, the diagnosis remains elusive in 10–15% of patients. In about 75%, the fever abates spontaneously and the clinician never knows the cause; in the remainder, more classic manifestations of the underlying disease appear

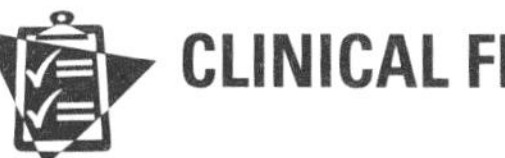

CLINICAL FINDINGS

SYMPTOMS AND SIGNS

- Document the fever in order to exclude factitious (self-induced) fever. Tachycardia, chills, and piloerection generally accompany fever
- Repeated physical examination may reveal subtle, evanescent clinical findings, such as a rash

DIFFERENTIAL DIAGNOSIS

- *Infection*: tuberculosis, endocarditis, osteomyelitis, urinary tract infection, sinusitis, occult abscess (eg, intra-abdominal, dental, brain), cholangitis, primary HIV, Epstein–Barr virus, CMV, systemic mycosis, toxoplasmosis, brucellosis, Q fever, cat scratch disease, salmonellosis, malaria
- *Neoplasm*: Hodgkin's and non-Hodgkin's lymphoma, leukemia, primary or metastatic liver cancer, renal cell carcinoma, atrial myxoma, post-transplant lymphoproliferative disease
- *Autoimmune:* adult Still's disease, systemic lupus erythematosus, cryoglobulinemia, polyarteritis nodosa, temporal (giant cell) arteritis, polymyalgia rheumatica, Wegener's granulomatosis
- *Miscellaneous causes:* drug fever, sarcoidosis, alcoholic or granulomatous hepatitis, Crohn's disease, ulcerative colitis, factitious fever, thyroiditis, hematoma, recurrent pulmonary emboli, hypersensitivity pneumonitis, familial Mediterra-

nean fever, Whipple's disease, transplant rejection, organ ischemia and necrosis, thrombophlebitis

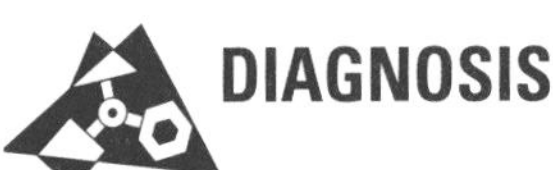

DIAGNOSIS

LABORATORY TESTS

- Blood culture all patients, and usually other fluids, ie, urine, sputum, stool, cerebrospinal fluid, and morning gastric aspirates (if one suspects tuberculosis), preferably when antibiotics have not been taken for several days, and hold in the laboratory for 2 weeks to detect slow-growing organisms
- Cultures on special media are requested for *Legionella*, *Bartonella*, or nutritionally deficient streptococci
- "Screening tests" with immunologic or microbiologic serologies ("febrile agglutinins") are not useful
- A single elevated titer rarely is diagnostic of an infection; a four-fold rise or fall in titer confirms a specific cause
- Direct examination of blood smears may establish a diagnosis of malaria or relapsing fever (*Borrelia*)

IMAGING STUDIES

- Chest x-ray in all patients
- Targeted studies (eg, sinus films, gallbladder studies) are best used when symptoms, signs, or a history suggest disease in these body regions
- CT scan of the abdomen and pelvis is particularly useful for looking at the liver, spleen, and retroperitoneum. A positive CT scan often leads to a specific diagnosis. A negative CT scan is not quite as useful
- MRI is generally better than CT for lesions of the nervous system and is useful in diagnosing some vasculitides
- Ultrasound is sensitive for lesions of the kidney, pancreas, and biliary tree
- Radionuclide scans are not very helpful when used as screening tests
- A gallium or PET scan may be more helpful than an indium-labeled white blood cell scan because gallium and (18)fluorodeoxyglucose detect infection, inflammation, and neoplasm whereas indium is only useful for infection

DIAGNOSTIC PROCEDURES

- Echocardiography if endocarditis or atrial myxoma is being considered: transesophageal echocardiography is more sensitive than surface echocardiography for detecting valvular lesions
- Invasive procedures are often required for diagnosis
- Any abnormal finding should be aggressively evaluated: headache calls for lumbar puncture; skin from a rash should be biopsied; and enlarged lymph nodes should be aspirated or biopsied for cytology and culture
- Bone marrow aspiration with biopsy is a relatively low-yield procedure (except in HIV-positive patients, in whom mycobacterial infection is a common cause of FUO), but is low-risk and should be done if other less invasive tests have not yielded a diagnosis
- Liver biopsy will yield a specific diagnosis in 10–15% of FUO patients
- Consider laparotomy or laparoscopy in the deteriorating patient if the diagnosis is elusive despite extensive evaluation

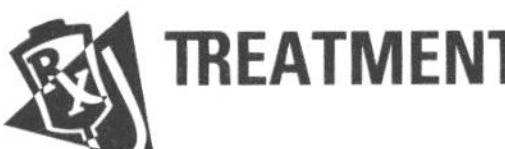

TREATMENT

MEDICATIONS

- Therapeutic trials are indicated if a diagnosis is strongly suspected—eg, antituberculous drugs. However, if there is no clinical response in several weeks, it is imperative to stop therapy and reevaluate the patient
- In the seriously ill or rapidly deteriorating patient, empiric therapy is often given. Antituberculosis medications (particularly in the elderly or foreign-born) and broad-spectrum antibiotics are reasonable in this setting (Table 128)
- Empiric administration of corticosteroids should be discouraged; they can suppress fever and exacerbate many infections that cause FUO

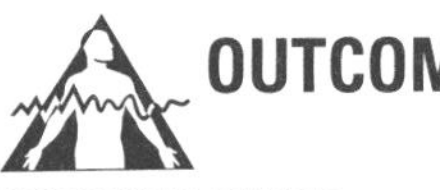

OUTCOME

WHEN TO REFER

- If patients remain symptomatic without a diagnosis after initial cultural and radiographic evaluation

WHEN TO ADMIT

- Patients who are clinically deteriorating with symptoms that are interfering with daily activity
- Progressive debilitating weight loss

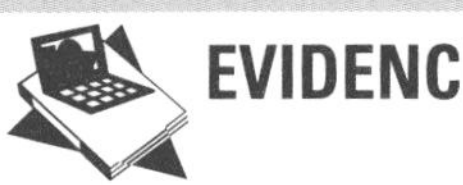

EVIDENCE

PRACTICE GUIDELINES

- American Academy of Family Physicians
  - http://www.aafp.org/afp/20031201/2223.html
- Infectious Diseases Society of America
  - http://www.journals.uchicago.edu/CID/journal/issues/v25n3/se34_551/se34_551.web.pdf
- Wade JC et al: NCCN Fever and Neutropenia Practice Guidelines Panel. NCCN: Fever and neutropenia. Cancer Control 2001;8(6 suppl 2):16. [PMID: 11760554]

INFORMATION FOR PATIENTS

- National Cancer Institute
  - http://www.cancer.gov/cancerinfo/pdq/supportivecare/fever/patient
- The National Institutes of Health
  - http://www.nlm.nih.gov/medlineplus/ency/article/003090.htm

REFERENCES

- Knockaert DE et al: Fever of unknown origin in adults: 40 years on. J Intern Med 2003;253:263. [PMID: 12603493]
- Tal S: Fever of unknown origin in the elderly. J Intern Med 2002;242:295. [PMID: 12366602]

Author(s)

Richard A. Jacobs, MD, PhD

Fibrocystic Condition, Breast

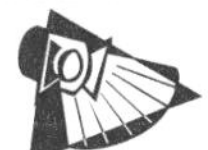

KEY FEATURES

ESSENTIALS OF DIAGNOSIS

- Painful, often multiple, often bilateral masses of the breasts
- Pain and size often increase premenstrually

GENERAL CONSIDERATIONS

- Most frequent lesion of the breast
- Estrogen hormone is considered a causative factor
- Encompasses a wide variety of pathological entities
- Always associated with benign changes in the breast epithelium
- Microscopic findings include cysts (gross and microscopic), papillomatosis, adenosis, fibrosis, and ductal epithelial hyperplasia
- Risk factor for breast cancer only if ductal epithelial hyperplasia is present, especially when atypia is present

DEMOGRAPHICS

- Occurs most commonly in women age 30–50
- Rare in postmenopausal women not receiving hormonal replacement therapy

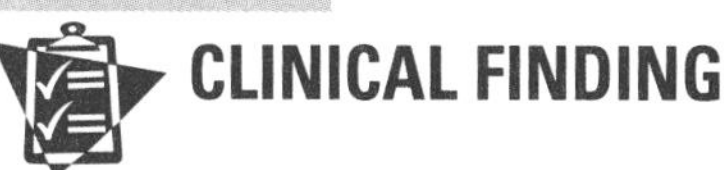

CLINICAL FINDINGS

SYMPTOMS AND SIGNS

- Generally painful lump or lumps, but may be asymptomatic
- Nipple discharge may be present
- Rapid fluctuation in size of masses is common

DIFFERENTIAL DIAGNOSIS

- Breast cancer
- Fibroadenoma
- Lipoma
- Breast abscess
- Intraductal papilloma

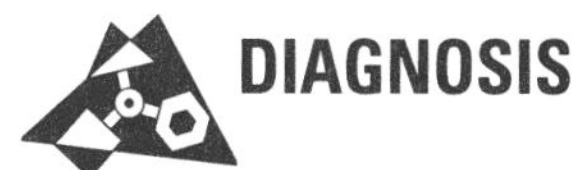

DIAGNOSIS

IMAGING STUDIES

- Mammography may be helpful, but is often limited due to radiodensity of breast tissue in young women
- Breast ultrasonography is useful in differentiating cystic from solid mass

DIAGNOSTIC PROCEDURES

- Suspicious lesions should be biopsied
- Fine-needle aspiration cytology may be used, but if mass does not resolve over several months, it must be excised

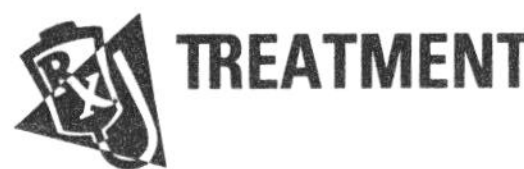

TREATMENT

MEDICATIONS

- Vitamin E, 400 IU PO QD (anecdotal data)
- Danazol, 100–200 mg PO QD, for severe pain, but is rarely used due to side effects (acne, hirsutism, edema)

SURGERY

- Total or subcutaneous mastectomy or extensive removal of breast tissue is rarely, if ever, indicated for fibrocystic breast disease

THERAPEUTIC PROCEDURES

- Aspiration of a discrete mass suggestive of a cyst is indicated in order to alleviate pain and, more importantly, to confirm the cystic nature of the mass

OUTCOME

FOLLOW-UP

- Reexamine at intervals
- Women with proliferative or atypical epithelium on biopsy should be monitored carefully by physical examination and mammography for development of breast cancer; consider tamoxifen chemoprevention
- The patient should be advised to examine her own breasts each month just after menstruation and to inform her physician if a mass appears
- Excisional biopsy should be performed if no fluid is obtained or if fluid is bloody on aspiration, if a mass persists after aspiration, or if at any time during follow-up a persistent lump is noted

COMPLICATIONS

- Risk of breast cancer in women with proliferative or atypical changes in the epithelium is higher than in women in general

PROGNOSIS

- Exacerbations of pain, tenderness, and cyst formation may occur at any time until menopause
- After menopause, symptoms usually subside, except in patients receiving hormone replacement therapy

PREVENTION

- Avoid trauma
- Avoid caffeine (anecdotal data)
- Wear supportive bra night and day

EVIDENCE

PRACTICE GUIDELINES

- Heisey R et al: Management of palpable breast lumps. Consensus guideline for family physicians. Can Fam Physician 1999;45:1926. [PMID: 10463093]

WEB SITE

- American Academy of Family Physicians: Breast Problems in Women Flowchart
  - http://familydoctor.org/519.xml

INFORMATION FOR PATIENTS

- American Cancer Society–Benign breast conditions
  - http://www.cancer.org/docroot/cri/content/cri_2_6x_benign_breast_conditions_59.asp
- American College of Obstetricians and Gynecologists: Fibrocystic Breast Changes
  - http://www.medem.com/MedLB/article_detaillb.cfm?article_ID=ZZZLF2SXODC&sub_cat=326
- MedlinePlus: Fibrocystic Breast Disease
  - http://www.nlm.nih.gov/medlineplus/ency/article/000912.htm
- National Cancer Institute: Understanding Breast Changes
  - http://www.cancer.gov/cancertopics/understanding-breast-changes/

REFERENCES

- Marchant DJ: Benign breast disease. Obstet Gynecol Clin North Am 2002;29:1. [PMID: 11892859]
- Morrow M: The evaluation of common breast problems. Am Fam Physician 2000;61:2371. [PMID: 10794579]
- Norlock FE: Benign breast pain in women: a practical approach to evaluation and treatment. J Am Med Womens Assoc 2002;57:85. [PMID: 11991427]

Author(s)

Armando E. Giuliano, MD

Filariasis

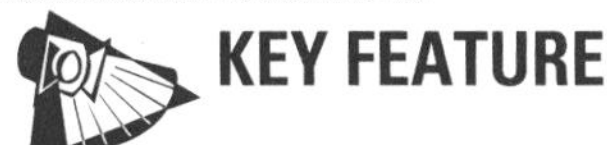

KEY FEATURES

ESSENTIALS OF DIAGNOSIS

- Acute disease has irregular episodes of fever (filarial fever), with or without inflammation of lymphatics
- Elephantiasis occurs in the chronic phase as a result of interference with normal lymphatic flow

GENERAL CONSIDERATIONS

- The disease is caused by three filarial nematodes: *Wuchereria bancrofti*, *Brugia malayi*, or *Brugia timori*
- Mosquitoes become infected by ingesting microfilariae with a blood meal; at subsequent feedings, they can infect new susceptible hosts
- Over months, adult worms (females, 8–9 cm × 0.2–0.3 mm) mature and live (up to 2 decades) in or near superficial and deep lymphatics and lymph nodes and produce large numbers of viviparous circulating microfilariae, which may be seen in the blood starting 6–12 months after infection
- Pathological changes in lymph vessels are due to host immunological reactions
- Living microfilariae generally cause no lesions, with the exception of tropical pulmonary eosinophilia. Rapid death of microfilariae, however, does produce findings, and an abscess may form at the site of a dying adult worm
- **Tropical pulmonary eosinophilia**: microfilariae of *W bancrofti* or *B malayi* are sequestered in the lungs but not found in the blood

DEMOGRAPHICS

- More than 80 million people are infected with lymphatic filariasis in 73 tropical and subtropical countries
- An estimated 1 million new persons are infected yearly

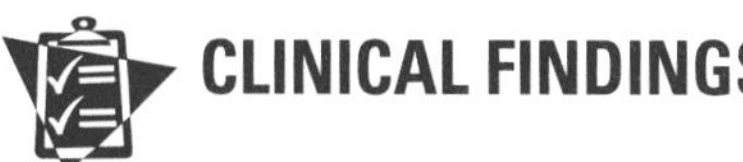

CLINICAL FINDINGS

SYMPTOMS AND SIGNS

- The incubation period is generally 8–16 months in expatriates but may be longer in indigenous persons
- Many infections remain asymptomatic

Acute disease

- Episodes of fever (filarial fever), with or without inflammation of lymphatics and nodes, occur at irregular intervals and last for several days
- Characteristically, the adenolymphangitis presents as retrograde extension from the affected node (unlike ascending bacterial lymphangitis)
- With disease progression, epididymitis and orchitis as well as involvement of pelvic, abdominal, or retroperitoneal lymphatics may occur intermittently
- In travelers, allergic-like findings (hives, rashes, eosinophilia) and lymphangitis and lymphadenitis are more likely

Chronic disease

- Obstruction occurs as a result of interference with normal lymphatic flow; this includes hydrocele, scrotal lymphedema, lymphatic varices and elephantiasis, particularly of the extremities, genitals, and breasts
- Extrapulmonary manifestations include splenomegaly and moderate hepatomegaly

Occult disease

- A few persons develop occult disease, in which the classic clinical manifestations and microfilaremia are not present but microfilariae are present in the tissues

Tropical pulmonary eosinophilia

- Episodic nocturnal coughing or wheezing, dyspnea, low-grade fever, scant expectoration

DIFFERENTIAL DIAGNOSIS

- Bacterial lymphangitis
- Loiasis (*Loa loa* infection)
- Idiopathic hydrocele
- Lower extremity edema due to other cause, eg, congestive heart failure, cirrhosis, nephrotic syndrome
- Lymphoma

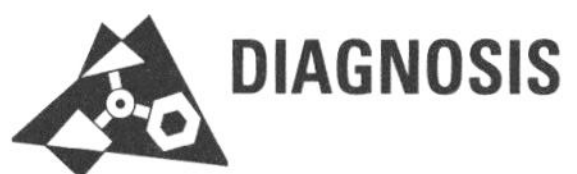

DIAGNOSIS

LABORATORY TESTS

- Diagnosis of active infection is made by finding microfilariae in blood (or hydrocele fluid), a positive antigen test (available only for *W bancrofti*), or by ultrasound
- In indigenous persons, microfilariae are rare in the first 2–3 years, abundant as the disease progresses, and again rare in the obstructive stage
- In persons from nonendemic areas, inflammatory reactions may be prominent in the absence of microfilariae
- Microfilariae of *W bancrofti* are found in the blood primarily at night (nocturnal periodicity 10 PM to 2 AM), except for a nonperiodic variety in the South Pacific. *B malayi* microfilariae are usually nocturnally periodic but in Southeast Asia may be present at all times, with a slight nocturnal rise
- Anticoagulated blood specimens are collected at times related to the periodicity of the local strain
  - Specimens may be stored at ambient temperatures until examined in the morning by wet film for motile larvae and by Giemsa-stained smears—thick for sensitivity and thin for specific morphology
  - A formalin-anionic detergent preservative can also be used. If these are negative, the blood specimens should be concentrated by the Knott concentration or membrane filtration technique
- ELISA and immunochromatographic card tests are sensitive (96–100%) and specific (nearly 100%)
  - Used for amicrofilaremic persons and for daytime examination of blood
  - A PCR assay is available for both *W bancrofti* and *B malayi*
- Serological tests may be helpful in screening
  - A negative test usually rules out present or past infection, but false-positive tests occur with other filarial and helminthic infections
  - An indirect hemagglutination titer of 1:128 and a bentonite flocculation titer of 1:5 in combination are considered the minimum significant titers
  - ELISA-IgG and -IgE tests are also available
- Eosinophil counts may be elevated
- **Tropical pulmonary eosinophilia**: hypereosinophilia, high filarial antibody titers, and IgE levels

IMAGING STUDIES

- Live adult worms can be detected by high-frequency ultrasound of the scrotum (up to 80% of infected men) and of the female breast
- Lymphangiography and radionuclide lymphoscintigraphy may be useful imaging methods
- Diffuse miliary lesions or increased bronchovascular markings on chest films in tropical pulmonary eosinophilia

TREATMENT

MEDICATIONS

- Diethylcarbamazine is the drug of choice
  - Cure may require multiple 12-day courses (2 mg/kg TID after meals, starting with small doses, and gradually increasing over 3–4 days)
  - Adverse immunological reactions to dying microfilariae and adult worms are common. Antipyretics and analgesics may be helpful
  - In the United States, the drug is available only from the Parasitic Diseases Drug Service, Centers for Disease Control and Prevention, Atlanta, GA
- In areas where onchocerciasis or loiasis is also prevalent, diethylcarbamazine is often contraindicated because of the potential for severe reactions to dying microfilariae of these parasites; instead, use albendazole plus ivermectin
- During acute inflammatory episodes, it is controversial whether to treat
- Ivermectin is effective only as a microfilaricide; it is given as a single 200-μg/kg PO dose and repeated in 6 months. Diethylcarbamazine, however, must be given to kill the adult worms, which are the cause of the pathological features
- Albendazole (400 mg PO twice daily) for 3 weeks has macrofilaricidal action. The drug is free of significant side effects but should not be used in pregnancy
- Tropical pulmonary eosinophilia should be treated with diethylcarbamazine (6 mg/kg daily for 21 days)

THERAPEUTIC PROCEDURES

- General measures include rest, antibiotics for secondary infections, use of postural drainage, elastic stockings and pressure bandages for leg edema, and suspensory bandaging for orchitis and epididymitis
- Small hydroceles may benefit from a locally injected sclerosing agent, or surgery may be indicated
- To manage elephantiasis, lymphovenous shunt procedures may be useful, combined with removal of excess subcutaneous fatty and fibrous tissue, postural drainage, and physiotherapy

OUTCOME

COMPLICATIONS

- Untreated tropical pulmonary eosinophilia can progress to chronic pulmonary fibrosis

PROGNOSIS

- The prognosis is good with treatment of early and mild cases (including low-grade lymphedema, chyluria, small hydrocele), but in advanced infection the prognosis is poor

WHEN TO REFER

- All patients should be referred to a specialist

WHEN TO ADMIT

- Debilitating filarial fever
- Progressive and disseminated disease

PREVENTION

- Mass treatment programs, in which albendazole is given once yearly with diethylcarbamazine or ivermectin, are being evaluated for their potential to interrupt lymphatic filariasis transmission

EVIDENCE

WEB SITES

- CDC—Division of Parasitic Diseases
  - http://www.cdc.gov/ncidod/dpd/parasites/lymphaticfilariasis/
- Filariasis.net
  - http://filariasis.net
- The Global Alliance to Eliminate Lymphatic Filariasis
  - http://www.filariasis.org

INFORMATION FOR PATIENTS

- Centers for Disease Control
  - http://www.cdc.gov/ncidod/dpd/parasites/lymphaticfilariasis/factsht_lymphatic_filar.htm
- National Institute of Allergy and Infectious Disease
  - http://www.niaid.nih.gov/newsroom/focuson/bugborne01/filar.htm

REFERENCES

- Dunyo SK et al: Ivermectin and albendazole alone and in combination for the treatment of lymphatic filariasis in Ghana: follow-up after re-treatment with the combination. Trans R Soc Trop Med Hyg 2002;96:189. [PMID: 12055812]
- Ravindran B: Mass drug administration to treat lymphatic filariasis. Lancet 2002;359:1948. [PMID: 12057582]

Focal Segmental Glomerular Sclerosis p. 1075. Folic Acid Deficiency p. 1075.

Folliculitis

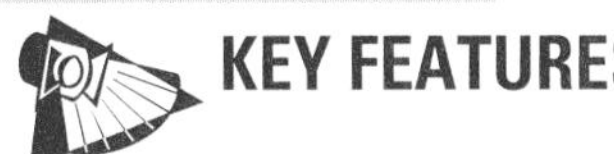

KEY FEATURES

ESSENTIALS OF DIAGNOSIS

- Itching and burning in hairy areas
- Pustules in the hair follicles

GENERAL CONSIDERATIONS

- May be more common in diabetic persons
- Multiple types
  - Bacterial (usually staphylococcal)
  - Sycosis (chronic on head and neck)
  - Gram-negative (eg, if on antibiotics for acne)
  - Hot tub folliculitis
  - Herpes folliculitis
  - Due to oils, occlusion, perspiration, or rubbing
  - *M furfur* (on back) "steroid acne"
  - Eosinophilic folliculitis (in AIDS)
- **Sycosis**
  - Deep-seated, chronic, recalcitrant lesion on the head and neck
  - Usually propagated by the autoinoculation and trauma of shaving; the upper lip is particularly susceptible to involvement in men
- **Gram-negative folliculitis**
  - May develop during antibiotic treatment of acne
  - May present as a flare of acne pustules or nodules
  - *Klebsiella*, *Enterobacter*, *Escherichia coli*, and *Proteus*
- **"Hot tub folliculitis"**
  - Caused by *Pseudomonas aeruginosa*
  - Characterized by pruritic or tender follicular or pustular lesions occurring within 1–4 days after bathing in a hot tub, whirlpool, or public swimming pool
  - Rarely, systemic infections may result
- **Nonbacterial folliculitis**
  - May be caused by oils that are irritating to the follicle
  - May be encountered in the workplace (machinists) or at home (various cosmetics and cocoa butter or coconut oils)
- Folliculitis may also be caused by occlusion, perspiration, and rubbing, such as that resulting from tight jeans and other heavy fabrics on the upper legs
- Folliculitis on the back that looks like acne but does not respond to acne therapy may be caused by the yeast *Malassezia furfur*; this infection may require biopsy for diagnosis
- Folliculitis—so-called steroid acne—may be seen during topical or systemic corticosteroid therapy
- **Eosinophilic folliculitis**
  - A form of sterile folliculitis
  - Consisting of urticarial papules with prominent eosinophilic infiltration
  - Common in patients with AIDS
- **Pseudofolliculitis**
  - Caused by ingrowing hairs in the beard area
  - In this entity, the papules and pustules are located at the side of and not in follicles
  - It may be treated by growing a beard, by using chemical depilatories, or by shaving with a foil-guard razor
  - Laser hair removal is dramatically beneficial in patients with pseudofolliculitis, requires limited maintenance, and can be done on patients of any skin color; pseudofolliculitis is a true medical indication for such a procedure and should not be considered cosmetic

CLINICAL FINDINGS

SYMPTOMS AND SIGNS

- The symptoms range from slight burning and tenderness to intense itching
- The lesions consist of pustules of hair follicles

DIFFERENTIAL DIAGNOSIS

- Acne vulgaris
- Miliaria (heat rash)
- Impetigo
- Tinea
- Pseudofolliculitis barbae (ingrown beard hairs)
- Hidradenitis suppurativa

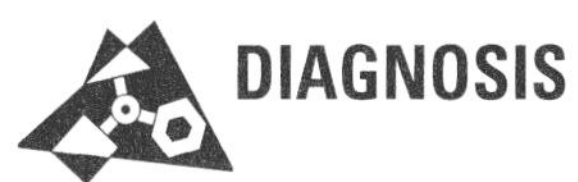

DIAGNOSIS

LABORATORY TESTS

- Clinical diagnosis

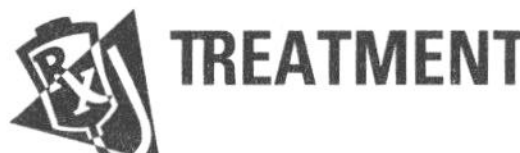

TREATMENT

MEDICATIONS

- See Table 6

Local measures

- Anhydrous ethyl alcohol containing 6.25% aluminum chloride (Xerac AC), applied to lesions and environs, may be helpful, especially for chronic folliculitis of the buttocks

Specific measures

- Systemic antibiotics may be tried if the skin infection is resistant to local treatment, if it is extensive or severe and accompanied by a febrile reaction, if it is complicated, or if it involves the nose or upper lip
- Extended periods of treatment (4–8 weeks or more) with antistaphylococcal antibiotics are required in some cases
- Hot tub *Pseudomonas* folliculitis virtually always resolves without treatment but may be treated with ciprofloxacin, 500 mg PO BID for 5 days
- Gram-negative folliculitis in acne patients may be treated with isotretinoin in compliance with all precautions for that medication
- Folliculitis due to *M furfur* is treated with topical 2.5% selenium sulfide, 15 min daily for 3 weeks, or with ketoconazole, 200 mg PO QD for 7–14 days
- Eosinophilic folliculitis may be treated initially by the combination of potent topical corticosteroids and oral antihistamines; in more severe cases, treatment is with one of the following: topical permethrin (application for 12 h every other night for 6 weeks); itraconazole, 200–400 mg daily; UVB or PUVA phototherapy; or isotretinoin, 0.5 mg/kg/day for up to 5 months; a remission may be induced by some of these therapies, but long-term treatment may be required

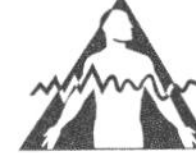

OUTCOME

COMPLICATIONS

- Abscess formation is the major complication of bacterial folliculitis

PROGNOSIS

- Bacterial folliculitis is occasionally stubborn and persistent, requiring prolonged or intermittent courses of antibiotics
- Steroid folliculitis is treatable by acne therapy and resolves as corticosteroids are discontinued

WHEN TO REFER

- If there is a question about the diagnosis, if recommended therapy is ineffective, or if specialized treatment is necessary

PREVENTION

- Correct any predisposing local causes (eg, irritations of a mechanical or chemical nature)
- Control of blood glucose in diabetes may reduce the number of these infections; be sure that the water in hot tubs and spas is treated properly with chlorine
- If staphylococcal folliculitis is persistent, treatment of nasal or perineal carriage with rifampin, 600 mg daily for 5 days, or with topical mupirocin ointment 2% twice daily for 5 days, may help
- Chronic oral clindamycin, 150–300 mg/day, is also effective in preventing recurrent staphylococcal folliculitis and furunculosis

EVIDENCE

WEB SITES

- American Academy of Dermatology
  - http://www.aad.org
- Dermatlas, Johns Hopkins University School of Medicine: Folliculitis Images
  - http://dermatlas.med.jhmi.edu/derm/result.cfm?Diagnosis=206

INFORMATION FOR PATIENTS

- American Academy of Family Physicians: *Staphylococcus aureus* Infections
  - http://www.kidshealth.org/PageManager.jsp?dn=familydoctor&lic=44&article_set=22940
- Mayo Clinic: Folliculitis
  - http://www.mayoclinic.com/invoke.cfm?id=DS00512
- MedlinePlus: Folliculitis
  - http://www.nlm.nih.gov/medlineplus/ency/article/000823.htm
- MedlinePlus: Hot Tub Folliculitis
  - http://www.nlm.nih.gov/medlineplus/ency/article/001460.htm

REFERENCES

- Cook-Bolden FE et al: Twice-daily applications of benzoyl peroxide 5%/clindamycin 1% gel versus vehicle in the treatment of pseudofolliculitis barbae. Cutis 2004;73:18. [PMID: 15228130]
- Stulberg DL et al: Common bacterial skin infections. Am Fam Physician 2002;66:119. [PMID: 12126026]

Author(s)

Timothy G. Berger, MD

Frostbite

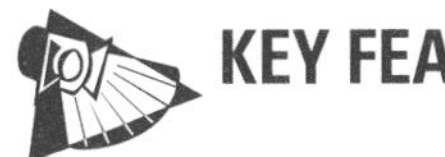

KEY FEATURES

ESSENTIALS OF DIAGNOSIS

- Injury is due to freezing and formation of ice crystals within tissues

GENERAL CONSIDERATIONS

- Localized hypothermia, vasoconstriction, and slowed metabolism occur as temperature falls below 25°C, although oxygen demand may increase if activity continues
- Once tissue is frozen it becomes pain free

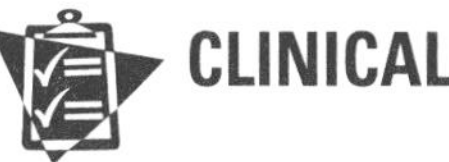

CLINICAL FINDINGS

SYMPTOMS AND SIGNS

Mild cases

- Only the skin and subcutaneous tissues are involved
- The symptoms are numbness, prickling, and itching

Severe cases

- With increasing severity, deep frostbite involves deeper structures
- There may be paresthesia and stiffness
- Thawing causes tenderness and burning pain; the skin is white or yellow, loses its elasticity, and becomes immobile
- Edema, blisters, necrosis, and gangrene may appear

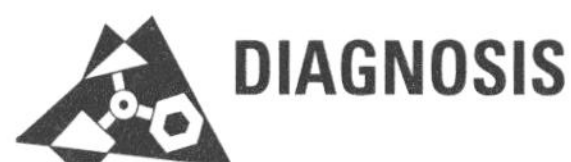

DIAGNOSIS

IMAGING STUDIES

- MRI with magnetic resonance angiography and triple-phase bone scanning can assess the degree of involvement and distinguish viable from nonviable tissue

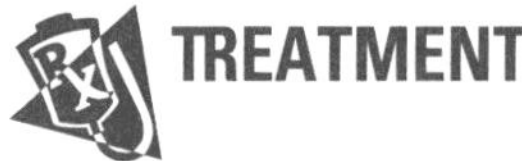

TREATMENT

MEDICATIONS

- Ibuprofen, 200 mg 4 × daily, and aloe vera may prevent dermal ischemia
- **Antiinfective measures**
  - Consider tetanus prophylaxis; frostbite increases susceptibility
  - Local infections should be treated with mild soapy water or povidone-iodine soaks
  - Antibiotics may be required for deep infections

THERAPEUTIC PROCEDURES

- Treat associated systemic hypothermia (see Hypothermia)
- For **superficial frostbite** (frostnip) of extremities:
  - In the field, apply firm steady pressure with warm hand (without rubbing)
  - Place fingers in the armpits
  - Remove footwear, dry the feet, rewarm, cover with adequate dry socks or other protective footwear
- For **deep frostbite**, rapid thawing at temperatures slightly above body heat may significantly decrease tissue necrosis
- If there is a possibility of refreezing, frostbitten part should not be thawed, even if it means prolonged walking on frozen feet; refreezing increases tissue necrosis

Rewarming

- Immerse the frozen extremity for several minutes in a moving-water bath heated to 40–42°C until the distal tip of the part being thawed flushes (water feels warm but not hot to the normal hand)
- Dry heat (eg, stove or open fire) is more difficult to regulate and is not recommended
- After thawing, and the part has returned to normal temperature (usually in ~30 min), discontinue external heat
- Avoid rewarming by exercise or thawing frozen tissues by rubbing with snow or ice water

Protection

- Avoid pressure, friction, physical therapy in early stage
- Do not apply casts, dressings, bandages
- Keep patient on bed rest, with affected parts elevated and uncovered at room temperature
- Protect skin blebs from physical contact
- Whirlpool therapy at 37–40°C 2 × daily for 15–20 min for ≥ 3 weeks helps cleanse skin and débrides superficial sloughing tissue

SURGERY

- Early regional sympathetic blockade can reduce symptoms; sympathectomy (in 36–72 h) is controversial; in general, avoid other surgical intervention
- Do not consider amputation until tissues are confirmed dead; tissue necrosis may be superficial; underlying skin may sometimes heal spontaneously, even after months

OUTCOME

FOLLOW-UP

- Gentle, progressive physical therapy to promote circulation should be instituted as tolerated

COMPLICATIONS

- Loss of fingers, toes, extremities, tip of nose
- There may be increased susceptibility to discomfort in the involved extremity upon reexposure to cold with pain, numbness, tingling, hyperhidrosis
- Cold sensitivity of the extremities and nerve conduction abnormalities may persist for years after the cold injury

PROGNOSIS

- Recovery from frostbite is most often complete

WHEN TO ADMIT

- Hypothermia
- Most cases, including all cases of deep frostbite

EVIDENCE

PRACTICE GUIDELINES

- Syme D et al: Position paper: on-site treatment of frostbite for mountaineers. High Alt Med Biol 2002;3:297. [PMID: 12396885]

INFORMATION FOR PATIENTS

- Centers for Disease Control and Prevention: Winter Weather FAQs
  - http://www.bt.cdc.gov/disasters/winter/faq.asp
- Mayo Clinic: Frostbite
  - http://www.mayoclinic.com/invoke.cfm?id=FA00023
- Mayo Clinic: Hypothermia
  - http://www.mayoclinic.com/invoke.cfm?id=DS00333
- Medline Plus: Frostbite
  - http://www.nlm.nih.gov/medlineplus/ency/article/000057.htm

REFERENCES

- Murphy JV et al: Frostbite: pathogenesis and treatment. J Trauma 2000;48:171. [PMID: 10647591]
- Petrone P et al: Surgical management and strategies in the treatment of hypothermia and cold injury. Emerg Med Clin North Am 2003;21:1165. [PMID: 14708823]

Author(s)

Richard Cohen, MD, MPH

Furunculosis

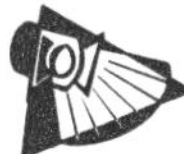

KEY FEATURES

ESSENTIALS OF DIAGNOSIS

- Extremely painful inflammatory swelling based on a hair follicle that forms an abscess
- Predisposing condition (diabetes mellitus, HIV disease, injection drug use) sometimes present
- Coagulase-positive *Staphylococcus aureus* is the causative organism

GENERAL CONSIDERATIONS

- A furuncle (boil) is a deep-seated infection (abscess) involving the entire hair follicle and adjacent subcutaneous tissue
- The most common sites of occurrence are the hairy parts exposed to irritation and friction, pressure, or moisture
- Because the lesions are autoinoculable, they are often multiple
- A carbuncle consists of several furuncles developing in adjoining hair follicles and coalescing to form a conglomerate, deeply situated mass with multiple drainage points

DEMOGRAPHICS

- Predisposing cause usually not found
- However, diabetes mellitus (especially if using insulin injections), injection drug use, allergy injections, and HIV disease all increase the risk of staphylococcal infections by increasing the rate of nasal carriage

CLINICAL FINDINGS

SYMPTOMS AND SIGNS

Furuncle

- Rounded or conical abscesses on the hairy parts exposed to irritation and friction, pressure, or moisture
- Lesions are often multiple and pain and tenderness may be prominent
- Gradually enlarges, becomes fluctuant, and then softens and opens spontaneously after a few days to 1–2 weeks to discharge a core of necrotic tissue and pus
- Infection of the soft tissue around the nails (paronychia) may be due to staphylococci when it is acute; other organisms may be involved, including *Candida* and herpes simplex (herpetic whitlow)

Carbuncle

- Consists of several furuncles in adjoining hair follicles and coalescing to form a deeply situated mass with multiple drainage points

DIFFERENTIAL DIAGNOSIS

- Inflamed sebaceous (epidermal inclusion) cyst—suddenly becomes red, tender, and expands greatly in size over 1 to a few days; history of prior cyst in the same location, the presence of a clearly visible cyst orifice, and the extrusion of malodorous cheesy rather than purulent material helps in the diagnosis
- Acne vulgaris
- Tinea profunda (deep tinea of hair follicle)
- Sporotrichosis
- Blastomycosis
- Hidradenitis suppurativa (recurrent tender sterile abscesses in the axillae, groin, on the buttocks, or below the breasts; presence of old scars or sinus tracts plus negative cultures suggests this diagnosis)
- Anthrax
- Tularemia

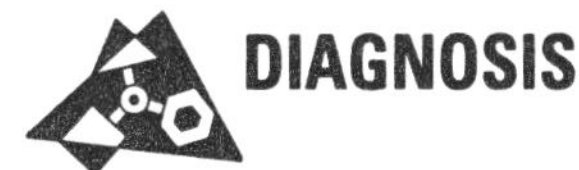

DIAGNOSIS

LABORATORY TESTS

- Leukocytosis may occur, but a white blood cell count is rarely required
- Although *S aureus* is almost always the cause, pus should be cultured, especially in immunocompromised patients, to rule out methicillin-resistant *S aureus* or other bacteria

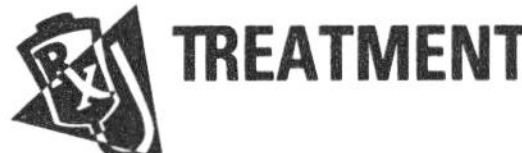

TREATMENT

MEDICATIONS

- Systemic antibiotics
  - Sodium dicloxacillin or cephalexin, 1 g daily in divided doses by mouth for 10 days, is usually effective
  - Erythromycin in similar doses may be used in penicillin-allergic individuals in communities with low prevalence of erythromycin-resistant staphylococci or if the particular isolate is sensitive
  - Ciprofloxacin, 500 mg twice daily, is effective against strains of staphylococci resistant to other antibiotics
- Recurrent furunculosis may be effectively treated with a combination of dicloxacillin, 250–500 mg four times daily for 2–4 weeks, and rifampin, 300 mg twice daily for 5 days, during this period
- Chronic clindamycin, 150–300 mg daily for 1–2 months, may also cure recurrent furunculosis
- Applications of topical 2% mupirocin to the nares, axillae, and anogenital areas twice daily for 5 days eliminates the staphylococcal carrier state

SURGERY

- Incision and drainage: recommended for all loculated collections; mainstay of therapy
- Use surgical incision and débridement **after** the lesions are "mature"
- It is not necessary to incise and drain an acute staphylococcal paronychia

THERAPEUTIC PROCEDURES

- Immobilize the part and avoid overmanipulation of inflamed areas
- Use moist heat to help larger lesions "localize"
- Inserting a flat metal spatula or sharpened hardwood stick into the nail fold where it adjoins the nail will release pus from a mature lesion

OUTCOME

FOLLOW-UP

Recurrent furunculosis

- Culture of the anterior nares may identify chronic staphylococcal carriage in recurrent infections
- Family members and intimate contacts may need evaluation for staphylococcal carrier state and perhaps concomitant treatment

PROGNOSIS

- Recurrent crops may occur for months or years

WHEN TO REFER

- If there is a question about the diagnosis, if recommended therapy is ineffective, or if specialized treatment is necessary

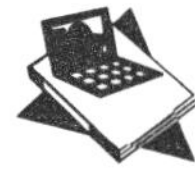

EVIDENCE

WEB SITE

- American Academy of Dermatology
  - http://www.aad.org

INFORMATION FOR PATIENTS

- American Osteopathic College of Dermatology: Boils
  - http://www.aocd.org/skin/dermatologic_diseases/boils.html
- Mayo Clinic: Boils and Carbuncles
  - http://www.mayoclinic.com/invoke.cfm?id=DS00466American
- MedlinePlus: Furuncle
  - http://www.nlm.nih.gov/medlineplus/ency/article/001474.htm
- MedlinePlus: Carbunculosis
  - http://www.nlm.nih.gov/medlineplus/ency/article/000825.htm

REFERENCES

- Baggett HC et al: Community-onset methicillin-resistant *Staphylococcus aureus* associated with antibiotic use and the cytotoxin Panton-Valentin leukocidin during a furunculosis outbreak in rural Alaska. J Infect Dis 2004;189:1565. [PMID: 15116291]
- Stulberg DL et al: Common bacterial skin infections. Am Fam Physician 2002;66:119. [PMID: 12126026]

Author(s)

Timothy G. Berger, MD

Galactorrhea p. 1076. Gamma Hydroxybutyrate Overdose p. 1076.

Gastric Cancer

KEY FEATURES

ESSENTIALS OF DIAGNOSIS

- Dyspeptic symptoms with weight loss in patients age >40
- Iron deficiency anemia; occult blood in stools
- Abnormality on upper gastrointestinal series or endoscopy

GENERAL CONSIDERATIONS

- Gastric adenocarcinoma is the most common cancer worldwide
- Most gastric cancers arise in the antrum
- Chronic *Helicobacter pylori* gastritis is a major risk factor; however, among individuals chronically infected with *H pylori*, < 1% will develop gastric carcinoma
- Other risk factors: gastric adenomas, chronic atrophic gastritis with intestinal metaplasia, pernicious anemia, and partial gastric resection >15 years previously

DEMOGRAPHICS

- Incidence in the United States has declined by two-thirds over the last 30 years
- Currently, 20,000 cases annually in the United States
- Uncommon under age 40; mean age at diagnosis is 63 years
- Men affected twice as often as women
- Incidence is higher in Hispanics, African Americans, and Asian Americans

CLINICAL FINDINGS

SYMPTOMS AND SIGNS

- Generally asymptomatic or nonspecific symptoms until advanced disease
- Dyspepsia, vague epigastric pain, anorexia, early satiety, and weight loss
- Acute upper gastrointestinal bleeding with hematemesis or melena
- Postprandial vomiting suggests gastric outlet obstruction
- Progressive dysphagia suggests lower esophageal obstruction
- Physical examination rarely helpful
- Gastric mass is palpated in less than 20%
- Lymphadenopathy: left supraclavicular lymph node (Virchow's node), umbilical nodule (Sister Mary Joseph nodule)
- Rigid rectal shelf (Blumer's shelf)
- Ovarian metastases (Krukenberg tumor)

DIFFERENTIAL DIAGNOSIS

- Benign gastric ulcers
- Lymphoma
- Menetrier's disease

DIAGNOSIS

LABORATORY TESTS

- Guaiac-positive stools
- Iron deficiency anemia or anemia of chronic disease
- Liver function test abnormalities if metastatic spread
- Serologic markers (eg, carcinoembryonic antigen) not helpful

IMAGING STUDIES

- Barium upper gastrointestinal series when endoscopy is not readily available
- Upper gastrointestinal series may not detect small or superficial lesions and cannot reliably distinguish benign from malignant ulcerations
- Preoperative evaluation with abdominal CT and endoscopic ultrasonography

DIAGNOSTIC PROCEDURES

- Upper endoscopy with biopsy and cytological brushings
- Staging by TNM system
  - Stage I: T1N0, T1N1, T2N0, all M0
  - Stage II: T1N2, T2N1, T3N0, all M0
  - Stage III: T2N2, T3N1, T4N0, all M0
  - Stage IV: T4N2M0, any M1
- After preoperative staging, about two-thirds found to have localized disease (ie, stages I–III)

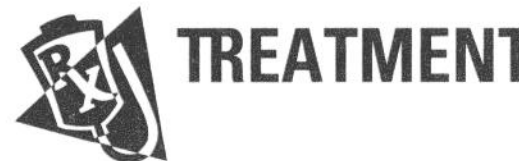

TREATMENT

MEDICATIONS

- Single-agent or combination chemotherapy with fluorouracil, doxorubicin, and cisplatin or mitomycin may provide palliation in up to 30%
- Patients with stage III tumors undergoing curative resection may be considered for postoperative adjuvant chemoradiotherapy

SURGERY

- For patients with clinically localized disease (stages I–III), surgical exploration
  - Patients with confirmed localized disease should undergo radical surgical resection with curative intent
  - Approximately 25% will be found to have locally unresectable tumors or peritoneal, hepatic, or distant lymph node metastases, and "curative" surgical resection is not warranted
- Palliative resection of the tumor
  - Can reduce the risk of bleeding and obstruction
  - Lead to improved quality of life
  - Improve survival
- For patients with unresectable disease, gastrojejunostomy can prevent obstruction

THERAPEUTIC PROCEDURES

- After careful staging (including endoscopic ultrasonography), small (< 3 cm), early intramucosal gastric cancers may be amenable to endoscopic mucosal resection
- Endoscopic laser or stent therapy, radiation therapy, or angiographic embolization can palliate bleeding or obstruction from unresected tumors

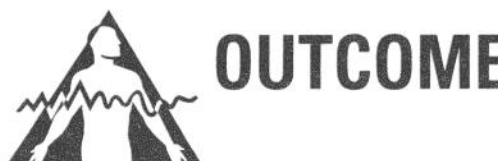

OUTCOME

FOLLOW-UP

- After surgical therapy, further follow-up is determined by clinical course
- Routine follow-up not recommended

COMPLICATIONS

- Acute or chronic gastrointestinal blood loss
- Gastric outlet obstruction
- Carcinomatosis with ascites, small bowel obstruction

PROGNOSIS

- Overall long-term survival is <15%
- Survival related to tumor stage, location, and histological features
- Stage I and stage II tumors resected for cure have a >50% long-term survival
- Patients with stage III tumors have a <20% long-term survival
- Tumors of the diffuse and signet ring type have a worse prognosis than those of the intestinal type
- Tumors of the proximal stomach (fundus and cardia) have 5-year survival of <15%, a far worse prognosis than distal lesions

WHEN TO REFER

- Patients with a confirmed diagnosis of gastric adenocarcinoma should be evaluated by a general surgeon or oncologist

WHEN TO ADMIT

- Acute upper gastrointestinal bleeding
- Vomiting and dehydration

PREVENTION

- In Japan, population-based endoscopic screening is performed
- At present, population-based testing and treating of *H pylori* as a chemopreventative measure to reduce the incidence of gastric adenocarcinoma is not recommended

EVIDENCE

PRACTICE GUIDELINES

- Allum WH et al: Guidelines for the management of oesophageal and gastric cancer. Gut 2002;50(50 Suppl 5):v1. [PMID:12049068]
- Earle CC et al: Neoadjuvant or adjuvant therapy for resectable gastric cancer? A practice guideline. Can J Surg 2002;45:438. [PMID:12500920]

WEB SITES

- WebPath GI Pathology Index
  - http://medstat.med.utah.edu/WebPath/GIHTML/GIIDX.html

INFORMATION FOR PATIENTS

- Cleveland Clinic—Stomach cancer
  - http://www.clevelandclinic.org/health/health-info/docs/1800/1813.asp?index=8105
- Mayo Clinic—Stomach cancer
  - http://www.mayoclinic.com/invoke.cfm?objectid=4545F9D7-17A0-4275-9C296401969A8E11
- MEDLINEplus—Gastric cancer
  - http://www.nlm.nih.gov/medlineplus/ency/article/000223.htm

REFERENCES

- Higuchi K et al: Gastric cancer: advances in adjuvant and adjunct therapy. Curr Treat Options Oncol 2003;4:413. [PMID:12941201]
- Hohenberger P et al: Gastric cancer. Lancet 2003;362:305. [PMID:12892963]
- McCulloch P et al: Extended versus limited lymph nodes dissection technique for adenocarcinoma of the stomach. Cochrane Database Syst Rev 2004;CD001964. [PMID:15495024]

Author(s)

Kenneth R. McQuaid, MD

Gastritis, Erosive & Hemorrhagic

Gastritis, Atrophic p. 1077

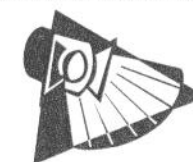

KEY FEATURES

ESSENTIALS OF DIAGNOSIS

- Hematemesis, "coffee grounds" emesis, or melena; usually not significant bleeding
- Often asymptomatic; may cause epigastric pain, anorexia, nausea, and vomiting
- Occurs most commonly in alcoholics, critically ill patients, or patients taking nonsteroidal anti-inflammatory drugs (NSAIDs)

GENERAL CONSIDERATIONS

- Most common causes
  - Drugs (especially NSAIDs)
  - Alcohol
  - Stress due to severe medical or surgical illness
  - Portal hypertension ("portal gastropathy")
- Uncommon causes
  - Caustic ingestion
  - Radiation

DEMOGRAPHICS

- Patients using acute or chronic NSAIDs, especially aspirin
- Heavy alcohol ingestion
- Critically ill ICU patients: major risk factors
  - Coagulopathy
  - Mechanical ventilation
  - Sepsis
  - Trauma
  - Burns
  - Central nervous system injury
  - Hepatic or renal failure

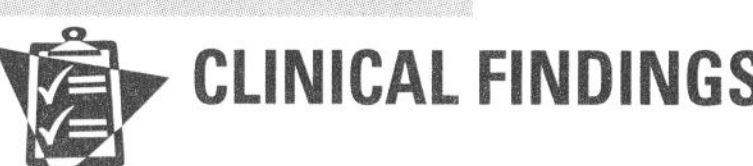

CLINICAL FINDINGS

SYMPTOMS AND SIGNS

- Often asymptomatic
- Symptoms, when they occur, include dyspepsia, anorexia, epigastric pain, nausea, and vomiting
- Upper gastrointestinal bleeding, hematemesis, "coffee grounds" emesis, or melena
  - Bleeding is not usually hemodynamically significant

DIFFERENTIAL DIAGNOSIS

- Epigastric pain suggests peptic ulcer, gastroesophageal reflux, gastric cancer, biliary tract disease, food poisoning, viral gastroenteritis, and functional dyspepsia
- Severe pain suggests a perforated or penetrating ulcer, pancreatic disease, esophageal rupture, ruptured aortic aneurysm, gastric volvulus, and myocardial ischemia
- Upper gastrointestinal bleeding suggests peptic ulcer disease, esophageal varices, Mallory-Weiss tear, and arteriovenous malformations

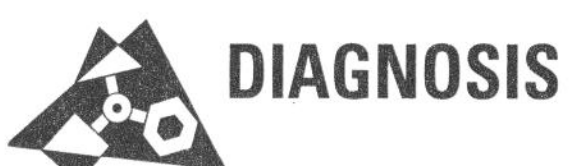

DIAGNOSIS

LABORATORY TESTS

- Hematocrit is low if significant bleeding
- Iron deficiency

IMAGING STUDIES

- Upper endoscopy for dyspepsia or upper gastrointestinal bleeding is diagnostic
  - Erythema
  - Subepithelial petechiae
  - Erosion
- Barium upper gastrointestinal series is insensitive because abnormalities are confined to the mucosa

DIAGNOSTIC PROCEDURES

- Nasogastric tube placement reveals bloody aspirate

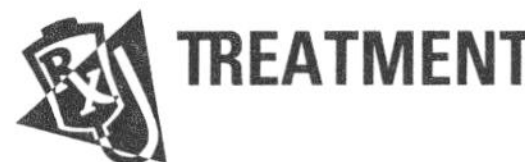

TREATMENT

MEDICATIONS

- Stress gastritis: continuous infusions of an H_2 receptor antagonist or proton pump inhibitor to raise intragastric pH >4.0
- NSAID gastritis: empirical treatment for dyspepsia alone (without bleeding) with H_2 receptor antagonist (cimetidine, 400 mg PO BID, ranitidine, 150 mg PO BID, or famotidine, 20 mg PO BID), or proton pump inhibitor (omeprazole 20 mg PO QD, rabeprazole, 20 mg PO QD, esomeprazole, 40 mg PO QD, pantoprazole, 40 mg PO QD, or lansoprazole, 30 mg PO QD)
- Alcoholic gastritis: H_2 receptor antagonists or sucralfate for 2–4 weeks
- Portal hypertensive gastropathy:
  - Nonselective β-blocker (propranolol or nadolol)
  - Dose adjusted to reduce resting heart rate to < 60/minute

THERAPEUTIC PROCEDURES

- Portal hypertensive gastropathy: portal decompressive procedures, eg, transvenous intrahepatic portosystemic shunts, are sometimes required for acute hemorrhage

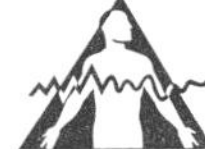

OUTCOME

COMPLICATIONS

- Acute upper gastrointestinal hemorrhage
- Chronic gastrointestinal blood loss with anemia

WHEN TO REFER

- NSAID gastritis: persistent dyspepsia despite discontinuation of NSAIDs or empirical therapy should be referred for endoscopy

WHEN TO ADMIT

- NSAID gastritis
  - Acute upper gastrointestinal (GI) hemorrhage
  - Severe dyspepsia with concern for complicated peptic ulcer disease or alternative diagnosis
- Alcoholic gastritis: protracted vomiting and/or acute upper GI hemorrhage or signs of alcohol withdrawal
- Portal hypertensive gastropathy

PREVENTION

- Stress gastritis: prophylactic therapy warranted in high-risk ICU patients only
- H_2 receptor antagonist infusions at a dose sufficient to maintain intragastric pH >4.0
- Cimetidine (900–1200 mg), ranitidine (150 mg), or famotidine (20 mg) by continuous IV infusion over 24 hours
- IV proton pump inhibitors (pantoprazole) are more expensive than H_2 receptor agonists; efficacy and optimal dosage not yet established
- NSAID gastritis
  - Patients at high risk for NSAID-induced complications should receive co-therapy with a proton pump inhibitor and/or misoprostol, 200 μg PO QID
  - Alternatively, a COX-2 selective agent should be used (celecoxib)
  - Use of low-dose aspirin negates safety of COX-2 selective agent
- High-risk patients should be tested for *Helicobacter pylori* and treated if positive

EVIDENCE

PRACTICE GUIDELINES

- National Guideline Clearinghouse
  - http://www.guideline.gov/summary/summary.aspx?ss=15&doc_id=2947&nbr=2173&string=gastritis
- Dubois RW et al: Guidelines for the appropriate use of non-steroidal anti-inflammatory drugs, cyclo-oxygenase-2-specific inhibitors and proton pump inhibitors in patients requiring chronic anti-inflammatory activity. Aliment Pharmacol Ther 2004;19:197. [PMID:14723611]
- Sharma P et al: Review article: *Helicobacter pylori* and reflux disease. Aliment Pharmacol Ther 2003;17:297. [PMID:12562442]

INFORMATION FOR PATIENTS

- Mayo Clinic
  - http://www.mayoclinic.com/invoke.cfm?id=DS00488
- MEDLINEplus—Acute gastritis
  - http://www.nlm.nih.gov/medlineplus/ency/article/000240.htm
- MEDLINEplus—Chronic gastritis
  - http://www.nlm.nih.gov/medlineplus/ency/article/000232.htm

REFERENCES

- Duerksen DR: Stress-related mucosal disease in critically ill patients. Best Pract Res Clin Gastroenterol 2003;17:327. [PMID:12763499]
- Jung R et al: Proton-pump inhibitors for stress ulcer prophylaxis in critically ill patients. Ann Pharmacother 2002;36:1929. [PMID:12452757]
- Marli M et al: The natural history of portal hypertensive gastropathy in patients with liver cirrhosis and mild portal hypertension. Am J Gastroenterol 2004;99:1959. [PMID:15447756]

Author(s)

Kenneth R. McQuaid, MD

Gastroesophageal Reflux Disease (GERD)

Gastroenteritis, *Escherichia coli* p. 1077.

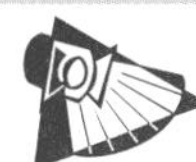

KEY FEATURES

ESSENTIALS OF DIAGNOSIS

- Heartburn exacerbated by meals, bending, or recumbency
- Endoscopy demonstrates esophageal abnormalities in <50% of patients

GENERAL CONSIDERATIONS

- Affects 20% of adults, who report at least weekly episodes of heartburn
- Up to 10% complain of daily symptoms
- Most patients have mild disease
- Up to 50% develop esophageal mucosal damage (reflux esophagitis)
- Few develop serious complications
- Uncomplicated patients treated empirically without diagnostic studies
- Investigation is required in complicated disease and those unresponsive to empirical therapy
- Pathogenesis includes
  - Relaxation or incompetence of lower esophageal sphincter
  - Hiatal hernia
  - Abnormal acid clearance (esophageal peristalsis), eg, scleroderma
  - Impaired salivation (exacerbates GERD), eg, Sjögren's syndrome, anticholinergics, radiation
  - Delayed gastric emptying (exacerbates GERD), eg, gastroparesis

DEMOGRAPHICS

- Increased in whites
- High prevalence in North America and Europe
- Chronic *Helicobacter pylori* infection may be protective in subset of patients with reduced acid secretion
- Increased in pregnancy

CLINICAL FINDINGS

SYMPTOMS AND SIGNS

- Heartburn, most often 30–60 minutes after meals and upon reclining, with relief from antacids
- Regurgitation—spontaneous reflux of sour or bitter gastric contents into the mouth
- Dysphagia common due to inflammation, impaired motility, or stricture
- Atypical manifestations: asthma, chronic cough, chronic laryngitis, sore throat, and noncardiac chest pain
- Gradual development of solid food dysphagia progressive over months to years suggests stricture formation
- Physical examination normal

DIFFERENTIAL DIAGNOSIS

- Peptic ulcer disease, gastritis, nonulcer dyspepsia, or cholelithiasis
- Angina pectoris
- Infectious esophagitis: *Candida*, herpes simplex virus, cytomegalovirus
- Pill-induced esophagitis
- Esophageal motility disorders, eg, achalasia, esophageal spasm, scleroderma
- Radiation esophagitis
- Zollinger-Ellison syndrome (gastrinoma) may cause severe esophagitis due to acid hypersecretion

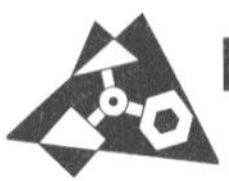

DIAGNOSIS

LABORATORY TESTS

- Laboratory tests are normal

IMAGING STUDIES

- Upper endoscopy with biopsy
- Endoscopy reveals visible mucosal abnormalities (erythema, friability, and erosions) in 50%
- Endoscopy is indicated
  - In patients who have not responded to empirical medical management
  - In patients with symptoms suggesting complicated disease (dysphagia, odynophagia, occult or overt bleeding, or iron deficiency anemia)
  - In patients who have longstanding (>5 years) symptoms
  - In patients who require continuous maintenance therapy
  - To look for Barrett's esophagus
  - To differentiate peptic stricture from other benign or malignant causes of dysphagia
- Barium esophagography seldom useful
  - Insensitive for detection of mucosal abnormalities
  - Useful for detection of esophageal stricture in patients with dysphagia

DIAGNOSTIC PROCEDURES

- Clinical diagnosis has sensitivity of 80%; specificity, 70%
- In patients with typical GERD symptoms without complications, empirical medical management recommended without diagnostic procedures
- Ambulatory esophageal pH monitoring: best study to document acid reflux, but unnecessary in most patients. Indicated:
  - To document abnormal esophageal acid exposure in a patient being considered for antireflux surgery who has a normal endoscopy
  - To evaluate patients with a normal endoscopy who have reflux symptoms unresponsive to proton pump inhibitor
  - To detect association between reflux and atypical symptoms

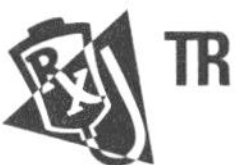

TREATMENT

MEDICATIONS

- Mild, occasional symptoms: Gaviscon alginate-antacid; other antacids provide rapid, short-term relief
- Nonprescription H_2 receptor antagonists: cimetidine, 200 mg, ranitidine and nizatidine, 75 mg, famotidine, 10 mg; taken before meals may prevent symptoms; if taken after symptoms develop, symptom relief within 60 minutes
- Moderate symptoms: H_2 receptor antagonist (nizatidine, 150 mg PO BID, famotidine, 20 mg PO BID, or cimetidine, 400–800 mg PO BID) or proton pump inhibitors (omeprazole or rabeprazole, 20 mg PO QD, lansoprazole, 30 mg PO QD, esomeprazole, 40 mg PO QD, or pantoprazole, 40 mg PO QD) for 8–12 weeks
- Promotility drugs (metoclopramide, bethanechol): reduce reflux, but side effects preclude use for reflux disease
- Severe symptoms and erosive disease
  - Proton pump inhibitors (omeprazole, 20 mg PO QD, or rabeprazole, 20 mg PO QD, lansoprazole, 30 mg PO QD, pantoprazole, 40 mg PO QD, or esomeprazole, 40 mg PO QD for 8–12 weeks) produce relief and healing in >80%; given BID, they provide relief in >95%
  - Patients with severe erosive esophagitis, Barrett's esophagus, or peptic stric-

ture should be maintained on chronic proton pump inhibitor therapy
- Relapse: treated with either continuous or intermittent courses of proton pump inhibitor therapy
- Unresponsive disease
  - Occurs in 10–20% of patients on once-daily doses of proton pump inhibitors and in 5% of those on twice-daily doses
  - Treated with higher proton pump inhibitor doses (eg, omeprazole 40 mg PO BID) or proton pump inhibitor BID (before breakfast and dinner) and a bedtime dose of an H_2 receptor antagonist
- Peptic stricture: chronic proton pump inhibitor therapy

SURGERY

- Surgical fundoplication produces relief in >85% of properly selected patients, 10-year success rates 60–90%
- Fundoplication may now be performed laparoscopically with low complication rates
- However, >50% of patients undergoing fundoplication require continued acid-suppression medication
- >30% develop new symptoms of dysphagia, bloating, increased flatulence, or dyspepsia
- Surgical treatment recommended
  - For otherwise healthy patients with extraesophageal manifestations of reflux
  - For those with severe reflux who are unwilling to accept lifelong medical therapy
  - For patients with erosive disease who are intolerant of or resistant to proton pump inhibitors

THERAPEUTIC PROCEDURES

- Lifestyle modifications
- Reduce meal size
- Avoid bending over after meals
- Avoid lying down within 3 hours after meals
- Avoid acidic foods (tomato, citrus, spicy foods, coffee) and agents that relax the lower esophageal sphincter or delay gastric emptying (fatty foods, peppermint, chocolate, alcohol, and smoking)
- Weight reduction
- Elevate the head of the bed
- Dilation of peptic stricture effective in up to 90% of symptomatic patients
- Endoscopic treatments to bolster gastroesophegeal junction now available
  - Endoscopic suturing device; short-term improvement in symptoms demonstrated in several studies, but long-term efficacy and safety unknown
  - Radiofrequency wave ablation of neural reflex pathways
  - Injection of nonresorbable polymers into muscularis

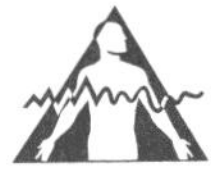

OUTCOME

FOLLOW-UP

- After discontinuation of therapy, relapse of symptoms occurs in 80% of patients within 1 year—most within the first 3 months
- Barrett's esophagus (intestinal metaplasia) is present in up to 10% of patients with chronic reflux
- Patients with Barrett's who are operative candidates should undergo endoscopic surveillance with mucosal biopsies every 3 years
- Patients with low-grade dysplasia are treated with aggressive medical management and endoscopic surveillance every 6–12 months
- For patients with high-grade dysplasia or frequent endoscopic surveillance (every 3 months), surgery is recommended; otherwise, photodynamic ablation or endoscopic mucosal resection
- Barrett's esophagus is treated long-term with proton pump inhibitors

COMPLICATIONS

- GERD
  - Stricture formation in ~10% (effectively treated with dilation)
  - Acid-peptic ulceration
  - Erosive, or hemorrhagic esophagitis
- Barrett's esophagus
  - Increased annual incidence of esophageal adenocarcinoma to 0.5%
  - A 40-fold risk compared with patients without Barrett's

PROGNOSIS

- Heartburn symptoms can be controlled in almost all patients with intermittent or chronic therapy
- Symptoms of regurgitation, bloating, dyspepsia may persist despite acid-reduction therapy

WHEN TO REFER

- Complicated disease: dysphagia, weight loss, fecal-occult positive stool, anemia
- Symptoms that persist despite proton pump inhibitor therapy
- Candidates for fundoplication

WHEN TO ADMIT

- Seldom required

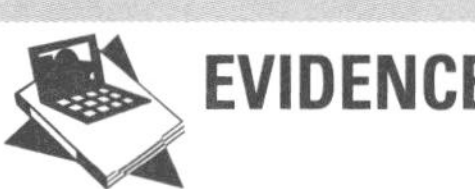

EVIDENCE

PRACTICE GUIDELINES

- National Guideline Clearinghouse
  - http://www.guideline.gov/summary/summary.aspx?doc_id=3147&nbr=2373&string=gastroesophageal+AND+reflux+AND+disease
  - http://www.guideline.gov/summary/summary.aspx?ss=15&doc_id=3372&nbr=2598&string=gastroesophageal%20AND%20reflux%20AND%20disease
- Sampliner RE: Practice Parameters Committee of the American College of Gastroenterology. Updated guidelines for the diagnosis, surveillance, and therapy of Barrett's esophagus. Am J Gastroenterol 2002;97:1888. [PMID:12190150]

INFORMATION FOR PATIENTS

- NIH Patient Education Institute—Gastroesophageal reflux disease
  - http://www.nlm.nih.gov/medlineplus/tutorials/gerd.html
- Society of Thoracic Surgeons
  - http://www.sts.org/doc/4119
- Mayo Clinic
  - http://www.mayoclinic.com/invoke.cfm?id=DS00095

REFERENCES

- Behm BW et al: Endoluminal therapies for gastroesophageal reflex disease. J. Clin Gastroenterol 2004;38:209. [PMID:15128065]
- Falk GW: Barrett's esophagus. Gastroenterology 2002;122:1569. [PMID: 12016424]
- Tack J et al: Gastroesophageal reflux disease poorly responsive to single-dose proton pump inhibitors in patients without Barrett's esophogus: acid reflex, bile reflux, or both? Am J Gastroenterol 2004;99:981. [PMID:15180713]
- Tytgat GN: Management of mild and severe gastro-oesophageal reflux disease. Aliment Pharmacol Ther 2003;17(Suppl 2):52. [PMID: 12786613]

Author(s)

Kenneth R. McQuaid, MD

Gastrointestinal Bleeding, Acute Lower

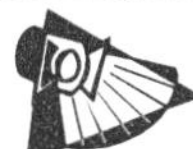

KEY FEATURES

ESSENTIALS OF DIAGNOSIS

- Hematochezia usually present
- Evaluation with colonoscopy in stable patients
- Massive active bleeding calls for evaluation with upper endoscopy, or nuclear bleeding scan, and/or angiography

GENERAL CONSIDERATIONS

- Lower gastrointestinal bleeding defined as that arising below the ligament of Treitz, ie, small intestine or colon; >95% of cases from the colon
- Lower tract bleeding
  - 25% less common than upper tract bleeding
  - Tends to have a more benign course
  - Is less likely to present with shock or orthostasis (< 20%) or to require transfusions (< 40%)
- Spontaneous cessation in >85%, hospital mortality in < 3%
- Most common cause
  - In patients < 50 years—infectious colitis, anorectal disease, and inflammatory bowel disease
  - In older patients—diverticulosis (50% of cases), vascular ectasias (5–10%), neoplasms (polyps or carcinoma) (10%), ischemia, radiation-induced proctitis, solitary rectal ulcer, nonsteroidal anti-inflammatory drug (NSAID)-induced ulcers, small bowel diverticula, and colonic varices
- In 20% no source of bleeding can be identified
- Diverticulosis
  - Acute, painless, large-volume maroon or bright red hematochezia occurs in 3–5%, associated with the use of NSAIDs
  - Bleeding more commonly originates on the right side
  - >95% require fewer than 4 units of blood transfusion
  - Bleeding subsides spontaneously in 80% but may recur in up to 25% of patients
- Vascular ectasias (angiodysplasias)
  - Painless bleeding ranging from melena or hematochezia to occult blood loss
  - Bleeding most commonly originates in the cecum and ascending colon
  - Causes: congenital, hereditary hemorrhagic telangiectasia, autoimmune disorders, typically scleroderma
- Neoplasms: benign polyps and carcinoma cause chronic occult blood loss or intermittent anorectal hematochezia
- Anorectal disease
  - Small amounts of bright red blood noted on the toilet paper, streaking of the stool, or dripping into the toilet bowl
  - Painless bleeding with internal hemorrhoids
  - Pain with bleeding suggests anal fissure
- Ischemic colitis: hematochezia or bloody diarrhea associated with mild cramps; in most, the bleeding is mild and self-limited

DEMOGRAPHICS

- Lower tract bleeding is more common in older men
- Diverticular bleeding is more common in patients >50 years
- Angiodysplasia bleeding is more common in patients >70 years and with chronic renal failure
- Ischemic colitis is most commonly seen
  - In older patients due to atherosclerotic disease—postoperatively after ileoaortic or abdominal aortic aneurysm surgery
  - In younger patients due to vasculitis, coagulation disorders, estrogen therapy, and long-distance running

CLINICAL FINDINGS

SYMPTOMS AND SIGNS

- Brown stools mixed or streaked with blood suggest rectosigmoid or anal source
- Painless large-volume bleeding suggests a colonic source (diverticular bleeding or vascular ectasias)
- Maroon stools suggest a right colon or small intestine source
- Black stools (melena) suggest a source proximal to the ligament of Treitz
- Bright red blood per rectum occurs uncommonly with upper tract bleeding and almost always in the setting of massive hemorrhage with shock
- Bloody diarrhea associated with cramping abdominal pain, urgency, or tenesmus suggests inflammatory bowel disease (especially ulcerative colitis), infectious colitis, or ischemic colitis

DIFFERENTIAL DIAGNOSIS

- Diverticulosis
- Vascular ectasias (angiodysplasias), eg, idiopathic arteriovenous malformation, CREST syndrome, hereditary hemorrhagic telangiectasias
- Colonic polyps
- Colorectal cancer
- Inflammatory bowel disease
- Hemorrhoids
- Anal fissure
- Ischemic colitis
- Infectious colitis
- Radiation colitis or proctitis
- NSAID-induced ulcers of small bowel or right colon

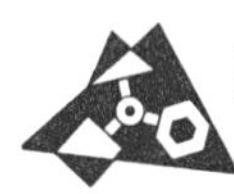

DIAGNOSIS

LABORATORY TESTS

- Complete blood cell count, platelet count, prothrombin time, INR, partial thomboplastin time
- Serum creatinine, blood urea nitrogen
- Type and cross-match

IMAGING STUDIES

- Nuclear bleeding scans: technetium-labeled red blood cell scan
- Selective mesenteric angiography in patients with massive bleeding or positive technetium scans

DIAGNOSTIC PROCEDURES

- Nasogastic tube aspiration to exclude upper tract source
- Anoscopy
- Colonoscopy in patients in whom bleeding has ceased or in patients with moderate active bleeding immediately after rapid purge with 4–12 L polyethylene glycol solution to clear colon (rapid purge colonoscopy)
- Small intestine push enteroscopy or video capsule imaging in patients with unexplained recurrent hemorrhage of obscure origin, suspected from the small intestine
- Upper endoscopy with massive hemotochezia to exclude upper gastrointestinal source

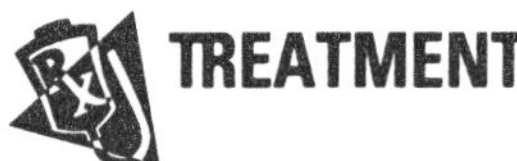

TREATMENT

MEDICATIONS

- Discontinue aspirin and other NSAIDs

SURGERY

- Surgery indicated in patients with ongoing bleeding that requires >4–6 units of blood transfusion within 24 hours or >10 total units
- Limited resection of the bleeding segment of small intestine or colon, if possible
- Total abdominal colectomy with ileorectal anastomosis, otherwise

THERAPEUTIC PROCEDURES

- Therapeutic colonoscopy: high-risk lesions (eg, diverticulum with active bleeding or a visible vessel, or a vascular ectasia) can be treated endoscopically with saline or epinephrine injection, cautery (bipolar or heater probe), or application of metallic clips
- Angiography: selective mesenteric arterial infusion of vasoconstrictors (eg, vasopressin) and/or embolization of actively bleeding arteriole controls hemorrhage in up to 90%

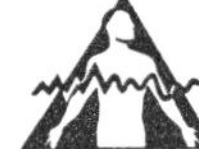

OUTCOME

COMPLICATIONS

- Complications of angiography in 3–10%, including atherosclerotic emboli, thrombosis, and localized bowel infarction
- Operative mortality for continuous or recurrent hemorrhage is 3–15% owing to comorbid illness

PROGNOSIS

- 25% with diverticular hemorrhage have recurrent bleeding

WHEN TO ADMIT

- Patients with mild, intermittent bleeding suggesting anorectal source (blood on toilet paper, dripping in bowl) may be evaluated as outpatients
- All patients with significant hematochezia require admission

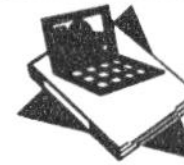

EVIDENCE

PRACTICE GUIDELINES

- Eisen GM et al: Standards of Practice Committee. An annotated algorithmic approach to acute lower gastrointestinal bleeding. Gastrointest Endosc 2001;53:859. [PMID:11375618]

INFORMATION FOR PATIENTS

- MEDLINEplus—Gastrointestinal bleeding
  - http://www.nlm.nih.gov/medlineplus/ency/article/003133.htm
- National Digestive Diseases Information Clearinghouse
  - http://digestive.niddk.nih.gov/ddiseases/pubs/bleeding/index.htm

REFERENCES

- Bezet A et al: Clinical impact of push enteroscopy in patients with gastrointestinal bleeding of unknown origin. Clin Gastroenterol Hepatol 2004;2:921. [PMID:15476156]
- Ellta GH: Urgent colonoscopy for acute lower-GI bleeding. Gastrointest Endosc 2004;59:402. [PMID:14997144]
- Enns R: Acute lower gastrointestinal bleeding: Part 1. Can J Gastroenterol 2001;15:509. [PMID:11544535]
- Enns R: Acute lower gastrointestinal bleeding: Part 2. Can J Gastroenterol 2001;15:517. [PMID:11544534]
- Strate LL et al: Early predictors of severity of acute lower gastrointestinal tract bleeding. Arch Intern Med 2003;163:838. [PMID:12695275]

Author(s)

Kenneth R. McQuaid, MD

Gastrointestinal Bleeding, Acute Upper

KEY FEATURES

ESSENTIALS OF DIAGNOSIS

- Hematemesis (bright red blood or "coffee grounds")
- Melena in most cases; hematochezia in massive upper gastrointestinal bleeds
- Volume status to determine severity of blood loss; hematocrit is a poor early indicator of blood loss
- Endoscopy is diagnostic and may be therapeutic

GENERAL CONSIDERATIONS

- Most common presentation is hematemesis or melena; hematochezia in 10% of cases
- Hematemesis is either bright red blood or brown "coffee grounds" material
- Melena develops after as little as 50–100 mL of blood loss
- Hematochezia requires a loss of >1000 mL
- Upper gastrointestinal bleeding is self-limited in 80% of cases, urgent medical therapy and endoscopic evaluation are required in the remainder
- Bleeding >48 hours prior to presentation carries a low risk of recurrent bleeding
- Peptic ulcers account for ~50%
- Portal hypertension bleeding (10–20% of cases) occurs from varices (most commonly esophageal)
- Mallory-Weiss tears are lacerations of the gastroesophageal junction (5–10% of cases)
- Vascular anomalies, vascular ectasias (angiodysplasias) (7% of cases) occur in hereditary hemorrhagic telangiectasia, CREST syndrome, or sporadically, with increased incidence in chronic renal failure
- Gastric neoplasms (1% of cases)
- Erosive gastritis (< 5% of cases) due to nonsteroidal antiinflammatory drugs (NSAIDs), alcohol, or severe medical or surgical illness (stress gastritis)

DEMOGRAPHICS

- 350,000 hospitalizations a year in the United States

CLINICAL FINDINGS

SYMPTOMS AND SIGNS

- Signs of chronic liver disease implicate bleeding due to portal hypertension, but a different lesion is identified in 25–50% of patients with cirrhosis
- Dyspepsia, NSAID use, or history of previous peptic ulcer suggests peptic ulcer disease
- Heavy alcohol ingestion or retching suggests a Mallory-Weiss tear

DIFFERENTIAL DIAGNOSIS

- Hemoptysis
- Peptic ulcer disease
- Esophageal varices
- Gastric or duodenal varices (rare)
- Erosive gastritis, eg, NSAIDs, alcohol, stress
- Mallory-Weiss syndrome
- Portal hypertensive gastropathy
- Vascular ectasias (angiodysplasias), eg, idiopathic arteriovenous malformation, CREST syndrome, hereditary hemorrhagic telangiectasias
- Gastric cancer
- Rare causes
  - Erosive esophagitis
  - Aortoenteric fistula
  - Dieulafoy's lesion (aberrant gastric submucosal artery)
  - Hemobilia (blood in biliary tree), eg, iatrogenic, malignancy
  - Pancreatic cancer
  - Hemosuccus pancreaticus (pancreatic pseudoaneurysm)

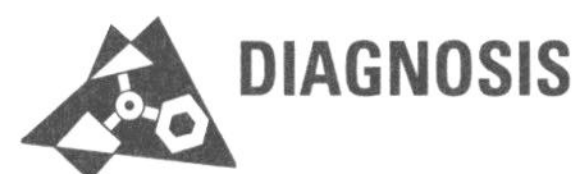

DIAGNOSIS

LABORATORY TESTS

- Obtain complete blood cell count, platelet count, prothrombin time, INR, partial thromboplastin time, serum creatinine, liver enzymes and serologies, and type and cross-matching for 2–4 units or more of packed red blood cells
- Hematocrit is not a reliable indicator of the severity of acute bleeding

DIAGNOSTIC PROCEDURES

- Assess hemodynamic status
  - Systolic blood pressure
  - Heart rate
  - Postural hypotension
- Upper endoscopy after the patient is hemodynamically stable
  - To identify the source of bleeding
  - To determine the risk of rebleeding
  - To render endoscopic therapy such as cautery or injection of a sclerosant or application of a rubber band, metallic clips, or epinephrine

TREATMENT

MEDICATIONS

- Intravenous proton pump inhibitor (eg, omeprazole or lansoprazole, 80-mg bolus, followed by 8 mg/hour continuous infusion for 72 hours) in patients admitted for active bleeding
- High doses of oral proton pump inhibitors (eg, omeprazole, 40 mg, or lansoprazole, 60 mg PO BID for 5 days) may also be effective; commonly administered in patients with suspected peptic ulcer bleeding in emergency room setting before endoscopy
- Octreotide, 100-μg bolus, followed by 50–100 μg/hour, for bleeding related to portal hypertension

SURGERY

- Surgery is required in < 5% of patients with peptic ulcer disease hemorrhage that cannot be controlled with endoscopic therapy

THERAPEUTIC PROCEDURES

- Insert two 18-gauge or larger intravenous lines
- In patients without hemodynamic compromise or overt active bleeding, aggressive fluid repletion can be delayed until extent of bleeding clarified
- Patients with hemodynamic compromise should be given 0.9% saline or lactated Ringer's injection and cross-matched blood
- Nasogastric tube placed for aspiration
- Blood replacement to maintain a hematocrit of 25–28%
- In the absence of continued bleeding, the hematocrit should rise 3% for each unit of transfused packed red cells
- Transfuse blood in patients with brisk active bleeding regardless of the hematocrit
- Transfuse platelets if platelet count < 50,000/μL or if impaired platelet function due to aspirin use
- Uremic patients with active bleeding should be given 1–2 doses of desmopressin (DDAVP), 0.3 μg/kg IV at 12- to 24-hour intervals
- Fresh frozen plasma should be given for actively bleeding patients with a coagulopathy and an INR >1.5
- In massive bleeding, 1 unit of fresh frozen plasma should be given for each 5 units of packed red blood cells transfused
- Intra-arterial embolization or vasopressin indicated (rarely) in patients with persistent bleeding from ulcers, angiomas, or Mallory-Weiss tears who have failed endoscopic therapy and are poor operative risks
- Transvenous intrahepatic portosystemic shunts (TIPS) provide effective decompression of the portal venous system and control of acute variceal bleeding and are indicated in patients in whom endoscopic modalities have failed

OUTCOME

PROGNOSIS

- Mortality rate is 10%, even higher in patients age >60
- Peptic ulcers have an overall acute mortality rate of 6–10%
- Portal hypertension has a hospital mortality rate of 15–40%; if untreated, 50% will rebleed during hospitalization; mortality rate of 60–80% at 1–4 years

WHEN TO REFER

- Refer to gastroenterologist for endoscopy (see below)
- Refer to surgeon for uncontrollable, life-threatening hemorrhage

WHEN TO ADMIT

- Very low risk—reliable patients without serious comorbid medical illnesses or advanced liver disease who have normal hemodynamics, no evidence of overt bleeding (hematemesis or melena) within 48 hours, a negative nasogastric lavage, and normal laboratory tests do not require hospital admission and further evaluation as outpatients
- Low to moderate risk—patients are admitted after appropriate stabilization for upper endoscopy and further treatment; based on the findings may be discharged and followed as outpatients
- High risk—patients with active bleeding manifested by hematemesis or bright red blood on nasogastric aspirate, an estimated loss of >5 units of blood, persistent hemodynamic derangement despite fluid resuscitation, serious comorbid medical illness, or evidence of advanced liver disease require ICU admission

EVIDENCE

PRACTICE GUIDELINES

- Adler DG: ASGE Guideline: the role of endoscopy in acute non-variceal hemorrhage. Gastrointest Endosc 2004;60:497. [PMID:14745397]
- Barkun A et el: A Canadian clinical practice algorithm for the management of patients with nonvariceal upper gastrointestinal bleeding. Can J Gastroenterol 2004;18:605. [PMID:15497000]
- Barkun A et al; Nonvariceal Upper GI Bleeding Consensus Conference Group: Consensus recommendations for managing patients with nonvariceal upper gastrointestinal bleeding. Ann Intern Med 2003;139:843.[PMID:14623622]
- Eisen GM et al; American Society for Gastrointestinal Endoscopy. Standards of Practice Committee: An annotated algorithmic approach to upper gastrointestinal bleeding. Gastrointest Endosc 2001;53:853. [PMID:11375617]

INFORMATION FOR PATIENTS

- American College of Gastroenterology
  - http://www.acg.gi.org/patients/gibleeding/index.asp
- MEDLINEplus—Gastrointestinal bleeding
  - http://www.nlm.nih.gov/medlineplus/ency/article/003133.htm
- National Digestive Diseases Information Clearinghouse
  - http://digestive.niddk.nih.gov/ddiseases/pubs/bleeding/index.htm

REFERENCES

- Das A et al: Prediction of outcome of acute GI hemorrhage: a review of risk scores and predictive models. Gastrointest Endosc 2004;60:85. [PMID:15229431]
- Exon DJ et al: Endoscopic therapy for upper gastrointestinal bleeding. Best Pract Res Clin Gastroenterol 2004;18:77. [PMID:15123086]
- Raju GS: Endoclips for GI endoscopy. Gastrointest Endosc 2004;59:267. [PMID:14745407]
- Sung JJ et al: The role of endoscopic therapy in patients receiving omeprazole for bleeding ulcers with nonbleeding visible vessels or adherent clots: a randomized comparison. Ann Intern Med 2003;139:237. [PMID:12965978]

Author(s)

Kenneth R. McQuaid, MD

Giardiasis

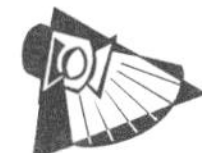

KEY FEATURES

ESSENTIALS OF DIAGNOSIS

- Most infections are asymptomatic
- If symptomatic, there is diarrhea, with greasy, malodorous stools
- Upper abdominal discomfort, excessive flatus, and lassitude
- Cysts and occasionally trophozoites in stools
- Trophozoites in duodenal fluid
- Positive immunoassays

GENERAL CONSIDERATIONS

- Infection of the upper small intestine is caused by the flagellate *Giardia lamblia* (also called *G intestinalis* and *G duodenalis*)
- The organism occurs in feces as a symmetric, heart-shaped flagellated trophozoite measuring 10–25 × 6–12 μm and as a cyst measuring 11–14 × 7–10 μm
- Only the cyst form is infectious by the oral route; trophozoites are destroyed by gastric acidity
- Humans are a reservoir for the infection; dogs, cats, beavers, and other mammals are implicated but are not confirmed reservoirs of infection
- Under moist, cool conditions, cysts can survive in the environment for weeks to months
- Hypogammaglobulinemia, low secretory IgA levels in the gut, achlorhydria, and malnutrition favor development of infection
- *Giardia* infections in AIDS may be more frequent and severe than previously thought
- Gastric giardiasis may represent reflux from the duodenum or localized infection

DEMOGRAPHICS

- The parasite occurs worldwide, especially in areas with poor sanitation
- Cysts are transmitted from fecal contamination of water or food, by person-to-person contact, or by anal-oral sexual contact
  - Multiple cases are common in households, children's day care centers (often the nidus for spread of organisms to the community), and mental institutions
  - Outbreaks occur from contamination of water supplies
- In the United States and Europe, the infection is the most common intestinal protozoal pathogen

CLINICAL FINDINGS

SYMPTOMS AND SIGNS

- Many persons remain asymptomatic cyst carriers, and their infection clears spontaneously
- Syndromes include acute or chronic diarrhea and malabsorption
- The incubation period is 1–3 weeks but may be longer
- The illness may begin gradually or suddenly
- The **acute phase** may last days or weeks, but it is usually self-limited, although cyst excretion may be prolonged
- Occasionally, the disorder may become **chronic** and last for years
- In both the acute and chronic forms, diarrhea ranges from mild to severe; most often it is mild
- There may be no complaints other than of one bulky, loose bowel movement a day, often after breakfast
- With larger numbers of movements, the stools become increasingly watery but are usually free of blood and pus; they are frothy, malodorous, and greasy
- The diarrhea may be daily or recurrent; if recurrent, stools may be normal to mushy during intervening days, or the patient may be constipated
- Other symptoms include anorexia, nausea, vomiting, midepigastric discomfort, cramps (often after meals), belching, flatulence, borborygmi, and abdominal discomfort
- Weight loss and weakness are frequent
- Malabsorption occasionally develops in the acute or chronic stage

DIFFERENTIAL DIAGNOSIS

- Viral or bacterial gastroenteritis
- Amebiasis
- Lactase deficiency
- Irritable bowel syndrome
- Malabsorption due to other causes, eg, celiac sprue
- Laxative abuse
- Crohn's disease
- Cryptosporidiosis

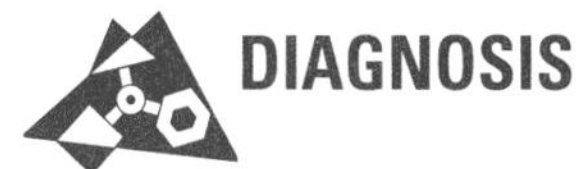

DIAGNOSIS

LABORATORY TESTS

- Using stool specimens, diagnosis is by **standard microscopy** to detect cysts and trophozoites or by **immunoassay** by two methods
  - One is to detect coproantigen by an enzyme immunoassay (sensitivity 94–97%, specificity 100%)
  - The other is to detect cysts by the direct fluorescent antibody assay (sensitivity and specificity, 96–100%)
- Although the coproantigen immunoassay is as sensitive and specific as microscopy and easier to perform, three stool specimens should be examined for ova and parasites if other organisms are being sought in addition to *Giardia*
- Some immunoassays require fresh or frozen stool and cannot be used with preserved specimens; additionally, some assays detect only cysts or only trophozoites
- Three stool specimens collected at intervals of 2 days or longer should be examined following concentration methods
  - One specimen will detect 50–75% of cases and three specimens about 90%
  - Unless the specimens can be submitted within an hour, they should be preserved immediately in a fixative
  - Purges do not increase the likelihood of finding the organism
  - Use of barium, antibiotics, antacids, kaolin products, or oily laxatives may temporarily (about 10 days) reduce the number of parasites
- Sometimes warranted is the search for trophozoites in the duodenum by the duodenal string test (Entero-Test), duodenal aspiration, endoscopic brush cytology, or duodenal biopsy (a mucosal imprint for staining should be made before sectioning)
- Tests for serum antibody are not recommended because of lack of sensitivity and specificity
- There is no eosinophilia, and the white blood cell count is normal

IMAGING STUDIES

- Radiological examination of the small bowel is usually normal

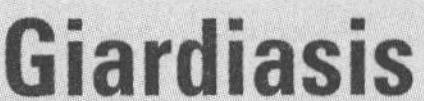

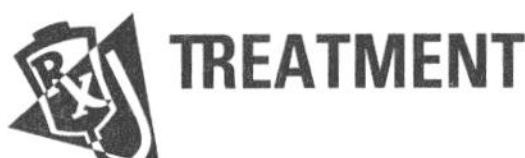

TREATMENT

MEDICATIONS

- Treatment is with tinidazole or metronidazole. Retreatment with an alternative drug may be needed, for which albendazole and paromomycin can be used
- Tinidazole 2 g PO given once is the drug of choice and has cure rates of 90–100%
- Metronidazole dose is 250 mg PO TID for 5–7 days
- Tinidazole and metronidazole may cause a metallic taste, gastrointestinal symptoms, and an antabuse-like reaction in alcohol users
- Furazolidone dose is 100 mg (in suspension) QID for 7–10 days. Gastrointestinal symptoms, fever, headache, rash, and a disulfiram-like reaction with alcohol occur. Furazolidone can cause mild hemolysis in glucose-6-phosphate dehydrogenase-deficient persons
- Albendazole (400 mg daily for 5 days) has cure rates of 10–95%
- Reports with paromomycin (25–35 mg/kg/day in three divided doses for 7 days) have been mixed; it may be useful in pregnancy
- Nitazoxamide, approved in the United States for children under 11 years (500 mg twice daily for 3 days), continues under study for adult treatment
- The potential for carcinogenicity of furazolidone, metronidazole, and tinidazole appears negligible. Because of limited availability and rare potential for severe toxicity, quinacrine is no longer recommended

THERAPEUTIC PROCEDURES

- All household contacts and children exposed in day care should be tested
- Treatment of asymptomatic patients should be considered since they can transmit the infection and may occasionally become symptomatic themselves
- In selected cases, it may be best to wait a few weeks before starting treatment, as some infections will clear spontaneously
- In the presence of a presumptive diagnosis but negative stool specimens, an empirical course of treatment is sometimes indicated

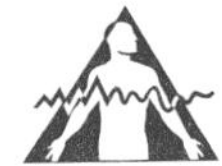

OUTCOME

FOLLOW-UP

- In follow-up, two or more stools are analyzed weekly starting 2 weeks after therapy
- With cure, the immunoasssay normally reverts to negative

COMPLICATIONS

- Extraintestinal manifestations (arthritis, anterior uveitis, urticaria) are unproven complications of giardiasis

PROGNOSIS

- With successful eradication of the infection, there are no sequelae
- Without treatment, severe malabsorption may rarely contribute to death from other causes

WHEN TO REFER

- Progressive diarrhea despite therapy
- To search for the organism in the duodenum

PREVENTION

- There is no effective chemoprophylaxis
- Since community water chlorination (0.4 mg/L) is relatively ineffective for inactivating cysts, filtration is required
- For hikers, bringing water to a boil for 1 min is adequate
  - Halogenation with iodine or filtration with a pore size less than 1 μm can also be used
  - Relying on iodine halogenation is no longer recommended by the Centers for Disease Control and Prevention
- In day care centers, appropriate disposal of diapers and frequent hand washing are essential

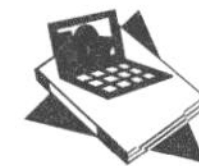

EVIDENCE

PRACTICE GUIDELINES

- National Guideline Clearinghouse
  - http://www.guideline.gov/summary/summary.aspx?doc_id=2791&nbr=2017&string=giardiasis

WEB SITE

- CDC—Division of Parasitic Diseases
  - http://www.cdc.gov/ncidod/dpd/parasites/giardiasis/default.htm

INFORMATION FOR PATIENTS

- American Academy of Family Physicians
  - http://familydoctor.org/078.xml
- Centers for Disease Control
  - http://www.cdc.gov/travel/diseases/giardiasis.htm
- CDC—Division of Parasitic Diseases
  - http://www.cdc.gov/ncidod/dpd/parasites/giardiasis/factsht_giardia.htm

REFERENCES

- Aziz H et al: A comparison study of different methods used in the detection of *Giardia lamblia.* Clin Lab Sci 2001;14:150. [PMID: 11517624]
- Gardner TB et al: Treatment of giardiasis. Clin Microbiol Rev 2001;14:114. [PMID: 11148005]

Glomerulonephritis

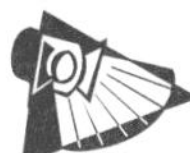

KEY FEATURES

ESSENTIALS OF DIAGNOSIS

- Acute renal insufficiency
- Edema
- Hypertension
- Hematuria (with or without dysmorphic red cells, red blood cell casts), and mild proteinuria

GENERAL CONSIDERATIONS

- A relatively uncommon cause of acute renal failure, ~5% of cases of intrinsic renal failure
- Acute glomerulonephritis usually signifies an inflammatory process causing renal dysfunction over days to weeks that may or may not resolve (Table 93)
- Inflammatory glomerular lesions include mesangioproliferative, focal and diffuse proliferative, and crescentic lesions
- Rapidly progressive acute glomerulonephritis can cause permanent damage to glomeruli if not identified and treated rapidly

Causes of glomerulonephritis

- Immune complex
  - IgA nephropathy
  - Endocarditis
  - Systemic lupus erythematosus
  - Cryoglobulinemia (often associated with hepatitis C)
  - Postinfectious glomerulonephritis
  - Membranoproliferative glomerulonephritis
- Pauci-immune (ANCA$^+$)
  - Wegener's granulomatosis
  - Churg-Strauss syndrome
  - Microscopic polyarteritis
- Antiglomerular basement membrane (GBM)
  - Goodpasture's disease
  - Anti-GBM glomerulonephritis

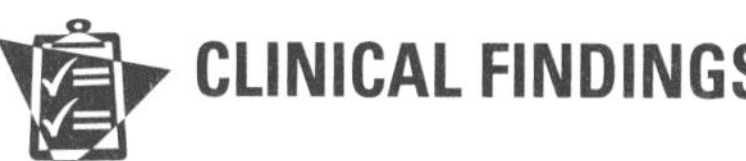

CLINICAL FINDINGS

SYMPTOMS AND SIGNS

- Hypertension
- Edema first in body parts with low tissue tension such as periorbital and scrotal regions
- Dark urine

DIFFERENTIAL DIAGNOSIS

- Acute interstitial nephritis (AIN)
- Acute tubular necrosis (ATN)

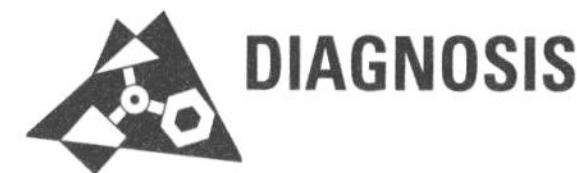

DIAGNOSIS

LABORATORY TESTS

- Urinalysis dipstick: hematuria, moderate proteinuria (usually < 2 g/day); microscopic: abnormal urinary sediment with cellular elements such as red cells, red cell casts, and white cells
- 24-h urine for protein excretion and creatinine clearance
- Urine creatinine clearance is an unreliable marker of glomerular filtration rate in cases of rapidly changing serum creatinine values
- Fractional excretion of sodium is usually low (< 1%), unless renal tubular dysfunction is marked
- Complement levels (C3, C4, CH50), ASO titer, anti-GBM antibody levels, ANA titers, cryoglobulins, hepatitis B surface antigen and hepatitis C virus antibody, C3 nephritic factor, ANCA

IMAGING STUDIES

- Renal ultrasound

DIAGNOSTIC PROCEDURES

- Renal biopsy: Type of glomerulonephritis can be categorized according to the light microscopy immunofluorescence pattern and electron microscopy appearance

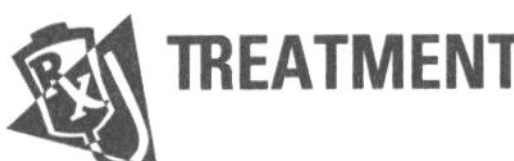

TREATMENT

MEDICATIONS

- Corticosteroids in high dose and cytotoxic agents such as cyclophosphamide, depending on the nature and severity of disease
- Antihypertensive agents
- Diuretics and salt and water restriction for fluid overload
- Angiotensin-converting enzyme inhibitors and angiotensin II receptor blockers

THERAPEUTIC PROCEDURES

- Specific therapies aimed at the underlying cause
- Dialysis as needed

OUTCOME

FOLLOW-UP

- With nephrologist as dictated by specific disease

COMPLICATIONS

- Chronic kidney disease

WHEN TO REFER

- Any evidence of possible glomerulonephritis

WHEN TO ADMIT

- Any acute or rapidly progressive symptoms (days to weeks) may be cause for admission depending on the disease

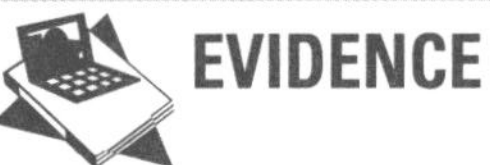

EVIDENCE

PRACTICE GUIDELINES

- Singapore Ministry of Health: Glomerulonephritis, 2001
  - http://www.guideline.gov/summary/summary.aspx?doc_id=2971&nbr=2197
- Tomino Y et al: Clinical guidelines for immunoglobulin A (IgA) nephropathy in Japan, second version. Clin Exp Nephrol 2003;7:93. [PMID: 14586726]

WEB SITE

- National Kidney and Urologic Diseases Information Clearinghouse
  - http://kidney.niddk.nih.gov/

INFORMATION FOR PATIENTS

- Mayo Clinic: Glomerulonephritis
  - http://www.mayoclinic.com/invoke.cfm?objectid=CAB55536-7CCC-44A4-832C420405FCCA39
- MedlinePlus: Glomerulonephritis
  - http://www.nlm.nih.gov/medlineplus/ency/article/000484.htm
- National Kidney Foundation: Glomerulonephritis
  - http://www.kidney.org/atoz/atozItem.cfm?id=65
- National Kidney and Urologic Diseases Information Clearinghouse: Glomerular Diseases
  - http://kidney.niddk.nih.gov/kudiseases/pubs/glomerular/index.htm

REFERENCE

- Hricik DE et al: Glomerulonephritis. N Engl J Med 1998;339:888. [PMID: 9744974]

Author(s)

Suzanne Watnick, MD
Gail Morrison, MD

Goiter, Endemic

Glomerulonephritis, Cryoglobulin-Associated p. 1082. Glomerulonephritis, Membranoproliferative p. 1082. Glomerulonephritis, Pauci-Immune p. 1083. Glomerulonephritis, Postinfectious p. 1083. Glossitis & Glossodynia p. 1084.

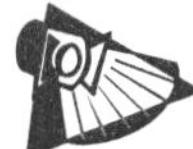

KEY FEATURES

ESSENTIALS OF DIAGNOSIS

- Common in regions of the world with low-iodine diets
- High rate of congenital hypothyroidism and cretinism
- Goiters may become multinodular and grow to great size
- Most adults with endemic goiter are euthyroid; however, some are hypothyroid or hyperthyroid
- Impaired cognition and hearing may be subtle or severe in congenital hypothyroidism

GENERAL CONSIDERATIONS

- Up to 0.5% of iodine-deficient populations have full-blown cretinism; less severe manifestations of congenital hypothyroidism more common
- Causes: iodine deficiency (most common); certain foods (eg, sorghum, millet, maize, cassava, turnip), mineral deficiencies (selenium, iron) and water pollutants; congenital partial defects in thyroid enzyme activity
- Increase in size of thyroid nodules and emergence of new nodules in pregnancy

DEMOGRAPHICS

- ~5% of world's population have goiters
- Of these, 75% occur in areas of iodine deficiency. Such areas found in 115 countries, mostly developing nations but also in Europe, eg, in Pescopagano, Italy, 60% of adults have goiters, with hyperthyroidism in 2.9%; overt hypothyroidism in 0.2% and subclinical hypothyroidism in 3.8%, thyroid cancer in < 0.1%

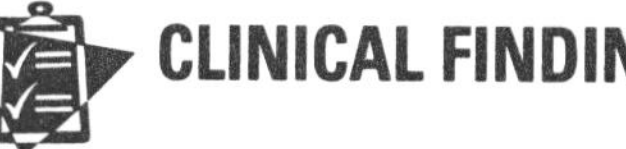

CLINICAL FINDINGS

SYMPTOMS AND SIGNS

- Thyroid may become multinodular and very large
- Growth often occurs during pregnancy and may cause compressive symptoms
- Substernal goiters usually asymptomatic but can cause tracheal compression, respiratory distress, dysphagia, superior vena cava syndrome, gastrointestinal bleeding from esophageal varices, phrenic or recurrent laryngeal nerve palsy, or Horner's syndrome, or pleural or pericardial effusions (rare)
- Cerebral ischemia and stroke can result from arterial compression or thyrocervical steal syndrome
- Malignancy in < 1%
- Some patients with goiter become hypothyroid; others become thyrotoxic as goiter grows and becomes more autonomous, especially if iodine added to diet
- Congenital hypothyroidism: isolated deafness, short stature, or impaired mentation

DIFFERENTIAL DIAGNOSIS

- Benign multinodular goiter
- Pregnancy (in areas of iodine deficiency)
- Graves' disease
- Hashimoto's thyroiditis
- Subacute (de Quervain's) thyroiditis
- Drugs causing hypothyroidism: lithium, amiodarone, propylthiouracil, methimazole, phenylbutazone, sulfonamides, interferon-α, iodide
- Infiltrating disease, eg, malignancy, sarcoidosis
- Suppurative thyroiditis
- Riedel's thyroiditis

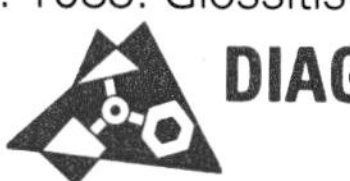

DIAGNOSIS

LABORATORY TESTS

- Serum thyroxine and thyroid-stimulating hormone (TSH) usually normal
- TSH low if multinodular goiter becomes autonomous in presence of sufficient iodine for thyroid hormone synthesis, causing hyperthyroidism
- TSH high in hypothyroidism
- Thyroid radioactive iodine uptake usually elevated, but may be normal if iodine intake has improved
- Serum levels of antithyroid antibodies usually undetectable or low
- Serum thyroglobulin often elevated

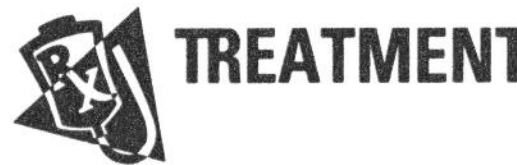

TREATMENT

MEDICATIONS

- Dietary iodine supplementation (eg, addition of potassium iodide to table salt) greatly reduces prevalence of endemic goiter and cretinism but is less effective in shrinking established goiter
- Dietary iodine supplementation increases risk of autoimmune thyroid dysfunction, which may result in hypothyroidism or hyperthyroidism
- Excessive iodine intake may increase risk of goiter
- Concurrent deficiencies in both vitamin A and iodine increase the risk of endemic goiter and concurrent repletion of both iodine and vitamin A reduces the risk of goiter in endemic regions
- Thyroxine supplementation can shrink goiters and reduce risk of further goiter growth, but may induce hyperthyroidism in individuals with autonomous multinodular goiters; thyroxine suppression should not be started in patients with suppressed TSH levels

SURGERY

- Thyroidectomy indicated for cosmesis, compressive symptoms, or thyrotoxicosis in adults with very large multinodular goiters

PROCEDURES

- Patients may be treated with ^{131}I for large compressive goiters

OUTCOME

FOLLOW-UP

- Partial thyroidectomy is followed by a high goiter recurrence rate in iodine-deficient geographic areas, so total thyroidectomy is preferred when surgery is indicated

COMPLICATIONS

- Initiating iodine supplementation in a geographic area causes increased frequency of hyperthyroidism in first year, followed by greatly reduced rates of toxic nodular goiter and Graves' disease thereafter
- Patients treated with ^{131}I may rarely develop Graves' disease 3–10 months after treatment
- Goiters may become multinodular and grow to great size

WHEN TO REFER

- Refer to endocrinologist for hyperthyroidism, enlarging goiter, suspicious nodules
- Refer to thyroid surgeon for thyroidectomy for cosmesis, compressive symptoms, or thyrotoxicosis in adults with very large multinodular goiters

WHEN TO ADMIT

- Thyroidectomy
- ^{131}I treatment

PREVENTION

- Dietary iodine supplementation started in Switzerland in 1922 with addition of potassium iodide to table salt
- Current level of supplementation in the United States is 20 mg potassium iodide per kg salt
- Iodized salt has greatly reduced incidence of endemic goiter. Unfortunately, many iodine-deficient countries have inadequate programs for iodine supplementation
- Minimum dietary requirement for iodine is about 50 µg daily; optimal iodine intake is 150–300 µg daily. Iodine sufficiency is demonstrated by urinary iodide excretion >10 µg/dL

EVIDENCE

PRACTICE GUIDELINES

- American Association of Clinical Endocrinologists medical guidelines for clinical practice for the evaluation and treatment of hyperthyroidism and hypothyroidism. American Association of Clinical Endocrinologists, American College of Endocrinology—Medical Specialty Society, 2002
  - http://www.aace.com/clin/guidelines/hypo_hyper.pdf

WEB SITES

- American Association of Clinical Endocrinologists
  - http://www.aace.com/clin/fcc/fcc-200009.php
- Thyroid Disease Manager site
  - http://www.thyroidmanager.org/Chapter20/20_cause.htm

INFORMATION FOR PATIENTS

- Merck Manual
  - http://www.merck.com/pubs/mmanual/section1/chapter4/4c.htm
- Program Against Micronutrient Malnutrition—Emory University
  - http://www.sph.emory.edu/PAMM/iodine.htm

REFERENCES

- Delange F: Iodine deficiency in Europe and its consequences: an update. Eur J Nucl Med Mol Imaging 2002;29 (Suppl 2):S404. [PMID: 12192540]
- Zimmermann MB et al: The effects of vitamin A deficiency and vitamin A supplementation on thyroid function in goitrous children. J Clin Endocrinol Metab 2004;89:5441. [PMID: 15531495]

Author(s)

Paul A. Fitzgerald, MD

Gonococcal Infections

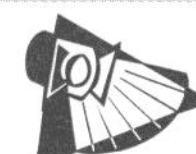

KEY FEATURES

ESSENTIALS OF DIAGNOSIS

- Purulent and profuse urethral discharge, especially in men, with dysuria, yielding positive smear
- In men
  - Epididymitis, prostatitis, periurethral inflammation, proctitis
- In women
  - Asymptomatic, or cervicitis with purulent discharge
  - Vaginitis, salpingitis, proctitis also occur
- Disseminated disease
  - Fever, rash, tenosynovitis, and arthritis
- Gram-negative intracellular diplococci seen in a smear or cultured from any site, particularly the urethra, cervix, pharynx, and rectum

GENERAL CONSIDERATIONS

- Gonorrhea is caused by *Neisseria gonorrhoeae*, a gram-negative diplococcus

DEMOGRAPHICS

- Gonorrhea is most commonly transmitted during sexual activity and has its greatest incidence in the 15- to 29-year-old age group

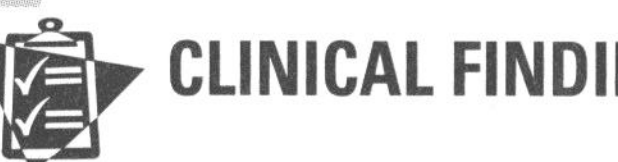

CLINICAL FINDINGS

SYMPTOMS AND SIGNS

- Asymptomatic infection is common and occurs in both sexes
- Atypical sites of primary infection (eg, the pharynx) must always be considered

Urethritis and cervicitis

- In men
  - Initially, burning on urination and a serous or milky discharge
  - One to 3 days later, more pronounced urethral pain and the discharge becomes yellow, creamy, and profuse, sometimes blood tinged
  - May regress and become chronic or progress to involve the prostate, epididymis, and periurethral glands with acute, painful inflammation
  - Rectal infection is common in homosexual men
- In women
  - Infection may be asymptomatic, with only slightly increased vaginal discharge and moderate cervicitis on examination
  - Infection often becomes symptomatic during menses
  - Women may have dysuria, urinary frequency, and urgency, with a purulent urethral discharge
  - Vaginitis and cervicitis with inflammation of Bartholin's glands are common
  - Infection may remain as a chronic cervicitis. It may progress to involve the uterus and tubes with acute and chronic salpingitis and with ultimate scarring of tubes and sterility
  - In pelvic inflammatory disease, anaerobes and chlamydiae often accompany gonococci

Conjunctivitis

- Direct inoculation of gonococci into the conjunctival sac occurs by autoinoculation from a genital infection
- The purulent conjunctivitis may rapidly progress to panophthalmitis and loss of the eye unless treated promptly

DIFFERENTIAL DIAGNOSIS

- Nongonococcal urethritis, eg, *Chlamydia, Ureaplasma urealyticum*
- Septic arthritis of other bacterial cause
- Reactive arthritis (Reiter's syndrome)
- Vaginal discharge due to candidiasis, bacterial vaginosis, or trichomoniasis
- Chronic meningococcemia

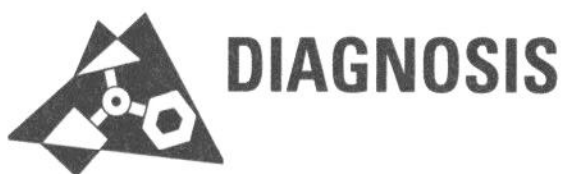

DIAGNOSIS

LABORATORY TESTS

- Gram stain
  - In men, gram stain of urethral discharge, especially during the first week after onset, typically shows gram-negative diplococci in polymorphonuclear leukocytes
  - Gram stain is less often positive in women
- Culture is the diagnostic gold standard, particularly when the Gram stain is negative
- A ligase chain reaction (LCR) assay that detects both *N gonorrhoeae* and *Chlamydia trachomatis* in cervical and urethral swab specimens and urine permits more rapid diagnosis of gonococcal infection. LCR also has improved sensitivity and high specificity compared with culture of swab specimens

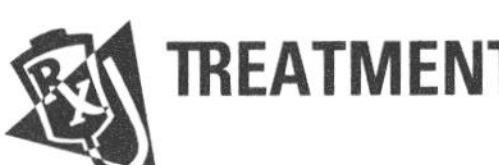

TREATMENT

MEDICATIONS

- For urethritis or cervicitis
  - Treatment of choice is either ceftriaxone, 125 mg IM, or cefixime, 400 mg PO as a single dose. Availability may be a problem; cefpodoxime, 200 mg as a single dose, can be substituted, but is slightly less efficacious
  - A single oral dose of ciprofloxacin 500 mg, ofloxacin 400 mg, or levofloxacin 250 mg is also effective
  - Since coexistent chlamydial infection is common, treat as well with doxycycline, 100 mg PO QD for 7 days, or a single 1-g oral dose of azithromycin
- Salpingitis, prostatitis, bacteremia, arthritis, and other complications due to susceptible strains
  - Treat with penicillin G, 10 million units IV QD for 5 days
  - Ceftriaxone, 1 g IV QD for 5 days, or an oral fluoroquinolone (ciprofloxacin, 500 mg BID, or levofloxacin, 500 mg QD) for 5 days is also effective

THERAPEUTIC PROCEDURES

- Therapy typically is administered before antimicrobial susceptibilities are known
- All sexual partners should be treated

OUTCOME

COMPLICATIONS

Disseminated disease

- Systemic complications follow the dissemination of gonococci from the primary site via the bloodstream
- Gonococcal bacteremia is associated with intermittent fever, arthralgia, and skin lesions ranging from maculopapular to pustular, which tend to be few in number and peripherally located

WHEN TO REFER

- Report to the public health department for tracing of contacts
- All suspected or proven ocular gonorrhea

WHEN TO ADMIT

- Most cases of pelvic inflammatory disease (perhaps not the mild cases)
- All cases of suspected or proven disseminated disease

PREVENTION

- The condom, if properly used, can reduce the risk of infection
- Effective drugs taken in therapeutic doses within 24 h of exposure can abort an infection

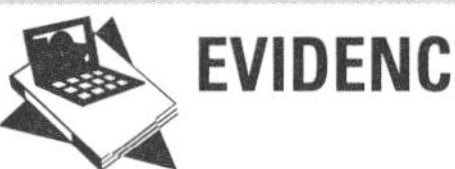

EVIDENCE

PRACTICE GUIDELINES

- Centers for Disease Control and Prevention. Sexually transmitted disease treatment guidelines 2002.
  - http://www.cdc.gov/STD/treatment/4-2002TG.htm
- National Guideline Clearinghouse
  - http://www.guideline.gov/summary/summary.aspx?doc_id=3031

WEB SITE

- Karolinska Institute—Directory of Bacterial Infections and Mycoses
  - http://www.mic.ki.se/Diseases/C01.html

INFORMATION FOR PATIENTS

- JAMA patient page: Sexually transmitted diseases. JAMA 1998;280:944.
- National Institute of Allergy and Infectious Diseases
  - http://www.niaid.nih.gov/factsheets/stdgon.htm

REFERENCE

- Centers for Disease Control and Prevention (CDC): Increases in fluoroquinolone-resistant *Neisseria gonorrhoeae* among men who have sex with men—United States, 2003, and revised recommendations for gonorrhea treatment, 2004. MMWR Morb Mortal Wkly Rep 2004;53:335. [PMID: 15123985]]

Author(s)

Henry F. Chambers, MD

Goodpasture's Syndrome, Pulmonary

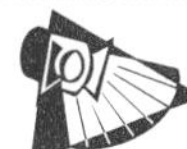

KEY FEATURES

ESSENTIALS OF DIAGNOSIS

- Triad of pulmonary hemorrhage, circulating anti-glomerulobasement membrane (GBM) antibody, and glomerulonephritis due to anti-GBM
- Up to one-third of patients with anti-GBM glomerulonephritis have no evidence of lung injury

GENERAL CONSIDERATIONS

- Clinical constellation of recurrent pulmonary alveolar hemorrhage with rapidly progressive glomerulonephritis
- Injury mediated by anti-GBM antibody
- ~5% of patients with rapidly progressive acute glomerulonephritis have anti-GBM
- Associated with influenza A infection, hydrocarbon solvent exposure, and HLA-DR2 and -B7 antigens

DEMOGRAPHICS

- Incidence in males ~6 times that in females
- Occurs most commonly in the second and third decades

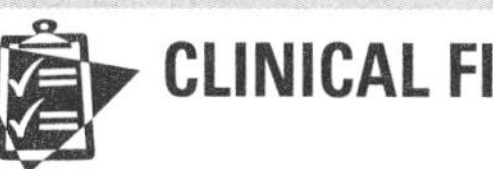

CLINICAL FINDINGS

SYMPTOMS AND SIGNS

- Usually presents with hemoptysis, though pulmonary hemorrhage may be occult
- Dyspnea, cough, hypoxemia, and bilateral pulmonary infiltrates are typical
- Iron deficiency anemia
- Microscopic hematuria
- Upper respiratory tract infection precedes onset in 20–60% of cases
- Possible respiratory failure
- Hypertension
- Edema

DIFFERENTIAL DIAGNOSIS

- Severe congestive heart failure (pulmonary edema and prerenal azotemia)
- Renal failure (with hypervolemia and pulmonary edema)
- Microscopic polyangiitis (polyarteritis nodosa)
- Systemic lupus erythematosus
- Henoch-Schönlein purpura
- Wegener's granulomatosis
- Legionnaire's disease
- Renal vein thrombosis with pulmonary embolism

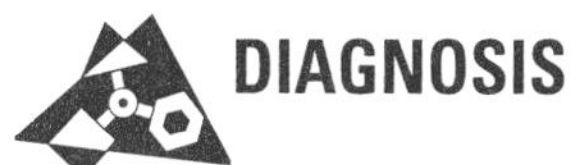

DIAGNOSIS

LABORATORY TESTS

- Circulating anti-GBM antibody in serum in > 90%
- Iron deficiency anemia
- Complement levels are normal
- Sputum contains hemosiderin-laden macrophages
- Diffusion capacity of carbon monoxide is markedly increased

IMAGING STUDIES

- Chest x-rays show shifting pulmonary infiltrates

DIAGNOSTIC PROCEDURES

- Biopsy demonstrates IgG deposits in glomeruli or alveoli

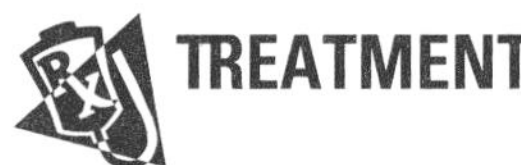

TREATMENT

MEDICATIONS

- Treatment is a combination of plasma exchange therapy to remove circulating antibodies and administration of immunosuppressive drugs (corticosteroids and cyclophosphamide) to prevent formation of new antibodies
- Give methylprednisolone, 30 mg/kg IV QD followed by oral prednisone at 1 mg/kg/day AND cyclophosphamide, 2 mg/kg/day PO

THERAPEUTIC PROCEDURES

- Plasmapheresis, performed daily for up to 2 weeks, in combination with the corticosteroids and cyclophosphamide

OUTCOME

FOLLOW-UP

- Anti-GBM antibody levels should decrease as the clinical course improves

COMPLICATIONS

- Renal failure
- Respiratory failure

PROGNOSIS

- Prognosis poor in patients with oliguria and serum creatinine > 6–7 mg/dL

WHEN TO REFER

- Patients should be referred to a pulmonologist, rheumatologist, or nephrologist

WHEN TO ADMIT

- Respiratory insufficiency
- Progressive or severe renal disease

EVIDENCE

INFORMATION FOR PATIENTS

- National Institutes of Health
  - http://www.nlm.nih.gov/medlineplus/ency/article/000142.htm
- National Kidney and Urologic Diseases Information Clearinghouse
  - http://kidney.niddk.nih.gov/kudiseases/pubs/goodpasture/index.htm

REFERENCES

- Hudson B et al: Alport's syndrome, Goodpasture's syndrome, and type IV collagen. N Engl J Med 2003;348:2543. [PMID: 12815141]
- Salama A et al: Goodpasture's disease in the absence of circulating anti-glomerular basement membrane antibodies as detected by standard techniques. Am J Kidney Dis 2002;39:1162. [PMID: 12046026]
- Shah M et al: Characteristics and outcomes of patients with Goodpasture's syndrome. South Med J 2002;95:1411. [PMID: 12597309]

Author(s)

Suzanne Watnick, MD
Gail Morrison, MD
Mark S. Chestnutt, MD
Thomas J. Prendergast, MD

Gouty Arthritis

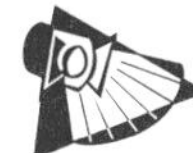

KEY FEATURES

ESSENTIALS OF DIAGNOSIS

- Acute onset, typically nocturnal
- Usually monarticular, often involving the first metatarsophalangeal (MTP) joint
- Polyarticular involvement more common with long-standing disease
- Hyperuricemia in most; identification of urate crystals in joint fluid or tophi is diagnostic
- Dramatic therapeutic response to nonsteroidal antiinflammatory drugs or colchicine

GENERAL CONSIDERATIONS

- A metabolic disease of heterogeneous nature, often familial, associated with abnormal amounts of urates in the body and characterized early by a recurring acute arthritis, usually monarticular, and later by chronic deforming arthritis
- **Secondary gout** is from acquired causes of hyperuricemia
  - Medication use (diuretics, cyclosporine, low-dose aspirin, and niacin)
  - Myeloproliferative disorders, multiple myeloma, hemoglobinopathies
  - Chronic renal disease
  - Hypothyroidism, psoriasis, sarcoidosis, and lead poisoning
- Alcohol ingestion promotes hyperuricemia by increasing urate production and decreasing the renal excretion of uric acid
- Hospitalized patients frequently suffer attacks of gout because of changes in diet (eg, inability to take oral feedings following abdominal surgery) or medications that lead either to rapid reductions or increases in the serum urate level

DEMOGRAPHICS

- Especially common in Pacific Islanders, eg, Filipinos and Samoans
- Rarely caused by a specifically determined genetic aberration (eg, Lesch-Nyhan syndrome)
- 90% of patients with primary gout are men, usually over 30 years of age
- In women the onset is typically postmenopausal

CLINICAL FINDINGS

SYMPTOMS AND SIGNS

- Sudden onset of arthritis, frequently nocturnal, either without apparent precipitating cause or following rapid fluctuations in serum urate levels
- The MTP joint of the great toe is the most susceptible joint ("podagra"), although others, especially those of the feet, ankles, and knees, are commonly affected
- May develop in periarticular soft tissues such as the arch of the foot
- As the attack progresses, the pain becomes intense. The involved joints are swollen and exquisitely tender and the overlying skin tense, warm, and dusky red. Fever is common
- Tophi may be found in cartilage, external ears, hands, feet, olecranon, prepatellar bursas, tendons and bone. They are usually seen only after several attacks of acute arthritis
- Asymptomatic periods of months or years commonly follow the initial attack
- After years of recurrent severe monarthritis attacks, gout can evolve into a chronic, deforming polyarthritis of upper and lower extremities that mimics rheumatoid arthritis

DIFFERENTIAL DIAGNOSIS

Arthritis

- Cellulitis
- Septic arthritis
- Pseudogout
- Rheumatoid arthritis
- Reactive arthritis
- Osteoarthritis
- Chronic lead poisoning (saturnine gout)
- Palindromic rheumatism

Podagra

- Trauma
- Cellulitis
- Sarcoidosis
- Pseudogout
- Psoriatic arthritis
- Bursitis of first MTP joint (inflamed bunion)

Tophi

- Rheumatoid nodules
- Erythema nodosum
- Gout
- Coccidioidomycosis
- Endocarditis (Osler nodes)
- Sarcoidosis
- Polyarteritis nodosa

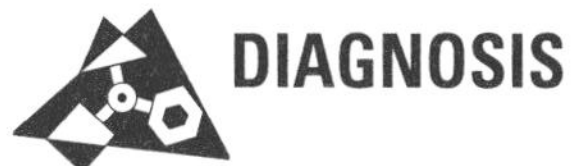

DIAGNOSIS

LABORATORY TESTS

- The serum uric acid is elevated (>7.5 mg/dL) in 95% of patients who have serial measurements during the course of an attack. However, a single uric acid determination is normal in up to 25% of cases, so it does not exclude gout

IMAGING STUDIES

- Early in the disease, radiographs show no changes
- Later, punched-out erosions with an overhanging rim of cortical bone ("rat bite") develop. When these are adjacent to a soft tissue tophus, they are diagnostic of gout

DIAGNOSTIC PROCEDURES

- Identification of sodium urate crystals by compensated polariscopic examination of joint fluid aspirates
- Crystals are negatively birefringent and needle-like and may be found free or in neutrophils

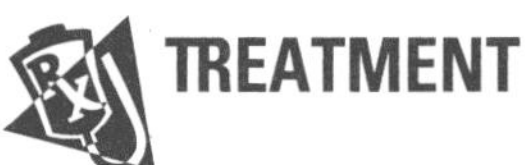

TREATMENT

MEDICATIONS

Acute attack

- **Nonsteroidal antiinflammatory** drugs are the treatment of choice
- The pain of an acute attack may require **opioids.** Aspirin should be avoided since it aggravates hyperuricemia
- For monarticular gout, **intraarticular corticosteroid administration** (eg, triamcinolone, 10–40 mg depending on the size of the joint) is most effective
- For polyarticular gout, **corticosteroids** may be given intravenously (eg, methylprednisolone, 40 mg/day tapered off over 7 days) or orally (eg, prednisone, 40–60 mg/day tapered off over 7 days)

SURGERY

- Surgical excision of large tophi rarely offers mechanical improvement in selected deformities

THERAPEUTIC PROCEDURES

- Corticosteroid injections for acute monarticular disease
- Bed rest is important and should be continued for about 24 h after the acute attack has subsided. Early ambulation may precipitate a recurrence
- Treat the acute arthritis first and hyperuricemia later, if at all. Sudden reduction of serum uric acid often precipitates further gouty arthritis

OUTCOME

FOLLOW-UP

- Maintain uric acid level within the normal range in nontophaceous gout
- Maintain serum uric acid below 6.5 mg/dL in tophaceous gout

COMPLICATIONS

- Chronic tophaceous arthritis can occur after repeated attacks of inadequately treated acute gout
- Uric acid kidney stones (5–10% of patients). Hyperuricemia correlates highly with the likelihood of developing stones; the risk of stone formation reaching 50% with a serum urate level above 13 mg/dL
- Chronic urate nephropathy. Although progressive renal failure occurs in a substantial percentage of patients with chronic gout, the etiological role of hyperuricemia is controversial, because there are numerous confounding risk factors for renal failure

PROGNOSIS

- Untreated, the acute attack may last from a few days to several weeks, but proper treatment quickly terminates the attack
- The intervals between acute attacks vary up to years, but the asymptomatic periods often become shorter if the disease progresses

WHEN TO REFER

- Refer to a rheumatologist if the patient has recurrent attacks despite treatment

WHEN TO ADMIT

- For suspected or proven superimposed septic arthritis

PREVENTION

- Asymptomatic hyperuricemia should not be treated
- Potentially reversible causes of hyperuricemia are a high-purine diet, obesity, frequent alcohol consumption, and use of certain medications (diuretics, niacin, low-dose aspirin)
- Colchicine, 0.6 mg orally QD or BID, can be used to prevent future attacks and is frequently prescribed to prevent attacks when probenecid or allopurinol is being initiated
- Two classes of drugs can lower uric acid levels in patients with frequent arthritis, tophaceous deposits, or renal damage
  - Probenicid, 1–2 g PO daily, is the principal uricosuric drug, which cannot be used if the creatinine is >2 mg/dL
  - Allopurinol (100–300 mg/day PO based on renal function) promptly lowers plasma urate and urinary uric acid concentrations and facilitates tophus mobilization. The commonest sign of hypersensitivity to allopurinol (occurring in 2% of cases) is a pruritic rash that may progress to toxic epidermal necrolysis. Vasculitis and hepatitis are other rare complications

EVIDENCE

PRACTICE GUIDELINES

- Pal B et al: How is gout managed in primary care? A review of current practice and proposed guidelines. Clin Rheumatol 2000;19:21. [PMID: 10752494]

WEB SITE

- American College of Rheumatology
  - http://www.rheumatology.org

INFORMATION FOR PATIENTS

- National Institute of Arthritis and Musculoskeletal and Skin Disease
  - http://www.niams.nih.gov/hi/topics/gout/gout.htm

REFERENCES

- Bieber JD: Gout: On the brink of novel therapeutic options for an ancient disease. Arthritis Rheum 2004;50:2400. [PMID: 15334451]
- Choi HK et al: Alcohol intake and risk of incident gout in men: a prospective study. Lancet 2004;363:1277. [PMID: 15094272]

Author(s)

David B. Hellmann, MD, FACP

John H. Stone, MD, MPH

Granuloma Inguinale p. 1086

Guillain-Barré Syndrome

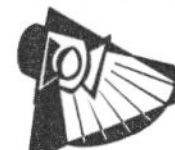

KEY FEATURES

ESSENTIALS OF DIAGNOSIS

- Acute or subacute progressive polyradiculoneuropathy
- Usually ascending, symmetric weakness
- Paresthesias are more variable

GENERAL CONSIDERATIONS

- A symmetric sensory, motor, or mixed deficit, often most marked distally
- Probably has an immunologic basis, but the mechanism is unclear

DEMOGRAPHICS

- Sometimes follows infective illness, innoculations, or surgical procedures
- There is an association with preceding *Campylobacter jejuni* enteritis

CLINICAL FINDINGS

SYMPTOMS AND SIGNS

Motor symptoms

- The main complaint is of weakness
  - Varies widely in severity in different patients
  - Often has a proximal emphasis and symmetric distribution
  - Usually begins in the legs, spreading to a variable extent but frequently involving the arms and often one or both sides of the face
  - The muscles of respiration or deglutition may also be affected

Sensory symptoms

- Sensory symptoms are usually less conspicuous than motor ones, but distal paresthesias and dysesthesias are common, and neuropathic or radicular pain is present in many patients

Autonomic symptoms

- Autonomic disturbances are common, may be severe, and are sometimes life-threatening; they include tachycardia, cardiac irregularities, hypotension or hypertension, facial flushing, abnormalities of sweating, pulmonary dysfunction, and impaired sphincter control

DIFFERENTIAL DIAGNOSIS

- Chronic inflammatory demyelinating polyneuropathy (CIDP)
- Porphyria
- Diphtheritic neuropathy
- Toxic neuropathy, eg, lead, mercury, organophosphates, hexacarbon solvents
- Poliomyelitis
- Botulism
- Tick paralysis
- Spinal cord lesion
- Transverse myelitis
- West Nile virus infection
- Periodic paralysis syndrome

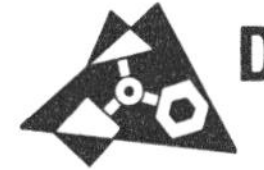

DIAGNOSIS

LABORATORY TESTS

- The cerebrospinal fluid characteristically contains a high protein concentration with a normal cell content, but these changes may take 2 or 3 weeks to develop

DIAGNOSTIC PROCEDURES

- Electrophysiologic (nerve conduction) studies may reveal marked abnormalities, which do not necessarily parallel the clinical disorder in their temporal course
- Pathologic examination has shown primary demyelination or, less commonly, axonal degeneration

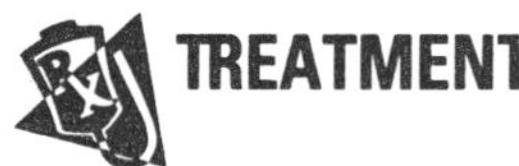

TREATMENT

MEDICATIONS

- Marked hypotension may respond to volume replacement or pressor agents
- IV immunoglobulin (400 mg/kg/day for 5 days) is helpful and imposes less stress on the cardiovascular system than plasmapheresis
- Low-dose heparin to prevent pulmonary embolism should be considered
- Prednisone is ineffective and may prolong recovery time

THERAPEUTIC PROCEDURES

- Respiratory toilet and chest physical therapy help prevent atelectasis
- Plasmapheresis is of value; it is best performed within the first few days of illness and is best reserved for clinically severe or rapidly progressive cases or those with ventilatory impairment

OUTCOME

FOLLOW-UP

- Monitor spirometry: patients should be admitted to intensive care units if their forced vital capacity is declining, and intubation is considered if the forced vital capacity reaches 15 mL/kg, dyspnea becomes evident, or the oxygen saturation declines

PROGNOSIS

- Most patients eventually make a good recovery, but this may take many months, and 10–20% of patients are left with persisting disability
- Approximately 3% of patients have one or more clinically similar relapses, sometimes several years after the initial illness

WHEN TO ADMIT

- All patients should be admitted to the hospital and may need intensive care unit admission if their forced vital capacity is declining

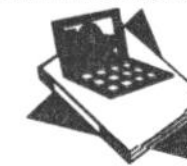

EVIDENCE

PRACTICE GUIDELINES

- National Guideline Clearinghouse
  - http://www.guideline.gov/summary/summary.aspx?doc_id=4110&nbr=3155&string=Guillain+AND+Barre

WEB SITE

- Neuromuscular Disease Center
  - http://www.neuro.wustl.edu/neuromuscular/antibody/gbs.htm#cgbs

INFORMATION FOR PATIENTS

- National Institute of Neurological Disorders and Stroke
  - http://www.ninds.nih.gov/disorders/gbs/gbs.htm
- The Mayo Clinic
  - http://www.mayoclinic.com/invoke.cfm?id=DS00413

REFERENCES

- Donofrio PD: Immunotherapy of idiopathic inflammatory neuropathies. Muscle Nerve 2003;28:273. [PMID: 12929187]
- Kieseier BC et al: Advances in understanding and treatment of immune-mediated disorders of the peripheral nervous system. Muscle Nerve 2004;30:131. [PMID: 15266629]
- Winer JB: Guillain-Barré syndrome. Mol Pathol 2001;54:381. [PMID: 11724912]

Author(s)

Michael J. Aminoff, MD, DSc, FRCP

Gynecomastia

KEY FEATURES

ESSENTIALS OF DIAGNOSIS

- Glandular enlargement of the male breast
- Often asymmetric or unilateral; may be tender
- Nipple discharge may be present
- Must be distinguished from tumors and fatty breast enlargement of obesity

GENERAL CONSIDERATIONS

Causes

- Endocrine: hyperprolactinemia of any cause, hyperthyroidism, Klinefelter's syndrome, hypogonadism
- Systemic disease: chronic liver or renal disease
- Neoplasms: testicular, adrenal, lung, liver
- Drugs (selected): alcohol, amiodarone, cimetidine, diazepam, digoxin, estrogens, finasteride, flutamide, isoniazid, ketoconazole, marijuana, omeprazole, opioids, progestins, protease inhibitors and antiretrovirals, spironolactone, testosterone, tricyclic antidepressants, eating necks of poultry that have been fed estrogen
- HIV infection treated with highly active antiretroviral therapy (HAART), especially efavirenz or didanosine; breast enlargement resolves spontaneously in 73% within 9 months

DEMOGRAPHICS

- Common in puberty, especially in boys taller and heavier than average
- Common among elderly men
- Common in obesity
- Develops in ~50% of athletes who abuse androgens and anabolic steroids
- Family history of malignancy

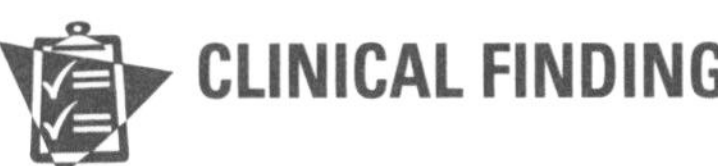

CLINICAL FINDINGS

SYMPTOMS AND SIGNS

- Breast enlargement, often asymmetric or unilateral, sometimes tender, with or without nipple discharge
- Pubertal gynecomastia: tender discoid enlargement of breast tissue beneath areola, 2–3 cm in diameter
- Testicular examination may reveal tumor

DIFFERENTIAL DIAGNOSIS

- Breast cancer
- Fatty breast enlargement of obesity
- Breast abscess (mastitis)
- Metastatic cancer, eg, prostate
- Treatment of prostate cancer with gonadotropin-releasing hormone agonists/antagonists or antiandrogens

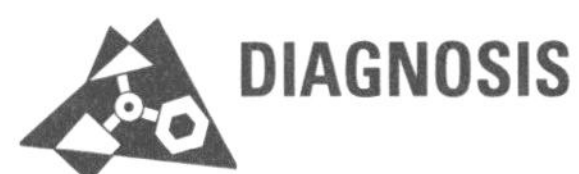

DIAGNOSIS

LABORATORY TESTS

- Serum prolactin elevated if gynecomastia caused by hyperprolactinemia
- Detectable serum β-human chorionic gonadotropin (hCG) implicates testicular tumor (germ cell or Sertoli cell) or other malignancy (usually lung or liver). However, low detectable levels (β-hCG < 5 mU/mL) may occur in primary hypogonadism if assay cross-reacts with luteinizing hormone (LH)
- Low serum testosterone, high serum LH in primary hypogonadism
- High testosterone, high LH in partial androgen resistance
- Serum estradiol usually normal but may be increased by testicular tumors, increased β-hCG, liver disease, obesity, adrenal tumors (rare)
- Serum thyroid-stimulating hormone low in hyperthyroidism
- Karyotype (for Klinefelter's syndrome) indicated in men with persistent gynecomastia without obvious cause

IMAGING STUDIES

- Chest x-ray or lung CT if lung cancer or metastases suspected
- Testicular ultrasound if detectable β-hCG or mass on examination
- CT or MRI of abdomen/pelvis if detectable β-hCG and no mass on testicular examination or ultrasound
- Mammography for large tumor to exclude breast cancer

DIAGNOSTIC PROCEDURES

- Fine needle aspiration of suspicious masses, especially when unilateral or asymmetric, to distinguish gynecomastia from cancer or mastitis

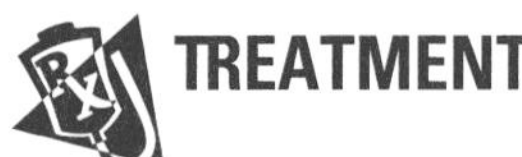

TREATMENT

MEDICATIONS

- Treatment of underlying condition
- Discontinue potentially offending medications if possible; discontinue spironolactone and substitute eplerenone
- Medications used to treat gynecomastia can produce adverse reactions; treat gynecomastia only if it is a troubling and persistent problem
- Raloxifene, 60 mg PO QD, may be the most effective drug
- Tamoxifen (an antiestrogen), 10 mg PO BID, may reduce pain and breast size in >50%; relapses occur in ~28% after tamoxifen is stopped
- Danazol, 400 mg PO QD, improves gynecomastia in 40%; relapses are uncommon after danazol is stopped. Liver enzymes must be monitored

SURGERY

- Surgery is reserved for persistent or severe gynecomastia, since results are often disappointing
- Endoscopically assisted transaxillary liposuction and subcutaneous mastectomy may produce acceptable results

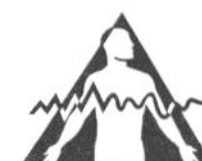

OUTCOME

PROGNOSIS

- Pubertal and idiopathic gynecomastia usually subside spontaneously within 1–2 years
- Drug-induced gynecomastia resolves after offending drug is discontinued

PREVENTION

- Avoidance of androgen and anabolic steroid abuse

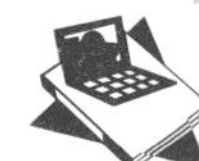

EVIDENCE

PRACTICE GUIDELINES

- Daniels IR et al: Gynaecomastia. Eur J Surg 2001;167:885. [PMID: 11841077]
- Dicker AP: The safety and tolerability of low-dose irradiation for the management of gynaecomastia caused by antiandrogen monotherapy. Lancet Oncol 2003;4:30. [PMID: 12517537]
- Fruhstorfer BH et al: A systematic approach to the surgical treatment of gynaecomastia. Br J Plast Surg 2003;56:237. [PMID: 12859919]

INFORMATION FOR PATIENTS

- American Academy of Family Physicians—Gynecomastia: when breasts form in males
  - http://familydoctor.org/handouts/080.html
- Mayo Clinic
  - http://www.mayoclinic.com/invoke.cfm?objectid=7BB5F30F-8628-4876-B280D38A83B9965B
- MEDLINEplus—Gynecomastia
  - http://www.nlm.nih.gov/medlineplus/ency/article/003165.htm
- University of Iowa Plastic Surgery
  - http://www.surgery.uiowa.edu/surgery/plastic/gyneco.html

REFERENCES

- Lawrence SE et al: Beneficial effects of tamoxifen and raloxifene in the treatment of pubertal gynecomastia. J Pediatr 2004;145:71. [PMID: 15238910]
- Mira JA et al: Gynaecomastia in HIV-infected men on highly active antiretroviral therapy: association with efavirenz and didanosine treatment. Antivir Ther 2004;9:511. [PMID: 15456082]

Author(s)

Paul A. Fitzgerald, MD

Haemophilus Infections p. 1086

Head & Neck Cancer

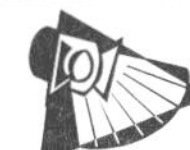

KEY FEATURES

ESSENTIALS OF DIAGNOSIS

- A firm, painless, and slowly enlarging mass is often neoplastic
- Persistent symptoms (more than 2 weeks duration) of one or more of the following:
  - Throat pain
  - Ear pain (referred otalgia, via branches of vagus nerve that innervate ear and pharynx)
  - Change in character of voice
  - Blood in the mouth or throat
  - Unexplained middle ear effusion, which may indicate nasopharyngeal mass
- Indirect or fiberoptic examination of the oropharynx by an experienced clinician as well as examination and palpation of the base of the tongue and tonsillar fossae and the neck
- Regional metastatic lymphadenopathy is common at presentation

GENERAL CONSIDERATIONS

- Head and neck examination in patients with concerning symptoms or signs or unexplained weight loss, especially in those over 45 who smoke tobacco or drink immoderately
- Examination components include the following:
  - A systematic intraoral, pharyngeal, and laryngeal examination (including the lateral tongue, floor of the mouth, gingiva, buccal area, palate, tonsillar fossae, and indirect or fiberoptic examination of the pharynx and larynx)
  - Palpation of the neck for enlarged lymph nodes

DEMOGRAPHICS

- Occurs predominantly in heavy smokers and/or those with significant alcohol use
- Most common between ages 50 and 70
- Incidence is 25/100,000
- Nasopharyngeal cancer most common in southern Chinese ancestry

CLINICAL FINDINGS

SYMPTOMS AND SIGNS

- Persistent (> 2 weeks) throat or ear pain (referred otalgia)
- Weight loss
- Blood in the throat or mouth
- Change in speech/voice quality (including hoarseness or dysarthria)
- Dysphagia
- Airway compromise
- Visible mass (as seen on oral examination or indirect or fiberoptic pharyngoscopy)
- Palpable mass in base of tongue or tonsil
- Neck adenopathy (usually hard)

DIFFERENTIAL DIAGNOSIS

Oropharynx mass

- Occasionally a tumor can be misdiagnosed as a peritonsillar abscess

Laryngeal mass

- Vocal cord nodules
- Papillomas or granulomas
- Leukoplakia, as in the oral cavity, requires clarification clinically or by biopsy as judged by an experienced clinician

Oral mass

- Aphthous ulcer (canker sore, ulcerative stomatitis)
- See Leukoplakia, erythroplakia, lichen planus, and oral cancer for additional differential diagnosis

Nasopharynx mass

- Occasional benign cysts can mimic a tumor

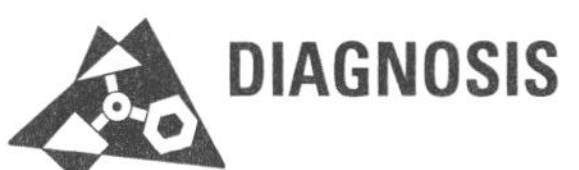

DIAGNOSIS

LABORATORY TESTS

- Complete blood cell count, liver function tests

IMAGING STUDIES

- MRI is preferred to CT for staging, except laryngeal lesions
- Chest x-ray
- Chest CT may be indicated if there is concern for a second primary mass in the lung or for lung metastases
- PET or PET-CT may be helpful

DIAGNOSTIC PROCEDURES

- Indirect or fiberoptic examination of the nasopharynx, oropharynx, hypopharynx, and larynx
- Fine-needle aspiration biopsy may confirm the presence of the carcinoma and the histological type, but caution and clinical judgment should be exercised in interpreting an apparently negative result

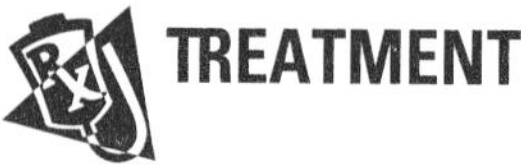

TREATMENT

MEDICATIONS

- Cisplatin as a radiosensitizer during radiation therapy
- Other chemotherapy agents, including 5-fluorouracil, taxanes, carboplatinol, as well as methotrexate
- Management of associated **pain** is critically important and often includes narcotics with short (3 h) and long (8–72 h) duration of effect, nonsteroidal anti-inflammatory agents, COX-II inhibitors, and gabapentin
- See Tables 153 and 154

SURGERY

- **Small tumors** are often best treated with a sole modality of either function-sparing surgery or radiation, depending on the site of the primary tumor
- **Large nonoropharyngeal tumors** often are best treated with surgery and postoperative irradiation

THERAPEUTIC PROCEDURES

- Treatment depends on tumor site, TNM stage, prior treatment, and patient comorbidities (such as cardiovascular and lung disease)
- There must be careful weighing of the side effects of treatment options
- **Oropharyngeal tumors** (eg, base of the tongue and tonsil fossa) are usually best treated with radiation and often concomitant chemotherapy regardless of extent of primary and nodal disease
- **T1–2 laryngeal tumors** are best treated with radiation, endoscopic resection, or open partial resection
- **More advanced laryngeal tumors** are treated with chemoradiation or extended partial laryngeal surgery, both intended to avoid a permanent laryngeal stoma
- For **unresectable recurrent disease** and distant metastases, weigh the benefits of chemotherapy and possibly palliative radiation therapy

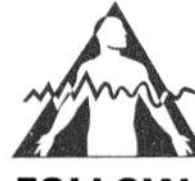

OUTCOME

FOLLOW-UP

- Early diagnosis of recurrent squamous cell carcinoma or new primary tumor is key; incidence of second tumors: ~3–4%/year
- Patient with prior cavity head and neck cancer is examined clinically q4–6 weeks in year 1, q8–10 weeks in year 2, q3–4 months thereafter for several years
- Periodic PET scans at 3 months postradiation therapy and baseline posttreatment MRIs for subsequent surveillance
- Strategies for DNA or protein molecular markers under investigation

COMPLICATIONS

- Airway compromise, requiring tracheotomy
- Bleeding associated with surface ulceration
- Erosion into major artery can lead to life-threatening oral or neck hemorrhage
- Dysphagia and odynophagia may lead to weight loss, requiring gastrostomy tube
- Failure to recognize early tumors results in more extensive intervention, with greater operative risks

PROGNOSIS

- Correlated with TNM staging, including specific site of disease, extent of primary tumor, nodal stage, presence of distant metastases
- Overall, 65% of head and neck cancers are cured; prognosis ranges from > 90% for early tongue and early larynx lesions to very poor for unresectable neck disease or distant metastases

WHEN TO REFER

- Specialty referral should be sought early for diagnosis and treatment
- Indirect or fiberoptic examination of the nasopharynx, oropharynx, hypopharynx, and larynx by otolaryngologist–head and neck surgeon should be considered with oral erythroplakia, unexplained throat or ear pain, unexplained oral or nasal bleeding, firm neck mass, or visible oral cavity or oropharyngeal mass

WHEN TO ADMIT

- Airway compromise, hemorrhage, dehydration
- Institute effective pain management regimen for severe pain

PREVENTION

- Smoking cessation and alcohol abatement programs helpful

EVIDENCE

PRACTICE GUIDELINES

- Forastiere AA et al; NCCN Head and Neck Cancers Practice Guidelines Panel. National Comprehensive Cancer Network: Head and Neck Cancers v.1.2004.
  - http://www.nccn.org/professionals/physician_gls/PDF/head-and-neck.pdf

WEB SITES

- Baylor College of Medicine Otolaryngology Resources: Head and Neck Oncology
  - http://www.bcm.edu/oto/othersa7.html
- National Cancer Institute: Head and Neck Cancers
  - http://www.cancer.gov/cancertopics/cancersbodylocation/page11

INFORMATION FOR PATIENTS

- American Cancer Society
  - www.cancer.org
- American Academy of Otolaryngology: Head and Neck Surgery: Head and Neck Cancer
  - http://www.entnet.org/healthinfo/tobacco/cancer.cfm
- National Cancer Institute: Head and Neck Cancer: Q & A
  - http://cis.nci.nih.gov/fact/6_37.htm

REFERENCES

- Brockstein B et al: Patterns of failure, prognostic factors and survival in locoregionally advanced head and neck cancer treated with concomitant chemoradiotherapy: a 9-year, 337-patient, multi-institutional experience. Ann Oncol 2004;15:1179. [PMID: 15277256]
- Cooper JS et al: Postoperative concurrent radiotherapy and chemotherapy for high-risk squamous-cell carcinoma of the head and neck. N Engl J Med 2004;305:1937. [PMID: 15128893]
- Ohizumi Y et al: Prognostic factors of reirradiation for recurrent head and neck cancer. Am J Clin Oncol 2002;25:408. [PMID: 12151975]
- Piccirillo JF et al: Development of a new head and neck cancer-specific comorbidity index. Arch Otolaryngol Head Neck Surg 2002;128:1172. [PMID: 12365889]
- Scarbrough TJ et al: Referred otalgia in head and neck cancer: a unifying schema. Am J Clin Oncol 2003;26:e157. [PMID: 14528091]

Author(s)

Robert K. Jackler, MD

Michael J. Kaplan, MD

Headache

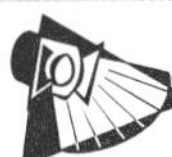

KEY FEATURES

ESSENTIALS OF DIAGNOSIS

- Severe headache in a previously well patient is more likely than chronic headache to relate to an intracranial disorder such as hemorrhage, meningitis, or mass lesion
- Headaches worse on awakening may indicate sinusitis or intracranial mass

GENERAL CONSIDERATIONS

- Chronic headaches are commonly due to migraine, tension, or depression, but may be related to intracranial pathology
- Possibility of underlying structural lesions is important because about one-third of patients with brain tumors have a primary complaint of headache

CLINICAL FINDINGS

SYMPTOMS AND SIGNS

Tension headache

- Often pulsating or throbbing
- Bandlike pain is common
- Sense of tightness or pressure is common
- Worsens with stress and at end of day

Migraine

- Often pulsating or throbbing
- May be ocular or periorbital ice pick–like pain
- Lateralized pain is common

Cluster headache

- Ocular or ice pick–like pain
- Lateralized pain is common
- Tends to occur at the same time each day or night

Neuritic causes

- Sharp lancinating pain may be suggestive
- Pain localized to one of the divisions of the trigeminal nerve or to the pharynx and external auditory meatus, respectively, in trigeminal or glossopharyngeal neuralgia

Sinusitis-related headache

- May cause tenderness of overlying skin and bone

Ophthalmic-related headache

- Ocular or periocular pain

Intracranial mass lesion-related headache

- Typically dull or steady pain
- Pain may be worse in the morning
- Pain may be localized or general

DIFFERENTIAL DIAGNOSIS

Intracranial

- Migraine
- Cluster headache
- Brain tumor
- Subarachnoid hemorrhage
- Meningitis
- Brain abscess
- Temporal (giant cell) arteritis
- Hypertension
- Caffeine, alcohol, or drug withdrawal
- Pseudotumor cerebri
- Subdural hemorrhage
- Cerebral ischemia
- Arterial dissection (carotid or vertebral)
- Arteriovenous malformation
- Head injury
- Lumbar puncture
- Venous sinus thrombosis (intracranial venous thrombosis)
- Postlumbar puncture
- Carbon monoxide poisoning

Extracranial

- Systemic infections
- Tension headache
- Cervical arthritis
- Glaucoma
- Dental abscess
- Sinusitis
- Otitis media
- Temporomandibular joint (TMJ) syndrome
- Depression
- Somatoform disorder (somatization)
- Trigeminal neuralgia
- Glossopharyngeal neuralgia

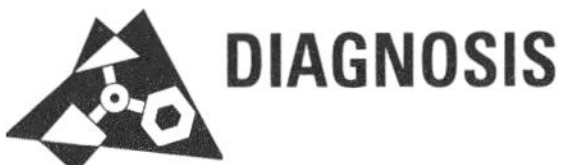

DIAGNOSIS

LABORATORY TESTS

- Cerebrospinal fluid examination if a meningeal infection or subarachnoid hemorrhage is considered

IMAGING STUDIES

- Cranial MRI or CT scan to exclude an intracranial mass lesion in patients with
  - A progressive headache disorder
  - New onset of headache in middle or later life
  - Headaches that disturb sleep or are related to exertion
  - Headaches that are associated with neurologic symptoms or a focal neurologic deficit

DIAGNOSTIC PROCEDURES

- Inquire about precipitating and exacerbating factors
- Precipitating factors include recent sinusitis or hay fever, dental surgery, head injury, and symptoms suggestive of a systemic viral infection
- Alcohol is a precipitating factor for cluster headache
- Chewing as a precipitating factor is associated with TMJ dysfunction, trigeminal or glossopharyngeal neuralgia, and giant cell arteritis
- Cough-induced headache occurs with structural lesions of the posterior fossa, but a specific cause is frequently unidentifiable
- Exacerbating factors for migraine include emotional stress, fatigue, foods containing nitrite or tyramine, and menses

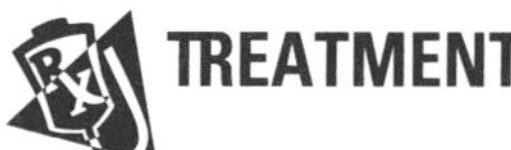

TREATMENT

- See specific headache disorder: Headache, Tension; Headache, Migraine; Polymyalgia Rheumatica and Giant Cell Arteritis; Posttraumatic; Cough

OUTCOME

WHEN TO REFER

- If expertise in evaluation or treatment is needed

WHEN TO ADMIT

- Depends on the underlying cause (eg, mass lesion, intracerebral bleed)

EVIDENCE

PRACTICE GUIDELINES

- American Academy of Neurology
  - http://www.aan.com/professionals/practice/pdfs/gl0085.pdf
- Lewis DW et al: Practice parameter: evaluation of children and adolescents with recurrent headaches: report of the Quality Standards Subcommittee of the American Academy of Neurology and the Practice Committee of the Child Neurology Society. Neurology 2002;59:490. [PMID: 12196640]
- National Guideline Clearinghouse
  - http://www.guideline.gov/summary/summary.aspx?doc_id=3298&nbr=2524&string=headache

INFORMATION FOR PATIENTS

- JAMA patient page: Headaches. JAMA 2003;289:1462. [PMID: 12636471]
- JAMA patient page: Tension headache. JAMA 2001;285:2282. [PMID: 11368044]
- National Institute of Neurological Disorders and Stroke
  - http://www.ninds.nih.gov/disorders/headache/headache.htm

REFERENCES

- Goadsby PJ: Mechanisms and management of headache. J R Coll Physicians Lond 1999;33:228. [PMID: 10402569]
- Kaniecki R: Headache assessment and management. JAMA 2003;289;1430. [PMID: 12636467]
- Schoenen J et al: Headache with focal neurological signs or symptoms: a complicated differential diagnosis. Lancet Neurol 2004;3:237. [PMID: 15039036]

Author(s)

Michael J. Aminoff, MD, DSc, FRCP

Headache, Acute

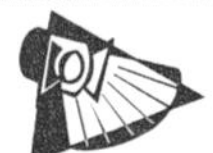

KEY FEATURES

ESSENTIALS OF DIAGNOSIS

- Age > 50 years
- Rapid onset with severe intensity
- History of hypertension or HIV
- Fever, hypertension
- Trauma
- Vision changes
- Neurological findings (mental status changes, motor or sensory deficits)

GENERAL CONSIDERATIONS

- In the emergency department, 1% of patients with acute headache have a life-threatening condition
- In the physician's office, the prevalence of life-threatening conditions is much lower

CLINICAL FINDINGS

SYMPTOMS AND SIGNS

- Sudden-onset headache that reaches maximal and severe intensity within seconds or a few minutes ("thunderclap headache") suggests subarachnoid hemorrhage
- Headache with uncontrolled hypertension should prompt search for other manifestations of "hypertensive urgency or emergency" (See Hypertensive Urgencies & Emergencies)
- Headache and hypertension in pregnancy may be due to preeclampsia
- Episodic headache with hypertension, palpitations, and sweats may be due to pheochromocytoma
- Physical examination should include vital signs, neurologic examination, vision/fundoscopic examination, and Kernig and Brudzinski signs
- Patients ≥ 60 years old should be examined for scalp or temporal artery tenderness
- Diminished visual acuity suggests glaucoma, temporal arteritis, or optic neuritis
- Ophthalmoplegia or visual field defects suggest venous sinus thrombosis, tumor, or aneurysm
- Afferent pupillary defects occur with intracranial masses or optic neuritis
- Ipsilateral ptosis and miosis (Horner's syndrome) occur with carotid artery dissection
- Papilledema and/or absent retinal venous pulsation occur with elevated intracranial pressure

DIFFERENTIAL DIAGNOSIS

- Causes of headache that require immediate treatment
  - Imminent or completed vascular events (intracranial hemorrhage, thrombosis, vasculitis, malignant hypertension, arterial dissection, or aneurysm)
  - Infections (abscess; encephalitis; meningitis)
  - Intracranial masses causing intracranial hypertension
  - Preeclampsia
  - Carbon monoxide poisoning

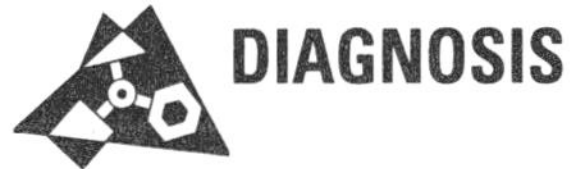

DIAGNOSIS

LABORATORY TESTS

- Cerebrospinal fluid (CSF) Gram stain, white blood cell count with differential, red blood cell count, glucose, total protein, bacterial culture, VDRL
- In suspected cases, obtain CSF polymerase chain reaction test for herpes simplex 2
- In HIV-infected patients, obtain CSF cryptococcal antigen, acid-fast bacillus stain and culture, and complement fixation and culture for coccidioidomycosis
- Erythrocyte sedimentation rate
- Urinalysis

IMAGING STUDIES

- Sinus CT scan or x-ray
- Noncontrast head CT immediately, followed by contrast head CT later
- In HIV-infected patients, new-onset headache warrants CT with and without contrast or MRI
- For clinical features associated with acute headache that warrant urgent or emergent neuroimaging (Table 94)
- Perform neuroimaging prior to lumbar puncture in acute headache with abnormal neurologic examination, abnormal mental status, abnormal fundoscopic examination (papilledema; loss of venous pulsations)
- Perform neuroimaging emergently in acute headache with abnormal neurologic examination, abnormal mental status, "thunderclap headache"
- Perform neuroimaging urgently in acute headache with HIV infection, age > 50 years (despite normal neurological examination)

DIAGNOSTIC PROCEDURES

- Lumbar puncture
- If high suspicion for subarachnoid hemorrhage or aneurysm, lumbar puncture followed by cerebral angiography

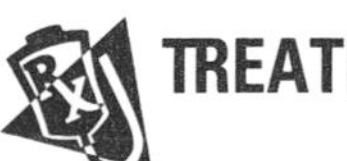

TREATMENT

- Treatment should be guided by the underlying etiology

MEDICATIONS

- Nonsteroidal anti-inflammatory drugs (Table 1)
- Opioid agonist analgesics (Table 2)
- Clinical response to analgesics does not exclude life-threatening causes of acute headache

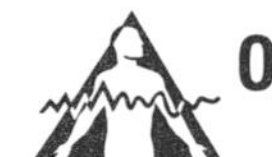

OUTCOME

WHEN TO REFER

- Refer to the emergency department patients with acute headache who have
  - Age > 50 years
  - Rapid onset with severe intensity
  - History of hypertension or HIV
  - Fever, hypertension
  - Trauma
  - Vision changes
  - Neurologic findings (mental status changes, motor or sensory deficits)

PREVENTION

- Prophylactic treatment of migraine (Table 95)

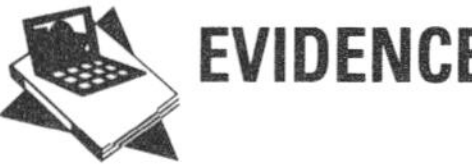

EVIDENCE

PRACTICE GUIDELINES

- American College of Emergency Physicians (ACEP). Clinical policy: critical issues in the evaluation and management of patients presenting to the emergency department with acute headache, 2002
  - http://www.acep.org/download.cfm?resource=673
- National Guideline Clearinghouse
  - http://www.guideline.gov/summary/summary.aspx?doc_id=3298&nbr=2524&string=acute+AND+headache

WEB SITES

- American Academy of Neurology
  - http://www.aan.com/professionals/
- Cleveland Clinic
  - http://www.clevelandclinicmeded.com/diseasemanagement/neurology/headache/headache.htm

INFORMATION FOR PATIENTS

- JAMA patient page: Headaches. JAMA 2003;289:1462. [PMID: 12636471]

REFERENCES

- Evans RW: New daily persistent headache. Curr Pain Headache Rep 2003;7:303. [PMID: 12828880]
- Ryan RE: Common headache misdiagnoses. Prim Care 2004;31:395. [PMID: 15172514]
- Silberstein SD: Migraine. Lancet 2004;363:381. [PMID: 15070571]

Author(s)

Ralph Gonzales, MD

Headache, Migraine

KEY FEATURES

ESSENTIALS OF DIAGNOSIS

- Headache, usually pulsatile
- May be accompanied by nausea, vomiting, photophobia, phonophobia
- Transient neurologic symptoms (typically visual) may precede the headache of classic migraine
- No preceding aura is common in migraines

GENERAL CONSIDERATIONS

- The pathophysiology probably relates to serotonin and to dilation and excessive pulsation of the branches of the external carotid artery
- Focal disturbances of neurologic function may precede or accompany the headaches (classic migraines) and have been attributed to constriction of branches of the internal carotid artery
- Attacks may be triggered by emotional or physical stress, lack or excess of sleep, missed meals, specific foods (eg, chocolate), alcoholic beverages, menstruation, or use of oral contraceptives

DEMOGRAPHICS

- Patients often give a family history of migraine

CLINICAL FINDINGS

SYMPTOMS AND SIGNS

Classic migraine

- Lateralized throbbing headache that occurs episodically following its onset in adolescence or early adult life
- Visual disturbances occur quite commonly and may consist of field defects; of luminous visual hallucinations such as stars, sparks, unformed light flashes (photopsia), geometric patterns, or zigzags of light; or of some combination of field defects and luminous hallucinations (scintillating scotomas)
- Other focal disturbances such as aphasia or numbness, tingling, clumsiness, or weakness in a circumscribed distribution may also occur

Common migraine

- Headaches commonly bilateral and periorbital
- Visual disturbances and other focal neurologic deficits do not occur

Basilar artery migraine

- Blindness or disturbances throughout both visual fields are accompanied or followed by dysarthria, dysequilibrium, tinnitus, and perioral and distal paresthesias
- Sometimes followed by transient loss or impairment of consciousness or by a confusional state. This, in turn, is followed by a throbbing (usually occipital) headache, often with nausea and vomiting

Ophthalmoplegic migraine

- Lateralized pain, often about the eye, is accompanied by nausea, vomiting, and diplopia due to transient external ophthalmoplegia
- Ophthalmic division of the fifth nerve has also been affected in some patients

Migraine equivalent

- In rare instances, the neurologic or somatic disturbance accompanying typical migrainous headaches becomes the sole manifestation of an attack ("migraine equivalent")

DIFFERENTIAL DIAGNOSIS

- Other causes of headache
- Cluster headache
- Brain tumor
- Temporal (giant cell) arteritis
- Sinusitis
- Subarachnoid hemorrhage
- Pseudotumor cerebri
- Transient ischemic attack

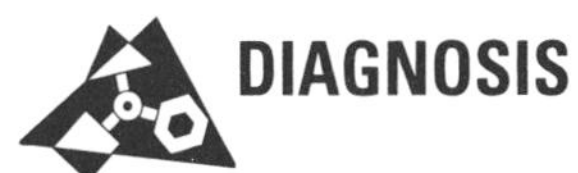

DIAGNOSIS

DIAGNOSTIC PROCEDURES

- Inquire about precipitating and exacerbating factors
- Inquire about family history

Headache, Cluster p. 1087

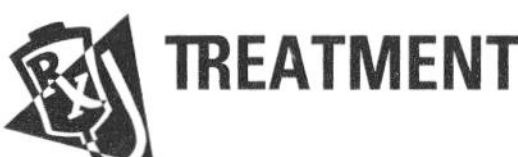

TREATMENT

MEDICATIONS

- A simple analgesic (eg, aspirin) taken right away often provides relief, but treatment with extracranial vasoconstrictors or other drugs is sometimes necessary
  - Cafergot, a combination of ergotamine tartrate (1 mg) and caffeine (100 mg), is often particularly helpful; one or two tablets are taken at the onset of headache or warning symptoms, followed by one tablet every 30 min, if necessary, up to six tablets per attack and ten tablets per week
  - Cafergot can be given rectally as suppositories (one-half to one suppository containing 2 mg of ergotamine)
  - Dihydroergotamine mesylate (0.5–1 mg IV or 1–2 mg SC or IM) may be useful in patients with nausea. Ergotamines should be avoided during pregnancy and in those with coronary artery disease
  - Sumatriptan is a rapidly effective agent for aborting attacks when given subcutaneously by an autoinjection device (6 mg)
  - Zolmitriptan is effective for acute treatment. The optimal initial oral dose is 5 mg, and relief usually occurs within 1 h. It can also be taken by nasal spray
  - Other triptans are available including rizatriptan, naratriptan, almotriptan, frovatriptan and eletriptan. Eletriptan (up to 80 mg over 24 h) is useful for acute therapy and frovatriptan, which has a longer half-life, helps patients with prolonged attacks (up to 7.5 mg over 24 h). Triptans should be avoided in pregnancy, are contraindicated by coronary or peripheral vascular disease, and may cause nausea or vomiting
  - Narcotic analgesics are needed in rare instances, such as meperidine 100 mg intramuscularly or butorphanol tartrate by nasal spray (1 mg/spray in one nostril, repeated after 3 or 4 h if necessary)

THERAPEUTIC PROCEDURES

- Management of migraine consists of avoidance of any precipitating factors, together with prophylactic or symptomatic pharmacologic treatment if necessary
- During acute attacks, many patients find it helpful to rest in a quiet, darkened room until symptoms subside

OUTCOME

COMPLICATIONS

- Very rarely, the patient may be left with a permanent neurologic deficit following a migrainous attack

PREVENTION

- Prophylactic treatment may be necessary if migrainous headaches occur more frequently than two or three times a month (see Table 95)
- Several drugs may have to be tried in turn before the headaches are brought under control. Once a drug has been found to help, it should be continued for several months
- If the patient remains headache free, the dose can then be tapered and the drug eventually withdrawn

EVIDENCE

PRACTICE GUIDELINES

- American Academy of Neurology
  - http://www.neurology.org/cgi/reprint/59/4/490.pdf
  - http://www.aan.com/professionals/practice/pdfs/gl0087.pdf
- National Guideline Clearinghouse
  - http://www.guideline.gov/summary/summary.aspx?doc_id=3592&nbr=2818&string=Migraine

INFORMATION FOR PATIENTS

- Parmet S et al: JAMA patient page: Headaches. JAMA 2003;289:1462. [PMID: 12636471]
- The Mayo Clinic
  - http://www.mayoclinic.com/invoke.cfm?id=DS00120
  - http://www.mayoclinic.com/invoke.cfm?id=AN00392

REFERENCES

- Ashkenazi A et al: The evolving management of migraine. Curr Opin Neurol 2003;16:341. [PMID: 12858071]
- Goadsby PJ et al: Drug therapy: migraine—current understanding and treatment. N Engl J Med 2002;346:257. [PMID: 11807151]
- Kaniecki R: Headache assessment and management. JAMA 2003;289:1430. [PMID: 12636467]
- Snow V et al: Pharmacologic management of acute attacks of migraine and prevention of migraine headache. Ann Intern Med 2002;137:840. [PMID: 12435222]

Author(s)

Michael J. Aminoff, DSc, MD, FRCP

Head Injury

Headache, Tension p. 1087

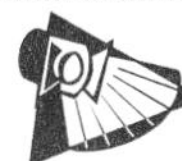

KEY FEATURES

ESSENTIALS OF DIAGNOSIS

- Absence of skull fracture does not exclude the possibility of severe head injury
- In many elderly patients, there may not be a known history of head trauma
- Occasionally, head injury, often trivial, precedes symptoms by several weeks

GENERAL CONSIDERATIONS

- Some guide to prognosis is provided by the mental status
  - Loss of consciousness for more than 1 or 2 min implies a worse prognosis than otherwise
- The degree of retrograde and posttraumatic amnesia provides an indication of the severity of injury and thus of the prognosis

DEMOGRAPHICS

- Trauma is the most common cause of death in young people, and head injury accounts for almost half of these trauma-related deaths

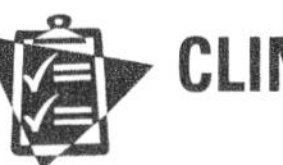

CLINICAL FINDINGS

SYMPTOMS AND SIGNS

- See Table 101
- Special attention should be given to the level of consciousness and extent of any brainstem dysfunction
- Clinical signs of basilar skull fracture
  - Bruising about the orbit (raccoon sign)
  - Blood in the external auditory meatus (Battle's sign)
  - Leakage of cerebrospinal fluid (which can be identified by its glucose content) from the ear or nose
- **Chronic subdural hemorrhage**
  - Head injury, often subtle, may precede the onset of symptoms by several weeks
  - Mental changes such as slowness, drowsiness, headache, confusion, memory disturbances, personality change, or even dementia may occur
  - Focal neurologic deficits such as hemiparesis or hemisensory disturbance are less common

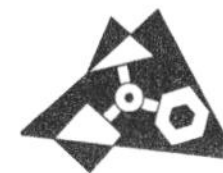

DIAGNOSIS

IMAGING STUDIES

- See Table 101
- Because injury to the spine may have accompanied head trauma, cervical spine radiographs (especially in the lateral projection) should always be obtained in comatose patients and in patients with severe neck pain or a deficit possibly related to cord compression
- CT scanning can demonstrate intracranial hemorrhage and may also provide evidence of cerebral edema and displacement of midline structures
- Skull radiographs or CT scans may provide evidence of fractures

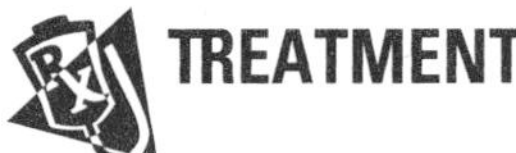

TREATMENT

MEDICATIONS

- Measures to reduce intracranial pressure include
  - Induced hyperventilation
  - Intravenous mannitol infusion
  - Intravenous furosemide
  - Corticosteroids provide no benefit in this context
- If there is any leakage of cerebrospinal fluid, conservative treatment, with elevation of the head, restriction of fluids, and administration of acetazolamide (250 mg four times daily), is often helpful
- Antibiotics if infection occurs
- No clear evidence that prophylactic anticonvulsant therapy reduces the incidence of posttraumatic seizures

SURGERY

- Scalp lacerations and depressed or compound depressed skull fractures should be treated surgically as appropriate
- Surgical evacuation of intracranial hematomas may be needed to prevent cerebral compression and herniation
- If leakage of cerebrospinal fluid continues for more than a few days, lumbar subarachnoid drainage may be necessary

THERAPEUTIC PROCEDURES

- Simple skull fractures require no specific treatment

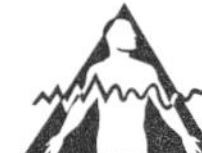

OUTCOME

FOLLOW-UP

- If admission to the hospital is declined, family members should be given clear instructions about the need for, and manner of, checking on them at regular (hourly) intervals and for obtaining additional medical help if necessary

COMPLICATIONS

- Increased intracranial pressure from
  - Seizures
  - Dilutional hyponatremia
  - Cerebral edema
  - Intracranial hematoma requiring surgical evacuation
- Chronic subdural hemorrhage
- Normal-pressure hydrocephalus
- Posttraumatic seizure disorder
- Posttraumatic headache

PROGNOSIS

- The prognosis depends on the site and severity of brain damage

WHEN TO ADMIT

- Patients who have lost consciousness for 2 min or more following head injury should be admitted to the hospital for observation
- Patients with focal neurologic deficits, lethargy, or skull fractures

EVIDENCE

PRACTICE GUIDELINES

- Kamerling SN et al: Mild traumatic brain injury in children: practice guidelines for emergency department and hospitalized patients. The Trauma Program, The Children's Hospital of Philadelphia, University of Pennsylvania School of Medicine. Pediatr Emerg Care 2003;19:431. [PMID: 14676497]
- National Guideline Clearinghouse
  - http://www.guideline.gov/summary/summary.aspx?doc_id=3794&nbr=3020&string=brain+AND+injury
  - http://www.guideline.gov/summary/summary.aspx?doc_id=3122&nbr=2348&string=brain+AND+injury
  - http://www.guideline.gov/summary/summary.aspx?doc_id=2272&nbr=1498&string=brain+AND+injury

INFORMATION FOR PATIENTS

- National Institute of Neurological Disorders and Stroke
  - http://www.ninds.nih.gov/disorders/tbi/tbi.htm
- Parmet S et al: JAMA patient page. Concussion in sports. JAMA 2003;290:2628. [PMID: 14625340]
- Torpy JM et al: Traumatic brain injury. JAMA 2003;289:3038. [PMID: 12799412]

REFERENCES

- Bavetta S et al: Assessment and management of the head-injured patient. Hosp Med 2002;63:289. [PMID: 12066348]
- Dutton RP et al: Traumatic brain injury. Curr Opin Crit Care 2003;9:503. [PMID: 14639070]
- Schierhout G et al: Prophylactic antiepileptic agents after head injury: a systematic review. J Neurol Neurosurg Psychiatry 1998;64:108. [PMID: 9436738]

Author(s)

Michael J. Aminoff, MD, DSc, FRCP

Hearing Loss

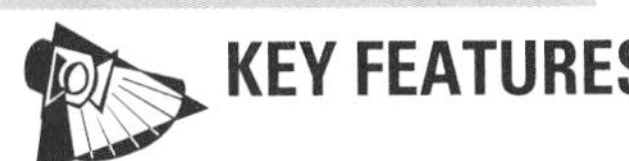

KEY FEATURES

ESSENTIALS OF DIAGNOSIS

- Three main types of hearing loss: conductive, sensory, and neural
- Most commonly caused by cerumen impaction or transient auditory tube dysfunction associated with upper respiratory tract infection

GENERAL CONSIDERATIONS

Conductive loss

- Four mechanisms, each resulting in impairment of the passage of sound vibrations to the inner ear: obstruction (eg, cerumen impaction), mass loading (eg, middle ear effusion), stiffness effect (eg, otosclerosis), and discontinuity (eg, ossicular disruption)
- Generally more correctable than sensory and neural losses

Sensory loss

- Common causes include excessive noise exposure, head trauma, and systemic diseases such as diabetes mellitus

Neural hearing loss

- Occurs with lesions involving the eighth nerve, auditory nuclei, ascending tracts, or auditory cortex
- It is the least common clinically recognized cause of hearing loss
- Causes include acoustic neuroma, multiple sclerosis, and cerebrovascular disease

DEMOGRAPHICS

- Nearly 30 million Americans have impaired hearing
- For the elderly—the largest group affected—excessive noise, drugs, toxins, and heredity are the most frequent contributing factors

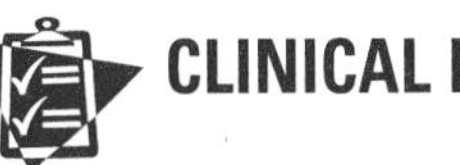

CLINICAL FINDINGS

SYMPTOMS AND SIGNS

- Reduction in hearing level
- **Weber test:** A 512-Hz tuning fork is placed on the forehead or front teeth; in conductive losses the sound appears louder in the poorer hearing ear, whereas in sensorineural losses it radiates to the better side
- **Rinne test:** A 512-Hz tuning fork is placed alternately on the mastoid bone and in front of the ear canal; in conductive losses bone conduction exceeds air conduction, whereas in sensorineural losses the opposite is true

DIFFERENTIAL DIAGNOSIS

Conductive (external or middle ear)

- Cerumen impaction (ear wax)
- Transient auditory tube dysfunction
- Acute or chronic otitis media
- Mastoiditis
- Otosclerosis
- Disruption of ossicles
- Trauma or barotrauma
- Glomus tympanicum (middle ear tumor)
- Paget's disease

Sensory

- Presbycusis (age related)
- Excessive noise exposure
- Ménière's disease (endolymphatic hydrops)
- Labyrinthitis
- Head trauma
- Ototoxicity
- Occlusion of ipsilateral auditory artery
- Hereditary hearing loss
- Autoimmune: systemic lupus erythematosus, Wegener's granulomatosis, Cogan's syndrome
- Other systemic causes: diabetes, hypothyroidism, hyperlipidemia, renal failure, infections

Neural

- Acoustic neuroma
- Multiple sclerosis
- Cerebrovascular disease

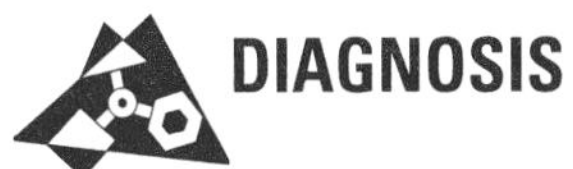

DIAGNOSIS

DIAGNOSTIC PROCEDURES

- Formal audiometric studies are performed in a soundproofed room
- Pure-tone thresholds in decibels (dB) are obtained over the range of 250–8000 Hz (the main speech frequencies are between 500 and 3000 Hz) for both air and bone conduction
- Conductive losses create a gap between the air and bone thresholds; in sensorineural losses both air and bone thresholds are equally diminished
- The threshold of normal hearing is from 0 to 20 dB, which corresponds to the loudness of a soft whisper
- Mild hearing loss is indicated by a threshold of 20–40 dB (soft spoken voice), moderate loss by a threshold of 40–60 dB (normal spoken voice), severe loss by a threshold of 60–80 dB (loud spoken voice), and profound loss by a threshold of 80 dB (shout)
- The clarity of hearing is often impaired in sensorineural hearing loss; this is evaluated by speech discrimination testing, which is reported as percentage correct (90–100% is normal)
- The site of the lesion responsible for sensorineural loss—whether it lies in the cochlea or in the central auditory system—may be determined with auditory brainstem-evoked responses

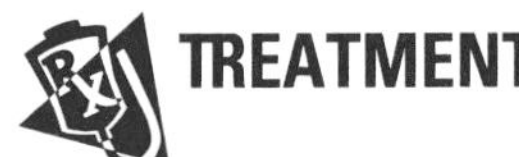

TREATMENT

SURGERY

- The cochlear implant—an electronic device that is surgically implanted to stimulate the auditory nerve—offers socially beneficial auditory rehabilitation to most adults with acquired deafness
- Many types of conductive hearing loss (eg, otosclerosis, tympanic membrane perforation, ossicular discontinuity) are surgically remediable

THERAPEUTIC PROCEDURES

- Hearing aids
- Assistive devices such as telephone amplifiers and infrared devices for use with TV, theaters, and auditoriums (eg, Senheiser)

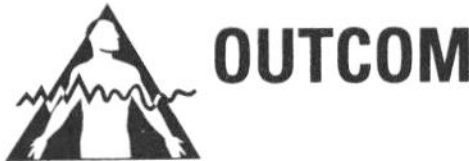

OUTCOME

WHEN TO REFER

- Every patient who complains of a hearing loss should be referred for audiological evaluation unless the cause is easily remediable (eg, cerumen impaction, otitis media)

EVIDENCE

PRACTICE GUIDELINES

- ACOEM Noise and Hearing Conservation Committee: ACOEM evidence-based statement: noise-induced hearing loss. J Occup Environ Med 2003;45:579. [PMID: 12802210]

WEB SITES

- American Academy of Otolaryngology—Head and Neck Surgery: Sensorineural Hearing Loss Interactive Module
  - http://www.entnet.org/education/COOL/snhl_intro.cfm
- Baylor College of Medicine Otolaryngology Resources
  - http://www.bcm.edu/oto/othersa3.html

INFORMATION FOR PATIENTS

- American Speech-Lauguage-Hearing Association: Types of Hearing Loss
  - http://www.asha.org/public/hearing/disorders/types.htm
- MedlinePlus: Hearing Loss Interactive Tutorial
  - http://www.nlm.nih.gov/medlineplus/tutorials/hearingloss/htm/index.htm
- NIH Senior Health: Hearing Loss
  - http://nihseniorhealth.gov/hearingloss/toc.html
- Occupation Safety & Health Administration: Noise and Hearing Conservation
  - http://www.osha-slc.gov/SLTC/noisehearingconservation/

REFERENCES

- Isaacson JE et al: Differential diagnosis and treatment of hearing loss. Am Fam Physician 2003;68:1125. [PMID: 14524400]
- Jackler RK: A 73-year-old man with hearing loss. JAMA 2003;289:1557. [PMID: 12672773]
- Parmet S et al: JAMA patient page. Adult hearing loss. JAMA 2003;289:2020. [PMID: 12697805]

Author(s)

Robert K. Jackler, MD
Michael J. Kaplan, MD

Heat Exposure Syndromes

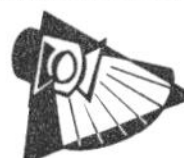

KEY FEATURES

ESSENTIALS OF DIAGNOSIS

- Four medical disorders can result: heat syncope, heat cramps, heat exhaustion, and heat stroke

GENERAL CONSIDERATIONS

Heat syncope

- Sudden unconsciousness from cutaneous vasodilation and volume depletion
- Typically occurs immediately following vigorous physical activity

Heat cramps

- Slow, painful muscle contractions of the skeletal muscles most heavily used
- Typically occurs immediately following vigorous physical activity
- Fluid and electrolyte depletion is cause

Heat exhaustion

- Results from prolonged strenuous activity with inadequate salt intake in a hot environment
- Characterized by dehydration, sodium depletion, or isotonic fluid loss with accompanying cardiovascular changes
- May progress to heat stroke if sweating ceases

Heat stroke

- A life-threatening medical emergency resulting from failure of the thermoregulatory mechanism
- Classic heat stroke occurs in patients with compromised homeostatic mechanisms
- Exertional heat stroke occurs in healthy persons undergoing strenuous exertion in a thermally stressful environment

DEMOGRAPHICS

- Persons at greatest risk for heat stroke are the very young, the elderly (age > 65), chronically infirm, and patients receiving medications (eg, anticholinergics, antihistamines, phenothiazines) that interfere with heat-dissipating mechanisms
- Heat stroke occurs in unconditioned amateurs participating in strenuous athletic activities

CLINICAL FINDINGS

SYMPTOMS AND SIGNS

Heat syncope

- Systolic blood pressure usually < 100 mm Hg; weak pulse
- Skin typically cool, moist

Heat cramps

- Muscle spasms last 1–3 min
- Muscles tender; may be twitching
- Skin moist, cool
- Victim alert, with stable vital signs, but may be agitated and complain of pain
- Body temperature may be normal or slightly increased

Heat exhaustion

- Prolonged symptoms and rectal temperature > 37.8°C, increased pulse (> 150% of patient's normal) and moist skin
- Symptoms associated with heat syncope and heat cramps may be present
- Patient may be thirsty and weak, with CNS symptoms (eg, headache, fatigue; in cases chiefly caused by water depletion, anxiety, paresthesias, impaired judgment, hysteria, psychosis)
- Hyperventilation secondary to heat exhaustion can lead to respiratory alkalosis

Heat stroke

- Core temperature usually > 41°C
- Cerebral dysfunction with impaired consciousness, fever, absence of sweating
- Skin hot; initially covered with perspiration, later dries
- Pulse initially strong
- Blood pressure may be slightly elevated at first, but hypotension develops later
- Hyperventilation may lead to respiratory alkalosis
- Exertional heat stroke may present with sudden collapse and loss of consciousness followed by irrational behavior
- 25% of victims have prodromal symptoms (dizziness, weakness, nausea, confusion, disorientation, drowsiness, irrational behavior)

DIFFERENTIAL DIAGNOSIS

Heat stroke

- Neuroleptic malignant syndrome
- Malignant hyperthermia (anesthetic associated)
- Serotonin syndrome (eg, selective serotonin reuptake inhibitors used with monoamine oxidase inhibitor [MAOI])
- Other drugs: anticholinergics, antihistamines, tricyclic antidepressants, MAOIs, salicylates, amphetamines, cocaine
- Thyrotoxicosis
- Prolonged seizures

DIAGNOSIS

LABORATORY TESTS

- For **muscle cramps**: low serum sodium, hemoconcentration, and elevated urea and creatinine may be seen
- For **heat stroke**: leukocytosis, elevated BUN, hyperuricemia, hemoconcentration, acid-base abnormalities (eg, lactic acidosis), and decreased serum potassium, sodium, calcium, and phosphorus
  - Urine is concentrated, with elevated protein, tubular casts, and myoglobinuria
  - Thrombocytopenia, increased bleeding and clotting times, fibrinolysis, and consumption coagulopathy may also be present
  - Rhabdomyolysis and myocardial, hepatic, or renal damage may be identified by elevated serum creatine kinase and aminotransferase levels and BUN and by the presence of anuria, proteinuria, and hematuria

IMAGING STUDIES

- In **heat stroke**, electrocardiographic findings may include ST–T changes consistent with myocardial ischemia

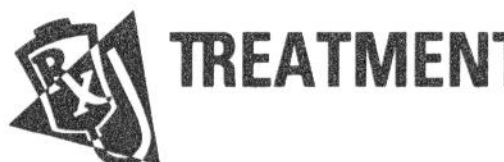

TREATMENT

MEDICATIONS

Heat stroke

- Chlorpromazine, 25–50 mg IV, or diazepam, 5–10 mg IV, can be given initially and then q4 h to control shivering
- Antipyretics (aspirin, acetaminophen) have no effect on environmentally induced hyperthermia and are contraindicated
- 5% dextrose in 0.45% or 0.9% saline should be administered for fluid replacement
- Fluid administration to ensure a high urine output (> 50 mL/h), mannitol administration (0.25 mg/kg), and alkalinizing the urine (IV bicarbonate administration, 250 mL of 4%) are recommended to reduce risk of renal failure from rhabdomyolysis

THERAPEUTIC PROCEDURES

Heat syncope

- Place patient at recumbency in a cool place, with fluids PO (or IV if necessary)

Heat cramps

- Place patient in a cool environment and give saline solution, 4 tsp of salt per gallon of water PO, to replace both salt and water. *Because of their slower absorption, salt tablets are not recommended.* The victim may have to rest for 1–3 days with continued dietary salt supplementation before returning to work or resuming strenuous activity in the heat

Heat exhaustion

- Place patient in a cool environment, provide adequate hydration (1–2 L over 2–4 h), salt replenishment—orally, if possible—and active cooling (eg, fans, ice packs) if necessary
- Physiological saline or isotonic glucose solution should be administered IV when oral administration is not appropriate. Intravenous 3% (hypertonic) saline may be necessary if sodium depletion is severe
- At least 24 h of rest is suggested

Heat stroke

- See Hyperthermia
- Aim to reduce the core temperature rapidly (within 1 h) and control the secondary effects
- Continue treatment until rectal temperature drops to 39°C
- Fluid output should be monitored by an indwelling urinary catheter

OUTCOME

FOLLOW-UP

- Because sensitivity to high environmental temperature may persist for prolonged periods following an episode of heat stroke, immediate reexposure should be avoided

COMPLICATIONS

- Hypovolemic and cardiogenic shock
- Renal failure from rhabdomyolysis, hypokalemia, cardiac arrhythmias, coagulopathy, and hepatic failure
- Hypokalemia may not appear until rehydration

PROGNOSIS

- In heat stroke, morbidity or even death can result from cerebral, cardiovascular, hepatic, or renal damage

WHEN TO ADMIT

- All patients with heat syncope, exhaustion, or stroke
- Patients with heat cramps if sustained fluid and electrolyte replacement is needed

PREVENTION

- Athletic competition is not recommended when the wet bulb globe temperature (WBGT) index exceeds 28°C
- Workers and athletes need acclimatization for hot temperatures and should drink water or balanced electrolyte fluids frequently
- Protective cooled suits have been used successfully in industry for prolonged work in environments up to 60°C

EVIDENCE

INFORMATION FOR PATIENTS

- American Red Cross: Heat-Related Illness
  - http://www.redcross.org/services/hss/tips/heat.html#termsl
- Centers for Disease Control
  - http://www.bt.cdc.gov/disasters/extremeheat/heattips.as
- MedlinePlus: Heat Emergencies
  - http://www.nlm.nih.gov/medlineplus/ency/article/000056.htm
- National Institute for Occupational Safety and Health: Working in Hot Environments
  - http://www.cdc.gov/niosh/hotenvt.html

REFERENCES

- Bouchama A et al: Heat stroke. N Engl J Med 2002;346:1978. [PMID: 12075060]
- Lugo-Amador NM et al: Heat-related illness. Emerg Med Clin North Am 2004;22:315. [PMID: 15163570]

Author(s)

Richard Cohen, MD, MPH

Helicobacter pylori Gastritis

Heavy Chain Disease p. 1087

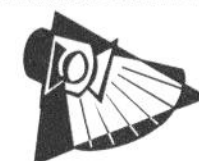

KEY FEATURES

ESSENTIALS OF DIAGNOSIS

- *Helicobacter pylori* is a spiral gram-negative rod that causes gastric mucosal inflammation

GENERAL CONSIDERATIONS

- Acute infection causes a transient illness of nausea and abdominal pain for several days associated with acute histologic gastritis with polymorphonuclear neutrophils
- After these symptoms resolve, the majority progress to chronic infection with chronic, diffuse mucosal inflammation characterized by polymorphonuclear neutrophils and lymphocytes
- Eradication achieved with antibiotics in >85% leads to resolution of the chronic gastritis
- Majority of those with chronic infection are asymptomatic and suffer no sequelae, but ~15% develop a peptic ulcer
- Risk of gastric adenocarcinoma and low-grade B cell gastric lymphoma (mucosa-associated lymphoid tissue lymphoma, or MALToma) is increased 2- to 6-fold

DEMOGRAPHICS

- Infection usually acquired in childhood through person-to-person spread
- In the United States, the prevalence of infection is < 10% in whites aged < 30 years to >50% in those aged >60 years
- Prevalence is higher in nonwhites and immigrants from developing countries

CLINICAL FINDINGS

SYMPTOMS AND SIGNS

- Acute infection: transient epigastric pain, nausea, vomiting
- Chronic infection: usually asymptomatic; symptoms arise in patients who develop peptic ulcer disease or gastric cancer; it is controversial whether chronic infection may cause dyspepsia

DIFFERENTIAL DIAGNOSIS

- Peptic ulcer disease
- Functional or nonulcer dyspepsia
- Gastroesophageal reflux disease or hiatal hernia
- Biliary disease or pancreatitis
- Gastric or pancreatic cancer
- Viral gastroenteritis
- "Indigestion" from overeating, high-fat foods, coffee
- Angina pectoris
- In patients aged < 50 years with dyspepsia without signs of complications (dysphagea, weight loss, vomiting, anemia), empirical testing and treating for *H pylori* are recommended
- In patients over age 50 years with chronic dyspepsia or signs of complications, endoscopy is recommended to exclude other organic disease

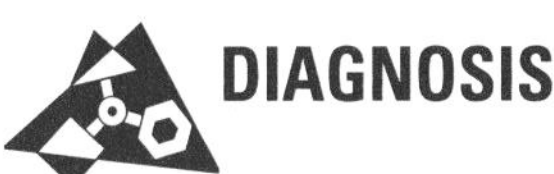

DIAGNOSIS

LABORATORY TESTS

***Noninvasive testing for* H pylori**

- Serological tests, urea breath tests, or fecal antigen tests are recommended as the most cost-effective initial tests
- Lab-based serologic ELISA test has sensitivity and specificity of >90%; positive test does not necessarily imply ongoing active infection
- Rapid (office-based) serologic tests have lower sensitivity and specificity (75–90%) but are less expensive and provide results within minutes
- After eradication with antibiotics, antibody levels decline to undetectable levels in 50% of patients by 12–18 months
- Fecal antigen immunoassay has sensitivity and specificity of 90%; positive test indicates active infection
- ^{13}C-urea breath tests have sensitivity and specificity of 90%; positive test indicates active infection
- Proton pump inhibitors significantly reduce the sensitivity of urea breath tests and fecal antigen assays (but not serologic tests) and should be discontinued 14 days prior to testing

***Endoscopic testing for* H pylori**

- Gastric biopsy specimens can detect *H pylori* organisms on histology and can be tested for active infection by urease production
- Urease test has sensitivity and specificity of 90%

DIAGNOSTIC PROCEDURES

- Upper endoscopy with biopsy is diagnostic

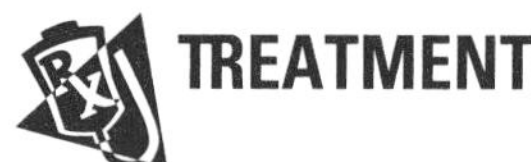

TREATMENT

MEDICATIONS

- Treat with anti–*H pylori* regimen for 10–14 days with one of the following
  - Triple-therapy: proton pump inhibitor: omeprazole 20 mg PO BID, rabeprazole 20 mg PO BID, lansoprazole 30 mg PO BID, pantoprazole 40 mg PO BID, or esomeprazole 40 mg PO QD, plus clarithromycin 500 mg PO BID, and amoxicillin 1 g PO BID *or* metronidazole 500 mg PO BID (in penicillin-allergic patients)
  - Quadruple-therapy: proton pump inhibitor: omeprazole 20 mg PO BID, rabeprazole 20 mg PO BID, lansoprazole 30 mg PO BID, or pantoprazole 40 mg PO BID, plus bismuth subsalicylate 2 tablets PO QID, plus tetracycline 500 mg PO QID, plus metronidazole 250 mg PO QID; this regimen is recommended for patients who failed initial attempt at eradication with triple-therapy regimen
- Proton pump inhibitors should be administered before meals
- Avoid metronidazole regimens in areas of known high resistance or in patients who have failed a course of treatment that included metronidazole

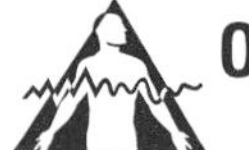

OUTCOME

FOLLOW-UP

- After antibiotic therapy, routine follow-up not recommended
- In patients with history of peptic ulcer disease with complications (bleeding) successful eradication should be confirmed with urea breath test or fecal antigen test

PROGNOSIS

- All recommended treatment regimens achieve >85% eradication
- Risk of reinfection with *H pylori* is only 1%/year

WHEN TO REFER

- Patients with persistent infection after one or two attempts at treatment should be referred to a gastroenterologist or infectious disease specialist

WHEN TO ADMIT

- Complications of *H pylori*-associated peptic ulcer disease

EVIDENCE

PRACTICE GUIDELINES

- Caselli M et al; Cervia Working Group: "Cervia Working Group Report": guidelines on the diagnosis and treatment of *Helicobacter pylori* infection. Dig Liver Dis 2001;33:75. [PMID: 11303980]
- Hunt R et al: Canadian Helicobacter Study Group Consensus Conference: update on the management of *Helicobacter pylori*—an evidence-based evaluation of six topics relevant to clinical outcomes in patients evaluated for *H pylori* infection. Can J Gastroenterol 2004;18:547. [PMID: 15457293]
- Malfertheiner P et al: Current concepts in the management of *Helicobacter pylori* infection—the Maastricht 2-2000 Consensus Report. Aliment Pharmacol Ther 2002;16:167. [PMID: 11860399]
- National Guideline Clearinghouse
  - http://www.guideline.gov/summary/summary.aspx?doc_id=2947&nbr=2173&string=Helicobacter+AND+Pylori

WEB SITE

- CDC—*H pylori*: The key to cure for most ulcer patients
  - http://www.cdc.gov/ulcer/keytocure.htm

INFORMATION FOR PATIENTS

- Uptodate—*Helicobacter pylori* infection and treatment
  - http://patients.uptodate.com/frames.asp?page=topic.asp&file=digestiv/8187&title=Helicobacter+pylori
- CDC—*H pylori*: The key to cure for most ulcer patients
  - http://www.cdc.gov/ulcer/keytocure.htm

REFERENCES

- Fischbach LA et al: Meta-analysis: the efficacy, adverse events, and adherence related to first-line anti-*Helicobacter pylori* quadruple therapies. Aliment Pharmacol Ther 2004;20:1071. [PMID: 15569109]
- Suerbaum S et al: *Helicobacter pylori* infection. N Engl J Med 2002;347:1175. [PMID: 12374879]
- Vaira D et al: Review article: diagnosis of *Helicobacter pylori* infection. Aliment Pharmacol Ther 2002;16(Suppl 1):16. [PMID: 11819423]

Author(s)

Kenneth R. McQuaid, MD

Hemochromatosis

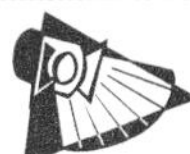

KEY FEATURES

ESSENTIALS OF DIAGNOSIS

- Usually diagnosed because of elevated iron saturation or serum ferritin or a family history
- Most patients are asymptomatic
- Hepatic abnormalities and cirrhosis, congestive heart failure, hypogonadism, and arthritis
- The disease is rarely recognized clinically before the fifth decade

GENERAL CONSIDERATIONS

- Autosomal recessive disease
- About 85% of persons with well-established hemochromatosis are homozygous for the *C282Y* mutation
- Increased accumulation of iron as hemosiderin in the liver, pancreas, heart, adrenals, testes, pituitary, and kidneys
- Heterozygotes do not develop cirrhosis in the absence of associated disorders such as viral hepatitis or nonalcoholic fatty liver disease; 1–2% of *C282Y/H63D* compound heterozygotes develop hemochromatosis

DEMOGRAPHICS

- The frequency of the gene mutation
  - Averages 7% in Northern European and North American white populations, resulting in a 0.5% frequency of homozygotes (of whom 40–70% will develop iron overload and even fewer will develop clinical symptoms)
  - Uncommon in African-American and Asian-American populations

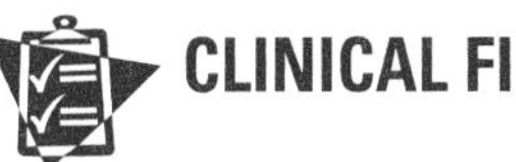

CLINICAL FINDINGS

SYMPTOMS AND SIGNS

- The onset is usually after age 50—earlier in men than in women
- Early symptoms are nonspecific (eg, fatigue, arthralgias)

Later clinical manifestations

- Arthropathy, hepatomegaly, and evidence of hepatic insufficiency (late finding)
- Skin pigmentation (combination of slate gray due to iron and brown due to melanin, sometimes resulting in a bronze color)
- Cardiac enlargement with or without heart failure or conduction defects, diabetes mellitus with its complications, and impotence in men
- Bleeding from esophageal varices
- A variant presentation in young patients is characterized by cardiac dysfunction, hypogonadotropic hypogonadism, and a high mortality rate and is not associated with the *C282Y* mutation

DIFFERENTIAL DIAGNOSIS

- Hepatomegaly due to other causes, eg, fatty liver
- Diabetes mellitus due to other causes, eg, Cushing's syndrome
- Cardiac infiltrative disease due to other causes, eg, amyloidosis, sarcoidosis
- Arthritis due to other causes, eg, rheumatoid arthritis, pseudogout
- Hyperpigmentation due to other causes, eg, hyperbilirubinemia
- Cirrhosis due to other causes

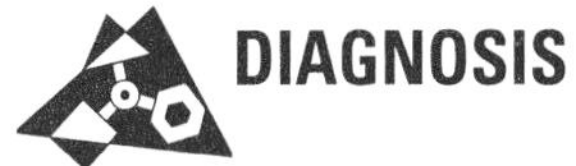

DIAGNOSIS

LABORATORY TESTS

- Mildly abnormal liver tests [aspartate aminotransferase (AST), alkaline phosphatase], an elevated plasma iron with greater than 50% saturation of the transferrin (after an overnight fast), and an elevated serum ferritin (although a normal iron saturation and a normal ferritin do not exclude the diagnosis)
- Testing for *HFE* mutations is indicated in any patient with evidence of iron overload and in siblings of patients with confirmed hemochromatosis

IMAGING STUDIES

- CT and MRI may show changes consistent with iron overload of the liver, but these techniques are not sensitive enough for screening

DIAGNOSTIC PROCEDURES

- The liver biopsy characteristically shows extensive iron deposition in hepatocytes and in bile ducts and the hepatic iron index—hepatic iron content per gram of liver converted to micromoles and divided by the patient's age—is generally greater than 1.9
- In patients who are homozygous for *C282Y*, liver biopsy is often indicated to determine whether cirrhosis is present. Biopsy can be deferred, however, in patients under age 40 in whom the serum ferritin level is < 1000 μg/L, serum AST level is normal, and no hepatomegaly is present. The likelihood of cirrhosis is low in these individuals
- Liver biopsy is also indicated when iron overload is suspected even though the patient is not homozygous for *C282Y*

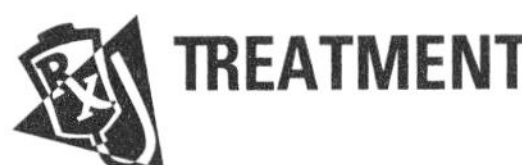

TREATMENT

MEDICATIONS

- The chelating agent deferoxamine
  - Indicated for patients with hemochromatosis and anemia or in those with secondary iron overload due to thalassemia who cannot tolerate phlebotomies
  - The drug is administered IV or SQ in a dose of 20–40 mg/kg/day infused over 24 h; treatment is painful and time consuming
  - Can mobilize 30 mg of iron per day

SURGERY

- Liver transplantation for advanced cirrhosis associated with severe iron overload, including hemochromatosis, has been reported to lead to survival rates that are lower than those for other types of liver disease because of cardiac complications and an increased risk of infections

THERAPEUTIC PROCEDURES

- Early diagnosis and treatment in the precirrhotic phase are of great importance
- Avoid foods rich in iron (such as red meat), alcohol, vitamin C, raw shellfish, and supplemental iron
- Phlebotomies
  - Initially, weekly 1 or 2 units of blood (each containing about 250 mg of iron)
  - Continue for up to 2–3 years to achieve depletion of iron stores
  - Process is monitored by hematocrit and serum iron determinations. When iron store depletion is achieved (iron saturation < 50% and serum ferritin level < 50 μg/L), maintenance phlebotomies (every 2–4 months) are continued
- Complications of hemochromatosis—arthropathy, diabetes, heart disease, portal hypertension, and hypopituitarism—also require treatment

OUTCOME

COMPLICATIONS

- Patients are at increased risk of infection with *Vibrio vulnificus, Listeria monocytogenes, Yersinia enterocolitica*, and other siderophilic organisms
- Arthropathy, diabetes, heart disease, portal hypertension, and hypopituitarism
- In patients who develop cirrhosis, there is a 15–20% incidence of hepatocellular carcinoma

PROGNOSIS

- The course of the disease is favorably altered by phlebotomy therapy. In precirrhotic patients, cirrhosis may be prevented
- Cardiac conduction defects and insulin requirements improve with treatment
- In patients with cirrhosis, varices may reverse, and the risk of variceal bleeding declines. However, cirrhotic patients must be monitored for the development of hepatocellular carcinoma

WHEN TO REFER

- All patients should be referred to a hepatologist or hematologist

PREVENTION

- Genetic testing is recommended for all first-degree family members of the proband; children of an affected person (*C282Y* homozygote) need to be screened only if the patient's spouse carries the *C282Y* or *H63D* mutation
- Screening all white men over age 30 or all adults over age 20 by measurement of the transferrin saturation or possibly the unbound iron-binding capacity has been recommended by some, but the value of screening is uncertain

EVIDENCE

PRACTICE GUIDELINES

- National Guideline Clearinghouse
  - http://www.guideline.gov/summary/summary.aspx?doc_id=3448&nbr=2674&string=hemochromatosis
  - http://www.guideline.gov/summary/summary.aspx?doc_id=3558&nbr=2784&string=hemochromatosis

WEB SITES

- Diseases of the Liver
  - http://cpmcnet.columbia.edu/dept/gi/disliv.html
- Hepatic Ultrasound Images
  - http://www.sono.nino.ru/english/hepar_en.html
- Liver Tutorials Visualization and Volume Measurement
  - http://dpi.radiology.uiowa.edu/nlm/app/livertoc/liver/liver.html
- Pathology Index
  - http://www-medlib.med.utah.edu/WebPath/LIVEHTML/LIVERIDX.html

INFORMATION FOR PATIENTS

- Mayo Clinic
  - http://www.mayoclinic.com/invoke.cfm?id=DS00455
- National Digestive Diseases Information Clearinghouse
  - http://digestive.niddk.nih.gov/ddiseases/pubs/hemochromatosis/index.htm

REFERENCES

- Dubois S et al: Review article: targeted screening for hereditary hemochromatosis in high-risk groups. Aliment Pharmacol Ther 2004;20:1. [PMID: 15225165]
- Limdi JK et al: Hereditary hemochromatosis. QJM 2004;97:315. [PMID: 15152104]
- Pietrangelo A: Hereditary hemochromatosis—a new look at an old disease. N Engl J Med 2004;350:2383. [PMID: 15175440]

Author(s)

Lawrence S. Friedman, MD

Hemolytic Uremic Syndrome

KEY FEATURES

ESSENTIALS OF DIAGNOSIS

- Microangiopathic hemolytic anemia
- Thrombocytopenia
- Renal failure
- Elevated serum lactate dehydrogenase (LDH)
- Normal coagulation tests
- Absence of neurological abnormalities

GENERAL CONSIDERATIONS

- Uncommon disorder consisting of microangiopathic hemolytic anemia, thrombocytopenia, and renal failure due to microangiopathy
- Cause is unknown
- Similar to thrombotic thrombocytopenic purpura (TTP) except different vascular beds involved; pathogenesis probably similar; platelet-agglutinating factor found in plasma may be involved
- In children, hemolytic uremic syndrome (HUS) frequently occurs after diarrheal illness due to *Shigella, Salmonella, Escherichia coli* strain O157:H7, or viruses
- In adults, often precipitated by estrogen use or postpartum state
- May occur as delayed complication of autologous bone marrow or stem cell transplantation, or of cyclosporine or tacrolimus as immunosuppression in allogeneic transplantation
- Familial (hereditary) HUS: family members have recurrent episodes over several years

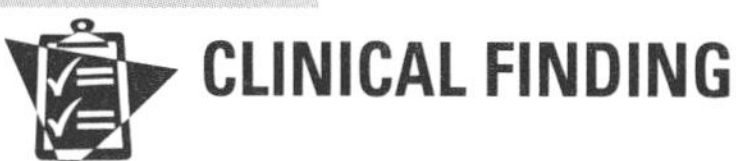

CLINICAL FINDINGS

SYMPTOMS AND SIGNS

- Symptoms of anemia, bleeding, or renal failure
- Renal failure may or may not be oliguric
- No neurological manifestations other than those due to uremia

DIFFERENTIAL DIAGNOSIS

- Disseminated intravascular coagulation
- TTP
- Preeclampsia-eclampsia
- Vasculitis
- Acute glomerulonephritis

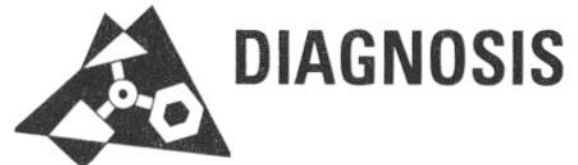

DIAGNOSIS

LABORATORY TESTS

- Microangiopathic hemolytic anemia
- Thrombocytopenia, but often less severe than in TTP
- Peripheral blood smear should show striking red blood cell fragmentation
- LDH usually elevated out of proportion to degree of hemolysis
- Coombs test negative
- Coagulation tests normal except elevated fibrin degradation products

DIAGNOSTIC PROCEDURES

- Kidney biopsy shows endothelial hyaline thrombi in afferent arterioles and glomeruli
- Ischemic necrosis in renal cortex may occur with obstruction from intravascular coagulation

Hemoglobinuria, Paroxysmal Nocturnal p. 1088. Hemolytic Disease in Newborn p. 1088. Hemolytic Transfusion Reactions p. 1088.

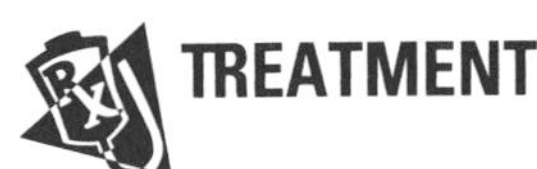

TREATMENT

THERAPEUTIC PROCEDURES

- Treatment of choice (as in TTP): large-volume plasmapheresis with fresh-frozen replacement (exchange of up to 80 mL/kg), repeated daily until remission is achieved
- In children, HUS is almost always self-limited and requires only conservative management of acute renal failure
- In adults, high rate of permanent renal insufficiency and death without treatment

OUTCOME

COMPLICATIONS

- Chronic renal insufficiency

PROGNOSIS

- Mortality rate of childhood form is low (< 5%)
- Prognosis in adults remains unclear; without effective therapy, up to 40% have died, and 80% have had chronic renal insufficiency
- Early institution of aggressive therapy with plasmapheresis promises to be beneficial
- Survival and correction of hematological abnormalities are the rule, but restoration of renal function requires early treatment

EVIDENCE

PRACTICE GUIDELINES

- Allford SL et al; Haemostasis and Thrombosis Task Force, British Committee for Standards in Haematology. Guidelines on the diagnosis and management of the thrombotic microangiopathic haemolytic anaemias. Br J Haematol 2003;120:556. [PMID: 12588343]

WEB SITES

- National Organization of Rare Disorders: Hemolytic Uremic Syndrome
  - http://www.rarediseases.org/search/rdbdetail_abstract.html?disname=Hemolytic%20Uremic%20Syndrome

INFORMATION FOR PATIENTS

- MedlinePlus: Hemolytic Uremic Syndrome
  - http://www.nlm.nih.gov/medlineplus/ency/article/000510.htm
- National Kidney and Urologic Diseases Information Clearinghouse: Hemolytic Uremic Syndrome
  - http://kidney.niddk.nih.gov/kudiseases/pubs/childkidneydiseases/hemolytic_uremic_syndrome/index.htm
- National Kidney Foundation: Hemolytic Uremic Syndrome
  - http://www.kidney.org/atoz/atozItem.cfm?id=72

REFERENCES

- Garg AX et al: Long-term renal prognosis of diarrhea-associated hemolytic uremic syndrome: a systematic review, meta-analysis, and meta-regression. JAMA 2003;290:1360. [PMID: 12966129]
- Vesely SK et al: ADAMTS13 activity in thrombotic thrombocytopenic purpura-hemolytic uremic syndrome: relation to presenting features and clinical outcomes in a prospective cohort of 142 patients. Blood 2003;102:60. [PMID: 12637323]

Author(s)

Charles A. Linker, MD

Hemophilia A

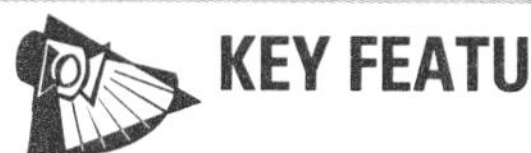

KEY FEATURES

ESSENTIALS OF DIAGNOSIS

- X-linked recessive pattern of inheritance with only males affected
- Factor VIII coagulant (VIII:C) activity low
- Factor VIII antigen normal
- Spontaneous hemarthroses

GENERAL CONSIDERATIONS

- Hemophilia A (classic hemophilia, factor VIII deficiency hemophilia) is a hereditary bleeding disorder caused by deficiency of coagulation factor VIII (VIII:C)
- Factor VIII coagulant protein usually quantitatively reduced, but defective coagulant protein is present on immunoassay in small number of cases
- Hemophilia classified as severe if factor VIII:C levels < 1%, moderate if 1–5%, and mild if levels > 5%
- X-linked recessive disease
- Families tend to breed true in severity of hemophilia
- Many hemophiliacs acquired HIV infection via factor VIII concentrate; many have developed AIDS
- HIV-associated immune thrombocytopenia may aggravate bleeding tendency

DEMOGRAPHICS

- Most common severe bleeding disorder and second most common congenital bleeding disorder, after von Willebrand's disease
- ~1 in 10,000 males affected
- Rarely, female carriers clinically affected if their normal X chromosomes are disproportionately inactivated
- Females may also be affected if they are offspring of hemophiliac father and carrier mother

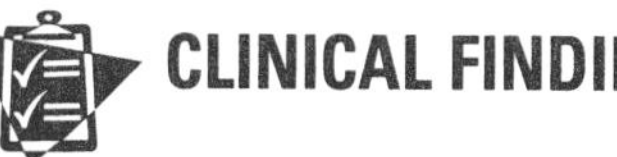

CLINICAL FINDINGS

SYMPTOMS AND SIGNS

- Bleeding tendency, with severity in proportion to factor VIII:C levels
- Mild hemophilia: bleeding only after major trauma or surgery
- Moderately severe hemophilia: bleeding with mild trauma or surgery
- Severe hemophilia: spontaneous bleeding
- Bleeding may occur anywhere, but most commonly into joints (knees, ankles, elbows), muscles, and gastrointestinal tract
- Spontaneous hemarthroses virtually diagnostic of hemophilia

DIFFERENTIAL DIAGNOSIS

- Hemophilia B
- von Willebrand's disease
- Disseminated intravascular coagulation
- Heparin administration
- Acquired factor deficiency or inhibitors (eg, paraproteins with anti-VIII or anti-IX activity)

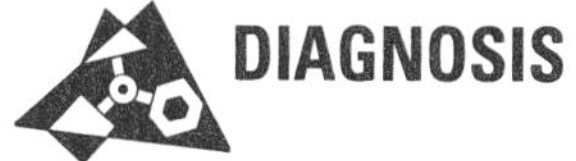

DIAGNOSIS

LABORATORY TESTS

- Partial thromboplastin time (PTT) prolonged
- Other coagulation tests, including prothrombin time, bleeding time, and serum fibrinogen level, are normal
- Factor VIII:C levels reduced, but measurements of von Willebrand factor are normal
- If plasma from a hemophiliac patient is mixed with normal plasma, PTT becomes normal; failure of PTT to normalize in such a mixing test is diagnostic of factor VIII inhibitor
- Platelet count below normal in a hemophiliac should raise suspicion of HIV-associated immune thrombocytopenia

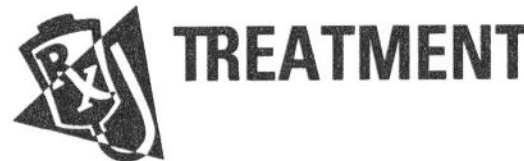

TREATMENT

MEDICATIONS

- Infusion of factor VIII concentrates, heat-treated to reduce likelihood of HIV transmission, is standard treatment
- Recombinant factor VIII appears safe and effective, though expensive, and imposes no risk of transmitting HIV or other viruses
- Desired plasma level of factor VIII depends on bleeding severity
  - For minor bleeding, raise factor VI-II:C levels to 25% with one infusion
  - For moderate bleeding (eg, deep muscle hematoma), raise level initially to 50% and maintain level > 25% with repeated infusion for 2–3 days
  - For major bleeding, raise level to 100% and maintain level > 50% continuously for 10–14 days
- Factor VIII concentrate dose is 60 U/kg (~4000 U for 70-kg individual); to raise level to 25% requires 1000 U; half-life of factor VIII:C is ~12 h
- To raise level to 100%, initial dose is 60 U/kg, followed by 30 U/kg Q12 h; during surgery, verify initial rise in factor VIII levels; if levels fail to rise, suspect presence of factor VIII inhibitor
- Desmopressin, 0.3 μg/kg IV Q24 h, may be useful in preparing patients with mild hemophilia for minor surgical procedures; causes release of factor VIII:C and raises factor VIII:C levels 2- to 3-fold for several hours
- For persistent bleeding after use of either desmopressin or factor VIII concentrate, use ε-aminocaproic acid (EACA; Amicar), 4 g PO Q4 h for several days
- Avoid aspirin

THERAPEUTIC PROCEDURES

- Treat patients with head injuries (with or without neurological signs) emergently as for major bleeding

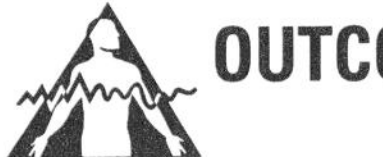

OUTCOME

COMPLICATIONS

- Arthritis from recurrent joint bleeding
- Hepatitis B and C and HIV infection from recurrent transfusion (incidence decreasing)

PROGNOSIS

- Prognosis markedly improved by availability of factor VIII replacement
- Major limiting factor is disability from recurrent joint bleeding
- Hemophiliacs with hepatitis B or C or HIV have worse prognosis associated with those disorders
- ~15% develop inhibitors to factor VIII and thus cannot be adequately supported with factor VIII

EVIDENCE

PRACTICE GUIDELINES

- Hay CR: The 2000 United Kingdom Haemophilia Centre Doctors' Organisation (UKHCDO) inhibitor guidelines. Pathophysiol Haemost Thromb 2002;32(Suppl 1):19. [PMID: 12214141]
- Kasper CK: Protocols for the treatment of haemophilia and von Willebrand disease. Haemophilia 2000;6(Suppl 1):84. [PMID: 10982273]
- United Kingdom Haemophilia Centre Doctors' Organisation: Guidelines on the selection and use of therapeutic products to treat haemophilia and other hereditary bleeding disorders. Haemophilia 2003;9:1. [PMID: 12558775]

WEB SITES

- National Library of Medicine Genetics Home Reference: Hemophilia
  - http://ghr.nlm.nih.gov/condition=hemophilia
- National Hemophilia Foundation
  - http://www.hemophilia.org
- World Federation of Hemophilia
  - http://www.wfh.org/

INFORMATION FOR PATIENTS

- National Heart, Lung, and Blood Institute: Hemophilia
  - http://www.nhlbi.nih.gov/health/dci/Diseases/hemophilia/hemophilia_what.html
- National Hemophilia Foundation: Hemophilia A
  - http://www.hemophilia.org/bdi/bdi_types1.htm
- World Federation of Hemophilia: What Is Hemophilia?
  - http://www.wfh.org/ShowDoc.asp?Rubrique=28&Document=402

REFERENCES

- Mannucci PM et al: The hemophilias—from royal genes to gene therapy. N Engl J Med 2001;344:1773. [PMID: 11396445]
- Nathwani AC et al: Current status of gene therapy for hemophilia. Curr Hematol Rep 2003;2:319. [PMID: 12901329]

Author(s)

Charles A. Linker, MD

Hemophilia B

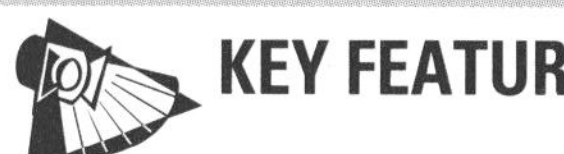

KEY FEATURES

ESSENTIALS OF DIAGNOSIS

- X-linked recessive inheritance, with only males affected
- Factor IX coagulant activity levels low
- Spontaneous hemarthroses

GENERAL CONSIDERATIONS

- Hemophilia B (Christmas disease, factor IX hemophilia) is a hereditary bleeding disorder caused by deficiency of coagulation factor IX
- Factor IX is usually quantitatively reduced, but an abnormally functioning molecule is detectable immunologically in one third of cases
- One seventh as common as hemophilia A (factor VIII deficiency) but otherwise clinically and genetically identical

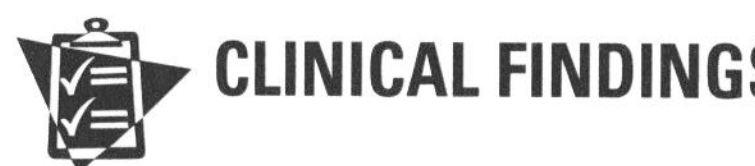

CLINICAL FINDINGS

SYMPTOMS AND SIGNS

- Bleeding tendency, with severity in proportion to factor IX levels
- Mild hemophilia: bleeding only after major trauma or surgery
- Moderately severe hemophilia: bleeding with mild trauma or surgery
- Severe hemophilia: spontaneous bleeding
- Bleeding may occur anywhere, but most commonly into joints (knees, ankles, elbows), muscles, and gastrointestinal tract
- Spontaneous hemarthroses virtually diagnostic of hemophilia

DIFFERENTIAL DIAGNOSIS

- Hemophilia A
- von Willebrand's disease
- Disseminated intravascular coagulation
- Heparin administration
- Acquired factor deficiency or inhibitor (eg, paraproteins with anti-VIII or anti-IX activity)

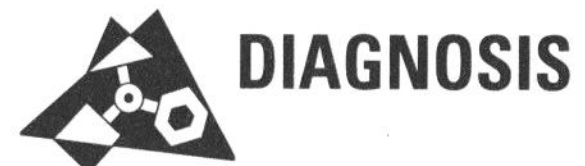

DIAGNOSIS

LABORATORY TESTS

- Partial thromboplastin time (PTT) prolonged
- Factor IX coagulant activity levels are low when measured by specific factor assays, but measurements of von Willebrand factor are normal
- Other coagulation tests, including prothrombin time, bleeding time, and serum fibrinogen level, are normal
- If plasma from hemophiliac patient is mixed with normal plasma, PTT becomes normal; failure of PTT to normalize in such a mixing test is diagnostic of factor IX inhibitor
- Platelet count below normal in a hemophiliac should raise suspicion of HIV-associated immune thrombocytopenia

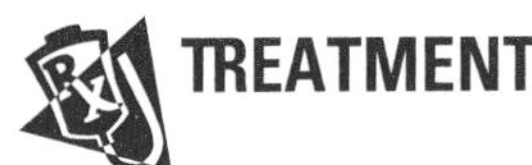

TREATMENT

MEDICATIONS

- Infusion of factor IX concentrates, heat-treated to reduce likelihood of HIV transmission, is standard treatment
- Factor VIII concentrates are ineffective
- Factor IX concentrate dose is 80 U/kg (~6000 units) to achieve 100% level; half-life is 18 h
- For major surgery, give 80 U/kg initially, followed by 40 U/kg Q18 h; measure factor IX levels to ensure that expected levels are achieved and that factor IX inhibitor is not present
- Unlike factor VIII concentrates, factor IX concentrates contain other proteins, including activated coagulating factors that appear to contribute to risk of thrombosis with recurrent usage; more care is thus needed in deciding to use these concentrates
- Desmopressin is not useful in hemophilia B
- Avoid aspirin

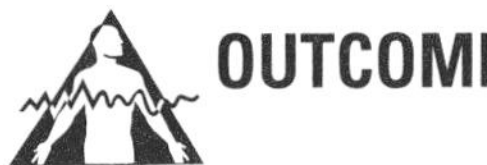

OUTCOME

COMPLICATIONS

- Risk of thrombosis with recurrent factor IX concentrate usage

PROGNOSIS

- Prognosis markedly improved by availability of factor IX replacement
- Major limiting factor is disability from recurrent joint bleeding
- Hemophiliacs with hepatitis B or C or HIV have worse prognosis associated with those disorders
- ~2.5% develop inhibitors to factor IX and thus cannot be adequately supported with factor IX

EVIDENCE

PRACTICE GUIDELINES

- Hay CR: The 2000 United Kingdom Haemophilia Centre Doctors' Organisation (UKHCDO) inhibitor guidelines. Pathophysiol Haemost Thromb 2002;32(Suppl 1):19. [PMID: 12214141]
- United Kingdom Haemophilia Centre Doctors' Organisation: Guidelines on the selection and use of therapeutic products to treat haemophilia and other hereditary bleeding disorders. Haemophilia 2003;9:1. [PMID: 12558775]

WEB SITES

- National Library of Medicine Genetics Home Reference: Hemophilia
  - http://ghr.nlm.nih.gov/condition=hemophilia
- National Hemophilia Foundation
  - http://www.hemophilia.org
- World Federation of Hemophilia
  - http://www.wfh.org/

INFORMATION FOR PATIENTS

- National Heart, Lung, and Blood Institute: Hemophilia
  - http://www.nhlbi.nih.gov/health/dci/Diseases/hemophilia/hemophilia_what.html
- National Hemophilia Foundation: Hemophilia B
  - http://www.hemophilia.org/bdi/bdi_types2.htm
- World Federation of Hemophilia: What Is Hemophilia?
  - http://www.wfh.org/ShowDoc.asp?Rubrique=28&Document=402

REFERENCE

- Bolton-Maggs PH et al: Haemophilias A and B. Lancet 2003;361:1801. [PMID: 12781551]

Author(s)

Charles A. Linker, MD

Hemorrhoids

Hemoptysis p. 1089. Hemorrhagic Fever & Hantavirus p. 1089.

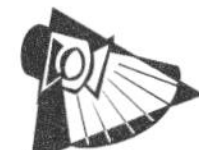

KEY FEATURES

ESSENTIALS OF DIAGNOSIS

- Bright red blood per rectum
- Protrusion of tissue from anus, with discomfort
- Characteristic findings on external anal inspection and anoscopy

GENERAL CONSIDERATIONS

- Internal hemorrhoids are a plexus of superior hemorrhoidal veins located above the dentate line that are covered by mucosa
- External hemorrhoids arise from the inferior hemorrhoidal veins located below the dentate line and are covered with squamous epithelium of the anal canal or perianal region
- Causes include straining at stool, constipation, prolonged sitting, pregnancy, obesity, and low-fiber diet

DEMOGRAPHICS

- Prevalence increases with
  - Advancing age
  - Chronic constipation with straining
  - Pregnancy
  - Weight-lifting

CLINICAL FINDINGS

SYMPTOMS AND SIGNS

- Bright red blood per rectum: streaks of blood visible on toilet paper or stool, or bright red blood that drips
- Rarely severe enough to cause anemia
- Mucoid discharge
- Internal hemorrhoids may gradually enlarge and protrude
- Discomfort and pain are unusual, occurring only with internal hemorrhoids when there is extensive inflammation and thrombosis of irreducible tissue, or with thrombosis of an external hemorrhoid
- External hemorrhoids readily visible on perianal inspection, or may protrude through the anus with gentle straining
- Prolapsed hemorrhoids appear as protuberant purple nodules covered by mucosa
- Thrombosed external hemorrhoid appears as an exquisitely painful, tense and bluish perianal nodule covered with skin that may be up to several centimeters in size

DIFFERENTIAL DIAGNOSIS

- Rectal prolapse
- Anal fissure
- Anal skin tag
- Perianal fistula or abscess, eg, Crohn's disease
- Infectious proctitis, eg, gonorrhea
- Anogenital warts (condyloma acuminata)
- Pruritus ani
- Proctalgia fugax or levator ani syndrome
- Lower gastrointestinal bleeding due to other cause, eg, diverticulosis, polyps, colorectal cancer

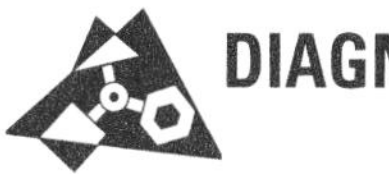

DIAGNOSIS

DIAGNOSTIC PROCEDURES

- Anoscopy: visualization of internal hemorrhoids
- Grading
  - I. No prolapse
  - II. Prolapse with defecation spontaneously reduces
  - III. Prolapse with defecation or other times; requires manual reduction
  - IV. Permanently prolapsed mucosal tissue; visible externally

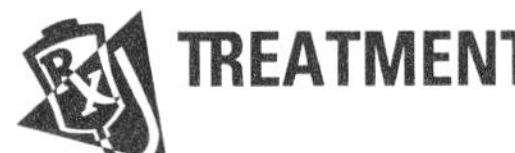

TREATMENT

SURGERY

- Surgical excision (hemorrhoidectomy) for patients with Grade IV hemorrhoids with persistent bleeding or discomfort

THERAPEUTIC PROCEDURES

- Injection sclerotherapy for symptomatic Grade I–II hemorrhoids
- Rubber band ligation, bipolar cautery or infrared photocoagulation for symptomatic Grade I–III hemorrhoids; choice dictated by operator preference

Conservative measures

- High-fiber diet
- Increase fluid intake
- Application of a cotton ball tucked next to the anal opening after bowel movements for mucoid discharge
- Symptomatic relief of prolapsed hemorrhoids by suppositories (eg, Anusol with or without hydrocortisone)
- Warm sitz baths

Thrombosed external hemorrhoid

- Warm sitz baths
- Analgesics
- Ointments
- Incision to remove the clot may hasten symptomatic relief

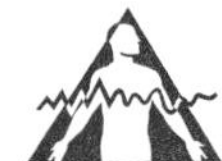

OUTCOME

FOLLOW-UP

- Bleeding usually subsides after 1–3 sessions of sclerotherapy or rubber band ligation

COMPLICATIONS

- Sclerotherapy or rubber band ligation rarely complicated by bleeding or life-threatening pelvic cellulitis; early signs are worsening anal pain radiating to legs, or difficulty with urination

PROGNOSIS

- Recurrence is common after injection sclerosis or banding

WHEN TO REFER

- Refer to surgeon or gastroenterologist for injection sclerosis, banding, or hemorrhoidectomy

WHEN TO ADMIT

- Severe bleeding with anemia (rare)
- Incarcerated, thrombosed Grade IV internal hemorrhoids
- Pelvic cellulitis after banding or sclerotherapy

PREVENTION

- High-fiber diet
- Stool softeners to prevent straining at stool

EVIDENCE

PRACTICE GUIDELINES

- Clinical Practice Committee, American Gastroenterological Association. American Gastroenterological Association medical position statement: Diagnosis and treatment of hemorrhoids. Gastroenterology 2004;126:1461. [PMID: 15131806]
- Madoff RD et al: American Gastroenterological Association technical review on the diagnosis and treatment of hemorrhoids. Gastroenterology 2004;126:1463. [PMID: 15131807]
- Surgical management of hemorrhoids. Society for Surgery of the Alimentary Tract, Inc., 2000
  – http://www.ssat.com/cgi-bin/hemorr.cgi?affiliation=student

INFORMATION FOR PATIENTS

- American Academy of Family Physicians
  – http://familydoctor.org/090.xml
- Mayo Clinic—Hemorrhoids
  – http://www.mayoclinic.com/invoke.cfm?objectid=37177394-6BD1-4401-AB747238D2AEBD84
- MEDLINEplus—Hemorrhoids
  – http://www.nlm.nih.gov/medlineplus/ency/article/000292.htm
- NIH Patient Education Institute – Hemorrhoid Surgery
  – http://www.nlm.nih.gov/medlineplus/tutorials/hemorrhoidsurgery.html

REFERENCES

- Berkelhammer C et al: Retroflexed endoscopic band ligation of bleeding internal hemorrhoids. Gastrointest Endosc 2002;55:532. [PMID: 11923767]
- Nisar PJ et al: Managing haemorrhoids. BMJ 2003;327:847. [PMID: 14551102]
- Sardinha T et al: Hemorrhoids. Surg Clin North Am 2002;82:1153. [PMID: 12516845]

Author(s)

Kenneth R. McQuaid, MD

Henoch-Schönlein Purpura p. 1090

Hepatic Encephalopathy

KEY FEATURES

ESSENTIALS OF DIAGNOSIS

- Stage 1: mild confusion, somnolence
- Stage 2: confusion
- Stage 3: stupor
- Stage 4: coma

GENERAL CONSIDERATIONS

- A state of disordered central nervous system function resulting from failure of the liver to detoxify noxious agents of gut origin because of hepatocellular dysfunction and portosystemic shunting
- Ammonia is the most readily identified toxin but is not solely responsible for the disturbed mental status
- Precipitants of hepatic encephalopathy
  - Gastrointestinal bleeding—increases the protein in the bowel and rapidly precipitates hepatic encephalopathy
  - Constipation
  - Alkalosis
  - Potassium deficiency induced by diuretics
  - Opioids, hypnotics, and sedatives
  - Medications containing ammonium or amino compounds
  - Paracentesis with attendant hypovolemia
  - Hepatic or systemic infection
  - Portosystemic shunts (including transjugular intrahepatic portosystemic shunts)

DEMOGRAPHICS

- Alcoholic liver disease and chronic hepatitis C are the most common etiologies of cirrhosis

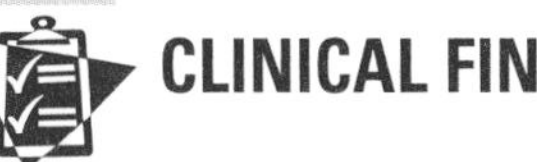

CLINICAL FINDINGS

SYMPTOMS AND SIGNS

- Metabolic encephalopathy characterized by
  - Day–night reversal
  - Asterixis, tremor, dysarthria
  - Delirium
  - Drowsiness and ultimately coma
- Symptoms occur late in liver disease except when precipitated by an acute hepatocellular insult or an episode of gastrointestinal bleeding
- Clinical diagnosis supported by asterixis, elevated serum ammonia with exclusion of other causes of delirium
- Minimal hepatic encephalopathy is characterized by mild cognitive and psychomotor deficits

DIFFERENTIAL DIAGNOSIS

- Metabolic encephalopathy, especially hyponatremia, hypoglycemia, or renal failure
- Central nervous system infection
- Altered mental status from medication effects, particularly if they are hepatically metabolized

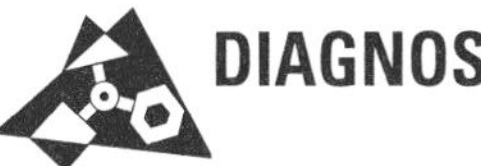

DIAGNOSIS

LABORATORY TESTS

- Liver function tests of advanced liver disease
- Serum and cerebrospinal fluid ammonia level is generally elevated

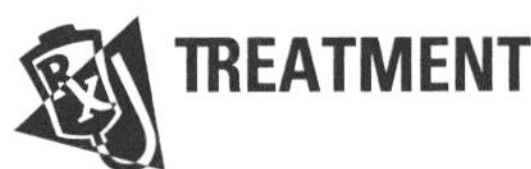

TREATMENT

MEDICATIONS

- Purge blood from the gastrointestinal tract with 120 mL of magnesium citrate by mouth or nasogastric tube every 3–4 h until the stool is free of gross blood, or by administration of lactulose
- Lactulose
  - Initial dose is 30 mL PO TID or QID
  - Titrate so that two or three soft stools per day are produced
  - When rectal use is indicated because of the patient's inability to take medicines orally, the dose is 300 mL of lactulose in 700 mL of saline or sorbitol as a retention enema for 30–60 min; it may be repeated every 4–6 h
- Neomycin sulfate, 0.5–1 g PO Q 6 or 12 h for 7 days
  - Controls the ammonia-producing intestinal flora
  - Side effects include diarrhea, malabsorption, superinfection, ototoxicity, and nephrotoxicity, usually only after prolonged use
- Alternative antibiotics are vancomycin, 1 g PO BID, or metronidazole, 250 mg PO TID. Patients who do not respond to lactulose alone may improve with a 1-week course of an antibiotic in addition to lactulose
- Avoid opioids, tranquilizers, and sedatives metabolized or excreted by the liver
- If agitation is marked, oxazepam, 10–30 mg, which is not metabolized by the liver, may be given cautiously by mouth or by nasogastric tube
- Correct zinc deficiency, if present, with oral zinc sulfate, 600 mg/day in divided doses. Eradication of *Helicobacter pylori*, which generates ammonia in the stomach, may improve encephalopathy
- Sodium benzoate, 10 g daily, and ornithine aspartate, 9 g three times daily, may lower blood ammonia levels, but less is known about these drugs than lactulose
- Flumazenil is effective in about 30% of severe hepatic encephalopathy, but the drug is short-acting and intravenous administration is required

THERAPEUTIC PROCEDURES

- Withhold dietary protein during acute episodes
- When the patient resumes oral intake, protein intake should be restricted to 60–80 g/day as tolerated, and vegetable protein is better tolerated than meat protein
- Use of special dietary supplements enriched with branched-chain amino acids is usually unnecessary except in occasional patients who are intolerant of standard protein supplements

OUTCOME

COMPLICATIONS

- Hypernatremia can develop from intensive lactulose use

WHEN TO ADMIT

- Inability to care for self or follow medical instructions

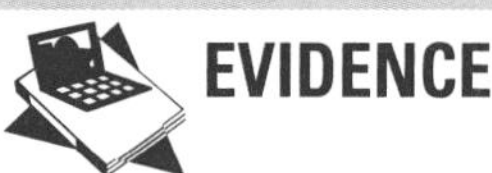

EVIDENCE

PRACTICE GUIDELINES

- Blei AT et al: Hepatic encephalopathy. Am J Gastrtoenterol 2001; 96:1968. [PMID:11467622]

WEB SITES

- Acute Liver Failure: Case study
  - http://path.upmc.edu/cases/case21.html
- Diseases of the Liver
  - http://cpmcnet.columbia.edu/dept/gi/disliv.html
- Hepatic Ultrasound Images
  - http://www.sono.nino.ru/english/hepar_en.html
- Pathology Index
  - http://www-medlib.med.utah.edu/WebPath/LIVEHTML/LIVERIDX.html

INFORMATION FOR PATIENTS

- National Institute of Neurological Disorders and Stroke
  - http://www.ninds.nih.gov/disorders/encephalopathy/encephalopathy.htm
- National Institutes of Health
  - http://www.nlm.nih.gov/medlineplus/ency/article/000302.htm

REFERENCE

- Ong JP: Correlation between ammonia levels and the severity of hepatic encephalopathy. Am J Med 2003;114:188. [PMID: 12637132]

Author(s)

Lawrence S. Friedman, MD

Hepatic Failure, Acute

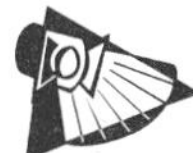

KEY FEATURES

ESSENTIALS OF DIAGNOSIS

- May be fulminant or subfulminant and both carry an equally poor prognosis
- Acetaminophen and idiosyncratic drug reactions are the most common causes

GENERAL CONSIDERATIONS

- In fulminant hepatic failure, encephalopathy and coagulopathy develop within 8 weeks after the onset of acute liver disease
- Subfulminant hepatic failure occurs when encephalopathy and coagulopathy appear between 8 weeks and 6 months after the onset of acute liver disease
- Acetaminophen toxicity accounts for 40% of cases. Idiosyncratic drug reactions are second
- In acute hepatic failure due to hepatitis or drug toxicity, extensive necrosis of the liver gives a typical pathological picture of acute liver atrophy

Etiology

- Acetaminophen toxicity
- Idiosyncratic drug reactions
- Poisonous mushrooms
- Viral hepatitis
- Shock
- Hyper- or hypothermia
- Budd-Chiari syndrome
- Malignancy (especially lymphomas)
- Wilson's disease
- Reye's syndrome
- Fatty liver of pregnancy and other disorders of fatty acid oxidation
- Autoimmune hepatitis
- Parvovirus B19 infection

DEMOGRAPHICS

- Most cases of acute hepatic failure in the United States are caused by acetaminophen toxicity, idiosyncratic drug reactions, and acute viral hepatitis, especially hepatitis B. Some cases are due to hepatitis A or unknown (non-ABCDE) viruses
- In endemic areas, hepatitis D and hepatitis E cause acute hepatic failure
- Hepatitis C is a rare cause of acute hepatic failure; acute hepatitis A or B superimposed on chronic hepatitis C has a high risk of fulminant hepatitis

CLINICAL FINDINGS

SYMPTOMS AND SIGNS

- Jaundice may be absent or minimal early
- Hepatic encephalopathy
- Coagulopathy
- Ultimately symptoms and signs of increased intracranial pressure may develop
- High risk of infection, especially with gram-positive organisms

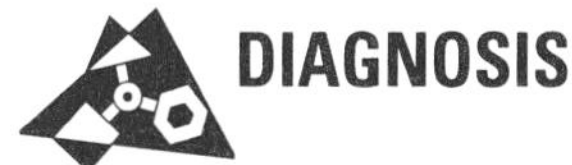

DIAGNOSIS

LABORATORY TESTS

- Severe hepatocellular damage (Table 60)
- Coagulopathy
- Elevated serum ammonia
- Low factor V levels (correlate with outcome)
- In acute hepatic failure due to microvesicular steatosis (eg, Reye's syndrome), serum aminotransferase elevations may be modest (< 300 units/L)

IMAGING STUDIES

- Head CT can help rule out or detect cerebral edema

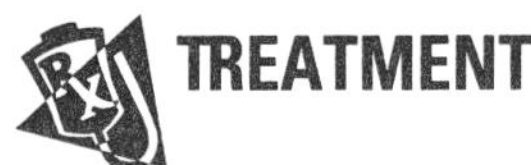

TREATMENT

MEDICATIONS

- Prophylactic antibiotic therapy decreases the risk of infection, observed in up to 90% of patients, but has no effect on survival and is not routinely recommended
- For suspected sepsis, broad coverage is indicated. The most frequent isolates are *Staphylococcus aureus*, *Streptococcus* species, coliforms, and, later in the course, *Candida* species
- Early administration of acetylcysteine (140 mg/kg orally followed by 70 mg/kg orally every 4 h for an additional 17 doses) is indicated for acetaminophen toxicity and improves cerebral blood flow and oxygenation in fulminant hepatic failure due to any cause. (Acetylcysteine treatment can prolong the prothrombin time leading to the erroneous perception that liver failure is worsening)
- Mannitol, 100–200 mL of a 20% solution by intravenous infusion over 10 min, may decrease cerebral edema but should be used with caution in renal failure; intravenous hypertonic saline may also reduce intracranial pressure. If these measures fail, hypothermia to 33.1°C may reduce intracranial pressure
- The value of hyperventilation and intravenous prostaglandin E_1 is uncertain

SURGERY

- Early transfer to a liver transplantation center is essential

THERAPEUTIC PROCEDURES

- The treatment is directed toward correcting metabolic abnormalities. These include coagulation defects; electrolyte and acid-base disturbances; renal failure; hypoglycemia; and encephalopathy
- Hepatic-assist devices using living hepatocytes, extracorporeal whole liver perfusion, hepatocyte transplantation, and liver xenografts have shown promise. The Molecular Adsorbents Recirculating System (MARS), which is based on extracorporeal albumin dialysis, is of uncertain benefit

OUTCOME

FOLLOW-UP

- Extradural sensors are placed to monitor intracranial pressure for impending cerebral edema
- Monitor for disseminated intravascular coagulopathy
- Monitor renal function, acid-base status

PROGNOSIS

- The mortality rate of fulminant hepatitis with severe encephalopathy is as high as 80%. The outlook is especially poor in patients younger than 10 and older than 40 years of age and in those with an idiosyncratic drug reaction
- Other adverse prognostic factors are a serum bilirubin level >18 mg/dL, INR >6.5, onset of encephalopathy more than 7 days after the onset of jaundice, and a low factor V level (< 20% of normal)
- For acetaminophen-induced fulminant hepatic failure, indicators of a poor outcome (which is less common than for other causes) are acidosis (pH < 7.3), INR >6.5, and azotemia (serum creatinine ≥3.4 mg/dL)
- Hyperphosphatemia (>1.2 mmol/L) and an elevated blood lactate level (>3.5 mmol/L) also predict poor survival
- Emergency liver transplantation is considered for patients with stage II to stage III encephalopathy and is associated with an 80% survival rate at 1 year

WHEN TO REFER

- Refer to a liver transplantation center early

WHEN TO ADMIT

- Any patient with acute liver disease and encephalopathy

EVIDENCE

PRACTICE GUIDELINES

- Blei AT et al: Practice Parameters Committee of the American College of Gastroenterology. Hepatic encephalopathy. Am J Gastroenterol 2001;96:1968. [PMID: 11467622]

WEB SITES

- Acute Liver Failure: Case study
  - http://path.upmc.edu/cases/case21.html
- Diseases of the Liver
  - http://cpmcnet.columbia.edu/dept/gi/disliv.html
- Hepatic Ultrasound Images
  - http://www.sono.nino.ru/english/hepar_en.html
- Liver Tutorials Visualization and Volume Measurement
  - http://dpi.radiology.uiowa.edu/nlm/app/livertoc/livertoc.html
- Pathology Index
  - http://www-medlib.med.utah.edu/WebPath/LIVEHTML/LIVERIDX.html

INFORMATION FOR PATIENTS

- National Institutes of Health
  - http://www.nlm.nih.gov/medlineplus/liverdiseases.html

REFERENCES

- Jalan R et al: Moderate hypothermia in patients with acute liver failure and uncontrolled intracranial hypertension. Gastroenterology 2004;127:1338. [PMID: 15521003]
- Lee WM: Acetaminophen and the U.S. Acute Liver Failure Study Group: lowering the risks of hepatic failure. Hepatology 2004;40:6. [PMID: 15239078]
- Murphy N et al: The effect of hypertonic sodium chloride on intracranial pressure in patients with acute liver failure. Hepatology 2004;39:464. [PMID: 14767999]

Author(s)

Lawrence S. Friedman, MD

Hepatic Vein Obstruction (Budd-Chiari Syndrome)

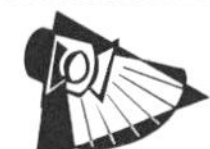

KEY FEATURES

ESSENTIALS OF DIAGNOSIS

- Right upper quadrant pain and tenderness
- Ascites
- Imaging study showing occlusion/absence of flow in the hepatic vein(s) or inferior vena cava
- Similar picture in venoocclusive disease but major hepatic veins are patent

GENERAL CONSIDERATIONS

- Occlusion of the hepatic veins may occur from a variety of causes
- In India, China, and South Africa, Budd-Chiari syndrome is often the result of occlusion of the hepatic portion of the inferior vena cava, presumably due to prior thrombosis, and the clinical presentation is mild but the course is frequently complicated by hepatocellular carcinoma
- Venoocclusive disease
  - Occlusion of terminal venules that mimics Budd-Chiari syndrome clinically
  - Is common in patients who have undergone bone marrow transplantation, particularly those with pretransplant aminotransferase elevations or fever during cytoreductive therapy with cyclophosphamide, azathioprine, carmustine, busulfan, or etoposide or those receiving high-dose cytoreductive therapy or high-dose total body irradiation
  - Can be caused by some cytotoxic agents and "bush teas" (pyrrolizidine alkaloids)

Etiologies

- Hypercoagulable state
- Caval webs
- Myeloproliferative disease, eg, polycythemia vera
- Right-sided congestive heart failure (CHF) or constrictive pericarditis
- Neoplasm compressing the hepatic vein
- Paroxysmal nocturnal hemoglobinuria
- Behçet's syndrome
- Oral contraceptives or pregnancy

CLINICAL FINDINGS

SYMPTOMS AND SIGNS

- The presentation may be fulminant, acute, subacute, or chronic; an insidious (subacute) onset is most common
- Tender, painful hepatic enlargement
- Jaundice; splenomegaly; and ascites
- With advanced disease, bleeding varices and hepatic coma may be evident
- Hepatopulmonary syndrome may occur

DIFFERENTIAL DIAGNOSIS

- Cholecystitis
- Shock liver
- Cirrhosis
- Hepatic congestion from right-sided CHF
- Metastatic cancer involving the liver

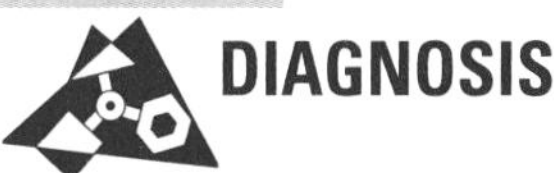

DIAGNOSIS

LABORATORY TESTS

- Liver function test abnormalities are nonspecific
- Jaundice may or may not be present
- Very high alanine aminotransferase/aspartate aminotransferase (ALT/AST) (>1000) suggests occlusion of hepatic and portal veins
- Signs of decompensated liver disease (low albumin, coagulopathy) indicate poor prognosis

IMAGING STUDIES

- Hepatic imaging studies may show a prominent caudate lobe, since its venous drainage may not be occluded
- The screening test of choice is duplex Doppler ultrasonography, which has a sensitivity of 85% for detecting evidence of hepatic venous or inferior vena caval thrombosis
- MRI and caval venography can delineate caval webs and occluded hepatic veins

DIAGNOSTIC PROCEDURES

- Percutaneous liver biopsy frequently shows a characteristic centrilobular congestion; it is frequently contraindicated because of thrombocytopenia, and the diagnosis is based on clinical findings

Hepatic Vein Obstruction (Budd-Chiari Syndrome)

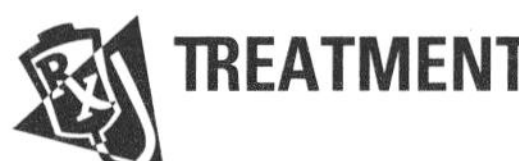

TREATMENT

MEDICATIONS

- Lifelong anticoagulation and treatment of the underlying myeloproliferative disease is often required; antiplatelet therapy with aspirin and hydroxyurea may be an alternative to coumadin in myeloproliferative disorders

SURGERY

- Surgical decompression (side-to-side portacaval, mesocaval, or mesoatrial shunt) of the congested liver may be required to relieve persistent hepatic congestion; TIPS may be attempted first
- Consider liver transplantation for fulminant hepatic failure, cirrhosis and hepatocellular dysfunction, and a failed portosystemic shunt

THERAPEUTIC PROCEDURES

- Treat ascites with fluid and salt restriction and diuretics (see *Ascites*)
- Treatable causes of Budd-Chiari syndrome should be sought
- Prompt recognition and treatment of an underlying hematological disorder may avoid the need for surgery
- Rarely, thrombolytic therapy may be attempted within 2 weeks of acute hepatic vein thrombosis
- In some cases, placement of a transjugular intrahepatic portosystemic shunt (TIPS) may be feasible, although late TIPS dysfunction is common
- Balloon angioplasty, in some cases with placement of an intravascular metallic stent, is preferred in inferior vena caval web and may be feasible when there is a short segment of thrombosis in the hepatic vein

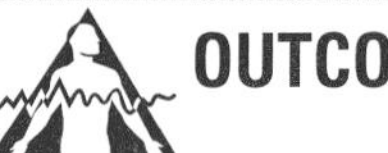

OUTCOME

COMPLICATIONS

- Liver failure
- Cirrhosis
- Spontaneous bacterial peritonitis (less common than in cirrhosis alone)

EVIDENCE

WEB SITES

- Diseases of the Liver
  - http://cpmcnet.columbia.edu/dept/gi/disliv.html
- Pathology Index
  - http://www-medlib.med.utah.edu/WebPath/LIVEHTML/LIVERIDX.html

INFORMATION FOR PATIENTS

- American Liver Foundation
  - http://www.liverfoundation.org/cgi-bin/dbs/articles.cgi?db=articles&uid=default&ID=1004&view_records=1
- National Institutes of Health
  - http://www.nlm.nih.gov/medlineplus/ency/article/000239.htm

REFERENCES

- Menon KVN et al: The Budd-Chiari syndrome. N Engl J Med 2004;350:578. [PMID: 14762185]
- Rössle M et al: The Budd-Chiari syndrome: outcome after treatment with the transjugular intrahepatic portosystemic shunt. Surgery 2004;135:394. [PMID: 15041963]

Author(s)

Lawrence S. Friedman, MD

Hepatitis, Autoimmune

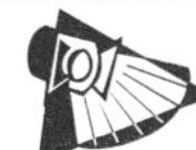

KEY FEATURES

ESSENTIALS OF DIAGNOSIS

- Usually young to middle-aged women
- Chronic hepatitis with high serum globulins
- Antinuclear antibody (+ANA) and/or smooth muscle antibody
- Responds to corticosteroids

GENERAL CONSIDERATIONS

- The onset is usually insidious, but up to 40% present with an acute attack of hepatitis and some cases follow a viral illness such as hepatitis A, Epstein-Barr infection, measles, or exposure to a drug or toxin such as nitrofurantoin
- There are at least three types of autoimmune hepatitis, distinguished by autoantibodies

DEMOGRAPHICS

- Though usually a disease of young women, autoimmune hepatitis can occur in either sex at any age
- Affected younger persons are often positive for HLA-B8 and -DR3; in older patients, HLA-DR4
- The principal susceptibility allele among white Americans and northern Europeans is HLA *DRB1*0301;* HLA *DRB1*0401* is a secondary but independent risk factor

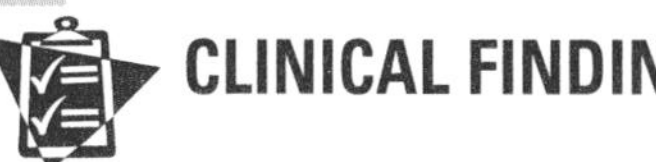

CLINICAL FINDINGS

SYMPTOMS AND SIGNS

- Typically, a healthy-appearing young woman with multiple spider nevi, cutaneous striae, acne, hirsutism, and hepatomegaly
- Amenorrhea may be a presenting feature
- Extrahepatic features include arthritis, Sjögren's syndrome, thyroiditis, nephritis, ulcerative colitis, and Coombs-positive hemolytic anemia

DIFFERENTIAL DIAGNOSIS

- Chronic viral hepatitis
- Primary biliary cirrhosis
- Primary sclerosing cholangitis
- Wilson's disease
- Hemochromatosis

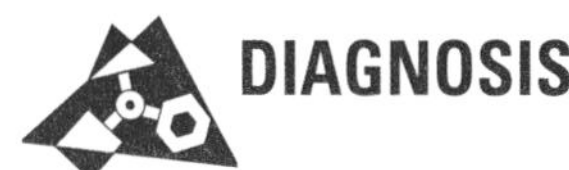

DIAGNOSIS

LABORATORY TESTS

- The serum bilirubin is usually increased, but 20% are anicteric; serum aminotransferase levels may be >1000 U/L
- In classic (type I) autoimmune hepatitis, ANA or smooth muscle antibody (either or both) is detected in serum
- Serum γ-globulin levels are typically elevated (up to 5–6 g/dL), and in this setting, the enzyme immunoassay for antibody to hepatitis C virus may be falsely positive. Other antibodies, including antineutrophil cytoplasmic antibodies (ANCA), may be found
- A second type, seen more often in Europe, is characterized by circulating antibody to liver–kidney microsomes (anti-LKM1)—directed against cytochrome P-450 2D6—or anti-liver cytosol type 1—directed against formiminotransferase—without anti-smooth muscle antibody or ANA. This type can be seen in patients with autoimmune polyglandular syndrome type 1
- A third variant is characterized by antibodies to soluble liver antigen/liver pancreas (anti-SLA/LP) and may represent a variant of type I autoimmune hepatitis characterized by severe disease, high relapse rate after treatment, and absence of the usual antibodies (ANA and smooth muscle antibody). Anti-SLA/LP antibodies appear to be directed against a transfer RNA complex responsible for incorporating selenocysteine into peptide chains

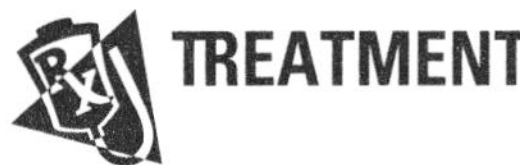

TREATMENT

MEDICATIONS

- Prednisone with or without azathioprine improves symptoms and reduces hepatic inflammation. The symptomatic patients optimal for therapy have at least a 10-fold elevation of aminotransferases (or 5-fold if the serum globulins are elevated at least 2-fold), and if asymptomatic but with modest enzyme elevations, treat on clinical grounds
- Initally, give prednisone, 30 mg orally daily, or an equivalent drug with azathioprine or mercaptopurine, 50 mg/day orally. Taper prednisone after 1 week to 20 mg/day and again after 2 or 3 weeks to 15 mg/day. Ultimately, a maintenance dose of 10 mg/day is achieved

SURGERY

- Liver transplantation may be required for treatment failures, and the disease has been recognized to recur in up to one-third of transplanted livers (and rarely to develop de novo) as immunosuppression is reduced

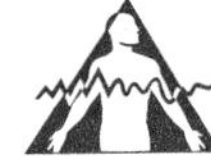

OUTCOME

FOLLOW-UP

- Blood cell counts are monitored weekly for the first 2 months of azathioprine therapy and monthly thereafter because of the small risk of bone marrow suppression
- The response rate to therapy with prednisone and azathioprine is 80%
- Fibrosis may reverse after apparent biochemical and histological remission
- Once remission is achieved, therapy may be withdrawn, but the subsequent relapse rate is 50–90%. Relapses may again be treated in the same manner as the initial episode, with the same remission rate
- After successful treatment of a relapse, treat indefinitely with azathioprine up to 2 mg/kg and the lowest dose of prednisone needed to maintain aminotransferase levels as close to normal as possible, although another attempt at withdrawing therapy may be considered in patients remaining in remission long term (eg, ≥4 years)
- Budesonide, a corticosteroid with less toxicity than prednisone, does not appear to be effective in maintaining remission
- Nonresponders to prednisone and azathioprine may be considered for a trial of cyclosporine, tacrolimus, or methotrexate. Mycophenolate mofetil is effective when azathioprine is not tolerated or there is no response to it

COMPLICATIONS

- Concurrent primary biliary cirrhosis or primary sclerosing cholangitis occurs in up to 15% of patients with autoimmune hepatitis. Liver biopsy is indicated to help establish the diagnosis, evaluate disease severity, and determine the need for treatment

PROGNOSIS

- With immunosuppressive therapy, there is prompt symptomatic improvement but biochemical improvement is more gradual, with normalization of serum aminotransferase levels after several months in many cases
- Histological resolution of inflammation may require 18–24 months, the time at which repeat liver biopsy is recommended
- The overall response rate is at least 80%
- Failure of aminotransferase levels to normalize invariably predicts lack of histological resolution

PREVENTION

- Monitor bone density, particularly with corticosteroid use, for osteoporosis

EVIDENCE

PRACTICE GUIDELINES

- Czaja AJ et al: American Association for the Study of Liver Disease. Diagnosis and treatment of autoimmune hepatitis. Hepatology 2002;36(2):479.
- National Guideline Clearinghouse
  - http://www.guideline.gov/summary/summary.aspx?doc_id=3447&nbr=2673&string=autoimmune+hepatitis

WEB SITES

- Diseases of the Liver
  - http://cpmcnet.columbia.edu/dept/gi/disliv.html
- Hepatic Ultrasound Images
  - http://www.sono.nino.ru/english/hepar_en.html
- Pathology Index
  - http://www-medlib.med.utah.edu/WebPath/LIVEHTML/LIVERIDX.html

INFORMATION FOR PATIENTS

- National Institute of Diabetes and Digestive and Kidney Diseases
  - http://digestive.niddk.nih.gov/ddiseases/pubs/autoimmunehep/index.htm
- National Institutes of Health
  - http://www.nlm.nih.gov/medlineplus/ency/article/000245.htm

REFERENCES

- Bridoux-Henno L et al: Features and outcome of autoimmune hepatitis type 2 presenting with isolated positivity for anti-liver cytosol antibody. Clin Gastroenterol Hepatol 2004;2:825. [PMID: 15354284]
- Czaja AJ et al: Progressive fibrosis during corticosteroid therapy of autoimmune hepatitis. Hepatology 2004;39:1631. [PMID: 15185304]
- Medina J et al: Review article: immunopathogenic and therapeutic aspects of autoimmune hepatitis. Aliment Pharmacol Ther 2003;17:1. [PMID: 12492728]

Author(s)

Lawrence S. Friedman, MD

Hepatitis, Drug- or Toxin-Induced

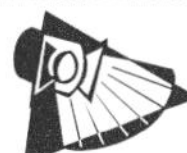

KEY FEATURES

ESSENTIALS OF DIAGNOSIS

- Drug-induced liver disease can mimic viral hepatitis, biliary tract obstruction, or other types of liver disease
- Clinicians must inquire about the use of many widely used therapeutic agents, including over-the-counter "natural" and "herbal" products in any patient with liver disease

GENERAL CONSIDERATIONS

- Drug toxicity may be categorized on the basis of pathogenesis or histological appearance

Direct hepatotoxic group

- Dose-related severity
- A latent period following exposure
- Susceptibility in all individuals. Examples include acetaminophen (toxicity enhanced by fasting and chronic alcohol use), alcohol, carbon tetrachloride, chloroform, heavy metals, mercaptopurine, niacin, plant alkaloids, phosphorus, tetracyclines, valproic acid, and vitamin A
- Coadministration of a second agent may increase the toxicity of the first (eg, isoniazid and rifampin, acetaminophen and alcohol)

Idiosyncratic reactions

- Reactions are sporadic, not dose-related, and occasionally are associated with fever and eosinophilia
- May have genetic predisposition
- Examples include amiodarone, aspirin, carbamazepine, chloramphenicol, diclofenac, flutamide, halothane, isoniazid, ketoconazole, lamotrigine, methyldopa, oxacillin, phenytoin, pyrazinamide, quinidine, streptomycin, troglitazone (withdrawn from the market in the United States), and less commonly other thiazolidinediones, and perhaps tacrine

Cholestatic reactions

- **Noninflammatory**
  - Direct effect of agent on bile secretory mechanisms: azathioprine, estrogens, or anabolic steroids containing an alkyl or ethinyl group at carbon 17, indinavir, mercaptopurine, methyltestosterone, cyclosporine
- **Inflammatory**
  - Inflammation of portal areas with bile duct injury (cholangitis), often with allergic features such as eosinophilia: amoxicillin-clavulanic acid, azithromycin, chlorothiazide, chlorpromazine, chlorpropamide, erythromycin, penicillamine, prochlorperazine, semisynthetic penicillins (eg, cloxacillin), and sulfadiazine

Acute or chronic hepatitis

- Can be clinically and histologically indistinguishable from autoimmune hepatitis: aspirin, isoniazid (increased risk in HBV carriers), methyldopa, minocycline, nitrofurantoin, nonsteroidal antiinflammatory drugs, and propylthiouracil
- Can occur with cocaine, ecstasy, efavirenz, nevirapine, ritonavir, sulfonamides, troglitazone (withdrawn from the market in the United States), zafirlukast, and various herbal and alternative remedies (eg, chaparral, germander, jin bu huan, skullcap)

Other reactions

- Fatty liver: macrovesicular: alcohol, amiodarone, corticosteroids, methotrexate
- Fatty liver: microvesicular: didanosine, stavudine, tetracyclines, valproic acid, zidovudine
- Granulomas: allopurinol, quinidine, quinine, phenylbutazone, phenytoin
- Fibrosis and cirrhosis: methotrexate, vitamin A
- Peliosis hepatis (blood-filled cavities): anabolic steroids, azathioprine, oral contraceptive steroids
- Neoplasms: oral contraceptive steroids, estrogens (hepatic adenoma but not focal nodular hyperplasia); vinyl chloride (angiosarcoma)

DIFFERENTIAL DIAGNOSIS

Causes of acute hepatitis

- Viral: hepatitis A, B, C, D (in presence of B), and E, infectious mononucleosis, cytomegalovirus, herpes simplex virus, parvovirus B19
- Other infections, eg, leptospirosis, secondary syphilis, brucellosis, Q fever
- Vascular: right-sided congestive heart failure, shock liver, portal vein thrombosis, Budd-Chiari syndrome
- Metabolic: Wilson's disease, acute fatty liver of pregnancy, Reye's syndrome
- Autoimmune hepatitis
- Lymphoma or metastatic cancer

Causes of cholestasis

- Extrahepatic: choledocholithiasis, pancreatic tumor, biliary stricture, primary sclerosing cholangitis (intra- and extrahepatic)
- Intrahepatic: primary biliary cirrhosis, autoimmune cholangitis, infiltrative disease (eg, TB, sarcoidosis, lymphoma, amyloidosis), drugs

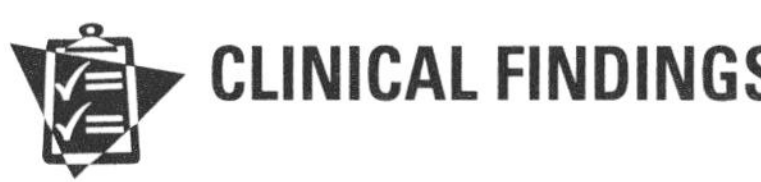

CLINICAL FINDINGS

SYMPTOMS AND SIGNS

- Can mimic all types of liver disease

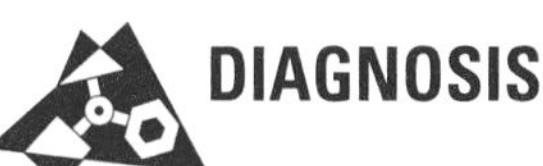

DIAGNOSIS

DIAGNOSTIC PROCEDURES

- Inquire about the use of potentially hepatotoxic drugs or exposure to hepatotoxins

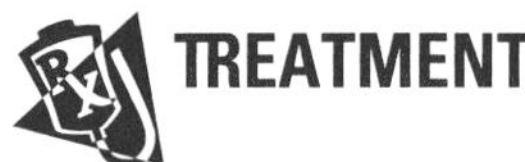

TREATMENT

MEDICATIONS

- Removing the offending agent is critical
- Corticosteroids are rarely, if ever, indicated

SURGERY

- Liver transplantation in rare instances of acute liver failure

THERAPEUTIC PROCEDURES

- Supportive treatment: see *Hepatitis*

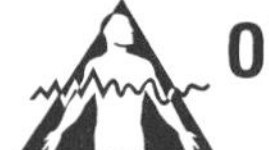

OUTCOME

FOLLOW-UP

- Monitor liver function tests until sustained improvement is seen

COMPLICATIONS

- Complications are those of liver disease of any etiology, and include hypoprothrombinemia, ascites, edema, portal hypertension, variceal bleeding, and spontaneous bacterial peritonitis

WHEN TO ADMIT

- Intractable nausea and vomiting and need for parenteral fluids
- Encephalopathy or severe coagulopathy indicates impending acute hepatic failure, and hospitalization is mandatory

EVIDENCE

PRACTICE GUIDELINES

- Centers for Disease Control and Prevention (CDC); American Thoracic Society. Update: adverse event data and revised American Thoracic Society/CDC recommendations against the use of rifampin and pyrazinamide for treatment of latent tuberculosis infection–United States, 2003. MMWR 2003;52:735.

WEB SITES

- Diseases of the Liver
  - http://cpmcnet.columbia.edu/dept/gi/disliv.html
- Pathology Index
  - http://www-medlib.med.utah.edu/WebPath/LIVEHTML/LIVERIDX.html

INFORMATION FOR PATIENTS

- National Institutes of Health
  - http://www.nlm.nih.gov/medlineplus/ency/article/000226.htm

REFERENCES

- Chalasani N et al: Patients with elevated liver enzymes are not at higher risk for statin hepatotoxicity. Gastoenterology 2004;126:1287. [PMID: 15131789]
- Rubenstein JH et al: Systematic review: the hepatotoxicity of non-steroidal anti-inflammatory drugs. Aliment Pharmacol Ther 2004;20:373. [PMID: 15298630]
- Rumack BH: Acetaminophen misconceptions. Hepatology 2004;40:10. [PMID: 15239079]

Author(s)

Lawrence S. Friedman, MD

Hepatitis A

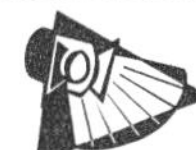

KEY FEATURES

ESSENTIALS OF DIAGNOSIS

- Prodrome of anorexia, nausea, vomiting, malaise, aversion to smoking
- Fever, enlarged and tender liver, jaundice
- Normal to low white blood cell count; abnormal liver tests, especially markedly elevated aminotransferases
- Hepatitis can be caused by many drugs, toxic agents, and viruses, and the clinical manifestations may be similar

GENERAL CONSIDERATIONS

- Transmission of hepatitis A virus (HAV) is by the fecal-oral route. The incubation period averages 30 days
- HAV is excreted in feces for up to 2 weeks before the clinical illness and rarely persists in feces after the first week of illness
- Chronic hepatitis A does not occur, and there is no carrier state

DEMOGRAPHICS

- HAV spread is favored by crowding and poor sanitation
- Common source outbreaks result from contaminated water or food

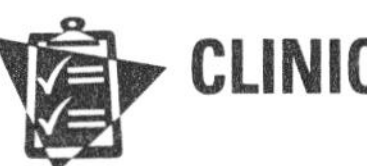

CLINICAL FINDINGS

SYMPTOMS AND SIGNS

Prodromal phase

- Onset may be abrupt or insidious, with general malaise, myalgia, arthralgia, easy fatigability, upper respiratory symptoms, and anorexia
- A distaste for smoking, paralleling anorexia, may occur early
- Nausea and vomiting are frequent, and diarrhea or constipation may occur
- Defervescence and a fall in pulse rate often coincide with the onset of jaundice
- Abdominal pain is usually mild and constant in the right upper quadrant or epigastrium, often aggravated by jarring or exertion, and rarely may be severe enough to simulate cholecystitis

Icteric phase

- Jaundice occurs after 5–10 days but may appear at the same time as the initial symptoms. Most never develop it
- With the onset of jaundice, there is often worsening of the prodromal symptoms, followed by progressive clinical improvement
- HAV is the only viral hepatitis that may be associated with spiking fevers
- Hepatomegaly—rarely marked—is present in over 50% of cases. Liver tenderness is usually present
- Splenomegaly is reported in 15% of patients, and soft, enlarged lymph nodes—especially in the cervical or epitrochlear areas—may occur

Convalescent phase

- There is an increasing sense of well-being and disappearance of symptoms

Course

- The acute illness usually subsides over 2–3 weeks with complete clinical and laboratory recovery by 9 weeks
- Clinical, biochemical, and serological recovery may be followed by one or two relapses, but recovery is the rule
- A protracted course has been reported to be associated with HLA *DRB1*1301*

DIFFERENTIAL DIAGNOSIS

- Hepatitis B, C, D (delta agent), E virus (an enterically transmitted hepatitis seen in epidemic form in Asia, North Africa, and Mexico)
- Hepatitis G virus (HGV) applies to an agent that rarely, if ever, causes frank hepatitis. Unidentified agents account for a small percentage of cases of apparent acute viral hepatitis
- A DNA virus designated the TT virus (TTV) is in up to 7.5% of blood donors and is readily transmitted by blood transfusions, but an association between this virus and liver disease has not been established. A related virus known as SEN-V has been found in 2% of U.S. blood donors, is transmitted by transfusion, and may account for some cases of transfusion-associated non-ABCDE hepatitis
- In immunocompromised and rare immunocompetent hosts, consider cytomegalovirus, Epstein-Barr virus, and herpes simplex virus
- Severe acute respiratory syndrome (SARS) may be associated with high serum aminotransferase elevations

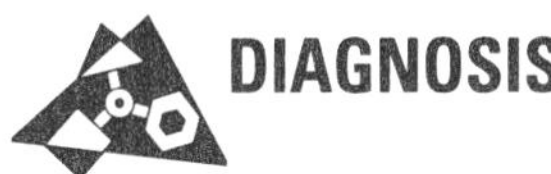

DIAGNOSIS

LABORATORY TESTS

- Antibody to hepatitis A (anti-HAV) appears early in the course of the illness. Both IgM and IgG anti-HAV are detectable in serum soon after the onset
- Peak titers of IgM anti-HAV occur during the first week of clinical disease and disappear within 3–6 months
- Detection of IgM anti-HAV is an excellent test for diagnosing acute hepatitis A
- Titers of IgG anti-HAV peak after 1 month of the disease and may persist for years
- IgG anti-HAV indicates previous exposure to HAV, noninfectivity, and immunity. In the United States, about 30% of the population have serological evidence of previous infection
- The white blood cell count is normal to low, especially in the preicteric phase. Large atypical lymphocytes may occasionally be seen
- Mild proteinuria is common, and bilirubinuria often precedes the appearance of jaundice. Acholic stools are often present during the icteric phase
- Strikingly elevated aspartate or alanine aminotransferases occur early, followed by elevations of bilirubin and alkaline phosphatase; in a minority of patients, the latter persist after aminotransferase levels have normalized
- Cholestasis is occasionally marked

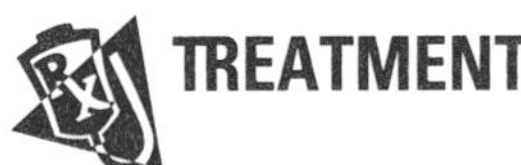

TREATMENT

MEDICATIONS

- If nausea and vomiting are pronounced or if oral intake is substantially decreased, intravenous 10% glucose is indicated
- Small doses of oxazepam are safe, as metabolism is not hepatic; morphine sulfate is avoided
- Corticosteroids produce no benefit

THERAPEUTIC PROCEDURES

- Bed rest is recommended only for marked symptoms
- Dietary management consists of palatable meals as tolerated, without overfeeding; breakfast is usually best tolerated. Strenuous physical exertion, alcohol, and hepatotoxic agents are avoided

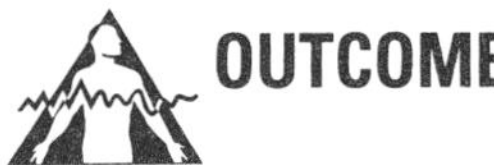

OUTCOME

COMPLICATIONS

- Fulminant hepatitis A is uncommon; it occurs rarely where hepatitis A occurs in chronic hepatitis C

PROGNOSIS

- Generally, clinical recovery is complete in 3–6 weeks
- Does not cause chronic liver disease, though it may persist for up to 1 year, and clinical and biochemical relapses may occur before full recovery. The mortality rate is less than 0.2%

WHEN TO ADMIT

- Intractable nausea and vomiting and need for parenteral fluids
- Severe coagulopathy (eg, prothrombin time >28 s)
- Encephalopathy

PREVENTION

- Strict isolation is not necessary, but hand washing after bowel movements is required. Thorough hand washing by anyone who may contact contaminated utensils, bedding, or clothing is essential

Immune globulin

- Give immune globulin to all *close* (eg, household) personal contacts and consider giving it to persons who consume food prepared by an infected food handler. The recommended dose, 0.02 mL/kg IM, is protective if administered during incubation

Vaccination

- Two effective inactivated hepatitis A vaccines are recommended for persons living in or traveling to endemic areas (including military personnel), patients with chronic liver disease on diagnosis, persons with clotting-factor disorders who are treated with concentrates, homosexual and bisexual men, animal handlers, illicit drug users, sewage workers, food handlers, and children and caregivers in day care centers and institutions
- Routine vaccination of all children has been recommended in states with a high incidence of hepatitis A
- HAV vaccine is effective in the prevention of secondary spread to household contacts of primary cases
- The recommended dose for adults is 1 mL (1440 ELISA units) of Havrix (GlaxoSmithKline) or 0.5 mL (50 units) of Vaqta (Merck) IM, followed by a booster dose at 6–12 months. A combined hepatitis A and B vaccine (Twinrix, GlaxoSmithKline) is available

EVIDENCE

PRACTICE GUIDELINES

- National Guideline Clearinghouse
  - http://www.guideline.gov/summary/summary.aspx?doc_id=3454&nbr=2680&string=hepatitis

INFORMATION FOR PATIENTS

- Centers for Disease Control
  - http://www.cdc.gov/ncidod/diseases/hepatitis/a/faqa.htm
  - http://www.cdc.gov/ncidod/diseases/hepatitis/index.htm
  - http://www.cdc.gov/ncidod/diseases/hepatitis/a/faqa.htm
- Hepatitis Information Network
  - http://www.hepnet.com/
- National Digestive Diseases Information Clearinghouse
  - http://digestive.niddk.nih.gov/ddiseases/pubs/viralhepatitis/index.htm

REFERENCE

- Fiore AE: Hepatitis A transmitted by food. Clin Infect Dis 2004;38:705. [PMID: 14986256]

Author(s)

Lawrence S. Friedman, MD

Hepatitis B, Acute

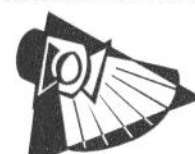

KEY FEATURES

ESSENTIALS OF DIAGNOSIS

- Prodrome of anorexia, nausea, vomiting, malaise, aversion to smoking
- Fever, tender hapatomegaly, jaundice
- Markedly elevated aminotransferases early in the course
- Liver biopsy shows hepatocellular necrosis and mononuclear infiltrate but is rarely indicated

GENERAL CONSIDERATIONS

- Hepatitis B virus (HBV) contains an inner core protein (hepatitis B core antigen, HBcAg) and outer surface coat (hepatitis B surface antigen, HBsAg)
- The incubation period is 6 weeks to 6 months (average 3 months)
- The onset of HBV is more insidious and the aminotransferase levels higher on average than in hepatitis A virus (HAV) infection
- Hepatitis can be caused by many drugs, toxic agents, and viruses, the clinical manifestations of which may be similar

DEMOGRAPHICS

- HBV is usually transmitted by infected blood or blood products or by sexual contact and is present in saliva, semen, and vaginal secretions
- HBsAg-positive mothers may transmit HBV at delivery; the risk of chronic infection in the infant approaches 90% if the mother is HBeAg positive (see below)
- HBV is prevalent in homosexuals and intravenous drug users, but most cases result from heterosexual transmission; the incidence has decreased by 75% since the 1980s
- Groups at risk include patients and staff at hemodialysis centers, physicians, dentists, nurses, and personnel working in clinical and pathology laboratories and blood banks
- The risk of HBV infection from a blood transfusion is less than one in 60,000 units transfused in the United States

CLINICAL FINDINGS

SYMPTOMS AND SIGNS

Prodromal phase

- The onset may be abrupt or insidious, with malaise, myalgia, arthralgia, fatigability, upper respiratory symptoms, anorexia, and a distaste for smoking
- Nausea and vomiting, diarrhea or constipation
- Low-grade fever is generally present; serum sickness may be seen
- Abdominal pain is usually mild and constant in the right upper quadrant or epigastrium
- Defervescence and a fall in pulse rate coincide with the onset of jaundice

Icteric phase

- Jaundice occurs after 5–10 days but may appear at the same time as the initial symptoms. Most never develop it
- Often worsening of the prodromal symptoms, followed by progressive clinical improvement

Convalescent phase

- Progressive sense of well-being

Course of illness

- The acute illness usually subsides over 2–3 weeks with complete clinical and laboratory recovery by 16 weeks
- In 5–10% of cases, the course may be more protracted, but less than 1% will have a fulminant course. Hepatitis B may become chronic

DIFFERENTIAL DIAGNOSIS

- Acute and chronic hepatitis ACDE
- The TT virus (TTV) is found in about 8% of blood donors and is readily transmitted by blood transfusions, but an association with liver disease is not established
- The SEN-V virus is found in 2% of U.S. blood donors, is transmitted by transfusion, and may account for transfusion-associated non-ABCDE hepatitis
- Cytomegalovirus, Epstein-Barr virus, and herpes simplex virus, particularly in immunocompromised hosts

DIAGNOSIS

LABORATORY TESTS

- See Table 61

HBsAg

- HBsAg appears before biochemical evidence of liver disease, and persists throughout the clinical illness; after the acute illness it may be associated with chronic hepatitis
- HBsAg establishes infection with HBV and implies infectivity

Anti-HBs

- Specific antibody to HBsAg (anti-HBs) appears after clearance of HBsAg and after successful vaccination against hepatitis B
- Appearance of anti-HBs signals recovery from HBV infection, noninfectivity, and immunity

Anti-HBc

- IgM anti-HBc appears shortly after HBsAg is detected. (HBcAg alone does not appear in serum)
- Its presence in acute hepatitis indicates a diagnosis of acute hepatitis B, and it fills the rare serological gap when HBsAg has cleared but anti-HBs is not yet detectable; it can persist for 6 months or more and reappear during flares of chronic hepatitis B
- IgG anti-HBc also appears during acute hepatitis B but persists indefinitely
- In asymptomatic blood donors, an isolated anti-HBc with no other positive HBV serological results may represent a falsely positive result or latent infection; HBV DNA is detectable only by PCR

HBeAg

- Found only in HBsAg-positive serum and indicates viral replication and infectivity
- Persistence in serum beyond 3 months indicates an increased likelihood of chronic hepatitis B
- Its disappearance is often followed by the appearance of anti-HBe, signifying diminished viral replication and decreased infectivity

HBV DNA

- Generally parallels the presence of HBeAg, though HBV DNA is a more sensitive and precise marker of viral replication and infectivity
- Very low levels of HBV DNA, detectable only by PCR, may persist in serum after recovery from acute hepatitis B, but the HBV DNA is bound to IgG and is rarely infectious
- Normal to low white blood cell count and large atypical lymphocytes
- Mild proteinuria is common, and bilirubinuria often precedes the appearance of jaundice. Elevated aspartate or alanine aminotransferase occurs early, followed by elevations of bilirubin and alkaline phosphatase
- Marked prolongation of the prothrombin time in severe hepatitis correlates with increased mortality

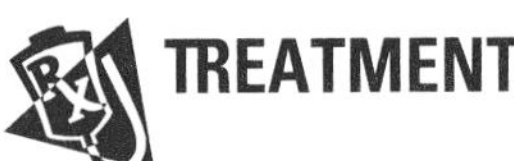

TREATMENT

MEDICATIONS

- If nausea and vomiting are pronounced or oral intake is substantially decreased, give 10% glucose IV
- Small doses of oxazepam are safe, as metabolism is not hepatic; morphine sulfate is avoided
- Corticosteroids have no benefit

THERAPEUTIC PROCEDURES

- Bed rest only for severe symptoms
- Dietary management consists of palatable meals as tolerated, without overfeeding
- Strenuous physical exertion, alcohol, and hepatotoxic agents are avoided

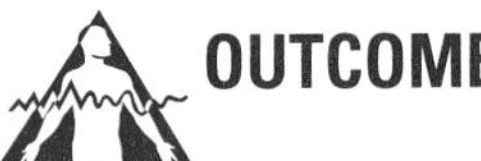

OUTCOME

COMPLICATIONS

- See *Hepatic failure, acute*
- See *Hepatitis B, chronic*

PROGNOSIS

- The risk of fulminant hepatitis is less than 1%, with a 60% mortality rate
- Following acute hepatitis B, HBV infection persists in 1–2% of immunocompetent hosts but is higher in immunocompromised hosts
- Chronic hepatitis B, particularly when HBV infection is acquired early in life and viral replication persists, confers a substantial risk of cirrhosis and hepatocellular carcinoma (up to 25–40%). Men are at greater risk than women
- HBV may be associated with serum sickness, glomerulonephritis, and polyarteritis nodosa
- Universal vaccination of neonates in countries endemic for HBV reduces the incidence of hepatocellular carcinoma

WHEN TO ADMIT

- Intractable nausea and vomiting and need for parenteral fluids
- Encephalopathy or severe coagulopathy, which indicates impending acute hepatic failure

PREVENTION

- Strict isolation of patients is not necessary, but thorough hand washing by medical staff is essential
- Screening of donated blood for HBsAg and anti-HBc has reduced the risk of transfusion-associated hepatitis markedly. Test pregnant women for HBsAg
- Practice safe sex
- Vaccinate against HAV (after prescreening for prior immunity) in those with chronic hepatitis B

Hepatitis B immune globulin (HBIG)

- May be protective, or attenuate the severity of illness, if given within 7 days after exposure (dose is 0.06 mL/kg body weight) followed by HBV vaccine
- Use this approach after exposure to HBsAg-contaminated material via mucous membranes, breaks in the skin, and after sexual contact

Vaccination

- The current vaccines are recombinant-derived
- CDC recommends universal vaccination of infants and children (Table 132)
- Over 90% of recipients mount protective antibody to hepatitis B
- Give 10–20 μg initially (depending on the formulation), repeated again at 1 and 6 months, but alternative schedules are approved
- Check postimmunization anti-HBs titers if need to document seroconversion
- Protection appears to be excellent even if the titer of anti-HBs wanes—at least for 15 years—and booster reimmunization is not routinely recommended but is advised for immunocompromised persons in whom anti-HBs titers fall below 10 mIU/mL
- For vaccine nonresponders, three additional vaccine doses may elicit seroprotective anti-HBs levels in 30–50%

EVIDENCE

PRACTICE GUIDELINES

- National Guideline Clearinghouse
  - http://www.guideline.gov/summary/summary.aspx?doc_id=3454&nbr=2680&string=hepatitis
  - http://www.guideline.gov/summary/summary.aspx?doc_id=3492&nbr=2718&string=hepatitis

INFORMATION FOR PATIENTS

- Hepatitis Information Network
  - http://www.hepnet.com/
- Mayo Clinic
  - http://www.mayoclinic.com/invoke.cfm?id=DS00398

REFERENCES

- Ganem D et al: Hepatitis B virus infection—natural history and clinical consequences. N Engl J Med 2004;350:1118. [PMID: 15014185]
- Tran TT et al (guest eds): Hepatitis B. Clin Liv Dis 2004;8:255.

Author(s)

Lawrence S. Friedman, MD

Hepatitis B, Chronic

KEY FEATURES

ESSENTIALS OF DIAGNOSIS

- Chronic inflammatory reaction of the liver of more than 3–6 months duration
- Persistently abnormal serum aminotransferase levels
- Liver biopsy shows features of chronic hepatitis, ground-glass hepatocytes

GENERAL CONSIDERATIONS

- Early in the course, hepatitis B e antigen (HBeAg) and hepatitis B virus (HBV) DNA are present in serum
  - Indicative of active viral replications and necroinflammatory activity in the liver
  - These persons are at risk for progression to cirrhosis and for hepatocellular carcinoma
  - Low-level IgM anti-HBc is also present in about 70%
- Clinical and biochemical improvement may coincide with the disappearance of HBeAg and HBV DNA from serum, appearance of anti-HBe, and integration of the HBV genome into the host genome in infected hepatocytes. If cirrhosis has not yet developed, such persons are at a lower risk for cirrhosis and hepatocellular carcinoma
- Histology
  - Traditional histology has been chronic persistent or chronic active hepatitis
  - More specific categorization is now possible, based on etiology; the grade of portal, periportal, and lobular inflammation (minimal, mild, moderate, or severe); and the stage of fibrosis (none, mild, moderate, severe, cirrhosis)

DEMOGRAPHICS

- Chronic hepatitis B afflicts nearly 400 million people worldwide and 1.25 million (predominantly males) in the United States

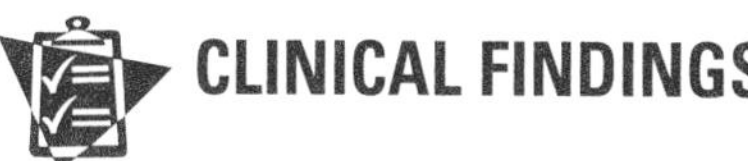

CLINICAL FINDINGS

SYMPTOMS AND SIGNS

- Clinically indistinguishable from chronic hepatitis due to other causes

DIFFERENTIAL DIAGNOSIS

- Hepatitis C and D (delta)
- Autoimmune hepatitis
- α_1-Antitrypsin deficiency
- Drug-induced chronic hepatitis
- Wilson's disease

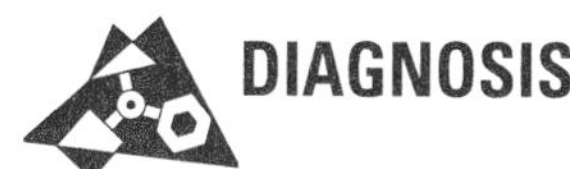

DIAGNOSIS

LABORATORY TESTS

- In approximately 40% of cases, serum aminotransferase levels remain normal

DIAGNOSTIC PROCEDURES

- Liver biopsy may be indicated for diagnosis, staging, and predicted response to therapy

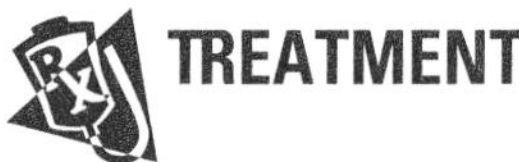

TREATMENT

MEDICATIONS

- Treat active viral replication (HBV DNA in serum, usually with HBeAg, except with precore mutant, when HBeAg is absent and anti-HBe is present) with recombinant human interferon alfa-2b, 5 million units a day or 10 million units three times a week intramuscularly for 4 months
- Lamivudine, 100 mg orally daily as a single dose, may be used instead of interferon and is much better tolerated; it can be used in decompensated cirrhosis and may be effective in rapidly progressive hepatitis B ("fibrosing cholestatic hepatitis") following organ transplantation
- Relapse is frequent when lamivudine is stopped, and long-term treatment is associated with a high rate of viral resistance. Combined use of interferon and lamivudine offers no advantage over the use of either drug alone
- Adefovir, 10 mg orally once a day, has activity against wild-type and lamivudine-resistant HBV. Resistance to this drug has not been reported. Nephrotoxicity can develop, especially if there is underlying renal dysfunction
- Tenofovir has activity against HBV
- Nucleoside analogs are recommended for inactive HBV carriers before starting immunosuppressive therapy or cancer chemotherapy to prevent reactivation
- Peginterferon may be more effective than interferon and lamivudine and is under study

THERAPEUTIC PROCEDURES

- Activity is modified according to symptoms; bed rest is not necessary
- The diet should be well balanced, without limitations other than sodium or protein restriction if dictated by fluid overload or encephalopathy

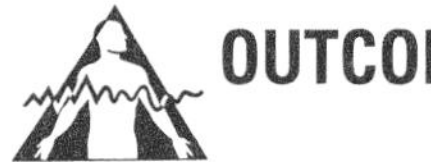

OUTCOME

COMPLICATIONS

- Cirrhosis
- Hepatocellular carcinoma

PROGNOSIS

- Interferon
  - About 40% of patients will respond with sustained normalization of aminotransferase levels, disappearance of HBeAg and HBV DNA from serum, appearance of anti-HBe, and improved survival
  - Response is most likely with a low HBV DNA level and high aminotransferase levels
  - Over 60% of the responders may eventually clear HBsAg from serum and liver, develop anti-HBs in serum, and be cured. Relapses are uncommon in such complete responders
  - HBeAg-negative chronic hepatitis B (precore mutant) has a durable sustained response rate of only 15–25% after 12 months of therapy
  - The response is poor in patients with HIV coinfection and autoimmune diseases
- Lamivudine
  - Reliably suppresses HBV DNA in serum
  - Improves liver histology in 60% of patients, and leads to normal alanine aminotransferase levels in over 40% and HBeAg seroconversion in 20% of patients after 1 year of therapy. However, 15–30% of responders experience a generally mild relapse during treatment as a result of mutation in the polymerase gene of HBV DNA that confers resistance to lamivudine
  - Hepatitis may recur when the drug is stopped, and perhaps indefinite treatment may be required when HBeAg seroconversion does not ensue. Rates of complete response—as well as resistance to lamivudine—increase with increasing duration of therapy

WHEN TO ADMIT

- Decompensated liver disease (eg, severe coagulopathy, variceal bleeding, severe ascites)

PREVENTION

- Strict isolation of patients is not necessary, but hand washing after bowel movements is required. Thorough hand washing by anyone who may contact contaminated utensils, bedding, or clothing is essential
- Screening of donated blood for HBsAg and anti-HBc has reduced the risk of transfusion-associated hepatitis markedly
- Pregnant women should be tested for HBsAg
- Persons with HBV should practice safe sex
- Vaccinate against HAV (after prescreening for prior immunity) in those with chronic hepatitis B

EVIDENCE

PRACTICE GUIDELINES

- National Guideline Clearinghouse
  - http://www.guideline.gov/summary/summary.aspx?doc_id=3454&nbr=2680&string=hepatitis
  - http://www.guideline.gov/summary/summary.aspx?doc_id=3242&nbr=2468&string=hepatitis
  - http://www.guideline.gov/summary/summary.aspx?doc_id=3492&nbr=2718&string=hepatitis

INFORMATION FOR PATIENTS

- Centers for Disease Control
  - http://www.cdc.gov/ncidod/diseases/hepatitis/index.htm
- Mayo Clinic
  - http://www.mayoclinic.com/invoke.cfm?id=DS00398
- Patient Information
  - http://patients.uptodate.com/topic.asp?file=livr_dis/4813&title=Hepatitis+B+virus

REFERENCES

- Aggarwal R et al: Preventing and treating hepatitis B infection. BMJ 2004;329:1080. [PMID: 15528620]
- Keeffe EB et al (guest eds): HBV kinetics and clinical management: key issues and current perspectives. Semin Liver Dis 2004;24(suppl 1):1.
- Keeffe EB et al: A treatment algorithm for the management of chronic hepatitis B virus infection in the United States. Clin Gastroenterol Hepatol 2004;2:87. [PMID: 15017613]

Author(s)

Lawrence S. Friedman, MD

Hepatitis C, Acute

KEY FEATURES

ESSENTIALS OF DIAGNOSIS

- Prodrome of anorexia, nausea, vomiting, malaise, aversion to smoking
- Fever, enlarged and tender liver, jaundice
- Markedly elevated aminotransferases early in the course
- Liver biopsy shows hepatocellular necrosis and mononuclear infiltrate
- Source of infection in many is unknown

GENERAL CONSIDERATIONS

- The hepatitis C virus (HCV) is a single-stranded RNA virus (hepacivirus) with properties similar to those of flavivirus. At least six major genotypes of HCV have been identified
- Coinfection is found in at least 30% of persons infected with HIV; HIV leads to more rapid progression of chronic hepatitis C to cirrhosis
- Anti-HCV is not protective, and in patients with acute or chronic hepatitis its presence in serum generally signifies that HCV is the cause

DEMOGRAPHICS

- There are more than 2.7 million HCV carriers in the United States and another 1.3 million previously exposed persons who have cleared the virus
- In the past, HCV caused over 90% of cases of posttransfusion hepatitis, yet only 4% of cases of hepatitis C were attributable to blood transfusions
- Over 50% of cases are transmitted by intravenous drug use. Intranasal cocaine use and body piercing also are risk factors
- The risk of sexual and maternal-neonatal transmission is low and may be greatest in those with high circulating levels of HCV RNA. Multiple sexual partners may increase the risk of HCV infection. Transmission via breast-feeding has not been documented

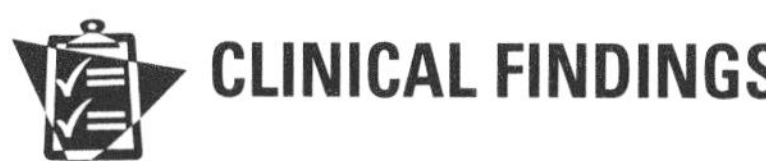

CLINICAL FINDINGS

SYMPTOMS AND SIGNS

- The incubation period averages 6–7 weeks
- Clinical illness is often mild, usually asymptomatic, and characterized by waxing and waning aminotransferase elevations and a high rate (>80%) of chronic hepatitis
- Slight neurocognitive impairment may occur with chronic hepatitis C
- Hepatic steatosis is a particular feature of infection with HCV genotype 3

DIFFERENTIAL DIAGNOSIS

- Hepatitis A, B, D, E virus
- Hepatitis G virus (HGV) rarely, if ever, causes frank hepatitis
- TT virus (TTV) is found in up to 7.5% of blood donors and is readily transmitted by blood transfusions, but an association between this virus and liver disease has not been established. A related virus known as SEN-V has been found in 2% of U.S. blood donors, is transmitted by transfusion, and may account for some cases of transfusion-associated non-ABCDE hepatitis
- Cytomegalovirus, Epstein-Barr virus, and herpes simplex virus, particularly in immunocompromised hosts

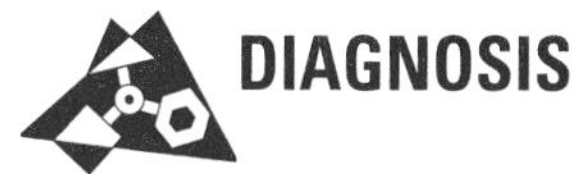

DIAGNOSIS

LABORATORY TESTS

- Antibodies to HCV
  - The immunoassay has moderate sensitivity (false-negatives) for the diagnosis early in the course and in healthy blood donors and low specificity (false-positives) in some persons with elevated γ-globulin levels. In these situations, a diagnosis of hepatitis C may be confirmed by use of an assay for HCV RNA and, in some cases, a supplemental recombinant immunoblot assay (RIBA) for anti-HCV
- Most RIBA-positive persons are potentially infectious, as confirmed by use of polymerase chain reaction-based tests to detect HCV RNA
- Occasional persons are found to have anti-HCV in serum, confirmed by RIBA, without HCV RNA in serum, suggesting recovery from HCV infection in the past
- In pregnant patients, serum aminotransferase levels frequently normalize despite persistence of viremia, only to increase again after delivery
- The white blood cell count is normal to low, especially in the preicteric phase. Large atypical lymphocytes may occasionally be seen
- Mild proteinuria is common, and bilirubinuria often precedes the appearance of jaundice. Acholic stools are often present during the icteric phase. Strikingly elevated aspartate or alanine aminotransferase occurs early, followed by elevations of bilirubin and alkaline phosphatase; in a minority of patients, the latter persist after aminotransferase levels have normalized
- Cholestasis is occasionally marked

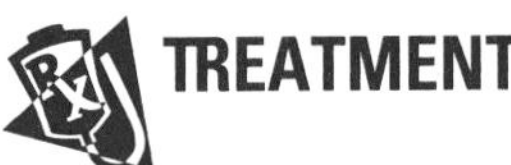

TREATMENT

MEDICATIONS

- If nausea and vomiting are pronounced or if oral intake is substantially decreased, intravenous 10% glucose is indicated
- Small doses of oxazepam are safe, as metabolism is not hepatic; morphine sulfate is avoided
- Corticosteroids have no benefit
- Treatment with interferon alfa or peginterferon can be considered when HCV RNA has not cleared from serum in 3–4 months. If HCV RNA has not cleared after 3 months of therapy, ribavirin can be added

THERAPEUTIC PROCEDURES

- Bed rest is recommended only if symptoms are marked
- Dietary management consists of palatable meals as tolerated, without overfeeding; breakfast is usually best tolerated
- Strenuous physical exertion, alcohol, and hepatotoxic agents are avoided

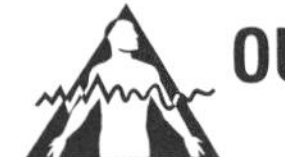

OUTCOME

COMPLICATIONS

- Mixed cryoglobulinemia and membranoproliferative glomerulonephritis
- Possibly lichen planus, autoimmune thyroiditis, lymphocytic sialadenitis, idiopathic pulmonary fibrosis, sporadic porphyria cutanea tarda, monoclonal gammopathies, and probably lymphoma
- The risk of type 2 diabetes mellitus may increase with chronic hepatitis C

PROGNOSIS

- In the majority, clinical recovery is complete in 3–6 weeks. Liver function returns to normal, though aminotransferase elevations persist in the majority of patients in whom chronic hepatitis C ensues
- The mortality rate is less than 1%, but the rate is higher in older people
- Fulminant hepatitis C is rare in the United States
- As many as 80% of all persons with acute hepatitis C develop chronic hepatitis, which in many cases progresses very slowly
- Cirrhosis develops in up to 30% of those with chronic hepatitis C; the risk is higher in patients coinfected with both viruses or with HIV
- Patients with cirrhosis are at risk of hepatocellular carcinoma at a rate of 3–5% per year

WHEN TO ADMIT

- Intractable nausea and vomiting and need for parenteral fluids
- Encephalopathy or severe coagulopathy indicate impending acute hepatic failure, and hospitalization is necessary

PREVENTION

- Strict isolation of patients is not necessary, but hand washing after bowel movements is required. Thorough hand washing by anyone who may contact contaminated utensils, bedding, or clothing is essential
- Testing blood for HCV has helped reduce the risk of transfusion-associated hepatitis C

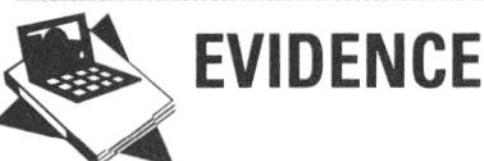

EVIDENCE

PRACTICE GUIDELINES

- National Guideline Clearinghouse
  - http://www.guideline.gov/summary/summary.aspx?doc_id=3416&nbr=2642&string=hepatitis
  - http://www.guideline.gov/summary/summary.aspx?doc_id=3454&nbr=2680&string=hepatitis

WEB SITE

- Hepatitis C: Case study
  - http://path.upmc.edu/cases/case17.html

INFORMATION FOR PATIENTS

- Centers for Disease Control
  - http://www.cdc.gov/ncidod/diseases/hepatitis/c/faq.htm
  - http://www.cdc.gov/ncidod/diseases/hepatitis/index.htm
- Torpy JM et al: JAMA Patient Page. Hepatitis C. JAMA 2003;289:2450. [PMID: 12746370]

REFERENCES

- Nomura H et al: Short-term interferon-alfa therapy for acute hepatitis C: a randomized controlled trial. Hepatology 2004;39:1201. [PMID: 15122749]
- Strader DB et al: Diagnosis, management, and treatment of acute hepatitis C. Hepatology 2004;39:1147. [PMID: 15057920]
- Vallet-Pichard A et al: Hepatitis viruses and human immunodeficiency virus co-infection: pathogenesis and treatment. J Hepatol 2004;41:156. [PMID: 15246224]

Author(s)

Lawrence S. Friedman, MD

Hepatitis C, Chronic

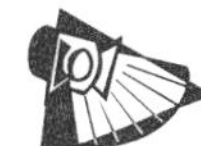

KEY FEATURES

ESSENTIALS OF DIAGNOSIS

- Chronic inflammatory reaction of the liver of more than 3–6 months duration, with persistently abnormal serum aminotransferase levels and characteristic histological findings
- May be made on initial presentation
- Liver biopsy shows features of chronic hepatitis, often with portal lymphoid nodules and interface hepatitis
- Source of infection often is unknown

GENERAL CONSIDERATIONS

- Chronic hepatitis has been categorized histologically as chronic persistent hepatitis and chronic active hepatitis. More specific categorization is possible, based on etiology; the grade of portal, periportal, and lobular inflammation (minimal, mild, moderate, or severe); and the stage of fibrosis (none, mild, moderate, severe, cirrhosis)
- May be the most common etiology of chronic hepatitis
- HCV coinfection is found in 30% of persons infected with HIV
- Anti-hepatitis C virus (HCV) is not protective; in chronic hepatitis its presence in serum signifies that HCV is the cause
- At least six major genotypes of HCV have been identified

DEMOGRAPHICS

- Up to 80% of patients with acute hepatitis C develop chronic hepatitis C
- There are more than 2.7 million HCV carriers in the United States and another 1.3 million previously exposed persons who have cleared the virus
- HCV was responsible for over 90% of cases of posttransfusion hepatitis; yet only 4% of cases of hepatitis C were attributable to blood transfusions
- Over 50% of cases are transmitted by intravenous drug use
- The risk of sexual and maternal-neonatal transmission is low and may be greatest in those with high circulating levels of HCV RNA. Multiple sexual partners may increase the risk of HCV infection

CLINICAL FINDINGS

SYMPTOMS AND SIGNS

- Clinically indistinguishable from chronic hepatitis due to other causes
- In approximately 40% of cases, serum aminotransferase levels are persistently normal
- Slight neurocognitive impairment has been reported

DIFFERENTIAL DIAGNOSIS

- Hepatitis B and D (delta agent)
- Autoimmune hepatitis
- α_1-Antitrypsin deficiency
- Drug-induced hepatitis
- Hemochromatosis
- Wilson's disease

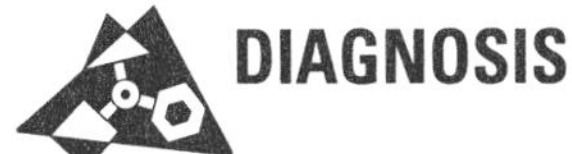

DIAGNOSIS

LABORATORY TESTS

- Serum anti-HCV by enzyme immunoassay (EIA) is present
- In rare cases of negative EIA, HCV RNA is detected by PCR
- Hepatic steatosis (fatty liver) is a particular feature of infection with HCV genotype 3

DIAGNOSTIC PROCEDURES

- Liver biopsy is indicated in patients offered treatment for diagnosis, staging, and predicted response to therapy

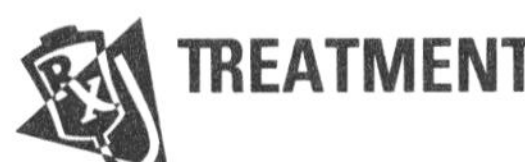

TREATMENT

MEDICATIONS

- Standard therapy is "pegylated" interferon (peginterferon) and ribavirin
  - Two peginterferon formulations are available: Pegintron (peginterferon alfa-2b) in a dose of 1.5 μg/kg weekly, and Pegasys (peginterferon alfa-2a) in a dose of 180 μg once per week for 48 weeks
  - When used with **peginterferon alfa-2b**, the dose of ribavirin is based on the patient's weight and may range from 800 mg to 1400 mg daily in two divided doses.
  - When used with **peginterferon alfa-2a**, the daily ribavirin dose is 1000 mg or 1200 mg depending on whether the patient's weight is less than or greater than 75 kg
- Treat cirrhosis or a high viral level in serum (>800,000 IU/mL) for 48 weeks
- Treat genotype 1a or 1b for 48 weeks if the level of viremia is reduced by 2 logs at 12 weeks
- Treat genotypes 2 or 3, without cirrhosis, and with low levels of viremia (< 2–3.5 × 10^6 copies/mL) for 24 weeks with a decreased dose of ribavirin of 800 mg in a split dose
- Peginterferon alfa with ribavirin may be effective treatment for cryoglobulinemia associated with chronic hepatitis C
- Asymptomatic "chronic carriers" with normal serum aminotransferase levels respond as well to treatment as do patients with elevated aminotransferase levels
- Coinfection of HCV and HIV may benefit from treatment of HCV if the CD4 count is not low

- Treatment with peginterferon alfa plus ribavirin is costly and side effects (flu-like symptoms) are almost universal; more serious toxicity includes psychiatric symptoms (irritability, depression), thyroid dysfunction, and bone marrow suppression
- Interferon is contraindicated with decompensated cirrhosis, profound cytopenias, severe psychiatric disorders, and autoimmune diseases
- Ribavirin should be avoided in persons over age 65 and in others in whom hemolysis could pose a risk of angina or stroke. Rash, itching, headache, cough, and shortness of breath also occur with the drug
- Lactic acidosis is a concern if also taking highly active antiretroviral therapy for HIV
- Occasionally, erythropoietin and granulocyte colony-stimulating factor are used to treat therapy-induced anemia and leukopenia, respectively

THERAPEUTIC PROCEDURES

- Activity is modified according to symptoms; bed rest is not necessary
- The diet should be well balanced, without limitations other than sodium or protein restriction if dictated by fluid overload or encephalopathy
- Generally offer treatment if less than age 70 and more than minor fibrosis on liver biopsy
- Because of high response rates to treatment with HCV genotype 2 or 3 infection, treatment may be initiated without a liver biopsy

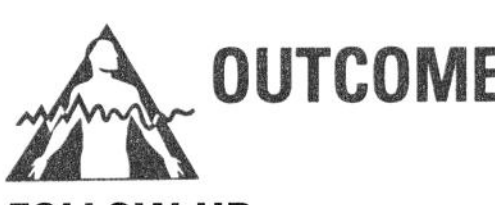

OUTCOME

FOLLOW-UP

- Obtain a blood cell count at weeks 1, 2, and 4 after peginterferon alfa plus ribavirin therapy is started and monthly thereafter
- Patients taking ribavirin must be monitored for hemolysis, and, because of teratogenic concerns, patients must practice strict contraception until 6 months after conclusion of therapy

COMPLICATIONS

- Cryoglobulinemia and membranoproliferative glomerulonephritis
- May be related to lichen planus, autoimmune thyroiditis, lymphocytic sialadenitis, idiopathic pulmonary fibrosis, porphyria cutanea tarda, lymphoma, and monoclonal gammopathy
- Type 2 diabetes mellitus may be increased

PROGNOSIS

- Up to 80% of acute hepatitis C becomes chronic hepatitis, which in many cases progresses very slowly
- Most with persistently normal serum aminotransferase levels have mild chronic hepatitis with slow or absent progression to cirrhosis; however, cirrhosis is present in 10% of these patients
- Progression to cirrhosis occurs in 20% of affected patients after 20 years, with an increased risk in men, those who drink more than 50 g of alcohol daily, and possibly those who acquire HCV infection after age 40
- Immunosuppressed persons (hypogammaglobulinemia, HIV infection with a low CD4 count, or organ transplant recipients receiving immunosuppressants) progress more rapidly to cirrhosis than immunocompetent persons
- Hepatocellular carcinoma develops in cirrhosis at a rate of 3–5% per year
- Peginterferon plus ribavarin probably improves survival and quality of life, are cost-effective, retard and even reverse fibrosis, and in responders may reduce the risk of hepatocellular carcinoma. Factors predicting an increased chance of response include no cirrhosis on liver biopsy (though treatment is not contraindicated by compensated cirrhosis), low serum HCV RNA levels, and infection by genotypes of HCV other than 1a, 1b, or 4

WHEN TO ADMIT

- Rarely necessary
- Only in advanced cirrhosis with decompensation

PREVENTION

- Strict isolation of patients is not necessary, but hand washing after bowel movements is required. Thorough hand washing by anyone who may contact contaminated utensils, bedding, or clothing is essential
- Testing of donated blood for HCV has helped reduce the risk of transfusion-associated hepatitis C from 10% a decade ago to about 1 in 2 million units today

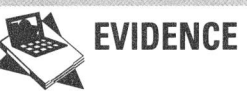

EVIDENCE

PRACTICE GUIDELINES

- National Guideline Clearinghouse
  - http://www.guideline.gov/summary/summary.aspx?doc_id=3243&nbr=2469&string=hepatitis
  - http://www.guideline.gov/summary/summary.aspx?doc_id=3416&nbr=2642&string=hepatitis
  - http://www.guideline.gov/summary/summary.aspx?doc_id=3454&nbr=2680&string=hepatitis
  - http://www.guideline.gov/summary/summary.aspx?doc_id=3454&nbr=2680&string=hepatitis

WEB SITES

- Hepatitis C: Case Study
  - http://path.upmc.edu/cases/case17.html
- Viral Hepatitis
  - http://www.cdc.gov/ncidod/diseases/hepatitis/index.htm

INFORMATION FOR PATIENTS

- Centers for Disease Control
  - http://www.cdc.gov/ncidod/diseases/hepatitis/index.htm
- Torpy JM et al: JAMA Patient Page. Hepatitis C. JAMA 2003;289:2450. [PMID: 12746370]

REFERENCES

- Chung RT et al: Peginterferon alfa-2a plus ribavirin versus interferon alfa-2a plus ribavirin for chronic hepatitis C in HIV-coinfected persons. N Engl J Med 2004;351:451. [PMID: 15282352]
- Davila JA et al: Hepatitis C infection and the increasing incidence of hepatocellular carcinoma: a population-based study. Gastroenterology 2004;127:1372. [PMID: 15521006]
- Farci P et al: Long-term benefit of interferon alpha therapy of chronic hepatitis D: regression of advanced hepatic fibrosis. Gastroenterology 2004;126:1740. [PMID: 15188169]
- Shiffman ML (ed): Chronic hepatitis C. Semin Liver Dis 2004;24(suppl 2):1. [PMID: 15346239]

Author(s)

Lawrence S. Friedman, MD

Hepatocellular Carcinoma

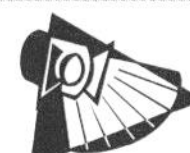

KEY FEATURES

ESSENTIALS OF DIAGNOSIS

- Hepatocellular carcinoma: malignant neoplasm of the liver that arises from parenchymal cells
- Cholangiocarcinoma: malignant neoplasm that originates in the ductular cells

GENERAL CONSIDERATIONS

- Risk factors
  - Cirrhosis in general, including nonalcoholic fatty liver disease, and hepatitis B or C in particular
  - In Africa and Asia, hepatitis B is of major etiological significance; in the west and Japan, hepatitis C and alcoholic cirrhosis are most common
  - Hemochromatosis, aflatoxin exposure (associated with mutation of the *p53* gene), α_1-antiprotease (α_1-antitrypsin) deficiency, and tyrosinemia
- Fibrolamellar variant of hepatocellular carcinoma
  - Occurs in young women
  - Characterized by a distinctive histological picture, absence of risk factors, and indolent course
- Histologically, hepatocellular carcinoma is made up of cords or sheets of cells that roughly resemble the hepatic parenchyma. Blood vessels such as portal or hepatic veins are commonly involved by tumor
- Staging in the TNM classification
  - T0: there is no evidence of primary tumor; T1: solitary tumor without vascular invasion; T2: solitary tumor with vascular invasion or multiple tumors none >5 cm; T3: multiple tumors >5 cm or a tumor involving a major branch of the portal or hepatic vein(s); and T4: tumor(s) with direct invasion of adjacent organs other than the gallbladder or with perforation of the visceral peritoneum

DEMOGRAPHICS

- Incidence is rising in the United States and western countries because of the high prevalence of chronic hepatitis C infection

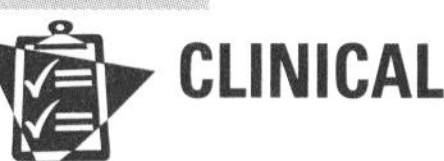

CLINICAL FINDINGS

SYMPTOMS AND SIGNS

- May be unsuspected until there is deterioration in a cirrhotic patient who was formerly stable
- Cachexia, weakness, and weight loss are associated symptoms
- The sudden appearance of ascites, which may be bloody, suggests portal or hepatic vein thrombosis by tumor or bleeding from the necrotic tumor
- There may be a tender enlargement of the liver, with an occasionally palpable mass
- In Africa, young patients typically present with a rapidly expanding abdominal mass. Auscultation may reveal a bruit over the tumor or a friction rub when the process has extended to the surface of the liver

DIFFERENTIAL DIAGNOSIS

- Metastatic cancer
- Benign liver tumors: hemangioma, adenoma, focal nodular hyperplasia
- Pyogenic or amebic liver abscess

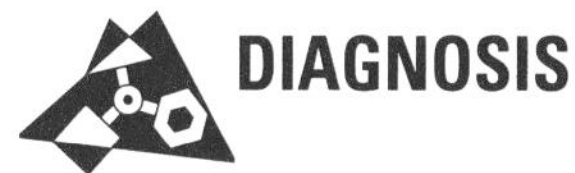

DIAGNOSIS

LABORATORY TESTS

- There may be leukocytosis, as opposed to the leukopenia that is frequently encountered in cirrhotic patients
- Anemia is common, but a normal or elevated hematocrit may be found in one-third of patients from tumor elaboration of erythropoietin
- Sudden and sustained elevation of the serum alkaline phosphatase in a formerly stable patient is common
- Hepatitis B surface antigen is found in most cases in endemic areas; in the United States, anti-hepatitis C virus (HCV) is found in up to 40% of cases
- α-Fetoprotein levels are elevated in up to 70% of patients in western countries (though the sensitivity is lower in African-Americans); however, mild elevations are also often seen in patients with chronic hepatitis
- Serum levels of des-γ-carboxy prothrombin are elevated in up to 90% of patients, but they may also be elevated in patients with vitamin K deficiency, chronic hepatitis, and metastatic cancer
- Cytological study of ascitic fluid rarely reveals malignant cells

IMAGING STUDIES

- Arterial-phase helical CT scanning with and without intravenous contrast or MRI is preferred for the location and vascularity of the tumor
- Ultrasound is less sensitive but is used to screen for hepatic nodules in high-risk patients
- Contrast-enhanced ultrasound has a sensitivity and specificity approaching those of arterial-phase helical CT

DIAGNOSTIC PROCEDURES

- Liver biopsy is diagnostic, though seeding of the needle tract by tumor is a potential risk (≤3%), and biopsy can be deferred if imaging studies and α-fetoprotein levels are diagnostic or if surgical resection is planned

Hepatitis D (Delta) p. 1090

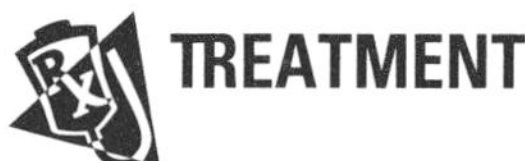

TREATMENT

MEDICATIONS

- Chemotherapy, hormonal therapy with tamoxifen, and long-activing octreotide have not been shown to prolong life
- Adaptive immunotherapy and treatment of underlying chronic viral hepatitis may lower postsurgical recurrence rates

SURGERY

- Liver transplantation may achieve a better recurrence-free survival than resection with well-compensated cirrhosis and small tumors (one tumor < 5 cm or three or fewer tumors each < 3 cm in diameter) but is often impractical because of the donor organ shortage; living donor liver transplantation may be considered in these cases
- Liver transplantation may be appropriate for small unresectable tumors in a patient with advanced cirrhosis, with reported 5-year survival rates of up to 75%
- Laparoscopic liver resection has been performed in selected cases

THERAPEUTIC PROCEDURES

- If the disease progresses despite treatment, meticulous efforts at palliative care are essential. Patients may develop severe pain due to expansion of the liver capsule by the tumor and require concerted efforts at pain management, including opioid use
- Chemoembolization via the hepatic artery may be palliative and may prolong survival
- Injection of absolute ethanol into, radiofrequency ablation of, or cryotherapy of small tumors (< 3 cm) may prolong survival; these are reasonable alternatives to surgical resection in some patients and may provide a "bridge" to liver transplantation

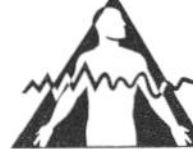

OUTCOME

PROGNOSIS

- In the United States, overall 1- and 5-year survival rates for hepatocellular carcinoma are 23% and 5%, respectively
- Attempts at surgical resection are usually fruitless if concomitant cirrhosis is present and if the tumor is multifocal
- Surgical resection of solitary hepatocellular carcinomas may result in cure if liver function is preserved (Child class A or possibly B)
- Five-year survival rates rise to 56% for patients with localized resectable disease (T1, T2, T3, selected T4; N0; M0) but are almost nil for those with localized unresectable or advanced disease
- The fibrolamellar variant has a better prognosis than conventional hepatocellular carcinoma

PREVENTION

- In chronic hepatitis B or cirrhosis caused by HCV or alcohol, surveillance should be considered with every 6-month α-fetoprotein testing and ultrasonography
- The risk of hepatocellular carcinoma with cirrhosis is 3–5% a year

EVIDENCE

PRACTICE GUIDELINES

- British Society of Gastroenterology
  - http://www.bsg.org.uk/pdf_word_docs/hcc.pdf

WEB SITES

- Diagnostic and Interventional Radiology of Hepatocellular Carcinoma
  - http://www.rad.unipi.it/works/hcc/presentation-hcc.html
- Hepatic Ultrasound Images
  - http://www.sono.nino.ru/english/hepar_en.html
- Liver Tutorials Visualization and Volume Measurement
  - http://dpi.radiology.uiowa.edu/nlm/app/livertoc/livertoc.html

INFORMATION FOR PATIENTS

- American Cancer Society
  - http://www.cancer.org/docroot/cri/content/cri_2_2_1x_what_is_liver_cancer_25.asp
- National Cancer Institute
  - http://www.cancer.gov/cancerinfo/wyntk/liver

REFERENCES

- Seeff LB et al (eds): Hepatocellular carcinoma: screening diagnosis and management. Gastroenterology 2004;127(suppl 1):S1.
- Sherman M et al: AASLD single-topic research conference on hepatocellular carcinoma: conference proceedings. Hepatology 2004;40:1465. [PMID:14999699]

Author(s)

Lawrence S. Friedman, MD

Herpes Simplex Virus Infections

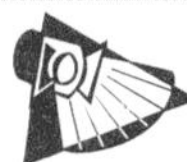

KEY FEATURES

ESSENTIALS OF DIAGNOSIS

- Recurrent small grouped vesicles, especially in the orolabial and genital areas
- May follow minor infections, trauma, stress, or sun exposure
- Tzanck smear is positive for multinucleated epithelial giant cells; viral cultures and direct fluorescent antibody tests are positive

GENERAL CONSIDERATIONS

- The patient may have recurrent self-limited attacks, provoked by sun exposure, orofacial surgery, fever, or a viral infection
- HSV-2 causes lesions whose morphology and natural history are similar to those caused by HSV-1 on the genitalia of both sexes; the infection is acquired by sexual contact

DEMOGRAPHICS

- Over 85% of adults have serologic evidence of herpes simplex type 1 (HSV-1) infections, most often acquired asymptomatically in childhood
- About 25% of the US population has serologic evidence of infection with herpes simplex type 2 (HSV-2)
- In monogamous heterosexual couples where one partner has HSV-2 infection, seroconversion of the noninfected partner occurs in 10% over a 1-year period
  - Up to 70% of such infections appeared to be transmitted during periods of asymptomatic shedding; uninfected female partners are at greater risk than males
- Owing to changes in sexual behavior, up to 40% of newly acquired cases of genital herpes are due to HSV-1

CLINICAL FINDINGS

SYMPTOMS AND SIGNS

- See Table 7
- The principal symptoms are burning and stinging; neuralgia may precede or accompany attacks
- The lesions consist of small, grouped vesicles on an erythematous base that can occur anywhere but that most often occur on the vermillion border of the lips, the penile shaft, the labia, the perianal skin, and the buttocks
- Regional lymph nodes may be swollen and tender
- The lesions usually crust and heal in 1 week
- Occasionally, primary infections may be manifested as severe gingivostomatitis

DIFFERENTIAL DIAGNOSIS

- Impetigo
- Varicella (chickenpox)
- Herpes zoster (shingles)
- Scabies
- Trauma
- Genital lesions
  - Syphilis
  - Chancroid
  - Lymphogranuloma venereum
  - Behçet's syndrome
  - Fixed drug eruption
- Oral lesions
  - Aphthous ulcers
  - Herpangina (coxsackievirus)
  - Erythema multiforme
  - Pemphigus
  - Primary HIV infection
  - Candidiasis
  - Reactive arthritis
  - Systemic lupus erythematosus
  - Behçet's syndrome
  - Bullous pemphigoid

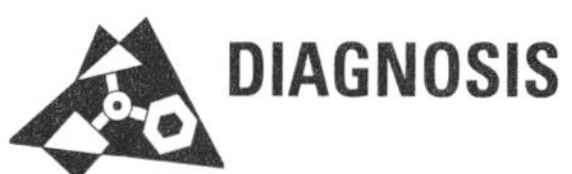

DIAGNOSIS

LABORATORY TESTS

- Direct immunofluorescent antibody slide tests offer rapid, sensitive diagnosis; viral culture may also be helpful
- Tzanck smear is positive for multinucleated epithelial giant cells; viral cultures and direct fluorescent antibody tests are positive
- Herpes serology
  - Not used in the diagnosis of an acute genital ulcer
  - Can determine who is HSV infected and potentially infectious
  - Such testing is very useful in couples in which only one partner reports a history of genital herpes
  - Beware of laboratory variations in type of HSV serologies

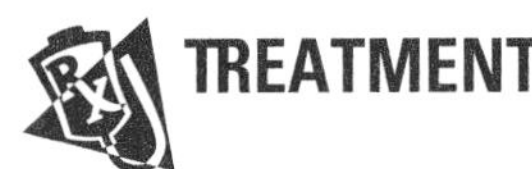

TREATMENT

MEDICATIONS

- **For first clinical episodes**
  - Acyclovir: 200 mg PO five times daily (or 800 mg three times daily)
  - Valacyclovir: 1000 mg twice daily
  - Famciclovir: 250 mg three times daily
  - Treatment is from 7–10 days depending on the severity of the outbreak
- **For recurrent herpes**
  - Generally milder symptoms than first episode and does not require therapy; when therapy is tried, it is of limited benefit, with studies finding a reduction in the average outbreak by only 12–24 h
  - Recurrent outbreaks may be treated with 5 days of acyclovir, 200 mg five times a day; 3 days of valacyclovir, 500 mg BID; or 5 days of famciclovir, 125 mg BID
  - For orolabial HSV, valacyclovir, 2 g BID for 1 day, is as effective as longer courses of therapy
  - The addition of a potent topical corticosteroid three times daily reduces the duration, size, and pain of orolabial herpes treated with an oral antiviral agent
- **For frequent or severe recurrences**
  - Suppressive treatment will reduce outbreaks by 85% and reduces viral shedding by more than 90%
  - The recommended suppressive doses, taken continuously, are acyclovir, 400 mg twice daily; valacyclovir, 500 mg once daily; or famciclovir, 125–250 mg twice daily
  - Long-term suppression appears very safe, and after 5–7 years a substantial proportion of patients can discontinue treatment
  - It is unknown if the suppression of outbreaks and asymptomatic shedding will reduce transmission
- **Local measures:** topical antiviral therapy is not significantly effective

OUTCOME

COMPLICATIONS

- Complications include
  - Pyoderma
  - Eczema herpeticum
  - Herpetic whitlow
  - Herpes gladiatorum (epidemic herpes in wrestlers transmitted by contact)
  - Esophagitis
  - Neonatal infection
  - Keratitis
  - Encephalitis
- Recurrent attacks lasting several days

PROGNOSIS

- Recurrent attacks last several days and patients generally recover without sequelae

WHEN TO REFER

- Refractory cases not responding to oral antiviral therapy

PREVENTION

- Sunscreens are very useful adjuncts in preventing sun-induced recurrences
- Prophylactic use of oral acyclovir
  - May prevent recurrence
  - Dosage is 200 mg five times daily beginning 24 h prior to ultraviolet light exposure, dental surgery, or orolabial cosmetic surgery; comparable doses are 500 mg twice daily for valacyclovir and 250 mg twice daily for famciclovir
- Barrier protection is not completely effective, since shedding occurs from widespread areas of the perineum not covered by condoms

EVIDENCE

PRACTICE GUIDELINES

- Association for Genitourinary Medicine, Medical Society for the Study of Venereal Disease (London). 2002 national guideline for the management of genital herpes
  - http://www.guideline.gov/summary/summary.aspx?doc_id=3035&nbr=2261
- Centers for Disease Control and Prevention: Diseases characterized by genital ulcers. Sexually transmitted diseases treatment guidelines. 2002
  - http://www.guideline.gov/summary/summary.aspx?doc_id=3233&nbr=2459

WEB SITES

- American Social Health Association: National Herpes Resource Center
  - http://www.ashastd.org/hrc
- Centers for Disease Control and Prevention
  - http://www.cdc.gov

INFORMATION FOR PATIENTS

- American Association of Family Physicians: Herpes: What It Is and How to Deal With It
  - http://familydoctor.org/091.xml
- American Social Health Association: Herpes: Get the Facts
  - http://www.ashastd.org/hrc/educate.html
- Mayo Clinic: Cold Sores
  - http://www.mayoclinic.com/invoke.cfm?id=DS00358
- National Institute of Allergy and Infectious Disease: Genital Herpes
  - http://www.niaid.nih.gov/factsheets/stdherp.htm

REFERENCES

- Corey L et al: Once-daily valacyclovir to reduce the risk of transmission of genital herpes. N Engl J Med 2004;350:67. [PMID: 14702423]
- Spruance SL et al: Combination treatment with famciclovir and a topical corticosteroid gel versus famciclovir alone for experimental ultraviolet radiation-induced herpes simplex labialis: a pilot study. J Infect Dis 2000;181:1906. [PMID: 10837169]

Author(s)

Timothy G. Berger, MD

Herpes Zoster

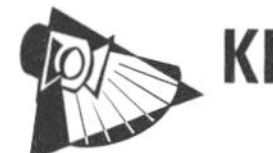

KEY FEATURES

ESSENTIALS OF DIAGNOSIS

- Pain along the course of a nerve followed by painful grouped vesicular lesions
- Involvement is unilateral; some lesions (fewer than 20) may occur outside the affected dermatome
- Lesions are usually on face or trunk
- Tzanck smear positive, especially in vesicular lesions

GENERAL CONSIDERATIONS

- An acute vesicular eruption due to the varicella-zoster virus
- It usually occurs in adults
- With rare exceptions, patients suffer only one attack
- Dermatomal herpes zoster does not imply the presence of a visceral malignancy
- Generalized disease, however, raises the suspicion of an associated immunosuppressive disorder such as Hodgkin's disease or HIV infection
- Early (within 72 h after onset) and aggressive antiviral treatment of herpes zoster reduces the severity and duration of postherpetic neuralgia

DEMOGRAPHICS

- HIV-infected patients are 20 times more likely to develop zoster, often before other clinical findings of HIV disease are present

CLINICAL FINDINGS

SYMPTOMS AND SIGNS

- See Table 7
- Pain usually precedes the eruption by 48 h or more and may persist and actually increase in intensity after the lesions have disappeared
- The lesions consist of grouped, tense, deep-seated vesicles distributed unilaterally along a dermatome
- The most common distributions are on the trunk or face
- Up to 20 lesions may be found outside the affected dermatomes
- Regional lymph glands may be tender and swollen

DIFFERENTIAL DIAGNOSIS

- Contact dermatitis (eg, poison oak or ivy)
- Herpes simplex
- Erysipelas
- Prodromal pain mimics angina, peptic ulcer, appendicitis, biliary or renal colic

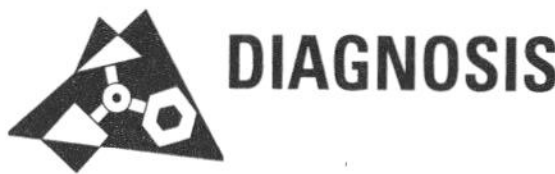

DIAGNOSIS

LABORATORY TESTS

- Clinical
- A history of HIV risk factors and HIV testing when appropriate should be considered, especially in zoster patients under 55 years of age

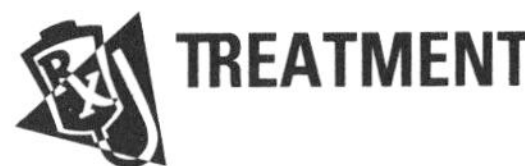

TREATMENT

MEDICATIONS

- See Table 6

Immunocompetent person

- Patients over age 55 should be treated with antiviral therapy; in addition, younger patients with acute moderate to severe pain may benefit from effective antiviral therapy
- Famciclovir, 500 mg PO TID; valacyclovir, 1 g PO TID; or acyclovir, 800 mg five times daily; all for 7 days
- The dose of antiviral should be adjusted for renal function
- Systemic corticosteroids are effective in reducing acute pain, improving quality of life, and returning patients to normal activities much more quickly; they do not increase the risk of dissemination in immunocompetent hosts
- If not contraindicated, a tapering 3-week course of prednisone, starting at 60 mg/day, for adjunctive benefit

Immunocompromised person

- Most immunocompromised patients are candidates for antiviral therapy
- The dosage schedule is as listed above, but treatment should be continued until the lesions have completely crusted and are healed or almost healed (up to 2 weeks)
- Corticosteroids should not be given adjunctively since they increase the risk of dissemination
- Progression of disease may necessitate IV therapy with acyclovir, 10 mg/kg TID; after 3–4 days, oral therapy may be substituted if there has been a good response to IV therapy; adverse effects include decreased renal function from crystallization, nausea and vomiting, and abdominal pain
- Foscarnet, administered in a dosage of 40 mg/kg two or three times daily IV, is indicated for treatment of acyclovir-resistant varicella-zoster virus infections

Local measures

- Calamine or starch shake lotions

Postherpetic neuralgia

- Capsaicin ointment, 0.025–0.075%, or lidocaine (Lidoderm) topical patches
- Chronic postherpetic neuralgia may be relieved by regional blocks (stellate ganglion, epidural, local infiltration, or peripheral nerve), with or without corticosteroids added to the injections
- Amitriptyline, 25–75 mg as a single nightly dose, is the first-line oral therapy beyond simple analgesics
- Gabapentin, up to 3600 PO mg daily (starting at 300 mg three times daily), may be added for additional pain relief

THERAPEUTIC PROCEDURES

- Nerve blocks may be important in the management of initial severe pain
- Patients should maintain good hydration, and elderly patients with reduced renal function should be followed closely

OUTCOME

COMPLICATIONS

- Sacral zoster may be associated with bladder and bowel dysfunction
- Persistent neuralgia, anesthesia or scarring of the affected area following healing, facial or other nerve paralysis, and encephalitis may occur
- Postherpetic neuralgia is most common after involvement of the trigeminal region, and in patients over 55
- Zoster ophthalmicus (V_1) can result in visual impairment

PROGNOSIS

- The eruption persists 2–3 weeks and usually does not recur
- Motor involvement in 2–3% may lead to temporary palsy
- Oral corticosteroids do not reduce the prevalence, severity, or duration of postherpetic neuralgia beyond that achieved by effective antiviral therapy

WHEN TO REFER

- Ophthalmologic consultation is vital for involvement of the first branch of the trigeminal nerve

PREVENTION

- The zoster vaccine markedly reduced morbidity from herpes zoster and postherpetic neuralgia among older adults
- Early and aggressive antiviral therapy for postherpetic neuralgia

EVIDENCE

PRACTICE GUIDELINES

- Gross G et al: Herpes zoster guideline of the German Dermatology Society. J Clin Virol 2003;26:277. [PMID: 12637076]

WEB SITES

- American Academy of Dermatology
  - http://www.aad.org
- National Institute of Allergy and Infectious Disease: Photos of Shingles
  - http://www.niaid.nih.gov/shingles/photos.htm

INFORMATION FOR PATIENTS

- American Academy of Dermatology: Herpes Zoster
  - http://www.aad.org/public/Publications/pamphlets/HerpesZoster.htm
- American Academy of Family Physicians: Shingles
  - http://familydoctor.org/574.xml
- MedlinePlus: Shingles Interactive Tutorial
  - http://www.nlm.nih.gov/medlineplus/tutorials/shingles.html
- National Institute on Aging: Shingles
  - http://www.niapublications.org/engagepages/shingles.asp

REFERENCES

- Oxman MN et al: A vaccine to prevent herpes zoster and postherpetic neuralgia in older adults. N Engl J Med 2005;352:2271. [PMID: 15930418]
- Vanhems P et al: The incidence of herpes zoster is less likely than other opportunistic infections to be reduced by highly active antiretroviral therapy. J Acquir Immune Defic Syndr 2005;38:111. [PMID: 15608535]
- Wareham D: Postherpetic neuralgia. Clin Evid 2003;10:942. [PMID: 15555130]
- Wassilew S; Collaborative Brivudin PHN Study Group: Brivudin compared with famciclovir in the treatment of herpes zoster: effects in acute disease and chronic pain in immunocompetent patients. A randomized, double-blind, multinational study. J Eur Acad Dermatol Venereol 2005;19:47. [PMID: 15649191]

Author(s)

Timothy G. Berger, MD

Hirsutism & Virilization

Hiccups p. 1091

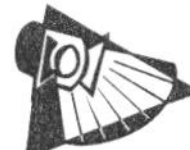

KEY FEATURES

ESSENTIALS OF DIAGNOSIS

- Menstrual disorders, hirsutism, acne
- Virilization: increased muscularity, androgenic alopecia, deepening of voice, enlargement of clitoris
- Occasionally, a palpable pelvic tumor
- Urinary 17-ketosteroids and serum dehydroepiandrosterone sulfate (DHEAS) and androstenedione elevated in adrenal disorders, variable in others
- Serum testosterone often elevated

GENERAL CONSIDERATIONS

- Major androgen is testosterone. If serum testosterone is normal, an endocrine cause for hirsutism is extremely unlikely
- In women, circulating testosterone is normally derived from ovarian secretion (60%) and peripheral conversion from androstenedione (40%)
- Androstenedione is secreted in equal amounts by adrenals and ovaries; DHEAS secreted only by adrenals

Causes of hirsutism

- Idiopathic or familial—most women with hirsutism or androgenic alopecia have no detectable hyperandrogenism. Often hirsutism is familial and may be normal for genetic background
- Polycystic ovary syndrome—accounts for >50% of cases. Affects 4–6% of premenopausal women in the United States. Associated with amenorrhea or oligomenorrhea, anovulation, and obesity. Insulin resistance and diabetes common
- Ovarian tumor (uncommon) and adrenal carcinoma (rare)
- Steroidogenic enzyme defects
  - Baby girls with "classic" 21-hydroxylase deficiency have ambiguous genitalia and may become virilized unless corticosteroids replaced
  - ~2% of adult-onset hirsutism is due to partial defect in adrenal 21-hydroxylase
  - Rare patients with hyperandrogenism and hypertension have 11-hydroxylase deficiency
  - Patients with XY karyotype and deficiency of 17α-hydroxysteroid dehydrogenase-3 or 5α-reductase-2 may present as phenotypic girls who develop virilization at puberty
- Other rare causes: acromegaly; ACTH-induced Cushing's syndrome; adrenal carcinoma, genetic cortisol resistance, maternal virilization during pregnancy due to luteoma of pregnancy, hyperreactio luteinalis, or diffuse stromal Leydig cell hyperplasia in postmenopausal women
- Pharmacologic causes: minoxidil, cyclosporine, phenytoin, anabolic steroids, diazoxide, some progestins

DEMOGRAPHICS

- Most common in women with some Mediterranean ancestry

CLINICAL FINDINGS

SYMPTOMS AND SIGNS

- Increased sexual hair (chin, upper lip, abdomen, and chest)
- Acne due to increased sebaceous gland activity
- Menstrual irregularities, anovulation, and amenorrhea common
- Defeminization (breast size decrease, loss of feminine adipose tissue) and virilization (frontal balding, muscularity, clitoromegaly, and deepening of voice) if androgen excess is pronounced
- Virilization implicates presence of testosterone-producing neoplasm
- Hypertension seen in rare conditions with Cushing's syndrome, adrenal 11-hydroxylase deficiency, or cortisol resistance syndrome
- Clitoromegaly
- Ovarian enlargement may be cystic or neoplastic
- Polycystic ovary syndome associated with hypertension and hyperlipidemia

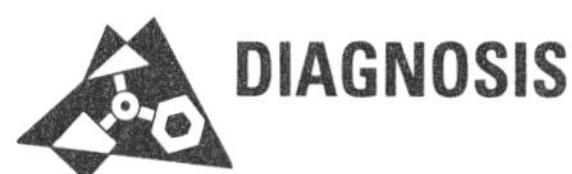

DIAGNOSIS

LABORATORY TESTS

- Serum androgens mainly useful to screen for rare occult adrenal or ovarian neoplasms
- Serum total testosterone and free testosterone. Some free testosterone assays are unreliable: free androgen index, analog free testosterone assay, electrochemical luminescence assay
- Serum testosterone >200 ng/dL or free testosterone >40 ng/dL indicates need for pelvic examination and ultrasound. If negative, perform adrenal CT scan
- Serum androstenedione >1000 ng/dL also implicates ovarian or adrenal neoplasm
- Milder elevations of testosterone or androstenedione are usually treated with oral contraceptives
- Markedly elevated serum DHEAS (>700 μg/dL) implies adrenal source of androgen, usually adrenal hyperplasia and rarely adrenal carcinoma. Perform adrenal CT scan
- Unclear which patients (if any) with hyperandrogenism should be screened for "late-onset" 21-hydroxylase deficiency, where baseline 17-hydroxyprogesterone is usually >300 ng/dL or stimulated level is >1000 ng/dL (30–60 min after 0.25 mg IM cosyntropin)
- Signs of Cushing's syndrome should prompt screening
- Follicle-stimulating hormone (FSH) and luteinizing hormone (LH) elevated if amenorrhea is due to ovarian failure
- LH:FSH ratio >2.0, hyperglycemia, and elevated fasting insulin level are common in polycystic ovary syndrome
- Selective venous sampling for testosterone may be required to diagnose small virilizing ovarian tumors not detected on ultrasound, MRI, or CT

IMAGING STUDIES

- Adrenal CT as described above
- Pelvic ultrasound or MRI to detect virilizing tumors of ovary
- Ultrasound shows polycystic ovaries in ~33% of normal young women, so test is not helpful in diagnosis of polycystic ovary syndrome

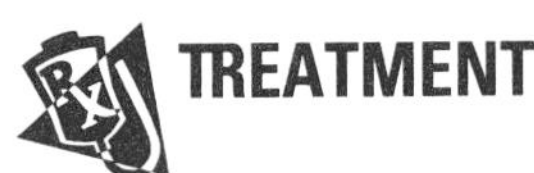

TREATMENT

MEDICATIONS

- Use medication if underlying cause not reversible
- Spironolactone, 50–100 mg PO BID on days 5–25 of menstrual cycle or QD if used concomitantly with oral contraceptive. Hyperkalemia or hyponatremia occur uncommonly
- Cyproterone acetate (not available in United States), 2 mg PO QD, is potent antiandrogen; usually given with oral contraceptive
- Finasteride, 5 mg PO QD inhibits 5α-reductase, which converts testosterone to active dihydrotestosterone in skin. Modestly reduces hirsutism over 6 months—comparable results to spironolactone. Finasteride ineffective for androgenic alopecia in women
- Flutamide, 250 mg PO QD inhibits androgen receptors and uptake. Used with oral contraceptive, likely more effective than spironolactone in improving hirsutism, acne, and male pattern baldness. Hepatotoxicity is rare
- Oral contraceptives stimulate menses, if desired, but less effective for hirsutism. Low-androgenic progestin (desogestrel, gestodene)-containing contraceptives are preferred
- Metformin, 500–1000 mg PO BID, for polycystic ovary syndrome with amenorrhea tends to restore normal menses and reduce hirsutism. Contraindicated in renal and liver disease. Does not cause hypoglycemia in nondiabetics
- Androgenic alopecia may be treated with topical minoxidil 2% solution applied BID chronically to a dry scalp. Hypertrichosis occurs in 3–5% (eg, on forehead, cheeks, upper lip, chin) and usually resolves 1–6 months after drug stopped
- **Note: Give antiandrogen treatments only to nonpregnant women—use during pregnancy causes malformations and pseudohermaphroditism in male infants. Women should take oral contraceptives when indicated and avoid pregnancy**

SURGERY

- Resection of any testosterone-secreting ovarian or adrenal tumor
- Laparoscopic bilateral oophorectomy (if CT scan of adrenals and ovaries normal) indicated in postmenopausal women with severe hyperandrogenism, since small hilar cell tumors of ovary may not be visible on scans

THERAPEUTIC PROCEDURES

- Treat underlying cause of hyperandrogenism if possible
- Discontinue any potentially offending drugs
- Encourage shaving, depilatories, waxing, electrolysis, or bleaching, and laser therapy for hirsutism

OUTCOME

FOLLOW-UP

- Check serum potassium and creatinine 1 month after starting spironolactone
- If testosterone elevated, follow serum testosterone during therapy or after surgery

PROGNOSIS

- Polycystic ovary syndrome: women frequently regain normal menstrual cycles with aging

EVIDENCE

PRACTICE GUIDELINES

- AACE Medical Guidelines for Clinical Practice: 2001 Hyperandrogenism
  - http://www.aace.com/clin/guidelines/hyperandrogenism2001.pdf
- Azziz R: The evaluation and management of hirsutism. Obstet Gynecol 2003;101(5 Pt 1):995. [PMID: 12738163]
- Claman P et al: SOGC clinical practice guidelines. Hirsutism: evaluation and treatment. J Obstet Gynaecol Can 2002;24:62. [PMID: 12196888]

WEB SITE

- University of Maryland Medicine—Hirsutism
  - http://www.umm.edu/altmed/ConsConditions/Hirsutismcc.html

INFORMATION FOR PATIENTS

- American Academy of Family Physicians—Hirsutism
  - http://familydoctor.org/handouts/210.html
- MEDLINEplus—Virilization
  - http://www.nlm.nih.gov/medlineplus/ency/article/002339.htm

REFERENCES

- Bayram F et al: Comparison of high-dose finasteride (5 mg/day) versus low-dose finasteride (2.5 mg/day) in the treatment of hirsutism. Eur J Endocrinol 2002;147:467. [PMID: 12370107]
- Farquhar C et al: Spironolactone versus placebo or in combination with steroids for hirsutism and/or acne (Cochrane Review). Cochrane Database Syst Rev 2001;4:CD000194. [PMID: 11687072]
- Ganic MA et al: Comparison of efficacy of spironolactone with metformin in the management of polycystic ovary syndrome: an open-label study. J Clin Endocrinol Metab 2004;89:2756. [PMID: 15181054]
- Kelly CJ et al: The effect of metformin on hirsutism in polycystic ovary syndrome. Eur J Endocrinol 2002;147:217. [PMID: 12153743]
- Mercke DP et al: NIH conference. Future directions in the study and management of congenital adrenal hyperplasia due to 21-hydroxylase deficiency. Ann Intern Med 2002;136:320. [PMID: 11848730]
- Venturoli S et al: Low-dose flutamide (125 mg/day) as maintenance therapy in the treatment of hirsutism. Horm Res 2001;56:25. [PMID: 11815724]

Author(s)

Paul A. Fitzgerald, MD

Histoplasmosis

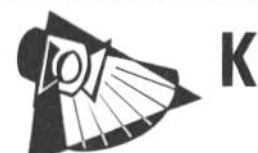

KEY FEATURES

ESSENTIALS OF DIAGNOSIS

- Infection caused by *Histoplasma capsulatum*, a dimorphic fungus isolated from soil contaminated with bird or bat droppings in endemic areas
- Most patients asymptomatic; if symptomatic, respiratory illness most common
- Dissemination in profoundly immunocompromised patients

GENERAL CONSIDERATIONS

- Acute histoplasmosis frequently occurs in epidemics, often when soil containing infected bird or bat droppings is disturbed
- Infection presumably occurs by inhalation
- The organism proliferates and is carried hematogenously from lungs to other organs
- Disseminated histoplasmosis occurs rarely in patients with normal immune function
- Dissemination common in AIDS patients, usually with CD4 counts < 100 cells/μL, and in other immunocompromised patients, with poor prognosis

DEMOGRAPHICS

- Endemic areas
  - Central and eastern United States (especially Ohio River and Mississippi River valleys)
  - Eastern Canada
  - Mexico
  - Central America
  - South America
  - Africa
  - Southeast Asia
- Disseminated disease most often occurs as reactivation of prior infection but may reflect acute infection
- Chronic progressive pulmonary histoplasmosis occurs in older patients with chronic obstructive pulmonary disease

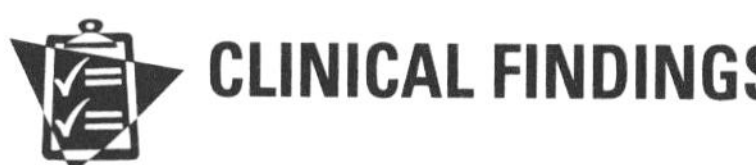

CLINICAL FINDINGS

SYMPTOMS AND SIGNS

- Most cases asymptomatic with no pulmonary symptoms or signs even in those who later have calcifications on chest x-ray
- Mild symptomatic illness: influenza-like illness, often lasting 1–4 days
- More severe illness: presents as atypical pneumonia, with fever, cough, and mild central chest pain for 5–15 days
- Physical examination usually normal
- Acute pulmonary histoplasmosis: marked prostration, fever, but few pulmonary complaints even when chest x-ray shows pneumonia
- Progressive pulmonary histoplasmosis occurs in patients with chronic pulmonary disease
  - Fever, weight loss, prostration
  - Dyspnea, cough
  - Upper lobe cavitation and fibrosis
- Mediastinal fibrosis thought to represent abnormal immune response to organisms in mediastinal lymph nodes
- Disseminated histoplasmosis occurs mainly in immunocompromised patients
  - Fever, weight loss, cough
  - Hepatomegaly, splenomegaly, lymphadenopathy
  - Gastrointestinal involvement with oral ulcers, intestinal lesions
  - Skin findings include papules, ulcers
  - Adrenal glands commonly involved
  - Meningitis and endocarditis rare
  - Shock occurs in severe cases

DIFFERENTIAL DIAGNOSIS

- Influenza
- Atypical pneumonia
- Tuberculosis
- Coccidioidomycosis
- Sarcoidosis
- Blastomycosis
- Pneumoconiosis
- *Pneumocystis jiroveci* pneumonia
- Lymphoma (including lymphocytic interstitial pneumonia)

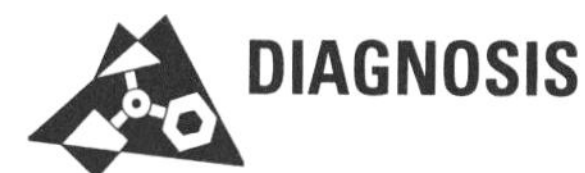

DIAGNOSIS

LABORATORY TESTS

- Elevations of alkaline phosphatase and lactate dehydrogenase (marked) and ferritin common
- Anemia of chronic disease in chronic progressive pulmonary histoplasmosis
- Sputum culture rarely positive except in chronic pulmonary histoplasmosis
- Pancytopenia from bone marrow involvement in disseminated disease
- Blood or bone marrow cultures positive in > 80% of disseminated disease in immunocompromised individuals
- Skin tests and serologic tests seldom diagnostic
- Positive histoplasmin skin test reflects past infection
- In acute pulmonary histoplasmosis: screening immunodiffusion test sensitivity 50%, complement fixation titers sensitivity ~80%, combination sensitivity up to 80% in immunocompromised
- Urine antigen test
  - Sensitivity > 90% for disseminated disease in AIDS
  - Useful to diagnose relapse
- Biopsy of affected organs with culture useful in disseminated disease

IMAGING STUDIES

- Lung and splenic calcifications on x-rays may reflect past infection
- Radiographic findings during acute illness are variable and nonspecific
- Disseminated disease in profoundly immunocompromised: chest x-ray may show a miliary pattern

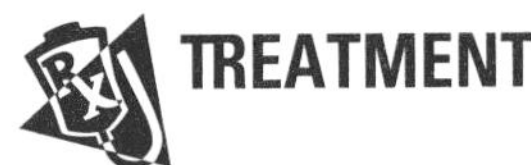

TREATMENT

MEDICATIONS

- Itraconazole is highly effective against *H capsulatum*
  - Oral itraconazole, 200-400 mg PO QD for weeks to months, can be used for progressive pulmonary disease, mild to moderate non-meningeal disease
  - Response rates of ~80% can be expected
  - Due to variable absorption, some experts recommend measuring drug levels with peak value of 4–10 μg/mL being sufficient
- Amphotericin B 0.7–1.0 mg/kg/day IV is used if patients
  - Cannot take amphotericin B orally
  - Have not responded to itraconazole
  - Have meningitis
  - Have severe disseminated disease
- Oral itraconazole can replace amphotericin once patient is stable and afebrile, which usually occurs in 3–7 days
- Relapse rates are high, especially among HIV patients in the absence of immune reconstitution so itraconazole 200 mg PO QD should be used in this situation indefinitely
  - After at least 12 months of itraconazole, secondary prophylaxis can be safely discontinued in HIV patients that have responded to antiretroviral therapy
- Treatment of endocarditis is difficult with removal of infected valve recommended along with maximal doses of amphotericin B and prolonged oral itraconazole
- Mediastinal fibrosis may not respond to antifungal therapy and itraconazole has shown the best efficacy in patients who have evidence of inflammation and not just fibrosis on biopsy of affected nodes
  - Surgery is not generally recommended in this condition because complications are common
  - Intravascular stents may be helpful in maintaining patency of central blood vessels

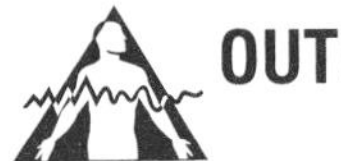

OUTCOME

PROGNOSIS

- Acute histoplasmosis: lasts from 1 week to 6 months but is almost never fatal
- Progressive disseminated histoplasmosis: usually fatal within 6 weeks or less; more rapidly in immunocompromised

PREVENTION

- Recurrence of AIDS-related histoplasmosis decreased with lifelong itraconazole, 200–400 mg PO QD; it is possible to discontinue secondary prophylaxis following adequate treatment of histoplasmosis and a sustained CD4 cell response (> 150/μL) to highly active antiretroviral therapy

EVIDENCE

PRACTICE GUIDELINES

- Practice Guidelines from the Infectious Diseases Society of America
  - http://www.journals.uchicago.edu/CID/journal/issues/v30n4/990670/990670.web.pdf2001
- USPHS/IDSA Guidelines for the Prevention of Opportunistic Infections in Persons Infected with Human Immunodeficiency Virus. US Department of Health and Human Services, Public Health Service
  - http://aidsinfo.nih.gov/guidelines/op_infectionsOI_112801.pdf

WEB SITE

- Centers for Disease Control and Prevention—Division of Bacterial and Mycotic Diseases
  - http://www.cdc.gov/ncidod/dbmd/diseaseinfo/histoplasmosis_g.htm

INFORMATION FOR PATIENTS

- Centers for Disease Control and Prevention—Division of Bacterial and Mycotic Diseases
  - http://www.cdc.gov/ncidod/dbmd/diseaseinfo/histoplasmosis_g.htm#What%20is%20histoplasmosis
- Cleveland Clinic—OHS
  - http://www.clevelandclinic.org/health/health-info/docs/0900/0998.asp?index=5635
- National Institute of Allergy and Infectious Diseases
  - http://www.aegis.com/news/niaid/1994/NA941102.html

REFERENCES

- Goldman M et al: Safety of discontinuation of maintenance therapy for disseminated histoplasmosis after immunologic response to antiretroviral therapy. Clin Infect Dis 2004;38:1485. [PMID: 15156489]
- Johnson PC et al: Safety and efficacy of liposomal amphotericin B compared with conventional amphotericin B for induction therapy of histoplasmosis in patients with AIDS. Ann Intern Med 2002;137:105. [PMID: 12118965]
- Mocherla S et al: Treatment of histoplasmosis. Semin Respir Infect 2001;16:141. [PMID: 11521246]

Author(s)

Richard J. Hamill, MD

Samuel A. Shelburne, MD

HIV Infection

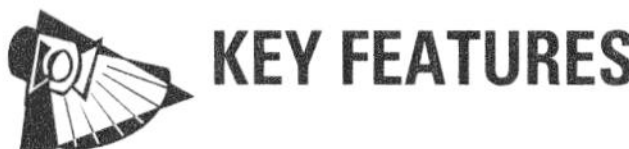

KEY FEATURES

ESSENTIALS OF DIAGNOSIS

- Risk factors: sexual contact with an infected person, parenteral exposure to infected blood by transfusion or needle sharing, perinatal exposure
- Opportunistic infections due to diminished cellular immunity—often life-threatening
- Aggressive cancers, particularly Kaposi's sarcoma and extranodal lymphoma
- Neurologic manifestations: dementia, aseptic meningitis, and neuropathy

GENERAL CONSIDERATIONS

- Definition: Centers for Disease Control and Prevention AIDS case definition (Table 120)
- Etiology: HIV-1, a retrovirus

DEMOGRAPHICS

- In 2002, HIV infection in
  - ~40 million persons worldwide
  - ~700,000 Americans
- In 2002, AIDS in ~384,000 Americans: 51% are gay or bisexual men; 26% are heterosexual injection drug users; 21% are heterosexual noninjection drug users; and 22% are women

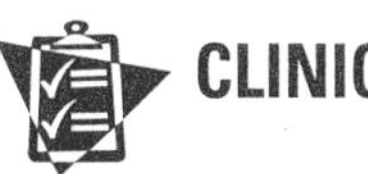

CLINICAL FINDINGS

SYMPTOMS AND SIGNS

- HIV-related infections and neoplasms affect virtually every organ
- Many HIV-infected persons remain asymptomatic for years even without antiretroviral therapy, with a mean time of approximately 10 years between exposure and development of AIDS
- Symptoms protean and nonspecific
- Fever, night sweats, and weight loss
- Shortness of breath, cough, and fever from pneumonia
- Anorexia, nausea and vomiting, and increased metabolic rate contribute to weight loss
- Diarrhea from infections with bacterial, viral, or parasitic agents
- Physical examination may be normal. Hairy leukoplakia of the tongue, disseminated Kaposi's sarcoma, and cutaneous bacillary angiomatosis are predictive of AIDS; cutaneous anergy is common
- Ocular: cytomegalovirus (CMV), herpesvirus, or toxoplasmosis retinitis
- Oral: candidiasis, pseudomembranous (removable white plaques) and erythematous (red friable plaques); hairy leukoplakia; angular cheilitis; gingivitis or periodontitis; aphthous ulcers; Kaposi's sarcoma (usually on the hard palate); and warts
- Sinuses: chronic sinusitis
- Lungs: bacterial (eg, *Steptococcus pneumoniae, Haemophilus influenzae*), mycobacterial [eg, *Mycobacterium tuberculosis, M avium* complex (MAC)], fungal (eg, *Pneumocystis jiroveci*), and viral pneumonias. Noninfectious: Kaposi's sarcoma, non-Hodgkin's lymphoma, and interstitial pneumonitis
- Gastrointestinal: esophagitis (*Candida*, herpes simplex, CMV); gastropathy and malabsorption. Enterocolitis: bacteria (*Campylobacter, Salmonella, Shigella*), viruses (CMV, adenovirus, HIV), and protozoans (*Cryptosporidium, Entamoeba histolytica, Giardia, Isospora, Microsporidia*)
- Hepatic: liver infections (mycobacterial, CMV, hepatitis B and C viruses) and neoplasms (lymphoma), and medication-related hepatitis
- Biliary: cholecystitis, sclerosing cholangitis, and papillary stenosis (CMV, *Cryptosporidium*, and *Microsporidia*)
- Central nervous system (CNS): intracerebral space-occupying lesions (eg, toxoplasmosis, bacterial and nocardia abscesses, cryptococcomas, tuberculomas), HIV encephalopathy, meningitis, CNS (non-Hodgkin's) lymphoma, progressive multifocal leukoencephalopathy (PML)
- Spinal cord: HIV myelopathy
- Peripheral nervous system: inflammatory polyneuropathies, sensory neuropathies, and mononeuropathies; CMV polyradiculopathy; transverse myelitis (herpes zoster or CMV)
- Endocrinologic: adrenal insufficiency from infection (eg, CMV and MAC), infiltration (Kaposi's sarcoma), hemorrhage, and presumed autoimmune injury; isolated mineralocorticoid defect; thyroid function test abnormalities (high T3, T4, and thyroxine-binding globulin, and low reverse-T3)
- Gynecologic: vaginal candidiasis, cervical dysplasia and carcinoma, and pelvic inflammatory disease
- Malignancies: Kaposi's sarcoma, non-Hodgkin's and Hodgkin's lymphoma, primary CNS lymphoma, cervical dysplasia and invasive cervical carcinoma, anal dysplasia and squamous cell carcinoma
- Skin: viral (herpes simplex, herpes zoster, *Molluscum contagiosum*), bacterial (*Staphylococcus* folliculitis, furuncles, bullous impetigo, dissemination with sepsis; bacillary angiomatosis caused by *Bartonella henselae* and *B quintana*), fungal (*Candida*, dermatophytes, *Malassezia furfur/Pityrosporum ovale* seborrheic dermatitis), neoplastic (Kaposi's sarcoma), and nonspecific (psoriasis, severe pruritus, xerosis) dermatitides
- Musculoskeletal: myopathy; arthritis of single or multiple joints, with or without effusions; reactive arthritis (Reiter's syndrome); psoriatic arthritis; sicca syndrome, and systemic lupus erythematosus

DIFFERENTIAL DIAGNOSIS

- Cancer; chronic infections, such as tuberculosis and endocarditis; endocrinologic diseases, such as hyperthyroidism; acute and chronic lung infections; diffuse interstitial pulmonary infiltrates; alcoholism; liver disease; renal dysfunction; vitamin deficiency; chronic meningitis; infectious enterocolitis; antibiotic-associated colitis; inflammatory bowel disease; and malabsorption syndromes

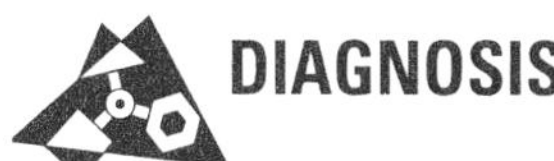

DIAGNOSIS

LABORATORY TESTS

- Lab findings in HIV infection (Table 121)
- HIV antibody by ELISA, confirmed by Western blot (sensitivity > 99.5%, specificity ~100%)
- ~95% of persons develop antibodies within 6 weeks after infection
- Absolute CD4 lymphocyte count: as counts decrease, risk of serious opportunistic infection over the subsequent 3–5 years increases

IMAGING STUDIES

- Tests for CNS toxoplasmosis: head CT scan, stereotactic brain biopsy
- Tests for HIV myelopathy: lumbar puncture and head MRI or CT scan

DIAGNOSTIC PROCEDURES

- For *P jiroveci* pneumonia: arterial blood gases, serum lactate dehydrogenase, chest x-ray, Wright-Giemsa stain of induced sputum, bronchoalveolar lavage
- For cryptococcal meningitis: cerebrospinal fluid (CSF) culture; CSF, serum CRAG
- For HIV meningitis: CSF cell count
- For AIDS dementia complex, depression: neuropsychiatric testing
- For myopathy: creatine kinase; muscle biopsy

- For hepatic dysfunction: percutaneous liver biopsy; blood culture, biopsy of a more accessible site
- For enterocolitis: stool culture and multiple ova and parasite examinations; colonoscopy and biopsy

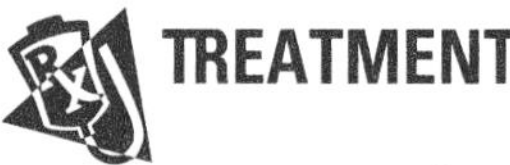

TREATMENT

MEDICATIONS

- Fever: antipyretics
- Anorexia: megestrol acetate, 80 mg QID or dronabinol, 2.5–5 mg TID
- Weight loss: food supplementation with high-calorie drinks; growth hormone, 0.1 mg/kg/day SQ for 12 weeks, or anabolic steroids—oxandrolone, 15–20 mg PO in 2–4 divided doses; testosterone enanthate or cypionate, 100–200 mg IM Q 2–4 weeks; or testosterone patches or gel
- Nausea: prochlorperazine, 10 mg PO TID QAC; metoclopramide, 10 mg PO TID QAC; or ondansetron, 8 mg PO TID QAC; empiric oral antifungal agent
- Antiretroviral treatment when CD4 count < 350 cells/μL (Table 124)
- Common opportunistic infections and malignancies (Table 123)

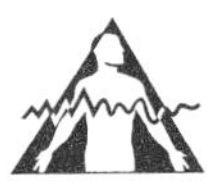

OUTCOME

FOLLOW-UP

- CD4 cell counts Q 3–6 months
- Viral load tests Q 3–6 months, and 1 month after change in therapy
- Health care maintenance (Table 122)

PROGNOSIS

- The efficacy of antiretroviral treatments—especially protease inhibitors or nonnucleoside reverse transcriptase inhibitors—has improved prognosis

WHEN TO REFER

- Refer for advice regarding change of antiretroviral therapy, including interpretation of resistance tests
- Refer for management of complicated opportunistic infections

WHEN TO ADMIT

- For new unexplained fever if bacterial infection requiring IV antibiotics is suspected
- As indicated by acute organ system dysfunction or acute change in mental status

PREVENTION

Primary prevention

- Precautions regarding sexual practices and injection drug use (safer sex, latex condoms, and clean needle use); perinatal HIV prophylaxis; screening of blood products; and infection control practices in the health care setting

Secondary prevention

- For *P jiroveci* pneumonia when CD4 counts < 200 cells/μL, a CD4 lymphocyte percentage < 14%, or weight loss or oral candidiasis: trimethoprim-sulfamethoxazole, aerosolized pentamidine, or dapsone (Table 125)
- For MAC infection when CD4 counts < 75–100 cells/μL: azithromycin (1200 mg PO Q week), clarithromycin (500 mg PO BID), or rifabutin (300 mg PO QD)
- For *M tuberculosis* infection when positive PPD reactions > 5 mm of induration: isoniazid, 300 mg PO QD plus pyridoxine, 50 mg PO QD for 9–12 months
- For toxoplasmosis when positive IgG toxoplasma serology: trimethoprim-sulfamethoxazole (1 DS tablet PO QD), or pyrimethamine, 25 mg PO Q week plus dapsone, 100 mg PO QD
- For cryptococcosis, candidiasis, other fungi: fluconazole, 200 mg PO QD

EVIDENCE

PRACTICE GUIDELINES

- Department of Health and Human Services: Guidelines for the use of antiretroviral agents in HIV-infected adults and adolescents. October 2004.
  - http://www.hivatis.org

WEB SITES

- AIDS Info—US Department of Health and Human Services
  - http://aidsinfo.nih.gov
- Center for HIV Information, University of California—San Francisco
  - http://hivinsite.ucsf.edu/
- Johns Hopkins AIDS Service
  - http://www.hopkins-aids.edu/
- National Institutes of Health—National Institute of Allergy and Infectious Diseases—Division of AIDS
  - http://www.niaid.nih.gov/daids/

INFORMATION FOR PATIENTS

- AIDS Info—US Department of Health and Human Services
  - http://aidsinfo.nih.gov/ed_resources/default.asp?Cat_ID=P
- CDC—American Social Health Association: Hotline information and FAQs
  - http://www.ashastd.org/nah/tty/ttyfaq.html
- CDC—National AIDS Hotline: 1-800-342-AIDS
- JAMA Patient Page. HIV Infection: The Basics. JAMA 2004;292:296. Available at
  - http://www.medem.com/medlb/article_detaillb.cfm?article_ID=ZZZN6UVAG3D&sub_cat=329 (nonsubscribers)
  - http://jama.ama-assn.org/cgi/reprint/292/2/296 (subscribers only)
- MedlinePlus: Interactive AIDS tutorial
  - http://www.nlm.nih.gov/medlineplus/tutorials/aids/htm/index.htm
- National Institutes of Health—National Institute of Allergy and Infectious Diseases
  - http://www.niaid.nih.gov/factsheets/hivinf.htm (basic HIV information)
  - http://www.niaid.nih.gov/factsheets/howhiv.htm (how HIV causes AIDS)
- Project Inform (nonprofit AIDS support organization)
  - http://www.projinf.org/
- The Body (AIDS resource clearinghouse)
  - http://www.thebody.com

REFERENCES

- Benson CA et al; CDC, National Institutes of Health; Infectious Diseases Society of America: Treating opportunistic infections among HIV-exposed and infected children: recommendations from CDC, the National Institutes of Health, and the Infectious Diseases Society of America. MMWR Recomm Rep 2004;53(RR-15):1. Erratum in MMWR Recomm Rep 2005;54:311. [PMID: 15841069]
- Yeni PG et al: Treatment for adult HIV infection: 2004 recommendations of the International AIDS Society USA-Panel. JAMA 2004;292:251. [PMID: 15249575]

Author(s)

Mitchell H. Katz, MD
Andrew R. Zolopa, MD
Harry Hollander, MD

Hoarseness, Dysphonia, & Stridor

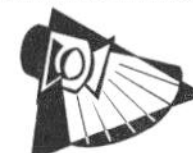

KEY FEATURES

ESSENTIALS OF DIAGNOSIS

- The primary symptoms of laryngeal disease are hoarseness and stridor

GENERAL CONSIDERATIONS

- Hoarseness is caused by an abnormal flow of air past the vocal cords
- Laryngitis, voice abuse, and vocal cord nodules are common causes of hoarseness

Acute hoarseness

- Acute laryngitis is thought to be viral in origin, although *Moraxella catarrhalis* and *Haemophilus influenzae* isolates from the nasopharynx occur at higher than expected frequencies

Persistent hoarseness

- Vocal cord nodules or polyps (from overuse of voice or improper use over extended periods of time) produce prolonged hoarseness
- Vocal cord polypoid changes (from vocal abuse, smoking, chemical industrial irritants, or hypothyroidism)
- Gastroesophageal reflux is a common cause of chronic hoarseness and should be considered if other causes of abnormal laryngeal airflow (such as tumor) have been excluded by laryngoscopy; less than 50% of patients have typical symptoms of heartburn and regurgitation
- In patients with a history of tobacco use, laryngeal cancer or lung cancer (leading to paralysis of a recurrent laryngeal nerve) must be strongly considered in persistent hoarseness

DEMOGRAPHICS

- Acute laryngitis is the most common cause of hoarseness

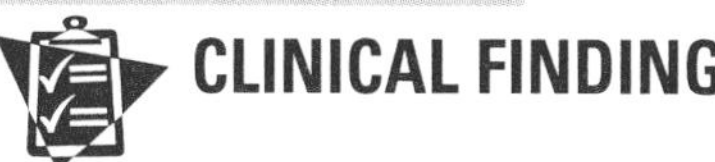

CLINICAL FINDINGS

SYMPTOMS AND SIGNS

- The voice is "breathy" when too much air passes incompletely apposed vocal cords, as in unilateral vocal cord paralysis
- The voice is harsh when turbulence is created by irregularity of the vocal cords, as in laryngitis or a mass lesion
- Stridor, a high-pitched sound, is produced by lesions that narrow the airway
  - Airway narrowing above the vocal cords produces predominantly inspiratory stridor
  - Airway narrowing below the vocal cords produces either expiratory or mixed stridor
- In gastroesophageal reflux-induced hoarseness, the voice is usually worse in the morning and improves during the day; associated symptoms include a feeling of a lump in the throat or an excessive desire for throat clearing

DIFFERENTIAL DIAGNOSIS

- Laryngitis
- Voice overuse
- Vocal cord nodules, polyps, or papillomas
- Intubation granulomas
- Laryngeal cancer
- Lung cancer
- Unilateral vocal cord paralysis
- Hypothyroidism
- Retrosternal goiter, thyroiditis, multinodular goiter, or thyroid carcinoma
- Gastroesophageal reflux
- Angioedema

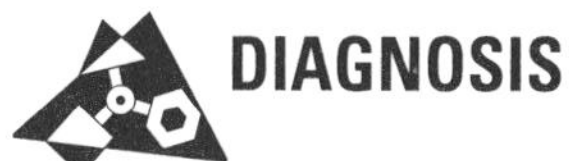

DIAGNOSIS

IMAGING STUDIES

- Consider chest x-ray for tumor

DIAGNOSTIC PROCEDURES

- Evaluation of an abnormal voice begins with obtaining a history of the circumstances preceding its onset and an examination of the airway
- Indirect or flexible laryngoscopy and at times videostrobolaryngoscopy
- In gastroesophageal reflux, nonresponders to medical management should undergo pH testing and manometry

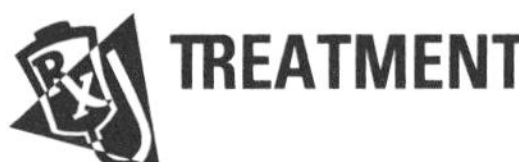

TREATMENT

MEDICATIONS

- Erythromycin may reduce the severity of hoarseness and cough in acute laryngitis

Vocal cord polypoid changes

- Attention to the underlying cause may resolve the problem
- Inhaled steroid spray (eg, beclomethasone, 42 μg/spray, or dexamethasone, 84 μg/spray, two or three times a day) may hasten resolution

Gastroesophageal reflux

- Empiric trial of a proton pump inhibitor at twice-daily dosing (eg, omeprazole, 20 mg PO twice daily) for 2–3 months as a practical alternative to an initial pH study
- If symptoms improve and cessation of therapy leads to recurrence of symptoms, resume a proton pump inhibitor at the lowest dose effective for remission, usually daily but at times on a demand basis
- H_2 receptor antagonists are generally less clinically effective

SURGERY

- Recalcitrant nodules or polyps may require excision

OUTCOME

COMPLICATIONS

- In hoarseness from acute laryngitis, patients should avoid vigorous use of the voice (singing, shouting) while laryngitis is present to avoid formation of vocal nodules

PROGNOSIS

Acute laryngitis

- Self-limited
- May persist for 1–2 weeks after other symptoms of upper respiratory tract infection have cleared

Vocal nodules

- Benign condition

WHEN TO REFER

- Refer to an otolaryngologist when hoarseness lasts longer than 2 weeks or has no obvious cause
- Refer to a speech therapist for modification of voice habits for vocal cord polyps

PREVENTION

- Prevent vocal abuse, particularly among singers
- Modification of voice habits to avoid formation of vocal cord nodules

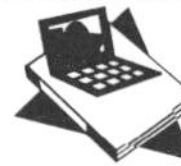

EVIDENCE

PRACTICE GUIDELINES

- Dejonckere PH et al: A basic protocol for functional assessment of voice pathology, especially for investigating the efficacy of (phonosurgical) treatments and evaluating new assessment techniques. Guideline elaborated by the Committee on Phoniatrics of the European Laryngological Society (ELS). Eur Arch Otorhinolaryngol 2001;258:77. [PMID: 11307610]

WEB SITES

- American Academy of Otolaryngology—Head and Neck Surgery: Hoarseness Interactive Module
  - http://www.entnet.org/education/COOL/hoarse_intro.cfm
- Baylor College of Medicine Otolaryngology Resources: Laryngology
  - http://www.bcm.edu/oto/othersa5.html

INFORMATION FOR PATIENTS

- American Academy of Otolaryngology—Head and Neck Surgery: Doctor, Why Am I Hoarse?
  - http://www.entnet.org/healthinfo/throat/hoarse.cfm
- American Academy of Otolaryngology—Head and Neck Surgery: Most Common Voice Disorders
  - http://www.entnet.org/healthinfo/throat/common-disorders.cfm
- American Academy of Otolaryngology—Head and Neck Surgery: Understanding Vocal Cord Lesions: Nodules, Polyps, and Cysts
  - http://www.entnet.org/healthinfo/throat/vocal-cord-lesions.cfm

REFERENCES

- Garrett CG et al: Hoarseness. Med Clin North Am 1999;83:115. [PMID: 9927964]
- MacKenzie K et al: Is voice therapy an effective treatment for dysphonia? A randomised controlled trial. BMJ 2001;323:658. [PMID: 11566828]
- Sataloff RT: Professional voice users: the evaluation of voice disorders. Occup Med 2001;16:633. [PMID: 11567923]

Author(s)

Robert K. Jackler, MD
Michael J. Kaplan, MD

Hodgkin's Disease

KEY FEATURES

ESSENTIALS OF DIAGNOSIS

- Painless lymphadenopathy
- Constitutional symptoms may or may not be present
- Pathological diagnosis by lymph node biopsy

GENERAL CONSIDERATIONS

- Group of cancers characterized by Reed-Sternberg cells in appropriate reactive cellular background
- Nature of the malignant cell is subject of controversy, probably B cells
- Divided into several subtypes: lymphocyte predominance, nodular sclerosis, mixed cellularity, and lymphocyte depletion
- Important feature of Hodgkin's disease: tendency to arise within single lymph node areas and spread in orderly fashion to contiguous lymph nodes
- Widespread hematogenous dissemination only late in course

DEMOGRAPHICS

- Bimodal age distribution: one peak at age 20–30 and second peak at age > 50

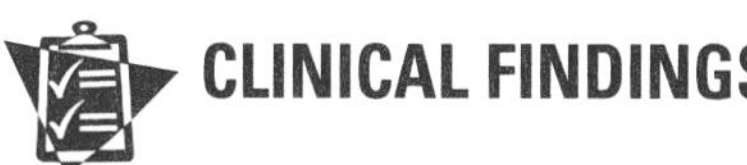

CLINICAL FINDINGS

SYMPTOMS AND SIGNS

- Painless lymphadenopathy (mass), commonly in neck
- Constitutional symptoms, eg, fever, weight loss, or drenching night sweats, or generalized pruritus
- Pain in involved lymph node after alcohol ingestion is an unusual symptom

DIFFERENTIAL DIAGNOSIS

- Non-Hodgkin's lymphoma
- Tuberculous lymphadenitis (scrofula)
- Cat-scratch disease
- Sarcoidosis
- Metastatic cancer
- Drug-induced pseudolymphoma (eg, phenytoin)

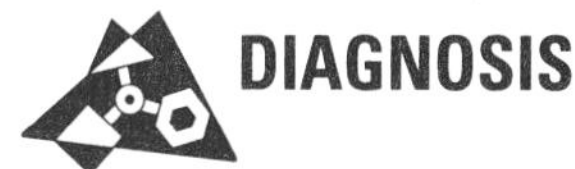

DIAGNOSIS

DIAGNOSTIC PROCEDURES

- Lymph node biopsy establishes pathological diagnosis
- Staging usually clinical; laparotomy no longer routinely performed
- Staging nomenclature (Ann Arbor): stage I, one lymph node region involved; stage II, involvement of two lymph node areas on one side of diaphragm; stage III, lymph node regions involved on both sides of diaphragm; stage IV, disseminated disease with bone marrow or liver involvement
- In addition, designated as stage A if there is a lack of constitutional symptoms and stage B if there is a 10% weight loss over 6 months, fever, or night sweats ("B symptoms")

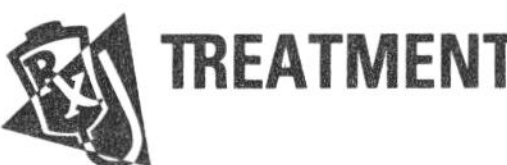

TREATMENT

MEDICATIONS

- Combination chemotherapy involving doxorubicin (Adriamycin), bleomycin, vincristine, and dacarbazine (ABVD) for most patients (including all stage IIIB and IV disease)
- Shorter and more intensive regimens have produced promising results and may supplant ABVD in treatment of advanced disease
- Addition of limited chemotherapy for some patients treated with radiation appears promising

THERAPEUTIC PROCEDURES

- All patients with both localized and disseminated disease should be treated with curative intent
- Radiation therapy is initial treatment only for patients with low-risk stage IA and IIA disease
- High-dose chemotherapy with autologous stem cell transplantation is treatment of choice for relapse after initial chemotherapy

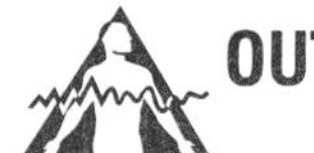

OUTCOME

PROGNOSIS

- Excellent prognosis for stage IA or IIA disease treated by radiotherapy: 10-year survival rates > 80%
- Disseminated disease (stage IIIB, IV): 5-year survival rates of 50–60%
- Prognosis is poorer in patients who are older, who have bulky disease, and who have lymphocyte depletion or mixed cellularity Hodgkin's
- Recurrent disease after initial radiotherapy may still be curable with chemotherapy
- High-dose chemotherapy with autologous stem cell transplantation for relapse offers 35–50% chance of cure if disease is still chemotherapy sensitive

EVIDENCE

PRACTICE GUIDELINES

- Ferme C et al: Hodgkin's disease. Br J Cancer 2001;84(Suppl 2):55. [PMID: 11355971]
- Hoppe RT et al: NCCN Hodgkins Disease Practice Guidelines Panel. National Comprehensive Cancer Network: Hodgkin's Disease v.2.2005
  - http://www.nccn.org/professionals/physician_gls/PDF/hodgkins.pdf

WEB SITES

- National Cancer Institute: Adult Hodgkins Lymphoma: Treatment
  - http://www.cancer.gov/cancertopics/pdq/treatment/adulthodgkins/HealthProfessional

INFORMATION FOR PATIENTS

- American Cancer Society: What Is Hodgkin's Disease?
  - http://www.cancer.org/docroot/cri/content/cri_2_4_1x_what_is_hodgkins_disease_20.asp?sitearea=cri
- Leukemia & Lymphoma Society: Hodgkin Lymphoma
  - http://www.leukemia-lymphoma.org/all_page?item_id=7085
- National Cancer Institute: Hodgkin's Disease
  - http://www.cancer.gov/cancerinfo/wyntk/hodgkins

REFERENCES

- Aleman BM et al: Involved-field radiotherapy for advanced Hodgkin's lymphoma. N Engl J Med 2003;348:2396. [PMID: 12802025]
- Bonadonna G et al: ABVD plus subtotal nodal versus involved-field radiotherapy in early-stage Hodgkin's disease: long-term results. J Clin Oncol 2004;22:2835. [PMID: 15199092]
- Diehl V et al: Standard and increased dose BEACOPP chemotherapy compared with COPP-ABUD for advanced Hodgkin's disease. N Engl J Med 2003;348:2386. [PMID: 12802024]

Author(s)

Charles A. Linker, MD

Hookworm Disease

KEY FEATURES

ESSENTIALS OF DIAGNOSIS

Early findings (not commonly recognized)

- Dermatitis: pruritic, erythematous, papulovesicular eruption at site of larval invasion
- Pulmonary migration of larvae: transient episodes of coughing, asthma, fever, blood-tinged sputum, marked eosinophilia

Later findings

- Intestinal symptoms: anorexia, diarrhea, abdominal discomfort
- Anemia (iron deficiency): fatigue, pallor, dyspnea on exertion, poikilonychia, heart failure
- Characteristic eggs and occult blood in the stool

GENERAL CONSIDERATIONS

- The disease, widespread in the moist tropics and subtropics and sporadically in southeastern United States, is caused by *Ancylostoma duodenale* and *Necator americanus*
- Infection is rare in regions with less than 40 inches of rainfall annually
- Humans are the only host for both species
- The worms suck blood at their attachment sites. Blood loss is proportionate to the worm burden. Over years—and depending on the host's dietary intake of iron—iron reserves can be depleted and severe anemia can result

DEMOGRAPHICS

- Probably 25% of the world's population is infected, and in many areas the infection is a major cause of general debility, retardation of growth and development of children, and increased susceptibility to infection
- Prevalence rates can reach 80% in the humid tropics under unsanitary conditions

CLINICAL FINDINGS

SYMPTOMS AND SIGNS

Ground itch

- The first manifestation of infection
- A pruritic erythematous dermatitis, either maculopapular or vesicular, that follows skin penetration of the infective larvae
- Severity is a function of the number of invading larvae and the sensitivity of the host
- Scratching may result in secondary infection

The pulmonary stage

- Occurs when there is larval migration through the lungs
- There may be a dry cough, wheezing, blood-tinged sputum, and low-grade fever
- In heavy infections, there may be anorexia, diarrhea, vague abdominal pain, and ulcer-like epigastric symptoms
- Severe anemia may result in pallor, deformed nails, pica, and cardiac decompensation
- Marked protein loss may also occur, resulting in hypoalbuminemia, with edema and ascites

DIFFERENTIAL DIAGNOSIS

- Ascariasis
- Strongyloidiasis
- Paragonimiasis
- Tapeworm (especially *Diphylobothrium latum* with associated anemia)
- Tuberculosis
- Allergic bronchopulmonary aspergillosis (ABPA)
- *Mycoplasma pneumoniae* infection
- Iron-deficiency anemia due to other causes, eg, gastrointestinal malignancy

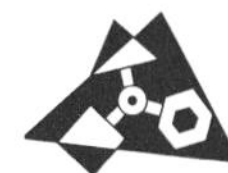

DIAGNOSIS

LABORATORY TESTS

- Diagnosis depends on demonstration of characteristic eggs in feces; a concentration method may be needed. The two species cannot be differentiated by the appearance of their eggs
- The stool usually contains occult blood
- Hypochromic microcytic anemia can be severe, with hemoglobin levels as low as 2 g/dL, a low serum iron and a high iron-binding capacity, and low serum ferritin
- Eosinophilia (as high as 30–60% of a total white blood cell count reaching 17,000/μL) is usually present in the pulmonary migratory stage of infection but is not marked in the chronic intestinal stage

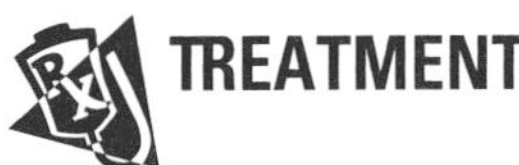

TREATMENT

MEDICATIONS

- Light infections may not need treatment
- Mebendazole, pyrantel, and albendazole are effective drugs for treatment of both hookworm species; mebendazole or albendazole can be used to treat concurrent trichuriasis, and all three drugs can be used to treat concurrent ascariasis. The drugs are given after meals, without purges. None of the three drugs should be used in pregnancy
- Albendazole (400 mg) PO or mebendazole (500 mg) PO is being used for repeated (up to 3 times yearly) mass treatment of children for intestinal parasites (hookworm, ascariasis, trichuriasis). Drug resistance may be emerging

Pyrantel pamoate

- In *A duodenale* infections, pyrantel given as a single oral dose, 10 mg (base)/kg (maximum 1 g), produces cures in 75–98% of cases and a marked reduction in the worm burden in the remainder
- For *N americanus* infections, a single dose may give a satisfactory cure rate in light infection, but for moderate or heavy infection a 3-day course is necessary
- If the species is unknown, treat as for necatoriasis
- Mild and transient drowsiness and headache may occur

Mebendazole

- Mebendazole 100 mg PO BID for 3 days produces cure rates of 35–95% from both hookworm species
- A single 500-mg dose may be sufficient for light infections

Albendazole

- Albendazole 400 mg PO given once results in the cure of 85–95% of patients with *Ancylostoma* infection and markedly reduces the worm burden in those not cured
- Treatment for *Necator* infection should be continued for 2–3 days, especially in heavy infections

Ferrous sulfate

- If anemia is present, give ferrous sulfate 200 mg PO TID for 2 months, then 200 mg QD for 4 months
- Include a diet high in protein and vitamins for at least 3 months after the anemia has been corrected to replace iron stores
- Parenteral iron is rarely indicated. Blood transfusion may be necessary if anemia is severe

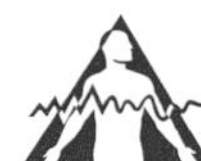

OUTCOME

FOLLOW-UP

- Eradication of infection is not essential, since light infections do not injure the well-nourished patient and iron loss is replaced if the patient is receiving adequate dietary iron
- Retreatment of heavy infections may be necessary at 2-week intervals until the worm burden is reduced to a low level as estimated by semiquantitative egg counts

EVIDENCE

WEB SITE

- CDC—Division of Parasitic Diseases
  - http://www.cdc.gov/ncidod/dpd/parasites/hookworm/default.htm

INFORMATION FOR PATIENTS

- Centers for Disease Control
  - http://www.cdc.gov/ncidod/dpd/parasites/hookworm/factsht_hookworm.htm
- National Institutes of Health
  - http://www.nlm.nih.gov/medlineplus/ency/article/000629.htm

REFERENCES

- Loukas A et al: Immune responses in hookworm infections. Clin Microbiol Rev 2001;14(4):689. [PMID: 11585781]
- Utzinger J et al: Reduction in the prevalence and intensity of hookworm infections after praziquantel treatment for schistosomiasis infection. Int J Parasitol 2002;32(6):759. [PMID: 12062494]

Huntington's Disease

KEY FEATURES

ESSENTIALS OF DIAGNOSIS

- Gradual onset and progression of chorea and dementia or behavioral change
- Family history of the disorder
- Responsible gene identified on chromosome 4

GENERAL CONSIDERATIONS

- Inherited in an autosomal dominant manner and occurs throughout the world, in all ethnic groups, with a prevalence rate of about 5 per 100,000
- The gene responsible for the disease has been located on the short arm of chromosome 4. At 4p16.3 there is an expanded and unstable CAG trinucleotide repeat
- Offspring should be offered genetic counseling. Genetic testing permits presymptomatic detection and definitive diagnosis of the disease

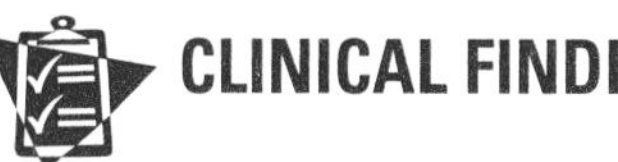

CLINICAL FINDINGS

SYMPTOMS AND SIGNS

- Clinical onset is usually between 30 and 50 years of age
- **Initial symptoms** may consist of either abnormal movements or intellectual changes, but ultimately both occur
- The earliest **mental changes** are often behavioral, with irritability, moodiness, antisocial behavior, or a psychiatric disturbance, but a more obvious dementia subsequently develops
- The **dyskinesia** may initially be no more than an apparent fidgetiness or restlessness, but eventually choreiform movements and some dystonic posturing occur
- **Progressive rigidity** and **akinesia** (rather than chorea) sometimes occur in association with dementia, especially in cases with childhood onset

DIFFERENTIAL DIAGNOSIS

- Chorea developing with no family history of choreoathetosis should not be attributed to Huntington's disease, at least not until other causes of chorea have been excluded clinically and by appropriate laboratory studies
- In younger patients, self-limiting Sydenham's chorea develops after group A streptococcal infections on rare occasions
- Other nongenetic causes of chorea include stroke, systemic lupus erythematosus and related disorders, paraneoplastic syndromes, infection with HIV, and various medications
- If a patient presents solely with progressive intellectual failure, it may not be possible to distinguish Huntington's disease from other causes of dementia unless there is a characteristic family history or a dyskinesia develops
- A clinically similar autosomal dominant disorder (dentatorubral-pallidoluysian atrophy), manifested by chorea, dementia, ataxia, and myoclonic epilepsy, is uncommon except in persons of Japanese ancestry. It is due to a mutant gene mapping to 12p13.31

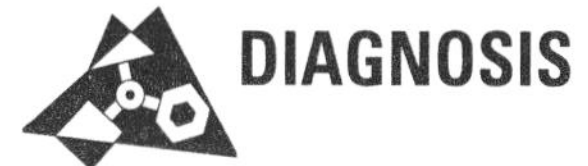

DIAGNOSIS

IMAGING STUDIES

- CT scanning usually demonstrates cerebral atrophy and atrophy of the caudate nucleus in established cases
- MRI and positron emission tomography (PET) have shown reduced glucose utilization in an anatomically normal caudate nucleus

Human T-Cell Lymphotrophic Virus (HTLV) p. 1092

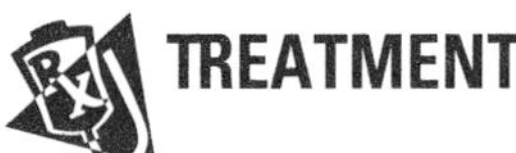

TREATMENT

MEDICATIONS

- Treatment with drugs blocking dopamine receptors, such as phenothiazines or haloperidol, may control the dyskinesia and any behavioral disturbances
- Initial haloperidol dose is 1 mg PO QD or BID, which is then increased every 3 or 4 days depending on the response
- Tetrabenazine, a drug that depletes central monoamines, is widely used in Europe to treat dyskinesia but is not available in the United States
- Reserpine is similar in its actions to tetrabenazine and may be helpful; the daily dose is built up gradually to between 2 and 5 mg PO, depending on the response
- Behavioral disturbances may respond to clozapine
- Attempts to compensate for the relative gamma-aminobutyric acid (GABA) deficiency by enhancing central GABA activity or to compensate for the relative cholinergic underactivity by giving choline chloride have not been therapeutically helpful
- The therapeutic response to cysteamine (a selective depleter of somatostatin in the brain) is currently under study

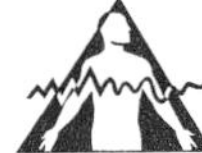

OUTCOME

PROGNOSIS

- There is no cure for Huntington's disease; progression cannot be halted; and treatment is purely symptomatic
- It usually leads to a fatal outcome within 15–20 years

WHEN TO REFER

- All patients may benefit from practitioners with particular expertise in this area
- Offspring should be offered genetic counseling

PREVENTION

- Genetic counseling is important

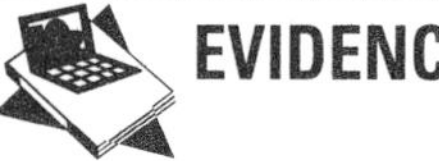

EVIDENCE

PRACTICE GUIDELINES

- International Huntington Association and the World Federation of Neurology Research Group on Huntington's Chorea. Guidelines for the molecular genetics predictive test in Huntington's disease. J Med Genet 1994;31:555. [PMID: 7966192]
- National Guideline Clearinghouse
  - http://www.guideline.gov/summary/summary.aspx?doc_id=1968&nbr=1194&string=huntingtons+disease

WEB SITE

- National Institute of Neurological Disorders and Stroke
  - http://www.ninds.nih.gov/health_and_medical/disorders/huntington.htm

INFORMATION FOR PATIENTS

- Huntington's Disease Society of America
  - http://www.hdsa.org/
- The Mayo Clinic
  - http://www.mayoclinic.com/invoke.cfm?id=DS00401

REFERENCES

- Cardosi F: Chorea: non-genetic causes. Curr Opin Neurol 2004;17:433. [PMID: 15247538]
- MacDonald ME et al: Huntington's disease. Neuromolecular Med 2003;4:7. [PMID: 14528049]
- Rosenblatt A et al: Predictors of neuropathological severity in 100 patients with Huntington's disease. Ann Neurol 2003;54:488. [PMID: 14520661]

Author(s)

Michael J. Aminoff, MD, DSc, FRCP

Hydatidiform Mole & Choriocarcinoma

KEY FEATURES

ESSENTIALS OF DIAGNOSIS

- Uterine bleeding
- Pathologic demonstration of choriocarcinoma in samples of a pelvic or vaginal mass, or in a metastatic tumor
- Hydatidiform mole
  - Amenorrhea
  - Irregular uterine bleeding
  - Serum human chorionic gonadotropin (hCG)-β subunit > 40,000 mU/mL
  - Passage of grape-like clusters of enlarged edematous villi per vagina
  - Ultrasound of uterus with characteristic "snowstorm" image and no fetus or placenta
  - Cytogenetic composition is 46,XX (85%) completely of paternal origin

GENERAL CONSIDERATIONS

- Hydatidiform mole, invasive mole, and choriocarcinoma comprise a spectrum of gestational trophoblastic neoplasia
- Partial moles generally show evidence of an embryo or gestational sac; are polypoid, slower-growing, and less symptomatic; and often present clinically as a missed abortion

DEMOGRAPHICS

- Highest rates of gestational trophoblastic neoplasia occur in some developing countries: 1/125 pregnancies in areas of Asia, 1/1500 pregnancies in the United States
- Risk factors include low socioeconomic status, a history of mole, and age below 18 or above 40

CLINICAL FINDINGS

SYMPTOMS AND SIGNS

- Excessive nausea and vomiting in over one-third of patients with **hydatidiform mole**
- Uterine bleeding beginning at 6–8 weeks is usual
- In 20% of cases, the uterus appears larger than would be expected
- Intact or collapsed grape-like clusters of enlarged villi (vesicles) may be passed
- Bilaterally enlarged cystic ovaries may be palpable
- Less commonly, preeclampsia-eclampsia may develop during the second trimester
- **Choriocarcinoma** may be manifested by continued or recurrent bleeding after evacuation of a mole or following delivery, abortion, or ectopic pregnancy
- An ulcerative vaginal tumor, pelvic mass, or evidence of distant metastatic tumor may be observed
- Diagnosis is established by pathologic examination of curettings or biopsy

DIFFERENTIAL DIAGNOSIS

- Similarly elevated levels of serum hCG-β subunit are seen in multiple gestation
  - Spontaneous abortion
  - Ectopic pregnancy
  - Prolapsed uterine fibroid
  - Uterine leiomyomas (fibroids), endometrial polyp, or adenomyosis (uterine endometriosis)
  - Ovarian tumor
  - Cervical neoplasm or lesion

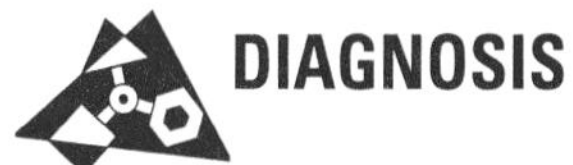

DIAGNOSIS

LABORATORY TESTS

- Serum hCG-β subunit value > 40,000 mU/mL or a urinary hCG > 100,000 over 24 h increases the likelihood of hydatidiform mole, though such values are occasionally seen with a normal pregnancy in multiple gestation

IMAGING STUDIES

- Ultrasound has replaced all other means of preoperative diagnosis of mole
- Ultrasound findings are multiple echoes indicating edematous villi within an enlarged uterus, and absent fetus and placenta
- Preoperative chest x-ray is required to evaluate for pulmonary metastases of trophoblast

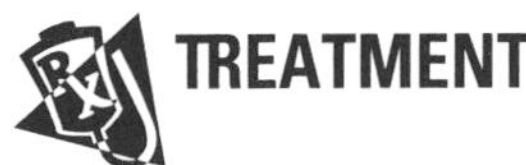

TREATMENT

MEDICATIONS

- Chemotherapy is indicated for mole if malignant tissue is discovered at surgery or during follow-up examination
- For low-risk patients with a good prognosis, methotrexate, 0.4 mg/kg IM over a 5-day period, or dactinomycin, 10–12 μg/kg/day IV over a 5-day period, is used (see Table 153). The side effects—anorexia, nausea and vomiting, stomatitis, rash, diarrhea, and bone marrow depression—usually are reversible in about 3 weeks and can be ameliorated by the administration of leucovorin (0.1 mg/kg)
- Repeated courses of methotrexate 2 weeks apart generally are required to destroy the trophoblast and maintain a zero chorionic gonadotropin titer, as indicated by β-hCG determination
- β-Blockers should be used preoperatively to stabilize patients who have thyrotoxicosis as a result of their mole

SURGERY

- The uterus should be emptied as soon as a mole is diagnosed, preferably by suction
- Ovarian cysts should not be resected nor ovaries removed; spontaneous regression of theca lutein cysts will occur with elimination of the mole

OUTCOME

FOLLOW-UP

- hCG levels should be negative for 1 year before conception is attempted
- In the pregnancy following a mole, hCG level should be checked 6 weeks postpartum
- Contraception should be prescribed to avoid the confusion of elevated hCG from a new pregnancy; oral contraceptive pills are preferred
- Weekly serum hCG levels are measured
- After two negative hCG levels are documented in succession, levels may be checked less frequently at intervals out to 1 year
- A plateau or rise in hCG levels mandates a repeat chest film and D&C before chemotherapy

COMPLICATIONS

- Approximately 10% of women require further treatment after evacuation of the mole; choriocarcinoma develops in 5%
- hCG has minimal TSH–like activity; at very high levels, release of T_3 and T_4 may occur and cause hyperthyroidism, which resolves promptly after resection

PROGNOSIS

- Partial moles tend to follow a benign course
- Complete moles have a greater tendency to become choriocarcinomas
- 5-year survival after courses of chemotherapy, even when metastases have been demonstrated, can be expected in at least 85% of cases of choriocarcinoma

WHEN TO REFER

- Patients with a poor prognosis should be referred to a cancer center, where multiple-agent chemotherapy probably will be given

WHEN TO ADMIT

- Patients with excessive vaginal bleeding
- Patients passing vesicular tissue
- Patients with thyrotoxicosis
- Patients with symptomatic metastatic disease

EVIDENCE

PRACTICE GUIDELINES

- Benedet JL et al: FIGO staging classifications and clinical practice guidelines in the management of gynecologic cancers. FIGO Committee on Gynecologic Oncology. Int J Gynaecol Obstet 2000;70:209. [PMID: 11041682]
- Soper JT et al; American College of Obstetricians and Gynecologists. Diagnosis and treatment of gestational trophoblastic disease: ACOG Practice Bulletin No. 53. Gynecol Oncol 2004;93:575. [PMID: 15196847]

WEB SITE

- National Cancer Institute: Gestational Trophoblastic Disease Information for Patients and Health Professionals
  - http://www.cancer.gov/cancertopics/types/gestationaltrophoblastic/

INFORMATION FOR PATIENTS

- American Cancer Society: Gestational Trophoblastic Disease
  - http://www.cancer.org/docroot/CRI/CRI_2_3x.asp?rnav=cridg&dt=49
- MedlinePlus: Gestational Trophoblastic Disease
  - http://www.nlm.nih.gov/medlineplus/ency/article/001496.htm

REFERENCES

- Fulop V et al: Molecular biology of gestational trophoblastic neoplasia: a review. J Reprod Med 2004;49:415. [PMID:15283047]
- Shapter AP et al: Gestational trophoblastic disease. Obstet Gynecol Clin North Am 2001;28:805. [PMID: 11766153]

Author(s)

William R. Crombleholme, MD

Hyperaldosteronism, Primary

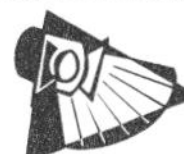

KEY FEATURES

ESSENTIALS OF DIAGNOSIS

- Hypertension, polyuria, polydipsia, muscular weakness
- Hypokalemia, alkalosis
- Plasma and urine aldosterone levels elevated and plasma renin level low

GENERAL CONSIDERATIONS

- Aldosterone stimulates renal tubule to reabsorb sodium and excrete potassium
- Primary hyperaldosteronism may be due to unilateral adrenocortical adenoma (Conn's syndrome, 73%) or to bilateral cortical hyperplasia (27%), which may be glucocorticoid suppressible due to an autosomal dominant genetic defect allowing ACTH stimulation of aldosterone production

DEMOGRAPHICS

- Classic hyperaldosteronism (with hypokalemia) accounts for ~0.7% of cases of hypertension
- Milder hyperaldosteronism, without hypokalemia, is more common, with a prevalence of 5–14% among hypertensives
- More common in women

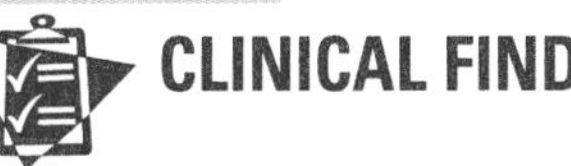

CLINICAL FINDINGS

SYMPTOMS AND SIGNS

- Hypertension ranging from mild to severe. Malignant hypertension rare
- Muscular weakness; episodic paralysis simulating periodic paralysis
- Fatigue and reduced stamina
- Paresthesias, sometimes with frank tetany
- Headache
- Polyuria and polydipsia
- Edema, common in secondary hyperaldosteronism, rare in primary hyperaldosteronism

DIFFERENTIAL DIAGNOSIS

- Essential hypertension
- Hypokalemic thyrotoxic periodic paralysis
- Renal vascular hypertension (hypertension and hypokalemia, but plasma renin activity is high)
- Hypokalemia due to other cause, eg, diuretics
- Secondary hyperaldosteronism (dehydration, heart failure)
- Congenital adrenal hyperplasia: 11β-hydroxylase deficiency, 17α-hydroxylase deficiency
- Cushing's syndrome
- Excessive real licorice ingestion
- Syndrome of cortisol resistance

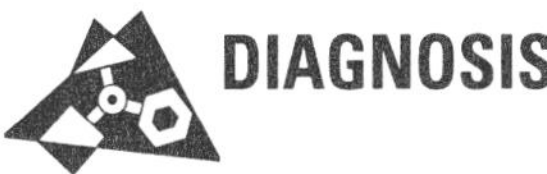

DIAGNOSIS

LABORATORY TESTS

- Discontinue all antihypertensives and remain off diuretics for 3 weeks
- Maintain high sodium intake (>120 mEq/day) during evaluation
- Hypokalemia, persistent even after potassium-wasting diuretics stopped
- Obtain 24-h urine aldosterone, free cortisol, and creatinine
- 24-h urine aldosterone >20 μg with low plasma renin activity (< 5 μg/dL) indicates hyperaldosteronism
- 24-h urine aldosterone is < 20 μg/day in rare adrenal or gonadal enzyme defects, eg, in 17α-hydroxylase (ambiguous genitalia or primary amenorrhea) or 11β-hydroxylase (virilization)
- Once hyperaldosteronism diagnosed, further testing to distinguish between resectable adrenal adenoma and nonsurgical adrenal hyperplasia
- Plasma 18-hydroxycorticosterone is >85 ng/dL with adrenal neoplasms; level < 85 ng/dL is nondiagnostic
- Plasma aldosterone is measured at 8 AM while patient is supine after overnight recumbency and again after 4 h upright. With adrenal adenoma, baseline aldosterone is usually >25 ng/dL (695 pmol/L) and does not rise during upright posture. With hyperplasia, baseline aldosterone usually is < 20 ng/dL and rises during upright posture

IMAGING STUDIES

- Thin-section CT suggests discrete (>1 cm diameter) adrenal adenoma in 60–80% of patients with laboratory findings suggesting adrenal adenoma

DIAGNOSTIC PROCEDURES

- Adrenal vein catheterization for aldosterone or during stimulation with cosyntropin. An adrenal vein to inferior vena cava gradient of >5:1 confirms the adrenal location of the adenoma
- Dexamethasone-suppressed adrenal scan using ^{131}I-labeled 6-iodomethyl-19-norcholesterol is recommended following CT

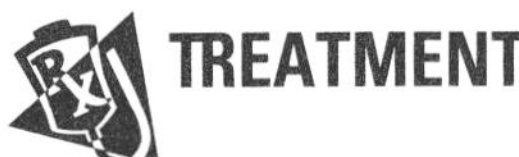

TREATMENT

MEDICATIONS

- Spironolactone is treatment of choice for bilateral adrenal hyperplasia
- Spironolactone therapy (lifelong) is an option for patients with unilateral adrenal adenoma (Conn's syndrome) who are poor surgical candidates
- Potassium supplements are required
- Antihypertensive medications for hypertension in bilateral adrenal hyperplasia: angiotensin receptor blockers or angiotensin-converting enzyme inhibitors preferred since they reduce renal potassium losses; thiazides aggravate potassium loss
- Low-dose dexamethasone suppression is an alternative for bilateral adrenal hyperplasia

SURGERY

- Surgical resection (laparoscopic adrenalectomy) is treatment of choice for unilateral adrenal adenoma secreting aldosterone (Conn's syndrome)
- Bilateral adrenalectomy corrects hypokalemia but not hypertension and should *not* be performed for bilateral adrenal hyperplasia

OUTCOME

FOLLOW-UP

- Monitor electrolytes, blood pressure, renal function

COMPLICATIONS

- Complications of chronic hypertension
- Progressive renal damage is less reversible than in essential hypertension
- Hyperkalemia and hypotension from temporary postoperative hypoaldosteronism can occur from suppression of contralateral adrenal gland following unilateral adrenalectomy for Conn's syndrome
- Surgical morbidity is 7.1%; < 4.1% in major centers. Surgical mortality is rare

PROGNOSIS

- Hypertension remits after surgery in about two-thirds of cases but persists or returns despite surgery in one-third
- Prognosis much improved by early diagnosis and treatment
- Only 2% of aldosterone-secreting adrenal tumors are malignant

EVIDENCE

PRACTICE GUIDELINES

- Foo R et al: Hyperaldosteronism: recent concepts, diagnosis, and management. Postgrad Med J 2001;77:639. [PMID: 11571370]
- Young WF Jr: Minireview: primary aldosteronism–changing concepts in diagnosis and treatment. Endocrinology 2003;144:2208. [PMID: 12746276]

WEB SITE

- Family Practice Notebook article on hyperaldosteronism
  - http://www.fpnotebook.com/END2.htm

INFORMATION FOR PATIENTS

- MEDLINEplus—Hyperaldosteronism—primary and secondary
  - http://www.nlm.nih.gov/medlineplus/ency/article/000330.htm
- National Adrenal Disease Foundation—Hyperaldosteronism
  - http://www.medhelp.org/nadf/nadf9.htm

REFERENCES

- Al Fehaily M, Duh QY: Clinical manifestations of aldosteronoma. Surg Clin North Am 2004;84:887. [PMID: 15145241]
- Espiner EA et al: Predicting surgically remedial primary aldosteronism: role of adrenal scanning, posture testing, and adrenal vein sampling. J Clin Endocrinol Metab 2003;88:3637. [PMID: 12915648]
- Sawka AM et al: Primary aldosteronism: factors associated with normalization of blood pressure after surgery. Ann Intern Med 2001;135:258. [PMID: 11511140]
- Schwartz GL et al: Screening for primary aldosteronism: implications of an increased plasma aldosterone/renin ratio. Clin Chem 2002;48:1919. [PMID: 12406976]
- Seiler L et al: Diagnosis of primary aldosteronism: value of different screening parameters, and influence of antihypertensive medication. Eur J Endocrinol 2004;150:329. [PMID: 15012618]
- Young WF Jr: Primary aldosteronism: management issues. Ann NY Acad Sci 2002;970:61. [PMID: 12381542]

Author(s)

Paul A. Fitzgerald, MD

Hypercalcemia

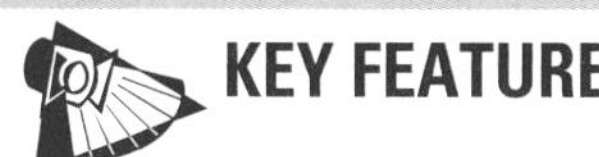

KEY FEATURES

ESSENTIALS OF DIAGNOSIS

- Malignancy-associated hypercalcemia and primary hyperparathyroidism are the most common causes
- Asymptomatic, mild hypercalcemia (≤11 mg/dL) is usually due to primary hyperparathyroidism
- Hypercalcemia of malignancy is usually symptomatic and severe (≥14 mg/dL)
- Hypercalciuria usually precedes hypercalcemia
- Hypophosphatemia suggests elevated parathyroid hormone (PTH) or parathyroid hormone–related protein (PTHrP)

GENERAL CONSIDERATIONS

- Primary hyperparathyroidism and malignancy account for 90% of all cases of hypercalcemia
- Primary hyperparathyroidism is the most common cause of hypercalcemia in ambulatory patients
- Tumor production of PTHrP is the most common paraneoplastic endocrine syndrome, accounting for most cases of hypercalcemia among inpatients. The neoplasm is clinically apparent in nearly all cases when hypercalcemia is detected
- Chronic hypercalcemia (> 6 months) or some manifestation such as nephrolithiasis suggests a benign cause
- Hypocalciuric hypercalcemia occurs in milk-alkali syndrome, thiazide diuretic use, and familial hypocalciuric hypercalcemia
- Hypercalcemia can cause nephrogenic diabetes insipidus and volume depletion, which further worsen hypercalcemia

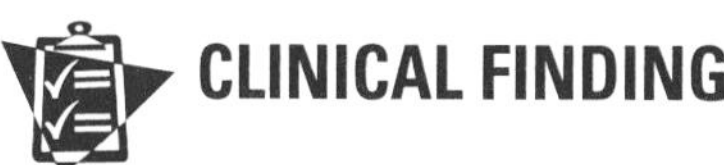

CLINICAL FINDINGS

SYMPTOMS AND SIGNS

- Determine duration of hypercalcemia and examine for evidence of a neoplasm
- Symptoms usually occur if the serum calcium is > 12 mg/dL and tend to be more severe in acute hypercalcemia
- Constipation and polyuria occur regardless of cause of hypercalcemia
- Stupor, coma, and azotemia may develop in severe hypercalcemia
- Polyuria is absent in familial hypocalciuric hypercalcemia
- Ventricular extrasystoles and idioventricular rhythm occur and can be accentuated by digitalis

DIFFERENTIAL DIAGNOSIS

- Increased intake or absorption
  - Milk-alkali syndrome
  - Vitamin D or A excess
- Endocrine disorders
  - Primary and secondary hyperparathyroidism
  - Renal failure
  - Acromegaly
  - Adrenal insufficiency
  - Hyperthyroidism
- Neoplastic diseases
  - Tumor production of PTHrP proteins (ovary, kidney, lung)
  - Multiple myeloma (osteoclast-activating factor)
- Other
  - Thiazide diuretics
  - Sarcoidosis
  - Paget's bone disease
  - Immobilization
  - Familial hypocalciuric hypercalcemia

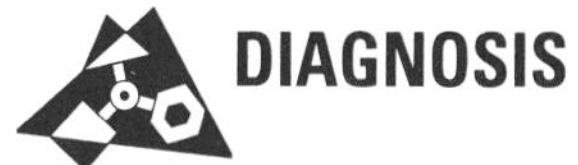

DIAGNOSIS

LABORATORY TESTS

- Serum calcium must be interpreted in relation to serum albumin level
- When albumin is low, serum Ca^{2+} concentration is depressed in a ratio of 0.8–1 mg/dL of Ca^{2+}:1 g/dL of albumin
- The highest serum calcium levels (> 15 mg/dL) generally occur in malignancy
- A high serum chloride concentration and a low serum phosphate concentration (ratio > 33:1) suggest primary hyperparathyroidism because PTH decreases proximal tubular phosphate reabsorption
- A low serum chloride concentration with a high serum bicarbonate concentration, along with blood urea nitrogen and serum creatinine elevations, suggests milk-alkali syndrome
- Urinary calcium excretion > 200 mg/day suggests hypercalciuria; < 100 mg/day, hypocalciuria
- Hypercalciuria from malignancy or from vitamin D therapy frequently results in hypercalcemia when volume depletion occurs
- Serum PTH and PTHrP levels help distinguish between malignancy-associated hypercalcemia (elevated PTHrP) and hyperparathyroidism (elevated PTH)
- Serum phosphate may or may not be low, depending on the cause
- A serum calcium × serum phosphorus product > 70 markedly increases the risk of nephrocalcinosis and soft tissue calcification

IMAGING STUDIES

- ECG: shortened QT interval
- Chest x-ray film: to exclude malignancy or granulomatous disease

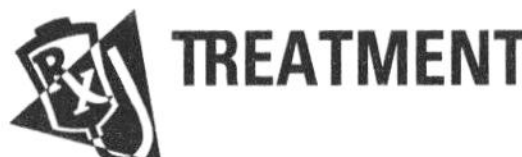

TREATMENT

MEDICATIONS

Emergency treatment

- Establish euvolemia to induce renal excretion of Na^+, which is accompanied by excretion of Ca^{2+}
- In dehydrated patients with normal cardiac and renal function, infuse 0.45% saline or 0.9% saline rapidly (250–500 mL/h)
- Intravenous furosemide (20–40 mg Q2 h) to prevent volume overload and enhance Ca^{2+} excretion
- Thiazides can actually worsen hypercalcemia (as can furosemide if inadequate saline is given)
- In the treatment of hypercalcemia of malignancy, bisphosphonates are the mainstay of treatment. Zoledronic acid, 4-mg single 15-min IV infusion, with adequate hydration normalizes serum calcium in 70% of patients in 3 days and can be repeated as necessary to control the hypercalcemia
- See Hyperparathyroidism

THERAPEUTIC PROCEDURES

- In emergency cases, dialysis with low or no calcium dialysate may be needed

OUTCOME

FOLLOW-UP

- Monitor serum calcium at least after 6 months of medical therapy for hyperparathyroidism

COMPLICATIONS

- Pathologic fractures are more common in individuals with hyperthyroidism than the general population
- Renal stones
- Renal failure
- Peptic ulcer disease
- Pancreatitis
- Precipitation of calcium throughout the soft tissues
- Gestational hypercalcemia produces neonatal hypocalcemia

PROGNOSIS

- Depends on the underlying disease
- Poor prognosis in malignancy

WHEN TO REFER

- Early referral to an oncologist or nephrologist may aid in management
- Persistent hypercalcemia > 10.5 mg/dL even without symptoms

WHEN TO ADMIT

- Altered mental status
- Marked dehydration and hypotension
- Severe renal insufficiency

PREVENTION

- Prevent dehydration that can further aggrevate hypercalcemia

EVIDENCE

WEB SITE

- National Cancer Institute: Hypercalcemia
  - http://www.cancer.gov/cancertopics/pdq/supportivecare/hypercalcemia/HealthProfessional

INFORMATION FOR PATIENTS

- American Association for Clinical Chemistry: Lab Tests Online: Calcium
  - http://www.labtestsonline.org/understanding/analytes/calcium/test.html
- Mayo Clinic: Hypercalcemia
  - http://www.mayoclinic.com/invoke.cfm?id=AN00342
- National Cancer Institute: Hypercalcemia
  - http://www.cancer.gov/cancerinfo/pdq/supportivecare/hypercalcemia/Patient

REFERENCES

- Bilezikian JP et al: Clinical practice. Asymptomatic primary hyperparathyroidism. N Engl J Med 2004;350:1746. [PMID: 15103001]
- Inzucchi SE: Management of hypercalcemia. Diagnostic workup, therapeutic options for hyperparathyroidism and other common causes. Postgrad Med 2004;115:27 [PMID: 15171076]
- Marx SJ: Hyperparathyroidism and hypoparathyroid disorders. N Engl J Med 2000;343:1863. [PMID: 11117980]
- Ziegler R: Hypercalcemic crisis. J Am Soc Nephrol 2001;12(Suppl 17):S3. [PMID: 11251025]

Author(s)

Masafumi Fukagawa, MD, PhD
Kiyoshi Kurokawa, MD, MACP
Maxine A. Papadakis, MD

Hypercoagulable States

Hypercalcemia, Malignant p. 1093

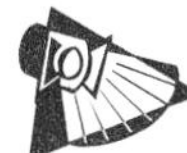

KEY FEATURES

ESSENTIALS OF DIAGNOSIS

- Thrombosis
- Erythromelalgia

GENERAL CONSIDERATIONS

- There are both acquired and congenital causes of thrombosis (see Differential Diagnosis)
- Family history usually present with congenital causes, often precipitated by trauma or pregnancy
- Cancer associated with increased risk of venous and arterial thrombosis
- Myeloproliferative disorders associated with high incidence of thrombosis due to qualitative platelet abnormalities
- Venous thrombosis may occur in unusual locations, eg, mesenteric, hepatic, or splenic venous beds
- Arterial thrombosis may manifest as large-vessel occlusion (stroke, myocardial infarction) or microvascular events (burning in hands and feet)
- Heparin associated with thrombocytopenia in ~10% of treatment courses; often modest and resolves spontaneously, but may be severe and complicated by arterial thrombosis
- Warfarin-induced skin necrosis may occur in patients with undiagnosed protein C deficiency
  - Warfarin, by creating a vitamin K–dependent state, transiently depletes protein C (which has a short half-life) before it leads to anticoagulation
  - During this period of hypercoagulability, thrombosis of skin vessels may lead to infarction and necrosis

DEMOGRAPHICS

- Congenital hypercoagulable states often present during early adulthood rather than childhood

CLINICAL FINDINGS

SYMPTOMS AND SIGNS

- Thrombosis
- Erythromelalgia (painful redness and burning of hands) in essential thrombocytosis

DIFFERENTIAL DIAGNOSIS

- Acquired causes of thrombosis
  - Immobility or postoperative state
  - Cancer
  - Inflammatory disorders, eg, ulcerative colitis
  - Myeloproliferative disorder, eg, polycythemia vera, essential thrombocytosis
  - Estrogens, pregnancy
  - Heparin-induced thrombocytopenia
  - Lupus anticoagulant
  - Anticardiolipin antibodies
  - Nephrotic syndrome
  - Paroxysmal nocturnal hemoglobinuria
  - Disseminated intravascular coagulation
  - Congestive heart failure
- Congenital causes of thrombosis
  - Activated protein C resistance, eg, factor V Leiden
  - Prothrombin 20210 mutation
  - Antithrombin III deficiency
  - Protein C deficiency
  - Protein S deficiency
  - Hyperhomocystinemia
  - Dysfibrinogenemia
  - Abnormal plasminogen

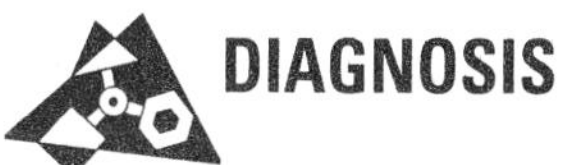

DIAGNOSIS

LABORATORY TESTS

- Dysfibrinogenemia is diagnosed by a prolonged reptilase time
- Assays of antithrombin III, protein S, and protein C

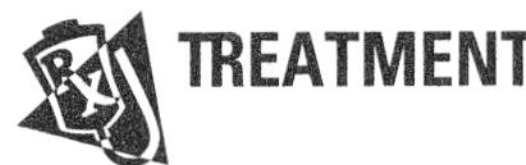

TREATMENT

MEDICATIONS

- Preoperative minidose heparin (5000 units SQ Q8–12 h) may reduce perioperative thrombosis risk
- Heparin, 10,000 units SQ Q12 h, may reduce thrombosis in hypercoagulable state associated with cancer
  - Low-molecular-weight heparin is more convenient, equally effective, and requires less laboratory monitoring
  - Warfarin is usually ineffective in cancer, most likely because of low-grade disseminated intravascular coagulation
- Antiplatelet therapy may be helpful for thrombosis in myeloproliferative disease, but may increase risk of bleeding
- Aspirin, 325 mg PO QD, is effective for erythromelalgia
- Warfarin is effective and given indefinitely in congenital defects such as deficiency of antithrombin III or vitamin K–dependent proteins C and S
- Warfarin-induced skin necrosis can be prevented by the use of heparin for 5–7 days until warfarin induces anticoagulation

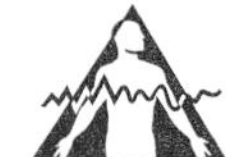

OUTCOME

FOLLOW-UP

- Screen family members for congenital defects (eg, deficiency of antithrombin III or vitamin K–dependent proteins C and S)

COMPLICATIONS

- Arterial thrombosis in heparin-induced thrombocytopenia

EVIDENCE

PRACTICE GUIDELINES

- American College of Chest Physicians: The Seventh ACCP Conference on Antithrombotic and Thrombolytic Therapy: Evidence-Based Guidelines. Chest 2004;126(suppl 3).
  - http://www.chestnet.org/education/hsp/guidelines.php
- College of American Pathologists Consensus Conference XXXVI: Diagnostic Issues in Thrombophilia. Arch Pathol Lab Med. 2002;126:1277. [PMID: 12421135]
  - http://arpa.allenpress.com/arpaonline/?request=get-abstract&issn=1543-2165&volume=126&page=1277
- Haemostasis and Thrombosis Task Force, British Committee for Standards in Haematology. Investigation and management of heritable thrombophilia. Br J Haematol 2001;114:512. [PMID: 11552975]

WEB SITE

- Deitcher SR, Gomes MPV: Hypercoagulable States. Cleveland Clinic 2003.
  - http://www.clevelandclinicmeded.com/diseasemanagement/hematology/hyperco/hyperco.htm

INFORMATION FOR PATIENTS

- American Academy of Family Physicians: Hypercoagulation
  - http://familydoctor.org/244.xml
- MedlinePlus: Hypercoagulable States
  - http://www.nlm.nih.gov/medlineplus/ency/article/001120.htm
- Parmet S et al: JAMA patient page. Pulmonary embolism. JAMA 2003;290:2898. [PMID: 14657080]

REFERENCES

- Kovalevsky G et al: Evaluation of the association between hereditary hemophilias and recurrent pregnancy loss: a meta-analysis. Arch Intern Med 2004;164:558. [PMID: 15006834]
- Mann KG et al: Factor V: a combination of Dr Jekyll and Mr Hyde. Blood 2003;101:20. [PMID: 12393635]
- Schulman S et al: Secondary prevention of venous thromboembolism with the oral direct thrombin inhibitor ximelagatran. N Engl J Med 2003;349:1713. [PMID: 14585939]

Author(s)

Charles A. Linker, MD

Hyperemesis Gravidarum p. 1093

Hyperglycemic Hyperosmolar State

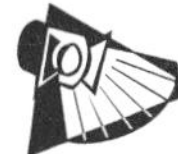

KEY FEATURES

ESSENTIALS OF DIAGNOSIS

- Hyperglycemia > 600 mg/dL
- Serum osmolality > 310 mOsm/kg
- No acidosis; blood pH above 7.3
- Serum bicarbonate > 15 mEq/L
- Normal anion gap (< 14 mEq/L)

GENERAL CONSIDERATIONS

- Frequently occurs with mild or occult diabetes
- Infection, myocardial infarction, stroke, or recent operation is often a precipitating event
- Drugs (phenytoin, diazoxide, glucocorticoids, and diuretics) or procedures associated with glucose loading such as peritoneal dialysis can also precipitate the syndrome
- Renal insufficiency develops from hypovolemia, leading to increasingly higher blood glucose concentrations
- Underlying renal insufficiency or congestive heart failure is common, and the presence of either worsens the prognosis

DEMOGRAPHICS

- Rarer than diabetic ketoacidosis even in older age groups
- Affects middle-aged to elderly

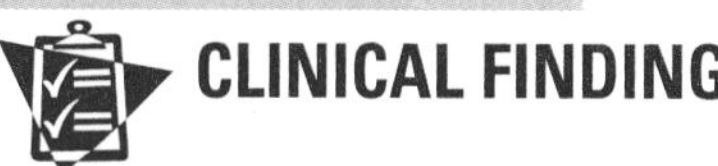

CLINICAL FINDINGS

SYMPTOMS AND SIGNS

- Onset may be insidious over days or weeks, with weakness, polyuria, and polydipsia
- The lack of features of ketoacidosis may retard recognition until dehydration becomes more profound than in ketoacidosis
- Fluid intake is usually reduced from inappropriate lack of thirst, nausea, or inaccessibility of fluids to bedridden patients
- Lethargy and confusion develop as serum osmolality exceeds 310 mOsm/kg; coma can occur if osmolality exceeds 320–330 mOsm/kg
- Physical examination shows profound dehydration, lethargy, or coma without Kussmaul respirations

DIFFERENTIAL DIAGNOSIS

- Diabetic ketoacidosis
- Cerebrovascular accident or head trauma
- Hypoglycemia
- Sepsis
- Diabetes insipidus

DIAGNOSIS

LABORATORY TESTS

- Severe hyperglycemia (600–2400 mg/dL)
- When dehydration is less severe, dilutional hyponatremia as well as urinary sodium losses may reduce serum sodium to 120–125 mEq/L
- As dehydration progresses, serum sodium can exceed 140 mEq/L, producing serum osmolality readings of 330–440 mOsm/kg
- Ketosis and acidosis are usually absent or mild
- Prerenal azotemia with serum urea nitrogen elevations > 100 mg/dL is typical

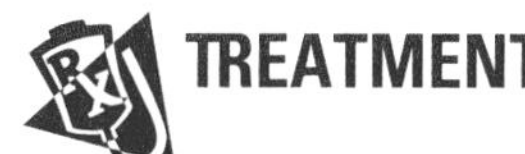

TREATMENT

MEDICATIONS

Saline

- Fluid replacement paramount to correct fluid deficits of 6–10 L
- In hypovolemic oliguric hypotension, initiate fluid resuscitation with isotonic 0.9% saline
- Otherwise, hypotonic (0.45%) saline preferred because of hyperosmolality
- As much as 4–6 L of fluid may be required in first 8–10 h
- Once blood glucose reaches 250 mg/dL, add 5% dextrose to either water, 0.45% saline solution, or 0.9% saline solution at a rate to maintain glycemic levels of 250–300 mg/dL to reduce risk of cerebral edema
- Goal of fluid therapy is to restore urine output to ≥ 50 mL/h

Insulin

- Less insulin is required than in diabetic ketoacidotic coma
- Fluid replacement alone can reduce hyperglycemia by increasing glomerular filtration and renal excretion of glucose
- Initial dose of 0.15 U/kg is followed by insulin infusion of 1–2 U/h, titrated to lower blood glucose levels by 50–70 mg/dL/h

Potassium

- Add potassium chloride (10 mEq/L) to initial fluids if serum potassium not elevated. Adjust subsequent potassium replacement based on serum potassium level

Phosphate

- If severe hypophosphatemia (serum phosphate < 1 mg/dL (0.35 mmol/L) develops during therapy, phosphate replacement can be given as potassium salt
- To minimize risk of tetany from phosphate replacement overload, average deficit of 40–50 mmol phosphate should be replaced by IV infusion not to exceed 3 mmol/h
  - A stock solution (Abbott) provides a mixture of 1.12 g KH_2PO_4 and 1.18 g K_2HPO_4 in a 5-mL single-dose vial representing 22 mEq potassium and 15 mmol phosphate (27 mEq)
  - 5 mL of this solution in 2 L of 0.45% saline or 5% dextrose in water, infused at 400 mL/h, will replace the phosphate at optimal rate of 3 mmol/h and provide 4.4 mEq potassium/h
- If serum phosphate remains < 0.35 mmol/L (1 mg/dL), repeat a 5-h infusion of potassium phosphate at 3 mmol/h

THERAPEUTIC PROCEDURES

- Using a flow sheet, document vital signs, time sequence of laboratory values (arterial pH, plasma glucose, acetone, bicarbonate, serum urea nitrogen, electrolytes, serum osmolality) in relation to therapy

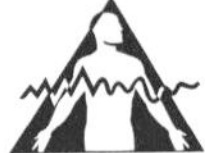

OUTCOME

PROGNOSIS

- The overall mortality rate is > 10 times that of diabetic ketoacidosis because of its higher incidence in older patients and greater dehydration
- When prompt therapy is instituted, the mortality rate can be reduced from nearly 50% to that related to the severity of coexistent disorders

WHEN TO ADMIT

- Altered mental status
- Severe volume depletion

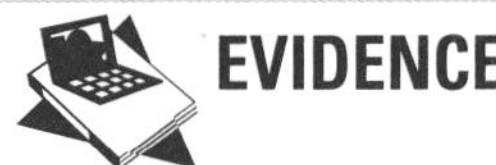

EVIDENCE

PRACTICE GUIDELINES

- American Diabetes Association: Hyperglycemic Crises in Patients With Diabetes Mellitus
  - http://care.diabetesjournals.org/cgi/content/full/26/suppl_1/s109
- Joslin Diabetes Center: Hyperglycemic Emergencies for Adults, 2004
  - https://diabetesmanagement.joslin.org/Guidelines/HyperglycemicGuide.pdf
- National Guideline Clearinghouse: Hyperglycemic Crises in Diabetes, 2001
  - http://www.guideline.gov/summary/summary.aspx?doc_id=4694

WEB SITES

- American Association of Diabetes Educators
  - http://www.aadenet.org/
- American Diabetes Association
  - http://www.diabetes.org
- CDC Diabetes Public Health Resource
  - http://www.cdc.gov/diabetes/

INFORMATION FOR PATIENTS

- American Diabetes Association: What Is Hyperosmolar Hyperglycemic Nonketotic Syndrome (HHNS)?
  - http://www.diabetes.org/type-2-diabetes/treatment-conditions/hhns.jsp
- National Institutes of Health: Diabetic Hyperglycemic Hyperosmolar Coma
  - http://www.nlm.nih.gov/medlineplus/ency/article/000304.htm
- Stevens LM: JAMA patient page: The ABCs of diabetes. JAMA 2002;287:2608. [PMID: 12025825]

REFERENCES

- American Diabetes Association: Hyperglycemic crises in patients with diabetes mellitus. Diabetes Care 2001;24:154. [PMID:11221603]
- Trence DL et al: Hyperglycemic crisis in diabetes mellitus type 2. Endocrinol Metab Clin North Am 2001;30:817. [PMID:11727401]

Author(s)

Umesh Masharani, MB, BS, MRCH (UK)

Hyperkalemia

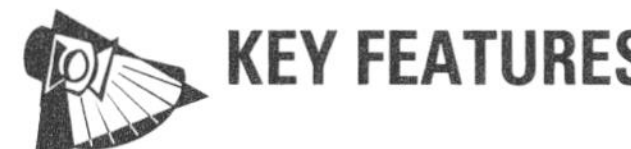

KEY FEATURES

ESSENTIALS OF DIAGNOSIS

- ECG may be normal despite life-threatening hyperkalemia
- Potassium release from blood cells should be ruled out in cases of clotting, leukocytosis, and thrombocytosis

GENERAL CONSIDERATIONS

- Serum potassium concentration rises about 0.7 mEq/L for every decrease of 0.1 pH unit during acidosis
- In the absence of acidosis, serum potassium concentration rises about 1 mEq/L when there is a total body potassium excess of 1–4 mEq/kg; however, the higher the serum potassium concentration, the smaller the excess necessary to raise the potassium levels further
- Hyperkalemia may develop with use of angiotensin-converting enzyme (ACE) inhibitors, angiotensin-receptor blockers, potassium-sparing diuretics, or their combination, even with normal or mild renal dysfunction
- Mild hyperkalemia that occurs in the absence of potassium-sparing drug therapy is usually due to type IV renal tubular acidosis
- Life-threatening hyperkalemia during combined therapy with ACE inhibitors and spironolactone occurs
- Hyperkalemia occurs commonly in AIDS
  - Impaired renal excretion of potassium can be due to use of pentamidine or trimethoprim-sulfamethoxazole or to hyporeninemic hypoaldosteronism
  - Also, an abnormality may occur in potassium redistribution between intracellular and extracellular compartments

Etiology

- **Spurious**
  - Leakage from erythrocytes, marked thrombocytosis or leukocytosis
  - Repeated fist clenching during phlebotomy
  - Specimen from arm with K^+ infusion
- **Decreased excretion**
  - Renal failure
  - Renal secretory defects, eg, interstitial nephritis, sickle cell disease
  - Hyporeninemic hypoaldosteronism (type IV renal tubular acidosis), eg, diabetic nephropathy, heparin, AIDS; adrenal insufficiency
  - Drugs that inhibit K^+ excretion (spironolactone, triamterene, ACE inhibitors, trimethoprim, nonsteroidal anti-inflammatory drugs)
- **Potassium shift out of cell**
  - Burns, rhabdomyolysis, hemolysis, severe infection, internal bleeding, vigorous exercise
  - Metabolic acidosis
  - Hypertonicity (solvent drag)
  - Insulin deficiency
  - Hyperkalemic periodic paralysis
  - Drugs: digitalis toxicity, β-adrenergic antagonists, succinylcholine, arginine
- **Excessive intake of K^+**
  - Ingestion or iatrogenic

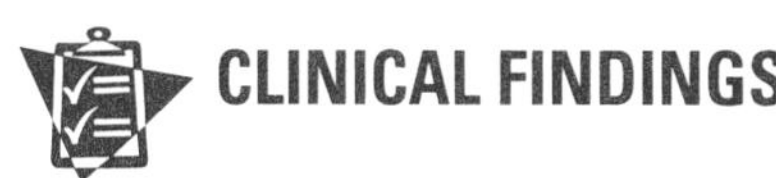

CLINICAL FINDINGS

SYMPTOMS AND SIGNS

- Frequently asymptomatic
- Muscle weakness and, rarely, flaccid paralysis
- Abdominal distention and diarrhea may occur

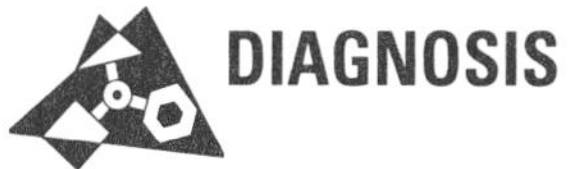

DIAGNOSIS

LABORATORY TESTS

- Confirm that the hyperkalemia is genuine by measuring plasma potassium rather than serum potassium
- Serum electrolytes and creatinine
- Consider arterial blood gas

IMAGING STUDIES

- ECG is not a sensitive method for detecting hyperkalemia, since nearly half of patients with a serum potassium level > 6.5 mEq/L will not manifest ECG changes

ECG changes

- Peaked T waves
- Widening of the QRS complex
- Biphasic QRS–T complexes
- Inhibition of atrial depolarization despite normal conduction through usual pathways may occur
- Slow heart rate; ventricular fibrillation and cardiac arrest are terminal events

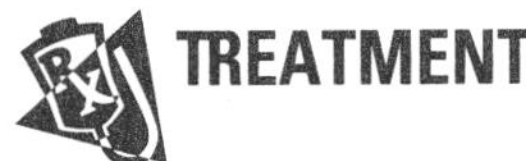

TREATMENT

MEDICATIONS

- Withhold potassium and give cation exchange resin (see Table 84)
- Emergent treatment is indicated if cardiac toxicity or muscular paralysis is present or if the hyperkalemia is severe ($K^+ > 6.5–7$ mEq/L) even in the absence of ECG changes

THERAPEUTIC PROCEDURES

- Hemodialysis or peritoneal dialysis may be required to remove K^+ in the presence of renal failure

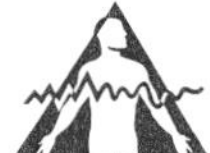

OUTCOME

FOLLOW-UP

- Monitor potassium frequently (every 1–4 h) during inpatient therapy for hyperkalemia

PROGNOSIS

- Depends on the underlying condition (renal failure)
- Drug-induced hyperkalemia is generally readily reversible with therapy

WHEN TO REFER

- Refer to a nephrologist if expertise is needed for treatment, particularly for emergent treatment or dialysis

WHEN TO ADMIT

- For serum potassium > 6.0 mg/dL
- For rapidly increasing serum potassium in the setting of acutely worsening comorbid condition (eg, acute renal failure, rhabdomyolysis)

PREVENTION

- Monitor serum potassium after administration of potassium-altering drugs in patients with renal insufficiency

EVIDENCE

WEB SITE

- National Kidney Foundation
  - http://www.kidney.org/

INFORMATION FOR PATIENTS

- Mayo Clinic: Hyperkalemia
  - http://www.mayoclinic.com/invoke.cfm?objectid=8D0B86A2-65A6-4D82-B4822110131E4C8D
- Mayo Clinic: Kidney Failure
  - http://www.mayoclinic.com/invoke.cfm?id=DS00280
- MedlinePlus: Hyperkalemia
  - http://www.nlm.nih.gov/medlineplus/ency/article/001179.htm
- National Kidney and Urologic Diseases Information Clearinghouse: Renal Tubular Acidosis
  - http://kidney.niddk.nih.gov/kudiseases/pubs/tubularacidosis/index.htm

REFERENCES

- Palmer BF: Managing hyperkalemia caused by inhibitors of the renin-angiotensin-aldosterone system. N Engl J Med 2004;351:585. [PMID: 15295051]
- Schepkens H et al: Life-threatening hyperkalemia during combined therapy with angiotensin-converting enzyme inhibitors and spironolactone: an analysis of 25 cases. Am J Med 2001;110:438. [PMID: 11331054]
- Schoolwerth AC et al: Renal considerations in angiotensin converting enzyme inhibitor therapy: a statement for healthcare professionals from the Council on the Kidney in Cardiovascular Disease and the Council for High Blood Pressure Research of the American Heart Association. Circulation 2001;104:1985. [PMID: 11602506]

Author(s)

Masafumi Fukagawa, MD, PhD
Kiyoshi Kurokawa, MD, MACP
Maxine A. Papadakis, MD

Hypernatremia

Hypermagnesemia p. 1093

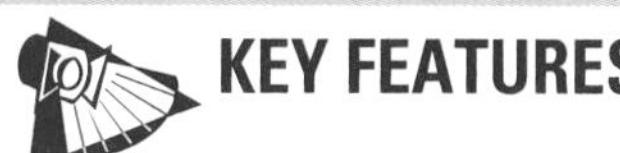

ESSENTIALS OF DIAGNOSIS

- Serum sodium > 145 mEq/L
- Occurs most commonly when water intake is inadequate, eg, with altered mental status
- Urine osmolality helps determine whether the water loss is renal or nonrenal

GENERAL CONSIDERATIONS

- An intact thirst mechanism usually prevents hypernatremia
- Excess water loss can cause hypernatremia only when water intake is inadequate
- Rarely, excessive sodium intake may cause hypernatremia
- Hypernatremia in the presence of salt and water overload is uncommon but has been reported in very ill patients in the course of therapy

Etiology

- **Urine osmolality > 400 mOsm/kg**
  - *Nonrenal losses*
  - Excessive sweating, burns
  - Insensible respiratory tract losses
  - Diarrhea, vomiting, nasogastric suctioning, osmotic cathartics (eg, lactulose)
  - *Renal losses*
  - Diuretics
  - Osmotic diuresis (eg, hyperglycemia, mannitol, urea)
  - Postobstructive diuresis
  - Diuretic phase of acute tubular necrosis
  - *Hypertonic sodium gain*
  - Salt intoxication (rare)
  - Hypertonic IV fluids, tube feeds, enemas
  - Primary hyperaldosteronism (hypernatremia usually mild and asymptomatic)
- **Urine osmolality < 250 mOsm/kg**
  - Central diabetes insipidus: idiopathic, head trauma, CNS mass
  - Nephrogenic diabetes insipidus: lithium, demeclocycline, prolonged urinary tract infections, interstitial nephritis, hypercalcemia, hypokalemia, congenital

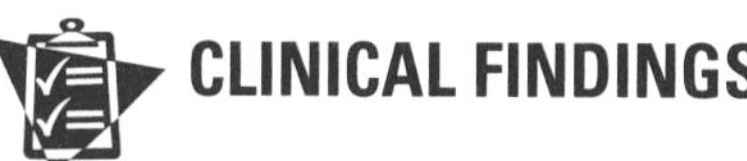

SYMPTOMS AND SIGNS

- With dehydration, orthostatic hypotension and oliguria are typical findings
- Altered mental status
- With severe hyperosmolality, hyperthermia, delirium, and coma may be seen

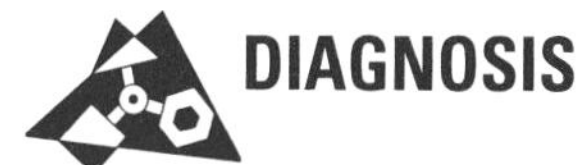

LABORATORY TESTS

- Urine osmolality > 400 mOsm/kg when renal water-conserving ability is functioning
- Urine osmolality < 250 mOsm/kg when renal water-conserving ability is impaired
- Serum osmolality invariably increased in the dehydrated state

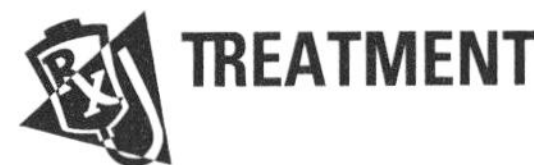

TREATMENT

MEDICATIONS

Type of fluid for replacement

- **Hypernatremia with hypovelemia**
  - Severe hypovolemia: give 0.9% saline (osmolality 308 mOsm/kg) to restore volume deficit and treat hyperosmolality, followed by 0.45% saline to replace any remaining free water deficit
  - Milder hypovolemia: give 0.45% saline and 5% dextrose in water
- **Hypernatremia with euvolemia**
  - Encourage water drinking or give 5% dextrose and water to cause excretion of excess sodium in urine
  - If GFR is decreased, give diuretics to increase urinary sodium excretion; however, they may impair renal concentrating ability, increasing quantity of water that needs to be replaced
- **Hypernatremia with hypervolemia**
  - Give 5% dextrose in water to reduce hyperosmolality, though this will expand vascular volume
  - Administer loop diuretic (eg, furosemide, 0.5–1 mg/kg) IV to remove excess sodium
  - In severe renal insufficiency, consider hemodialysis

Calculation of water deficit

- When calculating fluid replacement, add deficit and maintenance requirements to each 24-h replacement regimen
- **Acute hypernatremia**
  - In acute dehydration without much solute loss, free water loss is similar to weight loss
  - Initially, use 5% dextrose in water
  - As water deficit corrects, continue therapy with 0.45% saline with dextrose
- **Chronic hypernatremia**
  - Water deficit is calculated to restore normal osmolality for total body water (TBW)
  - TBW correlates with muscle mass and therefore decreases with advancing age, cachexia, and dehydration and is lower in women than men
  - Current TBW is 0.4–0.6 of current body weight

THERAPEUTIC PROCEDURES

- Correct the cause of fluid loss, and replace water and, as needed, electrolytes
- Administer fluid therapy over 48-h period, aiming for decrease in serum sodium of 1 mEq/L/h (1 mmol/L/h)
- Add potassium and phosphate as indicated by serum levels; monitor other electrolytes often

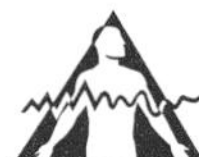

OUTCOME

COMPLICATIONS

- If hypernatremia is too rapidly corrected, the osmotic imbalance may cause water to preferentially enter brain cells, causing cerebral edema and potentially severe neurological impairment

WHEN TO REFER

- Hypernatremia > 150 mEq/L

WHEN TO ADMIT

- Altered mental status
- Marked dehydation
- Hypernatremia with hypervolemia

EVIDENCE

PRACTICE GUIDELINES

- American Medical Directors Association: Dehydration and Fluid Maintenance, 2001
  - http://www.guideline.gov/summary/summary.aspx?doc_id=3305&nbr=2531

WEB SITE

- Fall PJ: Hyponatremia and Hypernatremia: A Systematic Approach to Causes and Their Correction. Postgrad Med Online, 2000.
  - http://www.postgradmed.com/issues/2000/05_00/fall.htm

INFORMATION FOR PATIENTS

- MedlinePlus: Serum Sodium
  - http://www.nlm.nih.gov/medlineplus/ency/article/003481.htm
- National Kidney and Urologic Diseases Information Clearinghouse: Diabetes Insipidus
  - http://kidney.niddk.nih.gov/kudiseases/pubs/insipidus/index.htm

REFERENCES

- Adrogue HJ et al: Hypernatremia. N Engl J Med 2000;342:1493. [PMID: 10816188]
- Fall PJ: Hyponatremia and hypernatremia. A systematic approach to causes and their correction. Postgrad Med 2000;107:75. [PMID: 10844943]
- Kahn T: Hypernatremia with edema. Arch Intern Med 1999;159:93. [PMID: 9892337]
- Kugler JP et al: Hyponatremia and hypernatremia in the elderly. Am Fam Physician 2000;61:3623. [PMID: 10892634]

Author(s)

Masafumi Fukagawa, MD, PhD
Kiyoshi Kurokawa, MD, MACP
Maxine A. Papadakis, MD

Hyperparathyroidism

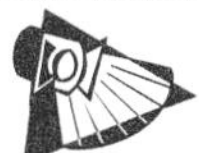

KEY FEATURES

ESSENTIALS OF DIAGNOSIS

- Primary hyperparathyroidism is characterized by chronic poorly regulated excessive secretion of parathyroid hormone (PTH) by one or more parathyroid glands that results in hypercalcemia
- Common disorder
- Patients frequently asymptomatic, hypercalcemia detected by screening
- Renal stones, polyuria, hypertension, constipation, fatigue, mental changes
- Bone pain; rarely, cystic lesions and pathological fractures
- Serum and urine calcium elevated; urine phosphate high with low or normal serum phosphate; alkaline phosphatase normal or elevated
- Elevated or high-normal serum (PTH) level

GENERAL CONSIDERATIONS

- PTH increases serum calcium and decreases serum phosphate via effects on bone osteoclastic activity and renal tubules
- PTH hypersecretion usually due to parathyroid adenoma, less commonly hyperplasia or carcinoma (rare)
- If age < 30 years, higher incidence of multiglandular disease (36%) and carcinoma (5%) responsible for hyperparathyroidism
- In chronic renal failure, hyperphosphatemia and decreased renal vitamin D production initially decrease ionized calcium, causing stimulation of parathyroids. Bone disease in this setting known as "renal osteodystrophy"

DEMOGRAPHICS

- Incidence of primary hyperparathyroidism in adults is 0.1%
- More common in persons age >50
- Ratio of M:F is 1:3
- Parathyroid adenomas or hyperplasia can be familial (about 5%) and may be part of multiple endocrine neoplasia (MEN) types 1, 2A, and 2B. In MEN 1, multiglandular hyperparathyroidism is usually the initial manifestation and ultimately occurs in over 90% of affected individuals. Hyperparathyroidism in MEN 2A is less frequent that in MEN 1 and is usually milder

CLINICAL FINDINGS

SYMPTOMS AND SIGNS

- Hypercalcemia usually discovered incidentally on routine laboratory testing
- Patients may be asymptomatic
- Symptomatic patients have problems with "bones, stones, abdominal groans, psychic moans, fatigue"
- Bone pain and arthralgias are common
- Chronic cortical bone resorption due to excess PTH (osteitis fibrosa cystica) may cause diffuse demineralization, pathological fractures, or cystic bone lesions (eg, "brown tumors" of jaw)
- Polyuria and polydipsia may result from hypercalcemia-induced nephrogenic diabetes insipidus
- Calcium-containing kidney stones
- Depression, intellectual weariness, and increased sleep requirement common
- Constipation, fatigue, anemia, weight loss, muscle weakness, easy fatigability, pruritus, and paresthesias
- Anorexia, nausea, and vomiting in severe cases
- Hypertension
- Parathyroid adenomas rarely palpable; palpable mass usually a thyroid nodule
- Parathyroid carcinomas often palpable (50%)
- Pancreatitis occurs in 3%
- Psychosis or even coma in severe hypercalcemia
- Calcium phosphate deposition in corneas or soft tissues

DIFFERENTIAL DIAGNOSIS

- Hypercalcemia of malignancy
- Multiple myeloma
- Vitamin D intoxication
- Sarcoidosis, tuberculosis
- Hyperthyroidism
- Vitamin D deficiency (serum 25-OH Vit D < 20 ng/ml) can cause high serum PTH with normal serum
- High-dose glucocorticoid therapy in patients taking thiazide diuretics

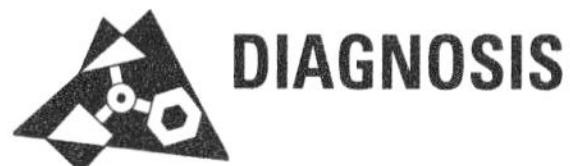

DIAGNOSIS

LABORATORY TESTS

- Serum calcium >10.5 mg/dL
- Elevated or high-normal PTH confirms the diagnosis. Immunoradiometric assay (IRMA) is most specific and sensitive
- Serum phosphate often low (< 2.5 mg/dL)
- Serum phosphate high in secondary hyperparathyroidism (renal failure)
- Urine calcium excretion high or normal (average 250 mg/g creatinine), but low for degree of hypercalcemia
- Screen for familial benign hypocalciuric hypercalcemia with 24-h urine for calcium and creatinine. Discontinue thiazide diuretics prior to this test
- Urine phosphate high despite low to low normal serum phosphate
- Serum alkaline phosphatase elevated only if bone disease present
- Plasma chloride and uric acid may be elevated

IMAGING STUDIES

- Preoperative imaging may be unsuccessful due to small size of gland, but if successful, may allow limited surgery
- ^{99m}Tc-sestamibi/Tc-pertechnetate subtraction scintigraphy with SPECT recommended; has sensitivity of 87%, specificity 95%
- Neck ultrasound has sensitivity of 80%
- Combination of both tests has sensitivity of 94%, but sensitivity only 55% if multiglandular disease
- MRI and CT not as sensitive as ultrasound
- MRI or ultrasound for hyperparathyroidism reveals incidental small benign thyroid nodules in ~50%
- Bone x-rays usually normal and not required, but may show demineralization, subperiosteal bone resorption, cysts throughout skeleton, mottling of skull, or pathological fractures
- In renal osteodystrophy, bone x-rays may show ectopic calcifications around joints or soft tissue, osteopenia, osteitis fibrosa, or osteosclerosis
- Bone densitometry of wrist, hip, and spine

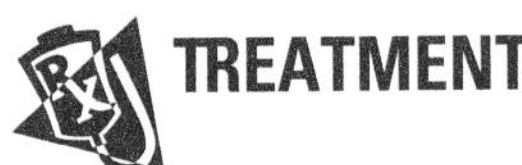

TREATMENT

MEDICATIONS

- Primary hyperparathyroidism: intravenous bisphosphonates can temporarily treat hypercalcemia and relieve bone pain. Pamidronate, 30–90 mg IV over 2–4 h, or zoledronic acid, 2–4 mg IV over 15 min (expensive). Oral bisphosphonates are ineffective
- Secondary or tertiary hyperparathyroidism of renal failure
  - Cinacalcet (Sesipar), a calcimimetic that stimulates the parathyroid glands calcium sensing receptor (CaSR) decreasing PTH secretion, given in doses of 30–250 mg PO QD, causes in a drop of serum PTH levels to < 250 pg/mL in 41%
  - Paricalcitol, 0.04–0.1 mg/kg IV TIW or doxercalciferol, 10 mg orally TIW after dialysis; increase to maximum of 20 mg TIW if PTH remains >400 ng/L. Hold for PTH < 100 ng/L
- Propranolol may prevent adverse cardiac effects of hypercalcemia
- Glucocorticoid therapy is ineffective for hypercalcemia in hyperparathyroidism

SURGERY

- Parathyroidectomy for patients with symptomatic hyperparathyroidism, kidney stones, or bone disease
- Consider surgery in asymptomatic patients with serum calcium 1 mg/dL above the upper limit of normal if urine calcium excretion >50 mg/24 h; urine calcium excretion >400 mg/24 h; cortical bone density >2 SD below normal; age < 50–60 years; difficulty ensuring medical follow-up; or pregnancy (second trimester)
- Minimally invasive parathyroid surgery usually sufficient if adenoma identified preoperatively
- Subtotal parathyroidectomy (3-1/2 glands removed) for patients with resistant parathyroid hyperplasia
- Postoperatively, keep patients hospitalized overnight
- Postoperative oral calcium and calcitriol 0.25 mg/day orally for 2 weeks helps prevent tetany

THERAPEUTIC PROCEDURES

- Patients with mild, asymptomatic hyperparathyroidism are advised to keep active, avoid immobilization, drink adequate fluids, and avoid thiazides, large doses of vitamins D and A, calcium-containing antacids or supplements, and digitalis (hypercalcemia predisposes to toxicity)

OUTCOME

FOLLOW-UP

- Check serum calcium and albumin twice yearly, renal function and urine calcium once yearly, and bone density (distal radius) every 2 years in mild, asymptomatic hyperparathyroidism
- Postoperatively, monitor serum calcium and PTH
- Symptomatic postoperative hypocalcemia is treated with liquid or chewable calcium carbonate and calcitriol 0.25–1 μg PO QD
- Postoperative secondary hyperparathyroidism (PTH rising above normal while serum calcium is normal or low due to "hungry bones") occurs in ~12% and is treated with calcium and vitamin D, usually for 3–6 months
- Hyperthyroidism immediately following parathyroid surgery may require short-term propranolol

COMPLICATIONS

- Forearm and hip fractures
- UTI due to obstruction by stones may lead to renal failure and uremia
- Clouding of sensorium, renal failure, and soft tissue calcinosis from rapidly rising serum calcium
- Peptic ulcer and pancreatitis
- Pseudogout before or after surgery
- Neonatal hypocalcemia and tetany from hypercalcemia during gestation
- In secondary hyperparathyroidism, disseminated calcification in skin, soft tissues, and arteries (calciphylaxis) can result in gangrene, arrhythmias, and respiratory failure

PROGNOSIS

- Asymptomatic mild hypercalcemia does not affect survival
- Surgical resection of sporadic parathyroid adenoma generally results in permanent cure
- Bones, despite severe cyst formation, deformity, and fracture, heal if parathyroid tumor removed
- Pancreatitis increases mortality rate
- Significant renal damage may progress even after adenoma removal
- Parathyroid carcinoma tends to invade local structures and may metastasize; repeat surgical resections and radiation therapy can prolong life

WHEN TO REFER

- Refer to parathyroid surgeon for parathyroidectomy

WHEN TO ADMIT

- Patients with severe hypercalcemia for IV hydration
- Prevent renal osteodystrophy (due to secondary hyperparathyroidism in renal failure) by avoiding hyperphosphatemia

EVIDENCE

PRACTICE GUIDELINES

- Malone JP et al: Hyperparathyroidism and multiple endocrine neoplasia. Otolaryngol Clin North Am 2004;37:715. [PMID: 15262511]

WEB SITES

- Allerheiligen D et al: Hyperthyroidism. American Family Physician, 1998.
  - http://www.aafp.org/afp/980415ap/allerhei.html
- National Institute of Diabetes and Digestive and Kidney Diseases (NIDDK)
  - http://www.niddk.nih.gov/health/endo/pubs/hyper/hyper.htm

INFORMATION FOR PATIENTS

- American Academy of Family Physicians—Hyperparathyroidism
  - http://familydoctor.org/handouts/251.html

REFERENCES

- Arciero CA et al: The utility of a rapid parathyroid assay for uniglandular, multiglandular, and recurrent parathyroid disease. Am Surg 2004;70:588. [PMID: 15279180]
- Caron NR et al: Persistent and recurrent hyperparathyroidism. Curr Treat Options Oncol 2004;5:335. [PMID: 15233910]
- Felderbauer P et al: Identification of a novel calcium-sensing gene mutation causing hypocalciuric hyercalcemia by single-strand conformation polymorphism analysis. Exp Clin Endocrinol Diabetes 2005;113:31. [PMID: 15662592]
- Peacock M et al: Cinacalcet hydrochloride maintains long-term normocalcemia in patients with primary hyperparathyroidism. J Clin Endocrinol Metab 2005;90:135. [PMID: 15522938]
- Rao DS et al: Randomized controlled clinical trial of surgery versus no surgery in patients with mild asymptomatic primary hyperparathyroidism. J Clin Endocrinol Metab 2004;89:5415. [PMID: 15531491]

Author(s)

Paul A. Fitzgerald, MD

Hyperprolactinemia

Hyperphosphatemia p. 1094

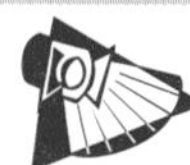

KEY FEATURES

ESSENTIALS OF DIAGNOSIS

- Women
  - Menstrual cycle disturbances (oligomenorrhea, amenorrhea)
  - Galactorrhea
  - Infertility
  - Gynecomastia
- Men
  - Hypogonadism
  - Decreased libido and erectile dysfunction
  - Infertility
- Serum prolactin elevated (Table 110)
- CT scan or MRI often demonstrates pituitary adenoma

GENERAL CONSIDERATIONS

- Prolactin's main role is to induce lactation
- During pregnancy, prolactin increases from normal (< 20 ng/mL) to as high as 600 ng/mL
- Suckling stimulates continued production of prolactin
- Prolactin is mainly under inhibitory control by dopamine
- Elevated serum prolactin can be caused by numerous conditions (see Differential Diagnosis)
- Most prolactinomas are microadenomas (< 1 cm in diameter) that usually do not grow, even with pregnancy or oral contraceptives
- However, macroadenomas occur and can spread into cavernous sinuses, suprasellar areas, and rarely into sinsuses by eroding the sella floor

DEMOGRAPHICS

- Prolactin-secreting pituitary tumors more common in women
- Usually sporadic but rarely familial as part of multiple endocrine neoplasia type 1 (MEN-1)

CLINICAL FINDINGS

SYMPTOMS AND SIGNS

- Hypogonadotropic hypogonadism
  - Men usually have erectile dysfunction, diminished libido, sometimes gynecomastia, but never galactorrhea
  - Women may have oligomenorrhea or amenorrhea, infertility, galactorrhea
- Of women with secondary amenorrhea and galactorrhea, 70% have hyperprolactinemia
- Large pituitary tumors may cause headaches, visual field defects
- Pituitary prolactinomas
  - May co-secrete growth hormone and cause acromegaly
  - Large tumors may cause pituitary insufficiency (hypogonadism), hypothyroidism, adrenal insufficiency, growth hormone deficiency

DIFFERENTIAL DIAGNOSIS

- See Table 110
- Causes of elevated prolactin
  - Pregnancy, postpartum, suckling, nipple stimulation, nipple rings
  - Macroprolactinemia (relatively inactive "big prolactin")
  - Exercise, sleep (REM phase), stress (trauma, surgery)
  - Idiopathic
  - Psychotropics, cimetidine, tricyclic antidepressants, oral contraceptives, marijuana
  - Prolactinoma
  - Hypothyroidism
  - Cirrhosis or renal failure
  - Acromegaly (pituitary tumor may co-secrete prolactin and growth hormone)
  - Hypothalamic disease
  - Tumor near pituitary
  - Systemic lupus erythematosus
  - Chronic chest wall stimulation
  - Multiple sclerosis, optic neuritis, spinal cord lesions

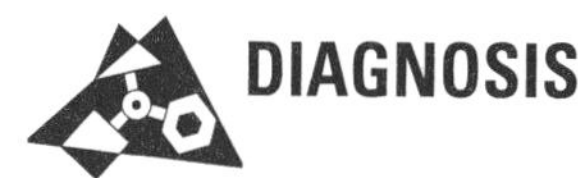

DIAGNOSIS

LABORATORY TESTS

- Urine or serum human chorionic gonadotropin to rule out pregnancy
- Serum thyroid-stimulating hormone high if hypothyroidism is cause
- Renal and liver chemistries abnormal in renal failure or cirrhosis
- Serum calcium elevated in hyperparathyroidism (MEN-1)
- Consider assay for macroprolactinemia if asymptomatic patient with no apparent cause for hyperprolactinemia

IMAGING STUDIES

- MRI of pituitary and hypothalamus indicated for nonpregnant patients
  - With prolactin >200 mg/dL
  - With headaches or visual field defects
  - With persistently elevated prolactin with no discernible cause
- Small prolactinomas may be demonstrated, but clear differentiation from normal variants not always possible

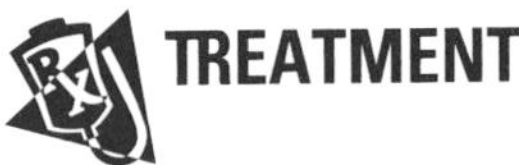

TREATMENT

MEDICATIONS

- Medical therapy is preferable to surgery or radiation, particularly for huge "macroprolactinomas"
- Discontinue medications known to increase prolactin, if possible, and recheck prolactin in a few weeks
- Dopamine agonists are initial treatment of choice for macroprolactinomas and to restore normal sexual function and fertility in hyperprolactinemia
- Cabergoline, 0.25 mg PO once weekly for 1 week, then 0.25 mg twice weekly for 1 week, then 0.5 mg twice weekly. Further increases may be required monthly, up to 1.5 mg twice weekly, based on serum prolactin
- Alternatives: bromocriptine (1.25–20 mg/day orally) and pergolide (0.125–2 mg/day orally)
- Quinagolide (not available in the United States) is a non–ergot-derived dopamine agonist for patients intolerant or resistant to other agents; dose: start at 0.075 mg/day PO, up to 0.6 mg/day
- Give dopamine agonists at bedtime to minimize side effects (fatigue, nausea, dizziness, and orthostatic hypotension), which usually improve with dosage reduction and continued use
  - Psychiatric side effects occur, are not dose related, and may take weeks to resolve after dopamine agonist is discontinued
- Treat hypothyroidism with thyroxine
- Oral contraceptives or estrogen replacement are safe for women with microprolactinomas who have amenorrhea or wish contraception; minimal risk of stimulating adenoma enlargement
- Estrogens and testosterone can stimulate macroprolactinomas and should not be used unless in full remission with medication or surgery

SURGERY

- Transsphenoidal resection of tumor may be urgently required for large tumors severely compromising visual fields or undergoing apoplexy
- Transsphenoidal selective resection of the pituitary adenoma is done electively for patients who do not tolerate or respond to dopamine agonists
- Craniotomy rarely indicated

THERAPEUTIC PROCEDURES

- Radiation therapy is reserved for macroadenomas that are growing despite dopamine agonist treatment
- Focused radiation therapy with gamma knife or cyber knife is preferable for certain patients, because it is generally safer and more convenient than conventional radiation therapy
- Conventional radiation therapy carries high risk of eventual hypopituitarism and may also cause memory impairment, second tumors, and small-vessel ischemic strokes
- After radiation therapy, patients should take low-dose aspirin for life to reduce risk of stroke

OUTCOME

FOLLOW-UP

- Women with microadenomas may have dopamine agonists safely withdrawn during pregnancy
- Macroadenomas may enlarge during pregnancy; if therapy is withdrawn, they must be followed up clinically and with computer-assisted visual field perimetry
- After pituitary surgery or radiation, monitor serum prolactin every 3 months

COMPLICATIONS

- Macroadenomas can impair visual fields and cause hypopituitarism
- Untreated hypogonadism increases risk of osteoporosis

PROGNOSIS

- Fertility is usually promptly restored with dopamine agonists
- Discontinuing dopamine agonists after months or years usually results in reappearance of hyperprolactinemia, galactorrhea, and amenorrhea
- With dopamine agonist treatment for prolactinoma
  - Nearly half—even massive tumors—shrink by >50%
  - Shrinkage of pituitary adenoma occurs early, but maximum effect may take up to a year
  - 90% have fall in serum prolactin to ≤10% pretreatment levels; 80% achieve normal serum prolactin level

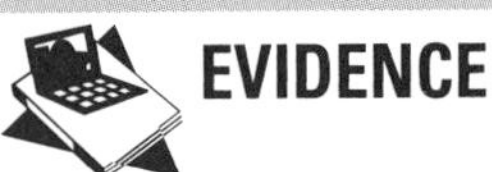

EVIDENCE

PRACTICE GUIDELINES

- Leung AK, Pacaud D: Diagnosis and management of galactorrhea. Am Fam Physician 2004;70:543. [PMID:15317441]
- Liu JK, Couldwell WT: Contemporary management of prolactinomas. Neurosurg Focus 2004;16:E2. [PMID:15191331]

WEB SITE

- E-Medicine Review Article
  - http://www.emedicine.com/med/topic1098.htm

INFORMATION FOR PATIENTS

- NIDDK—Prolactinoma
  - http://www.niddk.nih.gov/health/endo/pubs/prolact/prolact.htm

REFERENCES

- Colao A et al: Outcome of cabergoline treatment in men with prolactinoma: effects of a 24-month treatment on prolactin levels, tumor mass, recovery of pituitary function, and semen analysis. J Clin Endocrinol Metab 2004;89:1704. [PMID:15070934]
- Haddad PM, Wieck A: Antipsychotic-induced hyperprolactinaemia: mechanisms, clinical features and management. Drugs 2004;64:2291. [PMID:15456328]
- Toldy E et al: Macroprolactinemia: the consequences of a laboratory pitfall. Endocrine 2003;22:267. [PMID:14709800]

Author(s)

Paul A. Fitzgerald, MD

Hypersomnia p. 1094

Hypertension, Chronic

KEY FEATURES

ESSENTIALS OF DIAGNOSIS

- Usually asymptomatic
- Severe hypertension: occipital headache at awakening, blurry vision

GENERAL CONSIDERATIONS

- Mild to moderate hypertension nearly always asymptomatic
- Severe hypertension usually due to parenchymal renal disease, endocrine abnormalities, renal artery stenosis, drug use, or abrupt cessation of antihypertensive medications
- Table 42 provides classification based on blood pressure (BP) measurements
- Table 43 summarizes potential identifiable causes of hypertension
- Resistant hypertension is defined as failure to reach BP control in patients adherent to full doses of a 3-drug regimen (including a diuretic)
- Table 44 summarizes reasons for failure to reach BP control

DEMOGRAPHICS

- 50 million Americans affected
- 70% are aware of their condition
- 50% of those aware are receiving treatment
- 25% of all hypertensive patients have BP under control
- Incidence of hypertension increases with age
- More men than women in early life
- More women than men later in life
- More common in black Americans (up to 25%)

CLINICAL FINDINGS

SYMPTOMS AND SIGNS

- Usually asymptomatic
- Occipital headaches characteristic but uncommon
- Elevated BP
- Loud A_2 on cardiac examination
- Retinal arteriolar narrowing with "silver-wiring," arteriovenous nicking
- Flame-shaped hemorrhages
- Laboratory findings usually normal
- In severe hypertension, renal dysfunction and hemolysis

DIFFERENTIAL DIAGNOSIS

Primary (essential) hypertension

- "White-coat" hypertension
- BP cuff too small

Secondary hypertension

- See Table 43
- Adrenal
  - Primary hyperaldosteronism
  - Cushing's syndrome
  - Pheochromocytoma
- Renal
  - Chronic renal disease
  - Renal artery stenosis (atherosclerotic or fibromuscular dysplasia)
- Other
  - Oral contraceptives
  - Alcohol
  - Nonsteroidal anti-inflammatory drugs
  - Pregnancy associated
  - Hypercalcemia
  - Hyperthyroidism
  - Obstructive sleep apnea
  - Obesity
  - Coarctation of the aorta
  - Acromegaly
  - Increased intracranial pressure

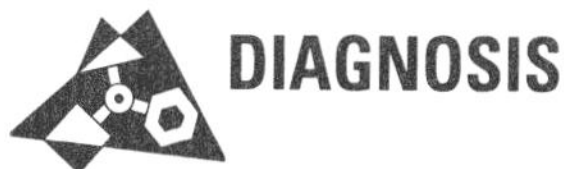

DIAGNOSIS

LABORATORY TESTS

- Hemoglobin
- Urinalysis
- Serum creatinine, blood urea nitrogen
- Serum potassium
- Fasting blood glucose
- Serum uric acid
- ECG
- When a secondary cause is suspected, consider
  - Chest x-ray
  - ECG
  - Plasma metanephrine levels
  - Plasma aldosterone concentration, plasma renin activity
  - Urine electrolytes

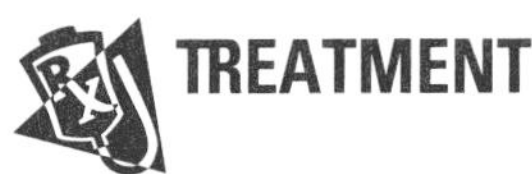

TREATMENT

MEDICATIONS

- Initiation of drug therapy based on level of BP, presence of target end-organ damage, and overall cardiovascular risk profile
- Major risk factors include
  - Smoking
  - Dyslipidemia
  - Diabetes mellitus
  - Age > 60 years
  - Family history of cardiovascular disease
- Specific choice of pharmacotherapeutic agent should be based on other risk factors, compliance, and cost
- Diuretics: Table 46
- β-Adrenergic blocking agents: Table 47
- Angiotensin-converting enzyme (ACE) inhibitors and angiotensin receptor blockers: Table 48
- Calcium channel-blocking agents: Table 49
- α-Adrenergic blockers, vasodilators, centrally acting agents: Table 50

THERAPEUTIC PROCEDURES

- See Table 41
- Dietary changes (DASH diet): high in fruits and vegetables, low fat, low salt
- Weight reduction
- Alcohol restriction
- Salt reduction
- Adequate potassium intake
- Adequate calcium intake
- Increase physical activity
- Smoking cessation
- Aggressive risk factor management should be considered in all patients with hypertension
- Antihypertensive medications should be individualized: Table 45
- Diabetics with hypertension should be treated aggressively, aiming for target BP < 130/80 mm Hg, given high risk of cardiovascular events, and ACE inhibitors or angiotensin receptor blockers should be part of regimen

OUTCOME

FOLLOW-UP

- Frequent visits until BP is controlled
- Once controlled, visits can be infrequent, limited laboratory tests
- Lipid monitoring every year
- ECG every 2–4 years, depending on initial ECG

COMPLICATIONS

- Stroke
- Dementia
- Myocardial infarction
- Congestive heart failure
- Retinal vasculopathy
- Aortic dissection
- Renal disease, including proteinuria and nephrosclerosis

WHEN TO REFER

- Refer if BP remains uncontrolled after three concurrent medications
- Refer if patient has uncontrolled BP and symptoms and signs of end-organ damage

WHEN TO ADMIT

- Consider hospitalization if symptoms and signs of a hypertensive emergency (see Hypertensive Urgencies & Emergencies) including, in the setting of very high BP, severe headache, neurologic symptoms, chest pain, altered mental status, or acutely worsening renal failure

EVIDENCE

PRACTICE GUIDELINES

- Seventh report of the Joint National Committee on Prevention, Detection, Evaluation, and Treatment of High Blood Pressure. 2003.
  - http://www.nhlbi.nih.gov/guidelines/hypertension/index.htm

WEB SITES

- American College of Cardiology
  - http://www.acc.org
- American Society for Hypertension
  - www.ash-us.org/
- Hypertension, Dialysis, and Clinical Nephrology, Renal Disease Electronic Journal
  - www.hdcn.com/free.htm
- National Heart, Lung, and Blood Institute
  - http://www.nhlbi.nih.gov/

INFORMATION FOR PATIENTS

- American Academy of Family Physicians: High Blood Pressure: Things You Can Do to Help Lower Yours
  - http://familydoctor.org/092.xml
- American Heart Association: High Blood Pressure
  - http://www.americanheart.org/presenter.jhtml?identifier=2112
- MedlinePlus: Hypertension Interactive Tutorial
  - http://www.nlm.nih.gov/medlineplus/tutorials/hypertension/htm/index.htm
- National Heart, Lung, and Blood Institute: Your Guide to Lowering High Blood Pressure
  - http://www.nhlbi.nih.gov/hbp/index.html
- National Heart, Lung, and Blood Institute: High Blood Pressure
  - http://www.nhlbi.nih.gov/health/dci/Diseases/Hbp/HBP_WhatIs.html

REFERENCES

- Chobanian AV et al: The Seventh Report of the Joint National Committee on prevention, detection, evaluation and treatment of high blood pressure: the JNC 7 report. JAMA 2003;289:2560. [PMID: 12748199]
- Sheridan S et al: Screening for high blood pressure: a review of the evidence for the U.S. Preventive Services Task Force. Am J Prev Med 2003;25:157. [PMID: 12880884]

Author(s)

Stephen J. McPhee, MD
Barry Massie, MD

Hypertensive Urgencies & Emergencies

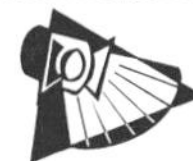

KEY FEATURES

ESSENTIALS OF DIAGNOSIS

- Important to differentiate hypertensive urgency (marked hypertension without end-organ damage) from hypertensive emergency (marked hypertension with end-organ damage)

GENERAL CONSIDERATIONS

- Hypertensive urgency usually has systolic blood pressure (BP) > 220 mm Hg or diastolic BP > 125 mm Hg without evidence of end-organ damage
- Hypertensive emergency defined by acute manifestations involving heart, brain, kidneys and/or retina

DEMOGRAPHICS

- Occurs in any age, gender, or racial/ethnic group
- Usually occurs in people with preexisting hypertension
- Often due to acute cessation of antihypertensive therapy
- Also occurs in setting of acute renal failure or use of high doses of sympathomimetics

CLINICAL FINDINGS

SYMPTOMS AND SIGNS

- Symptoms depend on the end organ involved
- Headaches, irritability, confusion, and somnolence are signs of encephalopathy
- Chest pain or dyspnea occurs with cardiopulmonary involvement
- Back pain occurs with aortic dissection
- Blurry or diminished vision occurs with retinal involvement
- Cardiac examination may reveal low A_2, an S_4, or a murmur of aortic regurgitation
- Papilledema, "silver-wiring" of retinal arterioles, and flame hemorrhages are indicative of elevation of intracranial pressure
- Crackles on lung examination occur with congestive heart failure
- Hematuria, proteinuria, or other evidence of renal dysfunction
- Hemolysis
- Elevated troponin or creatine kinase (CK) occurs with myocardial damage

DIFFERENTIAL DIAGNOSIS

- Adrenal
  - Primary hyperaldosteronism
  - Cushing's syndrome
  - Pheochromocytoma
- Renal
  - Chronic renal disease
  - Renal artery stenosis (atherosclerotic or fibromuscular dysplasia)
- Other
  - Oral contraceptives
  - Alcohol
  - Nonsteroidal anti-inflammatory drugs
  - Pregnancy associated
  - Hypercalcemia
  - Hyperthyroidism
  - Obstructive sleep apnea
  - Obesity
  - Coarctation of the aorta
  - Acromegaly
  - Increased intracranial pressure

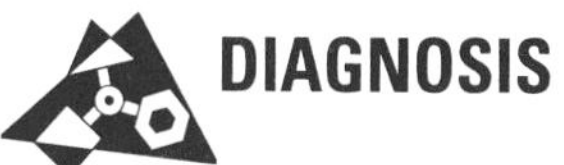

DIAGNOSIS

LABORATORY TESTS

- Hemoglobin
- Platelet count
- Urinalysis
- Serum creatinine, blood urea nitrogen, troponin, CK
- ECG
- Chest x-ray

DIAGNOSTIC PROCEDURES

- If central nervous system symptoms, head CT to rule out bleed
- If chest pain, ECG to rule out aortic dissection
- If nephropathy (hematuria, proteinuria, or renal dysfunction), renal ultrasound to rule out other causes of renal failure

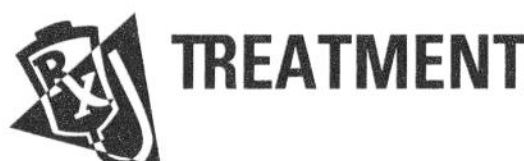

TREATMENT

MEDICATIONS

Hypertensive urgency

- Goal is to relieve symptoms and bring BP to reasonable level
- Clonidine, captopril, metoprolol, and hydralazine are effective oral agents
- Avoid β-blockers if cocaine use
- Avoid angiotensin-converting enzyme inhibitors if renal artery stenosis suspected
- Avoid short-acting dihydropyridine calcium channel blockers because BP reduction is often precipitous

Hypertensive emergency

- Treatment goal is to reduce mean arterial pressure by 25% in 1–2 h; then to reduce BP to 160/100 mm Hg over next 6–12 h
- Avoid excessive reduction in BP because this can lead to coronary, cerebral, or renal hypoperfusion
- Key to pharmacologic therapy is to use an agent with predictable, dose-dependent, transient effect
- Nitroprusside, labetalol, and nitroglycerin are most commonly used intravenously
- Fenoldopam, a peripheral dopamine agonist, is also effective

THERAPEUTIC PROCEDURES

- Treatment algorithm differs for hypertensive urgency and hypertensive emergency
- Goal is similar: reduce BP to "safe" range without causing end-organ damage
- Table 51 lists treatment options for hypertensive emergencies and urgencies
- In women who are pregnant or of childbearing age, preeclampsia or eclampsia should be excluded; if diagnosed, proper management plans should be instituted promptly

OUTCOME

FOLLOW-UP

- Patients with hypertensive urgency whose BP is brought under control should be seen within 48–72 h for a recheck of BP and tolerability of the antihypertensive regimen
- Patients with hypertensive emergency, once discharged from the hospital, should be followed-up in 48–72 h to ensure good compliance with BP medication and adequate BP control

COMPLICATIONS

- Stroke
- Myocardial infarction
- Congestive heart failure
- Retinal vasculopathy
- Aortic dissection
- Renal failure

WHEN TO REFER

- Refer patients with hypertensive urgency to expert in management of severe hypertension
- Refer patients with elevated BP and symptoms or signs of end-organ damage immediately for diagnostic workup and management

WHEN TO ADMIT

- Hospitalization for hypertensive urgency rarely needed
- Hypertensive emergency
  - Admit any patient with hypertensive emergency, in particular symptoms of encephalopathy, neurologic deficits, chest pain, dyspnea, or signs of papilledema, hematuria, renal dysfunction, or ECG changes
  - Usually need ICU admission for close monitoring of BP and clinical symptoms and signs

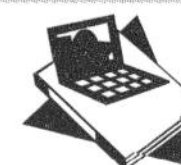

EVIDENCE

PRACTICE GUIDELINES

- American College of Obstetricians and Gynecologists. ACOG practice bulletin. Diagnosis and management of preeclampsia and eclampsia. Number 33, January 2002. Int J Gynaecol Obstet 2002;77:67. [PMID: 12094777]
- Seventh report of the Joint National Committee on Prevention, Detection, Evaluation, and Treatment of High Blood Pressure. 2003.
  - http://www.nhlbi.nih.gov/guidelines/hypertension/index.htm

WEB SITES

- American College of Cardiology
  - http://www.acc.org/
- Bales A: Hypertensive Crisis. Postgraduate Medicine Online 1999
  - http://www.postgradmed.com/issues/1999/05_01_99/bales.htm
- National Heart, Lung, and Blood Institute
  - http://www.nhlbi.nih.gov/

INFORMATION FOR PATIENTS

- Mayo Clinic: Hypertensive Crisis
  - http://www.mayoclinic.com/invoke.cfm?id=AN00626
- MedlinePlus: Hypertension Interactive Tutorial
  - http://www.nlm.nih.gov/medlineplus/tutorials/hypertension/htm/index.htm

REFERENCES

- Cherney D et al: Management of patients with hypertensive urgencies and emergencies. J Gen Intern Med 2002;17:947. [PMID: 12372930]
- Devlin JW et al: Fenoldopam versus nitroprusside for the treatment of hypertensive emergency. Ann Pharmacother 2004;38:755. [PMID: 15039472]
- Khanna A et al: Malignant hypertension presenting as hemolysis, thrombocytopenia, and renal failure. Rev Cardiovasc Med 2003;4:255. [PMID: 14674379]
- Phillips RA et al: Hypertensive emergencies: diagnosis and management. Prog Cardiovasc Dis 2002;45:33. [PMID: 12138413]

Author(s)

Stephen J. McPhee, MD

Barry Massie, MD

Hyperthyroidism

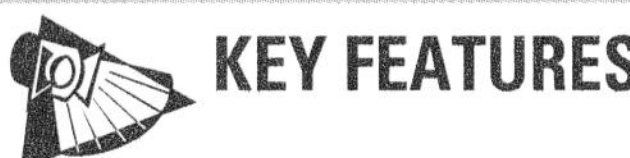

KEY FEATURES

ESSENTIALS OF DIAGNOSIS

- Sweating, weight loss (or gain), anxiety, loose stools, heat intolerance, irritability, fatigue, weakness, menstrual irregularity
- Tachycardia; warm, moist skin; stare; tremor
- In Graves' disease: goiter (often with bruit); ophthalmopathy
- Suppressed thyroid-stimulating hormone (TSH) in primary hyperthyroidism; increased free tetraiodothyronine (T_4) and triiodothyronine (T_3)

GENERAL CONSIDERATIONS

- Most common cause is Graves' disease
- Autonomous toxic adenomas, single or multiple
- Subacute de Quervain's thyroiditis: possibly viral, with hyperthyroidism followed by hypothyroidism
- Jodbasedow disease, or iodine-induced hyperthyroidism, may occur with multinodular goiters after significant iodine intake, radiographic contrast, or drugs, eg, amiodarone
- Amiodarone-induced hyperthyroidism: can occur 4 months to 3 years after initiation of amiodarone and after discontinuation. Thyrotoxicosis may cause angina or relapse of cardiac arrhythmia
- Thyrotoxicosis factitia: excessive exogenous thyroid hormone
- Hashimoto's thyroiditis may cause transient hyperthyroidism during initial phase and may occur postpartum
- High serum human chorionic gonadotropin levels in first 4 months of pregnancy, molar pregnancy, choriocarcinoma, and testicular malignancies may cause thyrotoxicosis

CLINICAL FINDINGS

SYMPTOMS AND SIGNS

- Nervousness, restlessness, heat intolerance, increased sweating, fatigue, weakness, muscle cramps, frequent bowel movements, weight loss (or gain), palpitations or angina pectoris
- Menstrual irregularities
- Stare and lid lag, tachycardia or atrial fibrillation, fine resting tremor, moist warm skin, hyperreflexia, fine hair, onycholysis, and (rarely) heart failure
- Goiter (often with a bruit) in Graves' disease
- Moderately enlarged, tender thyroid in subacute thyroiditis
- Ophthalmopathy (chemosis, conjunctivitis, and mild proptosis) in 20–40% of patients with Graves' disease
- Cardiac manifestations, eg, forceful heart beat, premature atrial contractions, sinus tachycardia, atrial fibrillation or atrial tachycardia, thyrotoxic cardiomyopathy due to thyrotoxicosis
- Diplopia may be due to coexistent myasthenia gravis
- Dermopathy (myxedema) in 3% of patients with Graves' disease
- Thyroid storm
- Hypokalemic paralysis (Asian or Native-American men)

DIFFERENTIAL DIAGNOSIS

- General anxiety or panic disorder
- Mania
- Other hypermetabolic state, eg, cancer, pheochromocytoma
- Exophthalmos due to other cause, eg, orbital tumor
- Atrial fibrillation due to other cause
- Acute psychiatric disorders (may falsely increase serum thyroxine)
- High estrogen states, eg, pregnancy
- Hypopituitarism
- Subclinical hyperthyroidism

DIAGNOSIS

LABORATORY TESTS

- Sensitive TSH assay best test for thyrotoxicosis
- Serum T_3 and free T_4 usually increased
- T_4 sometimes normal but T_3 elevated
- Serum FT_3 (rather than T_3) in women, pregnant or taking oral estrogen
- Serum TT_3 can be misleadingly elevated when blood collected in tubes using gel barrier
- Hypercalcemia
- Alkaline phosphatase increased
- Anemia, neutropenia
- TSH receptor antibody (TSH-R Ab) levels high in 75% of patients with Graves' disease
- Antithyroglobulin or antithyroperoxidase (anti-TPO, antimicrosomal) antimicrosomal antibodies usually elevated in Graves' disease, but nonspecific
- ANA and anti–double-stranded DNA antibodies usually elevated
- Erythrocyte sedimentation rate often elevated in subacute thyroiditis
- TSH elevated or normal despite thyrotoxicosis in TSH-secreting pituitary tumor
- Suppressed TSH and total T_4 >20 μg/dL or T_3 >200 ng/dL to diagnose amiodarone-induced hyperthyroidism because high total T_4 and free T_4 common on amiodarone
- Type I amiodarone-induced thyrotoxicosis, diagnosable by elevated serum levels of thyroperoxidase Ab and TSH-R Ab

IMAGING STUDIES

- Thyroid radioactive iodine uptake and scan usually indicated for hyperthyroid patients
- High ^{123}I uptake in Graves' disease and toxic nodular goiter. Scan can detect toxic nodule or multinodular goiter
- Low uptake characteristic of subacute thyroiditis and amiodarone-induced hyperthyroidism
- Color-flow Doppler: increased blood flow in type I and lower blood flow in type II amiodarone-induced thyrotoxicosis
- Thyroid ultrasound can detect multinodular goiter

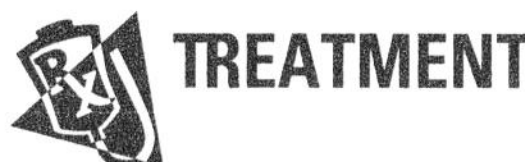

TREATMENT

MEDICATIONS

- **Graves' disease**
- Propranolol, 20 mg PO BID to start, increased until adequate response, usually 20–80 mg PO QID; improves tachycardia, tremor, diaphoresis, and anxiety of hyperthyroidism; may then use propranolol LA, 60, 80, 120, or 160 mg PO BID. Continue until hyperthyroidism resolved
- Thioureas: methimazole or propylthiouracil (PTU) generally used for young adults, those with mild thyrotoxicosis, small goiters, or fear of radioiodine; preparing patients for surgery, and elderly patients for ^{131}I treatment
- Methimazole preferred over PTU, because PTU can rarely cause acute hepatic necrosis. During pregnancy, use low doses of methimazole (5–15 mg/d) or PTU (50–150 mg/d) to avoid fetal hypothyroidism. During lactation, recommended doses are methimazole ≤20 mg/d and PTU ≤450 mg/d, taken just after breastfeeding
  - Methimazole may be used chronically for patients who are tolerating it well
- Agranulocytosis is an uncommon but serious complication of thioureas
- Goiter occurs if patient is allowed to develop prolonged hypothyroidism on

thioureas, but usually regresses rapidly with thyroid hormone replacement

- Methimazole, 10–30 mg BID, with dose reduced and given once daily as manifestations of hyperthyroidism resolve and free T_4 normalizes
- Propylthiouracil, 300–600 mg PO divided QID, with dose and frequency reduced as symptoms resolve and free T_4 normalizes
- Iodinated contrast agents [iopanoic acid (Telepaque) or ipodate sodium (Bilivist, Oragrafin)], 500 mg PO QD or BID. Begin after thiourea commenced
- **Subacute thyroiditis:** Propranolol for symptoms as above; ipodate sodium or iopanoic acid as above for 15–60 days
- **Amiodarone-induced thyrotoxicosis:** Methimazole, iopanoic acid, β-blockers, prednisone
- **Hypokalemic thyrotoxic paralysis:** Propranolol corrects hypokalemia, even in apathetic hyperthyroidism

SURGERY

- Patients treated preoperatively with methimazole; ipodate sodium or iopanoic acid (500 mg PO BID), commenced 6 hours after methimazole commenced, accelerates euthyroidism and reduces thyroid vascularity. Iodine (eg, Lugols solution, 2–3 gtts PO daily for several days) also reduces vascularity. Propranolol given until serum T_3 or free T_3 is normal preoperatively. For patients undergoing surgery while thyrotoxic, larger doses of propranolol required perioperatively to reduce possibility of thyroid crisis
- **Graves' disease:** thyroidectomy preferred over radioiodine for:
  - Pregnant women whose thyrotoxicosis is not controlled with low-dose thioureas
  - Women desiring pregnancy in very near future
  - Children
  - Patients with extremely large goiters
  - Those with suspected malignancy
- Hartley-Dunhill operation is procedure of choice for Graves' disease: total resection of one lobe and a subtotal resection of the other lobe, leaving about 4 g of thyroid tissue
- **Toxic solitary thyroid nodules:** partial thyroidectomy for patients aged < 40, ^{131}I for those aged >40 years

THERAPEUTIC PROCEDURES

- **Graves' disease, toxic multinodular goiter**
  - Radioactive iodine (^{131}I) therapy. Patients usually only on propranolol, but those with coronary disease, aged >65 years, or severe hyperthyroidism are usually first rendered euthyroid with methimazole. Contraindicated in pregnancy
  - Discontinue methimazole 4 days before ^{131}I treatment; methimazole given after ^{131}I for symptomatic hyperthyroidism until euthyroid

OUTCOME

FOLLOW-UP

- Check WBC periodically on thioureas, and for sore throat or febrile illness
- Free T_4 levels every 2–3 weeks during initial treatment
- Hypothyroidism common months to years after ^{131}I or subtotal thyroidectomy. Lifelong clinical follow-up, with TSH and free T_4 measurements

COMPLICATIONS

- Atrial fibrillation, congestive heart failure, cardiomyopathy
- Periodic hypokalemic paralysis
- Osteoporosis, hypercalcemia
- Temporary decreased libido, impotence, decreased sperm count, gynecomastia
- Diplopia or loss of vision
- Subtotal thyroidectomy of both lobes results in 9% recurrence of hyperthyroidism
- Total thyroidectomy of both lobes, increased risk for hypoparathyroidism and bilateral damage to the recurrent laryngeal nerves
- Complications of thiourea therapy: rash, nausea, agranulocytosis, rarely acute hepatic necrosis (PTU)
- Retrobulbar radiation, for Graves' exophthalmos, can cause radiation-induced retinopathy (usually subclinical) in about 5% of patients overall, mostly diabetics

PROGNOSIS

- Post-treatment hypothyroidism common, especially with ^{131}I or surgery
- Recurrence of hyperthyroidism occurs most commonly after thioureas (~50%)
- Subacute thyroiditis usually subsides spontaneously in weeks to months
- Graves' disease usually progresses, but may rarely subside spontaneously or even result in hypothyroidism
- Despite treatment, increased risk of death from cardiovascular disease, stroke, and femur fracture in women
- Mortality of thyroid storm is high
- Subclinical hyperthyroidism: good prognosis; increased risk for bone loss

WHEN TO ADMIT

- Thyroid storm
- Hyperthyroidism-induced atrial fibrillation with severe tachycardia
- ^{131}I therapy or thyroidectomy

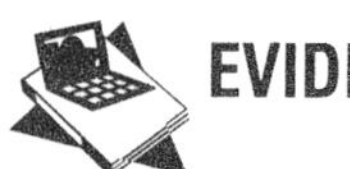

EVIDENCE

WEB SITES

- American Thyroid Association
  - http://www.thyroid.org/index.php3?M_Session=444ddf3f109e91628b84729a2dc7ca3a
- Thyroid Disease Manager site
  - http://www.thyroidmanager.org

REFERENCES

- Chi SY et al: A prospective, randomized comparison of bilateral subtotal thyroidectomy versus unilateral total and contralateral subtotal thyroidectomy for Graves disease. World J Surg 2005;29:160. [PMID:15650802]
- Cooper DS: Antithyroid drugs. N Engl J Med 2005;352:905. [PMID:15745981]
- Frost L et al: Hyperthyroidism and risk of atrial fibrillation or flutter: a population-based study. Arch Intern Med 2004;164:1675. [PMID:15302638]
- Read CH Jr et al: A 36-year retrospective analysis of the efficacy and safety of radioactive iodine in treating young Graves' patients. J Clin Endocrinol Metab 2004;89:4229. [PMID:15356012]
- Streetman DD et al: Diagnosis and treatment of Graves' disease. Ann Pharmacother 2003;37:1100. [PMID:12841824]
- Wakelkamp IM et al: Orbital irradiation for Graves' ophthalmopathy: Is it safe? A long-term follow-up study. Ophthalmology 2004;111:1557. [PMID:15288988]

Author(s)

Paul A. Fitzgerald, MD

Hypocalcemia

KEY FEATURES

ESSENTIALS OF DIAGNOSIS

- Frequently mistaken for a neurological disorder
- Mainly caused by insufficient action of parathyroid hormone (PTH) and/or vitamin D as well as magnesium difficiency
- If the ionized calcium is normal despite a low total serum calcium, calcium metabolism is usually normal

GENERAL CONSIDERATIONS

- True hypocalcemia (decreased ionized calcium) implies insufficient action of PTH or active vitamin D
- The most common cause of low total serum calcium is hypoalbuminemia, correction of which is needed to accurately reflect the ionized calcium concentration
- The most common cause of true hypocalcemia is renal failure, in which there is decreased production of active vitamin D_3 and hyperphosphatemia

Etiology

- **Decreased intake or absorption**
  - Malabsorption
  - Small bowel bypass
  - Vitamin D deficit, including 25-hydroxyvitamin D or 1,25-dihydroxyvitamin D
- **Increased loss**
  - Alcoholism
  - Chronic renal failure
  - Diuretic therapy
- **Endocrine disease**
  - Hypoparathyroidism
  - Sepsis
  - Pseudohypoparathyroidism
  - Calcitonin secretion from medullary carcinoma of the thyroid
  - Familial hypocalcemia
- **Physiological causes**
  - Decreased serum albumin but normal ionized calcium
  - Decreased end-organ response to vitamin D
  - Hyperphosphatemia
  - Loop diuretics

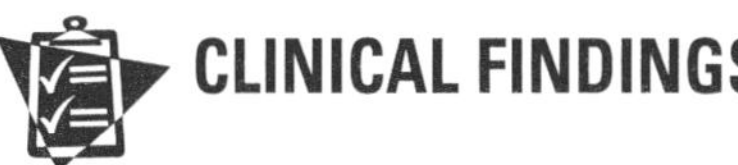

CLINICAL FINDINGS

SYMPTOMS AND SIGNS

- Extensive spasm of skeletal muscle causes cramps and tetany
- Laryngospasm with stridor can obstruct the airway
- Convulsions, paresthesias of lips and extremities, and abdominal pain
- Chvostek's sign (contraction of the facial muscle in response to tapping the facial nerve anterior to the ear)
- Trousseau's sign (carpal spasm occurring after occlusion of the brachial artery with a blood pressure cuff for 3 min) is usually readily elicited
- In chronic hypoparathyroidism, cataracts and calcification of basal ganglia of the brain may occur
- Ventricular arrhythmias if there is QT prolongation

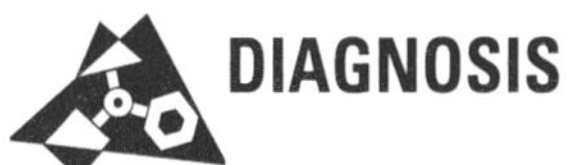

DIAGNOSIS

LABORATORY TESTS

- When albumin is low, serum Ca^{2+} concentration is depressed in a ratio of 0.8–1 mg/dL of Ca^{2+} to 1 g/dL of albumin, but the physiologically active ionized calcium is normal
- In true hypocalcemia, the ionized serum calcium concentration is low (< 4.7 mg/dL)
- Serum phosphate is usually elevated in hypoparathyroidism or end-stage renal disease, whereas it is suppressed in early-stage renal failure or vitamin D deficiency
- Serum Mg^{2+} is commonly low, and hypomagnesemia reduces both PTH release and tissue responsiveness to PTH, causing hypocalcemia
- In respiratory alkalosis, total serum calcium is normal but ionized calcium is low

IMAGING STUDIES

- ECG can show prolongation of the QT interval (as a result of lengthened ST segment)

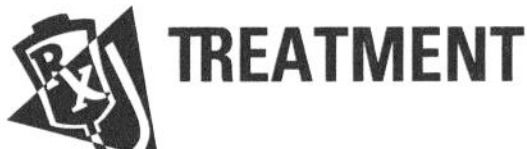

TREATMENT

MEDICATIONS

Severe, symptomatic hypocalcemia

- In the presence of tetany, arrhythmias, or seizures, administer calcium gluconate 10% (10–20 mL) IV over 10–15 min
- Because of the short duration of action, calcium infusion is usually required; add 10–15 mg of calcium per kilogram body weight, or six to eight 10-mL vials of 10% calcium gluconate (558–744 mg of calcium), to 1 L of D_5W and infuse over 4–6 h
- Adjust the infusion rate to maintain the serum calcium level at 7–8.5 mg/dL

Asymptomatic hypocalcemia

- Oral calcium (1–2 g) and vitamin D preparations (Table 88)
- Calcium carbonate is well tolerated and less expensive than many other calcium tablets
- The low serum Ca^{2+} associated with low serum albumin concentration does not require replacement therapy
- If serum Mg^{2+} is low, therapy must include replacement of magnesium, which by itself usually will correct hypocalcemia

OUTCOME

FOLLOW-UP

- Monitor the serum calcium level frequently (every 4–6 h) during calcium infusions for severe hypocalcemia

PROGNOSIS

- Depends on the underlying cause (eg, renal failure)

WHEN TO REFER

- Refer early to a nephrologist if renal failure is the underlying cause

WHEN TO ADMIT

- Admit all symptomatic patients. Intensive care unit admission may be needed
- Admit if parenteral therapy is needed

EVIDENCE

INFORMATION FOR PATIENTS

- American Association for Clinical Chemistry: Lab Tests Online: Calcium
  - http://www.labtestsonline.org/understanding/analytes/calcium/test.html
- Mayo Clinic: Hypoparathyroidism
  - http://www.mayoclinic.com/invoke.cfm?id=AN00718
- Mayo Clinic: Kidney Failure
  - http://www.mayoclinic.com/invoke.cfm?id=DS00280
- MedlinePlus: Calcium Supplements (Systemic)
  - http://www.nlm.nih.gov/medlineplus/druginfo/uspdi/202108.html
- MedlinePlus: Pseudohypoparathyroidism
  - http://www.nlm.nih.gov/medlineplus/ency/article/000364.htm
- NIH Office of Dietary Supplements: Calcium Fact Sheet
  - http://dietary-supplements.info.nih.gov/factsheets/calcium.asp#h7

REFERENCES

- Ariyan CE: Assessment and management of patients with abnormal calcium. Crit Care Med 2004;32:5146. [PMID: 15064673]
- Diercks DB et al: Electrocardiographic manifestations: electrolyte abnormalities. J Emerg Med 2004;27:153. [PMID: 15261358]
- Marx SJ: Hyperparathyroidism and hypoparathyroid disorders. N Engl J Med 2000;343:1863. [PMID: 11117980]
- Zivin JR et al: Hypocalcemia: a pervasive metabolic abnormality in the critically ill. Am J Kidney Dis 2001;37:689. [PMID: 11273867]

Author(s)

Masafumi Fukagawa, MD, PhD
Kiyoshi Kurokawa, MD, MACP
Maxine A. Papadakis, MD

Hypoglycemic Disorders

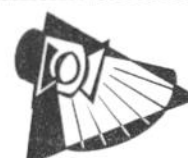

KEY FEATURES

ESSENTIALS OF DIAGNOSIS

- Symptoms begin at plasma glucose levels of ~60 mg/dL, brain function impairment at ~50 mg/dL
- Two types of spontaneous hypoglyemia: fasting and postprandial
- Fasting hypoglycemia often subacute or chronic; usually presents with neuroglycopenia
- Postprandial hypoglycemia relatively acute, with symptoms of neurogenic autonomic discharge (sweating, palpitations, anxiety, tremulousness)

GENERAL CONSIDERATIONS

Fasting hypoglycemia

- Endocrine disorders (eg, hypopituitarism, Addison's disease, myxedema)
- Liver malfunction (eg, acute alcoholism, liver failure)
- Renal failure on dialysis
- In absence of endocrine disorders, rule out hyperinsulinism from pancreatic B-cell tumors or surreptitious administration of insulin (or sulfonylureas) and hypoglycemia caused by non-insulin-producing extrapancreatic tumors

Postprandial (reactive) hypoglycemia

- Postprandial hypoglycemia is early (2–3 h after a meal) or late (3–5 h after eating)
- Early, or alimentary, hypoglycemia occurs when there is rapid discharge of ingested carbohydrate into the small bowel followed by rapid glucose absorption and hyperinsulinism
- Particularly associated with dumping syndrome after gastrectomy
- Rarely results from defective counterregulatory responses such as deficiencies of growth hormone, glucagon, cortisol, or autonomic responses
- Alcohol-related hypoglycemia is due to hepatic glycogen depletion combined with alcohol-mediated inhibition of gluconeogenesis. Most common in malnourished alcohol abusers but can occur in anyone unable to ingest food after an acute alcoholic episode followed by gastritis and vomiting
- Factitious hypoglycemia is due to surreptitious administration of insulin or sulfonylurea

CLINICAL FINDINGS

SYMPTOMS AND SIGNS

- Whipple's triad is characteristic of hypoglycemia regardless of the cause: a history of hypoglycemic symptoms, an associated fasting blood glucose of ≤ 40 mg/dL, and immediate recovery on administration of glucose

Fasting hypoglycemia

- Healthy-appearing person with fasting hypoglycemia and confusion or abnormal behavior
- Obesity can result from overeating to relieve symptoms
- Insulinoma
- Symptoms often develop in the early morning, after missing a meal, or occasionally after exercise
- Initial CNS symptoms include blurred vision or diplopia, headache, feelings of detachment, slurred speech, and weakness
- Convulsions or coma may occur; sweating and palpitations may not
- Personality changes vary from anxiety to psychotic behavior
- Hypoglycemic unawareness is very common

DIFFERENTIAL DIAGNOSIS

- Fasting hypoglycemia
  - Hyperinsulinism: pancreatic B-cell tumor and surreptitious insulin or sulfonylureas
  - Extrapancreatic tumors
- Postprandial hypoglycemia: early hypoglycemia (alimentary)
- Postgastrectomy
- Functional (increased vagal tone): late hypoglycemia (occult diabetes)
- Delayed insulin release resulting from B-cell dysfunction
  - Counterregulatory deficiency
  - Idiopathic
- Alcohol-related hypoglycemia
- Immunopathological hypoglycemia: antibodies to insulin receptors, which act as agonists
- Pentamidine-induced hypoglycemia
- Islet hyperplasia (noninsulinoma pancreatogenous hypoglycemia syndrome)

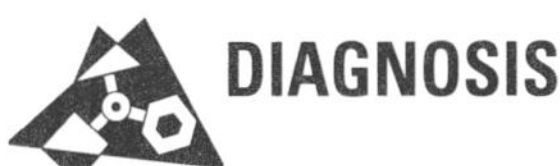

DIAGNOSIS

LABORATORY TESTS

- Serum insulin level ≥ 6 μU/mL in RIA assay (3 μU/mL ICMA assay) in the presence of blood glucose values < 40 mg/dL is diagnostic of inappropriate hyperinsulinism. Other causes of hyperinsulinemic hypoglycemia must be considered, including factitious administration of insulin or sulfonylureas
- An elevated circulating proinsulin level (> 5 pmol/L) in the presence of fasting hypoglycemia is characteristic of most B-cell adenomas and does not occur in factitious hyperinsulinism
- In patients with epigastric distress, history of renal stones, or menstrual or erectile dysfunction, serum calcium, gastrin, or prolactin level may be useful in screening for MEN-1 associated with insulinoma
- Prolonged fasting up to 72 h under hospital supervision until hypoglycemia is documented
- In normal men, the blood glucose does not fall below 55–60 mg/dL during a 3-day fast, whereas in normal premenopausal women who have fasted for only 24 h, the plasma glucose may fall normally to as low as 35 mg/dL. The women are not symptomatic, presumably owing to the development of sufficient ketonemia to supply energy needs to the brain
- Insulinoma patients become symptomatic when plasma glucose drops to subnormal levels, because inappropriate insulin secretion restricts ketone formation
- A high-carbohydrate breakfast can differentiate postprandial reactive hypoglycemia from normal states; half of patients with reactive hypoglycemia will have glucose levels as low as 59 mg/dL versus 2% of controls. This test is more sensitive than a standard mixed meal

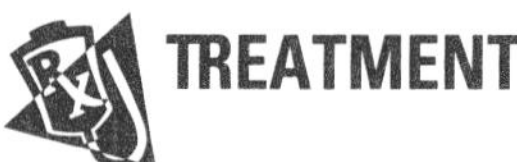

TREATMENT

MEDICATIONS

Inoperable pancreatic B-cell tumors

- Diazoxide, 300–600 mg PO QD (along with a thiazide diuretic to control sodium retention)
- Glucagon
- Octreotide, 50 μg SC BID

SURGERY

- Surgical treatment for endocrine tumors

THERAPEUTIC PROCEDURES

Inoperable pancreatic B-cell tumors

- Carbohydrate feeding every 2–3 h

Postprandial (reactive) hypoglycemia

- Frequent feedings with smaller portions of less rapidly assimilated carbohydrate combined with more slowly absorbed fat and protein

Functional alimentary hypoglycemia

- Support and mild sedation are mainstays of therapy
- Dietary manipulation is an adjunct: reduce proportion of carbohydrates in the diet, increase the frequency and reduce the size of the meals

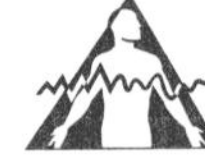

OUTCOME

COMPLICATIONS

- Indiscriminate use and overinterpretation of glucose tolerance tests have led to an overdiagnosis of functional hypoglycemia
- As many as one third or more of normal individuals have blood glucose levels as low as 40–50 mg/dL with or without symptoms during a 4-h glucose tolerance test

EVIDENCE

WEB SITES

- American Diabetes Association
  - http://www.diabetes.org/main/application/commercewf
- American Dietetic Association
  - http://www.eatright.org
- CDC Diabetes Public Health Resource
  - http://www.cdc.gov/diabetes/
- Joslin Diabetes Center
  - http://www.joslin.harvard.edu/

INFORMATION FOR PATIENTS

- Joslin Diabetes Center: Is Low Blood Glucose (Hypoglycemiz) Dangerous?
  - http://www.joslin.harvard.edu/education/library/low_bs_danger.shtml
- Mayo Clinic: Hypoglycemia
  - http://www.mayoclinic.com/invoke.cfm?id=DS00198
- National Diabetes Information Clearinghouse
  - http://diabetes.niddk.nih.gov/dm/pubs/hypoglycemia

REFERENCE

- Service FJ: Diagnostic approach to adults with hypoglycemic disorders. Endocrinol Metab Clin North Am 1999;28:519. [PMID: 10500929]

Author(s)

Umesh Masharani, MB, BS, MRCH (UK)

Hypogonadism, Male

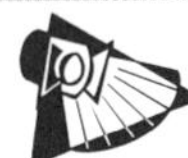

KEY FEATURES

ESSENTIALS OF DIAGNOSIS

- Diminished libido and erections
- Decreased growth of body hair
- Small or normal testes; serum or free testosterone decreased
- Serum gonadotropins [luteinizing hormone (LH) and follicle-stimulating hormone (FSH)] decreased in hypogonadotropic hypogonadism (insufficient gonadotropin secretion by pituitary) and increased in hypergonadotropic hypogonadism (testicular failure)

GENERAL CONSIDERATIONS

- Caused by deficient testosterone secretion by the testes
- In hypogonadotropic form, FSH and LH deficiency may be isolated or accompanied by other pituitary hormone abnormalities

Hypogonadotropic hypogonadism

- Pituitary adenoma or hypopituitarism causing hyperprolactinemia, Cushing's syndrome, adrenal insufficiency, growth hormone excess or deficiency, thyroid hormone excess or deficiency
- Hemochromatosis
- Estrogen-secreting tumor (testicular, adrenal)
- Gonadotropin-releasing hormone agonist therapy, eg, leuprolide
- Other drugs, eg, alcohol, ketoconazole, spironolactone, marijuana
- Anorexia nervosa, cirrhosis, other serious illness, or malnutrition
- Kallmann's or Prader-Willi syndrome
- Intrathecal opioid infusion
- Congenital adrenal hypoplasia
- Idiopathic

Hypergonadotropic hypogonadism

- Male climacteric (andropause)
- Klinefelter's syndrome: at least one Y chromosome and at least two X chromosomes (47,XXY et al)
- Orchitis, eg, mumps, gonorrhea, tuberculosis, leprosy
- Testicular failure secondary to radiation therapy or chemotherapy
- Autoimmune, uremia, testicular trauma or torsion, lymphoma, myotonic dystrophy, androgen insensitivity

CLINICAL FINDINGS

SYMPTOMS AND SIGNS

- Delayed puberty if congenital or acquired during childhood
- Decreased libido with acquired hypogonadism in most
- Erectile dysfunction, hot sweats, fatigue, or depression
- Infertility, gynecomastia, headache, or fracture
- Decreased body, axillary, beard, or pubic hair
- Loss of muscle mass and weight gain due to increased subcutaneous fat
- Testicular size, as assessed with orchidometer, may decrease but usually remains within normal range (normal volume about 10–25 mL; normal length usually >6 cm) in postpubertal hypogonadotropic hypogonadism
- In Klinefelter's syndrome, manifestations are variable
  - Generally, testes normal in childhood, but usually become small, firm, fibrotic, and nontender in adolescence
  - Normal onset of puberty, variable degree of virilization, gynecomastia at puberty, tall stature with increased arm span
  - Patients with >2 X or >1 Y chromosomes are more prone to mental deficiency, clinodactyly, synostosis, poor social skills
- Testicular mass (Leydig cell tumor), trauma, infiltrative lesions (eg, lymphoma), or chronic infection (eg, leprosy, tuberculosis)

DIFFERENTIAL DIAGNOSIS

- Erectile dysfunction due to other cause, eg, diabetes mellitus, atherosclerosis, stroke, or drugs
- Male infertility due to other cause, eg, cryptorchism, retrograde ejaculation
- Gynecomastia due to other cause, eg, puberty, chronic liver disease, drugs, malignancy
- Hypothyroidism (may also cause hypogonadism)
- Depression

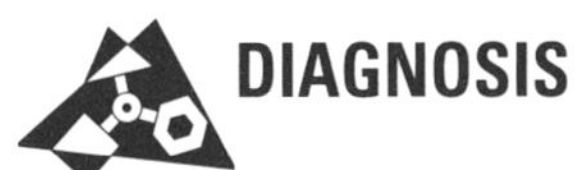

DIAGNOSIS

LABORATORY TESTS

- Total testosterone measured nonfasting in AM is low (may be 25–50% lower, below "normal range," if obtained fasting or in PM)
- Testosterone highest at age 20–30 years, slightly lower at 30–40 years; falls gradually but progressively after age 40
- Free testosterone useful in elderly men due to rising sex hormone-binding globulin (SHBG) with age
  - Equilibrium dialysis, calculated free testosterone, and non–HBG-bound testosterone assays are best
  - Free androgen index, direct radioimmunoassay, and analog free testosterone assays are inaccurate
- Check serum LH and FSH levels if serum testosterone is low or borderline–low
- LH and FSH high in hypergonadotropic hypogonadism and low or inappropriately normal in hypogonadotropic hypogonadism

Hypogonadotropic hypogonadism

- Check serum prolactin: elevated in prolactinoma
- If gynecomastia, check serum androstenedione and estrone: both elevated in partial 17-ketosteroid reductase deficiency
- Check serum estradiol: elevated in cirrhosis and rare estrogen-secreting tumors (testicular Leydig cell tumor or adrenal carcinoma)
- If no clear cause for hypogonadotropic hypogonadism, check serum ferritin: elevated in hemochromatosis

Hypergonadotropic hypogonadism

- Check karyotyping or measurement of leukocyte X-inactive-specific transcriptase (XIST) by PCR for Klinefelter's syndrome

IMAGING STUDIES

- MRI of pituitary to evaluate for tumor or other lesion when no clear cause of hypogonadotropic hypogonadism
- Bone densitometry: reduced bone density in long-standing male hypogonadism

DIAGNOSTIC PROCEDURES

- Testicular biopsy is usually reserved for younger patients when reason for primary hypogonadism is unclear

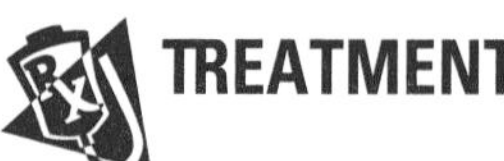

TREATMENT

MEDICATIONS

- Testosterone replacement to reverse sexual dysfunction and muscle atrophy is usually begun when hypogonadism is confirmed and cause determined
- Screen older men for prostate cancer before initiating testosterone therapy
- Topical testosterone 1% gel is available as Androgel (2.5-g and 5-g packets):
  - Starting dose is 5 g; dosage may be increased to maximum of 10 g/day if clinically indicated
  - Gel is applied QD to clean, dry skin of shoulders, upper arms, or abdomen, not genitals. **Note**: Hands must be washed after gel application, site allowed to dry 5 minutes before dressing, and clothing worn during contact with women or children
- Transdermal testosterone is available in patch formulations applied QD to different nongenital skin sites:
  - Testoderm II, 5 mg/day leaves sticky residue but causes little skin irritation
  - Androderm, 2.5–10 mg/day adheres more tightly but may cause skin irritation
- Parenteral testosterone (enanthate or cypionate), 300 mg IM Q 3 weeks or 200 mg IM Q 2 weeks, usually in gluteal area, with dose adjustment per patient response
- Oral androgens (eg, methyltestosterone and fluoxymesterone) should not be used because they predispose patients to peliosis hepatis, hepatic tumors, and hepatic dysfunction and are less effective than transdermal or parenteral testosterone

THERAPEUTIC PROCEDURES

- Men with mosaic Klinefelter's syndrome (eg, 46,XY/47,XXY) may be fertile. Otherwise, infertility may be overcome by in vitro intracytoplasmic sperm injection (ICSI) into an ovum

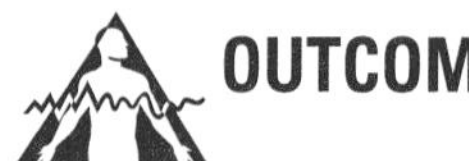

OUTCOME

FOLLOW-UP

- Reassess patient clinically and measure serum testosterone after initiation of testosterone replacement
  - If inadequate clinical response or serum testosterone below normal, increase dose
- Monitor hematocrit due to risk of polycythemia

COMPLICATIONS

- Complication of hypogonadism: osteoporosis
- Complications of Klinefelter's syndrome
  - Neoplasms including breast cancer
  - Chronic pulmonary disease
  - Varicosities of the legs
  - Diabetes mellitus (8%)
  - Impaired glucose tolerance without frank diabetes (19%)
- Side effects of testosterone replacement
  - Acne
  - Gynecomastia
  - Aggravation of sleep apnea
  - Reduced HDL cholesterol
- Side effects of oral androgens: cholestatic jaundice (1–2%), and liver tumors or peliosis hepatis rarely with long-term use
- Side effects of megestrol acetate: increased appetite, weight gain, hyperglycemia, and hypertriglyceridemia

PROGNOSIS

- Prognosis of hypogonadism due to pituitary lesion is that of primary disease (eg, tumor, necrosis)
- Prognosis for restoration of virility is good if testosterone replacement is given

EVIDENCE

PRACTICE GUIDELINES

- AACE Medical Guidelines for Clinical Practice: Hypogonadism, 2002
  - http://www.aace.com/clin/guidelines/hypogonadism.pdf
- Morales A et al: International Society for the Study of the Aging Male. Investigation, treatment and monitoring of late-onset hypogonadism in males. Official recommendations of ISSAM. Aging Male 2002;5:74. [PMID:12198738]

WEB SITES

- The Pituitary Foundation
  - http://www.pituitary.org.uk/resources/hypogon-m.htm
- Pituitary Network Association
  - http://www.pituitary.com/disorders/hypogonadism.php

INFORMATION FOR PATIENTS

- Mayo Clinic—Hypogonadism
  - http://www.mayoclinic.com/invoke.cfm?objectid=E97FDCB5-E617-4C36-859B911C11AOE9257
- MEDLINEplus—Hypogonadism
  - http://www.nlm.nih.gov/medlineplus/ency/article/001195.htm

REFERENCES

- Basaria S et al: Long-term effects of androgen deprivation therapy in prostate cancer patients. Clin Endocrinol (Oxf) 2002; 56:779. [PMID:12072048]
- Matsumoto AM et al: Serum testosterone assays—accuracy matters. J Clin Endocrinol Metab 2004;89:529. [PMID:14764756]
- Morley JE et al: Androgen treatment of male hypogonadism in older males. J Steroid Biochem Mol Biol 2003;85:367. [PMID:12943724]

Author(s)

Paul A. Fitzgerald, MD

Hypokalemia

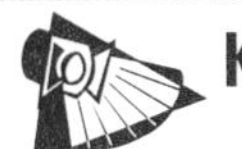

KEY FEATURES

ESSENTIALS OF DIAGNOSIS

- Serum K^+ < 3.5 mEq/L
- Severe hypokalemia may induce dangerous arrhythmias and even rhabdomyolysis
- Transtubular potassium concentration gradient (TTKG) can distinguish renal from nonrenal loss of potassium

GENERAL CONSIDERATIONS

- Total potassium content of the body is 50 mEq/kg, more than 95% of which is intracellular
- A deficit of about 4–5 mEq/kg occurs for each 1 mEq/L decrement in serum potassium concentration below a level of 4 mEq/L
- Potassium shift into the cell is transiently stimulated by insulin and glucose and facilitated by β-adrenergic stimulation
- α-Adrenergic stimulation blocks potassium shift into the cell
- Aldosterone, which facilitates urinary potassium excretion through enhanced potassium secretion at the distal renal tubules, is the most important regulator of body potassium content
- Magnesium is an important cofactor for potassium uptake and for maintenance of intracellular potassium levels

Etiology

- **Potassium shift into cell**
- Insulin excess, eg, postprandial
- Alkalosis
- β-Adrenergic agonists
- Trauma (via epinephrine release)
- Hypokalemic periodic paralysis
- **Renal potassium loss (urine K^+ > 40 mEq/L)**
- Barium or cesium intoxication
- Increased aldosterone (mineralocorticoid) effects
  - Primary hyperaldosteronism
  - Secondary hyperaldosteronism (dehydration, heart failure)
  - Renovascular or malignant hypertension
  - Cushing's syndrome
  - European licorice (inhibits cortisol)
  - Renin-producing tumor
  - Congenital abnormality of steroid metabolism (eg, adrenogenital syndrome, 17α-hydroxylase defect)
- Increased flow of distal nephron
  - Diuretics (furosemide, thiazides)
  - Salt-losing nephropathy
- Hypomagnesemia
  - Unreabsorbable anion
  - Carbenicillin, penicillin
- Renal tubular acidosis (type I or II)
  - Fanconi's syndrome
  - Interstitial nephritis
  - Metabolic alkalosis (bicarbonaturia)
- Genetic disorder of the nephron
  - Bartter's syndrome
  - Liddle's syndrome
- **Extrarenal potassium loss (urine K^+ < 20 mEq/L)**
- Vomiting, diarrhea, laxative abuse
- Villous adenoma, Zollinger-Ellison syndrome

CLINICAL FINDINGS

SYMPTOMS AND SIGNS

- Muscular weakness, fatigue, and muscle cramps are common in mild to moderate hypokalemia
- Constipation or ileus may result from smooth muscle involvement
- Flaccid paralysis, hyporeflexia, hypercapnia, tetany, and rhabdomyolysis may be seen with severe hypokalemia (< 2.5 mEq/L)

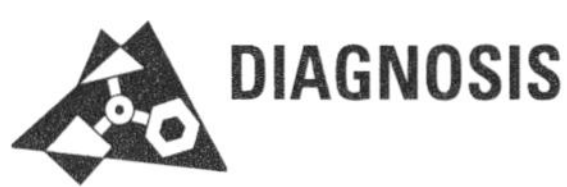

DIAGNOSIS

LABORATORY TESTS

- Urinary potassium concentration is low (< 20 mEq/L) as a result of extrarenal loss and inappropriately high (> 40 mEq/L) with urinary losses
- Calculating TTKG is a simple and rapid method to evaluate net potassium secretion

$$\text{TTKG} = \frac{\text{Urine K}^+/\text{Plasma K}^+}{\text{Urine osm}/\text{Plasma osm}}$$

- Hypokalemia with TTKG > 4 suggests renal potassium loss with increased distal K
  - In such cases, plasma renin and aldosterone levels are helpful in differential diagnosis
  - The presence of nonabsorbed anions, including bicarbonate, also increases the TTKG

IMAGING STUDIES

- ECG can show decreased amplitude and broadening of T waves, prominent U waves, premature ventricular contractions, and depressed ST segments

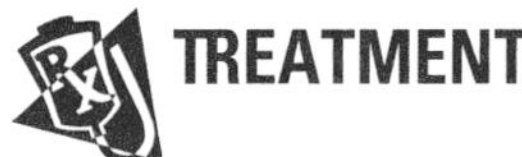

TREATMENT

MEDICATIONS

- Oral potassium is the safest way to treat mild to moderate deficiency
- All potassium formulations are easily absorbed
- Dietary potassium is almost entirely coupled to phosphate—rather than chloride—and does not correct potassium loss associated with chloride depletion, such as from diuretics or vomiting
- In the setting of abnormal renal function and mild to moderate diuretic dosage, 20 mEq/day of oral potassium is generally sufficient to prevent hypokalemia, but 40–100 mEq/day over a period of days to weeks is needed to treat hypokalemia and fully replete potassium stores
- Intravenous potassium replacement is indicated for patients with severe hypokalemia and for those who cannot take oral supplementation
- For severe deficiency, potassium may be given through a peripheral intravenous line in a concentration that should not exceed 40 mEq/L at rates of up to 40 mEq/L/h
- Coexisting magnesium and potassium depletion can result in refractory hypokalemia despite potassium repletion if there is no magnesium repletion

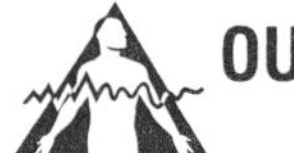

OUTCOME

FOLLOW-UP

- Continuous ECG monitoring indicated when infusing intravenous potassium for severe hypokalemia
- Check serum potassium level every 3–6 h

COMPLICATIONS

- Hypokalemia increases the likelihood of digitalis toxicity. Thus, hypokalemia induced by concomitant drugs such as β_2-adrenergic agonists and diuretics may impose a substantial risk

WHEN TO REFER

- Persistent hypokalemia ($K^+ < 3.0$ mEq/ L) or use of diuretics without any recent gastrointestinal losses

WHEN TO ADMIT

- For severe hypokalemia ($K^+ < 2.5$ mEq/ L)
- If intravenous potassium replacement is needed
- If cardiac monitoring is necessary during potassium replacement

PROGNOSIS

- Most hypokalemia will correct with replacement after 24–72 h

EVIDENCE

PRACTICE GUIDELINES

- Cohn JN et al: New guidelines for potassium replacement in clinical practice: a contemporary review by the National Council on Potassium in Clinical Practice. Arch Intern Med 2000;160:2429. [PMID: 10979053]

INFORMATION FOR PATIENTS

- MedlinePlus: Hyperaldosteronism
  - http://www.nlm.nih.gov/medlineplus/ency/article/000330.htm
- MedlinePlus: Hypokalemia
  - http://www.nlm.nih.gov/medlineplus/ency/article/000479.htm
- MedlinePlus: Potassium Drug Information
  - http://www.nlm.nih.gov/medlineplus/druginfo/medmaster/a601099.html
- National Kidney and Urologic Diseases Information Clearinghouse: Renal Tubular Acidosis
  - http://kidney.niddk.nih.gov/kudiseases/pubs/tubularacidosis/index.htm

REFERENCES

- Gennari FJ: Hypokalemia. N Engl J Med 1998;339:451. [PMID: 9700180]
- Loughrey CM: Serum magnesium must also be known in profound hypokalaemia. BMJ 2002;324:1039. [PMID: 11976255]
- Macdonald JE et al: What is the optimal serum potassium level in cardiovascular patients? J Am Coll Cardiol 2004;43:155. [PMID: 14736430]
- Rastegar A et al: Hypokalaemia and hyperkalaemia. Postgrad Med J 2001;77:759. [PMID: 11723313]
- Welfare W et al: Challenges in managing profound hypokalemia. BMJ 2002;324:269 [PMID: 11823358]

Author(s)

Masafumi Fukagawa, MD, PhD
Kiyoshi Kurokawa, MD, MACP
Maxine A. Papadakis, MD

Hypomagnesemia

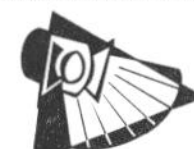

KEY FEATURES

ESSENTIALS OF DIAGNOSIS

- Causes neurological symptoms and arrhythmias
- Serum concentration may not be decreased even in the presence of magnesium deficiency
- Check urinary magnesium excretion if depletion is suspected
- Impairs release of parathyroid hormone (PTH)

GENERAL CONSIDERATIONS

- Magnesium acts directly on the myoneural junction
- Altered concentration of Mg^{2+} in the plasma usually provokes an associated alteration of Ca^{2+}
- Severe and prolonged magnesium depletion impairs secretion of PTH with consequent hypocalcemia
- Hypomagnesemia may impair end-organ response to PTH as well

Etiology

- **Diminished absorption or uptake**
- Malabsorption
- Chronic diarrhea
- Laxative abuse
- Prolonged gastrointestinal suction
- Malnutrition
- Alcoholism
- Parenteral alimentation with inadequate Mg^{+} content
- **Increased renal loss**
- Diuretic therapy
- Hyperaldosteronism
- Barrter's syndrome
- Hyperparathyroidism
- Hyperthyroidism
- Hypercalcemia
- Volume expansion
- Tubulointerstitial diseases
- Drugs (aminoglycoside, cisplatin, amphotericin B, pentamidine)
- **Others**
- Diabetes mellitus
- Postparathyroidectomy (hungry bone syndrome)
- Respiratory alkalosis
- Pregnancy

DEMOGRAPHICS

- Nearly half of hospitalized patients for whom serum electrolytes are ordered have unrecognized hypomagnesemia
- Common causes include use of large volumes of IV fluids, diuretics, cisplatin in cancer patients (with concomitant hypokalemia), and administration of nephrotoxic agents such as aminoglycosides and amphotericin B

CLINICAL FINDINGS

SYMPTOMS AND SIGNS

- Weakness, muscle cramps, and tremor
- Marked neuromuscular and central nervous system hyperirritability, with tremors, athetoid movements, jerking, nystagmus, and a positive Babinski response
- Confusion and disorientation
- Hypertension, tachycardia, and ventricular arrhythmias

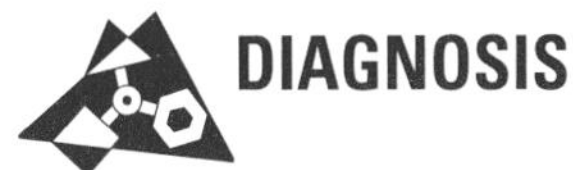

DIAGNOSIS

LABORATORY TESTS

- Urinary excretion of magnesium exceeding 10–30 mg/day or a fractional excretion more than 2% indicates renal magnesium wasting
- In calculating fractional excretion of magnesium, only 30% is protein bound, thus 70% of circulating magnesium is filtered by the glomerulus
- Up to 40% of patients have hypokalemia and up to 50% have hypocalcemia
- PTH secretion is often suppressed

IMAGING STUDIES

- ECG may show a prolonged QT interval because of lengthening of the ST segment

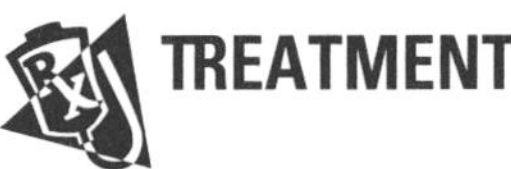

TREATMENT

MEDICATIONS

- Symptomatic hypomagnesemia: infuse 1–2 g of magnesium sulfate immediately, followed by an infusion of 6 g of magnesium sulfate in at least 1 L of fluid over 24 h, repeated for up to 7 days
- Magnesium sulfate may also be given IM in a dosage of 200–800 mg/day (8–33 mmol/day) in four divided doses
- In magnesium replacement in a patient with renal insufficiency, reduce dose of magesium sulfate by 50–75%
- Chronic hypomagnesemia: magnesium oxide, 250–500 mg PO once or twice daily, is useful for repleting stores
- Hypokalemia and hypocalcemia of hypomagnesemia do not recover without magnesium supplementation; thus, replacement of K^+ and Ca^{2+} are also required

OUTCOME

FOLLOW-UP

- Monitor serum magnesium levels and adjust dosage of magnesium supplementation to keep the level below 2.5 mmol/L; tendon reflexes can also be checked, because hypermagnesemia causes hyporeflexia
- In patients with renal insufficiency, replace magnesium cautiously to avoid hypermagnesemia. Frequent monitoring of serum levels (at least twice daily) is indicated

WHEN TO REFER

- Refer to an endocrinologist or nephrologist for consultation about repletion in the setting of marked neuromuscular symptoms or cardiac arrhythmia

WHEN TO ADMIT

- Confusion, disorientation
- Marked neuromuscular and central nervous system hyperirritability
- Need for intravenous replacement

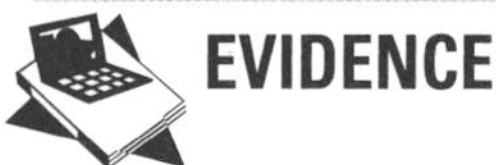

EVIDENCE

INFORMATION FOR PATIENTS

- American Association for Clinical Chemistry: Lab Tests Online: Magnesium
  - http://www.labtestsonline.org/understanding/analytes/magnesium/test.html
- MedlinePlus: Hypomagnesemia
  - http://www.nlm.nih.gov/medlineplus/ency/article/000315.htm
- MedlinePlus: Magnesium Supplements (Systemic)
  - http://www.nlm.nih.gov/medlineplus/druginfo/uspdi/202644.html
- NIH Office of Dietary Supplements: Magnesium
  - http://ods.od.nih.gov/factsheets/cc/magn.html

REFERENCES

- Dacey M: Hypomagnesemic disorders. Crit Care Clin 2001;17:155. [PMID: 11219227]
- Huijgen HJ et al: Magnesium levels in critically ill patients. What should we measure? Am J Clin Pathol 2000;114:688. [PMID: 11068541]

Author(s)

Masafumi Fukagawa, MD, PhD
Kiyoshi Kurokawa, MD, MACP
Maxine A. Papadakis, MD

Hyponatremia

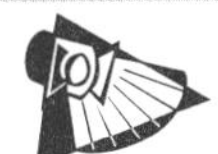

KEY FEATURES

ESSENTIALS OF DIAGNOSIS

- Serum sodium concentration < 130 mEq/L
- Mainly caused by abnormality of water balance, not salt balance
- Assessment of extracellular fluid (ECF) volume and measurement of serum osmolality are essential to determine cause of hyponatremia

GENERAL CONSIDERATIONS

- Hyponatremia is usually associated with abnormal serum osmolality
- Implies abnormal water balance rather than abnormal sodium balance
- Abnormal sodium balance is often associated with either volume depletion or edema formation
- Hospitalized patients treated with hypotonic fluid are at increased risk for hyponatremia

Etiology

- **Isotonic hyponatremia or pseudohyponatremia**
  - Normal serum osmolality; artifact corrected in most U.S. labs
  - Hyperlipidemia
  - Hyperproteinemia
- **Hypertonic hyponatremia**
  - Serum osmolality > 295 mOsm/kg
  - Hyperglycemia
  - Mannitol, sorbitol, glycerol, maltose
  - Radiocontrast agents
- **Hypotonic hyponatremia**
  - Serum osmolality < 280 mOsm/kg
- **Hypovolemic**
  - Extrarenal salt loss (U_{Na+} < 10 mEq/L): dehydration, diarrhea, vomiting, or third-spacing, as with ascites
  - Renal salt loss (U_{Na+} > 20 mEq/L): diuretics, angiotensin-correcting enzyme (ACE) inhibitors, salt-losing nephropathies, mineralocorticoid deficiency, cerebral sodium-wasting syndrome
- **Euvolemic**
  - Syndrome of inappropriate antidiuretic hormone
  - Postoperative hyponatremia
  - Hypothyroidism
  - Psychogenic polydipsia
  - Beer potomania
  - Idiosyncratic drug reaction (thiazides, ACE inhibitors)
  - Endurance exercise
- **Hypervolemic** (edematous states)
  - Congestive heart failure
  - Liver disease
  - Nephrotic syndrome (rare)
  - Advanced renal failure

CLINICAL FINDINGS

DEMOGRAPHICS

- Most common electrolyte abnormality observed in a general hospitalized population (~2% of patients)

SYMPTOMS AND SIGNS

- Frequently asymptomatic
- Symptomatic hyponatremia is usually seen with serum sodium levels < 120 mEq/L
- Usually, central nervous system (CNS) symptoms: lethargy, weakness, confusion, delirium, and seizures
- Symptoms are often mistaken for primary neurological or metabolic disorders

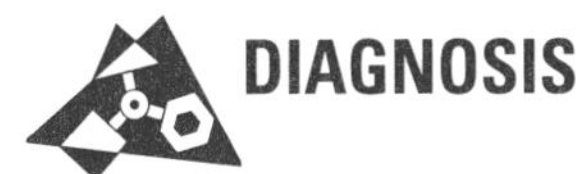

DIAGNOSIS

LABORATORY TESTS

- Measure serum and urine osmolality and assess patient's volume status
- Urine sodium helps distinguish renal from nonrenal causes of hyponatremia
- Urine sodium > 20 mEq/L implies renal salt wasting
- Urine sodium < 10 mEq/L or fractional excretion of sodium < 1% (unless diuretics have been given) implies avid sodium retention by the kidney because of extrarenal fluid losses

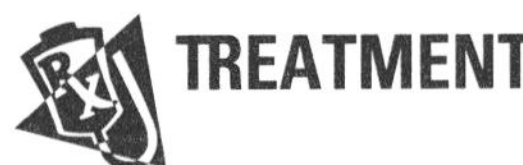

TREATMENT

MEDICATIONS

Hypovolemic hypotonic hyponatremia

- Replace lost volume with isotonic (0.9%) or half-normal (0.45%) saline or lactated Ringer's
- Adjust rate of correction to prevent permanent cerebral damage
- Administer corticosteroids empirically if hypocortisolism is possible

Euvolemic hyponatremia

- See Syndrome of Inappropriate Antidiuretic Hormone
- Symptomatic hyponatremia
  - If CNS symptoms, treat hyponatremia rapidly at any level of serum sodium concentration
  - Increase serum sodium concentration by ≤ 1–2 mEq/L/h and not > 25–30 mEq/L in the first 2 days to prevent central pontine myelinolysis; reduce rate to 0.5–1 mEq/L/h as neurological symptoms improve
  - Initial goal: serum sodium 125–130 mEq/L, guarding against overcorrection
  - Hypertonic (eg, 3%) saline plus furosemide (0.5–1 mg/kg IV)
  - To determine how much 3% saline (513 mEq/L) to administer, obtain spot urinary Na^+ after furosemide diuresis has begun. Excreted Na^+ is replaced with 3% saline, empirically begun at 1–2 mL/kg/h and then adjusted based on urinary output and urinary sodium (eg, after furosemide, urine volume may be 400 mL/h and sodium + potassium excretion 100 mEq/L; excreted Na^+ = 40 mEq/h, which is replaced with 78 mL/h of 3% saline [40 mEq/h divided by 513 mEq/L])
- Asymptomatic hyponatremia
  - Restrict water intake to 0.5–1 L/day; serum sodium will gradually increase occur over days
  - Correction rate: ≤ 0.5 mEq/L/h
  - No specific treatment needed for patients with reset osmostats
  - Isotonic 0.9% saline with furosemide in asymptomatic patients with serum sodium < 120 mEq/L. Replace urinary sodium and potassium losses as above
  - Demeclocycline, 300–600 mg PO BID, inhibits effect of ADH on distal tubule; is useful for patients who cannot adhere to water restriction or need additional therapy. Onset of action may be 1 week, and concentrating may be permanently impaired. Therapy with demeclocycline in cirrhosis appears to increase renal failure risk
  - Fludrocortisone for hyponatremia as part of cerebral salt-wasting syndrome

Hypervolemic hypotonic hyponatremia

- Treat underlying condition (eg, improving cardiac output in congestive heart failure) and restrict water (< 1–2 L daily)
- Diuretics to hasten water and salt excretion
- Diuretics may worsen hyponatremia; caution patient not to increase free water intake
  - Hypertonic 3.0% saline administration is potentially dangerous in volume-overloaded states, thus not generally recommended
  - In patients with severe hyponatremia (serum sodium < 110 mEq/L) and CNS symptoms, judicious administration of small amounts (100–200 mL) of 3% saline with diuretics may be necessary
  - Consider emergency dialysis

OUTCOME

FOLLOW-UP

- If symptomatic, measure plasma sodium ~Q4 h and observe patient closely

COMPLICATIONS

- Central pontine myelinolysis may occur from osmotically induced demyelination as a result of overly rapid correction of serum sodium (an increase of > 1 mEq/L/h, or ≥25 mEq/L within first 24 h of therapy)
- Hypoxic-anoxic episodes during hyponatremia may contribute to demyelination

PROGNOSIS

- Premenopausal women who develop hyponatremic encephalopathy from rapidly acquired hyponatremia (eg, postoperative hyponatremia) are about 25 times more likely than postmenopausal women to suffer permanent brain damage or die

WHEN TO REFER

- Persistent hyponatremia despite therapy

WHEN TO ADMIT

- Symptomatic hyponatremia
- Serum sodium < 120 mEq/L

EVIDENCE

WEB SITE

- Fall PJ: Hyponatremia and Hypernatremia, A Systematic Approach to Causes and Their Correction. Postgraduate Medicine Online, 2000
  - http://www.postgradmed.com/issues/2000/05_00/fall.htm

INFORMATION FOR PATIENTS

- American Association for Clinical Chemistry: Lab Tests Online: Sodium
  - http://labtestsonline.org/understanding/analytes/sodium/test.html
- Mayo Clinic: Low Blood Sodium in Older Adults
  - http://www.mayoclinic.com/invoke.cfm?id=AN00621
- MedlinePlus: Dilutional Hyponatremia (SIADH)
  - http://www.nlm.nih.gov/medlineplus/ency/article/000394.htm
- MedlinePlus: Serum Sodium
  - http://www.nlm.nih.gov/medlineplus/ency/article/003481.htm
- Penn State College of Medicine: Hyponatremia
  - http://www.hmc.psu.edu/healthinfo/h/hyponatremia.htm

REFERENCES

- Adrogue HJ et al: Hyponatremia. N Engl J Med 2000;342:1581. [PMID: 10824078]
- Decaux G et al: Treatment of symptomatic hyponatremia. Am J Med Sci 2003;326:25. [PMID: 12861122]
- Goh KP: Management of hyponatremia. Am Fam Physician 2004;69:2387. [PMID: 15168958]
- Izzedine H et al: Angiotensin-converting enzyme inhibitor-induced syndrome of inappropriate secretion of antidiuretic hormone: case report and review of the literature. Clin Pharmacol Ther 2002;71:503. [PMID: 12087354]

Author(s)

Masafumi Fukagawa, MD, PhD
Kiyoshi Kurokawa, MD, MACP
Maxine A. Papadakis, MD

Hypoparathyroidism & Pseudohypoparathyroidism

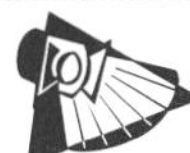

KEY FEATURES

ESSENTIALS OF DIAGNOSIS

- Tetany, carpopedal spasms, tingling of lips and hands, muscle and abdominal cramps, psychological changes
- Positive Chvostek's sign and Trousseau's phenomenon; defective nails and teeth; cataracts
- Serum calcium low; serum phosphate high; alkaline phosphatase normal; urine calcium excretion reduced
- Serum magnesium may be low

GENERAL CONSIDERATIONS

- Parathyroid hormone (PTH) increases serum calcium and decreases serum phosphate via effects on bone osteoclastic activity and renal tubules
- Hypoparathyroidism occurs most commonly after thyroidectomy; usually transient but may be permanent
- May occur after parathyroid adenoma removal due to suppression of remaining parathyroids
- May occur in DiGeorge's syndrome, with congenital cardiac and facial anomalies
- May result from damage to gland by heavy metals, eg, copper (Wilson's disease), iron (hemochromatosis, transfusion hemosiderosis); granulomas; sporadic autoimmunity; Riedel's thyroiditis; tumors; infection; or neck irradiation (rare)
- Magnesium deficiency, which prevents PTH secretion, may cause functional hypoparathyroidism
- Pseudohypoparathyroidism
  - Hypocalcemia and high PTH levels due to renal resistance to PTH from mutations in PTH receptor
  - Characterized by short stature, round face, obesity, short fourth metacarpals, ectopic bone formation, and mental retardation but without hypocalcemia
- Autosomal dominant hypocalcemia with hypocalciuria (ADHH)
  - Gain-of-function (constitutive activation) mutations of the calcium-sensing receptor (CaSR) gene essentially "fool" the parathyroid glands
  - Hypocalcemia without elevations in serum PTH hormone levels
  - Characterized by hypocalcemic seizures in infancy

CLINICAL FINDINGS

SYMPTOMS AND SIGNS

- Acute symptoms
  - Tetany, with muscle cramps, irritability, carpopedal spasm, and convulsions
  - Tingling of circumoral area, hands, and feet
- Chronic symptoms
  - Lethargy
  - Personality changes
  - Anxiety
  - Blurred vision due to cataracts
  - Parkinsonism
  - Mental retardation
- Chvostek's sign (facial muscle contraction on tapping facial nerve in front of the ear)
- Trousseau's phenomenon (carpal spasm after application of blood pressure cuff)
- Cataracts
- Nails thin and brittle; skin dry and scaly, at times with candidiasis; hair loss (eyebrows)
- Deep tendon reflexes hyperactive
- Papilledema and elevated cerebrospinal fluid pressure occasionally
- Defective teeth if onset in childhood

DIFFERENTIAL DIAGNOSIS

- Pseudohypoparathyroidism (renal resistance to PTH)
- Vitamin D deficiency
- Acute pancreatitis
- Chronic renal failure
- Hypoalbuminemia
- Paresthesias or tetany due to respiratory alkalosis
- Familial hypocalcemia with hypercalciuria (normal serum PTH)
- Hypomagnesemia

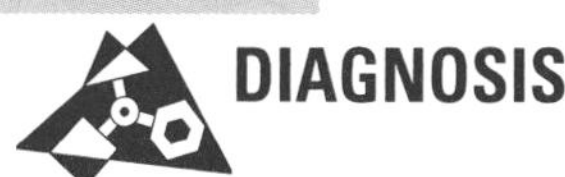

DIAGNOSIS

LABORATORY TESTS

- Serum calcium low
  - Note: serum calcium is largely bound to albumin. If hypoalbuminemia is present, obtain ionized calcium or correct calcium level for albumin level
  - Corrected Ca^{2+} = serum Ca^{2+} mg/dL + [0.8 × (4.0 – albumin g/dL)]
- Serum phosphate high
- Alkaline phosphatase normal
- Urinary calcium low
- PTH level low
- Obtain serum magnesium: hypomagnesemia frequently accompanies hypocalcemia and may decrease parathyroid gland function

IMAGING STUDIES

- Skull radiographs or head CT may show basal ganglia calcifications
- Bone x-rays may show increased bone density
- Other x-rays may show cutaneous calcifications

DIAGNOSTIC PROCEDURES

- Slit-lamp examination may show early posterior lenticular cataract formation
- ECG shows prolonged QT interval and T-wave abnormalities

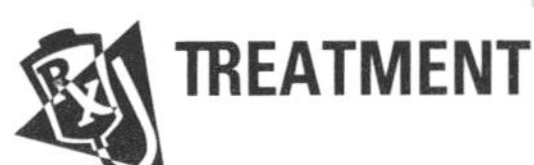

TREATMENT

MEDICATIONS

Emergency treatment for acute tetany

- Ensure adequate airway
- Calcium gluconate, 10–20 mL of 10% solution IV, given *slowly* until tetany ceases. Add 10–50 mL of calcium gluconate 10% to 1 L of D5W or saline by slow IV drip; titrate to serum calcium of 8–9 mg/dL
- Oral calcium, 1–2 g daily as soon as possible. Liquid calcium carbonate (Titralac Plus), 500 mg/5 mL is useful. Calcium citrate contains 21% calcium, but higher proportion is absorbed with less gastrointestinal intolerance
- Vitamin D derivatives to be given with oral calcium, include calcitriol (1,25-dihydroxycholecalciferol), 0.25 to 4 µg PO QD; ergocalciferol (vitamin D_2), 25,000–150,000 units PO QD, or calcifediol (25-hydroxyvitamin D_3), 20 µg PO QD; or dihydrotachysterol, 0.125–1 mg PO QD (Table 88)
- If hypomagnesemia is present, give $MgSO_4$ 1–2 g IV Q 6 h acutely; and magnesium oxide tablets, 600 mg 1–2 PO QD, or combined magnesium and calcium preparation (dolomite, others) chronically

Maintenance treatment

- Calcium (1–2 g/day) and vitamin D supplementation (see above) to achieve slightly low but asymptomatic serum calcium (8–8.6 mg/dL) to minimize hypercalciuria and provide margin of safety against overdosage and hypercalcemia
- Calcitriol, 0.25 µg PO QAM, titrated up to 0.5–2 µg PO QAM, to achieve near normocalcemia in patients with chronic hypocalcemia
- Avoid phenothiazines in hypocalcemia; may precipitate extrapyramidal symptoms
- Avoid furosemide; may worsen hypocalcemia

SURGERY

- Transplantation of cryopreserved parathyroid tissue from prior surgery restores normocalcemia in ~23%

OUTCOME

FOLLOW-UP

- Monitor serum calcium at regular intervals (at least every 3 months)
- Monitor "spot" urine calcium to keep level < 30 mg/dL if possible
- Hypercalciuria may respond to oral hydrochlorothiazide, usually given with a potassium supplement
- Hypercalcemia developing in patients with previously stable, treated hypoparathyroidism may signal new onset of Addison's disease

COMPLICATIONS

- Stridor, especially with vocal cord palsy, may cause respiratory obstruction requiring tracheostomy
- Chronic hypoparathyroidism may be associated with autoimmune diseases, eg, sprue, pernicious anemia, or Addison's disease
- Cataract formation and calcification of the basal ganglia occur in longstanding cases; parkinsonism or choreoathetosis occasionally develops
- Nerve root compression due to ossification of paravertebral ligaments
- Seizures in untreated patients
- Nephrocalcinosis and impaired renal function if overtreatment with calcium and vitamin D

PROGNOSIS

- Prognosis good with prompt diagnosis and treatment
- Dental changes, cataracts, and brain calcifications permanent

WHEN TO REFER

- Refer all patients to endocrinologist for stable regimen

WHEN TO ADMIT

- Any symptomatic hypocalcemia

EVIDENCE

INFORMATION FOR PATIENTS

- Mayo Clinic—Hypoparathyroidism
  - http://www.mayoclinic.com/invoke.cfm?id=AN00718
  - http://www.hypoparathyroid.com

REFERENCES

- Chan FK et al: Increased bone mineral density in patients with chronic hypoparathyroidism. J Clin Enocrinol Metab 2003;88:315. [PMID:12843159]
- Gunn IR, Gaffney D: Clinical and laboratory features of calcium-sensing receptor disorders: a systematic review. Ann Clin Biochem 2004;41:441. [PMID:15588433]
- Tfelt-Hansen J, Brown EM: The calcium-sensing receptor in normal physiology and pathophysiology: a review. Crit Rev Clin Lab Sci 2005;42:35. [PMID:15697170]

Author(s)

Paul A. Fitzgerald, MD

Hypophosphatemia

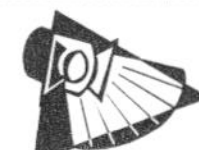

KEY FEATURES

ESSENTIALS OF DIAGNOSIS

- Serious depletion of body phosphate may exist with low, normal, or high concentrations of phosphorus in serum
- May cause hypooxygenation and even rhabdomyolysis
- Reduced maximal tubular reabsorption rate of phosphate (TmP/GFR) indicates urinary phosphate loss

GENERAL CONSIDERATIONS

- Cellular uptake is stimulated by alkalemia, insulin, epinephrine, feeding, post-parathyroidectomy (hungry bone syndrome), and accelerated cell proliferation
- Alcoholism
  - In acute alcohol withdrawal, increased plasma insulin and epinephrine along with respiratory alkalosis promote intracellular shift of phosphate
  - Vomiting, diarrhea, and poor dietary intake contribute to hypophosphatemia
  - In chronic alcohol use, there is a decreased renal threshold of phosphate excretion
- Parathyroid hormone (PTH) is one of the major factors that decrease TmP/GFR, leading to renal loss of phosphate
- In chronic obstructive pulmonary disease and asthma, hypophosphatemia can be attributed to xanthine derivatives causing shifts of phosphate intracellularly and the phosphaturic effects of β-adrenergic agonists, loop diuretics, xanthine derivatives, and corticosteroids
- Therapy of hyperglycemia causes phosphate to accompany glucose intracellularly
- Moderate hypophosphatemia (1.0–2.5 mg/dL) occurs commonly in hospitalized patients and may not reflect decreased phosphate stores

Etiology

- Diminished supply or absorption
  - Starvation
  - Parenteral alimentation with inadequate phosphate content
  - Malabsorption
  - Vitamin D–resistant osteomalacia
- Increased loss
  - Phosphaturic drugs (diuretics, theophylline, bronchodilators, corticosteroids)
  - Hyperparathyroidism, hyperthyroidism
  - Renal tubular acidosis (eg, monoclonal gammopathy)
  - Alcoholism
  - Hypokalemic nephropathy
- Intracellular shift of phosphorus
  - Glucose administration
  - Drugs (anabolic steroids, estrogen, oral contraceptives)
  - Respiratory alkalosis
  - Salicylate poisoning
- Electrolyte abnormalities
  - Hypercalcemia, hypomagnesemia, metabolic alkalosis
- Abnormal losses followed by inadequate repletion
  - Diabetes mellitus with acidosis, especially during aggressive therapy
  - Recovery from starvation
  - Chronic alcoholism
  - Severe burns

CLINICAL FINDINGS

SYMPTOMS AND SIGNS

- Moderate hypophosphatemia (1.0–2.5 mg/dL) is usually asymptomatic
- Severe hypophosphatemia (≤ 1 mg/dL) may cause muscle weakness
- Acute, severe hypophosphatemia (0.1–0.2 mg/dL)
  - Weakness from acute hemolytic anemia
  - Infection from impaired chemotaxis of leukocytes
  - Petechial hemorrhages from platelet dysfunction
  - Rhabdomyolysis
  - Encephalopathy (irritability, confusion, dysarthria, seizures, and coma)
  - Heart failure
- Chronic severe phosphate depletion causes anorexia, pain in muscles and bones, and fractures

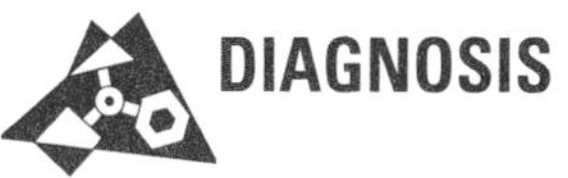

DIAGNOSIS

LABORATORY TESTS

- Spot urine phosphate > 20 mg/dL suggests renal phosphate loss
- Normal TmP/GFR is 2.5–4.5 mg/dL

$$\frac{\text{TmP}}{\text{GFR}} = \frac{\text{Serum Pi} - (\text{UPi} \times \text{UV})}{\text{GFR}}$$

The main factors regulating TmP/GFR are PTH and phosphate intake. Increases of PTH or phosphate intake decreases TmP/GFR, so that more phosphate is excreted in the urine

- Lower values indicate urinary phosphate loss
- Hemolytic anemia may be present
- Elevated serum creatine kinase and myoglobinuria from rhabdomyolysis
- Renal glycosuria and hypouricemia together with hypophosphatemia indicate Fanconi's syndrome

IMAGING STUDIES

- In chronic depletion, radiographs and biopsies of bones show changes resembling those of osteomalacia

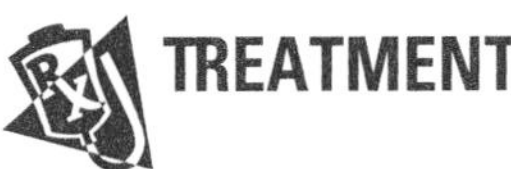

TREATMENT

MEDICATIONS

Oral replacement

- Acute hypocalcemia can occur with parenteral administration of phosphate; therefore, when possible, oral replacement of phosphate is preferable
- Oral phosphate used if the patient is asymptomatic and serum phosphorus is > 1 mg/dL
- Phosphate salts are available in skim milk (approximately 1 g/L [33 mmol/L])
- Sodium plus potassium phosphate tablets or capsules may be given to provide 0.5–1 g (18–32 mmol) per day
- Contraindications to phosphate salts include hypoparathyroidism, renal insufficiency, tissue damage and necrosis, and hypercalcemia

Intravenous replacement

- For asymptomatic patients with severe hypophosphatemia (serum phosphorus 0.7–1 mg/dL) who cannot eat, infuse 279–310 mg (9–10 mmol)/12 h until the serum phosphorus exceeds 1 mg/dL and then switch patient to oral therapy
- For symptomatic patients with severe hypophosphatemia (serum phosphorus < 0.5–1 mg/dL) who cannot eat, give intravenous phosphorus up to 1 g in 1 L of fluid over 8–12 h
- Slow the infusion rate if hypotension occurs
- 3 g or more of phosphorus may be required over several days to replete body stores
- Parenteral phosphorus replacement carries potential of precipitating soft tissue calcification and nephrocalcinosis. Serum calcium × serum phosphorus product > 70 markedly increases the risk
- A magnesium deficit often coexists and should be treated simultaneously

THERAPEUTIC PROCEDURES

- Mild hypophosphatemia usually resolves spontaneously with treatment of the underlying cause

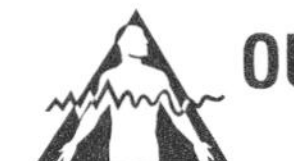

OUTCOME

FOLLOW-UP

- Response to phosphate supplementation is not predictable
- During intravenous replacement of phosphate, monitor plasma phosphate, calcium and potassium every 6 h

WHEN TO REFER

- For consultation about etiology
- If expertise in phosphate repletion is needed, particularly intravenous

WHEN TO ADMIT

- Symptomatic hypophosphatemia
- Need for parenteral replacement

PREVENTION

- Include phosphate in repletion and maintenance fluids
- For parenteral alimentation, 620 mg (20 mmol) of phosphorus is required for every 1000 nonprotein kcal to maintain phosphate balance and to ensure anabolic function. A daily ration for prolonged parenteral fluid maintenance is 620–1240 mg (20–40 mmol) of phosphorus

EVIDENCE

INFORMATION FOR PATIENTS

- American Association for Clinical Chemistry: Phosphorus Test
  - http://labtestsonline.org/understanding/analytes/phosphorus/test.html
- MedlinePlus: Hypophosphatemia
  - http://www.nlm.nih.gov/medlineplus/ency/article/000307.htm
- MedlinePlus: Phosphates Drug Information
  - http://www.nlm.nih.gov/medlineplus/druginfo/uspdi/202463.html
- National Institute on Alcoholism and Alcohol Abuse: Alcoholism—Getting the Facts
  - http://www.niaaa.nih.gov/publications/booklet.htm

REFERENCES

- Shiber JR et al: Serum phosphate abnormalities in the emergency room. J Emerg Med 2002;23:395. [PMID: 12480022]
- Subramian R et al: Severe hypophosphatemia: pathophysiologic implications, clinical presentations, and treatment. Medicine 2000;79:1. [PMID: 10670405]
- Taylor BE et al: Treatment of hypophosphatemia using a protocol based on patient weight and serum phosphorus level in a surgical intensive care unit. J Am Coll Surg 2004;198:198. [PMID: 14759775]

Author(s)

Masafumi Fukagawa, MD, PhD
Kiyoshi Kurokawa, MD, MACP
Maxine A. Papadakis, MD

Hypopituitarism

KEY FEATURES

ESSENTIALS OF DIAGNOSIS

- Loss of one, all, or any combination of pituitary hormones
- ACTH deficiency reduces adrenal secretion of cortisol and testosterone; aldosterone secretion remains intact
- Growth hormone (GH) deficiency causes short stature in children; adults experience asthenia and increased cardiovascular mortality
- Thyroid-stimulating hormone (TSH) deficiency causes secondary hypothyroidism
- Luteinizing hormone (LH) and follicle-stimulating hormone (FSH) are secreted by the same pituitary cells, and their loss causes hypogonadism in men and women
- Antidiuretic hormone deficiency results in central diabetes insipidus
- Oxytocin deficiency causes insufficient lactation in postpartum women

GENERAL CONSIDERATIONS

- Caused by hypothalamic or pituitary dysfunction, including mass lesions, such as pituitary adenomas, granulomas, Rathke's cleft cysts
- May have single or multiple hormonal deficiencies, such as those of anterior pituitary and posterior pituitary
- Pituitary tumor may be part of multiple endocrine neoplasia (type 1)
- Hypopituitarism without mass lesions may be idiopathic, genetic, cranial radiation, surgery, encephalitis, hemochromatosis, autoimmune, stroke, post-CABG, chronic epidural opioid infusion, X-linked congenital adrenal hypoplasia
- Moderate-to-severe traumatic brain injury (Glasgow coma scale ≤13/15)
- Isolated hypogonadotrophic hypogonadism can occur with severe illness, malnutrition, intrathecal opioids, methadone, and extreme prolonged exercise (women), and in obese type 2 diabetic patients and those with congenital adrenal hypoplasia
- Kallman's syndrome is the most common cause of congenital isolated gonadotropin deficiency
- Combined hypopituitarism can occur congenitally

CLINICAL FINDINGS

SYMPTOMS AND SIGNS

- Gonadotropin (LH and FSH) deficiency
  - Hypogonadism, delayed adolescence, infertility, decreased libido
  - Amenorrhea (women), decreased erections (men)
  - Loss of axillary, pubic, and body hair, especially with ACTH deficiency
  - Diminished beard growth (men)
  - Micropenis, cryptorchism
- TSH deficiency: fatigue, weakness, weight gain
- ACTH deficiency symptoms of decreased cortisol with normal mineralocorticoid secretion: weakness, fatigue, weight loss, hypotension
- Patients with partial ACTH deficiency have some cortisol secretion and may not have symptoms until stressed by illness or surgery. Hyponatremia may occur, especially with combined ACTH and TSH deficiencies
- Growth hormone (GH) deficiency: obesity, weakness, reduced cardiac output, feelings of social isolation
- ADH deficiency: central diabetes insipidus with polyuria and polydipsia
- Oxytocin deficiency: no lactation
- Panhypopituitarism
  - Dry, pale, finely textured skin
  - Fine facial wrinkles and an apathetic countenance
- Patients with congenital hypopituitarism due to *PROP1* gene mutations
  - Usually present with growth failure due to GH and TSH deficiency
  - Lack of pubertal development occurs due to lack of FSH and LH. ACTH-cortisol deficiency occurs later, typically requiring glucocorticoid therapy by age 18 years

DIFFERENTIAL DIAGNOSIS

- Anorexia nervosa (hypogonadotropic hypogonadism)
- Serious illness [hypogonadotropic hypogonadism, functional suppression of TSH and thyroxine (T_4)]
- Severe malnutrition (hypogonadotropic hypogonadism)
- Primary hypothyroidism causes low T_4, high prolactin
- Addison's disease
- High-dose glucocorticoids (secondary adrenal insufficiency)
- Low serum cortisol in critically ill patients due to low cortisol-binding globulin; free cortisol levels normal
- Cachexia due to other causes (eg, carcinoma, tuberculosis)
- Triiodothyronine (T_3) administration can cause low TSH and low serum free T_4

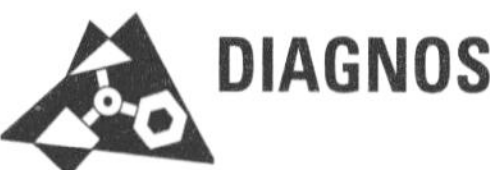

DIAGNOSIS

LABORATORY TESTS

- Serum sodium and fasting glucose may be low, potassium normal
- Low free T_4, TSH not elevated
- Low or low normal testosterone, estradiol, LH, FSH
- Elevated prolactin in prolactinoma, acromegaly, hypothalamic disease
- ACTH stimulation test: cosyntropin (synthetic ACTH analog), 0.25 mg IM or IV, normally causes cortisol to rise to >20 μg/dL (550 nmol/L) in 30–60 min; ACTH deficiency causes adrenal atrophy and a deficient response
- Baseline ACTH low or normal in secondary hypoadrenalism; ACTH high in primary adrenal disease
- Basal cortisol >19 μg/dL excludes adrenal insufficiency
- Metyrapone stimulation test used if cosyntropin test is normal but pituitary adrenal insufficiency is suspected. Metyrapone, 1.5 g PO, is given at 11 PM. In hypoadrenalism, 8 AM 11-deoxycortisol < 7 μg/dL and cortisol < 5 μg/dL
- IGF-1 levels are normal in 50% of adults with GH deficiency, but very low levels (< 84 μg/L) indicate GH deficiency except in conditions that suppress IGF-1 (malnutrition, oral estrogen, hypothyroidism, uncontrolled diabetes mellitus, liver failure)
- Low serum levels of epinephrine and DHEA with ACTH-cortisol deficiency
- Screen for hemochromatosis with serum Fe, transferrin saturation, ferritin

IMAGING STUDIES

- MRI scan shows parasellar lesions
- In hemochromatosis, MRI shows hypointense anterior lobe on T1-weighted images surrounded by hyperintense cerebrospinal fluid on T2-weighted images
- In central diabetes insipidus, the posterior pituitary "bright spot" is absent on MRI T1-weighted imaging

TREATMENT

MEDICATIONS

Secondary adrenal insufficiency

- Hydrocortisone, 15 mg PO Q AM and 5–10 mg PO Q PM, or prednisone, 3 mg Q AM and 2 mg Q PM PO QD, or dexamethasone, 0.25 mg PO QD
- Patients with partial ACTH deficiency (basal morning serum cortisol above 8 mg/dL [220 mmol/L]) require hydrocortisone replacement in maintenance doses of ~5 mg PO BID
- Some patients feel better with equivalent doses of prednisone 3–7.5 mg/day
- Monitor patients for manifestations of Cushing's syndrome or underreplacement. A serum WBC with a relative differential is useful, because a relative neutrophilia and lymphopenia can indicate overreplacement with glucocorticoid, and vice versa
- Fludrocortisone is rarely needed
- Give additional hydrocortisone during stress. For mild illness, doses should be doubled or tripled. For trauma or surgery, 50 mg IM or IV Q 6 h, then reduce to normal doses as stress subsides

Hypothyroidism

- Levothyroxine, 0.05–0.2 mg PO QD, for hypothyroidism only after assessment for cortisol deficiency, otherwise may precipitate adrenal crisis
- Optimal replacement doses of thyroxine must be assessed by careful clinical evaluation. Serum free thyroxine levels may need to be in the high-normal or mildly elevated range for adequate replacement. Serum TSH assays are useless because levels are always low

Hypogonadism

- Testosterone replacement for men (see Hypogonadism, Male)
- Estrogen replacement for women (see Amenorrhea, Secondary)
- Oral dehydroepiandrosterone (USP-grade DHEA; 30 mg/d orally) for women: increases sexual hair in 84%, improves stamina in 70% and sexual interest in 50%
- To improve spermatogenesis, human chorionic gonadotropin (hCG), 2000–3000 units IM 3 times weekly, may be used with no testosterone
- If sperm count remains low, FSH injections may be added
- Clomiphene can induce ovulation

Growth hormone deficiency

- Somatotropin or somatrem (hGH) for symptomatic adults with severe growth hormone deficiency, starting at 0.2 mg (0.6 IU) SC 3 × weekly or QD
- Women who receive hGH should not take oral estrogen because this reduces hGH effect; topical estrogen is preferred. Administer adequate hGH to maintain normal serum IGF-I levels
- Somatotropin discontinued if no improvement in energy, mentation, or visceral adiposity within 3–6 months at maximum tolerated dosage
- Do not administer hGH during major surgery or severe illness

Hyperprolactinemia

- Hypopituitarism from prolactin-secreting pituitary tumor may be reversible with bromocriptine, cabergoline, or quinagolide or with tumor resection (see Hyperprolactinemia)

Central diabetes insipidus

- Nasal desmopressin (DDAVP), 0.1 mL Q 12–24 h
- Oral desmopressin, 0.1 or 0.2 mg Q 12–24 h
- Parenteral desmopressin, 1–2 mg IV SQ Q 12–24 h

SURGERY

- Transsphenoidal hypophysectomy for pituitary tumors sometimes reverses hypopituitarism

THERAPEUTIC PROCEDURES

- Radiation therapy for GH-secreting tumors, but increases risk of hypopituitarism

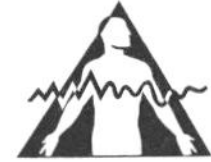

OUTCOME

FOLLOW-UP

- After pituitary surgery, check serum sodium frequently for 2 weeks, since postoperative hyponatremia is common
- If on somatotropin, careful monitoring for side effects including hypertension, proliferative retinopathy

COMPLICATIONS

- Mass lesions may cause visual field deficits
- Radiation therapy increases risk of small vessel ischemic strokes and second tumors
- In craniopharyngioma, 16% have diabetes insipidus preoperatively and 60% postoperatively
- Hypothalamic damage may cause morbid obesity, cognitive and emotional problems
- Growth hormone deficiency increases cardiovascular morbidity
- Rarely, acute hemorrhage occurs in large pituitary tumors (pituitary apoplexy) causing rapid loss of vision and headache, requiring emergent decompression

PROGNOSIS

- Prognosis depends on primary cause
- Patients can recover from functional hypopituitarism, eg, hypogonadism due to starvation or severe illness, ACTH suppression by glucocorticoids, TSH suppression by hyperthyroidism, or intrathecal opioids

PREVENTION

- Patients with adrenal insufficiency should wear a medical ID bracelet

EVIDENCE

PRACTICE GUIDELINES

- Smith JC: Hormone replacement therapy in hypopituitarism. Expert Opin Pharmacother 2004;5:1023. [PMID: 5155105]

WEB SITE

- Pituitary Network Association
  - http://www.pituitary.org.uk/disorders/hypopit.htm

INFORMATION FOR PATIENTS

- Mayo Clinic—Hypopituitarism
  - http://www.mayoclinic.com/invoke.cfm?id=DS00479

REFERENCES

- Agha A et al: Conventional glucocorticoid replacement overtreats adult hypopituitary patients with partial ACTH deficiency. Clin Endocrinol (Oxf) 2004;60:688. [PMID:15163331]
- Böttner A et al: *PROP1* mutations cause progressive deterioration of anterior pituitary function including adrenal insufficiency: a longitudinal analysis. J Clin Endocrinol Metab 2004;89:5256. [PMID:15472232]
- Johannsson G et al: Low dose dehydroepiandrosterone affects behavior in hypopituitary androgen-deficient women: a placebo-controlled trial. J Clin Endocrinol Metab 2002;87:2046.[PMID:11994339]
- Kreitschmann-Andermahr I et al: Prevalence of pituitary deficiency in patients after aneurysmal subarachnoid hemorrhage. J Clin Endocrinol Metab 2004;89:4986. [PMID:15472195]
- Verrees M et al: Pituitary tumor apoplexy: characteristics, treatment, and outcomes. Neurosurg Focus 2004;16:E6. [PMID:15191335]

Author(s)

Paul A. Fitzgerald, MD

Hypotension & Shock

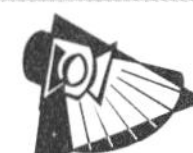

KEY FEATURES

ESSENTIALS OF DIAGNOSIS

- Hypotension, tachycardia, oliguria, altered mental status
- Peripheral hypoperfusion and hypoxia

GENERAL CONSIDERATIONS

- The rate of arterial blood flow and oxygen delivery is inadequate to meet tissue metabolic needs
- Shock can be classified as hypovolemic, cardiogenic, obstructive, and distributive (including septic and neurogenic)
- Hypovolemic: decreased intravascular volume resulting from loss of blood, plasma, or fluids and electrolytes; > 15% blood volume loss results in hypotension, increased peripheral resistance, collapse of capillary and venous beds, and progressive tissue hypoxia
- Cardiogenic: pump failure related to myocardial infarction, myocardial contusion, cardiomyopathy, valvular regurgitation or stenosis, or arrhythmias
- Obstructive: cardiac tamponade, tension pneumothorax, and massive pulmonary embolism
- Distributive: reduction in systemic vascular resistance from sepsis, anaphylaxis, systemic inflammatory response syndrome (SIRS) produced by severe pancreatitis or burns, or acute adrenal insufficiency
- Septic: most often caused by gram-negative bacteremia (*Escherichia coli, Klebsiella, Proteus*, and *Pseudomonas*); less often to gram-positive cocci and gram-negative anaerobes (*Bacteroides*)
- Neurogenic: resulting from traumatic spinal cord injury or effects of an epidural or spinal anesthetic; reflex vagal parasympathetic stimulation evoked by pain, gastric dilation, or fright

DEMOGRAPHICS

- Risk factors for septic shock: extremes of age, diabetes, immunosuppression, and recent urinary, biliary, or gynecological manipulation

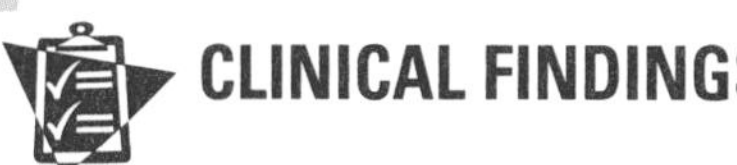

CLINICAL FINDINGS

SYMPTOMS AND SIGNS

- Hypotension: cool or mottled extremities and weak or absent peripheral pulses, delayed capillary refill
- Tachycardia
- Oliguria
- Bowel ischemia
- Hepatic dysfunction
- Altered mental status, increasing agitation
- Sepsis: fever, chills, hyperglycemia

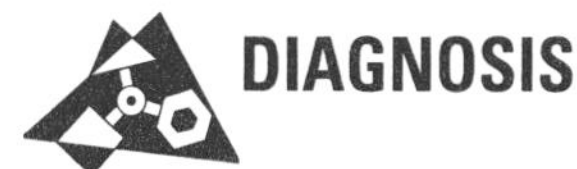

DIAGNOSIS

LABORATORY TESTS

- Check serial hematocrits, complete blood cell count, serum electrolytes, prothrombin time, partial thromboplastin time, ionized calcium, magnesium, phosphate, and cardiac enzymes
- Serum glucose to exclude hyperglycemia, reflecting insulin resistance
- Fecal occult blood test to exclude gastrointestinal hemorrhage
- Arterial blood gas determinations
- Type and cross-match, as indicated
- Urinalysis, urine culture, and blood cultures

IMAGING STUDIES

- Chest x-ray
- Electrocardiogram
- Echocardiogram
- Kidneys, ureters, and bladder x-ray or abdominal CT for abdominal pain

DIAGNOSTIC PROCEDURES

- Arterial line for continuous blood pressure measurement
- Foley catheter to measure urine output
- Central venous pressure (CVP) (right atrial pressure) or pulmonary capillary wedge pressure (PCWP) < 5 mm Hg suggests hypovolemia; CVP or PCWP > 18 mm Hg suggests volume overload, cardiac failure, tamponade, or pulmonary hypertension
- Pulmonary artery catheter for hemodynamic pressure measurements
- Low systemic vascular resistance (SVR) (< 800 dyne $\times$ s/cm^{-5}) suggests early sepsis and neurogenic shock; high SVR (> 1500 dyne $\times$ s/cm^{-5}) suggests hypovolemic and cardiogenic shock
- A high cardiac index (> 4 L/min/m^2) in a hypotensive patient suggests early septic shock

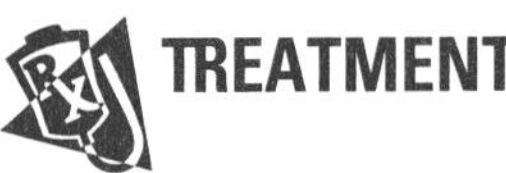

TREATMENT

MEDICATIONS

- Pressor medications
  - Dopamine, > 5 µg/kg/min
  - Dobutamine, 2–20 µg/kg/min
- Diuretics, thrombolytics, morphine, nitroglycerin, antiarrhythmics, and antiplatelet agents as indicated in acute myocardial infarction
- Peripheral vasoconstrictors such as epinephrine, 2–10 µg/min, or norepinephrine, 0.5–30 µg/min, in distributive or neurogenic shock
- Vasopressin (antidiuretic hormone)
- Broad-spectrum antibiotics in septic shock
- Corticosteroids in shock because of acute adrenal insufficiency
- Calcium gluconate to maintain an ionized calcium level > 1.0
- Sodium bicarbonate for arterial pH < 7.20

SURGERY

- Dependent on the cause of shock
- Cardiogenic shock: transcutaneous or transvenous pacing or intraaortic balloon pump, and emergent revascularization by stent angioplasty or coronary artery bypass grafting, as indicated
- Drainage or excision of source of sepsis

THERAPEUTIC PROCEDURES

- Treatment must be directed both at the manifestations of shock and at its cause
- Basic life support: airway maintenance, oxygen, cardiopulmonary resuscitation, IV access and fluid resuscitation with crystalloid or blood products
- Treatment is directed at maintaining a CVP of 8–12 mm Hg, a mean arterial pressure of 65–90 mm Hg, a cardiac index of 2–4 L/min/m^2, and central venous oxygen saturation of > 70%

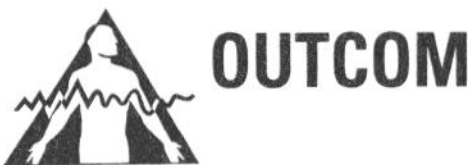

OUTCOME

PROGNOSIS

- Septic shock mortality is 40–80%

WHEN TO ADMIT

- Any patient presenting with shock

EVIDENCE

PRACTICE GUIDELINES

- Dellinger RP et al: Surviving Sepsis Campaign guidelines for management of severe sepsis and septic shock. Crit Care Med 2004;32:858. [PMID: 15090974]
- Guidelines for the management of severe sepsis and septic shock. The International Sepsis Forum. Intensive Care Med 2001;27(Suppl 1):S1. [PMID: 11519475]
- Martel MJ et al: Hemorrhagic shock. J Obstet Gynaecol Can 2002;24:504. [PMID: 12196857]

INFORMATION FOR PATIENTS

- Mayo Clinic: Shock
  - http://www.mayoclinic.com/invoke.cfm?id=FA00056

REFERENCES

- Bernard GR et al: Efficacy and safety of recombinant human activated protein C for severe sepsis. N Engl J Med 2001;344:699. [PMID: 11236773]
- Hochman JS et al: One-year survival following early revascularization for cardiogenic shock. JAMA 2001;285:190. [PMID: 11176812]
- Landry DW et al: The pathogenesis of vasodilatory shock. N Engl J Med 2001;345:588. [PMID: 11529214]
- Orlinsky M et al: Current controversies in shock and resuscitation. Surg Clin North Am 2001;81:1217. [PMID: 11766174]

Author(s)

Louis M. Messina, MD

Hypothermia

KEY FEATURES

ESSENTIALS OF DIAGNOSIS

- Systemic hypothermia is a reduction of core (rectal) body temperature below 35°C
- Oral temperatures are inaccurate; an esophageal or rectal probe that reads as low as 25°C is required

GENERAL CONSIDERATIONS

- In colder climates, elderly individuals living in inadequately heated housing are particularly susceptible
- Patients with comorbid conditions and those who are using sedating or tranquilizing drugs are more vulnerable to accidental hypothermia
- Prolonged postoperative hypothermia or administration of large amounts of refrigerated stored blood (without rewarming) can cause systemic hypothermia

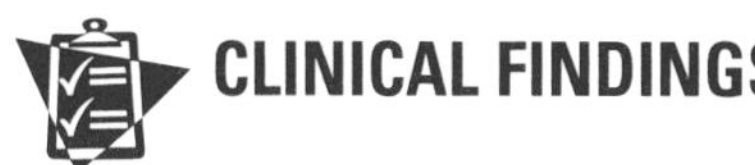

CLINICAL FINDINGS

SYMPTOMS AND SIGNS

Systemic hypothermia

- Early manifestations may include weakness, drowsiness, lethargy, irritability, confusion, shivering, and impaired coordination
- The skin may appear blue or puffy
- At core temperatures below 35°C, the patient may become delirious, drowsy, or comatose and may stop breathing
- The pulse and blood pressure may be unobtainable, leading one to believe the patient is dead

Hypothermia of the extremities

- Exposure of the extremities to cold produces immediate localized vasoconstriction followed by generalized vasoconstriction
- When the skin temperature falls to 25°C, the area becomes cyanotic
- At 15°C, there is a deceptively pink, well-oxygenated appearance to the skin. Tissue damage occurs at this temperature

DIFFERENTIAL DIAGNOSIS

- Infection
- Other cause of altered mental status (eg, hypoglycemia, drugs, stroke)
- Hypothyroidism
- Anorexia or malnutrition (poor fat stores)
- Adrenal insufficiency
- Burns
- Spinal cord injury

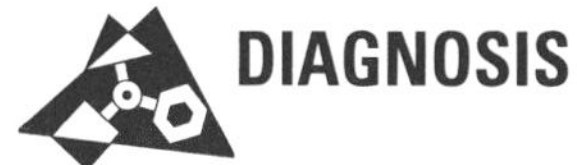

DIAGNOSIS

LABORATORY TESTS

- Obtain complete blood cell count, prothrombin time, partial thromboplastin time, electrolytes, blood urea nitrogen, serum creatinine, liver function tests, amylase, glucose, pH, blood gases, urinalysis, and urine volume

IMAGING STUDIES

- Cardiac arrhythmias and the pathognomonic J wave of Osborn, prominent in lateral precordial leads, can be seen on the electrocardiogram

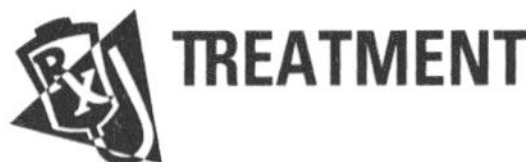

TREATMENT

THERAPEUTIC PROCEDURES

- **Mild hypothermia** (rectal temperature > 33°C) in healthy patients: warm bed or rapid passive rewarming with warm bath or warm packs and blankets
- **Moderate or severe hypothermia** (core temperatures of < 33°C): active rewarming with supportive care
- Establish cardiovascular support, acid-base balance, arterial oxygenation, and adequate intravascular volume before rewarming to minimize risk of organ infarction and "afterdrop" (recurrent hypothermia)
- Active rewarming: combination of active external and internal methods
- Aggressive rewarming attempted only by those with experience
- Once begun, CPR should continue until patient rewarmed to ≥ 32°C

Active external rewarming

- Heated blankets, warm baths, forced hot air
- Easier to monitor and perform diagnostic/therapeutic procedures using **heated blankets**
- **Warm bath** rewarming best done in tub of 40–42°C moving water (rewarming rate: ~1–2°C/h)
- When extracorporeal blood rewarming not an option, **forced air** rewarming (38–43°C) recommended
- Rewarming may cause marked peripheral dilation, predisposing to ventricular fibrillation and hypovolemic shock
- Antibiotics not routinely given

Active internal (core) rewarming

- Essential for severe hypothermia
- **Extracorporeal blood rewarming** (cardiopulmonary, venovenous, or arteriovenous femorofemoral bypass) treatment of choice, especially with cardiac arrest
- Without equipment for extracorporeal rewarming, left-sided thoracotomy followed by pericardial cavity irrigation with warmed saline and cardiac massage effective in systemic hypothermia < 28°C
- Repeated peritoneal dialysis with 2 L of warm (43°C) potassium-free dialysate solution exchanged every 10–12 min until core temperature raised to ~35°C
- Parenteral fluids (D_5 normal saline) warmed to 43°C
- Administer humidified air heated to 42°C through face mask or endotracheal tube
- Warm colonic and GI irrigations of less value
- Trachael intubation for patients who are comatose or in respiratory failure

OUTCOME

FOLLOW-UP

- Monitor cardiac rhythm
- Core temperature (esophageal preferred over rectal) should be monitored frequently during and after initial rewarming because of reports of recurrent hypothermia

COMPLICATIONS

- Metabolic acidosis, hyperkalemia, pneumonia, pancreatitis, ventricular fibrillation, hypoglycemia or hyperglycemia, coagulopathy, and renal failure may occur
- Cardiac arrhythmias may occur, especially during rewarming
- Death is usually from cardiac asystole or ventricular fibrillation

PROGNOSIS

- More than 75% of otherwise healthy patients may survive moderate or severe systemic hypothermia
- Prognosis is directly related to the severity of metabolic acidosis; if the pH is ≤ 6.6, the prognosis is poor
- The prognosis is grave if there are underlying predisposing causes or if treatment is delayed
- Neuropathic sequelae such as pain, numbness, tingling, hyperhidrosis, cold sensitivity of the extremities, and nerve conduction abnormalities may persist for many years after the cold injury

PREVENTION

- "Keep warm, keep moving, and keep dry"
- Tobacco and alcohol should be avoided
- Cardiac, central vascular, or chest trauma or stimulation (eg, catheter, cannulas) should be avoided unless essential because of the risk of inducing ventricular fibrillation

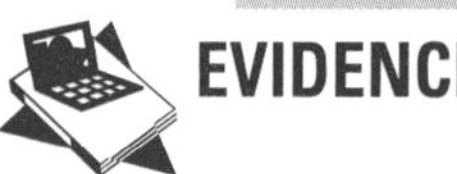

EVIDENCE

PRACTICE GUIDELINES

- Durrer B et al: The medical on-site treatment of hypothermia: ICAR-MEDCOM recommendation. High Alt Med Biol 2003;4:99. [PMID: 12713717]
- European Resuscitation Council: Part 8: advanced challenges in resuscitation. Section 3: special challenges in ECC. 3A: hypothermia. Resuscitation 2000;46:267. [PMID: 10978806]

INFORMATION FOR PATIENTS

- Centers for Disease Control and Prevention: Extreme Cold: A Prevention Guide to Promote Your Personal Health and Safety
  - http://www.bt.cdc.gov/disasters/winter/guide.asp
- Centers for Disease Control and Prevention: Winter Weather FAQs
  - http://www.bt.cdc.gov/disasters/winter/faq.asp
- Mayo Clinic: Hypothermia
  - http://www.mayoclinic.com/invoke.cfm?id=DS00333
- National Institute on Aging: Hypothermia: A Cold Weather Hazard
  - http://www.niapublications.org/engagepages/hypother.asp

REFERENCES

- Kempainen RR et al: The evaluation and management of accidental hypothermia. Respir Care 2004;49:192. [PMID: 14744270]
- Mattu A et al: Electrocardiographic manifestations of hypothermia. Am J Emerg Med 2002;20:314. [PMID: 12098179]
- Ulrich AS et al: Hypothermia and localized cold injuries. Emerg Med Clin North Am 2004;22:281. [PMID: 15163568]

Author(s)

Richard Cohen, MD, MPH

Hypothyroidism (Myxedema)

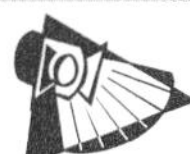

KEY FEATURES

ESSENTIALS OF DIAGNOSIS

- Weakness, fatigue, cold intolerance, constipation, weight change, depression, menorrhagia, hoarseness
- Dry skin, bradycardia, delayed return of deep tendon reflexes
- Anemia, hyponatremia
- Serum free tetraiodothyronine (T_4) low
- Thyroid-stimulating hormone (TSH) elevated in primary hypothyroidism

GENERAL CONSIDERATIONS

- Severity ranges from mild, unrecognized hypothyroidism, to striking myxedema and cretinism
- Hypothyroidism due first to thyroid gland disease or second to lack of pituitary TSH
- Maternal hypothyroidism during pregnancy results in cognitive impairment in child
- Causes of hypothyroidism with goiter: Hashimoto's thyroiditis; subacute (de Quervain's thyroiditis) (after initial hyperthyroidism); Riedel's thyroiditis; iodine deficiency; genetic thyroid enzyme defects; hepatitis C, drugs (lithium, amiodarone, propylthiouracil, methimazole, phenylbutazone, sulfonamides, interferon-α or β); food goitrogens in iodide-deficient areas; peripheral resistance to thyroid hormone; or infiltrating diseases.
- Causes of hypothyroidism without goiter: thyroid surgery, irradiation, or radioiodine treatment; deficient pituitary TSH; severe illness
- Radiation therapy to the head-neck-chest-shoulder region can cause hypothyroidism with or without goiter or thyroid cancer many years later
- "Subclinical" hypothyroidism, ie, clinically euthyroid individual with high TSH, normal T_4, occurs commonly in elderly women (~10% incidence)
- Amiodarone, due to high iodine content, causes clinical hypothyroidism in ~8%
- High iodine intake from other sources may also cause hypothyroidism, especially in those with underlying lymphocytic thyroiditis
- Myxedema is caused by interstitial accumulation of hydrophilic mucopolysaccharides, leading to fluid retention and lymphedema
- Hyponatremia occurs due to impaired renal tubular sodium reabsorption

CLINICAL FINDINGS

SYMPTOMS AND SIGNS

- Early symptoms: fatigue, lethargy, weakness, arthralgias, myalgias, muscle cramps, cold intolerance, constipation, dry skin, headache, menorrhagia
- Late symptoms: slow speech, constipation, peripheral edema, pallor, hoarseness, decreased senses of taste, smell, and hearing, muscle cramps, aches and pains, dyspnea, weight changes (usually gain, sometimes loss), amenorrhea or menorrhagia, galactorrhea, absent sweating
- Early signs: thin, brittle nails, thinning of hair, pallor, poor turgor of mucosa, delayed return of deep tendon reflexes
- Late signs: goiter, puffiness of face and eyelids, carotenemia, thinning of outer eyebrows, tongue thickening, hard pitting edema, pleural, peritoneal, pericardial, and joint effusions
- Myxedema coma: signs of hypothyroidism and impaired mentation
- Cardiac enlargement due to pericardial effusion, bradycardia
- Hypothermia
- Pituitary enlargement due to hyperplasia of TSH-secreting cells in long-standing cases

DIFFERENTIAL DIAGNOSIS

- Chronic fatigue syndrome
- Depression
- Congestive heart failure
- Irregular vaginal bleeding due to other cause
- Anemia due to other cause
- Amyloidosis (thick tongue)
- Pituitary adenoma (may have hyperprolactinemia and pituitary often enlarged due to reversible hyperplasia of TSH-secreting cells)
- Patients with TSH resistance, caused by a mutation in the gene encoding the TSH receptor, have high serum TSH levels despite usually being clinically and biochemically euthyroid.
- TSH-secreting pituitary tumor (serum TSH and FT_4 elevated). Rare: recheck lab tests in a reference lab before making diagnosis.
- TSH may be increased by phenothiazines and atypical antipsychotics without clinical hypothyroidism

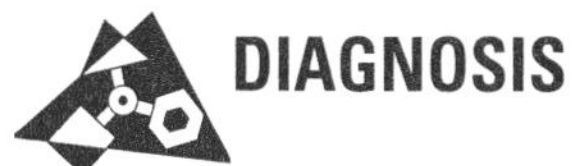

DIAGNOSIS

LABORATORY TESTS

- Serum TSH is increased in primary hypothyroidism but low or normal in secondary hypothyroidism (pituitary insufficiency)
- Free T_4 may be low or low normal
- Serum triiodothyronine (T_3) is not a good test for hypothyroidism
- Serum cholesterol, liver enzymes, creatine kinase, prolactin increased
- Hyponatremia
- Hypoglycemia
- Anemia (with normal or increased mean corpuscular volume)
- Thyroperoxidase or thyroglobulin antibody titers usually high in hypothyroidism due to Hashimoto's thyroiditis
- During pregnancy in women with hypothyroidism taking replacement thyroxine, check serum TSH frequently (eg, Q 1–2 months) to ensure adequate replacement

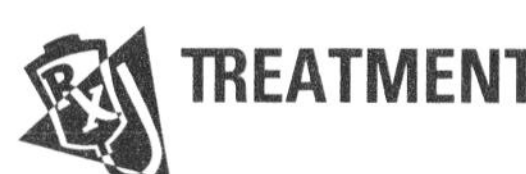

TREATMENT

MEDICATIONS

- Levothyroxine (T_4) is treatment of choice; T_4 is partially converted to T_3, the more active thyroid hormone
- Before levothyroxine started, exclude adrenal insufficiency, which would require concurrent treatment
- Levothyroxine starting dose: 50–100 μg PO Q AM if no coronary disease and age < 60 years; 100–150 μg PO Q AM if hypothyroid during pregnancy; and 25–50 μg PO Q AM if coronary disease or age >60 years. Dose titrated up by 25 μg Q 1–3 weeks until patient is euthyroid, usually at 100–250 μg Q AM
- Hypothyroid patients taking thyroxine typically have low serum T_3 levels (FT_3 levels during pregnancy or oral estrogen)
  - Addition of triiodothyronine (T_3, Cytomel) is controversial
  - Once a maintenance dose of thyroxine is determined, it is best to continue with the same brand owing to slight differences in absorption. Thyroxine requirements increase with oral estrogen therapy and pregnancy
  - Thyroxine requirements increase an average of 47% during the first half of pregnancy, with increased requirements seen as early as 5–8 weeks of gestation

   - Increase thyroxine dose 30% as soon as pregnancy is confirmed
   - Thyroxine requirements decrease postpartum, with menopause, or when switching from oral to transdermal estrogen therapy
- Elevated TSH usually indicates levothyroxine underreplacement. Before increasing T_4 dosage, assess for compliance and presence of angina, diarrhea, or malabsorption
- Avoid administration of levothyroxine concurrently with binding substances, eg, iron, sucralfate, aluminum hydroxide antacids, calcium supplements, or soy milk; or with bile acid-binding resins (eg, cholestyramine)
- Suppressed TSH may indicate levothyroxine overreplacement. Assess for severe nonthyroidal illness or medications (eg, nonsteroidal anti-inflammatory drugs, opioids, nifedipine, verapamil, corticosteroids)
- Amiodarone-induced hypothyroidism: treat with just enough levothyroxine to relieve symptoms
- Myxedema coma: levothyroxine sodium, 400 µg IV loading dose, then 100 µg IV QD. If hypothermic, warm only with blankets; if hypercapnic, mechanical ventilation. Treat infections aggressively
- If adrenal insufficiency suspected, give hydrocortisone, 100 mg IV, then 25–50 mg Q 8 h
- Myxedematous patients are unusually sensitive to opiates and may develop respiratory depression with typical doses
- Hypothyroid patients with ischemic heart disease should begin thyroxine therapy *after* coronary artery angioplasty or bypass. Thyroxine dosage requirements can rise, owing to increased hepatic metabolism of thyroxine induced by certain medications: carbamazepine, phenobarbitol, phenytoin, rifabutin, and rifampin

OUTCOME

FOLLOW-UP

- Continue levothyroxine for life; reassess dosage requirements periodically
- Surveillance for atrial arrhythmias and for osteoporosis, especially in patients who require high doses of levothyroxine
- Monitor patients with subclinical hypothyroidism for subtle signs (eg, fatigue, depression, hyperlipidemia). Clinical hypothyroidism later develops in ~18%

COMPLICATIONS

- Angina pectoris, congestive heart failure; may be precipitated by too rapid thyroid replacement
- Increased susceptibility to infection
- Megacolon in longstanding hypothyroidism
- Organic psychoses with paranoid delusions ("myxedema madness")
- Adrenal crisis precipitated by thyroid replacement
- Infertility (rare), miscarriage in untreated hypothyroidism
- Sellar enlargement and TSH-secreting tumors in untreated cases
- Myxedema coma: hypothermia, hypotension, hypoventilation, hypoxia, hypercapnia, hyponatremia, convulsions and abnormal CNS signs
   - Often induced by underlying infection; cardiac, respiratory, or CNS illness; cold exposure; or drug use

PROGNOSIS

- Excellent prognosis with early treatment, but relapses may occur if treatment is interrupted
- Mortality rate for myxedema coma is high

WHEN TO REFER

- Difficulty titrating levothyroxine replacement to normal TSH or clinically euthyroid state
- Any patient with significant coronary disease needing levothyroxine

WHEN TO ADMIT

- Suspected myxedema coma
- Hypercapnia

EVIDENCE

PRACTICE GUIDELINES

- AACE Medical Guidelines for Clinical Practice: Hyperthyroidism and Hypothyroidism, 2002
   - http://www.aace.com/clin/guidelines/hypo_hyper.pdf
- Roberts CG, Ladenson PW: Hypothyroidism. Lancet 2004;363:793. Comment in: Lancet 2004;363:1558. [PMID:15016491]

WEB SITES

- American Thyroid Association
   - http://www.thyroid.org/patients/brochures/Hypo_brochure.pdf
- Thyroid Disease Manager: http://www.thyroidmanager.org

INFORMATION FOR PATIENTS

- Mayo Clinic—Hypothyroidism
   - http://www.mayoclinic.com/invoke.cfm?id=DS00353
- JAMA patient page. Hypothyroidism. JAMA 2003;290:3024.

REFERENCES

- Alexander EK et al: Timing and magnitude of increases in levothyroxine requirements during pregnancy in women with hypothyroidism. N Engl J Med 2004;351:241. [PMID:15254282]
- Antonelli A, et al: Thyroid disorders in chronic hepatitis C. Am J Med 2004;117:10.[PMID:15210382]
- Indra R et al: Accuracy of physical examination in the diagnosis of hypothyroidism: a cross-sectional, double-blind study. J Postgrad Med 2004;50:7. [PMID:15047991]
- Rodriguez I et al: Factors associated with mortality of patients with myxoedema coma: prospective study in 11 cases treated in a single institution. J Endocrinol 2004;180:347. [PMID:14765987]
- Siegmund W et al: Replacement therapy with levothyroxine plus triiodothyronine (bioavailable molar ratio 14:1) is not superior to thyroxine alone to improve well-being and cognitive performance in hypothyroidism. Clin Endocrinol (Oxf) 2004;60:750. [PMID:15163340]
- Surks MI et al: Subclinical thyroid disease: scientific review and guidelines for diagnosis and management. JAMA 2004;29:228. [PMID:14722150]
- Tell R et al: Long-term incidence of hypothyroidism after radiotherapy in patients with head-and-neck cancer. Int J Radiat Oncol Biol Phys 2004;60:395

Author(s)

Paul A. Fitzgerald, MD

Idiopathic (Autoimmune) Thrombocytopenic Purpura

Hypoventilation, Primary Alveolar p. 1095

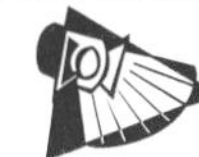

KEY FEATURES

ESSENTIALS OF DIAGNOSIS

- Isolated thrombocytopenia
- Other hematopoietic cell lines normal
- No systemic illness
- Spleen not palpable
- Normal bone marrow with normal or increased megakaryocytes

GENERAL CONSIDERATIONS

- Autoimmune disorder in which immunoglobulin G (IgG) autoantibody is formed that binds to platelets; unclear which antigen on platelet surface is involved
- Platelets are not destroyed by direct lysis; splenic macrophages bind to antibody-coated platelets
- Because spleen is major site of antibody production and platelet sequestration, splenectomy is highly effective therapy
- Hematologically identical to secondary thrombocytopenic purpura associated with systemic lupus erythematosus and chronic lymphocytic leukemia
- Childhood idiopathic thrombocytopenic purpura (ITP) frequently precipitated by viral infection and usually self-limited
- Adult form is usually chronic and infrequently follows viral infection
- Higher incidence with HIV infection

DEMOGRAPHICS

- Disease of young persons: peak incidence between ages 20 and 50
- 2:1 female predominance

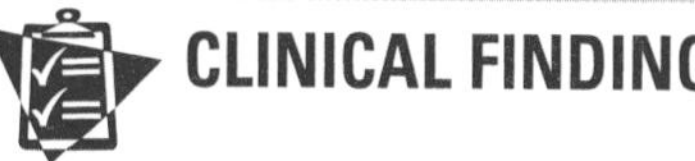

CLINICAL FINDINGS

SYMPTOMS AND SIGNS

- Patients are systemically well and usually not febrile
- Mucosal or skin bleeding: epistaxis, oral bleeding or hemorrhagic bullae, menorrhagia, purpura, or petechiae
- No other abnormal physical findings
- Splenomegaly should lead to consideration of an alternative diagnosis

DIFFERENTIAL DIAGNOSIS

- Thrombotic thrombocytopenic purpura
- Acute leukemia
- Myelodysplastic syndrome
- Disseminated intravascular coagulation
- Early aplastic anemia
- Drug toxicity (eg, heparin, sulfonamides, thiazides, quinine)
- Alcohol abuse
- Hypersplenism
- Systemic lupus erythematosus

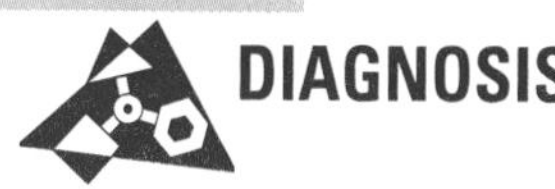

DIAGNOSIS

LABORATORY TESTS

- Thrombocytopenia, which may be severe (< 10,000/μL)
- Other counts are usually normal except for occasional anemia resulting from bleeding or associated hemolysis
- Peripheral blood smear shows normal cell morphology except for slightly enlarged platelets (megathrombocytes)
- Coexistent autoimmune hemolytic anemia (Evans's syndrome) in ~10%; associated with anemia, and peripheral smear showing reticulocytosis and spherocytes; red blood cell fragmentation should not be seen
- Coagulation studies entirely normal

DIAGNOSTIC PROCEDURES

- Bone marrow aspiration and biopsy are normal, with normal or increased number of megakaryocytes

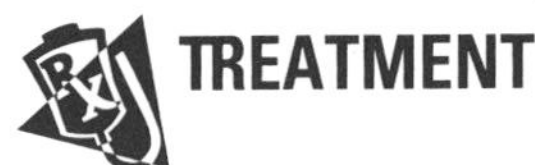

TREATMENT

MEDICATIONS

- Initial treatment: prednisone, 1–2 mg/kg/day, gradually tapered after platelet count normalizes; normal platelet count not necessary because risk of bleeding is small if platelet count is > 50,000/μL
- High-dose IVIG, 1 g/kg for 1 or 2 days, rapidly raises platelet count in 90%, and platelet count rises within 1–5 days; expensive and effect lasts only 1–2 weeks, so reserved for bleeding emergencies or preparing a severely thrombocytopenic patient for surgery
- Danazol, 600 mg/day, may be used if no response to prednisone and splenectomy
- Immunosuppressive agents used in refractory cases (eg, vincristine, azathioprine, cyclosporine, and cyclophosphamide)
- Rituximab benefits some with refractory disease

SURGERY

- Splenectomy is definitive treatment; most adults ultimately undergo splenectomy
- Splenectomy indications: no initial response to prednisone or unacceptably high doses required to maintain adequate platelet count, or patient prefers surgery
- Splenectomy can be performed safely even with platelet counts < 10,000/μL
- Splenectomy benefits 80% with either complete or partial remission
- ITP may recur in 10–20% of cases

THERAPEUTIC PROCEDURES

- Few adults with ITP have spontaneous remissions; most require treatment
- High-dose immunosuppression and autologous stem cell transplantation for rare patients with severe and refractory ITP
- Platelet transfusions are reserved for life-threatening bleeding and are rarely used because exogenous platelets survive no better than the patient's own (only a few hours)

OUTCOME

FOLLOW-UP

- With prednisone, bleeding often diminishes within 1 day; platelet count usually begins to rise within a week, and almost always within 3 weeks
- About 80% respond to prednisone, normalizing platelet count, but thrombocytopenia usually recurs if prednisone is completely withdrawn, so the aim is to find a dose that maintains adequate platelet count (> 50,000/μL)
- About 50% of patients respond to danazol

COMPLICATIONS

- Major initial concern is cerebral hemorrhage, a risk when platelet count is < 5000/μL
- Fatal bleeding is rare, even at very low platelet counts

PROGNOSIS

- Prognosis for remission is good
- Disease is usually initially controlled with prednisone; splenectomy offers definitive therapy

EVIDENCE

PRACTICE GUIDELINES

- British Committee for Standards in Haematology General Haematology Task Force: Guidelines for the investigation and management of idiopathic thrombocytopenic purpura in adults, children and in pregnancy. Br J Haematol 2003;120:574. [PMID: 12588344]
- George JN et al: Idiopathic Thrombocytopenic Purpura: A Practice Guideline Developed by Explicit Methods for The American Society of Hematology 1996, reviewed 2001.
  - http://www.hematology.org/practice/idiopathic.cfm

INFORMATION FOR PATIENTS

- National Heart, Lung, and Blood Institute: What Is Idiopathic Thrombocytopenic Purpura?
  - http://www.nhlbi.nih.gov/health/dci/Diseases/Itp/ITP_WhatIs.html
- Platelet Disorder Support Association: About ITP
  - http://www.itppeople.com/aboutitp.htm
- American Academy of Family Physicians: ITP
  - http://familydoctor.org/113.xml
- National Institute of Diabetes & Digestive & Kidney Diseases: Immune Thrombocytopenic Purpura
  - http://www.niddk.nih.gov/health/hematol/pubs/itp/itp.htm

REFERENCES

- Maloisel F et al: Danazol therapy in patients with chronic idiopathic thrombocytopenic purpura: long-term results. Am J Med 2004;716:590. [PMID: 15093754]
- Stasi R et al: Management of immune thrombocytopenic purpura in adults. Mayo Clin Proc 2004;79:504. [PMID: 15065616]
- Vesely SK et al: Management of adult patients with persistent idiopathic thrombocytopenic purpura following splenectomy: a systematic review. Ann Intern Med 2004;140:112. [PMID: 14734334]

Author(s)

Charles A. Linker, MD

Ileus, Acute Paralytic

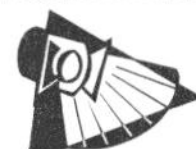

KEY FEATURES

ESSENTIALS OF DIAGNOSIS

- Precipitating factors: surgery, peritonitis, electrolyte abnormalities, severe medical illness
- Nausea, vomiting, obstipation, distention
- Minimal abdominal tenderness; decreased bowel sounds
- Plain abdominal radiography with gas and fluid distention in small and large bowel

GENERAL CONSIDERATIONS

- Neurogenic failure or loss of peristalsis in the intestine in the absence of any mechanical obstruction
- Common in hospitalized patients as a result of the following
  - Intraabdominal processes, such as recent gastrointestinal or abdominal surgery or peritoneal irritation (peritonitis, pancreatitis, ruptured viscus, hemorrhage)
  - Severe medical illness, such as pneumonia, respiratory failure requiring intubation, sepsis or severe infections, uremia, diabetic ketoacidosis, and electrolyte abnormalities (hypokalemia, hypercalcemia, hypomagnesemia, hypophosphatemia)
  - Medications, such as opioids, anticholinergics, phenothiazines

CLINICAL FINDINGS

SYMPTOMS AND SIGNS

- Mild diffuse, continuous abdominal discomfort
- Nausea and vomiting
- Generalized abdominal distention
- Minimal abdominal tenderness
- No signs of peritoneal irritation
- Bowel sounds are diminished to absent

DIFFERENTIAL DIAGNOSIS

- Mechanical obstruction of small intestine or proximal colon, eg, adhesions, volvulus, Crohn's disease
- Chronic intestinal pseudoobstruction

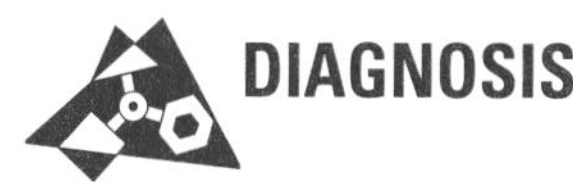

DIAGNOSIS

LABORATORY TESTS

- Obtain serum electrolytes, potassium, magnesium, phosphorus, and calcium

IMAGING STUDIES

- Plain abdominal radiography: air-fluid levels, distended gas-filled loops of small and large intestine
- Limited barium small bowel series or a CT scan can help to exclude mechanical obstruction

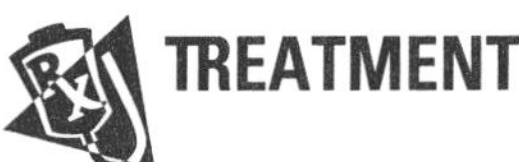

TREATMENT

THERAPEUTIC PROCEDURES

- Treat underlying primary medical or surgical illness
- Nasogastric suction for discomfort or vomiting
- Restrict oral intake, intravenous fluids
- Liberalize diet gradually as bowel function returns
- Minimize anticholinergic and opioid medications
- Peripheral nonopioid receptor antagonists reduce the duration of postoperative ileus; these agents are in clinical trials
- Severe or prolonged ileus requires nasogastric suction and infusion of parenteral fluids and electrolytes

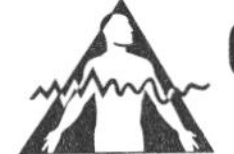

OUTCOME

FOLLOW-UP

- Return of bowel function usually heralded by return of appetite and passage of flatus
- Serial plain film radiography and/or abdominal CT warranted for persistent or worsening symptoms to distinguish from mechanical obstruction

COMPLICATIONS

- Metabolic disturbances due to prolonged nasogastric suction (hypokalemia, metabolic alkalosis)
- Delayed nutritional intake complication of prolonged postoperative immobility

PROGNOSIS

- Ileus usually resolves within 48–72 h
- Following surgery, small intestinal motility normalizes first (within hours), followed by stomach (24–48 h) and colon (48–72 h)

WHEN TO REFER

- Persistent ileus >3–5 days warrants further evaluation for underlying cause and to exclude mechanical obstruction

WHEN TO ADMIT

- All patients with ileus require admission for IV fluids

EVIDENCE

PRACTICE GUIDELINES

- Bauer AJ et al: Ileus in critical illness: mechanisms and management. Curr Opin Crit Care 2002;8:152. [PMID: 12386517]
- Holte K et al: Postoperative ileus: progress towards effective management. Drugs 2002;62:2603. [PMID: 12466000]

INFORMATION FOR PATIENTS

- MEDLINEplus—Intestinal obstruction
  - http://www.nlm.nih.gov/medlineplus/ency/article/000260.htm

REFERENCES

- Behm B et al: Postoperative ileus: etiologies and interventions. Clin Gastroenterol Hepatol 2003;1:71. [PMID: 15017498]
- Luckey A et al: Mechanisms and treatment of postoperative ileus. Arch Surg 2003;138:206. [PMID: 12578422]

Author(s)

Kenneth R. McQuaid, MD

Immobility in Elderly

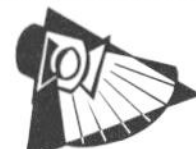

KEY FEATURES

ESSENTIALS OF DIAGNOSIS

- Weakness, stiffness, pain, imbalance, and comorbid illness

GENERAL CONSIDERATIONS

- Although common in older people, reduced mobility is never normal
- It is an important cause of hospital-induced functional decline
- The hazards of bed rest are multiple, serious, quick to develop, and slow to reverse
- Weakness may result from disuse of muscles, malnutrition, electrolyte disturbances, anemia, neurologic disorders, or myopathies
- The most common cause of pain and stiffness is osteoarthritis, but also consider Parkinson's disease, other arthritides such as rheumatoid arthritis, and polymyalgia rheumatica
- Pain, such as painful foot problems, may immobilize the patient
- Imbalance and fear of falling are major causes of immobilization
- Imbalance often results from
  - Neurologic disorders (eg, stroke, cervical myelopathy, peripheral neuropathy due to diabetes or alcohol, vestibulocerebellar abnormalities)
  - Orthostatic or postprandial hypotension
  - Drugs (eg, diuretics, antihypertensives, sedatives, neuroleptics, antidepressants)
  - Prolonged bed rest
- Psychological conditions such as severe anxiety or depression may contribute to immobilization

DEMOGRAPHICS

- Among hospitalized medical patients over age 70, about 10% experience a decline in their ability to perform activities of daily living (ADL)

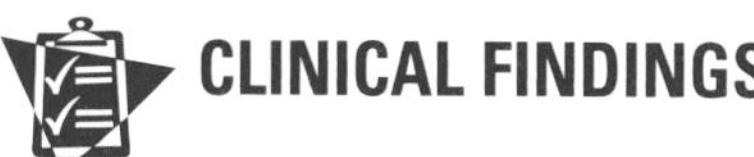

CLINICAL FINDINGS

SYMPTOMS AND SIGNS

- Older person who is weak, stiff, has pain, or imbalance with gait
- Orthostatic or postprandial hypotension
- Depression may manifest as immobility
- Depression and dementia frequently coexist

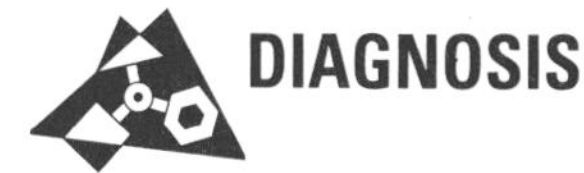

DIAGNOSIS

LABORATORY TESTS

- For a simple geriatric functional screening instrument, see Table 3

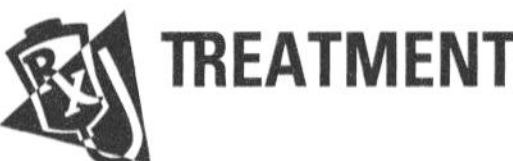

TREATMENT

MEDICATIONS

- For many cases of osteoarthritis, acetaminophen or glucosamine may be effective and safer than a nonsteroidal anti-inflammatory drug or COX-2 inhibitor
- If depression is preventing a patient from participating in physical activity, it may prove necessary to start with a short course of stimulant medication (eg, methylphenidate; see Depression or Depression in Elderly), at least until a more traditional antidepressant has had time to take effect

THERAPEUTIC PROCEDURES

- Reduced mobility in older people is often treatable if its causes are identified
- All patients should assist with their own positioning, transferring, and self-care whenever possible
- Install handrails, lower the bed, and provide chairs of proper height with arms and rubber skid guards
- A properly sized cane or walker may be useful
- Exercise is an effective treatment for both knee and hip osteoarthritis
- For hospitalized patients, activity should be initiated as soon as possible
  - To minimize cardiopulmonary deconditioning, position patients as close to the upright position as possible, several times daily
  - To reduce the risks of contracture and weakness, immediately begin range of motion and isometric and isotonic exercises while the patient is in bed
  - To encourage activity, avoid restraints and discontinue invasive devices (intravenous lines, urinary catheters)
- Immobilized patients should receive low-dose heparin or graduated compression stockings, or both, to reduce the risk of thromboembolism

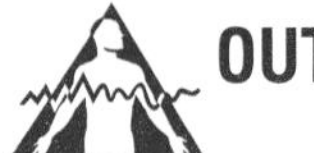

OUTCOME

COMPLICATIONS

- Deconditioning of the cardiovascular system occurs within days and involves fluid shifts, decreased cardiac output, decreased peak oxygen uptake, and increased resting heart rate
- Striking changes occur in skeletal muscle, with loss of contractile velocity and strength
- Pressure sores are a serious complication; mechanical pressure, moisture, friction, and shearing forces all predispose to their development
- Thrombophlebitis and pulmonary embolism are additional serious risks
- Within days after being confined to bed, the risk of postural hypotension, falls, skin breakdown, and pulmonary embolism rises rapidly

PROGNOSIS

- Among patients who decline in their ability to do their ADLs while hospitalized, about 50% will not recover by 3 months after discharge
- Decreased ambulation and impairments in the ability to independently perform ADLs are associated with higher rates of mortality

WHEN TO REFER

- Early referral to occupational or physical therapy is essential

PREVENTION

- In hospitalized patients, bed rest orders should be avoided as much as possible
- Devices that immobilize such as Foley catheters should be withdrawn as soon as possible
- Adequate nutrition should be ensured
- The skin over pressure points should be inspected frequently, and if the patient is unable, staff should reposition the patient every 2 h

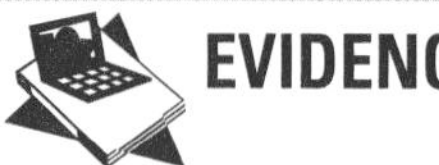

EVIDENCE

PRACTICE GUIDELINES

- National Guideline Clearinghouse
  - Constipation. Association of Rehabilitation Nurses, 2002
    - http://www.guideline.gov/summary/summary.aspx?doc_id=3687
  - Pressure ulcers. Wound, Ostomy, and Continence Nurses Society, 2003
    - http://www.guideline.gov/summary/summary.aspx?doc_id=3860
  - Venous thromboembolism. American College of Chest Physicians, 2001
    - http://www.guideline.gov/summary/summary.aspx?doc_id=2724

WEB SITES

- AARP Guide to Internet Resources on Aging
  - http://www.aarp.org/cyber/sd1_3.htm
- Administration on Aging
  - http://www.aoa.dhhs.gov
- The American Geriatrics Society
  - http://www.americangeriatrics.org

INFORMATION FOR PATIENTS

- American Academy of Family Physicians: Osteoarthritis
  - http://familydoctor.org/handouts/115.xml
- American Academy of Family Physicians: Deep Venous Thrombosis
  - http://familydoctor.org/800.xml
- Osteoporosis
  - http://www.fcmsdocs.org
- Wheelchairs
  - http://www.wheelchairnet.org/WCN_ProdServ/Products/mobility.html

REFERENCE

- van Baar ME: Effectiveness of exercise therapy in patients with osteoarthritis of the hip or knee. Arthritis Rheum 1999; 42:1361. [PMID: 104032263]

Author(s)

Helen Chen, MD

C. Bree Johnston, MD

Infection, Central Nervous System

Immunoglobulin A Deficiency, Selective p. 1096. Impetigo p. 1096.

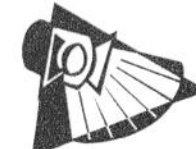

KEY FEATURES

ESSENTIALS OF DIAGNOSIS

- Central nervous system (CNS) infection is a medical emergency
- Immediate diagnostic steps must be instituted to establish the specific cause

GENERAL CONSIDERATIONS

- Infections can be caused by almost any infectious agent, including bacteria, mycobacteria, fungi, spirochetes, protozoa, helminths, and viruses

Etiologic classification

- CNS infections can be divided into several categories that are readily distinguished by cerebrospinal fluid examination as the first step toward diagnosis (Table 130)
- Purulent meningitis
  - 18–50 years: *Streptococcus pneumoniae, Neisseria meningitidis*
  - > 50 years: *S pneumoniae, N meningitidis, Listeria*, gram-negative bacilli
  - Impaired cellular immunity: *Listeria*, gram-negative bacilli, *S pneumoniae*
  - Postsurgical or posttraumatic: *Staphylococcus aureus, S pneumoniae*, gram-negative bacilli
- Chronic meningitis
  - Tuberculosis or atypical mycobacteria
  - Fungi: *Cryptococcus, Coccidioides, Histoplasma*
  - Spirochetes: syphilis, Lyme disease, leptospirosis
  - Other: brucellosis, HIV infection
- Aseptic meningitis
  - Mumps, coxsackievirus, echoviruses
  - Infectious mononucleosis
  - Leptospirosis, syphilis, Lyme disease
- Encephalitis
- Partially treated bacterial meningitis
- Neighborhood reaction
- Noninfectious meningeal irritation
- Brain abscess
- Amebic meningoencephalitis

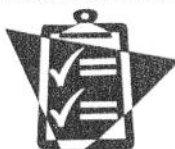

CLINICAL FINDINGS

SYMPTOMS AND SIGNS

- Symptoms and signs common in all types of CNS infection
  - Headache, fever, sensorial disturbances, neck and back stiffness, positive Kernig and Brudzinski signs
  - Cerebrospinal fluid abnormalities
- Although it is rare for all of these manifestations to be present in any one individual, the presence of even one should suggest the possibility of a CNS infection

DIFFERENTIAL DIAGNOSIS

- Subarachnoid hemorrhage
- Encephalitis
- "Neighborhood reaction" causing abnormal cerebrospinal fluid, eg, brain abscess, epidural abscess, vertebral osteomyelitis, mastoiditis, sinusitis, brain tumor
- Dural sinus thrombosis
- Noninfectious meningeal irritation
  - Carcinomatous meningitis
  - Sarcoidosis
  - Systemic lupus erythematosus
  - Drugs (eg, nonsteroidal anti-inflammatory drugs, trimethoprim-sulfamethoxazole)
  - Pneumonia
  - Shigellosis
- If fever and rash
  - Gonococcemia
  - Infective endocarditis
  - Thrombotic thrombocytopenic purpura
  - Rocky Mountain spotted fever
  - Viral exanthem
- Seizure due to other cause eg, febrile seizure
- Amebic meningoencephalitis (*Naegleria fowleri*)

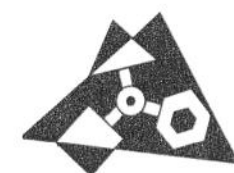

DIAGNOSIS

LABORATORY TESTS

- See Table 130
- Blood cell count, blood culture
- Lumbar puncture followed by careful study and culture of the cerebrospinal fluid
  - Fluid must be examined for cell count, glucose, and protein, and a smear stained for bacteria (and acid-fast organisms when appropriate) and cultured for pyogenic organisms and for mycobacteria and fungi when indicated
  - Latex agglutination tests can detect antigens of encapsulated organisms *(S pneumoniae, Haemophilus influenzae, N meningitidis*, and *Cryptococcus neoformans)* but are rarely used except for detection of *Cryptococcus* or in partially treated patients
  - Polymerase chain reaction (PCR) for herpes simplex and varicella-zoster is very sensitive (> 95%) and specific
  - PCR to detect other organisms may not be any more sensitive than culture, but the real value is the rapidity with which results are available, ie, hours compared with days or weeks
  - At present, with the exception of PCR for herpes simplex, PCR tests are performed only in reference laboratories

IMAGING STUDIES

- Chest x-ray
- Since performing a lumbar puncture in the presence of a space-occupying lesion (brain abscess, subdural hematoma, subdural abscess) may result in brainstem herniation, a CT scan is performed before lumbar puncture if a space-occupying lesion is suspected on the basis of papilledema, coma, seizures, or focal neurologic findings

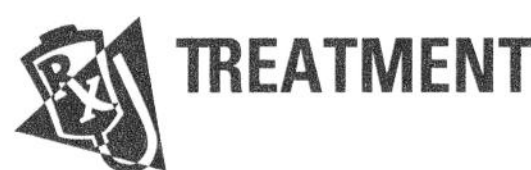

TREATMENT

MEDICATIONS

- If CT scan is delayed and bacterial meningitis is suspected, blood cultures should be drawn and antibiotics and corticosteroids administered even before cerebrospinal fluid is obtained to avoid delay in treatment (Table 129)
- Antibiotics given within 4 h before obtaining cerebrospinal fluid probably do not affect culture results
- Increased intracranial pressure due to brain edema often requires treatment with hyperventilation, mannitol (25–50 g bolus IV infusion), dexamethasone (4 mg Q 4–6 h)

Purulent meningitis

- Treat presumptive microorganism based on age group (Table 129). The identity of the causative microorganism may remain unknown for a few days
- The duration of therapy for bacterial meningitis varies depending on the etiological agent
  - *H influenzae,* 7 days
  - *N meningitidis,* 7 days
  - *S pneumoniae,* 10–14 days
  - *Listeria monocytogenes,* 14–21 days
  - Gram-negative bacilli, 21 days
- For pneumococcal meningitis, administer dexamethasone 10 mg IV 15–20 min before or simultaneously with the first dose of antibiotics and continue Q 6 h for 4 days

Brain abscess

- Therapy consists of drainage and 3–4 weeks of systemic antibiotics directed against organisms isolated
- A regimen often used includes metronidazole, 500 mg IV or PO Q 8 h, plus ceftizoxime, 2 g IV Q 8 h, or ceftriaxone, 2 g IV Q 12 h
- In cases where abscesses are < 2 cm in size, where there are multiple abscesses that cannot be drained, or if an abscess is located in an area where significant neurologic sequelae would result from drainage, antibiotics for 6–8 weeks without drainage can be used

Therapy of other types of meningitis

- See specific diagnoses

SURGERY

- Brain abscesses need drainage (excision or aspiration) if ≥ 4 cm in size, and systemic antibiotics

THERAPEUTIC PROCEDURES

- Treatment of cerebral edema and increased intracranial pressure may require drainage of cerebrospinal fluid by repeated lumbar puncture and placement of ventricular catheters

OUTCOME

FOLLOW-UP

- Monitor CNS pressures if extraventricular drain is in place

PROGNOSIS

- Prompt antibiotic therapy probably improves outcome in bacterial meningitis
- Dexamethasone therapy for pneumococcal meningitis decreases morbidity and mortality

WHEN TO ADMIT

- Acute CNS symptoms are emergencies
- All patients with meningitis, except viral, should be admitted
- Brain abscess and epidural abscess require admission

PREVENTION

Pneumococcal vaccine

- See MMWR 2000;49(No. RR-9):1.
- Recommended for patients with cerebrospinal fluid leaks
- Because of the apparent increased risk of developing pneumococcal meningitis following cochlear implants, patients receiving these implants should be vaccinated

Meningococcal vaccine

- Should be administered to asplenic patients or those with terminal complement deficiencies
- A new conjugated polysaccharide vaccine is now recommended as a routine vaccination for preadolescents aged 11–12 and as "catch-up" vaccination for previously unvaccinated teens entering high school or college
- Other groups recommended for vaccination include laboratory workers with exposures to *N meningitidis,* travelers to endemic regions (Nepal, sub-Saharan Africa, the "meningitis belt" from Sengal in the west to Ethiopia in the east, northern India)
- Vaccination of all persons previously vaccinated with the unconjugated product

EVIDENCE

PRACTICE GUIDELINES

- Infectious Diseases Society of America
  - http://www.journals.uchicago.edu/CID/journal/issues/v39n9/34796/34796.web.pdf
- National Guideline Clearinghouse:
  - Cryptococcal disease management. IDSA, 2000
    - http://www.guideline.gov/summary/summary.aspx?doc_id=2666&nbr=1892&string=meningitis
  - Imaging of intracranial infections. ACR, 2000
    - http://www.guideline.gov/summary/summary.aspx?doc_id=2446&nbr=1672&string=meningitis
  - Prevention and control of meningococcal disease. Advisory Committee on Immunization Practices, 2000
    - http://www.guideline.gov/summary/summary.aspx?doc_id=2364

INFORMATION FOR PATIENTS

- The Mayo Clinic
  - http://www.mayoclinic.com/invoke.cfm?id=DS00118
- National Institute of Neurological Disorders and Stroke
  - http://www.ninds.nih.gov/health_and_medical/disorders/encmenin_doc.htm

REFERENCES

- Bernardini GL: Diagnosis and management of brain abscess and subdural empyema. Curr Neurol Neurosci Rep 2004;4:448. [PMID: 15509445]
- De Gans J: Dexamethasone in adults with bacterial meningitis. N Engl J Med 2002;347:1549. [PMID: 11144034]
- Hussein AS: Acute bacterial meningitis in adults. A 12-year review. Medicine (Baltimore) 2000;79:360. [PMID: 11144034]
- Sinner SW et al: Antimicrobial agents in the treatment of bacterial meningitis. Infect Dis Clin North Am 2004;18:581. [PMID: 15308277]

Author(s)

Richard A. Jacobs, MD, PhD

Infection in the Immunocompromised Host

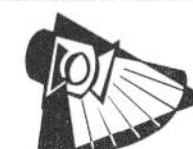

KEY FEATURES

ESSENTIALS OF DIAGNOSIS

- Clinical symptoms may be blunted because of immunosuppression
- Fever is often absent

GENERAL CONSIDERATIONS

Granulocytopenia

- Absolute granulocyte count below 1000/μL, and especially below 100/μL
- Increased infections with gram-negative enteric organisms
  - *Pseudomonas*
  - Gram-positive cocci (particularly *Staphylococcus aureus*, *Staphylococcus epidermidis*, and viridans streptococci)
  - *Candida*
  - *Aspergillus*
  - Other fungi such as *Trichosporon*, *Scedosporium*, *Fusarium*, and *Pseudallescheria*

Ineffective humoral immunity (eg, myeloma)

- Increased infections with encapsulated organisms such as *Haemophilus influenzae* and *Streptococcus pneumoniae*

Cellular immune deficiency

- HIV infection, lymphoreticular malignancies such as Hodgkin's disease, immunosuppressive medications
- Increased infections by a large number of organisms, such as *Listeria*, *Legionella*, *Salmonella*, and *Mycobacterium*; viruses such as herpes simplex, varicella, and cytomegalovirus (CMV); fungi such as *Cryptococcus*, *Coccidioides*, *Histoplasma*, and *Pneumocystis*; and protozoa such as *Toxoplasma*

Asplenic patients

- Increased risk of overwhelming bacteremia with encapsulated bacteria (primarily *S pneumoniae* but also *H influenzae* and *Neisseria meningitidis*)

Debilitating injury (severe burns or trauma)

- Increased infections from Foley catheters, dialysis catheters, central nervous system dysfunction (which predisposes to aspiration pneumonia and decubitus ulcers), obstructing lesions (eg, pneumonia due to an obstructed bronchus), and use of broad-spectrum antibiotics

Transplantation

- Infections immediately after transplant often involve the transplanted organ
  - Lung transplantation: pneumonia and mediastinitis
  - Liver transplantation: intra-abdominal abscess, cholangitis, and peritonitis
  - Renal transplantation: urinary tract infections, perinephric abscesses, and infected lymphoceles
- In contrast to solid organ transplants, in bone marrow transplants the source of fever cannot be found in 60–70% of patients
- Most infections that occur in the first 2–4 weeks are related to the operative procedure and to hospitalization itself (wound infection, IV catheter infection, urinary tract infection from a Foley catheter) or are related to the transplanted organ
- Infections that occur between the first and sixth months are often related to immunosuppression. Reactivated herpes simplex, varicella-zoster, and CMV infections are quite common. Opportunistic infections with fungi (*Candida*, *Aspergillus*, *Cryptococcus*, *Pneumocystis*, and others), *Listeria monocytogenes*, *Nocardia*, and *Toxoplasma* are also common
- After 6 months, when immunosuppression has been reduced to maintenance levels, infections that are found in any population occur

Other

- Organisms not usually pathogens in the immunocompetent person may cause serious life-threatening infection in the immunocompromised patient (eg, *S epidermidis*, *Corynebacterium jeikeium*, *Propionibacterium acnes*, *Bacillus* species). Therefore, interpret culture results with caution and do not disregard isolates as mere contaminants

CLINICAL FINDINGS

SYMPTOMS AND SIGNS

- Symptoms may be subtle because of the immunosuppression
- There may be increased insulin requirements in diabetics
- Fever is often absent

DIFFERENTIAL DIAGNOSIS

- Neutropenia
  - Gram-negative enteric organisms
  - *Pseudomonas*
  - Gram-positive cocci, eg, *S aureus*, *S epidermidis*
  - Canidida
  - *Aspergillus* and other fungi
- Cellular immune defect, eg, HIV, lymphoma, immunosuppressive drugs
  - Bacteria: *Listeria*, *Legionella*, *Salmonella*, *Mycobacterium*
  - Viruses: herpes simplex virus, varicella, CMV
  - Fungi: *Cryptococcus*, *Coccidioides*, *Histoplasma*, *Pneumocystis*
  - Protozoa: *Toxoplasma*
- Humoral immune defect, eg, congenital, multiple myeloma, chronic lymphocytic leukemia
  - Encapsulated organisms: *S pneumoniae*, *H influenzae*, *N meningitidis*
- Asplenia (functional or anatomic)
  - Encapsulated organisms: *S pneumoniae*, *H influenzae*, *N meningitidis*
- Noninfectious causes: transplant rejection, organ ischemia or necrosis, thrombophlebitis, and lymphoma

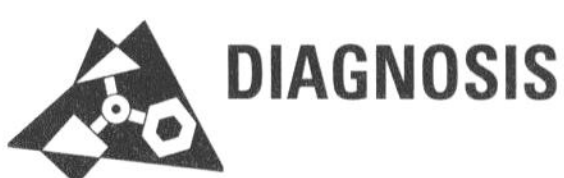

DIAGNOSIS

LABORATORY TESTS

- Complete blood cell count with differential and blood cultures
- Urine and sputum cultures should be obtained if indicated clinically or radiographically
- Any focal complaints (localized pain, headache, rash) should prompt culture and imaging appropriate to the site
- If fever persists without an obvious source, evaluate for viral infection (CMV blood cultures or antigen test), abscess (which usually occurs near previous operative sites), candidiasis involving the liver or spleen, or aspergillosis
- Serologic tests may be helpful if *Toxoplasma*, *Aspergillus* (galactomannin), *Cryptococcus*, or endemic fungi (*Coccidioides*, *Histoplasma*) are possible pathogens

IMAGING STUDIES

- Chest x-ray
- Other imaging tests depend on the clinical setting

DIAGNOSTIC PROCEDURES

- Sputum induction diagnoses *Pneumocystis* pneumonia in 50–80% of AIDS patients with this infection. In other situations, more invasive procedures may be required (bronchoalveolar lavage, transbronchial biopsy, or even open lung biopsy)
- Skin, liver, or bone marrow biopsy may be helpful in establishing a diagnosis

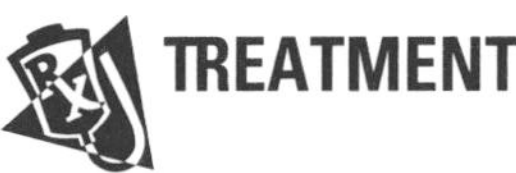

TREATMENT

MEDICATIONS

- Because infections can be rapidly progressive and life-threatening, diagnostic procedures must be done promptly, and empiric therapy is usually instituted before a specific agent has been isolated (Table 128)
- Reduction or discontinuation of immunosuppressive medication may be necesary in life-threatening infections
- Hematopoietic growth factors (granulocyte and granulocyte-macrophage colony-stimulating factors) in prolonged neutropenia (> 7 days) can reverse immunosuppression
- The antibiotics used depend on the type of immunocompromise and site of infection

Neutropenia

- Primarily bacterial and fungal infections
- Initial treatment is often directed at gram-positive and gram-negative organisms (Table 128)
- If the patient does not respond, broader-spectrum antibiotics and antifungal drugs are added
- Although different antibiotic agents can be used, choices should be based on local microbiological trends

Example of one algorithm

- Initiate therapy with a fluoroquinolone active against gram-positive organisms (such as levofloxacin, gatifloxacin, or moxifloxacin) when the absolute neutrophil count falls below 500/μL
- If fever develops, cultures are obtained and vancomycin, 10–15 mg/kg IV Q 12 h, is given (to cover methicillin-resistant *S aureus*, *S epidermidis*, and *Enterococcus*)
- If after 48–72 h fever continues, antifungal coverage can be increased by changing to voriconazole, 200 mg twice daily (if the patient received fluconazole prophylaxis), and broader-spectrum antibiotics can be added sequentially. For example, to better cover *Acinetobacter*, *Citrobacter*, and *Pseudomonas*, the fluoroquinolone may be switched to cefipime, 2 g IV Q 8 h; with continued fever, imipenem, 500 mg Q 6 h (or meropenem, 1 g Q 8 h), with or without tobramycin, 1.8 mg/kg Q 8 h, may be used in place of cefipime
- If fevers persist, trimethoprim-sulfamethoxazole at 10 mg/kg/day (of trimethoprim) in three divided doses can be added to cover *Stenotrophomonas*
- Regardless of whether the patient becomes afebrile, therapy must be continued until resolution of neutropenia
- Patients with fever and neutropenia at low risk for complications (neutropenia persisting for < 10 days, no comorbid complications requiring hospitalization, and cancer adequately treated) can be treated with oral antibiotic regimens (ciprofloxacin, 750 mg Q 12 h, plus amoxicillin-clavulanic acid, 500 mg Q 8 h)

Organ transplant

- For interstitial infiltrates, consider empiric treatment for *Pneumocystis* or *Legionella* species with trimethoprim-sulfamethoxazole and a macrolide
- If the patient does not respond, add more antimicrobial agents or undertake invasive procedures to make a specific diagnosis
- By making a specific diagnosis, therapy can be specific and polypharmacy with potentially toxic agents avoided

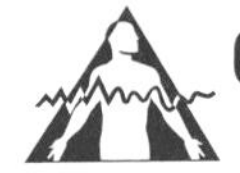

OUTCOME

WHEN TO REFER

- Infections can be rapidly progressive and any patient who does not respond to treatment in 2–3 days should be referred to a specialist and probably admitted to the hospital

PREVENTION

- See Table 134
- Hand washing is the simplest and most effective means of decreasing nosocomial infections in *all* patients
- Invasive devices such as central and peripheral lines and Foley catheters are a potential source of infection

EVIDENCE

PRACTICE GUIDELINES

- National Guideline Clearinghouse. Prevention of Opportunistic Infections in HIV+ Patients. USPHS/IDSA, 2001
  - http://www.guideline.gov/summary/summary.aspx?doc_id=3080

INFORMATION FOR PATIENTS

- American Academy of Family Physicians
  - http://familydoctor.org/248.xml
- Centers for Disease Control and Prevention
  - http://www.cdc.gov/ncidod/dpd/parasites/cryptosporidiosis/factsht_crypto_prevent_ci.htm
  - http://www.cdc.gov/travel/alteredimmun.htm

REFERENCES

- Simon DM et al: Infectious complications of solid organ transplantation. Infect Dis Clin North Am 2001;15:521. [PMID: 11447708]
- Viscoli C: Treatment of febrile neutropenia: what is new? Curr Opin Infect Dis 2002;15:377. [PMID: 12130933]

Author(s)

Richard A. Jacobs, MD, PhD

Infection, Nosocomial

KEY FEATURES

ESSENTIALS OF DIAGNOSIS

- Nosocomial infections are by definition acquired during the course of hospitalization
- Hand washing is the easiest and most effective means of prevention and should be done routinely even when gloves are utilized

GENERAL CONSIDERATIONS

- Although most fevers are due to infections, about 25% of patients will have fever of noninfectious origin
- Many infections are a direct result of the use of invasive devices for monitoring or therapy such as IV catheters, Foley catheters, catheters placed by interventional radiology for drainage, and orotracheal tubes for ventilatory support. Early removal reduces infection
- Patients in whom nosocomial infections develop are often critically ill, have been hospitalized for extended periods, and have received several courses of broad-spectrum antibiotic therapy
- As a result, the causative organisms are often multidrug resistant and different from those in community-acquired infections
  - *Staphylococcus aureus* and *Staphylococcus epidermidis* (a frequent cause of prosthetic device infection) may be resistant to nafcillin and cephalosporins and require vancomycin for therapy
  - *Enterococcus faecium* resistant to ampicillin and vancomycin
  - Gram-negative infections caused by *Pseudomonas*, *Citrobacter*, *Enterobacter*, *Acinetobacter*, and *Stenotrophomonas* may be sensitive only to fluoroquinolones, carbapenems, aminoglycosides, or trimethoprim-sulfamethoxazole

DEMOGRAPHICS

- In the United States, approximately 5% of patients who enter the hospital free of infection acquire a nosocomial infection resulting in prolongation of the hospital stay, increase in cost of care, significant morbidity, and a 5% mortality rate

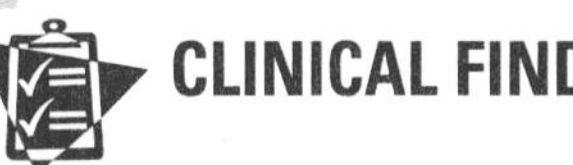

CLINICAL FINDINGS

SYMPTOMS AND SIGNS

- Those of the underlying disease

DIFFERENTIAL DIAGNOSIS

- Noninfectious
  - Drug fever
  - Postoperative atelectasis or tissue necrosis
  - Hematoma
  - Pancreatitis
  - Pulmonary embolus
  - Myocardial infarction
  - Ischemic bowel
- Urinary tract infections
- Pneumonia
- Bacteremia, eg, indwelling catheter, wound, abscess, pneumonia, genitourinary or gastrointestinal tract
- Wound infection, eg, decubitus ulcer, *Clostridium difficile* colitis

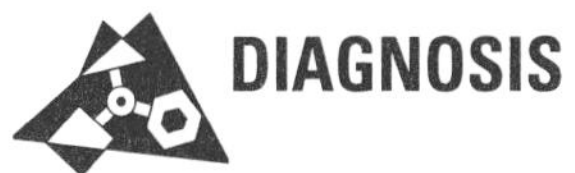

DIAGNOSIS

LABORATORY TESTS

- Unreliable or uninterpretable specimens are often obtained for culture that result in unnecessary use of antibiotics
  - The best example of this principle is the diagnosis of line-related or bloodstream infection in the febrile patient
  - Blood cultures from unidentified sites, a single blood culture from any site, or a blood culture through an existing line will often be positive for *S epidermidis* and will result in therapy with vancomycin
  - The likelihood that such a culture represents a true bacteremia is 10–20%
- Unless two separate venipuncture cultures are obtained—*not* through catheters—interpretation of results is impossible and unnecessary therapy is given
- A positive wound culture without signs of inflammation or infection, a positive sputum culture without pulmonary infiltrates on chest x-ray, or a positive urine culture in a catheterized patient without signs or symptoms of pyelonephritis are all likely to represent colonization, not infection

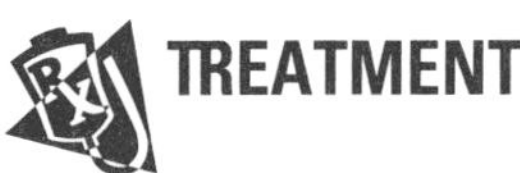

TREATMENT

MEDICATIONS

- When choosing antibiotics to treat the seriously ill patient, consider the previous antimicrobial therapy the patient has received as well as the "local ecology"
- It is often necessary to institute therapy with vancomycin, a carbapenem, an aminoglycoside, or a fluoroquinolone until a specific agent is isolated and sensitivities are known

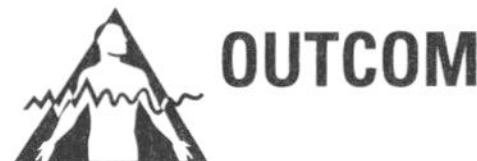

OUTCOME

FOLLOW-UP

- Monitoring of high-risk areas by hospital epidemiologists detects increases in infection rates early

WHEN TO REFER

- For persistent fevers or systemic toxicity despite treatment of underlying problem

PREVENTION

- Universal precautions against potential blood-borne transmissible disease
- Hepatitis A, hepatitis B, and varicella vaccines should be considered in the appropriate setting
- Peripheral IV lines should be replaced every 3 days and arterial lines every 4 days
- Lines in the central venous circulation (including those placed peripherally) can be left in indefinitely and are changed or removed when they are clinically suspected of being infected, when they are nonfunctional, or when they are no longer needed
- Silver alloy–impregnated Foley catheters reduce the incidence of catheter-associated bacteriuria, and antibiotic-impregnated (minocycline plus rifampin or chlorhexidine plus silver sulfadiazine) venous catheters reduce line infections and bacteremia
- Whether the increased cost of these devices justifies their routine use should be determined by individual institutions based on local infection rates
- Attentive nursing care (positioning to prevent decubitus ulcers, wound care, elevating the head during tube feedings to prevent aspiration) is critical

EVIDENCE

PRACTICE GUIDELINES

- American Thoracic Society; Infectious Diseases Society of America: Guidelines for the management of adults with hospital-acquired, ventilation-associated and healthcare-associated pneumonia. Am J Respir Crit Care Med 2005;171:388. [PMID: 15699079]
- National Guideline Clearinghouse:
  - Guidelines for preventing health-care–associated pneumonia, 2003: CDC and the Healthcare Infection Control Practices Advisory Committee
    - http://www.guideline.gov/summary/summary.aspx?doc_id=4872
  - Handwashing and antisepsis. APIC 1995.
    - http://www.guideline.gov/summary/summary.aspx?doc_id=2226
  - Hand hygiene. HICPAC/SHEA/APIC/IDSA, 2002
    - http://www.guideline.gov/summary/summary.aspx?doc_id=3484
  - Stem cell transplant and infection prevention. CDC, 2000
    - http://www.guideline.gov/summary/summary.aspx?doc_id=2573

WEB SITE

- Centers for Disease Control and Prevention—National Nosocomial Infections Surveillance System
  - http://www.cdc.gov/ncidod/hip/SURVEILL/NNIS.HTM

INFORMATION FOR PATIENTS

- National Institute of Allergy and Infectious Diseases
  - http://www.niaid.nih.gov/factsheets/antimicro.htm
- National Institutes of Health
  - http://www.nlm.nih.gov/medlineplus/ency/article/000146.htm

REFERENCES

- Kollef MH: Prevention of hospital-associated pneumonia and ventilation-associated pneumonia. Crit Care Med 2004;82:1396. [PMID: 15187525]
- Lorente C et al: Prevention of infection in the intensive care unit: current advances and opportunities for the future. Curr Opin Crit Care 2002;8:461. [PMID: 12357116]
- Safdar N et al: The commonality of risk factors for nosocomial colonization and infection with antimicrobial-resistant *Staphylococcus aureus,* enterococcus, gram-negative bacilli, *Clostridium difficile,* and *Candida.* Ann Intern Med 2002;136:834. [PMID: 12044132]

Author(s)

Richard A. Jacobs, MD, PhD

Infertility, Female

Infertility, Assisted Reproductive Technologies p. 1096

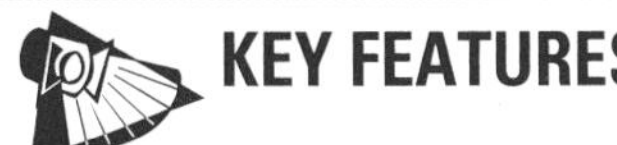

KEY FEATURES

ESSENTIALS OF DIAGNOSIS

- Pregnancy does not result after 6–12 months of normal sexual activity without contraceptives

GENERAL CONSIDERATIONS

- About 25% of couples experience infertility at some point
- The incidence increases with age
- The male partner contributes to about 40% of cases of infertility, and a combination of male and female factors is common

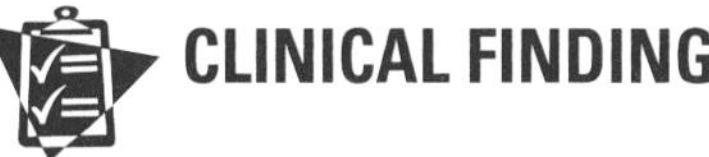

CLINICAL FINDINGS

SYMPTOMS AND SIGNS

- Obtain history of sexually transmitted disease or prior pregnancies
- Discuss ill effects of cigarettes, alcohol, and other drugs on male fertility
- Prescription drugs may impair male potency
- The gynecologic history should include the menstrual pattern
- The present history includes use and types of contraceptives, douches, libido, sex techniques, frequency and success of coitus, and correlation of intercourse with time of ovulation; the family history includes repeated abortions and maternal diethylstilbestrol use
- General physical and genital examinations for both partners

DIFFERENTIAL DIAGNOSIS

- Male factor (hypogonadism, varicocele, alcohol or drug use, immotile cilia syndrome)
- Polycystic ovary syndrome
- Premature ovarian failure
- Hyperprolactinemia
- Hypothyroidism
- Inadequate luteal progesterone or short luteal phase
- Endometriosis
- Uterine leiomyomas (fibroids) or polyps
- Prior pelvic inflammatory disease
- Pelvic adhesions, eg, pelvic surgery, therapeutic abortion, ectopic pregnancy, septic abortion, intrauterine device use

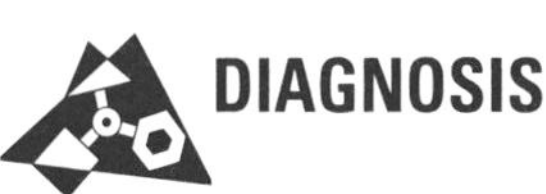

DIAGNOSIS

DIAGNOSTIC PROCEDURES

- Complete blood cell count, urinalysis, cervical culture for *Chlamydia*, serologic test for syphilis, rubella antibody determination, and thyroid function tests
- The woman should chart her oral basal body temperature daily on arising, record episodes of coitus and days of menstruation
- Self-performed urine tests for the midcycle luteinizing hormone (LH) surge can enhance temperature observations relating to ovulation. Coitus resulting in conception occurs during the 6-day period ending with the day of ovulation
- Before additional testing, an ejaculate for semen analysis is obtained after sexual abstinence for at least 3 days
- Semen should be examined within 1–2 h after collection. Normal semen: volume, 3 mL; concentration, 20 million sperm per milliliter; motility, 50% after 2 h; and normal forms, 60%. If the sperm count is abnormal, search for exposure to environmental and workplace toxins, alcohol or drug abuse, and hypogonadism

First testing cycle

- Perform a postcoital test just before ovulation (eg, Day 12 or 13 in an expected 28-day cycle). Preovulation timing can be enhanced by serial urinary LH tests
- Examine the patient within 6 h after coitus
  - The cervical mucus should be clear, elastic, and copious
  - A good spinnbarkeit (stretching to a fine thread 4 cm or more in length) is desirable
  - A small drop of cervical mucus should be obtained from within the cervical os and examined under the microscope
  - The presence of five or more active sperm per high-power field constitutes a satisfactory postcoital test
  - If no spermatozoa are found, the test should be repeated (assuming that active spermatozoa were present in the semen analysis)
  - Sperm agglutination and sperm immobilization tests should be considered if the sperm are immotile or show ineffective tail motility
- The presence of more than three white blood cells per high-power field in the postcoital test suggests cervicitis or prostatitis. When estrogen levels are normal, the cervical mucus dried on the slide will form a fern-like pattern when viewed with a low-power microscope
- Serum progesterone should be measured at the midpoint of the secretory phase (Day 21); a level of 10–20 ng/mL confirms adequate luteal function

Second testing cycle

- Hysterosalpingography is performed using oil dye within 3 days following the menstrual period
  - This x-ray study will demonstrate uterine abnormalities and tubal obstruction
  - A repeat x-ray film 24 h later will confirm tubal patency if there is wide pelvic dispersion of the dye
- If the woman has had prior pelvic inflammation, give doxycycline, 100 mg twice daily, beginning immediately before and for 7 days after the x-ray study

Further testing

- Gross deficiencies of sperm (number, motility, or appearance) require repeat analysis. Zona-free hamster egg penetration tests evaluate the ability of the human sperm to fertilize an egg

- Obvious obstruction of the uterine tubes requires assessment for microsurgery or in vitro fertilization
- Absent or infrequent ovulation requires additional laboratory evaluation. Elevated follicle-stimulating hormone (FSH) and LH levels indicate ovarian failure causing premature menopause. Elevated LH levels in the presence of normal FSH levels confirm the presence of polycystic ovaries. Elevation of blood prolactin (PRL) levels suggests pituitary microadenoma
- Major histocompatibility antigen typing of both partners will confirm HLA-B locus homozygosity, found in greater numbers among infertile couples
- Ultrasound monitoring of folliculogenesis may reveal unruptured luteinized follicles
- Endometrial biopsy in the luteal phase associated with simultaneous serum progesterone levels will rule out luteal phase deficiency

Laparoscopy

- Approximately 25% of women whose basic evaluation is normal will have findings on laparoscopy explaining their infertility (eg, peritubal adhesions)

TREATMENT

MEDICATIONS

- **Induction of ovulation**
  - Clomiphene citrate. After a normal menstrual period or induction of withdrawal bleeding with progestin, give 50 mg of clomiphene PO daily for 5 days. If ovulation does not occur, increase dosage to 100 mg PO daily for 5 days. If ovulation still does not occur, the course is repeated with 150 mg daily and then 200 mg daily for 5 days, with the addition of chorionic gonadotropin, 10,000 units IM, 7 days after clomiphene
  - In the presence of increased androgen production (DHEA-S > 200 μg/dL), the addition of dexamethasone, 0.5 mg PO, or prednisone, 5 mg PO, at bedtime, improves the response to clomiphene. Dexamethasone should be discontinued after pregnancy is confirmed
  - Bromocriptine is used only if PRL levels are elevated and there is no withdrawal bleeding following progesterone administration (otherwise, clomiphene is used). The initial dosage is 2.5 mg PO once daily, increased to two or three times daily in increments of 1.25 mg. The drug is discontinued once pregnancy has occurred
  - Human menopausal gonadotropins (hMG) or recombinant FSH is indicated in cases of hypogonadotropism and most other types of anovulation (exclusive of ovarian failure)
  - Gonadotropin-releasing hormone (GnRH)—hypothalamic amenorrhea unresponsive to clomiphene can be treated with subcutaneous pulsatile GnRH
  - See Endometriosis for treatment

SURGERY

- Fertility can be improved with excision of ovarian tumors or ovarian foci of endometriosis, and microsurgical relief of tubal obstruction due to salpingitis
- Some cornual or fimbrial block can be relieved. Peritubal adhesions or endometriotic implants often can be treated via laparoscopy or via laparotomy
- Sperm characteristics are often improved following surgical treatment of varicocele in the man

THERAPEUTIC PROCEDURES

- Treat hypothyroidism or hyperthyroidism. Give antibiotics for cervicitis if present. In women with abnormal postcoital tests and demonstrated antisperm antibodies causing sperm agglutination or immobilization, condom use for up to 6 months may result in lower antibody levels and improved pregnancy rates
- Women who engage in vigorous athletic training often have low sex hormone levels; fertility improves with reduced exercise and some weight gain
- Intrauterine insemination of concentrated washed sperm can bypass a poor cervical environment associated with scant or hostile cervical mucus
- For azoospermia, artificial insemination by a donor usually results in pregnancy if female function is normal

OUTCOME

PROGNOSIS

- The prognosis for normal pregnancy is good if minor disorders can be treated; it is poor if the causes of infertility are severe, untreatable, or of prolonged duration (over 3 years)
- In the absence of identifiable causes of infertility, 60% of couples will achieve a pregnancy within 3 years
- Couples with unexplained infertility who do not achieve pregnancy within 3 years should be offered ovulation induction, assisted reproductive technology, or information about adoption

WHEN TO REFER

- For induction of ovulation and procedures

EVIDENCE

PRACTICE GUIDELINES

- Brigham and Women's Hospital. Infertility. A guide to evaluation, treatment, and counseling. 2003
  - http://www.guideline.gov/summary/summary.aspx?doc_id=4742&nbr=3435
- Institute for Clinical Systems Improvement. Diagnosis and management of basic infertility. 2004
  - http://www.guideline.gov/summary/summary.aspx?doc_id=5567&nbr=3764

WEB SITE

- Centers for Disease Control and Prevention: Assisted Reproductive Technology Reports
  - http://www.cdc.gov/reproductivehealth/art.htm

INFORMATION FOR PATIENTS

- American Society for Reproductive Medicine: Patient Resources
  - http://www.asrm.org/Patients/mainpati.html
- Mayo Clinic: Infertility
  - http://www.mayoclinic.com/invoke.cfm?id=DS00310
- MedlinePlus: Infertility
  - http://www.nlm.nih.gov/medlineplus/ency/article/001191.htm
- National Infertility Association
  - http://www.resolve.org
- National Women's Health Information Center: Fertility Awareness and Infertility
  - http://www.4woman.gov/Pregnancy/infertility.htm

REFERENCE

- Rosene-Montella K et al: Evaluation and management of infertility in women: the internist's role. Ann Intern Med 2000;132:973. [PMID: 10858181]

Author(s)

H. Trent MacKay, MD, MPH

Infertility, Male

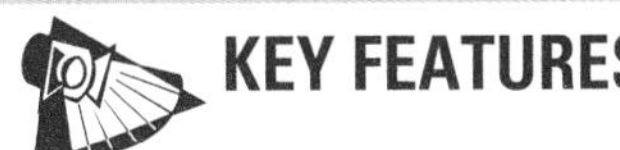

KEY FEATURES

GENERAL CONSIDERATIONS

- Primary infertility affects 15–20% of married couples: ~one-third of cases result from male factors, one-third from female factors, and one-third from combined factors
- Simultaneous evaluation of the female partner warranted (see Infertility, Female)
- Clinical evaluation is warranted following 6–12 months of unprotected intercourse

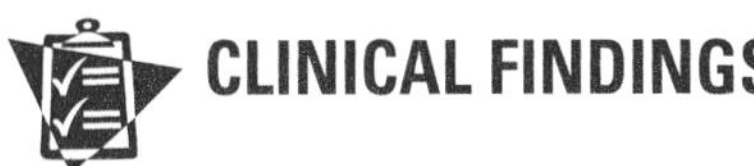

CLINICAL FINDINGS

SYMPTOMS AND SIGNS

- History
  - Prior testicular insults (torsion, cryptorchism, trauma)
  - Infections (mumps orchitis, epididymitis)
  - Environmental factors (excessive heat, radiation, chemotherapy)
  - Medications (anabolic steroids, cimetidine, and spironolactone may affect spermatogenesis; phenytoin may lower follicle-stimulating hormone [FSH]; sulfasalazine and nitrofurantoin affect sperm motility)
  - Drugs (alcohol, marijuana)
  - Sexual habits, frequency and timing of intercourse, use of lubricants, and each partner's previous fertility experiences are important
  - Loss of libido and headaches or visual disturbances
- Past medical or surgical history
  - Thyroid or liver disease (abnormalities of spermatogenesis)
  - Diabetic neuropathy (retrograde ejaculation)
  - Radical pelvic or retroperitoneal surgery (absent seminal emission secondary to sympathetic nerve injury)
  - Hernia repair (damage to the vas deferens or testicular blood supply)
- Physical examination: signs of hypogonadism, such as underdeveloped secondary sexual characteristics, diminished male pattern hair distribution (axillary, body, facial, pubic), eunuchoid skeletal proportions (arm span 2 inches > height; upper to lower body ratio < 1.0), and gynecomastia
- Evaluate testicular size (normal size ~4.5 × 2.5 cm, volume 18 mL)
- Examine for varicocele in the standing position, with Valsalva maneuver
- Palpate the vas deferens, epididymis, and prostate

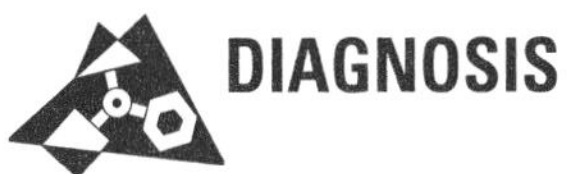

DIAGNOSIS

LABORATORY TESTS

- Semen analysis after 72 h of abstinence (see Infertility, Female)
- Endocrinological evaluation: serum FSH, luteinizing hormone (LH), and testosterone
- Elevated FSH and LH and low testosterone (hypergonadotropic hypogonadism) in primary testicular failure
- Low FSH and LH and low testosterone in secondary testicular failure (hypogonadotropic hypogonadism) of hypothalmic or pituitary origin—check serum prolactin

IMAGING STUDIES

- Scrotal ultrasound for varicocele
- Vasography for suspected ductal obstruction

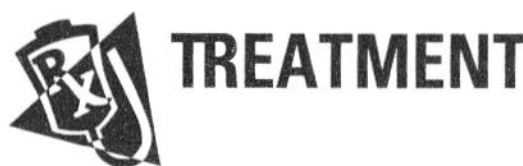

TREATMENT

MEDICATIONS

- Genitourinary tract infections should be treated with antibiotics

Endocrine therapy

- Hypogonadotropic hypogonadism
  - Chorionic gonadotropin, 2000 IU IM 3 times weekly, once primary pituitary disease has been excluded or treated
  - If sperm counts fail to rise after 12 months, FSH/LH therapy should be initiated
- Menotropins (Pergonal), 75 IU of FSH and 75 IU of LH, 0.5–1 vial IM 3 times weekly

Retrograde ejaculation therapy

- α-Adrenergic agonists (eg, pseudoephedrine, 60 mg PO TID) or imipramine, 25 mg PO TID
- Collect postmasturbation urine for intrauterine insemination
- Electroejaculation in cases of absent emission

SURGERY

- Varicocele: surgical repair by scrotal, inguinal, laparoscopic, or percutaneous venographic approaches
- Ductal obstruction: operative treatment for mechanical obstruction of the ejaculatory duct is transurethral resection and unroofing of the ducts in the prostatic urethra
- For obstruction of the vas deferens, microsurgical vasovasostomy or vasoepididymostomy

THERAPEUTIC PROCEDURES

- Education
- Proper timing for intercourse
- Avoidance of spermicidal lubricants
- Removal of toxins or medications

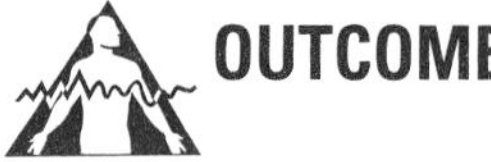

OUTCOME

WHEN TO REFER

- Assisted reproductive techniques: intrauterine insemination, in vitro fertilization, and gamete intrafallopian transfer

EVIDENCE

PRACTICE GUIDELINES

- Gangel EK: American Urological Association, Inc and American Society for Reproductive Medicine. AUA and ASRM produce recommendations for male infertility. Am Fam Physician 2002;65:2589. [PMID: 12086246]
- Jarow JP et al; Male Infertility Best Practice Policy Committee of the American Urological Association Inc. Best practice policies for male infertility. J Urol 2002;167:2138. [PMID: 11956464]
- Weidner W et al: EAU guidelines on male infertility. Eur Urol 2002;42:313. [PMID: 12361894]

INFORMATION FOR PATIENTS

- American Academy of Family Physicians
  - http://familydoctor.org/766.xml
- Mayo Clinic
  - http://www.mayoclinic.com/invoke.cfm?objectid=C9EBA8CE-D250-4AF0-B86F72A71D3DAB34

REFERENCES

- Boyle KE et al: Assisted reproductive technology in the new millennium: part I. Urology 2004;63:2. [PMID: 14751335]
- Brugh VM 3rd et al: Male factor infertility: evaluation and management. Med Clin North Am 2004;88:367. [PMID: 15049583]
- Vogt PH: Molecular genetics of human male infertility: from genes to new therapeutic perspectives. Curr Pharm Des 2004;10:471. [PMID: 14965334]

Author(s)

Marshall L. Stoller, MD
Peter R. Carroll, MD

Influenza

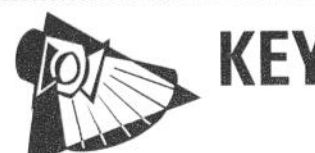

KEY FEATURES

ESSENTIALS OF DIAGNOSIS

- Abrupt onset of fevers, chills, malaise, cough, arthralgias, and myalgias
- Although sporadic cases do occur, most cases of influenza occur as part of epidemics or pandemics, usually in the fall or winter seasons

GENERAL CONSIDERATIONS

- An orthomyxovirus transmitted by respiratory droplets
- Three antigenic subtypes have been described: types A and B produce identical clinical symptoms, type C produces milder disease
- Pandemics usually due to type A infections with significant antigenic shift (large genetic recombination of the virus)
- Influenza is difficult to diagnose in the absence of the epidemic because it resembles other viral illnesses

DEMOGRAPHICS

- 5000–250,000 cases annually in the United States
- Incidence highest in school-age children and young adults, students, prisoners, day care and health care workers; asthmatics are at particular risk
- Complications occur most often in elderly, immunocompromised individuals

CLINICAL FINDINGS

SYMPTOMS AND SIGNS

- Abrupt onset
- Fevers, chills, malaise with myalgias and headaches are common
- Nasal congestion, substernal tenderness, and nausea are not uncommon
- Fever typically lasts 3–5 days (range 1 to 7 days)
- Sore throat, cervical lymphadenopathy, and nonproductive cough are usually present
- Leukopenia is common
- Leukocytosis may be a marker of secondary complications
- Proteinuria occasionally

DIFFERENTIAL DIAGNOSIS

- Common cold
- Primary bacterial pneumonia
- Infectious mononucleosis
- *Mycoplasma* infection
- Early Legionnaire's
- *Chlamydial pneumoniae* infection (TWAR)
- Acute HIV infection
- Meningitis
- In returning tropical traveler: malaria, dengue, typhoid

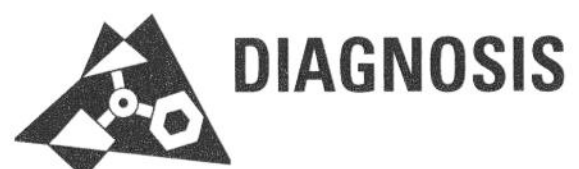

DIAGNOSIS

LABORATORY TESTS

- Influenza virus can be isolated from throat or nasal washings sent for tissue culture
- Direct fluorescent antibody staining of washings can also make the diagnosis, though it cannot identify subtypes

DIAGNOSTIC PROCEDURES

- Usually diagnosed clinically when characteristic symptoms are found in the setting of an epidemic

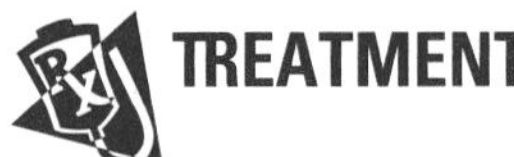

TREATMENT

MEDICATIONS

- When diagnosed early, amantadine or rimantadine can decrease the duration of symptoms and signs of influenza A but is ineffective during epidemics of influenza B
- Amantadine dose reduction is required in the elderly in whom CNS dysfunction develops
- Zanamivir (inhaled) or oseltamivir (oral) is also effective at reducing the duration and severity of symptoms of influenza A and B, but are costly and must be started within 48 h of onset of symptoms to be effective. Zanamivir may cause bronchospasm in asthmatics

THERAPEUTIC PROCEDURES

- Supportive measures with adequate hydration, analgesics, and rest

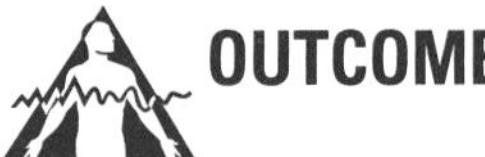

OUTCOME

COMPLICATIONS

- Influenza predisposes individuals to secondary bacterial infections of the respiratory tract, especially with pneumococcus and *Staphylococcus aureus*
- Pneumonia and purulent bronchitis are frequent complications
- Reye's syndrome, a severe form of hepatic failure, occurs rarely, particularly in young children given salicylates during influenza B or varicella infections

PROGNOSIS

- Most patients recover fully back to baseline health within 4–7 days
- Secondary complications can lengthen the course of illness and worsen the chances of a full recovery
- Poor outcomes usually occur in the elderly, often due to dehydration, exacerbations of comorbid conditions, or secondary complications

WHEN TO REFER

- Refer when signs of secondary complications occur

WHEN TO ADMIT

- Consider hospitalization for signs of significant secondary complications such as pneumonia or acute exacerbations of chronic bronchitis

PREVENTION

- Trivalent influenza vaccine is highly effective (85%) most years
- Vaccination is recommended for persons who are older than 50 years or who have heart, lung, or other chronic diseases
- Vaccine should be avoided in patients with known hypersensitivity to eggs or its components
- Vaccine is not contraindicated in patients on warfarin or corticosteroids, or in those with HIV infection
- The neuraminidase inhibitors (zanamivir or oseltamivir) can be used prophylactically for both influenza A and B
- Amantadine or rimantadine reduces the attack rate for influenza A

EVIDENCE

PRACTICE GUIDELINES

- National Guideline Clearinghouse
  - Prevention and control of influenza: recommendations of the Advisory Committee on Immunization Practices (ACIP)
  - Interim influenza vaccination recommendations—2004–05 influenza season
  - Influenza antiviral medications: 2004-05 interim chemoprophylaxis and treatment guidelines
  - http://www.guideline.gov/summary/summary.aspx?doc_id=5961

WEB SITE

- Centers for Disease Control and Prevention
  - http://www.cdc.gov/flu/

INFORMATION FOR PATIENTS

- Centers for Disease Control and Prevention Fact Sheet
  - http://www.cdc.gov/flu/keyfacts.htm
- Torpy JM et al: JAMA patient page. Influenza. JAMA 2004;292:2182. [PMID: 15523077]

REFERENCES

- Bridges CB et al: Prevention and control of influenza. Recommendations of the Advisory Committee on Immunization Practices (ACIP). MMWR Recomm Rep 2001;50(RR-4):1. [PMID: 11334444]
- Couch RB: Influenza: prospects for control. Ann Intern Med 2000;133:992. [PMID: 11119401]
- Jefferson TO et al: Amantadine and rimantadine for preventing and treating influenza A in adults. Cochrane Database Syst Rev 2002;3:CD001169. [PMID: 12137620]
- Monto AS et al: Zanamivir prophylaxis: an effective strategy for the prevention of influenza types A and B within households. J Infect Dis 2002;186:1582. [PMID: 12447733]

Author(s)

Wayne X. Shandera, MD

Ana Moran, MD

Insomnia

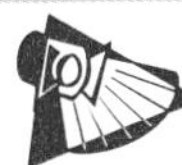

KEY FEATURES

ESSENTIALS OF DIAGNOSIS

- Transient episodes are usually of little significance
- Common factors
  - Stress
  - Caffeine
  - Physical discomfort
  - Daytime napping
  - Early bedtime
- Psychiatric disorders are often associated with persistent insomnia

GENERAL CONSIDERATIONS

- **Sleep** consists of two distinct states
  - REM (rapid eye movement) sleep, also called dream sleep, D state sleep, paradoxic sleep
  - NREM (non-REM) sleep, also called S stage sleep, which is divided into stages 1, 2, 3, and 4 recognizable by different electroencephalographic patterns. Stages 3 and 4 are "delta" sleep
  - **Dreaming** occurs mostly in REM and to a lesser extent in NREM sleep
  - Sleep is a cyclic phenomenon, with four or five REM periods during the night accounting for about one-fourth of the total night's sleep (1 1/2 –2 hours)
  - The first REM period occurs about 80–120 minutes after onset of sleep and lasts about 10 minutes
  - Later REM periods are longer (15–40 minutes) and occur mostly in the last several hours of sleep. Most stage 4 (deepest) sleep occurs in the first several hours
- **Age-related changes** in normal sleep include
  - An unchanging percentage of REM sleep
  - A marked decrease in stage 3 and stage 4 sleep
  - An increase in wakeful periods during the night
  - These normal changes, early bedtimes, and daytime naps play a role in the increased complaints of insomnia in older people
  - Variations in sleep patterns may be due to circumstances (eg, "jet lag") or to idiosyncratic patterns ("night owls") in persons who perhaps because of different "biological rhythms" habitually go to bed late and sleep late in the morning
  - Creativity and rapidity of response to unfamiliar situations are impaired by loss of sleep
  - There are rare individuals who have chronic difficulty in adapting to a 24-hour sleep-wake cycle (desynchronization sleep disorder), which can be resynchronized by altering exposure to light
- **Depression** is usually associated with
  - Fragmented sleep
  - Decreased total sleep time
  - Earlier onset of REM sleep
  - A shift of REM activity to the first half of the night
  - Loss of slow-wave sleep
- **Manic disorders**
  - Sleeplessness is a cardinal feature and an important early sign of impending mania in bipolar cases
  - Total sleep time is decreased
  - Shortened REM latency and increased REM activity
- Sleep-related panic attacks occur in the transition from stage 2 to stage 3 sleep in some patients with a longer REM latency in the sleep pattern preceding the attacks
- **Abuse of alcohol**
  - May cause or be secondary to the sleep disturbance
  - There is a tendency to use alcohol as a means of getting to sleep without realizing that it disrupts the normal sleep cycle
  - *Acute alcohol intake*
    - Produces a decreased sleep latency with reduced REM sleep during the first half of the night
    - REM sleep is increased in the second half of the night, with an increase in total amount of slow-wave sleep (stages 3 and 4)
    - Vivid dreams and frequent awakenings are common
  - *Chronic alcohol abuse*
    - Increases stage 1 and decreases REM sleep (most drugs delay or block REM sleep)
    - Symptoms persist for many months after the person has stopped drinking
  - *Acute alcohol or other sedative withdrawal*
    - Delayed onset of sleep and REM rebound
    - Intermittent awakening during the night
- **Heavy smoking** (more than a pack a day) causes difficulty falling asleep—apparently independently of the often associated increase in coffee drinking
- Excess intake of stimulants near bedtime of caffeine, cocaine, and other stimulants (eg, over-the-counter cold remedies) causes decreased total sleep time—mostly NREM sleep—with some increased sleep latency
- **Sedative-hypnotics**—specifically, the benzodiazepines, which are the prescription drugs of choice to promote sleep—tend to
  - Increase total sleep time
  - Decrease sleep latency
  - Decrease nocturnal awakening
  - Have variable effects on NREM sleep
  - Withdrawal of benzodiazepines causes just the opposite effects and results in continued use of the drug for the purpose of preventing withdrawal symptoms
- Antidepressants decrease REM sleep (with marked rebound on withdrawal in the form of nightmares) and have varying effects on NREM sleep
- REM sleep deprivation produces improvement in some depressions
- Persistent insomnias are also related to a wide variety of medical conditions, particularly delirium, pain, respiratory distress syndromes, uremia, asthma, and thyroid disorders
- Adequate analgesia and proper treatment of medical disorders reduce symptoms and decrease the need for sedatives

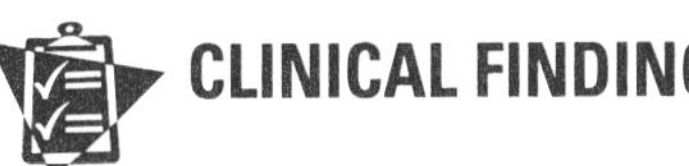

CLINICAL FINDINGS

SYMPTOMS AND SIGNS

- Difficulty getting to sleep or staying asleep
- Intermittent wakefulness during the night
- Early morning awakening
- Combinations of any of the latter

DIFFERENTIAL DIAGNOSIS

- Emotional stress, physical discomfort, jet lag
- Alcohol abuse
- Stimulants, eg, caffeine, nicotine, cocaine, pseudoephedrine
- Depression
- Poor sleep hygiene, eg, daytime naps, TV in bed
- Mania or bipolar disorder
- Medical illness, eg, chronic obstructive pulmonary disease, uremia, hyperthyroidism, hepatic encephalopathy, gastroesophageal reflux disease
- Nocturia, eg, diuretics, benign prostatic hyperplasia, incontinence, chronic heart failure
- Restless legs syndrome
- CNS disease, eg, complex partial seizures, tumor, neurosyphilis
- Medications, eg, corticosteroids, selective serotonin reuptake inhibitors, theophylline, benzodiazepine withdrawal
- Circadian rhythm disorder

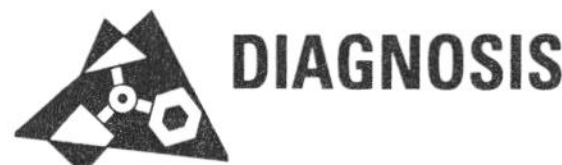

DIAGNOSIS

LABORATORY TESTS

- Consider thyroid-stimulating hormone

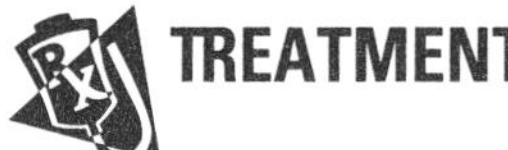

TREATMENT

MEDICATIONS

- There are two broad classes of treatment for insomnia, and the two may be combined
  - Psychological (cognitive-behavioral)
  - Pharmacologic
- Pharmacologic
  - In situations of acute distress, such as a grief reaction, pharmacologic measures may be most appropriate
  - These drugs are often effective for the elderly population and can be given in larger doses—twice what is prescribed for the elderly—in younger patients
    - Lorazepam 0.5 mg PO HS
    - Temazepam 7.5–15 mg PO HS
    - Zolpidem 5–10 mg PO HS
    - Zaleplon 5–10 mg PO HS
  - Longer-acting agents such as flurazepam (half-life of >48 h) may accumulate in the elderly and lead to cognitive slowing, ataxia, falls, and somnolence
  - In general, it is appropriate to use medications for short courses of 1–2 weeks
  - Antihistamines such as diphenhydramine 25 mg PO HS or hydroxyzine 25 mg PO HS may be useful
    - Their anticholinergic effects may produce confusion or urinary symptoms in the elderly
  - Trazodone 25–150 mg PO HS is a non–habit-forming effective sleep medication in lower than antidepressant doses
    - Priapism is a rare side effect requiring emergent treatment
  - Triazolam is popular because of its very short duration of action
    - Because it has been associated with dependency, transient psychotic reactions, anterograde amnesia, and rebound anxiety, triazolam has been removed from the market in several European countries
    - If used, it must be prescribed only for short periods of time

THERAPEUTIC PROCEDURES

- With primary insomnia initial efforts should be psychologically based, particularly in the elderly
- Psychological
  - Educate the patient regarding good sleep hygiene
    - Go to bed only when sleepy
    - Use the bed and bedroom only for sleeping and sex
    - If still awake after 20 minutes, leave the bedroom and return only when sleepy
    - Get up at the same time every morning, regardless of the amount of sleep during the night
    - Discontinue caffeine and nicotine, at least in the evening if not completely
    - Establish a daily exercise regimen
    - Avoid alcohol because it may disrupt continuity of sleep
    - Limit fluids in the evening
    - Learn and practice relaxation techniques
  - Cognitive behavioral therapy for insomnia may be efficacious
  - The clinician should also discuss any myths or misconceptions about sleep that the patient may hold

OUTCOME

PREVENTION

- Discontinue use of caffeine and nicotine
- Avoid alcohol
- Engage in regular exercise program

EVIDENCE

PRACTICE GUIDELINES

- National Guideline Clearinghouse: American Academy of Sleep Medicine, 2000
  - http://www.guideline.gov/summary/summary.aspx?doc_id=2276

WEB SITE

- National Institutes of Health—National Heart, Lung, and Blood Institute
  - http://www.nhlbi.nih.gov/health/prof/sleep/insom_pc.htm
- National Sleep Foundation
  - http://www.sleepfoundation.org

INFORMATION FOR PATIENTS

- American Academy of Family Physicians
  - http://familydoctor.org/healthfacts/110/
- JAMA patient page: Insomnia. JAMA 2003;289:2602. [PMID:12759329]
- National Inststutes of Health—National Heart, Lung, and Blood Institute
  - http://www.nhlbi.nih.gov/health/public/sleep/insomnia.pdf

REFERENCES

- Jacobs G et al: Cognitive behavioral therapy and pharmacotherapy for insomnia: a randomized controlled trial and direct comparison. Arch Intern Med 2004;164:1888. [PMID:15451764]
- Jindal RD, Thase ME: Treatment of insomnia associated with clinical depression. Sleep Med Rev 2004;8:19. [PMID:15062208]
- Simon GE et al: Prevalence, burden and treatment of insomnia in primary care. Am J Psychiatry 1997;154:1417. [PMID:9326825]

Author(s)

Stuart J. Eisendrath, MD

Jonathan E. Lichtmacher, MD

Insulinoma

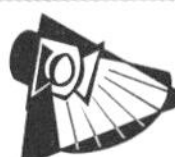

KEY FEATURES

ESSENTIALS OF DIAGNOSIS

- Fasting hypoglycemia rather than postprandial hypoglycemia
- Blood glucose < 40 mg/dL in an otherwise healthy-appearing person with central nervous dysfunction such as confusion or abnormal behavior
- Hypoglycemic unawareness is common

GENERAL CONSIDERATIONS

- Insulinoma is generally an adenoma of the islets of Langerhans
- Adenomas can be familial
- 90% of tumors are single and benign
- Multiple benign adenomas can occur as can malignant tumors with functional metastases
- Multiple adenomas can occur with tumors of parathyroids and pituitary [multiple endocrine neoplasia type 1 (MEN-1)]
- Rarely, B-cell hyperplasia can be a cause of fasting hypoglycemia
- Patients adapt to chronic hypoglycemia by increasing their efficiency in transporting glucose across the blood–brain barrier, which masks awareness that their blood glucose is approaching critically low levels
- Counterregulatory hormonal responses as well as neurogenic symptoms such as tremor, sweating, and palpitations are blunted during hypoglycemia

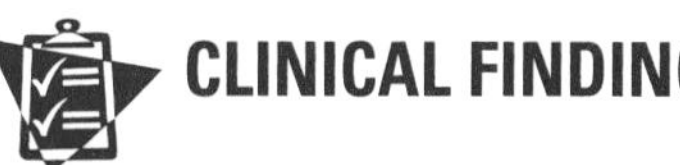

CLINICAL FINDINGS

SYMPTOMS AND SIGNS

- Whipple's triad is characteristic of hypoglycemia regardless of the cause: a history of hypoglycemic symptoms, an associated fasting blood glucose of ≤ 40 mg/dL, and immediate recovery on administration of glucose
- Symptoms often develop in the early morning, after missing a meal, or occasionally after exercise
- Initial CNS symptoms include blurred vision or diplopia, headache, feelings of detachment, slurred speech, and weakness
- Convulsions or coma may occur
- Personality changes vary from anxiety to psychotic behavior
- Hypoglycemic unawareness is very common

DIFFERENTIAL DIAGNOSIS

- Hyperinsulinism from surreptitious insulin or sulfonylureas
- Extrapancreatic tumors
- Postprandial hypoglycemia: early hypoglycemia (alimentary)
- Postgastrectomy
- Functional (increased vagal tone): late hypoglycemia (occult diabetes)
- Delayed insulin release resulting from B-cell dysfunction
  - Counterregulatory deficiency
  - Idiopathic
- Alcohol-related hypoglycemia
- Immunopathological hypoglycemia: antibodies to insulin receptors, which act as agonists
- Pentamidine-induced hypoglycemia

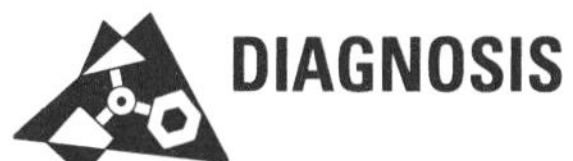

DIAGNOSIS

LABORATORY TESTS

- Serum insulin level ≥ 6 μU/mL in a radioimmunoassay (3 μU/mL ICMA) in the presence of blood glucose values < 40 mg/dL is diagnostic of inappropriate hyperinsulinism
- An elevated circulating proinsulin level (> 5 pmol/L) in the presence of fasting hypoglycemia is characteristic of most B-cell adenomas and does not occur in factitious hyperinsulinism
- In patients with epigastric distress, history of renal stones, or menstrual or erectile dysfunction, serum calcium, gastrin, or prolactin level may be useful in screening for MEN-1 associated with insulinoma
- Prolonged fasting up to 72 h under hospital supervision until hypoglycemia is documented
- In normal males, the blood glucose does not fall below 55–60 mg/dL during a 3-day fast
- In normal premenopausal women who have fasted for only 24 h, the plasma glucose may fall to as low as 35 mg/dL; these women are not symptomatic owing to the development of sufficient ketonemia to supply energy needs to the brain
- Insulinoma patients become symptomatic when plasma glucose drops to subnormal levels, because inappropriate insulin secretion restricts ketone formation

IMAGING STUDIES

- Radiographic and arteriographic techniques are seldom helpful in localizing insulinomas preoperatively owing to the small size of these tumors
- Intraoperative ultrasonography and palpation is the tumor localization method of choice
- CT scan or MRI can screen for hepatic metastases
- If insulinoma is not found at initial surgery: correlation of imaging from selective arteriography of segments of the pancreas with simultaneous hepatic vein sampling for insulin during a bolus of intraarterial calcium delivered selectively to these same pancreatic segments

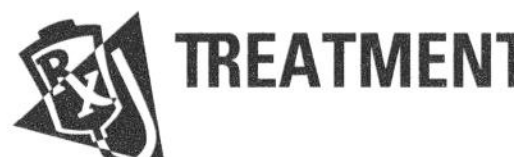

TREATMENT

MEDICATIONS

- Glucagon for hypoglycemic emergencies, but its benefit may be less than for diabetic hypoglycemia because of the concomitant insulin release from the tumor
- Diazoxide, 300–600 mg PO QD, along with thiazide to control sodium retention
- Verapamil may inhibit insulin release from insulinoma cells; use if intolerant to diazoxide
- Octreotide, 50 mg SC BID, is a synthetic analog of somatostatin; use when surgery fails to remove the source of hyperinsulinism
- Streptozocin can decrease insulin secretion in islet cell carcinomas; effective doses can be delivered via selective arterial catheter to decrease renal toxicity

SURGERY

- Laparoscopy using ultrasonography and denucleation can be successful with a single tumor of the body or tail of the pancreas, but open surgery is necessary for tumors in the head of the pancreas

THERAPEUTIC PROCEDURES

- In islet cell carcinoma and in 5–10% of MEN-1 cases when surgical resection has not been curative, frequent feedings are necessary. Because most tumors are not responsive to glucose, carbohydrate feedings every 2–3 h are usually effective in preventing hypoglycemia

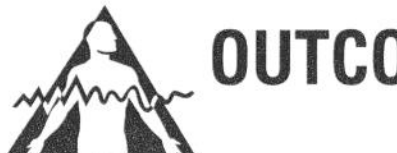

OUTCOME

COMPLICATIONS

- Irreversible brain damage from hypoglycemia
- Obesity may become a problem from frequent feeding
- Gastrointestinal upset, hirsutism, or edema from diazoxide

PROGNOSIS

- 90–95% cure at first surgical attempt for single benign adenoma when performed by a skilled surgeon
- Severe brain damage from severe prolonged hypoglycemia is irreversible
- Significant increase in survival in streptozocin-treated patients with islet cell carcinoma, with reduction in tumor mass and decrease in hyperinsulinism

WHEN TO REFER

- Refer to endocrinologist to perform inpatient 72-h fast
- Refer to skilled surgeon for resection

WHEN TO ADMIT

- For 72-h fast

EVIDENCE

INFORMATION FOR PATIENTS

- Mayo Clinic: Hyperinsulinemia
  - http://www.mayoclinic.com/invoke.cfm?id=HQ00896
- Medline Medical Encyclopedia: Insulinoma
  - http://www.nlm.nih.gov/medlineplus/ency/article/000387.htm

REFERENCES

- Boukhman MP et al: Localization of insulinomas. Arch Surg 1999;134:818. [PMID: 10443803]
- Grant CS: Surgical aspects of hyperinsulinemic hypoglycemia. Endocrinol Metab Clin North Am 1999;28:533. [PMID: 10500930]
- Hirshberg B et al: Forty-eight-hour fast: the diagnostic test for insulinoma. J Clin Endocrinol Metab 2000;85:3222. [PMID: 10999812]

Author(s)

Umesh Masharani, MB, BS, MRCP (UK)

Irritable Bowel Syndrome

Interstitial Lung Disease, Respiratory Bronchiolitis-Associated p. 1097. Intertrigo p. 1097. Iron Poisoning p. 1097.

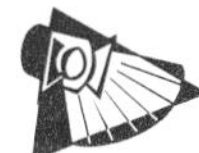

KEY FEATURES

ESSENTIALS OF DIAGNOSIS

- Common chronic functional disorder characterized by abdominal pain or discomfort with alterations in bowel habits
- Limited evaluation to exclude organic causes of symptoms

GENERAL CONSIDERATIONS

- No definitive diagnostic study
- Idiopathic clinical entity characterized by some combination of chronic (>3 months) lower abdominal symptoms and bowel complaints that may be continuous or intermittent
- Abdominal discomfort or pain that has two of the following three features: relieved with defecation; onset associated with a change in frequency of stool; onset associated with a change in form (appearance) of stool
- Other symptoms include abnormal stool frequency (more than three bowel movements per day or fewer than three per week); abnormal stool form (lumpy or hard; loose or watery); abnormal stool passage (straining, urgency, or feeling of incomplete evacuation); passage of mucus; and bloating or abdominal distention
- Other somatic or psychological complaints are common

DEMOGRAPHICS

- Affects up to 20% of the adult population
- Symptoms usually begin in late teens to early 20s

CLINICAL FINDINGS

SYMPTOMS AND SIGNS

- Symptoms for >3 months
- Subjective abdominal distention; visible distention not clinically evident
- Abdominal pain, intermittent, crampy, in the lower abdomen, relieved by defecation, worsened by stress, worse for 1–2 h after meals
- More frequent or less frequent stools with the onset of abdominal pain
- Looser stools or harder stools with the onset of pain
- Constipation, diarrhea, or alternating constipation and diarrhea
- Mucus is common
- Physical examination usually is normal
- Abdominal tenderness in the lower abdomen is common, but not pronounced; physical examination is otherwise normal

DIFFERENTIAL DIAGNOSIS

- Inflammatory bowel disease
- Colonic neoplasia
- Celiac disease, bacterial overgrowth, lactase deficiency, and endometriosis
- Depression and anxiety
- Sexual and physical abuse

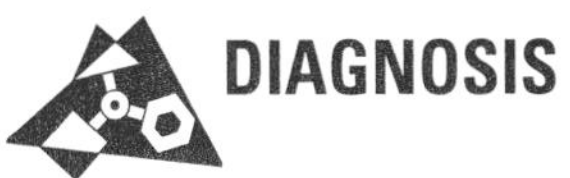

DIAGNOSIS

LABORATORY TESTS

- Obtain complete blood cell count, erythrocyte sedimentation rate, serum albumin, and thyroid-stimulating hormone
- Stool occult blood test
- Stool examination for ova and parasites if diarrhea

IMAGING STUDIES

- Barium enema or colonoscopy for patients aged >40–50 years

DIAGNOSTIC PROCEDURES

- Diagnosis is established with compatible symptoms and exclusion of organic disease
- Consider flexible sigmoidoscopy for patients aged <40 years
- Colonoscopy for patients aged >40–50 years

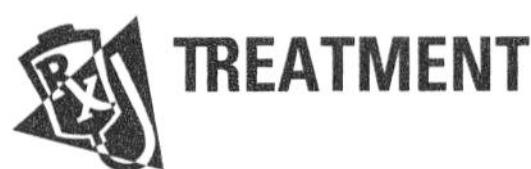

TREATMENT

MEDICATIONS

- Antispasmodic (anticholinergic) agents: dicyclomine, 10–20 mg PO TID–QID; hyoscyamine, 0.125 mg PO (or SL PRN), or sustained-release 0.037 mg or 0.75 mg PO BID
- Antidiarrheal agents: loperamide, 2 mg PO TID–QID, and diphenoxylate with atropine, 2.5 mg PO QID
- Fiber supplementation: bran, psyllium, methylcellulose, or polycarbophil
- Osmotic laxatives: milk of magnesia or polyethylene glycol
- Tricyclic antidepressants: nortriptyline, desipramine, imipramine, or trazodone; begin at 10 mg QHS; increase gradually to 25–50 mg as tolerated
- Serotonin reuptake inhibitors: sertraline, 50–150 mg PO QD, or fluoxetine, 20–40 mg PO QD
- Tegaserod, 6 mg PO BID, for constipation—predominant symptoms unresponsive to conservative measures
- Alosetran, 1 mg PO BID, for diarrhea—predominant symptoms unresponsive to other conventional therapies; may cause ischemic colitis in 4:1000 patients

THERAPEUTIC PROCEDURES

- Reassure patient
- Explain functional nature of the symptoms
- Exclude lactose intolerance by a breath hydrogen test or a trial of a lactose-free diet
- High-fiber (20–30 g/day) diet
- Behavioral modification with relaxation techniques, hypnotherapy

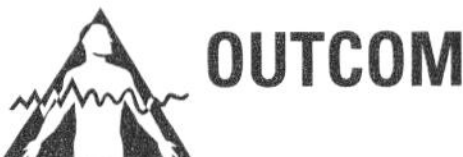

OUTCOME

FOLLOW-UP

- Regular visits helpful in reducing patient anxiety and overuse of the health care system

PROGNOSIS

- Symptoms usually chronic, but episodic; majority of affected patients learn to cope with their symptoms

WHEN TO REFER

- Persistent or worsening symptoms
- Signs of organic disease (blood per rectum, positive fecal occult blood, weight loss, severe pain)
- Signs of serious psychiatric disease or physical/sexual abuse

WHEN TO ADMIT

- Patients with irritable bowel syndrome have increased rate of hospitalizations and inappropriate abdominal surgeries for abdominal pain
- ER physicians and surgeons should avoid unnecessary hospitalizations and surgeries

EVIDENCE

PRACTICE GUIDELINES

- American College of Gastroenterology Functional Gastrointestinal Disorders Task Force: Evidence-based position statement on the management of irritable bowel syndrome in North America. Am J Gastroenterol 2002;97(11 Suppl):S1. [PMID: 12425585]
- American Gastroenterological Association medical position statement: irritable bowel syndrome. Gastroenteology 2002;123:2105. [PMID: 12454865]

WEB SITES

- American Academy of Family Physicians—Irritable bowel syndrome: tips on controlling your symptoms
  - http://familydoctor.org/healthfacts/112/
- Functional Brain-Gut Research Group
  - http://www.fbgweb.org
- International Foundation for Functional Gastrointestinal Disorders
  - http://www.iffgd/org

INFORMATION FOR PATIENTS

- American Gastroenterological Association Patient Resource Services: Irritable bowel syndrome
  - http://www.gastro.org/generalpublic.html
- International Foundation for Functional Gastrointestinal Disorders (IFFGD): About Irritable Bowel Syndrome
  - http://www.aboutibs.org/
- National Digestive Diseases Information Clearinghouse—What I Need to Know about Irritable Bowel Syndrome
  - http://digestive.niddk.nih.gov/ddiseases/pubs/ibs_ez/index.htm

REFERENCES

- Chey WD et al: Long-term safety and efficacy of alosetron in women with severe diarrhea-predominant irritable bowel syndrome. Am J Gastroenterol 2004;99:2195 [PMID: 1555502]
- Drossman DA: AGA technical review on irritable bowel syndrome. Gastroenterology 2002;123:2108. [PMID: 12454866]
- Mertz H: Irritable bowel syndrome. N Engl J Med 2003;349:22. [PMID: 14645642]
- Talley NJ: Pharmacologic therapy for irritable bowel syndrome. Am J Gastroenterol 2003;98:750. [PMID: 12738451]

Author(s)

Kenneth R. McQuaid, MD

Ischemia, Limb, Acute

KEY FEATURES

ESSENTIALS OF DIAGNOSIS

- Causes: arterial emboli, thrombosis, or trauma
- Bruit, abnormal contralateral pulse examination, or history of secondary skin changes or intermittent claudication suggests primary arterial thrombosis
- Valvular heart disease, atrial fibrillation, or myocardial infarction suggests embolism

GENERAL CONSIDERATIONS

Arterial embolism

- 80–90% arise from the heart
- Atrial fibrillation is present in 60–70%, rheumatic heart disease in < 20%
- Arterial emboli are associated with formation of thrombus in the left atrial appendage or within a postinfarct ventricular aneurysm
- Other cardiac causes: cardiac valvular prostheses and cardiac tumors (myxomas)
- Noncardiac causes: atherosclerotic lesions in proximal vessels, tumors, foreign bodies, and paradoxical emboli deriving from deep venous thrombosis in the leg
- Of emboli, 50% lodge in aortic bifurcation or the infrainguinal vessels, 30% in cerebrovascular vessels, 10% in visceral vessels, and 10% in upper extremity vessels
- Noncardiac emboli are usually small, giving rise to peripheral ulceration and digital ischemia or occasionally to a systemic illness resembling vasculitis
- Atheroemboli can also produce transient ischemic attacks, acute renal insufficiency, or bowel ischemia

Acute arterial thrombosis

- Most commonly a complication of chronic atherosclerotic occlusive disease, peripheral aneurysm, trauma, low-flow states such as hypovolemic or cardiogenic shock, or an inflammatory arteritis
- Other potential risk factors include polycythemia, dehydration, and hypercoagulable states
- Must be excluded with any knee or elbow dislocation

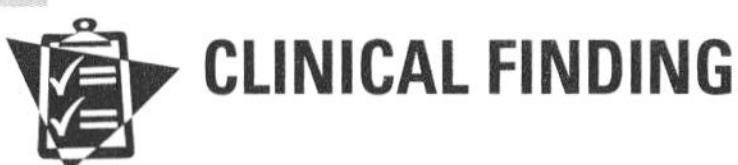

CLINICAL FINDINGS

SYMPTOMS AND SIGNS

- Symptoms and signs are related to the location of the occlusion, duration of ischemia, and degree of development of collateral circulation
- Six Ps: pain, pallor, pulselessness, paresthesias, poikilothermia, and paralysis

DIFFERENTIAL DIAGNOSIS

- Musculoskeletal injury
- Shock states
- Radiculopathy

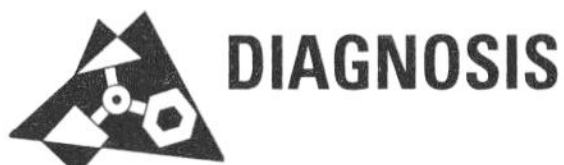

DIAGNOSIS

LABORATORY TESTS

- Microhematuria
- Eosinophilia
- Elevated sedimentation rate
- With atheroemboli, biopsy of the infarcted tissue reveals cholesterol clefts in the small vessels under polarized light

IMAGING STUDIES

- Surface or transesophageal echocardiography to evaluate for atrial thrombus, valvular disease, patent foramen ovale, or cardiac tumor

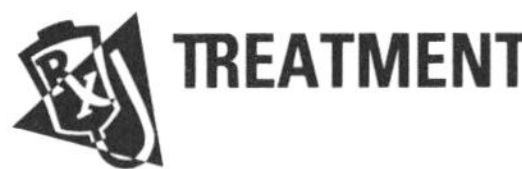

TREATMENT

MEDICATIONS

Arterial embolism

- Heparin given immediately and continued intraoperatively

Arterial thrombosis

- Catheter-directed thrombolysis (eg, instillation of alteplase, 0.5–1 mg/h), successful in 50–80% of cases, limb salvage rate 90%

SURGERY

- Treatment may include thromboendartерectomy, bypass, catheter-guided TPA thrombolysis, or a combination of these

Arterial embolism

- Acute emboli should be surgically treated
- Emergent embolectomy by balloon catheter through a small arteriotomy
- Percutaneous catheter techniques (aspiration, mechanical thrombolysis, or thrombolytic therapy)

Arterial thrombosis

- Surgical thromboendarterectomy or bypass

Arterial trauma

- Arterial thrombosis after penetrating trauma or blunt trauma requires surgical treatment

THERAPEUTIC PROCEDURES

- Acute thrombosis should be treated acutely if it causes limb-threatening symptoms and signs: rest pain, nerve or muscle dysfunction

OUTCOME

FOLLOW-UP

- Routine pulse examinations
- Ankle-brachial index

COMPLICATIONS

- Development of a compartment syndrome
- Myoglobinuria and renal failure from rhabdomyolysis
- Ischemic neuropathy

PROGNOSIS

Arterial embolism

- 5–25% risk of limb loss and 25–30% in-hospital mortality for arterial embolism

Arterial thrombosis

- Limb salvage usually possible with acute thrombosis of the iliac or superficial femoral arteries but is less likely with popliteal thrombosis
- Acute thrombosis of a popliteal aneurysm: 10–25% risk of limb loss

WHEN TO REFER

- All patients with symptoms or signs of acute limb ischemia

WHEN TO ADMIT

- All patients with symptoms and signs of limb-threatening ischemia

PREVENTION

- In atrial fibrillation, mechanical or pharmacological cardioversion may decrease the risk of further emboli
- Lifelong anticoagulation because of high frequency of recurrent emboli

EVIDENCE

PRACTICE GUIDELINES

- Betteridge DJ et al: Guidelines on the management of secondary prophylaxis of vascular events in stable patients in primary care. Int J Clin Pract 2004; 58:153. [PMID: 15055864]
- Clagett GP et al: Antithrombotic therapy in peripheral arterial occlusive disease: the Seventh ACCP Conference on Antithrombotic and Thrombolytic Therapy. Chest 2004;126(Suppl):609S. [PMID: 15383487]

WEB SITE

- The TransAtlantic Inter-Society Consensus: Acute Limb Ischemia
  - http://www.tasc-pad.org/html/journal/C4.pdf

INFORMATION FOR PATIENTS

- MedlinePlus: Arterial Embolism
  - http://www.nlm.nih.gov/medlineplus/ency/article/001102.htm

REFERENCES

- Canova CR et al: Long-term results of percutaneous thrombo-embolectomy in patients with infrainguinal embolic occlusions. Int Angiol 2001;20:66. [PMID: 11342998]
- Van Cott EM et al: Laboratory evaluation of hypercoagulability with venous or arterial thrombosis. Arch Pathol Lab Med 2002;126:1281. [PMID: 12421136]

Author(s)

Louis M. Messina, MD

Islet Cell Tumors

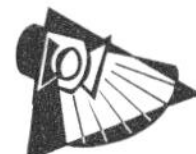

KEY FEATURES

ESSENTIALS OF DIAGNOSIS

- Half of pancreatic islet cell tumors are nonsecretory; patients present with weight loss, abdominal pain and jaundice
- Secretory tumors cause a variety of manifestations, depending on the hormones secreted

GENERAL CONSIDERATIONS

- Pancreatic islet cells are of several types: A cells (20%) secrete glucagon, B cells (70%) secrete insulin, D cells (5%) secrete somatostatin or gastrin, and F cells secrete pancreatic polypeptide
- Each cell type may give rise to benign or malignant neoplasms. Tumors usually present with a syndrome related to hormone hypersecretion
- Many tumors secrete two or more hormones
- Insulinomas are usually (82%) benign
  - May be multiple, especially in familial multiple endocrine neoplasia type 1 (MEN-1) (12% of cases)
  - Found in pancreatic head or neck (57%), body (15%), or tail (19%), or in duodenum (9%)
- Gastrinomas secrete excessive gastrin, stimulating stomach to hypersecrete acid and causing peptic ulceration (see Zollinger-Ellison Syndrome)
  - Most are benign, but a minority are malignant, metastasizing to liver
  - Typically found in duodenum (49%), pancreas (24%), or lymph nodes (11%)
  - Usually 5-year delay from symptom onset to diagnosis. Occur as part of MEN-1 in ~22%
- Glucagonomas are usually malignant and usually co-secrete other hormones, eg, gastrin
- Somatostatinomas and VIPomas (tumors secreting excessive vasoactive intestinal polypeptide) are very rare
- Islet cell tumors can also secrete ectopic hormones, eg, ACTH, producing Cushing's syndrome; or serotonin, producing atypical carcinoid syndrome
- Islet cell tumors may be part of MEN-1 (with pituitary and parathyroid adenomas)

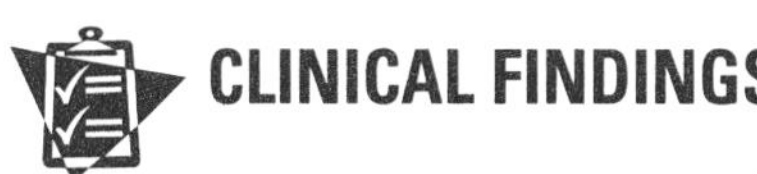

CLINICAL FINDINGS

SYMPTOMS AND SIGNS

- Insulinoma: hypoglycemic symptoms
- Gastrinoma
  - Abdominal pain (75%)
  - Diarrhea (73%)
  - Heartburn (44%)
  - Bleeding (25%)
  - Weight loss (17%)
- Glucagonoma
  - Diarrhea, nausea, peptic ulcer, or necrolytic migratory erythema
  - Weight loss and liver metastases usual at time of diagnosis
  - Diabetes mellitus develops in 35%
- Somatostatinoma
  - Weight loss
  - Diabetes mellitus
  - Malabsorption
- VIPoma
  - Profuse watery diarrhea
  - Hypokalemia
  - Acidosis (Verner-Morrison syndrome)

DIFFERENTIAL DIAGNOSIS

- Insulinoma: other cause of hypoglycemia, eg, surreptitious or excess use of insulin or sulfonylurea; liver failure; acute alcohol intoxication; sepsis; postprandial hypoglycemia (postgastrectomy, occult diabetes, idiopathic); or drugs (pentamidine, sulfamethoxazole, quinine)
- Gastrinoma: peptic ulcer disease due to other cause, eg, nonsteroidal anti-inflammatory drugs, *Helicobacter pylori*; gastroesophageal reflux disease; diarrhea due to other cause; hypergastrinemia due to other cause (atrophic gastritis, gastric outlet obstruction, pernicious anemia, chronic renal failure)
- Glucagonoma or somatostatinoma: other cause of weight loss, diarrhea, or diabetes mellitus

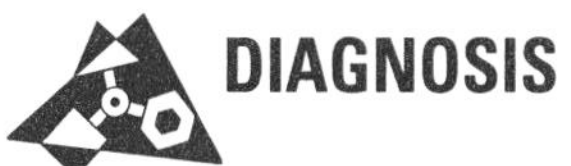

DIAGNOSIS

LABORATORY TESTS

- Insulinoma: serum glucose low with nonsuppressed insulin; elevated proinsulin level (see Hypoglycemic Disorders)
- Gastrinoma: serum gastrin elevated in normocalcemic patient not on a proton pump inhibitor
- Somatostatinoma: hypochlorhydria

IMAGING STUDIES

- Somatostatin receptor scintigraphy detects about 75% of noninsulinoma pancreatic cell islet tumors and their metastases
- CT and MRI also useful
- Preoperative localization for insulinomas are less successful, with low sensitivities
  - Ultrasonography, 25%
  - CT, 25%
  - Endoscopic ultrasonography, 27%
  - Transhepatic portal vein sampling, 40%
  - Arteriography, 45%
  - Intraoperative palpation, 55%
  - Intraoperative pancreatic ultrasound, 75%
- Combination of intraoperative palpation and ultrasound at surgery detects nearly all insulinomas

DIAGNOSTIC PROCEDURES

- Gastrinoma: endoscopy usually (94%) demonstrates prominent gastric folds

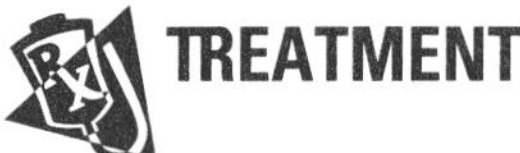

TREATMENT

MEDICATIONS

- Gastrinoma: high-dose proton pump inhibitors usually effective (see Zollinger-Ellison Syndrome)
- VIPoma
  - Octreotide improves symptoms but does not halt tumor growth
  - Calcitonin also may improve symptoms
- Antihormonal and anticancer chemotherapy for palliation of functioning malignant disease: Streptozocin, doxorubicin, and asparaginase produce encouraging results, especially for malignant insulinoma, but are quite toxic
- Hypoglycemia of insulinoma may be counteracted by verapamil or diazoxide
- Octreotide, a somatostatin analog, is used for noninsulinoma islet cell tumor

SURGERY

- Direct resection of tumor (or tumors), which often spreads locally, is primary therapy for all islet cell neoplasms except gastrinomas
- Surgery is not usually used for gastrinoma because of low cure rates, particularly with MEN-1
- Surgery is rarely curative for insulinomas in MEN-1, so is usually reserved for dominant masses

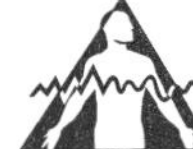

OUTCOME

COMPLICATIONS

- Pancreatic carcinoid tumors grow slowly but usually metastasize to local and distant sites, particularly to other endocrine organs

PROGNOSIS

- Surgical complication rate is ~40%; fistulas and infections occur commonly
- Extensive pancreatic resection may cause diabetes mellitus
- Overall 5-year survival higher with functional (77%) than nonfunctional (55%) tumors and higher with benign (91%) than malignant (55%) tumors
- Gastrinomas: 5-, 10-, and 20-year survival rates for gastrinomas in MEN-1 are 94%, 75%, and 58%, respectively, while survival rates for sporadic Zollinger-Ellison syndrome are 62%, 50%, and 31%, respectively
- Glucagonoma: median survival is 2.8 years after diagnosis

EVIDENCE

PRACTICE GUIDELINES

- Aldridge MC: Islet cell tumours: surgical treatment. Hosp Med 2000;61:830. [PMID:11211581]
- Azimuddin K et al: The surgical management of pancreatic neuroendocrine tumors. Surg Clin North Am 2001; 81:511. [PMID:11459268]
- Mullan MH et al: Endocrine tumours of the pancreas: review and recent advances. ANZ J Surg 2001;71:475. [PMID:11504292]

WEB SITE

- National Pancreas Foundation
  - http://www.pancreasfoundation.org

INFORMATION FOR PATIENTS

- National Cancer Institute—Islet cell carcinoma
  - http://www.cancer.gov/cancerinfo/pdq/treatment/isletcell/patient
- University of Maryland Medicine—Pancreatic islet cell tumor
  - http://www.umm.edu/ency/article/000393.htm
- Yale New Haven Health—Pancreatic islet cell tumor
  - http://yalenewhavenhealth.org/Library/HealthGuide/IllnessConditions/topic.asp?hwid=nord716

REFERENCES

- Finlayson E, Clark OH: Surgical treatment of insulinomas. Surg Clin North Am 2004;84:775. [PMID:15145234]
- Hochwald SN et al: Prognostic factors in pancreatic endocrine neoplasms: an analysis of 136 cases with a proposal for low-grade and intermediate-grade groups. Clin Oncol 2002;20:2633. [PMID:12039924]
- Li ML et al: Gastrinoma. Curr Treat Options Oncol 2001;2:337. [PMID:12057114]
- Matthews BD et al: Surgical experience with functioning pancreatic neuroendocrine tumors. Am Surg 2002;68:660. [PMID:12206598]
- Shojamanesh H et al: Prospective study of the antitumor efficacy of long-term octreotide treatment in patients with progressive metastatic gastrinoma. Cancer 2002;94:331. [PMID:11900219]

Author(s)

Paul A. Fitzgerald, MD

Isosporiasis

Isoniazid Poisoning p. 1098

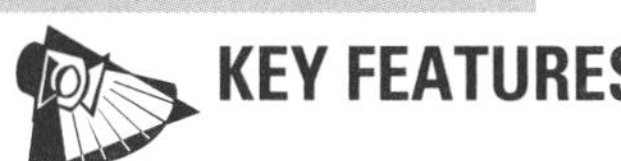

KEY FEATURES

ESSENTIALS OF DIAGNOSIS

In immunocompetent patients
- Mild to severe diarrhea. Mucus may be present in the stool but blood is absent
- Low-grade fever, vomiting, malaise

In immunodeficient patients
- Diarrhea may be profuse
- Occasionally, severe malabsorption and weight loss
- Blood and leukocytes are seldom present
- Serological tests sometimes available

GENERAL CONSIDERATIONS

- Coccidiosis is an intracellular infection of intestinal epithelial cells by spore-forming protozoa
- The causes of coccidiosis are *Cryptosporidium* spp, particularly *C parvum* and *C hominis*; *Isospora belli*; *Cyclospora cayetanensis; Sarcocystis bovihominis* and *S suihominis*; all but the sarcocystis species complete their life cycle in a single host. Diarrhea caused by any of these organisms is usually clinically similar
- The incubation period is 7–11 days
- The infectious agents are oocysts (spores) transmitted directly from person to person or by contaminated water or food
- The *Isospora* found in humans appear to be distinct to humans only
- The organism probably requires time outside the host to sporulate and become infectious
- The pathogenesis of the diarrhea is not well understood. No enterotoxin has been identified. Voluminous secretory or malabsorption diarrhea (including vitamin B_{12}, D-xylose, and fat absorption dysfunction) can result

DEMOGRAPHICS

- The infection occur worldwide, particularly in the tropics and in regions where hygiene is poor
- Clustering occurs in day care centers and mental institutions

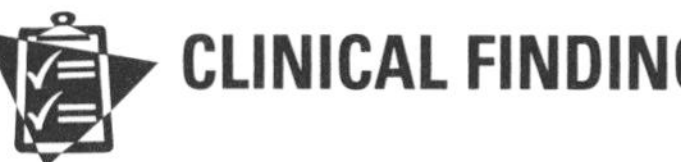

CLINICAL FINDINGS

SYMPTOMS AND SIGNS

- Generally, the diarrhea caused by the coccidial and microsporidial agents is clinically indistinguishable
- Infection varies from no symptoms, to a mild diarrhea with flatulence and bloating, to severe and frequent watery diarrhea in which the onset may be explosive
- Mucus may be present in the stools, but there is no microscopic or gross blood
- There may be low-grade fever, malaise, anorexia, abdominal cramps, vomiting, and myalgia
- These symptoms are generally self-limited, lasting weeks to months
- Weight loss can be marked

In immunodeficient patients
- The diarrhea can be profuse (up to 15 L daily has been reported), with cholera-like watery movements, accompanied by severe malabsorption, electrolyte imbalance, and marked weight loss; fever is uncommon
- Mucus is seen in the stools, but blood and leukocytes are seldom present
- The diarrhea may recur or persist
- Biliary tract infections can occur

DIFFERENTIAL DIAGNOSIS

- *C parvum, I belli, S bovihominis,* and *S suihominis*
- Giardiasis
- Viral gastroenteritis, eg, rotavirus
- Other traveler's diarrhea, eg, *Escherichia coli*
- Cholera
- Other causes of diarrhea in AIDS, eg, cytomegalovirus colitis

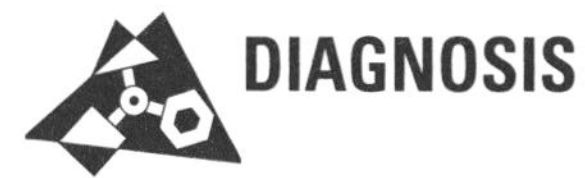

DIAGNOSIS

LABORATORY TESTS

- Three stool specimens should be collected over 5–7 days and saved both as fresh specimens and in preservative and processed by flotation or concentration methods to detect the distinctive oocysts (differences are based on size and intracellular location)
- Diagnosis by stool examination is often difficult, for the organisms may be scanty even in the presence of significant symptoms
- Eosinophilia and eosinophils in stools are sometimes present
- Because of their buoyancy, oocysts (20–30 × 10–20 μm) must be looked for just beneath the coverslip of the preparation. Confirmation is by acid-fast staining
- Serological tests are available

DIAGNOSTIC PROCEDURES

- Frequently, the diagnosis can be made only after duodenal aspiration or duodenal biopsy of multiple specimens

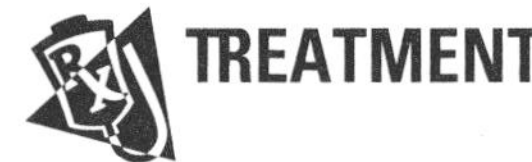

TREATMENT

MEDICATIONS

In immunocompetent patients

- Trimethoprim (160 mg) and sulfamethoxazole (800 mg) (TMP-SMX) PO QID for 10 days and then twice daily for 3 weeks; or sulfadiazine, 4 g, and pyrimethamine, 35–75 mg PO, in four divided doses daily, plus leucovorin calcium, 10–25 mg daily, for 3–7 weeks

In immunocompromised patients

- It may be necessary to continue a maintenance dose indefinitely with TMP-SMX three times weekly or Fansidar once weekly
- Efficacy in primary infection has also been reported for furazolidone (400 mg/day for 10 days), roxithromycin, ciprofloxacin, nitrofurantoin, metronidazole, quinacrine, pyrimethamine, albendazole with ornidazole, and diclazuril

THERAPEUTIC PROCEDURES

- Most acute infections in immunocompetent persons are self-limited and do not require treatment
- Supportive treatment for severe or chronic diarrhea includes fluid and electrolyte replacement and, in chronic cases, parenteral nutrition

OUTCOME

WHEN TO REFER

- Persistent symptoms despite therapy, particularly in immunocompromised patients

WHEN TO ADMIT

- Profuse diarrhea causing hypotension or electrolyte imbalance

PREVENTION

- Measures to reduce exposure to these organisms are recommended for immunocompromised patients. These include reduced exposure to swimming in fresh water and boiling of drinking water (1 min) or use of a filter that removes particles over 1 μm in size

EVIDENCE

WEB SITE

- CDC—Division of Parasitic Diseases
  - http://www.dpd.cdc.gov/dpdx/HTML/isosporiasis.htm

PRACTICE GUIDELINES

- National Guideline Clearinghouse
  - http://www.guideline.gov/summary/summary.aspx?doc_id=3080
  - http://www.guideline.gov/summary/summary.aspx?doc_id=2573

REFERENCE

- Ambroise-Thomas P: Parasitic diseases and immunodeficiencies. Parasitology 2001;122(Suppl):S65. [PMID: 11442198]

Jaundice

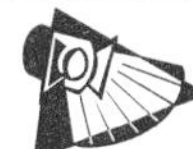

KEY FEATURES

ESSENTIALS OF DIAGNOSIS

- Results from accumulation of bilirubin in the body tissues; the cause may be hepatic or nonhepatic
- Hyperbilirubinemia may be due to abnormalities in the formation, transport, metabolism, and excretion of bilirubin
- Total serum bilirubin is normally 0.2–1.2 mg/dL, and jaundice may not be recognizable until levels are about 3 mg/dL

GENERAL CONSIDERATIONS

- Jaundice is caused by predominantly unconjugated or conjugated bilirubin in the serum (Table 58)
- In the absence of liver disease, hemolysis rarely elevates the serum bilirubin level to more than 7 mg/dL
- "Cholestasis" denotes retention of bile in the liver, and "cholestatic jaundice" implies conjugated hyperbilirubinemia from impaired bile flow

CLINICAL FINDINGS

SYMPTOMS AND SIGNS

- See Table 59

Unconjugated hyperbilirubinemia

- Normal stool and urine color—no bilirubin in the urine
- Mild jaundice
- Splenomegaly occurs in hemolytic disorders except in sickle cell anemia
- Abdominal or back pain may occur with acute hemolytic crises

Conjugated hyperbilirubinemia

- Hereditary cholestatic syndromes or intrahepatic cholestasis
  - May be asymptomatic
  - Intermittent cholestasis is often accompanied by pruritus, light-colored stools, and, occasionally, malaise
- Hepatocellular disease
  - Malaise, anorexia, low-grade fever, and right upper quadrant discomfort are frequent
  - Dark urine, jaundice, and, in women, amenorrhea occur
  - An enlarged, tender liver; vascular spiders; palmar erythema; ascites; gynecomastia; sparse body hair; fetor hepaticus; and asterixis may be present, depending on the cause, severity, and chronicity of liver dysfunction

Biliary obstruction

- Right upper quadrant pain, weight loss (suggesting carcinoma), jaundice, dark urine, and light-colored stools
- Symptoms and signs may be intermittent if caused by stone, carcinoma of the ampulla, or cholangiocarcinoma
- Pain may be absent early in pancreatic cancer
- Stool occult blood suggests cancer of the ampulla
- Hepatomegaly and a palpable gallbladder (Courvoisier's sign) are characteristic, but are neither specific nor sensitive of pancreatic head tumor
- Fever and chills are far more common in benign obstruction and associated cholangitis

DIFFERENTIAL DIAGNOSIS

- Obstructive hepatobiliary disease [γ-glutamyl transpeptidase (GGT) elevated]
- Hepatitis, eg, viral, alcoholic, toxic
- Hemochromatosis

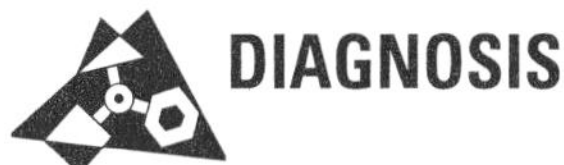

DIAGNOSIS

LABORATORY TESTS

- Table 60
- Elevated serum aspartate and alanine aminotransferase (AST, ALT) levels result from hepatocellular necrosis or inflammation, as in hepatitis; ALT is more specific for the liver than AST, but an AST level at least twice that of the ALT is typical of alcoholic liver injury
- The ALT level is greater than the AST level in nonalcoholic fatty liver disease prior to the development of cirrhosis
- An isolated elevation of serum ALT may be seen in celiac disease
- Elevated alkaline phosphatase levels are seen in cholestasis or infiltrative liver disease (such as tumor or granuloma)
- Alkaline phosphatase elevations of hepatic rather than bone, intestinal, or placental origin are confirmed by concomitant elevation of GTT or 5'-nucleotidase levels

IMAGING STUDIES

- Demonstration of dilated bile ducts by ultrasonography or CT scan indicates biliary obstruction (90–95% sensitivity). Ultrasonography, CT scan, and MRI may also demonstrate hepatomegaly, intrahepatic tumors, and portal hypertension
- Spiral arterial-phase and multislice CT scanning, in which the liver is imaged during peak hepatic enhancement while the patient holds one or two breaths, improves diagnostic accuracy
- Multiphasic spiral or multislice CT, CT arterial portography, in which imaging follows intravenous contrast infusion via a catheter placed in the superior mesenteric artery, MRI with use of ferumoxides as contrast agents, and intraoperative ultrasonography are the most sensitive techniques for detection of individual small hepatic lesions in patients eligible for resection of metastases
- Color Doppler ultrasound or contrast agents that produce microbubbles increase the sensitivity of transcutaneous ultrasound for detecting small neoplasms
- MRI is the most accurate technique for identifying isolated liver lesions such as hemangiomas, focal nodular hyperplasia, or focal fatty infiltration and for detecting hepatic iron overload
- Because of its much lower cost, ultrasonography is preferable to CT or MRI as a screening test

- Ultrasonography can detect gallstones with a sensitivity of 95%
- Magnetic resonance cholangiopancreatography (MRCP) appears to be a sensitive, noninvasive method of detecting bile duct stones, strictures, and dilation
- Endoscopic ultrasonography is the most sensitive test for detecting small lesions of the ampulla or pancreatic head and for detecting portal vein invasion by pancreatic cancer. It is also accurate in detecting or excluding bile duct stones

DIAGNOSTIC PROCEDURES

- Percutaneous liver biopsy is the definitive diagnostic method for determining the etiology and severity of the liver disease. It should be performed under ultrasound or CT guidance for suspected metastatic disease or a hepatic mass. A transjugular route can be used in patients with coagulopathy or ascites

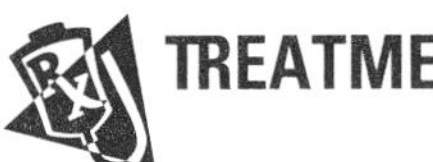

TREATMENT

THERAPEUTIC PROCEDURES

- Treatment of the causative etiology
- Uncomplicated obstructive jaundice responds to parenteral vitamin K
- Use endoscopic retrograde cholangiopancreatography (ERCP) or percutaneous transhepatic cholangiography (PTC) to demonstrate pancreatic or ampullary causes of jaundice, to perform papillotomy and stone extraction, or to insert a stent through an obstructing lesion

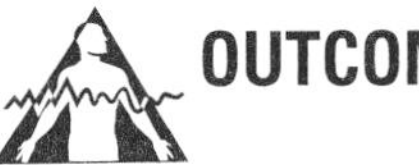

OUTCOME

COMPLICATIONS

- Complications of ERCP include pancreatitis in 5% of cases and, less commonly, cholangitis, bleeding, or duodenal perforation after papillotomy
- Severe complications of PTC occur in 3% of cases and include fever, bacteremia, bile peritonitis, and intraperitoneal hemorrhage

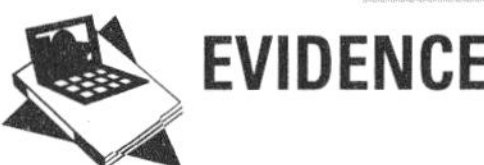

EVIDENCE

WEB SITES

- Diseases of the Liver
  - http://cpmcnet.columbia.edu/dept/gi/disliv.html
- Pathology Index
  - http://www-medlib.med.utah.edu/WebPath/LIVEHTML/LIVERIDX.html

INFORMATION FOR PATIENTS

- National Institutes of Health
  - http://www.nlm.nih.gov/medlineplus/ency/article/003243.htm

REFERENCES

- Adams PC et al: Screening for liver disease: report of an AASLD clinical workshop. Hepatology 2004;39:1204. [PMID: 15122748]
- Kim HC et al: Normal serum aminotransferase concentration and risk of mortality from liver diseases: prospective cohort study. BMJ 2004;328:983. [PMID: 15028636]
- Zucker SD et al: Serum bilirubin levels in the U.S. population: gender effect and inverse correlation with colorectal cancer. Hepatology 2004;40:827. [PMID: 15382174]

Author(s)

Lawrence S. Friedman, MD

Kaposi's Sarcoma

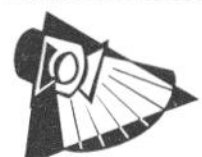

KEY FEATURES

ESSENTIALS OF DIAGNOSIS

- Human herpes virus 8 (HHV-8) or Kaposi's sarcoma–associated herpes virus (KSHV), is universally present in all forms of Kaposi's sarcoma
- It is a common infection in central Africa, is more common in Italy than in the United States, and is common in HIV-infected homosexual men and rare in HIV-infected hemophiliacs

GENERAL CONSIDERATIONS

- Before 1980 in the United States, this rare malignant skin lesion was seen mostly in elderly white men, had a chronic clinical course, and was rarely fatal
- Occurs endemically in an often aggressive form in young black men of equatorial Africa, but it is rare in American blacks
- The epidemiology of infection with HHV-8 or KSHV parallels the incidence of Kaposi's sarcoma in various risk groups and geographic regions
- The virus is present in the skin lesions and circulating B lymphocytes of persons with Kaposi's sarcoma but uncommonly in their normal skin

DEMOGRAPHICS

- The most common HIV-related malignancy

CLINICAL FINDINGS

SYMPTOMS AND SIGNS

- Red, purple, or dark plaques or nodules on cutaneous or mucosal surfaces
- Commonly involves the gastrointestinal tract, but in asymptomatic patients these lesions are not sought or treated

DIFFERENTIAL DIAGNOSIS

- Bacillary angiomatosis
- Hemangioma
- Vasculitis (palpable purpura)
- Dermatofibroma
- Pyogenic granuloma
- Prurigo nodularis
- Melanoma

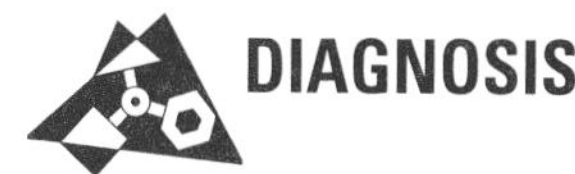

DIAGNOSIS

LABORATORY TESTS

- Based on appearance of skin lesions with confirmatory biopsy
- A low sensitivity serologic test is available to detect infection with HHV-8 but is not used to confirm the diagnosis

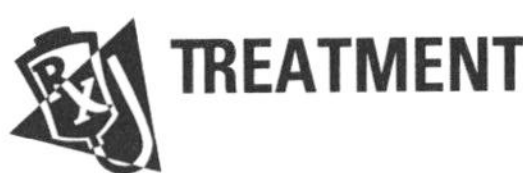

TREATMENT

MEDICATIONS

- Kaposi's sarcoma in the elderly
  - Palliative local therapy with intralesional chemotherapy or radiation is usually all that is required
- In the setting of iatrogenic immunosuppression
  - The treatment is primarily reduction of doses of immunosuppressive medications
- AIDS-associated Kaposi's
  - The patient should first be given effective anti-HIV antiretrovirals (including a protease inhibitor), because in most cases this treatment alone is associated with improvement (See HIV Infection)
- Other therapeutic options include cryotherapy or intralesional vinblastine (0.1–0.5 mg/mL) for cosmetically objectionable lesions
- Systemic chemotherapy
  - Indicated for rapidly progressive skin disease (more than 10 new lesions per month), with edema or pain, and with symptomatic visceral disease or pulmonary disease
  - Liposomal doxorubicin is highly effective in controlling these cases and has considerably less toxicity—and greater efficacy—than anthracycline monotherapy or combination chemotherapeutic regimens

SURGERY

- Laser surgery for certain intraoral and pharyngeal lesions

THERAPEUTIC PROCEDURES

- Radiation therapy for accessible and space-occupying lesions

OUTCOME

PROGNOSIS

- Pulmonary Kaposi's sarcoma may be life-threatening and is managed aggressively

WHEN TO REFER

- If there is a question about the diagnosis, if recommended therapy is ineffective, or if specialized treatment is necessary

WHEN TO ADMIT

- Respiratory insufficiency or other signs of systemic failure

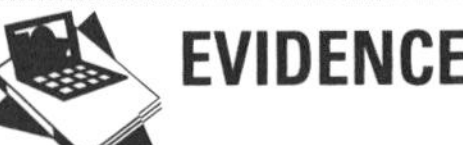

EVIDENCE

PRACTICE GUIDELINES

- Kaplan JE et al: Guidelines for preventing opportunistic infections among HIV-infected persons—2002. Recommendations of the U.S. Public Health Service and the Infectious Diseases Society of America. MMWR Recomm Rep 2002;51:1.
  - http://www.cdc.gov/mmwr/PDF/rr/rr5108.pdf

WEB SITES

- American Academy of Dermatology
  - http://www.aad.org
- National Cancer Institute: Kaposi's Sarcoma Treatment
  - http://www.cancer.gov/cancertopics/pdq/treatment/kaposis/healthprofessional

INFORMATION FOR PATIENTS

- American Cancer Society: Kaposi's Sarcoma
  - http://www.cancer.org/docroot/CRI/CRI_2_3x.asp?rnav=cridg&dt=21
- MedlinePlus: Kaposi's Sarcoma
  - http://www.nlm.nih.gov/medlineplus/ency/article/000661.htm
- National Cancer Institute: Kaposi's Sarcoma
  - http://www.cancer.gov/cancertopics/pdq/treatment/kaposis/patient

REFERENCES

- Antman K et al: Kaposi's sarcoma. N Engl J Med 2000;342:1027. [PMID: 10749966]
- Dezube BJ: Acquired immunodeficiency syndrome-related Kaposi's sarcoma: clinical features, staging, and treatment. Semin Oncol 2000;27:424. [PMID: 10950369]

Author(s)

Timothy G. Berger, MD

Larva Migrans, Visceral

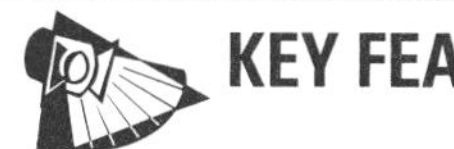

KEY FEATURES

ESSENTIALS OF DIAGNOSIS

Acute infection

- Cough, wheezing, fever
- Hepatosplenomegaly and lymphadenopathy

Ocular toxocariasis

- Most common in children
- Occurs years after the acute infection

GENERAL CONSIDERATIONS

- Most visceral larva migrans cases are due to *Toxocaracanis*, an ascarid of dogs and other canids; *Toxocaracati* in domestic cats has occasionally been implicated and rarely *Belascarisprocyonis* of raccoons
- The reservoir mechanism for *T canis* is latent infection in female dogs that is reactivated during pregnancy. Transmission from mother to puppies is via the placenta and milk. Most eggs passed to the environment are from puppies (2 weeks to 6 months) and lactating bitches. The life cycle of *T cati* is similar, but transplacental transmission does not occur
- Direct contact with infected animals does not produce infection, as the eggs require a 3- to 4-week extrinsic incubation period to become infective; thereafter, eggs in soil remain infective for months to years
- In humans, hatched larvae are unable to mature but continue to migrate through the tissues for up to 6 months. Eventually they lodge in various organs, particularly the lungs and liver and less often the brain, eyes, and other tissues, where they produce eosinophilic granulomas up to 1 cm in diameter

DEMOGRAPHICS

- Human infections are sporadic and probably occur worldwide
- In the United States, antibody seroprevalence is 5–7%
- Infection is generally in dirt-eating young children who ingest *T canis* or *T cati* eggs from soil or sand contaminated with animal feces, most often from puppies

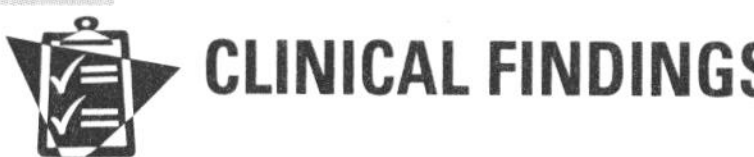

CLINICAL FINDINGS

SYMPTOMS AND SIGNS

Acute infection

- Migrating larvae may induce fever, cough, wheezing, hepatosplenomegaly, and lymphadenopathy
- Other symptoms depend on which organs are invaded, including myelitis, encephalitis, and carditis
- The acute phase may last 2–3 weeks, but resolution of all physical and laboratory findings may take up to 18 months

Ocular toxocariasis

- Generally occurs years after the acute infection
- Most cases occur in children, most commonly 5–10 years old, who present with visual impairment in one eye and sometimes leukocoria, squint, and red eye
- Other common findings are peripheral retinochoroiditis, a diffuse, painless endophthalmitis; posterior pole granuloma; and a peripheral inflammatory mass
- Uncommonly seen are an iris nodule, optic nerve granuloma, uniocular pars planitis, and a migrating retinal nematode

DIFFERENTIAL DIAGNOSIS

- Acute HIV infection
- Infectious mononucleosis
- Lymphoma
- Malaria
- Ascariasis
- Chagas' disease
- Retinoblastoma

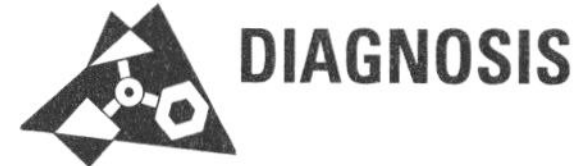

DIAGNOSIS

LABORATORY TESTS

Acute infection

- Leukocytosis is marked (may exceed 100,000/μL), with 30–80% due to eosinophils
- Hyperglobulinemia occurs when the liver is extensively invaded and is a useful clue in diagnosis
- An ELISA test is the most specific (92%) and sensitive (78%) serological test and may permit a presumptive diagnosis, although it does not distinguish acute from prior infection. However, rising or falling titers with twofold differences are consistent with the diagnosis
- Nonspecific isohemagglutinin titers (anti-A and anti-B) are usually greater than 1:102
- With central nervous system involvement, the cerebrospinal fluid may show eosinophils
- No parasitic forms can be found by stool examination

Ocular toxocariasis

- Generally not associated with peripheral eosinophilia, hypergammaglobulinemia, or isohemagglutinin elevation
- Serum ELISA tests may be positive, but a negative test does not rule out the diagnosis
- If doubt exists about whether a patient with a positive serum ELISA test has toxocariasis or retinoblastoma, examination of the vitreous humor for ELISA antibody and eosinophils can be helpful

IMAGING STUDIES

- In acute infection, chest radiographs may show infiltrates
- Ultrasonography may detect 1-cm hypoechoic lesions in the liver, each with a thread-like hyperechoic line
- High-resolution CT scanning of the orbit should be done for ocular symptoms

DIAGNOSTIC PROCEDURES

- Specific diagnosis can be made only by percutaneous liver biopsy or by direct biopsy of a granuloma at laparoscopy (mixed inflammatory infiltrate with numerous eosinophils), but these procedures are seldom justified and may not yield larvae

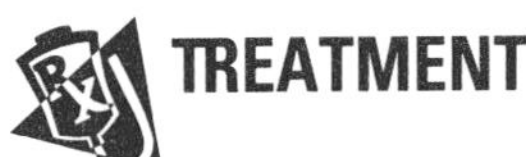

TREATMENT

MEDICATIONS

Acute infection

- Although there is no proved specific treatment, the following drugs can be tried: albendazole (400 mg PO BID for 21 days), mebendazole (200 mg PO BID for 21 days), thiabendazole (as used in strongyloidiasis), or ivermectin
- Corticosteroids, antibiotics, antihistamines, and analgesics may be needed to provide symptomatic relief

Ocular toxocariasis

- Treatment includes oral and subconjunctival corticosteroids, and an anthelmintic drug

SURGERY

- Treatment for ocular toxocariasis includes vitrectomy for vitreous traction and laser photocoagulation

THERAPEUTIC PROCEDURES

- Treatment of symptomatic persons is primarily supportive

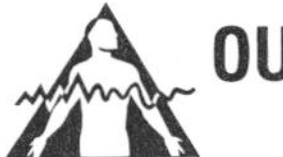

OUTCOME

PROGNOSIS

- Symptoms of the acute infection may persist for months but generally clear within 1–2 years
- The ultimate outcome is usually good, but permanent neuropsychological deficits have been seen
- Partial or total permanent visual impairment is rare

WHEN TO REFER

- Patients whose disease is progressive despite therapy
- All patients with ocular toxocariasis

WHEN TO ADMIT

- Progressive respiratory disease
- Patients with central nervous system involvement or carditis

PREVENTION

- Disease in humans is best prevented by periodic treatment of puppies, kittens, and nursing dog and cat mothers, starting at 2 weeks postpartum, repeating at weekly intervals for 3 weeks and then every 6 months

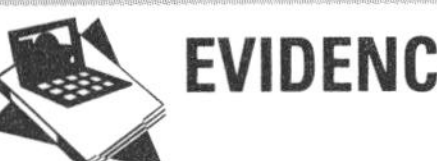

EVIDENCE

INFORMATION FOR PATIENTS

- National Institutes of Health
  - http://www.nlm.nih.gov/medlineplus/ency/article/000633.htm

REFERENCES

- Barisani-Asenbauer T et al: Treatment of ocular toxocariasis with albendazole. J Ocul Pharmacol Ther 2001;17:287. [PMID: 11436948]
- Hartleb M et al: Severe hepatic involvement in visceral larva migrans. Eur J Gastroenterol Hepatol 2001;13:1245. [PMID: 11711784]
- Pawlowski Z: Toxocariasis in humans: clinical expression and treatment dilemma. J Helminthol 2001;75:299. [PMID: 11818044]
- Sabrosa NA et al: Nematode infections of the eye: toxocariasis and diffuse unilateral subacute neuroretinitis. Curr Opin Ophthalmol 2001;12:450. [PMID: 11734685]

Legionnaire's Disease

Lactase Deficiency p. 1099. Larva Migrans, Cutaneous p. 1100. Lead Poisoning p. 1100.

KEY FEATURES

ESSENTIALS OF DIAGNOSIS

- Patients are often immunocompromised, smokers, or have chronic lung disease
- Scant sputum production, pleuritic chest pain, toxic appearance
- Chest x-ray shows focal patchy infiltrates or consolidation
- Gram's stain of sputum shows polymorphonuclear leukocytes and no organisms

GENERAL CONSIDERATIONS

- Ranks among the three or four most common causes of community-acquired pneumonia
- Classically, this pneumonia is caused by *Legionella pneumophila*, though other species can cause identical disease
- Is more common in immunocompromised persons, in smokers, and in those with chronic lung disease
- Outbreaks have been associated with contaminated water sources, such as shower heads and faucets in patient rooms, and air conditioning cooling towers

DEMOGRAPHICS

- An estimated 8,000–18,000 cases occur each year in the United States
- Most cases are sporadic; 10–20% can be linked to outbreaks, and about 20% are nosocomial

CLINICAL FINDINGS

SYMPTOMS AND SIGNS

- Many features of typical pneumonia, with high fevers, a toxic patient, pleurisy, and grossly purulent sputum

DIFFERENTIAL DIAGNOSIS

- Other infectious pneumonia
- Pulmonary embolism
- Aspiration pneumonia
- Myocardial infarction
- Pleurodynia (coxsackievirus)

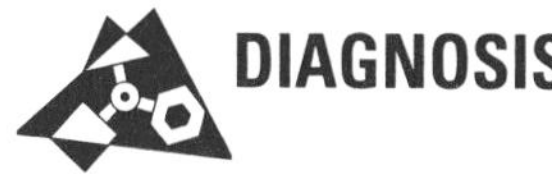

DIAGNOSIS

LABORATORY TESTS

- Is an atypical pneumonia, because a Gram-stained smear of sputum does not show organisms
- Culture onto charcoal-yeast extract agar or similar enriched medium is the most sensitive method (80–90% sensitivity) for diagnosis and permits identification of infections caused by species and serotypes other than *L pneumophila* serotype 1
- Dieterle's silver staining of tissue, pleural fluid, or other infected material is also a reliable method for detecting *Legionella* species
- Direct fluorescent antibody stains and serological testing are less sensitive because these will detect only *L pneumophila* serotype 1
- Serological diagnosis requires that the host respond with sufficient specific antibody production and be infected with a serotype 1 strain
- Urinary antigen tests, which are targeted for detection of *L pneumophila* serotype 1, are also less sensitive than culture

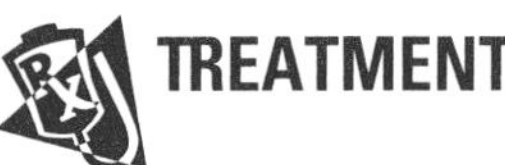

TREATMENT

MEDICATIONS

- Levofloxacin (500 mg once daily orally or intravenously), azithromycin (500 mg then 250 mg once daily, orally or intravenously), and clarithromycin (500 mg orally twice daily)—all administered for 10–14 days
- Azithromycin may be effective as a 5-day regimen
- A 21-day course of treatment and combination therapy (eg, addition of rifampin 300 mg twice daily or macrolide-fluoroquinolone) are recommended in the immunocompromised patient; improved outcome is not certain
- Tetracyclines and trimethoprim-sulfamethoxazole are used for the patient who cannot be treated with either a macrolide or a fluoroquinolone

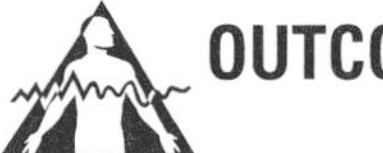

OUTCOME

PROGNOSIS

- Death occurs in 5–15% of cases: a substantially higher proportion of fatal cases occurs during nosocomial outbreaks

WHEN TO REFER

- For progressive respiratory failure or if expertise in management is needed

WHEN TO ADMIT

- For respiratory compromise or if supportive care if needed

PREVENTION

- Improved design and maintenance of cooling towers and plumbing systems to limit the growth and spread of *Legionella* organisms
- Person-to-person transmission does not occur

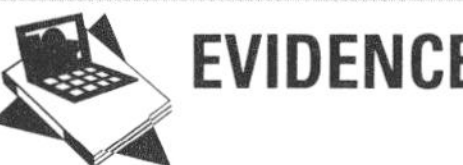

EVIDENCE

PRACTICE GUIDELINES

- National Guideline Clearinghouse
  - http://www.guideline.gov/summary/summary.aspx?doc_id=4546

WEB SITES

- CDC—Division of Bacterial and Mycotic Diseases
  - http://www.cdc.gov/ncidod/dbmd/
- Karolinska Institute—Directory of Bacterial Infections and Mycoses
  - http://www.mic.ki.se/Diseases/C01.html

INFORMATION FOR PATIENTS

- Centers for Disease Control
  - http://www.cdc.gov/ncidod/dbmd/diseaseinfo/legionellosis_g.htm
- JAMA patient page: Pneumonia. JAMA 2000;283:1922.
- National Institute of Environmental Health Sciences
  - http://www.niehs.nih.gov/external/faq/legion.htm
- National Institutes of Health
  - http://www.nlm.nih.gov/medlineplus/ency/article/000616.htm

REFERENCES

- Benin AL et al: Trends in legionnaires disease, 1980–1998: declining mortality and new patterns of diagnosis. Clin Infect Dis 2002;35:1039. [PMID: 12384836]
- Plouffe JF et al: Azithromycin in the treatment of Legionella pneumonia requiring hospitalization. Clin Infect Dis 2003;37:1475. [PMID: 14614670]
- Waterer GW et al: Legionella and community-acquired pneumonia: a review of current diagnostic tests from a clinician's viewpoint. Am J Med 2001;110:41. [PMID: 11152864]

Author(s)

Henry F. Chambers, MD

Leiomyoma of the Uterus

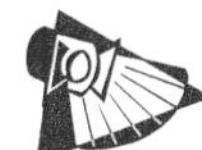

KEY FEATURES

ESSENTIALS OF DIAGNOSIS

- Irregular enlargement of the uterus (may be asymptomatic)
- Heavy or irregular vaginal bleeding, dysmenorrhea
- Acute and recurrent pelvic pain if the tumor becomes twisted on its pedicle or infarcted
- Symptoms due to pressure on neighboring organs (large tumors)

GENERAL CONSIDERATIONS

- Most common benign neoplasm of the female genital tract
- Tumor is discrete, round, firm, and often multiple, composed of smooth muscle and connective tissue
- The most convenient classification is by anatomic location:
  - Intramural
  - Submucous
  - Subserous
  - Intraligamentous
  - Parasitic (ie, deriving its blood supply from an organ to which it becomes attached)
  - Cervical
- A submucous myoma may become pedunculated and descend through the cervix into the vagina

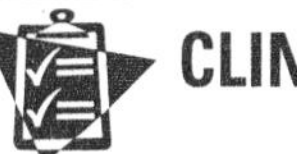

CLINICAL FINDINGS

SYMPTOMS AND SIGNS

- In nonpregnant women, myomas are frequently asymptomatic. However, they can cause urinary frequency, dysmenorrhea, heavy bleeding (often with anemia), or other complications due to the presence of an abdominal mass. Occasionally, degeneration occurs, causing intense pain

DIFFERENTIAL DIAGNOSIS

- Adenomyosis (uterine endometriosis)
- Pregnancy
- Ovarian tumor
- Endometrial polyp
- Endometrial cancer
- Leiomyosarcoma

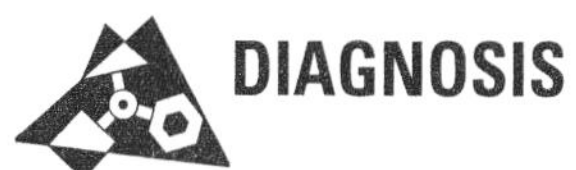

DIAGNOSIS

LABORATORY TESTS

- Anemia from blood loss may occur
- Rarely, polycythemia is present, presumably as a result of the production of erythropoietin by the myomas

IMAGING STUDIES

- Ultrasonography will confirm the presence of uterine myomas
- When multiple subserous or pedunculated myomas are being followed, ultrasonography is important to exclude ovarian masses
- MRI can delineate intramural and submucous myomas accurately

DIAGNOSTIC PROCEDURES

- Hysterography or hysteroscopy can confirm cervical or submucous myomas

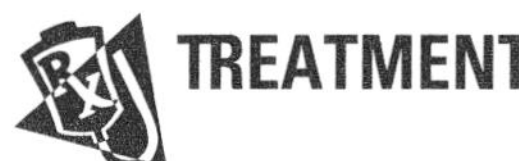

TREATMENT

MEDICATIONS

- For marked anemia as a result of long, heavy menstrual periods, preoperative treatment with depot medroxyprogesterone acetate, 150 mg IM every 28 days, or danazol, 400–800 mg PO daily, will slow or stop bleeding, and medical treatment of anemia can be given prior to surgery
- Because the risk of surgical complications increases with the increasing size of the myoma, preoperative reduction of myoma size is desirable
- Gonadotropin-releasing hormone analogs such as depot leuprolide, 3.75 mg IM monthly, or nafarelin, 0.2–0.4 mg intranasally twice a day, are used preoperatively for 3- to 4-month periods to induce reversible hypogonadism, which temporarily reduces the size of myomas, suppresses their further growth, and reduces surrounding vascularity

SURGERY

- Emergency surgery is required for acute torsion of a pedunculated myoma
- The only emergency indication for myomectomy during pregnancy is torsion; abortion is not inevitable
- Surgical measures: available for treatment are myomectomy and total or subtotal abdominal, vaginal, or laparoscopy-assisted vaginal hysterectomy
- Myomectomy is the treatment of choice during the childbearing years
- Myomas do not require surgery on an urgent basis unless they cause significant pressure on the ureters, bladder, or bowel or severe bleeding leading to anemia or unless they are undergoing rapid growth
- Cervical myomas larger than 3–4 cm in diameter or pedunculated myomas that protrude through the cervix must be removed
- Submucous myomas can be removed using a hysteroscope and laser or resection instruments
- Recent alternatives to myomectomy include transcatheter bilateral uterine artery embolization, myolysis with MRI-guided, high-frequency, focused ultrasound, and laser cauterization. However, randomized trials to compare long-term outcomes of the methods with conventional therapy are needed

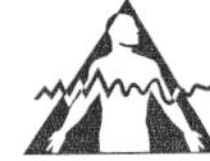

OUTCOME

FOLLOW-UP

- Women who have small asymptomatic myomas should be examined at 6-month intervals
- Ultrasound can be used sequentially to monitor growth

COMPLICATIONS

- Infertility may be due to a myoma that significantly distorts the uterine cavity

PROGNOSIS

- Surgical therapy is curative
- Future pregnancies are not endangered by myomectomy, although cesarean delivery may be necessary after wide dissection with entry into the uterine cavity

WHEN TO REFER

- Refer to gynecologist for surgical therapy of symptomatic leiomyomata

WHEN TO ADMIT

- For acute abdomen associated with an infracted leiomyoma (rare)

EVIDENCE

PRACTICE GUIDELINES

- Lefebvre G et al; Clinical Practice Gynaecology Committee, Society for Obstetricians and Gynaecologists of Canada. The management of uterine leiomyomas. J Obstet Gynaecol Can 2003;25:396. [PMID: 12738981]

WEB SITE

- National Uterine Fibroids Foundation
  - http://www.nuff.org/health.htm

INFORMATION FOR PATIENTS

- American Association of Family Physicians: Uterine Fibroid Embolization
  - http://familydoctor.org/601.xml
- MedlinePlus: Uterine Fibroids Interactive Tutorial
  - http://www.nlm.nih.gov/medlineplus/tutorials/uterinefibroids.html
- MedlinePlus: Uterine Fibroids
  - http://www.nlm.nih.gov/medlineplus/ency/article/000914.htm
- National Institute of Child Health & Human Development: Uterine Fibroids
  - http://www.nichd.nih.gov/publications/pubs/fibroids/index.htm

REFERENCES

- Beinfeld MT et al: Cost-effectiveness of uterine artery embolization and hysterectomy for uterine fibroids. Radiology 2004;230:207. [PMID: 14695395]
- Wallach EE et al: Uterine myomas: an overview of development, clinical features, and management. Obstet Gynecol 2004;104:393. [PMID: 15292018]

Author(s)

H. Trent MacKay, MD, MPH

Leishmaniasis

KEY FEATURES

ESSENTIALS OF DIAGNOSIS

- Four clinical syndromes occur
  - Visceral leishmaniasis (kala azar)
  - Cutaneous leishmaniasis
  - Mucocutaneous leishmaniasis (espundia)
  - Diffuse cutaneous leishmaniasis

GENERAL CONSIDERATIONS

- The disease is transmitted by bites of sand flies [phlebotomus (Old World leishmaniasis) and lutzomyia (New World leishmaniasis) species] from the wild animal reservoir (eg, rodents, marsupials) and domestic dogs (who can die from *Leishmania infantum* infections) to humans; kala azar is transmitted directly from humans to humans
- Leishmaniae have two distinct forms in their life cycle. In mammalian hosts, the parasite is found in its amastigote form (Leishman-Donovan bodies, 2–5 μm) within mononuclear phagocytes. When sand flies feed on an infected host, the parasitized cells are ingested with the blood meal. In the sand fly vector, the parasite converts to, multiplies, and is then transmitted during feeding as a flaggellated extracellular promastigote (10–15 μm)
- There is overlap between the four clinical syndromes, and each syndrome is caused by more than one species
- See Leishmaniasis, visceral (kala azar)
- See Leishmaniasis, cutaneous
- See Leishmaniasis, mucocutaneous
- Diffuse cutaneous leishmaniasis is a state of deficient cell-mediated immunity; skin lesions are generally progressive and refractory to treatment. The causative organisms are the *L mexicana* complex in the New World and *L aethiopica* in the Old World
- *Leishmania* results in lifelong latent infection
- Several hundred cutaneous and a few visceral leishmaniasis infections have been found in US military after exposure in Afghanistan and Iraq
- Leishmaniae can become opportunistic pathogens through reactivation or new infection; in southern Europe (France, Italy, Spain, Portugal), 2–9% of people with AIDS have coinfections

DEMOGRAPHICS

- In tropical and temperate zones, an estimated 12 million persons are infected with leishmaniasis; 1.5–2 million new cases occur yearly; >1 million are cutaneous and 500,000 visceral disease; approximately 50% are in children

CLINICAL FINDINGS

SYMPTOMS AND SIGNS

- Severity of infection ranges from subclinical or minimally pathological (self-curing or easily treated cutaneous lesions) to persistent, disfiguring cutaneous and mucocutaneous lesions to potentially fatal visceral disease
- See Leishmaniasis, visceral (kala azar)
- See Leishmaniasis, cutaneous
- See Leishmaniasis, mucocutaneous
- In diffuse cutaneous leishmaniasis, there are widespread, leprosy-like skin lesions
- In patients with AIDS who have coinfection with *Leishmania*, splenomegaly may not occur in visceral disease

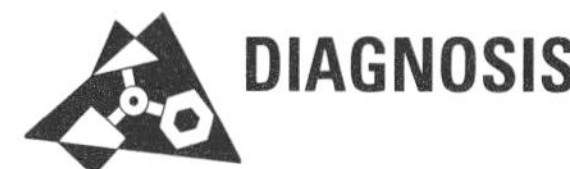

DIAGNOSIS

LABORATORY TESTS

- Definitive diagnosis is by finding the intracellular nonflagellated amastigote in Giemsa-stained biopsies from skin, mucosal lesions, liver, or lymph nodes; or from aspirates from spleen (the most sensitive site, but also a risky procedure), bone marrow, or lymph nodes; or by finding the flagellated promastigote state in culture of these tissues (requires up to 21 days)
- Occasionally, the organisms are seen in mononuclear cells of Giemsa-stained smears of the buffy coat
- In patients with AIDS who have *Leishmania* coinfections, diagnostic criteria may be altered (*Leishmania* antibodies become undetectable and, in visceral disease, splenomegaly may not occur)
- Golden hamster or BALB/c mouse inoculation of the nose, footpad, or tail base may be used and requires 2–12 weeks of observation
- Polymerase chain reaction has up to 100% specificity and sensitivity and can be performed on any type of biological specimen. Where available, species identification is by molecular, isoenzyme, and monoclonal antibody methods
- Serological tests (ELISA, indirect fluorescent antibody, direct agglutination, and others) and the leishmanin (Montenegro) skin test (not licensed in the United States) may facilitate diagnosis, but none is sufficiently sensitive or specific to be used alone, to speciate, or to distinguish current from past infection

DIAGNOSTIC PROCEDURES

- Specimens from skin lesions should be obtained through intact skin (cleansed with 70% alcohol) at a raised edge of an ulcer margin. Local anesthesia can be used. To obtain tissue fluid for staining, press blood out of the site with two fingers, incise a 3-mm slit, and then scrape with the blade
- When doing a biopsy, an impression smear is made, a portion is macerated for culture, and the remainder is reserved for pathological sections. For needle aspiration, sterile preservative-free saline is inserted with a 23- to 27-gauge needle; the aspirate is then cytospun at 800 × *g* for 5 min

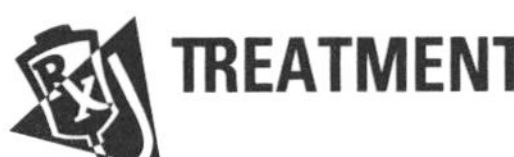

TREATMENT

- See Leishmaniasis, visceral (kala azar)
- See Leishmaniasis, cutaneous
- See Leishmaniasis, mucocutaneous

MEDICATIONS

- The drug of choice is a pentavalent antimonial, either sodium stibogluconate or meglumine antimoniate; resistance and treatment failures are increasing in frequency
- A generic formulation of sodium stibogluconate is equivalent in efficacy and safety to Pentostam. Treatment is started with a 200-mg Sb test dose followed by 20 mg Sb/kg/d. Intravenous is generally preferred to intramuscular administration
- Meglumine antimoniate (85 mg Sb/mL) is equal in efficacy and toxicity when used in equivalent Sb doses (20 mg Sb/kg/d)
- The selected drug is given on consecutive days: 28 days for visceral and mucocutaneous leishmaniasis and 20 days for cutaneous leishmaniasis. In certain regions of the world, because of resistance, longer courses are indicated. Side effects are more likely to appear with cumulative doses. Most common are gastrointestinal symptoms, fatigue, fever, myalgia, arthralgia, phlebitis, and rash; hemolytic anemia, hepatitis, renal and heart damage, and pancreatitis are rare
- Therapy is discontinued if the following occur: aminotransferases three to four times normal levels or significant arrhythmias, corrected QT intervals greater than 0.50 s, or concave ST segments
- Relapses should be treated at the same dosage level for at least twice the previous duration
- In the United States, only stibogluconate is available, obtainable from the Parasitic Drug Service, Centers for Disease Control and Prevention, Atlanta, GA 30333 (404-639-3670)
- Second-line drugs are amphotericin B and pentamidine. A lipid formulation, AmBisome, is considered by some workers to be the drug of choice for the treatment of visceral leishmaniasis

Amphotericin B

- For visceral leishmaniasis, the parenteral dosage of AmBisome is 3 mg/kg/d on days 1–5, 14, and 21 and may be repeated; the dosage for immunoincompetent persons is 4 mg/kg/d on days 1–5, 10, 17, 24, 31, and 38. There may be comparable effectiveness with cumulative doses of 3.75 or 7.5 mg/kg, given in five divided doses, over 5 days. Single-dose treatment is under evaluation
- Conventional amphotericin B deoxycholate, as given in India, is slow infusion (4–6 hours) of 1 mg/kg daily for 20 days

Pentamidine isethionate

- Pentamidine isethionate, 2–4 mg/kg IM (preferable) or IV, is given daily or on alternate days (15 doses for visceral and 4 doses for cutaneous leishmaniasis). For some forms of visceral leishmaniasis, it may be necessary to repeat treatment using up to twice the dose, but resistance may persist

Paromomycin (aminosidine)

- In cutaneous leishmaniasis, topical application in various formulations has variable success that differs by region
- One ointment is paromomycin 15%/methylbenzethonium chloride 12% in soft paraffin, applied BID for 15 days; skin reactions may occur. The ointment cannot be used in regions of mucocutaneous leishmaniasis as it does not prevent metastatic disease
- In parenteral treatment of refractory visceral leishmaniasis, paromomycin is promising but may cause renal or otic toxicity

Miltefosine

- Miltefosine, the first oral drug for the treatment of leishmaniasis, is approved in India for treatment of visceral leishmaniasis
- The daily dose of 2.5 mg/kg in two divided doses for 4 weeks has resulted in 95% cure rates
- Preliminary reports show efficacy in cutaneous leishmaniasis
- Side effects include vomiting (40%), diarrhea (20%), and occasional transient elevations of serum transaminases and creatinine and urea blood nitrogen
- It cannot be used in pregnancy due to teratogenic potential

Paromomycin (aminosidine)

- In cutaneous leishmaniasis, topical application in various formulations has variable success that differs by region

OUTCOME

FOLLOW-UP

- Patients should be monitored weekly for the first 3 weeks and twice weekly thereafter by serum chemistries, complete blood cell counts, and electrocardiography

PREVENTION

- Sand fly habitats are warm, humid, dark microclimates, including rodent burrows, rock piles, or tree holes; these are often in sylvatic areas near forests or semiarid ecosystems. Peridomestic sand flies are found on debris close to buildings. Biting is generally at twilight or at night but may occur in shaded areas during the day
- Partial protection is from permethrin applied to clothing, DEET repellent, avoidance of endemic areas (especially at night), use of mosquito coils, and use of fine-mesh insecticide-impregnated nets for sleeping (may be too warm for tropical use)

WHEN TO REFER

- All patients should be referred to a clinician with expertise in this disease

EVIDENCE

PRACTICE GUIDELINES

- National Guideline Clearinghouse
  - http://www.guideline.gov/summary/summary.aspx?doc_id=2573
  - http://www.guideline.gov/summary/summary.aspx?doc_id=3080

WEB SITE

- CDC—Division of Parasitic Diseases
  - http://www.cdc.gov/ncidod/dpd/parasites/leishmania/default.htm

INFORMATION FOR PATIENTS

- Centers for Disease Control
  - http://www.cdc.gov/ncidod/dpd/parasites/leishmania/factsht_leishmania.htm
- CDC Traveler's Health
  - http://www.cdc.gov/travel/diseases/leishmaniasis.htm
- National Institutes of Health
  - http://www.nlm.nih.gov/medlineplus/ency/article/001386.htm

REFERENCES

- Croft SL: Monitoring drug resistance in leishmaniasis. Trop Med Int Health 2001;6:899. [PMID: 11703844]
- Croft SL et al: Chemotherapy of leishmaniasis. Curr Pharm Des 2002;8:319. [PMID: 11860369]
- Desjeux P: The increase in risk factors for leishmaniasis worldwide. Trans R Soc Trop Med Hyg 2001;95:239. [PMID: 11490989]

Leishmaniasis, Cutaneous

KEY FEATURES

ESSENTIALS OF DIAGNOSIS

- **Old World cutaneous leishmaniasis**—moist or dry cutaneous leishmaniasis—is caused mainly by *Leishmania tropica, L major*, and *L aethiopica*, and is frequently self-healing
- **New World cutaneous leishmaniasis** is caused by *L mexicana* and *L amazonensis*

GENERAL CONSIDERATIONS

Agents of Old World cutaneous leishmaniasis

- *L tropica* is responsible for urban infections of dogs and humans
- It is found in the Middle East, India, East Africa, central Asian area of the former Soviet Union, Afghanistan, Pakistan, Turkey, Armenia, Greece, and southern France and Italy
- The incubation period is 2 months or longer, and healing is complete in 1–2 years
- *L major* infection causes lesions in dry or desert rural areas and is primarily a disease of desert rodents
- Human disease occurs in the Middle East, central Asian area of the former Soviet Union, Arabian peninsula, Afghanistan, and Africa (North, East, and sub-Saharan Africa from Senegal to Sudan and Kenya)
- *L aethiopica* infection occurs in the Ethiopian and Kenyan highlands
- In Afghanistan, Iraq, and Kuwait, the common agents are *L tropica* and *L major*, but *L infantum* has recently been isolated in Iraq. From 2002 to 2004, more than 600 cases of cutaneous leishmaniasis were confirmed in military personnel and 176 isolations of *L major* were made. In the US, for advice on treating such cases call 202-782-1663/8691

Agents of New World cutaneous leishmaniasis

- *L mexicana* (Texas, Oklahoma, Arizona, Mexico, Central America)
- *L amazonensis* (Amazonian basin, Venezuela, Panama)
- *L chagasi* (Central and South America)
- *L braziliensis* (Central and South America)

CLINICAL FINDINGS

SYMPTOMS AND SIGNS

- Cutaneous swellings appear 2 weeks to several months after sand fly bites and can be single or multiple
- Depending on the leishmanial species and host immune response, lesions begin as small papules and develop into nonulcerated dry plaques or large encrusted ulcers with well-demarcated raised and indurated margins
- Satellite lesions may be present
- The lesions are painless unless secondarily infected
- Local lymph nodes may be enlarged
- Systemic symptoms are rare, but a low-grade fever of short duration may be present at the onset
- For most species, healing usually occurs spontaneously from months to 1–3 years, starting with central granulation tissue that spreads peripherally

Old World cutaneous leishmaniasis

- The lesions of *L tropica* infection tend to be single and dry, to ulcerate slowly or not at all, and to persist for a year or longer
- Leishmaniasis recidivans is a relapsing form of *L tropica* infection in which the primary lesion nearly heals, lateral spread with central healing follows, and scarring can be extensive; it is associated with hypersensitivity and a strongly positive skin test but scarce amastigotes
- Visceral involvement by *L tropica* has been reported rarely (including after troop exposure in Operation Desert Storm) and is relatively resistant to antimony treatment
- *L major* lesions are characterized by multiple, wet, rapidly ulcerating sores with crusting. Spontaneous healing is generally complete in 6–12 months
- *L aethiopica* infection can cause ulceration, rarely. Spontaneous healing is slow over several years

New World cutaneous leishmaniasis

- The lesions are usually ulcers, but vegetative, verrucous, or nodular lesions may also occur
- *L mexicana* ("chiclero's ulcer") produces destructive lesions on the ear cartilage
- Up to 80% of *L braziliensis* cutaneous lesions progress to espundia (see Leishmaniasis, mucocutaneous); some *L braziliensis* complex strains also show a chain of palpable local lymph nodes, and some *L mexicana* and South American strains can cause diffuse cutaneous leishmaniasis

DIFFERENTIAL DIAGNOSIS

- Hansen's disease (leprosy)
- Fungal infection
- Cutaneous tuberculosis
- Neoplasm
- Syphilis
- Sarcoidosis
- Yaws
- *L donovani* [see Leishmaniasis, visceral (kala azar)] sometimes causes cutaneous disease with visceral manifestations

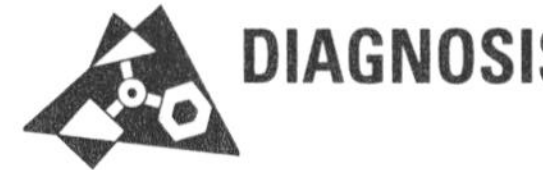

DIAGNOSIS

LABORATORY TESTS

- Definitive diagnosis is made by identification of the organisms
- Microscopic examination of skin scrapings has limited sensitivity, particularly in chronic infections
- Where available after culture, species identification should be done by molecular methods
- The skin test becomes positive within 3 months and remains positive for life; false positives occur
- Serological tests are unreliable. Antibody may be undetectable or appear only at low levels after 4–6 weeks; cross-reactions occur including with leprosy

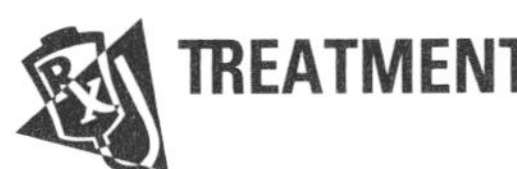

TREATMENT

MEDICATIONS

- **Old World leishmaniasis**, especially in the Middle East, is generally self-healing in about 6 months
  - No treatment may be needed for small, unobtrusive lesions that are healing
- Parenteral sodium stibogluconate (20–28 days) should be used to treat large or multiple lesions or lesions that are on cosmetically or functionally important areas (eg, the wrist)
- Complete healing may not be evident until weeks after the first or second course of treatment
- Amphotericin B desoxycholate and pentamidine are used for failures. Pentamidine is often effective against *L aethiopica* lesions and ketoconazole (400–600 mg/day for 4–6 weeks) against *L major* and *L* (*V*) *panamensis*
- Milefosine (2.5 mg/kg/d for 4 weeks), fluconazole (200 mg/kg/d for 6 weeks), and ketoconazole (600 mg/kg/d for 4 weeks) are under evaluation
- Paromomycin ointment may also be effective against *L tropica*
- In **New World** *L mexicana* infections from Mexico and Central America, solitary nodules or ulcers in inconspicuous sites generally heal spontaneously
- Variable success has been had with paromomycin ointment, ketoconazole, heat applications, or metronidazole (750 mg PO TID for 10 days)
- Preliminary trials with miltefosine (150 mg PO for 3–4 weeks) had reported cure rates of 94%
- Treat lesions on the ear, face, or hands with sodium stibogluconate
- Cutaneous lesions acquired in regions of mucocutaneous leishmaniasis may be due to *L braziliensis*, *L guyanensis*, or *L panamensis;* treat with a full course of sodium stibogluconate

THERAPEUTIC PROCEDURES

- Other treatments for less severe Old World disease are physical measures (local cryotherapy or heat therapy, electrocoagulation, surgical removal) and intralesional injection of sodium stibogluconate

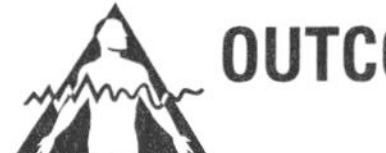

OUTCOME

COMPLICATIONS

- Pyogenic complications may be followed by lymphangitis or erysipelas
- Contraction of scars can cause deformities and disfigurement, especially if lesions are on the face

Diffuse cutaneous leishmaniasis

- An uncommon complication is diffuse cutaneous leishmaniasis, caused by the *L mexicana* complex and *L aethiopica*
- It is an anergic form with nodular lesions and high parasite count
- Nonulcerating lesions resembling lepromatous leprosy occur over the entire body
- The skin test is negative, but amastigotes are abundant
- In spite of repeated doses of antimony, pentamidiine, or amphotericin, cures are rare

WHEN TO REFER

- All patients should be referred to a clinician with expertise in this disease

EVIDENCE

WEB SITES

- Centers for Disease Control and Prevention: Leishmaniasis Professional Information
  - http://www.dpd.cdc.gov/dpdx/HTML/Leishmaniasis.htm
- World Health Organization: Leishmaniasis
  - http://www.who.int/leishmaniasis/en/

INFORMATION FOR PATIENTS

- Centers for Disease Control and Prevention: Leishmania Infection
  - http://www.cdc.gov/ncidod/dpd/parasites/leishmania/factsht_leishmania.htm
- Centers for Disease Control and Prevention: Protection Against Mosquitoes and Other Arthropods
  - http://www.cdc.gov/travel/bugs.htm
- MedlinePlus: Leishmaniasis Interactive Tutorial
  - http://www.nlm.nih.gov/medlineplus/tutorials/leishmaniasis.html
- MedlinePlus: Leishmaniasis
  - http://www.nlm.nih.gov/medlineplus/ency/article/001386.htm

REFERENCES

- Alrajhi AA et al: Fluconazole for the treatment of cutaneous leishmaniasis caused by *Leishmania major.* N Engl J Med 2002;346:891. [PMID: 11907288]
- Esfandiarpour I et al: Evaluating the efficacy of allopurinol and meglumine antimoniate (Glucantime) in the treatment of cutaneous leishmaniasis. Int J Dermatol 2002;41:521. [PMID: 12207774]
- Fisher C et al: Development status of miltefosine as first oral drug in visceral and cutaneous leishmaniasis. Med Microbiol Immunol 2001;190:85. [PMID: 11770118]
- Hepburn NC: Management of cutaneous leishmaniasis. Curr Opin Infect Dis 2001;14:151. [PMID: 11979125]

Leishmaniasis, Visceral (Kala Azar)

KEY FEATURES

ESSENTIALS OF DIAGNOSIS

- An infection of the reticuloendothelial system
- Symptoms include fever, hepatosplenomegaly, and pancytopenia, and leads to death without treatment

GENERAL CONSIDERATIONS

- The disease is caused mainly by the *Leishmania donovani* complex: *L donovani* (northeastern India, Bangladesh, Nepal, Southwest Asia, Sudan, Ethiopia, Kenya, Uganda, scattered foci in sub-Saharan Africa, and northern and eastern China); *L infantum* (Mediterranean littoral, Middle East, China, central and southwestern Asia, Ethiopia, Sudan, Afghanistan, Pakistan); and *L chagasi* (South America, Central America, Mexico)
- Two other species—*L tropica* in the Middle East, the Mediterranean littoral, Kenya, India, and western Asia and *L amazonensis* in the Amazon Basin—cause visceral leishmaniasis in a few patients, generally in a milder form
- Although humans are the major reservoir, animal reservoirs such as the dog, other canids, and rodents are important
- In the United States and Canada, foxhounds and other breeds of dogs and wild canids have been found to be serologically positive; *L infantum* has been isolated. There have been no findings in humans
- The incubation period is usually 4–6 months (range: 10 days to 24 months)
- In each locale, the disease has its own peculiar clinical and epidemiological features

DEMOGRAPHICS

- More than 500,000 cases occur yearly
- In HIV-infected persons—with or without AIDS—visceral leishmaniasis can be an opportunistic infection

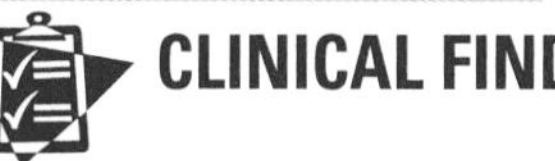

CLINICAL FINDINGS

SYMPTOMS AND SIGNS

- A local nonulcerating nodule at the site of the bite may precede systemic manifestations but usually is inapparent
- The onset may be acute (as early as 2 weeks after infection) or insidious
- Fever often peaks twice daily, with chills and sweats, weakness, weight loss, cough, and diarrhea
- The spleen progressively becomes huge, hard, and nontender; the liver is somewhat enlarged, and generalized lymphadenopathy is common
- Petechiae, bleeding from the nose and gums, jaundice, edema, and ascites may occur
- Hyperpigmentation, especially on the hands, feet, abdomen, and forehead, is marked in light-skinned patients
- In blacks, there may be warty eruptions or skin ulcers
- Wasting is progressive; death, often due to intercurrent infection, occurs within months to 1–2 years
- In some regions, oral and nasopharyngeal or cutaneous manifestations occur with or without visceral involvement

DIFFERENTIAL DIAGNOSIS

- Leukemia or lymphoma
- Cirrhosis
- Tuberculosis
- Histoplasmosis
- Infectious mononucleosis
- Brucellosis
- Malaria
- Typhoid fever
- Schistosomiasis
- African trypanosomiasis
- Tropical splenomegaly syndrome

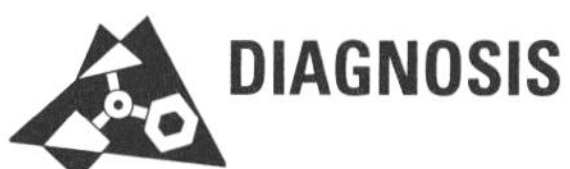

DIAGNOSIS

LABORATORY TESTS

- On occasion, the organism can be found in buffy coat preparations of blood, particularly obtained at night
- More commonly, the diagnosis depends on stained smears, touch preparations, culture, or animal inoculation of aspirated marrow, liver, enlarged lymph nodes, or spleen
- In immunocompetent persons, serological tests are sensitive (>90%) but false positives may occur, especially in malaria and typhoid fever
- The direct agglutination IgM test and the ELISAs become positive early; the immunofluorescent IgG test becomes positive in most persons at a titer of 1:256 or higher. After treatment, the tests remain positive for months, though in immunoincompetent persons titers may be low or undetectable
- The leishmanin skin test is always negative during active disease and becomes positive months to years after recovery. The polymerase chain reaction has excellent sensitivity and specificity
- Other characteristic findings are progressive leukopenia (seldom over 3000/μL after the first 1–2 months), with lymphocytosis and monocytosis, normochromic anemia, thrombocytopenia, and eosinophilia
- There is a marked increase in total protein up to or greater than 10 g/dL owing to an elevated IgG fraction; serum albumin is 3 g/dL or less
- Liver function tests show hepatocellular damage
- Proteinuria may be present

DIAGNOSTIC PROCEDURES

- Although splenic aspiration is the most sensitive test, because of its hazard (intraabdominal bleeding and death) it should be reserved for last and should be performed only by experienced persons; contraindications are a soft spleen in the acute phase, a prolonged prothrombin time, severe anemia, and platelet counts under 40,000/μL

Leishmaniasis, Mucocutaneous p. 1100

Leishmaniasis, Visceral (Kala Azar)

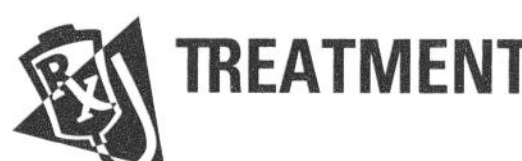

TREATMENT

MEDICATIONS

- See Leishmaniasis
- Sodium stibogluconate is the drug of choice; however, some prefer lipid formulations of amphotericin B (AmBisome)
- Whereas Mediterranean kala azar may respond to 10–15 doses of stibogluconate (one per day), the disease in Kenya, Sudan, and India requires at least 30 days of treatment. With incomplete response or relapse, the treatment should be repeated for up to 60 days
- Failure of stibogluconate or liposomal amphotericin B should lead to use of pentamidine
- Other drugs under evaluation individually or in combination with antimony, pentamidine, or amphotericin B are allopurinol, human gamma-interferon, atovaquone, and parenteral paromomycin (aminosidine)
- In Bihar, India, where the infection is becoming increasingly unresponsive to antimonials (currently 40%), liposomal amphotericin B is usually effective. Miltefosine, an oral treatment, shows high cure rates at a dosage of 100–150 mg daily for 4 weeks. Gastrointestinal side effects are frequent; the drug is contraindicated in pregnancy. It is not available in the United States

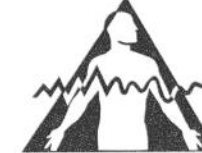

OUTCOME

COMPLICATIONS

- Post–kala azar dermal leishmaniasis may appear after apparent cure in the Indian subcontinent and east Africa. It may simulate leprosy, as multiple hypopigmented macules or nodules develop on preexisting lesions. Erythematous patches may appear on the face. Leishmaniae are present in the skin. Antimony treatment should be tried but is often ineffective

PROGNOSIS

- Without treatment, the fatality rate reaches 90%
- Early diagnosis and treatment reduce mortality to 2–5%
- Relapses (up to 10% in India and 30% in Kenya) are most likely to occur within 6 months after completion of treatment

WHEN TO REFER

- All patients
- For splenic aspiration

EVIDENCE

WEB SITE

- CDC—Division of Parasitic Diseases
  - http://www.cdc.gov/ncidod/dpd/parasites/leishmania/default.htm

PRACTICE GUIDELINES

- National Guideline Clearinghouse
  - http://www.guideline.gov/summary/summary.aspx?doc_id=2573
  - http://www.guideline.gov/summary/summary.aspx?doc_id=3080

INFORMATION FOR PATIENTS

- Centers for Disease Control
  - http://www.cdc.gov/ncidod/dpd/parasites/leishmania/factsht_leishmania.htm
- CDC Traveler's Health
  - http://www.cdc.gov/travel/diseases/leishmaniasis.htm
- National Institutes of Health
  - http://www.nlm.nih.gov/medlineplus/ency/article/001386.htm

REFERENCES

- Guerin PJ et al: Visceral leishmaniasis: current status of control, diagnosis, and treatment, and a proposed research and development agenda. Lancet Infect Dis 2002;2:494. [PMID: 12150849]
- Murray HW: Clinical and experimental advances in treatment of visceral leishmaniasis. Antimicrob Agents Chemother 2001;45:2185. [PMID: 11451673]
- Pintado V et al: HIV-associated visceral leishmaniasis. Clin Microbiol Infect 2001;7:291. [PMID: 11442562]
- Sundar S et al: Low-dose liposomal amphotericin B in refractory Indian visceral leishmaniasis: a multicenter study. Am J Trop Med Hyg 2002;66:143. [PMID: 12135284]

Leprosy

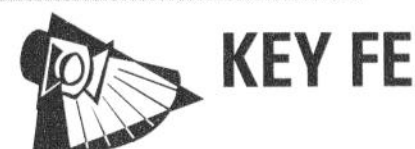

KEY FEATURES

ESSENTIALS OF DIAGNOSIS

- Pale, anesthetic macular—or nodular and erythematous—skin lesions
- Superficial nerve thickening with associated anesthesia
- History of residence in endemic area in childhood
- Acid-fast bacilli in skin lesions or nasal scrapings, or characteristic histological nerve changes

GENERAL CONSIDERATIONS

- A chronic infectious disease caused by the acid-fast rod *Mycobacterium leprae*
- The mode of transmission probably is respiratory droplets and involves prolonged exposure in childhood
- The disease is divided into two distinct types: lepromatous and tuberculoid
- The lepromatous type occurs in persons with defective cellular immunity
- In the tuberculoid type, cellular immunity is intact and the course is more benign

DEMOGRAPHICS

- The disease is endemic in tropical and subtropical Asia, Africa, Central and South America, and the Pacific regions
- India, Myanmar, and Nepal have 70% of the cases

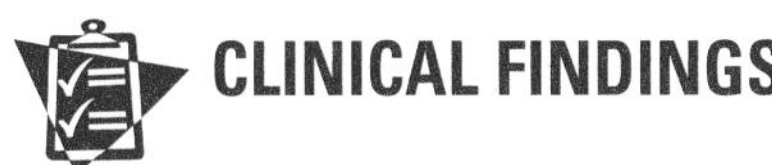

CLINICAL FINDINGS

SYMPTOMS AND SIGNS

- The onset is insidious
- The lesions involve the cooler body tissues: skin, superficial nerves, nose, pharynx, larynx, eyes, and testicles
- Skin lesions may occur as pale, anesthetic macular lesions 1–10 cm in diameter; discrete erythematous, infiltrated nodules 1–5 cm in diameter; or diffuse skin infiltration
- Neurological disturbances are caused by nerve infiltration and thickening, with resultant anesthesia, and motor abnormalities
- Bilateral ulnar neuropathy is highly suggestive

Lepromatous type

- The course is progressive and malignant, with nodular skin lesions and slow, symmetric nerve involvement

Tuberculoid type

- The course is more benign and less progressive, with macular skin lesions and severe asymmetric nerve involvement of sudden onset
- Intermediate ("borderline") cases are frequent. Eye involvement (keratitis and iridocyclitis), nasal ulcers, epistaxis, anemia, and lymphadenopathy may occur

DIFFERENTIAL DIAGNOSIS

- Systemic lupus erythematosus
- Sarcoidosis
- Syphilis
- Erythema nodosum
- Erythema multiforme
- Cutaneous tuberculosis
- Vitiligo
- Scleroderma
- Mycosis fungoides
- Diffuse cutaneous leishmaniasis
- Neuropathy due to other causes, eg, amyloidosis

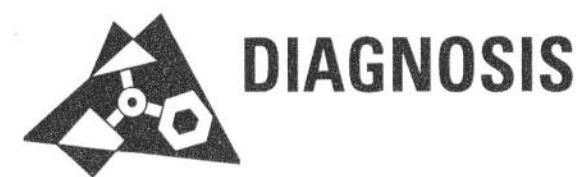

DIAGNOSIS

LABORATORY TESTS

- *M leprae* does not grow in artificial media but does grow in the footpads of armadillos
- The lepromatous type: abundant acid-fast bacilli in the skin lesions and a negative lepromin skin test
- The tuberculoid type: few bacilli present in the lesions and a positive lepromin skin test

DIAGNOSTIC PROCEDURES

- Laboratory confirmation requires the demonstration of acid-fast bacilli in a skin biopsy
- Biopsy of skin or of a thickened involved nerve also gives a typical histological picture

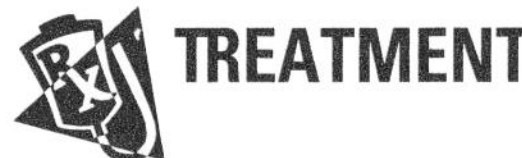

TREATMENT

MEDICATIONS

- Combination therapy is recommended for treatment of all types of leprosy
- For borderline and lepromatous cases, a three-drug regimen such as dapsone, 50–100 mg/day, clofazimine, 50 mg/day, and rifampin, 10 mg/kg/day (up to 600 mg/day), all given orally, should be used. The triple-drug combination should be administered for a minimum of 2–3 years and, ideally, until all biopsies are negative for acid-fast bacilli
- For indeterminate and tuberculoid leprosy, the dapsone-rifampin combination is recommended for 6–12 months, often followed by a course of dapsone alone for 2 or more years

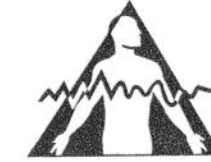

OUTCOME

COMPLICATIONS

- Renal failure and hepatomegaly from secondary amyloidosis may occur with long-standing disease
- Two reactional states—erythema nodosum leprosum and the reversal reaction—may occur as a consequence of therapy
- Erythema nodosum leprosum
  - Typical of lepromatous leprosy
  - Is a consequence of immune injury from antigen-antibody complex deposition in skin and other tissues (nerves)
  - Fever and systemic involvement may be seen
  - Prednisone, 60 mg/day, or thalidomide, 300 mg/day (in the nonpregnant patient only), is effective. Improvement is expected within a few days after initiating prednisone, and thereafter the dose may be tapered over several weeks to avoid recurrence. Thalidomide is also tapered over several weeks to a 100-mg bedtime dose
  - Usually confined to the first year of therapy, and prednisone or thalidomide can be discontinued after that
- The reversal reaction
  - Typical of borderline lepromatous leprosy
  - Probably results from enhanced host immunity
  - Skin lesions and nerves become swollen and tender, but systemic manifestations are not seen
  - Thalidomide is ineffective and prednisone, 60 mg/day, is indicated
  - Reversal reactions tend to recur, and the dose of prednisone should be slowly tapered over weeks to months
  - Therapy for leprosy should not be discontinued during treatment of reactional states

PROGNOSIS

- In untreated cases, disfigurement due to the skin infiltration and nerve involvement may be extreme, leading to trophic ulcers, bone resorption, and loss of digits

WHEN TO REFER

- Consultation with a physician experienced in the treatment of leprosy is suggested

PREVENTION

- Elimination efforts are to reach populations that have not yet received multidrug therapy services

EVIDENCE

WEB SITES

- CDC—Division of Bacterial and Mycotic Diseases
  - http://www.cdc.gov/ncidod/dbmd/
- Karolinska Institute—Directory of Bacterial Infections and Mycoses
  - http://www.mic.ki.se/Diseases/C01.html

INFORMATION FOR PATIENTS

- Centers for Disease Control
  - http://www.cdc.gov/ncidod/dbmd/diseaseinfo/hansens_t.htm
- National Institutes of Health
  - http://www.nlm.nih.gov/medlineplus/ency/article/001347.htm

REFERENCE

- Ustianowski AP et al: Leprosy: current diagnostic and treatment approaches. Curr Opin Infect Dis 2003;16:421. [PMID: 14501994]

Author(s)

Henry F. Chambers, MD

Leptospirosis

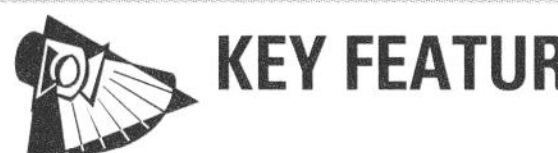

KEY FEATURES

ESSENTIALS OF DIAGNOSIS

- Leptospirosis is an acute and often severe infection caused by *Leptospira interrogans,* a diverse organism of 23 serogroups and over 200 serovars
- The three most common serovars are *Leptospira icterohaemorrhagiae* of rats, *Leptospira canicola* of dogs, and *Leptospira pomona* of cattle and swine
- *L icterohaemorrhagiae* causes the most severe illness
- Leptospirosis occurs worldwide, transmitted to humans by the ingestion of food and drink contaminated by the urine of the reservoir animal. The organism may also enter through minor skin lesions and probably via the conjunctiva
- The incubation period is 2–20 days

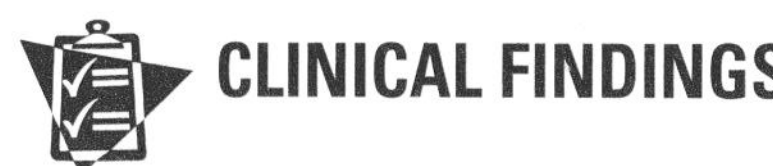

CLINICAL FINDINGS

SYMPTOMS AND SIGNS

- **Anicteric** leptospirosis is the more common and milder form of the disease and is often biphasic
- **Icteric** leptospirosis (Weil's syndrome) (usually caused by *L icterohaemorrhagiae*) is characterized by impaired renal and hepatic function, abnormal mental status, hemorrhagic pneumonia, and hypotension
- Initial or "septicemic" phase: abrupt fever to 39–40°C, chills, abdominal pain, severe headache, and myalgias, marked conjunctival suffusion
- Following a 1- to 3-day period of improvement, the second or "immune" phase begins
- Specific antibodies appear
- A recurrence of symptoms with the onset of meningitis
- Uveitis—unilateral or bilateral
- Rash and adenopathy
- Hemorrhagic pneumonia

DIFFERENTIAL DIAGNOSIS

- Bacterial meningitis
- Influenza
- Viral hepatitis
- Yellow fever
- Dengue
- Hemorrhagic fever, eg, hantavirus
- Relapsing fever

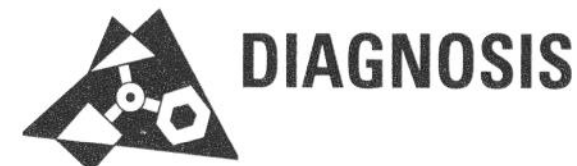

DIAGNOSIS

LABORATORY TESTS

- Anicteric leptospirosis: leptospires can be isolated from blood, cerebrospinal fluid, and tissues
- Leukocyte count may be normal or as high as 50,000/μL
- Urine bile, protein, casts, and red cells
- Uremia
- Elevated bilirubin and aminotransferases in 75%
- Elevated creatine kinase (> 1.5 mg/dL) in 50%
- Serum creatinine is usually elevated
- Organisms may be found in the cerebrospinal fluid. The organism may be identified by darkfield examination of the patient's blood or by culture on a semisolid medium (eg, Fletcher's EMJH). Takes 1–6 weeks to become positive. May be grown from the urine
- Diagnosis is usually made by serologic tests
- Agglutination tests show a four-fold or greater rise in titer
- Indirect hemagglutination, enzyme immunosorbent assay (EIA), and ELISA tests are also available. The IgM EIA is particularly useful [positive as early as 2 days into illness, extremely sensitive and specific (93%)]
- Polymerase chain reaction methods

IMAGING STUDIES

- Dictated by symptoms; hemorrhagic pneumonia has been described

DIAGNOSTIC PROCEDURES

- Lumbar puncture for central nervous system symptoms

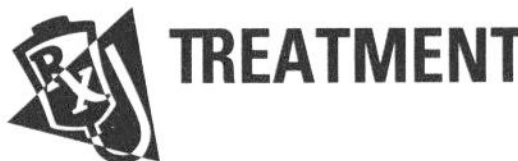

TREATMENT

MEDICATIONS

- Severe leptospirosis: penicillin, 6 million units IV QD, is the drug of choice
- Mild to moderate leptospirosis: doxycycline, 100 mg PO BID for 7 days, is effective if started early
- Jarisch-Herxheimer reactions may occur

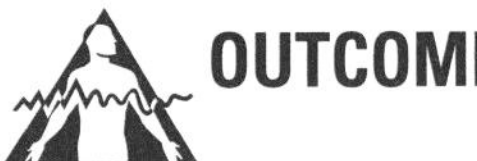

OUTCOME

FOLLOW-UP

- Routine

COMPLICATIONS

- Myocarditis, aseptic meningitis, renal failure, and pulmonary infiltrates with hemorrhage
- Iridocyclitis

PROGNOSIS

- Anicteric leptospirosis is usually self-limited, lasting 4–30 days, and almost never fatal. Complete recovery is the rule
- Icteric leptospirosis has symptoms and signs that often are continuous and not biphasic, and a 5–10% mortality rate (5% for those under age 30 and 30% for those over age 60)

WHEN TO REFER

- Refer for supportive care such as dialysis

WHEN TO ADMIT

- Admit for severe liver or renal disease

PREVENTION

- Prophylaxis: doxycycline, 200 mg PO once weekly during the risk of exposure

EVIDENCE

PRACTICE GUIDELINES

- Guidugli F et al: Antibiotics for preventing leptospirosis. Cochrane Database Syst Rev 2000;(4):CD001305. [PMID: 11034711]
- Guidugli F et al: Antibiotics for treating leptospirosis. Cochrane Database Syst Rev 2000;(2):CD001306. [PMID: 10796767]

WEB SITES

- Centers for Disease Control and Prevention Traveler's Information on Leptospirosis
  - http://www.cdc.gov/travel/diseases/lepto.htm
- Centers for Disease Control and Prevention—Division of Bacterial and Mycotic Diseases
  - http://www.cdc.gov/ncidod/dbmd/diseaseinfo/leptospirosis_t.htm

INFORMATION FOR PATIENTS

- Centers for Disease Control and Prevention Leptospirosis General Information
  - http://www.cdc.gov/ncidod/dbmd/diseaseinfo/leptospirosis_g.htm

REFERENCES

- Bharti AR et al: Leptospirosis: a zoonotic disease of global importance. Lancet Infect Dis 2003;3:757. [PMID: 14652202]
- Katz AR et al: Assessment of the clinical presentation and treatment of 353 cases of laboratory-confirmed leptospirosis in Hawaii, 1974–1998. Clin Infect Dis 2001;33:1834. [PMID: 11692294]
- Vinetz JM: Leptospirosis. Curr Opin Infect Dis 2001;14:527. [PMID: 11964872]

Author(s)

Richard A. Jacobs, MD, PhD

Leukemia, Acute

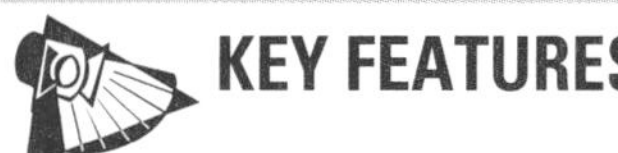

KEY FEATURES

ESSENTIALS OF DIAGNOSIS

- Short duration of symptoms, including fatigue, fever, and bleeding
- Cytopenias or pancytopenia
- > 20% blasts in bone marrow
- Blasts in peripheral blood in 90%

GENERAL CONSIDERATIONS

- A malignancy of the hematopoietic progenitor cell, which loses its ability to mature and differentiate; cells proliferate in uncontrolled fashion and replace normal bone marrow elements
- Most cases arise with no clear cause
- Radiation and some toxins (benzene) are leukemogenic; chemotherapeutic agents (procarbazine, melphalan, other alkylating agents, and etoposide) may cause leukemia
- Acute promyelocytic leukemia, characterized by chromosomal translocation t(15;17)
- Acute myelogenous leukemia (AML) usually categorized by morphology and histochemistry as acute undifferentiated leukemia (M0), acute myeloblastic leukemia (M1), acute myeloblastic leukemia with differentiation (M2), acute promyelocytic leukemia (M3), acute myelomonocytic leukemia (M4), acute monoblastic leukemia (M5), erythroleukemia (M6), or megakaryoblastic leukemia (M7)
- Acute lymphoblastic leukemia (ALL) classified by immunological phenotype as B- or T-cell lineage
- Cytogenetics are single most important prognostic factor

DEMOGRAPHICS

- ALL comprises 80% of acute leukemias of childhood; peak incidence between ages 3 and 7 years
- ALL also seen in adults, causing ~20% of adult acute leukemias
- AML chiefly occurs in adults with median age at presentation of 60 years and increasing incidence with advanced age

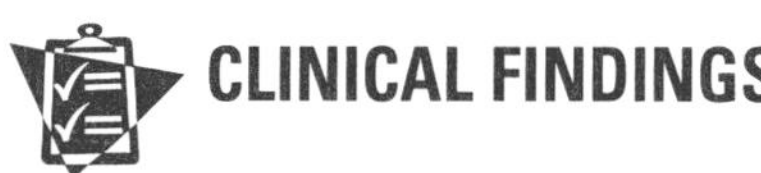

CLINICAL FINDINGS

SYMPTOMS AND SIGNS

- Clinical findings are due to replacement of normal bone marrow or infiltration of organs (skin, gastrointestinal tract, meninges)
- Gingival bleeding, epistaxis, or menorrhagia common
- Less commonly, widespread bleeding from disseminated intravascular coagulation (DIC) (in acute promyelocytic leukemia and monocytic leukemia)
- Increased susceptibility to infection with neutrophil count < 500/μL; infection (eg, cellulitis, pneumonia, and perirectal infections) within days is the rule when < 100/μL; death within a few hours may occur if treatment delayed; signs of infection may be absent; gram-negative bacteria or fungi (*Candida, Aspergillus*) are most common pathogens
- Gum hypertrophy
- Bone and joint pain
- Impaired circulation, causing headache, confusion, and dyspnea, with hyperleukocytosis (circulating blast count usually > 200,000/μL)
- Pallor, purpura, and petechiae common
- Hepatosplenomegaly and lymphadenopathy are variable
- Bone tenderness, particularly in sternum, tibia

DIFFERENTIAL DIAGNOSIS

Acute myelogenous leukemia

- Chronic myelogenous leukemia
- Myelodysplastic syndrome ("preleukemia")
- Left-shifted bone marrow recovering from toxic insult

Acute lymphoblastic leukemia

- Chronic lymphocytic leukemia
- Lymphoma
- Hairy cell leukemia
- Atypical lymphocytosis of mononucleosis or pertussis

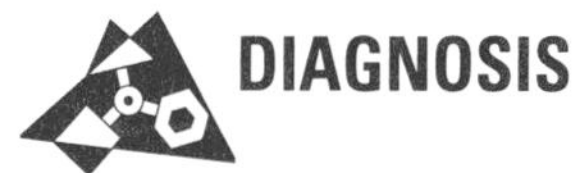

DIAGNOSIS

LABORATORY TESTS

- Combination of pancytopenia with circulating blasts on peripheral smear
- Blasts absent from peripheral smear in up to 10% ("aleukemic leukemia")
- Serum fibrinogen low, prothrombin time prolonged, and fibrin degradation products or fibrin D-dimers present if DIC
- Blasts in cerebrospinal fluid occur with meningeal leukemia in ~5% of cases at diagnosis
- Auer rod, an eosinophilic needle-like inclusion in cytoplasm of blasts, is pathognomonic of AML
- Lack of morphological or histochemical evidence of myeloid or monocytic lineage suggests diagnosis of ALL; demonstration of characteristic surface markers by immunophenotype confirms diagnosis of ALL
- In ALL, Philadelphia chromosome t(9;22) and t(4;11) has an unfavorable prognosis
- In AML, cytogenetic studies showing t(8;21), t(15;17), and inv(16)(p13;q22) have favorable prognosis; those showing monosomy 5 and 7 and complex abnormalities are unfavorable

IMAGING STUDIES

- Chest x-ray: mediastinal mass in ALL (especially T cell)

DIAGNOSTIC PROCEDURES

- Bone marrow is hypercellular, with > 20% blasts required for diagnosis of acute leukemia

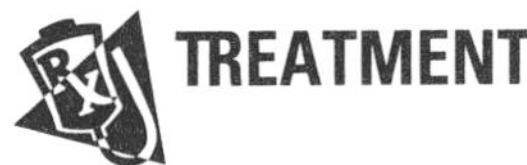

TREATMENT

MEDICATIONS

Remission induction therapy

- Initial treatment goal is to produce complete remission, defined as normal peripheral blood with resolution of cytopenias, normal bone marrow with no excess blasts, and normal clinical status
- AML: combination of an anthracycline (daunorubicin or idarubicin) plus cytarabine
- Acute promyelocytic leukemia: combination of all-*trans*-retinoic acid, a vitamin A analog that leads to terminal differentiation of acute promyelocytic leukemia cells, with anthracyclines
- ALL: combination chemotherapy, including daunorubicin, vincristine, prednisone, and asparaginase

Postremission therapy

- Once in remission, postremission therapy (chemotherapy or autologous or allogeneic transplantation, depending on age, clinical status, leukemia type) is given with curative intent
- Acute promyelocytic leukemia: chemotherapy plus retinoic acid
- AML and ALL (average-risk patients): chemotherapy, autologous transplantation, or allogeneic transplantation
- Antibiotics for infection

THERAPEUTIC PROCEDURES

- AML: Allogeneic transplantation is treatment of choice if no remission or high-risk cytogenetics, but cure rates only 20%
- ALL: Allogeneic transplantation if adverse cytogenetics or poor responses to chemotherapy; autologous transplantation is an option in patients without a suitable donor
- Emergent leukapheresis and chemotherapy for hyperleukocytosis

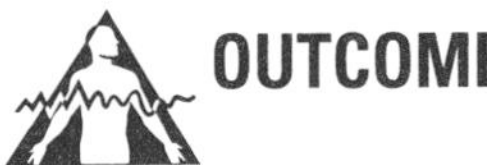

OUTCOME

FOLLOW-UP

- Repeat bone marrow

COMPLICATIONS

- Infection

PROGNOSIS

- AML: combination chemotherapy produces complete remissions in 70–80% of patients aged < 60 and 40–60% of patients aged > 60; postremission therapy leads to cure in 30–40% with chemotherapy, in 50% with autologous transplantation, and in 50–60% with allogeneic transplantation (for younger adults with HLA-matched siblings)
- Some AML types have better prognosis
- Acute promyelocytic leukemia: combination chemotherapy produces complete remissions in > 90%; postremission chemotherapy leads to cure in 60–70%
- ALL: combination chemotherapy produces complete remissions in 80–90%

WHEN TO REFER

- Refer all patients with acute leukemia to hematologist-oncologist

WHEN TO ADMIT

- Hyperleukocytosis (leukostasis syndrome)
- With initial diagnosis

EVIDENCE

PRACTICE GUIDELINES

- O'Donnell MR et al: NCCN Acute Myeloid Leukemia Practice Guidelines Panel. National Comprehensive Cancer Network: Acute Myeloid Leukemia v.2.2005
  - http://www.nccn.org/professionals/physician_gls/PDF/aml.pdf

WEB SITE

- National Cancer Institute: Leukemia
  - http://www.cancer.gov/cancertopics/types/leukemia

INFORMATION FOR PATIENTS

- American Cancer Society: Overview: Leukemia—Acute Lymphocytic
  - http://www.cancer.org/docroot/CRI/CRI_2_1x.asp?rnav=criov&dt=57
- American Cancer Society: Overview: Leukemia—Acute Myeloid
  - http://www.cancer.org/docroot/CRI/CRI_2_3x.asp?dt=82
- Leukemia & Lymphoma Society: Leukemia
  - http://www.leukemia-lymphoma.org/all_page?item_id=7026
- MedlinePlus: Leukemia Interactive Tutorial
  - http://www.nlm.nih.gov/medlineplus/tutorials/leukemia.html

REFERENCES

- Linker CA et al: Intensified and shortened cyclical chemotherapy for adult acute lymphoblastic leukemia. J Clin Oncol 2002;20:2464. [PMID: 12011123]
- Ruiz-Arguelles GJ et al: Allogeneic hematopoietic stem cell transplantation with non-myeloablative conditioning in patients with acute myelogenous leukemia eligible for conventional allografting: a prospective study. Leuk Lymphoma 2004;45:1191. [PMID: 15360000]
- Tallman MS et al: Acute promyelocytic leukemia: evolving therapeutic strategies. Blood 2002;99:759. [PMID: 11806975]

Author(s)

Charles A. Linker, MD

Leukemia, Chronic Lymphocytic

KEY FEATURES

ESSENTIALS OF DIAGNOSIS

- Most patients asymptomatic at presentation
- Splenomegaly typical
- Lymphocytosis > 5000/μL
- Mature appearance of lymphocytes
- Coexpression of CD19, CD5

GENERAL CONSIDERATIONS

- A clonal malignancy of B lymphocytes
- Usually indolent, with slowly progressive accumulation of long-lived small lymphocytes that are immunoincompetent
- Results in immunosuppression, bone marrow failure, and organ infiltration with lymphocytes
- Immunodeficiency also related to inadequate antibody production by abnormal B cells
- Prognostically useful staging system (Rai system): stage 0, lymphocytosis only; stage I, lymphocytosis plus lymphadenopathy; stage II, organomegaly; stage III, anemia; stage IV, thrombocytopenia

DEMOGRAPHICS

- Chronic lymphocytic leukemia (CLL) occurs mainly in older patients: 90% of cases occur at age > 50 and median age at presentation is 65

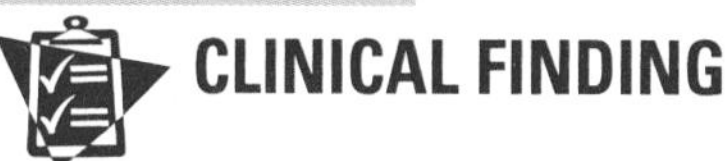

CLINICAL FINDINGS

SYMPTOMS AND SIGNS

- Incidentally discovered lymphocytosis in many
- Fatigue
- Lymphadenopathy in 80%
- Hepatomegaly or splenomegaly in 50%
- Occasionally, symptoms of hemolytic anemia or thrombocytopenia

DIFFERENTIAL DIAGNOSIS

- Atypical lymphocytosis of mononucleosis or pertussis
- Lymphoma in leukemic stage, especially mantle cell lymphoma
- Hairy cell leukemia

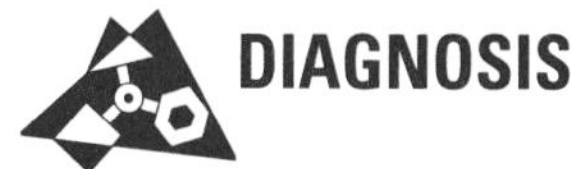

DIAGNOSIS

LABORATORY TESTS

- Isolated lymphocytosis
- White blood cell count usually > 20,000/μL and may be several hundred thousand
- Differential: usually 75–98% of circulating cells are lymphocytes
- Hematocrit and platelet count usually normal at presentation
- Autoimmune hemolytic anemia or thrombocytopenia present in 5–10%
- On peripheral smear, lymphocytes are small and mature, with condensed nuclear chromatin, and morphologically indistinguishable from normal small lymphocytes
- Larger and more immature cells in prolymphocytic leukemia (CLL variant)
- CLL is unusual in coexpressing B-lymphocyte lineage marker CD19 with T-lymphocyte marker CD5
- Hypogammaglobulinemia in half, becomes more common with advanced disease
- Serum protein electrophoresis: IgM paraprotein may be present in small amount

DIAGNOSTIC PROCEDURES

- Bone marrow is variably infiltrated with small lymphocytes
- Lymph node biopsy shows same pathological changes as in diffuse small cell lymphocytic lymphoma

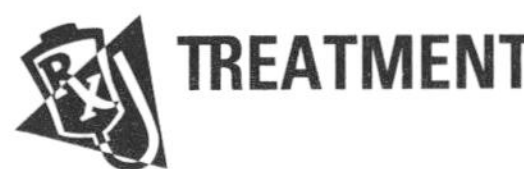

TREATMENT

MEDICATIONS

- Fludarabine IV infusion 5 days/week once a month for 4–6 months is first-line therapy; avoid in autoimmune hemolytic anemia (may exacerbate)
- Fludarabine plus rituximab produces better response rates and complete response
- Based on low toxicity and demonstrated survival benefit, fludarabine plus rituximab can be considered current standard of care
- Fludarabine plus cyclophosphamide and fludarabine plus cyclophosphamide plus rituximab also produce high response rates and are being studied
- Chlorambucil, 0.6–1 mg/kg PO q3 weeks for ~6 months, is a convenient, well-tolerated, and usually effective alternative for older patients
- Alemtuzumab for refractory CLL
- Prednisone for associated autoimmune hemolytic anemia or immune thrombocytopenia

SURGERY

- Splenectomy for associated autoimmune hemolytic anemia or immune thrombocytopenia

THERAPEUTIC PROCEDURES

- No specific therapy required in most cases of early indolent CLL
- Indications for treatment include progressive fatigue, symptomatic lymphadenopathy, or anemia or thrombocytopenia (symptomatic and progressive stage II disease or stage III/IV disease)
- Allogeneic transplantation potentially curative, but used only if CLL cannot be controlled by standard therapies
- Nonmyeloablative allogeneic transplantation is newer technique; may expand role of transplantation in CLL

OUTCOME

COMPLICATIONS

- Autoimmune hemolytic anemia or autoimmune thrombocytopenia in 5–10%
- Isolated lymph node transformation into aggressive large cell lymphoma (Richter's syndrome) despite stable systemic disease in ~5% of cases

PROGNOSIS

- CLL usually pursues an indolent course
- Overall, median survival is ~6 years, and 10-year survival is 25%
- Patients with stage 0 or stage I disease have median survival > 10 years
- Patients with stage III or stage IV disease have median survival of < 2 years
- Biological markers (eg, gene mutation status, CD38 expression, and cytogenetic abnormalities) useful in predicting outcomes of subsets of CLL patients
- Prolymphocytic leukemia, a variant of CLL, often pursues a more aggressive course

EVIDENCE

PRACTICE GUIDELINES

- Oscier D et al: Guidelines on the diagnosis and management of chronic lymphocytic leukaemia. Br J Haematol 2004;125:294. [PMID: 15086411]

WEB SITE

- National Cancer Institute: Chronic Lymphocytic Leukemia: Treatment
  - http://www.cancer.gov/cancertopics/pdq/treatment/CLL/healthprofessional

INFORMATION FOR PATIENTS

- American Cancer Society: Detailed Guide: Leukemia—Chronic Lymphocytic
  - http://www.cancer.org/docroot/CRI/CRI_2_3x.asp?rnav=cridg&dt=62
- Leukemia & Lymphoma Society: Chronic Lymphocytic Leukemia
  - http://www.leukemia-lymphoma.org/all_page?item_id=7059
- MedlinePlus: Leukemia Interactive Tutorial
  - http://www.nlm.nih.gov/medlineplus/tutorials/leukemia.html
- National Cancer Institute: Chronic Lymphocytic Leukemia: Treatment
  - http://www.cancer.gov/cancertopics/pdq/treatment/CLL/patient

REFERENCES

- Byrd JC et al: Randomized phase 2 study of fludarabine with concurrent versus sequential treatment with rituximab in symptomatic, untreated patients with B-cell chronic lymphocytic leukemia. Blood 2003;101:6. [PMID: 12393429]
- Keating M et al: Management guidelines for use of alemtuzumab in B-cell chronic lymphocytic leukemia. Clin Lymphoma 2004;4:220. [PMID: 15072613]

Author(s)

Charles A. Linker, MD

Leukemia, Chronic Myelogenous

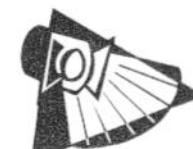

KEY FEATURES

ESSENTIALS OF DIAGNOSIS

- Strikingly elevated white blood cell count
- Markedly left-shifted myeloid series but low percentage of promyelocytes and blasts
- Presence of Philadelphia chromosome or *bcr/abl* gene

GENERAL CONSIDERATIONS

- Myeloproliferative disorder characterized by overproduction of myeloid cells
- Associated with characteristic chromosomal abnormality, the Philadelphia chromosome, a reciprocal translocation between long arms of chromosomes 9 and 22
- Translocated portion of 9q contains *abl*, a protooncogene, which is received on 22q, at the break point cluster (bcr) site
- The fusion gene *bcr/abl* produces a novel protein that possesses tyrosine kinase activity, leading to leukemia
- Approximately 5% of cases are Philadelphia chromosome negative by light microscope cytogenetics, though molecular studies demonstrate *bcr/abl* fusion gene and such patients have similar clinical outcomes as those with Philadelphia chromosome
- Entity formerly known as Philadelphia chromosome–negative chronic myelogenous leukemia (CML), now recognized as chronic myelomonocytic leukemia (CMML), a subtype of myelodysplasia
- "Chronic phase" of CML usually stable for years with normal bone marrow function
- Disease may progress to accelerated phase and after several years to blast crisis
- Progression often associated with added chromosomal defects superimposed on Philadelphia chromosome
- Blast crisis CML is morphologically indistinguishable from acute leukemia

DEMOGRAPHICS

- CML occurs mainly in middle age; median age at presentation is 42 years

CLINICAL FINDINGS

SYMPTOMS AND SIGNS

- Fatigue, night sweats, and low-grade fever
- Abdominal fullness related to splenomegaly
- Leukostasis clinical syndrome with blurred vision, respiratory distress, or priapism (rare)
- Splenomegaly (often marked)
- Sternal tenderness
- Fever in absence of infection, bone pain, and splenomegaly may mark disease acceleration
- Bleeding and infection related to bone marrow failure in blast crisis

DIFFERENTIAL DIAGNOSIS

- Reactive leukocytosis resulting from infection, inflammation, or cancer
- Other myeloproliferative disorder: essential thrombocytosis, polycythemia vera, or myelofibrosis

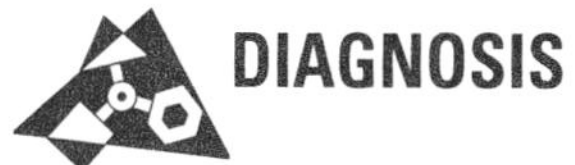

DIAGNOSIS

LABORATORY TESTS

- Markedly elevated white blood cell (WBC) count; median WBC at diagnosis is 150,000/μL, although some cases are discovered when WBC is only modestly increased
- WBC usually > 500,000/μL in rare cases of symptomatic leukostasis
- Peripheral blood smear: myeloid series left-shifted with mature forms dominating; blasts usually < 5%
- Basophilia and eosinophilia may be present
- Hematocrit is usually normal at presentation
- Red blood cell (RBC) morphology normal; nucleated RBCs rarely seen
- Platelet count may be normal or elevated (sometimes strikingly elevated)
- Platelet morphology usually normal, but sometimes abnormally large forms
- The Philadelphia chromosome may be detected in peripheral blood or bone marrow
- The *bcr-abl* gene is reliably found in peripheral blood by molecular techniques
- Progressive anemia and thrombocytopenia occur in accelerated and blast phases, and percentage of blasts in blood and bone marrow increases

DIAGNOSTIC PROCEDURES

- Bone marrow aspirate and biopsy: hypercellular, with left-shifted myelopoiesis
- Myeloblasts comprise < 5% of marrow cells in CML
- When blasts comprise > 20% of bone marrow cells, blast phase of CML is diagnosed

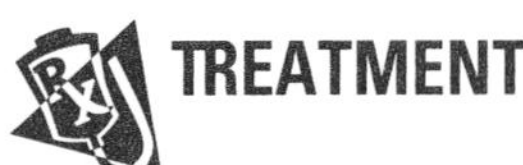

TREATMENT

MEDICATIONS

- Imatinib mesylate (Gleevec), an inhibitor of tyrosine kinase activity of the *bcr/abl* oncogene, 400 mg PO QD, for chronic phase CML; well tolerated; most common toxicities are mild nausea, periorbital swelling, rash, and myalgia
- Hydroxyurea, 0.5–2.5 g PO QD, is an alternative if imatinib is not tolerated
- Hydroxyurea is given without interruption because of rapid WBC rebound and dose adjusted to keep WBC count > 2000/μL and ideally near 5000/μL

THERAPEUTIC PROCEDURES

- Treatment usually not emergent even with WBC > 200,000/μL
- Allogeneic bone marrow transplantation indicated if age < 60 with HLA-matched sibling or if no cytogenetic response to imatinib after 6 months
- Chronic-phase disease, which recurs after allogeneic transplantation, can usually be reversed without additional chemotherapy by infusion of T lymphocytes from initial bone marrow donor
- Emergent leukapheresis is performed in conjunction with myelosuppressive therapy in rare instances of symptomatic leukostasis

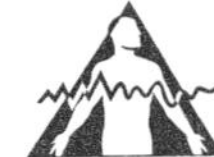

OUTCOME

FOLLOW-UP

- Response is assessed by (1) hematologic complete remission, with normalization of blood counts and splenomegaly, usually within several weeks to 3 months; (2) cytogenetic remission within 6–12 months; (3) quantitative assessment of the *bcr/abl* gene by PCR assay
- Bone marrow cytogenetics after 6 months of imatinib treatment to assess hematologic and cytogenetic remission

COMPLICATIONS

- Leukostasis clinical syndrome

PROGNOSIS

- Patients with complete cytogenetic response and > 3 log reduction in *bcr/abl* appear to have excellent prognosis, with 100% remaining in control at > 4 years
- Long-term data not yet available
- In the past, median survival was 3–4 years
- Imatinib mesylate results in hematologic control of chronic-phase disease in 98% of cases and may lead to marked improvements in survival rates
- Allogeneic bone marrow transplantation produces overall long-term disease-free survival in 60% and cure in 80% if patient age < 40 and transplant occurs within 1 year after diagnosis
- Infusion of T lymphocytes from initial bone marrow donor in recurrent disease can produce long-term remission in 50–70%

EVIDENCE

PRACTICE GUIDELINES

- O'Brien S et al: NCCN Chronic Myelogenous Leukemia Practice Guidelines Panel. National Comprehensive Cancer Network: Chronic myelogenous leukemia v.2.2005.
  - http://www.nccn.org/professionals/physician_gls/PDF/cml.pdf

WEB SITE

- National Cancer Institute: Chronic Myelogenous Leukemia: Treatment
  - http://www.cancer.gov/cancertopics/pdq/treatment/CML/HealthProfessional

INFORMATION FOR PATIENTS

- American Cancer Society: Detailed Guide: Leukemia—Chronic Myeloid
  - http://www.cancer.org/docroot/CRI/CRI_2_3x.asp?dt=83
- Leukemia & Lymphoma Society: Chronic Myelogenous Leukemia
  - http://www.leukemia-lymphoma.org/all_page?item_id=8501
- MedlinePlus: Leukemia Interactive Tutorial
  - http://www.nlm.nih.gov/medlineplus/tutorials/leukemia.html
- National Cancer Institute: Chronic Myelogenous Leukemia: Treatment
  - http://www.cancer.gov/cancerinfo/pdq/treatment/CML/patient/

REFERENCES

- Crossman LC et al: Imatinib therapy in chronic myeloid leukemia. Hematol Oncol Clin North Am 2004;18:605. [PMID: 15271395]
- Kalidas M et al: Chronic myelogenous leukemia. JAMA 2001;286:895. [PMID: 11509034]
- Kantarjian HM et al: Long-term survival benefit and improved complete cytogenetic and molecular response rates wih imatinib mesylate in Philadelphia chromosome-positive chronic-phase chronic myeloid leukemia after failure of interferon-alpha. Blood 2004;104:1979. [PMID: 15198956]
- Or R et al: Nonmyeloablative allogeneic stem cell transplantation for the treatment of chronic myeloid leukemia in first chronic phase. Blood 2003;101:441. [PMID: 12393604]

Author(s)

Charles A. Linker, MD

Leukemia, Hairy Cell

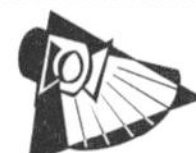

KEY FEATURES

ESSENTIALS OF DIAGNOSIS

- Pancytopenia
- Splenomegaly, often massive
- Hairy cells present on blood smear and especially in bone marrow biopsy

GENERAL CONSIDERATIONS

- Indolent cancer of B lymphocytes
- An uncommon form of leukemia

DEMOGRAPHICS

- Characteristically presents in middle-aged men
- Median age at presentation is 55 years
- Striking 5:1 male predominance

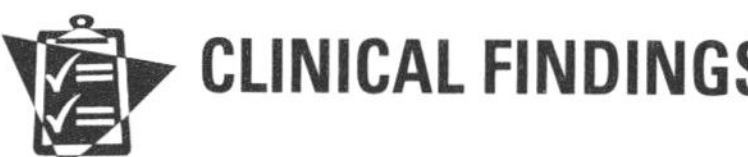

CLINICAL FINDINGS

SYMPTOMS AND SIGNS

- Gradual onset of fatigue
- Symptoms related to markedly enlarged spleen
- Increased susceptibility to infection
- Splenomegaly almost invariably present and may be massive
- Hepatomegaly in 50% of cases
- Lymphadenopathy uncommon

DIFFERENTIAL DIAGNOSIS

- Myelofibrosis
- Chronic lymphocytic leukemia
- Waldenström's macroglobulinemia
- Non-Hodgkin's lymphoma
- Aplastic anemia
- Other cause of bone marrow infiltration, eg, metastatic cancer, infection

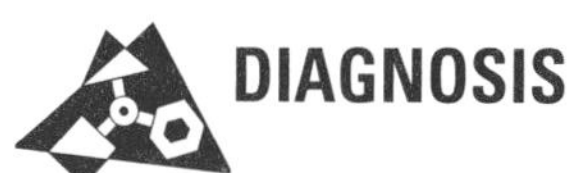

DIAGNOSIS

LABORATORY TESTS

- Complete blood count
  - Pancytopenia
  - Anemia nearly universal
  - Thrombocytopenia and neutropenia in 75% of patients
- Striking monocytopenia in nearly all, which is encountered in almost no other condition
- Peripheral blood smear: "hairy cells," with numerous characteristic cytoplasmic projections, usually present in small numbers
- Hairy cells have characteristic histochemical staining pattern, with tartrate-resistant acid phosphatase
- Hairy cells coexpress CD11c and CD22 on immunophenotyping

DIAGNOSTIC PROCEDURES

- Bone marrow aspirate: usually inaspirable (dry tap)
- Bone marrow biopsy establishes diagnosis made by characteristic morphology
- Pathologic examination of spleen shows marked infiltration of red pulp with hairy cells (in contrast to usual predilection of lymphomas to involve white pulp)

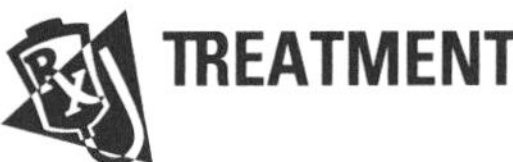

TREATMENT

MEDICATIONS

- Cladribine (2-chlorodeoxyadenosine; CdA), 0.14 mg/kg daily for 7 days; relatively nontoxic; produces benefit in 95% of cases
- Treatment with pentostatin produces similar results but more cumbersome to administer

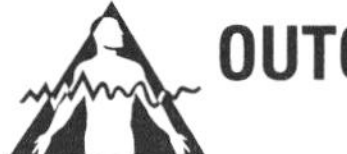

OUTCOME

PROGNOSIS

- Hairy cell leukemia usually indolent disorder; course dominated by pancytopenia and recurrent infections, including mycobacterial infections
- Formerly, median survival was 6 years, and only one-third survived > 10 years
- Development of new therapies has changed the prognosis
- Now, most live > 10 years
- With current trends in treatment, prognosis appears open-ended at this time
- Cladribine produces complete remission in > 80%; response long-lasting, with few patients relapsing in first few years

EVIDENCE

WEB SITE

- National Cancer Institute: Hairy Cell Leukemia Treatment
  - http://www.cancer.gov/cancertopics/pdq/treatment/hairy-cell-leukemia/HealthProfessional

INFORMATION FOR PATIENTS

- American Cancer Society: Treatment of Hairy Cell Leukemia
  - http://www.cancer.org/docroot/CRI/content/CRI_2_4_4X_Treatment_of_Hairy_Cell_Leukemia_HCL_62.asp?sitearea=
- Leukemia & Lymphoma Society: Hairy Cell Leukemia
  - http://www.leukemia-lymphoma.org/all_page?item_id=8507
- MedlinePlus: Leukemia Interactive Tutorial
  - http://www.nlm.nih.gov/medlineplus/tutorials/leukemia.html
- National Cancer Institute: Hairy Cell Leukemia
  - http://www.cancer.gov/cancerinfo/pdq/treatment/hairy-cell-leukemia/patient

REFERENCES

- Goodman GR et al: Extended follow-up of patients with hairy cell leukemia after treatment with cladribine. J Clin Oncol 2003;201:891. [PMID: 12610190]
- Jehn U et al: An update: 12-year follow-up of patients with hairy cell leukemia following treatment with 2-chlorodeoxyadenosine. Leukemia 2004;18:1476. [PMID: 15229616]
- Robak T: Monoclonal antibodies in the treatment of chronic lymphoid leukemias. Leuk Lymphoma 2004;45:205. [PMID: 15101704]

Author(s)

Charles A. Linker, MD

Leukoplakia & Erythroplakia

KEY FEATURES

ESSENTIALS OF DIAGNOSIS

Leukoplakia

- A white lesion that, unlike oral candidiasis, cannot be removed by rubbing the mucosal surface

Erythroplakia

- Similar to leukoplakia except that it has a definite erythematous component

Oral lichen planus

- Most commonly presents as lacy leukoplakia but may be erosive; definitive diagnosis requires biopsy

Oral cancer

- Early lesions appear as leukoplakia or erythroplakia; more advanced lesions are larger, with invasion into tongue such that a mass lesion is palpable; ulceration may be present

GENERAL CONSIDERATIONS

Leukoplakia

- About 5% represent either dysplasia or early invasive squamous cell carcinoma
- Histologically, there is often hyperkeratoses, occurring in response to chronic irritation

Erythroplakia

- Distinction from leukoplakia is important, because about 90% of cases of erythroplakia are either dysplasia or carcinoma

Oral lichen planus

- An inflammatory pruritic disease of the skin and mucous membranes
- Mucosal lichen planus must be differentiated from leukoplakia
- Erosive oral lesions require biopsy and often direct immunofluorescence for diagnosis because lichen planus may simulate other erosive diseases
- There is a low risk (1%) of squamous cell carcinoma arising within lichen planus

DEMOGRAPHICS

- Alcohol and tobacco use are the major etiological risk factors for oral carcinoma

CLINICAL FINDINGS

SYMPTOMS AND SIGNS

- Intraoral examination (lateral tongue, floor of the mouth, gingiva, buccal area, palate, and tonsillar fossae) and palpation of the neck for enlarged lymph nodes in patients over 45 who smoke tobacco or drink immoderately

Leukoplakia

- Any white lesion that, unlike oral candidiasis, cannot be removed by rubbing the mucosal surface
- Usually small

Erythroplakia

- A white lesion with an erythematous component that cannot be removed by rubbing the mucosal surface

Oral lichen planus

- Lacy leukoplakia but may be erosive
- Reticular pattern mimics candidiasis
- Erosive pattern mimics carcinoma

Oral cancer

- Early lesions appear as leukoplakia or erythroplakia; advanced lesions larger
- Invasion into tongue leads to palpable mass; ulceration may be present
- Biopsy essential for diagnosis
- Metastases to submandibular and jugulodigastric neck nodes are common

DIFFERENTIAL DIAGNOSIS

Oral leukoplakia

- Hyperkeratosis resulting from irritation
- Dysplasia or carcinoma
- Lichen planus
- Oral candidiasis
- Oral hairy leukoplakia

Erythroplakia

- Dysplasia or carcinoma
- Necrotizing sialometaplasia (when on hard palate)
- Ulcerative lichen planus

Oral lichen planus

- Oral cancer
- Candidiasis
- Erythema multiforme
- Pemphigus vulgaris
- Bullous pemphigoid
- Inflammatory bowel disease

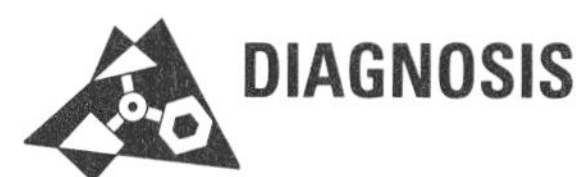

DIAGNOSIS

IMAGING STUDIES

- If squamous cell carcinoma is suspected, then metastatic evaluation of neck and imaging deep extent in oral cavity is warranted
- May include PET and MRI

DIAGNOSTIC PROCEDURES

- Any erythroplakic or enlarging leukoplakic area, and any mass lesion, should undergo incisional biopsy or exfoliative cytological examination
- Intraoral staining with 1% toluidine blue may aid in selection of the most suspicious biopsy site
- Fine-needle aspiration biopsy may be indicated if an enlarged lymph node is found

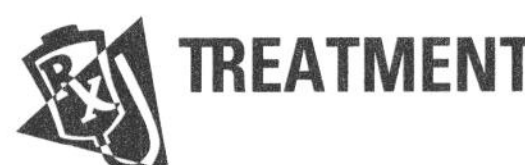

TREATMENT

MEDICATIONS

Lichen planus

- Therapy for confirmed diagnoses is management of pain
- Local and, if needed, systemic steroids are widely used

SURGERY

Oral cancer

- Small lesions are best treated surgically, often with a laser; if the tumor invades more than a few millimeters into the tongue, then consideration of the neck is important
- Larger tumors of the oral cavity are usually treated wth resection of the primary tumor, neck dissection, and postoperative irradiation
- Reconstruction, when needed, is done at the time of initial surgery
  - Vascularized free flaps, with bone if needed, are commonly used
  - Myocutaneous flaps may also be used

THERAPEUTIC PROCEDURES

- Small lesions may be treated with radiation therapy (external beam, often supplemented with an implant)
- Intraoral radiation is associated with dry mouth (xerostomia) and a low risk of osteoradionecrosis of the mandible
- Use of radiation limits future treatment options because a curative dose of radiation cannot be used again within the treatment field
- Tumors of the tonsillar fossa and base of tongue are usually best treated with radiation, often with concomitant chemotherapy, reserving surgery for salvage

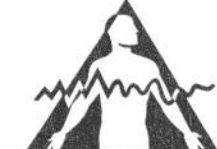

OUTCOME

FOLLOW-UP

- Leukoplakia, erythroplakia, lichen planus, and oral cancer require monitoring; early diagnosis of recurrent squamous cell carcinoma or a new primary lesion is key to management
- Commonly a patient with a prior malignancy is examined every 4–6 weeks in the first year, every 8–10 weeks in the second year, and every 3–4 months thereafter for several additional years; the incidence of second tumors is about 3–4% annually, likely associated with prior use of tobacco and/or alcohol
- Periodic PET scans and baseline post-treatment MRIs are frequently used in subsequent tumor surveillance

COMPLICATIONS

- Failure to recognize early tumors contributes to the need for more extensive intervention

PROGNOSIS

- Squamous cell carcinoma that invades less than 4–5 mm into the tongue has a < 10% rate of nodal metastasis
- Floor of mouth and alveolar ridge are associated with neck metastases
- Base of tongue and tonsillar fossa are usually associated with nodal metastases; late distant metastases may occur in as many as 30%
- Early-stage tumors (< 2 cm without nodal involvement) have cure rates above 90%

WHEN TO REFER

- Specialty referral should be sought early for both diagnosis and treatment
- Consider indirect or fiberoptic examination of the nasopharynx, oropharynx, hypopharynx, and larynx by an otolaryngologist–head and neck surgeon when there is oral erythroplakia, unexplained throat or ear pain, or unexplained oral or nasal bleeding

PREVENTION

- Smoking cessation and alcohol abatement programs

EVIDENCE

PRACTICE GUIDELINES

- Forastiere AA et al: NCCN Head and Neck Cancers Practice Guidelines Panel. National Comprehensive Cancer Network: Head and Neck Cancers v.1.2004.
  - http://www.nccn.org/professionals/physician_gls/PDF/head-and-neck.pdf

WEB SITE

- Baylor College of Medicine Otolaryngology Resources
  - http://www.bcm.tmc.edu/oto/othersa.html

INFORMATION FOR PATIENTS

- Mayo Clinic: Leukoplakia
  - http://www.mayoclinic.com/invoke.cfm?id=DS00458
- MedlinePlus: Leukoplakia
  - http://www.nlm.nih.gov/medlineplus/ency/article/001046.htm
- MedlinePlus: Lichen Planus
  - http://www.nlm.nih.gov/medlineplus/ency/article/000867.htm
- National Cancer Institute: Oral Cancer
  - http://www.cancer.gov/cancertopics/wyntk/oral

REFERENCES

- Bromwich M: Retrospective study of the progression of oral premalignant lesions to squamous cell carcinoma: a South Wales experience. J Otolaryngol 2002;31:150. [PMID: 12121018]
- Hegarty AM et al: Fluticasone propionate spray and betamethasone sodium phosphate mouthrinse: a randomized crossover study for the treatment of symptomatic oral lichen planus. J Am Acad Dermatol 2002;47:271. [PMID: 12140475]
- Neville BW et al: Oral cancer and precancerous lesions. CA Cancer J Clin 2002;52:195. [PMID: 12139232]
- Rosin MP et al: 3p14 and 9p21 loss is a simple tool for predicting second oral malignancy at previously treated oral cancer sites. Cancer Res 2002;62:6447. [PMID: 12438233]
- Sudbo J et al: Which putatively premalignant oral lesions become oral cancers? J Oral Pathol Med 2003;32:63. [PMID: 12542827]

Author(s)

Robert K. Jackler, MD
Michael J. Kaplan, MD

Lichen Planus

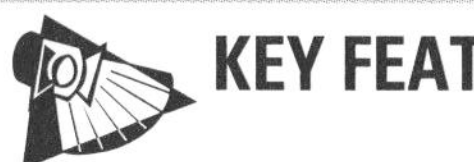

KEY FEATURES

ESSENTIALS OF DIAGNOSIS

- Pruritic, violaceous, flat-topped papules with fine white streaks and symmetric distribution
- Lacy lesions of the buccal mucosa
- Commonly seen along linear scratch marks (Koebner phenomenon) on anterior wrists, penis, legs
- Histopathologic examination is diagnostic

GENERAL CONSIDERATIONS

- An inflammatory pruritic disease of the skin and mucous membranes characterized by distinctive papules with a predilection for the flexor surfaces and trunk
- Three cardinal findings
  - Typical skin lesions
  - Mucosal lesions
  - Histopathologic features of band-like infiltration of lymphocytes and melanophages in the dermis

Oral lichen planus

- A relatively common (0.5–2% of the population) chronic inflammatory autoimmune disease
- May be difficult to diagnose clinically because of its numerous distinct phenotypic subtypes, eg, the reticular pattern may mimic candidiasis or hyperkeratosis, while the erosive pattern may mimic squamous cell carcinoma
- There is probably a low rate (1%) of squamous cell carcinoma arising within lichen planus (in addition to the possibility of clinical misdiagnosis)
- Drugs causing lichen planus–like reactions include
  - Gold
  - Streptomycin
  - Tetracycline
  - Iodides
  - Chloroquine
  - Quinacrine
  - Quinidine
  - Nonsteroidal anti-inflammatory drugs
  - Phenothiazines
  - Hydrochlorothiazide
- Hepatitis C infection is found with greater frequency in lichen planus patients than in controls in Europe and the United States
- A benign disease, but it may persist for months or years and may be recurrent

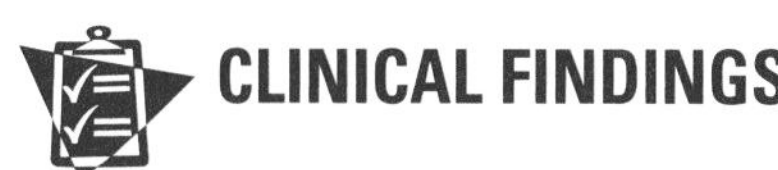

CLINICAL FINDINGS

SYMPTOMS AND SIGNS

- Itching is mild to severe
- The lesions are
  - Violaceous, flat-topped, angulated papules, 1–4 mm in diameter
  - Discrete or in clusters
  - Contain very fine white streaks on the surface (Wickham's striae) on the flexor surfaces of the wrists and on the penis, lips, tongue, and buccal and vaginal mucous membranes
- In the oral mucosa lichen planus may be confused with leukoplakia
- Mucosal lichen planus in the oral, genital, and anorectal areas may be erosive and painful
- The papules may become bullous
- The disease may be generalized
- The Koebner phenomenon (appearance of lesions in areas of trauma) may be seen

DIFFERENTIAL DIAGNOSIS

- Lichenoid drug eruption
- Psoriasis
- Lichen simplex chronicus
- Secondary syphilis
- Pityriasis rosea
- Discoid lupus erythematosus
- Graft-versus-host disease
- Mucosal lesions
  - Leukoplakia
  - Candidiasis
  - Erythema multiforme
  - Pemphigus vulgaris
  - Bullous pemphigoid
  - Lichen sclerosus
- Lichen planus on the mucous membranes must be differentiated from leukoplakia; erosive oral lesions require biopsy and often direct immunofluorescence for diagnosis since lichen planus may simulate other erosive diseases

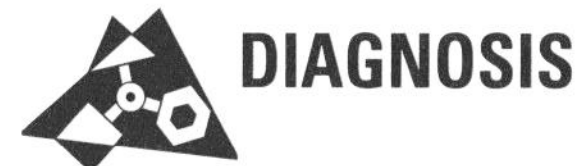

DIAGNOSIS

LABORATORY TESTS

- Confirmed by biopsy showing a band-like infiltration of lymphocytes and melanophages in the dermis

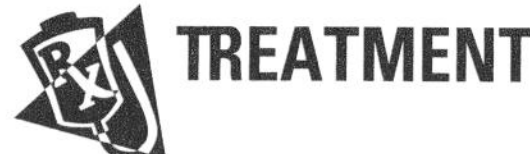

TREATMENT

MEDICATIONS

Topical therapy

- See Table 6
- Superpotent topical corticosteroid ointments
  - Examples are betamethasone dipropionate in optimized vehicle, diflorasone diacetate, clobetasol propionate, and halobetasol propionate
  - Apply twice daily for localized disease in nonflexural areaa
  - Aternatively, high-potency corticosteroid cream or ointment may be used nightly under thin pliable plastic film
- Tretinoin cream 0.05%: applied to mucosal lichen planus, followed by a corticosteroid ointment, may be helpful
- Topical tacrolimus
  - Appears effective in oral and vaginal erosive lichen planus, but long-term therapy is required to prevent relapse
  - Concern regarding absorption suggests monitoring blood counts when treating mucosal lesions

Systemic therapy

- Corticosteroids may be required in severe cases, or where the most rapid response to treatment is desired
- Unfortunately, relapse almost always occurs as the corticosteroids are tapered
- Isotretinoin and acitretin by mouth appear to be effective in some cases of oral and cutaneous lichen planus
- Psoralens plus long-wave ultraviolet light (PUVA)

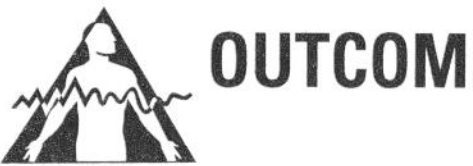

OUTCOME

PROGNOSIS

- Benign disease, but it may persist for months or years
- May be recurrent
- Hypertrophic lichen planus and oral lesions tend to be especially persistent, and neoplastic degeneration has been described in chronically eroded lesions

WHEN TO REFER

- If there is a question about the diagnosis, if recommended therapy is ineffective, or specialized treatment is necessary

EVIDENCE

WEB SITE

- American Academy of Dermatology
  - http://www.aad.org

INFORMATION FOR PATIENTS

- American Association of Family Physicians: Lichen Planus
  - http://familydoctor.org/600.xml
- American Academy of Dermatology: Lichen Planus
  - http://www.aad.org/public/Publications/pamphlets/LichenPlanus.htm
- Mayo Clinic: Lichen Planus
  - http://www.mayoclinic.com/invoke.cfm?objectid=0043F225-E973-4B80-9BE1ADC5EF8483B2
- MedlinePlus: Lichen Planus
  - http://www.nlm.nih.gov/medlineplus/ency/article/000867.htm

REFERENCES

- Katta R: Lichen planus. Am Fam Physician 2000;61:3319. [PMID: 10865927]
- Mignogna MD et al: Oral lichen planus: different clinical features in HCV-positive and HCV-negative patients. Int J Dermatol 2000;39:134. [PMID: 10692063]

Author(s)

Timothy G. Berger, MD

Lichen Simplex Chronicus

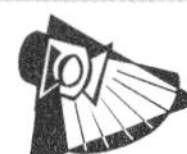

KEY FEATURES

ESSENTIALS OF DIAGNOSIS

- Chronic itching
- Dry, leathery, hypertrophic, lichenified plaques
- Appear on the neck, ankles, perineum, or almost anywhere

GENERAL CONSIDERATIONS

- A self-perpetuating scratch-itch cycle
- Intermittent itching incites the patient to scratch the lesions
- Itching may be so intense as to interfere with sleep

CLINICAL FINDINGS

SYMPTOMS AND SIGNS

- See Table 7
- Lichenified lesions with exaggerated skin lines overlying a thickened, well-circumscribed scaly plaque
- Predilection for nape of neck, wrists, external surfaces of forearms, lower legs, popliteal and antecubital areas, scrotum, and vulva
- The patches are rectangular, thickened, and pigmented

DIFFERENTIAL DIAGNOSIS

- Psoriasis (redder lesions having whiter scales on the elbows, knees, and scalp and nail findings)
- Lichen planus (violaceous, usually smaller polygonal papules)
- Atopic dermatitis (eczema)
- Nummular eczema or dermatitis (coin-shaped)
- Tinea corporis
- Chronic atopic dermatitis

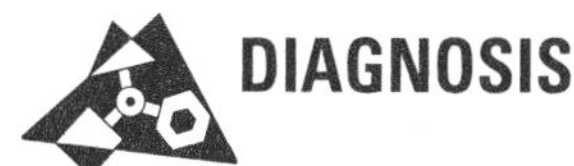

DIAGNOSIS

LABORATORY TESTS

- Clinical diagnosis

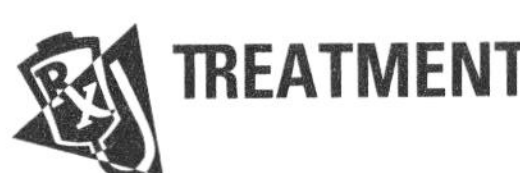

TREATMENT

MEDICATIONS

- See Table 6
- Clobetasol, halobetasol, diflorasone, and betamethasone dipropionate in augmented vehicle are effective without occlusion and are used twice daily for several weeks
- In some patients, flurandrenolide (Cordran) tape may be more effective, since it prevents scratching and rubbing of the lesion
- These superpotent corticosteroids are probably the treatment of choice but must be used with careful follow-up to avoid local side effects
- The injection of triamcinolone acetonide suspension (5–10 mg/mL) into the lesions may occasionally be curative

THERAPEUTIC PROCEDURES

- Use of tars, such as 10% LCD (liquor carbonis detergens) in triamcinolone 0.1% ointment, or continuous occlusion with DuoDerm (occlusive flexible hydrocolloid dressing) for 7 days at a time for 1–2 months, may also be helpful; the area should be protected and the patient encouraged to become aware of when he or she is scratching

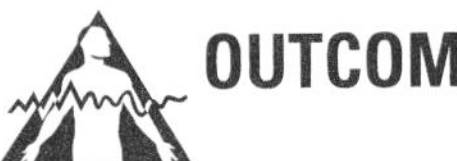

OUTCOME

PROGNOSIS

- The disease tends to remit during treatment but may recur or develop at another site

WHEN TO REFER

- If there is a question about the diagnosis, if recommended therapy is ineffective, or if specialized treatment is necessary

EVIDENCE

WEB SITES

- American Academy of Dermatology
  - http://www.aad.org
- MedlinePlus: Lichen Simplex Chronicus Image
  - http://www.nlm.nih.gov/medlineplus/ency/imagepages/2494.htm

INFORMATION FOR PATIENTS

- MedlinePlus: Lichen Simplex Chronicus
  - http://www.nlm.nih.gov/medlineplus/ency/article/000872.htm
- University of Michigan Health System: Neurodermatitis
  - http://www.med.umich.edu/1libr/aha/umskin18.htm

REFERENCE

- Novick CL: Unilateral, circumscribed, chronic dermatitis of the papillary-areolar complex: case report and review of the literature. Mt Sinai J Med 2001;68:321. [PMID: 11514919]

Author(s)

Timothy G. Berger, MD

Lipid Abnormalities

KEY FEATURES

ESSENTIALS OF DIAGNOSIS

- Elevated serum total cholesterol or low-density lipoprotein (LDL) cholesterol, low serum high-density lipoprotein (HDL) cholesterol, or elevated serum triglycerides
- Usually asymptomatic
- In severe cases associated with metabolic abnormalities, superficial lipid deposition occurs

GENERAL CONSIDERATIONS

- Cholesterol and triglycerides are the two main circulating lipids
- Elevated levels of LDL cholesterol are associated with increased risk of atherosclerotic heart disease
- High levels of HDL cholesterol are associated with lower risk of atherosclerotic heart disease
- The exact mechanism by which LDL and HDL affect atherosclerosis is not fully delineated
- Familial genetic disorders are an uncommon, but often lethal, cause of elevated cholesterol
- Familial genetic disorders should be considered in patients who have onset of atherosclerosis in their 20s or 30s

DEMOGRAPHICS

- More common in men than women before age 50
- More common in women than men after age 50
- More common in whites and Hispanics than among blacks
- Up to 25% of Americans have the metabolic syndrome that consists of a large waist circumference, elevated blood pressure, elevated triglycerides, low HDL cholesterol, and elevated serum glucose

CLINICAL FINDINGS

SYMPTOMS AND SIGNS

- Usually asymptomatic
- Extremely high levels of chylomicrons or VLDL particles are associated with eruptive xanthomas
- Very high LDL levels are associated with tendinous xanthomas
- Very high triglycerides (> 2000 mg/dL) are associated with lipemia retinalis (cream-colored vessels in the fundus)

DIFFERENTIAL DIAGNOSIS

- See Table 117

Hypercholesterolemia (cholesterol, elevated)

- Idiopathic
- Hypothyroidism
- Nephrotic syndrome
- Chronic renal insufficiency
- Obstructive liver disease
- Diabetes mellitus
- Anorexia nervosa
- Cushing's syndrome
- Familial, eg, familial hypercholesterolemia
- Drugs: oral contraceptives, thiazides (short-term effect), β-blockers (short-term effect), corticosteroids, cyclosporine

Hypertriglyceridemia (triglycerides, elevated)

- Alcohol
- Obesity
- Metabolic syndrome (insulin resistance, low HDL)
- Diabetes mellitus
- Chronic renal insufficiency
- Lipodystrophy, eg, protease inhibitors
- Pregnancy
- Familial
- Drugs: oral contraceptives, isotretinoin, thiazides (short-term effect), β-blockers (short-term effect), corticosteroids, bile-acid binding resins

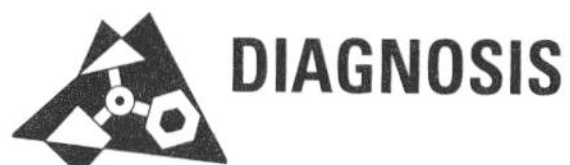

DIAGNOSIS

- Screen for lipid disorders in
  - Patients with coronary heart disease, peripheral vascular disease, aortic aneurysm, or carotid artery disease
  - Men older than 35 years and women older than 45 years if asymptomatic or no striking family history
  - Obtain fasting serum total cholesterol, HDL cholesterol, and triglyceride levels
  - LDL cholesterol can be estimated by the following formula: LDL cholesterol = (Total cholesterol) – (HDL) – (Triglycerides/5)
- Serum thyroid-stimulating hormone to screen for hypothyroidism
- Other tests only as indicated by symptoms and signs suggestive of a secondary cause
- LDL cholesterol (mg/dL) is classified into 5 categories: optimal, < 100; near optimal, 100–129; borderline high, 130–159; high, 160–189; very high, ≥ 190

TREATMENT

MEDICATIONS

- See Table 119
- Choice of whether to initiate drug therapy should be based on overall risk profile and LDL cholesterol level
- LDL cholesterol threshold for treatment depends on risk factors
- Presence of coronary heart disease (CHD), diabetes, cerebral vascular disease, peripheral vascular disease, or 10-year risk > 20% requires most aggressive therapy
- Presence of 2 or more risk factors, including smoking, hypertension, older age, and family history of CHD, and 10-year risk 10–20%, requires treatment at LDL ≥130 mg/dL
- Presence of 2 or more risk factors and 10-year risk < 10% requires treatment above LDL ≥ 160 mg/dL
- Presence of 1 or no risk factors requires treatment above LDL ≥190 mg/dL
- See Table 118
- **HMG-CoA reductase inhibitors** (statins)
  - Potent impact on LDL
  - Minimal impact on HDL
  - Best data for reducing coronary events, mortality
- **Niacin**
  - Moderate impact on LDL and HDL
  - Reduces triglycerides and has mortality benefit
  - High rates of intolerance, which can be improved with concomitant aspirin use
- **Bile acid binding resins** (eg, cholestyramine)
  - Moderate impact on LDL
  - Minimal impact on HDL
  - Reduce coronary events but not mortality
  - Mainly gastrointestinal side effects and can block the absorption of fat-soluble vitamins
  - Safe in pregnancy
- **Fibric acid derivatives** (eg, gemfibrozil)
  - Moderate impact on LDL and HDL
  - Reduce triglycerides
  - Reduce coronary events but not mortality
  - Side effects increased when taken with statins

THERAPEUTIC PROCEDURES

- For hypercholesterolemia, low-fat diets may produce a moderate (5–10%) decrease in LDL cholesterol
- Low-fat diet may also lower HDL cholesterol
- Substituting monounsaturated fats for saturated fats can lower LDL without affecting HDL
- In diabetics, control of hyperglycemia can improve lipid profile
- Exercise and moderate alcohol consumption can increase HDL levels
- For hypertriglyceridemia, primary therapy is dietary, including reducing alcohol, reducing fatty foods and excess dietary carbohydrates, and controlling hyperglycemia in diabetics

OUTCOME

- Fasting lipid panel 3–6 months after initiation of therapy
- Annual or biannual screening depending on risk factors
- Monitoring for side effects of therapy, such as liver enzyme elevation or myopathy in those on statins
- Atherosclerotic: myocardial infarction, stroke, and other vascular diseases
- Nonatherosclerotic: xanthomas and pancreatitis
- Metabolic syndrome patients are at increased risk for cardiovascular events
- Very high triglyceride levels (fasting triglyceride > 500 mg/dL) increase the risk of pancreatitis
- Refer patients with evidence of genetic disorders such as very high LDL or triglycerides to a lipid specialist
- Acute pancreatitis

EVIDENCE

- Update (2004) of the Third Report of the National Cholesterol Education Program Expert Panel on Detection, Evaluation, and Treatment of High Blood Cholesterol in Adults (2001)
  - http://www.guideline.gov/summary/summary.aspx?doc_id=5503&nbr=3746

WEB SITES

- American College of Cardiology
  - http://www.acc.org/
- National Heart, Lung, and Blood Institute
  - http://www.nhlbi.nih.gov/about/ncep/index.htm

INFORMATION FOR PATIENTS

- American Academy of Family Physicians: Cholesterol: What You Can Do to Lower Your Level
  - http://familydoctor.org/029.xml
- American Heart Association: Cholesterol
  - http://www.americanheart.org/presenter.jhtml?identifier=4488
- National Cholesterol Education Program: High Blood Cholesterol
  - http://www.nhlbi.nih.gov/health/public/heart/chol/wyntk.htm

REFERENCES

- Birjmohun RS et al: Efficacy and safety of high-density lipoprotein cholesterol-increasing compounds: a meta-analysis of randomized controlled trials. J Am Coll Cardiol 2005;45:185. [PMID: 15653014]
- Grundy SM et al; National Heart, Lung, and Blood Institute; American College of Cardiology Foundation; American Heart Association: Implications of recent clinical trials for the National Cholesterol Education Program Adult Treatment Panel III guidelines. Circulation 2004;110:227. [PMID: 15249516]
- Jenkins DJ et al: Direct comparison of a dietary portfolio of cholesterol-lowering foods with a statin in hypercholesterolemic participants. Am J Clin Nutr 2005;81:380. [PMID: 15699225]
- Mosca L et al; American Heart Association: Evidence-based guidelines for cardiovascular disease in women. Circulation 2004;109:672. [PMID: 14761900]
- Nissen SE et al: Effect of intensive compared with moderate lipid-lowering therapy on progression of coronary atherosclerosis: a randomized controlled trial. JAMA 2004;291:1071. [PMID: 14996776]
- Szapary PO et al: The triglyceride-high-density lipoprotein axis: an important target of therapy? Am Heart J 2004;148:211. [PMID: 15308990]
- Walsh JM et al: Drug treatment of hyperlipidemia in women. JAMA 2004;291:2243. [PMID: 15138247]
- Whitney EJ et al: A randomized trial of a strategy for increasing high-density lipoprotein cholesterol levels: effects on progression of coronary heart disease and clinical events. Ann Intern Med 2005;142:95. [PMID: 15657157]

Author(s)

Robert B. Baron, MS, MD

Liver Abscess, Pyogenic

KEY FEATURES

ESSENTIALS OF DIAGNOSIS

- Fever, right upper quadrant pain, jaundice
- Often in setting of biliary disease but up to 40% cryptogenic abscesses are seen on imaging study

GENERAL CONSIDERATIONS

- The liver can be invaded by bacteria via the portal vein (pylephlebitis); the common duct (ascending cholangitis); the hepatic artery, secondary to bacteremia; direct extension from an infectious process; and traumatic implantation of bacteria through the abdominal wall
- Ascending cholangitis resulting from biliary obstruction due to a stone, stricture, or neoplasm is the most common identifiable cause of hepatic abscess in the United States
- In 10% of cases, liver abscess is secondary to appendicitis or diverticulitis
- Up to 40% of abscesses have no demonstrable cause and are classified as cryptogenic. A dental source is identified in some such cases
- The most frequently encountered organisms are *Escherichia coli, Klebsiella pneumoniae, Proteus vulgaris, Enterobacter aerogenes,* and multiple anaerobic species. *Staphylococcus aureus* is usually the causative organism in chronic granulomatous disease
- Hepatic candidiasis is seen in immunocompromised patients and those with hematological malignancies
- Rarely, hepatocellular carcinoma can present as a pyogenic abscess because of tumor necrosis, biliary obstruction, and superimposed bacterial infection
- The possibility of an amebic liver abscess must always be considered

CLINICAL FINDINGS

SYMPTOMS AND SIGNS

- The presentation is often insidious
- Fever is almost always present and may antedate other symptoms or signs
- Pain may be a prominent complaint and is localized to the right hypochondrium or epigastric area
- Jaundice, tenderness in the right upper abdomen, and either steady or swinging fever are the primary physical findings

DIFFERENTIAL DIAGNOSIS

- Cholecystitis
- Cholangitis
- Acute hepatitis
- Amebic liver abscess
- Appendicitis
- Right lower lobe pneumonia
- Pancreatitis
- Echinococcosis (hydatid disease)
- Liver mass, eg, hepatocellular carcinoma

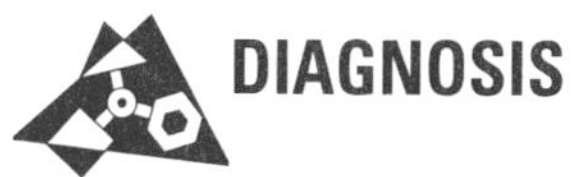

DIAGNOSIS

LABORATORY TESTS

- Leukocytosis with a shift to the left
- Liver function studies are nonspecifically abnormal

IMAGING STUDIES

- Chest roentgenograms usually reveal elevation of the diaphragm if the abscess is on the right side
- Ultrasound, CT, or MRI may reveal the presence of intrahepatic defects
- On MRI, characteristic findings include high signal intensity on T2-weighted images and rim enhancement
- Hepatic candidiasis is seen usually in the setting of systemic candidiasis, and on CT scan the characteristic appearance is that of multiple "bulls-eyes," but imaging studies may be negative in neutropenic patients

Listeriosis p. 1101. Lithium Toxicity p. 1101.
Livedo Reticularis p. 1101.

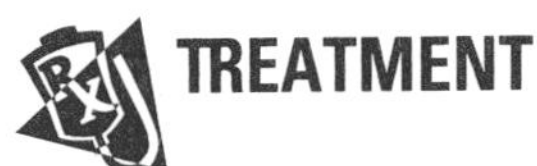

TREATMENT

MEDICATIONS

- Use antimicrobial agents (a third-generation cephalosporin and metronidazole) that are effective against coliform organisms and anaerobes
- Hepatic candidiasis often responds to intravenous amphotericin B (total dose of 2–9 g)

SURGERY

- If the abscess is at least 5 cm in diameter or the response to antibiotic therapy is not rapid, repeated needle aspiration or catheter or surgical (eg, laparoscopic) drainage should be undertaken
- Fungal abscesses require drainage

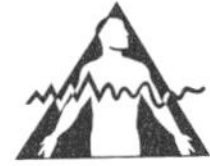

OUTCOME

PROGNOSIS

- The mortality rate is still substantial (≥8%) and is highest in underlying biliary malignancy or severe multiorgan dysfunction
- Fungal abscesses are associated with mortality rates of up to 50%

WHEN TO ADMIT

- All patients

EVIDENCE

PRACTICE GUIDELINES

- National Guideline Clearinghouse
  - http://www.guideline.gov/summary/summary.aspx?doc_id=3258&nbr=2484&string=liver+abscess

PATIENT INFORMATION

- National Institutes of Health
  - http://www.nlm.nih.gov/medlineplus/ency/article/000261.htm

REFERENCE

- Rahimian J et al: Pyogenic liver abscess: recent trends in etiology and mortality. Clin Infect Dis 2004;39:1654. [PMID: 15578367]

Author(s)

Lawrence S. Friedman, MD

Liver Disease, Alcoholic

KEY FEATURES

ESSENTIALS OF DIAGNOSIS

- >80 g/day intake of alcohol in men and 30–40 g/day intake in women
- Fatty liver is often asymptomatic
- Fever, right upper quadrant pain, tender hepatomegaly, and jaundice but the patient may also be asymptomatic
- Aspartate aminotransferase (AST) is usually elevated but rarely above 300 units/L. AST is greater than alanine aminotransferase (ALT), usually by a factor of 2 or more
- Often reversible, but it is the most common precursor of cirrhosis in the United States

GENERAL CONSIDERATIONS

- Excessive alcohol intake can lead to fatty liver, hepatitis, and cirrhosis
- Alcoholic hepatitis is characterized by acute or chronic inflammation and parenchymal necrosis
- Can appear within a year but usually decades after onset of excessive drinking
- Many of the adverse effects of alcohol are probably mediated by the oxidative metabolite acetaldehyde, which contributes to lipid peroxidation and induction of an immune response
- Concurrent hepatitis B or C virus infection and heterozygosity for the *HFE* gene mutation for hemochromatosis increase the severity of alcoholic liver disease

DEMOGRAPHICS

- Over 80% of patients have been drinking 5 years or more before developing any liver symptoms
- The longer the duration of drinking (10–15 or more years) and the larger the alcoholic consumption, the greater the probability of developing alcoholic hepatitis and cirrhosis

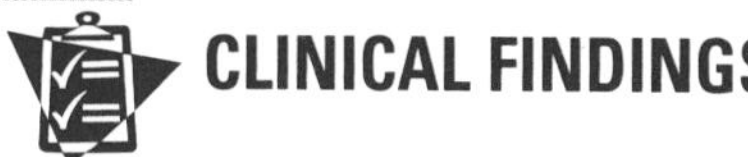

CLINICAL FINDINGS

SYMPTOMS AND SIGNS

- Can vary from asymptomatic with an enlarged liver to a critically ill individual who dies quickly
- Recent period of heavy drinking
- Anorexia and nausea
- Hepatomegaly and jaundice
- Abdominal pain and tenderness, splenomegaly, ascites, fever, and encephalopathy may be present

DIFFERENTIAL DIAGNOSIS

- Nonalcoholic fatty liver disease
- Viral hepatitis
- Drug-induced hepatitis
- Cirrhosis
- Biliary tract disease
- Pneumonia

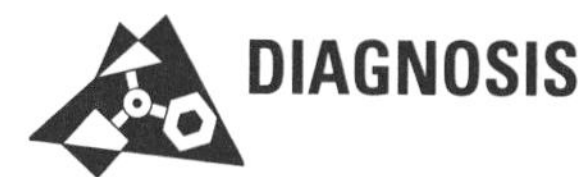

DIAGNOSIS

LABORATORY TESTS

Liver panel

- AST is usually elevated up to 300 units/L, but not higher
- AST is greater than ALT, usually by a factor of 2 or more
- Serum alkaline phosphatase is generally elevated, but seldom more than three times the normal value
- Serum bilirubin is increased in 60–90% of patients with alcoholic hepatitis

Complete blood cell count

- Anemia (usually macrocytic) may be present
- Leukocytosis with shift to the left is common with severe alcoholic hepatitis
- Leukopenia is occasionally seen and disappears after cessation of drinking
- About 10% of patients have thrombocytopenia related to a direct toxic effect of alcohol on megakaryocyte production or to hypersplenism

Other labs

- Serum γ-glutamyl transpeptidase, carbohydrate-deficient transferrin, and mitochondrial AST may be elevated, but these tests lack both sensitivity and specificity
- The serum albumin is depressed, and the γ-globulin level is elevated in 50–75% of individuals with alcoholic hepatitis, even in the absence of cirrhosis
- Increased transferrin saturation and hepatic iron stores are found in many due to sideroblastic anemia
- Folic acid deficiency may coexist

IMAGING STUDIES

- Imaging studies may show steatosis but are generally not helpful in the diagnosis of alcoholic hepatitis
- Ultrasound helps exclude biliary obstruction and identifies subclinical ascites
- CT scanning with intravenous contrast or MRI may be indicated in selected cases to evaluate patients for collateral vessels, space-occupying lesions of the liver, or concomitant disease of the pancreas

DIAGNOSTIC PROCEDURES

- Liver biopsy, if done, demonstrates various combinations of macrovesicular fat, polymorphonuclear neutrophil infiltration with hepatic necrosis, and Mallory bodies (alcoholic hyaline), and perivenular and perisinusoidal fibrosis. Micronodular cirrhosis may be present as well. The findings are identical to those of nonalcoholic steatohepatitis

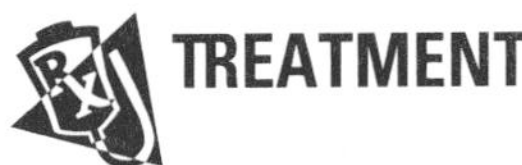

TREATMENT

MEDICATIONS

- Give **vitamins,** particularly folic acid and thiamin; glucose administration increases the vitamin B_1 requirement and can precipitate Wernicke-Korsakoff syndrome if thiamin is not coadministered

Corticosteroids

- Methylprednisolone, 32 mg/day for 1 month or the equivalent, may reduce short-term mortality and either encephalopathy or a greatly elevated bilirubin concentration and prolonged prothrombin time

Experimental therapies

- Pentoxifylline—an inhibitor of tumor necrosis factor—400 mg orally three times daily for 4 weeks, may reduce 1-month mortality rates in severe disease, primarily by decreasing the risk of hepatorenal syndrome
- Other experimental therapies include propylthiouracil, oxandrolone, and *S*-adenosyl-*l*-methionine

THERAPEUTIC PROCEDURES

- Abstinence from alcohol is essential; fatty liver is quickly reversible
- Provide sufficient carbohydrates and calories in anorectic patients to reduce endogenous protein catabolism, promote gluconeogenesis, and prevent hypoglycemia
- Nutritional support (40 kcal/kg with 1.5–2 g/kg as protein) improves survival in malnutrition. Use of liquid formulas rich in branched-chain amino acids does not improve survival beyond that achieved with less expensive caloric supplementation

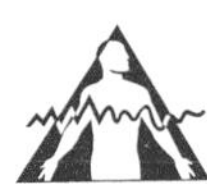

OUTCOME

COMPLICATIONS

Alcoholic cirrhosis

- Occurs in about 10–15% of persons who consume over 50 g of alcohol (4 oz of 100-proof whiskey, 15 oz of wine, or four 12-oz cans of beer) daily for over 10 years (the risk may be lower for wine than for comparable intake of beer or spirits)
- The risk of cirrhosis is lower (5%) in the absence of other cofactors such as chronic viral hepatitis
- There are associations with polymorphisms of the genes encoding for tumor necrosis factor-α and cytochrome P-450 2E1
- Women appear to be more susceptible than men, in part because of lower gastric mucosal alcohol dehydrogenase levels

PROGNOSIS

Short term

- A prothrombin time short enough to permit liver biopsy (< 3 s above control) has a 1-year mortality rate of 7%, rising to 20% if there is progressive prolongation of the prothrombin time during hospitalization
- If the prothrombin time prohibits liver biopsy, there is a 40% 1-year mortality rate
- Other unfavorable prognostic factors are hepatic encephalopathy, azotemia, little steatosis on a liver biopsy specimen, and reversal of portal blood flow on Doppler ultrasound
- Serum bilirubin levels greater than 10 mg/dL and marked prolongation of the prothrombin time (≥6 s above control) indicate severe hepatitis with a mortality rate as high as 50%

Long term

- In the United States, the 3-year mortality rate after recovery from acute alcoholic hepatitis is 10 times that of controls
- Histologically severe disease is associated with continued excessive mortality rates after 3 years, whereas the death rate is not increased after the same period in those whose liver biopsies show only mild alcoholic hepatitis
- Complications of portal hypertension (ascites, variceal bleeding, hepatorenal syndrome), coagulopathy, following recovery from acute alcoholic hepatitis suggest a poor long-term prognosis
- The most important prognostic consideration is continued excessive drinking. A 6-month period of abstinence is generally required before liver transplantation can be considered

PREVENTION

- Abstinence from alcohol

EVIDENCE

WEB SITES

- Diseases of the Liver
  - http://cpmcnet.columbia.edu/dept/gi/disliv.html
- Hepatic Ultrasound Images
  - http://www.sono.nino.ru/english/hepar_en.html
- Pathology Index
  - http://www-medlib.med.utah.edu/WebPath/LIVEHTML/LIVERIDX.html

INFORMATION FOR PATIENTS

- Alcoholics Anonymous
  - http://www.alcoholics-anonymous.org/
- Mayo Clinic
  - http://www.mayoclinic.com/invoke.cfm?id=HQ00200

REFERENCES

- Duvoux C et al: Low-grade steatosis and major changes in portal flow as new prognostic factors in steroid-treated alcoholic hepatitis. Hepatology 2004;40:1370. [PMID: 15565651]
- Tome S et al: Review article: current management of alcoholic liver disease. Aliment Pharmacol Ther 2004;19:707. [PMID: 15043511]

Author(s)

Lawrence S. Friedman, MD

Loiasis

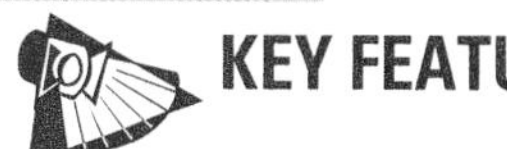

KEY FEATURES

ESSENTIALS OF DIAGNOSIS

- Worms make temporary appearances beneath the skin, eyes, or by Calabar swellings
- Calabar swellings are subcutaneous edematous reactions (up to 10 cm) to the worms and may migrate or be stationary

GENERAL CONSIDERATIONS

- This filarial disease is caused by infection with *Loa loa*
- The adult worms live in the subcutaneous tissues for up to 12 years
- Gravid females release microfilariae into the bloodstream, which subsequently are ingested in a blood meal by the vector-intermediate host, female chrysops species, day-biting flies. When the fly feeds again, the larval stage can infect a new host or cause superinfection
- The time to worm maturity and detection of new microfilariae is 6 months to several years

DEMOGRAPHICS

- The infection occurs in humans and monkeys in rain and swamp forest areas of West Africa from Nigeria to Angola and throughout the Congo River watershed of central Africa eastward to southwestern Sudan and western Uganda
- An estimated 3–13 million persons are infected

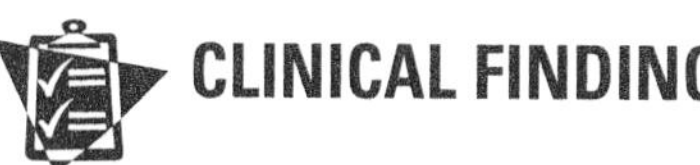

CLINICAL FINDINGS

SYMPTOMS AND SIGNS

- Many infected persons are asymptomatic
- In symptomatic persons, the worms (females, 4–7 cm × 0.5 mm) are evidenced by their temporary appearance beneath the skin or conjunctiva, by unilateral edema of an extremity, or by Calabar swellings
- Natives generally have a mild form of the infection or are asymptomatic. The disease among visitors, however, is often characterized by more pronounced frequent and debilitating Calabar swellings

Calabar swellings

- Subcutaneous edematous reactions, 3–10 cm in diameter, nonpitting and nonerythematous
- At times associated with low-grade fever, local pain, and pruritus
- The swellings may migrate a few centimeters for 2–3 days or stay in place before they subside
- At irregular intervals, they recur at the same or different sites, but only one appears at a time
- When near joints, they may be temporarily disabling
- Migration across the eye may be asymptomatic or may produce pain, intense conjunctivitis, and eyelid edema
- Dying adult worms may elicit small nodules or local sterile abscesses, and dead worms may result in radiologically detectable calcification

Microfilariae

- Do not induce symptoms if in the blood
- Rarely they enter the central nervous system and may cause encephalitis, myelitis, or jacksonian seizures
- Can also induce lesions and complications in the retina, heart, lungs, kidneys, and other tissues

DIFFERENTIAL DIAGNOSIS

- Dracunculiasis
- Cutaneous larva migrans
- Gnathostomiasis
- Myiasis
- Filariasis
- Onchocerciasis (river blindness)
- Bacterial pyoderma
- Cysticercosis (with ophthalmic involvement)

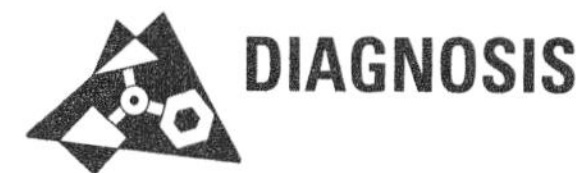

DIAGNOSIS

LABORATORY TESTS

- Specific diagnosis is made by finding characteristic microfilariae in daytime (10 AM to 4 PM) blood specimens by concentration methods; in order of increasing sensitivity, they are thick films, Knott's concentration, and Nuclepore filtration
- Presumptive diagnosis that permits treatment is based on Calabar swellings or eye migration, a history of residence in an endemic area, and marked eosinophilia (40% or greater)
- Serological tests may be positive, but cross-reactions occur with other filarial diseases and sometimes with other nematode infections
- A polymerase chain reaction test, highly sensitive and specific, can detect the organism in some amicrofilaremic persons
- Natives generally are microfilaremic and serologically positive. Visitors often have more pronounced immunologically mediated findings (elevated leukocyte and eosinophil counts, hypergammaglobulinemia, increased polyclonal IgE) and frequently a positive serological test but nondetectable microfilaremia

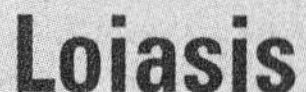

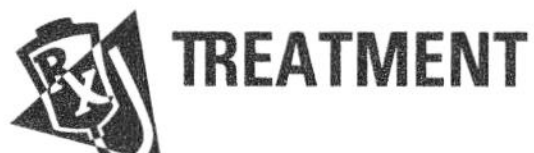

TREATMENT

MEDICATIONS

- See specialized sources for details on proper use of **diethylcarbamazine** (drug of choice both as a micro- and macrofilaricide), since side effects to dying microfilariae may be severe, and life-threatening encephalitis can occur rarely. The dosage is 50 mg once (Day 1), 50 mg three times daily (Day 2), 100 mg three times daily (Day 3), and 3 mg/kg three times daily (Days 4–21)
- One course of treatment cures about 50% of patients; three courses cure 90%
- Reactions are more likely with pretreatment microfilaria counts greater than 25/μL
- Prednisone (40–60 mg daily) is sometimes indicated in heavily infected persons to minimize reactions
- In the United States, diethylcarbamazine is available only from the Parasitic Diseases Drug Service, Centers for Disease Control and Prevention, Atlanta, GA 30333, telephone 404-639-3670

SURGERY

- Surgical removal of adult worms from the eye or skin is not recommended

THERAPEUTIC PROCEDURES

- Cytapheresis has been used to reduce parasite loads before starting diethylcarbamazine

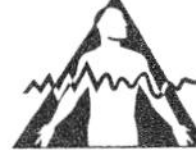

OUTCOME

COMPLICATIONS

- When ivermectin was used in treatment of 1.1 million persons with onchocerciasis in the presence of endemic loiasis, 28 neurological reactions occurred (some severe) from death of *Loa loa* microfilariae. The risk of these reactions was high when the *L loa* microfilaria load exceeded 8/μL and very high above 50/μL; albendazole at a dosage of 200 mg twice daily for 3 weeks is being evaluated as a safe way to reduce the level of *L loa* microfilariae

PROGNOSIS

- Most infections run a benign course, but some are accompanied by severe and temporarily disabling symptoms
- The prognosis is excellent with treatment

WHEN TO REFER

- Refer symptomatic patients to a specialist with expertise in this problem
- Refer all patients with ocular symptoms to an ophthalmologist

WHEN TO ADMIT

- Patients with debilitating Calabar swellings

PREVENTION

- Individual protection is facilitated by daytime use of insect repellent and by wearing light-colored clothing with long sleeves and trousers
- Diethylcarbamazine prophylaxis, 300 mg weekly, may be useful if the risk of exposure is high. It is not indicated, however, for the casual traveler or for persons who might previously have acquired any of the filarial infections

EVIDENCE

WEB SITE

- CDC—Division of Parasitic Diseases
  - http://www.cdc.gov/ncidod/dpd/parasites/lymphaticfilariasis/
  - default.htm

INFORMATION FOR PATIENTS

- CDC—Traveler's Health
  - http://www.cdc.gov/travel/diseases/filariasis.htm

REFERENCES

- Kamgno J et al: Effect of a single dose (600 mg) of albendazole on *Loa loa* microfilaraemia. Parasite 2002;9:59. [PMID: 11938697]
- Nutman TB et al: Case records of the Massachusetts General Hospital. Weekly clinicopathological exercises. Case 1-2002. A 24-year-old woman with paresthesias and muscle cramps after a stay in Africa. N Engl J Med 2002;346:115. [PMID: 11784879]

Low Back Pain

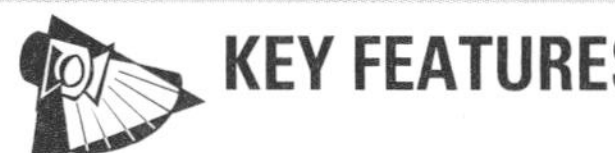

KEY FEATURES

ESSENTIALS OF DIAGNOSIS

- A precise diagnosis cannot be made in the majority of cases
- Even when anatomic defects—such as vertebral osteophytes or a narrowed disk space—are present, clinical disease cannot be assumed since such defects are common in asymptomatic patients
- The majority of patients will improve in 1–4 weeks and need no evaluation beyond the initial history and physical examination

GENERAL CONSIDERATIONS

- Exceedingly common, experienced at some time by up to 80% of the population

DEMOGRAPHICS

- Chronic low back pain from degenerative joint disease is rare before age 40

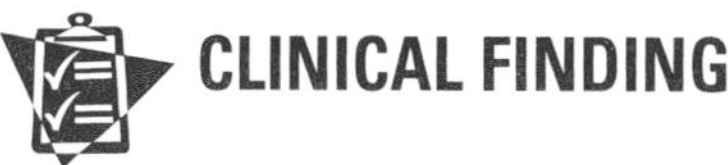

CLINICAL FINDINGS

SYMPTOMS AND SIGNS

- Pattern of pain
  - **Radiation down the buttock** and below the knee suggests nerve root irritation from a herniated disc
  - **Pain that worsens with rest** and improves with activity is characteristic of ankylosing spondylitis or other seronegative spondyloarthropathies, especially when the onset begins before age 40. Most degenerative back diseases produce precisely the opposite pattern, with rest alleviating and activity aggravating the pain
  - **Low back pain at night,** unrelieved by rest or the supine position, suggests the possibility of malignancy
  - Symptoms of **large or rapidly evolving neurological** deficits identify patients who need urgent evaluation for possible cauda equina tumor, epidural abscess, or, rarely, massive disk herniation
  - **Bilateral leg weakness** (from multiple lumbar nerve root compressions) or saddle area anesthesia, bowel or bladder incontinence, or impotence (indicating sacral nerve root compressions) indicates a cauda equina process
- Positive straight leg raising test indicates nerve root irritation. The examiner performs the test on the supine patient by passively raising the patient's leg. The test is positive if radicular pain is produced with the leg raised 60 degrees or less. The test has a specificity of 40% but is 95% sensitive with herniation at the L4–5 or L5–S1 level (the sites of 95% of disk herniations)
- The crossed straight leg sign has a sensitivity of 25% but is 90% specific for disk herniation and is positive when raising the contralateral leg reproduces the sciatica
- Disk herniation produces deficits predictable for the site involved (Table 79)
- Deficits of multiple nerve roots suggest a cauda equina tumor, an epidural abscess, or some other important process that requires urgent evaluation and treatment
- Palpation of the spine usually does not yield diagnostic information. Point tenderness over a vertebral body may suggest osteomyelitis

DIFFERENTIAL DIAGNOSIS

- Muscular strain
- Herniated disk
- Lumbar spinal stenosis
- Compression fracture
- Degenerative joint disease
- Infectious diseases (eg, osteomyelitis, epidural abscess, subacute bacterial endocarditis)
- Neoplastic disease (vertebral metastases)
- Seronegative spondylarthopathies, eg, ankylosing spondylitis
- Leaking abdominal aortic aneurysm
- Renal colic

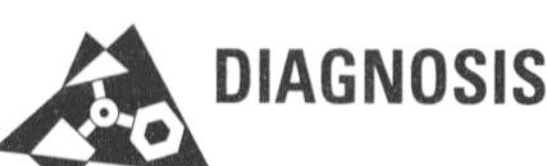

DIAGNOSIS

IMAGING STUDIES

- Plain x-rays are warranted promptly for suspected infection, cancer, fractures, or inflammation; selected other patients who fail to improve after 2–4 weeks of conservative therapy are also candidates
- MRI is needed urgently in any patient suspected of having an epidural mass or cauda equina tumor but not if a patient is felt to have a routine disk herniation, since most will improve over 4–6 weeks of conservative therapy

DIAGNOSTIC PROCEDURES

- If the history and physical examination do not suggest the presence of infection, cancer, inflammatory back disease, major neurological deficits, or pain referred from abdominal or pelvic disease, further evaluation can be deferred while conservative therapy is tried

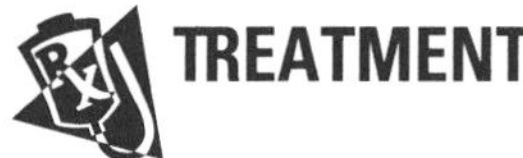

TREATMENT

MEDICATIONS

- Nonsteroidal antiinflammatory drugs (NSAIDs) for analgesia, but severe pain may require opioids
- Limited evidence supports the use of "muscle relaxants" such as diazepam, cyclobenzaprine, carisoprodol, and methocarbamol. These drugs should be reserved for patients who fail NSAIDs and should also be limited to courses of 1–2 weeks

SURGERY

- Surgical consultation is needed urgently for any patient with a large or evolving neurological deficit
- Surgery for disk disease is indicated when there is documentation of herniation by some imaging procedure, a consistent pain syndrome, and a consistent neurological deficit that has failed to respond to 4–6 weeks of conservative therapy

THERAPEUTIC PROCEDURES

- All patients should be taught how to protect the back in daily activities
- Rest and back exercises, once thought to be cornerstones of conservative therapy, are now known to be ineffective for acute back pain
- Epidural corticosteroid injections can provide short-term relief of sciatica but do not improve functional status or reduce the need for surgery
- Corticosteroid injections into facet joints are ineffective for chronic low back pain

OUTCOME

PROGNOSIS

- The great majority of patients will spontaneously improve with conservative care over 1–4 weeks

WHEN TO REFER

- Refer to neurosurgeon or orthopedist if patient has disk herniation that does not respond after 4–6 weeks of conservative therapy or sooner if patient has important neurological deficits

WHEN TO ADMIT

- Admit if symptoms and signs suggest epidural or spinal abscess, cauda equina syndrome, or new metastatic cancer

EVIDENCE

PRACTICE GUIDELINES

- National Guideline Clearinghouse
  - http://www.guideline.gov/summary/summary.aspx?doc_id=5883

INFORMATION FOR PATIENTS

- American Academy of Family Physicians
  - http://familydoctor.org/healthfacts/117/
- JAMA patient page. Low back pain. JAMA 1998;279:1846. [PMID: 9628721]

REFERENCES

- Assendelft WJ et al: Spinal manipulative therapy for low back pain. A meta-analysis of effectiveness relative to other therapies. Ann Intern Med 2003;138:871. [PMID: 12779297]
- Cherkin DC et al: A review of the evidence for the effectiveness, safety, and cost of acupuncture, massage therapy, and spinal manipulation for back pain. Ann Intern Med 2003;138:898. [PMID: 12779300]
- Hagen K et al: Bed rest for acute low-back pain and sciatica. Cochrane Database Syst Rev 2004:4;CD001254. [PMID: 15495012]
- Jarvik JG et al: Diagnostic evaluation of low back pain with emphasis on imaging. Ann Intern Med 2002;137:586. [PMID: 12353946]
- Speed C: Low back pain. BMJ 2004;328:1119. [PMID: 15130982]

Author(s)

David B. Hellmann, MD, FACP

John H. Stone, MD, MPH

Lung Cancer, Secondary

LSD & Hallucinogens p. 1102

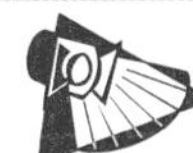

KEY FEATURES

ESSENTIALS OF DIAGNOSIS

- Identification of a primary tumor
- Radiographic findings consistent with pulmonary metastases
- Exclusion of other diseases in the differential diagnosis for multiple pulmonary nodules

GENERAL CONSIDERATIONS

- Represent metastases from extrapulmonary malignancies
- Almost any cancer can spread to the lung, usually hematogenously via the pulmonary artery
- Lung metastases are found in 20–55% of patients dying of various cancers

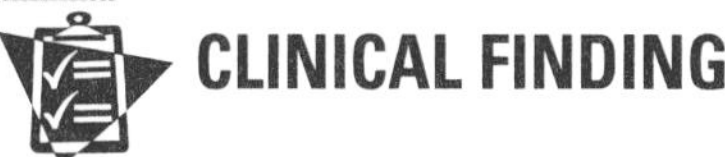

CLINICAL FINDINGS

SYMPTOMS AND SIGNS

- Symptoms are uncommon, but include cough, hemoptysis, and dyspnea in advanced cases
- Symptoms are most commonly referrable to the primary tumor

DIFFERENTIAL DIAGNOSIS

- Bronchogenic carcinoma
- Lymphoproliferative cancer
- Tuberculosis
- Lung abscess
- Granulomas (eg, tuberculous, fungal)
- Coccidioidomycosis
- Histoplasmosis
- Sarcoidosis
- Silicosis
- Coal worker's pneumoconiosis
- *Mycobacterium avium* complex
- Arteriovenous malformations
- Rheumatoid nodules
- Hamartomas
- Wegener's granulomatosis
- Methotrexate-induced

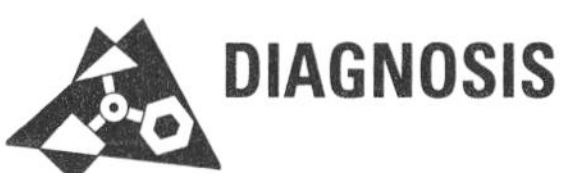

DIAGNOSIS

LABORATORY TESTS

- Appropriate studies should be ordered in a search for the primary tumor
- Occasionally, cytologic studies of pleural fluid or pleural biopsy are diagnostic
- Sputum cytology is rarely helpful

IMAGING STUDIES

- Chest CT is more sensitive than chest x-ray in detecting pulmonary metastases
- Chest x-ray usually shows multiple spherical densities with sharp margins, nearly all < 5 cm
- Lesions are usually bilateral, pleural, or subpleural, and are more common in lower lung zones
- Mammography should be performed in a search for the primary tumor

DIAGNOSTIC PROCEDURES

- If a primary tumor cannot be found, tissue from lung lesions may be obtained by bronchoscopy, percutaneous biopsy, or thoracotomy

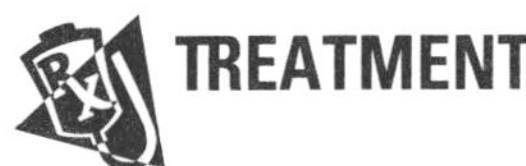

TREATMENT

SURGERY

- Resection of a solitary pulmonary nodule is often prudent in a patient with known current or prior extrapulmonary cancer
- Local resection of one or more pulmonary metastases is feasible in a few carefully selected patients

THERAPEUTIC PROCEDURES

- Management consists of treatment of the primary malignancy and any pulmonary complications

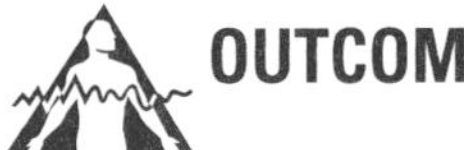

OUTCOME

PROGNOSIS

- Overall 5-year survival rate in secondary lung cancer treated surgically is 20–35%

WHEN TO REFER

- All patients deserve an evaluation by a multidisciplinary lung cancer evaluation and treatment program
- For bronchoscopy or thoracotomy
- A palliative care specialist should be involved in advanced disease care

WHEN TO ADMIT

- Respiratory distress, altered mental status, pain control

EVIDENCE

PRACTICE GUIDELINES

- National Guideline Clearinghouse
  - http://www.guideline.gov/summary/summary.aspx?doc_id=3639&nbr=2865&string=secondary+AND+lung+AND+cancer
  - http://www.guideline.gov/summary/summary.aspx?doc_id=3641&nbr=2867&string=secondary+AND+lung+AND+cancer

INFORMATION FOR PATIENTS

- National Cancer Institute
  - http://cis.nci.nih.gov/fact/6_20.htm
- National Institutes of Health
  - http://www.nlm.nih.gov/medlineplus/ency/article/000097.htm

REFERENCE

- Greelish JP et al: Secondary pulmonary malignancy. Surg Clin North Am 2000;80:633. [PMID:10836010]

Author(s)

Mark S. Chesnutt, MD
Thomas J. Prendergast, MD

Lupus Anticoagulant p. 1103

Lyme Disease

KEY FEATURES

ESSENTIALS OF DIAGNOSIS

- Erythema migrans, a flat or slightly raised red lesion that expands with central clearing
- Headache or stiff neck
- Arthralgias, arthritis, and myalgias; arthritis is often chronic and recurrent
- Wide geographic distribution, with most cases in the northeast, mid-Atlantic, upper midwest, and Pacific coastal regions of the United States

GENERAL CONSIDERATIONS

- Illness caused by the spirochete *Borrelia burgdorferi* is transmitted to humans by ixodid ticks in North America, Europe, Australia, and Asia
- Ticks must feed for 24 h or longer to transmit infections
- Incidence of disease is significantly higher when tick attachment is for longer than 72 h
- The percentage of ticks infected varies on a regional basis. In the northeast and midwest, 15–65%, in the west, only 2%
- Congenital infection has been documented

DEMOGRAPHICS

- In 2002, there were 23,763 cases reported but the true incidence is not known; overreporting remains a problem
- Most cases (over 95%) were reported from the mid-Atlantic, northeastern, and north central regions of the country
- Cases of Lyme disease reported in the midwest and southern areas are probably due to the Lone Star tick, *Amblyomma americanum*, which produces a Lyme-disease–like illness referred to as Southern tick-associated rash illness (STARI)
- Most infections occur in the spring and summer

CLINICAL FINDINGS

SYMPTOMS AND SIGNS

- **Stage 1, early localized infection:** flu-like symptoms, erythema migrans, fever, chills, and myalgia in about half
- **Stage 2, early disseminated infection** (weeks to months later): skin (50% of patients), cardiac (4–10%), neurologic (10–20%), and musculoskeletal system manifestations
- *Borrelia* lymphocytoma is a rare skin lesion
- Myopericarditis, with atrial or ventricular arrhythmias and heart block
- Headache, stiff neck
- Aseptic meningitis, Bell's palsy, or encephalitis
- Peripheral neuropathy (sensory or motor), transverse myelitis, and mononeuritis multiplex
- Conjunctivitis, keratitis
- Migratory pains in joints, muscles, and tendons; fatigue and malaise
- **Stage 3, late persistent infection** (months to years later): musculoskeletal (up to 60%), neurologic, and skin disease
- Musculoskeletal manifestations: joint and periarticular pain; frank arthritis, mainly of large joints, chronic or recurrent; and chronic synovitis
- Subacute encephalopathy (memory loss, mood changes, and sleep disturbance), axonal polyneuropathy (distal sensory paresthesias or radicular pain), rare leukoencephalitis (cognitive dysfunction, spastic paraparesis, ataxia, and bladder dysfunction)
- Acrodermatitis chronicum—lesions atrophic and sclerotic, resemble localized scleroderma
- **Great overlap between stages**; the skin, central nervous system, and musculoskeletal system can be involved early or late

DIFFERENTIAL DIAGNOSIS

- Babesiosis
- Ehrlichiosis
- *Amblyomma americanum* (Lone Star tick) bite-related illness
- Urticaria, reaction to arthropod bite, cellulitis, erythema multiforme, granuloma annulare
- Rocky Mountain spotted fever
- Primary HIV infection
- Parvovirus B19 infection
- Rheumatic fever, Still's disease, gonococcal arthritis, sarcoidosis, systemic lupus erythematosus
- Viral meningitis
- Bell's palsy

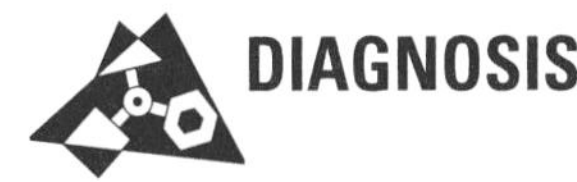

DIAGNOSIS

LABORATORY TESTS

- Elevated sedimentation rate of > 20 mm/h seen in 50% of cases and mildly abnormal liver function tests in 30%
- Mild anemia, leukocytosis, and microscopic hematuria in 10% or less
- Detection of specific antibodies to *B burgdorferi* in serum, either by indirect immunofluorescence assay (IFA) or ELISA; both false-positive and false-negative reactions occur
- A Western blot assay that can detect both IgM and IgG antibodies is used as a confirmatory test
- A two-test approach is now recommended
- Polymerase chain reaction (PCR) test is very specific for detecting *Borrelia* DNA, but sensitivity is variable and depends on which body fluid is tested and which stage of disease
- Up to 85% of synovial fluid samples are PCR positive in active arthritis
- 38% of cerebrospinal fluid samples are PCR positive in acute neuroborreliosis, but only 25% are positive in chronic neuroborreliosis

DIAGNOSTIC PROCEDURES

- Diagnosis is based on both clinical manifestations and laboratory findings. A person with exposure to a potential tick habitat (within the 30 days just prior to developing erythema migrans) with erythema migrans diagnosed by a physician or at least one late manifestation of the disease and laboratory confirmation
- Positive cultures for *B burgdorferi* can be obtained early in the course of disease. Aspiration of erythema migrans lesions is positive in up to 30% of cases, 2-mm punch biopsy is positive in 50–70%, blood cultures positive in up to 50%, cerebrospinal fluid positive in 1–10%
- Peripheral neuropathy may be detected by electromyography

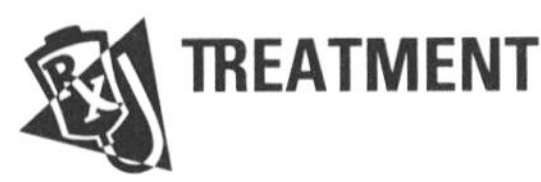

TREATMENT

MEDICATIONS

- See Table 142
- Erythema migrans: doxycycline, 100 mg PO BID for 2–3 weeks; or amoxicillin, 500

mg PO TID for 2–3 weeks; or cefuroxime axetil, 500 mg PO BID for 2–3 weeks
- Bell's palsy: doxycycline, 100 mg PO BID for 2–3 weeks; or amoxicillin, 500 mg PO TID for 2–3 weeks
- Other central nervous system disease: ceftriaxone, 2 g IV QD for 2–4 weeks; or penicillin G, 20 million units daily IV in 6 divided doses for 2–4 weeks; or cefotaxime, 2 g IV q8h for 2–4 weeks
- First-degree block (PR < 0.3 s): doxycycline, 100 mg PO BID for 3–4 weeks; or amoxicillin, 500 mg PO TID for 3–4 weeks
- High-degree atrioventricular block: ceftriaxone, 2 g IV once daily for 2–4 weeks; or penicillin G, 20 million units daily IV in 6 divided doses for 2–4 weeks
- Arthritis
  - Oral: doxycycline, 100 mg PO BID for 4 weeks; or amoxicillin, 500 mg PO TID for 4 weeks; if this fails (persistent or recurrent joint swelling), retreat with oral agent for 8 weeks or switch to IV agent for 2–4 weeks
  - Parenteral: ceftriaxone, 2 g IV QD for 2–4 weeks; or penicillin G, 20 million units daily IV in 6 divided doses for 2–4 weeks
- Acrodermatitis chronicum atrophicans: doxycycline, 100 mg PO BID for 3–4 weeks; or amoxicillin, 500 mg PO TID for 4 weeks

THERAPEUTIC PROCEDURES

- Tick bite: no treatment in most circumstances; observe
- If acute arthritis, need aspiration to rule out pyogenic arthritis
- If neurologic symptoms, need lumbar puncture because drug and duration of therapy are unique for neuroborreliosis
- If suspect peripheral neuropathy, nerve conduction studies

OUTCOME

FOLLOW-UP

- Routine follow-up
- Complete recovery in 4–6 weeks after therapy of early disease
- Fatigue, arthralgias, myalgias may persist for weeks or months, but do not require antimicrobial therapy
- After treatment of arthritis, arthralgias may persist and be severe; if not resolved after 3 months, re-treat with antibiotics; if arthralgias still persist treat symptomatically

COMPLICATIONS

- Rarely, residual facial nerve palsy, synovitis or heart block requiring a pacemaker

PROGNOSIS

- With appropriate therapy symptoms usually resolve within 4 weeks
- The long-term outcome of adult patients with Lyme disease is not clear
- Long-term sequelae are uncommon

WHEN TO REFER

- If persistent symptoms after initial appropriate therapy; usually continued symptoms are part of the natural history of the disease and not reinfection or indication for prolonged use of antibiotics

WHEN TO ADMIT

- For serious complications such as high-degree heart block

PREVENTION

- Avoiding tick-infested areas, covering exposed skin, using repellents, and inspecting for ticks after exposure
- Prophylactic antibiotics following tick bites are not recommended

EVIDENCE

PRACTICE GUIDELINES

- American Academy of Pediatrics. Committee on Infectious Diseases. Prevention of Lyme disease. Pediatrics 2000;105(1 Pt 1):142. [PMID: 10617720]
  - Guideline summary available at National Guideline Clearinghouse
  - http://www.guideline.gov/summary/summary.aspx?doc_id=2767
- Centers for Disease Control and Prevention—Advisory Committee on Immunization Practices. Recommendations for the Use of Lyme Disease Vaccine. MMWR Recomm Rep 1999;48(No. RR-7).
  - http://www.cdc.gov/mmwr/PDF/RR/RR4807.pdf
- Wormser GP et al: Practice guidelines for the treatment of Lyme disease. The Infectious Diseases Society of America. Clin Infect Dis 2000;31(Suppl 1):1. [PMID: 10982743]
  - Guideline summary available at National Guideline Clearinghouse
  - http://www.guideline.gov/summary/summary.aspx?doc_id=2672

WEB SITES

- Lyme Disease Network
  - http://www.lymenet.org/
- American Lyme Disease Foundation
  - http://www.aldf.com/
- The Lyme Disease Foundation
  - http://www.lyme.org/
- Centers for Disease Control and Prevention: Lyme Disease Home Page
  - http://www.cdc.gov/ncidod/dvbid/lyme/index.htm

INFORMATION FOR PATIENTS

- American College of Physicians: Lyme Disease, A Patient's Guide, Diagnosis
  - http://www.acponline.org/lyme/patient/diagnosis.htm
- American College of Physicians: Lyme Disease, A Patient's Guide, Treatment
  - http://www.acponline.org/lyme/patient/treatment.htm
- Centers for Disease Control and Prevention—Division of Vector Borne Infectious Diseases. Lyme Disease: A Public Information Guide
  - http://www.cdc.gov/ncidod/dvbid/lyme/lyme_brochure.pdf

REFERENCES

- Coyle PK et al: Neurologic aspects of Lyme disease. Med Clin North Am 2002;86:261. [PMID: 11982301]
- Halperin JJ: Central nervous system Lyme disease. Curr Infect Dis Rep 2004;6:298. [PMID: 15265459]
- Hayes ET et al: How can we prevent Lyme disease? N Engl J Med 2003;348:2424. [PMID: 12802029]
- Hengge UR et al: Lyme borreliosis. Lancet Infect Dis 2003;3:489. [PMID: 12901891]
- Klempner MS et al: Two controlled trials of antibiotic treatment in patients with persistent symptoms and a history of Lyme disease. N Engl J Med 2001;345:85. [PMID: 11450676]
- Massarotti EM: Lyme arthritis. Med Clin North Am 2002;86:297. [PMID: 11982303]
- Pinto DS: Cardiac manifestations of Lyme disease. Med Clin North Am 2002;86:285. [PMID: 11982302]
- Poland GA: Prevention of Lyme disease: a review of the evidence. Mayo Clin Proc 2001;76:713. [PMID: 11444404]
- Steere AC: Lyme disease. N Engl J Med 2001;345:115. [PMID: 11450660]

Author(s)

Richard A. Jacobs, MD, PhD

Lymphangitis & Lymphadenitis

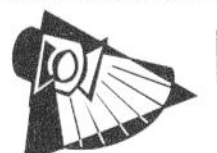

KEY FEATURES

ESSENTIALS OF DIAGNOSIS

- Red streak extending from an infected area toward enlarged, tender regional lymph nodes

GENERAL CONSIDERATIONS

- Lymphangitis and lymphadenitis frequently accompany a streptococcal or staphylococcal infection in the distal arm or leg
- Inciting wound can be a superficial scratch or insect bite with cellulitis or an established abscess
- Systemic manifestations: fever, chills, tachycardia, and malaise
- If untreated, infection can progress rapidly

CLINICAL FINDINGS

SYMPTOMS AND SIGNS

- Throbbing pain at the site of the inciting wound
- Temperature of 37.8–40°C
- Chills
- Sweats
- Malaise
- Anorexia
- Regional lymph nodes significantly enlarged and tender
- Red streak extending toward regional lymph nodes

DIFFERENTIAL DIAGNOSIS

- Superficial thrombophlebitis
- Cat-scratch disease caused by *Bartonella henselae*
- Acute streptococcal hemolytic gangrene
- Superficial thrombophlebitis
- Cellulitis
- Necrotizing fasciitis
- Filariasis (acute)
- *Nocardia brasiliensis* infection

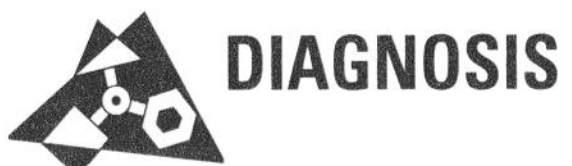

DIAGNOSIS

LABORATORY TESTS

- Leukocytosis with a left shift
- Blood cultures often positive for *Staphylococcus* or *Streptococcus*

IMAGING STUDIES

- Consider plain film if concerned about possible retained foreign body or necrotizing infection

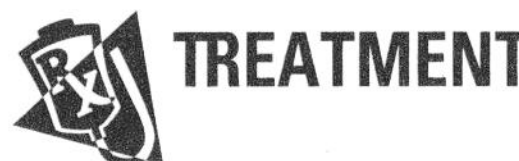

TREATMENT

MEDICATIONS

- Analgesics
- Antibiotics: penicillin G, 4 million units IV Q6 h; or cefazolin, 1 g every IV Q8 h; or clindamycin, 600 mg IV Q12 h

SURGERY

- Incision and drainage of abscess, excision of necrotic tissue or foreign body

THERAPEUTIC PROCEDURES

- Elevation of extremity
- Warm compresses

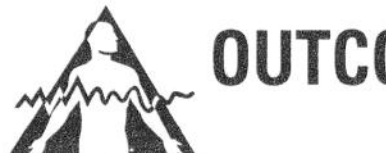

OUTCOME

FOLLOW-UP

- Wound examination to determine the need for débridement or incision and drainage of an abscess

COMPLICATIONS

- Wound-healing problems
- Sepsis

PROGNOSIS

- Early institution of antibiotic therapy and wound care usually controls the infection in 48–72 h
- Delayed or inadequate therapy can result in rapidly progressive infection, septicemia, and death

WHEN TO REFER

- Lymphangitis complicated by abscess, nonhealing wound, sepsis

WHEN TO ADMIT

- Signs of sepsis
- Failed outpatient management

EVIDENCE

INFORMATION FOR PATIENTS

- Cleveland Clinic: Lymphedema
  - http://www.clevelandclinic.org/health/health-info/docs/1800/1896.asp?index=8353
- Mayo Clinic: Swollen Lymph Glands (Lymphadenitis)
  - http://www.mayoclinic.com/invoke.cfm?objectid=799E8349-32F2-40FE-94FAC192833334E6
- MedlinePlus: Lymphadenitis and Lymphangitis
  - http://www.nlm.nih.gov/medlineplus/ency/article/001301.htm

Author(s)

Louis M. Messina, MD

Lymphedema

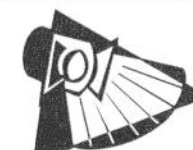

KEY FEATURES

ESSENTIALS OF DIAGNOSIS

- Painless edema of upper or lower extremities
- Involves the dorsal surfaces of the hands and fingers or the feet and toes
- Developmental or acquired
- Unilateral or bilateral
- Edema initially pitting; with time, becoming brawny and nonpitting
- No ulceration, varicosities, or stasis pigmentation
- Episodes of lymphangitis and cellulitis

GENERAL CONSIDERATIONS

- Primary lymphedema is due to congenital developmental abnormalities consisting of hypoplastic or hyperplastic changes of the proximal or distal lymphatics
- Familial lymphedema developing before age 1 is Milroy's disease; usually bilateral, it affects boys more often than girls
- Lymphedema developing during adolescence (lymphedema praecox) is unilateral; 3.5:1 female predominance
- Lymphedema after age 35 is lymphedema tarda
- Secondary lymphedema results from an inflammatory or mechanical obstruction of the lymphatics after trauma, regional lymph node resection, irradiation, bacterial or fungal infections, lymphoproliferative diseases, or filariasis

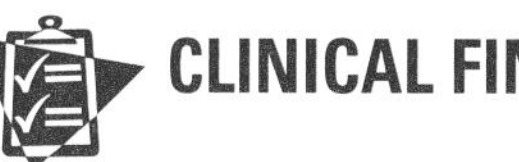

CLINICAL FINDINGS

SYMPTOMS AND SIGNS

- Slowly progressive, painless edema
- Edema usually centered around the ankle and involves the toes and dorsum
- Hypertrophy of the limb
- Markedly thickened skin and subcutaneous tissue
- Rarely, lymphangiosarcoma or angiosarcoma (Stewart-Treves syndrome)
- Secondary fibrosis is exacerbated by superimposed episodes of acute infection

DIFFERENTIAL DIAGNOSIS

- Venous insufficiency
- Chronic venous stasis disease
- Edema secondary to congestive heart failure
- Cellulitis

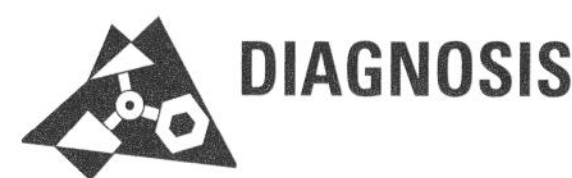

DIAGNOSIS

IMAGING STUDIES

- Venous duplex ultrasonography to exclude venous insufficiency or vascular malformations
- Lymphangiography and radioactive isotope studies if surgical reconstruction (rare)

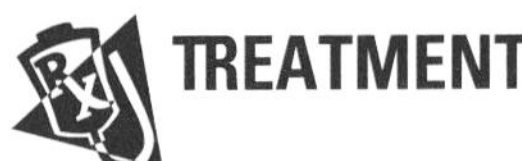

TREATMENT

MEDICATIONS

- No effective drug therapy
- Diuretics are not recommended for long-term use but can be useful for acute exacerbation of edema secondary to infection or for coexisting venous stasis disease

SURGERY

- Primary treatment is nonsurgical
- Surgery to reduce limb bulk, either by ablative techniques (excision of excess tissue) or by physiological techniques (lymphatic reconstruction), in carefully selected cases
- Microsurgical lymphaticovenous anastomosis, although long-term efficacy is unknown

THERAPEUTIC PROCEDURES

- Meticulous skin care
- Moisturizing lotions
- Frequent leg elevation
- Manual lymphatic drainage massage
- External compression with fitted graduated (20–30 mm Hg) compression stockings
- Sequential pneumatic compression devices
- Reid sleeves for postmastectomy arm lymphedema
- Avoidance of trauma to the affected extremity

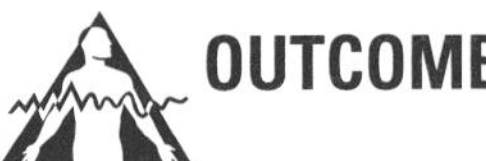

OUTCOME

COMPLICATIONS

- Secondary infection and ulceration

PROGNOSIS

- Good with vigorous skin care regimen

WHEN TO REFER

- Refer for early intervention and counseling

WHEN TO ADMIT

- Lymphedema complicated by infection

EVIDENCE

PRACTICE GUIDELINES

- Harris SR et al: Clinical practice guidelines for the care and treatment of breast cancer: 11. Lymphedema. CMAJ 2001;164:191. [PMID: 11332311]
- Surgical management of early-stage invasive breast cancer. Practice Guidelines Initiative, 2003
  - http://www.cancercare.on.ca/pdf/pebc1-1f.pdf

INFORMATION FOR PATIENTS

- Cleveland Clinic: Lymphedema
  - http://www.clevelandclinic.org/health/health-info/docs/1800/1896.asp?index=8353
- MedlinePlus: Lymphatic Obstruction
  - http://www.nlm.nih.gov/medlineplus/ency/article/001117.htm

REFERENCES

- Campisi C et al: Long-term results after lymphatic-venous anastomoses for the treatment of obstructive lymphedema. Microsurgery 2001;21:135. [PMID: 11494379]
- Ko DS et al: Effective treatment of lymphedema of the extremities. Arch Surg 1998;133:452. [PMID: 9565129]

Author(s)

Louis M. Messina, MD

Lymphoma, Cutaneous T Cell

Lymphocytic Choriomeningitis p. 1103.
Lymphogranuloma Venereum p. 1103.

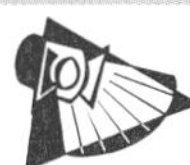

KEY FEATURES

ESSENTIALS OF DIAGNOSIS

- Localized or generalized erythematous scaling plaques
- Pruritus
- Lymphadenopathy
- Distinctive histology

GENERAL CONSIDERATIONS

- A cutaneous T cell lymphoma that begins on the skin and may involve only the skin for years or decades
- Certain medications (including selective serotonin reuptake inhibitors) may produce eruptions clinically and histologically identical to those of mycosis fungoides, so this possibility must always be considered
- Lymph node enlargement may be due to benign expansion of the node (dermatopathic lymphadenopathy) or by specific involvement with mycosis fungoides

CLINICAL FINDINGS

SYMPTOMS AND SIGNS

- See Table 7
- Localized or generalized erythematous patches or plaques, usually on the trunk
- Plaques are almost always over 5 cm in diameter
- Pruritus is a frequent complaint
- The lesions often begin as nondescript or nondiagnostic patches, and it is not unusual for the patient to have skin lesions for more than a decade before the diagnosis can be confirmed
- In more advanced cases, tumors appear
- Lymphadenopathy may occur locally or widely

DIFFERENTIAL DIAGNOSIS

- Psoriasis
- Drug eruption
- Atopic dermatitis (eczema)
- Hansen's disease (leprosy)
- Tinea corporis (body ringworm)

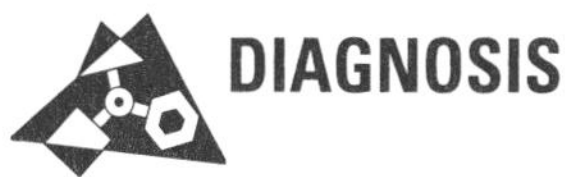

DIAGNOSIS

LABORATORY TESTS

- Circulating atypical cells (Sézary cells) can be detected in the blood by sensitive methods
- Eosinophilia may be present

THERAPEUTIC PROCEDURES

- The skin biopsy remains the basis of diagnosis, though at times numerous biopsies are required before the diagnosis can be confirmed

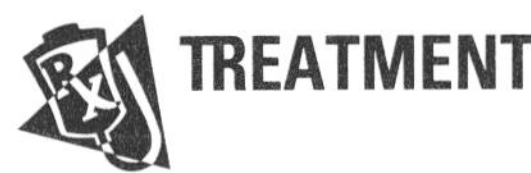

TREATMENT

MEDICATIONS

- The treatment is complex
- Topical mechlorethamine ointment or solution, topical corticosteroids and PUVA are all used for early patches and plaques
- Radiation therapy for local lesions and systemic agents such as retinoids, antitumor chemotherapeutic drugs, and alpha interferon are used alone or in various combinations for more advanced disease or in patients who do not respond to topical therapy

OUTCOME

COMPLICATIONS

- Overly aggressive treatment may lead to complications and premature demise

PROGNOSIS

- Usually slowly progressive (over decades)
- Early and aggressive treatment has not been proved to cure or prevent progression of the disease
- Prognosis is better in patients with patch or plaque stage disease and worse in patients with erythroderma, tumors, and lymphadenopathy
- Survival is not reduced in patients with limited patch disease
- Elderly patients with patch and plaque stage disease commonly die of other causes

WHEN TO REFER

- All patients with suspected or proven diagnosis

EVIDENCE

PRACTICE GUIDELINES

- Whittaker SJ et al; British Association of Dermatologists; U.K. Cutaneous Lymphoma Group. Joint British Association of Dermatologists and U.K. Cutaneous Lymphoma Group guidelines for the management of primary cutaneous T-cell lymphomas. Br J Dermatol 2003; 149:1095. [PMID: 14696593]
- Zelentz AD et al; NCCN Non-Hodgkin's Lymphoma Practice Guidelines Panel. National Comprehensive Cancer Network: Non-Hodgkin's Lymphoma v.1.2005
  - http://www.nccn.org/professionals/physician_gls/PDF/nhl.pdf

WEB SITES

- American Academy of Dermatology
  - http://www.aad.org
- American Cancer Society: Treatment of Extranodal Non-Hodgkin's Lymphoma
  - http://www.cancer.org/docroot/CRI/content/CRI_2_4_4X_Treatment_of_Extranodal_Non-Hodgkins_Lymphoma_32.asp
- National Cancer Institute: Non-Hodgkin's Lymphoma
  - http://www.cancer.gov/cancertopics/types/non-hodgkins-lymphoma/

INFORMATION FOR PATIENTS

- Leukemia & Lymphoma Society: Cutaneous T Cell Lymphoma
  - http://www.leukemia-lymphoma.org/all_mat_toc.adp?item_id=9846&cat_id=1215
- National Cancer Institute: Mycosis Fungoides and Sézary Syndrome
  - http://www.cancer.gov/cancertopics/pdq/treatment/mycosisfungoides/patient

REFERENCES

- Kim YH et al: Mycosis fungoides and the Sézary syndrome. Semin Oncol 1999;26:276. [PMID: 10375085]
- Siegel RS et al: Primary cutaneous T-cell lymphoma: review and current concepts. J Clin Oncol 2000;18:2908. [PMID: 10920140]
- van Doorn R et al: Mycosis fungoides: disease evolution and prognosis of 309 Dutch patients. Arch Dermatol 2000;136:504. [PMID: 1076864]

Author(s)

Timothy G. Berger, MD

Malaria

KEY FEATURES

ESSENTIALS OF DIAGNOSIS

- History of exposure in a malaria-endemic area
- Periodic attacks of sequential chills, fever, and sweating
- Headache, myalgia, nausea, vomiting, splenomegaly; anemia, leukopenia
- Characteristic parasites in erythrocytes, identified in thick or thin blood films
- Complications of *Plasmodium falciparum* malaria: cerebral findings (mental disturbances, neurological signs, convulsions), prostration, hemolytic anemia, hyperpyrexia, hypotension, secretory diarrhea or dysentery, dark urine, hepatic or renal failure

GENERAL CONSIDERATIONS

- Four species of the genus *Plasmodium* are responsible for human malaria: *P vivax, P malariae, P ovale*, and *P falciparum*
- Transmitted from human to human by the bite of infected female mosquitoes. Transmission congenitally and by blood transfusion occurs
- The incubation period after exposure or after stopping chemoprophylaxis is, for *P falciparum*, approximately 12 days (range: 9–60 days); for *P vivax* and *P ovale*, 14 days [range: 8–27 days (initial attacks for some temperate strains may not occur for up to 8 months)]; and for *P malariae*, 30 days (range: 16–60 days)
- Untreated *P falciparum* infections can persist for up to 1.5 years but usually end in 6–8 months; *P vivax* and *P ovale* infections persist for as long as 5 years; and *P malariae* infections have lasted for as long as 50 years
- Protective immunity results from infection but decays after several years

DEMOGRAPHICS

- Annually worldwide, malaria causes 300–500 million new cases and over 1 million deaths
- About 30,000 travelers from the developed world are infected yearly, and several hundred die
- Malaria transmission occurs in large parts of Central and South America, Hispaniola, Africa, Asia, the Middle East, eastern Europe, and the South Pacific. Travel to urban areas of Central and South America and Southeast Asia entails minimal risk

CLINICAL FINDINGS

SYMPTOMS AND SIGNS

- Typical attacks show sequential symptoms over 4–6 h
  - Shaking chills (the **cold stage**)
  - Fever (the **hot stage**) to 41°C or higher
  - Marked diaphoresis (the **sweating stage**)
- Associated symptoms
  - Malaise, headache, dizziness
  - Gastrointestinal symptoms (anorexia, nausea, slight diarrhea, vomiting, abdominal cramps)
  - Myalgias, arthralgia, backache
  - Dry cough
- The attacks may show an every-other-day (tertian) periodicity in *P vivax, ovale*, or *falciparum* malaria or an every-third-day (quartan) periodicity in *P malariae* malaria
- Splenomegaly usually appears 4 or more days after the onset of acute symptoms; there may be mild hepatomegaly
- Presence of rash or lymphadenopathy suggests an additional or other diagnosis
- Between attacks, the patient feels fine
- After the primary episode, recurrences are common, each separated by a latent interval
- The severely ill patient may present with hyperpyrexia, prostration, impaired consciousness, agitation, hyperventilation, and bleeding

DIFFERENTIAL DIAGNOSIS

- Influenza
- Typhoid fever
- Viral hepatitis
- Dengue
- Visceral leishmaniasis (kala azar)
- Amebic liver abscess
- Babesiosis
- Leptospirosis
- Relapsing fever

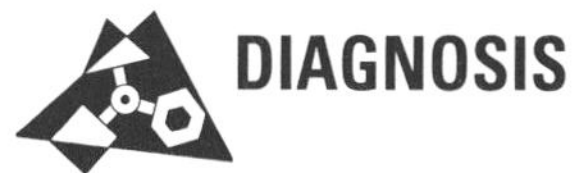

DIAGNOSIS

LABORATORY TESTS

- Thick and thin blood films, Giemsa stained, are the mainstay of diagnosis—clinical diagnosis is only 20–60% reliable compared with microscopy
- Blood from finger sticks or from the earlobe is preferred but should be free-flowing and uncontaminated by alcohol; if venipuncture blood is used, it should be examined shortly after it is drawn to avoid changes in morphology. Specimens should be obtained at about 8-h intervals for 3 days, including during and between febrile periods
- Serological tests are not commonly used in the diagnosis of initial acute attacks since antibody becomes detectable only 8–10 days after onset of symptoms. Antibody persists for 10 or more years, so it does distinguish between current and past infection
- A variety of serological tests—rapid antigen detection methods (including a dipstick format), fluorescent antibody methods, and polymerase chain reaction—are not satisfactory for field use or for establishing cure due to cost, need for expert interpretation or specialized equipment, or inability to differentiate malarial species
- During paroxysms, there may be transient leukocytosis. A marked anemia (normochromic, normocytic with reticulocytosis) may develop

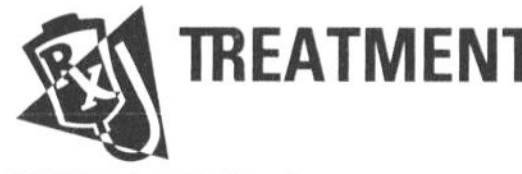

TREATMENT

MEDICATIONS

- See Table 144

Antimalarial drugs

- **4-Aminoquinolines**—chloroquine, hydroxychloroquine, amodiaquine
- **Diaminopyrimidines**—pyrimethamine, trimethoprim
- **Biguanides**—proguanil (chlorguanide, chlorproguanil)
- **8-Aminoquinolines**—primaquine
- **Cinchona alkaloids**—quinine, quinidine
- **Sulfonamides**—sulfadoxine, sulfadiazine, sulfamethoxazole
- **Sulfones**—dapsone
- **4-Quinoline-carbinolamines**—mefloquine
- **Antibiotics**—tetracycline, doxycycline, clindamycin

- **Others**—halofantrine, artemisinin (qinghaosu) and its derivatives, and atovaquone
- Pyrimethamine and proguanil are known as **antifolates**, since they inhibit dihydrofolate reductase of plasmodia
- **Drug combinations** used to treat chloroquine-resistant *P falciparum* malaria include Fansidar (pyrimethamine plus sulfadoxine), Maloprim (pyrimethamine plus dapsone), and Malarone (atovaquone plus proguanil)
- Resistance has developed to all classes of antimalarial drugs except the artemisinins. To slow the development of resistance, the antimalarial drugs are increasingly being evaluated in combinations with an artemisinin derivative
- Seek additional information on individual drug adverse reactions, cautions, contraindications, and parasitic resistance

THERAPEUTIC PROCEDURES

Management of severe* P falciparum *malaria

- Indications for parenteral treatment are failure to ingest or retain drugs, cerebral malaria, complications, and peripheral asexual parasitemia of 5% (250,000/μL) or more
- Black urine suggests hemoglobinuria. Renal failure, metabolic acidosis, severe anemia, pulmonary edema, gram-negative sepsis, and shock may ensue
- Rehydrate cautiously, particularly in the first 24 h, since overhydration may precipitate noncardiogenic pulmonary edema. Usually, 2–3 L of fluid is needed the first day, followed by 10–20 mL/kg/day
- Early dialysis may be necessary
- Blood glucose levels should be monitored every 6 h during the acute and early convalescent period
- Treat convulsions with diazepam (0.15 mg/kg intravenously or 0.5 mg/kg rectally) or with paraldehyde (0.1 mL/kg intramuscularly from a glass syringe)
- Keep the temperature below 38.5°C using acetaminophen (paracetamol) plus tepid sponging and fanning
- Significant disseminated intravascular coagulation should be treated with fresh whole blood, clotting factors, or platelets. Transfuse fresh whole blood or packed cells for hematocrits below 20%
- Consider exchange transfusion (5–10 L) when more than 10% of red blood cells are parasitized (5% if severe dysfunction of other organs is present)

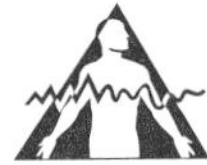

OUTCOME

FOLLOW-UP

- Blood films should be checked daily until parasitemia clears in *P falciparum*; check weekly thereafter for 4 weeks to observe for recrudescence of infection

COMPLICATIONS

***From* P falciparum**

- Cerebral malaria with edema, hyperpyrexia, hemolytic anemia, noncardiogenic pulmonary edema, or acute respiratory distress syndrome
- Bleeding, hypotension, or shock
- Acute tubular necrosis and renal failure, which is rarely associated with blackwater fever (dark urine), most commonly due to severe hemolysis following quinine treatment
- Acute hepatopathy, with centrilobular necrosis and jaundice
- Hypoglycemia, cardiac dysrhythmias, gastrointestinal syndromes, lactic acidosis; water and electrolyte disorders, disseminated intravascular coagulation

PROGNOSIS

- With prompt antimalarial treatment, the prognosis is generally good, except in *P falciparum* complications, when mortality may reach about 15%
- The prognosis is poor if more than 20% of infected red cells contain mature parasites, if more than 5% of neutrophils contain pigment, or if parasitemia is > 500,000/μL. Gram-negative bacteremia may contribute to death

WHEN TO REFER

- All patients should be referred to a provider with expertise in this area

WHEN TO ADMIT

- Severe *P falciparum* malaria is a medical emergency that requires hospitalization, intensive care with monitoring of electrolytes and acid-base balance, and immediate treatment without waiting for all laboratory results to be available

PREVENTION

- See Table 145 for chemoprophylaxis
- All persons who will be exposed should receive chemoprophylaxis. (See CDC information sites below)
- When out of doors between dusk and dawn, use protective measures. Clothing should cover most of the body, and DEET mosquito repellent should be applied to exposed areas every 3–4 h. To minimize the slight risk of toxic encephalopathy from DEET, it should be applied sparingly and only to exposed skin and outer clothing; the Ultrathon formulation provides a reduced concentration of DEET (33%) with extended protection (12 h)
- Emergency ("standby") self-treatment may be necessary when medical attention is unavailable within 24 h. Such persons may want to carry medications for self-treatment if they develop fever or flu-like symptoms (Table 144). It is imperative that medical follow-up be sought promptly

EVIDENCE

WEB SITES

- http://www.who.int/ith/chapter07_01.html
- http://www.cdc.gov/travel/diseases/htm#malaria
- www.malaria.org

INFORMATION FOR PATIENTS

- Centers for Disease Control
  – http://www.cdc.gov/malaria/faq.htm
- JAMA patient page. Malaria. JAMA 2005;293:1542. PMID: 15784878

REFERENCES

- Goldsmith RS: Infectious diseases: protozoal & helminthic. *Current Medical Diagnosis and Treatment*. Tierney LM, McPhee SJ, Papadakis, MA (editors). McGraw-Hill, 2005.
- Malarial Branch, Centers for Disease Control and Prevention (CDC), Atlanta, Georgia. For recorded information on prophylaxis: fax response, 888-232-3299; Internet. For additional information on prophylaxis or for management of acute attacks, phone 770-488-7788; after business hours, 404-639-2888.

Mallory-Weiss Syndrome

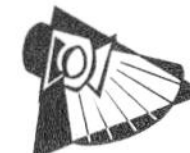

KEY FEATURES

ESSENTIALS OF DIAGNOSIS

- Defined as nonpenetrating mucosal tear at the gastroesophageal junction
- Hematemesis; usually self-limited
- Prior history of vomiting, retching, straining, lifting in 50%
- Endoscopy establishes diagnosis

GENERAL CONSIDERATIONS

- Accounts for ~5% of upper gastrointestinal bleeding

DEMOGRAPHICS

- Hiatal hernia present in majority; with vomiting, increased risk of tear
- Heavy alcohol use with vomiting or retching in 50% of patients
- Other risk factors: age, hiccups

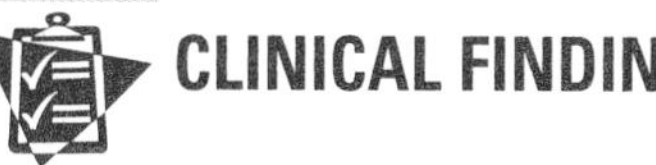

CLINICAL FINDINGS

SYMPTOMS AND SIGNS

- History of vomiting, retching, straining, lifting in 50%
- Hematemesis with or without melena

DIFFERENTIAL DIAGNOSIS

Other causes of hematemesis

- Hemoptysis
- Peptic ulcer disease
- Esophageal varices
- Gastric or duodenal varices (rare)
- Erosive gastritis, eg, nonsteroidal antiinflammatory drugs, alcohol, stress
- Portal hypertensive gastropathy
- Vascular ectasias (angiodysplasias)
- Gastric cancer

Rare causes

- Erosive esophagitis
- Aortoenteric fistula
- Dieulafoy's lesion (aberrant gastric submucosal artery)
- Hemobilia (blood in biliary tree), eg, iatrogenic, malignancy
- Pancreatic cancer
- Hemosuccus pancreaticus (pancreatic pseudoaneurysm)

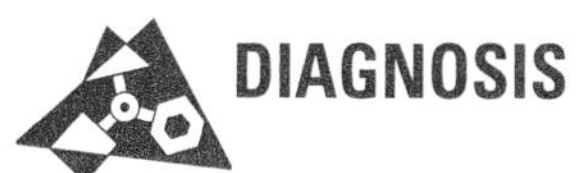

DIAGNOSIS

LABORATORY TESTS

- Obtain complete blood cell count, platelet count, prothrombin time, partial thromboplastin time, serum creatinine, liver enzymes and serologies, and type and cross-matching for 2–4 units or more of packed red blood cells
- Hematocrit is not a reliable indicator of the severity of acute bleeding

DIAGNOSTIC PROCEDURES

- Upper endoscopy is diagnostic: identification of a 0.5–4 cm linear mucosal tear usually located either at the gastroesophageal junction or, more commonly, just below the junction in the gastric mucosa of a hiatal hernia at the level of the diaphragm
- Assess hemodynamic status: systolic blood pressure; heart rate; postural hypotension

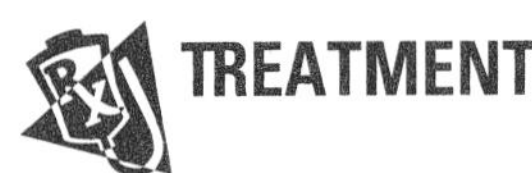

TREATMENT

MEDICATIONS

- Proton pump inhibitors to accelerate mucosal healing: omeprazole or rabeprazole, 20 mg PO QD, esomeprazole or pantoprazole, 40 mg PO QD

SURGERY

- Surgery with oversew of bleeding vessel rarely necessary

THERAPEUTIC PROCEDURES

- In patients without hemodynamic compromise or overt active bleeding, delay aggressive fluid repletion until extent of bleeding clarified
- For those with continuing active bleeding, insert two 18-gauge or larger intravenous lines
- Patients with hemodynamic compromise should be given 0.9% saline or lactated Ringer's injection and cross-matched blood
- Blood replacement to maintain a hematocrit of 25–28%
- In the absence of continued bleeding, the hematocrit should rise 3% for each unit of transfused packed red cells
- Transfuse blood in patients with brisk active bleeding regardless of the hematocrit
- Transfuse platelets if platelet count < 50,000/μL or if impaired platelet function due to aspirin use
- Uremic patients with active bleeding should be given 1–2 doses of desmopressin (DDAVP), 0.3 μg/kg IV at 12- to 24-h intervals
- Fresh frozen plasma should be given for actively bleeding patients with a coagulopathy and INR >1.5
- In massive bleeding, give 1 unit of fresh frozen plasma for each 5 units of packed red blood cells transfused
- Endoscopic hemostatic therapy for those with continuing active bleeding
- Epinephrine 1:10,000 injection, cautery with a bipolar or heater probe coagulation device or application of metallic clip is effective in 90–95% of cases
- Angiographic arterial embolization or operative intervention is required in patients who fail endoscopic therapy

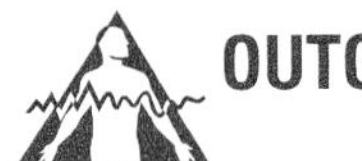

OUTCOME

FOLLOW-UP

- None required

COMPLICATIONS

- Persistent bleeding

PROGNOSIS

- Most Mallory-Weiss bleeds stop spontaneously with rapid healing of mucosal tears
- Persistent or recurrent bleeding most likely in patients with concomitant portal hypertension or coagulopathy

WHEN TO ADMIT

- All patients with significant hematemesis warrant admission
- Patients without active bleeding and without portal hypertension or coagulopathy may be discharged after 24 h
- Patients with active bleeding requiring hemostasis therapy should be observed in hospital at least 48 h

EVIDENCE

PRACTICE GUIDELINES

- Adler DG: ASGE Guideline: the role of endoscopy in acute non-variceal hemorrhage. Gastrointest Endosc 2004;60:497. [PMID: 14623622]
- Barkus A et al: A Canadian clinical practice algorithm for the management of patients with nonvariceal upper gastrointestinal bleeding. Can J Gastroenterol 2004;18:605. [PMID: 15497000]

INFORMATION FOR PATIENTS

- Medline Plus Medical Encyclopedia
  - http://www.nlm.nih.gov/medlineplus/ency/article/000269.htm
  - http://home.mdconsult.com/das/book/30975174/view/891?sid=204180645
- National Digestive Diseases Information Clearinghouse
  - http://digestive.niddk.nih.gov/ddiseases/pubs/bleeding/

REFERENCES

- Kortas D et al: Mallory-Weiss tear: predisposing factors and predictors of a complicated course. Am J Gastroenterol 2001;96:2863. [PMID: 11693318]
- Park CH et al: A prospective, randomized trial of endoscopic band ligation vs. epinephrine injection for actively bleeding Mallory-Weiss syndrome. Gastrointest Endosc 2004;60:22. [PMID: 15229420]

Author(s)

Kenneth R. McQuaid, MD

Mania

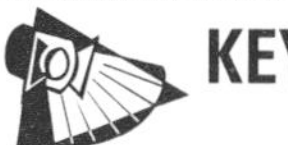

KEY FEATURES

ESSENTIALS OF DIAGNOSIS

- Mood ranging from euphoria to irritability
- Sleep disruption
- Hyperactivity
- Racing thoughts
- Grandiosity
- Variable psychotic symptoms

GENERAL CONSIDERATIONS

- Often combined with depression
- May occur alone, together with mania in a mixed episode, or in cyclic fashion with depression
- In almost all cases, the manic episode is part of a broader bipolar (manic-depressive) disorder

DEMOGRAPHICS

- Spring and summer tend to be the peak periods

CLINICAL FINDINGS

SYMPTOMS AND SIGNS

- Mood change characterized by
  - Elation with hyperactivity
  - Overinvolvement in life activities
  - Increased irritability
  - Flight of ideas
  - Easy distractibility
  - Little need for sleep
- The overenthusiastic quality of the mood and the expansive behavior initially attract others
- The irritability, mood lability with swings into depression, aggressive behavior, and grandiosity usually lead to marked interpersonal difficulties
- Activities may occur that are later regretted, eg
  - Excessive spending
  - Resignation from a job
  - A hasty marriage
  - Sexual acting out
  - Exhibitionistic behavior
  - Alienation of friends and family
- A typical manic episode can include
  - Gross delusions
  - Paranoid ideation of severe proportions
  - Auditory hallucinations usually related to some grandiose perception
- The episodes begin abruptly (sometimes precipitated by life stresses) and may last from several days to months
- Manic patients differ from schizophrenics in that the former use more effective interpersonal maneuvers, are more sensitive to the social maneuvers of others, and are more able to utilize weakness and vulnerability in others to their own advantage

DIFFERENTIAL DIAGNOSIS

- Bipolar disorder (manic-depression)
- Substance abuse, eg, cocaine
- Hypomania
- Cyclothymic disorder (depression and hypomania)
- Schizophrenia
- Hyperthyroidism
- Substance abuse, eg, cocaine, amphetamines
- Medications, eg, corticosteroids, thyroxine
- CNS disease, eg, complex partial seizures, tumor, neurosyphilis, HIV
- Personality disorder, eg, borderline, narcissistic

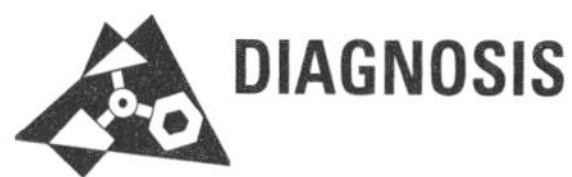

DIAGNOSIS

LABORATORY TESTS

- Thyroid-stimulating hormone
- Complete blood cell count
- Blood urea nitrogen
- Serum creatinine
- Serum electrolyte determinations
- Urinalysis

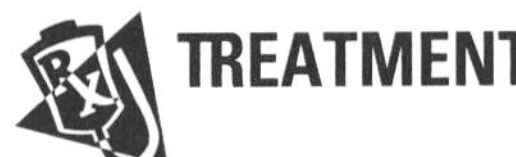

TREATMENT

MEDICATIONS

- Mania due to bipolar disorder
  - Acute manic or hypomanic symptoms respond to lithium therapy after several days of treatment
    - It is common to use neuroleptic drugs or high-potency benzodiazepines (eg, clonazepam) to immediately treat the excited or psychotic manic stage
  - Atypical neuroleptics (olanzapine 5–20 mg PO) along with a benzodiazepine, if indicated, may be used initially to treat agitation and psychosis
  - For immediate behavioral control, when necessary, olanzapine (2.5–10 mg IM) or haloperidol (5–10 mg orally or IM) may be used
  - Clonazepam (1–2 mg PO Q 4–6 h) may be used instead of or in conjunction with a neuroleptic agent to control acute behavioral symptoms
  - Lithium (1200–1800 mg/day targeted to therapeutic serum level) is effective in acute mania or hypomania, but takes several days to take effect
  - Valproic acid (750 mg/day PO divided and titrated to therapeutic levels) can be loaded to therapeutic levels in 2–3 days
  - Carbamazepine (800–1600 mg/day PO) is used in patients intolerant or unresponsive to lithium
  - Calcium channel blockers (verapamil) have been used in refractory patients
  - Anticonvulsants such as lamotrigine (25–50 mg/day titrated slowly upward) and topiramate are beginning to be used

THERAPEUTIC PROCEDURES

- Mania secondary to other conditions
  - The underlying condition needs to be treated as well

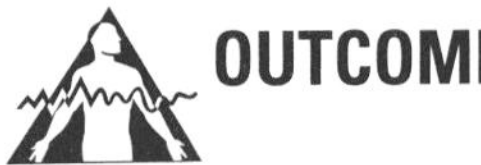

OUTCOME

WHEN TO REFER

- Patients should be under the care of a psychiatrist

WHEN TO ADMIT

- Most patients with mania should be admitted for monitoring until the symptoms are brought under control

PREVENTION

- Lithium (1200–1800 mg/day targeted to therapeutic serum level) as prophylaxis can limit the frequency and severity of mood swings in 70% of patients

EVIDENCE

PRACTICE GUIDELINES

- American Psychiatric Association. Practice guideline for the treatment of patients with bipolar disorder (revision). Am J Psychiatry 2002;159(4 Suppl):1. [PMID:11958165]
- Goodwin G et al: Evidence-based guidelines for treating bipolar disorder: recommendations from the British Association for Psychopharmacology. J Psychopharmacol 2003;1:149. [PMID: 12870562]
- National Guideline Clearinghouse: American Psychiatric Association. Bipolar disorder guidelines, 2002
  - http://www.guideline.gov/summary/summary.aspx?doc_id=3302

WEB SITES

- American Psychiatric Association
  - http://www.psych.org/
- Internet Mental Health
  - http://www.mentalhealth.com/
- National Institutes of Health—National Institute of Mental Health
  - http://www.nimh.nih.gov

INFORMATION FOR PATIENTS

- Depression and Bipolar Support Alliance
  - http://www.dbsalliance.org/info/bipolar.html
- National Institute of Mental Health
  - http://www.nimh.nih.gov/publicat/bipolar.cfm
  - http://www.nimh.nih.gov/publicat/manic.cfm

REFERENCE

- Hirschfeld RM et al: Rapid antimanic effect of risperidone monotherapy: a 3-week multicenter, double blind, placebo-controlled study. Am J Psychiatry 2004;161:1057. [PMID:15169694]
- Keck PE Jr et al: Ziprasidone in the treatment of acute bipolar mania: a 3-week placebo-controlled, double-blind, randomized trial. Am J Psychiatry 2003;160:741. [PMID:12668364]
- Sato T et al: Syndromes and phenomenological subtypes underlying acute mania: a factor analytic study of 576 manic patients. Am J Psychiatry 2000;159:968. [PMID:12042185]

Author(s)

Stuart J. Eisendrath, MD

Jonathan E. Lichtmacher, MD

Marfan's Syndrome

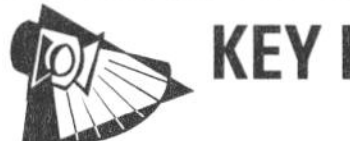

KEY FEATURES

ESSENTIALS OF DIAGNOSIS

- Marfan's syndrome is a systemic connective tissue disease, characterized by abnormalities of skeletal, ocular, and cardiovascular systems
- Disproportionately tall stature, thoracic deformity, and joint laxity or contractures
- Ectopia lentis and myopia
- Aortic dilation and dissection; mitral valve prolapse
- Autosomal dominant inheritance

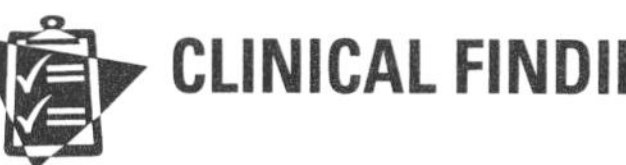

CLINICAL FINDINGS

SYMPTOMS AND SIGNS

- Wide variability in clinical presentation
- Affected patients typically are tall, with particularly long arms, legs, and digits (arachnodactyly)
- Commonly, joint dislocations and pectus excavatum
- Ectopia lentis, severe myopia, and retinal detachment
- Aortic and mitral valve regurgitation occur often from elongated chordae tendineae, which on occasion may rupture
- Mitral valve prolapse in about 85%
- Ascending aortic involvement produces a dilated aortic root, aortic regurgitation, and aortic dissection
- Spontaneous pneumothorax
- Dural ectasia
- Striae atrophicae

DIFFERENTIAL DIAGNOSIS

- Tall stature (normal)
- Homocystinuria (with lens dislocation) as a result of cystathionine synthase deficiency
- Aortic root disease resulting from other cause, eg, ankylosing spondylitis, syphilis, temporal (giant cell) arteritis, Takayasu's arteritis
- Ehlers-Danlos syndrome
- Idiopathic mitral valve prolapse

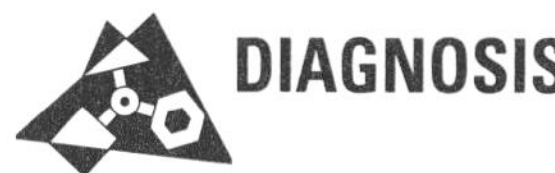

DIAGNOSIS

LABORATORY TESTS

- No simple laboratory test
- DNA analysis can detect mutations in the fibrillin gene on chromosome 15

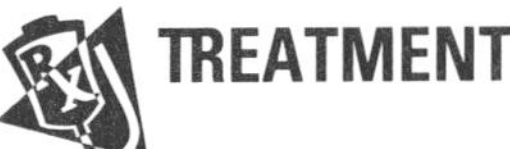

TREATMENT

MEDICATIONS

- Standard endocarditis prophylaxis
- Chronic β-adrenergic blockade (eg, atenolol, 1–2 mg/kg) retards the rate of aortic dilation

SURGERY

- Prophylactic replacement of the aortic root (and, if necessary, aortic valve) when the diameter reaches 50–55 mm (normal: < 40 mm) prolongs life
- Annual orthopedic consultation if scoliosis

THERAPEUTIC PROCEDURES

- Regular ophthalmological surveillance to correct visual acuity and thus prevent amblyopia
- Restriction of vigorous physical exertion

OUTCOME

FOLLOW-UP

- Echocardiography at least annually to monitor aortic diameter and aortic and mitral valve function

PROGNOSIS

- Untreated, Marfan's syndrome patients commonly die in the fourth or fifth decade from aortic dissection or congestive heart failure secondary to aortic regurgitation

PREVENTION

- Prenatal and presymptomatic diagnosis for patients in whom a molecular defect in fibrillin has been found and for families in whom linkage analysis using polymorphic markers around the fibrillin gene can be performed

EVIDENCE

PRACTICE GUIDELINES

- European Society of Cardiology: Management of grown up congenital heart disease, 2003
  - http://www.guideline.gov/summary/summary.aspx?doc_id=3826&nbr=3051

WEB SITES

- National Center for Biotechnology Information: Online Mendelian Inheritance in Man
  - http://www.ncbi.nlm.nih.gov/entrez/dispomim.cgi?id=154700
- National Marfan Foundation
  - http://www.marfan.org/

INFORMATION FOR PATIENTS

- Dolan DNA Learning Center: Marfan Syndrome
  - http://www.yourgenesyourhealth.org/marfan/whatisit.htm
- Mayo Clinic: Marfan Syndrome
  - http://www.mayoclinic.com/invoke.cfm?id=DS00540
- National Institute of Arthritis and Musculoskeletal and Skin Diseases: Questions and Answers About Marfan Syndrome
  - http://www.niams.nih.gov/hi/topics/marfan/marfan.htm
- National Library of Medicine: Marfan Syndrome
  - http://ghr.nlm.nih.gov/condition=marfansyndrome

REFERENCES

- Dean JC: Management of Marfan syndrome. Heart 2002;88:97. [PMID: 12067963]
- Erkula G et al: Growth and maturation in Marfan syndrome. Am J Med Genet 2002;109:100. [PMID: 11977157]
- Gott VL et al: Replacement of the aortic root in patients with Marfan's syndrome. N Engl J Med 1999;340:1307. [PMID: 10219065]
- Miller DC: Valve-sparing aortic root replacement in patients with the Marfan syndrome. J Thorac Cardiovasc Surg 2003;125:773. [PMID: 12698136]
- Pyeritz RE: The Marfan syndrome. Annu Rev Med 2000;51:481. [PMID: 10774478]

Author(s)

Reed E. Pyeritz, MD, PhD

Melanoma, Malignant

KEY FEATURES

ESSENTIALS OF DIAGNOSIS

- The American Cancer Society has proposed the mnemonic "ABCD = Asymmetry, Border irregularity, Color variegation, and Diameter greater than 6 mm"
- Should be suspected in any pigmented skin lesion with recent change in appearance
- Examination with good light may show varying colors, including red, white, black, and bluish
- Borders typically irregular

GENERAL CONSIDERATIONS

- Leading cause of death due to skin disease
- Melanoma favors fair-skinned whites with a history of significant (blistering) sun exposure before the age of 18
- 10% of melanomas occur in "melanoma prone kindreds," ie, familial

Classification

- Lentigo maligna melanoma (arising on sun-exposed skin of older individuals)
- Superficial spreading malignant melanoma (the most common type, occurring in two-thirds of individuals developing melanoma, largely a disease of whites)
- Nodular malignant melanoma
- Acral lentiginous melanomas (arising on palms, soles, and nail beds); occur in nonwhites primarily); may be a difficult diagnosis because benign pigmented lesions of the hands, feet, and nails occur commonly in more darkly pigmented persons and clinicians may hesitate to biopsy the palms and especially the soles and nail beds; as a result, the diagnosis is often delayed until the tumor has become clinically obvious and histologically thick; clinicians should give special attention to new or changing lesions in these areas
- Malignant melanomas on mucous membranes
- Miscellaneous forms such as amelanotic (nonpigmented) melanoma and melanomas arising from blue nevi (rare) and congenital nevi

DEMOGRAPHICS

- One in four cases of melanoma occur before the age of 40
- Melanoma is the most common cancer of women between the ages of 25 and 29 and the second most common cause in women ages 30–34
- There are about 51,000 cases of melanoma in the United States annually, with 7800 deaths

CLINICAL FINDINGS

SYMPTOMS AND SIGNS

- An irregular notched border where the pigment appears to be leaking into the normal surrounding skin
- Topography may be irregular, ie, partly raised and partly flat
- Color variegation, and colors such as pink, blue, gray, white, and black are indications for referral
- Bleeding and ulceration
- A mole that stands out from the patient's other moles (the "ugly duckling sign")
- A patient with a large number of moles is at increased risk for melanoma
- The history of a changing mole (evolution) is the single most important historical reason for close evaluation and possible referral
- Acral lentiginous melanomas: dark, sometimes irregularly shaped lesions on the palms and soles and new, often broad and solitary, darkly pigmented longitudinal streaks in the nails

DIFFERENTIAL DIAGNOSIS

- Acquired nevus (mole), eg, junctional nevus, compound nevus
- Seborrheic keratosis
- Lentigo, eg, solar lentigo
- Dermatofibroma
- Basal cell carcinoma (pigmented type)
- Congenital nevus
- Atypical (dysplastic) nevus
- Blue nevus
- Halo nevus
- Pyogenic granuloma
- Kaposi's sarcoma
- Pregnancy-associated darkening of nevi

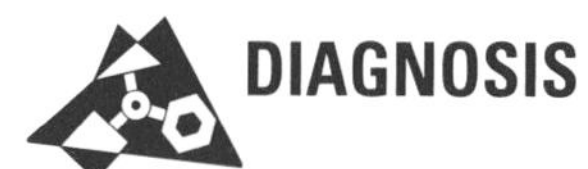

DIAGNOSIS

LABORATORY TESTS

- Skin biopsies

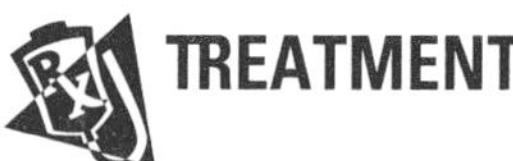

TREATMENT

MEDICATIONS

- Alpha interferon and vaccine therapy may reduce recurrences in patients with high-risk melanomas

SURGERY

- Treatment consists of excision once a histologic diagnosis is made
- The area is usually excised with margins dictated by the thickness of the tumor; large margins (radius ≥ 5 cm) are no longer indicated; thin low-risk and intermediate-risk tumors require only conservative margins of 1–3 cm; more specifically, surgical margins of 0.5 cm for melanoma in situ and 1 cm for lesions < 1 mm in thickness are most often recommended
- Sentinel lymph node biopsy (selective lymphadenectomy) using preoperative lymphoscintigraphy and intraoperative lymphatic mapping is effective for staging melanoma patients with intermediate risk without clinical adenopathy and is recommended for all patients with lesions over 1 mm in thickness or with high-risk histologic features

OUTCOME

PROGNOSIS

- Tumor thickness is the single most important prognostic factor
- 10-year survival rates—related to thickness in millimeters—are as follows:
  - < 0.76 mm, 96%
  - 0.76–1.69 mm, 81%
  - 1.7–3.6 mm, 57%
  - > 3.6 mm, 31%
- With lymph node involvement, the 5-year survival rate is 30%; and with distant metastases, it is < 10%; more accurate prognoses can be made on the basis of thickness, site, histologic features, and sex of the patient
- Overall survival for melanomas in whites rose from 60% in 1960–1963 to 85% in 1983–1990, due primarily to earlier detection of lesions

WHEN TO REFER

- Any pigmented lesion with suspicious features should be referred to a dermatologist for possible biopsy

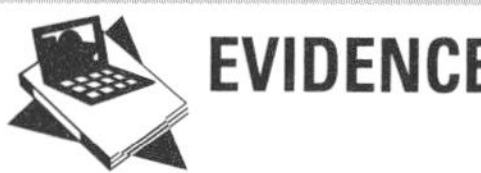

EVIDENCE

PRACTICE GUIDELINES

- Houghton AN et al; NCCN Melanoma Practice Guidelines Panel. National Comprehensive Cancer Network: Melanoma v.1.2004
  - http://www.nccn.org/professionals/physician_gls/PDF/melanoma.pdf
- Scottish Intercollegiate Guidelines Network. Cutaneous melanoma. A national clinical guideline. 2003
  - http://www.guideline.gov/summary/summary.aspx?ss=15&doc_id=3877&nbr=3086

WEB SITES

- American Academy of Dermatology
  - http://www.aad.org
- National Cancer Institute: Melanoma Information for Patients and Health Professionals
  - http://www.cancer.gov/cancertopics/types/melanoma

INFORMATION FOR PATIENTS

- American Academy of Family Physicians: Melanoma: A Kind of Skin Cancer
  - http://familydoctor.org/666.xml
- American Cancer Society: Melanoma
  - http://www.cancer.org/docroot/CRI/CRI_2_3x.asp?rnav=cridg&dt=39
- MedlinePlus: Melanoma Interactive Tutorial
  - http://www.nlm.nih.gov/medlineplus/tutorials/melanoma.html
- Skin Cancer Foundation: Melanoma
  - http://www.skincancer.org/melanoma/index.php

REFERENCES

- Bafounta M et al: Is dermoscopy (epiluminescence microscopy) useful for the diagnosis of melanoma? Arch Dermatol 2001;137:1343. [PMID: 11594860]
- Balch CM et al: A new American Joint Committee on Cancer staging system for cutaneous melanoma. Cancer 2000;88:1484. [PMID: 10717634]
- Goldstein BG et al: Diagnosis and management of malignant melanoma. Am Fam Physician 2001;63:1359. [PMID: 11310650]
- Rigel DS et al: Malignant melanoma: prevention, early detection, and treatment in the 21st century. CA Cancer J Clin 2000;50:215. [PMID: 10986965]

Author(s)

Timothy G. Berger, MD

Meningitis, Meningococcal

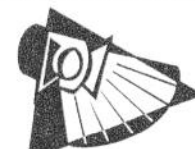

KEY FEATURES

ESSENTIALS OF DIAGNOSIS

- Fever, headache, vomiting, confusion, delirium, convulsions
- Petechial rash of skin and mucous membranes
- Neck and back stiffness
- Purulent spinal fluid with gram-negative intracellular and extracellular diplococci
- Culture of cerebrospinal fluid, blood, or petechial aspiration confirms the diagnosis

GENERAL CONSIDERATIONS

- Caused by *Neisseria meningitidis* of groups A, B, C, Y, W-135, and others
- Infection is transmitted by droplets
- The clinical illness may take the form of meningococcemia (a fulminant form of septicemia) without meningitis, meningococcemia with meningitis, or predominantly meningitis
- Chronic recurrent meningococcemia with fever, rash, and arthritis can occur, particularly in those with terminal complement deficiencies

DEMOGRAPHICS

- College freshmen—particularly those living in dormitories—have been shown to have a modestly increased risk of invasive meningococcal disease

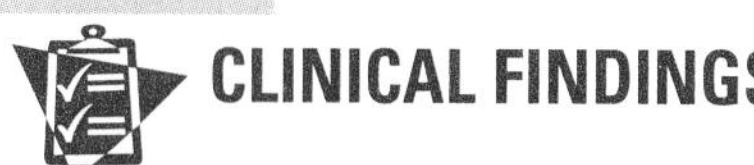

CLINICAL FINDINGS

SYMPTOMS AND SIGNS

- High fever, chills, and headache; back, abdominal, and extremity pains; and nausea and vomiting are typical
- In severe cases, rapidly developing confusion, delirium, seizures, and coma occur
- Nuchal and back rigidity are typical
- A petechial rash often first appearing in the lower extremities and at pressure points is found in most cases. Petechiae may vary from pinhead sized to large ecchymoses or even areas of skin gangrene that may later slough if the patient survives

DIFFERENTIAL DIAGNOSIS

- Meningitis due to other causes, eg, pneumococcus, *Listeria*, aseptic
- Rickettsial or echovirus infection and other bacterial infections (eg, staphylococcal infections, scarlet fever) may also produce a petechial rash
- Subarachnoid hemorrhage
- Encephalitis
- Petechial rash due to gonococcemia, infective endocarditis, thrombotic thrombocytopenic purpura, Rocky Mountain spotted fever, or viral exanthem
- "Neighborhood reaction" causing abnormal cerebrospinal fluid, eg, brain abscess, epidural abscess, vertebral osteomyelitis, mastoiditis, sinusitis, brain tumor
- Dural sinus thrombosis
- Noninfectious meningeal irritation: carcinomatous meningitis, sarcoidosis, systemic lupus erythematosus, drugs (eg, nonsteroidal antiinflammatory drugs, trimethoprim-sulfamethoxazole), pneumonia, shigellosis

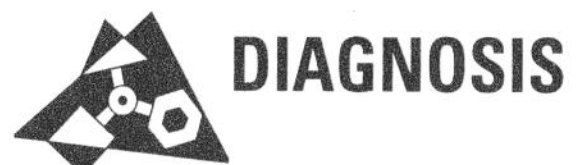

DIAGNOSIS

LABORATORY TESTS

- The organism is usually found by smear or culture of the cerebrospinal fluid, oropharynx, blood, or aspirated petechiae
- Prothrombin time and partial thromboplastin time are prolonged, fibrin dimers are elevated, fibrinogen is low, and the platelet count is depressed if disseminated intravascular coagulation is present

Cerebrospinal fluid analysis

- See Table 130
- Typically, a cloudy or purulent fluid, with elevated pressure, increased protein, and decreased glucose content
- Usually contains more than 1000 cells/μL, with polymorphonuclear cells predominating and containing gram-negative intracellular diplococci
- The absence of organisms in a Gram-stained smear does not rule out the diagnosis
- The capsular polysaccharide can often be demonstrated in cerebrospinal fluid or urine by latex agglutination; this is especially useful in partially treated patients, though sensitivity is only 60–80%

IMAGING STUDIES

- For neurological defects or signs of elevated intracranial pressure, MRI or CT imaging can exclude mass lesions

DIAGNOSTIC PROCEDURES

- Lumbar puncture

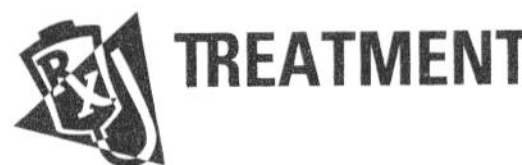

TREATMENT

MEDICATIONS

- See Table 128
- Intravenous antimicrobial therapy should be started immediately after blood cultures are obtained in all acutely ill patients and before proceeding with imaging studies, if these are indicated
- Aqueous penicillin G is the antibiotic of choice (24 million units/24 h) in divided doses every 4 h
- In penicillin-allergic patients or those in whom pneumococcal or gram-negative meningitis is a consideration, ceftriaxone, 4 g intravenously once a day, should be used
- Chloramphenicol, 1 g every 6 h, is an alternative in the severely penicillin- or cephalosporin-allergic patient
- In critically ill patients with evidence of increased intracranial pressure, administration of dexamethasone (0.6 mg/kg/day in four divided doses) may help
- Duration of therapy: 10–14 days (with ceftriaxone a 5-day regimen has been reported to be effective)

THERAPEUTIC PROCEDURES

- Lumbar puncture should be performed in all patients with suspected meningococcal meningitis; imaging prior to lumbar puncture to rule out mass lesions is indicated if papilledema, other evidence of increased intracranial pressure, or focal neurological deficits are present

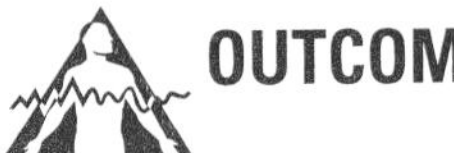

OUTCOME

COMPLICATIONS

- Obtundation or deterioration in mental status may result from cerebral edema and increased intracranial pressure
- Disseminated intravascular coagulation
- Ischemic necrosis of digits, distal extremities

PROGNOSIS

- Mortality <5% with early therapy of patients with meningitis
- Meningococcemia associated with a 20% mortality

WHEN TO ADMIT

- All patients in whom meningococcal meningitis is suspected should be admitted for observation and empirical therapy

PREVENTION

- Effective polysaccharide vaccines for groups A, C, Y, and W-135 are available
- The Advisory Committee on Immunization Practices now recommends immunization with a single dose of polyvalent vaccine (active against meningococcal groups A, C, Y, and W-135) for college freshmen
- Outbreaks in closed populations are best controlled by eliminating nasopharyngeal carriage of meningococci. Rifampin is the drug of choice, in a dosage of 600 mg twice a day for 2 days. A single 500-mg oral dose of ciprofloxacin or one intramuscular 250-mg dose of ceftriaxone in adults is also effective

EVIDENCE

PRACTICE GUIDELINES

- National Guideline Clearinghouse
  - http://www.guideline.gov/summary/summary.aspx?doc_id=2364
  - http://www.guideline.gov/summary/summary.aspx?doc_id=2365

WEB SITES

- CDC—Division of Bacterial and Mycotic Diseases
  - http://www.cdc.gov/ncidod/dbmd/
- Meningococcemia Case Study
  - http://path.upmc.edu/cases/case53.html
  - http://path.upmc.edu:80/cases/case53.html

INFORMATION FOR PATIENTS

- CDC—Division of Bacterial and Mycotic Diseases
  - http://www.cdc.gov/ncidod/dbmd/diseaseinfo/meningococcal_g.htm
  - http://www.cdc.gov/nip/publications/VIS/vis-mening.pdf
- JAMA patient page: Lumbar puncture. JAMA 2002;288:2056.
- JAMA patient page: Meningitis. JAMA 1999;281:1560.

REFERENCES

- Harrison LH et al: Risk of meningococcal infection in college students. JAMA 1999;281:1906. [PMID: 10349894]
- Van de Beek D et al: Clinical features and prognostic factors in adults with bacterial meningitis. N Engl J Med 2004;351:1849. [PMID: 1550981]

Author(s)

Henry F. Chambers, MD

Meningitis, Pneumococcal

KEY FEATURES

ESSENTIALS OF DIAGNOSIS

- Fever, headache, altered mental status
- Meningismus
- Gram-positive diplococci on Gram stain of cerebrospinal fluid; counterimmunoelectrophoresis may be positive in partially treated cases

GENERAL CONSIDERATIONS

- *Streptococcus pneumoniae* is the most common cause of meningitis in adults and the second most common cause of meningitis in children over the age of 6 years
- Head trauma, with cerebrospinal fluid leaks, sinusitis, and pneumonia may precede it
- Up to 40% of infections are caused by pneumococci resistant to at least one drug and 15% are due to a strain resistant to three or more drugs

DEMOGRAPHICS

- Until 2000, *S pneumoniae* infections caused 100,000–135,000 hospitalizations for pneumonia, 6 million cases of otitis media, and 60,000 cases of invasive disease, including 3300 cases of meningitis
- Disease figures are now changing due to conjugate vaccine introduction

CLINICAL FINDINGS

SYMPTOMS AND SIGNS

- Rapid onset, with fever, headache, and altered mentation
- Pneumonia may be present
- Compared with meningitis caused by the meningococcus, pneumococcal meningitis lacks a rash, and focal neurological deficits, cranial nerve palsies, and obtundation are more prominent features

DIFFERENTIAL DIAGNOSIS

- Meningitis due to other causes, eg, meningococcus, *Listeria*, aseptic
- Subarachnoid hemorrhage
- Encephalitis
- "Neighborhood reaction" causing abnormal cerebrospinal fluid, eg, brain abscess, epidural abscess, vertebral osteomyelitis, mastoiditis, sinusitis, brain tumor
- Dural sinus thrombosis
- Noninfectious meningeal irritation: carcinomatous meningitis, sarcoidosis, systemic lupus erythematosus, drugs (eg, nonsteroidal antiinflammatory drugs, trimethoprim-sulfamethoxazole), pneumonia, shigellosis

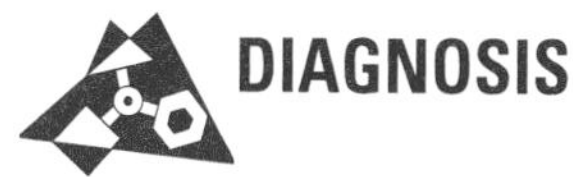

DIAGNOSIS

LABORATORY TESTS

- See Table 130
- Cerebrospinal fluid
  - Typically has more than 1000 white blood cells per microliter, over 60% of which are polymorphonuclear leukocytes
  - Glucose concentration is less than 40 mg/dL, or less than 50% of the simultaneous serum concentration
  - Protein usually exceeds 150 mg/dL
  - Gram stain shows gram-positive cocci in up to 80–90% of cases
- In untreated cases, blood or cerebrospinal fluid cultures are almost always positive
- Fifty percent rate of bacteremia
- Antigen detection tests may occasionally be helpful in establishing the diagnosis in the patient who has been partially treated and in whom cultures and stains are negative

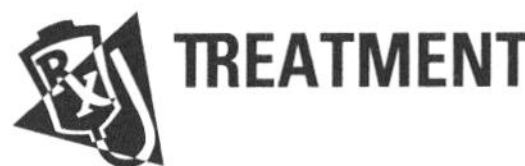

TREATMENT

MEDICATIONS

- See Tables 128 and 129
- Give antibiotics as soon as the diagnosis is suspected
- If lumbar puncture must be delayed (eg, while awaiting results of an imaging study to exclude a mass lesion), ceftriaxone, 4 g, is given intravenously after blood cultures (positive in 50% of cases) have been obtained
- If gram-positive diplococci are present on the Gram stain, then vancomycin, 30 mg/kg/day intravenously in two divided doses, should be administered in addition to ceftriaxone until the isolate is confirmed not to be penicillin-resistant
- Once susceptibility to penicillin has been confirmed, penicillin, 24 million units daily in six divided doses, or ceftriaxone, 4 g/day as a single dose or as two divided doses, is recommended
- For severe penicillin allergy chloramphenicol, 50 mg/kg every 6 h, is an alternative (failures have occurred with penicillin-resistant strains)
- Duration of therapy is 10–14 days in documented cases
- The best therapy for penicillin-resistant strains is not known. Susceptibility testing is essential
- If the minimum inhibitory concentration (MIC) of ceftriaxone or cefotaxime is ≤0.5 μg/mL, single-drug therapy with either of these cephalosporins is likely to be effective; when the MIC is ≥1 μg/mL, treatment with a combination of ceftriaxone, 2 g every 12 h, plus vancomycin, 30 mg/kg/day in two divided doses, is recommended
- Give 10 mg of dexamethasone intravenously immediately prior to or concomitantly with the first dose of appropriate antibiotic and every 6 h thereafter for a total of 4 days. The antiinflammatory activity could impair penetration of some drugs into the cerebrospinal fluid, particularly vancomycin, and cause a potential treatment failure

OUTCOME

FOLLOW-UP

- If a patient with a penicillin-resistant organism has not responded to a third-generation cephalosporin, repeat lumbar puncture is indicated to assess the bacteriological response

COMPLICATIONS

- Hearing loss
- Residual neurological deficit

PROGNOSIS

- Patients presenting with depressed levels of consciousness have a worse outcome
- Dexamethasone administered with antibiotic to adults has been associated with a 60% reduction in mortality and a 50% reduction in unfavorable outcome

WHEN TO REFER

- Consider early referral to an infectious disease specialist

WHEN TO ADMIT

- All patients with suspected bacterial meningitis

PREVENTION

- Pneumococcal vaccine recommendations (Table 132)

EVIDENCE

PRACTICE GUIDELINES

- National Guideline Clearinghouse
  - http://www.guideline.gov/summary/summary.aspx?doc_id=2773

WEB SITES

- CDC—Division of Bacterial and Mycotic Diseases
  - http://www.cdc.gov/ncidod/dbmd/
- Karolinska Institute—Directory of Bacterial Infections and Mycoses
  - http://www.mic.ki.se/Diseases/C01.html

INFORMATION FOR PATIENTS

- CDC—Division of Bacterial and Mycotic Diseases
  - http://www.cdc.gov/ncidod/dbmd/diseaseinfo/meningococcal_g.htm
- JAMA patient page: Lumbar puncture. JAMA 2002;288:2056.
- JAMA patient page: Meningitis. JAMA 1999;281:1560.
- National Institutes of Health
  - http://www.nlm.nih.gov/medlineplus/ency/article/000607.htm

REFERENCES

- de Gans J et al: Dexamethasone in adults with bacterial meningitis. N Engl J Med 2002;347:1549. [PMID: 12432041]
- Tunkel AR, Scheld WM: Treatment of bacterial meningitis. Curr Infect Dis Rep 2002;4:7. [PMID 11853652]
- van de Beek D et al: Clinical features and prognostic factors in adults with bacterial meningitis. N Engl J Med 2004;351:1849. [PMID: 15509818]

Author(s)

Henry F. Chambers, MD

Menopausal Syndrome

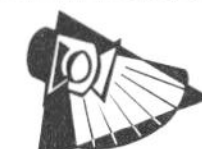

KEY FEATURES

ESSENTIALS OF DIAGNOSIS

- Cessation of menses due to aging or to bilateral oophorectomy
- Elevation of follicle-stimulating hormone (FSH) and luteinizing hormone (LH) levels
- Hot flushes and night sweats (in 80% of women)
- Decreased vaginal lubrication; thinned vaginal mucosa with or without dyspareunia

GENERAL CONSIDERATIONS

- Menopause denotes a 1- to 3-year period during which a woman adjusts to a diminishing and then absent menstrual flow and the physiologic changes that may be associated—hot flushes, night sweats, and vaginal dryness
- Premature menopause is defined as ovarian failure and menstrual cessation before age 40; this often has a genetic or autoimmune basis
- Surgical menopause due to bilateral oophorectomy is common and can cause more severe symptoms owing to the sudden rapid drop in sex hormone levels
- Cessation of ovarian function is not associated with severe emotional disturbance or personality changes. The time of menopause often coincides with other major life changes, such as departure of children from the home, a midlife identity crisis, or divorce

DEMOGRAPHICS

- The average age at menopause in Western societies today is 51 years

CLINICAL FINDINGS

SYMPTOMS AND SIGNS

- Menstrual cycles generally become irregular as menopause approaches
- Anovular cycles occur more often, with irregular cycle length and occasional menorrhagia
- Menstrual flow amount diminishes
- Finally, cycles become longer, with missed periods or episodes of spotting only
- When no bleeding has occurred for 1 year, the menopausal transition has occurred
- Hot flushes (feelings of intense heat over the trunk and face, with flushing of the skin and sweating)
- Hot flushes can begin before the cessation of menses and are more severe after surgical menopause
- Flushing is more pronounced late in the day, during hot weather, after ingestion of hot foods or drinks, or during periods of tension. Occurring at night, they often cause sweating and insomnia and result in fatigue on the following day
- Vaginal atrophy and decreased vaginal lubrication
- The introitus decreases in diameter
- Pelvic examination reveals pale, smooth vaginal mucosa and a small cervix and uterus
- The ovaries are not normally palpable after the menopause

DIFFERENTIAL DIAGNOSIS

- Pregnancy
- Premature ovarian failure
- Hypothyroidism or hyperthyroidism
- Hyperprolactinemia
- Polycystic ovary syndrome
- Hypothalamic amenorrhea, eg, stress, weight change, exercise
- Other endocrine causes: Cushing's syndrome, Addison's disease, androgen-secreting tumor (adrenal, ovarian), congenital adrenal hyperplasia, acromegaly
- Depression

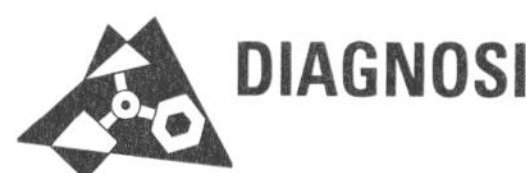

DIAGNOSIS

LABORATORY TESTS

- Serum FSH and LH levels are elevated
- Vaginal cytologic examination will show a low estrogen effect with predominantly parabasal cells

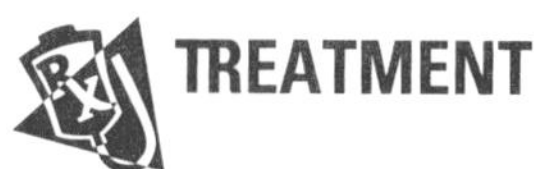

TREATMENT

MEDICATIONS

Natural menopause

- **Vasomotor symptoms**
- Oral conjugated estrogens, 0.3 mg or 0.625 mg; estradiol, 0.5 or 1 mg; or estrone sulfate, 0.625 mg; or estradiol can be given transdermally as skin patches that are changed once or twice weekly and secrete 0.05–0.1 mg of hormone daily
- When either form of estrogen is used, add a progestin (medroxyprogesterone acetate) to prevent endometrial hyperplasia or cancer
  - Give estrogen on Days 1–25 of each calendar month, with 5–10 mg of medroxyprogesterone acetate added on Days 14–25. Withhold hormones from Day 26 until the end of the month, which will produce a light, generally painless monthly period
  - Alternatively, give the estrogen along with 2.5 mg of medroxyprogesterone acetate daily, without stopping. This causes initial bleeding or spotting, but within a few months it produces an atrophic endometrium that will not bleed
- If the patient has had a hysterectomy, a progestin need not be used
- Explain that hot flushes will probably return if the hormone is discontinued
- Data from the Womens Health Initiative (WHI) study
  - Women should not use combination progestin-estrogen therapy for more than 3 or 4 years
  - The increased risk of cardiovascular disease, cerebrovascular disease, and breast cancer with this regimen outweighed the benefits
  - Women who cannot find relief with alternative approaches may wish to consider continuing use of combination therapy after a thorough discussion of the risks and benefits
  - Alternatives to hormone therapy for vasomotor symptoms include

1. Selective serotonin reuptake inhibitors such as paroxetine 12.5 mg or 25 mg/day, or venlafaxine 75 mg/day
2. Gabapentin, an antiseizure medication, is also effective at 900 mg/day
3. Clonidine given orally or transdermally, 100–150 μg daily, also may reduce the frequency of hot flushes, but its use is limited by side effects, including dry mouth, drowsiness, and hypotension

- **Vaginal atrophy**
- Estradiol vaginal ring, left in place for 3 months, is suitable for long-term use. Progestin therapy to protect the endometrium is unnecessary
- Short-term use of estrogen vaginal cream will relieve symptoms of atrophy, but because of variable absorption, therapy with either systemic hormone replacement or the vaginal ring is preferable
- Testosterone propionate, 1–2%, 0.5–1 g, in a vanishing cream base used in the same manner is also effective if estrogen is contraindicated
- A bland lubricant such as unscented cold cream or water-soluble gel can be helpful at the time of coitus
- **Osteoporosis**
- Women should ingest at least 800 mg of calcium daily and 1 g of elemental calcium should be taken as a daily supplement at the time of the menopause and thereafter; calcium supplements should be taken with meals to increase their absorption. Vitamin D, 400 units/day from food, sunlight, or supplements, enhances calcium absorption
- Daily energetic walking and exercise help maintain bone mass
- **Advantages and risks of hormone therapy**
- The use of long-term hormone replacement therapy for prevention is no longer indicated. Clinicians should review with women and carefully consider the risks and benefits
- Current indications for hormone therapy (estrogen and progestin) are for treatment of vasomotor symptoms, which resolve within several months to a few years

Surgical menopause

- Estrogen replacement is generally started immediately after surgery
- Conjugated estrogens 1.25 mg, estrone sulfate 1.25 mg, or estradiol, 2 mg is given for 25 days of each month
- After age 45–50 years, this dose can be tapered to 0.625 mg of conjugated estrogens or equivalent

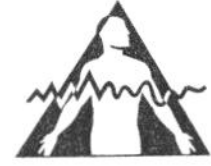

OUTCOME

FOLLOW-UP

- Annual visit to monitor symptoms and need for therapy
- Any bleeding after cessation of menses warrants investigation by endometrial curettage or aspiration to rule out endometrial cancer
- For women who are receiving hormone replacement therapy for vasomotor symptoms, an attempt should be made at least every 6 months to taper the dose and to discontinue therapy

COMPLICATIONS

- Dyspareunia from vaginal atrophy and decreased vaginal lubrication
- Overall health risks exceed benefits from use of both combined estrogen plus progestin and estrogen alone for an average of 5 years
  - For combination therapy, these risks include increased coronary heart disease events, cerebral vascular accidents, pulmonary emboli, invasive breast cancer, gallbladder disease, and mild cognitive impairment and dementia
  - For estrogen alone, the risks included an increased risk of stroke, no evidence of protection from coronary heart disease, and an increase in the combined risk of mild cognitive impairment and dementia compared with placebo

PREVENTION

- Continued sexual activity will help prevent vaginal shrinkage

EVIDENCE

PRACTICE GUIDELINES

- Institute for Clinical Systems Improvement. Menopause and Hormone Therapy: Collaborative Decision Making and Management, 2004.
  - http://www.icsi.org/knowledge/detail.asp?catID=29&itemID=172

WEB SITE

- North American Menopause Society
  - http://www.menopause.org/

INFORMATION FOR PATIENTS

- American Academy of Family Physicians: Menopause
  - http://familydoctor.org/125.xml
- MedlinePlus: Menopause Interactive Tutorial
  - http://www.nlm.nih.gov/medlineplus/tutorials/menopause.html
- National Women's Health Information Center: Menopause
  - http://www.4woman.gov/faq/menopaus.htm

REFERENCES

- American College of Obstetricians and Gynecologists: Hormone therapy. Obstet Gynecol 2004;104(Suppl):1S. [PMID: 15458927–15458942]
- Anderson GL: Effects of conjugated equine estrogen in postmenopausal women with hysterectomy: the Women's Health Initiative randomized controlled trial. JAMA 2004;291:1701. [PMID: 15082697]
- Rapp SR et al: Effect of estrogen plus progestin on global cognitive function in postmenopausal women: the Women's Health Initiative Memory Study: a randomized controlled trial. JAMA 2003;289:2663. [PMID: 12771113]
- Rossouw JE et al: Risks and benefits of estrogen plus progestin in healthy postmenopausal women: principal results from the Women's Health Initiative randomized controlled trial. JAMA 2002;288:321. [PMID: 12117397]
- Shumaker SA et al: Conjugated equine estrogens and incidence of probable dementia and mild cognitive impairment in postmenopausal women: Women's Health Initiative Memory Study. JAMA 2004;291:2947. [PMID: 15213206]

Author(s)

H. Trent MacKay, MD, MPH

Mesothelioma

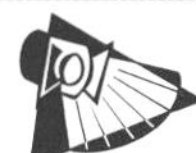

KEY FEATURES

ESSENTIALS OF DIAGNOSIS

- Chronic progressive chest pain and dyspnea
- Pleural effusion and/or pleural thickening on chest radiographs
- Malignant cells in pleural fluid or tissue

GENERAL CONSIDERATIONS

- Primary tumors arising from the mesothelial surfaces of the pleura (80% of cases), peritoneum, pericardium, or tunica vaginalis
- 75% of pleural mesotheliomas are diffuse (usually malignant)
- Mean age at symptom onset is 60 years with time between exposure and symptoms 20–40 years

DEMOGRAPHICS

- Men outnumber women 3:1
- Malignant pleural mesothelioma is associated with asbestos exposure (70% of cases), with a lifetime risk to asbestos workers of 8%
- Cigarette smoking significantly increases the risk of bronchogenic carcinoma in asbestos workers and aggravates asbestosis, but there is no association between smoking and mesothelioma independent of asbestos
- Asbestos exposure occurs through
  - Mining
  - Milling
  - Manufacturing
  - Shipyard work
  - Insulation
  - Brake linings
  - Building construction and demolition
  - Roofing materials
  - Other asbestos-containing products

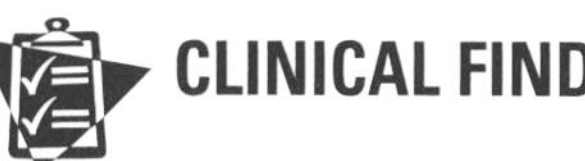

CLINICAL FINDINGS

SYMPTOMS AND SIGNS

- Insidious onset of shortness of breath, nonpleuritic chest pain, and weight loss
- Physical findings include
  - Dullness to percussion
  - Diminished breath sounds
  - Finger clubbing in some cases
- Malignant pleural mesothelioma progresses rapidly as the tumor spreads along the pleural surface to involve the pericardium, mediastinum, and contralateral pleura
- Tumor may eventually extend beyond the thorax to involve abdominal lymph nodes and organs

DIFFERENTIAL DIAGNOSIS

- Chronic organized empyema
- Sarcoma
- Metastatic tumor to the pleura, especially adenocarcinoma
- Malignant fibrosing histiocytoma
- Other causes of pleural effusion (see Pleural Effusion)

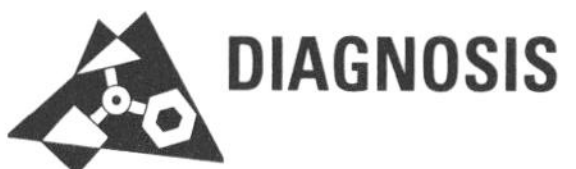

DIAGNOSIS

LABORATORY TESTS

- Pleural fluid analysis often reveals a hemorrhagic exudate

IMAGING STUDIES

- Radiographic findings
  - Nodular, irregular, unilateral pleural thickening
  - Varying degrees of unilateral pleural effusion
- CT helps determine the extent of pleural and extrapleural involvement

DIAGNOSTIC PROCEDURES

- Thoracentesis
- Closed pleural biopsy
- Open pleural biopsy may be necessary to obtain an adequate specimen for histological diagnosis

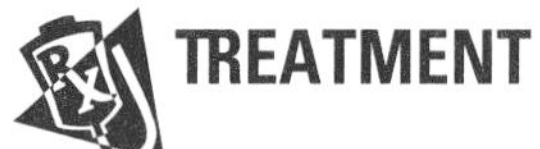

TREATMENT

SURGERY

- Some surgeons believe that extrapleural pneumonectomy is the preferred approach for patients with early-stage disease
- Resection may offer palliative benefit in some cases

THERAPEUTIC PROCEDURES

- Treatment with surgery, radiation, chemotherapy, or a combination of methods is generally unsuccessful
- Drainage of effusions, pleurodesis, and radiation therapy may offer palliative benefit

OUTCOME

COMPLICATIONS

- Local invasion of thoracic structures with superior vena caval syndrome, hoarseness, Horner's syndrome, dysphagia
- Paraneoplastic syndrome
  - Thrombocytosis
  - Hemolytic anemia
  - Disseminated intravascular coagulopathy
  - Migratory thrombophlebitis
- Metastatic disease

PROGNOSIS

- Median survival from symptom onset ranges from 5 months in extensive disease to 16 months in localized disease
- 75% of patients are dead 1 year from diagnosis
- Most patients die of respiratory failure and complications of local extension

WHEN TO REFER

- Upon diagnosis, refer to a pulmonologist, oncologist, or possibly a thoracic surgeon who can evaluate the patient for multidisciplinary treatment

WHEN TO ADMIT

- For pleural fluid drainage
- For severe dyspnea
- For pain management

PREVENTION

- Avoidance of tobacco smoke (primary or secondary) in those with a history of asbestos exposure

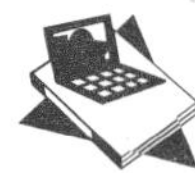

EVIDENCE

PRACTICE GUIDELINES

- National Guideline Clearinghouse
  - http://www.guideline.gov/summary/summary.aspx?doc_id=3637&nbr=2863&string=lung+cancer
- Detterbeck FC et al: Lung cancer. Invasive staging: the guidelines. Chest 2003;123(1 Suppl):167S. [PMID:12527576]
- Rivera MP et al: Diagnosis of lung cancer: the guidelines. Chest 2003;123(1 Suppl):129S. [PMID:12527572]

INFORMATION FOR PATIENTS

- National Cancer Institute
  - http://cis.nci.nih.gov/fact/6_36.htm
- National Institutes of Health
  - http://www.nlm.nih.gov/medlineplus/ency/article/000115.htm
  - http://www.nlm.nih.gov/medlineplus/ency/article/000116.htm

REFERENCES

- Pistolesi M et al: Malignant pleural mesothelioma: update, current management, and newer therapeutic strategies. Chest 2004;126:1318. [PMID:15486399]
- van Ruth S et al: Surgical treatment of malignant pleural mesothelioma: a review. Chest 2003;123:551. [PMID:12576380]

Author(s)

Mark S. Chesnutt, MD
Thomas J. Prendergast, MD

Mononeuropathies

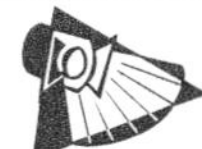

KEY FEATURES

ESSENTIALS OF DIAGNOSIS

- Focal motor or sensory deficit that conforms to the territory of an individual peripheral nerve

GENERAL CONSIDERATIONS

- Injury of an individual nerve along its course
- Possible compression, angulation, or stretching of an individual nerve by neighboring anatomic structures
- Nerve affected at a point where it passes through a narrow space (entrapment neuropathy)

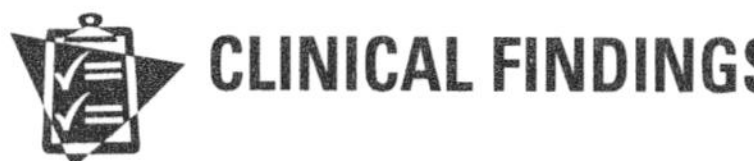

CLINICAL FINDINGS

SYMPTOMS AND SIGNS

- Entrapment neuropathies
  - May be asymptomatic
  - Symptoms may resolve rapidly and spontaneously
  - Symptoms may become progressively more disabling and distressing
  - Precise neurologic deficit depends on the nerve involved
- Involvement of a sensory or mixed nerve commonly results in pain distal to the lesion
- Percussion of the nerve at the site of the lesion may lead to paresthesias in its distal distribution
- There are several syndromes
  - See Carpal Tunnel Syndrome
  - See Femoral Neuropathy
  - See Meralgia Paresthetica
  - See Ulnar Neuropathy
- **Pronator teres syndrome** affects the anterior interosseous nerve, a motor branch of the median nerve, that arises below the elbow between the two heads of the pronator teres muscle
  - A lesion may result after trauma or from compression, eg, from a fibrous band
  - Weakness is confined to the pronator quadratus, flexor pollicis longus, and the flexor digitorum profundus to the second and third digits
- **Sciatic and common peroneal nerve palsies**
  - Most common etiology for sciatic nerve palsy is probably a misplaced deep intramuscular injection
  - Trauma to the buttock, hip, or thigh may also be responsible
  - The common peroneal nerve itself may be compressed or injured in the region of the head and neck of the fibula, eg, by sitting with crossed legs or wearing high boots
  - Common peroneal involvement causes weakness of dorsiflexion and eversion of the foot, accompanied by numbness or blunted sensation of the anterolateral aspect of the calf and dorsum of the foot
- In **tarsal tunnel syndrome** compression of the posterior tibial nerve or its branches between the bony floor and ligamentous roof of the tarsal tunnel leads to pain, paresthesias, and numbness over the bottom of the foot, especially at night, with sparing of the heel
- In **facial neuropathy,** an isolated facial palsy may occur with HIV seropositivity, sarcoidosis, Lyme disease, or most often, idiopathic (see Bell's palsy)

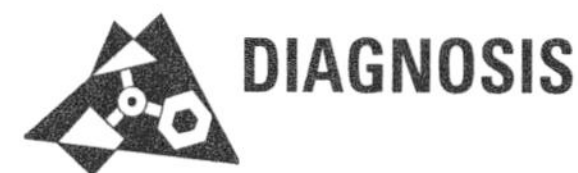

DIAGNOSIS

DIAGNOSTIC PROCEDURES

- EMG can be indispensable for the accurate localization of the focal lesion
- Entrapment neuropathy may be the sole manifestation of subclinical polyneuropathy, which can be excluded by nerve conduction studies
- Peripheral nerve tumors may be distinguishable from entrapment neuropathy only by
  - Noting the presence of a mass along the course of the nerve
  - Demonstrating the precise site of the lesion with appropriate electrophysiologic studies

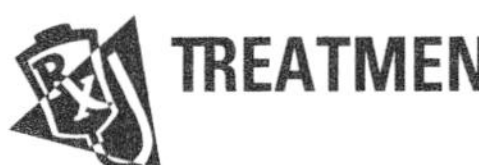

TREATMENT

MEDICATIONS

- In some neuropathies, local infiltration of the region about the nerve with corticosteroids may be of value

SURGERY

- Surgical decompression may help when there is a progressively increasing neurologic deficit or electrodiagnostic studies show evidence of partial denervation in weak muscles
- In the rare peripheral nerve tumors, symptomatic lesions are surgically removed when possible

THERAPEUTIC PROCEDURES

- When repetitive mechanical trauma is responsible, avoid by occupational adjustment or job retraining
- When acute compression is the cause such as may occur in intoxicated individuals ("Saturday night palsy"), no treatment is needed in most cases
- In chronic compressive or entrapment neuropathies, avoid aggravating factors and correct any underlying systemic conditions

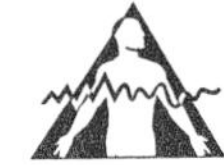

OUTCOME

PROGNOSIS

- In patients with acute compression neuropathy, complete recovery generally occurs within 2 months without treatment, presumably because the underlying pathology is demyelination
- Axonal degeneration can occur in severe cases, and then recovery takes longer and may be partial

EVIDENCE

PRACTICE GUIDELINES

- Jablecki CK et al; American Association of Electrodiagnostic Medicine; American Academy of Neurology; American Academy of Physical Medicine and Rehabilitation: Practice parameter: Electrodiagnostic studies in carpal tunnel syndrome. Report of the American Association of Electrodiagnostic Medicine, American Academy of Neurology, and the American Academy of Physical Medicine and Rehabilitation. Neurology 2002;58:1589. [PMID: 12058083]

INFORMATION FOR PATIENTS

- The Mayo Clinic
  - http://www.mayoclinic.com/invoke.cfm?id=DS00131
- National Institutes of Health
  - http://www.nlm.nih.gov/medlineplus/ency/article/000780.htm

REFERENCE

- Brown WF, Bolton CF, Aminoff MJ (eds): *Neuromuscular Function and Disease*, 2 vols. Saunders, 2002.

Author(s)

Michael J. Aminoff, MD, DSc, FRCP

Motor Neuron Disease, Degenerative

Mitral Valve Prolapse p. 1109. Molluscum Contagiosum p. 1110.

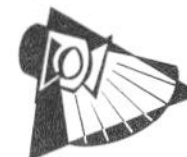

KEY FEATURES

ESSENTIALS OF DIAGNOSIS

- Variable weakness and wasting of muscles without sensory changes
- Progressive course
- No identifiable underlying cause other than genetic basis in familial cases

GENERAL CONSIDERATIONS

- There is degeneration of the anterior horn cells in the spinal cord, the motor nuclei of the lower cranial nerves, and the corticospinal and corticobulbar pathways
- Five varieties have been characterized on clinical grounds

Progressive bulbar palsy

- Bulbar involvement predominates
- Disease processes affect primarily the motor nuclei of the cranial nerves

Pseudobulbar palsy

- Bulbar involvement predominates
- Due to bilateral corticobulbar disease and thus reflects upper motor neuron dysfunction

Progressive spinal muscular atrophy

- A lower motor neuron deficit in the limbs
- Due to degeneration of the anterior horn cells in the spinal cord

Primary lateral sclerosis

- There is a purely upper motor neuron deficit in the limbs

Amyotrophic lateral sclerosis

- A mixed upper and lower motor neuron deficit is found in the limbs and bulbar muscles
- This disorder is sometimes associated with dementia or parkinsonism

DEMOGRAPHICS

- Symptoms generally begin between 30 and 60 years of age
- The disease is usually sporadic, but familial cases may occur

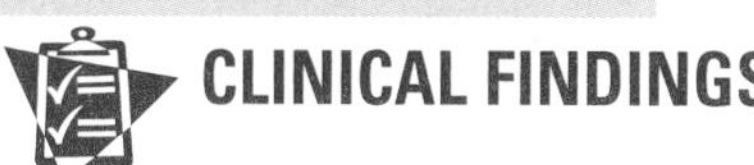

CLINICAL FINDINGS

SYMPTOMS AND SIGNS

- Difficulty in swallowing, chewing, coughing, breathing, and talking (dysarthria) occur with bulbar involvement
- In **progressive bulbar palsy**, there is drooping of the palate, a depressed gag reflex, pooling of saliva in the pharynx, a weak cough, and a wasted, fasciculating tongue
- In **pseudobulbar palsy**, the tongue is contracted and spastic and cannot be moved rapidly from side to side
- Limb involvement is characterized by motor disturbances (weakness, stiffness, wasting, fasciculations) reflecting lower or upper motor neuron dysfunction
- There are no objective changes on sensory examination, though there may be vague sensory complaints
- The sphincters are generally spared

DIFFERENTIAL DIAGNOSIS

Upper motor neuron disease

- Stroke
- Space-occupying lesion
- Compressive spinal cord lesion
- Multiple sclerosis

Lower motor neuron disease

- Infections of anterior horn cells (eg, poliovirus or West Nile virus)
- Radiculopathy, plexopathy, peripheral neuropathy, and myopathy are distinguished by clinical examination
- Pure motor syndromes resembling motor neuron disease may occur in association with monoclonal gammopathy or multifocal motor neuropathies with conduction block. Multifocal motor neuropathy is distinguished by electrodiagnostic studies
- A motor neuronopathy may develop in Hodgkin's disease and has a relatively benign prognosis

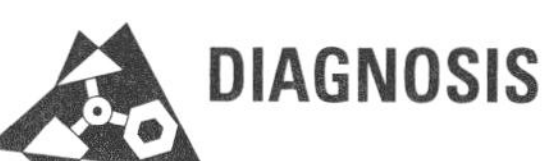

DIAGNOSIS

LABORATORY TESTS

- The serum creatine kinase may be slightly elevated but never reaches the extremely high values seen in some of the muscular dystrophies
- The cerebrospinal fluid is normal

DIAGNOSTIC PROCEDURES

- Electromyography may show changes of chronic partial denervation, with abnormal spontaneous activity in the resting muscle and a reduction in the number of motor units under voluntary control
- In patients with suspected spinal muscular atrophy or amyotrophic lateral sclerosis, the diagnosis should not be made with confidence unless such changes are found in at least three extremities
- Motor conduction velocity is usually normal but may be slightly reduced, and sensory conduction studies are also normal
- Biopsy of a wasted muscle shows the histologic changes of denervation

Monoamide Oxidase Inhibitor Overdose p. 1110. Monoclonal Gammopathy of Uncertain Significance (MGUS) p. 1110.

Motor Neuron Disease, Degenerative

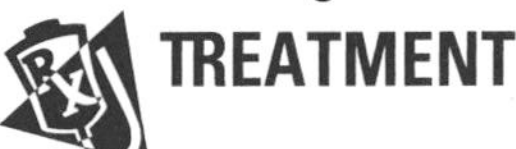

TREATMENT

MEDICATIONS

- Riluzole, 100 mg PO QD, reduces the presynaptic release of glutamate and may slow progression of amyotrophic lateral sclerosis
- There is otherwise no specific treatment except in patients with gammopathy, in whom plasmapheresis and immunosuppression may lead to improvement
- Multifocal motor neuropathy is treated by intravenous immunoglobulin therapy or with cyclophosphamide
- Symptomatic and supportive measures may include prescription of anticholinergic drugs (such as trihexyphenidyl, amitriptyline, or atropine) if drooling is troublesome, braces or a walker to improve mobility, and physical therapy to prevent contractures
- Spasticity may be helped by baclofen or diazepam

SURGERY

- Gastrostomy or cricopharyngomyotomy is sometimes resorted to in extreme cases of predominant bulbar involvement, and tracheostomy may be necessary if respiratory muscles are severely affected; however, in the terminal stages of these disorders, the aim of treatment should be to keep patients as comfortable as possible

THERAPEUTIC PROCEDURES

- A semiliquid diet or nasogastric tube feeding may be needed if dysphagia is severe

OUTCOME

PROGNOSIS

- The disorder is progressive, and amyotrophic lateral sclerosis is usually fatal within 3–5 years; death usually results from pulmonary infections
- Patients with bulbar involvement generally have the poorest prognosis

WHEN TO REFER

- All patients should be referred to a physician with expertise in the diagnosis and treatment of these disorders

EVIDENCE

PRACTICE GUIDELINES

- Brooks BR et al; World Federation of Neurology Research Group on Motor Neuron Diseases. El Escorial revisited: revised criteria for the diagnosis of amyotrophic lateral sclerosis. Amyotroph Lateral Scler Other Motor Neuron Disord 2000;1:293. [PMID: 11464847]
- National Guideline Clearinghouse
  - http://www.guideline.gov/summary/summary.aspx?doc_id=3259&nbr=2485&string=ALS

WEB SITE

- Neuromuscular Disease Center
  - http://www.neuro.wustl.edu/neuromuscular/

INFORMATION FOR PATIENTS

- National Institute of Neurological Disorders and Stroke
  - http://www.ninds.nih.gov/disorders/amyotrophiclateralsclerosis/detail_amyotrophiclateralsclerosis.htm
  - http://www.ninds.nih.gov/disorders/motor_neuron_diseases/motor_neuron_diseases.htm

REFERENCES

- Benditt JO et al: Empowering the individual with ALS at the end-of-life: disease-specific advance care planning. Muscle Nerve 2001;24:1706. [PMID: 11745983]
- Parton MJ et al: Motor neuron disease and its management. J R Coll Physicians Lond 1999;33:212. [PMID: 10402566]
- Rowland LP et al: Amyotrophic lateral sclerosis. N Engl J Med 2001;344:1688. [PMID: 11386269]

Author(s)

Michael J. Aminoff, MD, DSc, FRCP

Mountain Sickness

KEY FEATURES

ESSENTIALS OF DIAGNOSIS

- Mountain sickness disorders include acute mountain sickness, acute high-altitude pulmonary edema, subacute mountain sickness, and chronic mountain sickness

GENERAL CONSIDERATIONS

- Lack of sufficient time for acclimatization, increased physical activity, and varying degrees of health may be responsible for the acute, subacute, and chronic disturbances that result from hypoxia at altitudes greater than 2000 m (6560 ft)

Acute mountain sickness

- The severity correlates with altitude and rate of ascent

Acute high-altitude pulmonary edema

- This serious complication usually occurs at levels above 3000 m (9840 ft)

Acute high-altitude encephalopathy

- Appears to be an extension of the central nervous system symptoms of acute mountain sickness
- It usually occurs at elevations above 2500 m (8250 ft)
- More common in the unacclimatized
- Clinical findings are due largely to hypoxemia and cerebral edema

Subacute mountain sickness

- Occurs most frequently in unacclimatized individuals at altitudes above 4500 m (14,764 ft)

Chronic mountain sickness (Monge's disease)

- Chronic hypoxia and polycythemia in residents of high-altitude communities who have lost their acclimatization to such an environment
- May be difficult to differentiate from chronic pulmonary disease
- Uncommon condition

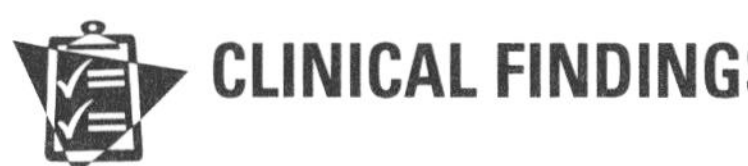

CLINICAL FINDINGS

SYMPTOMS AND SIGNS

Acute mountain sickness

- Initially, headache (most severe and persistent symptom), lassitude, drowsiness, dizziness, chilliness, nausea and vomiting, dyspnea, and cyanosis
- Later, facial flushing, irritability, difficulty in concentrating, vertigo, tinnitus, visual disturbances, auditory disturbances, anorexia, insomnia, increased dyspnea and weakness on exertion, increased headaches (from cerebral edema), palpitations, tachycardia, Cheyne-Stokes breathing, and weight loss
- More severe manifestations include pulmonary edema and encephalopathy

Acute high-altitude pulmonary edema

- Early symptoms may appear within 6–36 h
- Incessant dry cough, shortness of breath, headache, fatigue, dyspnea at rest, and chest tightness
- Later, wheezing, orthopnea, and hemoptysis may occur
- Tachycardia, mild fever, tachypnea, cyanosis, prolonged respiration, and rales and rhonchi
- Confusion or coma
- May resemble severe pneumonia

Acute high-altitude encephalopathy

- Altered consciousness, severe headaches, confusion, truncal ataxia, staggering gait, focal deficits, nausea and vomiting, and seizures may progress to obtundation and coma
- High-altitude retinopathy can include dilated vessels, retinal hemorrhage, vitreous hemorrhage, and papilledema

Subacute mountain sickness

- Dyspnea and cough
- Dehydration, skin dryness, and pruritus

Chronic mountain sickness

- Somnolence, mental depression, hypoxemia, cyanosis, finger clubbing
- Right ventricular failure

DIFFERENTIAL DIAGNOSIS

- Migraine or tension headache
- Stroke or intracerebral bleed
- Congestive heart failure
- Alcohol or drug intoxication
- Sepsis

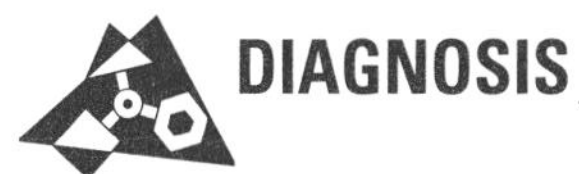

DIAGNOSIS

LABORATORY TESTS

Acute high-altitude pulmonary edema

- Hypoxia
- The white cell count is often slightly elevated, but the erythrocyte sedimentation rate is usually normal
- Elevated pulmonary arterial blood pressure; normal wedge pressure

Subacute mountain sickness

- Hypoxia
- The hematocrit may be elevated

Chronic mountain sickness

- Polycythemia; hemoglobin > 22 g/dL (hematocrit often > 75%)
- Pulmonary function tests usually disclose alveolar hypoventilation and elevated Pco_2 but fail to reveal defective oxygen transport

IMAGING STUDIES

Acute high-altitude pulmonary edema

- Chest x-ray findings vary from irregular patchy infiltration in one lung to nodular densities bilaterally or with transient prominence of the central pulmonary arteries
- Transient nonspecific electrocardiographic changes, occasional right ventricular strain

Subacute and chronic mountain sickness

- There may be ECG changes of right axis deviation and right atrial and ventricular hypertrophy
- X-ray evidence of right-sided heart enlargement and central pulmonary vessel prominence

Mononucleosis p. 1111. *Moraxella Catarrhalis* Infection p. 1111.

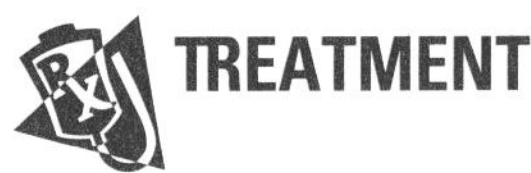

TREATMENT

MEDICATIONS

Acute mountain sickness

- Acetazolamide, 125–250 mg PO Q 12 h, or dexamethasone, 8 mg PO initially followed by 4 mg Q 6 h, while symptoms persist

Acute high-altitude pulmonary edema

- Nifedipine, 10 mg PO Q 4 h, for symptomatic relief
- Dexamethasone, 4 mg PO Q 6 h, for CNS symptoms
- Acetazolamide, 125–250 mg PO Q 12 h, if acute mountain sickness suspected
- For bacterial pneumonia, give appropriate antibiotics

Acute high-altitude encephalopathy

- Dexamethasone, 4–8 mg PO Q 6 h

THERAPEUTIC PROCEDURES

Acute mountain sickness

- Voluntary periodic hyperventilation
- Symptoms generally clear in 24–48 h; if they persist or are severe, patient must return to lower altitudes
- Definitive treatment is immediate descent (essential if reduced consciousness, ataxia, or pulmonary edema occurs)
- 100% O_2, 1–2 L/min, may relieve acute symptoms
- If immediate descent not possible, portable hyperbaric chambers may provide symptomatic relief

Acute high-altitude pulmonary edema

- Rest in semi-Fowler position (head raised) and administration of 100% O_2 by mask 4–6 L/min for 15–30 min; to conserve O_2, use lower flow rates (2–4 L/min)
- Immediate descent [≥ 610 m (2000 ft)] essential
- Recompression in portable hyperbaric bag will temporarily reduce symptoms if immediate descent not possible
- Treatment for acute respiratory distress syndrome may be required

Acute high-altitude encephalopathy

- Treatment is immediate descent of ≥ 610 m (2000 ft) until symptoms improve
- Administer O_2 (100%) (2–4 L/min) by mask
- If immediate descent impossible, use portable hyperbaric chamber

Subacute mountain sickness

- Treatment: rest, oxygen administration, diuretics, return to lower altitudes

Chronic mountain sickness

- Almost all abnormalities disappear when patient returns to sea level

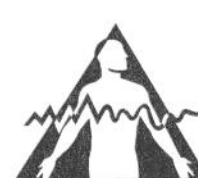

OUTCOME

PREVENTION

- Persons with symptomatic cardiac or pulmonary disease should avoid high altitudes
- Slow ascent: 300 m (984 ft) per day
- Adequate rest the day before travel, reduced food intake, and avoidance of alcohol, tobacco
- Avoid unnecessary physical activity during travel
- A period of rest and inactivity for 1–2 days after arrival at high altitudes
- Acetazolamide, 125–250 mg PO Q 12 h, beginning the day before ascent and continuing for 48–72 h at altitude, may be used as prophylaxis
- Dexamethasone, 4 mg PO Q 12 h beginning on the day of ascent, continuing for 3 days at the higher altitude, and then tapering over 5 days, is an alternative
- Prompt medical attention with rest and high-flow oxygen if respiratory symptoms develop may prevent progression to frank pulmonary edema
- Mountaineering parties at levels of 3000 m (9840 ft) or higher should carry a supply of oxygen and equipment sufficient for several days
- An early descent of even 500 or 1000 m may result in symptomatic improvement

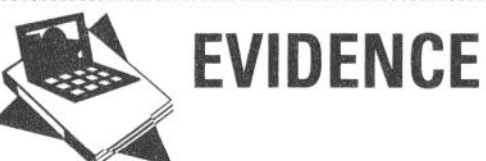

EVIDENCE

INFORMATION FOR PATIENTS

- American Academy of Family Physicians: High-Altitude Illness: How to Avoid It and How to Treat It
  - http://familydoctor.org/247.xml
- Mayo Clinic: High Altitude Sickness (Acute Mountain Sickness)
  - http://www.mayoclinic.com/invoke.cfm?objectid=8C687929-E677-44CF-9C04A16461FFBBC1
- MedlinePlus: Acute Mountain Sickness
  - http://www.nlm.nih.gov/medlineplus/ency/article/000133.htm

REFERENCE

- Gallagher SA et al: High altitude illness. Emerg Med Clin North Am 2004;22:329. [PMID: 15163571]

Author(s)

Richard Cohen, MD, MPH

Multiple Endocrine Neoplasia, Types 1 & 2

Mucormycosis p. 1112

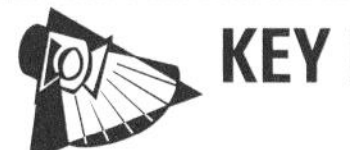

KEY FEATURES

ESSENTIALS OF DIAGNOSIS

Multiple endocrine neoplasia (MEN)

- Rare familial autosomal dominant multiglandular syndromes

GENERAL CONSIDERATIONS

MEN 1 (Wermer's syndrome)

- Parathyroid, enteropancreatic, and pituitary tumors
- Nonendocrine tumors
  - Subcutaneous lipomas
  - Facial angiofibromas
  - Collagenomas
- Caused by mutations in 1 of the 10 exons of the *menin* gene (11q13); mutations detectable in 60–95%
- Variants of MEN 1 also occur, eg, kindreds with MEN 1 Burin have a high prevalence of prolactinomas, late-onset hyperparathyroidism, and carcinoid tumors, but rarely enteropancreatic tumors
- In patients with MEN 1 gastrinomas, depending on the kindred, hepatic metastases tend to be less aggressive than sporadic gastrinomas

MEN 2A (Sipple's syndrome)

- Medullary thyroid carcinoma, hyperparathyroidism, pheochromocytomas
- Nonendocrine: Hirschsprung's disease
- Caused by a mutation of the *ret* protooncogene (*RET*) on chromosome 10 (95%)
- Each kindred has a certain *ret* codon mutation that correlates with the particular variation in the MEN 2 syndrome, such as the age of onset and aggressiveness of medullary thyroid cancer

MEN 2B

- Adrenal pheochromocytomas, medullary thyroid carcinoma, mucosal neuromas
- Nonendocrine manifestations
  - Intestinal ganglioneuromas
  - Marfan-like habitus
  - Skeletal abnormalities
  - Delayed puberty

DEMOGRAPHICS

- MEN 1 has a prevalence of 2–10 per 100,000

CLINICAL FINDINGS

SYMPTOMS AND SIGNS

MEN 1

- Tumors may develop in childhood or adulthood; presentation variable, even in same kindred
- Hyperparathyroidism in > 90%
  - Initial presentation of MEN 1 in two-thirds of patients
  - Hypercalcemia, caused by hyperplasia or adenomas of several parathyroid glands
- Enteropancreatic tumors in ~ 75%
  - Gastrinomas in 35%; gastrin secretion causes severe gastric hyperacidity (Zollinger-Ellison syndrome) with peptic ulcer disease or diarrhea
  - Gastrinomas tend to be small, multiple and ectopic; are frequently found outside the pancreas, usually in the duodenum; and can metastasize to the liver
  - Concurrent hyperparathyroidism stimulates gastrin and gastric acid secretion
- Insulinomas in ~15% of patients cause hyperinsulinism and fasting hypoglycemia
- Glucagonomas (1.6%) secrete glucagon and cause diabetes mellitus and migratory necrolytic erythema
- VIPomas (1%) secrete vasoactive intestinal polypeptide and cause profuse watery diarrhea, hypokalemia, and achorhydria (WDHA, Verner-Morrison syndrome)
- Somatostatinomas (0.7%) can cause diabetes mellitus, steatorrhea, and cholelithiasis
- Pituitary adenomas in 42%; presenting tumor in 17%
- Adrenal adenomas or hyperplasia in ~37%; bilateral in 50%; generally benign and nonfunctional
- Nonendocrine tumors are common
  - Small facial angiofibromas and subcutaneous lipomas
  - Collagenomas (firm skin nodules)
  - Malignant melanomas can occur

MEN 2A

- Pheochromocytomas are often bilateral
- Calcitonin levels rise in the presence of medullary thyroid carcinoma to levels > 80 pg/ mL in women or > 190 pg/mL in men

MEN 2B

- Medullary thyroid carcinoma is aggressive and presents early in life
- Mucosal neuromas (> 90%) with bumpy and enlarged lips and tongue
- Marfan-like habitus (75%)
- Adrenal pheochromocytomas (60%), often bilateral and rarely malignant
- Medullary thyroid carcinoma (80%)
- Intestinal abnormalities, eg, ganglioneuromas, in 75%
- Skeletal abnormalities (87%)
- Delayed puberty (43%)

DIFFERENTIAL DIAGNOSIS

- Sporadic or familial tumors of pituitary, parathyroids, or pancreatic islets
- Other causes of hypercalcemia, may increase gastrin levels, simulating gastrinoma

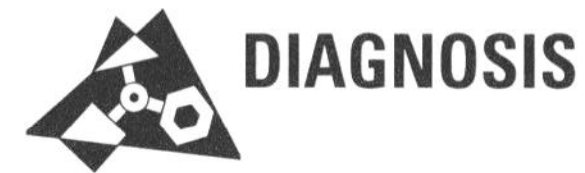

DIAGNOSIS

LABORATORY TESTS

MEN 1

- Genetic linkage analysis can be done if there are several affected members in the kindred
- *Menin* mutation genetic testing permits the rest of the kindred to be tested for the specific gene defect and allows informed genetic counseling

MEN 2A

- *RET* mutation genetic testing permits first-degree relatives to be tested for the specific gene defect and allows informed genetic counseling
- Serum calcitonin level drawn after 3 days of omeprazole, 20 mg PO BID, enables screening for medullary thyroid carcinoma

MEN 2B

- Genetic testing of infants who have a parent with MEN 2B is possible

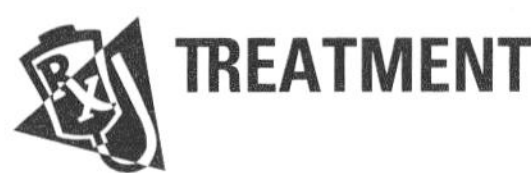

TREATMENT

MEDICATIONS

MEN 1

- Cinacalcet orally is effective for hyperparathyroidism
- Conservative treatment for patients with gastrinomas in MEN 1
  - High-dose proton pump inhibitor therapy
  - Control of hypercalcemia

SURGERY

MEN 1

- Parathyroidectomy (3 1/2 glands resected, along with thymectomy) for patients with hyperparathyroidism is effective in 62%
- Surgery for gastrinomas is palliative and usually reserved for aggressive gastrinomas and those tumors arising in the duodenum
- Surgical resection is usually attempted for insulinomas, but the tumors can be small, multiple, and difficult to detect

MEN 2A

- Prophylactic total thyroidectomy for children with a MEN 2A *RET* gene mutation, usually by age 6, though ~30% never manifest endocrine tumors
- Screen MEN 2 mutation carriers for pheochromocytoma before any surgical procedure

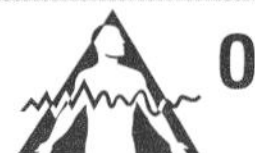

OUTCOME

COMPLICATIONS

MEN 1

- Aggressive parathyroid resection can cause permanent hypoparathyroidism
- Control of the hypercalcemia can reduce serum gastrin levels, gastric acidity, and frequency of peptic ulcer disease

PROGNOSIS

MEN 1

- Hyperparathyroidism recurrence rate is 16%, with hypercalcemia often recurring many years after neck surgery

EVIDENCE

PRACTICE GUIDELINES

- Brandi ML et al: Guidelines for diagnosis and therapy of MEN type 1 and type 2. J Clin Endocrinol Metab. 2001;86:5658. [PMID: 11739416]
- Lips CJ et al: Counselling in multiple endocrine neoplasia syndromes: from individual experience to general guidelines. J Intern Med 2005;257:69. [PMID: 15606378]

WEB SITES

- National Cancer Institute
  - http://www.nci.nih.gov/cancer_information/doc.aspx?viewid=F442B3FF-3213-40D9-8D90-7F6CAAA3AB10&version=1
- National Institute of Diabetes and Digestive and Kidney Diseases
  - http://www.niddk.nih.gov/health/endo/pubs/men1/men1.htm

INFORMATION FOR PATIENTS

- MedlinePlus: Multiple Endocrine Neoplasia
  - http://www.ncbi.nlm.nih.gov/disease/MEN.html
- NIDDK MEN 1
  - http://www.niddk.nih.gov/health/endo/pubs/men1/men1.htm

REFERENCES

- Agarwal SK et al: Molecular pathology of the MEN1 gene. Ann NY Acad Sci 2004;1014:189. [PMID: 15153434]
- Ebeling T et al: Effect of multiple endocrine neoplasia type 1 (MEN1) gene mutations on premature mortality in familial MEN1 syndrome with founder mutations. J Clin Endocrinol Metab 2004;89:3392. [PMID: 15240620]
- Gertner ME et al: Multiple endocrine neoplasia 2. Curr Treat Options Oncol 2004;5:315. [PMID: 15233908]
- Levy-Bohbot N et al: Prevalence, characteristics and prognosis of MEN 1-associated glucagonomas, VIPomas, and somatostatinomas: study from the GTE (Groupe des Tumeurs Endocrines) registry. Gastroenterol Clin Biol 2004;28:1075. [PMID: 15657529]
- Malone JP et al: Hyperparathyroidism and multiple endocrine neoplasia. Otolaryngol Clin North Am 2004;37:715. [PMID: 15262511]
- Verges B et al: Pituitary disease in MEN type 1 (MEN 1): data from the France-Belgium MEN 1 multicenter study. J Clin Endocrinol Metab 2002;87:457. [PMID: 11836268]

Author(s)

Paul A. Fitzgerald, MD

Multiple Myeloma

KEY FEATURES

ESSENTIALS OF DIAGNOSIS

- Bone pain, often in lower back
- Monoclonal paraprotein by serum and urine protein electrophoresis or immunoelectrophoresis
- Replacement of bone marrow by malignant plasma cells

GENERAL CONSIDERATIONS

- Malignancy of plasma cells characterized by replacement of bone marrow, bone destruction, and paraprotein formation
- Replacement of bone marrow initially causes anemia and later general bone marrow failure
- Malignant plasma cells can form tumors (plasmacytomas) that may cause spinal cord compression
- Bone involvement causes bone pain, osteoporosis, lytic lesions, pathologic fractures, and hypercalcemia
- Light chain component of immunoglobulin often leads to renal failure
- Light chain components may be deposited in tissues as amyloid, worsening renal failure and causing systemic symptoms
- Failure of antibody production in response to antigen challenge makes myeloma patients especially prone to infections with encapsulated organisms, eg, *Streptococcus pneumoniae* and *Haemophilus influenzae*

DEMOGRAPHICS

- Occurs most commonly in older adults: median age at presentation is 65 years

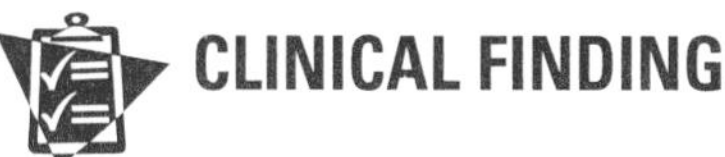

CLINICAL FINDINGS

SYMPTOMS AND SIGNS

- Symptoms of anemia
- Increased susceptibility to infection
- Bone pain most common in back or ribs or may present as pathologic fracture, especially of femoral neck
- Symptoms of renal failure
- Neuropathy or spinal cord compression
- Pallor
- Bone tenderness
- Soft tissue masses
- Enlarged tongue, neuropathy, congestive heart failure, or hepatosplenomegaly in amyloidosis
- Fever occurs only with infection

DIFFERENTIAL DIAGNOSIS

- Monoclonal gammopathy of uncertain significance (MGUS)
- Reactive polyclonal hypergammaglobulinemia
- Waldenström's macroglobulinemia
- Metastatic cancer
- Primary hyperparathyroidism
- Lymphoma or leukemia
- Primary amyloidosis

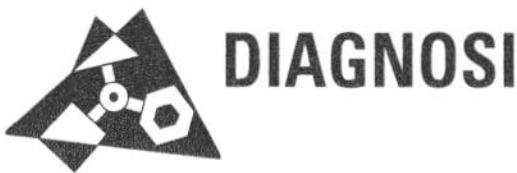

DIAGNOSIS

LABORATORY TESTS

- Anemia nearly universal
- Red blood cell morphology normal, but rouleau formation common and may be marked
- Neutrophil and platelet counts usually normal at presentation
- Hypercalcemia
- Proteinuria
- Erythrocyte sedimentation rate elevated
- Peripheral blood smear: plasma cells rarely visible (plasma cell leukemia)
- Serum protein electrophoresis (SPEP) demonstrates paraprotein, in the majority demonstrable as a monoclonal spike in β- or γ-globulin region
- Immunoelectrophoresis (IEP) reveals this to be monoclonal protein; 60% are IgG, 25% IgA, and 15% light chains only
- Urine IEP may reveal either complete immunoglobulin or light chains in ~15% who have no demonstrable paraprotein in serum
- β_2-Microglobulin level > 3 mg/L associated with poor survival
- Urinalysis may reveal proteinuria, but dipstick test (detects primarily albumin) unreliable for light chains
- Proximal renal tubular acidosis, with phosphaturia, glycosuria, uricosuria, and aminoaciduria
- Anion gap often narrow when paraprotein is cationic (70% of cases)

IMAGING STUDIES

- Bone x-rays: lytic lesions, especially in axial skeleton (skull, spine, proximal long bones, and ribs); or generalized osteoporosis
- Radionuclide bone scan: not useful in detecting bone lesions in myeloma, since usually no osteoblastic component

DIAGNOSTIC PROCEDURES

- Bone marrow biopsy: infiltration by variable numbers of plasma cells (5% to 100%); dismal outcome if bone marrow cytogenetic analysis shows deletions of chromosome 13q

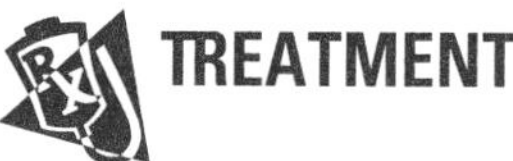

TREATMENT

MEDICATIONS

- Combination chemotherapy with vincristine, doxorubicin (Adriamycin), and dexamethasone (VAD)
- Thalidomide and thalidomide derivatives and experimental agents CC-5013 and PS-341 (Velcade, a protease inhibitor) for refractory disease
- Thalidomide, berexomib (PS-341, Velcade), and the experimental agent CC-5013 (Revimid) for refractory disease
- Mobilization, hydration, and bisphosphonates for hypercalcemia
- Bisphosphonates (eg, pamidronate, 90 mg, or zoledronic acid, 4 mg IV Q month) to reduce pathologic fractures in patients with significant bony disease

THERAPEUTIC PROCEDURES

- Observe without therapy if minimal disease or unclear whether paraproteinemia is benign (MGUS) or malignant, since no advantage to early treatment of asymptomatic multiple myeloma
- Autologous stem cell transplantation in patients aged < 70
- Autologous transplantation useful in relapse if disease still chemotherapy-sensitive
- Allogeneic transplantation potentially curative, but role limited by unusually high mortality rate (40–50%) in myeloma patients
- Less toxic forms of allogeneic transplantation using nonmyeloablative regimens have produced encouraging results

OUTCOME

FOLLOW-UP

- Follow height of paraprotein spike on SPEP as a useful marker for monitoring response to therapy

COMPLICATIONS

- Bony fractures
- Hypercalcemia

PROGNOSIS

- Median survival for myeloma has been 3 years, but is improving with new treatments
- Median survival is 5–6 years if low tumor burden (IgG spike < 5 g/dL, no more than one lytic bone lesion, and no hypercalcemia or renal failure)
- Median survival was 1–2 years if high tumor burden (IgG spike > 7 g/dL, hematocrit < 25%, calcium > 12 mg/dL, or > 3 lytic bone lesions), but survival is now 5–6 years with early autologous stem cell transplantation. Immunotherapy with allogeneic transplantation and investigational agent CC-5013 (Revimid) and PS-341 (Velcade) may improve outlook further

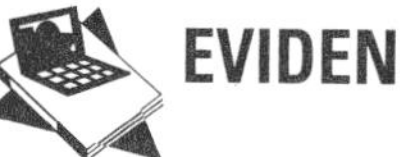

EVIDENCE

PRACTICE GUIDELINES

- Anderson KC et al; NCCN Multiple Myeloma Practice Guidelines Panel. National Comprehensive Cancer Network: Multiple Myeloma v.1.2005.
  - http://www.nccn.org/professionals/physician_gls/PDF/myeloma.pdf
- Durie BG et al; Scientific Advisors of the International Myeloma Foundation: Myeloma management guidelines: a consensus report from the Scientific Advisors of the International Myeloma Foundation. Hematol J 2003;4:379. [PMID: 14671610] Erratum in: Hematol J 2004;5:285.

WEB SITES

- International Myeloma Foundation
  - http://myeloma.org
- Multiple Myeloma Research Foundation
  - http://www.multiplemyeloma.org/
- National Cancer Institute: Multiple Myeloma Treatment
  - http://www.cancer.gov/cancertopics/pdq/treatment/myeloma/HealthProfessional

INFORMATION FOR PATIENTS

- American Cancer Society: Multiple Myeloma
  - http://www.cancer.org/docroot/CRI/CRI_2_3x.asp?rnav=cridg&dt=30
- MedlinePlus: Multiple Myeloma Interactive Tutorial
  - http://www.nlm.nih.gov/medlineplus/tutorials/multiplemyeloma.html
- National Cancer Institute: Multiple Myeloma
  - http://www.cancer.gov/cancerinfo/wyntk/myeloma

REFERENCES

- Badros A et al: Improved outcome of allogeneic transplantation in high-risk multiple myeloma patients after non-myeloablative conditioning. J Clin Oncol 2002;20:1295. [PMID: 11870172]
- Weber D et al: Thalidomide alone or with dexamethasone for previously untreated multiple myeloma. J Clin Oncol 2003;21:16. [PMID: 12506164]

Author(s)

Charles A. Linker, MD

Multiple Sclerosis

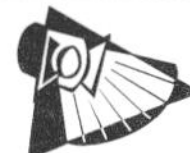

KEY FEATURES

ESSENTIALS OF DIAGNOSIS

- Episodic neurologic symptoms
- Usually under 55 years of age at onset
- Single pathologic lesion cannot explain clinical findings
- Multiple foci best visualized by MRI

GENERAL CONSIDERATIONS

- Should not be diagnosed unless there is evidence that two or more different regions of the central white matter have been affected at different times
- A diagnosis of clinically definite disease can be made in patients with a relapsing-remitting course and evidence on examination of at least two lesions involving different regions of the central white matter
- The diagnosis is probable in patients with multifocal white matter disease but only one clinical attack, or with a history of at least two clinical attacks but signs of only a single lesion

DEMOGRAPHICS

- Common disorder, probably an autoimmune basis, with its greatest incidence in young adults
- Much more common in persons of western European lineage who live in temperate zones. No population with a high risk for multiple sclerosis exists between latitudes 40°N and 40°S. Genetic, dietary, and climatic factors cannot account for these differences. Nevertheless, a genetic susceptibility to the disease is likely, based on twin studies, familial cases, and an association with specific HLA antigens (HLA-DR2)

CLINICAL FINDINGS

SYMPTOMS AND SIGNS

- Common **initial presentation**
  - Weakness, numbness, tingling, or unsteadiness in a limb
  - Spastic paraparesis
  - Retrobulbar neuritis
  - Diplopia
  - Dysequilibrium
  - Sphincter disturbance, such as urinary urgency or hesitancy
- Symptoms may disappear after a few days or weeks, although examination often reveals a residual deficit

Relapsing-remitting disease

- Symptoms occur months or years after initial presentation
- Eventually relapses and usually incomplete remissions lead to increasing disability, with weakness, spasticity, and ataxia of the limbs, impaired vision, and urinary incontinence
- The findings on examination commonly include optic atrophy; nystagmus; dysarthria; and pyramidal, sensory, or cerebellar deficits in some or all of the limbs

Secondary progressive disease

- In some of the relapsing-remitting patients, the clinical course changes to steady deterioration, unrelated to acute relapses

Primary progressive disease

- Less common
- Symptoms steadily progress from their onset, and disability develops at a relatively early stage
- The diagnosis cannot be made unless the total clinical picture indicates involvement of different parts of the CNS at different times
- A number of factors (eg, infection, trauma) may precipitate or trigger exacerbations. Relapses are also more likely during the 2 or 3 months following pregnancy

DIFFERENTIAL DIAGNOSIS

- Acute disseminated encephalomyelitis
- Foramen magnum lesion (Arnold-Chiari malformation)
- Progressive multifocal leukoencephalopathy
- Subacute combined degeneration of the spinal cord (B_{12} deficiency)
- Spinal cord tumor
- Vasculitis
- Neurosyphilis
- Lyme disease
- Syringomyelia
- HIV-associated myelopathy
- Human T cell lymphotropic virus-I myelopathy

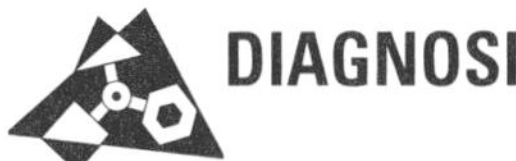

DIAGNOSIS

LABORATORY TESTS

- A definitive diagnosis can never be based solely on the laboratory findings
- Cerebrospinal fluid may reveal
  - Mild lymphocytosis or a slightly increased protein concentration, especially after an acute relapse
  - Elevated IgG and discrete bands of IgG (oligoclonal bands), which are not specific, having been found in a variety of inflammatory neurologic disorders and occasionally in patients with vascular or neoplastic disorders of the nervous system

IMAGING STUDIES

- MRI of the brain or cervical cord is often helpful in demonstrating the presence of a multiplicity of lesions
- In patients presenting with myelopathy alone and in whom there is no clinical or laboratory evidence of more widespread disease, myelography or MRI may be necessary to exclude a congenital or acquired surgically treatable lesion. The foramen magnum region must be visualized to exclude the possibility of Arnold-Chiari malformation, in which part of the cerebellum and the lower brainstem are displaced into the cervical canal and produce mixed pyramidal and cerebellar deficits in the limbs

DIAGNOSTIC PROCEDURES

- The electrocerebral responses evoked by monocular visual stimulation with a checkerboard pattern stimulus, by monaural click stimulation, and by electrical stimulation of a sensory or mixed peripheral nerve have been used to detect subclinical involvement of the visual, brainstem auditory, and somatosensory pathways, respectively

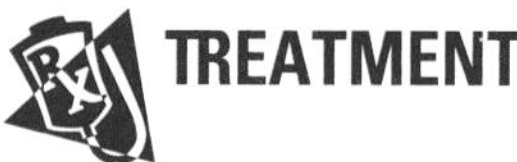

TREATMENT

MEDICATIONS

- Recovery from acute relapses may be hastened by corticosteroids, but the extent of recovery is unchanged. A high dose (eg, prednisone, 60 or 80 mg PO) is given daily for 1 week; medication is then tapered over the following 2 or 3 weeks. Such a regimen is often preceded by methylprednisolone, 1 g IV for 3 days
- Long-term treatment with corticosteroids provides no benefit and does not prevent further relapses
- In patients with relapsing-remitting or secondary progressive disease, β-interferon or daily subcutaneous administration of glatiramer acetate reduces the frequency of exacerbations
- Immunosuppressive therapy with cyclophosphamide, azathioprine, methotrexate, cladribine, or mitoxantrone may help arrest the course of secondary progressive multiple sclerosis. The evidence of benefit is incomplete, however
- Treatment with natalizumab, an alpha4 integrin antagonist that reduces the development of brain lesions in experimental models, has recently been shown to reduce the relapse rate
- There is little evidence that plasmapheresis enhances any beneficial effects of immunosuppression in multiple sclerosis
- Intravenous immunoglobulins may reduce the clinical attack rate in relapsing-remitting disease, but the available studies are inadequate to permit treatment recommendations

THERAPEUTIC PROCEDURES

- Treatment for spasticity and for neurogenic bladder may be needed in advanced cases
- Excessive fatigue must be avoided, and patients should rest during periods of acute relapse

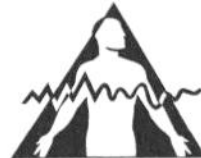

OUTCOME

PROGNOSIS

- At least partial recovery from acute exacerbations can reasonably be expected, but further relapses may occur without warning, and there is no means of preventing progression of the disorder. Some disability is likely to result eventually, but about half of all patients are without significant disability even 10 years after onset of symptoms

WHEN TO REFER

- If confirmation of the diagnosis is needed, or if the disease is progressive despite standard therapy
- For expertise in the use of immunotherapy

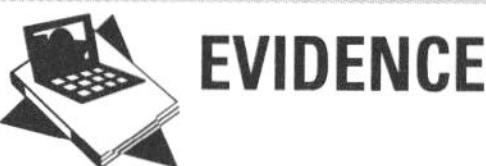

EVIDENCE

PRACTICE GUIDELINES

- American Academy of Neurology
  - http://www.aan.com/professionals/practice/pdfs/immunizations_ms.pdf
- Goodin DS et al: Disease modifying therapies in multiple sclerosis: subcommittee of the American Academy of Neurology and the MS Council for Clinical Practice Guidelines. Neurology 2002;58;169. [PMID: 11805241]

WEB SITE

- National Institute of Neurological Disorders and Stroke
  - http://www.ninds.nih.gov/disorders/multiple_sclerosis/multiple_sclerosis.htm

INFORMATION FOR PATIENTS

- The Mayo Clinic
  - http://www.mayoclinic.com/invoke.cfm?id=DS00188
- National Multiple Sclerosis Society
  - http://www.nmss.org/
  - http://www.nationalmssociety.org/Brochures-Guide%20for.asp

REFERENCES

- Filippini G et al: Interferons in relapsing remitting multiple sclerosis: a systematic review. Lancet 2003;361:545. [PMID: 12598138]
- Goodin DS et al: Disease modifying therapies in multiple sclerosis: subcommittee of the American Academy of Neurology and the MS Council for Clinical Practice Guidelines. Neurology 2002;58;169. [PMID: 11805241]
- Miller DH et al: A controlled trial of natalizumab for relapsing multiple sclerosis. N Engl J Med 2003;348:15. [PMID: 12510038]
- Rutschmann OT: Immunization and MS: a summary of published evidence and recommendations. Neurology 2002;59:1837. [PMID: 12499473]
- Vartanian T: An examination of the results of the EVIDENCE, INCOMIN, and phase III studies of interferon beta products in the treatment of multiple sclerosis. Clin Ther 2003;25:105. [PMID: 12637114]

Author(s)

Michael J. Aminoff, MD, DSc, FRCP

Mushroom Poisoning

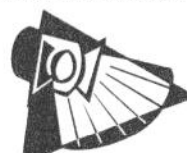

KEY FEATURES

ESSENTIALS OF DIAGNOSIS

- Vomiting, diarrhea, and abdominal cramps after ingestion of toxic mushrooms
- Amatoxin-type: Elevated hepatic transaminases and evidence of heptic dysfunction

GENERAL CONSIDERATIONS

- There are thousands of toxic mushroom species
- Ingestion of even a portion of an amatoxin-containing mushroom may be sufficient to cause death
- Cooking amatoxin-type cyclopeptides does not prevent the poisoning

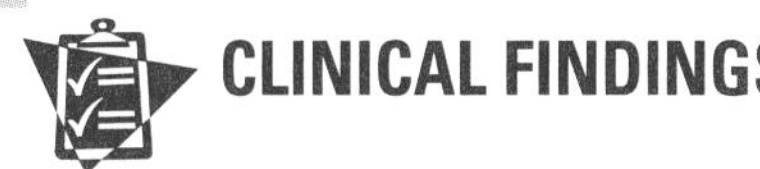

CLINICAL FINDINGS

SYMPTOMS AND SIGNS

- **Amatoxin-type** cyclopeptides (*Amanita phalloides, Amanita verna, Amanita virosa*, and *Galerina* species)
  - After a latent interval of 8–12 h, severe abdominal cramps and vomiting begin and progress to profuse diarrhea
  - Hepatic necrosis, hepatic encephalopathy, and frequently renal failure occur in 1–2 days
- **Gyromitrin** type (*Gyromitra* and *Helvella* species)
  - Toxicity is more common following ingestion of uncooked mushrooms
  - Vomiting, diarrhea, hepatic necrosis, convulsions, coma, and hemolysis may occur after a latent period of 8–12 h
- **Muscarinic** type (*Inocybe* and *Clitocybe* species)
  - Vomiting, diarrhea, bradycardia, hypotension, salivation, miosis, bronchospasm, and lacrimation occur shortly after ingestion
  - Cardiac arrhythmias may occur
- **Anticholinergic** type (*Amanita muscaria, Amanita pantherina*)
  - A variety of symptoms that may be atropine like, including excitement, delirium, flushed skin, dilated pupils, and muscular jerking tremors
  - Symptoms begin 1–2 h after ingestion
- **Gastrointestinal irritant** type (*Boletus, Cantharellus*)
  - Nausea, vomiting, and diarrhea occur shortly after ingestion
- **Disulfiram** type (*Coprinus* species)
  - Disulfiram-like sensitivity to alcohol may persist for several days
  - Toxicity is characterized by flushing, hypotension, and vomiting after co-ingestion of alcohol
- **Hallucinogenic** (*Psilocybe* and *Panaeolus* species)
  - Mydriasis, nausea and vomiting, and intense visual hallucinations occur 1–2 h after ingestion
- *Cortinarius orellanus*
  - May cause acute renal failure due to tubulointerstitial nephritis

DIFFERENTIAL DIAGNOSIS

- Acetaminophen poisoning
- Acute viral hepatitis

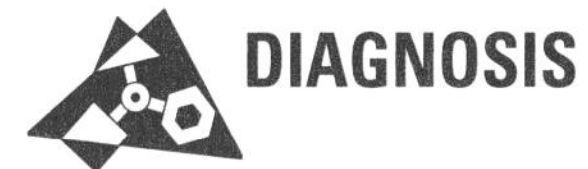

DIAGNOSIS

DIAGNOSTIC PROCEDURES

- Hepatic transaminases elevated
- Necrosis of the liver, massive and acute

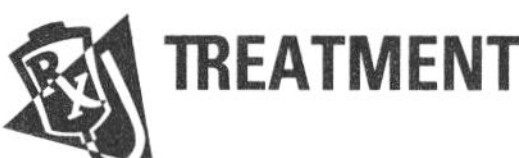

TREATMENT

MEDICATIONS

Emergency measures

- Administer activated charcoal for any recent ingestion
- Administer activated charcoal, 60–100 g PO or via gastric tube, mixed in aqueous slurry
- Repeated doses may be given to enhance removal of the toxin (uncertain benefit)
- After the onset of symptoms, efforts to remove the toxic agent are probably useless, especially in cases of amatoxin or gyromitrin poisoning, in which there is usually a delay of 12 h or more before symptoms occur

General measures

- **Amatoxin-type** cyclopeptides: aggressive fluid replacement for diarrhea and intensive supportive care for hepatic failure are the mainstays of treatment; antidote efficacy (eg, silibinin, penicillin, corticosteroids) is uncertain
- **Gyromitrin type:** pyridoxine, 25 mg/kg IV
- **Muscarinic type:** give atropine, 0.005–0.01 mg/kg IV, and repeat as needed
- **Anticholinergic type:** physostigmine, 0.5–1 mg IV, may calm extreme agitation and reverse peripheral anticholinergic manifestations, but it may also cause bradycardia, asystole, and seizures
- **Gastrointestinal irritant type:** treat with antiemetics and IV or oral fluid
- **Disulfiram type:** avoid alcohol and treat alcohol reaction with fluids and supine position
- **Hallucinogenic type:** provide a quiet, supportive atmosphere; diazepam or haloperidol may be used for sedation
- *Cortinarius*: provide supportive care and hemodialysis as needed for renal failure

OUTCOME

PROGNOSIS

- The fatality rate of amatoxin-type cyclopeptides is about 10–20% without liver transplant
- The fatality rate of gyromitrin-type mushrooms is less than 10%
- Fatalities are rare with muscarinic type, anticholingeric type, gastrointestinal irritant type, and hallucinogenic mushrooms

WHEN TO REFER

- Liver transplant may be necessary, particularly for amatoxin-type cyclopeptides
- Contact a transplant center early

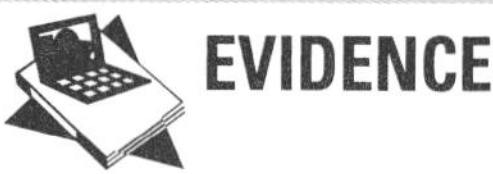

EVIDENCE

WEB SITES

- eMedicine: Toxicology Articles
  - http://www.emedicine.com/emerg/toxicology.htm
- Karolinska Institute: Diseases and Disorders: Links Pertaining to Poisoning
  - http://www.mic.ki.se/Diseases/C21.613.html#C21.613.415
- North American Mycological Association: Mushroom Poisoning Case Registry
  - http://www.sph.umich.edu/~kwcee/mpcr/index.htm
- U.S. Food and Drug Administration: Mushroom Toxins
  - http://vm.cfsan.fda.gov/~mow/Chap40.html

INFORMATION FOR PATIENTS

- American Academy of Family Physicians: Mushroom Poisoning in Children
  - http://familydoctor.org/handouts/129.html
- California Poison Control System: Mushrooms
  - http://www.calpoison.org/public/mushrooms.html
- MedlinePlus: Poisoning First Aid
  - http://www.nlm.nih.gov/medlineplus/ency/article/000003.htm

REFERENCES

- Enjalbert F et al: Treatment of amatoxin poisoning: 20-year retrospective analysis. J Toxicol Clin Toxicol 2002;40:715. [PMID: 12475187]
- Rengstorff DS et al: Recovery from severe hepatitis caused by mushroom poisoning without liver transplantation. Clin Gastroenterol Hepatol 2003;1:392. [PMID: 15017659]

Author(s)

Kent R. Olson, MD

Myasthenia Gravis

KEY FEATURES

ESSENTIALS OF DIAGNOSIS

- Fluctuating weakness of voluntary muscles, producing symptoms such as diplopia, ptosis, and difficulty in swallowing
- Activity increases weakness of affected muscles
- Short-acting anticholinesterases transiently improve the weakness

GENERAL CONSIDERATIONS

- Occurs at all ages, sometimes in association with a thymic tumor, thyrotoxicosis, rheumatoid arthritis, or lupus erythematosus
- Onset is usually insidious, but the disorder is sometimes unmasked by a coincidental infection
- Exacerbations may occur before the menstrual period and during or shortly after pregnancy
- Symptoms are due to blocks of neuromuscular transmission caused by autoantibodies binding to acetylcholine receptors
- The external ocular muscles and certain other cranial muscles, including the masticatory, facial, and pharyngeal muscles, are especially likely to be affected, and the respiratory and limb muscles may also be involved

DEMOGRAPHICS

- Most common in young women with HLA-DR3; if thymoma is associated, older men are more commonly affected

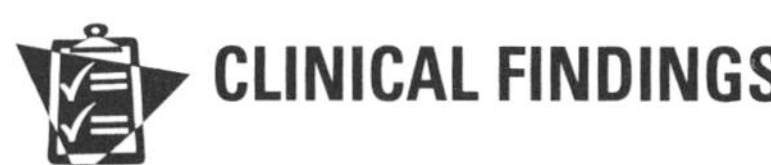

CLINICAL FINDINGS

SYMPTOMS AND SIGNS

- Initial symptoms
  - Ptosis
  - Diplopia
  - Difficulty in chewing or swallowing
  - Respiratory difficulties
  - Limb weakness
  - Some combination of these problems
- Weakness may remain localized to a few muscle groups, especially the ocular muscles, or may become generalized
- Symptoms often fluctuate in intensity during the day, and this diurnal variation is superimposed on a tendency to longer-term spontaneous relapses and remissions that may last for weeks
- Clinical examination confirms the weakness and fatigability of affected muscles
- Extraocular palsies and ptosis, often asymmetric, are common
- Pupillary responses are normal
- The bulbar and limb muscles are often weak, but the pattern of involvement is variable
- Sustained activity of affected muscles increases the weakness, which improves after a brief rest
- Sensation is normal, and there are usually no reflex changes

DIFFERENTIAL DIAGNOSIS

- Lambert-Eaton myasthenic syndrome (usually paraneoplastic)
- Botulism
- Aminoglycoside-induced neuromuscular weakness

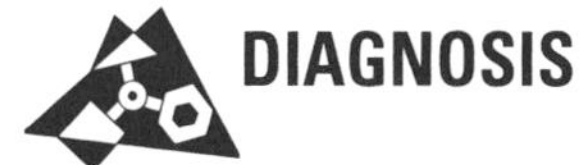

DIAGNOSIS

LABORATORY TESTS

- Elevated level of serum acetylcholine receptor antibodies has a sensitivity of 80–90%
- Certain patients have serum antibodies to muscle-specific tyrosine kinase (MuSK), which should be determined

IMAGING STUDIES

- Lateral and anteroposterior x-rays of the chest and CT scans should be obtained to demonstrate a coexisting thymoma, but normal studies do not exclude this possibility

DIAGNOSTIC PROCEDURES

- Response to **short-acting anticholinesterase** can confirm diagnosis
  - Edrophonium can be given IV in a dose of 10 mg (1 mL), 2 mg being given initially and the remaining 8 mg about 30 s later if the test dose is well tolerated
  - In myasthenic patients, there is an obvious improvement in strength of weak muscles lasting for about 5 min
  - Alternatively, 1.5 mg of neostigmine can be given IM, and the response then lasts for about 2 h; atropine sulfate (0.6 mg) should be available to reverse muscarinic side effects
- **Electrophysiologic** demonstration of a decrementing muscle response to repetitive 2- or 3-Hz stimulation of motor nerves indicates a disturbance of neuromuscular transmission. Such an abnormality may even be detected in clinically strong muscles with certain provocative procedures
- **Needle electromyography** of affected muscles shows a marked variation in configuration and size of individual motor unit potentials, and single-fiber electromyography reveals an increased jitter, or variability, in the time interval between two muscle fiber action potentials from the same motor unit

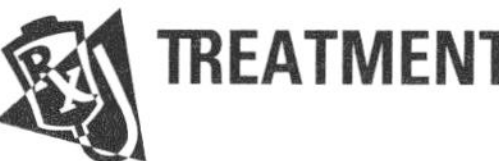

TREATMENT

MEDICATIONS

- Medication such as aminoglycosides that may exacerbate myasthenia gravis should be avoided
- Anticholinesterase drugs provide symptomatic benefit without influencing the course of the disease
- Neostigmine, pyridostigmine, or both can be used, the dose being determined on an individual basis
- The usual dose of neostigmine is 7.5–30 mg PO QID (average, 15 mg); of pyridostigmine, 30–180 mg PO QID (average, 60 mg). Overmedication may temporarily increase weakness, which is then unaffected or enhanced by IV edrophonium
- Corticosteroids are indicated if there has been a poor response to anticholinesterase drugs and the patient has had thymectomy. Start while the patient is in the hospital, since weakness may initially be aggravated. The dose of corticosteroids is determined on an individual basis
- Treatment with azathioprine may also be effective. The usual dose is 2–3 mg/kg PO daily after a lower initial dose
- Early reports on the use of mycophenolate mofetil, an immunosuppressant, indicate that it may provide symptomatic relief and allow for steroid dose reduction
- In patients with major disability in whom conventional treatment is either unhelpful or contraindicated, plasmapheresis or intravenous immunoglobulin therapy may be beneficial. It may also be useful for stabilizing patients before thymectomy and for managing acute crisis

SURGERY

- Thymectomy usually leads to symptomatic benefit or remission and should be considered in all patients younger than age 60, unless weakness is restricted to the extraocular muscles
- If the disease is of recent onset and only slowly progressive, operation is sometimes delayed for a year or so, in the hope that spontaneous remission will occur

OUTCOME

COMPLICATIONS

- Aspiration pneumonia

PROGNOSIS

- The disorder follows a slowly progressive course and may have a fatal outcome owing to respiratory complications such as aspiration pneumonia

WHEN TO REFER

- Most patients with a suspected or proven diagnosis should be referred to a clinician with expertise in managing this disorder

EVIDENCE

PRACTICE GUIDELINES

- National Guideline Clearinghouse
  - http://www.guideline.gov/summary/summary.aspx?doc_id=3347&nbr=2573&string=MYASTHENIA+GRAVIS

INFORMATION FOR PATIENTS

- The Mayo Clinic
  - http://www.mayoclinic.com/invoke.cfm?id=DS00375
- National Institute of Neurological Disorders and Stroke
  - http://www.ninds.nih.gov/disorders/myasthenia_gravis/detail_myasthenia_gravis.htm

REFERENCES

- Keesey JC: Clinical evaluation and management of myasthenia gravis. Muscle Nerve 2004;29:484. [PMID: 15052614]
- Palace J et al: Myasthenia gravis: diagnostic and management dilemmas. Curr Opin Neurol 2001;14:583. [PMID: 11562569]
- Vincent A et al: Myasthenia gravis. Lancet 2001;357:2122. [PMID: 11445126]

Author(s)

Michael J. Aminoff, MD, DSc, FRCP

Mycobacterial Pulmonary Infections, Nontuberculous

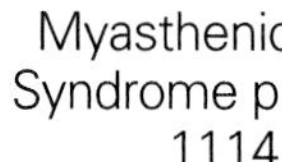
Myasthenic Syndrome p. 1114.

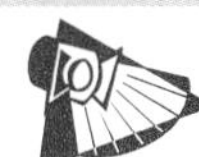

KEY FEATURES

ESSENTIALS OF DIAGNOSIS

- Chronic cough, sputum production, and fatigue
- Less commonly, malaise, dyspnea, fever, hemoptysis, and weight loss
- Parenchymal infiltrates on chest radiograph, often with thin-walled cavities, that spread contiguously and often involve overlying pleura
- Isolation of nontuberculous mycobacteria in a sputum culture

GENERAL CONSIDERATIONS

- Nontuberculous mycobacteria (NTM) or atypical mycobacteria are ubiquitous in water and soil
- NTM may colonize the airways or appear in cultures due to environmental contamination
- Organisms are not communicable from person to person
- NTM are often resistant to most antituberculous drugs
- Complementary data are important for diagnosis, as NTM can reside or colonize airways without causing clinical disease
- *Mycobacterium avium* complex (MAC) is the most common cause of NTM pulmonary disease in the United States
- *M kansasii* is the second most frequent pulmonary pathogen
- Other NTM that can cause pulmonary disease are *M abscessus, M xenopi,* and *M malmoense*
- Most organisms cause a chronic progressive pulmonary infection similar to tuberculosis, but more slowly progressive
- Many patients have AIDS or preexisting lung disease
- Disseminated disease is rare in immunocompetent patients
- Disseminated MAC infection is common in patients with AIDS

CLINICAL FINDINGS

SYMPTOMS AND SIGNS

- Chronic cough, sputum production, and fatigue
- Malaise, dyspnea, fever, hemoptysis, and weight loss are less common
- Symptoms from coexisting lung disease can confound the evaluation

DIFFERENTIAL DIAGNOSIS

- Postviral
- Bronchitis, especially in smokers
- Bronchiectasis
- Tuberculosis
- Cystic fibrosis
- Pertussis
- *Mycoplasma*
- *Chlamydia*
- Respiratory syncytial virus

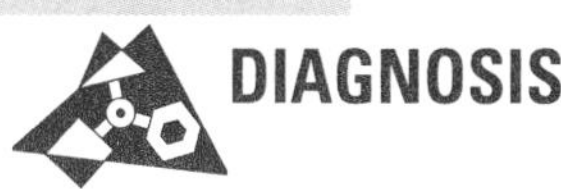

DIAGNOSIS

LABORATORY TESTS

- Diagnosis rests on recovery of the pathogen from cultures
- Bronchial washings are considered more sensitive than expectorated sputum, but their specificity for clinical disease is unknown
- Bacteriologic diagnostic criteria in HIV-negative or immunocompetent hosts require
  - Either three positive sputum culture specimens or two positive sputum cultures and one positive acid-fast bacillus (AFB) sputum smear within a 1-year period
  - A single bronchial wash culture with a 2+ to 4+ growth, or any positive culture with a 2+ to 4+ AFB smear
- DNA probes or HPLC allow rapid species identification of NTM
- Criteria for infection in HIV-positive patients is less stringent
- Drug susceptibility testing is recommended only as follows:
  - *M kansasii* and rifampin
  - Rapid growers (*M fortuitum, abscessus,* and *chelonei*) and amikacin, doxycycline, impipenem, fluoroquinolones, clarithromycin, cefoxitin, and a sulfonamide

IMAGING STUDIES

- Chest x-ray with progressive or persistent infiltrates for 2 months, cavitary lesions, and multiple nodular densities
- Cavities are usually thin walled and with less surrounding infiltrate than seen in *M tuberculosis*
- HRCT may show multiple small nodules with or without multiple foci of bronchiectasis
- Infiltrates clear slowly

DIAGNOSTIC PROCEDURES

- Lung biopsy demonstrating NTM with granulomatous inflammation can be diagnostic

Mycetoma p. 1114.

Mycobacterial Pulmonary Infections, Nontuberculous

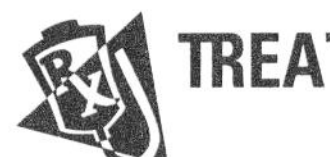

TREATMENT

MEDICATIONS

- See Tables 23, 24, and 127
- *M kansasii* responds well to therapy with daily rifampin, isoniazid, and ethambutol for at least 18 months
- Treatment of immunocompromised patients is controversial and largely empirical
- Non-HIV patients with MAC pulmonary disease usually receive a combination of daily clarithromycin or azithromycin, rifampin or rifabutin, and ethambutol; streptomycin is considered for the first 2 months
- Optimal duration of therapy is unknown, but it should be continued for at least 12 months after sputum is documented negative

SURGERY

- Surgical resection is an option for progressive disease that responds poorly to chemotherapy

OUTCOME

FOLLOW-UP

- Monitor serial chest x-rays and sputum cultures
- Follow drug-specific biochemical tests for toxicity

PROGNOSIS

- Medical treatment is initially successful in two-thirds of non-HIV patients with MAC, but relapses are common

WHEN TO REFER

- Nontuberculous mycobacterium disease other than MAC should be managed with the assistance of an infectious disease or pulmonary medicine expert

EVIDENCE

INFORMATION FOR PATIENTS

- National Institutes of Health
  - http://www.nlm.nih.gov/medlineplus/ency/article/000640.htm

REFERENCES

- Anonymous: Diagnosis and treatment of disease caused by nontuberculous mycobacteria. Am J Respir Crit Care Med 1997;156(2 Part 2):S1. [PMID:9279284]
- Field SK et al: *Mycobacterium avium* complex pulmonary disease in patients without HIV infection. Chest 2004;126:566 [PMID: 15302746]
- Holland SM: Nontuberculous mycobacteria. Am J Med Sci 2001;321:49. [PMID:11202480]

Author(s)

Mark S. Chesnutt, MD
Thomas J. Prendergast, MD

Mycobacterium Infection, Atypical

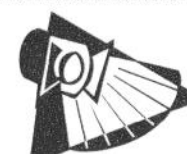

KEY FEATURES

ESSENTIALS OF DIAGNOSIS

- Lymphadenopathy and fever in disseminated disease in HIV-infected patients with CD4 < 50/μL
- Pulmonary infections similar to tuberculosis in patients with chronic lung disease
- Cervical adenopathy with mild or moderate inflammation

GENERAL CONSIDERATIONS

- About 10% of mycobacterial infections are not caused by *Mycobacterium tuberculosis* but by atypical mycobacteria
- Occur ubiquitously in the environment
- Are not communicable from person to person
- Are among the most common opportunistic infections in advanced HIV disease

Disseminated* Mycobacterium avium *infection

- *Mycobacterium avium* complex (MAC) produces asymptomatic colonization and a wide spectrum of diseases, including coin lesions, and in patients with chronic lung disease, bronchitis and invasive pulmonary disease that is often cavitary
- A common cause of disseminated disease in the late stages of HIV infection, when the CD4 cell count is less than 50–100/μL

Pulmonary infections

- MAC causes a chronic, slowly progressive pulmonary infection resembling tuberculosis in immunocompetent patients who typically have underlying pulmonary disease
- *Mycobacterium kansasii* infection can resemble tuberculosis, but the illness progresses more slowly. About 60% of infections occur in patients with preexisting lung disease

Lymphadenitis

- Most cases of lymphadenitis (scrofula) in adults are caused by *M tuberculosis* and can be a manifestation of disseminated disease
- In children, the majority of mycobacterial lymphadenitis cases are due to nontuberculous species, with *M scrofulaceum* and MAC most common

Skin and soft tissue infections

- Abscesses, septic arthritis, and osteomyelitis can result from direct inoculation or hematogenous dissemination or may occur as a complication of surgery
- *M chelonei* and *M fortuitum* are frequent causes of this type of infection
- *M marinum* infection ("swimming pool granuloma") follows exposure to nonchlorinated water

CLINICAL FINDINGS

SYMPTOMS AND SIGNS

Disseminated* Mycobacterium avium *infection

- Persistent fever and weight loss are the most common symptoms

Pulmonary infections

- Resembles tuberculosis

Lymphadenitis

- Swollen, somewhat tender lymph node

Skin and soft tissue infections

- Most cases occur in the extremities and initially present as nodules
- Ulceration with abscess formation often follows

DIFFERENTIAL DIAGNOSIS

- Tuberculosis
- Lymphoma (disseminated disease)
- Fungal infection (cryptococcosis, histoplasmosis, coccidioidomycosis)
- Cervical lymphadenitis due to *M tuberculosis*, cat-scratch, or other bacterial causes

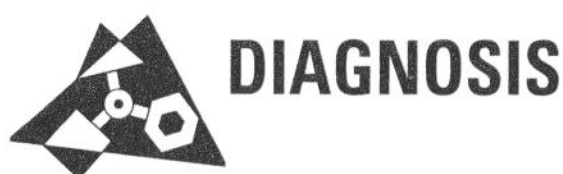

DIAGNOSIS

LABORATORY TESTS

Disseminated* Mycobacterium avium *infection

- The organism can usually be cultured from multiple sites, including blood, liver, lymph node, or bone marrow
- Blood culture is the preferred means of establishing the diagnosis and has a sensitivity of 98%

Pulmonary infections

- Sputum or bronchoalveolar lavage mycobacterial culture

Lymphadenitis

- Mycobacterial culture of lymph node aspirate or surgical specimen

Skin and soft tissue infections

- Mycobacterial culture of nodule

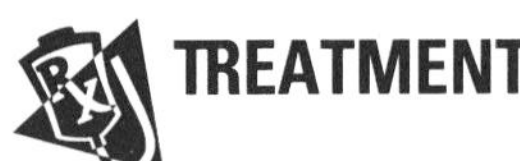

TREATMENT

MEDICATIONS

Disseminated* Mycobacterium avium *infection

- Clarithromycin, 500 mg orally twice daily, plus ethambutol, 15 mg/kg/day as a single dose, with or without rifabutin, 300 mg/day, is the treatment of choice
- Azithromycin, 500 mg once daily, may be used instead of clarithromycin

Pulmonary infections

- Rifampin, 600 mg once daily, plus ethambutol, 15–25 mg/kg/day, plus streptomycin, 1 g intramuscularly three to five times a week for the first 4–6 months, have been used
- Inclusion of clarithromycin in the initial treatment regimen of immunocompetent patients should be strongly considered. Therapy is continued for a total of 18–24 months
- Microbiologically, *M kansasii* is similar to *M tuberculosis* and is sensitive to the same drugs except pyrazinamide, to which it is resistant. Therapy with isoniazid, ethambutol, and rifampin for 2 years (or 1 year after sputum conversion) has been highly successful

Skin and soft tissue infections

- The organisms are resistant to the usual antituberculous drugs but may be sensitive to a variety of antibiotics, including erythromycin, doxycycline, amikacin, cefoxitin, sulfonamides, imipenem, and ciprofloxacin
- Initially, parenteral drugs are given for several weeks, and this is followed by an oral regimen to which the organism is sensitive
- The duration of therapy is variable but usually continues for several months after the soft tissue lesions have healed

SURGERY

Lymphadenitis

- Unlike disease caused by *M tuberculosis*, which requires systemic therapy for 6 months, infection with nontuberculous mycobacteria can be successfully treated by surgical excision without antituberculous therapy

Skin and soft tissue infections

- Therapy includes surgical debridement along with drug therapy

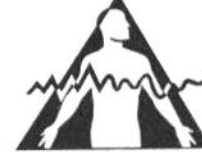

OUTCOME

WHEN TO REFER

- Early referral to an infectious disease specialist if the diagnosis is in question or to an HIV specialist for treatment

WHEN TO ADMIT

- To expedite a diagnostic workup or for respiratory insufficiency

PREVENTION

- Antimicrobial prophylaxis of MAC prevents disseminated disease and prolongs survival in HIV-infected patients with CD4 counts ≤50/μL
- Single-drug regimens of clarithromycin, 500 mg twice daily, azithromycin, 1200 mg once weekly, or rifabutin, 300 mg once daily, have been shown to be effective

EVIDENCE

PRACTICE GUIDELINES

- National Guideline Clearinghouse
  - http://www.guideline.gov/summary/summary.aspx?doc_id=3080

WEB SITES

- CDC—Division of Bacterial and Mycotic Diseases
  - http://www.cdc.gov/ncidod/dbmd/
- Karolinska Institute—Directory of Bacterial Infections and Mycoses
  - http://www.mic.ki.se/Diseases/C01.html

INFORMATION FOR PATIENTS

- JAMA patient page: HIV/AIDS. JAMA 1999;282:606. [PMID: 10450724]
- National Institutes of Health
  - http://www.nlm.nih.gov/medlineplus/ency/article/000640.htm

REFERENCES

- Kaplan JE et al: Guidelines for preventing opportunistic infections among HIV-infected persons–2002. Recommendations of the U.S. Public Health Service and the Infectious Diseases Society of America. MMWR Recomm Rep 2002;51(RR-8):1. [PMID: 12081007]
- Kovacs J et al: Prophylaxis against opportunistic infection in patients with human immunodeficiency virus infection. N Engl J Med 2000;342:1416. [PMID: 10805828]

Author(s)

Henry F. Chambers, MD

Myelodysplastic Syndromes

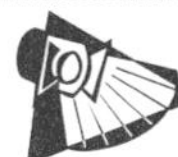

KEY FEATURES

ESSENTIALS OF DIAGNOSIS

- Cytopenias with hypercellular bone marrow
- Morphological abnormalities in two or more hematopoietic cell lines

GENERAL CONSIDERATIONS

- Group of acquired clonal disorders of hematopoietic stem cell, characterized by cytopenias, hypercellular marrow, and morphological and cytogenetic abnormalities
- "Ineffective hematopoiesis" occurs despite adequate numbers of hematopoietic stem cells
- No specific chromosomal abnormality seen, but abnormalities in chromosomes 5 and 7 common
- Causes: idiopathic (most common); postcytotoxic chemotherapy, especially mechlorethamine or procarbazine for Hodgkin's disease and melphalan for multiple myeloma or ovarian carcinoma
- May evolve into acute myelogenous leukemia (AML); has been termed "preleukemia"
- Myelodysplasia encompasses several heterogeneous syndromes
  - Refractory anemia (with or without ringed sideroblasts): no excess bone marrow blasts
  - Refractory anemia with excess blasts (RAEB): 5–19% blasts
  - Chronic myelomonocytic leukemia (CMML): proliferative syndrome, including peripheral blood monocytosis > 1000/μL

DEMOGRAPHICS

- Occurs most often in patients aged > 60

CLINICAL FINDINGS

SYMPTOMS AND SIGNS

- Asymptomatic, with incidentally found cytopenias
- Fatigue, infection, or bleeding related to bone marrow failure
- Wasting, fever, weight loss, and general debility
- Splenomegaly
- Pallor
- Bleeding
- Signs of infection

DIFFERENTIAL DIAGNOSIS

- AML (≥ 20% blasts)
- Aplastic anemia
- Anemic of chronic disease
- Vitamin B_{12} or folate deficiency

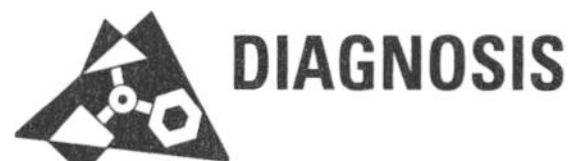

DIAGNOSIS

LABORATORY TESTS

- Anemia may be marked
- Mean cell volume is normal or increased
- Peripheral blood smear: macroovalocytes
- White blood cell count usually normal or reduced; neutropenia common
- Neutrophils may exhibit morphological abnormalities, including deficient numbers of granules, or bilobed nucleus (Pelger-Huet anomaly)
- Myeloid series may be left shifted with small numbers of promyelocytes or blasts
- Platelet count normal or reduced; hypogranular platelets may be present

DIAGNOSTIC PROCEDURES

- Bone marrow aspirate and biopsy characteristically hypercellular
- Erythroid hyperplasia common
- Signs of abnormal erythropoiesis include megaloblastic features, nuclear budding, and multinucleated erythroid precursors
- Prussian blue stain may demonstrate ringed sideroblasts
- Myeloid series often left shifted with variable increases in blasts
- Deficient or abnormal granules may be seen
- A characteristic abnormality is dwarf megakaryocytes with unilobed nucleus

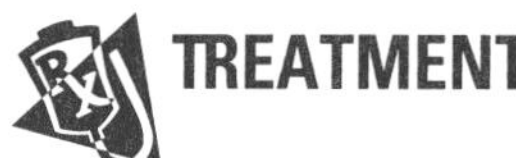

TREATMENT

MEDICATIONS

- Erythropoietin, 30,000 U SC weekly, reduces red blood cell transfusion requirement in ≤ 20%
- Granulocyte or granulocyte-macrophage colony-stimulating factor myeloid growth factors indicated in those with severe neutropenia
- Combination of high-dose erythropoietin and myeloid growth factors produces higher response rate, but cost is prohibitive
- Azacitidine (5-azacytidine) improves both symptoms and blood counts and prolongs time to conversion to acute leukemia
- In low-risk myelodysplasia (especially chromosome 5q-syndrome), lenalidomide can produce consistent and significant responses

THERAPEUTIC PROCEDURES

- Red blood cell transfusions indicated for severe anemia
- Allogeneic bone marrow transplantation in patients aged < 60 with matched sibling donors produces cure in 30–50%

OUTCOME

COMPLICATIONS

- Infection and bleeding

PROGNOSIS

- Myelodysplasia is ultimately fatal, most commonly because of infections or bleeding
- Risk of transformation to AML depends on percentage of blasts in bone marrow
- Patients with refractory anemia may survive many years, with low risk of leukemia (< 10%)
- Patients with excess blasts or CMML have short survivals (usually < 2 years) and higher (20–50%) risk of developing acute leukemia
- Deletions of chromosomes 5 and 7 associated with poor prognosis

EVIDENCE

PRACTICE GUIDELINES

- Bowen D et al: Guidelines for the diagnosis and therapy of adult myelodysplastic syndromes. Br J Haematol 2003;120:187. [PMID: 12542475]
- Greenberg PL et al: NCCN Myelodysplastic Syndromes Practice Guidelines Panel. National Comprehensive Cancer Network: Myelodysplastic Syndromes v.1.2005
  - http://www.nccn.org/professionals/physician_gls/PDF/mds.pdf

WEB SITE

- National Cancer Institute: Myelodysplastic Syndromes: Treatment
  - http://www.cancer.gov/cancertopics/pdq/treatment/myelodysplastic/HealthProfessional

INFORMATION FOR PATIENTS

- American Cancer Society: Myelodysplastic Syndrome
  - http://www.cancer.org/docroot/CRI/CRI_2_3x.asp?dt=65
- Leukemia & Lymphoma Society: Detailed Guide: Myelodysplastic Syndrome
  - http://www.leukemia-lymphoma.org/all_mat_toc.adp?item_id=54083
- National Cancer Institute: Myelodysplastic Syndromes: Treatment
  - http://www.cancer.gov/cancertopics/pdq/treatment/myelodysplastic/patient

REFERENCES

- Castro-Malaspina H et al: Unrelated donor marrow transplantation for myelodysplastic syndromes: outcome analysis in 510 transplants facilitated by the National Marrow Donor Program. Blood 2002;99:1943. [PMID: 11877264]
- Cutler CS et al: A decision analysis of allogeneic bone marrow transplantation for the myelodysplastic syndromes: delayed transplantation for low-risk myelodysplasia is associated with improved outcome. Blood 2004;104:579. [PMID: 15039286]
- Faderl S et al: Novel therapies for myelodysplastic syndromes. Cancer 2004;101:226. [PMID: 15241818]
- Silverman LR et al: Randomized controlled trial of azacitidine in patients with the myelodysplastic syndrome: a study of the cancer and leukemia group B. J Clin Oncol 2002;20:2429. [PMID: 12011120]

Author(s)

Charles A. Linker, MD

Myocardial Infarction, Acute

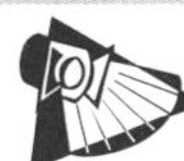

KEY FEATURES

ESSENTIALS OF DIAGNOSIS

- Sudden, but not instantaneous, development of prolonged (> 30 min) anterior chest discomfort (sometimes felt as "gas" or pressure) that may produce arrhythmias, hypotension, shock, or congestive heart failure (CHF)
- Pain likely to be diminished or absent in the very elderly and long-term diabetics
- ECG: ST-segment elevation or depression, evolving Q waves, symmetric inversion of T waves
- Cardiac enzyme (CK-MB, troponin T, or troponin I) elevation
- Appearance of segmental wall motion abnormality by echocardiography

GENERAL CONSIDERATIONS

- Results from prolonged myocardial ischemia, due most often to an occlusive thrombus in a coronary artery at the site of a preexisting atherosclerotic plaque
- The location and extent of infarction depend on the anatomic distribution of the occluded vessel, the presence of additional stenotic lesions, and the adequacy of collateral circulation
- Atrioventricular (AV) block and sinus node dysfunction occur during inferior or right ventricular (RV) infarctions
- Preferred classification of infarction type is Q-wave versus non-Q-wave myocardial infarction (MI)
- Q-wave infarctions are transumural
- Non-Q-wave infarctions are predominantly subendocardial and result from incomplete occlusion or spontaneous lysis of a thrombus, often signifying the presence of additional jeopardized myocardium and associated with a higher incidence of reinfarction and recurrent ischemia
- In small infarctions, cardiac function is normal; with more extensive damage, early heart failure and hypotension (cardiogenic shock) may appear
- Consider RV infarction when patients with inferior infarction exhibit low cardiac output and raised venous pressure, confirmed by echocardiography or hemodynamic measurements

CLINICAL FINDINGS

SYMPTOMS AND SIGNS

- Recent onset of angina or alteration in the pattern of angina or chest pressure, squeezing or "indigestion"
- Pain similar to angina in location and radiation, but more severe, usually occurs at rest, often in the early morning, builds rapidly, and is minimally responsive to nitroglycerin and even opioids
- Associated symptoms: diaphoresis, weakness, apprehensiveness, aversion to lying quietly, light-headedness, syncope, dyspnea, orthopnea, cough, wheezing, nausea and vomiting, or abdominal bloating
- ~20% of patients die before reaching the hospital, usually of ventricular fibrillation
- Marked bradycardia (inferior infarction) to tachycardia (increased sympathetic activity, low cardiac output, or arrhythmia)
- Blood pressure elevated (pain) to low (shock)
- Basilar rales are common and do not necessarily indicate heart failure
- Diffuse rales, wheezing, or respiratory distress usually indicate pulmonary edema and CHF
- Jugular venous distention indicates right atrial hypertension, often from right ventricular infarction or elevated left ventricular (LV) filling pressures
- Soft heart sounds may indicate LV dysfunction
- S_4 is common; S_3 indicates significant LV dysfunction
- Mitral regurgitation murmur usually indicates papillary muscle dysfunction or, rarely, rupture

DIFFERENTIAL DIAGNOSIS

- Aortic dissection, pulmonary embolism, tension pneumothorax, pericarditis, esophageal rupture

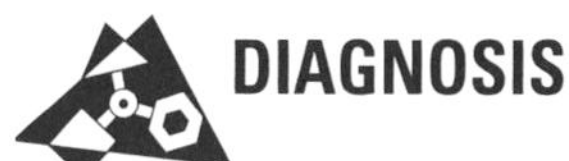

DIAGNOSIS

LABORATORY TESTS

- Quantitative CK-MB, troponin I, and troponin T elevations as early as 4–6 h after onset; almost always abnormal by 8–12 h
- Troponins more specific than CK-MB
- Troponins may remain elevated for ≥ 5–7 days

IMAGING STUDIES

- Chest x-ray: signs of CHF, often lagging behind the clinical findings
- Echocardiography: assesses global and regional LV function, wall motion
- Doppler echocardiography: can diagnose postinfarction mitral regurgitation or ventricular septal defect
- Thallium-201 or technetium scintigraphy does not distinguish recent from old MI

DIAGNOSTIC PROCEDURES

- Angiography: can demonstrate akinesis or dyskinesis and measure ejection fraction
- Swan-Ganz hemodynamic measurements: can be invaluable in managing the patient with suspected cardiogenic shock
- ST-segment elevation (> 0.1 mV) in two inferior or lateral leads or two contiguous precordial leads, or with new-onset LBBB
- Q-wave MI: classic evolution of changes (hours to days) from peaked ("hyperacute") T waves, to ST-segment elevation, to Q wave development, to T wave inversion
- Non-Q-wave MI: characteristic MI presentation, elevated cardiac enzymes, and ST-segment changes (usually depression) or T wave inversion lasting ≥48 hours, *without* development of Q waves

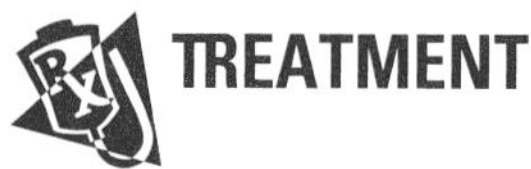

TREATMENT

MEDICATIONS

- Aspirin, 162 mg or 325 mg PO QD, begin immediately
- Clopidogrel, 300 mg PO QD, in patients with a definite aspirin allergy
- Metoprolol, 5 mg IV Q 5 min, for up to 3 doses, or an oral β-blocker, for a goal heart rate of 60/bpm; avoid in decompensated CHF, decompensated asthma, or high degrees of AV block
- Nitroglycerin (TNG), for chest pain to lower blood pressure, sublingually, topically, or IV if inadequate response (start 10 μg/min, then titrate up by 1 μg/kg/min over 30–60 min, higher doses PRN)
- Morphine sulfate, 4–8 mg IV, or meperidine, 50–75 mg IV, if TNG alone does not relieve pain
- Benzodiazepines for anxiety
- Thrombolytic therapy indicated in patients with > 1 mm ST-segment elevations in two contiguous leads or new LBBB, and no prior coronary artery bypass grafting (see Table 39)
- Thrombolysis is most beneficial when initiated within first 3 h, not given after 12 h of onset of chest pain
- RV MI: Treat with fluid loading, inotropic agents

THERAPEUTIC PROCEDURES

- In MI with ST-segment elevation, immediate coronary angiography and percutaneous transluminal coronary angioplasty or stenting of the infarct-related artery is an alternative to thrombolysis
- In MI with cardiogenic shock, early catheterization and percutaneous or surgical revascularization is the preferred management

OUTCOME

FOLLOW-UP

- For nonhypotensive patients with low ejection fractions, large infarctions, or clinical evidence of heart failure, start angiotensin-converting enzyme inhibitor on first postinfarction day; titrate and continue long-term
- Diltiazem appears to prevent reinfarction and ischemia in patients with non-Q-wave infarctions
- Patients with recurrent ischemic pain prior to discharge should undergo catheterization and, if indicated, revascularization

COMPLICATIONS

- Myocardial dysfunction, CHF, and hypotension
- Postinfarction ischemia
- Sinus bradycardia, sinus tachycardia, supraventricular premature beats, atrial fibrillation, ventricular premature beats, ventricular tachycardia, ventricular fibrillation, accelerated idioventricular rhythm, RBBB or LBBB or fascicular blocks, second- or third-degree AV block
- Rupture of a papillary muscle, interventricular septum, or LV free wall
- LV aneurysm
- Pericarditis, Dressler's syndrome
- Mural thrombi

PROGNOSIS

- Patients with a normal blood pressure, no signs of heart failure, and normal urinary output have a good prognosis

WHEN TO REFER

- Obtain immediate cardiology consultation for patients with new MI

WHEN TO ADMIT

- Admit all patients with possible MI to the CCU

PREVENTION

- Control of LDL-cholesterol and blood pressure, β-blockers, and antiplatelet agents
- Exercise training and cardiac rehabilitation programs

EVIDENCE

PRACTICE GUIDELINES

- ACC/AHA guidelines for the management of patients with ST-elevation myocardial infarction—executive summary. A report of the American College of Cardiology/American Heart Association Task Force on Practice Guidelines, 2004.
  - http://qc.acc.org/clinical/guidelines/stemi/exec_summ/index.pdf
- Institute for Clinical Systems Improvement: Diagnosis and Treatment of Acute Coronary Syndrome and Chest Pain, 2004.
  - http://www.icsi.org/knowledge/detail.asp?catID=29&itemID=1938

WEB SITES

- American College of Cardiology
  - http://www.acc.org/
- National Heart, Lung, and Blood Institute
  - http://www.nhlbi.nih.gov/health/prof/heart/index.htm#ami

INFORMATION FOR PATIENTS

- American Academy of Family Physicians: Heart Attack
  - http://familydoctor.org/291.xml
- American Heart Association: Heart Attack
  - http://www.americanheart.org/presenter.jhtml?identifier=4578
- MedlinePlus: Heart Attack Interactive Tutorial
  - http://www.nlm.nih.gov/medlineplus/tutorials/heartattack/htm/index.htm
- National Heart, Lung, and Blood Institute: Heart Attack
  - http://www.nhlbi.nih.gov/actintime/index.htm

REFERENCES

- Eagle KA et al: GRACE Investigators: A validated prediction model for all forms of acute coronary syndrome: estimating the risk of 6-month post discharge death in an international registry. JAMA 2004;291:2727. [PMID: 15187054]
- Granger CB et al: Global Registry of Acute Coronary Events. Investigators: Predictors of hospital mortality in the global registry of acute coronary events. Arch Intern Med 2003;163:2345. [PMID: 14581255]
- Keeley EC et al: Primary coronary intervention for acute myocardial infarction. JAMA 2004;291:736. [PMID: 14871919]
- Myocardial infarction redefined—a consensus document of The Joint European Society of Cardiology/American College of Cardiology Committee for the redefinition of myocardial infarction. J Am Coll Cardiol 2000;36:959. [PMID: 10987628]
- Ryan TJ: Percutaneous coronary intervention in ST-elevation myocardial infarction. Curr Cardiol Rep 2001;3:273. [PMID: 11406084]
- Zimetbaum PJ et al: Current concepts. Use of the electrocardiogram in acute myocardial infarction. N Engl J Med 2003;348:933. [PMID: 12621138]

Author(s)

Thomas M. Bashore, MD
Christopher B. Granger, MD

Myopathies: Dermatomyositis & Polymyositis

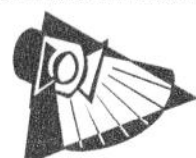

KEY FEATURES

ESSENTIALS OF DIAGNOSIS

- Bilateral proximal muscle weakness
- Characteristic cutaneous manifestations in dermatomyositis (Gottron's papules, heliotrope rash)
- Diagnostic tests: elevated creatine kinase and other muscle enzymes, muscle biopsy, electromyography
- Increased risk of malignancy, particularly in adult dermatomyositis

GENERAL CONSIDERATIONS

- An autoimmune disease of unknown cause characterized primarily by inflammation of muscles
- Five clinically defined subsets
  - Juvenile dermatomyositis
  - Dermatomyositis
  - Polymyositis
  - Myositis associated with malignancy
  - Myositis associated with another connective tissue disease [especially systemic lupus erythematosus (SLE)]
- Disorders of the peripheral and central nervous systems (eg, chronic inflammatory polyneuropathy, multiple sclerosis, myasthenia gravis, Eaton-Lambert disease, and amyotrophic lateral sclerosis) can produce weakness but are distinguished from inflammatory myopathies by characteristic symptoms and neurological signs and often by distinctive electromyographic abnormalities
- Inclusion body myositis can mimic polymyositis but is less responsive to treatment and has different epidemiological features
- Patients with polymyalgia rheumatica are over the age of 50 and—in contrast to patients with polymyositis—have pain but no objective weakness

DEMOGRAPHICS

- Peak incidence: fifth and sixth decades
- Women are affected twice as commonly as men
- The typical inclusion body myositis patient is white, male, and over age 50

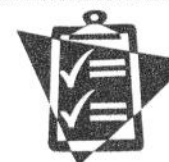

CLINICAL FINDINGS

SYMPTOMS AND SIGNS

- Gradual and progressive muscle weakness of the proximal muscle groups of the upper and lower extremities
- Leg weakness (eg, difficulty in rising from a chair or climbing stairs) typically precedes arm symptoms
- No facial or ocular muscle weakness
- Pain and tenderness of affected muscles (25%)

In dermatomyositis

- The characteristic rash is dusky red and may appear in malar distribution mimicking the classic rash of SLE
- Erythema also occurs over other areas of the face, neck, shoulders, and upper chest and back ("shawl sign")
- Periorbital edema and a purplish (heliotrope) suffusion over the eyelids are typical signs
- Periungual erythema, dilations of nailbed capillaries, and scaly patches over the dorsum of proximal interphalangeal and metacarpophalangeal joints (Gottron's sign) are highly suggestive
- A subset of patients with polymyositis and dermatomyositis develops the "antisynthetase syndrome," a group of findings including inflammatory arthritis, Raynaud's phenomenon, interstitial lung disease, and often severe muscle disease associated with certain autoantibodies (eg, anti-Jo-1 antibodies)

DIFFERENTIAL DIAGNOSIS

Muscle inflammation

- Polymyositis
- Dermatomyositis
- SLE
- Scleroderma
- Sjögren's syndrome
- Inclusion body myositis
- Trichinosis

Other causes of proximal muscle weakness

- Polymyalgia rheumatica
- Endocrine: hypothyroidism, hyperthyroidism, Cushing's syndrome
- Alcoholism
- Drugs: corticosteroids, statins, clofibrate, colchicine, chloroquine, emetine, aminocaproic acid, bretylium, penicillamine, drugs causing hypokalemia
- HIV myopathy
- Hyperparathyroidism
- Spinal stenosis
- Osteomalacia
- Mitochondrial myopathy

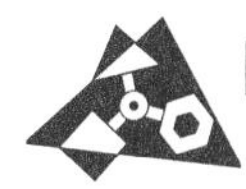

DIAGNOSIS

LABORATORY TESTS

- Serum levels of muscle enzymes, especially creatine kinase and aldolase, are elevated
- Antinuclear antibodies are present in many patients, and anti-Jo-1 antibodies are seen in the subset of patients that has associated interstitial lung disease

DIAGNOSTIC PROCEDURES

- Biopsy of clinically involved muscle is the only specific diagnostic test. The pathology findings in polymyositis and dermatomyositis are distinct, although both include lymphoid inflammatory infiltrates
- Electromyographic abnormalities consisting of polyphasic potentials, fibrillations, and high-frequency action potentials are helpful in establishing the diagnosis. None of the studies is specific

Myopathies: Dermatomyositis & Polymyositis

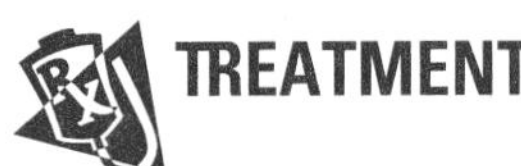

TREATMENT

MEDICATIONS

- Most patients respond to corticosteroids: 40–60 mg or more of prednisone is required initially daily. The dose is then adjusted downward according to the response of sequentially observed serum levels of muscle enzymes
- In patients resistant or intolerant to corticosteroids, therapy with methotrexate or azathioprine may be helpful

OUTCOME

FOLLOW-UP

- Up to one patient in four with dermatomyositis has an occult malignancy that may not be detected until months afterward in some cases
- Search for an occult malignancy should include age- and risk-appropriate cancer screening tests. If these evaluations are unrevealing, then a more invasive or extensive laboratory evaluation is probably not cost effective

COMPLICATIONS

- Hypercapnea and respiratory failure can develop from weakness of respiratory muscles
- Rhabdomyolysis with renal failure can complicate very severe muscle inflammation

PROGNOSIS

- Patients with an associated neoplasm have a poor prognosis, although remission may follow treatment of the tumor; steroids may or may not be effective in these patients

WHEN TO REFER

- Refer to a rheumatologist if the patient develops respiratory weakness or rhabdomyolysis

WHEN TO ADMIT

- Admit for airway protection and urgent treatment if the patient develops weakness of respiratory muscles
- Admit for rhabdomyolysis

EVIDENCE

PRACTICE GUIDELINES

- National Guideline Clearinghouse (chronic pain)
  - http://www.guideline.gov/summary/summary.aspx?doc_id=3415

WEB SITE

- The Myositis Association
  - http://www.myositis.org

INFORMATION FOR PATIENTS

- American Academy of Orthopaedic Surgeons
  - http://orthoinfo.aaos.org/fact/thr_report.cfm?Thread_ID=266&topcategory=About%20Orthopaedics
- Arthritis Foundation
  - http://www.arthritis.org/conditions/diseasecenter/myositis.asp
  - http://www.arthritis.org/conditions/diseasecenter/dermatomyositis.asp
- National Institutes of Health
  - http://www.nlm.nih.gov/medlineplus/ency/article/000839.htm

REFERENCES

- Dalakas MC et al: Polymyositis and dermatomyositis. Lancet 2003;362:971. [PMID: 14511932]
- Danko K et al: Long-term survival of patients with idiopathic inflammatory myopathies according to clinical features: a longitudinal study of 162 cases. Medicine 2004;83:35. [PMID: 14747766]

Author(s)

David B. Hellmann, MD, FACP
John H. Stone, MD, MPH

Nausea & Vomiting

KEY FEATURES

ESSENTIALS OF DIAGNOSIS

- Nausea is a vague, intensely disagreeable sensation of sickness or "queasiness"
- Distinguished from anorexia
- Retching (spasmodic respiratory and abdominal movements) often follows
- Vomiting may or may not follow
- Vomiting should be distinguished from regurgitation, the effortless reflux of liquid or solid (food) stomach contents

GENERAL CONSIDERATIONS

- May be caused by wide variety of conditions that stimulate the vagal afferent receptors, the brainstem vomiting center, or the chemoreceptor trigger zone (Table 52)
- May lead to serious complications, including electrolyte disturbances (hypokalemia, metabolic alkalosis), dehydration, aspiration pneumonia, Mallory-Weiss tear, and esophageal rupture

CLINICAL FINDINGS

SYMPTOMS AND SIGNS

- Acute symptoms without abdominal pain suggest food poisoning, infectious gastroenteritis, or drugs
- Acute pain with vomiting suggests peritoneal irritation, acute gastric or intestinal obstruction, or pancreaticobiliary disease
- Persistent vomiting suggests pregnancy, gastric outlet obstruction, gastroparesis, intestinal dysmotility, psychogenic disorders, and central nervous system or systemic disorders
- Vomiting immediately after meals suggests bulimia or psychogenic causes
- Vomiting of undigested food suggests gastroparesis or a gastric outlet obstruction; physical examination reveals a succussion splash
- Inquire about neurologic symptoms such as headaches, stiff neck, vertigo, and focal paresthesias or weakness

DIFFERENTIAL DIAGNOSIS

- Nausea and vomiting, causes (Table 52)

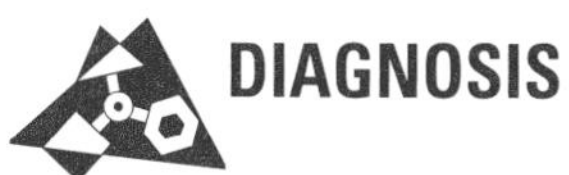

DIAGNOSIS

LABORATORY TESTS

- Obtain serum electrolytes, glucose, creatinine, calcium, amylase, liver enzymes, thyroid-stimulating hormone
- Obtain urine or serum pregnancy test

IMAGING STUDIES

- Flat and upright abdominal radiographs
- Ultrasound of abdomen or CT scan
- Barium upper gastrointestinal series
- Nuclear scintigraphic study for gastroparesis

DIAGNOSTIC PROCEDURES

- Nasogastric tube suction for patients with vomiting due to gastrointestinal obstruction, gastroparesis, ileus, or peritonitis
- Saline load test: formerly used to distinguish gastric outlet obstruction from delayed gastric emptying; this test is seldom used in era of endoscopy
- Upper endoscopy

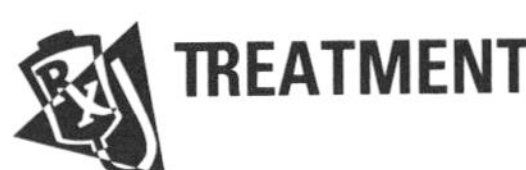

TREATMENT

MEDICATIONS

- Antiemetic medications (Table 53) given to control vomiting
- Combinations of drugs from different classes may provide better control
- Avoid antiemetic medications in pregnancy

THERAPEUTIC PROCEDURES

- For mild, self-limited, acute vomiting: no specific treatment, clear liquids and small quantities of dry foods
- For moderate to severe vomiting, nothing by mouth, give intravenous saline 0.45% solution with 20 mEq/L of potassium chloride
- Nasogastric suction for gastric decompression in patients with gastrointestinal obstruction, ileus or gastroparesis, or peritonitis

OUTCOME

COMPLICATIONS

- Dehydration, hypokalemia, metabolic alkalosis, aspiration, rupture of the esophagus (Boerhaave's syndrome), and bleeding secondary to a mucosal tear at the gastroesophageal junction (Mallory-Weiss syndrome)

WHEN TO ADMIT

- Hospitalize patient for severe acute vomiting, for rehydration, evaluation, and specific therapy

PREVENTION

- Antiemetic medications (especially 5-HT_3 antagonists) can be given to prevent vomiting in patients undergoing chemotherapy and abdominal surgery

EVIDENCE

PRACTICE GUIDELINES

- National Guideline Clearinghouse
  - http://www.guideline.gov/summary/summary.aspx?doc_id=3060&nbr=2286&string=nausea+and+vomiting

INFORMATION FOR PATIENTS

- American Academy of Family Physicians
  - http://familydoctor.org/529.xml
- National Digestive Diseases Information Clearinghouse
  - http://digestive.niddk.nih.gov/ddiseases/pubs/cvs/index.htm
  - http://familydoctor.org/flowcharts/529.html

REFERENCES

- Apfel CC et al: A factorial trial of six interventions in the prevention of postoperative nausea and vomiting. N Engl J Med 2004;350:2441. [PMID: 15190136]
- Gan TJ: Postoperative nausea and vomiting—can it be eliminated? JAMA 2002;287:1233. [PMID: 11886298]
- Hasler WL et al: Nausea and vomiting. Gastroenterology 2003;125:1860. [PMID: 14724837]
- Tramer MR: Treatment of postoperative nausea and vomiting. BMJ 2003;327:762. [PMID: 14525850]

Author(s)

Kenneth R. McQuaid, MD

Neck Masses

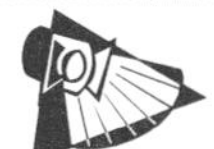

KEY FEATURES

ESSENTIALS OF DIAGNOSIS

- Rapid growth and tenderness suggest an inflammatory process
- Firm, painless, and slowly enlarging masses are often neoplastic

GENERAL CONSIDERATIONS

- In young adults, most neck masses are benign (branchial cleft cyst, thyroglossal duct cyst, reactive lymphadenitis), though malignancy should always be considered (lymphoma, metastatic thyroid carcinoma)
- Lymphadenopathy is common in HIV-positive individuals, but a growing or dominant mass may well be malignant
- In adults over 40, cancer is the most common cause of persistent neck mass
- A metastasis from squamous cell carcinoma arising within the mouth, pharynx, larynx, or upper esophagus should be suspected, especially if there is a history of tobacco or significant alcohol use
- An enlarged node unassociated with an obvious infection should be further evaluated, especially if the patient has a history of smoking or alcohol use or a history of cancer

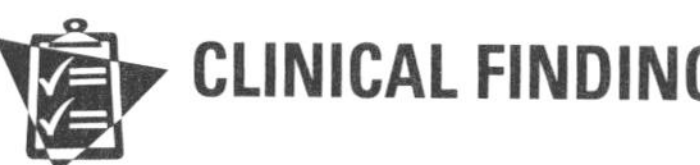

CLINICAL FINDINGS

SYMPTOMS AND SIGNS

Congenital lesions

- Branchial cleft cysts
  - Soft cystic mass on anterior border of sternocleidomastoid muscle, present with sudden swelling or infection at age 10–30
  - First branchial cleft cysts present high in neck, just below ear
  - Fistulous connection with external auditory canal floor may occur
  - Second branchial cleft cysts more common, may communicate with tonsillar fossa
  - Third branchial cleft cysts rare, may communicate with piriform sinus
- Thyroglossal duct cysts
  - Most common at age < 20
  - Midline neck mass, often just below hyoid bone, that moves on swallowing

Reactive lymphadenopathy

- Tender enlargement of neck nodes caused by pharynx, salivary gland, and scalp or HIV infection

Tuberculous and nontuberculous mycobacterial lymphadenitis

- Single or matted nodes
- Can drain externally (scrofula)

Neoplastic

- In older adults, 80% of firm, persistent, enlarging neck masses are metastases
- Most metastases arise from squamous cell carcinoma of upper aerodigestive tract
- Complete head and neck examination indicated
- Other than thyroid carcinoma, non-squamous cell metastases to neck are infrequent
- Except for lung and breast tumors, non-head and neck tumors seldom metastasize to middle or upper neck
- Except for renal cell carcinoma, infradiaphragmatic tumors rarely metastasize to neck

Lymphoma

- About 10% present in head and neck
- A growing concern in AIDS patients
- Multiple rubbery nodes, especially in young adults

DIFFERENTIAL DIAGNOSIS

- Reactive lymphadenopathy
- Lymphoma
- Skin abscess
- Parotitis
- Goiter
- Thyroiditis, thyroid carcinoma
- Branchial cleft or thyroglossal duct cyst
- Squamous cell carcinoma of upper aerodigestive tract
- Sarcoidosis
- Autoimmune adenopathy
- Kikuchi's disease

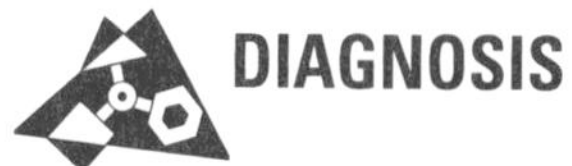

DIAGNOSIS

IMAGING STUDIES

- An MRI or PET scan before open biopsy may yield valuable information about a possible presumed primary site or another site for fine-needle aspiration (FNA) biopsy

DIAGNOSTIC PROCEDURES

- Common indications for FNA biopsy of a node include persistence or continued enlargement, particularly if an obvious primary tumor is not visible or palpable on physical examination

Tuberculous and nontuberculous mycobacterial lymphadenitis

- FNA is usually the best initial diagnostic approach: send specimens for cytology, smear for acid-fast bacilli, culture and sensitivity, and polymerase chain reaction (PCR), as indicated

Infectious, inflammatory, and neoplastic neck masses

- Examination under anesthesia with direct laryngoscopy, esophagoscopy, and bronchoscopy is usually required to fully evaluate the tumor and exclude second primaries

Lymphoma

- FNA may be diagnostic, but open biopsy is often required

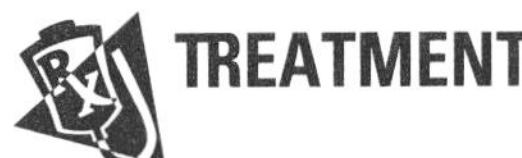

TREATMENT

SURGERY

Branchial cleft cysts

- To prevent recurrent infection and possible carcinoma, branchial cleft cysts should be completely excised, along with their fistulous tracts

Thyroglossal duct cysts

- Surgical excision is recommended to prevent recurrent infection

Reactive cervical lymphadenopathy

- Except for the occasional node that suppurates and requires incision and drainage, treatment is directed against the underlying infection

Infectious, inflammatory, and neoplastic neck masses

- Treat the underlying pathology

OUTCOME

PROGNOSIS

- Prognosis is that of the underlying pathology

WHEN TO REFER

- When the diagnosis is in question or for specialized treatment, particularly for a malignancy

EVIDENCE

PRACTICE GUIDELINES

- Forastiere AA et al: NCCN Head and Neck Cancers Practice Guidelines Panel. National Comprehensive Cancer Network: Head and Neck Cancers v.1.2005.
  - http://www.nccn.org/professionals/physician_gls/PDF/head-and-neck.pdf
- Sherman SI et al: NCCN Thyroid Carcinoma Practice Guidelines Panel. National Comprehensive Cancer Network: Thyroid Carcinoma v.1.2005.
  - http://www.nccn.org/professionals/physician_gls/PDF/thyroid.pdf

WEB SITES

- Baylor College of Medicine Otolaryngology Resources
  - http://www.bcm.tmc.edu/oto/othersa.html
- Lymphoma of the Head and Neck Demonstration Case
  - http://www.brighamrad.harvard.edu/Cases/bwh/hcache/47/full.html

INFORMATION FOR PATIENTS

- Mayo Clinic: Swollen Lymph Glands
  - http://www.mayoclinic.com/invoke.cfm?id=HQ01039
- MedlinePlus: Neck Lump
  - http://www.nlm.nih.gov/medlineplus/ency/article/003098.htm
- Medline Plus: Branchial Cleft Cyst
  - http://www.nlm.nih.gov/medlineplus/ency/article/001396.htm
- National Cancer Institute: Head and Neck Cancer: Q & A
  - http://cis.nci.nih.gov/fact/6_37.htm

REFERENCES

- Dedivitis RA et al: Thyroglossal duct: a review of 55 cases. J Am Coll Surg 2002;194:274. [PMID: 11893130]
- Handa U et al: Fine needle aspiration diagnosis of tuberculous lymphadenitis. Trop Doct 2002;32:147. [PMID: 12141296]
- Prakash PK et al: Differential diagnosis of neck lumps. Practitioner 2002;246:252. [PMID: 11961991]
- Schwetschenau E et al: The adult neck mass. Am Fam Physician 2002;66:831. [PMID: 12322776]

Author(s)

Robert K. Jackler, MD

Michael J. Kaplan, MD

Neck Pain

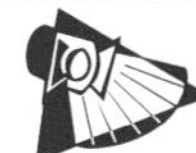

KEY FEATURES

ESSENTIALS OF DIAGNOSIS

- Most chronic neck pain is caused by degenerative joint disease and responds to conservative approaches

GENERAL CONSIDERATIONS

- A large group of articular and extraarticular disorders is characterized by pain that may involve simultaneously the neck, shoulder girdle, and upper extremity. Diagnostic differentiation among these disorders may be difficult

Etiology

- Cervical strain is generally caused by mechanical postural disorders, overexertion, or injury (eg, whiplash)
- Cervical spondylosis (degenerative arthritis) is a collective term describing degenerative changes that occur in the apophysial joints and intervertebral disk joints, with or without neurological signs

DEMOGRAPHICS

- Degeneration of cervical disks and joints may occur in adolescents but is more common after age 40

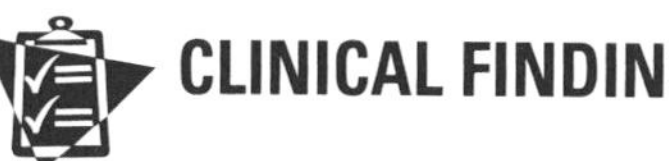

CLINICAL FINDINGS

SYMPTOMS AND SIGNS

- Pain may be limited to the posterior neck region or, depending on the level of the symptomatic joint, may radiate segmentally to the occiput, anterior chest, shoulder girdle, arm, forearm, and hand
- Radiating pain in the upper extremity is often intensified by hyperextension of the neck and deviation of the head to the involved side
- Limitation of cervical movements is the most common objective finding
- Neurological signs depend on the extent of compression of nerve roots or the spinal cord. Compression of the spinal cord may cause long-tract involvement resulting in paraparesis or paraplegia

Acute or chronic cervical musculotendinous strain

- Acute episodes are associated with pain, decreased cervical spine motion, and paraspinal muscle spasm, resulting in stiffness of the neck and loss of motion
- Local tenderness is often present in acute but not chronic strain

Herniated nucleus pulposus

- Rupture or prolapse of the nucleus pulposus of the cervical disks into the spinal canal causes pain that radiates to the arms at the level of C6–C7
- When intraabdominal pressure is increased by coughing, sneezing, or other movements, symptoms are aggravated, and cervical muscle spasm may often occur
- Neurological abnormalities may include decreased reflexes of the deep tendons of the biceps and triceps and decreased sensation and muscle atrophy or weakness in the forearm or hand

Arthritic disorders

- Osteoarthritis of the cervical spine is often asymptomatic but may cause diffuse neck pain, radicular pain, or myelopathy
- Myelopathy develops insidiously and is manifested by numb, clumsy hands
- Some patients also complain of unsteady walking, urinary frequency and urgency, or electrical shock sensations with neck flexion or extension (Lhermitte's sign)
- Weakness, sensory loss, and spasticity with exaggerated reflexes develop below the level of spinal cord compression

DIFFERENTIAL DIAGNOSIS

- Acute or chronic cervical musculotendinous strain
- Herniated nucleus pulposus
- Degenerative arthritides (eg, osteoarthritis)
- Inflammatory arthritides (eg, rheumatoid arthritis, ankylosing spondylitis)
- Infections (eg, meningitis, osteomyelitis)
- Cancer (eg, cervical spine metastases)
- Fibromyalgia

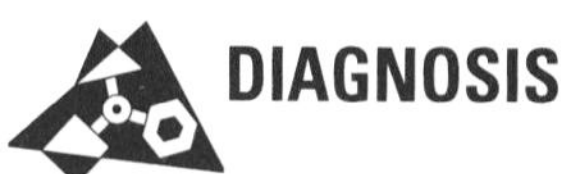

DIAGNOSIS

IMAGING STUDIES

- Plain x-rays are often completely normal in an acute cervical strain
- In osteoarthritis, comparative reduction in height of the involved disk space is a frequent finding. The most common late x-ray finding is osteophyte formation
- Use of MRI or CT is indicated in the patient who has severe pain of unknown cause that fails to respond to conservative therapy or in the patient who has evidence of myelopathy
- MRI is more sensitive than CT in detecting disk disease, extradural compression, and intramedullary cord disease
- CT is more sensitive for demonstration of fractures

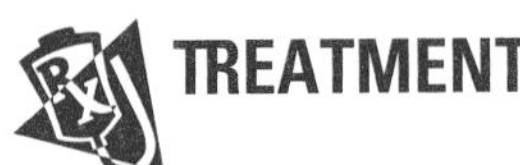

TREATMENT

MEDICATIONS

Acute or chronic cervical musculotendinous strain

- Analgesics and early mobilization (including whiplash)

Herniated nucleus pulposus

- Cervical traction, bed rest, and analgesics are usually successful for pain and radicular symptoms
- Cervical epidural steroid injections may help those who fail to improve

SURGERY

- Surgery is indicated for unremitting pain and progressive weakness from a herniated nucleus pulposus despite a full trial of conservative therapy and if a surgically correctable abnormality is identified by MRI or CT myelography. Surgical decompression achieves excellent results in 70–80% of such patients
- Surgical treatment may involve stabilization of the cervical spine when atlantoaxial subluxation occurs in patients with rheumatoid arthritis

THERAPEUTIC PROCEDURES

- Chronic pain in the zygapophysial joints resulting from whiplash injuries may benefit from percutaneous radiofrequency neurotomy

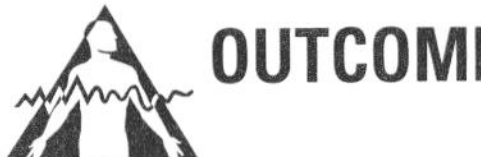

OUTCOME

COMPLICATIONS

- Progressive degenerative disease of the cervical spine can cause cervical myelopathy with weakness and spasticity of the legs
- Serious erosive disease of joints may lead to neurological complications as sometimes occurs in rheumatoid arthritis and occasionally in ankylosing spondylitis; the usual joint involved in these disorders is the atlantoaxial joint (C1–C2)

WHEN TO REFER

- Refer to a neurosurgeon for indications described under Surgery

EVIDENCE

PRACTICE GUIDELINES

- Gross AR et al: Clinical practice guideline on the use of manipulation or mobilization in the treatment of adults with mechanical neck disorders. Man Ther 2002;7:193. [PMID: 12419654]

INFORMATION FOR PATIENTS

- American Academy of Orthopedic Surgeons
  - http://orthoinfo.aaos.org/brochure/thr_report.cfm?Thread_ID=11&topcategory=Neck
- American Physical Therapy Association
  - http://www.apta.org/brochures/NeckPain.pdf

REFERENCES

- Hardin J: Pain and the cervical spine. Bull Rheum Dis 2001;50:1. [PMID: 11688257]
- Hoving JL et al: Manual therapy, physical therapy, or continued care by a general practitioner for patients with neck pain. A randomized, controlled trial. Ann Intern Med 2002;136:713. [PMID: 12020139]

Author(s)

David B. Hellmann, MD, FACP

John H. Stone, MD, MPH

Neck Pain, Discogenic

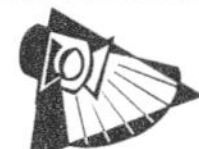

KEY FEATURES

ESSENTIALS OF DIAGNOSIS

- Neck pain, sometimes radiating to arms
- Restricted neck movements
- Motor, sensory, or reflex changes in arms with root involvement
- Neurologic deficit in legs, gait disorder, or sphincter disturbance with cord involvement

GENERAL CONSIDERATIONS

Acute cervical disk protrusion

- Acute cervical disk protrusion leads to pain in the neck and radicular pain in the arm, exacerbated by head movement

Cervical spondylosis

- Results from chronic cervical disk degeneration, with herniation of disk material, secondary calcification, and associated osteophytic outgrowths
- One or more of the cervical nerve roots may be compressed, stretched, or angulated; and myelopathy may also develop as a result of compression, vascular insufficiency, or recurrent minor trauma to the cord

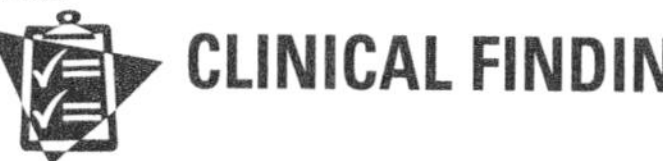

CLINICAL FINDINGS

SYMPTOMS AND SIGNS

Acute cervical disk protrusion

- With lateral disk herniation, motor, sensory, or reflex changes are in a radicular (usually C6 or C7) distribution on the affected side
- With more centrally directed herniations, the spinal cord may also be involved, leading to spastic paraparesis and sensory disturbances in the legs, sometimes accompanied by impaired sphincter function

Cervical spondylosis

- Neck pain and restricted head movement, occipital headaches, radicular pain and other sensory disturbances in the arms, weakness of the arms or legs, or some combination of these symptoms
- Examination generally reveals that lateral flexion and rotation of the neck are limited
- A segmental pattern of weakness or dermatomal sensory loss (or both) may be found unilaterally or bilaterally in the upper limbs, and tendon reflexes mediated by the affected root or roots are depressed
- The C5 and C6 nerve roots are most commonly involved; then, examination frequently reveals weakness of muscles supplied by these roots (eg, deltoids, supraspinatus and infraspinatus, biceps, brachioradialis), pain or sensory loss about the shoulder and outer border of the arm and forearm, and depressed biceps and brachioradialis reflexes
- Spastic paraparesis may also be present if there is an associated myelopathy, sometimes accompanied by posterior column or spinothalamic sensory deficits in the legs

DIFFERENTIAL DIAGNOSIS

- Congenital abnormalities may involve the cervical spine and lead to neck pain (eg, hemivertebrae, fused vertebrae, basilar impression, instability of the atlantoaxial joint)
- Traumatic, degenerative, infective, and neoplastic disorders may also lead to pain in the neck
- Spinal rheumatoid arthritis tends to affect especially the cervical region, leading to pain, stiffness, and reduced mobility; displacement of vertebrae or atlantoaxial subluxation may lead to cord compression that can be life-threatening if not treated by fixation

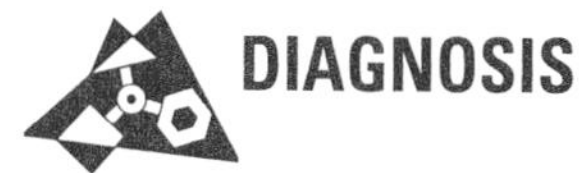

DIAGNOSIS

IMAGING STUDIES

Acute cervical disk protrusion

- The diagnosis is confirmed by MRI or CT myelography

Cervical spondylosis

- Plain radiographs of the cervical spine show osteophyte formation, narrowing of disk spaces, and encroachment on the intervertebral foramina, but such changes are common in middle-aged persons and may be unrelated to the presenting complaint
- CT or MRI helps confirm the diagnosis and exclude other structural causes of the myelopathy

TREATMENT

SURGERY

Acute cervical disk protrusion

- If other measures are unsuccessful or the patient has a significant neurologic deficit, surgical removal of the protruding disk may be necessary

Cervical spondylosis

- Operative treatment may be necessary to prevent further progression if there is a significant neurologic deficit or if root pain is severe, persistent, and unresponsive to conservative measures

THERAPEUTIC PROCEDURES

Acute cervical disk protrusion

- In mild cases, bed rest or intermittent neck traction may help, followed by immobilization of the neck in a collar for several weeks

Cervical spondylosis

- Restriction of neck movements by a cervical collar may relieve pain

OUTCOME

PROGNOSIS

- Self-limited

WHEN TO REFER

- Ergonomic consultation may improve symptoms

EVIDENCE

PRACTICE GUIDELINES

- National Guideline Clearinghouse
  - http://www.guideline.gov/summary/summary.aspx?doc_id=2803
- Philadelphia Panel evidence-based clinical practice guidelines on selected rehabilitation interventions for neck pain. Phys Ther 2001;81:1701. [PMID: 11589644]

INFORMATION FOR PATIENTS

- JAMA patient page: Neck injuries. JAMA 2001;286:1928. [PMID: 11680473]
- American Academy of Orthopaedic Surgeons
  - http://orthoinfo.aaos.org/fact/thr_report.cfm?Thread_ID=11&topcategory=Neck

REFERENCES

- Harris G: Managing musculoskeletal complaints with rehabilitation therapy: summary of the Philadelphia Panel evidence-based clinical practice guidelines on musculoskeletal rehabilitation interventions. J Fam Pract 2002;51:1042. [PMID: 12540330]
- Niemisto L: Radiofrequency denervation for neck and back pain. A systematic review of randomized controlled trials. Cochrane Database Syst Rev 2003;CD004058. [PMID: 12535508]
- Schonstein E: Work conditioning, work hardening and functional restoration for workers with back and neck pain. Cochrane Database Syst Rev 2003;CD001822. [PMID: 12535416]

Author(s)

Michael J. Aminoff, MD, DSc, FRCP

Non-Hodgkin's Lymphoma

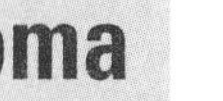

KEY FEATURES

GENERAL CONSIDERATIONS

- Heterogeneous group of cancers of lymphocytes
- Disorders vary in clinical presentation and course from indolent to rapidly progressive
- Indolent lymphomas often disseminated at diagnosis, and bone marrow involvement frequent
- In Burkitt's lymphoma, a protooncogene c-*myc* is translocated from chromosome 8 to heavy chain locus on chromosome 14, where c-*myc* overexpression is likely related to malignant transformation
- In follicular lymphomas, translocation of possible oncogene *bcl*-2 from chromosome 8 to the heavy chain locus on chromosome 14 causes *bcl*-2 overexpression, which appears to protect the lymphoma cell against apoptosis

REAL/WHO proposed classification of lymphomas

- B cell lymphomas
  - Precursor B cell lymphoblastic lymphoma
  - Small lymphocytic lymphoma/chronic lymphocytic leukemia
  - Marginal zone lymphomas: nodal marginal zone lymphoma, extranodal MALT, splenic
  - Hairy cell leukemia
  - Follicular lymphoma
  - Mantle cell lymphoma
  - Diffuse large B cell lymphoma
  - Burkitt's lymphoma
- T cell lymphomas
  - Anaplastic large cell lymphoma
  - Peripheral T cell lymphoma
  - Mycosis fungoides

CLINICAL FINDINGS

SYMPTOMS AND SIGNS

- Painless lymphadenopathy, isolated or widespread (retroperitoneal, mesenteric, and pelvic)
- Constitutional symptoms, eg, fever, drenching night sweats, or weight loss
- Extranodal sites of disease (skin, gastrointestinal tract) sometimes found on examination
- Abdominal pain or abdominal fullness in Burkitt's lymphoma because of predilection for abdomen

DIFFERENTIAL DIAGNOSIS

- Hodgkin's disease
- Metastatic cancer
- Infectious mononucleosis
- Cat-scratch disease
- Sarcoidosis
- Drug-induced pseudolymphoma (eg, phenytoin)

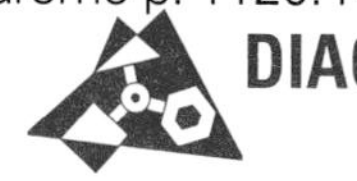

DIAGNOSIS

LABORATORY TESTS

- Peripheral blood usually normal, but some lymphomas may present in leukemic phase
- Cerebrospinal fluid cytology shows malignant cells in some high-grade lymphomas with meningeal involvement
- Serum lactate dehydrogenase is a useful prognostic marker and is now incorporated in risk stratification of treatment

IMAGING STUDIES

- Chest x-ray: mediastinal mass in lymphoblastic lymphoma, others
- CT scan of chest, abdomen, pelvis

DIAGNOSTIC PROCEDURES

- Needle aspiration biopsy may yield suspicious results, but lymph node biopsy (or biopsy of involved extranodal tissue) required for diagnosis and staging
- Bone marrow involvement manifested as paratrabecular lymphoid aggregates
- Staging after pathological diagnosis is established involves chest x-ray and CT of abdomen and pelvis; bone marrow biopsy; and in selected cases with high-risk morphology, lumbar puncture

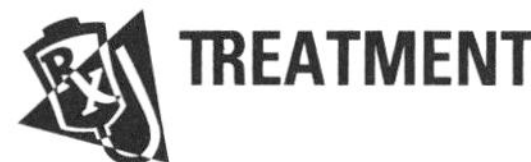

TREATMENT

MEDICATIONS

- Chemotherapy with alkylating agents, eg, chlorambucil, 0.6–1 mg/kg Q 3 weeks, or combination chemotherapy with cyclophosphamide, vincristine, and prednisone (CVP)
- Fludarabine may produce equivalent results
- Rituximab (monoclonal antibody directed against B cell surface antigen CD20) is effective as salvage therapy for relapsed low-grade B cell lymphomas and may improve outcomes when added to initial chemotherapy
- Chemotherapy with cyclophosphamide, doxorubicin [hydroxydaunomycin; adriamycin], vincristine [Oncovin], and prednisone [CHOP]) for 3 cycles plus localized radiation for localized intermediate-grade lymphomas
- Chemotherapy with CHOP for 6–8 cycles for more advanced intermediate-grade lymphomas
- Addition of rituximab to CHOP for older patients with diffuse large cell lymphomas

THERAPEUTIC PROCEDURES

- Most indolent lymphomas are disseminated at diagnosis
  - If not bulky and patient is asymptomatic, no initial therapy is required
  - Spontaneous remission in some
- Localized radiation therapy for patients who have limited indolent disease
- Radioimmunoconjugates, eg, yttrium-90 ibritumomab, which fuse anti-B cell antibodies with radiation, may produce improved results compared with antibody alone
- Special forms of lymphoma require individualized therapy
  - Burkitt's lymphoma
  - Lymphoblastic lymphoma
  - Mantle cell lymphoma
- Intensive initial therapy including autologous stem cell transplantation has been shown to improve outcomes and is now the standard of care
- Allogeneic transplantation for patients with clinically aggressive low-grade lymphomas
- Autologous stem cell transplantation early in course for high-risk lymphoma; or for intermediate-grade lymphoma that relapses after initial chemotherapy

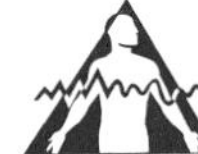

OUTCOME

PROGNOSIS

- Median survival with indolent lymphomas is 6–8 years; disease ultimately becomes refractory to chemotherapy
- For intermediate-grade lymphoma, the International Prognostic Index is widely used to categorize patients into prognostic groups
- Worse prognosis if age over 60, elevated serum LDH, stage III or stage IV disease, or poor performance status
- **0–1 risk factor**
  - 80% complete response rate to standard chemotherapy
  - Most responses (80%) durable
- **2 risk factors**
  - 70% complete response rate
  - 70% durable
- **> 2 risk factors**
  - Lower response rates and poor survival with standard regimens
  - Early treatment with high-dose therapy and autologous stem cell transplantation may improve outcome
- With relapse after initial chemotherapy, if lymphoma still partially sensitive to chemotherapy, autologous transplantation offers 50% chance of long-term salvage

EVIDENCE

PRACTICE GUIDELINES

- Zelenetz AD et al; NCCN Non-Hodgkin's Lymphoma Practice Guidelines Panel. National Comprehensive Cancer Network: Non-Hodgkin's Lymphoma v.1.2005.
  - http://www.nccn.org/professionals/physician_gls/PDF/nhl.pdf

WEB SITE

- National Cancer Institute: Adult Non-Hodgkin's Lymphoma Treatment
  - http://www.cancer.gov/cancertopics/pdq/treatment/adult-non-hodgkins/HealthProfessional

INFORMATION FOR PATIENTS

- American Cancer Society
  - http://www.cancer.org/docroot/cri/content/cri_2_4_1x_what_is_non_hodgkins_lymphoma_32.asp
- Leukemia & Lymphoma Society
  - http://www.leukemia-lymphoma.org/all_page?item_id=7087
- National Cancer Institute
  - http://www.cancer.gov/cancerinfo/wyntk/non-hodgkins-lymphoma

REFERENCES

- Cheson BB: Radioimmunotherapy of non-Hodgkin lymphomas. Blood 2003;101:391. [PMID: 12393555]
- Escalon MP et al: Nonmyeloablative allogeneic hematopoietic transplantation: a promising salvage therapy for patients with non-Hodgkin's lymphoma whose disease has failed a prior autologous transplantation. J Clin Oncol 2004;22:2419. [PMID: 15197204]
- Zinzani PL et al: Fludarabine plus mitoxantrone with and without rituximab versus CHOP with and without rituximab as front-line treatment for patients with follicular lymphoma. J Clin Oncol 2004;22:2654. [PMID: 15159414]

Author(s)

Charles A. Linker, MD

Obesity

Nevi, Dysplastic or Atypical p. 1121. Niacin Deficiency p. 1121. Nipple Discharge p. 1121. Nocardiosis p. 1122.

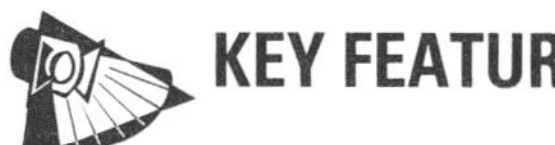

KEY FEATURES

ESSENTIALS OF DIAGNOSIS

- Excess adipose tissue, resulting in body mass index (BMI) > 30
- Upper body obesity (abdomen and flank) of greater health consequence than lower body obesity (buttocks and thighs)

GENERAL CONSIDERATIONS

- Quantitative evaluation involves determination of BMI
- BMI accurately reflects the presence of excess adipose tissue; it is calculated by dividing measured body weight in kilograms by the height in meters squared
- Normal: BMI = 18.5–24.9
- Overweight: BMI = 25–29.9
- Class I obesity: BMI = 30–34.9
- Class II obesity: BMI = 35–39.9
- Class III (extreme) obesity: BMI > 40
- Increased abdominal circumference (> 102 cm in men and > 88 cm in women) or high waist/hip ratios (> 1.0 in men and > 0.85 in women) confers greater risk of diabetes mellitus, stroke, coronary artery disease, and early death
- Associated with significant increases in morbidity and mortality
- Surgical and obstetric risks greater
- The relative risk associated with obesity decreases with age, and excess weight is no longer a risk factor in adults aged > 75
- 65% of Americans are overweight
- 30.4% of Americans are obese
- As much as 50% of obesity may be explained by genetic influences

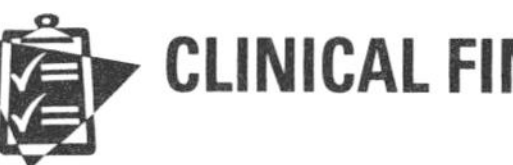

CLINICAL FINDINGS

SYMPTOMS AND SIGNS

- Assess degree and distribution of body fat
- Assess overall nutritional status
- Signs of secondary causes of obesity (hypothyroidism and Cushing's syndrome) are found in < 1%

DIFFERENTIAL DIAGNOSIS

- Increased caloric intake
- Fluid retention: congestive heart failure, cirrhosis, nephrotic syndrome
- Cushing's syndrome
- Hypothyroidism
- Diabetes mellitus (type 2)
- Drugs, eg, antipsychotics, antidepressants, corticosteroids
- Insulinoma
- Depression
- Binge eating disorder

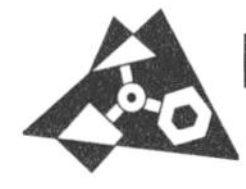

DIAGNOSIS

LABORATORY TESTS

- Endocrinologic evaluation, including serum thyroid-stimulating hormone and dexamethasone suppression test in obese patients with unexplained recent weight gain
- Assessment for medical consequences and metabolic syndrome: blood pressure and fasting glucose, cholesterol, and triglyceride levels

DIAGNOSTIC PROCEDURES

- Calculation of BMI
- Measurement of abdominal circumference (waist/hip ratio)

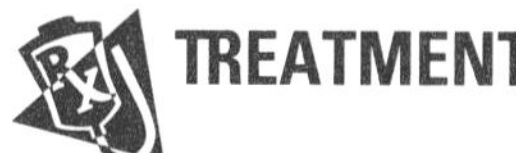

TREATMENT

MEDICATIONS

- Catecholaminergic or serotonergic medications: sometimes used in patients with BMI > 30 or patients with BMI > 27 who have obesity-related health risks
- Catecholaminergic medications
  - Amphetamines (high abuse potential)
  - Nonamphetamine schedule IV appetite suppressants (phentermine, diethylpropion, and mazindol) are approved for short-term use only and have limited utility
- Serotonergic medications
  - Selective serotonin reuptake inhibitor antidepressants (eg, fluoxetine and sertraline) have serotonergic activity though FDA-approved for weight loss
- Sibutramine (10 mg PO QD)
  - Blocks uptake of both serotonin and norepinephrine in the central nervous system
  - Side effects include dry mouth, anorexia, constipation, insomnia, dizziness, and increased blood pressure (< 5%)
- Orlistat (120 mg PO TID with meals)
  - Reduces fat absorption in the gastrointestinal tract by inhibiting intestinal lipase
  - Side effects include diarrhea, gas, and cramping and perhaps reduced absorption of fat-soluble vitamins

SURGERY

- Consider for patients with BMI > 40, or BMI > 35 if obesity-related comorbidities

- Effective surgical procedures include Roux-en-Y gastric bypass, vertical banded gastroplasty, and gastric banding; each can be done laparoscopically
- Surgical complications are common and include
  - Peritonitis due to anastomotic leak
  - Abdominal wall hernias
  - Staple line disruption
  - Gallstones
  - Neuropathy
  - Marginal ulcers
  - Stomal stenosis
  - Wound infections
  - Thromboembolic disease
  - Nutritional deficiencies
  - Gastrointestinal symptoms
- Surgical mortality ranges from 0.1% to 1.1%

THERAPEUTIC PROCEDURES

- Multidisciplinary approach, including hypocaloric diets, behavior modification, aerobic exercise, and social support
- Limit foods that provide large amounts of calories without other nutrients, ie, fat, sucrose, and alcohol
- No special advantage to carbohydrate-restricted or high-protein or high-fat diets, nor to ingestion of foods one at a time
- Plan and keep records of menus and exercise sessions; provide rewards such as refundable financial contracts
- Aerobic exercise useful for long-term weight maintenance
- For BMI > 35, consider very low-calorie diets (< 800 kcal/day) for 4–6 months; side effects include fatigue, orthostatic hypotension, cold intolerance, and fluid and electrolyte disorders; less common complications include gout, gallbladder disease, and cardiac arrhythmias

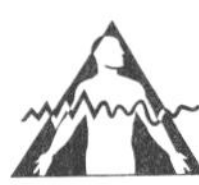

OUTCOME

COMPLICATIONS

- Hypertension
- Type 2 diabetes mellitus
- Hyperlipidemia
- Coronary artery disease
- Degenerative joint disease
- Psychosocial disability
- Cancers (colon, rectum, prostate, uterus, biliary tract, breast, ovary)
- Thromboembolic disorders
- Digestive tract diseases (gallstones, reflux esophagitis)
- Skin disorders

PROGNOSIS

- Only 20% of patients will lose 20 lb and maintain the loss for > 2 years; only 5% will maintain a 40-lb loss
- With very low-calorie diets, patients lose an average of 2–4 lb per week; long-term weight maintenance is less predictable and requires concurrent behavior modification and exercise
- Sibutramine, 10 mg PO QD, for 6–12 months results in average weight losses of 3–5 kg more than placebo
- Orlistat, 120 mg PO TID with meals, for up to 2 years results in 2–4 kg greater weight loss than placebo
- Surgical procedures lead to substantial weight loss—20–40% of initial body weight

WHEN TO REFER

- Refer for bariatric surgery for BMI > 40

WHEN TO ADMIT

- For bariatric surgery

EVIDENCE

PRACTICE GUIDELINES

- Cummings S et al: Position of the American Dietetic Association: weight management. J Am Diet Assoc 2002;102:1145. [PMID: 12171464]

WEB SITE

- American Obesity Association
  - http://www.obesity.org/

INFORMATION FOR PATIENTS

- American Obesity Association
  - http://www.obesity.org/
- Cleveland Clinic—Obesity
  - http://www.clevelandclinic.org/health/health-info/docs/2400/2435.asp?index=9468

REFERENCES

- American Medical Association: Assessment and Management of Adult Obesity: A Primer for Physicians, 2003. www.ama-assn.org/ama/pub/category/10931.html.
- Avenell A et al: What are the long-term benefits of weight reducing diets in adults? A systematic review of randomized controlled trials. J Hum Nutr Diet 2004;17:317. [PMID: 15250842]
- Buchwald H et al: Bariatric surgery: a systematic review and meta-analysis. JAMA 2004;292:1724. [PMID: 15479938]
- Dansinger ML et al: Comparison of the Atkins, Ornish, Weight Watchers, and Zone diets for weight loss and heart disease risk reduction: a randomized trial. JAMA 2005;293:43. [PMID: 15632335]
- Dietz WH: Overweight in childhood and adolescence. N Engl J Med 2004;350:855. [PMID: 14985480]
- Hedley AA et al: Prevalence of overweight and obesity among US children, adolescents, and adults, 1999–2002. JAMA 2004;291:2847. [PMID: 15199035]
- Katzmarzyk PT et al: Metabolic syndrome, obesity, and mortality: impact of cardiorespiratory fitness. Diabetes Care 2005;28:391. [PMID: 15677798]
- Norris S et al: Pharmacotherapy for weight loss in adults with type 2 diabetes mellitus. Cochrane Database Syst Rev 2005;(1):CD004096. [PMID: 15674929]
- Sjostrom L et al; Swedish Obese Subjects Study Scientific Group: Lifestyle, diabetes, and cardiovascular risk factors 10 years after bariatric surgery. N Engl J Med 2004;351:2683. [PMID: 15616203]
- Tsai AG et al: Systematic review: an evaluation of major commercial weight loss programs in the United States. Ann Intern Med 2005;142:56. [PMID: 15630109]

Author(s)

Robert B. Baron, MD, MS

Onchocerciasis

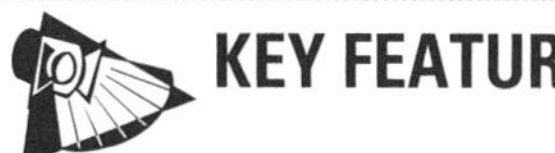

KEY FEATURES

ESSENTIALS OF DIAGNOSIS

- Primary findings are subcutaneous nodules that contain adult worms and skin and eye changes that result from dead or dying microfilariae
- Heavy infection leads to chronic pruritus, disfiguring skin lesions, visual impairment, and debility

GENERAL CONSIDERATIONS

- The infection is a chronic filarial disease caused by *Onchocerca volvulus*
- Humans are the only important host
  - The vector and intermediate host are *Simulium* flies, day biters that breed in rivers and fast-flowing streams and become infected by ingesting microfilariae with a human blood meal
  - At subsequent feedings, they can infect new susceptible hosts
- Female worms release motile microfilariae into the skin, subcutaneous tissues, lymphatics, and eyes; microfilariae are occasionally seen in the urine but rarely in blood or cerebrospinal fluid

DEMOGRAPHICS

- An estimated 18 million persons are infected, of whom 3–4 million have skin disease, 0.3 million are blinded, and 0.5 million are severely visually impaired
- In hyperendemic areas, more than 40% of inhabitants over 40 years of age are blind
- The infection, predominant in West Africa, also occurs in many other parts of tropical Africa and in localized areas of the southwestern Arabian peninsula, southern Mexico, Guatemala, Venezuela, Colombia, and northwestern Brazil
- The West African savanna strain is especially associated with severe blinding eye lesions

CLINICAL FINDINGS

SYMPTOMS AND SIGNS

- The interval from exposure to onset of symptoms can be as long as 1–3 years
- **Nodules**
  - Adult worms, which can live for up to 15 years, typically are in fibrous subcutaneous nodules that are painless, freely movable, and 0.5–1 cm in size
  - Many nodules are deep in the muscular tissues and nonpalpable
- **Pruritus**
  - May be severe, leading to skin excoriation and lichenification; other findings include pigmentary changes, papules, scaling, atrophy, pendulous skin, and acute inflammation
  - May occur without skin lesions
- **Dermatitis**
  - Infected visitors, as compared with indigenous persons, may show a more prominent dermatitis despite a low to nondetectable microfiladerma or eosinophilia and an absence of nodules and eye disease
- **Lymphadenopathy**
  - There may be marked enlargement of femoral and inguinal nodes and generalized lymph node enlargement
- **Eye**
  - Microfilariae in the eye may lead to visual impairment and blindness
  - Findings include itching, photophobia, anterior segment changes (limbitis, punctate and sclerosing keratitis, iritis, secondary glaucoma, cataract), and posterior segment changes (optic neuritis, optic atrophy, chorioretinitis, and other retinal findings)

DIFFERENTIAL DIAGNOSIS

- Glaucoma
- Loiasis (*Loa loa* infection)
- Gnathostomiasis
- Cysticercosis (with ophthalmic involvement)
- Sporotrichosis
- Coccidioidomycosis

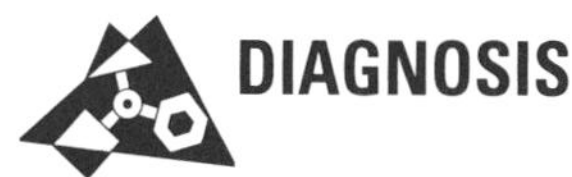

DIAGNOSIS

LABORATORY TESTS

- Traditional serological tests are usually positive, but cross-reactions occur with other forms of filariasis, and the tests do not distinguish current from past infection
- Immunoblot analysis of IgG_4 antibodies and an ELISA appear to be more sensitive than skin snips early in infection, but occasional cross-reactions also occur with other filarial infections
- PCR (on skin snips and urine) and antigen detection (in blood and urine) have the advantage over serology in that they are positive only in people who have active infection
- Eosinophilia (15–50%), polyclonal hypergammaglobulinemia, and elevated IgE levels are common

IMAGING STUDIES

- Ultrasound has been used to detect nonpalpable onchocercomas and to distinguish them from other lesions (lipomas, fibromas, lymph nodes, foreign body granulomas)

DIAGNOSTIC PROCEDURES

- Diagnosis is made by demonstrating microfilariae in skin snips (usually obtained with a punch biopsy instrument), identifying them in the cornea or anterior chamber by slitlamp examination (after the patient has sat with head lowered between knees for 2 min), or by nodule aspiration or excision
- Skin snips placed in saline are incubated for 2–4 h before examination, or overnight for low-intensity infections
- Adult worms may be recovered in excised nodules
- The Mazzotti oral test is based on the ingestion of diethylcarbamazine (0.5–1.0 mg/kg); a skin reaction or pruritus within several hours is highly suggestive of the infection

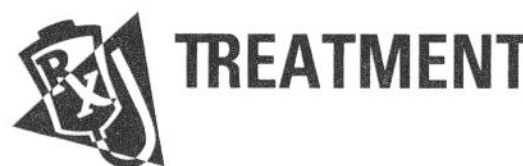

TREATMENT

MEDICATIONS

- Drug treatment is with ivermectin (a microfilaricide) as a single oral dose of 150 µg/kg given with water on an empty stomach; the patient should remain fasting for 2 more hours
  - The number of microfilariae in the skin diminishes markedly within 2–3 days, remains low for about 6 months, and then gradually increases
  - Microfilariae in the anterior chamber of the eye decrease slowly in number over months, eventually disappear, and then gradually return
  - The optimum frequency of treatment to control symptoms and prevent disease progression remains to be determined
- To initiate treatment, three schedules have been proposed
  - An initial and repeat dose at 6 months
  - Repeated doses at 3-month intervals for a year or
  - Repeated doses at monthly intervals for a total of three doses
- Thereafter, treatment is repeated at intervals of 6 months for 2 years and yearly thereafter until the adult worms die, which may take 12–15 years or longer
- With the initial treatment only, patients with microfilariae in the cornea or anterior chamber may benefit from several days of prednisone treatment (1 mg/kg/day) to avoid inflammatory eye reactions. Although single-dose ivermectin does not kill the adult worms, with repeated doses, increasing evidence suggests that the drug has a low-level macrofilaricidal action
- Adverse reactions, which are more marked with the first dose, are mild in 9% of patients and severe in 0.2%
  - These include edema (face and limbs), fever, pruritus, lymphadenitis, malaise, and hypotension
  - Ivermectin does not cause a severe reaction in the eyes or skin as occurs with diethylcarbamazine
- Ivermectin should not be used in the presence of concurrent *Loa loa* infections or pregnancy, or in patients with central nervous system diseases in which increased penetration may occur of ivermectin into the central nervous system (eg, meningitis)
- For selected patients in whom repeated ivermectin treatments do not control symptoms, suramin can be given for its macrofilaricidal action; however, because of suramin's toxicity and complex administration, it should be administered only by experts
- Doxycycline for 6 weeks has some macrofilaricidal action
- Diethylcarbamazine is no longer recommended for treatment

SURGERY

- In Latin America only, nodulectomy continues to be used for nodules on or near the head

OUTCOME

PROGNOSIS

- With treatment, some skin and ocular lesions improve and ocular progression is prevented
- The prognosis is unfavorable only for those patients who are seen for the first time with already far-advanced ocular onchocerciasis

WHEN TO REFER

- All patients should be referred to a clinician who has expertise in the diagnosis and treatment of this disease
- All patients with ocular involvement should be referred to an ophthalmologist

PREVENTION

- Mass treatment and control programs are underway since the advent of the safe drug ivermectin

EVIDENCE

WEB SITES

- CDC—Division of Parasitic Diseases
  - http://www.cdc.gov/ncidod/dpd/parasites/onchocerciasis/default.htm
- World Health Organization
  - http://www.who.int/tdr/diseases/oncho/default.htm

INFORMATION FOR PATIENTS

- National Institute of Allergy and Infectious Diseases
  - http://www2.niaid.nih.gov/newsroom/focuson/bugborne01/onchoc.htm

REFERENCES

- Gardon J et al: Effects of standard and high doses of ivermectin on adult worms of *Onchocerca volvulus*: a randomised controlled trial. Lancet 2002;360:203. [PMID: 12133654]
- Onchocerciasis (river blindness). Report from the eleventh InterAmerican conference on onchocerciasis, Mexico City, Mexico. Wkly Epidemiol Rec 2002;77:249. [PMID: 12221990]
- Pennisi E: Infectious disease. New culprit emerges in river blindness. Science 2002;295:1809. [PMID: 11884722]
- Unnasch TR: River blindness. Lancet 2002;360:182. [PMID: 12133647]

Onychomycosis

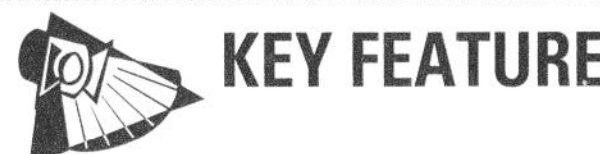

KEY FEATURES

ESSENTIALS OF DIAGNOSIS

- A trichophyton infection of one or more fingernails or toenails
- Yellowish discoloration with heaping of keritin
- Separation of the nail bed

GENERAL CONSIDERATIONS

- The species most commonly found is *Trichophyton rubrum*
- "Saprophytic" fungi may rarely (< 5%) cause onychomycosis
- Onycholysis (distal separation of the nail plate from the nail bed, usually of the fingers) is caused by excessive exposure to water, soaps, detergents, alkalies, and industrial cleaning agents
- Candidal infection of the nail folds and subungual area, nail hardeners, and drug-induced photosensitivity may cause onycholysis, as may hyperthyroidism and hypothyroidism and psoriasis

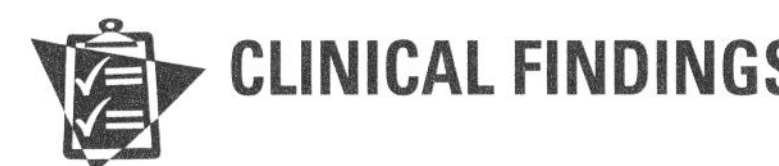

CLINICAL FINDINGS

SYMPTOMS AND SIGNS

- The nails are lusterless, brittle, and hypertrophic
- The substance of the nail is friable

DIFFERENTIAL DIAGNOSIS

- Psoriasis
- Candidal onychomycosis
- Lichen planus
- Allergy to nail polish or nail glue

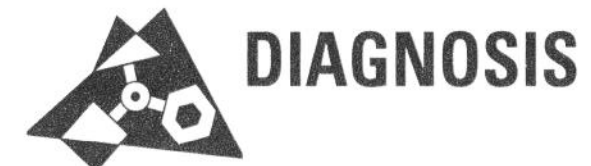

DIAGNOSIS

LABORATORY TESTS

- Laboratory diagnosis is mandatory since only 50% of dystrophic nails are due to dermatophytosis
- Portions of the nail should be cleared with 10% potassium hydroxide and examined under the microscope for hyphae
- Fungi may also be cultured

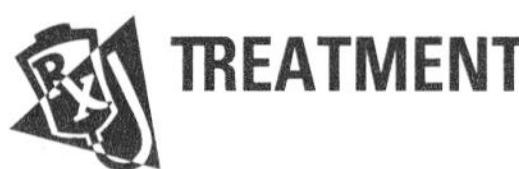

TREATMENT

MEDICATIONS

- Difficult to treat because of the long duration of therapy required and the frequency of recurrences
- Fingernails respond more readily than toenails
- For toenails, it is in some situations best to discourage therapy and to control discomfort by paring the thickened nail plate

Topical treatment

- Has relatively low efficacy (10% or less), but in well-motivated patients with minimally thickened nails it can be useful
- Naftifine gel 1% or ciclopirox nail lacquer (Penlac) 8% applied twice daily may clear fingernails in 4–6 months and toenails in 12–18 months

Systemic therapy

- Is generally required for the treatment of nail onychomycosis; fingernails can virtually always be cleared, whereas toenails respond in about 60% of cases
- Fingernails
  - Ultramicrosize griseofulvin, 250 mg PO TID for 6 months, is often effective
  - Treatment alternatives, in order of preference, are terbinafine, 250 mg QD for 6 weeks, itraconazole, 400 mg/day PO for 7 days each month for 2 months, and itraconazole, 200 mg/day PO for 2 months
- Toenails
  - Neither griseofulvin nor ketoconazole are recommended
  - Terbinafine pulse therapy (250 mg PO daily for 1 week every 2 to 3 months) for 12 months or 250 mg PO QD for 12 weeks
  - If terbinafine cannot be used, itraconazole 400 mg/day PO for 1 week per month for 3 months
  - For recurrent disease, terbinafine pulse therapy (250 mg daily for 7 days per month) every 2–3 months for 1 year, or give the standard 3-month daily treatment and repeat 6 months following first course (treat months 1 to 3 and 9 to 12)

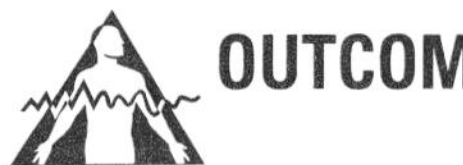

OUTCOME

FOLLOW-UP

- No matter which therapy is used, constant topical treatment for any coexisting tinea pedis is mandatory and should probably be continued for life to attempt to prevent recurrence

PROGNOSIS

- Once clear, fingernails often remain free of disease for years
- About 60% of patients will have substantial improvement with oral itraconazole, and 25–35% will be mycologically and clinically cured at 1 year

WHEN TO REFER

- If there is a question about the diagnosis, if recommended therapy is ineffective, or if specialized treatment is necessary

EVIDENCE

PRACTICE GUIDELINES

- Roberts DT et al; British Association of Dermatologists. Guidelines for treatment of onychomycosis. Br J Dermatol 2003;148:402. [PMID: 12653730]
- University of Texas at Austin: Recommendations for the management of onychomycosis in adults. 2003
  - http://www.guideline.gov/summary/summary.aspx?doc_id=4367&nbr=3289

WEB SITE

- American Academy of Dermatology
  - http://www.aad.org

INFORMATION FOR PATIENTS

- American Academy of Family Physicians: Fungal Infections of Fingernails and Toenails
  - http://familydoctor.org/663.xml
- American Osteopathic College of Dermatology: Fungus Infections: Preventing Recurrence
  - http://www.aocd.org/skin/dermatologic_diseases/fungus_preventing.html
- Mayo Clinic: Nail Fungal Infection
  - http://www.mayoclinic.com/invoke.cfm?id=DS00084
- MedlinePlus: Fungal Nail Infection
  - http://www.nlm.nih.gov/medlineplus/ency/article/001330.htm

REFERENCES

- Evans EG et al: Double blind, randomised study of continuous terbinafine compared with intermittent itraconazole in treatment of toenail onychomycosis. The LION Study Group. BMJ 1999;318:1031. [PMID: 10205099]
- Mayeaux EJ Jr: Nail disorders. Prim Care 2000;27:333. [PMID: 10815047]

Author(s)

Timothy G. Berger, MD

Opioid Dependency

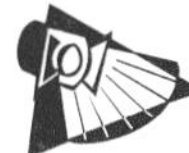

KEY FEATURES

ESSENTIALS OF DIAGNOSIS

- Dependency is a major concern when continued use of narcotics occurs
- Withdrawal causes only moderate morbidity (similar in severity to a bout of "flu")
- Addicted patients sometimes consider themselves more addicted than they really are and may not require a withdrawal program

GENERAL CONSIDERATIONS

- The terms "opioids" and "narcotics" are used interchangeably and include a group of drugs with actions that mimic those of morphine
  - Natural derivatives of opium (opiates)
  - Synthetic surrogates (opioids)
  - A number of polypeptides, some of which have been discovered to be natural neurotransmitters
- The principal narcotic of abuse is heroin (metabolized to morphine), which is not used as a legitimate medication
- Other common narcotics are prescription drugs, which differ in milligram potency, duration of action, and agonist and antagonist capabilities (Table 2)
- The incidence of snorting and inhaling heroin ("smoking") is increasing, particularly among cocaine users

DEMOGRAPHICS

- In the United States, lifetime prevalence for heroin abuse in people age 12 and over is approximately 1.4%

CLINICAL FINDINGS

SYMPTOMS AND SIGNS

- Mild narcotic intoxication
  - Changes in mood
  - Feelings of euphoria
  - Drowsiness
  - Nausea with occasional emesis
  - Needle tracks
  - Miosis
- Overdosage
  - Respiratory depression
  - Peripheral vasodilation
  - Pinpoint pupils
  - Pulmonary edema
  - Coma
  - Death
- Grades of withdrawal
  - Grade 0—craving and anxiety
  - Grade 1—yawning, lacrimation, rhinorrhea, and perspiration
  - Grade 2—previous symptoms plus mydriasis, piloerection, anorexia, tremors, and hot and cold flashes with generalized aching
  - Grades 3 and 4—increased intensity of previous symptoms and signs, with increased temperature, blood pressure, pulse, and respiratory rate and depth
  - In withdrawal from the most severe addiction, vomiting, diarrhea, weight loss, hemoconcentration, and spontaneous ejaculation or orgasm commonly occur

DIFFERENTIAL DIAGNOSIS

- Other drug dependence, eg, alcohol, amphetamines
- Underlying psychiatric disease, eg, depression, personality disorder
- Other drug withdrawal, eg, alcohol, benzodiazepines, amphetamines, cocaine
- Nausea or vomiting due to other cause
- Influenza or other viral syndrome

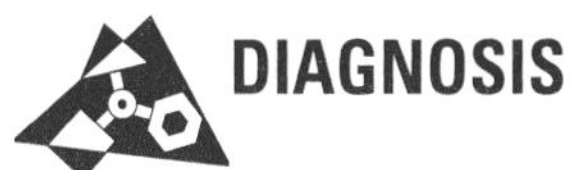

DIAGNOSIS

LABORATORY TESTS

- Serum or urine toxicology

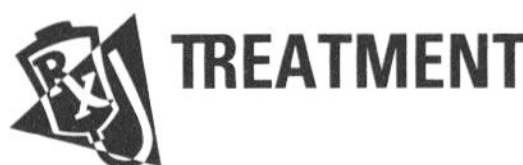

TREATMENT

MEDICATIONS

- Treatment for withdrawal begins if grade 2 signs develop
- Methadone
  - If a withdrawal program is necessary, use methadone, 10 mg PO (use parenteral administration if the patient is vomiting), and observe
  - If signs (piloerection, mydriasis, cardiovascular changes) persist for more than 4–6 hours, give another 10 mg
  - Continue to administer methadone at 4- to 6-hour intervals until signs are not present (rarely more than 40 mg of methadone in 24 hours)
  - Divide the total amount of drug required over the first 24-hour period by 2 and give that amount every 12 hours
  - Each day reduce the total 24-hour dose by 5–10 mg; thus, a moderately addicted patient initially requiring 30–40 mg of methadone could be withdrawn over a 4- to 8-day period
- Clonidine
  - 0.1 mg PO several times daily over a 10- to 14-day period
  - Is an alternative and an adjunct to methadone detoxification
  - It is not necessary to taper the dose
  - Helpful in alleviating cardiovascular symptoms
  - Does not significantly relieve anxiety, insomnia, or generalized aching
- Alternative strategies include rapid and ultrarapid detoxification techniques
  - In rapid detoxification, withdrawal is precipitated by opioid antagonists followed by naltrexone maintenance
- Narcotic antagonists (eg, naltrexone)
  - Can be used for treatment of the patient who has been free of opioids for 7–10 days
  - Blocks the narcotic "high" of heroin when 50 mg is given orally every 24 hours initially for several days and then 100 mg is given every 48–72 hours
  - Liver disorders are a major contraindication
  - Compliance tends to be poor, partly because of the dysphoria that can persist long after opioid discontinuance

THERAPEUTIC PROCEDURES

- Ultrarapid detoxification precipitates withdrawal with opioid antagonists under general anesthesia in a hospital and remains experimental

OUTCOME

FOLLOW-UP

- Methadone maintenance programs are of some value in chronic recidivism
- Under carefully controlled supervision, the narcotic addict is maintained on fairly high doses of methadone (40–120 mg/day) that satisfy craving and block the effects of heroin to a great degree

COMPLICATIONS

- Treatment for overdosage (or suspected overdosage) is naloxone, 2 mg intravenously
- Complications of heroin administration
  - Infections (eg, pneumonia, septic emboli, hepatitis)
  - HIV infection from using nonsterile needles), traumatic insults (eg, arterial spasm due to drug injection, gangrene)
  - Pulmonary edema

PROGNOSIS

- There is a protracted abstinence syndrome of metabolic, respiratory, and blood pressure changes over a period of 3–6 months
- The research on the impact of rapid detoxification on relapse rates, compared with more traditional methods, is limited at this time

WHEN TO REFER

- All opioid-dependent patients should be referred to an addiction specialist unless the primary caregiver has sufficient experience with this population

WHEN TO ADMIT

- For some patients residential treatment offers the best chance for recovery
- Some patients are able to enter recovery in a structured, supportive outpatient program

EVIDENCE

PRACTICE GUIDELINES

- American Academy of Family Physicians: Identification and Mangement of the Drug-Seeking Patient
  - http://www.aafp.org/afp/20000415/2401.html
- National Guideline Clearinghouse: VHA/DOD substance disorder guidelines, 2001
  - http://www.guideline.gov/summary/summary.aspx?doc_id=3169
- National Guideline Clearinghouse: Washington State Department of Labor and Industries: opioid prescription guidelines, 2002
  - http://www.guideline.gov/summary/summary.aspx?doc_id=4218

WEB SITE

- American Psychiatric Association
  - http://www.psych.org/
- National Institutes of Health—National Institute of Drug Abuse
  - http://www.drugabuse.gov

INFORMATION FOR PATIENTS

- JAMA patient page: Treating drug dependency. JAMA 2000;283:1378. [PMID:10714739]
- JAMA patient page: Opioid abuse. JAMA 2004;292:1394. [PMID:15367561]
- National Institute on Drug Abuse
  - http://www.nida.nih.gov/Infofax/heroin.html
  - http://www.nida.nih.gov/MOM/OP/MOMOP1.html

REFERENCES

- Fudala PJ et al: Office-based treatment of opiate addiction with sublingual-tablet formulation of buprenorphine and naloxone. N Engl J Med 2003;349:949. [PMID:12954743]
- Hamilton RJ et al: Complications of ultrarapid opioid detoxification with subcutaneous naltrexone pellets. Acad Emerg Med 2002;9:63. [PMID:11772672]

Author(s)

Stuart J. Eisendrath, MD

Jonathan E. Lichtmacher, MD

Osteoarthritis

Opioid Poisoning p. 1123. Osmolar Gap p. 1123.

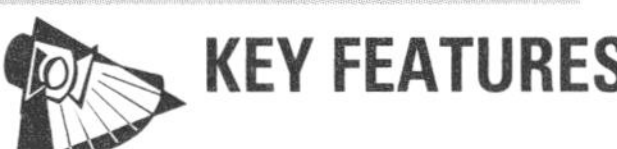

KEY FEATURES

ESSENTIALS OF DIAGNOSIS

- A degenerative disorder without systemic manifestations
- Pain relieved by rest; morning stiffness brief; articular inflammation minimal
- X-ray findings: narrowed joint space, osteophytes, increased density of subchondral bone, bony cysts

GENERAL CONSIDERATIONS

- Degeneration of cartilage and hypertrophy of bone at the articular margins
- Inflammation is usually minimal

Primary

- Most commonly affects some or all of the following—the distal interphalangeal joints and less commonly the proximal interphalangeal joints, the metacarpophalangeal and carpometacarpal joints of the thumb, the hip, the knee, the metatarsophalangeal joint of the big toe, and the cervical and lumbar spine

Secondary

- May occur in any joint as a sequela to articular injury resulting from either intraarticular or extraarticular causes
- Causes of articular injury that lead to secondary degenerative arthritis include trauma, gout, rheumatoid arthritis, hyperparathyroidism, hemochromatosis, Charcot joint

DEMOGRAPHICS

- The most common form of joint disease
- 90% of all people will have radiographic features of osteoarthritis in weight-bearing joints by age 40
- Obesity is a risk factor for knee osteoarthritis and probably for the hip

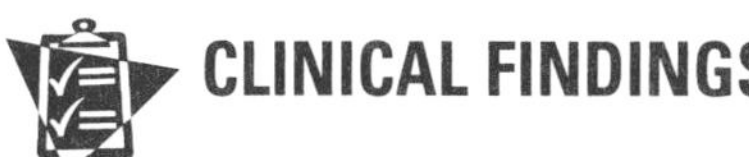

CLINICAL FINDINGS

SYMPTOMS AND SIGNS

- Insidious onset
- Pain is made worse by activity or weight bearing and relieved by rest
- Deformity may be absent or minimal; however, bony enlargement of the interphalangeal joints is occasionally prominent: DIP (Heberden's nodes) and PIP (Bouchard's nodes)
- Coarse crepitus may often be felt in the joint
- Joint effusion and other articular signs of inflammation are mild
- Because articular inflammation is minimal and systemic manifestations are absent, degenerative joint disease should seldom be confused with other arthritides
- The distribution of joint involvement in the hands also helps distinguish osteoarthritis from rheumatoid arthritis. Osteoarthritis primarily affects the distal and proximal interphalangeal joints and spares the wrist and metacarpophalangeal joints (except at the thumb); rheumatoid arthritis involves the wrists and metacarpophalangeal joints and spares the distal interphalangeal joints
- No systemic manifestations

DIFFERENTIAL DIAGNOSIS

- Rheumatoid arthritis
- Seronegative spondyloarthropathy, eg, psoriatic arthritis
- Gout
- Chondrocalcinosis, eg, pseudogout, Wilson's disease
- Other bone disease, eg, osteoporosis, metastatic cancer, multiple myeloma

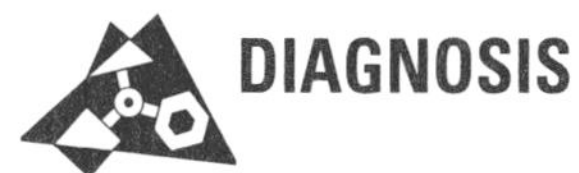

DIAGNOSIS

LABORATORY TESTS

- No laboratory evidence of inflammation such as elevated erythrocyte sedimentation rate

IMAGING STUDIES

- Radiographs may reveal narrowing of the joint space, sharpened articular margins, osteophyte formation and lipping of marginal bone, and thickened, dense subchondral bone, or bone cysts
- The correlation between radiographic findings and symptoms is poor

DIAGNOSTIC PROCEDURES

- Aspiration of effusions for pain relief
- Corticosteroid injections for pain relief

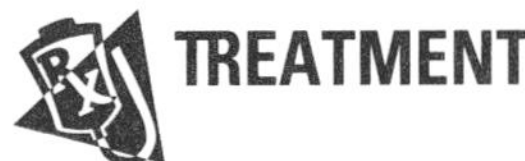

TREATMENT

MEDICATIONS

- Patients with mild disease should start with acetaminophen (2.4–4 g/day)
- Nonsteroidal antiinflammatory drugs (NSAIDs) should be considered for patients who fail to respond to acetaminophen, chondroitin sulfate, and glucosamine
- High doses of NSAIDs, as used in more inflammatory arthritides, are unnecessary

SURGERY

- Total hip and knee replacement provides excellent symptomatic and functional improvement when that joint is seriously afflicted, as indicated by severely restricted walking and pain at rest, particularly at night
- Although arthroscopic surgery for knee osteoarthritis is commonly performed, its long-term efficacy is unestablished

THERAPEUTIC PROCEDURES

- For patients with mild to moderate osteoarthritis of weight-bearing joints, a supervised walking program may result in clinical improvement of functional status without aggravating the joint pain. Weight loss can also improve the symptoms
- For patients with knee osteoarthritis and effusion, intraarticular injection of triamcinolone (20–40 mg) may obviate the need for analgesics or NSAIDs but should not be repeated more than two or three times in a year

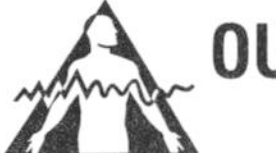

OUTCOME

WHEN TO REFER

- When other inflammatory arthritides cannot be confidently excluded
- For joint replacement

PROGNOSIS

- Symptoms may be quite severe and limit activity considerably (especially with involvement of the hips, knees, and cervical spine)

PREVENTION

- Weight reduction in women reduces the risk of developing symptomatic knee osteoarthritis

EVIDENCE

PRACTICE GUIDELINES

- National Guideline Clearinghouse
  - http://www.guideline.gov/summary/summary.aspx?doc_id=4610
  - http://www.guideline.gov/summary/summary.aspx?doc_id=3188

WEB SITE

- Arthritis Foundation
  - http://www.arthritis.org

INFORMATION FOR PATIENTS

- Arthritis Foundation
  - http://www.arthritis.org/conditions/DiseaseCenter/oa.asp
- National Institute of Arthritis and Musculoskeletal and Skin Diseases
  - http://www.niams.nih.gov/hi/topics/arthritis/oahandout.htm

REFERENCES

- Bjordal JM et al: Non-steroidal anti-inflammatory drugs, including cyclo-oxygenase-2 inhibitors in osteoarthritis knee pain: meta-analysis of randomised placebo controlled trials. BMJ 2004;329:1317. [PMID: 15561731]
- Fransen M: Dietary weight loss and exercise for obese adults with knee osteoarthritis: modest weight loss targets, mild exercise, modest effects. Arthritis Rheum 2004;50:1366. [PMID: 15146405]
- Lo GH et al: Intra-articular hyaluronic acid in treatment of knee osteoarthritis: a meta-analysis. JAMA 2003;290:3115. [PMID: 14679274]
- Moseley JB: A controlled trial of arthroscopic surgery for osteoarthritis of the knee. N Engl J Med 2002;347:81. [PMID: 12110735]
- Wegman A et al: Nonsteroidal antiinflammatory drugs or acetaminophen for osteoarthritis of the hip or knee? A systematic review of evidence and guidelines. J Rheumatol 2004;31:344. [PMID: 14760807]

Author(s)

David B. Hellmann, MD, FACP
John H. Stone, MD, MPH

Osteomalacia

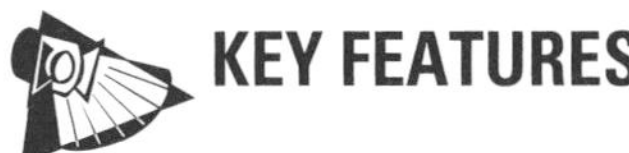

KEY FEATURES

ESSENTIALS OF DIAGNOSIS

- Painful proximal muscle weakness (especially pelvic girdle); bone pain and tenderness
- Decreased bone density from diminished mineralization of osteoid
- Laboratory abnormalities may include increased alkaline phosphatase, decreased 25-hydroxyvitamin D [25(OH)D_3], hypocalcemia, hypocalciuria, hypophosphatemia, secondary hyperparathyroidism
- Classic radiologic features may be present

GENERAL CONSIDERATIONS

- Defective mineralization of growing skeleton in children producing permanent bone deformities is known as rickets
- Defective skeletal mineralization in adults is known as osteomalacia
- Osteomalacia is caused by any condition that results in inadequate calcium or phosphate mineralization of bone
- Most common cause is deficiency of vitamin D, whose main function is to increase intestinal absorption of calcium
- Ergocalciferol (vitamin D_2) is derived from plants and used in most pharmaceutical vitamin D preparations
- Cholecalciferol (vitamin D_3) is synthesized in skin under the influence of ultraviolet radiation
- Two sequential hydroxylations are necessary for full biological activity: first occurs in liver—to 25(OH)D_3; second in kidney—to 1,25$(OH)_2D_3$
- Some degree of vitamin D deficiency was found in 24% of postmenopausal women
  - The incidence varies among regions: < 1% in Southeast Asia, 29.3% in the United States, and 36% in Italy. Incidence of severe vitamin D deficiency (serum 25[OH]D < 25 nmol/L or < 10 ng/mL) is 3.5% in the US and 12.5% in Italy
  - Vitamin D deficiency is found in 60% of the institutionalized elderly not receiving vitamin D supplementation. In one study of individuals age 98 years or older, 95% had undetectable levels of vitamin D
  - May arise from insufficient sun exposure, malnutrition, malabsorption, severe nephrotic syndrome
- Cholestyramine, orlistat, and anticonvulsants decrease vitamin D levels
- Dietary calcium deficiency, eg, in malnourished, elderly patients can also cause rickets and osteomalacia
  - Milk, especially skim milk, is a poor source of vitamin D
  - Breast-fed infants can develop rickets if they receive no sun exposure or vitamin D supplement
- Phosphate deficiency, eg, due to nutritional deficiency, malabsorption, phosphate-binding antacids, genetic disorders (vitamin D–resistant rickets), renal tubular acidosis, Fanconi's syndrome, can cause osteomalacia
- Aluminum toxicity due to chronic hemodialysis with tap water dialysate or from aluminum-containing phosphate binders can cause osteomalacia
- Vitamin D-dependent rickets type I
  - Caused by a rare autosomal recessive defect in renal synthesis of 1,25(OH)2D
  - Presents in childhood with rickets; adults develop osteomalacia
- Vitamin D-dependent rickets type II (hereditary 1,25[OH]2D-resistant rickets)
  - Caused by a genetic defect in the 1,25(OH)2D receptor
  - Presents in childhood with rickets and alopecia
- Oncogenic osteomalacia is caused by excessive production of phosphatonin by a wide variety of soft tissue tumors (87% benign). Manifestations
  - Hypophosphatemia
  - Excessive phosphaturia
  - Reduced serum 1,25$(OH)_2D_3$ concentrations
  - Osteomalacia
- X-linked hypophosphatemic rickets is caused by high levels of phosphatonin due to familial or sporadic mutations in PHEX endopeptidase, which fails to cleave phosphatonin
- Other causes
  - Disorders of bone matrix, eg, hypophosphatasia (deficient alkaline phosphatase)
  - Fibrogenesis imperfecta

CLINICAL FINDINGS

SYMPTOMS AND SIGNS

- Initially asymptomatic in adults
- Eventually, bone pain, simulating fibromyalgia
- Muscle weakness due to calcium deficiency
- Fractures with little or no trauma
- Infants and children may exhibit restlessness, interrupted sleep, bowing of legs, kyphoscoliosis, hypertrophy of epiphygeal cartilage (eg, costochondral beading)

DIFFERENTIAL DIAGNOSIS

- Osteoporosis
- Hypophosphatemia due to hyperparathyroidism
- Renal osteodystrophy
- Multiple myeloma, metastatic cancer
- Chronic hyperthyroidism
- Hypophosphatasia
  - Hypophosphatasia is a rare genetic cause of osteomalacia that is commonly misdiagnosed as osteoporosis
  - Incidence in the United States is about 1:100,000 live births; about 1:300 adults is a carrier
  - Transmission can be autosomal recessive or dominant. Phenotypic presentation of hypophosphatasia is variable
  - At its worst, it can present as a stillborn without dentition or calcified bones
  - At its mildest, it can present in middle age with premature loss of teeth, foot pain (due to metatarsal stress fractures), thigh pain (due to femoral pseudofractures), or arthritis (due to chondrocalcinosis)

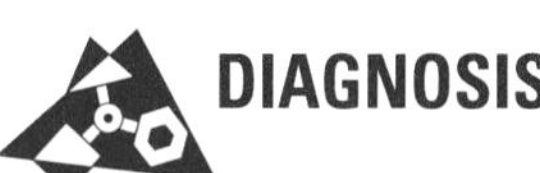

DIAGNOSIS

LABORATORY TESTS

- Alkaline phosphatase (age-adjusted) may be elevated
- 25(OH)D_3 typically low < 20 ng/mL (< 50 nmol/L)
- Calcium or phosphate (age-adjusted) may be low
- Phosphate low in 47%
- Parathyroid hormone may be increased due to secondary hyperparathyroidism
- Urinary calcium may be low
- 1,25$(OH)_2D_3$ may be low even when 25(OH)D_2 levels are normal
- Screen for hypophosphatasia
  - Serum alkaline phosphatase (collected in a non-EDTA tube) is low-for-age in patients with hypophosphatasia
  - Confirm diagnosis with a 24-hour urine assayed for phosphoethanolamine, a substrate for alkaline phosphatase, whose excretion is always elevated in patients with hypophosphatasia

IMAGING STUDIES

- Bone densitometry helps document the degree of osteopenia

- X-rays may show diagnostic features: cortical bone thinning, looser lines, stress or pathologic fractures
- Whole-body MRI may be required to search for occult tumors in sporadic adult-onset hypophosphatemia, hyperphosphaturia, and low serum $1,25(OH)_2D$ levels

DIAGNOSTIC PROCEDURES

- Bone biopsy not usually necessary but is diagnostic of osteomalacia if it shows significant unmineralized osteoid
- Prenatal genetic testing, by way of chorionic villus biopsy, is available for the infantile form of hypophosphatasia

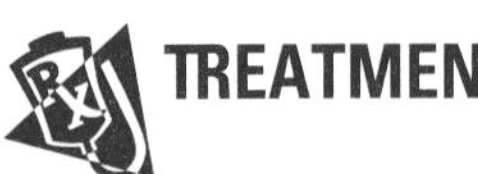

TREATMENT

MEDICATIONS

- Vitamin D deficiency
  - Treated with ergocalciferol (D_2), 50,000 IU PO once weekly for 6–12 months, followed by at least 1000 IU PO QD
  - May also be given 50,000 IU PO Q 2 months
- In intestinal malabsorption
  - 25,000–100,000 IU of vitamin D_2 may be required daily
  - Some patients with steatorrhea respond better to 25(OH)D (calcifediol), 50–100 µg PO QD or calcitriol 0.25–0.5 µg daily
- Oral calcium supplements with meals: calcium citrate (eg, Citracal) to provide 0.4–0.6 g elemental calcium per day; or calcium carbonate (eg, OsCal, Tums), 1–1.5 g elemental calcium per day
- Correct nutritional deficiencies in hypophosphatemic osteomalacia
  - Discontinue aluminum-containing antacids
  - Give bicarbonate therapy to patients with renal tubular acidosis
- Oral phosphate supplements given chronically for X-linked or idiopathic hypophosphatemia and hyperphosphaturia, along with calcitriol, 0.25–0.5 µg PO QD, to improve impaired calcium absorption caused by oral phosphate
  - Consider addition of human recombinant growth hormone to reduce phosphaturia
- Patients with vitamin D-dependent rickets type I are treated with oral calcitriol in doses of 0.5–1 µg daily
- Patients with hereditary 1,25[OH]2D-resistant rickets respond variably to oral calcitriol in very large doses (2–6 µg daily)
- Hypophosphatasia
  - No proven therapy except for supportive care
  - Teriparatide, a useful therapy for osteoporosis, has been administered to some patients with hypophosphatasia, but its long-term efficacy is unknown

THERAPEUTIC PROCEDURES

- Sun exposure, without SPF, stimulates vitamin D_3 production in skin, except in dark-skinned Africans

OUTCOME

COMPLICATIONS

- Fractures

PREVENTION

- Prevention of vitamin D deficiency by adequate sunlight exposure and vitamin D supplements
- US recommended daily allowance (RDA) of vitamin D is at least 10 µg (400 IU) daily
  - In sunlight-deprived individuals (eg, veiled women, confined patients, or residents of higher latitudes during winter), RDA should be 25 µg (1000 IU) daily
- Patients on chronic phenytoin may be treated prophylactically with vitamin D, 50,000 IU PO Q 2–4 weeks

EVIDENCE

PRACTICE GUIDELINES

- Hanley DA, Davison KS: Vitamin D insufficiency in North America. J Nutr 2005;135:332. [PMID:15671237]
- Mawer EB et al: Vitamin D nutrition and bone disease in adults. Rev Endocr Metab Disord 2001;2:153. [PMID:11705321]
  - http://content.kluweronline.com/article/320630/fulltext.pdf
- National Kidney Foundation
  - http://www.kidney.org/professionals/kdoqi/guidelines_bone/Guide13B.htm

INFORMATION FOR PATIENTS

- The Magic Foundation
  - http://www.magicfoundation.org/brochure/hypophosphatasia.htm
- MEDLINEplus—Osteomalacia
  - http://www.nlm.nih.gov/medlineplus/ency/article/000376.htm
- MEDLINEplus—Rickets
  - http://www.nlm.nih.gov/medlineplus/ency/article/000344.htm
- Tayside University Hospitals—Osteomalacia and rickets
  - http://www.dundee.ac.uk/medicine/tayendoweb/images/osteomalacia_and_rickets.htm

REFERENCES

- De Beur SM et al: Tumors associated with oncogenic osteomalacia express genes important in bone and mineral metabolism. Bone Miner Res 2002;17:1102. [PMID:12054166]
- Lyman D: Undiagnosed vitamin D deficiency in the hospitalized patient. Am Fam Physician 2005;71:299. [PMID:15686300]
- Passeri G et al: Low vitamin D status, high bone turnover, and bone fractures in centarians. J Clin Endocrinol Metab 2003;88:5109. [PMID:14602735]
- Plotnikoff GA et al: Prevalence of severe hypovitaminosis D in patients with persistent, nonspecific musculoskeletal pain. Mayo Clin Proc 2003;78:1463. [PMID:14661675]

Author(s)

Paul A. Fitzgerald, MD

Osteomyelitis, Acute Pyogenic

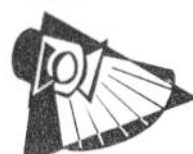

KEY FEATURES

ESSENTIALS OF DIAGNOSIS

- Fever and chills associated with pain and tenderness of involved bone
- Culture of blood or bone is essential for precise diagnosis
- Radiographs early in the course are typically negative

GENERAL CONSIDERATION

- Occurs as a consequence of hematogenous dissemination of bacteria, invasion from a contiguous focus of infection, or skin breakdown in the setting of vascular insufficiency
- In sickle cell anemia, *Salmonella* is the most common pathogen
- In intravenous drug users, *Staphylococcus aureus* is most common, also gram-negative infections (eg, *Pseudomonas aeruginosa* and *Serratia*)
- Contiguous focus infections are usually due to *S aureus* and *S epidermidis*

CLINICAL FINDINGS

SYMPTOMS AND SIGNS

Hematogenous osteomyelitis

- Associated with sickle cell disease, intravenous drug users, or the elderly
- High fever, chills, and pain and tenderness of the involved bone

Osteomyelitis from a contiguous focus of infection

- Prosthetic joint replacement, decubitus ulcer, neurosurgery, and trauma are common sources of infection
- Localized signs of inflammation are usually evident, but high fever and other signs of toxicity are usually absent

Osteomyelitis associated with vascular insufficiency

- Infection originates from an ulcer or other break in the skin may appear disarmingly unimpressive
- Bone pain is often absent or muted by the associated neuropathy
- Fever is also commonly absent

DIFFERENTIAL DIAGNOSIS

- Acute hematogenous osteomyelitis should be distinguished from suppurative arthritis, rheumatic fever, and cellulitis
- More subacute forms must be differentiated from tuberculosis or mycotic infections of bone or tumors
- When osteomyelitis involves the vertebrae, it commonly traverses the disk—a finding not observed in tumor
- Cellulitis
- Septic arthritis
- Gout
- Diabetic or arterial insufficiency ulcer
- Tuberculous or mycotic bone infection
- Rheumatic fever
- Metastatic cancer
- Multiple myeloma
- Ewing's sarcoma
- Avascular necrosis

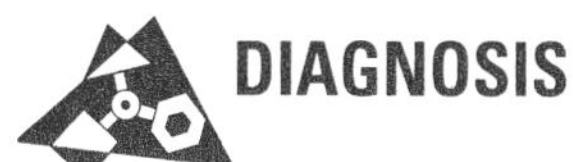

DIAGNOSIS

LABORATORY TESTS

- Blood cultures
- Cultures from overlying ulcers, wounds, or fistulas are unreliable
- Anemia of chronic disease and a markedly elevated erythrocyte sedimentation rate (ESR) are characteristic

IMAGING STUDIES

- Early radiographic findings may include soft tissue swelling, loss of tissue planes, and periarticular demineralization of bone
- About 2 weeks after onset of symptoms, erosion and alterations of bone appear, followed by periostitis
- MRI, CT, and nuclear medicine bone scanning are more sensitive than conventional radiography

DIAGNOSTIC PROCEDURES

- One of the best bedside clues to osteomyelitis is the ability to easily advance a sterile probe through a skin ulcer to bone
- Bone biopsy for culture is essential except in those with hematogenous osteomyelitis with positive blood cultures

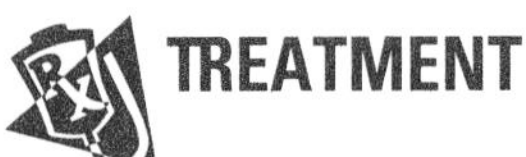

TREATMENT

MEDICATIONS

- Most patients require both debridement of necrotic bone and prolonged administration of antibiotics
- Traditionally, antibiotics have been administered parenterally for at least 4–6 weeks
- Oral therapy with quinolones (eg, ciprofloxacin, 750 mg twice daily) for 6–8 weeks is as effective as standard parenteral antibiotic therapy for chronic osteomyelitis with susceptible organisms
- When treating *S aureus*, quinolones are usually combined with rifampin, 300 mg twice daily

SURGERY

- Debridement of necrotic bone is usually necessary
- Revascularization of the extremity is required when osteomyelitis of a foot is accompanied by decreased perfusion due to large artery disease

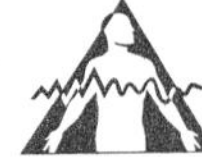

OUTCOME

FOLLOW-UP

- ESR should fall by 50% after 1 month of antibiotic therapy

COMPLICATIONS

- Inadequate treatment of bone infections results in chronic infection
- Squamous cell transformation within the chronic fistula tract

PROGNOSIS

- A good result can be expected in most cases if there is no compromise of the patient's immune system
- Progression of the disease to a chronic form may occur, especially in the lower extremities and in patients in whom circulation is impaired (eg, diabetics)

WHEN TO REFER

- Urgent consultation with a neurosurgeon or orthopedist is required for vertebral osteomyelitis associated with neurological findings

WHEN TO ADMIT

- Admit to establish the diagnosis and begin intravenous antibiotic therapy

EVIDENCE

INFORMATION FOR PATIENTS

- Mayo Clinic
  - http://www.mayoclinic.com/invoke.cfm?objectid=FD59F887-9E24-4A0D-883E01D48DC117C8
- National Institutes of Health
  - http://www.nlm.nih.gov/medlineplus/ency/article/000437.htm

REFERENCE

- Lew D et al: Osteomyelitis. Lancet 2004:24;364:369. [PMID: 15276398]

Author(s)

David B. Hellmann, MD, FACP
John H. Stone, MD, MPH

Osteoporosis

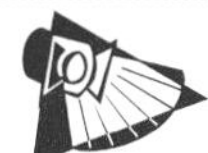

KEY FEATURES

ESSENTIALS OF DIAGNOSIS

- Symptoms range from none to severe back pain from vertebral fractures
- Spontaneous fractures are often discovered incidentally on radiography; loss of height
- Low bone density usually indicates osteoporosis, but may also indicate osteomalacia
- Osteoporosis: bone densitometry T score (standard deviations below young normal mean) ≤ –2.5
- Osteopenia (at risk for osteoporosis): bone densitometry T score –1.5 to –2.4
- Serum parathyroid hormone (PTH), 25-hydroxyvitamin D [25(OH)D_3], calcium, phosphorus, and alkaline phosphatase usually normal

GENERAL CONSIDERATIONS

- Estimated to cause 1.5 million fractures annually in the United States, mainly of the vertebrae
- Morbidity and indirect mortality rates very high
- Rate of bone formation often normal, but bone resorption rate is increased
- Reduction in bone matrix (osteoid); remaining osteoid is mineralized, unless osteomalacia is also present
- Osteogenesis imperfecta, due to major mutation in type I collagen, results in severe osteoporosis. Spontaneous fractures occur in utero or during childhood
- Causes of osteoporosis include
  - Estrogen (women) or androgen (men) deficiency
  - Cushing's syndrome (eg, glucocorticoid administration)
  - Hyperthyroidism
  - Hyperparathyroidism
  - Drugs (eg, alcohol, tobacco, excessive vitamin D or A, heparin)
  - Immobilization
  - Genetic disorders (eg, aromatase deficiency, type I collagen mutations)
  - Malignancy, especially multiple myeloma
  - Liver disease
- Celiac disease (3.4%)

DEMOGRAPHICS

- Clinically evident in middle life and beyond
- Women more frequently affected than men

CLINICAL FINDINGS

SYMPTOMS AND SIGNS

- Usually asymptomatic until fractures occur
- May present as back pain of varying degrees of severity or as spontaneous fracture or collapse of a vertebra
- Loss of height common
- Fractures of femoral neck and distal radius also common
- Once osteoporosis is identified, careful history and physical examination are required to determine its cause

DIFFERENTIAL DIAGNOSIS

- Osteomalacia or rickets
- Inadequate mineralization of existing bone matrix (osteoid)
- Osteomalacia results from inadequate calcium (usually due to vitamin D deficiency) or inadequate phosphate
- Multiple myeloma
- Metastatic cancer
- Paget's disease of bone
- Renal osteodystrophy

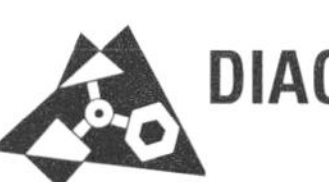

DIAGNOSIS

LABORATORY TESTS

- Serum calcium, phosphate, and PTH: normal
- Alkaline phosphatase: usually normal but may be slightly elevated, especially following fracture
- Once osteoporosis is identified, obtain serum thyroid-stimulating hormone, luteinizing hormone/follicle-stimulating hormone, testosterone (men), and 25(OH)D_3 level; when appropriate, screen for hypogonadism in men and women
- Screen for celiac disease with serum IgA anti-tissue transglutanimase and IgA anti-endomysial antibodies

IMAGING STUDIES

- X-rays of spine and pelvis, especially femoral neck and head, the principal areas of demineralization; in skull and extremities, demineralization is less marked
  - X-rays of spine commonly also show compression of vertebrae
- Bone densitometry permits screening for osteopenia in high-risk individuals and allows assessment of response to therapy
- Bone densitometry screening recommended for
  - All white and Asian women ≥55 years
  - All patients taking chronic prednisone
  - All patients with neurologic disorder (eg, paraplegia); prior pathologic fractures; family history of osteoporosis; alcoholism, anorexia, or malnutrition
- Osteoporosis: bone densitometry T score ≤ –2.5; osteopenia: T score ≤ –1.5 to –2.4
- Dual-energy x-ray absorptiometry (DEXA) can determine density of any bone, is quite accurate, and delivers negligible radiation
- CT bone densitometry: highly accurate and reproducible
  - More costly than DEXA
  - Reserved for assessing spinal bone density in patients with severe osteoporosis

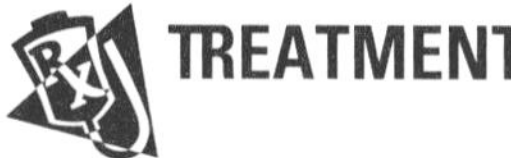

TREATMENT

MEDICATIONS

- Supplemental calcium and vitamin D is given to prevent or treat any concurrent osteomalacia
  - Give calcium citrate (0.4–0.7 g elemental calcium PO QD) or calcium carbonate (1–1.5 g elemental calcium PO QD). Calcium citrate causes less gastrointestinal intolerance
  - Give vitamin D_2 400–1000 IU PO QD
- Bisphosphonates for osteoporosis in patients taking high-dose glucocorticoids
  - Taken in morning with ≥ 8 oz water, 30–60 minutes before any other food or liquid
  - Must remain upright for 30 minutes after taking to reduce risk of pill-induced esophagitis
  - All patients on bisphosphonates should receive oral calcium with evening meal and vitamin D
- Pamidronate or zoledronic acid IV, or nasal calcitonin-salmon (Miacalcin) if unable to tolerate bisphosphonates
- Alendronate, 10 mg PO QAM or 70 mg PO Q week; 5 mg PO QAM or 35 mg PO Q week for prevention of osteoporosis
- Risedronate, 5 mg PO QAM; or 35 mg PO Q week for treatment or prevention of osteoporosis
- Consider estrogen or raloxifene (selective estrogen receptor modulator or SERM) for women with hypogonadism (see Menopausal Syndrome); osteoporosis can be prevented by low-dose estrogen
- Consider teriparatide (Forteo, PTH analog) 20 μg SC QD for ≤2 years for severe osteoporosis
- Strontium ranelate may be administered in daily oral doses of 2 g (680 mg elemental strontium)

- In one study, strontium was administered to women with osteoporosis and vertebral fractures and reduced fractures by >40% and increased bone density in the lumbar spine and femoral neck compared with placebo
- Side effects were reported to be negligible

THERAPEUTIC PROCEDURES

- Diet adequate in protein, total calories, calcium, and vitamin D
- Discontinue or reduce doses of glucocorticoids, if possible
- High-impact physical activity (eg, jogging), stair-climbing, and weight training increase bone density
- Fall-avoidance measures
- Balance exercises can reduce fall risk
- Avoid alcohol and smoking
- Verterobroplasty, kyphoplasty are investigational procedures for pain relief following vertebral compression fractures

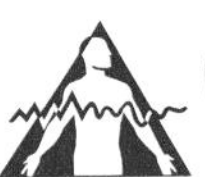

OUTCOME

FOLLOW-UP

- DEXA bone densitometry every 2–3 years
- Monitor patients on glucocorticoids or thiazides for development of hypercalcemia when given calcium supplements
- Reduce bisphosphonate dosage in renal insufficiency, and monitor serum phosphate

COMPLICATIONS

- Fractures common, especially femur, vertebrae, and distal radius
- Calcium supplementation for patients receiving thiazide diuretics and glucocorticoids can cause hypercalcemia; calcium taken by patients in renal failure can cause calciphylaxis
- Nasal calcitonin-salmon can cause bronchospasm and allergic reactions, rhinitis, epistaxis, back pain, and arthralgias
- Raloxifene
  - Increases the risk for thromboembolism
  - Aggravates hot flashes
  - Has been associated with nausea, weight gain, depression, insomnia, leg cramps, and rash
- Estrogen replacement
  - Increases the risk for thromboembolism and myocardial infarction, breast cancer, and endometrial cancer
  - Has been associated with cholestatic jaundice, worsening hypertriglyceridemia, and pancreatitis
  - Enlargement of uterine fibroids, migraines, edema, weight changes, rash, and gastrointestinal intolerance have been reported
- Bisphosphonates (oral) can cause esophagitis, gastritis, and abdominal pain
- Oral and IV bisphosphonates can cause bone, joint, or muscle pain as well as fatigue
  - Pains can be migratory or diffuse and can vary in severity from mild to incapacitating
  - Onset of pain may occur from 1 day to 1 year after therapy is initiated, with a mean of 14 days
  - The pain can be transient, lasting several days and resolving spontaneously but typically recurs with subsequent doses
  - When the bisphosphonate is discontinued, most patients experience gradual pain relief
- Teriparitide
  - May cause orthostatic hypotension, asthenia, nausea, and leg cramps
  - Must not be given to patients with Paget's disease or a history of osteosarcoma or chondrosarcoma

PROGNOSIS

- Bisphosphonates, calcitonin, and teriparitide can reverse osteoporosis and decrease fracture risk
- Prognosis good for preventing postmenopausal osteoporosis if estrogen therapy, raloxifene, or bisphosphonates started early and maintained for years
- Bone pain reduction may be noted within 2–4 weeks on nasal calcitonin
- Diet adequate in protein, calories, calcium, and vitamin D
- Calcium and vitamin D supplements and exercise for those at risk
- Consider hormone replacement therapy for hypogonadal men and women
- Consider bisphosphonate if patient on corticosteroids >2 weeks and for prevention of osteoporosis
- Raloxifene, 60 mg PO QD, can be used by postmenopausal women in place of estrogen for osteoporosis prevention
- Give calcium supplements with meals to reduce risk of calcium oxalate nephrolithiasis

EVIDENCE

PRACTICE GUIDELINES

- AACE Practice Guidelines for osteoporosis:
  - http://www.aace.com/clin/guidelines/osteoporosis2001Revised.pdf
- NIH Current Bibliographies in Medicine:
  - http://www.nlm.nih.gov/pubs/cbm/osteoporosis.pdf

WEB SITE

- National Osteoporosis Foundation
  - www.nof.org

INFORMATION FOR PATIENTS

- JAMA patient page: Osteoporosis. JAMA 1999;282:1396. [PMID:10527188]
- NIH Osteoporosis Resource Center
  - http://www.osteo.org/osteolinks.asp

REFERENCES

- Black DM et al: The effects of parathyroid hormone and alendronate alone or in combination in postmenopausal osteoporosis. N Engl J Med 2003;349:1207. [PMID:14500804]
- Bone HG et al: Ten years experience with alendronate for osteoporosis in postmenopausal women. N Engl J Med 2004;18:1189. [PMID:15028823]
- Finkelstein JS et al: The effects of parathyroid hormone, alendronate, or both in men with osteoporosis. N Engl J Med 2003;349:1216. [PMID:14500805]
- Johnell O et al: Raloxifene reduces risk of vertebral fractures and breast cancer in postmenopausal women regardless of prior hormone therapy. J Fam Pract 2004;53:789. [PMID:15469774]
- McClung MR et al: Prevention of postmenopausal bone loss: six-year results from the Early Postmenopausal Intervention Cohort Study. J Clin Endocrinol Metab 2004;89:4879. [PMID:15472179]
- Meunier PJ et al: The effects of strontium ranelate on the risk of vertebral fracture in women with postmenopausal osteoporosis. N Engl J Med 2004;350:504. [PMID:14749454]
- Saag KG: Glucocorticoid-induced osteoporosis. Endocrinol Metab Clin North Am 2003;32:135. [PMID:12699296]
- Shea B et al: Calcium supplementation on bone loss in postmenopausal women. Cochrane Database Syst Rev 2004(1):CD004526
- Stenson WF et al: Increased prevalence of celiac disease and need for routine screening among patients with osteoporosis. Arch Intern Med 2005;165:393

Author(s)

Paul A. Fitzgerald, MD

Otitis, External

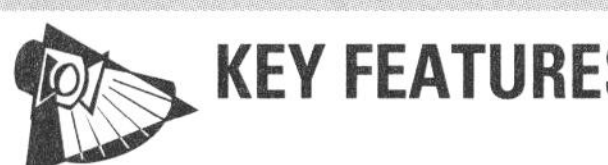

KEY FEATURES

ESSENTIALS OF DIAGNOSIS

- Erythema and edema of the ear canal skin
- Often with a purulent exudate
- Persistent external otitis in the diabetic or immunocompromised patient may evolve into osteomyelitis of the skull base, often called malignant external otitis

GENERAL CONSIDERATIONS

External otitis

- There is often a history of recent water exposure ("swimmer's ear") or mechanical trauma (eg, scratching, cotton applicators)
- Otitis externa is usually caused by gram-negative rods (eg, *Pseudomonas, Proteus*) or fungi (eg, *Aspergillus*), which grow in the presence of excessive moisture

Malignant external otitis

- Usually caused by *Pseudomonas aeruginosa*
- Osteomyelitis begins in the floor of the ear canal and may extend into the middle fossa floor, the clivus, and even the contralateral skull base

CLINICAL FINDINGS

SYMPTOMS AND SIGNS

External otitis

- Presents with otalgia, frequently accompanied by pruritus and purulent discharge
- Examination reveals erythema and edema of the ear canal skin, often with a purulent exudate
- Manipulation of the auricle often elicits pain
- Because the lateral surface of the tympanic membrane is ear canal skin, it is often erythematous
- In contrast to acute otitis media, the tympanic membrane in otitis externa moves normally with pneumatic otoscopy
- When the canal skin is very edematous, it may be impossible to visualize the tympanic membrane

Malignant external otitis

- Presents with persistent, refractory otalgia
- Granulation tissue in ear canal
- Cranial neuropathies (especially VII, IX, X)

DIFFERENTIAL DIAGNOSIS

- Otitis media
- Skin cancer
- Traumatic auricular hematoma
- Cellulitis
- Chondritis or perichondritis
- Relapsing polychondritis
- Chondrodermatitis nodularis helicis

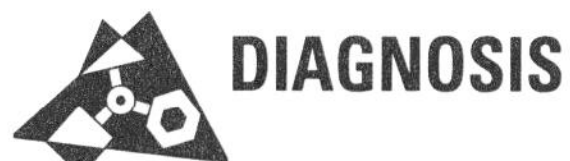

DIAGNOSIS

LABORATORY TESTS

- Persistent discharge unresponsive to treatment should be cultured

IMAGING STUDIES

- Diagnosis of malignant otitis externa is confirmed by demonstration of osseous erosion on CT and radioisotope scanning

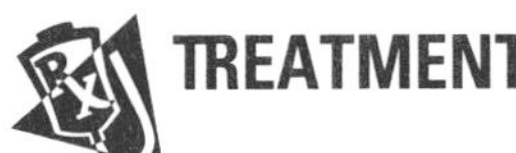

TREATMENT

MEDICATIONS

External otitis

- Otic drops containing a mixture of aminoglycoside antibiotic and antiinflammatory corticosteroid in an acid vehicle are generally very effective (eg, neomycin sulfate, polymyxin B sulfate, and hydrocortisone)
- Drops should be used abundantly (five or more drops three or four times a day) to penetrate the depths of the canal
- In recalcitrant cases, particularly when cellulitis of the periauricular tissue has developed, oral fluoroquinolones (eg, ciprofloxacin, 500 mg twice daily for 1 week) are the drugs of choice because of their effectiveness against *Pseudomonas* species

Malignant external otitis

- Prolonged antipseudomonal antibiotic administration, often for several months

SURGERY

- Surgical débridement of infected bone is reserved for cases of malignant external otitis that have worsened despite medical therapy or when material is needed for culture

THERAPEUTIC PROCEDURES

- Fundamental to the treatment of external otitis is protection of the ear from additional moisture and avoidance of further mechanical injury by scratching
- Purulent debris filling the ear canal should be gently removed to permit entry of the topical medication
- When substantial edema of the canal wall prevents entry of drops into the ear canal, a wick is placed to facilitate entry of the medication

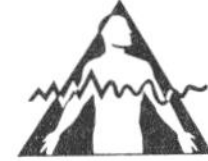

OUTCOME

FOLLOW-UP

Malignant external otitis

- To avoid relapse, antibiotic therapy should be continued, even in the asymptomatic patient, until gallium scanning indicates a marked reduction in the inflammatory process

WHEN TO REFER

- Any cases of suspected malignant external otitis should be referred to an otolaryngologist

EVIDENCE

WEB SITE

- Baylor College of Medicine Otolaryngology Resources on the Internet
  - http://www.bcm.tmc.edu/oto/othersa.html

INFORMATION FOR PATIENTS

- American Academy of Family Physicians: Otitis Externa
  - http://familydoctor.org/657.xml
- Centers for Disease Control and Prevention: Swimmer's Ear
  - http://www.cdc.gov/healthyswimming/swimmers_ear.htm
- MedlinePlus: Malignant Otitis Externa
  - http://www.nlm.nih.gov/medlineplus/ency/article/000672.htm

REFERENCES

- Roland PS et al: Ciprodex Otic AOE Study Group. Efficacy and safety of topical ciprofloxacin/dexamethasone versus neomycin/polymyxin B/hydrocortisone for otitis externa. Curr Med Res Opin 2004;20:1175. [PMID: 15324520]
- Roland PS et al: Microbiology of acute otitis externa. Laryngoscope 2002;112:1166. [PMID: 12169893]
- Rubin Grandis J et al: The changing face of malignant (necrotising) external otitis: clinical, radiological, and anatomic correlations. Lancet Infect Dis 2004;4:34. [PMID: 14720566]
- van Balen FA et al: Clinical efficacy of three common treatments in acute otitis externa in primary care: randomised controlled trial. BMJ 2003;327:1201. [PMID: 14630756]

Author(s)

Robert K. Jackler, MD
Michael J. Kaplan, MD

Otitis Media, Acute

KEY FEATURES

ESSENTIALS OF DIAGNOSIS

- Otalgia, often with an upper respiratory tract infection
- Erythema and hypomobility of tympanic membrane

GENERAL CONSIDERATIONS

- Bacterial infection of the mucosally lined air-containing spaces of the temporal bone
- Purulent material forms within not only the middle ear cleft but also the mastoid air cells and petrous apex when they are pneumatized
- Usually precipitated by a viral upper respiratory tract infection that causes auditory tube edema, resulting in accumulation of fluid and mucus, which become secondarily infected by bacteria
- Nasotracheal intubation can cause otitis media
- The most common pathogens are *Streptococcus pneumoniae, Haemophilus influenzae*, and *Streptococcus pyogenes*
- Chronic otitis media is usually not painful except during acute exacerbations

DEMOGRAPHICS

- Most common in infants and children, although it may occur at any age
- External otitis and acute otitis media are the most common causes of earache

CLINICAL FINDINGS

SYMPTOMS AND SIGNS

- Otalgia, aural pressure, decreased hearing, and often fever
- Typically, erythema and decreased mobility of the tympanic membrane
- Occasionally, bullae will be seen on the tympanic membrane, but these rarely indicate *Mycoplasma* infection
- When middle ear empyema is severe, the tympanic membrane can be seen to bulge outward
- In external otitis the ear canal skin is erythematous, whereas in acute otitis media this generally occurs only if the tympanic membrane has ruptured, spilling purulent material into the ear canal
- Persistent otorrhea despite topical and systemic antibiotic therapy

DIFFERENTIAL DIAGNOSIS

- Otitis externa
- Auditory (eustachian) tube dysfunction
- Mastoiditis
- Tympanosclerosis (scarred tympanic membrane)
- Referred pain: pharyngitis, sinusitis, tooth pain
- Glossopharyngeal neuralgia
- Temporomandibular joint syndrome
- Foreign body
- Cholesteatoma
- Bullous myringitis
- Herpes zoster oticus, especially when vesicles appear in the ear canal or concha

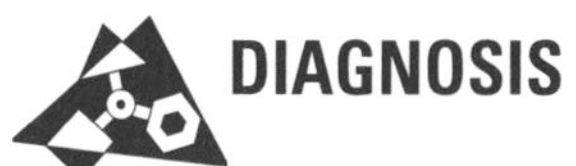

DIAGNOSIS

LABORATORY TESTS

- Tympanocentesis and culture of middle ear fluid (see below)

DIAGNOSTIC PROCEDURE

- Clinical diagnosis

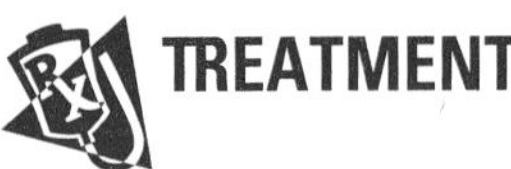

TREATMENT

MEDICATIONS

- Either amoxicillin (20–40 mg PO/kg/day) or erythromycin (50 mg PO/kg/day) plus sulfonamide (150 mg PO/kg/day) for 10 days
- Alternatives useful in resistant cases are cefaclor (20–40 mg PO/kg/day) or amoxicillin-clavulanate (20–40 mg PO/kg/day) combinations
- Nasal decongestants, if symptomatic
- Recurrent acute otitis media can be managed with long-term antibiotic prophylaxis: single oral daily doses of sulfamethoxazole (500 mg) or amoxicillin (250 or 500 mg) are given over a period of 1–3 months
- Failure of the regimen for recurrent acute otitis media is an indication for insertion of ventilating tubes

SURGERY

- Surgical drainage of the middle ear (myringotomy) is reserved for patients with severe otalgia or when complications of otitis (eg, mastoiditis, meningitis) have occurred

THERAPEUTIC PROCEDURES

- Tympanocentesis is useful for otitis media in immunocompromised patients and when infection persists or recurs despite multiple courses of antibiotics

OUTCOME

COMPLICATIONS

- Tympanic membrane rupture
- Chronic otitis media
  - Medical treatment includes regular removal of infected debris, use of earplugs to protect against water exposure, and topical antibiotic drops for exacerbations
  - Ciprofloxacin may help to dry a chronically discharging ear when given in a dosage of 500 mg PO twice a day for 1–6 weeks
  - Definitive management is surgical in most cases
- Mastoiditis
- Meningitis
  - The most common intracranial complication of ear infection
  - In acute otitis media, it arises from hematogenous spread of bacteria, most commonly *H influenzae* and *S pneumoniae*
  - In chronic otitis media, it results either from passage of infections along preformed pathways or from direct extension
- Epidural or brain abscess (temporal lobe or cerebellum)
- Facial palsy
- Sigmoid sinus thrombosis

WHEN TO REFER

- Persistent earache demands specialty referral to exclude cancer of the upper aerodigestive tract

EVIDENCE

PRACTICE GUIDELINES

- American Academy of Pediatrics, American Academy of Family Physicians: Diagnosis and Management of Acute Otitis Media, 2004.
  - http://www.guideline.gov/summary/summary.aspx?doc_id=4859&nbr=3500

WEB SITE

- Baylor College of Medicine Otolaryngology Resources on the Internet
  - http://www.bcm.tmc.edu/oto/othersa.html

INFORMATION FOR PATIENTS

- National Institute on Deafness and Other Communication Disorders: Otitis Media
  - http://www.nidcd.nih.gov/health/hearing/otitism.asp
- Nemours Foundation: Middle Ear Infections (Otitis Media)
  - http://kidshealth.org/parent/infections/bacterial_viral/otitis_media.html
- MedlinePlus: Otitis Media Interactive Tutorial
  - http://www.nlm.nih.gov/medlineplus/tutorials/otitismedia/htm/index.htm
- Parmet S et al: Patient page: acute otitis media. JAMA 2003;290:1666. [PMID:14506125]

REFERENCES

- Penido Nde O et al: Intracranial complications of otitis media: 15 years of experience in 33 patients. Otolaryngol Head Neck Surg 2005;132:37. [PMID: 15632907]
- Rovers MM et al: Otitis media. Lancet 2004;363:465. [PMID: 14962529]

Author(s)

Robert K. Jackler, MD
Michael J. Kaplan, MD

Otitis Media, Serous

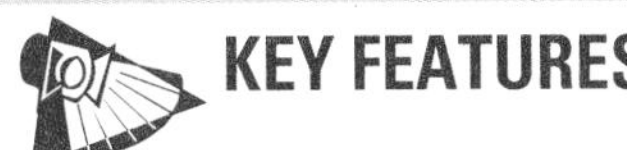

KEY FEATURES

ESSENTIALS OF DIAGNOSIS

- Blocked auditory tube remains for a prolonged period
- Resultant negative pressure will cause transudation of fluid

GENERAL CONSIDERATIONS

- Especially common in children because their auditory tubes are narrower and more horizontal in orientation than adults
- It is less common in adults, in whom it usually follows an upper respiratory tract infection or barotrauma
- In an adult with persistent unilateral serous otitis media, nasopharyngeal carcinoma must be excluded

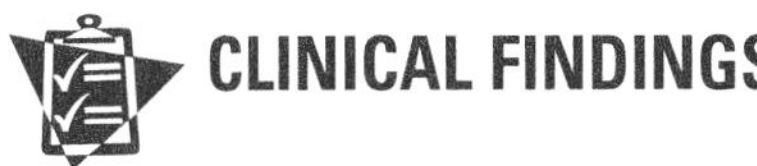

CLINICAL FINDINGS

SYMPTOMS AND SIGNS

- The tympanic membrane is dull and hypomobile
- Occasionally accompanied by air bubbles in the middle ear and conductive hearing loss

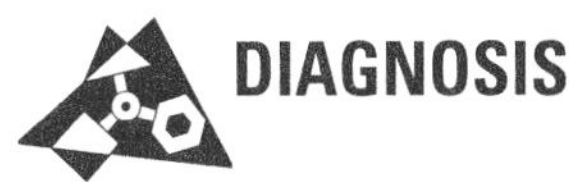

DIAGNOSIS

LABORATORY TESTS

- Clinical diagnosis

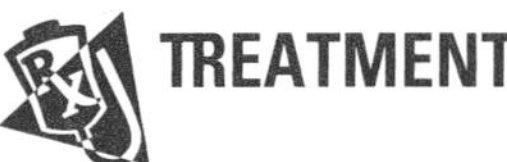

TREATMENT

MEDICATIONS

- A short course of oral corticosteroids (eg, prednisone, 40 mg/day for 7 days)
- Oral antibiotics (eg, amoxicillin, 250 mg PO three times daily for 7 days)
- A combination of oral corticosteroids and antibiotics
- The role of these regimens remains controversial, but they are probably of little lasting benefit

SURGERY

- When medication fails to bring relief after several months, a ventilating tube placed through the tympanic membrane may restore hearing and alleviate the sense of aural fullness

THERAPEUTIC PROCEDURES

- Similar to that for auditory tube dysfunction

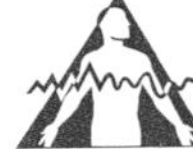

OUTCOME

WHEN TO REFER

- For persistent or recurrent symptoms

PREVENTION

Plane travel

- The patient should be advised to swallow, yawn, and autoinflate frequently during descent, which may be painful if the auditory tube collapses
- Systemic decongestants (eg, pseudoephedrine, 60–120 mg) should be taken several hours before anticipated arrival time so that they will be maximally effective during descent
- Topical decongestants such as 1% phenylephrine nasal spray should be administered 1 h before arrival
- Repeated episodes of barotrauma in persons who must fly frequently can be alleviated by insertion of ventilating tubes

Scuba diving

- Problem occurs most commonly during the descent phase, when pain develops within the first 15 feet if inflation of the middle ear via the auditory tube has not occurred
- Divers must descend slowly and equilibrate in stages to avoid severely negative pressures in the tympanum, which may result in hemorrhage (hemotympanum) or perilymphatic fistulization, in which the oval or round window ruptures, resulting in sensory hearing loss and acute vertigo
- Emesis resulting from acute labyrinthine dysfunction can be dangerous during an underwater dive
- Tympanic membrane perforation is an absolute contraindication to diving because the patient will experience an unbalanced thermal stimulus to the semicircular canals, possibly leading to vertigo, disorientation, and even emesis
- Individuals with only one hearing ear should be discouraged from diving because of the significant risk of otologic injury

EVIDENCE

PRACTICE GUIDELINES

- American Academy of Family Physicians, American Academy of Otolaryngology—Head and Neck Surgery, American Academy of Pediatrics: Otitis Media With Effusion, 2004.
  - http://www.guideline.gov/summary/summary.aspx?doc_id=5089&nbr=3556

WEB SITE

- Baylor College of Medicine Otolaryngology Resources on the Internet
  - http://www.bcm.tmc.edu/oto/othersa.html

INFORMATION FOR PATIENTS

- American Academy of Family Physicians: Otitis Media With Effusion
  - http://familydoctor.org/330.xml
- Centers for Disease Control and Prevention: Otitis Media With Effusion
  - http://www.cdc.gov/antibioticresistance/files/ome.pdf
- National Institute on Deafness and Other Communication Disorders: Otitis Media
  - http://www.nidcd.nih.gov/health/hearing/otitism.asp
- University of Minnesota Department of Otolaryngology: Serous Otitis Media
  - http://www.med.umn.edu/otol/library/serousot.htm

REFERENCES

- Becker GD et al: Barotrauma of the ears and sinuses after scuba diving. Eur Arch Otorhinolaryngol 2001;258:159. [PMID: 11407445]
- Kujawski OB et al: Laser eustachian tuboplasty. Otol Neurotol 2004;25:1. [PMID: 14724483]
- Newbegin C et al: Ear barotrauma after flying and diving. Practitioner 2000;244:96. [PMID: 10892042]
- Satre TJ et al: Treatments for persistent otitis media with effusion. Am Fam Physician 2005;71:529. [PMID: 15712626]

Author(s)

Robert K. Jackler, MD
Michael J. Kaplan, MD

Ovarian Tumors

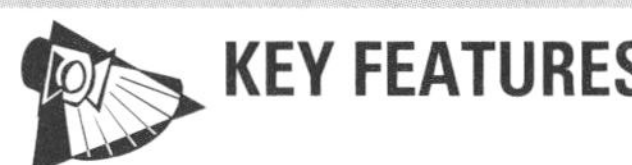

KEY FEATURES

ESSENTIALS OF DIAGNOSIS

- Vague gastrointestinal discomfort
- Pelvic pressure and pain
- Many cases of early-stage cancer are asymptomatic
- Pelvic examination, CA 125, and ultrasound are mainstays of diagnosis

GENERAL CONSIDERATIONS

- Ovarian tumors are common. Most are benign, but malignant ovarian tumors are the leading cause of death from reproductive tract cancer
- The wide range of types and patterns of ovarian tumors is due to the complexity of ovarian embryology and differences in tissues of origin (Table 67)

DEMOGRAPHICS

- In women with no family history of ovarian cancer, the lifetime risk is 1.6%, whereas a woman with one affected first-degree relative has a 5% lifetime risk. With two or more affected first-degree relatives, the risk is 7%
- Approximately 3% of women with two or more affected first-degree relatives will have a hereditary ovarian cancer syndrome with a lifetime risk of 40%
- Women with a *BRCA1* gene mutation have a 45% lifetime risk of ovarian cancer and those with a *BRAC2* mutation have a 25% risk

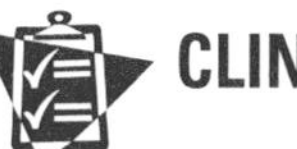

CLINICAL FINDINGS

SYMPTOMS AND SIGNS

- Both benign and malignant ovarian neoplasms are either asymptomatic or experience only mild nonspecific gastrointestinal symptoms or pelvic pressure
- Early disease is typically detected on routine pelvic examination
- In advanced malignant disease, women may experience abdominal pain and bloating, and a palpable abdominal mass with ascites is often present

DIFFERENTIAL DIAGNOSIS

- Benign ovarian tumor, eg, follicle cyst, corpus luteum cyst
- Malignant ovarian tumor
- Teratoma (usually benign)
- Tuboovarian abscess
- Endometriosis
- Colon cancer
- Ectopic pregnancy
- Metastases to ovary, eg, gastrointestinal, breast

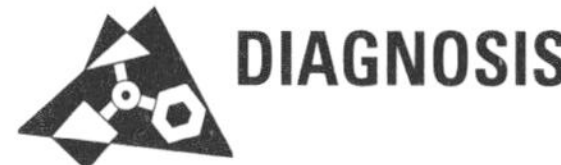

DIAGNOSIS

LABORATORY TESTS

- An elevated serum CA 125 (> 35 units) indicates a greater likelihood that an ovarian tumor is malignant
- CA 125 is elevated in 80% of women with epithelial ovarian cancer overall but in only 50% of women with early disease
- Serum CA 125 may be elevated in premenopausal women with benign disease such as endometriosis

IMAGING STUDIES

- Transvaginal sonography (TVS) is useful for screening high-risk women but has inadequate sensitivity for screening low-risk women
- Ultrasound is helpful in differentiating ovarian masses that are benign and likely to resolve spontaneously from those with malignant potential
- Color Doppler imaging may further enhance the specificity of ultrasound diagnosis

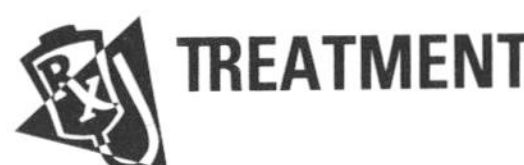

TREATMENT

MEDICATIONS

- Except for women with low-grade ovarian cancer in an early stage, postoperative chemotherapy is indicated. Several chemotherapy regimens are effective, such as the combination of cisplatin or carboplatin with paclitaxel, with clinical response rates of up to 60–70% (Table 153)

SURGERY

- Most ovarian masses in postmenopausal women require surgical evaluation
- However, a postmenopausal woman with an asymptomatic unilateral simple cyst < 5 cm in diameter and a normal CA 125 level may be monitored closely with TVS. All others require surgical evaluation
- Exploratory laparotomy has been the standard approach in postmenopausal women
- For ovarian cancer in an early stage, the standard therapy is complete surgical staging followed by abdominal hysterectomy and bilateral salpingo-oophorectomy with omentectomy and selective lymphadenectomy
- With more advanced disease, removal of all visible tumor improves survival
- For benign neoplasms, tumor removal or unilateral oophorectomy is usually performed

THERAPEUTIC PROCEDURES

- In a premenopausal woman, an asymptomatic, mobile, unilateral, simple cystic mass < 8–10 cm may be observed for 4–6 weeks. Most will resolve spontaneously. If the mass is larger or unchanged on repeat pelvic examination and TVS, surgical evaluation is required
- Laparoscopy may be considered for a small ovarian mass in a premenopausal woman
- If malignancy is suspected in a premenopausal woman, preoperative workup should include chest x-ray, evaluation of liver and kidney function, and hematologic indices

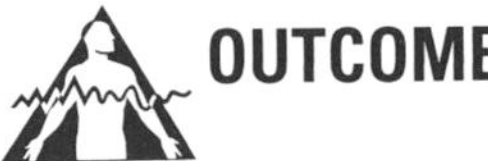

OUTCOME

PROGNOSIS

- Approximately 75% of women with ovarian cancer are diagnosed with advanced disease after regional or distant metastases have become established
- The overall 5-year survival is approximately 17% with distant metastases, 36% with local spread, and 89% with early disease

WHEN TO REFER

- If a malignant ovarian mass is suspected, surgical evaluation should be performed by a gynecologic oncologist

PREVENTION

- Women with a *BRCA1* gene mutation should be screened annually with TVS and CA 125 testing, and prophylactic oophorectomy is recommended by age 35 or whenever childbearing is completed because of the high risk of disease
- The benefits of such screening for women with one or no affected first-degree relatives are unproved, and the risks associated with unnecessary surgical procedures may outweigh the benefits in low-risk women

EVIDENCE

PRACTICE GUIDELINES

- Morgan R et al; NCCN Ovarian Cancer Practice Guidelines Panel. National Comprehensive Cancer Network: Ovarian Cancer v.1.2005.
  - http://www.nccn.org/professionals/physician_gls/PDF/ovarian.pdf
- US Preventive Services Task Force. Screening for ovarian cancer: recommendation statement. 2004
  - http://www.ahrq.gov/clinic/uspstf/uspsovar.htm

WEB SITES

- Cystic Teratoma Demonstration Case
  - http://www.brighamrad.harvard.edu/Cases/bwh/hcache/62/full.html
- Hemorrhagic Corpus Luteum Demonstration Case
  - http://www.brighamrad.harvard.edu/Cases/bwh/hcache/26/full.html
- National Cancer Institute: Ovarian Cancer Information for Patients and Health Professionals
  - http://www.cancer.gov/cancertopics/types/ovarian

INFORMATION FOR PATIENTS

- American Academy of Family Physicians: Ovarian Cyst
  - http://familydoctor.org/279.xml
- American Cancer Society: Ovarian Cancer
  - http://www.cancer.org/docroot/CRI/CRI_2_3x.asp?rnav=cridg&dt=33
- MedlinePlus: Ovarian Cancer Interactive Tutorial
  - http://www.nlm.nih.gov/medlineplus/tutorials/whatisovariancancer.html
- MedlinePlus: Ovarian Cancer
  - http://www.nlm.nih.gov/medlineplus/ency/article/000889.htm
- National Women's Health Information Center: Ovarian Cysts
  - http://www.4woman.gov/faq/ovarian_cysts.htm

REFERENCE

- Cannistra SA: Cancer of the ovary. N Engl J Med 2004;351:2519. [PMID: 15590954]

Author(s)

H. Trent MacKay, MD, MPH

Paget's Disease of Bone

KEY FEATURES

ESSENTIALS OF DIAGNOSIS

- Often asymptomatic
- Bone pain may be first symptom
- Kyphosis, bowed tibias, large head, deafness, and frequent fractures that vary with location of process
- Serum calcium and phosphate normal; alkaline phosphatase elevated; urinary hydroxyproline elevated
- Dense, expanded bones on x-ray

GENERAL CONSIDERATIONS

- Common condition manifested by one or more bony lesions having high bone turnover and disorganized osteoid formation
- Involved bones become vascular, weak, and deformed
- Usually discovered incidentally during radiographic imaging or evaluation of serum alkaline phosphatase elevation
- Familial Paget's disease is unusual but generally more severe

DEMOGRAPHICS

- Present in 1–2% of US adults, especially those of northern European ancestry; highest prevalence in northeastern United States (1.5%) and lowest in the South (0.3%)
- Usually diagnosed in patients age >40; highest prevalence is among persons aged 65–75 (2.3%); a rare form occurs in young people
- More common in elderly
- Slightly more common in men, with near-equal racial distribution

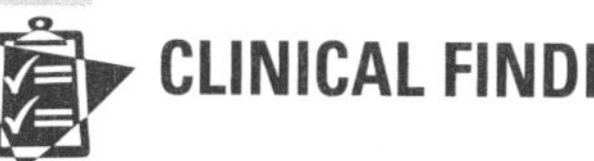

CLINICAL FINDINGS

SYMPTOMS AND SIGNS

- Often mild and asymptomatic; only 27% symptomatic at diagnosis
- Can involve just one bone (monostotic) or multiple bones (polyostotic), particularly skull, femur, tibia, pelvis, and humerus
- Pain is usual first symptom
- Bones become soft, leading to bowed tibias, kyphosis, and frequent fractures with slight trauma
- If skull is involved, patient may report headaches, increased hat size, and deafness
- Increased vascularity over involved bones causes increased warmth
- Sarcomatous change suggested by marked increase in bone pain

DIFFERENTIAL DIAGNOSIS

- Bone tumor, eg, osteosarcoma
- Multiple myeloma
- Metastatic cancer
- Fibrous dysplasia
- Osteitis fibrosa cystica (hyperparathyroidism)
- Fibrogenesis imperfecta ossium

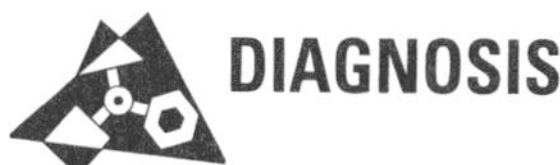

DIAGNOSIS

LABORATORY TESTS

- Serum alkaline phosphatase markedly elevated
- Serum calcium and phosphorus typically normal
- Serum calcium may be elevated, particularly if patient is at bed rest
- Urinary hydroxyproline elevated in active disease
- Sarcomatous change suggested by sudden rise in serum alkaline phosphatase

IMAGING STUDIES

- Bone radiographs show involved bones as expanded and denser than normal
- Multiple fissure fractures in long bones
- Initial lesion may be destructive and radiolucent, especially in skull ("osteoporosis circumscripta")
- Sarcomatous change suggested by appearance of new lytic lesion
- Technetium pyrophosphate bone scans helpful in delineating activity of bone lesions even before radiological changes are apparent

DIAGNOSTIC PROCEDURES

- Bone biopsy in suspected sarcomatous change

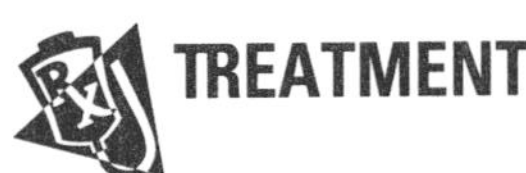

TREATMENT

MEDICATIONS

- Bisphosphonates are treatment of choice
- Therapeutic response is evidenced by normalization of serum alkaline phosphatase. Therapy is then discontinued for ~3 months or until alkaline phosphatase rises; then another cycle commenced
- Tiludronate, 400 mg PO QD for 3 months, is effective in reducing activity of bone lesions
  - May be taken in evening or day, but should not be taken within 2 hours of meals, aspirin, indomethacin, calcium, magnesium, or aluminum-containing antacids
  - Esophagitis is uncommon (avoidance of recumbency after dosing not required)
  - Abdominal pain and nausea are common
- Alendronate, 20–40 mg PO QAM (or 70 mg PO Q week) for 3-month cycles
- Risedronate, 30 mg PO QAM for 3-month cycles
- Patient must remain upright after taking alendronate and risedronate to reduce risk of pill-induced esophagitis. Taken in AM with ≥8 oz water, at least 30–60 min before any other food or liquid
- Zoledronic acid 4 mg IV over 20–30 minutes every 6 months
- Pamidronate, 60–120 mg IV over 2–4 hours
- Nasal calcitonin-salmon (Miacalcin), 200 IU one spray QD, alternating nostrils. Used less often than bisphosphonates

THERAPEUTIC PROCEDURES

- Asymptomatic patients require no treatment unless there is extensive skull involvement, in which prophylactic treatment may prevent deafness and stroke

OUTCOME

FOLLOW-UP

- Monitor alkaline phosphatase

COMPLICATIONS

- Fractures frequently occur with minimal trauma
- If patient is immobilized and has excessive calcium intake, hypercalcemia and kidney stones may develop
- Vertebral collapse may lead to spinal cord compression
- Osteosarcoma may develop in long-standing lesions (rare)
- Increased vascularity may cause high-output congestive heart failure
- Arthritis frequently develops in joints adjacent to involved bone
- Extensive skull involvement may cause cranial nerve palsies. Deafness may result from entrapment of cranial nerve VIII (and from conductive hearing loss). Tinnitus and vertigo occasionally occur
- Ischemic neurologic events may result form vascular "steal" phenomenon
- In severe forms, marked deformity, intractable pain, and congestive heart failure occur
- After bisphosphonates therapy, patients commonly experience fatigue, myalgia, and bone pain
  - Symptom onset may be anywhere from 1 day to months after institution of therapy and usually improve with discontinuation of therapy or with time after intermittent intravenous therapy
  - Symptoms can vary from nonexistent to incapacitation
  - Potent intravenous bisphosphonates, such as zoledronate, can cause fever

PROGNOSIS

- Prognosis generally good
- Most patients treated with bisphosphonates have normalization of serum alkaline phosphatase within 6 months, most maintaining this biochemical remission for several years
- Sarcomas, which occur in 1–3%, have poor prognosis
- In general, the prognosis of Paget's disease is worse the earlier in life the disease starts
- Fractures usually heal well

PREVENTION

- Prompt bisphosphonate treatment markedly reduces occurrence of complications of severe Paget's disease

EVIDENCE

PRACTICE GUIDELINES

- Lyles KW et al: A clinical approach to diagnosis and management of Paget's disease of bone. J Bone Miner Res 2001;16:1379. [PMID:11499860]

WEB SITES

- National Osteoporosis Foundation
  - http://www.nof.org
- The Paget Foundation
  - http://www.paget.org/

INFORMATION FOR PATIENTS

- MEDLINEplus—Paget's Disease
  - http://www.nlm.nih.gov/medlineplus/ency/article/000414.htm
- The National Institutes of Health Osteoporosis and Related Bone Diseases—National Resource Center—Information for patients about Paget's disease of bone
  - http://www.osteo.org/newfile.asp?doc=p110iYOURMOMMAdoctitle=Information+for+Patients+about+Paget%27s+Disease+of+Bone

REFERENCES

- Keen RW: The current status of Paget's disease of the bone. Hosp Med 2003;63:230. [PMID:12731136]
- Schneider D et al: Diagnosis and treatment of Paget's disease of bone. Am Fam Physician 2002;65:2069. [PMID:12046775]
- Vasireddy S et al: Patterns of pain in Paget's disease of bone and their outcomes on treatment with pamidronate. Clin Rheumatol 2003;22:376. [PMID:14677009]
- Walsh JP: Paget's disease of bone. Med J Aust 2004;181:262. [PMID:15347275]
- Whittern CR et al: MRI of Paget's disease of bone. Clin Radiol 2003;58:763. [PMID:14521884]

Author(s)

Paul A. Fitzgerald, MD

Pain Disorders, Chronic

KEY FEATURES

ESSENTIALS OF DIAGNOSIS

- Chronic complaints of pain
- Symptoms frequently exceed signs
- Minimal relief with standard treatment
- History of having seen multiple clinicians
- Frequent use of several nonspecific medications

GENERAL CONSIDERATIONS

- Components of the syndrome
  - Anatomic changes
  - Chronic anxiety and depression
  - Anger
  - An altered lifestyle
- Importance of psychological factors increases over time
- Often involves secondary gain for the patient via financial compensation or maintaining the sick role
- Clinicians unwittingly reinforce the sick role, since the nature of medical practice is to respond to complaints of illness
- It is counterproductive for the clinician to speculate whether the patient's pain is "real"
- Acceptance of the problem must precede attempts to reduce symptoms and improve function

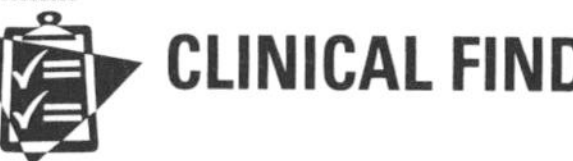

CLINICAL FINDINGS

SYMPTOMS AND SIGNS

- Patients often take multiple medications, stay in bed a great deal, and experience little joy in work or play
- Typically, the anatomic problem related to the pain is irreversible
- Marked decrease in pain threshold is apparent
- Chronic anxiety and depression produce heightened irritability and overreaction to stimuli
- Patients often have a hypochondriacal preoccupation with the body and a need for reassurance
- History of many interventions with unsatisfactory results
- Treatment failures may provoke anger, depression, and exacerbations of the chronic pain
- Relationships are impaired, including those with clinicians
- Clinicians develop covert rejection devices, such as being unavailable or making referrals to other physicians

DIFFERENTIAL DIAGNOSIS

- Somatoform disorders
- Malingering

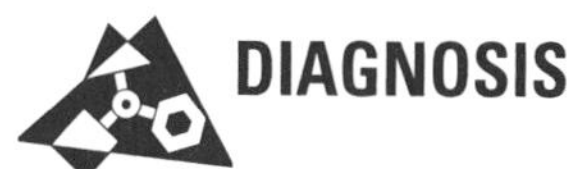

DIAGNOSIS

LABORATORY TESTS

- See Figure 8 (page 1261)

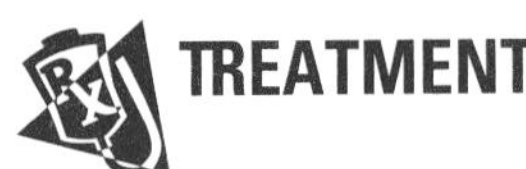

TREATMENT

MEDICATIONS

- Analgesics and sedatives are used only on a fixed-dose schedule to reduce their conditioning effects
- Tricyclic antidepressants and venalafaxine in doses used for depression can be helpful (see Table 108)
- Gabapentin can be helpful for neuropathic pain

THERAPEUTIC PROCEDURES

- A single clinician should direct treatment
- The physician should adopt an attitude of hopefulness for control of pain and improved function—but not for cure

Behavioral

- Behavioral approach to identify and eliminate pain reinforcers, decrease drug use, and shift focus from the pain
- Goal is to shift from a paradigm directed at biomedical cure to one of ongoing care
- Patient should discuss pain only with the physician
- Patient should be assigned self-help tasks graded toward maximal activity
- Patient should keep a self-rating chart of accomplishments and degrees of pain
- Emphasize a positive response to activities, which shift focus away from pain
- Avoid sympathy and attention to pain, which are positive reinforcers of this behavior
- Biofeedback and hypnosis

Social

- Family and significant others should be involved in care so that a physician's efforts are not undermined

Psychological

- Family therapy can help identify and eliminate "pain games" that facilitate the sick role
- Group therapy can help obtain patient involvement in care
- Individual therapy to strengthen defenses and build self-esteem

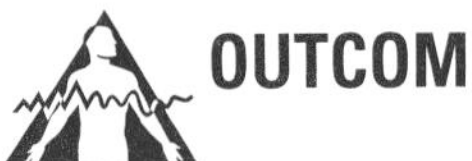

OUTCOME

COMPLICATIONS

- Sedative and analgesic dependency
- Substance abuse
- Unemployment
- Depression

WHEN TO REFER

- Refer to a chronic pain center if specialized consultation is needed

EVIDENCE

PRACTICE GUIDELINES

- National Guideline Clearinghouse: Siskin Hospital for Physical Rehabilitation: guidelines for management of non-malignant pain syndrome patients, 1999
  - http://www.guideline.gov/summary/summary.aspx?doc_id=2812
- National Guideline Clearinghouse: VHA/DoD clinical practice guideline for the management of medically unexplained symptoms: chronic pain and fatigue, 2001
  - http://www.guideline.gov/summary/summary.aspx?doc_id=3415

WEB SITES

- American Academy of Family Physicians
  - http://aafp.org/afp/20000301/1331.html
- American Psychiatric Association
  - http://www.psych.org/

INFORMATION FOR PATIENTS

- American Academy of Family Physicians: Chronic Pain Medicines
  - http://familydoctor.org/handouts/122.html
- JAMA patient page: Pain management. JAMA 2003;290:2504. [PMID: 14612487]
- National Institute of Neurological Disorders and Stroke
  - http://www.ninds.nih.gov/disorders/chronic_pain/chronic_pain.htm

REFERENCES

- Eisendrath SJ: Psychiatric aspects of chronic pain. Neurology 1995;45(Suppl 9):S26. [PMID:8538883]
- Evers AW et al: Tailored cognitive-behavioral therapy in early rheumatoid arthritis for patients at risk: a randomized controlled trial. Pain 2002; 100:141. [PMID:12435467]
- Garcia-Campayo J et al: Gabapentin for the treatment of patients with somatization disorder. J Clin Psychiatry 2001;62:474. [PMID:11465526]

Author(s)

Stuart J. Eisendrath, MD
Jonathan E. Lichtmacher, MD

Pancreatic Cancer

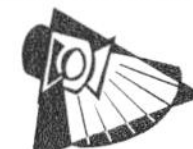

KEY FEATURES

ESSENTIALS OF DIAGNOSIS

- Obstructive jaundice (may be painless)
- Enlarged gallbladder (may be painful)
- Upper abdominal pain with radiation to back, weight loss, and thrombophlebitis are usually late manifestations

GENERAL CONSIDERATIONS

- Carcinoma is the commonest pancreatic neoplasm. About 75% are in the head and 25% in the body and tail of the organ
- Carcinomas involving the head of the pancreas, the ampulla of Vater, the distal common bile duct, and the duodenum are considered together, because they are usually indistinguishable clinically; of these, carcinomas of the pancreas constitute over 90%. They comprise 2% of all cancers and 5% of cancer deaths
- Neuroendocrine tumors account for 2–5% of pancreatic neoplasms
- Cystic neoplasms account for only 1% of pancreatic cancers, but they are often mistaken for pseudocysts. A cystic neoplasm should be suspected when a cystic lesion in the pancreas is found in the absence of a history of pancreatitis. Whereas serous cystadenomas are benign, mucinous cystadenomas, intraductal papillary mucinous tumors, and papillary cystic neoplasms are premalignant, though their prognoses are better than the prognosis of adenocarcinoma of the pancreas
- Staging by the TNM classification: Tis, carcinoma in situ; T1: tumor limited to the pancreas, ≤2 cm in greatest dimension; T2, tumor limited to the pancreas, >2 cm in greatest dimension; T3, tumor extends beyond the pancreas but without involvement of the celiac axis or the superior mesenteric artery; T4, tumor involves the celiac axis or the superior mesenteric artery

DEMOGRAPHICS

- Risk factors include age, obesity, tobacco use, chronic pancreatitis, prior abdominal radiation, and family history
- About 7–8% of pancreatic cancer patients have a first-degree relative with pancreatic cancer, compared with 0.6% of control subjects

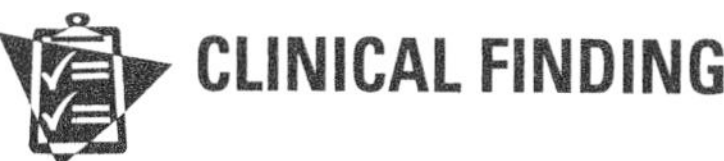

CLINICAL FINDINGS

SYMPTOMS AND SIGNS

- Pain is present in over 70% and is often vague, diffuse, and located in the epigastrium or left upper quadrant when the lesion is in the tail
- Radiation of pain into the back is common and sometimes predominates. Sitting up and leaning forward may afford some relief, which usually indicates extrapancreatic spread and inoperability
- Diarrhea, perhaps from maldigestion, is an occasional early symptom
- Migratory thrombophlebitis is a rare sign
- Weight loss commonly occurs late and may be associated with depression
- Occasionally acute pancreatitis is the presentation
- Jaundice is usually due to biliary obstruction in the pancreatic head
- A palpable gallbladder is indicative of obstruction by neoplasm (Courvoisier's law), but there are frequent exceptions
- A hard, fixed, occasionally tender mass may be present
- In advanced cases, a hard periumbilical (Sister Mary Joseph's) nodule may be palpable

DIFFERENTIAL DIAGNOSIS

- Choledocholithiasis
- Pancreatic pseudocyst or cystic neoplasm
- Carcinoma of the biliary tract
- Biliary stricture
- Hepatocellular carcinoma
- Primary sclerosing cholangitis
- Primary biliary cirrhosis

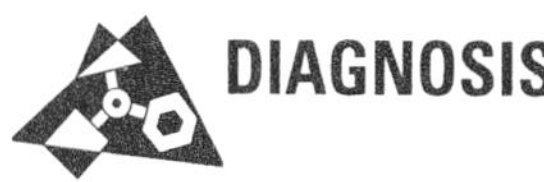

DIAGNOSIS

LABORATORY TESTS

- There may be mild anemia. Glycosuria, hyperglycemia, and impaired glucose tolerance or true diabetes mellitus are found in 10–20% of cases
- The serum amylase or lipase level is occasionally elevated
- Liver function tests may suggest obstructive jaundice
- Steatorrhea in the absence of jaundice is uncommon
- Occult blood in the stool is suggestive of ampulla of Vater carcinoma (the combination of biliary obstruction and bleeding may give the stools a distinctive silver appearance)
- CA 19-9, with a sensitivity of 70% and a specificity of 87%, is not sensitive enough for early detection; increased values are also found in acute and chronic pancreatitis and cholangitis

IMAGING STUDIES

- With carcinoma of the head of the pancreas, the upper gastrointestinal series may show a widened duodenal loop, mucosal abnormalities in the duodenum ranging from edema to invasion, or spasm or compression
- Ultrasound is not reliable because of interference by intestinal gas
- Multiphase thin-cut spiral CT detects a mass in over 80% of cases and can delineate the extent of the tumor and allow for percutaneous fine-needle aspiration for cytological studies; MRI is an alternative to CT
- Positron emission tomography appears to be a sensitive technique for detecting pancreatic cancer and metastases

DIAGNOSTIC PROCEDURES

- Selective mesenteric arteriography may demonstrate vessel invasion by a tumor, thus inoperable, but is being replaced by multiphase spiral CT
- Endoscopic ultrasonography is more sensitive than CT in diagnosing pancreatic cancer and is equivalent for determining nodal involvement and resectability. It can guide fine-needle aspiration for tissue diagnosis and tumor markers
- Endoscopic retrograde cholangiopancreatography (ERCP) may clarify an ambiguous CT or MRI study by delineating the pancreatic duct system or confirming an ampullary or biliary neoplasm
- Magnetic resonance cholangiopancreatography (MRCP) is as sensitive as ERCP in diagnosing pancreatic cancer
- Pancreatoscopy or intraductal ultrasonography can evaluate filling defects in the pancreatic duct and assess resectability of intraductal papillary mucinous tumors
- With obstruction of the splenic vein, splenomegaly or gastric varices are present, the latter delineated by endoscopy, endoscopic ultrasonography, or angiography
- Cystic neoplasms can be distinguished by their appearance on CT, endoscopic ultrasonography, and ERCP and features of the cyst fluid on gross and cytological analysis

Panbronchiolitis, Diffuse p. 1124

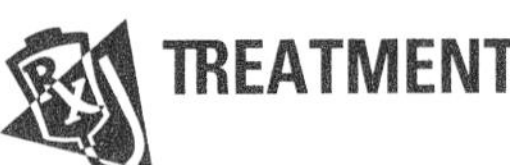

TREATMENT

MEDICATIONS

- Combined irradiation and chemotherapy may be used for palliation of unresectable cancer confined to the pancreas
- Chemotherapy with fluorouracil and gemcitabine has been disappointing in metastatic pancreatic cancer, though improved response rates have been reported with gemcitabine
- Adjuvant fluorouracil-based chemotherapy or gemcitabine has some benefit

SURGERY

- In about 30% of cases, abdominal exploration is necessary when cytological diagnosis cannot be made or if resection is attempted
- If a mass is localized in the head of the pancreas and there is no jaundice, laparoscopy may detect tiny peritoneal or liver metastases and thereby avoid resection in about 10% of patients
- Radical pancreaticoduodenal (Whipple) resection is indicated for lesions strictly limited to the head of the pancreas, periampullary zone, and duodenum
- Surgical resection is indicated for all mucinous cystic neoplasms, symptomatic serous cystadenomas, and cystic tumors that remain undefined after helical CT, endoscopic ultrasound, and diagnostic aspiration

THERAPEUTIC PROCEDURES

- When resection is not feasible, endoscopic stenting of the bile duct, or cholecystojejunostomy, is performed to relieve jaundice. A gastrojejunostomy is also done if duodenal obstruction is expected to develop later; alternatively, endoscopic placement of a self-expandable duodenal stent may be feasible
- Celiac plexus nerve block or thoracoscopic splanchnicectomy may improve pain control. Photodynamic therapy is under study

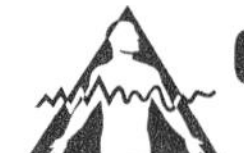

OUTCOME

PROGNOSIS

- Carcinoma of the pancreas, especially in the body or tail, has a poor prognosis. Reported 5-year survival rates range from 2% to 5%
- Jaundice and lymph node involvement are adverse prognostic factors
- Lesions of the ampulla have a better prognosis, with reported 5-year survival rates of 20–40% after resection
- In carefully selected patients, resection of cancer of the pancreatic head is feasible and results in reasonable survival
- In a person whose disease progresses with treatment, meticulous efforts at palliative care are essential

PREVENTION

- In persons with a family history of pancreatic cancer, screening with spiral CT and endoscopic ultrasonography should be considered beginning 10 years before the age at which pancreatic cancer was diagnosed in a family member

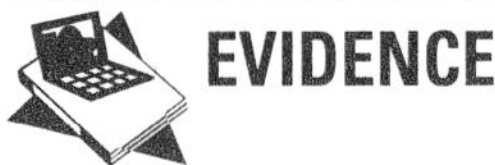

EVIDENCE

PRACTICE GUIDELINES

- Earle CC et al: Cancer Care Ontario Practice Guidelines Initiatives Gastrointestinal Cancer Disease Site Group. The treatment of locally advanced pancreatic cancer: a practice guideline. Can J Gastroenterol 2003;17:161. [PMID: 12677264]
- National Guideline Clearinghouse
  - http://www.guideline.gov/summary/summary.aspx?doc_id=5689&nbr=3827&string=pancreatic+AND+cancer

WEB SITE

- Cystic and Papillary Epithelial Neoplasm of the Pancreas Demonstration Case
  - http://www.brighamrad.harvard.edu/Cases/bwh/hcache/159/full.html

INFORMATION FOR PATIENTS

- Mayo Clinic
  - http://www.mayoclinic.com/invoke.cfm?id=DS00357
- National Cancer Institute
  - http://www.cancer.gov/cancerinfo/wyntk/pancreas

REFERENCES

- Bettschart V et al: Presentation, treatment and outcome in patients with ampullary tumours. Br J Surg 2004;91:1600. [PMID: 15515106]
- Brugge WR et al: Cystic neoplasms of the pancreas. N Engl J Med 2004;351:1218. [PMID: 15371579]
- Li D et al: Pancreatic cancer. Lancet 2004;363:1049. [PMID: 15051286]
- Takhar AS et al: Recent developments in diagnosis of pancreatic cancer. BMJ 2004;329:668. [PMID: 15374918]

Author(s)

Lawrence S. Friedman, MD

Pancreatitis, Acute

KEY FEATURES

ESSENTIALS OF DIAGNOSIS

- Abrupt onset of deep epigastric pain, often with radiation to the back
- Nausea, vomiting, sweating, weakness, fever
- Leukocytosis, elevated serum amylase
- History of previous episodes, often related to alcohol intake

GENERAL CONSIDERATIONS

- Most often due to passed gallstone, usually < 5 mm in diameter, or heavy alcohol intake
- Rarely, may be the initial manifestation of a pancreatic neoplasm
- The pathogenesis may include edema or obstruction of the ampulla of Vater, resulting in bile reflux into pancreatic ducts, or direct injury to the acinar cells. Pathological changes vary from edema to necrosis, hemorrhage, and intra- and extrapancreatic fat necrosis. All or part of the pancreas may be involved

CLINICAL FINDINGS

SYMPTOMS AND SIGNS

- There may be a history of alcohol intake or a heavy meal immediately preceding the attack, or a history of milder similar episodes or biliary colic in the past

Pain

- Severe, steady, boring epigastric pain, generally abrupt in onset. Usually radiates into the back but may radiate to the right or left
- Often made worse by walking and lying and better by sitting and leaning forward
- The upper abdomen is tender, most often without guarding, rigidity, or rebound
- There may be distention and absent bowel sounds from paralytic ileus
- Nausea and vomiting
- Weakness, sweating, and anxiety in severe attacks
- Fever of 38.4–39°C, tachycardia, hypotension (even true shock), pallor, and cool clammy skin are often present
- Mild jaundice is common
- Occasionally, an upper abdominal mass may be palpated
- Acute renal failure (usually prerenal) may occur early in the course

DIFFERENTIAL DIAGNOSIS

- Acute cholecystitis or cholangitis
- Penetrating duodenal ulcer
- Pancreatic pseudocyst
- Ischemic bowel
- Small bowel obstruction
- Abdominal aortic aneurysm
- Kidney stone

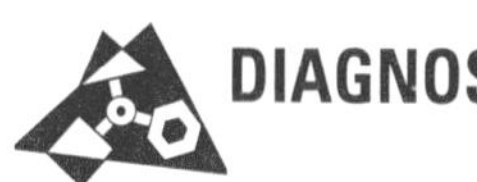

DIAGNOSIS

LABORATORY TESTS

- Serum amylase and lipase increase, usually in excess of three times normal, within 24 h in 90% of cases; lipase remains elevated longer than amylase
- Leukocytosis (10,000–30,000/μL), proteinuria, granular casts, glycosuria (10–20% of cases), hyperglycemia, and elevated serum bilirubin may be present
- Blood urea nitrogen (BUN) and serum alkaline phosphatase may be elevated and coagulation tests abnormal
- A serum alanine aminotransferase level of more than 80 units/L suggests biliary pancreatitis
- Decrease in serum calcium correlates well with severity of disease. Levels lower than 7 mg/dL (when serum albumin is normal) are associated with tetany
- Early hemoconcentration, hematocrit value above 47%, predicts severe disease
- An elevated C-reactive protein concentration after 48 h suggests the development of pancreatic necrosis
- The fluid amylase content is high in ascites or left pleural effusions

IMAGING STUDIES

- Plain abdominal radiographs may show gallstones, a "sentinel loop" (a segment of air-filled left upper quadrant small intestine), the "colon cutoff sign"—a gas-filled segment of transverse colon abruptly ending at the pancreatic inflammation—or linear focal atelectasis of the lower lobe of the lungs with or without pleural effusion
- CT scan can demonstrate an enlarged pancreas and pseudocysts, and can differentiate pancreatitis from other possible intraabdominal catastrophes
- Dynamic intravenous contrast-enhanced CT is of particular value after the first 3 days of severe disease to identify necrotizing pancreatitis and assess prognosis (Table 64); avoid intravenous contrast when the serum creatinine level is >1.5 mg/dL (order MRI instead)
- Ultrasonography is less reliable, but is the initial imaging study required if gallstones are a consideration
- Endoscopic ultrasonography is useful for occult biliary disease (eg, small stones, sludge)

DIAGNOSTIC PROCEDURES

- CT-guided needle aspiration of necrotizing pancreatitis may diagnose infection
- Endoscopic retrograde cholangiopancreatography (ERCP) is generally not indicated after a first attack unless there is associated cholangitis or jaundice. However, aspiration of bile for crystal analysis may demonstrate microlithiasis in apparently idiopathic acute pancreatitis

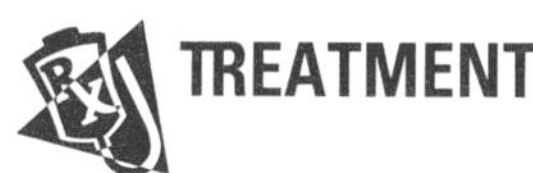

TREATMENT

MEDICATIONS

- Treat pain with meperidine, up to 100–150 mg IM Q 3–4 h as necessary; reduce dose for severe hepatic or renal dysfunction
- No fluid or foods should be given orally until the patient is largely free of pain and has bowel sounds. Begin with clear liquids and gradually advance to a low-fat diet, guided by the patient's tolerance and by absence of pain
- For **severe pancreatitis** large amounts of intravenous fluids are needed to maintain intravascular volume
- Give calcium gluconate intravenously for hypocalcemia with tetany
- Infusions of fresh frozen plasma or serum albumin may be needed for coagulopathy or hypoalbuminemia
- If shock persists after adequate volume replacement (including packed red cells), pressors may be required
- Consider total parenteral nutrition (including lipids) for ileus when there will be no nutrition for at least a week. Enteral nutrition via a jejunal tube is preferable if tolerated
- Imipenem (500 mg every 8 h IV) or possibly cefuroxime (1.5 g IV TID, then 250 mg PO BID), given for sterile pancreatic necrosis, may reduce the risk of pancreatic infection
- The role of intravenous somatostatin is uncertain, but octreotide is not beneficial

SURGERY

- For mild pancreatitis with cholelithiasis, cholecystectomy or cholecystotomy may be justified
- Infected pancreatic necrosis is an absolute indication for surgery
- Operation may improve survival of necrotizing pancreatitis and clinical deterioration with multiorgan failure or lack of resolution by 4–6 weeks

THERAPEUTIC PROCEDURES

- Usually a mild disease that subsides spontaneously within several days
- The pancreatic rest program includes nothing by mouth, bed rest, and nasogastric suction for moderately severe pain, vomiting, or abdominal distention
- When severe pancreatitis results from choledocholithiasis—particularly if jaundice (serum total bilirubin >5 mg/dL) or cholangitis is present—ERCP with endoscopic sphincterotomy and stone extraction is indicated

OUTCOME

FOLLOW-UP

- Close follow-up of white blood cell count, hematocrit, serum electrolytes, serum calcium, serum creatinine, BUN, serum aspartate aminotransferase and lactate dehydrogenase (LDH), and arterial blood gases is mandatory for severely ill patients
- Cultures of blood, urine, sputum, and pleural effusion (if present) and needle aspirations of pancreatic necrosis (with CT guidance) should be obtained
- Following recovery from acute biliary pancreatitis, laparoscopic cholecystectomy is generally performed, although endoscopic sphincterotomy alone may be done

COMPLICATIONS

- Acute tubular necrosis
- Necrotizing pancreatitis
- Acute respiratory distress syndrome (ARDS); cardiac dysfunction may be superimposed
- Pancreatic abscess may develop after 6 or more weeks. It requires prompt percutaneous or surgical drainage
- Treat pancreatic infections with imipenem, 500 mg every 8 h IV
- Pseudocysts less than 6 cm in diameter often resolve spontaneously. They are multiple in 14% of cases. They may become secondarily infected and need drainage. Drainage may also help persisting pain or pancreatitis. Erosion into a blood vessel can result in a major hemorrhage into the cyst
- Pancreatic ascites may present after recovery from acute pancreatitis with absence of frank abdominal pain. Marked elevations in the ascitic protein (>3 g/dL) and amylase (>1000 units/L) levels are typical
- Chronic pancreatitis develops in about 10% of cases. Permanent diabetes mellitus and exocrine pancreatic insufficiency occur uncommonly after a single acute episode

PROGNOSIS

Ranson's criteria

- Helps assess disease severity
- When three or more of the following are present on admission, a severe course complicated by pancreatic necrosis can be predicted with a sensitivity of 60–80%: age over 55 years; white blood cell count over 16,000/μL; blood glucose over 200 mg/dL; serum LDH over 350 units/L; AST over 250 units/L
- Development of the following in the first 48 h indicates a worsening prognosis: hematocrit drop of more than 10 percentage points; BUN rise greater than 5 mg/dL; arterial pO_2 of less than 60 mm Hg; serum calcium of less than 8 mg/dL; base deficit over 4 mEq/L; estimated fluid sequestration of more than 6 L
- Mortality rates correlate with the number of criteria present on admission and within the first 48 h: 0–2, 1%; 3–4, 16%; 5–6, 40%; 7–8, 100%
- Severity can also be assessed using the Acute Physiology and Chronic Health (APACHE) II or III scoring system as well as the CT scan index (Table 64)

WHEN TO REFER

- A surgeon should be consulted in all cases of severe acute pancreatitis

WHEN TO ADMIT

- The patient with severe pancreatitis requires treatment in an intensive care unit

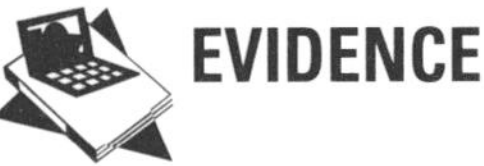

EVIDENCE

PRACTICE GUIDELINES

- National Guideline Clearinghouse
  - http://www.guideline.gov/summary/summary.aspx?doc_id=3257&nbr=2483&string=acute+AND+pancreatitis
- Toouli J et al: Working Party of the Program Committee of the Bangkok World Congress of Gastroenterology 2002. Guidelines for the management of acute pancreatitis. J Gastroenterol Hepatol 2002;17(Suppl):S15. [PMID: 12000591]
- Uhl W et al: International Association of Pancreatology. IAP guidelines for the surgical management of acute pancreatitis. Pancreatology 2002;2:565. [PMID: 12435871]

INFORMATION FOR PATIENTS

- Mayo Clinic
  - http://www.mayoclinic.com/invoke.cfm?id=DS00371
- National Digestive Diseases Information Clearinghouse
  - http://digestive.niddk.nih.gov/ddiseases/pubs/pancreatitis/index.htm
- National Pancreas Association
  - http://www.pancreasfoundation.org/cgi/csNews/csNews.cgi?database=faq%2edb&command=viewone&id=1&op=t

REFERENCES

- Arvanitakis M et al: Computed tomography and magnetic resonance imaging in the assessment of acute pancreatitis. Gastroenterology 2004;126:175. [PMID: 14988825]
- Swaroop VS et al: Severe acute pancreatitis. JAMA 2004;291:2865. [PMID: 15199038]
- Whitcomb DC et al (eds): Pancreatic diseases: novel mechanisms and management. Gastroenterol Clin North Am 2004;33:717.

Author(s)

Lawrence S. Friedman, MD

Pancreatitis, Chronic

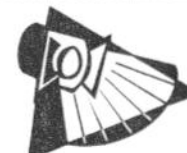

KEY FEATURES

ESSENTIALS OF DIAGNOSIS

- Epigastric pain, steatorrhea, weight loss, abnormal pancreatic imaging
- A mnemonic for the predisposing factors of chronic pancreatitis is TIGAR-O
  - Toxic-metabolic
  - Idiopathic
  - Genetic
  - Autoimmune
  - Recurrent and severe acute pancreatitis
  - Obstructive

GENERAL CONSIDERATIONS

- Occurs most often with alcoholism (70–80% of all cases). The risk of chronic pancreatitis increases with the duration and amount of alcohol consumed, but only 5–10% of heavy drinkers develop pancreatitis
- About 2% of patients with hyperparathyroidism develop pancreatitis
- In tropical Africa and Asia, tropical pancreatitis, related in part to malnutrition, is the most common cause of chronic pancreatitis
- A stricture, stone, or tumor obstructing the pancreas can lead to obstructive chronic pancreatitis
- Autoimmune chronic pancreatitis is associated with hypergammaglobulinemia and is responsive to corticosteroids
- About 10–20% of cases are idiopathic
- The pathogenesis of chronic pancreatitis may be explained by the SAPE (sentinel acute pancreatitis event) hypothesis; a first episode of acute pancreatitis initiates an inflammatory process that results in injury fibrosis

DEMOGRAPHICS

- Genetic factors may predispose to chronic pancreatitis in some of these cases. For example, mutations of the cystic fibrosis transmembrane conductance regulator *(CFTR)* gene have been identified in as many as 50% of patients with idiopathic chronic pancreatitis and no other clinical features of cystic fibrosis, and mutations in the trypsinogen gene (*PRSS 1*) cause hereditary pancreatitis

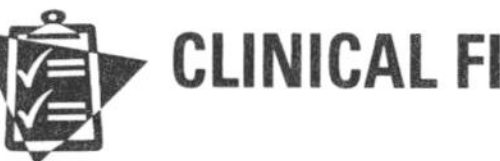

CLINICAL FINDINGS

SYMPTOMS AND SIGNS

- Persistent or recurrent episodes of epigastric and left upper quadrant pain with referral to the upper left lumbar region are typical
- Anorexia, nausea, vomiting, constipation, flatulence, and weight loss are common
- Abdominal signs during attacks consist primarily of tenderness over the pancreas, mild muscle guarding, and paralytic ileus
- Attacks may last only a few hours or as long as 2 weeks; pain may eventually be almost continuous
- Steatorrhea (as indicated by bulky, foul, fatty stools) may occur late in the course

DIFFERENTIAL DIAGNOSIS

- Cholelithiasis
- Diabetes mellitus
- Malabsorption due to other causes
- Intractable duodenal ulcer
- Pancreatic cancer
- Irritable bowel syndrome

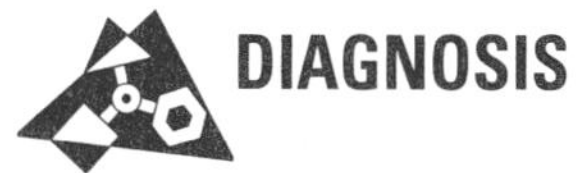

DIAGNOSIS

LABORATORY TESTS

- Serum amylase and lipase may be elevated during acute attacks; normal amylase does not exclude the diagnosis
- Serum alkaline phosphatase and bilirubin may be elevated owing to compression of the common duct
- Glycosuria may be present
- Excess fecal fat may be demonstrated in the stool; pancreatic insufficiency may be confirmed by response to therapy with pancreatic enzyme supplements or a secretin stimulation test if available
- Where available, detection of decreased fecal chymotrypsin or elastase levels may be used to diagnose pancreatic insufficiency, though the tests lack sensitivity and specificity
- Vitamin B_{12} malabsorption is detectable in about 40% of patients, but clinical deficiency of vitamin B_{12} and fat-soluble vitamins is rare
- Accurate genetic tests are available for the major trypsinogen gene mutations

IMAGING STUDIES

- Plain films show calcifications due to pancreaticolithiasis in 30% of patients
- CT may show calcifications not seen on plain films as well as ductal dilation and heterogeneity or atrophy of the gland
- Magnetic resonance cholangiopancreatography (MRCP) and endoscopic ultrasonography (with pancreatic tissue sampling) are promising diagnostic tools
- In autoimmune chronic pancreatitis imaging shows diffuse enlargement of the pancreas and irregular narrowing of the main pancreatic duct

DIAGNOSTIC PROCEDURES

- Endoscopic retrograde cholangiopancreatography is the most sensitive imaging study for chronic pancreatitis and may show dilated ducts, intraductal stones, strictures, or pseudocysts, but the results may be normal in patients with so-called minimal change pancreatitis
- Endoscopic ultrasonography can detect changes of chronic pancreatitis

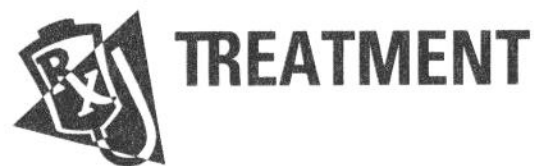

TREATMENT

MEDICATIONS

- Steatorrhea
  - Treat with pancreatic supplements, total dose of 30,000 units of lipase
  - The tablets should be taken at the start of, during, and at the end of a meal
  - Higher doses may be required in some cases
  - Concurrent administration of H_2 receptor antagonists (eg, ranitidine, 150 mg PO twice daily), or a proton pump inhibitor (eg, omeprazole, 20–60 mg daily), or sodium bicarbonate, 650 mg PO before and after meals, decreases the inactivation of lipase by acid and may thereby further decrease steatorrhea
- In selected cases of alcoholic pancreatitis and in cystic fibrosis, enteric-coated microencapsulated preparations may help. However, in cystic fibrosis, high-dose pancreatic enzyme therapy has been associated with strictures of the ascending colon
- Pain secondary to idiopathic chronic pancreatitis may be alleviated by the use of pancreatic enzymes (not enteric-coated) or octreotide, 200 μg subcutaneously three times daily
- Associated diabetes should be treated
- Autoimmune chronic pancreatitis is treated with prednisone 40 mg PO/day for 1–2 months, followed by a taper of 5 mg every 2–4 weeks

SURGERY

- Correctable coexistent biliary tract disease should be treated surgically
- Surgery may be indicated to drain persistent pseudocysts, treat other complications, or relieve pain
- When the pancreatic duct is diffusely dilated, anastomosis between the duct after it is split longitudinally and a defunctionalized limb of jejunum (modified Puestow procedure), in some cases combined with local resection of the head of the pancreas, is associated with relief of pain in 80% of cases
- In advanced cases, subtotal or total pancreatectomy may be considered as a last resort but has variable efficacy and is associated with a high rate of pancreatic insufficiency and diabetes
- Endoscopic or surgical drainage is indicated for symptomatic pseudocysts and those over 6 cm in diameter

THERAPEUTIC PROCEDURES

- A low-fat diet should be prescribed. Alcohol is forbidden because it frequently precipitates attacks. Narcotics should be avoided if possible
- When obstruction of the duodenal end of the duct can be demonstrated by endoscopic retrograde cholangiopancreatography, dilation of the duct or resection of the tail of the pancreas with implantation of the duct may be successful
- Pancreatic ascites or pancreaticopleural fistulas due to a disrupted pancreatic duct can be treated with endoscopic placement of a stent across the duct
- Fragmentation of pancreatic duct stones by lithotripsy and endoscopic removal of stones from the duct, pancreatic sphincterotomy, or pseudocyst drainage may relieve pain in selected patients
- For patients with chronic pain and nondilated ducts, a percutaneous celiac plexus nerve block may be considered under either CT or endoscopic ultrasound guidance, with pain relief in approximately 50% of patients

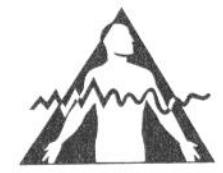

OUTCOME

COMPLICATIONS

- Opioid addiction is common
- Brittle diabetes mellitus, pancreatic pseudocyst or abscess, cholestatic liver enzymes with or without jaundice, common bile duct stricture, steatorrhea, malnutrition, and peptic ulcer
- Pancreatic cancer develops in 4% of patients after 20 years; the risk may relate to tobacco and alcohol use

PROGNOSIS

- In many cases, it is a self-perpetuating disease characterized by chronic pain or recurrent episodes of acute pancreatitis and ultimately by pancreatic exocrine or endocrine insufficiency
- After many years, chronic pain may resolve spontaneously or as a result of surgery tailored to the cause of pain
- Over 80% of adults develop diabetes 25 years after the clinical onset of chronic pancreatitis
- The prognosis is best with recurrent acute pancreatitis caused by a remediable condition such as cholelithiasis, choledocholithiasis, stenosis of the sphincter of Oddi, or hyperparathyroidism
- In alcoholic pancreatitis, pain relief is most likely when a dilated pancreatic duct can be decompressed. In patients with disease not amenable to decompressive surgery, addiction to narcotics is a frequent outcome

PREVENTION

- Abstinence from alcohol
- Medical management of the hyperlipidemia frequently associated with the condition may prevent recurrent attacks of pancreatitis

EVIDENCE

WEB SITE

- Pancreatic Diseases
  - http://chorus.rad.mcw.edu/index/48.html

INFORMATION FOR PATIENTS

- National Digestive Diseases Clearinghouse
  - http://digestive.niddk.nih.gov/ddiseases/pubs/pancreatitis/index.htm
- National Pancreas Foundation
  - http://www.pancreasfoundation.org/cgi/csNews/csNews.cgi?database=faq%2edb&command=viewone&id=2&op=t

REFERENCES

- Baillie J: Pancreatic pseudocysts (Parts I and II). Gastrointest Endosc 2004;59:873 and 2004;60:105. [PMID: 15229441; 15173808]
- Howes N et al: Clinical and genetic characteristics of hereditary pancreatitis in Europe. Clin Gastroenterol Hepatol 2004;2:252. [PMID: 15017610]
- Kim K et al: Autoimmune chronic pancreatitis. Am J Gastroenterol 2004;99:1605. [PMID: 15307882]
- Whitcomb DC: Value of genetic testing in the management of pancreatitis. Gut 2004;53:1710. [PMID: 15479696]

Author(s)

Lawrence S. Friedman, MD

Paragonimiasis

Paracoccidioidomycosis p. 1124. Paralysis, Periodic p. 1125.

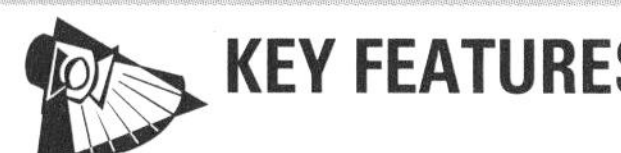

KEY FEATURES

ESSENTIALS OF DIAGNOSIS

- Lung flukes can present with pleuritic pain and hemoptysis
- Acute cerebral infection usually presents as meningitis
- Seizures, cranial neuropathies, and meningoencephalitis can occur from chronic central nervous system infection

GENERAL CONSIDERATIONS

- Many carnivores and omnivores in addition to humans serve as reservoir hosts for the adult fluke (8–16 × 4–8 × 3–5 mm)
- Eggs reaching water, either in sputum or feces, hatch in 3–6 weeks. Released miracidia penetrate and develop in snails. Emergent cercariae encyst as metacercariae in the tissues of crabs and crayfish. Human infection results if metacercariae are ingested when the crustaceans are eaten raw or pickled
- The metacercariae excyst in the small intestine and penetrate the peritoneal cavity. Most migrate through the diaphragm and enter the peripheral lung parenchyma; some may lodge in the brain (about 1% of all cases) or at other ectopic sites
- In the lungs, the parasite becomes encapsulated by granulomatous fibrous tissue, reaching up to 2 cm in diameter. The lesion may rupture, resulting in expectoration of eggs, blood, and inflammatory cells. The prepatent period until appearance of expectorated eggs is about 6 weeks

DEMOGRAPHICS

- *Paragonimus westermani*, the lung fluke, commonly infects humans (estimated 20 million) throughout the Far East; foci are also present in West Africa, South and Southeast Asia, the Pacific Islands, Indonesia, and New Guinea

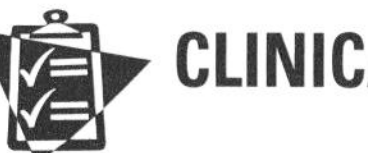

CLINICAL FINDINGS

SYMPTOMS AND SIGNS

- Most pulmonary infections are asymptomatic
- In symptomatic cases, low-grade fever and dry cough are present initially; subsequently, pleuritic pain is common, and a rusty, blood-flecked, viscous sputum or frank hemoptysis may occur
- Acute cerebral infection is uncommon, usually manifested by meningitis
- In chronic central nervous system disease, seizures, cranial neuropathies, or meningoencephalitis may occur; death can follow
- Peritoneal cavity or the intestinal wall infection may cause abdominal pain, diarrhea or dysentery, and a palpable tumor mass
- Migratory subcutaneous nodules (a few millimeters to 1 cm in diameter) occur with about 10% of *P westermani* infections and up to 60% of *Paragonimus skrjabini* infections

DIFFERENTIAL DIAGNOSIS

- Tuberculosis
- *Mycoplasma pneumoniae* infection
- Bacterial pneumonia
- Legionnaire's disease (legionella)
- Amebic lung abscess

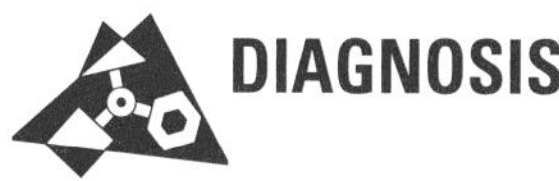

DIAGNOSIS

LABORATORY TESTS

- Pulmonary disease
  - Diagnosed by finding characteristic eggs in sputum (rusty sputum is nearly pathognomonic), feces, bronchoscopic washings, biopsy specimens, or pleural fluid; or adult flukes in subcutaneous nodules or other surgical specimens
  - Eggs not found after multiple direct sputum examinations may be detectable in a 24-h sputum collection processed by alkaline sodium hypochlorite concentration
- Stool examination for eggs has low sensitivity
- Serum and cerebrospinal fluid serological tests (ELISA, 99% sensitivity, 97% specificity; and immunoblot, 96% sensitivity and 99% specificity) do not differentiate active from prior infection; an IgM test may do so
- Most cured patients become seronegative
- Eosinophilia (sometimes marked) and low-grade leukocytosis are common
- Cerebrospinal fluid may be turgid or bloody, with numerous eosinophils, and eggs may be found
- Paragonimiasis and tuberculosis must be differentiated
  - Chest x-ray findings do not make the distinction
  - Since *Paragonimus* ova are destroyed by Ziehl-Neelsen stain for acid-fast bacilli, the sputum should first be examined for the eggs
  - Large number of eosinophils or Charcot-Leyden crystals in sputum suggests paragonimiasis

IMAGING STUDIES

- Pulmonary infection
  - Chest X-ray may show infiltrates, fibrosis, nodules, cavitary lesions, pleural thickening or effusion, or calcifications
  - CT may show round, cystic lesions (5–15 mm) filled with fluid or gas
- Acute cerebral disease
  - CT shows multilocular, ring-like enhancement with surrounding low-density areas
- Chronic cerebral disease
  - Plain skull films often show round or oval-shaped calcifications, sometimes surrounded by low-density areas
- The EEG is almost always abnormal

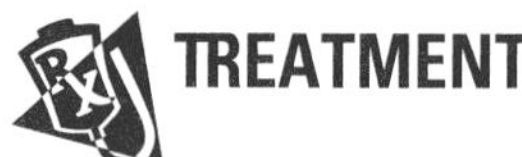

TREATMENT

MEDICATIONS

Pulmonary infection

- Praziquantel is the drug of choice (25 mg/kg PO after meals TID for 3 days, with a 4- to 6-h interval between doses)
- Praziquantel should not be used in regions where there may be concurrent cysticercosis
- Bithionol is the alternative drug [30–50 mg/kg, given on alternate days for 10–15 doses (20–30 days); the daily dose should be divided into a morning and evening dose]
- For both praziquantel and bithionol, gastrointestinal symptoms, headache, and skin rashes may occur but are mild. Serial liver function tests should be done with bithionol treatment
- Bithionol is available in the United States only from the Parasitic Disease Drug Service, Centers for Disease Control, Atlanta, GA 30333
- Antibiotics may be necessary for secondary pulmonary infection
- Triclabendazole, a veterinary fasciolicide that continues under clinical trials, is the second alternative drug for pulmonary disease. Cure rates reach 91% with a dosage of 10 mg/kg daily for 2 days; if treatment is repeated in 3 months, 100% cure rates have been reported

Cerebral infection

- In the acute stage of cerebral paragonimiasis, particularly meningitis, praziquantel or bithionol may be effective
- In the chronic stage, both surgical removal of the parasites and drug usage are likely to be ineffective in diminishing neurological symptoms
- With death of parasites, severe local reactions may occur; corticosteroids should therefore be given as in cerebral cysticercosis

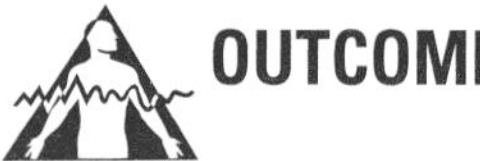

OUTCOME

COMPLICATIONS

- Bronchitis, bronchiectasis, bronchopneumonia, lung abscess, fibrosis, and pleural thickening or effusion may appear

PROGNOSIS

- Cure rates of over 90% can be anticipated for both praziquantel and bithionol

WHEN TO REFER

- All patients should be referred to a clinician with expertise in the diagnosis and management of this disease

WHEN TO ADMIT

- Patients with presumed or confirmed central nervous system infection

EVIDENCE

INFORMATION FOR PATIENTS

- Centers for Disease Control and Prevention
  - http://www.dpd.cdc.gov/dpdx/HTML/Paragonimiasis.htm

REFERENCES

- DeFrain M et al: North American paragonimiasis: case report of a severe clinical infection. Chest 2002;121:1368. [PMID: 11948081]
- Meehan AM et al: Severe pleuropulmonary paragonimiasis 8 years after emigration from a region of endemicity. Clin Infect Dis 2002;35:87. [PMID: 12060881]

Parkinsonism

Paraneoplastic Syndromes p. 1125. Paraphilias p. 1126. Paraquat Poisoning p. 1126. Parasomnias p. 1126.

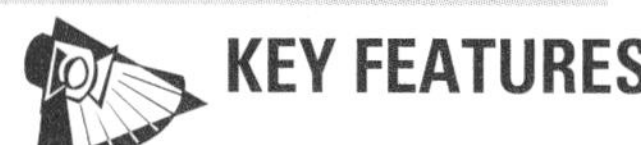

KEY FEATURES

ESSENTIALS OF DIAGNOSIS

- Any combination of tremor, rigidity, bradykinesia, progressive postural instability
- Mild intellectual deterioration may occur

GENERAL CONSIDERATIONS

- Dopamine depletion due to degeneration of the dopaminergic nigrostriatal system leads to an imbalance of dopamine and acetylcholine
- Exposure to toxins can lead to parkinsonism
  - Manganese dust
  - Carbon disulfide
  - Severe carbon monoxide poisoning
  - 1-methyl-4-phenyl-1,2,5,6-tetrahydropyridine (MPTP) for recreational purposes
  - Neuroleptic drugs
  - Reserpine
  - Metoclopramide
- Postencephalitic parkinsonism is becoming increasingly rare
- Only rarely is hemiparkinsonism the presenting feature of a space-occupying lesion

DEMOGRAPHICS

- Common disorder that occurs in all ethnic groups, with an approximately equal sex distribution
- The most common variety, idiopathic Parkinson's disease (paralysis agitans), begins most often in people between ages 45 and 65 years
- May rarely occur on a familial basis

CLINICAL FINDINGS

SYMPTOMS AND SIGNS

- Cardinal features
  - Tremor
  - Rigidity
  - Bradykinesia
  - Postural instability
- Mild decline in intellectual function
- Tremor
  - Four to six cycles per second
  - Most conspicuous at rest
  - Enhanced by stress
  - Often less severe during voluntary activity
  - Commonly confined to one limb or to one side for months or years before becoming more generalized
  - Occasionally involves the lower jaw
- Rigidity causes the flexed posture
- Bradykinesia is the most disabling symptom, ie, a slowness of voluntary movement and a reduction in automatic movements such as swinging of the arms while walking
- The face
  - Relatively immobile with widened palpebral fissures
  - Infrequent blinking
  - A fixity of facial expression
- Mild blepharoclonus
- Repetitive tapping (about twice per second) over the bridge of the nose producing a sustained blink response (Myerson's sign)
- Other findings
  - Saliva drooling from the mouth
  - Soft and poorly modulated voice
  - A variable rest tremor and rigidity in some or all of the limbs
  - Slowness of voluntary movements
  - Impairment of fine or rapidly alternating movements
  - Micrographia
- Typically no muscle weakness and no alteration in the tendon reflexes or plantar responses
- Difficulty rising from a sitting position and beginning to walk
- Gait
  - Small shuffling steps and a loss of the normal automatic arm swing
  - There may be unsteadiness on turning, difficulty in stopping, and a tendency to fall

DIFFERENTIAL DIAGNOSIS

- Different causes of parkinsonism
- Essential tremor
- Depression
- Wilson's disease
- Huntington's disease
- Normal pressure hydrocephalus
- Shy-Drager syndrome
- Progressive supranuclear palsy
- Cortical-basal ganglionic degeneration
- Creutzfeldt-Jakob disease
- Drugs causing parkinsonism: antipsychotic agents, reserpine, metoclopramide

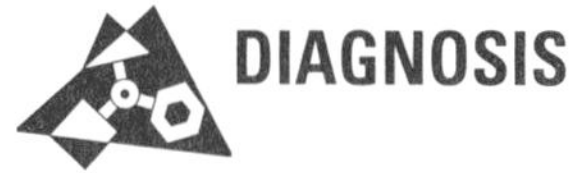

DIAGNOSIS

DIAGNOSTIC PROCEDURES

- Diagnosis is primarily clinical

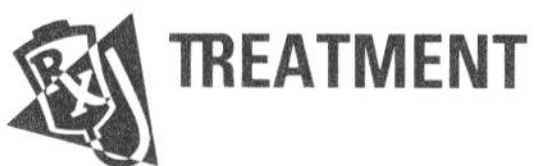

TREATMENT

MEDICATIONS

- **Amantadine,** usual dose (100 mg PO twice daily), may improve all of the clinical features of parkinsonism
- **Anticholinergics** are more helpful for tremor and rigidity than bradykinesia
  - Start with a small dose (Table 100)
  - Contraindicated in patients with prostatic hypertrophy, narrow-angle glaucoma, or obstructive intestinal disease
  - Often tolerated poorly by the elderly
- **Sinemet** is a combination of carbidopa and levodopa in a fixed ratio (1:10 or 1:4)
  - Start with small dose, eg, 1 tablet of Sinemet 25/100 (containing 25 mg of carbidopa and 100 mg of levodopa) three times daily, and gradually increase depending on the response
- Sinemet CR is a controlled-release formulation (containing 25 or 50 mg of carbidopa and 100 or 200 mg of levodopa)
  - Sometimes helpful in reducing fluctuations in clinical response and in reducing the frequency with which medication must be taken
- Pramipexole and ropinirole are two newer dopamine agonists that are not ergot derivatives. In each, the daily dose is built up gradually
  - **Pramipexole**
    - Started at 0.125 mg PO three times daily, doubled after 1 week, and again after another week

- The daily dose is then increased by 0.75 mg at weekly intervals depending on response and tolerance
- Most patients require between 0.5 and 1.5 mg three times daily

– **Ropinirole**
- Begun at 0.25 mg PO three times daily
- The total daily dose is increased at weekly intervals by 0.75 mg until the fourth week and increased by 1.5 mg thereafter
- Most patients require between 2 and 8 mg three times daily

- **Selegiline** is a monoamine oxidase B inhibitor
  - Improves fluctuations or declining response to levodopa
  - Data are inconclusive, but may arrest the progression of Parkinson's disease, which remains an important consideration for patients who are young or have mild disease
- Two catecholamine-*O*-methyltransferase inhibitors, **entacapone** and **tolcapone,** may be used as an adjunct to Sinemet when there are response fluctuations or inadequate responses
  - Entacapone is given as 200 mg PO with each dose of Sinemet
  - Entacapone is generally preferred over tolcapone because acute hepatic failure has occurred with tolcapone
  - Tolcapone is given in a dosage of 100 mg or 200 mg PO three times daily
  - With either preparation, the dose of Sinemet taken concurrently may have to be reduced by up to one-third to avoid side effects
- Confusion and psychotic symptoms often respond to atypical antipsychotic agents, such as olanzapine, quetiapine, risperidone, or clozapine
- **Clozapine** may rarely cause marrow suppression, and weekly blood cell counts are therefore necessary for patients taking it
  - The patient is started on 6.25 mg PO at bedtime
  - The dosage is increased to 25–100 mg/day as needed
  - In low doses, clozapine may also improve iatrogenic dyskinesias
- Bromocriptine and pergolide are dopamine agonists and ergot derivatives. They were widely used until recently, but have been replaced by newer agents because of rare reports of pericardial, pleural, or pulmonary fibrosis, and increasing concerns about cardiac valvopathy associated with pergolide use

SURGERY

- Thalamotomy or pallidotomy may be helpful for patients unresponsive to medical treatment or who have intolerable side effects
- High-frequency bilateral stimulation of the subthalamic nuclei or globus pallidus internus may benefit all the major features of the disease, and it has a lower morbidity than lesion surgery

THERAPEUTIC PROCEDURES

- Drug therapy may not be required early
- Physical and speech therapy and simple aids to daily living may help, such as
  - Rails or banisters placed strategically about the home
  - Special table cutlery with large handles
  - Nonslip rubber table mats
  - Devices to amplify the voice

OUTCOME

COMPLICATIONS

- Levodopa-induced dyskinesias may take any form, including chorea, athetosis, dystonia, tremor, tics, and myoclonus
- Later complications of the drug include the "on-off phenomenon"
  - Abrupt but transient fluctuations in the severity of parkinsonism occur unpredictably but frequently during the day
  - The "off" period of marked bradykinesia has been shown to relate in some instances to falling plasma levels of levodopa.
  - During the "on" phase, dyskinesias are often conspicuous but mobility is increased
  - Because of this complication, levodopa therapy should be postponed and dopamine agonists used instead, except in the elderly

WHEN TO REFER

- When expertise is needed to determine when to begin therapy
- Consultation with a practitioner with expertise in management may help when there is progressive disease despite appropriate therapy
- For physical and speech therapy

EVIDENCE

PRACTICE GUIDELINES

- Miyasaki JM et al: Practice parameter: initiation of treatment for Parkinson's disease: an evidence-based review: report of the Quality Standards Subcommittee of the American Academy of Neurology. Neurology 2002;58(1):11

INFORMATION FOR PATIENTS

- JAMA patient page: Parkinson disease. JAMA 2004;291:390
- National Institute of Neurological Disorders and Stroke
  - http://www.ninds.nih.gov/disorders/parkinsons_disease/parkinsons_disease.htm

REFERENCES

- Christine CW et al: Clinical differentiation of parkinsonian syndromes: prognostic and therapeutic relevance. Am J Med 2004;117:412. [PMID:15380498]
- Krack P et al: Five-year follow-up of bilateral stimulation of the subthalamic nucleus in advanced Parkinsons disease. N Engl J Med 2003;349:1925. [PMID:14614167]
- Miyasaki JM et al: Practice parameter: initiation of treatment for Parkinson's disease. An evidence-based review. Neurology 2002;58:11. [PMID:11781398]
- Samii A et al: Parkinson's disease. Lancet 2004;363:1783. [PMID:15172778]
- Siderowf A et al: Update on Parkinson disease. Ann Intern Med 2003;138:651. [PMID:12693888]

Author(s)

Michael J. Aminoff, MD, DSc, FRCP

Pediculosis

Parvovirus p. 1127. Patellofemoral Syndrome p. 1127. Patent Ductus Arteriosus p. 1127.

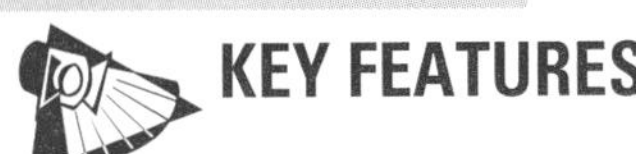

KEY FEATURES

ESSENTIALS OF DIAGNOSIS

- Pruritus with excoriation
- Nits on hair shafts; lice on skin or clothes
- Occasionally, sky-blue macules (maculae ceruleae) on the inner thighs or lower abdomen in pubic louse infestation

GENERAL CONSIDERATIONS

- A parasitic infestation of the skin of the scalp, trunk, or pubic areas
- **Head lice**
  - May be transmitted by shared use of hats or combs
  - Are epidemic among children of all socioeconomic classes in elementary schools
  - Very uncommon among black children
  - Adults with head lice almost always acquire their infestation from elementary school-aged children, so a source of infection must always be sought
- **Body lice**
  - Usually occur among people who live in overcrowded dwellings with inadequate hygiene facilities
  - Trench fever, relapsing fever, and typhus are transmitted by the body louse in countries where those diseases are endemic
- **Pubic lice** may be acquired by sexual transmission

CLINICAL FINDINGS

SYMPTOMS AND SIGNS

- See Table 7
- Head and body lice are similar in appearance and are 3–4 mm long
- **Head lice**
  - Can be found on the scalp or may be manifested as small nits resembling pussy willow buds on the scalp hairs close to the skin
  - They are easiest to see above the ears and at the nape of the neck
- **Body lice**
  - Itching may be very intense
  - Scratching may result in deep excoriations, especially over the upper shoulders, posterior flanks, and neck
  - In some cases, only itching is present, with few excoriations seen

DIFFERENTIAL DIAGNOSIS

- **Head lice**
  - Seborrheic dermatitis
  - Impetigo
  - Hair casts (hair debris)
- **Body lice**
  - Scabies
  - Impetigo
  - Dermatitis herpetiformis
  - Urticaria
- **Pubic lice**
  - Anogenital pruritus
  - Scabies
  - Atopic dermatitis (eczema)

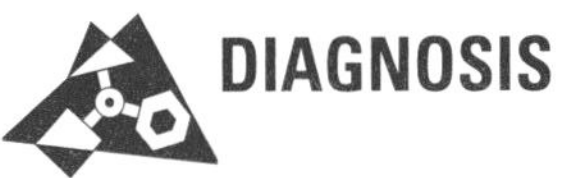

DIAGNOSIS

LABORATORY TESTS

- Relies on an index of suspicion and isolating the organism
- The body louse can seldom be found on the body, because the insect comes onto the skin only to feed and must be looked for in the seams of the clothing

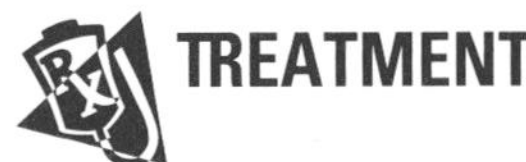

TREATMENT

MEDICATIONS

- See Table 6

Head lice

- Permethrin 1% cream rinse (Nix) is the treatment of choice; it is applied to the scalp and hair and left on for 30 min to 8 h before being rinsed off; treatment should be repeated in 1 week
- Five percent permethrin lotion may be used in refractory cases
- Permethrin 1% cream (Nix) is more effective than synergized pyrethrins (RID), OTC products that are applied undiluted until the infested areas are entirely wet; after 10 min, the areas are washed thoroughly with warm water and soap and then dried
- Malathion lotion 1% (Ovide) is very effective, but it is highly volatile and flammable, so application must be done in a well-ventilated room or outdoors
- For involvement of eyelashes, petrolatum is applied thickly twice daily for 8 days, and remaining nits are then plucked off

Pubic lice

- Lindane lotion or cream (Kwell, Scabene) is used; a thin layer is applied to the infested and adjacent hairy areas; it is removed after 8 h by thorough washing
- Permethrin rinse 1% for 10 min and permethrin cream 5% applied for 8 h are effective alternatives

THERAPEUTIC PROCEDURES

- Body lice are treated by disposing of the infested clothing
- Sexual contacts should be treated
- Clothes and bedclothes should be washed and dried at high temperature if possible

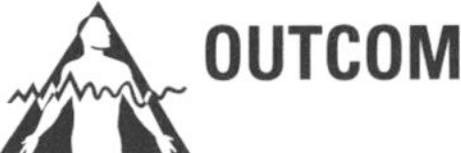

OUTCOME

WHEN TO REFER

- If there is a question about the diagnosis, if recommended therapy is ineffective, or specialized treatment is necessary

EVIDENCE

PRACTICE GUIDELINES

- Centers for Disease Control and Prevention: Ectoparasitic infections. Sexually transmitted diseases treatment guidelines, 2002
  - http://www.guideline.gov/summary/summary.aspx?doc_id=3245&nbr=2471
- National Guideline Clearinghouse
  - http://www.guideline.gov/summary/summary.aspx?d

WEB SITE

- Centers for Disease Control and Prevention: Head Lice Professional Information
  - http://www.dpd.cdc.gov/dpdx/HTML/HeadLice.htm

INFORMATION FOR PATIENTS

- Centers for Disease Control and Prevention: Body Lice
  - http://www.cdc.gov/ncidod/dpd/parasites/lice/factsht_body_lice.htm
- Centers for Disease Control and Prevention: Head Lice Infestation
  - http://www.cdc.gov/ncidod/dpd/parasites/headlice/factsht_head_lice.htm
- Centers for Disease Control and Prevention: Pubic Lice Infestation
  - http://www.cdc.gov/ncidod/dpd/parasites/lice/factsht_pubic_lice.htm
- Medline Plus: Head Lice
  - http://www.nlm.nih.gov/medlineplus/ency/article/000840.htm
- Medline Plus: Pubic Lice
  - http://www.nlm.nih.gov/medlineplus/ency/article/000841.htm

REFERENCES

- Dodd CS: Interventions for treating headlice. Cochrane Database Syst Rev 2001;(3):CD001165. [PMID: 11686980]
- Huynh TH et al: Scabies and pediculosis. Dermatol Clin 2004;22:7. [PMID: 15018005]

Author(s)

Timothy G. Berger, MD

Pelvic Inflammatory Disease (PID)

KEY FEATURES

ESSENTIALS OF DIAGNOSIS

- Lower abdominal, adnexal, or cervical motion tenderness
- Absence of a competing diagnosis

GENERAL CONSIDERATIONS

- A polymicrobial infection of the upper genital tract associated with the sexually transmitted organisms *Neisseria gonorrhoeae* and *Chlamydia trachomatis*, endogenous organisms, including anaerobes, *Haemophilus influenzae*, enteric gram-negative rods, and streptococci
- Tuberculous salpingitis is rare in the United States but more common in developing countries; it is characterized by pelvic pain and irregular pelvic masses not responsive to antibiotic therapy. It is not sexually transmitted

DEMOGRAPHICS

- Most common in young, nulliparous, sexually active women with multiple partners
- Other risk markers include nonwhite race, douching, and smoking
- The use of oral contraceptives or barrier methods of contraception may provide significant protection

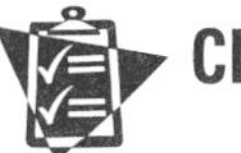

CLINICAL FINDINGS

SYMPTOMS AND SIGNS

- Symptoms may include lower abdominal pain, chills and fever, menstrual disturbances, purulent cervical discharge, and cervical and adnexal tenderness
- Right upper quadrant pain (Fitz-Hugh and Curtis syndrome) may indicate an associated perihepatitis
- Diagnosis is complicated by the fact that many women have mild symptoms, not readily recognized as PID

Minimum diagnostic criteria

- Lower abdominal, adnexal, or cervical motion tenderness should be treated as PID with antibiotics unless there is a competing diagnosis such as ectopic pregnancy or appendicitis
- The following criteria may be used to enhance the specificity of the diagnosis
  - Oral temperature > 38.3°C
  - Abnormal cervical or vaginal discharge with white cells on saline microscopy
  - Elevated erythrocyte sedimentation rate
  - Elevated C-reactive protein
  - Laboratory documentation of cervical infection with *N gonorrhoeae* or *C trachomatis* awaiting results

Definitive criteria

- When the clinical or laboratory evidence is uncertain, the following criteria may be used:
  - Histopathologic evidence of endometritis on endometrial biopsy
  - Transvaginal sonography or other imaging techniques showing thickened fluid-filled tubes with or without free pelvic fluid or tuboovarian complex
  - Laparoscopic abnormalities consistent with PID

DIFFERENTIAL DIAGNOSIS

- Ectopic pregnancy
- Appendicitis
- Septic abortion
- Ruptured ovarian cyst or tumor
- Ovarian torsion
- Tuboovarian abscess
- Degeneration of leiomyoma (fibroid)
- Diverticulitis
- Cystitis
- Tuberculous salpingitis
- Actinomycosis with prolonged intrauterine device use

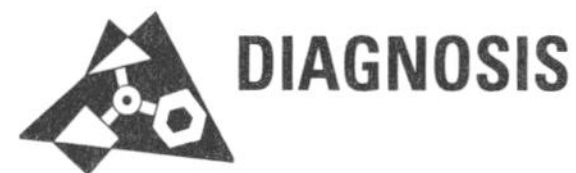

DIAGNOSIS

LABORATORY TESTS

- Abnormal cervical or vaginal discharge may show white blood cells on saline microscopy
- Endocervical culture for *N gonorrhoeae* and saline wet mount for *C trachomatis*
- Erythrocyte sedimentation rate and C-reactive protein may be elevated

IMAGING STUDIES

- Pelvic and vaginal ultrasound can differentiate ectopic pregnancy of over 6 weeks

DIAGNOSTIC PROCEDURES

- Culdocentesis will differentiate hemoperitoneum (ruptured ectopic pregnancy or hemorrhagic cyst) from pelvic sepsis (salpingitis, ruptured pelvic abscess, or ruptured appendix)
- Laparoscopy can diagnose PID, and it is imperative if the diagnosis is not certain or if the patient has not responded to antibiotic therapy after 48 h. The appendix should be visualized at laparoscopy to rule out appendicitis. Cultures obtained at the time of laparoscopy are often helpful

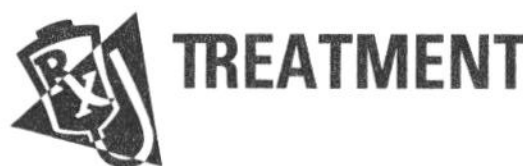

TREATMENT

MEDICATIONS

- Antibiotic treatment should not be delayed while awaiting culture results
- The sexual partner should be examined and treated appropriately

Inpatient regimens

- Cefoxitin, 2 g IV Q 6 h, or cefotetan, 2 g Q 12 h, plus doxycycline, 100 mg IV or PO Q 12 h. This regimen is continued for at least 24 h after there is significant clinical improvement. Doxycycline, 100 mg twice daily, should be continued to complete a total of 14 days of therapy
- Clindamycin, 900 mg IV Q 8 h, plus gentamicin IV in a loading dose of 2 mg/kg followed by 1.5 mg/kg Q 8 h. This regimen is continued for at least 24 h after there is significant clinical improvement and is followed by either clindamycin, 450 mg four times daily, or doxycycline, 100 mg twice daily, to complete a total of 14 days of therapy

Outpatient regimens

- Ofloxacin, 400 mg PO BID for 14 days, or levofloxacin, 500 mg PO QD for 14 days, plus metronidazole, 500 mg PO BID, for 14 days
- Either a single dose of cefoxitin, 2 g IM, with probenecid, 1 g PO, or ceftriaxone, 250 mg IM, plus doxycycline, 100 mg PO BID, for 14 days with or without metronidazole, 500 mg PO BID for 14 days

SURGERY

- Tuboovarian abscesses may require surgical excision or transcutaneous or transvaginal aspiration
- Unilateral adnexectomy is acceptable for unilateral abscess
- Hysterectomy and bilateral salpingo-oophorectomy may be necessary for overwhelming infection or in cases of chronic disease with intractable pelvic pain

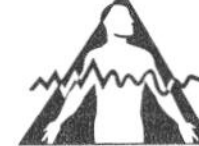

OUTCOME

FOLLOW-UP

- Inpatient therapy for tuboovarian abscess should be monitored by ultrasound

COMPLICATIONS

- In spite of treatment, one-fourth of women with acute disease develop long-term sequelae, including repeated episodes of infection, chronic pelvic pain, dyspareunia, ectopic pregnancy, or infertility
- The risk of infertility increases with repeated episodes of salpingitis: it is estimated at 10% after the first episode, 25% after a second episode, and 50% after a third episode

PROGNOSIS

- Early treatment with effective antibiotcs is essential to prevent long-term sequelae
- For tuboovarian abscess, unless rupture is suspected, high-dose antibiotic therapy in the hospital is effective in 70% of cases. In 30%, there is inadequate response in 48–72 h, and surgical intervention is required

WHEN TO ADMIT

- Admit for IV antibiotic therapy if
  - Surgical emergencies, such as appendicitis, cannot be ruled out
  - Patient has a tuboovarian abscess
  - Patient is pregnant
  - Patient is unable to follow or tolerate an outpatient regimen
  - Patient has not responded clinically to outpatient therapy
  - Patient has severe illness, nausea and vomiting, or high fever
  - Patient is immunodeficient (ie, has HIV infection with low CD4 counts, is taking immunosuppressive therapy, or has another immunosuppressing disease)
- Outpatient parenteral therapy is available in some settings and may be an acceptable alternative
- Patients with tuboovarian abscesses should have direct inpatient observation for at least 24 h prior to switching to outpatient parenteral therapy

EVIDENCE

PRACTICE GUIDELINES

- Centers for Disease Control and Prevention. Pelvic inflammatory disease. Sexually transmitted diseases treatment guidelines. MMWR Recomm Rep 2002;51:48-52.
  - http://www.guideline.gov/summary/summary.aspx?doc_id=3238&nbr=2464

INFORMATION FOR PATIENTS

- American Academy of Family Physicians: Pelvic Inflammatory Disease
  - http://familydoctor.org/213.xml
- American College of Obstetricians and Gynecologists: Pelvic Inflammatory Disease
  - http://www.medem.com/MedLB/article_detaillb.cfm?article_ID=ZZZAB51P97C&sub_cat=9
- MedlinePlus: Pelvic Inflammatory Disease
  - http://www.nlm.nih.gov/medlineplus/ency/article/000888.htm
- National Women's Health Information Center: Pelvic Inflammatory Disease
  - http://www.4woman.gov/faq/stdpids.htm

REFERENCES

- Ness RB et al: Effectiveness of outpatient strategies for women with pelvic inflammatory disease: results from the Pelvic Inflammatory Disease Evaluation and Clinical Health (PEACH) Randomized Trial. Am J Obstet Gynecol 2002;186:929. [PMID: 12015517]
- Sexually transmitted disease treatment guidelines 2002. Centers for Disease Control and Prevention. MMWR Recomm Rep 2002;51(RR-6):1. [PMID: 12184549]

Author(s)

H. Trent MacKay, MD, MPH

Pemphigus

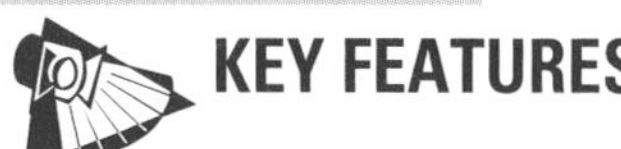

KEY FEATURES

ESSENTIALS OF DIAGNOSIS

- Relapsing crops of skin bullae
- Often preceded by mucous membrane bullae, erosions, and ulcerations
- Superficial detachment of the skin after pressure or trauma variably present (Nikolsky's sign)
- Acantholysis on biopsy
- Immunofluorescence studies are confirmatory

GENERAL CONSIDERATIONS

- There are several forms of pemphigus
  - Pemphigus vulgaris and its variant, pemphigus vegetans
  - Pemphigus foliaceus, which is more superficially blistering, and its variant, pemphigus erythematosus
- Pemphigus is an uncommon intraepidermal blistering disease occurring on skin and mucous membranes
- Caused by autoantibodies to adhesion molecules in the desmosomal complex expressed in the skin and mucous membranes
- Autoantibodies cause acantholysis, the separation of epidermal cells from each other
- The cause is unknown
- Drug-induced autoimmune pemphigus from drugs including penicillamine and captopril has been reported
- More than 95% of patients with pemphigus vulgaris are positive for HLA-DR4/DQw3 or HLA-DRw6/DQw1

DEMOGRAPHICS

- All forms may occur at any age but most commonly in middle age

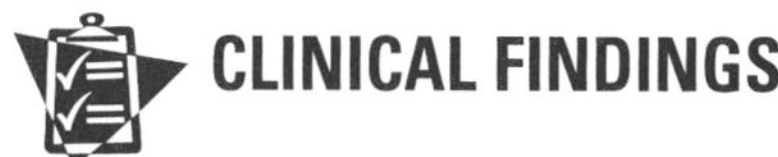

CLINICAL FINDINGS

SYMPTOMS AND SIGNS

- See Table 7
- An insidious onset of flaccid bullae in crops or waves
- The bullae appear spontaneously and are tender and painful when they rupture
- In pemphigus vulgaris, lesions often appear first on the oral mucous membranes, and these rapidly become erosive
- In some cases, erosions and crusts predominate over blisters
- The scalp is another site of early involvement
- Rubbing a cotton swab or finger laterally on the surface of uninvolved skin may cause easy separation of the epidermis (Nikolsky's sign)
- If the lesions become extensive, the complications of the disease lead to great toxicity and debility

DIFFERENTIAL DIAGNOSIS

- Erythema multiforme major or toxic epidermal necrolysis
- Drug eruptions
- Bullous impetigo
- Contact dermatitis
- Dermatitis herpetiformis
- Bullous pemphigoid
- Cicatricial pemphigoid
- Paraneoplastic pemphigus
- Linear IgA dermatosis
- Pemphigus foliaceus
- Porphyria cutanea tarda
- Epidermolysis bullosa
- Staphylococcus scalded skin syndrome
- Herpes gestationis
- Graft-versus-host disease

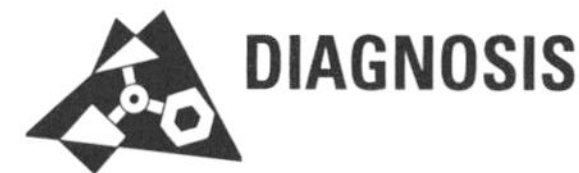

DIAGNOSIS

LABORATORY TESTS

- The diagnosis is made by light microscopy and by direct and indirect immunofluorescence microscopy
- Microscopically, acantholysis is the hallmark of pemphigus, but in some patients there may be eosinophilic spongiosis initially
- Immunofluorescence microscopy shows deposits of IgG intercellularly in the epidermis; C3 and other immunoglobulins and complement components may be present on occasion
- Indirect immunofluorescence microscopy to detect circulating pemphigus antibodies is not necessary for the diagnosis, but antibody titers in some patients may correspond with disease activity and might help in management

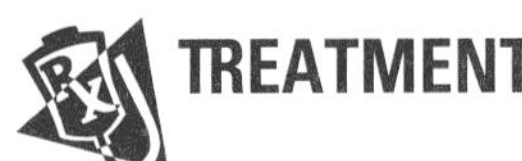

TREATMENT

MEDICATIONS

- See Table 6
- Local measures
  - In patients with limited disease, skin and mucous membrane lesions should be treated with topical corticosteroids
  - Complicating infection requires appropriate systemic and local antibiotic therapy
- Systemic measures
  - Initial therapy is with systemic steroids: prednisone, 60–80 mg daily
  - In all but the most mild cases, a steroid-sparing agent is added from the beginning, since the course of the disease is long and the steroid-sparing agents take several weeks to exert their activity
  - Azathioprine (100 mg daily) or mycophenolate mofetil (1 g twice daily) is used most frequently, the latter seeming to be the most reliable and recommended for most cases
- In refractory cases, monthly IGIV at 2 g/kg intravenously over 3 days is useful and has replaced high-dose steroids plus cyclophosphamide and pulse intravenous steroids as rescue therapy
- In pemphigus foliaceus and mild cases of pemphigus vulgaris, tetracycline, 500 mg, and nicotinamide, 500 mg, three times daily, may be tried
- Dapsone may also be tried as a steroid-sparing agent, especially in pemphigus foliaceus

THERAPEUTIC PROCEDURES

- When the disease is severe, hospitalize the patient at bed rest and provide antibiotics and intravenous feedings as indicated
- Anesthetic troches used before eating ease painful oral lesions

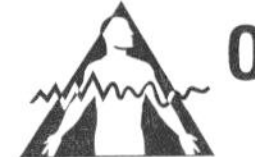

OUTCOME

COMPLICATIONS

- Secondary infection is a major cause of morbidity and mortality
- Disturbances of fluid and electrolyte balance can occur owing to losses through the involved skin in severe cases

PROGNOSIS

- The course tends to be chronic in most patients, though some appear to experience remission
- Infection is the most frequent cause of death, usually from *Staphylococcus aureus* septicemia

WHEN TO REFER

- If there is a question about the diagnosis, if recommended therapy is ineffective, or if specialized treatment is necessary

WHEN TO ADMIT

- For severe disease

EVIDENCE

PRACTICE GUIDELINES

- Harman KE et al: British Association of Dermatologists. Guidelines for the management of pemphigus vulgaris. Br J Dermatol 2003;149:926. [PMID: 14632796]

WEB SITE

- American Academy of Dermatology
  - http://www.aad.org

INFORMATION FOR PATIENTS

- International Pemphigus Foundation: What is Pemphigus?
  - http://www.pemphigus.org/whatisgus.html
- MedlinePlus: Pemphigus Vulgaris
  - http://www.nlm.nih.gov/medlineplus/ency/article/000882.htm

REFERENCES

- Bystryn JC et al: Treatment of pemphigus with intravenous immunoglobulin. J Am Acad Dermatol 2002;47:358. [PMID: 12196744]
- Sami N et al: Influence of IVIG therapy on autoantibody titers to desmoglein 1 in patients with pemphigus foliaceus. Clin Immunol 2002;105:192. [PMID: 12482393]

Author(s)

Timothy G. Berger, MD

Penicillium marneffei Infection p. 1128

Peptic Ulcer Disease

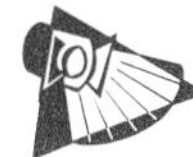

KEY FEATURES

ESSENTIALS OF DIAGNOSIS

- Peptic ulcer is a break in the gastric or duodenal mucosa, extending through the muscularis mucosae, and usually >5 mm in diameter
- Nonspecific epigastric pain in 80–90% with variable relationship to meals
- Ulcer symptoms characterized by rhythmicity and periodicity
- Ulcer complications without antecedent symptoms in 10–20%
- Of nonsteroidal antiinflammatory drug (NSAID)-induced ulcers, 30–50% are asymptomatic
- Upper endoscopy with antral biopsy for *Helicobacter pylori* is diagnostic
- Gastric ulcer biopsy or documentation of complete healing is necessary to exclude gastric malignancy

GENERAL CONSIDERATIONS

- Ulcers are 5 times more common in the duodenum than in the stomach
- In the stomach, benign ulcers are most common in the antrum (60%) and at the junction of the antrum and body on the lesser curvature (25%)
- Major causes of peptic ulcer disease: NSAIDs, chronic *H pylori* infection, and acid hypersecretory states such as Zollinger-Ellison syndrome
- Up to 10% of ulcers are idiopathic
- Prevalence of *H pylori* infection in duodenal ulcer patients is ~75–90%, but only ~1 in 6 chronically infected persons develops an ulcer
- Prevalence of gastric ulcers is 10–20% and duodenal ulcers is 2–5% in chronic NSAID users
- In NSAID users, relative risk of gastric ulcers is increased 40-fold, but risk of duodenal ulcers is only slightly increased
- *H pylori* infection increases risk of NSAID-induced ulcers and complications

DEMOGRAPHICS

- In the United States, ~500,000 new cases and 4 million ulcer recurrences per year
- Incidence of duodenal ulcers is declining, while that of gastric ulcers is increasing
- Lifetime prevalence of ulcers in adults is ~10%
- Gastric ulcers are slightly more common in men than in women (1.3:1)
- Duodenal ulcers are most common between the ages of 30 and 55
- Gastric ulcers are most common between the ages of 55 and 70
- Peptic ulcers are more common in smokers

CLINICAL FINDINGS

SYMPTOMS AND SIGNS

- Epigastric pain (dyspepsia), not severe, in 80–90%
- Ulcer complications such as bleeding with no antecedent symptoms ("silent ulcers") in 20%
- Pain is relieved by food or antacids in ~50%
- Nocturnal pain awakens two-thirds of patients with duodenal ulcers and one-third of patients with gastric ulcers
- Most patients have symptomatic periods lasting several weeks with intervals of months to years in which they are pain free (periodicity)
- Nausea and anorexia
- Significant vomiting and weight loss suggest gastric outlet obstruction or gastric malignancy
- Physical examination often normal
- Mild, localized epigastric tenderness to deep palpation

DIFFERENTIAL DIAGNOSIS

- Functional or nonulcer dyspepsia
- Gastritis, eg, NSAIDs, alcohol, stress, *H pylori*, pernicious anemia
- Biliary disease or pancreatitis
- Gastroesophageal reflux disease or reflux esophagitis
- "Indigestion" from overeating, high-fat foods, coffee
- Gastric or pancreatic cancer
- Angina pectoris
- Severe pain: esophageal rupture, gastric volvulus, ruptured aortic aneurysm

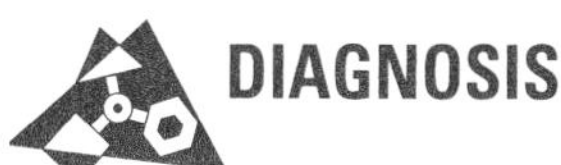

DIAGNOSIS

LABORATORY TESTS

- Anemia from acute blood loss with bleeding ulcer
- Fecal occult blood test positive in one-third
- Leukocytosis suggests ulcer penetration or perforation
- Elevated serum amylase suggests ulcer penetration into the pancreas
- Obtain fasting serum gastrin level to screen for Zollinger-Ellison syndrome

***Noninvasive testing for* H pylori**

- Serological, fecal antigen, or urea breath tests
- Rapid, office-based serological tests have lower sensitivity and specificity (75–90%) than laboratory-based serological ELISA test (sensitivity and specificity of >90%), but positive ELISA test does not necessarily indicate active infection
- After eradication with antibiotics, ELISA antibody levels decline to undetectable in 50% of patients by 12–18 months
- Fecal antigen immunoassay has sensitivity and specificity of 90%; positive test indicates active infection
- ^{13}C-urea breath test has sensitivity and specificity of 90%; positive test indicates active infection
- Proton pump inhibitors significantly reduce the sensitivity of fecal antigen and urea breath tests (but not serological tests); discontinue 14 days prior to testing

***Endoscopic testing for* H pylori**

- Gastric biopsy specimens can detect *H pylori* organisms by histology and active infection by urease production
- Urease test has sensitivity and specificity of 90%

IMAGING STUDIES

- Barium upper gastrointestinal series has limited accuracy in distinguishing benign from malignant gastric ulcers

DIAGNOSTIC PROCEDURES

- Upper endoscopy has better diagnostic accuracy than barium radiography
- Biopsy indicated for the presence of *H pylori* infection and malignancy
- With benign-appearing gastric ulcers, cytological brushings and biopsies of the ulcer margin reveal that 3–5% are malignant
- Nonhealing gastric ulcers may be malignant
- Duodenal ulcers are rarely malignant and do not require biopsy

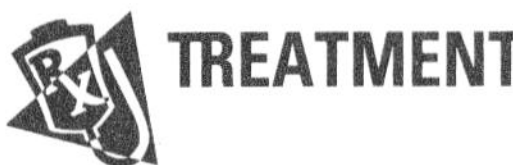

TREATMENT

MEDICATIONS

- See Table 55

Peptic ulcers with active* H pylori *infection

- Acute treatment for 10–14 days with one of the following
- "Triple-therapy" regimens
  - Proton pump inhibitor before meals: omeprazole, 20 mg PO BID, rabeprazole, 20 mg PO BID, lansoprazole, 30 mg PO BID, pantoprazole, 40 mg PO BID, or esomeprazole, 40 mg PO QD plus clarithromycin, 500 mg PO BID, and amoxicillin, 1 g PO BID *or* metronidazole, 500 mg PO BID (in penicillin-allergic patients)
- "Quadruple-therapy" regimens
  - Proton pump inhibitor before meals: omeprazole, 20 mg PO BID, rabeprazole, 20 mg PO BID, lansoprazole, 30 mg PO BID, pantoprazole, 40 mg PO BID, or esomeprazole 40 mg QD, plus bismuth subsalicylate, 2 tablets PO QID, plus tetracycline, 500 mg PO QID, plus metronidazole 250 mg PO QID; recommended for patients who fail an initial attempt at eradication with triple therapy
- Continue treatment for 4–8 weeks with proton pump inhibitor: omeprazole, 20 mg PO QD, rabeprazole, 20 mg PO QD, lansoprazole, 30 mg PO QD, or pantoprazole, 40 mg PO QD or esomeprazole, 40 mg QD

Peptic ulcers with no* H pylori *infection

- Proton pump inhibitors—omeprazole or rabeprazole, 20 mg PO QD, lansoprazole, 15–30 mg PO QD, pantoprazole, 40 mg PO QD, or esomeprazole, 40 mg QD given 30 min before breakfast heals >90% of duodenal ulcers after 4 weeks and 90% of gastric ulcers after 8 weeks
- H_2 receptor antagonists may be used as a less expensive alternative to proton pump inhibitors—ranitidine, 300 mg PO QHS, nizatidine, 300 mg PO QHS, famotidine, 40 mg PO QHS, or cimetidine, 800 mg PO QHS heals 85–90% of duodenal and gastric ulcers within 6 and 8 weeks, respectively
- Chronic "maintenance" therapy indicated in patients with recurrent ulcers who are *H pylori* negative, who have failed attempts at eradication therapy, or who require chronic therapy with NSAIDs or low dose aspirin; proton pump inhibitors: omeprazole, 20 mg PO QD, rabeprazole, 20 mg PO QD, lansoprazole, 30 mg PO QD, esomeprazole, 40 mg PO QD, pantoprazole, 40 mg PO QD; or H_2 receptor antagonist: cimetidine, 400–800 mg PO QHS, nizatidine or ranitidine, 150–300 mg PO QHS, famotidine, 20–40 mg PO QHS

SURGERY

- For complications of peptic ulcer disease, including perforation, penetration, gastric outlet obstruction, and bleeding that cannot be controlled with endoscopic therapy

THERAPEUTIC PROCEDURES

- Moderate alcohol intake
- Discontinue smoking
- Discontinue NSAIDs when possible

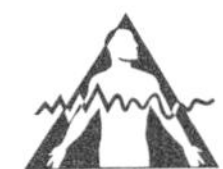

OUTCOME

FOLLOW-UP

- Repeat biopsies after 2–3 months of therapy if gastric ulcers do not heal

COMPLICATIONS

- See Peptic Ulcer Disease, Complications

PROGNOSIS

- If *H pylori* is not eradicated, 85% of patients will have ulcer recurrence within 1 year, half symptomatic; if successfully eradicated, recurrence rates are reduced dramatically to 5–20% at 1 year

WHEN TO REFER

- Patients with persistent dyspepsia after 1–2 weeks of medical treatment
- Complications of peptic ulcer disease

WHEN TO ADMIT

- Complications of peptic ulcer disease

PREVENTION

- To prevent NSAID-induced ulcers: consider the following options
  - Co-therapy with proton pump inhibitors: omeprazole 20 mg PO QD, rabeprazole, 20 mg PO QD, lansoprazole, 30 mg PO QD, pantoprazole 40 mg PO QD, or esomeprazole, 40 mg PO QD
  - Co-therapy with misoprostol, 100–200 μg PO QID; causes diarrhea in 10–20%
  - Substitute COX-2 selective NSAID (celecoxib, meloxicam, etodolac) for nonselective NSAID; may be associated with higher risk of cardiovascular disease

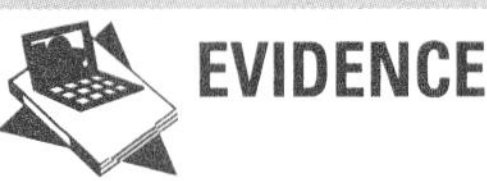

EVIDENCE

PRACTICE GUIDELINES

- Dubois RW et al: Guidelines for the appropriate use of non-steroidal anti-inflammatory drugs, cyclo-oxygenase-2-specific inhibitors and proton pump inhibitors in patients requiring chronic anti-inflammatory therapy. Aliment Pharmacol Ther 2004;20:1. [PMID: 14723611]
- National Guideline Clearinghouse
  - http://www.guideline.gov/summary/summary.aspx?doc_id=2947&nbr=2173&string=peptic+AND+ulcer+AND+disease
  - http://www.guideline.gov/summary/summary.aspx?doc_id=3557&nbr=2783&string=ulcer

WEB SITES

- National Digestive Diseases Information Clearinghouse
  - http://digestive.niddk.nih.gov/ddiseases/pubs/bleeding/index.htm
- WebPath Gastrointestinal Pathology Index
  - http://medstat.med.utah.edu/WebPath/GIHTML/GIIDX.html

INFORMATION FOR PATIENTS

- JAMA Patient Page: Peptic ulcers. JAMA 2001;286:2052. [PMID: 11693148]
- Mayo Clinic
  - http://www.mayoclinic.com/invoke.cfm?id=DS00242
- Medline Plus Medical Encyclopedia
  - http://www.nlm.nih.gov/medlineplus/ency/article/000213.htm

REFERENCES

- Chan FK et al: Peptic-ulcer disease. Lancet 2002;360:933. [PMID: 12354485]
- Fitzgerald GA: Coxibs and cardiovascular disease. N Engl J Med 2004;351:1709. [PMID: 15470192]
- Vaira D et al: Review article: *Helicobacter pylori* infection from pathogens to treatment. A critical appraisal. Aliment Pharmacol Ther 2002;16(Suppl 4):105. [PMID: 12030945]

Author(s)

Kenneth R. McQuaid, MD

Peptic Ulcer Disease, Complications

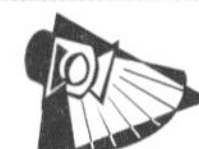

KEY FEATURES

ESSENTIALS OF DIAGNOSIS

- Upper gastrointestinial hemorrhage, with "coffee grounds" emesis, hematemesis, melena, or hematochezia
- Perforation, with severe pain and peritonitis
- Penetration, with severe pain and pancreatitis
- Gastric outlet obstructon, with vomiting
- Emergent upper endoscopy is usually diagnostic and sometimes therapeutic

GENERAL CONSIDERATIONS

Upper gastrointestinal hemorrhage

- ~50% of upper gastrointestinal bleeding is due to peptic ulcer disease
- Bleeding occurs in 10–20% of ulcer patients
- About 80% stop bleeding spontaneously; the remainder have severe bleeding
- Overall mortality rate for ulcer bleeding is 6–10%, higher in the elderly, in those with comorbid medical problems, and in those with nosocomial bleeding, persistent hypotension or shock, bright red blood in the vomitus or nasogastric lavage fluid, or severe coagulopathy

Ulcer perforation

- Perforations develop in 5%
- May be increasing due to use of nonsteroidal antiinflammatory drugs and cocaine
- Consider Zollinger-Ellison disease

Ulcer penetration

- Penetration occurs into contiguous structures such as the pancreas, liver, or biliary tree

Gastric outlet obstruction

- Occurs in 2% of patients with ulcer disease causing obstruction of pylorus or duodenum by scarring and inflammation

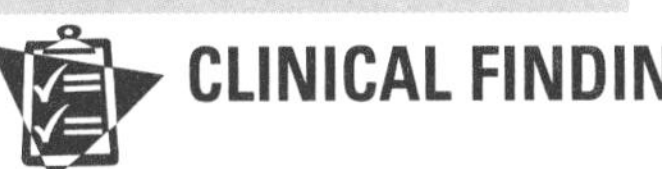

CLINICAL FINDINGS

SYMPTOMS AND SIGNS

Upper gastrointestinal hemorrhage

- Up to 20% have no antecedent symptoms of pain
- "Coffee grounds" emesis, hematemesis, melena, or hematochezia

Ulcer perforation

- Sudden, severe abdominal pain
- Elderly or debilitated patients and those receiving chronic corticosteroid therapy may have minimal initial symptoms, presenting late with bacterial peritonitis, sepsis, and shock
- Patients appear ill, with a rigid, quiet abdomen and rebound tenderness, hypotension

Ulcer penetration

- Pain is severe and constant, may radiate to the back, and is unresponsive to antacids or food
- Physical examination nonspecific

Gastric outlet obstruction

- Early satiety, vomiting, and weight loss
- Early symptoms: epigastric fullness or heaviness after meals
- Later symptoms: vomiting after eating of partially digested food contents
- Chronic obstruction may result in a grossly dilated, atonic stomach, severe weight loss, and malnutrition, dehydration
- Succussion splash in the epigastrium

DIFFERENTIAL DIAGNOSIS

- Upper gastrointestinal bleeding: bleeding esophageal varices, Mallory-Weiss tear, vascular ectasias, Dieulafoy's lesion, malignancy, aortoenteric fistula, hepatic or pancreatic lesions bleeding into pancreatobiliary system
- Severe epigastric pain: esophageal rupture, gastric volvulus, cholecystitis, acute pancreatitis, small bowel obstruction, appendicitis, ureteral colic, splenic rupture

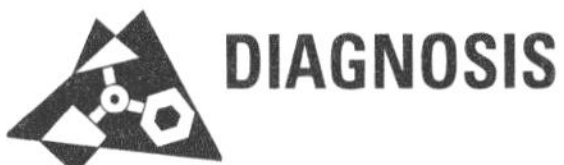

DIAGNOSIS

LABORATORY TESTS

- Upper gastrointestinal hemorrhage: anemia, positive fecal occult blood test
- Ulcer perforation: leukocytosis, and mildly elevated serum amylase
- Ulcer penetration: laboratory tests are nonspecific; elevated serum amylase
- Gastric outlet obstruction: metabolic alkalosis, hypokalemia

IMAGING STUDIES

Ulcer perforation

- Upright or decubitus films of the abdomen reveal free intraperitoneal air in 75%
- Upper gastrointestinal radiography with water-soluble contrast useful
- Abdominal CT increasingly used to establish diagnosis and exclude other causes of abdominal pain

Ulcer penetration

- Barium x-ray studies and endoscopy confirm ulceration but are not diagnostic of an actual penetration

Gastric outlet obstruction

- Endoscopy is preferred diagnostic study

DIAGNOSTIC PROCEDURES

Upper gastrointestinal hemorrhage

- Nasogastric lavage demonstrates "coffee grounds" or bright red blood; lavage fluid negative for blood does not exclude active bleeding from a duodenal ulcer
- Endoscopy should be performed within 12–24 h in most cases
- It is possible to predict which patients are at a higher risk of rebleeding (see When to Admit)

Gastric outlet obstruction

- Nasogastric aspiration evacuation of a large amount (>200 mL) of foul-smelling fluid establishes the diagnosis
- Saline load test seldom used

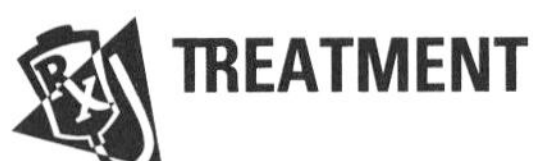

TREATMENT

MEDICATIONS

Upper gastrointestinal hemorrhage

- Antisecretory agents: intravenous proton pump inhibitors or oral proton pump inhibitors, with or without endoscopic therapy, reduce rebleeding, transfusions, and the need for further endoscopic therapy
- Octreotide (100 μg bolus; 50 μg/h) useful in patients in whom endoscopic therapy is unsuccessful in controlling bleeding

Ulcer perforation

- Initial nonoperative management for patients whose onset of symptoms is less than 12 h and whose upper gastrointestinal series with water-soluble contrast medium does not demonstrate leakage
- For patients who are poor operative candidates, fluids, nasogastric suction, antisecretory agents, and broad-spectrum antibiotics
- Up to 40% of ulcer perforations seal spontaneously
- For all others, emergency laparotomy or laparoscopy
- Postoperative treatment of *Helicobacter pylori*

Ulcer penetration

- Intravenous pantoprazole or lansoprazole (80 mg IV bolus; 8 mg/h) until able to take oral proton pump inhibitor

Gastric outlet obstruction

- Intravenous isotonic saline and KCl, intravenous pantoprazole or lansoprazole (80 mg IV bolus; 8 mg/h) continuous infusion, and nasogastric decompression of the stomach
- Severely malnourished patients should receive total parenteral nutrition

SURGERY

Upper gastrointestinal hemorrhage

- Patients with high-risk endoscopic lesions or in whom bleeding cannot be controlled with endoscopic treatment should be evaluated by a surgeon
- < 10% of patients treated with hemostatic therapy require surgery

Ulcer perforation

- Closure of the perforation with an omental ("Graham") patch, at emergency laparotomy or laparoscopy

Gastric outlet obstruction

- Vagotomy and either pyloroplasty or antrectomy

THERAPEUTIC PROCEDURES

- Gastric outlet obstruction: upper endoscopy with dilation by hydrostatic balloons achieves success in two-thirds of patients; surgery for those who fail to respond

OUTCOME

PROGNOSIS

Upper gastrointestinal hemorrhage

- The risk of rebleeding or continued bleeding in ulcers with a nonbleeding visible vessel is 50%, and with active bleeding it is 80–90%
- Endoscopic therapy with injection thermocoagulation or application of metallic clip for such lesions reduces the risk of rebleeding, the number of transfusions, and the need for subsequent surgery
- Surgical mortality for emergency ulcer bleeding is < 6%

Ulcer perforation

- Surgical mortality for emergency ulcer perforation is 5%

WHEN TO ADMIT

Upper gastrointestinal hemorrhage

- Nonbleeding ulcers < 2 cm in size with a base that is clean have a < 5% chance of rebleeding; young (< age 60) otherwise healthy patients who are stable hemodynamically may be discharged from the hospital or emergency room after endoscopy; others may be observed for 24 h
- Ulcers that have only a flat red or black spot have a < 10% chance of significant rebleeding; hospitalization for 24–72 h usually recommended
- Patients with high-risk ulcers requiring endoscopic therapy (active bleeding, visible vessel, adherent clot) should be monitored in an ICU setting for at least 24 h and in hospital for 72 h; rebleeding occurs in 10–20%

PREVENTION

- Upper gastrointestinal hemorrhage: long-term prevention of rebleeding: *H pylori* eradication; or in those with non-*H pylori*-associated ulcers, chronic bedtime dose of an H_2 antagonist or once daily dose of a proton pump inhibitor

EVIDENCE

PRACTICE GUIDELINES

- ASGE Guideline: the role of endoscopy in acute non-variceal upper GI hemorrhage. Gastrointest Endosc 2004;60:497. [PMID: 15472669]
- Barkun A et al: Consensus recommendations for managing patients with nonvariceal upper gastrointestinal bleeding. Ann Intern Med 2003;139:843. [PMID: 14623622]
- National Guideline Clearinghouse
  - http://www.guideline.gov/summary/summary.aspx?doc_id=2947&nbr=2173&string=peptic+AND+ulcer+AND+disease
  - http://www.guideline.gov/summary/summary.aspx?doc_id=3557&nbr=2783&string=ulcer

INFORMATION FOR PATIENTS

- American Gastroenterological Association Patient Information Resources
  - www.gastro.org/generalPublic.html
- JAMA Patient Page: Peptic ulcers. JAMA 2001;286:2052. [PMID: 11693148]
- Mayo Clinic
  - http://www.mayoclinic.com/invoke.cfm?id=DS00242
- Medline Plus Medical Encyclopedia
  - http://www.nlm.nih.gov/medlineplus/ency/article/000213.htm
- National Digestive Diseases Information Clearinghouse
  - http://digestive.niddk.nih.gov/ddiseases/pubs/bleeding/index.htm

REFERENCES

- Jensen D et al: Randomized trial of medical or endoscopic therapy to prevent recurrent ulcer hemorrhage in patients with adherent clots. Gastroenterology 2002;123:407. [PMID: 12145792]
- Lee K et al: Cost-effectiveness analysis of high-dose omeprazole infusion as adjuvant therapy to endoscopic treatment of bleeding ulcer. Gastrointest Endosc 2003;57:160. [PMID: 12556776]
- Paimela H et al: Surgery for peptic ulcer today. A study on the incidence, methods, and mortality in surgery for peptic ulcer in Finland between 1987 and 1999. Dig Surg 2004;21:185. [PMID: 15249752]

Author(s)

Kenneth R. McQuaid, MD

Peritonitis, Spontaneous Bacterial

Perianal Abscess & Fistula p. 1128. Pericardial Effusion p. 1128. Pericarditis, Acute p. 1129. Pericarditis, Constrictive p. 1129.

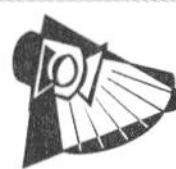

KEY FEATURES

ESSENTIALS OF DIAGNOSIS

- Spontaneous bacterial infection of ascitic fluid in the absence of an apparent intraabdominal source of infection
- A history of chronic liver disease and ascites
- Fever and abdominal pain
- Neutrocytic ascites [>250 white blood cells (WBCs)/µL] with neutrophilic predominance

GENERAL CONSIDERATIONS

- Occurs with few exceptions in patients with chronic liver disease
- Affects ~20–30% of cirrhotic patients
- Most common pathogens are enteric gram-negative bacteria (*Escherichia coli, Klebsiella pneumoniae*, enterococcus) or gram-positive bacteria (*Streptococcus pneumoniae*, viridans streptococci)

DEMOGRAPHICS

- Occurs in patients with ascites secondary to portal hypertension, usually with chronic liver disease
- Patients with serum ascites total protein of <1 g/dL at increased risk

CLINICAL FINDINGS

SYMPTOMS AND SIGNS

- Symptoms in 80–90%; asymptomatic in 20%
- Fever and abdominal pain present in two-thirds
- Change in mental status due to exacerbation or precipitation of hepatic encephalopathy
- Signs of chronic liver disease with ascites
- Abdominal tenderness in <50%

DIFFERENTIAL DIAGNOSIS

- Secondary bacterial peritonitis, eg, appendicitis, diverticulitis, perforated peptic ulcer, perforated gallbladder
- Peritoneal carcinomatosis
- Pancreatic ascites
- Tuberculous ascites

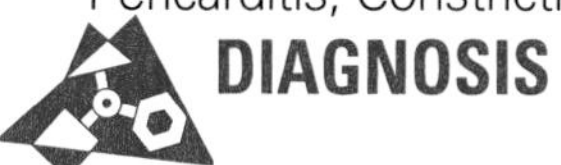

DIAGNOSIS

LABORATORY TESTS

- Renal dysfunction, abrupt worsening of renal function
- Ascitic fluid polymorphonuclear neutrophil (PMN) count of >250 cells/µL (neutrocytic ascites) or percentage of PMNs greater than 50–70% of the ascitic fluid WBC count is presumptive evidence of bacterial peritonitis
- Ascitic fluid Gram stain is insensitive
- Ascitic fluid cultures should be obtained by inoculating count blood culture bottles at the bedside
- 10–30% of patients with neutrocytic ascites have negative ascitic bacterial cultures ("culture-negative neutrocytic ascites"), but are presumed nonetheless to have bacterial peritonitis and treated empirically
- Blood cultures occasionally are positive, helping to identify the organism when ascitic fluid culture is negative

IMAGING STUDIES

- Abdominal ultrasound helpful in locating optimal site for paracentesis

DIAGNOSTIC PROCEDURES

- Abdominal paracentesis

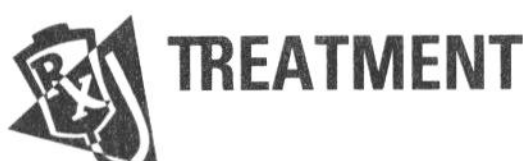

TREATMENT

MEDICATIONS

- Patients with neutrocytic ascites are presumed infected and should be started—regardless of symptoms—on antibiotics
- Empirical therapy usually employs a third-generation cephalosporin, such as cefotaxime, 2 g IV Q 8–12 h (depending on renal function)
- If enterococcus infection is suspected, ampicillin is added
- Recommended duration of antibiotic is 5–10 days or until the ascites fluid PMN count decreases to < 250 cells/μL
- Intravenous albumin, 1.5 g/kg on day 1 and day 3, is recommended to reduce the development of renal failure and mortality

SURGERY

- Liver transplant is the most effective treatment for spontaneous bacterial peritonitis

OUTCOME

FOLLOW-UP

- Repeat paracentesis at 5 days after start of antibiotic therapy if there is persistent fever, pain, or clinical deterioration

COMPLICATIONS

- Renal failure develops in up to 40% of patients and is a major cause of death

PROGNOSIS

- Mortality of spontaneous bacterial peritonitis exceeds 30%, but if recognized and treated early, mortality is < 10%
- Causes of death include liver failure, hepatorenal syndrome, or bleeding complications

WHEN TO REFER

- Patients failing to improve within 3–5 days of initial therapy
- Patients with possible secondary peritonitis, ie, ascites infected by an intraabdominal infection (appendicitis, diverticulitis); consider secondary peritonitis in patients with ascites total protein < 1 g/dL, glucose < 50 mg/dL, or LDH > upper limit of normal for serum; in patients with polymicrobial infection; and in patients with high ascitic neutrophil counts (>10,000/μL)

WHEN TO ADMIT

- Symptomatic patients require admission for intravenous antibiotics
- Selected asymptomatic patients may be treated with oral antibiotics with close follow-up

PREVENTION

- Up to 70% of patients who survive an episode of spontaneous bacterial peritonitis will have another episode within 1 year
- Secondary prophylaxis is recommended with norfloxacin, 400 mg PO QD; ciprofloxacin, 750 mg PO once weekly; or trimethoprim-sulfamethoxazole, 1 double-strength tablet PO QD
- Secondary prophylaxis reduces the rate of recurrent infections to < 20%
- Primary prophylaxis is also recommended in patients with no history of spontaneous bacterial peritonitis but who are at increased risk of infection due to low-protein ascites (total ascitic protein < 1 g/dL); antibiotics as above

EVIDENCE

PRACTICE GUIDELINES

- American Association for the Study of Liver Diseases (AASLD) Practice Guideline: management of adult patients with ascites due to cirrhosis. Hepatology 2004;39:841. [PMID: 14999706]
- Mowat C et al: Review article: spontaneous bacterial peritonitis—diagnosis, treatment and prevention. Aliment Pharmacol Ther 2001;15:1851. [PMID: 11736714]

WEB SITES

- American Association for the Study of Liver Diseases (AASLD): Practice Guidelines: portal hypertension
  - http://www.aasld.org/eweb/DynamicPage.aspx?siteAASLD3&webcode=portalhypertension
- Family Practice Handbook—Ascites and spontaneous bacterial peritonitis
  - http://www.vh.org/adult/provider/familymedicine/FPHandbook/Chapter05/18-5.html

INFORMATION FOR PATIENTS

- MEDLINEplus—Peritonitis, spontaneous
  - http://www.nlm.nih.gov/medlineplus/ency/article/000648.htm

REFERENCES

- Garcia-Tsao G: Current management of the complications of cirrhosis and portal hypertension: variceal hemorrhage, ascites, and spontaneous bacterial peritonitis. Gastroenterology 2001;1220:726. [PMID: 11179247]
- Gines P et al: Management of cirrhosis and ascites. N Engl J Med 2004;350:1646. [PMID: 15084697]
- Runyon BA: The evolution of ascitic fluid analysis in the diagnosis of spontaneous bacterial peritonitis. Am J Gastroenterol 2003;98:1675. [PMID: 12907318]

Author(s)

Kenneth R. McQuaid, MD

Personality Disorders

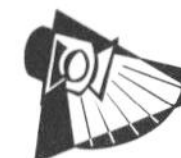

KEY FEATURES

ESSENTIALS OF DIAGNOSIS

- Long history dating back to childhood
- Recurrent maladaptive behavior
- Low self-esteem and lack of confidence
- Minimal introspective ability with a tendency to blame others for all problems
- Major difficulties with interpersonal relationships or society
- Depression with anxiety when maladaptive behavior fails

GENERAL CONSIDERATIONS

- Personality results from the interaction of a genetic substrate with personal drives and outside influences
- Classification of disorder subtypes depends on the predominant symptoms and their severity
- The most severe disorders are those that bring the patient into greatest conflict with society and tend to be classified as antisocial or borderline
- Types of personality disorders
  - Paranoid
  - Schizoid (introverted, withdrawn)
  - Obsessive-compulsive
  - Histrionic (dependent, immature, seductive, egocentric, emotionally labile)
  - Schizotypal (socially isolated, suspicious, eccentric behaviors)
  - Narcissistic
  - Avoidant (fear rejection, low self-esteem)
  - Dependent (passive, unable to make decisions, poor self-esteem)
  - Antisocial (selfish, callous, promiscuous, impulsive)
  - Borderline (impulsive, unstable and intense relationships, affective instability, suicidal)

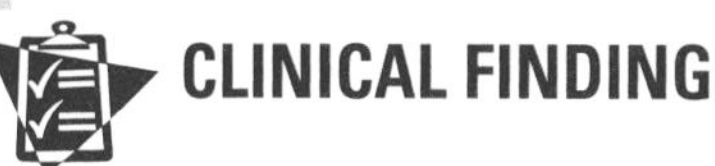

CLINICAL FINDINGS

SYMPTOMS AND SIGNS

- See Table 104

DIFFERENTIAL DIAGNOSIS

- Anxiety disorder, eg, general anxiety disorder
- Major depressive disorder
- Psychotic disorder, eg, schizophrenia
- Substance abuse
- Bipolar disorder
- Personality change due to medical illness, eg, CNS tumor, stroke

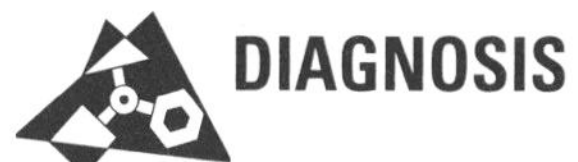

DIAGNOSIS

LABORATORY TESTS

- These are mainly clinical diagnoses

IMAGING STUDIES

- Consider head CT if there is an abrupt personality change

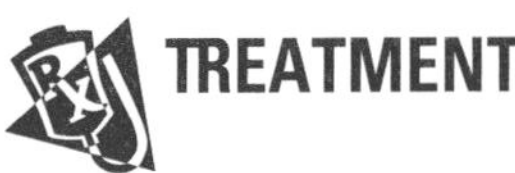

TREATMENT

MEDICATIONS

- Antipsychotic agents may be required for short periods when conditions have temporarily decompensated into transient psychoses. Options include
  - Haloperidol, 2–5 mg PO Q 3–4 h
  - Olanzapine, 2.5–10 mg PO QD
  - Risperidone, 0.5–2 mg PO QD with lorazepam, 1–2 mg PO Q 4 h
- Carbamazepine, 400–800 mg PO QD in divided doses decreases severity of behavioral dyscontrol
- Antidepressants have improved anxiety, depression, and sensitivity to rejection in some borderline patients
- Selective serotonin reuptake inhibitors may have a role in reducing aggressive behavior in impulsive aggressive patients

THERAPEUTIC PROCEDURES

- Social
  - Day hospitals, halfway houses, and self-help communities use peer pressure to modify self-destructive behavior
- Behavioral
  - Operant and aversive conditioning use reinforcement and punishment to change behavior
  - Dialectical behavioral therapy uses a cognitive-behavioral model to address self-awareness, interpersonal functioning, affective lability, and reactions to stress
- Psychological
  - Best conducted in group settings and helpful when specific behaviors need to be improved
  - Individual therapy should initially be supportive, to restabilize and mobilize defenses
  - Long-term introspective therapy may be warranted if the patient has the ability to observe his or her own behavior

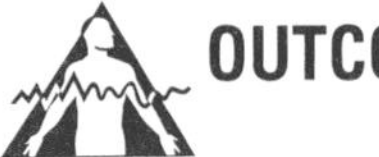

OUTCOME

COMPLICATIONS

- Up to 80% of hospitalized borderline patients make a suicide attempt at some time during treatment
- Drug abuse is common among borderline patients

PROGNOSIS

- Antisocial and borderline categories have a guarded prognosis
- Patients with poor outcomes are more likely to have a hisory of parental abuse and a family history of mood disorder
- Mild schizoid or passive-aggressive tendencies have a better prognosis

WHEN TO REFER

- When patient distress or second psychotic illness is present

WHEN TO ADMIT

- Hospitalization is rarely indicated except in cases of suicidal risk

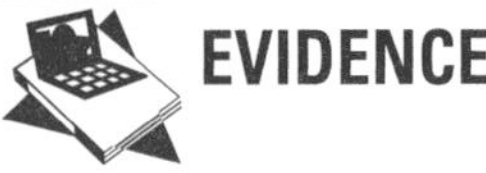

EVIDENCE

PRACTICE GUIDELINES

- American Academy of Family Physicians
  - http://www.aafp.org/afp/20041015/1505.html
- American Psychiatric Association: psychiatric evaluation guidelines, 1995
  - http://www.guideline.gov/summary/summary.aspx?doc_id=1407
- APA: Borderline personality disorder treatment, 2001
  - http://www.guideline.gov/summary/summary.aspx?doc_id=2972

WEB SITES

- American Psychiatric Association
  - http://www.psych.org/
- Borderline Personality Disorder Research Foundation
  - http://www.borderlineresearch.org/
- National Institutes of Health—National Institute of Mental Health
  - http://www.nimh.nih.gov

INFORMATION FOR PATIENTS

- National Institutes of Health
  - http://www.nlm.nih.gov/medlineplus/ency/article/000939.htm

REFERENCES

- Schultz S et al: Olanzapine safety and efficacy in patients with borderline personality disorder and comorbid dysthymia. Biol Psychiatry 1999;46:1429. [PMID:10578457]
- Swenson CR et al: Implementing dialectical behavioral therapy. Psychiatr Serv 2002;53:171. [PMID:11821547]

Author(s)

Stuart J. Eisendrath, MD
Jonathan E. Lichtmacher, MD

Pertussis, *Bordetella*

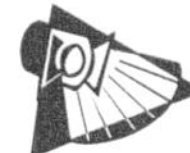

KEY FEATURES

ESSENTIALS OF DIAGNOSIS

- Predominantly in infants under age 2 years
- Adults are an important reservoir of infection
- Two-week prodromal catarrhal stage of malaise, cough, coryza, and anorexia
- Paroxysmal cough ending in a high-pitched inspiratory "whoop"
- Absolute lymphocytosis, often striking; culture confirms diagnosis

GENERAL CONSIDERATIONS

- An acute infection of the respiratory tract caused by *Bordetella pertussis*, a gram-negative coccobacillus
- Infection is transmitted by respiratory droplets
- Neither immunization nor disease confers lasting immunity to pertussis
- Adults are an important reservoir of this highly contagious disease
- The diagnosis often is not considered in adults, who may not have atypical presentation. Cough persisting more than 2 weeks is suggestive of pertussis

DEMOGRAPHICS

- This disease causes high morbidity and mortality in many countries
- In the United States, 5000–7000 cases are reported each year
- Incidence of pertussis has increased steadily since the 1980s

CLINICAL FINDINGS

SYMPTOMS AND SIGNS

- Symptoms of classic pertussis last about 6 weeks and are divided into three consecutive stages
- The **catarrhal stage**
  - Characterized by its insidious onset
  - Lacrimation, sneezing, and coryza, anorexia, and malaise
  - Hacking night cough that tends to become diurnal
- The **paroxysmal stage**
  - Characterized by bursts of rapid, consecutive coughs followed by a deep, high-pitched inspiration (whoop)
- The **convalescent stage**
  - Usually begins 4 weeks after onset of the illness with a decrease in the frequency and severity of paroxysms of cough

DIFFERENTIAL DIAGNOSIS

- Viral or bacterial pneumonia
- Asthma
- Other causes of chronic cough in adults, eg, postnasal drip, gastroesophageal reflux disease, tuberculosis, *Mycobacterium avium* complex
- Bronchiolitis, eg, respiratory syncytial virus (children)
- Croup (children)

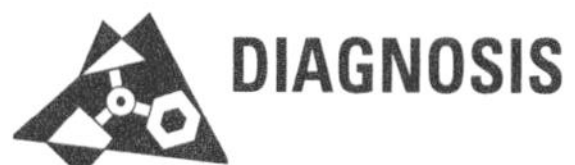

DIAGNOSIS

LABORATORY TESTS

- The white blood cell count is usually 15,000–20,000/μL (rarely, as high as 50,000/μL or more), 60–80% of which are lymphocytes
- The diagnosis is established by isolating the organism from nasopharyngeal culture. A special medium (eg, Bordet-Gengou agar) must be requested

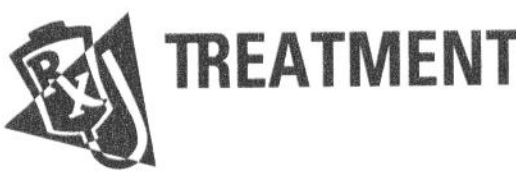

TREATMENT

MEDICATIONS

- Erythromycin, 500 mg PO QID for 10 days, shortens the duration of carriage. It also may diminish the severity of coughing paroxysms
- Azithromycin, 500 mg PO QD for 3 days, or clarithromycin, 500 mg PO TID for 7 days, is probably as effective as erythromycin and likely to be better tolerated
- Active immunization with pertussis vaccine is recommended for all infants, usually combined with diphtheria and tetanus toxoids (DTP) (Table 132)

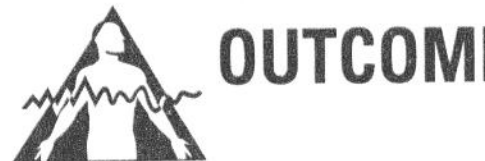

OUTCOME

WHEN TO REFER

- Pertussis is a disease that should be reported to the public health authorities

WHEN TO ADMIT

- Adults must be admitted if respiratory insufficiency (eg, hypoxia) is present

PREVENTION

- Immunizations (Table 132)
- Pertussis vaccine is recommended for all infants, combined with DTP
- Infants and susceptible adults with significant exposure should receive prophylaxis with erythromycin (40 mg/kg PO/day, up to 2 g/day, for 10 days)
- Booster doses of pertussis vaccine have not been recommended after age 6 except in outbreaks

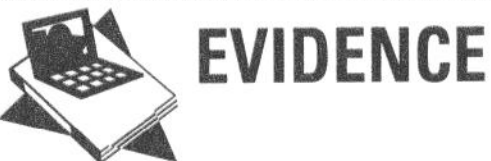

EVIDENCE

PRACTICE GUIDELINES

- National Guideline Clearinghouse
  - http://www.guideline.gov/summary/summary.aspx?doc_id=3376

WEB SITES

- CDC—Division of Bacterial and Mycotic Diseases
  - http://www.cdc.gov/ncidod/dbmd/
- CDC—National Immunization Program
  - http://www.cdc.gov/nip/publications/pink/pert.pdf

INFORMATION FOR PATIENTS

- American Medical Association
  - http://www.medem.com/medlb/article_detaillb.cfm?article_ID=ZZZPWVII1AC&sub_cat=286
- JAMA patient page: Immunizations. JAMA 1999;282:102. [PMID: 10404918]

REFERENCES

- Cherry JD: Epidemiological, clinical, and laboratory aspects of pertussis in adults. Clin Infect Dis 1999;28(Suppl 2):S112. [PMID: 10447028]
- Von Konig C et al: Pertussis of adults and infants. Lancet Infect Dis 2002;2:744. [PMID: 12467690]

Author(s)

Henry F. Chambers, MD

Pesticide Poisoning p. 1130. Petroleum Distillate Poisoning p. 1131.

Pharyngitis & Tonsillitis

KEY FEATURES

ESSENTIALS OF DIAGNOSIS

- Sore throat
- Fever
- Anterior cervical adenopathy
- Tonsillar exudate
- Focus is to treat group A β-hemolytic streptococcus infection to prevent rheumatic sequelae

GENERAL CONSIDERATIONS

- Group A β-hemolytic streptococci (*Streptococcus pyogenes*) are the most common bacterial cause of exudative pharyngitis
- Transmission is by droplets of infected secretions
- The main concern is to determine whether the cause is group A β-hemolytic streptococcal infection (GABHS), because of the complications of rheumatic fever and glomerular nephritis
- A second public health policy concern is to reduce the extraordinary cost (in both dollars and the development of antibiotic-resistant *Streptococcus pneumoniae* in the United States associated with unnecessary and unrecommended antibiotic use)
- Group A streptococci producing erythrogenic toxin may cause scarlet fever rashes in susceptible persons
- About one third of patients with infectious mononucleosis have secondary streptococcal tonsillitis, requiring treatment
- Ampicillin should routinely be avoided if mononucleosis is suspected because it induces a rash

DEMOGRAPHICS

- Pharyngitis and tonsillitis account for more than 10% of all office visits to primary care clinicians and 50% of outpatient antibiotic use

CLINICAL FINDINGS

SYMPTOMS AND SIGNS

- Centor diagnostic criteria
  - Fever > 38°C
  - Tender anterior cervical adenopathy
  - Lack of cough
  - Pharyngotonsillar exudate
- Sore throat may be severe, with odynophagia, tender adenopathy, and a scarlatiniform rash
- Hoarseness, cough, and coryza are not suggestive of this disease
- Marked lymphadenopathy and a shaggy white-purple tonsillar exudate, often extending into the nasopharynx, suggest mononucleosis, especially if present in a young adult

DIFFERENTIAL DIAGNOSIS

- Viral pharyngitis
- Epstein–Barr virus/infectious mononucleosis
- Primary HIV infection
- Candidiasis
- Necrotizing ulcerative gingivostomatitis (Vincent's fusospirochetal disease)
- Retropharyngeal abscess
- Diphtheria
- *Neisseria gonorrhoeae*
- Mycoplasma
- Anaerobic streptococci
- *Corynebacterium haemolyticum*
- Epiglottitis

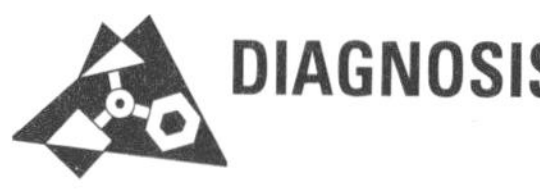

DIAGNOSIS

LABORATORY TESTS

- The presence of the four Centor diagnostic criteria strongly suggests GABHS, and some would treat regardless of laboratory results
- When three of the four Centor criteria are present, laboratory sensitivity of rapid antigen testing exceeds 90%
- When only one Centor criterion is present, GABHS is unlikely
- The sensitivity of current GABHS rapid antigen tests is now excellent, exceeding 90% in appropriately selected patients
- Routine throat cultures are not needed
- Leukocytosis with neutrophil predominance is common

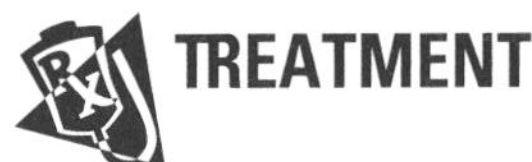

TREATMENT

MEDICATIONS

- One benzathine penicillin or procaine penicillin injection, 1.2 million U, optimal but painful; use for noncompliance
- Analgesic, antiinflammatory drugs (aspirin, acetaminophen)
- Oral antibiotics
  - Penicillin V potassium (250 mg PO TID or 500 mg BID for 10 days) or cefuroxime axetil (250 mg PO BID, 5–10 days)
  - Efficacy of 5-day penicillin V similar to 10-day course: 94% clinical response, 84% eradication
  - Erythromycin (500 mg PO QID) or azithromycin (500 mg PO QD for 3 days) for penicillin-allergic patients
  - Macrolides not as effective as penicillins
    - Macrolide resistance in group A streptococci strains as high as 25–40%
    - Macrolides are second-line agents because of treatment failure risk
  - Macrolide-resistant strains susceptible to clindamycin (10-day course of 300 mg PO TID)
  - Cephalosporins more effective than penicillin for bacterial cure (eg, cefpodoxime and cefuroxime for 5 days)
- Treatment failure
  - Second course with same drug
  - Penicillin alternatives: cephalosporins (eg, cefuroxime), dicloxacillin, amoxicillin-clavulanate
  - Erythromycin resistance (failure rates of ~25%) increasing
  - With severe penicillin allergy, avoid cephalosporins; cross-reaction common (≥ 8%)

SURGERY

- Remove tonsils in cases of recurrent abscess

THERAPEUTIC PROCEDURES

Strategies based on Centor criteria

- Test with GABHS rapid antigen tests patients with ≥ 2 criteria; treat those with positive results
- Test with current GABHS rapid antigen tests patients with 2–3 criteria; treat those with positive results
- Test no one and treat all with 4 criteria

Ancillary

- Salt-water gargling may be soothing
- Anesthetic gargles and lozenges (eg, benzocaine) for additional symptomatic relief

OUTCOME

FOLLOW-UP

- Patients who have had rheumatic fever should be treated with a continuous course of antimicrobial prophylaxis (erythromycin, 250 mg PO BID, or penicillin G, 500 mg PO QD) for at least 5 years

COMPLICATIONS

- Low (10–20%) incidence of treatment failures (positive culture after treatment despite symptomatic resolution) and recurrences

Suppurative

- Sinusitis, otitis media, mastoiditis, peritonsillar abscess, suppuration of cervical lymph nodes

Nonsuppurative

- Rheumatic fever may follow recurrent episodes of pharyngitis 1–4 weeks after onset of symptoms
- Glomerulonephritis follows a single infection with a nephritogenic strain of streptococcus group A (eg, types 4, 12, 2, 49, and 60), more commonly on the skin than in the throat, and begins 1–3 weeks after onset of infection
- Toxic shock syndrome
- Scarlet fever

PROGNOSIS

- Streptococcal pharyngitis usually resolves after 1 week
- Spontaneous resolution of symptoms without treatment still leaves the risk of rheumatic complications

WHEN TO REFER

- Peritonsillar abscess

WHEN TO ADMIT

- Occasionally, odynophagia is so intense that hospitalization for intravenous hydration and antibiotics is necessary
- Suspected or known epiglottitis

EVIDENCE

PRACTICE GUIDELINES

- Institute for Clinical Systems Improvement: Acute Pharyngitis, 2003.
  - http://www.icsi.org/knowledge/detail.asp?catID=29&itemID=147
- Infectious Diseases Society of America: Practice Guidelines for the Diagnosis and Management of Group A Streptococcal Pharyngitis, 2002.
  - http://www.journals.uchicago.edu/CID/journal/issues/v35n2/020429/020429.html

WEB SITE

- Baylor College of Medicine Otolaryngology Resources on the Internet
  - http://www.bcm.tmc.edu/oto/othersa.html

INFORMATION FOR PATIENTS

- American Academy of Family Physicians: Sore Throat: Easing the Pain of a Sore Throat
  - http://familydoctor.org/163.xml
- American Academy of Otolaryngology—Head and Neck Surgery: Sore Throats
  - http://www.entlink.org/healthinfo/throat/sore_throat.cfm
- Mayo Clinic: Tonsillitis
  - http://www.mayoclinic.com/invoke.cfm?id=DS00273

REFERENCES

- Bisno AL et al: Practice guidelines for the diagnosis and management of group A streptococcal pharyngitis. Infectious Diseases Society of America. Clin Infect Dis 2002;35:113. [PMID: 12087516]
- Hirschmann JV: Antibiotics for common respiratory tract infections in adults. Arch Intern Med 2002;162:256. [PMID: 11822917]
- Johnson BC et al: Cost-effective workup for tonsillitis. Testing, treatment, and potential complications. Postgrad Med 2003;113:115. [PMID: 12647478]
- Steinman MA et al: Predictors of broad-spectrum antibiotic prescribing for acute respiratory tract infections in adult primary care. JAMA 2003;289:719. [PMID: 12585950]

Author(s)

Robert K. Jackler, MD
Michael J. Kaplan, MD

Pheochromocytoma

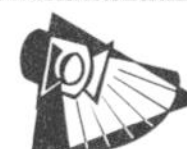

KEY FEATURES

ESSENTIALS OF DIAGNOSIS

- Attacks of headache, perspiration, palpitations
- Hypertension, frequently sustained but often paroxysmal, especially during surgery or obstetric delivery
- Attacks of nausea, abdominal pain, chest pain, weakness, dyspnea, tremor, visual disturbance
- Anxiety, tremor, weight loss, or heat intolerance
- Elevated urinary catecholamines or metanephrines. Normal serum tetraiodothyronine (T_4) and thyroid-stimulating hormone (TSH)

GENERAL CONSIDERATIONS

- Hypertension caused by excessive secretion of norepinephrine or neuropeptide Y
- Tumor located in either or both adrenals or along sympathetic chain
- Rule of tens: 10% in children; 10–15% familial; 10% without hypertension; 10% extra-adrenal, and of those, 10% extra-abdominal, location; 10% bilateral adrenal location (more frequent in familial cases); 10% metastatic at diagnosis. Metastases later discovered in another 5%
- Familial pheochromocytomas, bilateral (70%) and associated with
  - Calcitonin-secreting medullary thyroid carcinoma and hyperparathyroidism (MEN-2a)
  - Medullary thyroid carcinoma and syndrome of multiple mucosal neuromas (MEN-2b)
  - Neurofibromatosis (Recklinghausen's disease)
  - von Hippel-Lindau disease (hemangiomas of retina and CNS; pancreatic cysts; renal cysts, adenomas and carcinomas)
  - Islet cell tumors (rare)
- Germline mutations causing some hereditary forms of paraganglioma and pheochromocytoma identified in genes encoding certain mitochondrial proteins—succinate dehydrogenase subunit B (SDHB), D (SDHD), and rarely C (SDHC)
  - Paragangliomas associated with SDHB mutations tend to be malignant; all tend to develop multifocal tumors
  - Predisposition to tumors is inherited in autosomal dominant fashion with SDHB mutations. Only those who inherit SDHD mutations from their father are at risk for paragangliomas, but asymptomatic patients who inherit SDHD mutations from their mother can pass mutation to children (genetic imprinting)
  - Sequence analysis of these genes (from peripheral blood) performed in all patients with paragangliomas or pheochromocytomas, because patients with apparently sporadic tumors often harbor unsuspected germline mutations

DEMOGRAPHICS

- Pheochromocytomas rare: < 0.3% of hypertensive patients
- Incidence higher with moderate to severe hypertension
- Annually, ~2 cases per million population diagnosed clinically, but 250–1300 cases per million in autopsy series, indicating most cases are not diagnosed during life

CLINICAL FINDINGS

SYMPTOMS AND SIGNS

- Some are normotensive and asymptomatic
- Typically causes attacks of severe headache (80%), perspiration (70%), and palpitations (60%)
- May cause anxiety (50%), sense of impending doom, or tremor (40%)
- Hypertension in 90%; paroxysms of severe hypertension in 50%
- Vasomotor changes during attack include mottled cyanosis and facial pallor; facial flushing may occur as attack subsides
- May have angina, abdominal pain, vomiting, increased appetite, and weight loss
- May have cardiac enlargement; postural tachycardia, postural hypotension; mild elevation of basal body temperature
- Retinal hemorrhage or cerebrovascular hemorrhage occurs occasionally
- Other possible findings: psychosis or confusion, seizures, hyperglycemia, bradycardia, constipation, paresthesias, Raynaud's phenomenon, pulmonary edema and heart failure, syncope, abdominal discomfort due to mass
- Pheochromocytomas may secrete other peptides causing Cushing's syndrome (ACTH), erythrocytosis (erythropoietin), or hypercalcemia (parathyroid-related peptide; PTHrP)

DIFFERENTIAL DIAGNOSIS

- Other cause of secondary hypertension, eg, primary hyperaldosteronism, Cushing's syndrome, renal artery stenosis
- Panic attacks
- Thyrotoxicosis
- Acute intermittent porphyria
- Carcinoid syndrome
- Paroxysmal tachycardia
- Preeclampsia-eclampsia

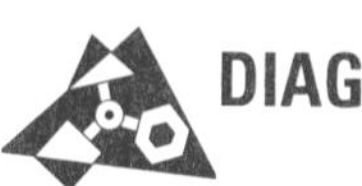

DIAGNOSIS

LABORATORY TESTS

- TSH, free T_4, and triiodothyronine (T_3) normal
- WBC and glucose elevations common
- A 24-hour urine specimen is collected with acid preservative and assayed for total and fractional catecholamines, metanephrines, and creatinine
- 24-hour urine or "spot" urine: >2.2 μg total metanephrine per mg creatinine and >135 μg total catecholamines per gram creatinine usual in pheochromocytoma
- Urinary total metanephrines has test sensitivity of 97%. Urine vanillylmandelic acid (VMA) has sensitivity of 89%. VMA not usually required
- Some drugs, foods, medical conditions, and stress interfere with assays
  - Drugs: acetaminophen, amphetamines, bronchodilators, captopril, cocaine, contrast media (meglumine, acetrizoate, or diatrizoate), cimetidine, codeine, decongestants, levodopa, labetalol, metoclopramide
  - Foods: bananas, caffeine, coffee
  - Conditions: acute illness, vigorous exercise, severe emotion, carcinoid, brain lesions, renal failure
- ~10% of hypertensive patients have misleadingly elevated level of tests
- High plasma and urine catcholamine and metanephrine levels during or after attack are sensitive tests for pheochromocytoma associated with paroxysmal hypertension. Proper collection essential
- Serum chromogranin A elevated in 90% and can serve as tumor marker
- Genetic testing for patients or relatives suspected of having von Hippel-Lindau disease, MEN-2a or -2b, or familial paraganglioma

IMAGING STUDIES

- Thin-section CT of adrenals. Glucagon and IV contrast agents should not be used during scanning, because they can

provoke hypertensive crisis; especially with uncontrolled hypertension
- MRI does not require IV contrast; lack of radiation during pregnancy
- CT and MRI have sensitivity of ~90% for adrenal pheochromocytoma and 95% for adrenal tumors >0.5 cm
- Incidental adrenal adenomas (2–4% of scans) can be misleading
- If no adrenal tumor found, CT scan extended to abdomen, pelvis, and chest
- Whole-body ^{123}I metaiodobenzylguanidine (MIBG) scan can localize tumors with 85% sensitivity and 99% specificity
- Drugs reducing MIBG uptake by pheochromocytoma
  - Tricyclic antidepressants, cyclobenzaprine (for 6 weeks)
  - Amphetamines, phenylpropanolamine, phenothiazines, haloperidol, thiothixene, diet pills, nasal decongestants, cocaine (for 2 weeks)
  - Selective serotonin reuptake inhibitors (for an unknown duration)

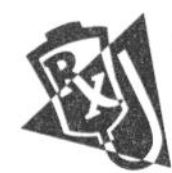

TREATMENT

MEDICATIONS

- Preoperative α-adrenergic blockade: phenoxybenzamine, 10 mg PO Q 12 h, increasing about every 3 days until hypertension is controlled. Usual maintenance dose is 20–60 mg PO BID. Optimal blockade achieved when supine BP < 160/90 mm Hg and standing BP >80/45 mm Hg
- Calcium channel blockers also effective and better tolerated than α-blockers
- Propranolol, 10–40 mg PO QID, to control tachycardia and other arrhythmias after BP is controlled
- Maintain BP control at least 4–7 days or until optimal cardiac status established
- Preoperative autotransfusion and generous intraoperative IV fluid reduces risk of postresection hypotension
- Postoperative shock treated with IV saline or colloid and high doses of IV norepinephrine
- Metyrosine, 250 mg PO QID; increase daily by increments of 250–500 mg to maximum 4 g/day to reduce catecholamine synthesis for inoperable or metastatic tumors
- Combination chemotherapy (eg, cyclophosphamide, vincristine, and dacarbazine) for metastatic pheochromocytomas

SURGERY

- Laparoscopic removal of tumor or tumors is treatment of choice
- Open laparotomy for large tumors
- Nicardipine, 2–6 μg/kg/min, or nitroprusside, 0.5–10 μg/kg/min, continuous IV infusion, for severe intraoperative hypertension
- Atenolol (1 mg boluses), esmolol, or lidocaine IV for tachyarrhythmias

THERAPEUTIC PROCEDURES

- ^{131}I-MIBG for metastatic pheochromocytomas

OUTCOME

FOLLOW-UP

- Recheck urinary catecholamine levels 2 weeks after surgery to exclude multiple or metastatic tumors
- Check ^{131}I -MIBG whole-body scan 2–3 months postoperatively
- Thereafter, recheck symptoms and BP regularly
- Lifetime clinical surveillance for recurrence or metastases
- Follow chromogranin A if elevated before surgery

COMPLICATIONS

- Complications of severe hypertension
- Catecholamine-induced cardiomyopathy
- Sudden death from cardiac arrhythmia
- Hypertensive crises with sudden blindness or stroke
- Decongestants, bladder catheterization, needle biopsy, anesthesia, intubation, unopposed β-blockade, and surgical manipulation of tumor may induce hypertensive paroxysms
- Metyrosine causes CNS side effects and crystalluria; hydration must be ensured

PROGNOSIS

- Malignancy determined by whether metastases are present or develop
- Complete cure usually achieved if tumor successfully removed before irreparable cardiovascular damage
- In about 25%, hypertension persists or returns in spite of successful surgery
- Surgical mortality rate < 3%
- Death may occur from hypertensive crisis induced by intravenous contrast, glucagons, or needle biopsy
- Patients with metastatic pheochromocytoma have 5-year survival rate of 50%, but prolonged survival does occur
- D_5W infusion postoperatively to prevent hypoglycemia

EVIDENCE

PRACTICE GUIDELINES

- Bravo EL: Pheochromocytoma: an approach to antihypertensive management. Ann NY Acad Sci 2002;970:1. [PMID:12381537]

INFORMATION FOR PATIENTS

- National Cancer Institute—Pheochromocytoma
  - http://www.cancer.gov/cancerinfo/pdq/treatment/pheochromocytoma/patient/

REFERENCES

- Bravo EL: Pheochromocytoma: an approach to antihypertensive management. Ann N Y Acad Sci 2002;970:1. [PMID:12381537]
- Goldstein DS et al: Diagnosis and localization of pheochromocytoma. Hypertension 2004;43:907. [PMID: 15023935]
- Ilias I et al: Current approaches and recommended algorithm for the diagnostic localization of pheochromocytoma. J Clin Endocrinol Metab 2004;89:479. [PMID:14764749]
- Khorram-Manesh A et al: Mortality associated with pheochromocytoma in a large Swedish cohort. Eur J Surg Oncol 2004;30:556. [PMID:15135486]
- Kudva YC et al: Clinical review 163: the laboratory diagnosis of adrenal pheochromocytoma: the Mayo Clinic experience. J Clin Endocrinol Metab 2003;88:4533.[PMID:14557417]
- Manger WM: Editorial: in search of pheochromocytoma. J Clin Endocrinol Metab 2003;88:4080. [PMID:11821644]
- Neumann HP et al: Distinct clinical features of paraganglioma syndromes associated with SDHB and SDHD gene mutations. JAMA 2004;292:943. [PMID:15328326]
- Rose B et al: High-dose ^{131}I-metaiodobenzylguanadine therapy for 12 patients with malignant pheochromocytoma. Cancer 2003;98:239. [PMID:12872341]
- Safford DS et al: Iodine-131 metaiodobenzylguanadine is an effective treatment for malignant pheochromocytoma and paraganglioma. Surgery 2003;134:956. [PMID:14668728]

Author(s)

Paul A. Fitzgerald, MD

Photodermatitis

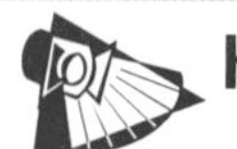

KEY FEATURES

ESSENTIALS OF DIAGNOSIS

- Painful or pruritic erythema, edema, or vesiculation on sun-exposed surfaces: the face, neck, hands, and "V" of the chest
- Inner upper eyelids spared, as is the area under the chin

GENERAL CONSIDERATIONS

- Acute or chronic inflammatory skin reaction due to
  - Hypersensitivity to sunlight or other sources of actinic rays
  - Photosensitization of the skin by certain drugs
  - Idiosyncrasy to actinic light as seen in some constitutional disorders including the porphyrias and many hereditary disorders (phenylketonuria, xeroderma pigmentosum, and others)
- Contact photosensitivity may occur with perfumes, antiseptics, and other chemicals
- Photodermatitis is manifested most commonly as phototoxicity—a tendency for the individual to sunburn more easily than usual—or, more rarely, as photoallergy, a true immunological reaction that often presents with papular or vesicular lesions

Etiology

- Medications
  - Phenothiazines, sulfones, chlorothiazides, griseofulvin, sulfonylureas, NSAIDs, antibiotics (eg, tetracycline)
- Systemic disease
  - Systemic lupus erythematosus, porphyria cutanea tarda, variegate porphyria
- Polymorphous light eruption (idiopathic)

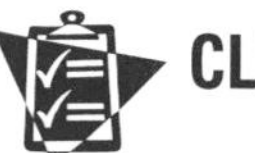

CLINICAL FINDINGS

SYMPTOMS AND SIGNS

- See Table 7
- Acute inflammatory skin reaction, which, if severe enough, is accompanied by pain, fever, gastrointestinal symptoms, malaise, and even prostration, but this is very rare
- Erythema, edema, and possibly vesiculation and oozing on exposed surfaces
- Peeling of the epidermis and pigmentary changes often result
- Inner upper eyelids spared, as is the area under the chin
- The lips are commonly involved in hereditary polymorphous light eruption, a disorder seen in persons of Native American descent

DIFFERENTIAL DIAGNOSIS

- Contact dermatitis

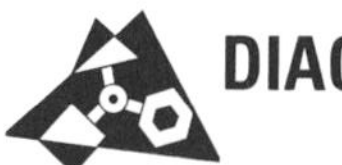

DIAGNOSIS

LABORATORY TESTS

- The key to diagnosis is localization of the rash to photoexposed areas, though these eruptions may become generalized with time to involve even photoprotected areas
- Blood and urine tests are not helpful in diagnosis unless porphyria cutanea tarda is suggested by the presence of blistering, scarring, milia (white cysts 1–2 mm in diameter) and skin fragility of the dorsal hands, and facial hypertrichosis

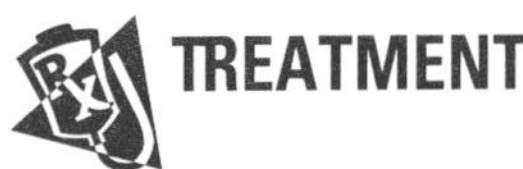

TREATMENT

MEDICATIONS

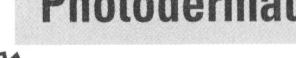

- Drugs should be suspected in cases of photoallergy even if the particular medication (such as hydrochlorothiazide) has been used for months

Local measures

- When the eruption is vesicular or weepy, treatment is similar to that of any acute dermatitis, using cooling and soothing wet dressing
- Mid-potency to high-potency topical steroids are of limited benefit in phototoxic reactions but may help in polymorphous light eruption and photoallergic reactions

Systemic measures

- Aspirin may have some value for fever and pain of acute sunburn, as prostaglandins appear to play a pathogenetic role in the early erythema
- Systemic corticosteroids in doses as described for acute contact dermatitis may be required for severe photosensitivity reactions
- Immunosuppressives may be indicated for severe photosensitivity, such as azathioprine, in the range of 50–150 mg/d; or cyclosporine, 3–5 mg/kg/d

PREVENTION

- While sunscreens are useful agents in general and should be used by persons with photosensitivity, patients may react to such low amounts of energy that sunscreens alone may not be sufficient
- Sunscreens with an SPF of 30–50, usually containing avobenzone (Parasol 1789), titanium dioxide, and micronized zinc oxide, are especially useful in patients with photoallergic dermatitis

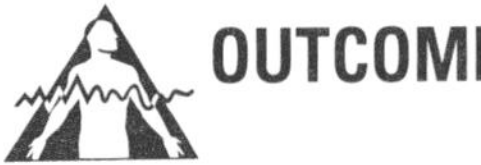

OUTCOME

PROGNOSIS

- The most common phototoxic reactions are usually benign and self-limiting except when the burn is severe or when it occurs as an associated finding in a more serious disorder
- Polymorphous light eruption and some cases of photoallergy can persist for years

WHEN TO REFER

- If there is a question about the diagnosis, if recommended therapy is ineffective, or if specialized treatment is necessary

EVIDENCE

WEB SITES

- American Academy of Dermatology
  - http://www.aad.org
- JAMA & Archives: Photosensitivity Disorders Article Collection
  - http://pubs.ama-assn.org/cgi/collection/photosensitivity_disorders_?page=1

INFORMATION FOR PATIENTS

- American Osteopathic College of Dermatology: Polymorphous Light Eruption
  - http://www.aocd.org/skin/dermatologic_diseases/polymorphous_light_eruption.html
- Centers for Disease Control and Prevention: Sun Exposure Prevention
  - http://www.cdc.gov/ChooseYourCover/qanda.htm
- Iron Disorders Institute: Porphyria Cutanea Tarda
  - http://www.irondisorders.org/disorders/pct/index.htmLupus
- Lupus Foundation of America: Photosensitivity and Lupus
  - http://www.lupus.org/education/brochures/photosensitivity.html
- U.S. Food and Drug Administration: Chemical Photosensitivity: Another Reason to Be Careful in the Sun
  - http://www.fda.gov/fdac/features/496_sun.html

REFERENCES

- Bilu D et al: Clinical and epidemiologic characterization of photosensitivity in HIV-positive individuals. Photodermatol Photoimmunol Photomed 2004;20:175. [PMID: 15238095]
- Brunner KL et al: Extreme photosensitivity. Mayo Clin Proc 2004;79:1316. [PMID: 15473416]
- Millard TP et al: Photodermatoses in the elderly. Clin Geriatr Med 2001;17:691. [PMID: 11535424]
- Morison WL: Clinical practice. Photosensitivity. N Engl J Med 2004;350:1111. [PMID: 15014184]

Author(s)

Timothy G. Berger, MD

Pityriasis Rosea

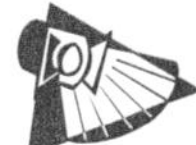

KEY FEATURES

ESSENTIALS OF DIAGNOSIS

- Oval, fawn-colored, scaly eruption following cleavage lines of trunk
- Herald patch precedes eruption by 1–2 weeks
- Occasional pruritus

GENERAL CONSIDERATIONS

- Common mild, acute inflammatory disease that is 50% more common in women
- The eruption usually lasts 4–8 weeks and heals without scarring

DEMOGRAPHICS

- Young adults are principally affected, mostly in the spring or fall

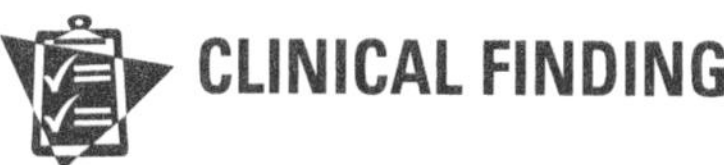

CLINICAL FINDINGS

SYMPTOMS AND SIGNS

- See Table 7
- Diagnosis is made by finding one or more classic lesions
- The lesions consist of oval, fawn-colored plaques up to 2 cm in diameter. The centers of the lesions have a crinkled or "cigarette paper" appearance and a collarette scale, ie, a thin bit of scale that is bound at the periphery and free in the center
- Only a few lesions in the eruption may have this characteristic appearance, however
- Lesions follow cleavage lines on the trunk (so-called Christmas tree pattern), and the proximal portions of the extremities are often involved
- Herald patch precedes eruption by 1–2 weeks
- Pruritus, if present, is usually mild
- Variants that affect the flexures (axillae and groin), so-called inverse pityriasis rosea, and papular variants, especially in black patients, also occur

DIFFERENTIAL DIAGNOSIS

- Secondary syphilis
- Tinea corporis (body ringworm)
- Seborrheic dermatitis
- Tinea versicolor (pityriasis versicolor)
- Lichen planus
- Psoriasis
- Nummular eczema
- Drug eruption
- Viral exanthem

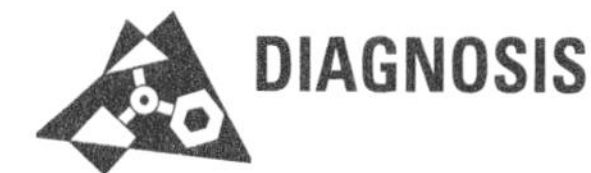

DIAGNOSIS

LABORATORY TESTS

- Clinical diagnosis

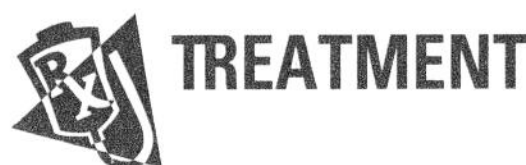

TREATMENT

MEDICATIONS

- See Table 6
- Often requires no treatment
- In Asians, Hispanics, or blacks, in whom lesions may remain hyperpigmented for some time, more aggressive management may be indicated
- The most effective management consists of daily UVB treatments for a week, or prednisone as used for contact dermatitis. Topical steroids of medium strength (triamcinolone 0.1%) may also be used if pruritus is bothersome
- Oral erythromycin for 14 days was reported to clear 73% of patients within 2 weeks (compared with none of the patients on placebo)

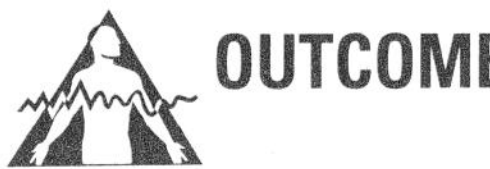

OUTCOME

WHEN TO REFER

- If there is a question about the diagnosis, if recommended therapy is ineffective, or if specialized treatment is necessary

EVIDENCE

WEB SITES

- American Academy of Dermatology
  - http://www.aad.org
- Dermatlas, Johns Hopkins University School of Medicine: Pityriasis Rosea Images
  - http://dermatlas.med.jhmi.edu/derm/result.cfm?Diagnosis=115
  - http://www.vh.org/Providers/ClinRef/FPHandbook/17.html

INFORMATION FOR PATIENTS

- American Academy of Dermatology: Pityriasis Rosea
  - http://www.aad.org/public/Publications/pamphlets/PityriasisRosea.htm
- American Academy of Family Physicians: Pityriasis Rosea
  - http://familydoctor.org/808.xml
- Mayo Clinic: Christmas Tree Rash
  - http://www.mayoclinic.com/invoke.cfm?objectid=DD0B41A0-CAFF-4AC1-9B0F334ED578DEB7
- MedlinePlus: Pityriasis Rosea
  - http://www.nlm.nih.gov/medlineplus/ency/article/000871.htm

REFERENCES

- Eslick GD: Atypical pityriasis rosea or psoriasis guttata? Early examination is the key to a correct diagnosis. Int J Dermatol 2002;41:788. [PMID: 12453007]
- Karnath B et al: Pityriasis rosea. Appearance and distribution of macules aid diagnosis. Postgrad Med 2003;113:93. [PMID: 12764899]
- Stulberg DL et al: Pityriasis rosea. Am Fam Physician 2004;69:87. [PMID: 14727822]

Author(s)

Timothy G. Berger, MD

Plague

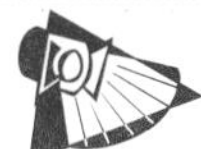

KEY FEATURES

ESSENTIALS OF DIAGNOSIS

- History of exposure to rodents in endemic area
- Sudden onset of high fever, malaise, muscular pains, and prostration
- Axillary or inguinal lymphadenitis (bubo)
- Bacteremia, pneumonitis, and meningitis may occur
- Positive smear and culture from bubo and positive blood culture

GENERAL CONSIDERATIONS

- An infection of wild rodents with *Yersinia pestis*, a small bipolar-staining gram-negative rod
- It is transmitted among rodents and to humans by the bites of fleas or from contact with infected animals
- Following the flea bite, the organisms spread through the lymphatics to the lymph nodes, which become greatly enlarged (bubo). They may then reach the bloodstream to involve all organs
- If a plague victim develops pneumonia, the infection can be transmitted by droplets to other individuals
- The incubation period is 2–10 days
- Because of its extreme virulence, its potential for dissemination and person-to-person transmission, and efforts to develop the organism as an agent of biowarfare, plague bacillus is considered a high-priority agent for bioterrorism

DEMOGRAPHICS

- It is endemic in California, Arizona, Nevada, and New Mexico

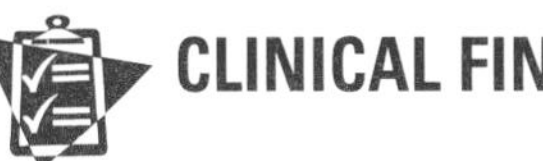

CLINICAL FINDINGS

SYMPTOMS AND SIGNS

- The onset is sudden, with high fever, malaise, tachycardia, intense headache, and severe myalgias
- The patient appears profoundly ill. Delirium may ensue
- A pustule or ulcer at the site of inoculation and lymphangitis may be observed
- Axillary, inguinal, or cervical lymph nodes become enlarged and tender and may suppurate and drain
- Signs of meningitis may develop
- With hematogenous spread, the patient may rapidly become toxic and comatose, with purpuric spots (black plague) appearing on the skin
- Primary plague pneumonia is a fulminant pneumonitis with bloody, frothy sputum and sepsis
- If pneumonia develops, tachypnea, productive cough, blood-tinged sputum, and cyanosis also occur

DIFFERENTIAL DIAGNOSIS

- Tularemia
- Lymphadenopathy of extremity due to bacterial infection
- Genital lymphadenopathy due to lymphogranuloma venereum, syphilis
- Typhoid fever
- Influenza
- Rickettsial disease, eg, epidemic typhus, Q fever
- Anthrax
- Other bacterial pneumonia
- Hantavirus pulmonary syndrome
- Sepsis due to other causes

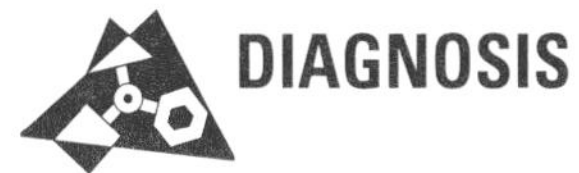

DIAGNOSIS

LABORATORY TESTS

- The plague bacillus may be found in smears from aspirates of buboes examined with Gram's stain
- Cultures from bubo aspirate or pus and blood are positive but may grow slowly
- In convalescing patients, an antibody titer rise may be demonstrated by agglutination tests

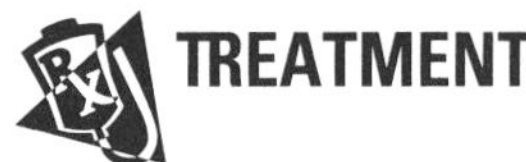

TREATMENT

MEDICATIONS

- Therapy should be started immediately once plague is suspected
- Either streptomycin (the agent with which there is greatest experience), 1 g every 12 h intravenously, or gentamicin, administered as a 2 mg/kg loading dose, then 1.7 mg/kg every 8 h intravenously, is effective
- Alternatively, doxycycline, 100 mg twice daily orally or intravenously, may be used
- The duration of therapy is 10 days

THERAPEUTIC PROCEDURES

- Patients with plague pneumonia are placed in strict respiratory isolation

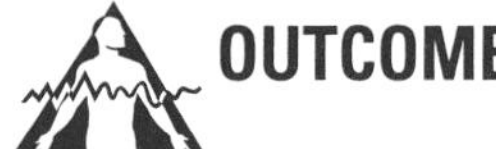

OUTCOME

PROGNOSIS

- Pneumonia or meningitis is usually fatal

WHEN TO REFER

- All suspected cases should be referred to an infectious disease specialist
- All cases must be reported to the public health authorities

WHEN TO ADMIT

- All suspected or known cases

PREVENTION

- Drug prophylaxis may provide temporary protection for persons exposed to plague, particularly by the respiratory route. Tetracycline hydrochloride, 500 mg orally once or twice daily for 5 days, is effective
- The efficacy of plague vaccines—both live and killed—is not clearly established

EVIDENCE

PRACTICE GUIDELINES

- National Guideline Clearinghouse
  - http://www.guideline.gov/summary/summary.aspx?doc_id=2983

WEB SITES

- CDC Bioterrorism
  - http://www.bt.cdc.gov/agent/plague/index.asp
- CDC—Division of Bacterial and Mycotic Diseases
  - http://www.cdc.gov/ncidod/dbmd/
- CDC—Division of Vector-Borne Infectious Disease
  - http://www.cdc.gov/ncidod/dvbid/plague
- Karolinska Institute—Directory of Bacterial Infections and Mycoses
  - http://www.mic.ki.se/Diseases/C01.html

INFORMATION FOR PATIENTS

- National Insitute of Allergy and Infectious Diseases
  - http://www.niaid.nih.gov/factsheets/plague.htm

REFERENCE

- Boulanger LL et al: Gentamicin and tetracyclines for the treatment of human plague: review of 75 cases in New Mexico, 1985–1999. Clin Infect Dis 2004;38:663. [PMID: 14986250]
- Koornhof HJ et al: Yersiniosis. II: The pathogenesis of *Yersinia* infections. Eur J Clin Microbiol Infect Dis 1999;18:87. [PMID: 0219573]

Author(s)

Henry F. Chambers, MD

Pleural Effusion

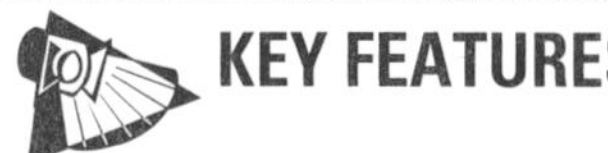

KEY FEATURES

ESSENTIALS OF DIAGNOSIS

- May be asymptomatic
- Chest pain seen in the setting of pleuritis, trauma, or infection
- Dyspnea is common with large effusions
- Dullness to percussion and decreased breath sounds over the effusion
- Radiographic evidence of pleural effusion
- Diagnostic findings on thoracentesis

GENERAL CONSIDERATIONS

- Pleural fluid is produced at 0.01 mL/kg/body weight/hour; a normal volume in the pleural space is 5–15 mL
- **Transudative** effusions (see Laboratory Tests) occur in the absence of pleural disease; 90% of cases result from congestive heart failure
- **Exudative** effusions are most commonly due to pneumonia (parapneumonic effusions) and malignancy (malignant effusions)
- Analysis of pleural fluid allows for identification of the pathophysiologic process leading to accumulation of pleural fluid
  - Increased production due to increased hydrostatic or decreased oncotic pressures (transudates)
  - Increased production due to abnormal capillary permeability (exudates)
  - Decreased lymphatic clearance of fluid (exudates)
  - Infection in the pleural space (empyema)
  - Bleeding into the pleural space (hemothorax)
- A definitive diagnosis is made through cytology or identification of causative organism in 25% of cases
- In 50–60% of cases, classification of the effusion leads to a presumptive diagnosis

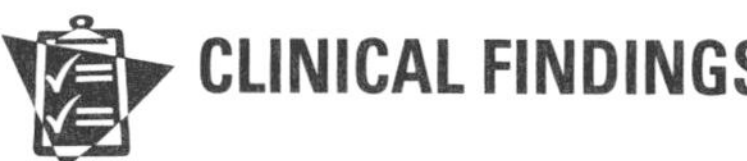

CLINICAL FINDINGS

SYMPTOMS AND SIGNS

- Dyspnea, cough, or chest pain with respirations
- Symptoms are more common in patients with underlying cardiopulmonary disease
- Large effusions are more likely to be symptomatic
- Bronchial breath sounds and egophony above the effusion are caused by compressive atelectasis
- Massive effusions may cause contralateral shift of the trachea and bulging of intercostal spaces
- A pleural friction rub indicates infarction or pleuritis

DIFFERENTIAL DIAGNOSIS

- Atelectasis
- Chronic pleural thickening
- Lobar consolidation
- Subdiaphragmatic process
- Table 36

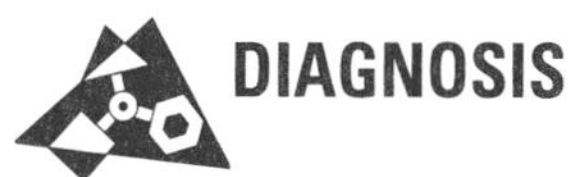

DIAGNOSIS

LABORATORY TESTS

- See Table 37
- Pleural fluid should be sent for protein, glucose, LDH, cell count, Gram stain, and culture
- Grossly purulent fluid signifies empyema; Gram stain and culture are confirmatory
- **Exudates** have one of the following
  - Pleural fluid protein/serum protein >0.5
  - Pleural fluid LDH/serum LDH >0.6
  - Pleural fluid LDH more than two-thirds of the upper limit of normal serum LDH
- **Transudates** lack any of these features
- **Hemothorax** is defined as a pleural fluid hematocrit/peripheral hematocrit ratio >0.5
- Elevated pleural fluid amylase suggests pancreatitis, pancreatic pseudocyst, adenocarcinoma of the lung, or esophageal rupture
- Pleural fluid triglyceride level >100 mg/dL suggests disruption of the thoracic duct
- Pleural fluid cytology has a sensitivity of 50–65% for detecting malignancy
- Repeat cytologic examination, followed by thoracoscopy or video-assisted thoracoscopic surgery (VATS), is indicated if suspicion is high and cytology is negative

IMAGING STUDIES

- Chest x-rays can detect as little as 175–200 mL of pleural fluid on a frontal and 75–100 mL on a lateral view
- Chest CT can identify as little as 10 mL of pleural fluid
- Lateral decubitus chest films can determine whether blind thoracentesis may be performed; a minimum 1 cm of fluid must be seen for the procedure to be done safely
- Ultrasonography should be used to safely guide thoracentesis of small effusions

DIAGNOSTIC PROCEDURES

- Diagnostic paracentesis should be performed for any new pleural effusion without apparent cause
- Pleural biopsy should be performed in cases of suspected tuberculous effusion
- Pleural fluid culture is only 44% sensitive for tuberculous effusion; culture and histologic examination of pleural tissue increases this to 70–90%

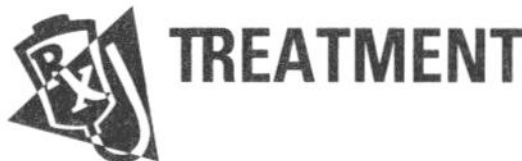

TREATMENT

MEDICATIONS

- Appropriate antibiotics for pleural infections (see Tables 127 and 128)

SURGERY

- Thoracotomy may be required in hemothorax to control hemorrhage, remove clot, and treat complications
- Chest tube insertion (tube thoracostomy)
  - Rarely indicated for transudates
  - May be useful in malignant effusions
  - Indicated for some complicated parapneumonic effusions and empyema

THERAPEUTIC PROCEDURES

- Pleurodesis involves placing an irritant into the pleural space to obliterate it by producing adhesions; side effects are pain and fever; premedication is necessary
  - Doxycycline is 70–75% effective
  - Talc is 90% effective
  - Rarely indicated for transudates
  - Often used for recurrent malignant effusions
- Intrapleural fibrinolysis
  - Streptokinase, 250,000 units or urokinase 100,000 units in 100 mL of saline can improve drainage of empyema or complicated parapneumonic effusions with loculations

Transudative effusions

- Treatment is directed at the underlying cause
- Therapeutic thoracentesis may offer only transient relief from dyspnea
- Tube thoracostomy and pleurodesis are rarely indicated

Malignant effusion

- Systemic therapy may address the underlying malignancy
- Repeated thoracentesis or chest tube insertion (tube thoracostomy) may be needed as local therapy to relieve symptoms related to the effusion itself
- Pleurodesis can reduce reaccumulation of fluid

Parapneumonic effusion

- Simple effusions (free-flowing, sterile) will resolve with treatment of the pneumonia and do not require drainage
- Complicated effusions should be drained via chest tube if fluid analysis reveals pH < 7.2 *or* glu < 60; drainage should be considered for pH 7.2–7.3 or LDH >1000 mg/dL
- Empyema should be drained via chest tube

Hemothorax

- If small-volume and stable, observation is adequate
- All other cases should be treated with immediate drainage via a large-bore chest tube

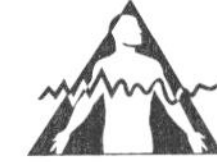

OUTCOME

FOLLOW-UP

- Serial chest x-rays to ensure resolution

COMPLICATIONS

- Fibrothorax can occur if hemothorax is not evacuated

PROGNOSIS

- Depends on the cause of the effusion

WHEN TO REFER

- All large effusions, exudative effusions, and complicated transudative effusions should be evaluated with the assistance of a pulmonologist

WHEN TO ADMIT

- For large-volume thoracentesis, chest tube placement, or complicated closed pleural biopsy

EVIDENCE

PRACTICE GUIDELINES

- Antunes G et al: BTS guidelines for the management of malignant pleural effusions. Thorax 2003;58(Suppl 2):ii29.
- Maskell NA et al: BTS guidelines for the investigation of a unilateral pleural effusion in adults. Thorax. 2003;58(Suppl 2):ii8.

INFORMATION FOR PATIENTS

- National Institutes of Health
  - http://www.nlm.nih.gov/medlineplus/ency/article/000086.htm

REFERENCE

- Colice GL et al: Medical and surgical treatment of parapneumonic effusions: an evidence-based guideline. Chest 2000;118:1158. [PMID:11035692]
- Light RW. Clinical practice. Pleural effusion. N Engl J Med 2002;346:1971. [PMID:12075059]
- Shaw P et al: Pleurodesis for malignant pleural effusions. Cochrane Database Syst Rev (1):CD002916, 2004. [PMID:14973997]

Author(s)

Mark S. Chesnutt, MD
Thomas J. Prendergast, MD

Pleuritis p. 1131. Plexopathies p. 1132.

Pneumocystis Pneumonia

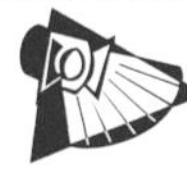

KEY FEATURES

ESSENTIALS OF DIAGNOSIS

- *Pneumocystis carinii* is a fungus found in lungs of many domesticated and wild mammals and *Pneumocystis jiroveci* in humans worldwide
- Infection causes pneumonia, with fever, dyspnea, nonproductive cough
- Bibasilar crackles on auscultation in many cases, others have no findings
- Bilateral diffuse interstitial disease without hilar adenopathy on chest x-ray
- Reduced partial pressure of oxygen
- *P jiroveci* in sputum, bronchoalveolar lavage fluid, or lung tissue

GENERAL CONSIDERATIONS

- Based on serology, asymptomatic infections occur at a young age in most persons
- Whether disease in adults represents reinfection or reactivation of existing infection is debated

DEMOGRAPHICS

- Most common in patients with AIDS, also occurs in patients with cancer, severe malnutrition, or in those undergoing immunosuppressive or radiation therapy (eg, for organ transplants, cancer)
- Mode of transmission unknown but likely airborne
- *Pneumocystis* pneumonia occurs in up to 80% of AIDS patients not on prophylaxis, usually at CD4 cell counts < 200/μL
- Infection outside of the lungs is rare, unless patient is receiving aerosolized pentamidine prophylaxis
- In non-AIDS patients taking immunosuppressives, symptoms often begin when corticosteroids are tapered or discontinued

CLINICAL FINDINGS

SYMPTOMS AND SIGNS

- Fever; tachypnea; shortness of breath; and cough, usually nonproductive
- Normal lung examination or bibasilar crackles; findings may be slight compared with degree of illness and chest x-ray abnormality
- Spontaneous pneumothorax may occur if patient had previous episodes or received aerosolized pentamidine prophylaxis
- In AIDS: fever, fatigue, and weight loss may occur weeks or months before pulmonary symptoms

DIFFERENTIAL DIAGNOSIS

- Bacterial pneumonia
- Tuberculosis
- Coccidioidomycosis
- Histoplasmosis
- Cytomegalovirus
- Kaposi's sarcoma
- Lymphoma (including lymphocytic interstitial pneumonitis)
- Pulmonary embolism

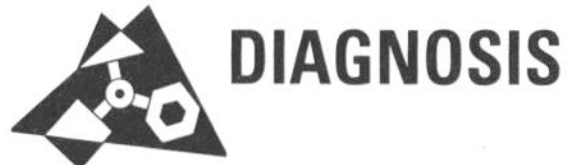

DIAGNOSIS

LABORATORY TESTS

- Lactate dehydrogenase elevation sensitive but not specific
- Lymphopenia with low CD4 count common
- Arterial blood gas shows hypoxemia and hypocarbia; peripheral oxygen saturation may be normal at rest but decreases rapidly with exercise
- Serologic tests not helpful
- Culture not possible
- Specimens of induced sputum can be stained to demonstrate cysts
- If induced sputum is negative and suspicion is high, diagnostic specimens may be obtained by bronchoalveolar lavage (sensitivity 86–97%) or, if necessary, by transbronchial lung biopsy (sensitivity 85–97%)
- Polymerase chain reaction test for *P jiroveci* appears sensitive but does not provide more rapid diagnosis

IMAGING STUDIES

- Chest x-ray usually shows diffuse "interstitial" infiltrates, but early in infection, these may be heterogeneous, miliary, or patchy; may also show diffuse or focal consolidation, cystic changes, nodules, or cavitation within nodules
- Pleural effusions not seen
- Chest x-ray normal in 5–10%; high-resolution chest CT better able to demonstrate mild disease
- Upper lobe infiltrates common if patient received aerosolized pentamidine prophylaxis
- Pulmonary function tests (PFTs) show reduced vital capacity, total lung capacity, and diffusing capacity
- Gallium lung scanning shows diffuse uptake. While sensitivity is high (> 95%), specificity is low (20–40%), so test usually obtained only if high suspicion and normal chest x-ray and PFTs

DIAGNOSTIC PROCEDURES

- Fine-needle aspiration and open lung biopsy are infrequently done

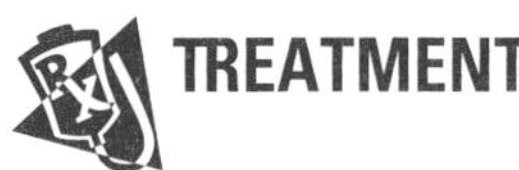

TREATMENT

MEDICATIONS

- If disease suspected clinically, initiate empiric therapy while work-up proceeds
- Trimethoprim-sulfamethoxazole (TMP-SMX) is preferred therapy when tolerated and no sulfa allergy
- Oral TMP-SMX generates same blood levels as IV and should be used when gastrointestinal tract is functioning
- Dose is based on TMP: 15–20 mg/kg QD divided TID or QID for 14–21 days; usual adult dose is two double-strength tablets three times daily
- Hypersensitivity to sulfonamide is especially common in AIDS patients
- Symptoms often persist for 4–6 days after starting therapy and may worsen in first 3–5 days presumably due to immune response to dying organisms
- If $PaO_2 < 70$ mm Hg: add prednisone 40 mg BID for 5 days, then 40 mg QD for 5 days, then 20 mg QD until therapy complete
- For severe cases where TMP-SMX is not tolerated, then pentamidine 3 mg/kg IV/IM QD for 14–21 days
- For mild to moderate disease in patients intolerant or not responding to TMP-SMX:
  - Clindamycin 600 mg PO TID plus primaquine 15 mg PO QD
  - Dapsone 100 mg PO QD plus trimethoprim 15 mg/kg/day divided TID
  - Atovaquone 750 mg PO QD
  - Trimetrexate 45 mg/m^2 IV QD plus high-dose leucovorin (salvage therapy)
- If patient with known *P jiroveci* is not responding to therapy after 4–6 days then:
  - Need to assess for other concomitant infectious or noninfectious pulmonary processes (cytomegalovirus, tuberculosis, atypical pneumonia, congestive heart failure)
  - Add prednisone if not added at baseline
  - If taking TMP-SMX, consider switch to alternative therapy
  - If not taking TMP-SMX because of allergy, consider desensitization and use of TMP-SMX

OUTCOME

PROGNOSIS

- Without treatment, mortality of pneumocytosis approaches 100%
- With treatment, survival is most closely correlated with pretreatment arterial-alveolar gradient
- Early treatment reduces mortality to 10–20% in AIDS and to 30–50% in other immunodeficient patients
- Recurrence is common without prophylaxis
- In patients who have *P jiroveci* pneumonia associated with AIDS, initiation of highly active antiretroviral treatment may result in "paradoxical deterioration" presumably due to increased immune response against residual microbial antigens

PREVENTION

- Primary prophylaxis is indicated for all AIDS patients with CD4 < 200/ μL
- Secondary prophylaxis indicated for AIDS patients until durable response to antiretroviral therapy has increased CD4 to > 200/μL on two occasions
- Primary prophylaxis also indicated in bone marrow transplant patients and in stem cell transplant patients who are receiving conditioning regimens; therapy usually continued for 6 months after transplant or longer for those with graft-versus-host disease
- First-line prophylaxis is TMP-SMX one double-strength tablet three times weekly or QD. Hypersensitivity is common but if mild may be able to continue therapy through to resolution
- Alternative to TMP-SMX for prevention:
  - Dapsone, 50–100 mg PO QD; need to check glucose-6-phosphate dehydrogenase levels prior to initiation
  - Oral atovaquone 1500 mg PO QD has some efficacy but also much more expensive than other regimens
  - Aerosolized pentamidine 300 mg monthly less effective compared with TMP-SMX and predisposes to extrapulmonary pneumocystosis and pneumothorax

EVIDENCE

PRACTICE GUIDELINES

- Centers for Disease Control and Prevention—Guidelines for PCP prophylaxis
  - http://www.cdc.gov/mmwr/preview/mmwrhtml/00001409.htm
- Infectious Diseases Society of America—Summary of the guidelines for preventing opportunistic infections among hematopoietic stem cell transplant recipients
  - http://www.journals.uchicago.edu/CID/journal/issues/v33n2/001547/001547.web.pdf
- 2001 USPHS/IDSA Guidelines for the Prevention of Opportunistic Infections in Persons Infected with Human Immunodeficiency Virus. US Department of Health and Human Services, Public Health Service
  - http://aidsinfo.nih.gov/guidelines/op_infectionsOI_112801.pdf

WEB SITES

- AIDS Info by the USDHHS
  - http://aidsinfo.nih.gov/
- Project Inform
  - http://www.projectinform.org/

INFORMATION FOR PATIENTS

- Centers for Disease Control and Prevention
  - http://www.cdc.gov/hiv/pubs/brochure/pcpb.htm
- JAMA patient page: HIV infection: the basics. JAMA 2002;288:268. [PMID: 12123237]
- MedlinePlus
  - http://www.nlm.nih.gov/medlineplus/ency/article/000671.htm

REFERENCE

- Stringer JR et al: A new name *(Pneumocystis jiroveci)* for pneumocystis from humans. Emerg Infect Dis 2002;8:891. [PMID: 12194762]

Author(s)

Samuel A. Shelburne, MD

Richard J. Hamill, MD

Pneumonia, Anaerobic, & Lung Abscess

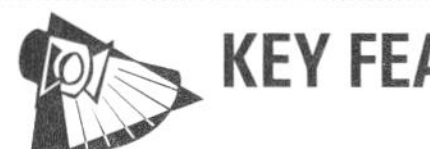

KEY FEATURES

ESSENTIALS OF DIAGNOSIS

- History of or predisposition to aspiration
- Indolent symptoms, including fever, weight loss, malaise
- Poor dentition
- Foul-smelling purulent sputum (in many patients)
- Infiltrate in dependent lung zone, with single or multiple areas of cavitation or pleural effusion

GENERAL CONSIDERATIONS

- Nocturnal aspiration of small amounts of oropharyngeal secretions is typically not pathologic
- Larger aspirations may cause
  - Nocturnal asthma
  - Chemical pneumonitis
  - Bronchiectasis
  - Mechanical obstruction
  - Pleuropulmonary infection
- Predisposing factors include
  - Drug or alcohol use
  - Seizures
  - Anesthesia
  - Central nervous system disease
  - Trachea or nasogastric tubes
- Periodontal disease and poor oral hygiene are associated with a greater likelihood of pleuropulmonary infection
- Disease usually occurs in dependent lung zones
- Most infections include multiple anaerobic bacteria: *Prevotella melaninogenica,* peptostreptococcus, *Fusobacterium nucleatum,* and *Bacteroides*

DEMOGRAPHICS

- Risk factors are poor dentition, heavy alcohol use, and aspiration

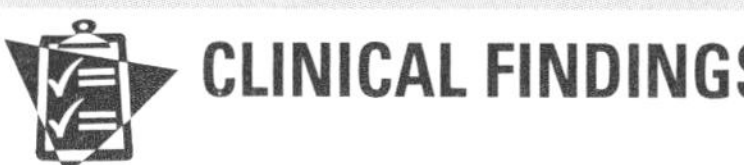

CLINICAL FINDINGS

SYMPTOMS AND SIGNS

- Onset is insidious; necrotizing pneumonia, abscess, or empyema may be apparent at presentation
- Constitutional symptoms of fever, malaise, and weight loss are common
- Cough with foul-smelling expectorant suggests anaerobic infection
- Poor dentition is typical
- Patients are rarely edentulous; this finding suggests an obstructing bronchial lesion

DIFFERENTIAL DIAGNOSIS

- Other causes of cavitary lung disease
  - Tuberculosis
  - Fungal infection
  - Bronchogenic cancer
  - Pulmonary infarction
  - Wegener's granulomatosis
  - Cavitary bacterial pneumonia
- Fungal infection, eg, histoplasmosis
- Bronchiectasis

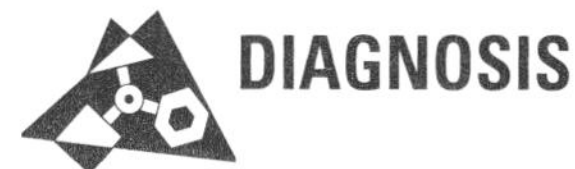

DIAGNOSIS

LABORATORY TESTS

- Culture of expectorated sputum is not useful due to contamination with oral flora

IMAGING STUDIES

- The chest x-ray in a lung abscess will show a thick-walled cavity surrounded by consolidation, occasionally with an air-fluid level
- Necrotizing pneumonia demonstrates multiple areas of cavitation within an area of consolidation
- Empyema is characterized by purulent pleural fluid and may accompany the findings of abscess or necrotizing pneumonia
- Ultrasonography may identify loculations or help localize fluid for safe thoracentesis

DIAGNOSTIC PROCEDURES

- Thoracentesis with pleural fluid analysis should be performed on all effusions

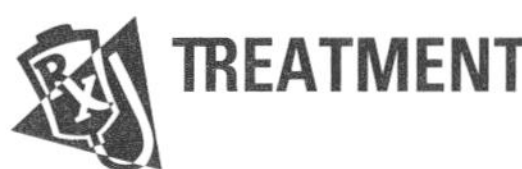

TREATMENT

MEDICATIONS

- Clindamycin (600 mg IV Q 8 h, then 300 mg PO Q 6 h after initial improvement)
- Amoxicillin-clavulanate (875 mg PO Q 12 h)
- Penicillin (amoxicillin 500 mg PO TID or penicillin G 1–2 million units IV Q 4–6 h) plus metronidazole 500 mg PO or IV Q 8–12 h
- Therapy should be continued until the chest x-ray improves, usually for a month or more

SURGERY

- Open pleural drainage is sometimes needed because of loculations associated with a parapneumonic effusion

THERAPEUTIC PROCEDURES

- Thoracentesis
- Anaerobic pleuropulmonary infection requires drainage with a thoracostomy tube for empyema

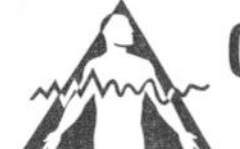

OUTCOME

FOLLOW-UP

- Monitor chest x-ray; if it does not improve, consider other causes

COMPLICATIONS

- Sepsis
- Parapneumonic effusion
- Empyema with loculations and/or pleural scarring and the need for surgical decortication via thoracotomy

PROGNOSIS

- Excellent with appropriate antimicrobial therapy

WHEN TO REFER

- Refer to infectious disease expert, pulmonary specialist, or thoracic surgeon if no response to antibiotic therapy or concern about the presence of another process (eg, cancer)

WHEN TO ADMIT

- Hypoxia
- Severe malnutrition
- Marked systemic symptoms

PREVENTION

- Good dental hygiene

EVIDENCE

PRACTICE GUIDELINES

- Tablan OC et al: Guidelines for preventing health-care–associated pneumonia, 2003: recommendations of CDC and the Healthcare Infection Control Practices Advisory Committee. MMWR Recomm Rep 2004 Mar 26;53(RR-3):1

INFORMATION FOR PATIENTS

- Mayo Clinic
  - http://www.mayoclinic.com/invoke.cfm?id=DS00135
- National Institutes of Health
  - http://www.nlm.nih.gov/medlineplus/ency/article/000121.htm

REFERENCES

- Levinson ME: Anaerobic pleuropulmonary infection. Curr Opin Infect Dis 2001;14:187. [PMID:11979131]
- Mansharamani N: Lung abscess in adults: clinical comparison of immunocompromised to non-immunocompromised patients. Respir Med 2002;96:178. [PMID:11905552]

Author(s)

Mark S. Chesnutt, MD
Thomas J. Prendergast, MD

Pneumonia, Chlamydial p. 1132

Pneumonia, Community-Acquired

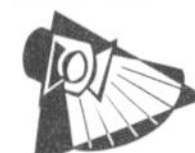

KEY FEATURES

ESSENTIALS OF DIAGNOSIS

- Symptoms and signs of an acute lung infection
  - Fever or hypothermia
  - Cough with or without sputum
  - Dyspnea
  - Chest discomfort
  - Sweats or rigors
- Bronchial breath sounds or rales are common auscultatory findings
- Parenchymal infiltrate on chest radiograph
- Occurs outside of the hospital or less than 48 hours after admission in a patient who has not been hospitalized or residing in a long-term care facility for 14 days or more before the onset of symptoms

GENERAL CONSIDERATIONS

- Defined as beginning outside the hospital or being diagnosed within 48 hours of admission
- The most deadly infectious disease in the United States and the sixth leading cause of death overall
- Mortality rate is 14% among hospitalized patients and 1% among outpatients
- Prospective studies fail to identify the cause in 40–60% of cases, although bacteria are more commonly identified than viruses
- The most common bacterial pathogens
  - *Streptococcus pneumoniae* (two-thirds of cases)
  - *Haemophilus influenzae*
  - *Mycoplasma pneumoniae*
  - *Chlamydia pneumoniae*
  - *Staphylococcus aureus*
  - *Neisseria meningitidis*
  - *Moraxella catarrhalis*
  - *Klebsiella pneumoniae*
- Common viral causes
  - Influenza
  - Respiratory syncytial virus
  - Adenovirus
  - Parainfluenza virus
- Assessment of epidemiologic risk factors may help in diagnosing pneumonia due to the following
  - *Chlamydia psittaci* (psittacosis)
  - *Coxiella burnetii* (Q fever)
  - *Francisella tularensis* (tularemia)
  - Endemic fungi (blastomyces, coccidioides, histoplasma)
  - Sin Nombre virus (hantavirus pulmonary syndrome)

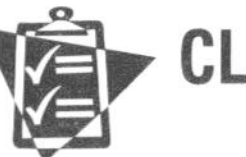

CLINICAL FINDINGS

SYMPTOMS AND SIGNS

- Acute or subacute onset of fever, cough with or without sputum, and dyspnea
- Rigors, sweats, chills, pleurisy, and chest discomfort are common
- Fatigue, anorexia, headache, myalgias, and abdominal pain can be present
- Physical findings include
  - Fever or hypothermia
  - Tachypnea
  - Tachycardia
  - Mild oxygen desaturation
- Altered breath sounds or rales are common
- Dullness to percussion may be present with a parapneumonic effusion

DIFFERENTIAL DIAGNOSIS

- Bacterial pneumonia
- Viral pneumonia
- Aspiration pneumonia
- *Pneumocystis jiroveci* pneumonia
- Bronchitis
- Lung abscess
- Tuberculosis
- Pulmonary embolism
- Myocardial infarction
- Sarcoidosis
- Lung neoplasm
- Hypersensitivity pneumonitis
- Bronchiolitis, BOOP

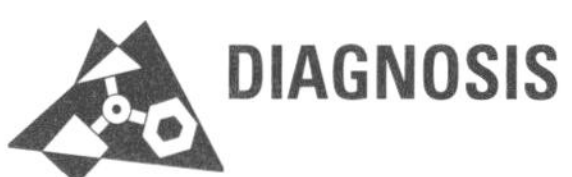

DIAGNOSIS

LABORATORY TESTS

- See Table 19
- Gram stain and culture of sputum are controversial, but recommended in hospitalized patients
- Preantibiotic blood cultures are generally recommended for hospitalized patients
- Recommended for all hospitalized patients
  - Arterial blood gases
  - Complete blood cell count
  - A comprehensive metabolic panel
- HIV serology should be considered in hospitalized patients

IMAGING STUDIES

- Chest x-ray can confirm the diagnosis and detect associated lung diseases
- Findings range from patchy airspace infiltrates to diffuse alveolar or interstitial infiltrates
- Clearing of infiltrates can take 6 weeks

DIAGNOSTIC PROCEDURES

- Sputum induction is reserved for patients who cannot provide expectorated samples or may have *Pnuemocystis carinii* or *Mycobacterium tuberculosis* pneumonia
- Thoracentesis with pleural fluid analysis should be performed in all patients with effusions

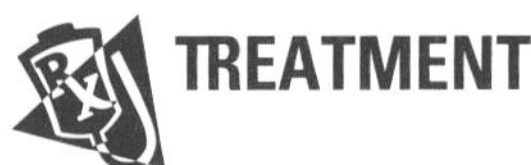

TREATMENT

MEDICATIONS

- See Table 19
- Outpatient therapy
  - Macrolides: clarithromycin, 500 mg PO BID, azithromycyin, 500 mg PO initially, then 250 mg QD for 4 days
  - Doxycycline, 100 mg PO BID
  - Fluoroquinolones with enhanced *S pneumoniae* activity: gatifloxacin, 400 mg PO QD, levofloxacin, 500 mg PO QD, or moxifloxacin 400 mg PO QD
  - Alternatives are erythromycin, amoxicillin-clavulanate, and some second- or third-generation cephalosporins
- Hospitalized patients on a general medical ward
  - Extended-spectrum β-lactam (ceftriaxone or cefotaxime) with a macrolide (clarithromycin or azithromycin)
  - Fluoroquinolones with enhanced *S pneumoniae* activity (gatifloxicin, levofloxacin, moxifloxacin)
  - β-Lactam/β-lactamase inhibitor (ampicillin-sulbactam or piperacillin-tazobactam) with a macrolide
- Patients in intensive care unit
  - Macrolide or fluoroquinolone plus an extended-spectrum cephalosporin or β-lactam/β-lactamase inhibitor
  - Penicillin-allergic patients may receive a fluoroquinolone with or without clindamycin
  - Suspected aspiration pneumonia should be treated with fluoroquinolone with or without clindamycin, metronidazole, or β-lactam/β-lactamase inhibitor
- Patients with cystic fibrosis or bronchiectasis should receive empiric antipseudomonal therapy
- Duration of therapy
  - Influenced by the severity of illness, the etiological agent, response to therapy, and other medical problems
  - For *S pneumoniae,* treat for 72 hours after the patient becomes afebrile
  - 2 weeks is minimum for pneumonia due to *S aureus, P aeruginosa, Klebsiella,* anaerobes, *M pneumoniae, C pneumoniae,* or *Legionella*

OUTCOME

FOLLOW-UP

- Chest x-ray 6 weeks after therapy

COMPLICATIONS

- Parapneumonic effusion—simple or complicated
- Empyema
- Sepsis
- Respiratory failure and/or ARDS
- Pneumotocele
- Lung abscess
- Focal bronchiectasis

PROGNOSIS

- Excellent with appropriate antimicrobial and supportive care

WHEN TO REFER

- Extensive disease and/or seriously ill
- Progression of disease or failure to improve on antibiotics

WHEN TO ADMIT

- The PORT score stratifies patients by mortality and can assist in decisions regarding admission (Tables 20 and 21)

PREVENTION

- Polyvalent pneumococcal vaccine
  - Can prevent or lessen the severity of pneumococcal infections
  - Indications are age >65 or any chronic illness increasing the risk of community-acquired pneumonia
- Influenza vaccine
  - Effective at preventing primary influenza pneumonia and secondary bacterial pneumonia
  - Given annually to patients who are >65, are residents of chronic care facilities, have cardiopulmonary disease, or were recently hospitalized with chronic metabolic disorders
- Hospitalized patients who would benefit from vaccine should receive it in hospital
- Pneumococcal and influenza vaccines can be given simultaneously and are not contraindicated immediately after a pneumonia

EVIDENCE

PRACTICE GUIDELINES

- American College of Emergency Physicians. Clinical policy for the management and risk stratification of community-acquired pneumonia in adults in the emergency department. Ann Emerg Med 2001;38:107. [PMID:11859897]
- Mandell LA et al: Infectious Diseases Society of American. Update of practice guidelines for the management of community-acquired pneumonia in immunocompetent adults. Clin Infect Dis 2003;37:1405. Epub 2003 Nov 03. [PMID:14614663]

INFORMATION FOR PATIENTS

- American Lung Association
  - http://www.lungusa.org/site/pp.asp?c=dvLUK9O0E&b=35692
- Mayo Clinic
  - http://www.mayoclinic.com/invoke.cfm?id=DS00135

REFERENCES

- de Roux A et al: Viral community-acquired pneumonia in nonimmunocompromised adults. Chest 2004;125:1343. [PMID:15078744]
- File TM Jr. Guidelines for empiric antimicrobial prescribing in community-acquired pneumonia. Chest 2004;125:1888. [PMID:15136404]
- Halm EA et al: Clinical practice. Management of community-acquired pneumonia. N Engl J Med 2002;347:2039. [PMID:12490686]
- Metlay JP et al: Testing strategies in the initial management of patients with community-acquired pneumonia. Ann Intern Med 2003;138:109. [PMID:12529093]
- Niederman MS et al: Guidelines for the management of adults with community-acquired pneumonia. Diagnosis, assessment of severity, antimicrobial therapy, and prevention. Am J Respir Crit Care Med 2001;163:1730. [PMID:11401897]

Author(s)

Mark S. Chesnutt, MD

Thomas J. Prendergast, MD

Pneumonia, Eosinophilic p. 1132

Pneumonia, Hospital-Acquired

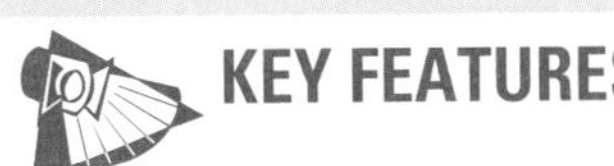

KEY FEATURES

ESSENTIALS OF DIAGNOSIS

- Occurs more than 48 hours after admission to the hospital and excludes any infection present at the time of admission
- At least **two** of the following are present
  - Fever
  - Cough
  - Leukocytosis
  - Purulent sputum
- New or progressive parenchymal infiltrate on chest radiograph
- Especially common in patients requiring intensive care or mechanical ventilation

GENERAL CONSIDERATIONS

- Second most common form of hospital-acquired infection
- Leading cause of deaths due to nosocomial infections
- Mortality rates range from 20% to 50%
- Highest morbidity and mortality occur in ICU and mechanically ventilated patients
- Most common organisms
  - *Pseudomonas aeruginosa*
  - *Staphylococcus aureus*
  - *Enterobacter*
  - *Klebsiella pneumoniae*
  - *Escherichia coli*
- Anaerobic organisms, when isolated, are commonly part of a polymicrobial flora
- Colonization of the pharynx with bacteria is the most important step in pathogenesis and is promoted by instrumentation, contamination, and patient factors
- Increased gastric pH leading to bacterial overgrowth has been suggested as a possible risk factor

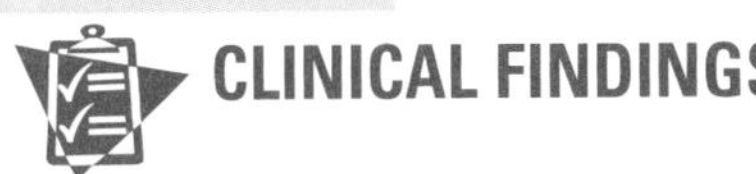

CLINICAL FINDINGS

SYMPTOMS AND SIGNS

- Presentation is nonspecific, but includes the findings seen in community-acquired pneumonia
- Fever, leukocytosis, purulent sputum, or a new or progressive infiltrate on chest x-ray is usually seen

DIFFERENTIAL DIAGNOSIS

- Congestive heart failure
- Atelectasis
- Aspiration
- Acute respiratory distress syndrome
- Pulmonary thromboembolism
- Pulmonary hemorrhage
- Drug reactions

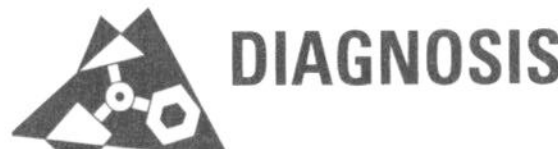

DIAGNOSIS

LABORATORY TESTS

- Blood cultures identify the pathogen in up to 20% of cases
- Arterial blood gases help define illness severity and the need for supplemental oxygen
- Complete blood cell count and chemistry tests are not helpful in identifying the etiologic agent, but can assist in determining illness severity and complications
- Examination of sputum and sputum cultures is controversial, but may be useful in guiding antibiotic therapy
- Direct fluorescent antibody staining for *Legionella* can be helpful when this organism is suspected
- Sputum stains and cultures for mycobacteria and fungi may be diagnostic

IMAGING STUDIES

- X-ray findings are nonspecific and range from patchy infiltrates to lobar consolidation to diffuse alveolar or interstitial infiltrates
- Progression of infiltrates and lack of improvement during antibiotic therapy are poor prognostic signs and may put the diagnosis in question

DIAGNOSTIC PROCEDURES

- Thoracentesis with pleural fluid analysis is indicated for any effusion
- Endotracheal aspiration and fiberoptic bronchoscopy with lavage or use of a protected specimen brush are used most commonly in patients with ventilator-associated pneumonia (VAP)
- A recent trial using quantitative culture of bronchoalveolar lavage or protected specimen brush samples in suspected VAP reduced antibiotic use, shortened the duration of organ dysfunction, and decreased mortality

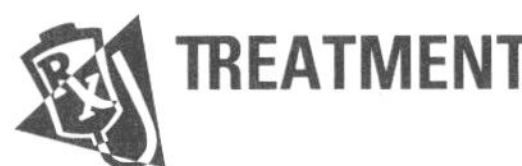

TREATMENT

MEDICATIONS

- See Table 128
- Treatment is usually empirical and should be started as soon as the diagnosis is suspected
- Initial regimens should be broad and tailored to the specific clinical setting
- No consensus regimens exist, but guidelines separate patients by disease severity
- **Mild-to-moderate disease** with early onset (< 5 days after hospitalization) or without unusual risk factors
  - Second-generation cephalosporin or nonantipseudomonal third-generation cephalosporin or
  - Combination of a β-lactam/β-lactamase inhibitor
- **Severe, late-onset disease** (>5 days after hospitalization), or with ICU-acquired disease or VAP
  - Combination of antibiotics against *P aeruginosa*, *Acinetobacter,* and *Enterobacter* species
  - Include aminoglycoside or fluoroquinolone plus one of the following: antipseudomonal penicillin, antipseudomonal cephalosporin, imipenem-cilastin, or aztreonam
  - Vancomycin is added for concern for methicillin-resistant *S aureus* (patients with head trauma, coma, diabetes, renal failure, or ICU stay)
  - Anaerobic coverage with clindamycin, or a β-lactam/β-lactamase inhibitor is added for patients with aspiration, recent thoracoabdominal surgery, or airway obstruction
  - Macrolide is added where there is risk for *Legionella* (patients on high-dose steroids)
- Duration of therapy should be individualized, but at least 14–21 days for gram-negative bacterial pneumonia

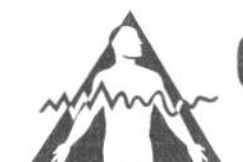

OUTCOME

COMPLICATIONS

- Parapneumonic effusion—simple or complicated
- Empyema
- Sepsis
- Respiratory failure and/or ARDS
- Pneumotocele
- Lung abscess
- Focal bronchiectasis

PROGNOSIS

- Mortality rates range from 20% to 50% and are highest in mechanically ventilated patients

WHEN TO REFER

- Extensive disease
- Seriously ill patient, particularly in the setting of comorbid conditions (eg, liver disease)
- Progression of disease or failure to improve on antibiotics

PREVENTION

- Sucralfate use for gastric ulcer prophylaxis (rather than H_2-receptor antagonists or proton-pump inhibitors) may reduce the incidence of VAP

EVIDENCE

INFORMATION FOR PATIENTS

- American Lung Association
  - http://www.lungusa.org/site/pp.asp?c=dvLUK9O0E&b=35692
- Mayo Clinic
  - http://www.mayoclinic.com/invoke.cfm?id=DS00135
- National Institutes of Health
  - http://www.nlm.nih.gov/medlineplus/ency/article/000146.htm

REFERENCES

- Chastre J et al: Ventilator-associated pneumonia. Am J Respir Crit Care Med 2002;165:867. [PMID:11934711]
- Fagon JY. Hospital-acquired pneumonia: diagnostic strategies: lessons from clinical trials. Infect Dis Clin N Am 2003;17:1717. [PMID:15008594]
- Mehta RM et al: Nosocomial pneumonia in the intensive care unit: controversies and dilemmas. J Intens Care Med 2003;18:175. [PMID:15035764]
- Sopena N et al: Multicenter study of hospital-acquired pneumonia in non-ICU patients. Chest 2005;127:213. [PMID:15653986]

Author(s)

Mark S. Chesnutt, MD

Thomas J. Prendergast, MD

Pneumonia, Idiopathic Fibrosing Interstitial

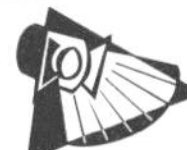

KEY FEATURES

ESSENTIALS OF DIAGNOSIS

- Progressive dyspnea and cough
- Diffuse dry rales on ausculation of the chest
- Restrictive ventilatory defect and abnormal gas exchange
- Bibasilar, peripheral interstitial fibrosis on chest x-ray or CT
- Exclusion of known causes of interstitial lung disease

GENERAL CONSIDERATIONS

- Formerly known as idiopathic pulmonary fibrosis (IPF) and in Britain as cryptogenic fibrosing alveolitis
- Historically, diagnosis was based on clinical and radiographic criteria, with lung biopsy uncommon
- Several histologic patterns once grouped together as IPF are now recognized to be associated with different natural histories and responses to therapy
- Evaluation must first identify patients whose disease is truly idiopathic
- Most identifiable causes of interstitial lung diseases
  - Infectious
  - Drug-related
  - Exposures
  - Associated with other medical conditions
- A specific diagnosis allows providers to give accurate information on natural history and to distinguish patients most likely to benefit from treatment
- See Table 29

DEMOGRAPHICS

- Age range usually 40–70 years
- Slight male predominance
- More common in cigarette smokers than nonsmokers

CLINICAL FINDINGS

SYMPTOMS AND SIGNS

- Insidious dry cough and exertional dyspnea lasting months
- Diffuse, fine late inspiratory crackles on auscultation of the lungs
- Clubbing is present at the time of diagnosis in 25–50%

DIFFERENTIAL DIAGNOSIS

- Bronchiolitis obliterans with organizing pneumonia (BOOP)
- Interstitial lung disease due to infection (eg, fungal, viral, *Pneumocystis jiroveci*, tuberculosis)
- Drug-induced fibrosis (eg, amiodarone, bleomycin)
- Sarcoidosis
- Pneumoconiosis
- Hypersensitivity pneumonitis
- Asbestosis
- See Table 28

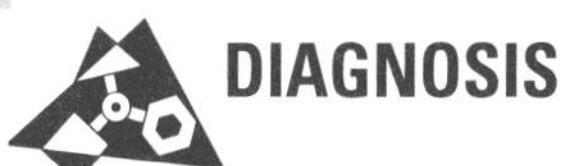

DIAGNOSIS

LABORATORY TESTS

- To exclude other causes
  - ANA, RF
  - Erythrocyte sedimentation rate
  - Aldolase, anti-Jo-1 antibody

IMAGING STUDIES

- Chest x-ray and HRCT classically demonstrate low lung volumes and diffuse, patchy fibrosis with pleural-based honeycombing

DIAGNOSTIC PROCEDURES

- Transbronchial biopsy cannot be used to definitively diagnose usual interstitial pneumonitis, though it may exclude it by confirming an alternative diagnosis
- Restrictive physiology with decreased diffusing capacity on pulmonary function testing

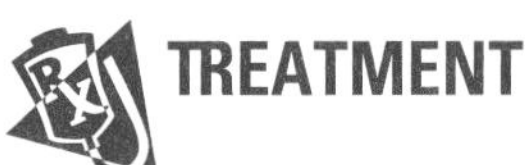

TREATMENT

MEDICATIONS

- Treatment is controversial: no randomized study has demonstrated that treatment improves survival

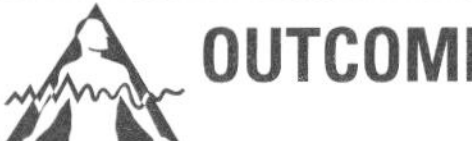

OUTCOME

FOLLOW-UP

- Serial pulmonary function tests and assessment of gas exchange

COMPLICATIONS

- Hypoxemia requiring oxygen therapy
- Respiratory failure

PROGNOSIS

- Median survival approximately 3 years, depending on stage at presentation

WHEN TO REFER

- All patients should be evaluated by a pulmonologist at the time of diagnosis to assist with diagnosis, consider treatment options, and evaluate for lung transplantation

WHEN TO ADMIT

- Progressive respiratory failure

EVIDENCE

INFORMATION FOR PATIENTS

- Coalition for Pulmonary Fibrosis
  - http://www.coalitionforpf.org/Patients/whatyoucando.asp

REFERENCES

- American Thoracic Society; European Respiratory Society: American Thoracic Society/European Respiratory Society International Multidisciplinary Consensus Classification of the Idiopathic Interstitial Pneumonias. Am J Respir Crit Care Med 2002;165:277. [PMID:11790668]
- Collard HR et al: Demystifying idiopathic interstitial pneumonia. Arch Intern Med 2003;163:17. [PMID: 12523913]
- Gross TJ et al: Idiopathic pulmonary fibrosis. N Engl J Med 2001;345:517. [PMID:11519507]
- Leslie KO. Pathology of interstitial lung disease. Clin Chest Med 2004;25:657. [PMID:15564015]
- Raghu G et al: Idiopathic pulmonary fibrosis: current trends in management. Clin Chest Med 2004;25:621. [PMID:15564012]
- Swigris JJ et al: Idiopathic pulmonary fibrosis: challenges and opportunities for the clinician and investigator. Chest 2005;127:275. [PMID:15653995]

Author(s)

Mark S. Chesnutt, MD

Thomas J. Prendergast, MD

Pneumonia, Pneumococcal

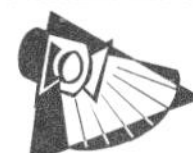

KEY FEATURES

ESSENTIALS OF DIAGNOSIS

- Productive cough, fever, rigors, dyspnea, early pleuritic chest pain
- Consolidating lobar pneumonia on chest x-ray
- Lancet-shaped gram-positive diplococci on Gram stain of sputum

GENERAL CONSIDERATIONS

- The most common cause of community-acquired pyogenic bacterial pneumonia
- Alcoholism, HIV infection, sickle cell disease, splenectomy, and hematological disorders are predisposing factors
- Up to 40% of infections are caused by pneumococci resistant to at least one drug and 15% are due to a strain resistant to three or more drugs

DEMOGRAPHICS

- Until 2000, *Streptococcus pneumoniae* infections caused 100,000–135,000 hospitalizations for pneumonia, 6 million cases of otitis media, and 60,000 cases of invasive disease, including 3300 cases of meningitis
- Disease figures are now changing due to conjugate vaccine introduction

CLINICAL FINDINGS

SYMPTOMS AND SIGNS

- High fever, productive cough, occasionally hemoptysis, and pleuritic chest pain
- Rigors can occur within the first few hours of infection
- Bronchial breath sounds are an early sign
- Differentiating pneumococcal from other bacterial pneumonias is not possible clinically or radiographically because of significant overlap in presentations

DIFFERENTIAL DIAGNOSIS

- Pneumonia due to other causes, eg, *Haemophilus influenzae*, influenza
- Aspiration pneumonia or lung abscess
- Pulmonary embolism
- Myocardial infarction
- Acute exacerbation of chronic bronchitis
- Acute bronchitis
- Hypersensitivity pneumonitis

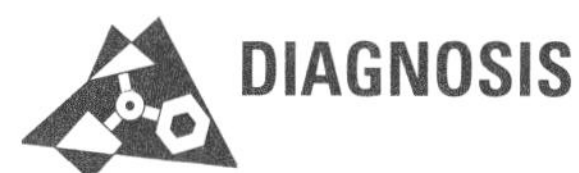

DIAGNOSIS

LABORATORY TESTS

- A good-quality sputum sample (less than 10 epithelial cells and more than 25 polymorphonuclear leukocytes per high-power field) shows gram-positive diplococci in 80–90% of cases
- Blood cultures are positive in up to 25% of selected cases and much more commonly so in HIV-positive patients

IMAGING STUDIES

- Chest x-ray shows findings of consolidation, often with a lobar distribution, infiltrates, pleural effusion

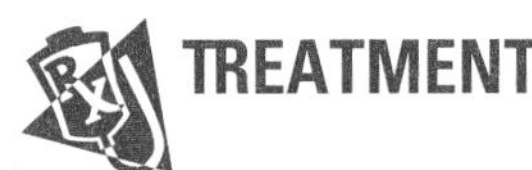

TREATMENT

MEDICATIONS

- Initial antimicrobial therapy of pneumonia is empirical pending isolation and identification of the causative agent (Table 19)

Outpatient

- Amoxicillin, 750 mg twice daily for 7–10 days
- Alternatives are azithromycin, one 500 mg dose on the first day and 250 mg for the next 4 days; clarithromycin, 500 mg twice daily for 10 days; or doxycycline, 100 mg twice daily for 10 days

Inpatient

- Aqueous penicillin G (susceptible strains), 2 million units intravenously every 4 h
- Ceftriaxone, 1 g intravenously every 24 h
- For a highly penicillin-resistant strain, vancomycin, 1 g every 12 h
- Fluoroquinolones with enhanced gram-positive activity (eg, levofloxacin, 500 mg once daily; moxifloxacin, 400 mg once daily; or gatifloxacin, 400 mg once daily) are effective oral alternatives

THERAPEUTIC PROCEDURES

- Pleural effusions developing after initiation of antimicrobial therapy usually are sterile, and thoracentesis need not be performed if the patient is otherwise improving
- Thoracentesis is indicated for an effusion present prior to initiation of therapy and in the patient who has not responded to antibiotics after 3–4 days

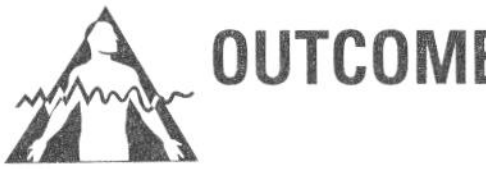

OUTCOME

FOLLOW-UP

- Repeat chest x-ray 6–8 weeks after treatment to ensure resolution of infiltrate

COMPLICATIONS

- Parapneumonic (sympathetic) effusion is common and may cause recurrence or persistence of fever
- Empyema occurs in ≤5% and contains organisms on gram-stained or positive pleural fluid cultures (unlike sympathetic effusion)
- Pneumococcal pericarditis (rare)
- Pneumococcal arthritis (rare)
- Pneumococcal endocarditis usually involves the aortic valve and often occurs in association with meningitis and pneumonia

PROGNOSIS

- The mortality rate remains high in the setting of advanced age, multilobar disease, severe hypoxemia, extrapulmonary complications, and bacteremia

WHEN TO REFER

- Early referral to a pulmonologist for management of seriously ill patients

WHEN TO ADMIT

- The Pneumonia Patient Outcomes Research Team (PORT) model can be used along with clinical judgment in the initial decision on whether to hospitalize a patient (Tables 20 and 21)
- Patients under 50 years old without comorbid conditions or physical examination abnormalities listed in Table 20 have the lowest risk

PREVENTION

Pneumococcal vaccine

- Contains purified polysaccharide from 23 of the most common strains of *S pneumoniae*, which cause 90% of bacteremic episodes in the United States
- Is about 60–70% effective in preventing bacteremic disease in immunocompetent patients
- Is about 50% effective in preventing bacteremic disease in patients with underlying diseases (not severely compromised) and only about 10% effective in immunocompromised patients
- Current recommendations
  - Table 132
  - Patients at increased risk of developing severe pneumococcal disease, especially asplenic patients and those with sickle cell disease
  - Chronic illnesses (eg, cardiopulmonary disease, alcoholism, renal disease, cancer)
  - All individuals over 65 years of age
  - Elderly individuals with unknown immunization status should be immunized once
- Revaccination
  - Recommended every 5 years, regardless of age, for those with the highest risk of fatal pneumococcal disease (eg, asplenic patients, nephrotic syndrome or renal failure, HIV, leukemia, lymphoma, myeloma, immunosuppressive medications, transplant patients)
  - 65 years of age if primary vaccine was at least 5 years before
  - High-risk individuals previously immunized with the 14-valent vaccine

EVIDENCE

PRACTICE GUIDELINES

- National Guideline Clearinghouse
  - http://www.guideline.gov/summary/summary.aspx?doc_id=4546
  - http://www.guideline.gov/summary/summary.aspx?doc_id=2773

WEB SITES

- CDC—Division of Bacterial and Mycotic Diseases
  - http://www.cdc.gov/ncidod/dbmd/
- Karolinska Institute—Directory of Bacterial Infections and Mycoses
  - http://www.mic.ki.se/Diseases/C01.html

INFORMATION FOR PATIENTS

- JAMA patient page: Pneumonia. JAMA 2000;283:1922. [PMID: 10683063]
- JAMA patient page: Immunizations. JAMA 1999;282:102. [PMID: 10404918]
- NIH—National Institute of Allergy and Infectious Disease
  - http://www.niaid.nih.gov/factsheets/pneumonia.htm

REFERENCES

- Aspa J et al; Pneumococcal Pneumonia in Spain Study Group: Drug-resistant pneumococcal pneumonia: clinical relevance and related factors. Clin Infect Dis 2004;38:787. [PMID: 14999620]
- Whitney CG et al: Rethinking recommendations for use of pneumococcal vaccines in adults. Clin Infect Dis 2001;33:662. [PMID: 11486289]
- Yu VL et al: An international prospective study of pneumococcal bacteremia: correlation with in vitro resistance, antibiotics administered, and clinical outcome. Clin Infect Dis 2003;37:230. [PMID: 12856216]

Author(s)

Henry F. Chambers, MD

Pneumonitis, Hypersensitivity

Pneumonia, Usual Interstitial p. 1133. Pneumonitis, Acute Interstitial p. 1133.

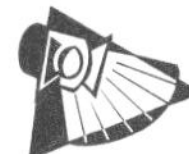

KEY FEATURES

ESSENTIALS OF DIAGNOSIS

- A link between symptoms and exposure may be obtained from work or environmental history
- Antigen can be microbial agents, animal proteins, or chemical sensitizers
- Presentation can be acute or a subacute illness

GENERAL CONSIDERATIONS

- A nonatopic, nonasthmatic allergic pulmonary disease
- Manifested mainly as occupational disease where exposure to an inhaled organic agent leads to acute and eventually chronic pulmonary disease
- Causes
  - See Table 35
  - Farmer's lung (moldy hay)
  - "Humidifier" lung (contaminated humidifier, heating, or air conditioning)
  - Bird fancier's lung ("pigeon breeder's disease")
  - Bagassosis (moldy sugar cane fiber)
  - Sequoiosis (moldy redwood sawdust)
  - Maple bark stripper's disease
  - Mushroom picker's disease (moldy compost)
  - Suberosis (moldy cork dust)
  - Detergent worker's lung (enzyme additives)

CLINICAL FINDINGS

SYMPTOMS AND SIGNS

- Acute illness 4–8 hours after exposure characterized by
  - Malaise
  - Chills
  - Fever
  - Cough
  - Dyspnea
  - Nausea
- Bibasilar crackles, tachypnea, tachycardia, and (occasionally) cyanosis are found
- Subacute illness (15% of cases)
  - Insidious onset of chronic cough and progressive dyspnea
  - Anorexia
  - Weight loss

DIFFERENTIAL DIAGNOSIS

- Sarcoidosis
- Asthma
- Atypical pneumonia
- Collagen vascular disease, eg, systemic lupus erythematosus
- Idiopathic pulmonary fibrosis
- Lymphoma

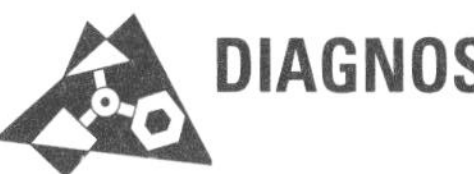

DIAGNOSIS

LABORATORY TESTS

- Pulmonary function studies show a restrictive pattern with decreased diffusion capacity
- Leukocytosis with a left shift
- Arterial blood gases show hypoxemia
- Hypersensitivity pneumonitis antibody panels are available and may reveal precipitating antibodies to the offending allergen in serum

IMAGING STUDIES

- Chest x-ray classically shows small nodular densities sparing the apices and bases
- Pulmonary fibrosis may be found with repeated exposure to the offending agent

DIAGNOSTIC PROCEDURES

- Bronchoscopy with bronchoalveolar lavage
- Surgical lung biopsy is occasionally necessary

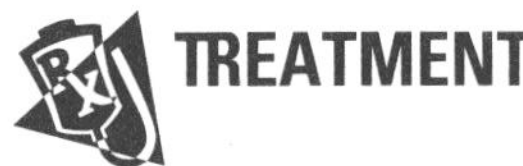

TREATMENT

MEDICATIONS

- Corticosteroids (prednisone, 0.5 mg/kg/day, tapered over 4–6 weeks) are typically used despite the lack of a placebo-controlled trial

THERAPEUTIC PROCEDURES

- Identification of the offending agent with removal or avoidance
- Change in occupation is often unavoidable

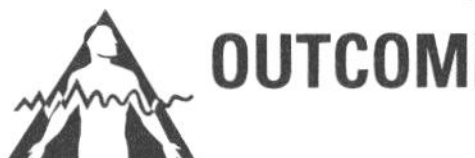

OUTCOME

FOLLOW-UP

- Monitor serial chest x-rays and pulmonary function tests

COMPLICATIONS

- Progressive pulmonary fibrosis and respiratory failure

PROGNOSIS

- Good if diagnosed early and offending agent is avoided

WHEN TO REFER

- For assistance in diagnosis, treatment, and follow-up

WHEN TO ADMIT

- Hypoxemic respiratory failure

EVIDENCE

INFORMATION FOR PATIENTS

- American Academy of Family Physicians
  - http://familydoctor.org/handouts/134.html
- Mayo Clinic
  - http://www.mayoclinic.com/invoke.cfm?objectid=98F1BC84-428A-43CF-B8E1372CAB04F7BB
- National Institutes of Health
  - http://www.nlm.nih.gov/medlineplus/ency/article/000109.htm

REFERENCES

- Lacasse Y et al: Clinical diagnosis of hypersensitivity pneumonitis. Am J Respir Crit Care Med 2003;168:952. [PMID:12842854]
- Patel AM et al: Hypersensitivity pneumonitis: current concepts and future questions. J Allergy Clin Immunol 2001;108:661. [PMID:11692086]

Author(s)

Mark S. Chesnutt, MD
Thomas J. Prendergast, MD

Pneumothorax, Spontaneous

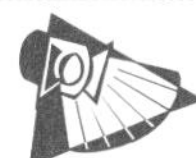

KEY FEATURES

ESSENTIALS OF DIAGNOSIS

- Acute onset of unilateral chest pain and dyspnea
- Minimal physical findings in mild cases
  - Unilateral chest expansion
  - Decreased tactile fremitus
  - Hyperresonance
  - Diminished breath sounds may occur
- Tension pneumothorax
  - Mediastinal shift
  - Cyanosis
  - Hypotension
- Pleural air on chest radiograph

GENERAL CONSIDERATIONS

- Traumatic pneumothorax occurs as a result of penetrating or blunt trauma
- Iatrogenic pneumothorax may follow procedures such as central line placement and transbronchial biopsy
- Tension pneumothorax usually occurs in the setting of
  - Penetrating trauma
  - Lung infection
  - Cardiopulmonary resuscitation
  - Positive-pressure ventilation
- Spontaneous pneumothorax occurs without trauma and is classified as
  - Secondary—complicating preexisting lung disease
  - Primary—no prior lung disease
- Risk factors for secondary pneumothorax include
  - Chronic obstructive pulmonary disease (COPD)
  - Asthma
  - Cystic fibrosis
  - Tuberculosis
  - Prior pneumocystis pneumonia
  - Menstruation (catemenial pneumothorax)
  - Many interstitial lung diseases

DEMOGRAPHICS

- Primary pneumothorax affects mainly tall, thin males between 10 and 30 years of age
- Family history and smoking may be contributing factors in primary spontaneous pneumothorax

CLINICAL FINDINGS

SYMPTOMS AND SIGNS

- Chest pain ranges from minimal to severe
- Dyspnea is almost always present
- Symptoms usually begin at rest and resolve within 24 hours, even if the pneumothorax persists
- In the setting of COPD or asthma, patients may present with life-threatening respiratory failure
- Often seen with large pneumothoraces
  - Unilateral chest expansion
  - Hyperresonance
  - Diminished breath sounds
  - Decreased tactile fremitus
  - Decreased movement of the chest
- Physical findings may be absent in small (< 15%) pneumothoraces
- Tension pneumothorax should be suspected if marked tachycardia, mediastinal or tracheal shift, or hypotension is present
- Crepitus may be found over the chest wall and adjacent structures

DIFFERENTIAL DIAGNOSIS

- Emphysematous bleb mimicking loculated pneumothorax
- Myocardial infarction
- Pneumonia
- Pulmonary embolus
- Pneumomediastinum can be caused by rupture of the esophagus or bronchus
- Upper respiratory tract infection
- Rib fracture
- Pericarditis
- Mesothelioma

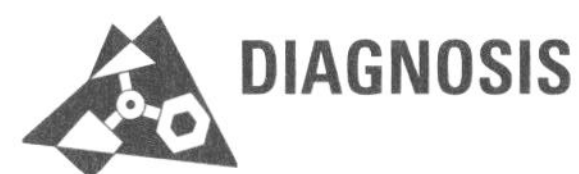

DIAGNOSIS

LABORATORY TESTS

- Arterial blood gas usually reveals hypoxemia and acute respiratory alkalosis
- QRS axis and precordial T-wave changes may mimic acute myocardial infarction in left-sided pneumothorax

IMAGING STUDIES

- A visceral pleural line on chest x-ray is diagnostic; an expiratory film will increase sensitivity
- Secondary pleural effusion can occur
- Supine patients may demonstrate the "deep sulcus sign"—an abnormally radiolucent costophrenic angle
- Large amounts of subpleural air with contralateral mediastinal shift are present in tension pneumothorax

Pneumonitis, Nonspecific Interstitial p. 1133.
Pneumonitis, Radiation p. 1134.

Pneumothorax, Spontaneous

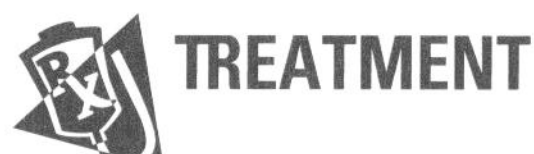

TREATMENT

MEDICATIONS

- Symptomatic treatment for cough and chest pain is appropriate
- Supplemental oxygen may increase the rate of reabsorption of pleural air
- Reliable patients with small (< 15%), primary pneumothoraces may be observed

SURGERY

- Simple aspiration of pleural air through a small-bore catheter can be performed for large or progressive pneumothoraces
- Placement of a small-bore chest tube (7F–14F) attached to a one-way Heimlich valve protects against development of a tension pneumothorax and may permit observation from home
- Chest tube placement (tube thoracostomy) may be indicated
  - For secondary, large, or tension pneumothorax
  - For severe symptoms or mechanically ventilated patients
- Thoracoscopy or open thoracotomy for removal of blebs or pleurodesis may be indicated in recurrent primary pneumothorax, failed tube thoracostomy

THERAPEUTIC PROCEDURES

- Pleurodesis is indicated in recurrent or refractory cases

OUTCOME

FOLLOW-UP

- Serial chest x-rays should be obtained at 24-hour intervals
- Chest tubes may be removed when the air leak subsides

COMPLICATIONS

- Tension pneumothorax, which may be life-threatening
- Pneumomediastinum and subcutaneous emphysema

PROGNOSIS

- 50% recurrence rate in smokers
- 30% risk of recurrence in spontaneous pneumothorax treated with observation or chest tube placement
- Recurrence after surgical therapy is less common

WHEN TO ADMIT

- Large, severely symptomatic, or progressive primary pneumothorax
- Secondary pneumothorax

PREVENTION

- Smokers should be counseled to quit
- Future exposure to high altitudes, unpressurized flight, and scuba diving should be avoided

EVIDENCE

PRACTICE GUIDELINES

- Baumann MH et al: AACP Pneumothorax Consensus Group Management of spontaneous pneumothorax: an American College of Chest Physicians Delphi consensus statement. Chest 2001;119:590. [PMID:11171742]
- Henry M et al: BTS guidelines for the management of spontaneous pneumothorax. Thorax 2003;58(Suppl 2):ii39. [PMID:12728149]

INFORMATION FOR PATIENTS

- American Lung Association
  - http://www.lungusa.org/site/pp.asp?c=dvLUK9O0E&b=35772#primary
- The Mayo Clinic
  - http://www.mayoclinic.com/invoke.cfm?id=HQ01228

REFERENCES

- Baumann MH et al: Management of spontaneous pneumothorax: an American College of Chest Physicians Delphi concensus statement. Chest 2001;119:590. [PMID:11171742]
- Sahn SA et al: Spontaneous pneumothorax. N Engl J Med 2000;342:868. [PMID:10727592]

Author(s)

Mark S. Chesnutt, MD

Thomas J. Prendergast, MD

Polyarteritis Nodosa & Microscopic Polyangiitis

KEY FEATURES

ESSENTIALS OF DIAGNOSIS

- Classic polyarteritis nodosa (PAN) involves medium-sized vessels (but substantial overlap occurs)
- Microscopic polyangiitis (MPA) may involve small blood vessels (capillaries, arterioles, venules) as well as medium-sized vessels
- Classic PAN is often associated with hypertension but spares the lung
- 10–30% of PAN are associated with hepatitis B or C

Etiology

- Idiopathic
- Hepatitis B or C
- Drugs, eg, propylthiouracil, hydralazine, allopurinol, penicillamine, sulfasalazine

GENERAL CONSIDERATIONS

- PAN is a medium-sized necrotizing arteritis with a predilection for involving peripheral nerves, mesenteric vessels (including renal arteries), heart, and brain but the capability of involving most organs
- MPA is a nongranulomatous vasculitis involving small blood vessels; it is often associated with antineutrophil cytoplasmic antibodies (ANCAs) that produce a perinuclear p-ANCA pattern on immunofluorescence testing and are directed against myeloperoxidase, a constituent of neutrophil granules
- Clinical findings depend on the arteries involved

CLINICAL FINDINGS

SYMPTOMS AND SIGNS

- Common symptoms of both disorders
  - Insidious onset
  - Fever and other constitutional symptoms
  - Abdominal pain, particularly diffuse periumbilical pain precipitated by eating. Nausea and vomiting are frequently associated
  - Livedo reticularis
- Pain in the extremities is often a prominent early feature caused by arthralgia, myalgia (particularly affecting the calves), or neuropathy
- Mononeuritis multiplex (most common: foot-drop)
- MPA
  - Pulmonary hemorrhage and glomerulonephritis
- PAN
  - Skin: livedo reticularis, subcutaneous nodules, and skin ulcers
  - Involvement of the renal arteries leads to a renin-mediated hypertension
  - Seldom involves the lung
- Infarction compromises the function of major viscera and may lead to acalculous cholecystitis or appendicitis
- Some patients present dramatically with an acute abdomen caused by mesenteric vasculitis and gut perforation or with hypotension resulting from rupture of a microaneurysm in the liver, kidney, or bowel

DIFFERENTIAL DIAGNOSIS

- Wegener's granulomatosis
- Churg-Strauss syndrome
- Endocarditis
- Cryoglobulinemia
- Cholesterol atheroembolic disease
- Other systemic causes of peripheral neuropathy, eg, rheumatoid arthritis, diabetes mellitus, amyloidosis, sarcoidosis, multiple myeloma
- Other causes of mesenteric ischemia, eg, embolism, atherosclerosis

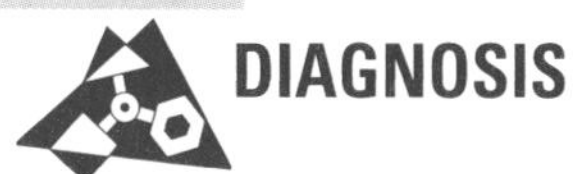

DIAGNOSIS

LABORATORY TESTS

- Anemia, and a sedimentation rate that is almost always elevated, often strikingly so
- Leukocytosis is common
- 75% of patients with MPA are ANCA positive (usually with antibodies directed against myeloperoxidase, causing a p-ANCA pattern on immunofluorescence testing)
- Patients with classic PAN are ANCA negative
- Serological tests for hepatitis B or C are positive in 10–30% of patients with polyarteritis nodosa
- MPA: hematuria, proteinuria, and red blood cell casts in the urine

IMAGING STUDIES

- Mesenteric angiogram revealing microaneurysms is diagnostic

DIAGNOSTIC PROCEDURES

- Biopsies of symptomatic sites (eg, nerve, muscle, lung, or kidney) have high sensitivities and specificities
- The diagnosis of both of these disorders requires confirmation with either a tissue biopsy or, in the case of polyarteritis nodosa, an angiogram
- Patients suspected of having polyarteritis nodosa—eg, on the basis of mesenteric ischemia or new-onset hypertension occurring in the setting of a systemic illness—may be diagnosed by the angiographic finding of aneurysmal dilations in the renal, mesenteric, or hepatic arteries

Polyarteritis Nodosa & Microscopic Polyangiitis

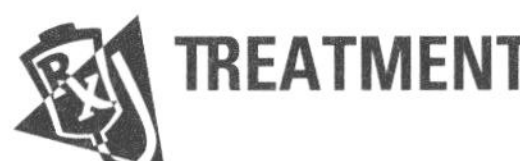

TREATMENT

MEDICATIONS

- For polyarteritis nodosa, corticosteroids in high doses (up to 60 mg of prednisone daily) may control fever and constitutional symptoms and heal vascular lesions
- Pulse methylprednisolone (eg, 1 g intravenously daily for 3 days) may be necessary for patients who are critically ill at presentation
- Immunosuppressive agents, especially cyclophosphamide, appear to improve the survival of patients when given with steroids
- In microscopic polyangiitis, patients are more likely to require cyclophosphamide because of the urgency in treating pulmonary hemorrhage and glomerulonephritis

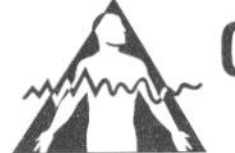

OUTCOME

COMPLICATIONS

- Mesenteric vasculitis can cause bowel ischemia with bleeding or perforation

PROGNOSIS

- Without treatment, the 5-year survival rate in these disorders is poor—on the order of 20%
- With appropriate therapy, remissions are possible in many cases and the 5-year survival rate has improved to 60–90%
- Relapses may occur in both disorders—approximately 35% among patients with microscopic polyangiitis and perhaps less in those with polyarteritis nodosa

WHEN TO REFER

- Refer to a rheumatologist to assist with establishing the diagnosis and planning therapy

WHEN TO ADMIT

- Admit for therapy whenever the patient develops new visceral complications such as bowel ischemia, cardiomyopathy, or rapidly progressive neuropathy

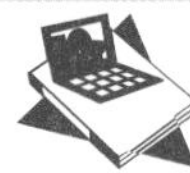

EVIDENCE

INFORMATION FOR PATIENTS

- Cleveland Clinic Foundation
  - http://www.clevelandclinic.org/arthritis/treat/facts/vasculitis.htm
- Johns Hopkins University
  - http://vasculitis.med.jhu.edu/typesof/polyarteritis.html
- National Institutes of Health
  - http://www.nlm.nih.gov/medlineplus/ency/article/001438.htm

REFERENCES

- Guillevin L et al: Short-term corticosteroids then lamivudine and plasma exchanges to treat hepatitis B virus-related polyarteritis nodosa. Arthritis Rheum 2004;5:482. [PMID: 15188337]
- Mahr A et al: Prevalences of polyarteritis nodosa, microscopic polyangiitis, Wegener's granulomatosis, and Churg-Strauss syndrome in a French urban multiethnic population in 2000: a capture-recapture estimate. Arthritis Rheum 2004;51:92. [PMID: 14872461]
- Stone JH: Polyarteritis nodosa. JAMA 2002;288(13):1632. [PMID: 12350194]

Author(s)

David B. Hellmann, MD, FACP
John H. Stone, MD, MPH

Polycystic Ovary Syndrome (Persistent Anovulation)

Polychondritis, Relapsing p. 1134.

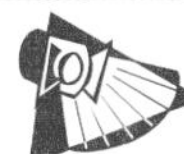

KEY FEATURES

ESSENTIALS OF DIAGNOSIS

- Chronic anovulation
- Infertility
- Elevated plasma testosterone and luteinizing hormone (LH) values and a reversed follicle-stimulating hormone (FSH) /LH ratio
- Hirsutism (in 70% of patients)

GENERAL CONSIDERATIONS

- The primary lesion is unknown
- There is a steady state of elevated estrogen (estrone), androgen, and LH levels rather than the fluctuating levels in ovulating women
- Increased estrone comes from conversion of androgens to estrone in body fat or from excessive levels of androgens seen in some women of normal weight. High estrone levels may cause suppression of pituitary FSH and a relative increase in LH
- Constant LH stimulation of the ovary results in anovulation, multiple cysts, and theca cell hyperplasia with excess androgen output
- The polycystic ovary has a thickened, pearly white capsule and may not be enlarged

DEMOGRAPHICS

- Affects 4% of women of reproductive age

CLINICAL FINDINGS

SYMPTOMS AND SIGNS

- Hirsutism (50% of cases)
- Obesity (40%)
- Virilization (20%)
- Amenorrhea (50% of cases) and abnormal uterine bleeding (30%); 20% have normal menstruation
- Women are generally infertile, although they may ovulate occasionally

DIFFERENTIAL DIAGNOSIS

- Hypothalamic amenorrhea, eg, stress, weight change, exercise
- Obesity
- Hypothyroidism
- Hyperprolactinemia
- Premature ovarian failure
- Cushing's syndrome
- Congenital adrenal hyperplasia
- Androgen-secreting tumor (adrenal, ovarian)
- Pregnancy

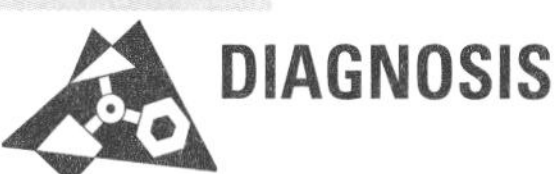

DIAGNOSIS

LABORATORY TESTS

- Check FSH, LH, prolactin, TSH, and dehydroepiandrosterone sulfate (DHEAS) when amenorrhea has persisted for 6 months
- 2-h glucose tolerance test
- Lipoprotein profile

IMAGING STUDIES

- Pelvic ultrasound may document polycystic ovaries (not necessary for diagnosis)

Polycystic Kidney Disease p. 1135.

Polycystic Ovary Syndrome (Persistent Anovulation)

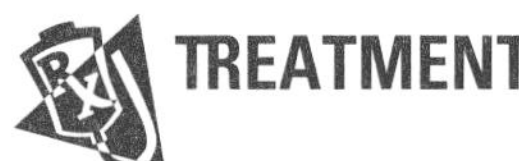

TREATMENT

MEDICATIONS

- **If the patient wishes to become pregnant**
  - Clomiphene or other drugs can be used for ovulatory stimulation
  - The addition of dexamethasone, 0.5 mg PO at bedtime, to a clomiphene regimen may increase the likelihood of ovulation
  - If unresponsive to clomiphene, 3- to 6-month courses of metformin, 500 mg PO TID, may bring resumption of regular cycles and ovulation
- **If the patient does not desire pregnancy**
  - Medroxyprogesterone acetate, 10 mg PO/day for the first 10 days of each month
  - If contraception is desired, a low-dose combination oral contraceptive can be used; this is also useful in controlling hirsutism, for which treatment must be continued for 6–12 months before results are seen
- Dexamethasone, 0.5 mg PO each night, is helpful in women with excess adrenal androgen secretion. If hirsutism is severe, some patients will elect to have a hysterectomy and bilateral oophorectomy followed by estrogen replacement therapy. Spironolactone, an aldosterone antagonist, is also useful for hirsutism in doses of 25 mg PO three or four times daily

THERAPEUTIC PROCEDURES

- In obese patients with polycystic ovaries, weight reduction is often effective; a decrease in body fat will lower the conversion of androgens to estrone and thereby help restore ovulation
- Hirsutism may be managed with epilation and electrolysis

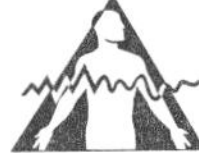

OUTCOME

FOLLOW-UP

- In long-term anovular patients over age 35, it is wise to search for an estrogen-stimulated cancer with mammography and endometrial aspiration

PROGNOSIS

- Women have insulin resistance and hyperinsulinemia when infused with glucose and are at increased risk for early-onset type 2 diabetes mellitus
- Women have an increased long-term risk of cancer of the breast and endometrium because of unopposed estrogen secretion

WHEN TO REFER

- If expertise in diagnosis is needed
- If the patient is having infertility problems

EVIDENCE

PRACTICE GUIDELINES

- American College of Obstetricians and Gynecologists. ACOG practice bulletin. Polycycstic ovary syndrome.
  - http://www.guideline.gov/summary/summary.aspx?doc_id=3989&nbr=3128
- American Association of Clinical Endocrinologists medical guidelines for clinical practice for the diagnosis and treatment of hyperandrogenic disorders.
  - http://www.guideline.gov/summary/summary.aspx?doc_id=2847&nbr=2073

WEB SITE

- Lakhani K et al: Polycystic Ovaries. Br J Radiol 2002;75:9. [PMID: 11806952]
  - http://bjr.birjournals.org/cgi/content/full/75/889/9

INFORMATION FOR PATIENTS

- National Women's Health Information Center: Polycystic Ovarian Syndrome
  - http://www.4woman.gov/faq/pcos.htm
- American Association of Family Physicians: Polycystic Ovary Syndrome
  - http://familydoctor.org/620.xml
- MedlinePlus: Ovarian Cysts Interactive Tutorial
  - http://www.nlm.nih.gov/medlineplus/tutorials/ovariancysts.html
- American Society for Reproductive Medicine: Hirsutism and Polycystic Ovarian Syndrome
  - http://www.asrm.org/Patients/patientbooklets/hirsutismPCOS.pdf
- International Council on Infertility Information Dissemination: PCOS FAQ
  - http://www.inciid.org/faq.php?cat=infertility101&id=2

REFERENCE

- Guzick DS: Polycystic ovarian syndrome. Obstet Gynecol 2004;103:181. [PMID: 14704263]

Author(s)

H. Trent MacKay, MD, MPH

Polymyalgia Rheumatica & Giant Cell Arteritis

KEY FEATURES

ESSENTIALS OF DIAGNOSIS

- Giant cell arteritis is characterized by headache, jaw claudication, polymyalgia rheumatica, visual abnormalities, and a markedly elevated erythrocyte sedimentation rate (ESR)
- The hallmark of polymyalgia rheumatica is pain and stiffness in shoulders and hips

GENERAL CONSIDERATIONS

- Polymyalgia rheumatica and giant cell arteritis probably represent a spectrum of one disease and frequently coexist
- The important difference between the two conditions is that polymyalgia rheumatica alone does not cause blindness and responds to low-dose (10–20 mg/day) prednisone therapy, whereas giant cell arteritis can cause blindness and large artery complications and requires high-dose therapy (40–60 mg/day)

DEMOGRAPHICS

- Both affect patients over age 50
- Giant cell arteritis is more common in northern Europeans and their descendants

CLINICAL FINDINGS

SYMPTOMS AND SIGNS

Polymyalgia rheumatica

- Pain and stiffness of the shoulder and pelvic girdle areas
- Fever, malaise, and weight loss
- Anemia and a markedly elevated sedimentation rate are almost always present
- Muscle pain much greater than muscle weakness

Giant cell arteritis

- Headache, scalp tenderness, visual symptoms, jaw claudication, or throat pain
- The temporal artery is usually normal on physical examination but may be nodular, enlarged, tender, or pulseless
- Blindness results from occlusive arteritis of the posterior ciliary branch of the ophthalmic artery; the ischemic optic neuropathy of giant cell arteritis may produce no funduscopic findings for the first 24–48 h after the onset of blindness
- Asymmetry of pulses in the arms, a murmur of aortic regurgitation, or bruits heard near the clavicle resulting from subclavian artery stenoses identify an affected aorta or its major branches
- Forty percent of patients with giant cell arteritis have nonclassic symptoms at presentation, primarily respiratory tract problems (most frequently dry cough), mononeuritis multiplex (most frequently with painful paralysis of a shoulder), or fever of unknown origin
- The fever can be as high as 40°C and is frequently associated with rigors and sweats
- Unexplained head or neck pain in an older patient may signal the presence of giant cell arteritis

DIFFERENTIAL DIAGNOSIS

Polymyalgia rheumatica

- Rheumatoid arthritis
- Polymyositis
- Chronic infection, eg, endocarditis
- Multiple myeloma
- Malignancy
- Fibromyalgia
- Polyarteritis nodosa

Giant cell (temporal) arteritis

- Migraine
- Glaucoma
- Takayasu's arteritis
- Uveitis
- Carotid plaque with embolic amaurosis fugax
- Trigeminal neuralgia

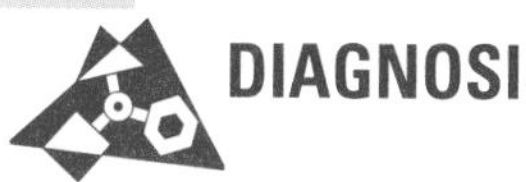

DIAGNOSIS

LABORATORY TESTS

- An elevated ESR, with a median result of about 65 mm/h, occurs in more than 90% of patients with polymyalgia rheumatica or giant cell arteritis
- Most patients also have a mild normochromic, normocytic anemia and thrombocytosis

IMAGING STUDIES

- Role of ultrasonography of temporal arteries is controversial
- Angiography is helpful in the subset of patients that has large-artery disease (especially the subclavian artery)

DIAGNOSTIC PROCEDURES

- Temporal artery biopsy
- Diagnostic findings of giant cell arteritis may still be present 2 weeks (or even considerably longer) after starting corticosteroids
- An adequate biopsy specimen (2 cm in length) is essential, because the disease may be segmental

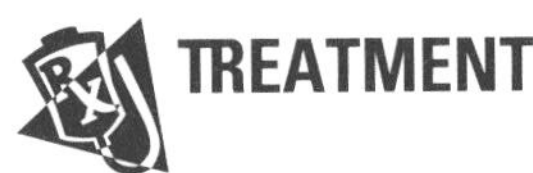

TREATMENT

MEDICATIONS

Polymyalgia rheumatica

- Prednisone, 10–20 mg PO/day; if no dramatic improvement within 72 h, the diagnosis should be revisited
- Weekly methotrexate may increase the chance of successfully tapering prednisone in some patients

Giant cell arteritis

- The urgency of early diagnosis and treatment in giant cell arteritis relates to the prevention of blindness
- When a patient has symptoms and findings suggestive of temporal arteritis, therapy with prednisone, 60 mg PO daily, is initiated immediately
- Prednisone should be continued in a dosage of 60 mg/day for 1–2 months before tapering
- Low-dose aspirin (~81 mg PO/day) may reduce the risk of visual loss or stroke and should be added to prednisone

OUTCOME

FOLLOW-UP

- Course is monitored by a composite of the patient's symptoms and laboratory markers of inflammation (ie, hematocrit, ESR, and C-reactive protein)
- In adjusting the dosage of steroid, the ESR is a useful but not absolute guide to disease activity. A common error is treating the ESR rather than the patient
- Within 1–2 months after beginning treatment, the patient's symptoms and laboratory abnormalities will resolve
- Disease flares are common (50% or more) as prednisone is tapered
- The total duration of treatment varies considerably but ranges from 6 months to more than 2 years

COMPLICATIONS

- Blindness; once blindness develops, it is usually permanent
- Thoracic aortic aneurysms occur 17 times more frequently in patients with giant cell arteritis than in normal individuals

PROGNOSIS

- Impact on survival appears small

WHEN TO REFER

- Refer to a rheumatologist to establish the diagnosis, plan therapy, and monitor treatment
- Consult an ophthalmologist for visual changes

WHEN TO ADMIT

- Admit for evaluation and high-dose intravenous methylprednisolone if the patient acutely develops visual loss

EVIDENCE

PRACTICE GUIDELINES

- American Academy of Family Physicians
  - http://www.aafp.org/afp/20000401/2061.html
- National Guideline Clearinghouse
  - http://www.guideline.gov/summary/summary.aspx?doc_id=3415

INFORMATION FOR PATIENTS

- American Academy of Family Physicians
  - http://www.aafp.org/afp/20000401/2073ph.html
- National Institute of Arthritis and Musculoskeletal and Skin Diseases
  - http://www.niams.nih.gov/hi/topics/polymyalgia/index.htm
- National Institutes of Health
  - http://www.nlm.nih.gov/medlineplus/ency/article/000415.htm
  - http://www.nlm.nih.gov/medlineplus/ency/article/000415.htm

REFERENCES

- Caporali R et al: Prednisone plus methotrexate for polymyalgia rheumatica: a randomized, double-blind, placebo-controlled trial. Ann Intern Med 2004;141:493. [PMID: 15466766]
- Nesher G et al: Low-dose aspirin and prevention of cranial ischemic complications in giant cell arteritis. Arthritis Rheum 2004;50:1332. [PMID: 15077317]
- Salvarani C et al: Polymyalgia rheumatica and giant cell arteritis. N Engl J Med 2002;347:261. [PMID: 12140303]
- Seo P et al: Large-vessel vasculitis. Arthritis Care Res 2004;51:128. [PMID: 14872466]
- Smetana GW et al: Does this patient have temporal arteritis? JAMA 2002;287:92. [PMID: 11754714]
- Stone JH: Methotrexate in polymyalgia rheumatica: kernel of truth or curse of Tantalus? Ann Intern Med 2004;141:568. [PMID: 15466775]

Author(s)

David B. Hellmann, MD, FACP

John H. Stone, MD, MPH

Polyneuropathies

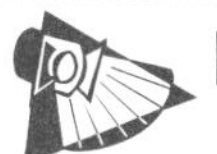

KEY FEATURES

ESSENTIALS OF DIAGNOSIS

- Weakness, sensory disturbances, or both in the extremities
- Pain sometimes common
- Depressed or absent tendon reflexes
- May have family history of neuropathy
- May have history of systemic illness or toxic exposure

GENERAL CONSIDERATIONS

- Categorized as axonal or demyelinating based on neurophysiologic findings
- The cause is suggested by the history, mode of onset, and predominant clinical manifestations
- In about 50% of cases, no specific cause can be established; of these, slightly less than half are found to be heredofamilial

Inherited neuropathies

- Charcot-Marie-Tooth disease
- Dejerine-Sottas disease (HMSN type III)
- Friedreich's ataxia
- Refsum's disease (HMSN type IV)
- Porphyria (axonal)
  - Motor symptoms usually occur first, and weakness is often most marked proximally and in the upper limbs
  - Sensory symptoms and signs may be proximal or distal in distribution
  - Autonomic involvement is sometimes pronounced

Neuropathies associated with systemic and metabolic disorders

- Diabetes mellitus
  - Symmetric sensory or mixed polyneuropathy
  - Asymmetric motor radiculoneuropathy or plexopathy (diabetic amyotrophy)
  - Thoracoabdominal radiculopathy
  - Autonomic neuropathy
  - Isolated lesions of individual nerves may occur singly or in any combination
- Uremia
  - Symmetric sensorimotor polyneuropathy
  - Tends to affect the lower limbs more than the upper limbs
  - More marked distally than proximally
- Alcoholism and nutritional deficiency (thiamin, and B_{12})
  - Axonal distal sensorimotor polyneuropathy
  - Frequently accompanied by painful cramps, muscle tenderness, and painful paresthesias
  - Often more marked in legs than arms
  - Symptoms of autonomic dysfunction may be conspicuous
  - A similar distal sensorimotor polyneuropathy is a well-recognized feature of beriberi (thiamine deficiency)
  - In vitamin B_{12} deficiency, distal sensory polyneuropathy may develop but is usually overshadowed by CNS manifestations
- Paraproteinemias, especially multiple myeloma, but also with macroglobulinemia and cryoglobulinemia
  - A gradual onset, progressive, symmetric sensorimotor neuropathy
  - Often accompanied by pain and dysesthesias in the limbs
  - Carpal tunnel syndrome may be seen in generalized amyloidosis

Neuropathies associated with infectious and inflammatory diseases

- Leprosy
  - Sensory disturbances from involvement of intracutaneous nerves
  - Motor deficits from involvement of superficial nerves where their temperature is lowest, eg, the ulnar nerve in the region proximal to the olecranon groove
- AIDS
  - Chronic symmetric sensorimotor axonal polyneuropathy with normal cerebrospinal fluid (CSF) findings
  - Progressive polyradiculopathy or radiculomyelopathy that leads to leg weakness and urinary retention (CSF may show mononuclear pleocytosis and increased protein and low glucose concentrations); cytomegalovirus is responsible in at least some cases
  - An inflammatory demyelinating polyradiculoneuropathy with weakness more obvious distally than proximally and depressed or absent tendon reflexes (CSF shows an increased cell count and protein concentration)
- Lyme borreliosis
- Sarcoidosis
- Polyarteritis
- Rheumatoid arthritis

Critical illness neuropathy (axonal)

- Initial manifestation may be difficulty in weaning from a mechanical ventilator
- In more advanced cases, there is wasting and weakness of the extremities and loss of tendon reflexes
- Sensory abnormalities are relatively inconspicuous
- Good prognosis if patients recover from the underlying critical illness

Other neuropathies

- Toxic neuropathies
- Neuropathies associated with malignant diseases (see Table 156)
- Acute idiopathic polyneuropathy (Guillain-Barré syndrome)
- Chronic inflammatory polyneuropathy

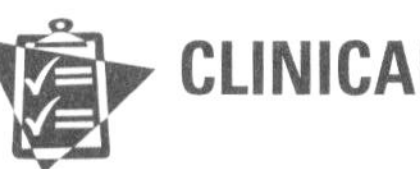

CLINICAL FINDINGS

SYMPTOMS AND SIGNS

- Weakness
- Sensory disturbance
- Pain

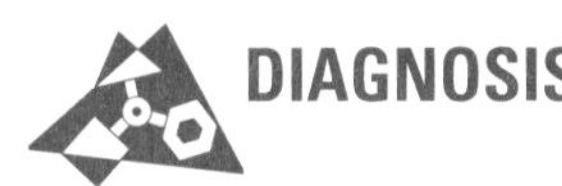

DIAGNOSIS

LABORATORY TESTS

- These tests should be ordered *selectively*, as guided by symptoms and signs
  - Fasting blood glucose
  - Plasma urea and electrolytes
  - Liver and thyroid function tests
  - Complete blood cell count and sedimentation rate
  - Serum protein electrophoresis
  - Tests for rheumatoid factor and antinuclear antibody
  - HBsAg determination
  - Serologic test for syphilis
  - Urinary heavy metal levels
  - CSF examination
  - Chest radiography

DIAGNOSTIC PROCEDURES

- In **axonal** neuropathies
  - Nerve conduction velocity is normal or reduced only mildly
  - Needle electromyography (EMG) shows denervation in affected muscles
- In **demyelinating** neuropathies
  - Conduction may be slowed considerably, or even blocked completely, without EMG signs of denervation
- Cutaneous nerve biopsy may help establish a precise diagnosis (eg, polyarteritis, amyloidosis)

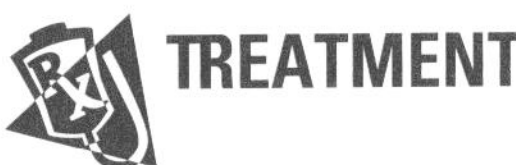

TREATMENT

MEDICATIONS

- Neuropathic pain may respond to simple analgesics such as aspirin
- Narcotics or narcotic substitutes may be necessary for severe hyperpathia or pain induced by minimal stimuli, but their use should be avoided as far as possible
- Episodic stabbing pains may respond to any of the following
  - Phenytoin
  - Carbamazepine
  - Gabapentin
  - Tricyclic antidepressants
- Postural hypotension
  - Often helped by wearing waist-high elastic stockings and sleeping in a semierect position at night
  - Fludrocortisone reduces postural hypotension, but doses as high as 1 mg PO/day are sometimes necessary in diabetics and may lead to recumbent hypertension
  - Midodrine, an α-agonist, is sometimes helpful in a dose of 2.5–10 mg PO three times daily
- Impotence and diarrhea are difficult to treat
- A flaccid neuropathic bladder may respond to parasympathomimetic drugs such as bethanechol chloride, 10–50 mg three or four times daily

THERAPEUTIC PROCEDURES

- Treatment of the underlying cause

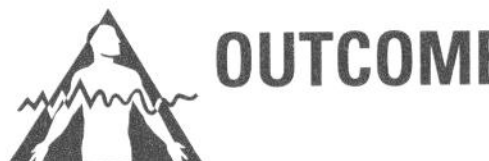

OUTCOME

WHEN TO REFER

- When the diagnosis is uncertain
- For specialized diagnostic tests or for nerve biopsy
- For physical therapy

PREVENTION

- Physical therapy helps prevent contractures
- Splints can maintain a weak extremity in a position of useful function
- Anesthetic extremities must be protected from injury
- To guard against burns, patients should do one of the following
  - Check the temperature of water and hot surfaces with a portion of skin that has normal sensation
  - Measure water temperature with a thermometer
  - Use cold water for washing or lower the temperature setting of their hot-water heaters
- Shoes should be examined frequently for grit or foreign objects to prevent pressure lesions
- Patients should avoid leaning on elbows or sitting with crossed legs for lengthy periods
- The use of a frame or cradle to reduce contact with bedclothes may be helpful for pain or dysesthesias

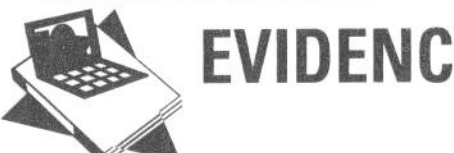

EVIDENCE

PRACTICE GUIDELINES

- National Guideline Clearinghouse
  - http://www.guideline.gov/summary/summary.aspx?doc_id=3550&nbr=2776&string=polyneuropathy

INFORMATION FOR PATIENTS

- Beth Israel Medical Center
  - http://stoppain.org/pain_medicine/polyneuropathy.html
- The Mayo Clinic
  - http://www.mayoclinic.com/invoke.cfm?id=DS00131

REFERENCES

- Donofrio PD: Immunotherapy of idiopathic inflammatory neuropathies. Muscle Nerve 2003;28:273. [PMID:12929187]
- Kieseier BC et al: Advances in understanding and treatment of immune-mediated disorders of the peripheral nervous system. Muscle Nerve 2004;30:131. [PMID:15266629]
- Mendell JR et al: Clinical practice. Painful sensory neuropathy. N Engl J Med 2003;348:1243. [PMID:12660389]
- Polydefkis M et al: New insights into diabetic polyneuropathy. JAMA 2003;290:1371. [PMID:12966130]
- Saperstein DS et al: Clinical spectrum of chronic acquired demyelinating polyneuropathies. Muscle Nerve 2001;24;311. [PMID:11353415]
- Wicklund MP et al: Paraproteinemic neuropathy. Curr Treat Options Neurol 2001;3:147. [PMID:11180752]
- Wolfe GI et al: Painful peripheral neuropathy and its nonsurgical treatment. Muscle Nerve 2004;30:3. [PMID:15221874]

Author(s)

Michael J. Aminoff, MD, DSc, FRCP

Polyneuropathy, Chronic Inflammatory p. 1135

Polyps, Colonic & Small Intestinal

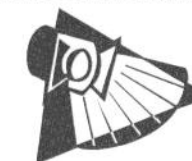

KEY FEATURES

ESSENTIALS OF DIAGNOSIS

- Discrete mass lesions that are flat or protrude into the intestinal lumen
- Most commonly sporadic, may be inherited as part of familial polyposis syndrome
- Three major pathological groups: mucosal neoplastic (adenomatous) polyps, mucosal nonneoplastic polyps (hyperplastic, juvenile polyps, hamartomas, inflammatory polyps), and submucosal lesions (lipomas, lymphoid aggregates, carcinoids, pneumatosis cystoides intestinalis)
- Nonneoplastic mucosal polyps have no malignant potential; adenomatous polyps do
- Of polyps removed at colonoscopy, over 70% are adenomatous; most of the remainder are hyperplastic; distinguished by histology

GENERAL CONSIDERATIONS

- Adenomatous polyps are tubular, villous, or tubulovillous; sessile or pedunculated
- >95% of adenocarcinoma arise from adenomas
- Small adenomas (< 1 cm) have a low risk of being malignant; larger adenomas (>1 cm) have a much higher risk (>10%) of harboring malignancy or high-grade dysplasia

DEMOGRAPHICS

- Adenomatous polyps are present in 35% of adults aged >50 years

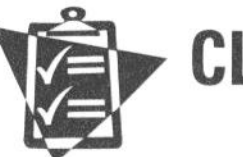

CLINICAL FINDINGS

SYMPTOMS AND SIGNS

- Usually asymptomatic
- Chronic occult blood loss may lead to iron deficiency anemia
- Large polyps may ulcerate, resulting in intermittent hematochezia

DIFFERENTIAL DIAGNOSIS

- Colorectal cancer
- Nonneoplastic polyp, eg, hyperplastic, inflammatory
- Submucosal polyp, eg, lipoma, lymphoid aggregate
- Other causes of occult gastrointestinal bleeding, eg, arteriovenous malformation, inflammatory bowel disease

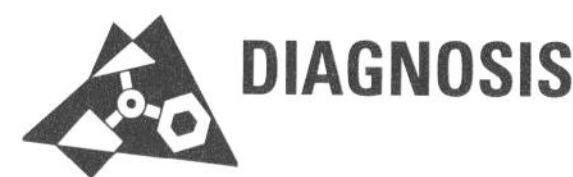

DIAGNOSIS

LABORATORY TESTS

- Fecal occult blood tests detect < 20% of adenomas >1 cm in diameter

IMAGING STUDIES

- Barium enema, whether single- or double-contrast, has unacceptably low sensitivity (~50%) and specificity for the detection of colorectal polyps
- Spiral CT colonography ("virtual colonoscopy") detects over 80–90%

DIAGNOSTIC PROCEDURES

- Flexible sigmoidoscopy: about one-half to two-thirds of colonic adenomas are within the reach of the flexible sigmoidoscope
- Colonoscopy is best means of detecting and removing adenomatous polyps

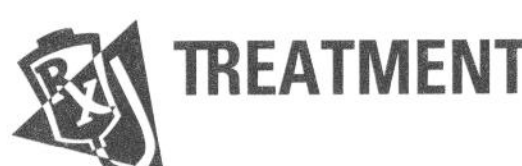

TREATMENT

SURGERY

- Primary surgical resection may be required for large (>2–3 cm) sessile polyps
- Malignant polyps are adenomas that appear grossly benign at endoscopy but on histological assessment are found to contain cancer
- Malignant polyps (termed "favorable") are adequately treated by polypectomy alone if the polyp is completely excised, well differentiated, the margin is not involved, and there is no vascular or lymphatic invasion
- Risk of residual cancer or nodal metastasis is 0.3% for pedunculated malignant polyps and 1.5% for sessile malignant polyps
- Surgical resection for "unfavorable" malignant polyps

THERAPEUTIC PROCEDURES

- Colonoscopic polypectomy is possible for most polyps, particularly pedunculated polyps

OUTCOME

FOLLOW-UP

- Periodic colonoscopic surveillance is recommended to detect "metachronous" adenomas
- In high-risk patients, colonoscopy is recommended at 3 years after the initial colonoscopy and polypectomy; in low-risk patients, at 5 years
- Excision site of "favorable" malignant polyps should be checked in 3 months for residual tissue

COMPLICATIONS

- Complications of colonoscopic polypectomy include perforation in 0.2%, bleeding in 1%

PREVENTION

- Nonsteroidal antiinflammatory drugs (NSAIDs), aspirin, and COX-2 selective NSAIDs may decrease the incidence of colorectal adenomas and the progression to cancer; due to their other side effects, routine prophylaxis with these agents is not currently recommended

EVIDENCE

PRACTICE GUIDELINES

- Atkin WS et al: Surveillance guidelines after removal of colorectal adenomatous polyps. Gut 2002;51(Suppl 5):V6. [PMID: 12221031]
- Jenkins PJ et al: Screening guidelines for colorectal cancer and polyps in patients with acromegaly. Gut 2002;51(Suppl 5):V13.
- National Guideline Clearinghouse
  - http://www.guideline.gov/summary/summary.aspx?ss=15&doc_id=4006&nbr=3135&string=polyps

INFORMATION FOR PATIENTS

- Mayo Clinic
  - http://www.mayoclinic.com/invoke.cfm?id=DS00511
- National Institute of Diabetes and Digestive and Kidney Diseases—What I need to know about colon polyps
  - http://digestive.niddk.nih.gov/ddiseases/pubs/colonpolyps_ez/index.htm
- Torpy JM et al: JAMA Patient Page. Colon cancer screening. JAMA 2003;289:1334. [PMID: 12633198]

REFERENCES

- Bond JH: Colon polyps and cancer. Endoscopy 2003;35:27. [PMID: 12510223]
- Schoen R: Surveillance after positive and negative colonoscopy examinations: issues, yields, and use. Am J Gastroenterol 2003;98:1237. [PMID: 12818263]
- Ueno H et al: Risk factors for an adverse outcome in early invasive colorectal carcinoma. Gastroenterology 2004;127:385. [PMID: 15300569]
- Van Dam J et al: AGA future trends report: CT colonography. Gastroenterology 2004;127:970. [PMID: 15362051]

Author(s)

Kenneth R. McQuaid, MD

Porphyria, Acute Intermittent

Pompholyx (Dyshidrotic Eczema) p. 1136. Popliteal Aneurysm p. 1136. Popliteal Artery Occlusion p. 1136.

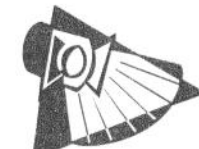

KEY FEATURES

ESSENTIALS OF DIAGNOSIS

- Unexplained abdominal crisis, generally in young women
- Acute central or peripheral nervous system dysfunction
- Recurrent psychiatric illnesses
- Hyponatremia
- Porphobilinogen in the urine during an attack

GENERAL CONSIDERATIONS

- Acute intermittent porphyria is caused by deficiency of porphobilinogen deaminase activity, leading to increased excretion of aminolevulinic acid and porphobilinogen in the urine
- Genetics: mutation in the porphobilinogen deaminase gene
- Autosomal dominant inheritance
- It remains clinically silent in the majority of patients who carry the trait
- Characteristic abdominal pain may be due to abnormalities in autonomic innervation in the gut
- Cutaneous photosensitivity is absent
- Attacks precipitated by numerous factors, including drugs and intercurrent infections
- Hyponatremia resulting from inappropriate release of antidiuretic hormone and gastrointestinal loss of sodium

DEMOGRAPHICS

- Usually presents in adulthood and has serious consequences
- Women usually develop clinical illness
- Symptoms beginning in the teens or 20s, but in rare cases after menopause

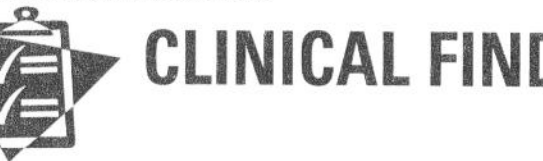

CLINICAL FINDINGS

SYMPTOMS AND SIGNS

- Intermittent abdominal pain of varying severity, sometimes simulating an acute abdomen
- Absence of fever and leukocytosis
- Complete recovery between attacks
- Autonomic neuropathy
- Peripheral neuropathy, symmetric or asymmetric, mild or profound
- Central nervous system manifestations include seizures, psychosis, and abnormalities of the basal ganglia

DIFFERENTIAL DIAGNOSIS

- Acute abdominal pain resulting from other cause (eg, appendicitis, peptic ulcer disease, cholecystitis, diverticulitis, ruptured ectopic pregnancy, familial Mediterranean fever)
- Polyneuropathy resulting from other cause
- Guillain-Barré syndrome
- Lead or other heavy metal poisoning
- Psychosis resulting from other cause
- Syndrome of inappropriate antidiuretic hormone resulting from other cause
- Dark urine resulting from other cause (eg, alkaptonuria)

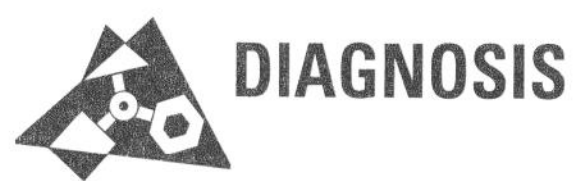

DIAGNOSIS

LABORATORY TESTS

- Hyponatremia, often profound
- Freshly voided urine is of normal color but may turn dark upon standing in light and air
- Urine porphobilinogen increased during an acute attack
- Mutation detection in the gene for porphobilinogen deaminase

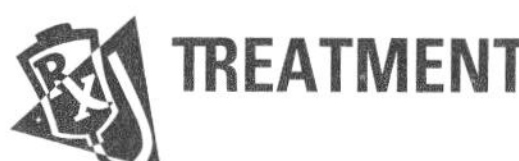

TREATMENT

MEDICATIONS

- Analgesics
- IV glucose
- High-carbohydrate intake, a minimum of 300 g carbohydrate/day PO or IV
- Hematin up to 4 mg/kg IV QD or BID
- Adverse consequences of hematin therapy include phlebitis and coagulopathy

THERAPEUTIC PROCEDURES

- High-carbohydrate diet diminishes the number of attacks
- Withdrawal of the inciting agent
- Liver transplantation for extreme cases

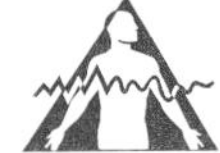

OUTCOME

FOLLOW-UP

- ECG
- Electrolytes
- Glucose
- Mental status

PROGNOSIS

- Acute attacks may be life threatening and require prompt diagnosis

WHEN TO REFER

- Genetic counseling

WHEN TO ADMIT

- Abdominal crisis
- Marked hyponatremia
- Acute CNS dysfunction

PREVENTION

- Avoidance of factors known to precipitate attacks, especially drugs (Table 149)
- Starvation diets must be avoided

EVIDENCE

WEB SITES

- American Porphyria Foundation
  - http://www.porphyriafoundation.com
- National Center for Biotechnology Information: Online Mendelian Inheritance in Man
  - http://www.ncbi.nlm.nih.gov/entrez/dispomim.cgi?id=176000

INFORMATION FOR PATIENTS

- American Porphyria Foundation: Acute Intermittent Porphyria (AIP)
  - http://www.porphyriafoundation.com/about_por/types/types01.html
- National Digestive Diseases Information Clearinghouse: Porphyria
  - http://digestive.niddk.nih.gov/ddiseases/pubs/porphyria/index.htm
- National Library of Medicine: Acute Intermittent Porphyria
  - http://ghr.nlm.nih.gov/condition=acuteintermittentporphyria

REFERENCES

- Badminton MN et al: Management of acute and cutaneous porphyrias. Int J Clin Pract 2002;56:272. [PMID: 12074210]
- Desnick RJ et al: Inherited porphyrias. In: *Emery and Rimoin's Principles and Practice of Medical Genetics,* ed 4. Rimoin DL et al (editors). Churchill Livingstone, 2002.
- Grandchamp B: Acute intermittent porphyria. Semin Liver Dis 1998;18:17. [PMID: 9516674]
- Kauppinen R: Molecular diagnostics of acute intermittent porphyria. Expert Rev Mol Diagn 2004;4(2):243. [PMID: 14995910]
- Soonawalla ZF et al: Liver transplantation as a cure for acute intermittent porphyria. Lancet 2004;363(9410):705. [PMID: 15001330]

Author(s)

Reed E. Pyeritz, MD, PhD

Porphyria Cutanea Tarda p. 1137.
Postherpetic Neuralgia p. 1137.

Posttraumatic Stress Disorder

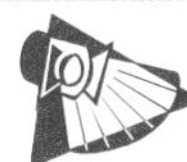

KEY FEATURES

ESSENTIALS OF DIAGNOSIS

- A syndrome characterized by
  - "Reexperiencing" a traumatic event (eg, rape, severe burns, military combat)
  - Decreased responsiveness and avoidance of current events associated with the trauma
- Alcohol and other drugs are commonly used in self-treatment

GENERAL CONSIDERATIONS

- Included among the anxiety disorders in *DSM-IV*
- The symptoms may be precipitated or exacerbated by events that are a reminder of the original stress
- Symptoms frequently arise after a long latency period (eg, child abuse can result in later-onset posttraumatic stress syndrome)

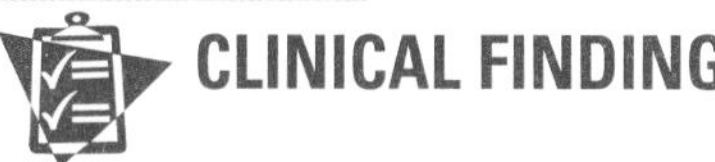

CLINICAL FINDINGS

SYMPTOMS AND SIGNS

- Physiologic hyperarousal
  - Startle reactions
  - Intrusive thoughts
  - Illusions
  - Overgeneralized associations
  - Sleep problems
  - Nightmares
  - Dreams about the precipitating event
  - Impulsivity
  - Difficulties in concentration
  - Hyperalertness

DIFFERENTIAL DIAGNOSIS

- Anxiety disorders
- Affective disorders
- Personality disorders exacerbated by stress
- Somatic disorders with psychic overlay

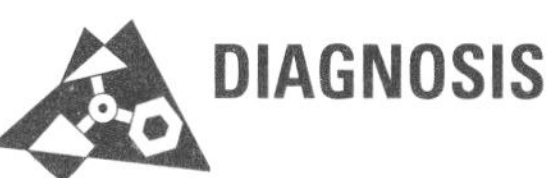

DIAGNOSIS

LABORATORY TESTS

- Thyroid-stimulating hormone
- Complete blood cell count
- Toxicology screen (if suspected)
- Glucose

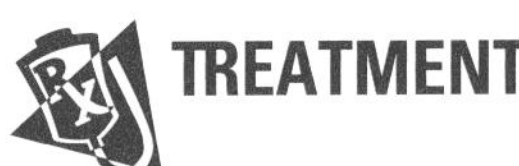

TREATMENT

MEDICATIONS

- Early treatment of anxious arousal with β-blockers (eg, propranolol, 80–160 mg PO daily)
  - May lessen the peripheral symptoms of anxiety (eg, tremors, palpitations)
  - May help prevent the development of the disorder
- Antidepressant drugs—particularly selective serotonin reuptake inhibitors (SSRIs)—in full dosage
  - Helpful in ameliorating depression, panic attacks, sleep disruption, and startle responses in chronic PTSD
  - Sertraline and paroxetine are FDA approved for this purpose
- Antiseizure medications such as carbamazepine (400–800 mg PO daily) often mitigate impulsivity and difficulty with anger management
- Benzodiazepines (Table 105) such as clonazepam (1–4 mg PO daily)
  - Reduce anxiety and panic attacks when used in adequate dosage
  - Dependency problems are a concern, particularly when the patient has had such problems in the past

THERAPEUTIC PROCEDURES

- The therapeutic approach is to facilitate the normal recovery that was blocked at the time of the trauma
  - Therapy close to the event should be brief and simple (catharsis and working through of the traumatic experience), expecting quick recovery and promoting a sense of mastery and acceptance over the traumatic event
- Early cognitive-behavioral interventions can also speed recovery
- Treatment initiated later, when symptoms have crystallized, includes
  - Programs for cessation of alcohol and other drug abuse
  - Group and individual psychotherapy
  - Improved social support systems
- Psychological debriefing in a single session, once considered a mainstay in prevention of PTSD, is under scrutiny

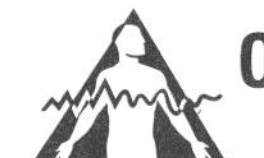

OUTCOME

PROGNOSIS

- The sooner the symptoms arise after the initial trauma and the sooner therapy is initiated, the better the prognosis
- Resolution may be delayed if others' responses to the patient's difficulties are thoughtlessly harmful or if the secondary gains outweigh the advantages of recovery
- The longer the symptoms persist, the worse the prognosis

WHEN TO REFER

- Marital problems are a major area of concern, and it is important that the clinician have available a dependable referral source when marriage counseling is indicated

EVIDENCE

PRACTICE GUIDELINES

- American Academy of Family Physicians
  - http://www.aafp.org/afp/20031215/2401.html
- National Guideline Clearinghouse: VHA/DoD, 2004
  - http://www.guideline.gov/summary/summary.aspx?doc_id=5187

WEB SITES

- American Psychiatric Association
  - http://www.psych.org/
- Internet Mental Health
  - http://www.mentalhealth.com/
- National Center for Posttraumatic Stress Disorder
  - http://www.ncptsd.org
- Posttraumatic stress disorder alliance
  - http://www.ptsdalliance.org

INFORMATION FOR PATIENTS

- American Psychiatric Association
  - http://www.psych.org/public_info/ptsd.cfm
- JAMA patient page: Posttraumatic strerss disorder. JAMA 2001;286:630. [PMID: 11508286]
- National Institute of Mental Health
  - http://www.nimh.nih.gov/publicat/nimhptsd.pdf

REFERENCES

- Brady K et al: Efficacy and safety of sertraline treatment of posttraumatic stress disorder, a randomised control trial. JAMA 2000;283:1837. [PMID:10770145]
- Pitman RK et al: Pilot study of secondary prevention of PTSD with propranolol. Biol Psychiatry 2002;51:189. [PMID:11822998]

Author(s)

Stuart J. Eisendrath, MD
Jonathan E. Lichtmacher, MD

Preeclampsia & Eclampsia

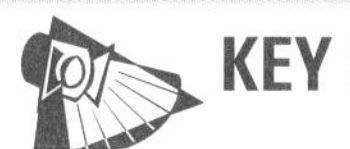

KEY FEATURES

ESSENTIALS OF DIAGNOSIS

- Preeclampsia
  - Blood pressure of ≥ 140 mm Hg systolic or ≥ 90 mm Hg diastolic after 20 weeks gestation
  - Proteinuria of ≥ 0.3 g in 24 h
- Severe preeclampsia
  - Blood pressure of ≥ 160 mm Hg systolic or ≥ 110 mm Hg diastolic
  - Proteinuria ≥ 5 g in 24 h or 4+ on dipstick
  - Oliguria of < 500 mL in 24 h
  - Thrombocytopenia
  - Hemolysis elevated liver enzymes low platelets (HELLP)
  - Pulmonary edema
- Fetal growth restriction

GENERAL CONSIDERATIONS

- Cause is unknown, but an immunologic cause is suspected
- The only cure is delivery of the fetus and placenta
- Uncontrolled eclampsia is a significant cause of maternal death
- Use of diuretics, dietary changes, aspirin, and vitamin-mineral supplements have not been shown to be effective
- Early diagnosis is the key to treatment
- Many cases are asymptomatic early
- 5% of women with preeclampsia progress to eclampsia

DEMOGRAPHICS

- Occurs in 7% of pregnant women in the United States
- Higher incidence in primiparas
- Other risk factors
  - Multiple gestations
  - Chronic hypertension
  - Diabetes
  - Renal disease
  - Collagen-vascular and autoimmune disease
  - Gestational trophoblastic disease

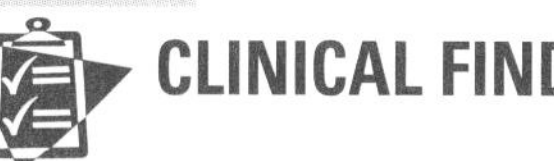

CLINICAL FINDINGS

SYMPTOMS AND SIGNS

- See Table 72
- Hypertension, proteinuria, and edema are classically required for the diagnosis, but presentation varies greatly
- Can occur any time after 20 weeks' gestation and up to 6 weeks postpartum
- Severity can be assessed with reference to the six sites where disease has its effects: CNS, kidneys, liver, hematologic and vascular systems, and the fetal placental unit
- Few complaints are present in mild disease; antepartum fetal testing is reassuring
- Symptoms are dramatic and persist in severe disease; thrombocytopenia may progress to disseminated intravascular coagulation

DIFFERENTIAL DIAGNOSIS

- Essential hypertension or other cause of secondary hypertension
- Chronic renal failure or proteinuria due to other cause
- Primary seizure disorder
- Thrombotic thrombocytopenic purpura
- Other cause of abdominal pain, eg, cholecystitis, appendicitis, acute fatty liver of pregnancy
- Gallbladder and pancreatic disease
- Hemolytic uremic syndrome

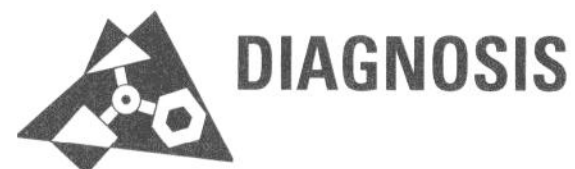

DIAGNOSIS

LABORATORY TESTS

- See Table 72
- Platelet count is over 100,000/μL in mild to moderate disease
- Thrombocytopenia seen in severe disease
- Hemolysis, elevated liver enzymes, and low platelets describe the HELLP syndrome
- Hyperuricemia is helpful in diagnosis, as in pregnancy, it is seen only with gout, renal failure, or preeclampsia-eclampsia

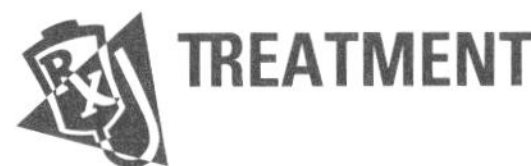

TREATMENT

MEDICATIONS

- Sedatives and opiates should be avoided, as they interfere with fetal assessment
- Two doses of corticosteroids IM (betamethasone, 12 mg or dexamethasone, 16 mg) 12–24 h apart should be given if fetal immaturity is present
- Diazepam (5–10 mg IV over 4 minutes) or magnesium sulfate (4 g over 4 minutes, then 2–3 g/h unless abnormal renal function is present) is used to stop seizures
- Hydralazine, 5–10 mg IV every 20 min, nifedipine, 10 mg SL or PO, or labetalol, 10–20 mg IV every 20 min can be used
- Oxytocin may be used to induce or augment labor
- Magnesium sulfate infusion should be continued postpartum until preeclampsia-eclampsia begins to resolve (1–7 days), as indicated by the onset of diuresis (100–200 mL/h)
- Antihypertensive therapy is used if diastolic blood pressure > 110 mm Hg, with a target of 90–100 mm Hg

SURGERY

- Cesarean section is reserved for the usual fetal indications or when rapid delivery is needed
- Regional anesthesia or analgesia is acceptable

THERAPEUTIC PROCEDURES

- Nonstress and stress fetal testing or a biophysical profile should be obtained initially and then serially to confirm fetal well-being
- Daily fetal kick counts can be recorded by the mother
- Amniocentesis should be considered to evaluate lung maturity if hospitalization occurs at 30–37 weeks

Preeclampsia

- Disease of any severity at 36 weeks or later is managed by delivery
- Prior to 36 weeks, severe disease requires delivery except with extreme fetal prematurity
- Bed rest is the cornerstone of therapy for mild to moderate preeclampsia; it may be attempted at home or in the hospital depending on the degree of organ system involvement
- Epigastric pain, thrombocytopenia, and visual disturbances are strong indications for delivery

Eclampsia

- Seizing patients are placed on their side to increase placental blood flow and avoid aspiration
- Maternal and fetal status determine the method of delivery

OUTCOME

FOLLOW-UP

- Blood pressure, reflexes, proteinuria, and fetal monitoring are required regularly in hospitalized patients
- Blood cell count, electrolytes, proteinuria, and liver enzymes should be checked every 1–2 days in hospitalized patients
- 24-h urine protein and creatinine clearance on admission and as indicated
- Magnesium levels are checked every 4–6 h and infusions titrated to serum levels of 4–6 mEq/L
- Urinary output is checked hourly in severe disease or eclampsia
- Patients receiving magnesium infusions are monitored for signs of toxicity such as loss of deep tendon reflexes or respiratory depression; calcium gluconate can be used for reversal

WHEN TO ADMIT

- Moderate or severe preeclampsia or an unreliable home situation warrants hospitalization

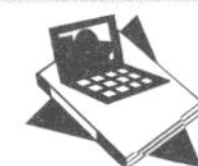

EVIDENCE

PRACTICE GUIDELINES

- ACOG Committee on Obstetrics Practice. ACOG practice bulletin. Diagnosis and management of preeclampsia and eclampsia. Number 33, January 2002. American College of Obstetricians and Gynecologists.Int J Gynaecol Obstet 2002;77:67. [PMID: 12094777]
- Roberts JM et al; NHLBI. Report of the Working Group on Research on Hypertension During Pregnancy, 2001.
  - http://www.nhlbi.nih.gov/resources/hyperten_preg/

WEB SITES

- Guidelines, Recommendations, and Evidence-Based Medicine in Obstetrics
  - http://matweb.hcuge.ch/matweb/endo/cours_4e_MREG/obstetrics_gynecology_guidelines.htm
- National Heart, Lung, and Blood Institute: Prevention of Preeclampsia
  - http://hin.nhlbi.nih.gov/nhbpep_slds/hbppreg_ss/download/preclmp.pdf

INFORMATION FOR PATIENTS

- American Academy of Family Physicians: Preeclampsia
  - http://familydoctor.org/064.xml
- MedlinePlus: Preeclampsia
  - http://www.nlm.nih.gov/medlineplus/ency/article/000898.htm
- MedlinePlus: Eclampsia
  - http://www.nlm.nih.gov/medlineplus/ency/article/000899.htm
- National Heart, Lung, and Blood Institute: High Blood Pressure in Pregnancy
  - http://www.nhlbi.nih.gov/health/public/heart/hbp/hbp_preg.htm

REFERENCE

- Lain KY et al: Contemporary concepts of the pathogenesis and management of pre-eclampsia. JAMA 2002;287:3183. [PMID: 12076198]

Author(s)

William R. Crombleholme, MD

Pregnancy

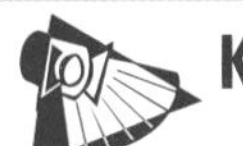

KEY FEATURES

ESSENTIALS OF DIAGNOSIS

- Amenorrhea, weight gain, nausea and vomiting, and breast changes
- Positive pregnancy test

GENERAL CONSIDERATIONS

- Prompt diagnosis of pregnancy allows early prenatal care and avoidance of harmful activities or exposures
- In the event of an unwanted pregnancy, early diagnosis allows for counseling regarding adoption or termination

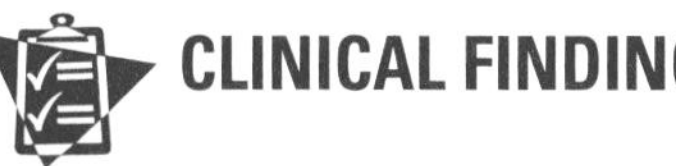

CLINICAL FINDINGS

SYMPTOMS AND SIGNS

- No symptoms or signs are diagnostic
- Amenorrhea, weight gain
- Nausea and vomiting
- Breast tenderness and tingling
- Urinary frequency and urgency
- "Quickening" (perception of the first fetal movement) is noted at about 18 weeks' gestation
- Signs
  - Breast changes, abdominal enlargement, and cyanosis of the vagina and cervical portio (week 7)
  - Softening of the cervix (week 7)
  - Generalized enlargement and softening of the corpus (post-week 8)
  - Uterine fundus is palpable above the pubic symphysis by 12–15 weeks from last menstrual period
  - Fundus reaches the umbilicus by 20–22 weeks
  - Fetal heart tones heard by Doppler at 10 to 12 weeks

DIFFERENTIAL DIAGNOSIS

- Myomas can be confused with a gravid uterus
- A midline ovarian tumor may displace a nonpregnant uterus
- Ectopic pregnancies may show lower levels of human chorionic gonadotropin (hCG) that level off or fall
- Premature menopause

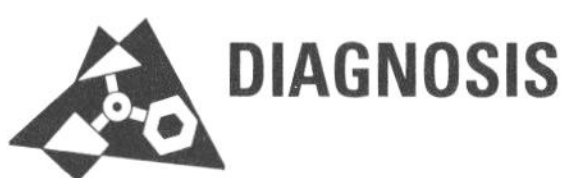

DIAGNOSIS

LABORATORY TESTS

Diagnostic tests

- All urine or blood pregnancy tests rely on detection of placental hCG and are accurate at the time of a missed period or shortly after it
- Laboratory and home assays use monoclonal antibodies specific for hCG
- hCG levels increase shortly after implantation, double every 48 h, peak at 50–75 days, and fall in second and third trimesters

Screening at the time of diagnosis

- Urinalysis, culture of a mid-stream urine sample, complete blood count (CBC), serologic test for syphilis, rubella antibody titer, blood group and Rh type, atypical antibody screening, and hepatitis B surface antigen testing are recommended
- HIV testing should be encouraged
- Cervical cultures for *Neisseria gonorrhoea* and *Chlamydia*, as well as Pap smear, are indicated
- Testing for abnormal hemoglobins should be done in patients at risk for sickle cell or thalassemia traits
- Tuberculosis skin testing is recommended for high-risk groups
- Tay-Sachs screening should be offered to
  - Jewish women with Jewish partners (especially those of Ashkenazi descent)
  - Couples of French-Canadian or Cajun ancestry
- Hepatitis C screening should be offered to mothers at high risk

Screening during pregnancy

- Maternal serum α-fetoprotein (AFP) is offered to all women to screen for neural tube defects and is mandatory in some states (16–20 weeks)
- hCG and estriol levels are combined with AFP (triple screen) for detection of fetal Down's syndrome
- Screening for gestational diabetes by checking glucose 1 h post a 50-g glucose load (26–28 weeks)
- 3-h glucose tolerance test follows up an abnormal 1-h glucose load test
- Repeat Rh testing for negative patients [28 weeks, though result is not required before Rho(D) Ig is given]
- CBC to evaluate for anemia of pregnancy (28–32 weeks)

- Repeat tests for syphilis, HIV, and cervical cultures in at-risk patients (36 weeks to delivery)
- Screening for group B streptococcal (GBS) colonization can be done by rectovaginal culture at 35–37 weeks
  - If negative, no prophylaxis is given
  - Intrapartum prophylaxis with penicillin or clindamycin is given if screening cultures are positive
  - Patients with risk factors for GBS or who deliver at < 37 weeks receive intrapartum prophylaxis
  - Patients without a culture at 35–37 weeks receive prophylaxis only for a history of GBS bacteriuria or prior GBS disease in an infant, intrapartum fevers, or membrane rupture > 18 h

IMAGING STUDIES

- X-rays should be avoided unless essential and approved by a physician
- Fetal ultrasound for accurate dating and to evaluate fetal anatomy is usually done at 18–20 weeks' gestation
- In multiple pregnancies, ultrasound is repeated every 4 weeks to identify discordant growth

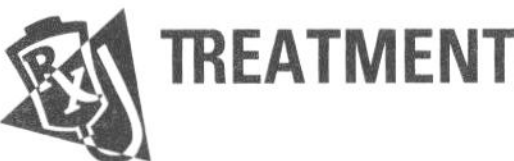

TREATMENT

MEDICATIONS

- Prenatal vitamins with iron and folic acid are indicated
- Medications should not be taken unless prescribed or authorized by the patient's provider (Tables 71 and 74)
- Penicillin (5 million units followed by 2.5 million units Q 4 h until delivery), or clindamycin (900 mg IV Q 8 h) are given for prophylaxis of group B streptococcal infection with susceptible isolates

THERAPEUTIC PROCEDURES

- Genetic counseling with the option of chorionic villous sampling or amniocentesis should be offered to women 35 or older at delivery, a family history of congenital abnormalities, or previous child with a metabolic disease, chromosomal abnormality, or neural tube defect

OUTCOME

FOLLOW-UP

- Prenatal visits should be scheduled
  - Every 4 weeks from 0–28 weeks
  - Every 2 weeks from 28–36 weeks
  - Weekly from 36 weeks to delivery

COMPLICATIONS

- Fetal alcohol syndrome: no safe level of alcohol intake has been established for pregnancy
- Cigarette smoking increases risk of abruptio placentae, placenta previa, and premature rupture of the membranes
- Premature delivery and lower birth weights are more common in children born to smokers
- Maternal cocaine, amphetamine, and opioid use in pregnancy is associated with numerous complications

WHEN TO REFER

- If the practitioner has no training or experience in prenatal care

WHEN TO ADMIT

- For any major medical or pregnancy-related complication

PREVENTION

- Hepatitis B vaccination for women with potential occupational exposure or household contacts
- Live virus immunizations (measles, rubella, varicella, yellow fever) are contraindicated during pregnancy
- Influenza vaccine is indicated in all women who will be in their second or third trimester during "flu season"
- Decrease caffeine intake
- Avoid ingestion of raw meat, all tobacco, alcohol, and recreational drugs, exposure to environmental tobacco smoke, excessive heat, hot tubs, and saunas, and handling of cat feces or litter
- Exercise should be mild to moderate, with heart rate kept below 140 bpm

EVIDENCE

PRACTICE GUIDELINES

- American College of Obstetricians and Gynecologists. Immunization during pregnancy. Int J Gynaecol Obstet 2003;81:123. [PMID: 12737148]
- National Collaborating Centre for Women's and Children's Health. Antenatal care: routine care for the healthy pregnant woman. 2003.
  - http://www.guideline.gov/summary/summary.aspx?doc_id=4808&nbr=3470

WEB SITES

- Guidelines, Recommendations, and Evidence-Based Medicine in Obstetrics
  - http://matweb.hcuge.ch/matweb/endo/cours_4e_MREG/obstetrics_gynecology_guidelines.htm
- Obstetric Ultrasound
  - http://www.ob-ultrasound.net

INFORMATION FOR PATIENTS

- National Women's Health Information Center: Pregnancy and a Healthy Diet
  - http://www.4woman.gov/faq/preg-nutr.htm
- Nemours Foundation: Medical Care During Pregnancy
  - http://kidshealth.org/parent/pregnancy_newborn/pregnancy/medical_care_pregnancy.html
- Nemours Foundation: Staying Healthy During Pregnancy
  - http://kidshealth.org/parent/pregnancy_newborn/pregnancy/preg_health.html
- New York Online Access to Health: Pregnancy
  - http://www.noah-health.org/en/pregnancy/index.html

REFERENCES

- Haertsch M et al: What is recommended for healthy women during pregnancy? A comparison of seven prenatal clinical practice guideline documents. Birth 1999;26:24. [PMID: 10352052]
- Jacqz-Aigrain E et al: Effects of drugs on the fetus. Semin Fetal Neonatal Med 2005;10:139. [PMID: 15701579]
- Schrag S et al: Prevention of perinatal group B streptococcal disease. Revised guidelines from CDC. MMWR Recomm Rep 2002;51(RR-11):1. [PMID: 12211284]

Author(s)

William R. Crombleholme, MD

Premenstrual Syndrome

Pregnancy, Third-Trimester Bleeding p. 1137.
Pregnancy, Thyroid Disease p. 1138.

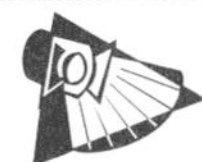

KEY FEATURES

ESSENTIALS OF DIAGNOSIS

- Recurrent, variable cluster of troublesome physical and emotional symptoms that develops during the 7–14 days before the onset of menses
- Symptoms subside when menstruation occurs
- In about 10% of affected women, the syndrome may be severe

GENERAL CONSIDERATIONS

- The pathogenesis is still uncertain. Psychosocial factors may play a role
- Suppression of ovulation with an oral contraceptive is sometimes helpful, but the patient often complains that she still has premenstrual syndrome

DEMOGRAPHICS

- Intermittently affects about one-third of all premenopausal women, primarily those 25–40 years of age

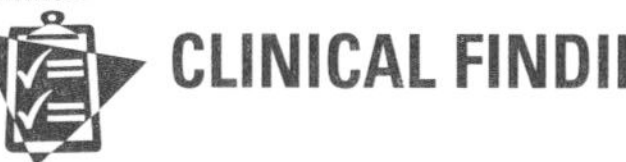

CLINICAL FINDINGS

SYMPTOMS AND SIGNS

- Women may not experiences all the symptoms or signs at one time
- Bloating
- Breast pain
- Ankle swelling
- A sense of increased weight
- Skin disorders
- Irritability, aggressiveness, depression, inability to concentrate, libido change, lethargy, and food cravings

DIFFERENTIAL DIAGNOSIS

- Depression
- Premenstrual dysphoric disorder
- Endometriosis
- Uterine leiomyomas (fibroids)
- Pregnancy
- Anxiety disorder
- Hypothyroidism

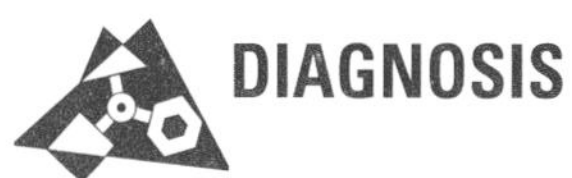

DIAGNOSIS

DIAGNOSTIC PROCEDURES

- Careful evaluation of the patient
- History of symptoms

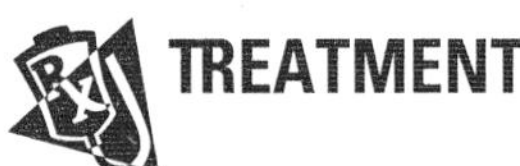

TREATMENT

MEDICATIONS

- Serotonin reuptake inhibitors such as fluoxetine, 20 mg PO/day, are effective in relieving tension, irritability, and dysphoria with few side effects
- When physical symptoms predominate
  - Spironolactone, 100 mg PO daily during the luteal phase, is effective for reduction of bloating and breast tenderness
  - Oral contraceptives or DMPA will decrease breast pain and cramping
  - Nonsteroidal anti-inflammatory drugs—eg, mefenamic acid, 500 mg PO three times a day—will reduce a number of symptoms, although not breast pain
- Suppression of ovarian function with DMPA or a gonadotropin-releasing hormone (GnRH) agonist diminishes all symptoms during therapy. "Add-back therapy" to provide the hormones suppressed by the GnRH agonist with low-dose estrogen and progestin may allow extended use of a GnRH agonist

THERAPEUTIC PROCEDURES

- Current treatment methods are mainly empiric
- Provide support for the emotional and physical distress
- Advise the patient to keep a daily diary of all symptoms for 2–3 months to help in evaluating the timing and characteristics of the syndrome. If her symptoms occur throughout the month rather than in the 2 weeks before menses, she may be depressed or may have other emotional problems in addition to premenstrual syndrome
- A diet emphasizing complex carbohydrates can be recommended
  - Foods high in sugar content and alcohol should be avoided to minimize reactive hypoglycemia
  - Use of caffeine should be minimized whenever tension and irritability predominate
- A program of regular conditioning exercise, such as jogging, can decrease depression, anxiety, and fluid retention

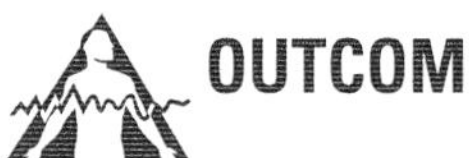

OUTCOME

PROGNOSIS

- Symptom-specific therapy is usually helpful in ameliorating symptoms

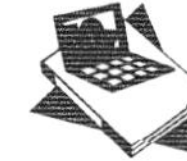

EVIDENCE

PRACTICE GUIDELINES

- American College of Obstetricians and Gynecologists: Premenstrual syndrome. 2000.
  - http://www.guideline.gov/summary/summary.aspx?doc_id=3965&nbr=3103

INFORMATION FOR PATIENTS

- American Academy of Family Physicians: PMS: What You Can Do To Ease Your Symptoms
  - http://familydoctor.org/141.xml
- American Academy of Family Physicians: Premenstrual Dysphoric Disorder
  - http://familydoctor.org/752.xml
- Mayo Clinic: Premenstrual Syndrome
  - http://www.mayoclinic.com/invoke.cfm?id=DS00134
- National Women's Health Information Center: Premenstrual Syndrome
  - http://www.4woman.gov/faq/pms.htm

REFERENCES

- Johnson SR: Premenstrual syndrome, premenstrual dysphoric disorder, and beyond: a clinical primer for practitioners. Obstet Gynecol 2004;104:845. [PMID: 15458909]

Author(s)

H. Trent MacKay, MD, MPH

Prostate Cancer

KEY FEATURES

ESSENTIALS OF DIAGNOSIS

- Prostatic induration on digital rectal examination (DRE) or elevation of prostate-specific antigen (PSA)
- Most often asymptomatic
- Rarely: systemic symptoms (weight loss, bone pain)

GENERAL CONSIDERATIONS

- Most common cancer detected in American men
- Second leading cause of cancer-related death
- In 2001, 198,000 new cases of prostate cancer, about 31,500 deaths
- At autopsy, > 40% of men aged > 50 years have prostatic carcinoma, most often occult
- Incidence increases with age: autopsy incidence ~30% of men aged 60–69 versus 67% in men aged 80–89 years
- Risk factors: black race, men with a family history of prostatic cancer, history of high dietary fat intake
- A 50-year-old American man has a lifetime risk of 40% for latent cancer, of 9.5% for clinically apparent cancer, and of 2.9% for death from prostatic cancer
- Majority of prostatic cancers are adenocarcinomas

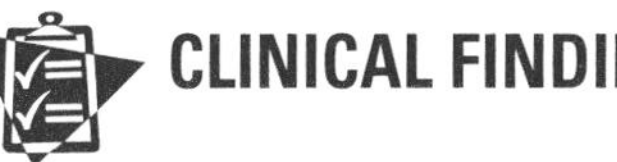

CLINICAL FINDINGS

SYMPTOMS AND SIGNS

- Focal nodules or areas of induration within the prostate on DRE
- Obstructive voiding symptoms
- Lymph node metastases
- Lower extremity lymphedema
- Back pain or pathologic fractures
- Rarely, signs of urinary retention (palpable bladder) or neurologic symptoms as a result of epidural metastases and cord compression

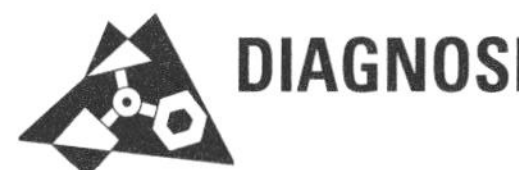

DIAGNOSIS

LABORATORY TESTS

- Elevations in serum PSA (normal < 4 ng/mL)
- PSA correlates with the volume of both benign and malignant prostatic tissue
- 18–30% of men with PSA 4.1–10 ng/mL have prostatic cancer
- Age-specific PSA reference ranges exist
- Most organ-confined cancers have PSA levels < 10 ng/mL
- Advanced disease (seminal vesicle invasion, lymph node involvement, or occult distant metastases) have PSA levels > 40 ng/mL
- Elevations in serum urea nitrogen or creatinine in patients with urinary retention or those with ureteral obstruction due to locally or regionally advanced prostatic cancers
- Elevations in alkaline phosphatase or hypercalcemia in patients with bony metastases
- Disseminated intravascular coagulation (DIC) in patients with advanced prostatic cancers

IMAGING STUDIES

- Transrectal ultrasound (TRUS): most prostatic cancers are hypoechoic
- MRI of the prostate
- Positive predictive value for detection of both capsular penetration and seminal vesicle invasion is similar for both TRUS and MRI

DIAGNOSTIC PROCEDURES

- TRUS-guided biopsy from the apex, mid portion, and base of the prostate
  - Done in men who have an abnormal DRE or an elevated PSA
  - Systematic rather than only lesion-directed biopsies are recommended
- Fine-needle aspiration biopsies should be considered in patients at an increased risk for bleeding

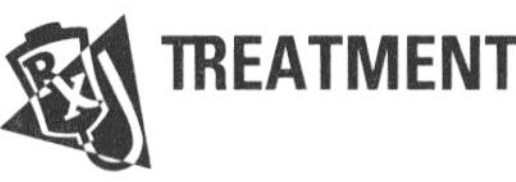

TREATMENT

MEDICATIONS

- Adrenal
  - Ketoconazole, 400 mg TID PO (adrenal insufficiency, nausea, rash, ataxia)
  - Aminoglutethimide, 250 mg QID (adrenal insufficiency, nausea, rash, ataxia)

- Corticosteroids: prednisone, 20–40 mg QD (gastrointestinal bleeding, fluid retention)

- Pituitary, hypothalamus
  - Estrogens, 1–3 mg QD (gynecomastia, hot flushes, thromboembolic disease, erectile dysfunction)
  - Luteinizing hormone-releasing hormone (LHRH) agonists, monthly or 3-monthly depot injection (erectile dysfunction, hot flushes, gynecomastia, rarely anemia)
- Prostate cell
  - Antiandrogens: flutamide, 250 mg TID, or bicalutamide, 50 mg QD (no erectile dysfunction when used alone; nausea, diarrhea)
- Testis
  - Orchiectomy (gynecomastia, hot flushes, impotence)
  - Ketoconazole for patients with advanced prostatic cancer who present with spinal cord compression, bilateral ureteral obstruction, or DIC
  - Complete androgen blockade by combining an antiandrogen with use of an LHRH agonist or orchiectomy

THERAPEUTIC PROCEDURES

- Patients need to be advised of all treatment options (including surveillance), benefits, risks, and limitations
- For minimal capsular penetration, standard irradiation or surgery
- For locally extensive cancers, including seminal vesicle and bladder neck invasion, combination therapy (androgen deprivation combined with surgery or irradiation)
- Androgen deprivation for metastatic disease
- Localized disease
  - Optimal form of treatment controversial
  - Selected patients may be candidates for surveillance; patients with an anticipated survival of > 10 years should be considered for treatment with radical prostatectomy, radiation therapy
- Radical prostatectomy
  - For stages T1 and T2 prostatic cancers, local recurrence is uncommon after radical prostatectomy; organ-confined cancers rarely recur; cancers locally extensive (capsular penetration, seminal vesicle invasion) have higher local (10–25%) and distant (20–50%) relapse rates
  - Adjuvant therapy (radiation for patients with positive surgical margins or androgen deprivation for lymph node metastases)
- Radiation therapy: external beam radiotherapy and transperineal implantation of radioisotopes
- Morbidity is limited; survival with localized cancers is 65% at 10 years
- Newer techniques of radiation (implantation, conformal therapy using three-dimensional reconstruction of CT-based tumor volumes, heavy particle, charged particle, and heavy charged particle) improve local control rates
- Brachytherapy, the implantation of permanent or temporary radioactive sources (palladium, iodine, or iridium)

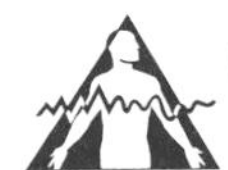

OUTCOME

FOLLOW-UP

- Surveillance alone may be appropriate for patients who are older and have very small and well-differentiated cancers

PREVENTION

Screening for prostatic cancer

- Screening tests currently available include DRE, PSA testing, TRUS
- Detection rates of DRE vary from 1.5% to 7%
- TRUS has low specificity (and therefore high biopsy rate). TRUS increases the detection rate very little when compared with the combined use of DRE and PSA testing
- With PSA testing, 2–2.5% of men older than age 50 have prostatic cancer compared with a rate of 1.5% using DRE screening alone. However, PSA is not specific for cancer
- Age-specific reference ranges for PSA have been established and increase specificity
  - For men aged 40–49 years, range is < 2.5 ng/mL
  - For men 50–59, < 3.5 ng/mL
  - For men 60–69, < 4.5 ng/mL
  - For men 70–79, < 6.5 ng/mL
- PSA velocity (serial measurement of PSA), PSA density (serum PSA/volume of the prostate as measured by ultrasound), and PSA transition zone density (the zone of the prostate that undergoes enlargement during development of benign prostatic hyperplasia)
- Free and protein-bound PSA levels can be measured: cancer patients have a lower percentage of free serum PSA
- PSA testing should be performed yearly in men with a normal DRE and a PSA > 2.5 ng/mL and biennially in those with a normal DRE and serum PSA < 2.5 ng/mL

EVIDENCE

PRACTICE GUIDELINES

- Loblaw DA et al; American Society of Clinical Oncology: American Society of Clinical Oncology recommendations for the initial hormonal management of androgen-sensitive metastatic, recurrent, or progressive prostate cancer. J Clin Oncol 2004;22:2927. Epub 2004 Jun 07. Erratum in: J Clin Oncol 2004;22:4435.
- Scher HI et al: Eligibility and outcomes reporting guidelines for clinical trials for patients in the state of a rising prostate-specific antigen: recommendations from the Prostate-Specific Antigen Working Group. J Clin Oncol 2004;22:537. Erratum in: J Clin Oncol 2004;22:3205.
- Villers A et al: Summary of the Standards, Options and Recommendations for the management of patients with nonmetastatic prostate cancer (2001). Br J Cancer 2003;89(Suppl 1):S50. [PMID: 12915903]

INFORMATION FOR PATIENTS

- Cleveland Clinic—Prostate cancer
  - http://www.clevelandclinic.org/health/health-info/docs/1900/1932.asp?index=8634
- Mayo Clinic
  - http://www.mayoclinic.com/invoke.cfm?id=DS00043

REFERENCES

- Arredondo SA et al: Watchful waiting and health related quality of life for patients with localized prostate cancer: data from CaPSURE. J Urol 2004;172(5 Pt 1):1830. [PMID: 15540732]
- Canto EI et al: Effects of systematic 12-core biopsy on the performance of percent free prostate specific antigen for prostate cancer detection. J Urol 2004;172:900. [PMID: 15310993]
- Catalona WJ: Prostate cancer screening. BJU Int 2004;94:964. [PMID: 15541107]
- Chan JM et al: The relative impact and future burden of prostate cancer in the United States. J Urol 2004;172(5 Pt 2):S13. [PMID: 15535436]

Author(s)

Marshall L. Stoller, MD

Peter R. Carroll, MD

Prostatitis, Acute Bacterial

KEY FEATURES

ESSENTIALS OF DIAGNOSIS

- Fever
- Irritative voiding symptoms
- Perineal or suprapubic pain
- Exquisite tenderness on rectal examination
- Positive urine culture

GENERAL CONSIDERATIONS

- Usual causative organisms: *Escherichia coli* and *Pseudomonas*
- Less common: *Enterococcus*

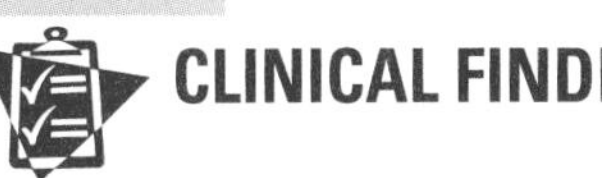

CLINICAL FINDINGS

SYMPTOMS AND SIGNS

- Perineal, sacral, or suprapubic pain
- Fever
- Irritative voiding complaints
- Obstructive symptoms
- Urinary retention
- Exquisitely tender prostate

DIFFERENTIAL DIAGNOSIS

- Epididymitis
- Diverticulitis
- Urinary retention from benign or malignant prostatic enlargement
- Chronic bacterial prostatitis
- Nonbacterial prostatitis
- Prostatodynia

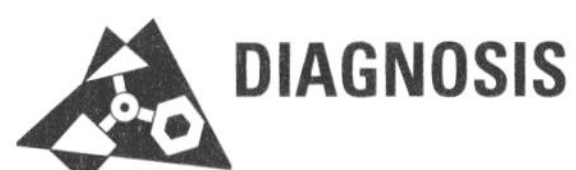

DIAGNOSIS

LABORATORY TESTS

- Complete blood cell count: leukocytosis and a left shift
- Urinalysis: pyuria, bacteriuria, hematuria
- Urine culture: positive

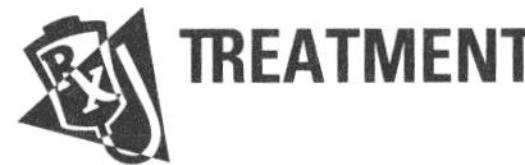

TREATMENT

MEDICATIONS

- IV ampicillin and an aminoglycoside until afebrile for 24–48 h, then PO quinolone for 4–6 weeks
- Ampicillin, IV 1 g Q 6 h, and gentamicin, IV 1 mg/kg Q 8 h for 21 days
- Ciprofloxacin, PO 750 mg Q 12 h for 21 days
- Ofloxacin, PO 200–300 mg Q 12 h for 21 days
- Trimethoprim-sulfamethoxazole, PO 160/800 mg Q 12 h for 21 days—increasing resistance noted (up to 20%)

THERAPEUTIC PROCEDURES

- Suprapubic drainage if urinary retention
- Urethral catheterization, instrumentation, and prostatic massage is contraindicated

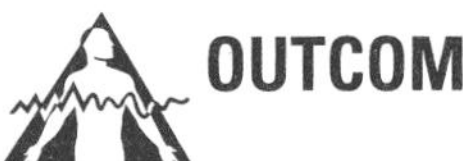

OUTCOME

FOLLOW-UP

- Posttreatment urine culture
- Posttreatment examination of expressed prostatic secretions after completion of therapy

PROGNOSIS

- With effective treatment, chronic bacterial prostatitis is rare

EVIDENCE

PRACTICE GUIDELINES

- 2002 National Guideline for the Management of Prostatitis. Association for Genitourinary Medicine. Medical Society for the Study of Venereal Diseases, 2002.
  - http://www.agum.org.uk/ceg2002/prostatitis0601.htm
- Naber KG et al: EAU guidelines for the management of urinary and male genital tract infections. Urinary Tract Infection (UTI) Working Group of the Health Care Office (HCO) of the European Association of Urology (EAU). Eur Urol 2001;40:576. [PMID: 11752870]
- National Guideline Clearinghouse
  - http://www.guideline.gov/summary/summary.aspx?doc_id=3041&nbr=2267&string=acute+AND+bacterial+AND+prostatitis.

INFORMATION FOR PATIENTS

- American Urological Association
  - http://www.urologyhealth.org/search/index.cfm?topic=115&search=Cystitis%20AND%20acute&searchtype=and
- Cleveland Clinic—Prostatitis
  - http://www.clevelandclinic.org/health/health-info/docs/1900/1962.asp?index=8527
- Mayo Clinic—Prostatitis
  - http://www.mayoclinic.com/invoke.cfm?objectid=8754C233-295A-4871-BB6EAE0904F9233A

REFERENCE

- Schaeffer AJ: NIDDK-sponsored chronic prostatitis collaborative research network (CPCRN) 5-year data and treatment guidelines for bacterial prostatitis. Int J Antimicrob Agents 2004;24(Suppl 1):S49. [PMID: 15364307]

Author(s)

Marshall L. Stoller, MD
Peter R. Carroll, MD

Pruritus, Anogenital

Prostatitis, Chronic Bacterial p. 1138. Prostatodynia p. 1139.
Pruritus p. 1139.

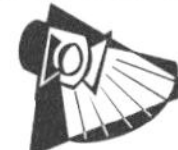

KEY FEATURES

ESSENTIALS OF DIAGNOSIS

- Itching, chiefly nocturnal, of the anogenital area
- Examination is highly variable, ranging from no skin findings to excoriations and inflammation of any degree, including lichenification

GENERAL CONSIDERATIONS

- May be due to intertrigo, psoriasis, lichen simplex chronicus, or seborrheic or contact dermatitis (from soaps, colognes, douches, contraceptives, and perhaps scented toilet tissue)
- May be due to irritating secretions, as in diarrhea, leukorrhea, or trichomoniasis, or to local disease (candidiasis, dermatophytosis, erythrasma)
- Uncleanliness may be at fault
- In pruritus ani, hemorrhoids are often found, and leakage of mucus and bacteria from the distal rectum onto the perianal skin may be important in cases in which no other skin abnormality is found
- **In women**, pruritus ani by itself is rare, and pruritus vulvae does not usually involve the anal area, though anal itching will usually spread to the vulva
- **In men**, pruritus of the scrotum is most commonly seen in the absence of pruritus ani
- When all possible known causes have been ruled out, the condition is diagnosed as idiopathic or essential pruritus—by no means rare

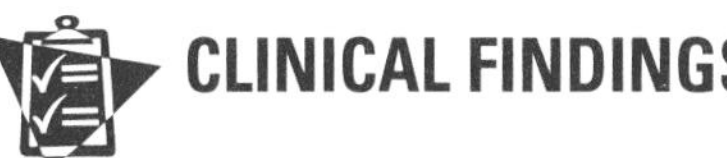

CLINICAL FINDINGS

SYMPTOMS AND SIGNS

- The only symptom is itching, which is primarily nocturnal
- Physical findings are usually not present, but there may be erythema, fissuring, maceration, lichenification, excoriations, or changes suggestive of candidiasis or tinea

DIFFERENTIAL DIAGNOSIS

- Idiopathic
- Intertrigo
- Psoriasis
- Hemorrhoids
- Lichen simplex chronicus
- Seborrheic dermatitis
- Contact dermatitis
- Candidiasis
- Tinea
- Erythrasma
- Irritants: diarrhea, vaginal discharge
- Lichen sclerosis et atrophicus
- Pinworm

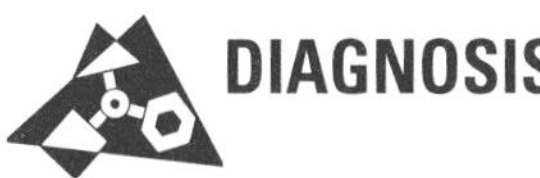

DIAGNOSIS

LABORATORY TESTS

- Urinalysis and blood glucose testing may lead to a diagnosis of diabetes mellitus
- Microscopic examination or culture of tissue scrapings may reveal yeasts or fungi
- Stool examination may show pinworms

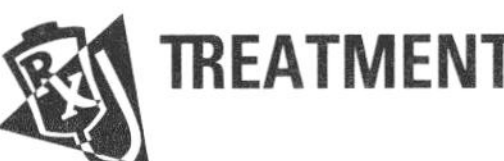

TREATMENT

MEDICATIONS

General measures

- Treating constipation, preferably with high-fiber management (psyllium), may help

Local measures

- Pramoxine cream or lotion or hydrocortisone-pramoxine (Pramosone), 1% or 2.5% cream, lotion, or ointment, is helpful in managing pruritus in the anogenital area; the ointment or cream should be applied after a bowel movement
- Potent fluorinated topical corticosteroids may lead to atrophy and striae if used for more than a few days and should in general be avoided; this includes combinations with antifungals
- The use of strong steroids on the scrotum may lead to persistent severe burning on withdrawal of the drug
- Soaks with aluminum subacetate solution, 1:20, are of value if the area is acutely inflamed and oozing
- Affected areas may be painted with Castellani's solution, Balneol Perianal Cleansing Lotion, or Tucks premoistened pads, ointment, or cream (all Tucks preparations contain witch hazel) may be very useful for pruritus ani

THERAPEUTIC PROCEDURES

- Instruct the patient to use very soft or moistened tissue or cotton after bowel movements and to clean the perianal area thoroughly with cool water if possible
- Women should use similar precautions after urinating
- Instruct the patient regarding the harmful and pruritus-inducing effects of scratching
- Underclothing should be changed daily

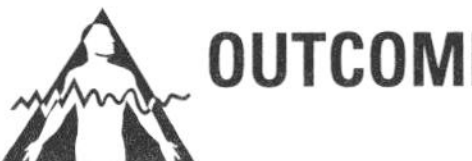

OUTCOME

PROGNOSIS

- Although benign, anogenital pruritus may be persistent and recurrent

WHEN TO REFER

- If there is a question about the diagnosis, if recommended therapy is ineffective, or if specialized treatment is necessary

PREVENTION

- Instruct the patient in proper anogenital hygiene after treating systemic or local conditions

EVIDENCE

WEB SITE

- American Academy of Dermatology
  - http://www.aad.org

INFORMATION FOR PATIENTS

- American Academy of Family Physicians: Fiber: How to Increase the Amount in Your Diet
  - http://familydoctor.org/099.xml
- American Society of Colon and Rectal Surgeons: Pruritus Ani
  - http://www.fascrs.org/displaycommon.cfm?an=1&subarticlenbr=17
- Mayo Clinic: Anal Itch
  - http://www.mayoclinic.com/invoke.cfm?id=DS00453
- MedlinePlus: Vaginal Itching
  - http://www.nlm.nih.gov/medlineplus/ency/article/003159.htm

REFERENCES

- Heard S: Pruritus ani. Aust Fam Physician 2004;33:511. [PMID: 15301168]
- Pfenniger JL et al: Common anorectal conditions: Part I. Symptoms and complaints. Am Fam Physician 2001;63:2391. [PMID: 11430454]
- Welsh B et al: Vulval itch. Aust Fam Physician 2004;33:505. [PMID: 15301167]

Author(s)

Timothy G. Berger, MD

Pseudotumor Cerebri

Pseudoallergic Reactions p. 1139. Pseudogout & Chondrocalcinosis p. 1140.

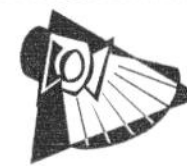

KEY FEATURES

ESSENTIALS OF DIAGNOSIS

- Headache, worse on straining
- Visual obscurations or diplopia may occur
- Level of consciousness may be impaired
- Other deficits depend on cause of intracranial hypertension or on herniation syndrome
- Examination reveals papilledema

GENERAL CONSIDERATIONS

- Pseudotumor cerebri is a diagnosis of exclusion in the setting of elevated intracranial pressure and normal cerebrospinal fluid
- Thrombosis of the transverse venous sinus as a noninfectious complication of otitis media or chronic mastoiditis is one cause, and sagittal sinus thrombosis may lead to a clinically similar picture
- Other causes
  - Chronic pulmonary disease
  - Endocrine disturbances such as hypoparathyroidism or Addison's disease
  - Vitamin A toxicity
  - Use of tetracycline or oral contraceptives
- Cases have also followed withdrawal of corticosteroids after long-term use

DEMOGRAPHICS

- Most patients are young, frequently obese, women

CLINICAL FINDINGS

SYMPTOMS AND SIGNS

- Symptoms
  - Headache
  - Diplopia
  - Other visual disturbances due to papilledema and abducens nerve dysfunction
- Examination reveals
  - Papilledema
  - Some enlargement of the blind spots
  - Abducens palsy is common
  - Patients otherwise look well

DIFFERENTIAL DIAGNOSIS

- Venous sinus thrombosis
- Dural arteriovenous malformation
- Space-occupying lesion, eg, brain tumor
- Meningitis
- Systemic hypertension
- Migraine
- Glaucoma
- Associated conditions
  - Hypoparathyroidism
  - Addison's disease
  - Chronic pulmonary disease
- Associated drugs
  - Vitamin A
  - Tetracycline
  - Minocycline
  - Oral contraceptives
  - Corticosteroid withdrawal
  - Isotretinoin
  - Danazol

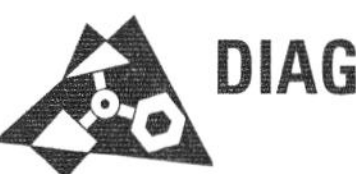

DIAGNOSIS

LABORATORY TESTS

- Lumbar puncture confirms intracranial hypertension, but the cerebrospinal fluid is normal

IMAGING STUDIES

- CT scan shows small or normal ventricles and no evidence of a space-occupying lesion
- MR venography can help to detect thrombosis of the transverse venous sinus and sagittal sinus thrombosis

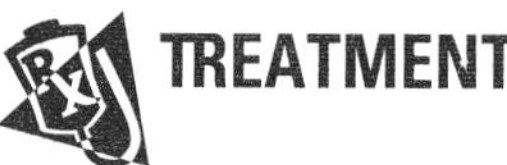

TREATMENT

MEDICATIONS

- Acetazolamide (250 mg PO three times daily) reduces formation of cerebrospinal fluid and can be initial therapy
- Oral corticosteroids (eg, prednisone, 60–80 mg daily) may also be necessary
- Any specific cause of pseudotumor cerebri requires appropriate treatment
  - Hormone therapy should be initiated if there is an underlying endocrine disturbance
  - Discontinue the use of tetracycline, oral contraceptives, or vitamin A
  - If corticosteroid withdrawal is responsible, the medication should be reintroduced and then tapered more gradually

SURGERY

- If medical treatment fails to control the intracranial pressure, surgical placement of a lumboperitoneal or other shunt—or subtemporal decompression or optic nerve sheath fenestration—should be undertaken to preserve vision

THERAPEUTIC PROCEDURES

- Obese patients should be advised to lose weight
- Repeated lumbar puncture to lower the intracranial pressure by removal of cerebrospinal fluid is effective on a short-term basis
- Pharmacologic approaches to treatment are also necessary

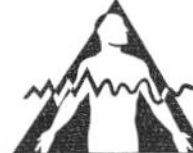

OUTCOME

FOLLOW-UP

- Treatment is monitored by checking visual acuity and visual fields, funduscopic appearance, and pressure of the cerebrospinal fluid

COMPLICATIONS

- Untreated pseudotumor cerebri can lead to secondary optic atrophy and permanent visual loss

PROGNOSIS

- Discontinuing the use of tetracycline, oral contraceptives, or vitamin A allows for resolution of pseudotumor cerebri due to these agents
- In many instances. no specific cause is found, and the disorder remits spontaneously after several months

WHEN TO REFER

- All patients benefit from specialist referral to exclude specific causes and from specialized care to monitor treatment response with visual acuity and field checks, and from funduscopic examination

WHEN TO ADMIT

- Need for surgical placement of a device to reduce intracranial hypertension

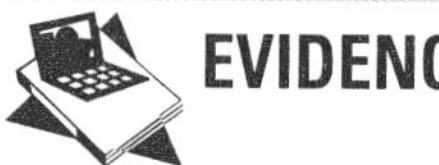

EVIDENCE

INFORMATION FOR PATIENTS

- National Institute of Neurological Diseases and Stroke
  - http://www.ninds.nih.gov/health_and_medical/disorders/pseudotumorcerebri_doc.htm
- National Institutes of Health
  - http://www.nlm.nih.gov/medlineplus/ency/article/000351.htm

REFERENCES

- Friedman DI: Pseudotumor cerebri. Neurol Clin 2004;22:99. [PMID:15062530]
- Krajewski KJ: Idiopathic intracranial hypertension: pseudotumor cerebri. Optometry 2002;73:546. [PMID: 12387561]

Author(s)

Michael J. Aminoff, DSc, MD, FRCP

Psittacosis

KEY FEATURES

ESSENTIALS OF DIAGNOSIS

- Fever, chills, and cough; headache common
- Atypical pneumonia with slightly delayed appearance of signs of pneumonitis
- Contact with infected bird (psittacine, pigeons, many others) 7–15 days previously
- Isolation of chlamydiae or rising titer of complement-fixing antibodies

GENERAL CONSIDERATIONS

- Etiological agent is *Chlamydia psittaci*, a bacterium
- Infection is acquired by inhaling dried secretions from infected birds (parrots, parakeets, pigeons, chickens, ducks, and many others), which may or may not appear ill
- The incubation period is 6–19 days
- The history may be difficult to obtain if the patient acquired infection from an illegally imported bird

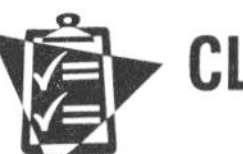

CLINICAL FINDINGS

SYMPTOMS AND SIGNS

- The onset is usually rapid, with fever, chills, myalgia, dry cough, and headache
- Signs include temperature-pulse dissociation, dullness to percussion, and rales
- Pulmonary findings may be absent early
- Dyspnea and cyanosis may occur later
- Endocarditis, which is culture negative, may occur

DIFFERENTIAL DIAGNOSIS

- Other atypical pneumonia (eg, viral pneumonia, *Mycoplasma pneumoniae*, *Chlamydia pneumoniae*)
- Unusual presentations of typical bacterial pneumonia
- Hypersensitivity pneumonitis
- Other cause of culture-negative endocarditis

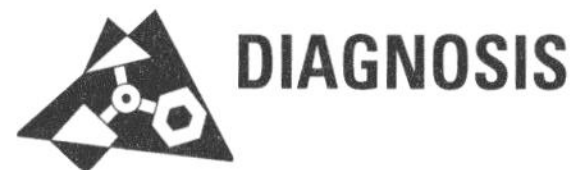

DIAGNOSIS

LABORATORY TESTS

- The diagnosis is usually made serologically
- Acute and convalescent serology demonstrating a rise in titer of complement-fixing antibody
- Antibodies appear during the second week
- Antibody response may be suppressed by early chemotherapy

IMAGING STUDIES

- The radiographic findings are those of atypical pneumonia, which tends to be interstitial and diffuse in appearance, though consolidation can occur
- Psittacosis is indistinguishable from other bacterial or viral pneumonias by radiography

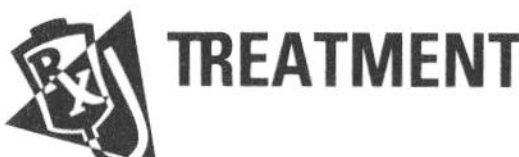

TREATMENT

MEDICATIONS

- Doxycycline 100 mg orally every 12 h or intravenously every 12 h, for 14–21 days
- Macrolides are also effective

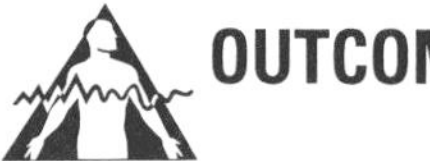

OUTCOME

COMPLICATIONS

- Endocarditis, hepatitis, and neurological complications may occasionally occur
- Severe pneumonia requiring intensive care support may also occur
- Fatal cases have been reported

PROGNOSIS

- Excellent with early treatment

WHEN TO REFER

- Early referral to an infectious disease specialist for severe disease may aid in management

WHEN TO ADMIT

- Respiratory compromise
- Rapidly deteriorating clinical course
- Suspected or proven endocarditis

PREVENTION

- Traceback of infected birds to distributors and breeders often is not possible because of limited regulation of the pet bird industry

EVIDENCE

PRACTICE GUIDELINES

- Centers for Disease Control and Prevention. Compendium of measures to control *Chlamydia psittaci* infection among humans (psittacosis) and pet birds (avian chlamydiosis), 2000. MMWR Recomm Rep 2000;49(RR-8):3.
  - http://www.cdc.gov/mmwr/preview/mmwrhtml/rr4908a1.htm

WEB SITES

- CDC—Division of Bacterial and Mycotic Diseases
  - http://www.cdc.gov/ncidod/dbmd/diseaseinfo/psittacosis_t.htm
- Karolinska Institute—Directory of Bacterial Infections and Mycoses
  - http://www.mic.ki.se/Diseases/C01.html

INFORMATION FOR PATIENTS

- National Institutes of Health
  - http://www.nlm.nih.gov/medlineplus/ency/article/000088.htm

REFERENCES

- Elliott JH: Psittacosis. A flu like syndrome. Aust Fam Physician 2001;30:739. [PMID: 11681143]
- Kalayoglu MV et al: Chlamydia pneumoniae as an emerging risk factor in cardiovascular disease. JAMA 2002;288:2724. [PMID: 12460096]

Author(s)

Henry F. Chambers, MD

Psoriasis

KEY FEATURES

ESSENTIALS OF DIAGNOSIS

- Silvery scales on bright red, well-demarcated plaques, usually on the knees, elbows, and scalp
- Nail findings include pitting and onycholysis (separation of the nail plate from the bed)
- Mild itching (usually)
- May be associated with psoriatic arthritis
- Histopathology is not often useful and can be confusing

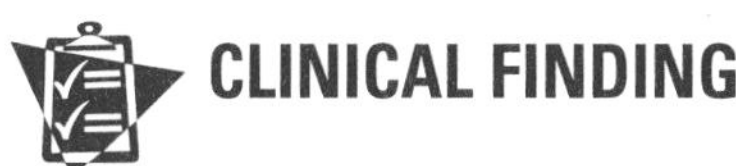

CLINICAL FINDINGS

GENERAL CONSIDERATIONS

- A common benign, acute or chronic inflammatory skin disease based on a genetic predisposition
- Injury or irritation of normal skin tends to induce lesions of psoriasis at the site (Koebner's phenomenon)
- Psoriasis has several variants—the most common is the plaque type
- See Table 7
- There are often no symptoms, but itching may occur
- Although psoriasis may occur anywhere, examine the scalp, elbows, knees, palms and soles, and nails
- The lesions are red, sharply defined plaques covered with silvery scales; the glans penis and vulva may be affected; occasionally, only the flexures (axillae, inguinal areas) are involved
- Fine stippling ("pitting") in the nails is highly suggestive
- Psoriatics often have a pink or red intergluteal fold
- There may be associated seronegative arthritis, often involving the distal interphalangeal joints
- Eruptive (guttate) psoriasis consisting of myriad lesions 3–10 mm in diameter occurs occasionally after streptococcal pharyngitis
- Plaque type or extensive erythrodermic psoriasis with abrupt onset may accompany HIV infection

DIFFERENTIAL DIAGNOSIS

- Atopic dermatitis (eczema)
- Contact dermatitis
- Nummular eczema (discoid eczema, nummular dermatitis)
- Tinea
- Candidiasis
- Intertrigo
- Seborrheic dermatitis
- Pityriasis rosea
- Secondary syphilis
- Pityriasis rubra pilaris
- Onychomycosis (nail findings)
- Cutaneous features of reactive arthritis
- Cutaneous T cell lymphoma (mycosis fungoides)

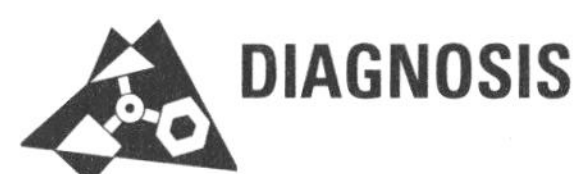

DIAGNOSIS

DIAGNOSTIC PROCEDURES

- The combination of red plaques with silvery scales on elbows and knees, with scaliness in the scalp or nail findings, is diagnostic
- Psoriasis lesions are well demarcated and affect extensor surfaces—in contrast to atopic dermatitis, with poorly demarcated plaques in flexural distribution
- In body folds, scraping and culture for *Candida* and examination of scalp and nails will distinguish psoriasis from intertrigo and candidiasis

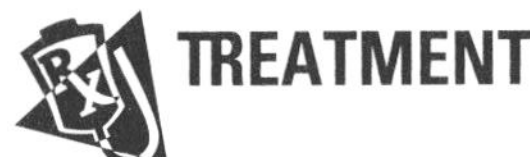

TREATMENT

MEDICATIONS

- See Table 6

Limited disease (mild to moderate)

- Topical steroid cream or ointment
  - Restrict the highest-potency steroids to 2–3 weeks of twice-daily use; then three or four times on weekends or switch to a midpotency corticosteroid
  - Rarely induces a lasting remission
- Calcipotriene ointment 0.005%, a vitamin D analog, is used twice daily
  - It is the second most commonly used topical treatment (after topical steroids)
  - Substitute calcipotriene once the topical steroids have controlled the lesions; once- or twice-daily calcipotriene is then continued chronically
  - It usually cannot be applied to the groin or the face because of irritation
  - Incompatible with many topical steroids; it must be applied at a different time
- Tazarotene gel
  - A topical retinoid for mild to moderate plaque psoriasis is available in 0.05% and 0.1% formulations; the 0.05% is less effective when used once daily
  - It is more expensive than calcipotriene and more irritating
  - May be applied with topical steroids
  - Anthralin may be used, but is irritating and may stain the skin
- Oclusion alone clears isolated plaques in 30–40% of patients
  - Duoderm is placed on the lesions and left undisturbed for a minimum of 5 days, up to 7 days and then replaced; responses may be seen within several weeks
- For the scalp
  - Start with a tar shampoo, daily
  - For thick scales, use 6% salicylic acid gel (eg, Keralyt), P & S solution (phenol, mineral oil, and glycerin), or oil-based fluocinolone acetonide 0.01% (Derma-Smoothe/FS) under a shower cap at night, and shampoo in the morning
  - In order of increasing potency, triamcinolone 0.1%, or fluocinolone, betamethasone dipropionate, fluocinonide or amcinonide, and clobetasol are available in solution form for use on the scalp twice daily
- Psoriasis in the body folds
  - Potent steroids cannot be used
  - Tacrolimus (protopic 0.1% or 0.03%) ointment or pimecrolimus (Elidel 1%) cream applied BID can be effective in intertriginous psoriasis (but not plaques type); burning may be a complication and may be avoided by applying mild steroid (hydrocortisone 1–2.5%) BID for the week of treatment

Moderate to severe disease (more than 30% of the body surface)

- Parenteral corticosteroids should not be used because of possible induction of pustular lesions
- Methotrexate is very effective in doses up to 25 mg once weekly
- Acitretin, a synthetic retinoid, is most effective for pustular psoriasis at 0.5–1 mg/kg/day, but it also improves erythrodermic and plaque types and psoriatic arthritis; liver enzymes and serum lipids must be checked periodically; because acitretin is a teratogen women must wait at least 3 years after completing treatment before considering pregnancy
- Cyclosporine dramatically improves psoriasis in severe cases
- Systemic immunomodulators (etanercept, alefacept) can be effective

THERAPEUTIC PROCEDURES

- Moderate to severe disease
  - The treatment of choice is narrow-band UVB light exposure three times weekly; clearing usually occurs around 7 weeks, and maintenance may be needed since relapses are frequent
  - Severe disease unresponsive to ultraviolet light may be treated in a psoriasis day care center with the Goeckerman regimen, using crude coal tar for many hours and exposure to UVB light; this offers the best chance for prolonged remissions
  - PUVA (psoralen plus ultraviolet A) may be effective even if standard UVB treatment has failed; may be used with other therapy, eg, acitretin

OUTCOME

COMPLICATIONS

- Treatment with calcipotriene may result in hypercalcemia
- Long-term use of PUVA is associated with an increased risk of skin cancer (especially squamous cell carcinoma and perhaps melanoma)

PROGNOSIS

- The course tends to be chronic and unpredictable, and the disease may be refractory to treatment

WHEN TO REFER

- If there is a question about the diagnosis, if recommended therapy is ineffective, or if specialized treatment is necessary

EVIDENCE

PRACTICE GUIDELINES

- Finnish Medical Society Duodecim. Psoriasis. 2002
  - http://www.guideline.gov/summary/summary.aspx?doc_id=3388&nbr=2614

WEB SITE

- American Academy of Dermatology
  - http://www.aad.org

INFORMATION FOR PATIENTS

- American Academy of Dermatology: What is Psoriasis?
  - http://www.skincarephysicians.com/psoriasisnet/whatis.html
- MedlinePlus: Psoriasis Interactive Tutorial
  - http://www.nlm.nih.gov/medlineplus/tutorials/psoriasis.html
- National Institute of Arthritis and Musculoskeletal and Skin Diseases: Psoriasis
  - http://www.niams.nih.gov/hi/topics/psoriasis/psoriafs.htm

REFERENCES

- Lebwohl M et al: Psoriasis treatment: traditional therapy. Ann Rheum Dis 2005;64:ii83. [PMID: 15708945]
- Mallbris L et al: Psoriasis phenotype at disease onset: clinical characterization of 400 adult cases. J Invest Dermatol 2005;124:499. [PMID: 15737189]
- Mason J et al: Topical preparations for the treatment of psoriasis: a systematic review. Br J Dermatol 2002:146:351. [PMID: 11952534]
- Yosipovitch G et al: Practical management of psoriasis in the elderly: epidemiology, clinical aspects, quality of life, patient education and treatment options. Drugs Aging 2002;19:847. [PMID: 12428994]

Author(s)

Timothy G. Berger, MD

Psoriatic Arthritis

KEY FEATURES

ESSENTIALS OF DIAGNOSIS

- Psoriasis precedes onset of arthritis in 80% of cases
- Arthritis usually asymmetric, with "sausage" appearance of fingers and toes
- Resembles rheumatoid arthritis; rheumatoid factor is negative
- Sacroiliac joint involvement common; ankylosis of the sacroiliac joints may occur

GENERAL CONSIDERATIONS

Patterns or subsets of arthritis accompanying psoriasis

- Joint disease that resembles rheumatoid arthritis with symmetric polyarthritis
- An oligoarticular form that may lead to considerable destruction of the affected joints
- Predominant involvement of the distal interphalangeal joints; pitting of the nails and onycholysis are frequently associated
- A severe deforming arthritis (arthritis mutilans) with marked osteolysis
- A spondylitic form in which sacroiliitis and spinal involvement predominate; 50% of these patients are HLA-B27 positive

DEMOGRAPHICS

- Arthritis is at least five times more common in patients with severe skin disease than in those with only mild skin findings

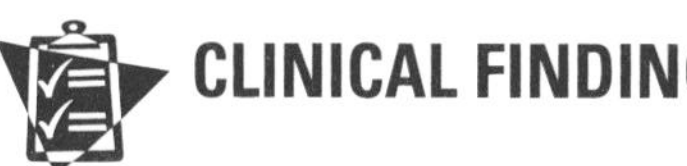

CLINICAL FINDINGS

SYMPTOMS AND SIGNS

- Although psoriasis usually precedes the onset of arthritis, arthritis precedes or occurs simultaneously with the skin disease in approximately 20% of cases
- May be a single patch of psoriasis (typically hidden in the scalp, gluteal cleft, or umbilicus)
- Nail pitting, a residue of previous psoriasis, is sometimes the only clue

DIFFERENTIAL DIAGNOSIS

- Rheumatoid arthritis
- Gout
- Osteoarthritis
- Other causes of sacroiliitis: reactive arthritis (Reiter's syndrome), ankylosing spondylitis, inflammatory bowel disease

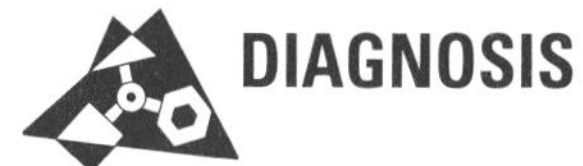

DIAGNOSIS

LABORATORY TESTS

- Elevation of the sedimentation rate
- Rheumatoid factor is not present

IMAGING STUDIES

- Radiographic findings are most helpful in distinguishing the disease from other forms of arthritis
- There are marginal erosions of bone and irregular destruction of joint and bone, which, in the phalanx, may give the appearance of a sharpened pencil ("pencil-in-cup")
- Fluffy periosteal new bone may be marked, especially at the insertion of muscles and ligaments into bone. Such changes will also be seen along the shafts of metacarpals, metatarsals, and phalanges
- Asymmetric sacroiliitis

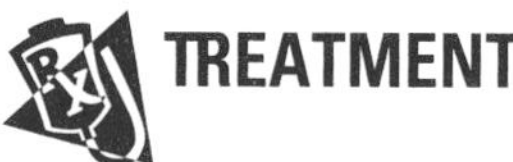

TREATMENT

MEDICATIONS

- Nonsteroidal antiinflammatory drugs (NSAIDs) are usually sufficient for mild cases
- Corticosteroids are less effective in psoriatic arthritis than in other forms of inflammatory arthritis
- In resistant cases, methotrexate may be helpful
- For cases with disease that is refractory to methotrexate, etanercept or infliximab is usually effective for both arthritis and psoriatic skin disease
- Successful treatment of the skin lesions (eg, by PUVA therapy) commonly—though not invariably—is accompanied by an improvement in peripheral articular symptoms

THERAPEUTIC PROCEDURES

- Treatment regimens are symptomatic

OUTCOME

COMPLICATIONS

- Fusion of peripheral or spinal joints

PROGNOSIS

- Generally better than rheumatoid arthritis, but severe cases occur

WHEN TO REFER

- Refer when joint disease does not respond to NSAIDs or when skin disease is severe

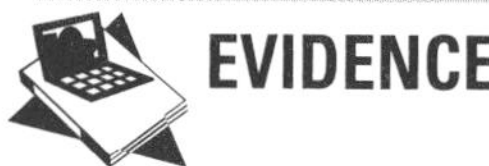

EVIDENCE

PRACTICE GUIDELINES

- American Academy of Dermatology
  - http://www.aadassociation.org/Guidelines/psoriasis.html

WEB SITES

- American College of Rheumatology
  - http://www.rheumatology.org
- Arthritis Foundation
  - http://www.arthritis.org

INFORMATION FOR PATIENTS

- Arthritis Foundation
  - http://www.arthritis.org/conditions/diseasecenter/juvenilepsoriaticarthritis.asp
- National Institutes of Health
  - http://www.nlm.nih.gov/medlineplus/ency/article/000413.htm
- National Psoriasis Foundation
  - http://www.psoriasis.org/facts/psa/

REFERENCE

- Mease PJ et al: Etanercept treatment of psoriatic arthritis: safety, efficacy, and effect on disease progression. Arthritis Rheum 2004;50:2264. [PMID: 15248226]

Author(s)

David B. Hellmann, MD, FACP
John H. Stone, MD, MPH

Pulmonary Embolism

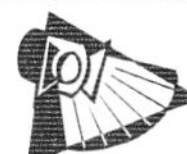

KEY FEATURES

ESSENTIALS OF DIAGNOSIS

- Predisposition to venous thrombosis, usually of the lower extremities
- Usually either dyspnea, chest pain, hemoptysis, or syncope
- Tachypnea and a widened alveolar–arterial P_{O_2} difference
- Characteristic defects on ventilation-perfusion lung scan, spiral CT scan of the chest, or pulmonary angiogram

GENERAL CONSIDERATIONS

- Cause of an estimated 50,000 deaths annually in the United States and the third most common cause of death in hospitalized patients
- Most cases are not recognized antemortem: < 10% with fatal emboli receive specific treatment
- Pulmonary thromboembolism (PE) and deep venous thrombosis (DVT) are manifestations of the same disease, with the same risk factors
  - Immobility (bed rest, stroke, obesity)
  - Hyperviscosity (polycythemia)
  - Increased central venous pressures (low cardiac output, pregnancy)
  - Vessel damage (prior DVT, orthopedic surgery, trauma)
  - Hypercoagulable states, either acquired or inherited
- Pulmonary thromboemboli most often originate in deep veins of the major calf muscles
- 50–60% of patients with proximal lower extremity DVT develop PE; 50% of these events are asymptomatic
- Hypoxemia results from vascular obstruction leading to dead space ventilation, right-to-left shunting, and decreased cardiac output
- Types of pulmonary emboli
  - Fat embolism
  - Air embolism
  - Amniotic fluid embolism
  - Septic embolism (eg, endocarditis)
  - Tumor embolism (eg, renal cell carcinoma)
  - Foreign body embolism (eg, talc in IV drug use)
  - Parasite egg embolism (schistosomiasis)

CLINICAL FINDINGS

SYMPTOMS AND SIGNS

- See Table 30
- Clinical findings depend on the size of the embolus and the patient's preexisting cardiopulmonary status
- Dyspnea occurs in 75–85% and pain in 65–75% of patients
- Tachypnea is the only sign reliably found in more than 50% of patients
- 97% of patients in the PIOPED study had **at least one** of the following
  - Dyspnea
  - Tachypnea
  - Chest pain with breathing

DIFFERENTIAL DIAGNOSIS

- Myocardial infarction (heart attack)
- Pneumonia
- Pericarditis
- Congestive heart failure
- Pleuritis (pleurisy)
- Pneumothorax
- Pericardial tamponade

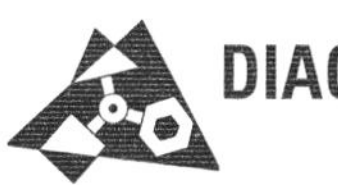

DIAGNOSIS

LABORATORY TESTS

- ECG is abnormal in 70% of patients
  - Sinus tachycardia and nonspecific ST-T changes are the most common findings
- Acute respiratory alkalosis, hypoxemia, and widened arterial–alveolar O_2 gradient (A–a D_{O_2}), but these findings are not diagnostic (Table 30)
- A normal D-dimer level by the ELISA assay virtually rules out DVT (sensitivity is 97%); however, many hospitals use a less-sensitive latex-agglutination assay

IMAGING STUDIES

- Chest x-ray—most common findings
  - Atelectasis
  - Infiltrates
  - Pleural effusions
  - Westermark's sign is focal oligemia with a prominent central pulmonary artery
  - Hampton's hump is a pleural-based area of increased intensity from intraparenchymal hemorrhage
- Lung scanning (V/Q scan)
  - A normal scan can exclude PE
  - A high-probability scan is sufficient to make the diagnosis in most cases
  - Indeterminate scans are common and do not further refine clinical pretest probabilities
- Helical CT arteriography is supplanting V/Q scanning as the initial diagnostic study
  - It requires administration of intravenous radiocontrast dye but is otherwise noninvasive
  - It is very sensitive for the detection of thrombus in the proximal pulmonary arteries but less so in the segmental and subsegmental arteries
- Venous thrombosis studies
  - Venous ultrasonography is the test of choice in most centers
  - Diagnosing DVT establishes the need for treatment and may preclude invasive testing in patients in whom there is a high suspicion for PE
- In the setting of a nondiagnostic V/Q scan, negative serial DVT studies over 2 weeks predict a low risk (< 2%) of subsequent DVT over the next 6 weeks
- Pulmonary angiography is the reference standard for the diagnosis of PE
  - Invasive, but safe—minor complications in < 5%
  - Role in the diagnosis of PE controversial, but generally used when there is a high clinical probability and negative noninvasive studies
- MRI is a primary research tool for the diagnosis of PE
- Integrated approach (Figure 2)

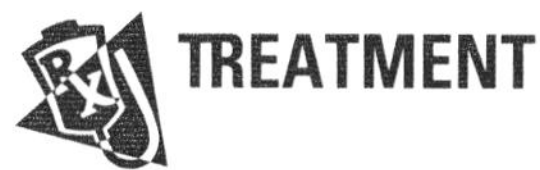

TREATMENT

MEDICATIONS

- See Tables 33 and 34
- **Anticoagulation** regimen use unfractionated heparin (UFH) followed by warfarin to maintain the INR 2.0–3.0
- Compared with UFH, low-molecular-weight heparins (LMWH) are
  - Easier to dose and require no monitoring
  - Have similar hemorrhage rates
  - Are at least as effective
- LMWH enables home-based therapy in selected patients
- Warfarin is contraindicated in pregnancy; LMWH can be used instead
- Guidelines for the duration of full anticoagulation
  - 6 months for an initial episode with a reversible risk factor
  - 12 months after an initial, idiopathic episode

  - 6–12 months to indefinitely in patients with irreversible risk factors or recurrent disease
- Recent data support the use of long-term low-intensity warfarin (INR 1.5–2.0) after full anticoagulation is completed
- **Thrombolytic therapy** accelerates resolution of thrombi when compared with heparin, but does not improve mortality
  - Carries 10-fold greater risk of intracranial hemorrhage compared with heparin (0.2–2.1%)
  - Indicated in patients who are hemodynamically unstable while on heparin
- **Venal caval interruption** (IVC filters) may be indicated when a significant contraindication to anticoagulation exists or when recurrence occurs despite adequate anticoagulation
- IVC filters decrease the short-term incidence of PE, but increase the rate of recurrent DVT

SURGERY

- Pulmonary embolectomy is an emergency procedure with a high mortality rate performed at few centers

THERAPEUTIC PROCEDURES

- Catheter devices that fragment and extract thrombus have been used on small numbers of patients
- Platelet counts should be monitored for the first 14 days of UFH due to the risk of immune-mediated thrombocytopenia
- Warfarin has interactions with many drugs

OUTCOME

COMPLICATIONS

- Immune-mediated thrombocytopenia in 3% of patient on UFH
- The major complication of anticoagulation with heparin is hemorrhage; risk of any hemorrhage is 0–7%; 0–2% for fatal hemorrhage
- The risk of hemorrhage on warfarin is 3–4% per patient year, but correlates with INR
- Approximately 1% of patients have chronic thromboembolic pulmonary hypertension; selected patients may benefit from pulmonary endarterectomy

PROGNOSIS

- Overall prognosis depends on the underlying disease rather than the thromboembolic event
- Death from recurrent PE occurs in only 3% of cases; 6 months of anticoagulation therapy reduces the risk of recurrent thrombosis and death by 80–90%
- Perfusion defects resolve in most survivors

WHEN TO REFER

- All patients evaluated for or diagnosed with a PE should be evaluated by an expert (typically a pulmonologist, hematologist, or internist)

WHEN TO ADMIT

- Patients with an acute PE should be admitted for stabilization, initiation of therapy, evaluation of cause of PE, and education

PREVENTION

- See Tables 31 and 32

EVIDENCE

PRACTICE GUIDELINES

- American College of Emergency Physicians Clinical Policies Committee; Clinical Policies Committee Subcommittee on Suspected Pulmonary Embolism. Clinical policy: critical issues in the evaluation and management of adult patients presenting with suspected pulmonary embolism. Ann Emerg Med 2003;41:257. [PMID:12548278]
- British Thoracic Society Standards of Care Committee Pulmonary Embolism Guideline Development Group. British Thoracic Society guidelines for the management of suspected acute pulmonary embolism. Thorax 2003;58:470
- Buller HR et al: Antithrombotic therapy for venous thromboembolic disease: the Seventh ACCP Conference on Antithrombotic and Thrombolytic Therapy. Chest 2004;126:401S. [PMID: 15383479]

INFORMATION FOR PATIENTS

- JAMA patient page: Pulmonary embolism. JAMA 2003;290:2828. [PMID:14657080]
- Mayo Clinic
  - http://www.mayoclinic.com/invoke.cfm?id=DS00429

REFERENCES

- Blom JW et al: Malignancies, prothrombotic mutations, and the risk of venous thrombosis. JAMA 2005;293:715. [PMID: 15701913]
- Buller HR et al: Antithrombotic therapy for venous thromboembolic disese: the Seventh ACCP Conference on Antithrombotic and Thrombolytic Therapy. Chest 2004;126(3 Suppl):401S. [PMID: 15383479]
- Fedullo PF et al: Clinical practice. The evaluation of suspected pulmonary embolism. N Engl J Med 2003;349:1247. [PMID: 14507950]
- Geerts WH et al: Prevention of venous thromboembolism: the Seventh ACCP Conference on Antithrombotic and Thrombolytic Therapy. Chest 2004;126(3 Suppl):338S. [PMID: 15383478]
- Hirsh J et al: New anticoagulants. Blood 2005;105:453. [PMID: 15191946]
- Moores LK et al: Meta-analysis: outcomes in patients with suspected pulmonary embolism managed with computed tomographic pulmonary angiography. Ann Intern Med 2004;141:866. [PMID: 15583229]
- Stein PD et al: D-dimer for the exclusion of acute venous thrombosis and pulmonary embolism: a systemic review. Ann Intern Med 2004;140:589. [PMID: 15096330]
- Tamariz LJ et al: Usefulness of clinical prediction rules for the diagnosis of venous thromboembolism: a systemic review. Am J Med 2004;117:676. [PMID: 15501206]
- Value of the ventilation/perfusion scan in acute pulmonary embolism. Results of the prospective investigation of pulmonary embolism diagnosis (PIOPED). The PIOPED Investigators. JAMA 1990;263:2753. [PMID: 2332918]

Author(s)

Mark S. Chesnutt, MD
Thomas J. Prendergast, MD

Pulmonary Hypertension

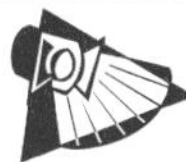

KEY FEATURES

ESSENTIALS OF DIAGNOSIS

- Dyspnea, fatigue, chest pain, and exertional syncope
- Narrow splitting of second heart sound with loud pulmonary component; findings of right ventricular hypertrophy and cardiac failure in advanced disease
- Hypoxemia and increased wasted ventilation on pulmonary function tests
- ECG evidence of right ventricular strain or hypertrophy and right atrial enlargement
- Enlarged central pulmonary arteries on chest x-ray

GENERAL CONSIDERATIONS

- The normal pulmonary circulation is unique in that it has low pressure and resistance, but high flow
- Pulmonary hypertension is present when pulmonary artery pressure rises to a level inappropriate for cardiac output
- Pulmonary hypertension is self-perpetuating, introducing changes in pulmonary vessels that further narrow the vascular bed, increasing pressures
- Primary (idiopathic) pulmonary hypertension is a rare disorder of young and middle-aged women
- Causes of secondary pulmonary hypertension
  - Chronic pulmonary embolism
  - Chronic obstructive pulmonary disease (COPD)
  - Interstitial lung disease
  - Scleroderma
  - Left-to-right intracardiac shunt
  - Drugs
    - Fenfluramine
    - Dexfenfluramine
    - Phentermine
    - Bleomycin
    - Amiodarone
    - Talc (via IV drug use)
  - Pulmonary venoocclusive disease
  - Valve disease
    - Mitral stenosis
    - Mitral regurgitation
    - Aortic stenosis
  - Left-sided heart failure
  - Atrial myxoma
  - Polycythemia vera
  - Cirrhosis with portal hypertension
  - HIV
  - Schistosomiasis
  - Sickle cell disease

CLINICAL FINDINGS

SYMPTOMS AND SIGNS

- In its early stages, symptoms are due primarily to the underlying disease
- Progressive dyspnea
- Dull retrosternal chest pain
- Fatigue and exertional syncope
- Narrow splitting of S_2, accentuation of P_2, and a systolic click may be heard
- Tricuspid and pulmonic insufficiency with signs of right ventricular failure and cor pulmonale are found in advanced disease

DIFFERENTIAL DIAGNOSIS

- Primary pulmonary hypertension
- Secondary pulmonary hypertension
- Cor pulmonale (right heart failure due to pulmonary disease)
- Congestive heart failure
- Right-sided valve disease
- Mitral stenosis

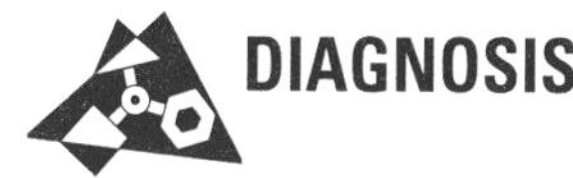

DIAGNOSIS

LABORATORY TESTS

- Polycythemia is found in cases resulting from chronic hypoxemia
- ECG findings
  - Right-axis deviation
  - Right ventricular hypertrophy
  - Right ventricular strain
  - Right atrial enlargement
- Routine pulmonary function tests are typically unrevealing, but can show a reduction in the single breath diffusion capacity
- HIV tests, collagen vascular serologic studies, and liver function tests can help rule out selected secondary causes

IMAGING STUDIES

- Chest x-rays may show
  - Pulmonary artery dilation
  - Right atrial and ventricular enlargement in advanced cases
  - "Pruning" of peripheral pulmonary arteries in cases associated with COPD
- Echocardiography can be used
  - To estimate pulmonary artery systolic pressure
  - To give information about cardiac valvular disease
- Ventilation-perfusion scanning can identify cases due to chronic thromboemboli

DIAGNOSTIC PROCEDURES

- Right-heart catheterization allows for precise hemodynamic measurements and identifies postcapillary disease, intracardiac shunting, or thromboembolic disease
- Polysomnography may be required to exclude ventilatory disorders
- Open-lung biopsy may be required to diagnose pulmonary venoocclusive disease

Pulmonary Hemosiderosis, Idiopathic p. 1141

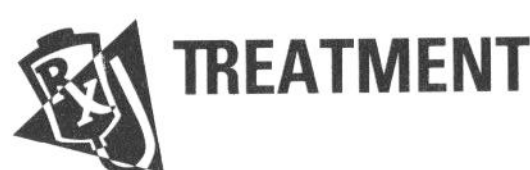

TREATMENT

MEDICATIONS

- Supplemental oxygen for at least 15 hours per day has been shown to slow the progression of pulmonary hypertension due to COPD
- Inhaled nitric oxide is effective in lowering pulmonary pressures transiently in patients with asthma and ARDS
- Anticoagulation has been used in cases of unknown etiology, because multiple small emboli may be responsible
- Vasodilator therapy has been disappointing in both primary and secondary disease
- Continuous long-term prostacyclin infusion may confer benefit in selected cases of secondary disease
- Diuretics along with salt restriction help treat cor pulmonale
- Digitalis use in cor pulmonale is controversial

SURGERY

- Single- or double-lung transplantation may be performed on patients with end-stage disease; 2-year survival is 50%

THERAPEUTIC PROCEDURES

- Phlebotomy for patients with hematocrit >60% will reduce blood viscosity

OUTCOME

FOLLOW-UP

- Periodic reassessment of pulmonary artery pressures to determine progression and/or response to thearpy

COMPLICATIONS

- Cor pulmonale

PROGNOSIS

- Depends on the severity of the underlying disease
- Disease due to a fixed obliteration of the pulmonary vascular bed responds poorly to therapy

WHEN TO REFER

- When considering the diagnosis or therapeutic options

WHEN TO ADMIT

- For initiation of vasodilator therapy
- For carefully monitored diuresis
- For debilitating peripheral edema

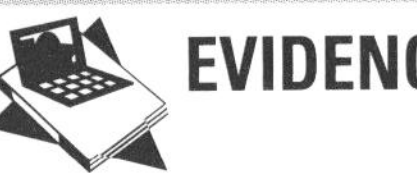

EVIDENCE

PRACTICE GUIDELINES

- Badesch DB et al: American College of Chest Physicians. Medical therapy for pulmonary arterial hypertension: ACCP evidence-based clinical practice guidelines. Chest 2004;126(1 Suppl):35S. [PMID:15249494]
- Doyle RL et al: American College of Chest Physicians. Surgical treatments/interventions for pulmonary arterial hypertension: ACCP evidence-based clinical practice guidelines. Chest 2004;126(1 Suppl):63S. [PMID:15249495]
- McGoon M et al: Screening, early detection, and diagnosis of pulmonary arterial hypertension: ACCP evidence-based clinical practice guidelines. Chest 2004;126(1 Suppl):14S. [PMID:15249493]

INFORMATION FOR PATIENTS

- American Heart Association
  - http://circ.ahajournals.org/cgi/reprint/106/24/e192.pdf
- Cleveland Clinic
  - http://www.clevelandclinic.org/health/health-info/docs/0600/0622.asp?index=6530
- Mayo Clinic
  - http://www.mayoclinic.com/invoke.cfm?id=DS00430

REFERENCES

- Chatterjee K et al: Pulmonary hypertension: hemodynamic diagnosis and management. Arch Intern Med 2002;162:1925. [PMID:12230414]
- Doyle RL et al: American College of Chest Physicians. Surgical treatments/interventions for pulmonary arterial hypertension: ACCP evidence-based clinical practice guidelines. Chest 2004;126(1 Suppl):63S. [PMID:15249495]
- Pengo V et al: Thromboembolic Pulmonary Hypertension Study Group. Incidence of chronic thromboembolic pulmonary hypertension after pulmonary embolism. N Engl J Med 2004;350:2257. [PMID:15163775]
- Runo JR et al: Primary pulmonary hypertension. Lancet 2003;361:1533. [PMID:12737878]

Author(s)

Mark S. Chesnutt, MD

Thomas J. Prendergast, MD

Pulmonary Nodule, Solitary

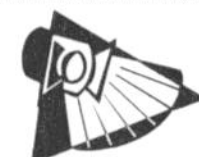

KEY FEATURES

ESSENTIALS OF DIAGNOSIS

- An isolated, < 3-cm rounded opacity on chest radiograph that is outlined by normal lung and not associated with infiltrate, atelectasis, or adenopathy

GENERAL CONSIDERATIONS

- Most are asymptomatic and represent an unexpected radiographic finding
- Associated with a 10–68% risk of malignancy
- Most benign nodules are infectious granulomas; benign neoplasms such as hamartomas account for 5% of solitary nodules
- Symptoms alone rarely establish etiology, but can be used with radiographic data to assess the probability of malignancy
- The goal of evaluation is to determine the probability of malignancy in any nodule in order to justify resection or biopsy versus observation

DEMOGRAPHICS

- Malignant nodules are rare in persons under age 30
- Over age 30, risk for malignancy increases with age
- Smokers are at increased risk, with the likelihood of cancer increasing with the number of daily cigarettes
- A history of malignancy increases the likelihood that a nodule represents cancer

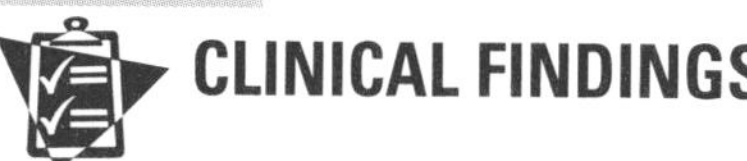

CLINICAL FINDINGS

SYMPTOMS AND SIGNS

- Solitary nodules are discovered incidentally on radiographic studies

DIFFERENTIAL DIAGNOSIS

- Granulomatous disease
- Benign neoplasm
- Bronchogenic carcinoma
- Granuloma (tuberculous, fungal)
- Lung abscess
- Hamartoma
- Metastatic cancer
- Arteriovenous malformation
- Resolving pneumonia
- Rheumatoid nodule
- Pulmonary infarction
- Carcinoid
- Pseudotumor (loculated fluid in a fissure)

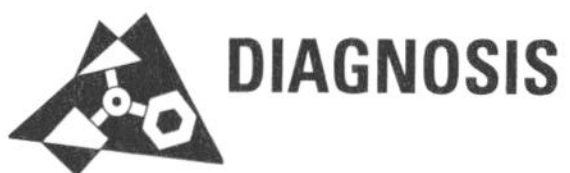

DIAGNOSIS

LABORATORY TESTS

- Sputum cytology is highly specific, but insensitive for detecting malignant nodules

IMAGING STUDIES

- Comparison with prior radiographic studies allows estimation of doubling time: rapid doubling time (< 30 days) suggests infection; slow doubling time (< 465 days) suggests benignity
- HRCT for any nodule
- Increasing size on CT scan correlates with malignancy
  - 1% malignancy rate for 2–5 mm
  - 33% for 11–20 mm
  - 80% for 21–45 mm
- CT features suggesting malignancy
  - Spiculations or a peripheral halo
  - Sparse stippled or eccentric calcifications
  - Thick-walled (>16 mm) cavitary lesions
- CT features associated with benign processes
  - Smooth, well-defined margins
  - Dense central or laminar calcifications
- Positron emission tomography (PET) is highly sensitive (85–95%) and specific (70–85%) for detecting malignant nodules and is incorporated in many diagnostic algorithms with HRCT

DIAGNOSTIC PROCEDURES

- In patients with a high probability of malignancy, biopsies rarely yield a specific benign diagnosis
- Bronchoscopy yields a diagnosis in 10–80%, depending on the size and location of the nodule; complications are rare
- Transthoracic needle aspiration (TTNA) has a diagnostic yield of 50–97%, with a 30% risk of pneumothorax
- Video-assisted thoracoscopic surgery (VATS) is used for initial evaluation of intermediate risk nodules; frozen sections can direct treatment in the operating room

Pulmonary Hypertension, Primary p. 1141

Pulmonary Nodule, Solitary

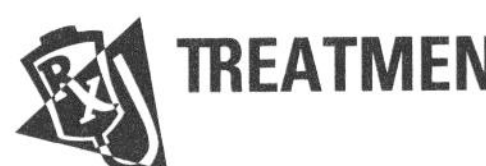

SURGERY

- Surgical resection via open thoracotomy or VATS is indicated for
  - Proven malignancies
  - Nodules likely to be malignant
  - Certain intermediate risk nodules

THERAPEUTIC PROCEDURES

- A probability of malignancy should be assigned to each nodule based on clinical and radiographic features
- Watchful waiting is appropriate for patients with low probability (< 8%) of malignancy (2 years, benign calcification pattern)
- Resection is indicated for patients with a high probability (>70%) of malignancy and no contraindications to surgery
- Optimal management of patients with an intermediate probability (8–70%) of malignancy is controversial; bronchoscopy, transthoracic needle biopsy, VATS, PET scan, and contrast-enhanced HRCT are used

FOLLOW-UP

- Patients being followed up for a nodule with a low probability of malignancy should get chest x-rays every 3 months for 1 year, then every 6 months for 1 year

WHEN TO REFER

- For specialized diagnostic procedures such as bronchoscopy, transthoracic needle aspiration, or thoracoscopic surgery

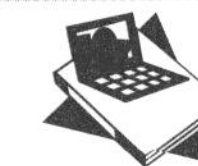

PRACTICE GUIDELINES

- National Guideline Clearinghouse
  - http://www.guideline.gov/summary/summary.aspx?doc_id=3638&nbr=2864&string=solitary+pulmonary+nodule
  - http://www.guideline.gov/summary/summary.aspx?doc_id=2570&nbr=1796&string=solitary+pulmonary+nodule

INFORMATION FOR PATIENTS

- National Institutes of Health
  - http://www.nlm.nih.gov/medlineplus/ency/article/000071.htm

REFERENCES

- Gould MK et al: Accuracy of positron emission tomography for diagnosis of pulmonary nodules and mass lesions. A meta-analysis. JAMA 2001;285:914. [PMID:11180735]
- Gurney JW: Determining the likelihood of malignancy in solitary pulmonary nodules with Bayesian analysis. Part I. Theory. Radiology 1993;186:405. [PMID:8421743]
- Ost D et al: Evaluation and management of the solitary pulmonary nodule. Am J Respir Crit Care Med 2000;162:782. [PMID:10988081]
- Ost D et al: Clinical practice. The solitary pulmonary nodule. N Engl J Med 2003;348:2535. [PMID:12815140]

Author(s)

Mark S. Chesnutt, MD
Thomas J. Prendergast, MD

Pyelonephritis, Acute

Pulmonary Radiation Fibrosis p. 1141. Pulmonary Stenosis p. 1142.
Pulmonary Veno-occlusive Disease p. 1142.

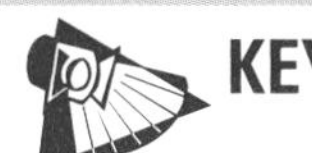

KEY FEATURES

ESSENTIALS OF DIAGNOSIS

- Fever
- Flank pain
- Irritative voiding symptoms
- Positive urine culture

GENERAL CONSIDERATIONS

- Acute pyelonephritis is an infectious inflammatory disease involving the kidney parenchyma and renal pelvis
- Most common causative organisms
  - *Escherichia coli*
  - *Proteus*
  - *Klebsiella*
  - *Enterobacter*
  - *Pseudomonas*
- Less common causative organisms
  - *Enterococcus faecalis*
  - *Staphylococcus aureus*

CLINICAL FINDINGS

SYMPTOMS AND SIGNS

- Fever
- Flank pain
- Shaking chills
- Urgency, frequency, dysuria
- Nausea, vomiting, diarrhea
- Tachycardia
- Costovertebral angle tenderness

DIFFERENTIAL DIAGNOSIS

- Appendicitis
- Cholecystitis
- Pancreatitis
- Diverticulitis
- Lower lobe pneumonia

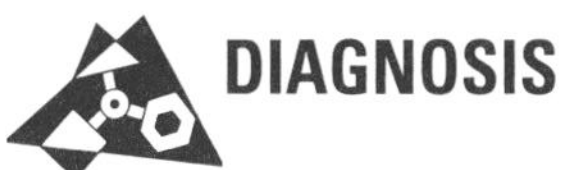

DIAGNOSIS

LABORATORY TESTS

- Complete blood cell count: leukocytosis and a left shift
- Urinalysis: pyuria, bacteriuria, hematuria, white blood cell casts
- Urine (and sometimes blood) culture positive

IMAGING STUDIES

- Renal ultrasound or abdominal CT (in complicated cases) to evaluate for hydronephrosis from stone or other obstruction

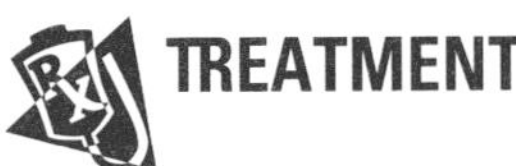

TREATMENT

MEDICATIONS

- Inpatients: IV ampicillin and an aminoglycoside until afebrile for 24 h, then PO antibiotics for 3 weeks
- Outpatients: quinolones or nitrofurantoin

Regimens

- Ampicillin, 1 g Q 6 h, and gentamicin, 1 mg/kg Q 8 h IV for 21 days
- Ciprofloxacin, 750 mg Q 12 h PO for 21 days
- Ofloxacin, 200–300 mg Q 12 h PO for 21 days
- Trimethoprim-sulfamethoxasole, 160/800 mg Q 12 h PO for 21 days [increasing resistance noted (up to 20%)]

SURGERY

- Nephrostomy drainage or double-J ureteral stent if ureteral obstruction

THERAPEUTIC PROCEDURES

- Failure to respond warrants abdominal imaging to exclude obstruction
- Catheter drainage

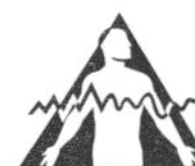

OUTCOME

FOLLOW-UP

- Follow-up urine cultures after completion of treatment

PROGNOSIS

- With prompt diagnosis and treatment, good prognosis
- Complicating factors, underlying renal disease, and increasing patient age, less favorable

WHEN TO ADMIT

- Admit if severe infections or complicating factors; obtain urine and blood cultures

EVIDENCE

PRACTICE GUIDELINES

- Bass PF 3rd et al: Urinary tract infections. Prim Care 2003;30:41. [PMID: 12838910]
- National Guideline Clearinghouse
  - http://www.guideline.gov/summary/summary.aspx?doc_id=3265&nbr=2491&string=pyelonephritis

INFORMATION FOR PATIENTS

- American College of Obstetricians and Gynecologists
  - http://www.medem.com/MedLB/article_detaillb.cfm?article_ID=ZZZ1LJ5770D&sub_cat-2008
- Mayo Clinic—Urinary tract infection
  - http://www.mayoclinic.com/invoke.cfm?objectid=364657CC-439E-4166-843C62403DD3A8D9
- National Kidney and Urologic Diseases Information Clearinghouse
  - http://kidney.niddk.nih.gov/kudiseases/pubs/pyelonephritis/index.htm

REFERENCES

- Efstathiou SP et al: Acute pyelonephritis in adults: prediction of mortality and failure of treatment. Arch Intern Med 2003;163:1206. [PMID: 12767958]
- Kawashima A et al: Radiologic evaluation of patients with renal infections. Infect Dis Clin North Am 2003;17:433. [PMID: 12848478]
- Velasco M et al: Blood cultures for women with uncomplicated acute pyelonephritis: are they necessary? Clin Infect Dis 2003;37:1127. [PMID: 14523779]

Author(s)

Marshall L. Stoller, MD
Peter R. Carroll, MD

Radiation Reactions

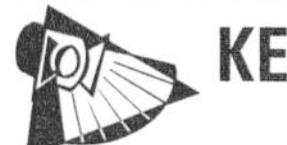

KEY FEATURES

ESSENTIALS OF DIAGNOSIS

- Damage depends on
  - The quantity of radiation delivered to the body
  - The dose rate
  - The organs exposed
  - The type of radiation (x-rays, neutrons, gamma-rays, α or β particles)
  - The duration of exposure
  - The energy transfer from the radioactive wave or particle to the exposed tissue

GENERAL CONSIDERATIONS

- The National Committee on Radiation Protection has established the maximum permissible radiation exposure for occupationally exposed workers over age 18 as 0.1 rem per week for the whole body (but not to exceed 5 rem per year) and 1.5 rem per week for the hands
- For purposes of comparison, routine chest x-rays deliver 0.1–0.2 rem

Radiation terminology

- Roentgen (R) refers to the amount of radiation dose delivered to the body
- A rad is the unit of absorbed dose
- A rem is the unit of any radiation dose to body tissue in terms of its estimated biological effect
- For x-ray or gamma-ray radiation, roentgens, rems, and rads are virtually the same
- For particulate radiation from radioactive materials, these terms may differ greatly (eg, for neutrons, 1 rad equals 10 rems)
- In the Système International (SI) nomenclature, the rad has been replaced by the gray (Gy), and 1 rad equals 0.01 Gy = 1 cGy
- The SI replacement for the rem is the Sievert (Sv), and 1 rem equals 0.01 Sv

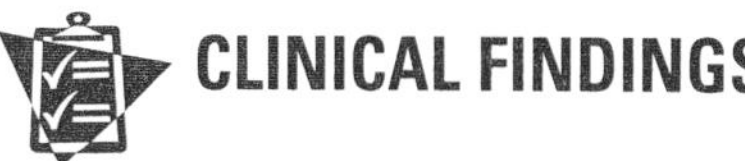

CLINICAL FINDINGS

SYMPTOMS AND SIGNS

Skin and mucous membranes

- Erythema, epilation, fingernail destruction, epidermolysis

Hematopoietic tissues

- Damage to blood-forming organs may vary from transient depression of ≥ 1 blood elements to complete destruction

Cardiovascular system

- Pericarditis with effusion or constrictive pericarditis after months or years
- Myocarditis less common
- Smaller vessels (the capillaries and arterioles) more readily damaged than larger ones

Reproductive effects

- In **males**, small single dose (200–300 cGy) cause temporary aspermatogenesis; larger doses (600–800 cGy), permanent sterility
- In **females**, single dose of 200 cGy may cause temporary cessation of menses; 500–800 cGy, permanent castration
- Moderate–heavy irradiation of embryo in utero results in injury to fetus (eg, mental retardation) or embryonic death/abortion

Respiratory tract

- High or repeated moderate doses may cause pneumonitis, often delayed for weeks or months

Mouth, pharynx, esophagus, and stomach

- Mucositis with edema and painful swallowing may occur within hours or days after exposure
- Gastric secretion may be inhibited by high doses

Intestines

- Inflammation and ulceration may follow moderately large doses

Endocrine glands and viscera

- Hepatitis and nephritis may be delayed effects of therapeutic radiation
- The normal thyroid, pituitary, pancreas, adrenals, and bladder relatively resistant to low or moderate doses of radiation; parathyroid glands especially resistant

Nervous system

- Brain and spinal cord are more sensitive to acute exposures than peripheral nerves

Systemic reaction (radiation sickness)

- Anorexia, nausea, vomiting, weakness, exhaustion, lassitude, and prostration may occur, singly or in combination
- Dehydration, anemia, and infection may follow

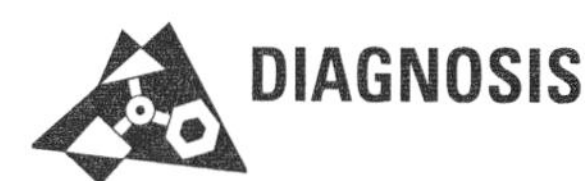

DIAGNOSIS

LABORATORY TESTS

- Serial lymphocyte counts are useful for dose estimation and monitoring of the clinical impact of exposure

Q Fever p. 1142. Rabies p. 1143. Radial Neuropathy p. 1143.

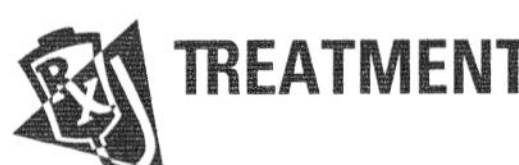

TREATMENT

MEDICATIONS

- Ondansetron, 8 mg PO twice or three times daily, for nausea and vomiting
- Alternatives include chlorpromazine, 25–50 mg given deeply IM Q 4–6 h as necessary or 10–25 mg PO Q 4–6 h as necessary; and dimenhydrinate, 50–100 mg, or perphenazine, 4–8 mg, 1 h before and 1 and 4 h after radiation therapy
- Blood and platelet transfusions, blood stem cell transplantation, bone marrow transplants, antibiotics, fluid and electrolyte maintenance, and other supportive measures may be useful
- Recombinant hematopoietic growth factors (filgrastim and sargramostim or molgramostim) can accelerate hematopoietic recovery

THERAPEUTIC PROCEDURES

- Particulate or radioisotope exposures should be decontaminated in designated confined areas
- For many radioisotopes, chelation, blocking, or dilution therapy is indicated
- Treatment of systemic reactions is symptomatic and supportive

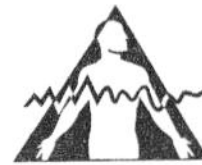

OUTCOME

COMPLICATIONS

- Skin scarring, atrophy, and telangiectasis; cataract, dry eye syndrome, retinopathy; neuropathy, myelopathy, cerebral injury; obliterative endarteritis, coronary artery disease, pericarditis; thyroid disease; pulmonary fibrosis, hepatitis, intestinal stenosis, and nephritis
- Neoplastic disease, including leukemia and cancers of the skin, breast, lung, and thyroid, is increased after exposure to radiation at relatively low doses (< 0.2 Gy)
- High-dose radon exposure is associated with an increased risk of lung cancer
  - Association of ionizing radiation with several other cancers is not well quantified
- Prenatal irradiation may increase the risk of congenital abnormalities and childhood cancer
- Carcinogenesis from low-dose (< 10 rem) exposure to adults can occur

PROGNOSIS

- Death after acute lethal radiation exposure is due to hematopoietic failure, gastrointestinal mucosal damage, central nervous system damage, widespread vascular injury, or secondary infection
- 400–600 cGy of x-ray or gamma-ray radiation applied to the entire body at one time may be fatal within 60 days; death is usually due to hemorrhage, anemia, and infection secondary to hematopoietic injury
- Levels of 1000–3000 cGy to the entire body destroy gastrointestinal mucosa; this leads to toxemia and death within 2 weeks
- Total-body doses above 3000 cGy cause widespread vascular damage, cerebral anoxia, hypotensive shock, and death within 48 h

EVIDENCE

PRACTICE GUIDELINES

- National Guideline Clearinghouse
  - http://www.guideline.gov/summary/summary.aspx?doc_id=3089&nbr=2315&string=radiation+exposure

WEB SITE

- Radiation Emergency Assistance Center/Training Site (REAC/TS)
  - http://www.orau.gov/reacts/guidance.htm

INFORMATION FOR PATIENTS

- Centers for Disease Control and Prevention: Acute Radiation Syndrome
  - http://www.bt.cdc.gov/radiation/ars.asp
- Mayo Clinic: Radiation Sickness
  - http://www.mayoclinic.com/invoke.cfm?objectid=1B032CE8-CC84-448C-99E45014638A72CE
- National Institutes of Health: What We Know About Radiation
  - http://www.nih.gov/health/chip/od/radiation/
- U.S. Environmental Protection Agency: Understanding Radiation
  - http://www.epa.gov/radiation/understand/index.html
- U.S. Nuclear Regulatory Commission: Fact Sheet on Biological Effects of Radiation
  - http://www.nrc.gov/reading-rm/doc-collections/fact-sheets/bio-effects-radiation.html

REFERENCES

- Gusev I et al: *Medical Management of Radiation Accidents.* CRC Press, 2001.
- Mettler FA et al: Major radiation exposure—what to expect and how to respond. N Engl J Med 2002;346:1554. [PMID: 12015396]

Author(s)

Richard Cohen, MD, MPH

Rape

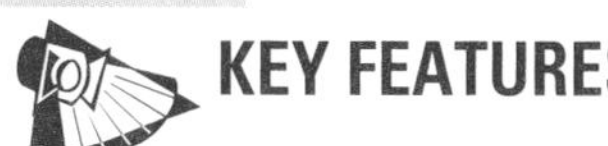

KEY FEATURES

ESSENTIALS OF DIAGNOSIS

- Women neither secretly want to be raped nor do they expect, encourage, or enjoy rape
- Rape is always a terrifying experience in which most victims fear for their lives
- The rapist is usually a hostile man who uses sexual intercourse to terrorize and humiliate a woman

GENERAL CONSIDERATIONS

- Rape, or sexual assault, is legally defined in different ways in various jurisdictions
- Clinicians and emergency department personnel who deal with rape victims should be familiar with the laws pertaining to sexual assault in their own state
- From a medical and psychological viewpoint, it is essential that persons treating rape victims recognize the nonconsensual and violent nature of the crime
- Penetration may be vaginal, anal, or oral and may be by the penis, hand, or a foreign object
- The absence of genital injury does not imply consent by the victim
- The assailant may be unknown to the victim or, more frequently, may be an acquaintance or even the spouse
- "Unlawful sexual intercourse," or statutory rape, is intercourse with a female before the age of majority even with her consent

DEMOGRAPHICS

- About 95% of reported rape victims are women
- Rape involves severe physical injury in 5–10% of cases

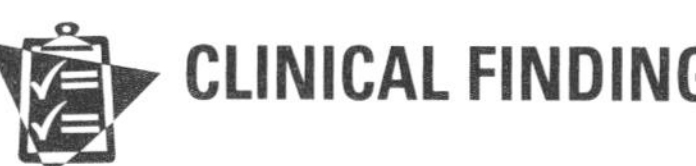

CLINICAL FINDINGS

SYMTOMS AND SIGNS

- Each patient will react differently to this personal crisis

Rape trauma syndrome

- Immediate or acute
  - Shaking, sobbing, and restless activity may last from a few days to a few weeks
  - The patient may experience anger, guilt, or shame or may repress these emotions
  - Reactions vary depending on the victim's personality and the circumstances of the attack
- Late or chronic
  - Problems related to the attack may develop weeks or months later
  - The lifestyle and work patterns of the individual may change
  - Sleep disorders or phobias often develop
  - Loss of self-esteem can in rare cases lead to suicide

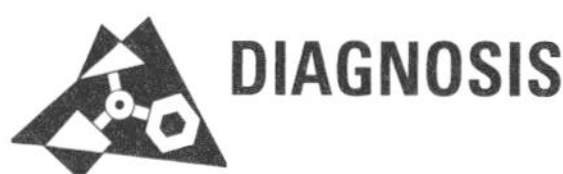

DIAGNOSIS

LABORATORY TESTS

- Culture the vagina, anus, or mouth (as appropriate) for *Neisseria gonorrhoeae* and *Chlamydia*
- Perform a Papanicolaou smear of the cervix, a wet mount for *Trichomonas vaginalis*, a baseline pregnancy test, and VDRL test
- A confidential test for HIV antibody can be obtained if desired by the patient and repeated in 2–4 months if initially negative
- Repeat the pregnancy test if the next menses is missed, and repeat the VDRL test in 6 weeks
- Obtain blood (10 mL without anticoagulant) and urine (100 mL) specimens if there is a history of forced ingestion or injection of drugs or alcohol

DIAGNOSTIC PROCEDURES

- The clinician who first sees the alleged rape victim should be empathetic. Begin with a statement such as, "This is a terrible thing that has happened to you. I want to help"
- Secure written consent from the patient, guardian, or next of kin for gynecologic examination and for photographs if they are likely to be useful as evidence. If police are to be notified, do so, and obtain advice on the preservation and transfer of evidence
- Obtain and record the history in the patient's own words. The sequence of events, ie, the time, place, and circumstances, must be included. Note the date of the last menstrual period, whether or not the woman is pregnant, and the time of the most recent coitus prior to the sexual assault. Note the details of the assault such as body cavities penetrated, use of foreign objects, and number of assailants
- Note whether the victim is calm, agitated, or confused (drugs or alcohol may be involved). Record whether the patient came directly to the hospital or whether she bathed or changed her clothing. Record findings but do not issue even a tentative diagnosis lest it be erroneous or incomplete
- Have the patient disrobe while standing on a white sheet. Hair, dirt, and leaves; underclothing; and any torn or stained clothing should be kept as evidence. Scrape material from beneath fingernails and comb pubic hair for evidence. Place all evidence in separate clean paper bags or envelopes and label carefully

- Examine the patient, noting any traumatized areas that should be photographed. Examine the body and genitals with a Wood light to identify semen, which fluoresces; positive areas should be swabbed with a premoistened swab and air-dried in order to identify acid phosphatase. Colposcopy can be used to identify small areas of trauma from forced entry, especially at the posterior fourchette
- Perform a pelvic examination, explaining all procedures and obtaining the patient's consent before proceeding gently with the examination
  - Use a narrow speculum lubricated with water only
  - Collect material with sterile cotton swabs from the vaginal walls and cervix and make two air-dried smears on clean glass slides
  - Wet and dry swabs of vaginal secretions should be collected and refrigerated for subsequent acid phosphatase and DNA evaluation
  - Swab the mouth (around molars and cheeks) and anus in the same way, if appropriate
  - Label all slides carefully
  - Collect secretions from the vagina, anus, or mouth with a premoistened cotton swab, place at once on a slide with a drop of saline, and cover with a coverslip
  - Look for motile or nonmotile sperm under high, dry magnification, and record the percentage of motile forms
- Perform appropriate laboratory tests
- Transfer clearly labeled evidence, eg, laboratory specimens, directly to the clinical pathologist in charge or to the responsible laboratory technician, in the presence of witnesses (never via messenger), so that the rules of evidence will not be breached

TREATMENT

MEDICATIONS

- Give analgesics or sedatives if indicated
- Administer tetanus toxoid if deep lacerations contain soil or dirt particles
- Give ceftriaxone, 125 mg IM, to prevent gonorrhea. In addition, give metronidazole, 2 g as a single dose, and doxycycline, 100 mg twice daily for 7 days to treat chlamydial infection. Incubating syphilis will probably be prevented by these medications, but the VDRL test should be repeated 6 weeks after the assault

THERAPEUTIC PROCEDURES

- Prevent pregnancy by using one of the methods discussed in *Contraception, emergency*, if necessary
- Vaccinate against hepatitis B
- Consider HIV prophylaxis
- Make sure the patient and her family and friends have a source of ongoing psychological support

OUTCOME

FOLLOW-UP

- Clinicians and emergency department personnel who deal with rape victims should work with community rape crisis centers whenever possible to provide ongoing support and counseling

COMPLICATIONS

- All victims suffer some psychological aftermath
- Some rape victims may acquire sexually transmissible disease or become pregnant

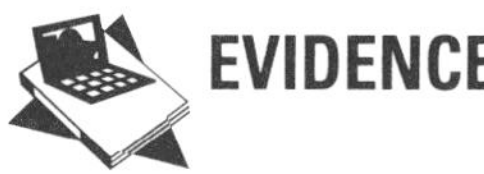

EVIDENCE

PRACTICE GUIDELINES

- Association for Genitourinary Medicine, Medical Society for the Study of Venereal Disease (London). 2002 national guidelines on the management of adult victims of sexual assault
  - http://www.guideline.gov/summary/summary.aspx?doc_id=3050&nbr=2276
- Centers for Disease Control and Prevention. Sexually transmitted diseases treatment guidelines 2002
  - http://www.cdc.gov/mmwr/preview/mmwrhtml/rr5106a1.htm

WEB SITES

- National Women's Health Information Center: Sexual Assault and Abuse
  - http://www.4woman.gov/violence/sexual.cfm
- National Women's Health Information Center: State Domestic Violence Resources
  - http://www.4woman.gov/violence/state.cfm
- National Sexual Violence Resource Center
  - http://www.nsvrc.org/

INFORMATION FOR PATIENTS

- American Academy of Family Physicians: What to Do if You're Raped
  - http://familydoctor.org/314.xml
- Department of Justice, Office on Violence Against Women: Myths and Facts about Sexual Violence
  - http://www.ojp.usdoj.gov/vawo/MythsFactSexualViolence.htm
- National Center for Victims of Crime: Sexual Assault
  - http://www.ncvc.org/ncvc/main.aspx?dbName=DocumentViewer&DocumentID=32369
- National Women's Health Information Center: Sexual Assault
  - http://www.4woman.gov/faq/sexualassault.htm

REFERENCE

- Cantu M et al: Evaluation and management of the sexually assaulted woman. Emerg Med Clin North Am 2003;21:737. [PMID: 12962356]

Author(s)

H. Trent MacKay, MD, MPH

Rash, Drug

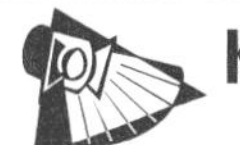

KEY FEATURES

ESSENTIALS OF DIAGNOSIS

- Usually, abrupt onset of widespread, symmetric erythematous eruption
- May mimic any inflammatory skin condition
- Constitutional symptoms (malaise, arthralgia, headache, and fever) may be present

GENERAL CONSIDERATIONS

- Only a minority of cutaneous drug reactions result from allergy
- True allergic drug reactions involve
  - Prior exposure
  - An "incubation" period
  - Reactions to doses far below the therapeutic range
  - Restriction to a limited number of syndromes (anaphylactic and anaphylactoid, urticarial, vasculitic, etc)
  - Reproducibility
- Amoxicillin, trimethoprim-sulfamethoxazole, and ampicillin or penicillin are the commonest causes of urticarial and maculopapular reactions
- Toxic epidermal necrolysis and Stevens-Johnson syndrome are most commonly produced by sulfonamides and anticonvulsants
- Phenolphthalein, pyrazolone derivatives, tetracyclines, NSAIDs, trimethoprim-sulfamethoxazole, and barbiturates are the major causes of *fixed drug eruptions*

DEMOGRAPHICS

- Rashes are among the most common adverse reactions to drugs and occur in 2–3% of hospitalized patients

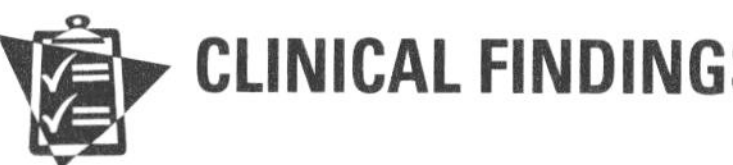

CLINICAL FINDINGS

SYMPTOMS AND SIGNS

- The onset is usually abrupt, with bright erythema and often severe itching, but may be delayed
- Fever and other constitutional symptoms may be present
- The skin reaction usually occurs in symmetric distribution
- Table 8 summarizes the types of skin reactions, their appearance and distribution, and the common offenders in each case

DIFFERENTIAL DIAGNOSIS

- Viral exanthem
- Early erythema multiforme major
- Other causes of erythema nodosum, eg, infection, sarcoidosis
- Atopic dermatitis (eczema)
- Secondary syphilis
- Systemic lupus erythematosus
- Acute HIV infection
- Scarlet fever
- Toxic shock syndrome
- Lichen planus

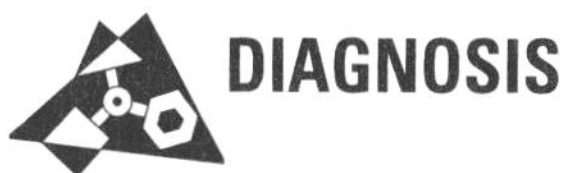

DIAGNOSIS

LABORATORY TESTS

- Routinely ordered blood work is of no value in the diagnosis of drug eruptions
- Observation after discontinuation, which may be a slow process, helps establish the diagnosis
- Rechallenge, though of theoretical value, may pose a danger to the patient and is best avoided

PROCEDURES

- Skin biopsies may be helpful in making the diagnosis

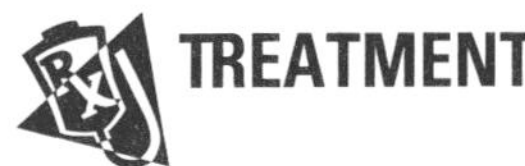

TREATMENT

General Measures

- Systemic manifestations are treated as they arise (eg, anemia, icterus, purpura)
- Antihistamines may be of value in urticarial and angioneurotic reactions
- Epinephrine 1:1000, 0.5–1 mL intravenously or subcutaneously, should be used as an emergency measure
- In severe cases, corticosteroids may be used at doses similar to those used for acute contact dermatitis

Local Measures

- The varieties and stages of dermatitis are treated according to the major dermatitis present

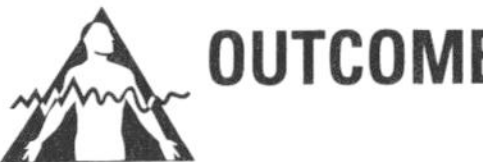

OUTCOME

COMPLICATIONS

- Some cutaneous drug reactions may be associated with a clinical complex involving other organs (complex drug reactions). Most common is an infectious mononucleosis-like illness and hepatitis associated with administration of anticonvulsants

PROGNOSIS

- Drug rash usually disappears upon withdrawal of the drug and proper treatment

WHEN TO REFER

- If there is a question about the diagnosis, if recommended therapy is ineffective, or if specialized treatment is necessary

WHEN TO ADMIT

- Extensive blistering eruptions resulting in erosions and superficial ulcerations demand hospitalization and nursing care as for burn patients

EVIDENCE

WEB SITES

- American Academy of Dermatology: Cutaneous Adverse Drug Reaction
  - http://www.aad.org/professionals/pracmanage/guidelines/CutaneousAdverseReactions.htm
- Reidl MA et al: Adverse drug reactions: types and treatment options. Am Fam Physician 2003;68,1781.
  - http://www.aafp.org/afp/20031101/1781.html

INFORMATION FOR PATIENTS

- American Academy of Allergy, Asthma & Immunology: Adverse Reactions to Medications
  - http://www.aaaai.org/patients/publicedmat/tips/adversereactions.stm
- American Academy of Family Physicians: Drug Reactions
  - http://familydoctor.org/231.xml
- Mayo Clinic: Penicillin Allergy
  - http://www.mayoclinic.com/invoke.cfm?id=HQ01195
- MedlinePlus: Drug Allergies
  - http://www.nlm.nih.gov/medlineplus/ency/article/000819.htm

REFERENCES

- Lerch M: The immunological and clinical spectrum of delayed drug-induced exanthems. Curr Opin Allergy Clin Immunol 2004;4:411. [PMID: 15349041]
- Wolf R et al: Treatment of toxic epidermal necrolysis syndrome with "disease-modifying" drugs: the controversy goes on. Clin Dermatol 2004;22:267. [PMID: 15262313]

Author(s)

Timothy G. Berger, MD

Raynaud's Disease & Phenomenon

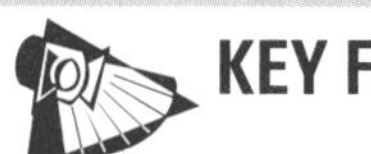

KEY FEATURES

ESSENTIALS OF DIAGNOSIS

- Episodic bilateral digital pallor, cyanosis, and rubor
- Precipitated by cold or emotional stress; relieved by warmth

GENERAL CONSIDERATIONS

- An episodic vasospastic disorder characterized by digital color change (white-blue-red) with exposure to cold or emotional stress
- Called Raynaud's disease if symptoms persist for > 3 years without evidence of an associated disease
- Called Raynaud's phenomenon if associated with autoimmune diseases, myeloproliferative disorders, multiple myeloma, cryoglobulinemia, myxedema, macroglobulinemia, or arterial occlusive disease
- Occurs in 10% of the general population
- Other vasospastic disorders (eg, variant angina and migraine headache) are common in patients with Raynaud's

DEMOGRAPHICS

- 70–80% of patients are women
- Raynaud's disease usually appears first between ages 15 and 45, almost always in women

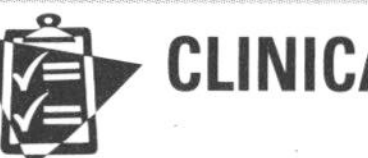

CLINICAL FINDINGS

SYMPTOMS AND SIGNS

- Mild discomfort, paresthesias, numbness, and trace edema often accompany the color changes
- The affected extremities may be entirely normal between attacks
- Raynaud's disease is symmetric
- Raynaud's phenomenon infrequently involves the feet and toes
- Raynaud's disease is benign and entirely reversible
- Raynaud's phenomenon may progress to atrophy of the terminal fat pads and development of fingertip gangrene

DIFFERENTIAL DIAGNOSIS

- Neurogenic thoracic outlet syndrome or carpal tunnel syndrome
- Frostbite, ergotamine toxicity, and chemotherapeutic agents
- Bleomycin and vincristine chemotherapy
- Atherosclerosis, Buerger's disease, embolic disease, repetitive motion injury
- Vasospasm with contrast injection
- Acrocyanosis
- Livedo reticularis

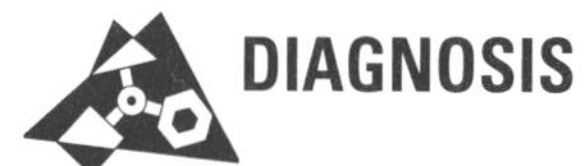

DIAGNOSIS

LABORATORY TESTS

- Complete blood cell count
- Autoimmune workup, if suspected

IMAGING STUDIES

- Conventional digital angiography is indicated only in cases of tissue loss or to rule out atheroemboli, atheroocclusive disease, or arterial trauma

DIAGNOSTIC PROCEDURES

- Diagnosis is based on clinical criteria

Rash, Heat p. 1143. Rat-Bite Fever p. 1144.

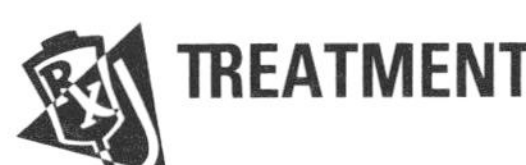

MEDICATIONS

- Aspirin
- Vasodilators
- Nifedipine, sustained-release 30 mg PO QD, or diltiazem, sustained-release 30 mg PO QD
- Fluoxetine, 20 mg PO QD
- Discontinue oral contraceptives, β-blockers, and ergotamine

SURGERY

- Bypass surgery for severe Raynaud's phenomenon associated with reconstructible arterial occlusive disease
- Sympathectomy for unreconstructible occlusive disease or pure vasospastic disease refractory to medical management

THERAPEUTIC PROCEDURES

- Warmth and protection of the hands
- Moisturizing lotion
- Smoking cessation
- Stress management

OUTCOME

PROGNOSIS

- Raynaud's disease usually benign
- Raynaud's phenomenon prognosis is that of the associated disease

WHEN TO REFER

- Raynaud's syndrome with tissue loss
- Severe arterial insufficiency from atheroocclusive disease

PREVENTION

- Avoidance of cold exposure
- Stress reduction

EVIDENCE

INFORMATION FOR PATIENTS

- Cleveland Clinic: Raynaud's Phenomenon
  - http://www.clevelandclinic.org/health/health-info/docs/3100/3132.asp?index=9849
- Mayo Clinic: Raynaud's Disease
  - http://www.mayoclinic.com/invoke.cfm?objectid=BEC8E664-5EE6-41C1-8955642FA71A0EEF
- MedlinePlus: Raynaud's Phenomenon
  - http://www.nlm.nih.gov/medlineplus/ency/article/000412.htm

REFERENCES

- Coleiro B et al: Treatment of Raynaud's phenomenon with the selective serotonin reuptake inhibitor fluoxetine. Rheumatology (Oxford) 2001;40:1038. [PMID: 11561116]
- Pache M et al: Cold feet and prolonged sleep-onset latency in vasospastic syndrome. Lancet 2001;358:125. [PMID: 11463418]

Author(s)

Louis M. Messina, MD

Reflex Sympathetic Dystrophy

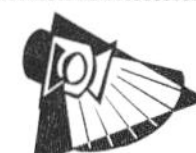

KEY FEATURES

ESSENTIALS OF DIAGNOSIS

- Burning or aching pain in an injured extremity more severe than would be expected given the inciting trauma
- Localized vasomotor instability

GENERAL CONSIDERATIONS

- Occurs equally in all age groups and both sexes
- Can involve either the arms or the legs
- Causes include trauma, closed fractures, simple lacerations, burns, operative procedures, and myocardial infarction

CLINICAL FINDINGS

SYMPTOMS AND SIGNS

- Early stages: pain, tenderness, and hyperesthesia localized to the injured area; extremity is warm, dry, swollen, and red or slightly cyanotic; with time, muscle spasm and joint stiffness limit mobility; the nails may become ridged
- Advanced stages: pain is more diffuse, nocturnal pain; extremity is cool, clammy, and intolerant of temperature changes
- Patient concerned to avoid external stimuli
- Pain and disuse lead to loss of function

DIFFERENTIAL DIAGNOSIS

- Acute limb ischemia
- Thoracic outlet syndrome
- Nerve root compression or radiculopathy

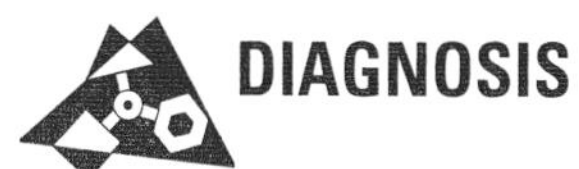

DIAGNOSIS

IMAGING STUDIES

- Bone radiographs: asymmetric osteopenia more severe than anticipated from immobility alone

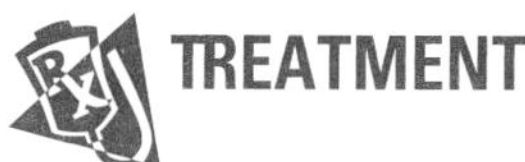

TREATMENT

MEDICATIONS

- Diazepam, 2 mg PO BID, or alprazolam, 0.125–0.25 mg PO QD
- Opioids
- Gabapentin

SURGERY

- Sympathectomy
- Implantable spinal cord biostimulator devices have had limited success

THERAPEUTIC PROCEDURES

- Early physical therapy involving active and passive exercises
- Protection from further injury
- Avoidance of irritating stimuli
- Sympathetic (stellate ganglion or lumbar) blocks

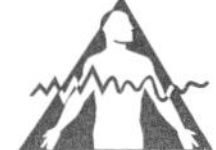

OUTCOME

COMPLICATIONS

- Chronic pain syndrome
- Disability

PROGNOSIS

- Good with early diagnosis and appropriate intervention

WHEN TO REFER

- Symptoms and signs of reflex sympathetic dystrophy

WHEN TO ADMIT

- Intractable pain

PREVENTION

- Avoid trauma to peripheral nerves during surgery
- After injury to an extremity, splinting and adequate analgesia followed by early mobilization

EVIDENCE

PRACTICE GUIDELINES

- Greipp ME: Complex regional pain syndrome—type I: research relevance, practice realities. J Neurosci Nurs 2003;35:16. [PMID: 12789717]
- Turner-Stokes L: Reflex sympathetic dystrophy—a complex regional pain syndrome. Disabil Rehabil 2002;24:939. [PMID: 12523947]

INFORMATION FOR PATIENTS

- Mayo Clinic: Complex Regional Pain Syndrome
  - http://www.mayoclinic.com/invoke.cfm?objectid=8F3237C2-D7C0-4063-AE87DC86D78085FE
- MedlinePlus: Complex Regional Pain Syndrome
  - http://www.nlm.nih.gov/medlineplus/ency/article/007184.htm
- National Institute of Neurological Disorders and Stroke: Complex Regional Pain Syndrome Information Page
  - http://www.ninds.nih.gov/disorders/reflex_sympathetic_dystrophy/reflex_sympathetic_dystrophy_pr.htm

REFERENCES

- Kemler MA et al: Impact of spinal cord stimulation on sensory characteristics in complex regional pain syndrome type 1: a randomized trial. Anesthesiology 2001;95:72. [PMID: 11465587]
- Wasner G et al: Vascular abnormalities in reflex sympathetic dystrophy (CPRS 1): mechanisms and diagnostic value. Brain 2001;124:587. [PMID: 11222458]

Author(s)

Louis M. Messina, MD

Renal Artery Stenosis

Relapsing Fever p. 1144. Renal Artery Aneurysm p. 1145.

KEY FEATURES

ESSENTIALS OF DIAGNOSIS

- Produced predominantly by atherosclerotic occlusive disease (80–90% of patients) or fibromuscular dysplasia (10–15%)
- Patients with occlusive disease have common risk factors for atherosclerosis, lesions are focal proximal or ostial calcific plaques, "spillover" aortic disease
- Patients with fibromuscular dysplasia are usually women 30–50 years old with distal renal artery disease that often extends into the branch vessels in a classic "string of beads" pattern of alternating stenoses and dilations

GENERAL CONSIDERATIONS

- Of patients with hypertension ~5% have renal artery stenosis
- Of patients aged > 60 with diastolic blood pressure > 105 mm Hg and serum creatinine > 2 mg/dL, 70% have renovascular disease
- In hypertensive children aged < 5 years with hypertension, 80% have renovascular disease
- Consider renal artery stenosis
  - In patients with poorly controlled or acutely worsening hypertension on three or more antihypertensive medications, particularly when presenting in conjunction with renal insufficiency, lateral abdominal bruit, or noncardiogenic "flash" pulmonary edema
  - In patients with a history of acute renal failure when starting an angiotensin-converting enzyme (ACE) inhibitor
- Renal artery stenosis is noted in as many as 45% of patients undergoing angiography for aortoiliac occlusive disease
- Suspect in patients with rapidly progressive renal insufficiency and no evidence of obstructive uropathy or intrinsic renal disease (no proteinuria, no polycystic disease)

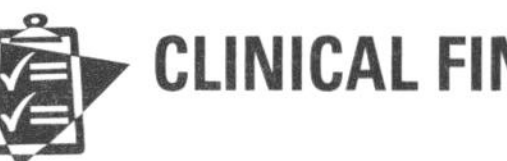

CLINICAL FINDINGS

SYMPTOMS AND SIGNS

- Hypertension, often severe and refractory to antihypertensive medications
- Lateral abdominal bruit

DIFFERENTIAL DIAGNOSIS

- Essential hypertension
- Hypertensive nephrosclerosis
- Primary hyperaldosteronism
- Cushing's syndrome
- Coarctation of the aorta

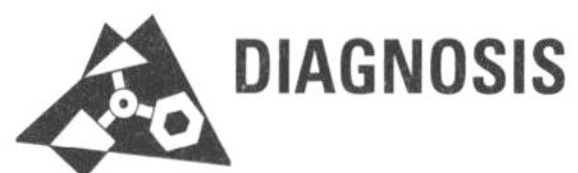

DIAGNOSIS

LABORATORY TESTS

- Serum creatinine > 2 mg/dL
- Urinalysis: no proteinuria

IMAGING STUDIES

- Initial screening tests: duplex ultrasonogram, captopril renal scintigraphy, and MRA, each of which has sensitivity and specificity > 90%
- Ultrasonography and MRA can assess renal size, cortical thickness, and presence of infarcts but can miss small accessory renal arteries, which when diseased can contribute to renovascular hypertension
- Angiography: indicated for treatment by percutaneous angioplasty and stenting or surgery

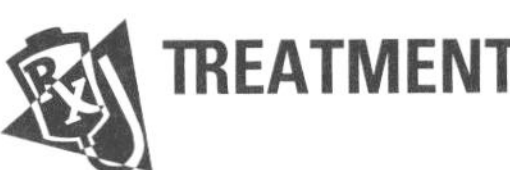

TREATMENT

MEDICATIONS

- Antihypertensive drug therapy, individualizing (Table 45)
- α-Adrenoreceptor blocking agents, sympatholytic agents, and vasodilator agents (Table 50)
- β-Adrenergic blocking agents (Table 47)
- Calcium channel-blocking agents (Table 49)
- Diuretics (Table 46)
- Hypertensive emergencies and urgencies (Table 51)
- Avoid ACE inhibitors and ACE receptor blockers

SURGERY

- For hypertension refractory to aggressive medical management or renal artery stenosis with progressive renal failure or sudden-onset noncardiogenic pulmonary edema
- For patients with lesions refractory to angioplasty, complex lesions extending into the branch vessels, or concomitant aortic disease requiring surgical reconstruction
- Superior long-term patency
- Transaortic renal endarterectomy, renal artery bypass, or extraanatomic (hepatorenal, splenorenal, or iliorenal) bypass
- Nephrectomy for patients with renovascular hypertension and irreversible renal atrophy
- Endarterectomy and aortorenal bypass have 5-year patency > 80%, beneficial blood pressure response in 70–90%, and improvement or stabilization in renal function in 70–80%

THERAPEUTIC PROCEDURES

- Endovascular treatment (angioplasty and stenting) for focal, proximal plaques that do not extend into the branch vessels
- Angioplasty alone effective for fibromuscular dysplasia
- Primary stenting for stenoses in renal arteries > 6 mm yields improved patency over angioplasty alone

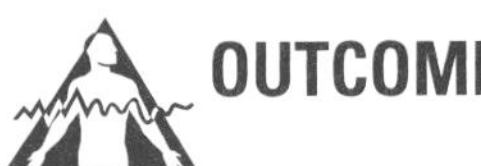

OUTCOME

FOLLOW-UP

- Careful blood pressure monitoring

COMPLICATIONS

- Renal failure

PROGNOSIS

- The long-term patency of renal artery stents is yet undefined, but a 20% restenosis rate from intimal hyperplasia is noted at 6–36 months
- Overall, 3–13% of initially stented patients ultimately require surgery

WHEN TO REFER

- Renal artery stenosis with poorly controlled hypertension or renal insufficiency

WHEN TO ADMIT

- Malignant hypertension

PREVENTION

- Antilipidemic, antihypertensive therapy to prevent atherosclerosis

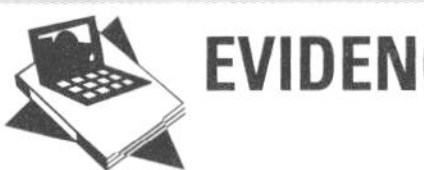

EVIDENCE

PRACTICE GUIDELINES

- Martin LG et al: Quality improvement guidelines for angiography, angioplasty, and stent placement in the diagnosis and treatment of renal artery stenosis in adults. J Vasc Interv Radiol 2002;13:1069. [PMID: 12427805]

INFORMATION FOR PATIENTS

- American College of Physicians: Summaries for Patients: Diagnosis of Renal Artery Stenosis
  - http://www.annals.org/cgi/content/full/141/9/I-66
- MedlinePlus: Renal Artery Stenosis
  - http://www.nlm.nih.gov/medlineplus/ency/article/001273.htm

REFERENCES

- Paty PS et al: Is prosthetic renal artery reconstruction a durable procedure? An analysis of 489 bypass grafts. J Vasc Surg 2001;34:127. [PMID: 11436085]
- Safian R: Renal-artery stenosis. N Engl J Med 2001;344:431. [PMID: 11172181]
- van de Ven PJ et al: Arterial stenting and balloon angioplasty in ostial atherosclerotic renovascular disease: a randomised trial. Lancet 1999;353:282. [PMID: 9929021]

Author(s)

Louis M. Messina, MD

Renal Cell Carcinoma

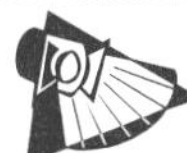

KEY FEATURES

ESSENTIALS OF DIAGNOSIS

- Gross or microscopic hematuria
- Flank pain or mass in some patients
- Systemic symptoms such as fever, weight loss may be prominent
- Solid renal mass on imaging

GENERAL CONSIDERATIONS

- ~2.3% of all adult cancers
- In 2001, ~30,800 cases of renal cell carcinoma and ~12,100 deaths in the United States

DEMOGRAPHICS

- Peak incidence in sixth decade of life
- Male-to-female ratio = 2:1
- Cause is unknown
- Risk factor: cigarette smoking
- Familial: von Hippel-Lindau syndrome
- Association with dialysis-related acquired cystic disease

CLINICAL FINDINGS

SYMPTOMS AND SIGNS

- Hematuria (gross or microscopic) in 60% of cases
- Flank pain or an abdominal mass in ~30%
- Triad of flank pain, hematuria, and mass in ~10–15%, often a sign of advanced disease
- Symptoms of metastatic disease (cough, bone pain) in ~20–30% at presentation
- Often detected incidentally

DIFFERENTIAL DIAGNOSIS

- Angiomyolipomas (fat density usually visible by CT)
- Transitional cell cancers of the renal pelvis (more centrally located, involvement of the collecting system, positive urinary cytology reports)
- Adrenal tumors (superoanterior to the kidney)
- Oncocytomas
- Renal abscesses

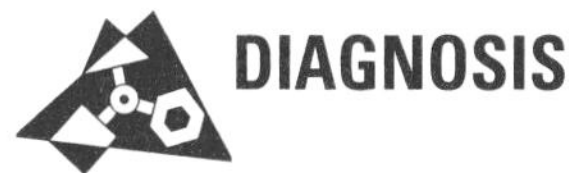

DIAGNOSIS

LABORATORY TESTS

- Hematuria in 60%
- Paraneoplastic syndromes
- Erythrocytosis from increased erythropoietin production in ~5% (anemia far more common)
- Hypercalcemia in 10%
- Stauffer's syndrome, a reversible syndrome of hepatic dysfunction

IMAGING STUDIES

- Renal mass on intravenous urography, ultrasound, CT or MRI scan

DIAGNOSTIC PROCEDURES

- CT scanning is the most valuable imaging test; it confirms character of the mass, stages the lesion
- Chest radiographs for pulmonary metastases
- Bone scans for large tumors, bone pain, elevated alkaline phosphatase levels
- MRI and duplex Doppler ultrasonography can assess for the presence and extent of tumor thrombus within the renal vein or vena cava in selected patients

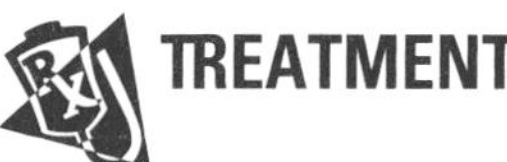

TREATMENT

MEDICATIONS

- For metastatic renal cell carcinoma, no effective chemotherapy is available
- Vinblastine yields short-term partial response rates of 15%
- Biological response modifiers: α-interferon yields partial response rate of 15–20% and interleukin-2, partial response rate of 15–35%

SURGERY

- Laparoscopic or open radical nephrectomy for localized renal cell carcinoma
- Partial nephrectomy for patients with a small cancer, single kidney, bilateral lesions, or significant medical renal disease

THERAPEUTIC PROCEDURES

- Cell type and histological pattern do not affect treatment
- Patients with metastatic disease usually should be considered for palliative therapy with surgery followed by systemic therapy—biological response modifiers

OUTCOME

PROGNOSIS

- For patients with solitary resectable metastases, radical nephrectomy with resection of the metastasis has resulted in 5-year disease-free survival rates of 15–30%

EVIDENCE

PRACTICE GUIDELINES

- Mickisch G et al: Guidelines on renal cell cancer. Eur Urol 2001;40:252. [PMID: 11684839]
- Motzer RJ et al: NCCN Kidney Cancer Practice Guidelines Panel. National Comprehensive Cancer Network: Kidney Cancer v.1.2005.
  - http://www.nccn.org/professionals/physician_gls/PDF/kidney.pdf

WEB SITE

- National Cancer Institute: Kidney Cancer Information for Patients and Health Professionals
  - http://www.cancer.gov/cancertopics/types/kidney

INFORMATION FOR PATIENTS

- American Cancer Society: Kidney Cancer
  - http://www.cancer.org/docroot/CRI/CRI_2_3x.asp?rnav=cridg&dt=22
- JAMA Patient Page: Kidney Cancer. JAMA 2004;292:134
  - http://www.medem.com/medlb/article_detaillb.cfm?article_ID=ZZZ8VD9OGXD&sub_cat=263
- Mayo Clinic: Kidney Cancer
  - http://www.mayoclinic.com/invoke.cfm?id=DS00360
- National Cancer Institute: Kidney Cancer
  - http://www.cancer.gov/cancerinfo/wyntk/kidney

REFERENCES

- McDermott DF et al: Randomized phase III trial of high-dose interleukin-2 versus subcutaneous interleukin-2 and interferon in patients with metastatic renal cell carcinoma. J Clin Oncol 2005;23:133. [PMID: 15625368]
- Lam JS et al: Tissue array-based predictions of pathobiology, prognosis, and response to treatment for renal cell carcinoma therapy. Clin Cancer Res 2004;10(18 Pt 2):6304S. [PMID: 15448022]
- Shirasaki Y et al: Long-term consequence of renal function following nephrectomy for renal cell cancer. Int J Urol 2004;11:704. [PMID: 15379932]

Author(s)

Marshall L. Stoller, MD
Peter R. Carroll, MD

Renal Failure, Acute

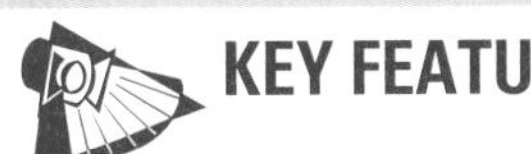

KEY FEATURES

ESSENTIALS OF DIAGNOSIS

- Defined as a sudden decrease in renal function, resulting in an inability to maintain fluid and electrolyte balance and to excrete nitrogenous wastes
- Sudden increase in blood urea nitrogen (BUN) or serum creatinine
- Oliguria often associated
- Symptoms and signs depend on cause

GENERAL CONSIDERATIONS

- 5% of hospital admissions and 30% of ICU admissions have acute renal failure
- 25% of hospitalized patients develop acute renal failure
- Serum creatinine concentration can typically increase 1–1.5 mg/dL daily
- Three categories of acute renal failure: prerenal azotemia, intrinsic renal failure, and postrenal azotemia

CLINICAL FINDINGS

SYMPTOMS AND SIGNS

- Nausea, vomiting
- Malaise
- Hypertension
- Pericardial friction rub, effusions, and cardiac tamponade
- Arrhythmias
- Rales
- Abdominal pain and ileus
- Bleeding secondary to platelet dysfunction
- Encephalopathy, altered sensorium, asterixis, seizures
- Oliguria, defined as urine output < 500 mL/day

DIFFERENTIAL DIAGNOSIS

Prerenal azotemia

- Dehydration
- Hemorrhage (eg, gastrointestinal bleeding)
- Congestive heart failure
- Renal artery stenosis, including fibromuscular dysplasia
- Nonsteroidal antiinflammatory drugs (NSAIDs), angiotensin-converting enzyme inhibitors

Postrenal azotemia

- Obstruction (eg, benign prostatic hyperplasia, bladder tumor)

Intrinsic renal disease

- Acute tubular necrosis
  - Toxins: NSAIDs, antibiotics, contrast, multiple myeloma, rhabdomyolysis, hemolysis, chemotherapy, hyperuricemia, cyclosporine
  - Ischemia (eg, prolonged prerenal azotemia)
- Acute glomerulonephritis
  - Immune complex: IgA nephropathy, endocarditis, systemic lupus erythematosus (SLE), cryoglobulinemia, postinfectious, membranoproliferative
  - Pauci-immune ($ANCA^+$): Wegener's granulomatosis, Churg-Strauss syndrome, microscopic polyarteritis
  - Antiglomerular basement membrane (GBM): Goodpasture's disease, anti-GBM glomerulonephritis
- Vascular
  - Malignant hypertension
  - Thrombotic thrombocytopenia purpura
  - Atheroembolism
- Acute interstitial nephritis
  - Drugs: β-lactams, sulfa, diuretics, NSAIDs, rifampin, phenytoin, allopurinol
  - Infections: *Streptococcus*, leptospirosis, cytomegalovirus, histoplasmosis, Rocky Mountain spotted fever
  - Immune: SLE, Sjögren's syndrome, sarcoidosis, cryoglobulinemia

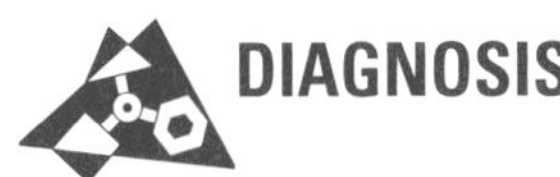

DIAGNOSIS

LABORATORY TESTS

- Serum creatinine and BUN elevated
- BUN–creatinine ratio > 20:1 in prerenal and postrenal azotemia, and acute glomerulonephritis; < 20:1 in acute tubular necrosis and acute interstitial nephritis
- Hyperkalemia
- Anion gap metabolic acidosis
- Hyperphosphatemia
- Hypocalcemia
- Anemia
- Fractional excretion of sodium (FE_{Na}) can be useful
  - FE_{Na} = clearance of Na^+/GFR = clearance of Na^+/creatinine clearance
  - FE_{Na} = (urine Na^+/plasma Na^+)/(urine Cr/plasma Cr) × 100
- FE_{Na} low (< 1%) in prerenal azotemia; high (> 1%) in acute tubular necrosis; variable in postrenal azotemia, acute interstitial nephritis, acute glomerulonephritis

IMAGING STUDIES

- Bladder ultrasonography
- CT or MRI if retroperitoneal fibrosis from tumor or radiation suspected
- Renal ultrasonography to exclude obstruction

DIAGNOSTIC PROCEDURES

- ECG: peaked T waves, PR prolongation, and QRS widening in hyperkalemia, long QT interval with hypocalcemia

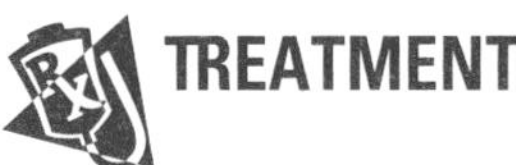

TREATMENT

THERAPEUTIC PROCEDURES

- Prerenal azotemia: treatment depends on cause; maintenance of euvolemia, attention to serum potassium, avoidance of nephrotoxic drugs
- Postrenal azotemia: relief of obstruction if present
  - Catheters or stents to treat obstruction
  - Bladder catheterization if hydroureter and hydronephrosis are present with an enlarged bladder on ultrasonography
- Intrinsic renal failure: treatment depends on cause (see Tubular Necrosis, Acute); hold offending agents
- Hemodialysis, peritoneal dialysis: indications include
  - Uremic symptoms such as pericarditis, encephalopathy, or coagulopathy
  - Fluid overload unresponsive to diuresis
  - Refractory hyperkalemia
  - Severe metabolic acidosis (pH < 7.20)
  - Neurological symptoms such as seizures or neuropathy

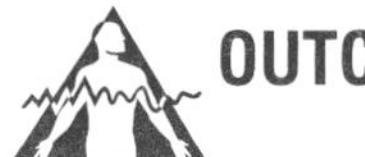

OUTCOME

WHEN TO REFER

- Persistence of acute renal failure for 2–4 weeks

WHEN TO ADMIT

- Significant acid–base, fluid, or electrolyte abnormalities or uremia

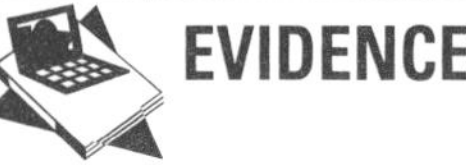

EVIDENCE

PRACTICE GUIDELINES

- American College of Radiology, Expert Panel on Urologic Imaging: ARC Appropriateness Criteria for Radiologic Investigation of Causes of Renal Failure, 2001
  - http://www.guideline.gov/summary/summary.aspx?doc_id=3271&nbr=2497

WEB SITE

- National Kidney and Urologic Diseases Information Clearinghouse
  - http://kidney.niddk.nih.gov/

INFORMATION FOR PATIENTS

- JAMA Patient Page: Acute Renal Failure. JAMA 2002;288:2634
  - http://www.medem.com/medlb/article_detaillb.cfm?article_ID=ZZZCFVFA09D&sub_cat=323
- Mayo Clinic: Kidney Failure
  - http://www.mayoclinic.com/invoke.cfm?id=DS00280
- MedlinePlus: Kidney Failure
  - http://www.nlm.nih.gov/medlineplus/tutorials/kidneyfailure/htm/index.htm

REFERENCES

- Albright RC Jr: Acute renal failure: a practical update. Mayo Clin Proc 2001;76:67. [PMID: 11155415
- Holt SG et al: Pathogenesis and treatment of renal dysfunction in rhabdomyolysis. Intensive Care Med 2001;27:803. [PMID: 11430535]
- Mehta R et al: Diuretics, mortality, and nonrecovery of renal function in acute renal failure. JAMA 2002;288:2547. [PMID: 12444861]
- Sauret JM et al: Rhabdomyolysis. Am Fam Physician 2002;65:907. [PMID: 11898964]
- Singri N et al: Acute renal failure. JAMA 2003;289:747. [PMID: 12585954]

Author(s)

Suzanne Watnick, MD
Gail Morrison, MD

Renal Failure, Chronic

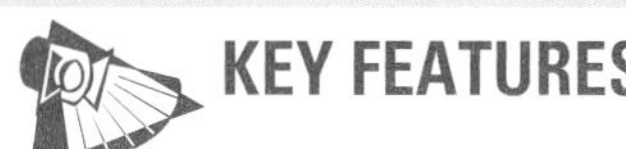

KEY FEATURES

ESSENTIALS OF DIAGNOSIS

- Progressive azotemia over months to years
- Symptoms and signs of uremia when nearing end-stage disease
- Hypertension in the majority
- Isosthenuria and broad casts in urinary sediment are common
- Bilateral small kidneys on ultrasonogram are diagnostic

GENERAL CONSIDERATIONS

- Major causes (> 50% of cases) are diabetes mellitus and hypertension
- Glomerulonephritis, cystic diseases, and other urological diseases account for another 20–25%, unknown causes (~15%) (Table 91)
- Rarely reversible
- Progressive decline in renal function

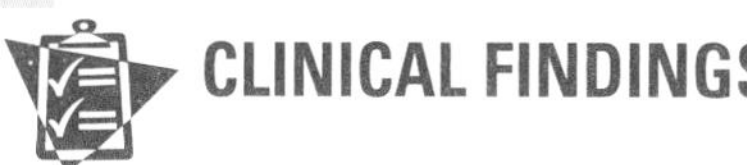

CLINICAL FINDINGS

SYMPTOMS AND SIGNS

- Symptoms develop slowly and are nonspecific
- Asymptomatic until renal failure is far advanced [glomerular filtration rate (GFR) < 10–15 mL/min]
- Fatigue, weakness, and malaise
- Gastrointestinal complaints such as anorexia, nausea, vomiting, a metallic taste in the mouth, and hiccups
- Neurological irritability, difficulty concentrating, insomnia, restless legs, and twitching
- Pruritus
- Decreased libido, menstrual irregularities
- Chest pain from pericarditis
- Renal osteodystrophy (osteitis fibrosa cystica), osteomalacia, and adynamic bone disease

DIFFERENTIAL DIAGNOSIS

- See Table 92

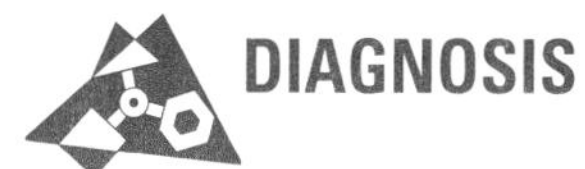

DIAGNOSIS

LABORATORY TESTS

- Serum creatinine and blood urea nitrogen (BUN) elevated; evidence of previously elevated creatinine and BUN, abnormal prior urinalyses help to differentiate between acute and chronic renal failure
- Plot of the inverse of serum creatinine ($1/S_{Cr}$) versus time if 3 or more prior measurements are available helps to estimate time to end-stage renal disease
- Anemia
- Platelet dysfunction, bleeding time prolongation
- Metabolic acidosis
- Hyperphosphatemia, hypocalcemia
- Hyperkalemia
- Isosthenuria
- Urinary sediment: broad waxy casts

IMAGING STUDIES

- Renal ultrasonogram for anatomic abnormalities, kidney size, and echogenicity

DIAGNOSTIC PROCEDURES

- Possible renal biopsy

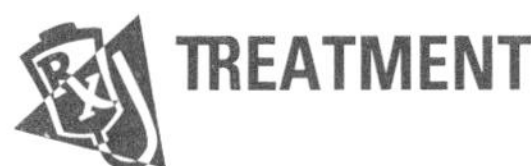

TREATMENT

MEDICATIONS

- Acute hyperkalemia: calcium chloride or gluconate IV, insulin administration with glucose IV, bicarbonate IV, and ion exchange resin (sodium polystyrene sulfonate) PO or PR, cardiac monitoring
- Chronic hyperkalemia: dietary potassium restriction, sodium polystyrene sulfonate, 15–30 g PO QD in juice or sorbitol
- Acid–base disorders: sodium bicarbonate, calcium bicarbonate, or sodium citrate 20–30 mmol/day divided into 2 doses, titrated to maintain serum bicarbonate at > 20 mEq/L
- Hypertension: salt and water restriction, weight loss, decreased salt diet (4–6 to 2 g/day), angiotensin-converting enzyme (ACE) inhibitors or angiotensin II receptor blockers (if serum potassium and GFR permit), calcium channel-blocking agents, diuretics, and β-blocking agents; clonidine, hydralazine, minoxidil as adjunctive drugs
- Congestive heart failure: salt and water restriction, loop diuretics; avoid ACE inhibitors if serum creatinine > 3 mg/dL
- Anemia
  - Recombinant erythropoietin, 50 U/kg (3000–4000 U/dose) 1× or 2× week IV or SC
  - Ferrous sulfate, 325 mg QD–TID if serum ferritin < 100 ng/mL or if iron saturation < 20–25%
- Coagulopathy: dialysis
  - Desmopressin, 25 μg IV Q 8–12 h for 2 doses for surgery
  - Conjugated estrogens, 0.6 mg/kg diluted in 50 mL of 0.9% sodium chloride infused over 30–40 min QD, or 2.5–5 mg PO QD for 5–7 days; effect lasts several weeks
- Renal osteodystrophy, osteomalacia
  - Dietary phosphorus restriction
  - Oral phosphorus-binding agents such as calcium carbonate or calcium acetate given in divided doses 3–4× daily with meals titrated to a serum calcium of 10 mg/dL and serum phosphorus ≤ 4.5 mg/dL
  - Vitamin D or vitamin D analogs (if iPTH > 2–3× normal), serum phosphate and calcium adequately low
  - Calcitriol 0.25–0.5 μg QD or QOD

THERAPEUTIC PROCEDURES

- Renal transplantation
- Hemodialysis, peritoneal dialysis
  - Uremic symptoms (eg, pericarditis, encephalopathy, coagulopathy)
  - Fluid overload unresponsive to diuresis
  - Refractory hyperkalemia
  - Severe metabolic acidosis (pH < 7.20)
  - Neurological symptoms (eg, seizures, neuropathy)
- Dialysis Outcomes Quality Initiative guidelines: Begin dialysis in nondiabetics at GFR of 10 mL/min or serum creatinine of 8 mg/dL, in diabetics at GFR of 15 mL/min or serum creatinine of 6 mg/dL

Diet

- Protein restriction to < 1 g/kg/day; if beneficial, < 0.6 g/kg/day
- Salt restriction to ≤ 2 g/day sodium for nondialysis patient approaching end-stage renal disease
- Water restriction to < 1–2 L /day
- Potassium restriction to < 60–70 mEq/day
- Phosphorus restriction to < 5–10 mg/kg/day
- Magnesium-containing laxatives and antacids contraindicated

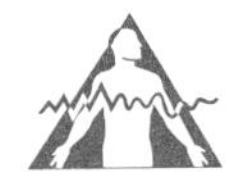

OUTCOME

FOLLOW-UP

- Check serum creatinine and potassium within 9–10 days if ACE inhibitors used

PROGNOSIS

- Mortality is higher for patients on dialysis than for age-matched controls; annual mortality rate is 22.4 deaths per 100 patient years
- Common causes of death: cardiac dysfunction (48%), infection (15%), cerebrovascular disease (6%), and malignancy (4%)

WHEN TO REFER

- Refer to nephrologist when GFR ≤ 60 mL/min for comanagement

WHEN TO ADMIT

- Congestive heart failure, pericarditis
- Severe acid–base or electrolyte disturbances or uremia

EVIDENCE

PRACTICE GUIDELINES

- Locatelli F et al: Revised European best practice guidelines for the management of anaemia in patients with chronic renal failure. Nephrol Dial Transplant 2004;19(Suppl 2):ii1. [PMID: 15206425]
- National Kidney Foundation: Kidney Disease Outcomes Quality Initiative (K/DOQI) Practice Guidelines
  - http://www.kidney.org/professionals/kdoqi/guidelines.cfm
- Parker TF III et al: The chronic kidney disease initiative. J Am Soc Nephrol 2004;15:708. [PMID: 14978173]

WEB SITE

- National Kidney Foundation
  - http://www.kidney.org/

INFORMATION FOR PATIENTS

- Mayo Clinic: Kidney Failure
  - http://www.mayoclinic.com/invoke.cfm?id=DS00280
- MedlinePlus: Kidney Failure
  - http://www.nlm.nih.gov/medlineplus/tutorials/kidneyfailure/htm/index.htm
- National Kidney Foundation: Dialysis
  - http://www.kidney.org/atoz/atozItem.cfm?id=39

REFERENCES

- Barry JM: Current status of renal transplantation. Patient evaluations and outcomes. Urol Clin North Am 2001;28:677. [PMID: 11791486]
- McCarthy JR: A practical approach to the management of patients with chronic renal failure. Mayo Clin Proc 1999;74:269. [PMID: 10089997]
- Ramanathan V et al: Renal transplantation. Semin Nephrol 2001;21:213. [PMID: 112457820]
- Ruggenenti P et al: Progression, remission, regression of chronic renal diseases. Lancet 2001;357:1601. [PMID: 11377666]

Author(s)

Suzanne Watnick, MD
Gail Morrison, MD

Respiratory Syncytial Virus p. 1145. Retinal Detachment p. 1146.

Rhabdomyolysis

KEY FEATURES

ESSENTIALS OF DIAGNOSIS

- Necrosis of skeletal muscle
- Can be encountered in a wide variety of clinical settings, alone or in concert with other disorders of muscle

GENERAL CONSIDERATIONS

- Rhabdomyolysis is generally seen with concomitant myopathy, though the term rhabdomyolysis refers only to a test abnormality
- Commonly due to a syndrome of crush injury to muscle, associated with myoglobinuria, renal insufficiency, markedly elevated creatine kinase (CK) levels, and, frequently, multiorgan failure as a consequence of other complications of the trauma

Causes

- Crush injury
- Prolonged immobility, eg, drug overdose, exposure, hypothermia
- Statin use
- Myositis, eg, polymyositis, dermatomyositis
- Seizure
- Strenuous exercise or heat stroke
- Hypokalemia or hypophosphatemia
- Severe volume contraction
- Acute alcoholic intoxication (rare)

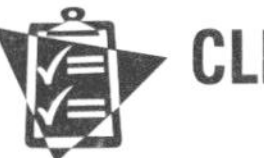

CLINICAL FINDINGS

SYMPTOMS AND SIGNS

- Often there is little evidence for muscle injury on external examination of these patients—and specifically, neither myalgia nor myopathy is present
- Can be associated with myopathy (objective weakness of muscle) or myalgias (pain in the muscle)

DIFFERENTIAL DIAGNOSIS

- Myopathy without muscle necrosis or elevated creatine phosphokinase, eg, endocrine causes of hyperthyroidism, Cushing's syndrome
- Other cause of myalgia, eg, influenza
- Polymyalgia rheumatica
- A simple intramuscular injection may cause some elevation of CK

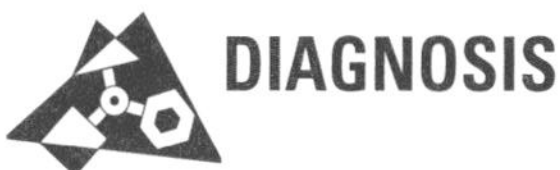

DIAGNOSIS

LABORATORY TESTS

- Elevated serum CK is the biochemical indicator of skeletal muscle necrosis
- A urinary dipstick testing positive for blood (due to myoglobinuria) in the absence of red blood cells in the sediment
- Elevations of alanine aminotransferase and lactate dehydrogenase may be present, and may have been obtained for other reasons, such as suspected liver disease or hemolysis. When these tests are disproportionately elevated, confirm that they are not of muscle origin with a CK determination

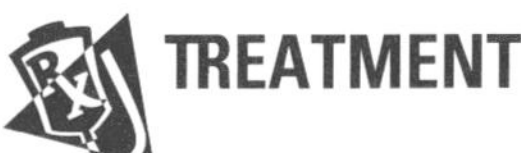

TREATMENT

MEDICATIONS

- Vigorous fluid resuscitation
- Mannitol 100 mg IV QD for 3 days
- Alkalinization of the urine with 2 ampules of sodium bicarbonate in 1 L D_5 1/2 normal saline

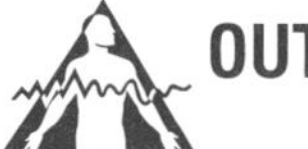

OUTCOME

COMPLICATIONS

- Renal insufficiency due to myoglobinuria is caused by tubular damage resulting from filtered myoglobin and is nearly always associated with hypovolemia

PROGNOSIS

- Renal insufficiency is usually reversible with hydration. The role of urine alkalinization is unproven

EVIDENCE

PRACTICE GUIDELINES

- American Academy of Family Physicians
  - http://www.aafp.org/afp/20020301/907.html

INFORMATION FOR PATIENTS

- National Institutes of Health
  - http://www.nlm.nih.gov/medlineplus/ency/article/000473.htm

REFERENCES

- Allison RC et al: The other medical causes of rhabdomyolysis. Am J Med Sci 2003;326:79. [PMID: 12920439]
- Thompson PD et al: Statin-associated myopathy. JAMA 2003;289:1681. [PMID: 12672737]

Author(s)

David B. Hellmann, MD, FACP
John H. Stone, MD, MPH

Rheumatoid Arthritis

Rheumatic Manifestations of Cancer p. 1146. Rheumatic Manifestations of HIV p. 1146. Rheumatism, Palindromic p. 1147.

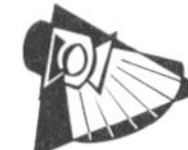

KEY FEATURES

ESSENTIALS OF DIAGNOSIS

- Prodromal systemic symptoms of malaise, fever, weight loss, and morning stiffness
- Onset usually insidious and in small joints; progression is centripetal and symmetric; deformities common
- Radiographic findings: juxtaarticular osteoporosis, joint erosions, and narrowing of the joint spaces
- Rheumatoid factor usually present
- Anti-cyclic citrullinated peptide (CCP) test also usually positive
- Extraarticular manifestations: subcutaneous nodules, pleural effusion, pericarditis, lymphadenopathy, splenomegaly with leukopenia, and vasculitis

GENERAL CONSIDERATIONS

- A chronic systemic inflammatory disease of unknown cause, primarily affecting synovial membranes of multiple joints
- The pathological findings in the joint include chronic synovitis with pannus formation. The pannus erodes cartilage, bone, ligaments, and tendons

DEMOGRAPHICS

- Female patients outnumber males almost 3:1
- Usual age at onset is 20–40 years

CLINICAL FINDINGS

SYMPTOMS AND SIGNS

- Prodromal symptoms of malaise, weight loss, and vague periarticular pain or stiffness
- Characteristically symmetric joint swelling with associated warmth, tenderness, and pain
- Prominent morning stiffness persisting for over 30 min that subsides during the day
- Proximal interphalangeal (PIP) and metacarpophalangeal (MCP) joints of the fingers, wrists, knees, ankles, and toes are the most often involved joint
- Entrapment syndromes—particularly of the median nerve at the carpal tunnel
- Subcutaneous nodules (20% of patients); most commonly over bony prominences but also in the bursas and tendon sheaths
- After months or years, deformities may occur; the most common are ulnar deviation of the fingers, boutonniere deformity [hyperextension of the distal interphalangeal (DIP) joint with flexion of the PIP joint], "swan-neck" deformity (flexion of the DIP joint with extension of the PIP joint), and valgus deformity of the knee
- Dryness of the eyes, mouth, and other mucous membranes, especially in advanced disease
- Eye: episcleritis, scleritis, peripheral ulcerative keratitis, and in severe cases, the corneal melt syndrome of scleromalacia perforans

DIFFERENTIAL DIAGNOSIS

- Gout with tophi (mistaken for nodules)
- Systemic lupus erythematosus
- Parvovirus B19 infection
- Osteoarthritis or inflammatory osteoarthritis
- Septic arthritis
- Polymyalgia rheumatica
- Hemochromatosis (MCP and wrist joints)
- Lyme disease
- Rheumatic fever
- Rubella arthritis
- Hepatitis B or C
- Palindromic rheumatism
- Hypertrophic pulmonary osteoarthropathy (paraneoplastic)
- Systemic vasculitis, especially polyarteritis nodosa, mixed cryoglobulinemia, and antineutrophil cytoplasmic antibody-associated vasculitides

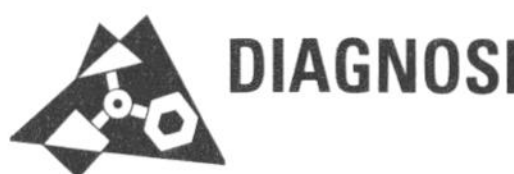

DIAGNOSIS

LABORATORY TESTS

- Rheumatoid factor, an IgM antibody directed against the Fc fragment of IgG, is present in the sera of more than 75% of patients
- Tests for anti–CCP antibody may be even more sensitive
- During both the acute and chronic phases, the erythrocyte sedimentation rate and the γ-globulins (most commonly IgM and IgG) are typically elevated
- A moderate hypochromic normocytic anemia is common
- The white blood cell count is normal or slightly elevated, but leukopenia may occur, often in the presence of splenomegaly (eg, Felty's syndrome)
- The platelet count is often elevated, roughly in proportion to the severity of overall joint inflammation
- Joint fluid examination is valuable, reflecting abnormalities that are associated with varying degrees of inflammation (see Tables 77 and 78)

IMAGING STUDIES

- X-ray changes are the most specific for rheumatoid arthritis. X-rays, however, are not sensitive in that most of those taken during the first 6 months are read as normal
- The earliest changes occur in the wrists or feet and consist of soft tissue swelling and juxtaarticular demineralization. Later, diagnostic changes of uniform joint space narrowing and erosions develop

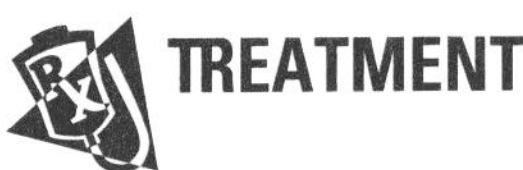

TREATMENT

MEDICATIONS

- Nonsteroidal antiinflammatory drugs (NSAIDs) are the first-line drugs. They have analgesic and antiinflammatory effects but do not prevent erosions or alter the progression of the disease
- Cyclooxygenase (COX)-2 inhibitors are just as effective and less likely to cause clinically significant upper gastrointestinal hemorrhage or ulceration
- Long-term use of COX-2 inhibitors, particularly in the absence of concomitant aspirin use, has been associated with increased risk of cardiovascular events
- Disease-modifying antirheumatic drugs (DMARDs) should be started as soon as the diagnosis is certain
- Methotrexate is the treatment of choice for patients who fail to respond to NSAIDs. It is generally well tolerated and often produces a beneficial effect in 2–6 weeks
- Tumor necrosis factor inhibitors work faster than methotrexate and may replace that drug as the remitting agent of first choice
- Hydroxychloroquine is useful for patients with mild disease
- Corticosteroids usually produce an immediate and dramatic antiinflammatory effect, and they may slow the rate of bony destruction
- Corticosteroids may be used on a short-term basis to tide patients over acute disabling episodes, to facilitate other treatment measures (eg, physical therapy), or to manage serious extraarticular manifestations (eg, pericarditis, perforating eye lesions)
- Corticosteroids may also be indicated for active and progressive disease that does not respond favorably to conservative management and when there are contraindications to or therapeutic failure of other agents
- Leflunomide, a pyrimidine synthesis inhibitor, is also FDA approved for treatment of rheumatoid arthritis (RA)
- Anakinra, a recombinant form of human interleukin-1 receptor antagonist, may be given to adult patients who have failed one or more DMARDs

SURGERY

- Long-standing, severe, erosive disease may benefit from joint replacements
- Hips, knees, shoulders, and metacarpophalangeal joints may benefit from replacement in cases of advanced destruction

THERAPEUTIC PROCEDURES

- Nonpharmacological: physical therapy, occupational therapy, joint rest, exercise, splinting, heat and cold, assist devices, and splints
- Intraarticular corticosteroids (triamcinolone, 10–40 mg) may be helpful if one or two joints are the primary source of difficulty

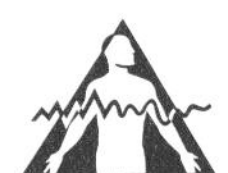

OUTCOME

FOLLOW-UP

- Frequent follow-up early after diagnosis to ensure appropriate patient education and response to treatment
- Patients on DMARDs require monitoring of blood cell counts and hepatic and renal function every 6–8 weeks

COMPLICATIONS

- Joint destruction
- Rheumatoid vasculitis (eg, skin ulcers, vasculitic neuropathy, pericarditis)
- Osteoporosis
- Cushing's syndrome from corticosteroids

PROGNOSIS

- Patients who present with polyarthritis that appears to be (but probably is not) RA experience remission 50–75% within 2 years
- Patients whose joint symptoms persist beyond 2 years die, on average, 10–15 years earlier than people without RA
- Patients who have polyarthritis lasting more than 12 weeks are at greatest risk for persistent disease and are candidates for aggressive therapy

WHEN TO REFER

- Progressive disease despite therapy
- Refer early to a physical or occupational therapist

WHEN TO ADMIT

- Admission is sometimes required at diagnosis to exclude other entities
- Superimposed septic arthritis
- Rheumatoid vasculitis
- Severe ocular inflammatory disease (eg, impending corneal melt)

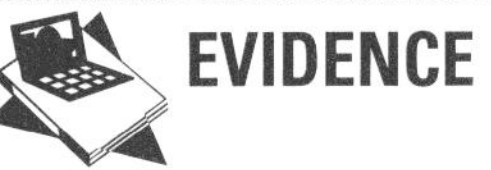

EVIDENCE

PRACTICE GUIDELINES

- American College of Rheumatology
  - http://www.rheumatology.org/publications/guidelines/raguidelines02.asp?aud=mem

WEB SITES

- American College of Rheumatology
  - http://www.rheumatology.org
- Arthritis Foundation
  - http://www.arthritis.org

INFORMATION FOR PATIENTS

- Arthritis Foundation
  - http://www.arthritis.org/conditions/DiseaseCenter/ra.asp
- National Institute of Arthritis and Musculoskeletal and Skin Diseases
  - http://www.niams.nih.gov/hi/topics/arthritis/rahandout.htm

REFERENCES

- Edwards JC et al: Efficacy of B cell-targeted therapy with rituximab in patients with rheumatoid arthritis. N Engl J Med 2004;350:2572. [PMID: 15201414]
- Kremer JM et al: Treatment of rheumatoid arthritis by selective inhibition of T-cell activation with fusion protein CTLA4Ig. N Engl J Med 2003;349: 1907. [PMID: 14614165]
- O'Dell JR: Therapeutic strategies for rheumatoid arthritis. N Engl J Med 2004;350:2591. [PMID: 15201416]
- Quinn MA et al: Very early treatment with infliximab in addition to methotrexate in early, poor-prognosis rheumatoid arthritis. Arthritis Rheum 2005;52:27. [PMID: 15641102]
- van Everdingen AA et al: Low-dose prednisone therapy for patients with early active rheumatoid arthritis: clinical efficacy, disease-modifying properties, and side effects. A randomized, double-blind, placebo-controlled clinical trial. Ann Intern Med 2002;136:1. [PMID: 11777359]

Author(s)

David B. Hellmann, MD, FACP

John H. Stone, MD, MPH

Rhinitis, Allergic

KEY FEATURES

ESSENTIALS OF DIAGNOSIS

- Seasonal occurrence of watery eyes, sneezing, itchy nose and eyes
- May be associated with lower respiratory symptoms
- Environmental aeroallergen exposure
- An inflammatory response orchestrated by an allergen-specific IgE antibody
- Eosinophilia of nasal secretions and occasionally of blood
- Skin tests usually of little value

GENERAL CONSIDERATIONS

- "Hay fever" symptoms are similar to those of viral rhinitis but are usually persistent and show seasonal variation and are not associated with constitutional symptoms of fever or myalgia
- Nasal symptoms are often accompanied by eye irritation (allergic conjunctivitis), which causes pruritus, erythema, and excessive tearing
- Up to 40% of patients manifest lower respiratory symptoms: cough, wheezing, chest tightness, or dyspnea
- Can be associated with eczematous dermatitis, pruritis

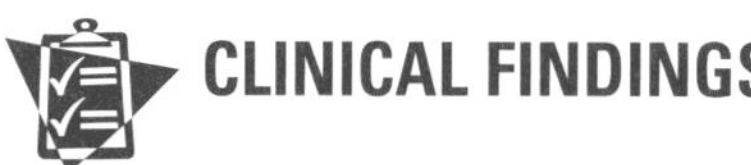

CLINICAL FINDINGS

SYMPTOMS AND SIGNS

- Physical examination may reveal inflamed, edematous, or even pale boggy nasal mucosa
- The mucosa of the turbinates is usually pale or violaceous because of venous engorgement; this is in contrast to the erythema of viral rhinitis
- Nasal polyps, which are yellowish boggy masses of hypertrophic mucosa, may be seen

DIFFERENTIAL DIAGNOSIS

- Viral rhinitis (common cold)
- Viral conjunctivitis
- Vasomotor rhinitis (eg, cold air or irritant-induced)
- Acute or chronic sinusitis
- Rhinitis medicamentosa (drug-induced rhinitis)
- Nasal polyposis
- Foreign body
- Wegener's granulomatosis

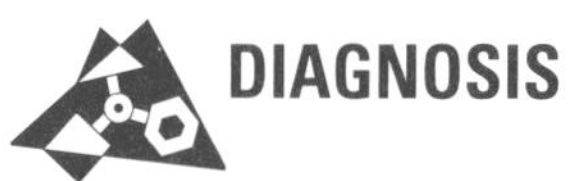

DIAGNOSIS

LABORATORY TESTS

- Usually a clinical diagnosis
- Confirmation of IgE-mediated hypersensitivity to aeroallergens is occasionally indicated
- Allergy skin tests or radioallergosorbent testing (RAST) or enzyme-linked immunosobent assay (ELISA) are available to detect specific IgE

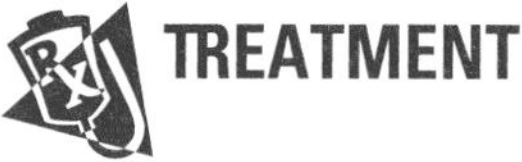

TREATMENT

MEDICATIONS

- The choice of medications is guided by the predominant symptoms (Table 75)

Intranasal corticosteroid sprays

- Mainstay of treatment
- More effective—and frequently less expensive—than nonsedating antihistamines
- There may be a delay in onset of relief of 1–2 weeks
- May also shrink nasal polyps, thereby providing an improved nasal airway and delaying or eliminating the indications for endoscopic sinus surgery
- Beclomethasone (42 μg/spray BID each nostril), flunisolide (25 μg/spray BID each nostril), mometasone furoate (200 μg QD per nostril), and fluticasone propionate (200 μg QD per nostril); the latter two synthetic glucocorticoids appear to have higher topical potencies and lipid solubility and reduced systemic bioavailability, suggesting possible practical advantages

Over-the-counter antihistamines

- Loratidine, 10 mg QD (less sedating than other OTC antihistamines)
- Brompheniramine or chlorpheniramine (4 mg PO Q 6–8 h, or 8–12 mg PO Q 8–12 h as a sustained-release tablet)
- Clemastine (1.34–2.68 mg PO BID)

H_1 receptor antagonists

- Cetirizine (10 mg PO QD), fexofenadine (60 mg PO BID or 120 mg PO QD); fexofenadine appears to be nonsedating and cetirizine mildly sedating; ebastine (10–20 mg PO QD) and misolastine (10 mg PO QD)
- H_1 receptor antagonist antihistamine nasal sprays include levocabastine (0.2 mg BID) and azelastine (two sprays per nostril, 1.1 mg/day)

Anticholinergic agents

- Intranasal anticholinergic agents such as ipratropium bromide 0.03% (42 μg per nostril TID) sprays when rhinorrhea is a major symptom
- Intranasal cromolyn spray prior to the onset of seasonal symptoms

Sympathomimetics

- Particularly effective for nasal symptoms, but prolonged topical use may lead to rebound vasodilation, called rhinitis medicamentosa

Cromolyn sodium and sodium nedocromil

- Pretreatment with these drugs prevents response to allergen
- Action is short-lived, so they need to be taken TID to QID
- Much less potent than topical corticosteroids, but these drugs have very few side effects

Immunotherapy

- Repeated long-term injection of allergen is an effective method for reducing or eliminating symptoms and signs of allergic disorders
- Recommended for patients with severe allergic rhinitis who respond poorly to medications or whose allergens are not avoidable
- Unequivocally effective in allergic rhinitis and allergic conjunctivitis

OUTCOME

WHEN TO REFER

- Moderate to severe cases, when avoidance measures, antihistamine administration, and nasal corticosteroids do not adequately control symptoms
- Associated persistent asthma
- Recurrent sinusitis
- Nasal polyposis

PREVENTION

- Allergen avoidance is most important, including staying indoors when pollen counts are high, avoiding pets, and reducing indoor dust and mold
- Washing or otherwise treating the fur of a live pet animal does not reduce allergenicity
- Maintaining an allergen-free environment by covering pillows and mattresses with plastic covers, substituting synthetic materials (foam mattress, acrylics) for animal products (wool, horsehair) and removing dust-collecting household fixtures (carpets, drapes, bedspreads, wicker) is worth the attempt to help more troubled patients
- Air purifiers and dust filters (such as Bionair models) may also aid in maintaining an allergen-free environment

EVIDENCE

PRACTICE GUIDELINES

- National Guideline Clearinghouse: Allergic Rhinitis
  - http://www.guideline.gov/summary/summary.aspx?doc_id=3373&nbr=2599&string=allergic+AND+rhinitis
- van Cauwenberge P et al: Consensus statement on the treatment of allergic rhinitis. European Academy of Allergology and Clinical Immunology. Allergy 2000;55:116. [PMID: 10726726]

WEB SITES

- Allergy, Asthma & Immunology Online: Rhinitis
  - http://allergy.mcg.edu/advice/rhin.html
- American Academy of Allergy, Asthma and Immunology
  - http://www.aaaai.org

INFORMATION FOR PATIENTS

- American Academy of Allergy, Asthma and Immunology: Allergic Rhinitis
  - http://www.aaaai.org/patients/resources/easy_reader/rhinitis.pdf
- JAMA patient page: Seasonal allergic rhinitis. JAMA 2001;286:3038.
- MedlinePlus: Allergic Rhinitis
  - http://www.nlm.nih.gov/medlineplus/ency/article/000813.htm

REFERENCES

- Abramson MJ et al: Allergen immunotherapy for asthma. Cochrane Database Syst Rev 2000;(2):CD001186. Update in Cochrane Database Syst Rev 2003;(4):CD001186. [PMID: 10796617]
- Finegold I: Immunotherapy in the age of anti-IgE. Clin Rev Allergy Immunol 2004;27:75. [PMID: 15576891]
- Iglesias-Cadarso A et al: A prospective safety study of allergen immunotherapy in daily clinical practice. Allergol Immunopathol (Madr) 2004;32:278. [PMID: 15456624]
- Moller C et al: Pollen immunotherapy reduces the development of asthma in children with seasonal rhinoconjunctivitis (the PAT-study). J Allergy Clin Immunol 2002;109:251. [PMID: 11842293]

Author(s)

Jeffrey L. Kishiyama, MD
Daniel C. Adelman, MD
Michael J. Kaplan, MD

Rosacea

Riboflavin Deficiency p. 1147. Right Middle Lobe Syndrome p. 1147.
Rocky Mountain Spotted Fever. p. 1148.

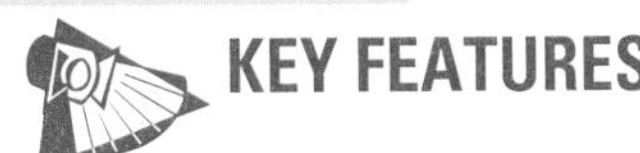

KEY FEATURES

ESSENTIALS OF DIAGNOSIS

- A chronic facial disorder of middle-aged and older people
- A vascular component (erythema and telangiectasis) and a tendency to flush easily
- An acneiform component (papules and pustules) may also be present
- A glandular component accompanied by hyperplasia of the soft tissue of the nose (rhinophyma)

GENERAL CONSIDERATIONS

- Rosacea is usually a lifelong affliction, so maintenance therapy is required
- A chronic facial disorder of middle-aged and older people

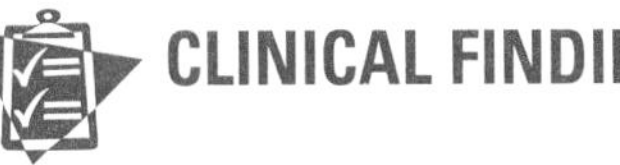

CLINICAL FINDINGS

SYMPTOMS AND SIGNS

- See Table 7
- The cheeks, nose, and chin—at times the entire face—may have a rosy hue
- No comedones
- Inflammatory papules are prominent, and there may be pustules
- Associated seborrhea may be found
- The patient often complains of burning or stinging with episodes of flushing
- It is not uncommon for patients to have associated ophthalmic disease, including blepharitis and keratitis

DIFFERENTIAL DIAGNOSIS

- Acne vulgaris
- Seborrheic dermatitis
- Topical steroid use
- Perioral dermatitis
- Systemic lupus erythematosus
- Carcinoid
- Dermatomyositis
- Rosacea is distinguished from acne by age, the presence of the vascular component, and the absence of comedones
- The rosy hue of rosacea is due to inflammation and telangiectases and generally will pinpoint the diagnosis
- Topical steroids can change trivial dermatoses of the face into perioral dermatitis and steroid rosacea

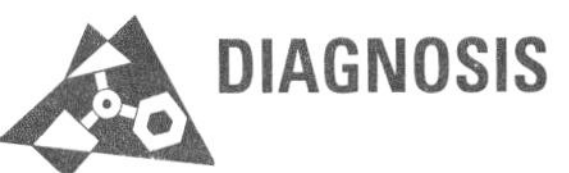

DIAGNOSIS

LABORATORY TESTS

- Clinical diagnosis

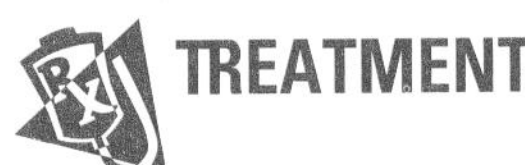

TREATMENT

MEDICATIONS

- See Table 6
- Medications are directed only at the inflammatory papules and pustules and the erythema that surrounds them

Local therapy

- Metronidazole, 0.75% gel applied twice daily or 1% cream once daily, is the topical treatment of choice
- If metronidazole is not tolerated, topical clindamycin (solution, gel, or lotion) used twice daily is effective
- Erythromycin as described above may be helpful (see *Acne vulgaris*)
- Five to eight weeks of treatment may be needed for significant response

Systemic therapy

- Tetracycline or erythromycin, 250 or 500 mg PO BID on an empty stomach, should be used when topical therapy is inadequate
- Minocycline or doxycycline, 50–100 mg PO QD or BID, may work in refractory cases
- Isotretinoin may succeed where other measures fail; a dosage of 0.5–1 mg/kg/day orally for 12–28 weeks is recommended
- Metronidazole, 250 mg PO BID for 3 weeks, may be worth trying but is seldom required; side effects are few, though metronidazole may produce a disulfiram-like effect when the patient ingests alcohol

SURGERY

- The only satisfactory treatment for the telangiectasias is laser surgery
- Rhinophyma (soft tissue and sebaceous hyperplasia of the nose) responds to surgical debulking

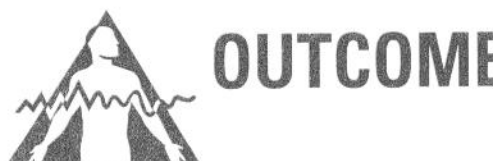

OUTCOME

PROGNOSIS

- Rosacea tends to be a stubborn and persistent process
- With the regimens described above, it can usually be controlled adequately

WHEN TO REFER

- If there is a question about the diagnosis, if recommended therapy is ineffective, or if specialized treatment is necessary

EVIDENCE

PRACTICE GUIDELINES

- Wilkin J et al: Standard classification of rosacea: Report of the National Rosacea Society Expert Committee on the Classification and Staging of Rosacea. J Am Acad Dermatol 2002;46:584. [PMID: 11907512]

WEB SITES

- American Academy of Dermatology
  - http://www.aad.org
- National Rosacea Society: Physician Information
  - http://www.rosacea.org/physicians/index.html

INFORMATION FOR PATIENTS

- American Academy of Dermatology: What is Rosacea?
  - http://www.skincarephysicians.com/rosaceanet/whatis.html
- American Academy of Family Physicians: Rosacea and Its Treatment
  - http://familydoctor.org/155.xml
- National Institute for Arthritis and Musculoskeletal and Skin Diseases: Questions and Answers About Rosacea
  - http://www.niams.nih.gov/hi/topics/rosacea/rosacea.htm
- National Rosacea Society: Frequently Asked Questions
  - http://www.rosacea.org/patients/faq.html

REFERENCE

- Powell FC: Rosacea. N Engl J Med 2005;352:793. [PMID: 15728812]

Author(s)

Timothy G. Berger, MD

Salicylate Poisoning

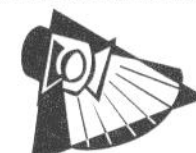

KEY FEATURES

ESSENTIALS OF DIAGNOSIS

- Tachypnea, altered mental status
- Metabolic acidosis
- Typical arterial blood gases reveal respiratory alkalosis and metabolic acidosis
- Elevated salicylate level diagnostic

GENERAL CONSIDERATIONS

- Salicylates (eg, aspirin, methyl salicylate) are found in a variety of over-the-counter and prescription medications
- Salicylates uncouple cellular oxidative phosphorylation, resulting in anaerobic metabolism and excessive production of lactic acid and heat, and interfere with several Krebs cycle enzymes
- A single ingestion of more than 200 mg/kg of salicylate is likely to produce significant acute intoxication
- Poisoning may also occur as a result of chronic excessive dosing over several days
- Although the half-life of salicylate is 2–3 h after small doses, it may increase to 20 h or more in patients with intoxication

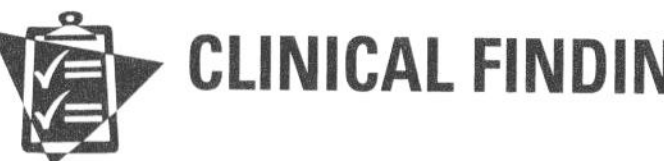

CLINICAL FINDINGS

SYMPTOMS AND SIGNS

- **Acute ingestion**
  - Nausea and vomiting, occasionally with gastritis
- **Moderate intoxication**
  - Hyperpnea (deep and rapid breathing), tachycardia, and tinnitus
- **Serious intoxication**
  - Agitation, confusion, seizures, coma
  - Cardiovascular collapse, pulmonary edema, hyperthermia
  - Death

DIFFERENTIAL DIAGNOSIS

- Other causes of anion gap acidosis (eg, alcoholic ketoacidosis, metformin toxicity, isoniazid poisoning, iron poisoning, methanol or ethylene glycol toxicity, carbon monoxide poisoning)
- Acetaminophen poisoning (common coingestion)

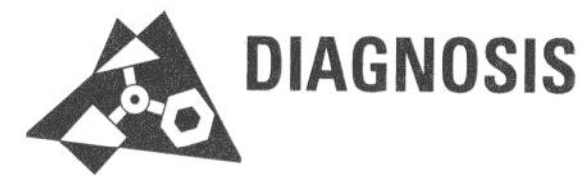

DIAGNOSIS

LABORATORY TESTS

- Diagnosis is suspected in any patient with metabolic acidosis and is confirmed by measuring the stat serum salicylate level
- Patients with levels greater than 100 mg/dL (1000 mg/L) after an acute overdose are more likely to have severe poisoning
- Patients with subacute or chronic intoxication may suffer severe symptoms with levels of only 60–70 mg/dL
- The arterial blood gas typically reveals a respiratory alkalosis with an underlying metabolic acidosis
- Anion gap metabolic acidosis
- The prothrombin time is often elevated owing to salicylate-induced hypoprothrombinemia

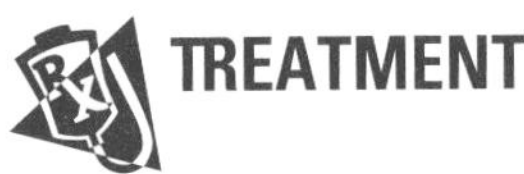

TREATMENT

MEDICATIONS

Emergency and supportive measures

- Administer activated charcoal, 60–100 g PO or via gastric tube, mixed in aqueous slurry
- Repeated doses may be given to ensure gastrointestinal adsorption or enhance elimination of the drug
- Do not use for comatose or convulsing patients unless it can be given by gastric tube and the airway is protected by a cuffed endotracheal tube
- Extra doses of activated charcoal may be needed in patients who ingest more than 10 g of aspirin (desired ratio of charcoal to aspirin: ~10:1 by weight); although this cannot always be given as a single dose, it may be administered over the first 24 h in divided doses every 2–4 h
- Treat metabolic acidosis with IV sodium bicarbonate; this is critical because acidosis (acidemia, pH < 7.40) promotes greater entry of salicylate into cells, worsening toxicity

Specific treatment

- Alkalinization of the urine enhances renal salicylate excretion by trapping the salicylate anion in the urine. Add 100 mEq (2 ampules) of sodium bicarbonate to 1 L of 5% dextrose in 0.2% saline, and infuse IV at a rate of ~150–200 mL/h
- Unless the patient is oliguric, add 20–30 mEq of potassium chloride to each liter of IV fluid
- Patients who are volume depleted often fail to produce an alkaline urine (paradoxical aciduria) unless potassium is given

THERAPEUTIC PROCEDURES

- Hemodialysis may be lifesaving and is indicated for patients with severe metabolic acidosis, markedly altered mental status, or significantly elevated salicylate levels [> 100–120 mg/dL (1000–1200 mg/L) after acute overdose or > 60–70 mg/dL (600–700 mg/L) with subacute or chronic intoxication]

OUTCOME

FOLLOW-UP

- Monitor serum salicylate level every 2 h initially to determine if it is continuing to rise
- Patients with massive ingestion (eg, > 100 tablets) may have delayed absorption and require prolonged observation until levels fall into normal range

COMPLICATIONS

- Intubation and controlled ventilation may cause sudden and severe deterioration in patients with marked respiratory alkalosis, if the P_{CO_2} rises and the pH is allowed to fall

WHEN TO ADMIT

- Suicidal ingestion
- History of massive ingestion with rising levels
- Evidence of significant intoxication (altered mental status, metabolic acidosis, elevated salicylate level)

PROGNOSIS

- Good if blood pH is maintained above 7.4 and hemodialysis is promptly performed in patients with serious toxicity

EVIDENCE

PRACTICE GUIDELINES

- Position statement and practice guidelines on the use of multi-dose activated charcoal in the treatment of acute poisoning. American Academy of Clinical Toxicology; European Association of Poisons Centres and Clinical Toxicologists. J Toxicol Clin Toxicol 1999;37:731. [PMID: 10584586]

WEB SITE

- eMedicine: Toxicology Articles
  - http://www.emedicine.com/emerg/toxicology.htm

INFORMATION FOR PATIENTS

- American Association of Poison Control Centers: What Is a Poison Center?
  - http://www.1-800-222-1222.info/poisonCenter/home.asp
- Mayo Clinic: Child Safety: Prevent Poisoning
  - http://www.mayoclinic.com/invoke.cfm?id=HQ01263

REFERENCES

- Chan TY: Ingestion of medicated oils by adults: the risk of severe salicylate poisoning is related to the packaging of these products. Hum Exp Toxicol 2002;21:171. [PMID: 12099617]
- Rivera W et al: Delayed salicylate toxicity at 35 hours without early manifestations following a single salicylate ingestion. Ann Pharmacother 2004;38:1186. [PMID: 15173556]

Author(s)

Kent R. Olson, MD

Sarcocystosis

KEY FEATURES

ESSENTIALS OF DIAGNOSIS

- Two syndromes in humans
  - Enteric form with mild, protracted diarrhea
  - Muscle form with tender swelling over the muscle involvment, fever, eosinophilia

GENERAL CONSIDERATIONS

- The causes of coccidiosis are *Cryptosporidium* spp., particularly *C parvum* and *C hominis, Isospora belli, Cyclospora cayetanensis, Sarcocystis bovihominis,* and *S suihominis*; all but the sarcocystis species complete their life cycle in a single host
- *Sarcocystis* is a two-host coccidian. Human disease occurs as two syndromes, both rare: an enteric infection in which humans are the definitive host and a muscle infection in which humans are an intermediate host

Enteric form

- Sporocysts (9–16 μm) passed in human feces are not infective for humans but must be ingested by cattle or pigs
- Humans become infected by eating poorly cooked beef or pork containing oocysts of *S bovihominis* or *S suihominis*, respectively
- Organisms enter intestinal epithelial cells and are transformed into oocysts that release sporocysts into the feces
- Although the small bowel is the usual location of infection, other sites can be involved

Muscle form

- Results when humans ingest sporocysts in feces from an infected carnivore that has eaten prey that harbored sarcocysts
- The sporocysts liberate sporozoites that invade the intestinal wall and are disseminated to skeletal muscle

DEMOGRAPHICS

- The muscle form occurs worldwide, particularly in the tropics and in regions where hygiene is poor
- The intestinal form has been reported only from Asia

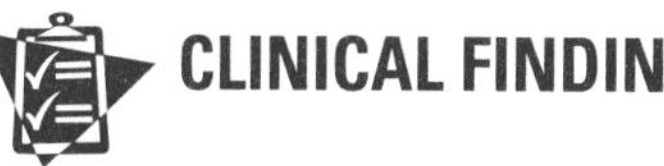

CLINICAL FINDINGS

SYMPTOMS AND SIGNS

- Generally, the forms of diarrhea caused by the coccidial and microsporidial agents are clinically indistinguishable from each other

Intestinal form

- Often asymptomatic or causes mild but protracted diarrhea
- Eosinophilic necrotizing enteritis has been reported

Muscle form

- Subcutaneous and muscular inflammation lasting several days to 2 weeks
- Swellings at the muscle sites, sometimes associated with local erythema, tenderness and myalgia
- Fever
- Eosinophilia
- Sarcocysts are often asymptomatic and are found incidentally at autopsy in cardiac muscle

DIFFERENTIAL DIAGNOSIS

- *Isospora belli, Cyclospora cayetanensis*, and *Sarcocystis*
- Giardiasis
- Viral gastroenteritis, eg, rotavirus
- Other traveler's diarrhea, eg, *Escherichia coli*
- Cryptosporidiosis
- Other causes of diarrhea in AIDS, eg, cytomegalovirus colitis
- Trichinosis

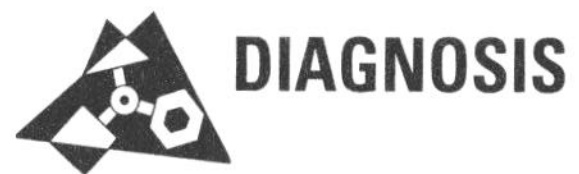

DIAGNOSIS

LABORATORY TESTS

- Diagnosis is by stool examination for oocysts and by biopsy of subcutaneous lesions

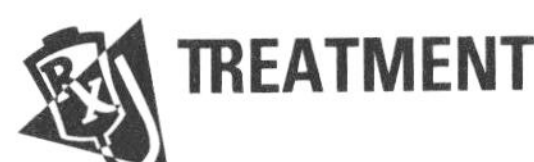

TREATMENT

MEDICATIONS

- No antibiotic treatment is consistently successful; sulfadiazine and tinidazole can be tried

THERAPEUTIC PROCEDURES

- Most acute infections in immunocompetent persons are self-limited and do not require treatment

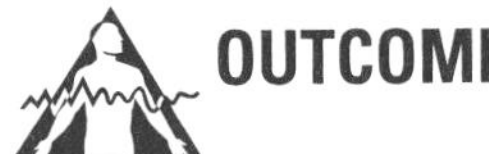

OUTCOME

WHEN TO REFER

- Refer all confirmed or suspected cases with protracted diarrhea, particularly in immunocompromised patients
- Refer all cases of sarcocyst muscle disease

EVIDENCE

INFORMATION FOR PATIENTS

- Department of Natural Resources, Michigan
  - http://www.michigan.gov/dnr/0,1607,7-153-10370_12150_12220-27272--,00.html

REFERENCES

- Ambroise-Thomas P: Parasitic diseases and immunodeficiencies. Parasitology 2001;122(Suppl):S65. [PMID: 11442198]
- Arness MK et al: An outbreak of acute eosinophilic myositis attributed to human *Sarcocystis* parasitism. Am J Trop Med Hyg 1999;61:548. [PMID: 10548287]

Sarcoidosis

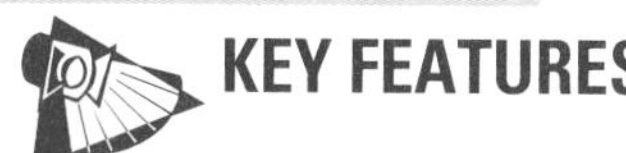

KEY FEATURES

ESSENTIALS OF DIAGNOSIS

- Symptoms related to
  - Lung
  - Skin
  - Eyes
  - Peripheral nerves
  - Liver
  - Kidney
  - Heart
  - Other tissues
- Demonstration of noncaseating granulomas in biopsy specimen
- Exclusion of other granulomatous disorders

GENERAL CONSIDERATIONS

- A systemic disease of unknown etiology
- Granulomatous inflammation of the lungs is present in 90% of cases

DEMOGRAPHICS

- Highest incidence in North American blacks and northern European whites
- Among blacks, women are more frequently affected than men
- Disease onset is usually in the third or fourth decade

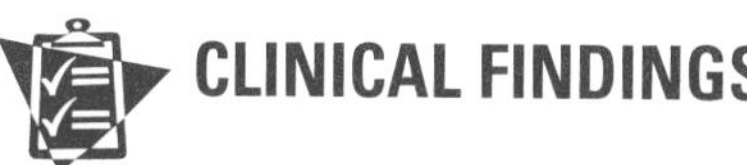

CLINICAL FINDINGS

SYMPTOMS AND SIGNS

- Malaise, fever, and insidious dyspnea
- Symptoms referable to the skin, eyes, peipheral nerves, liver, kidney, or heart may also prompt initial evaluation
- Some patients are asymptomatic and are diagnosed after abnormal findings are noted on chest x-ray
- Crackles are uncommon on chest examination
- Erythema nodosum, parotid gland enlargement, hepatosplenomegaly, and lymphadenopathy may be noted
- Myocardial sarcoidosis is found in 5% of patients and can lead to
  - Restrictive cardiomyopathy
  - Arrhythmias
  - Conduction disturbances

DIFFERENTIAL DIAGNOSIS

- Other granulomatous diseases must be excluded
- Tuberculosis
- Lymphoma (including lymphocytic interstitial pneumonitis)
- Histoplasmosis
- Coccidioidomycosis
- Idiopathic pulmonary fibrosis
- Pneumoconiosis (especially berylliosis)
- Syphilis

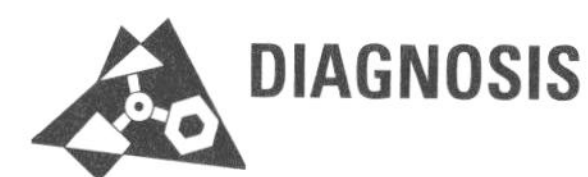

DIAGNOSIS

LABORATORY TESTS

- Leukopenia
- Elevation of erythrocyte sedimentation rate
- Hypercalcemia in 5%, hypercalciuria in 20%
- Angiotensin-converting enzyme (ACE) levels are commonly elevated in active disease; this finding is neither sensitive nor specific enough to be of diagnostic value
- Pulmonary function tests may show obstruction or restriction, with diminished diffusion capacity

IMAGING STUDIES

- Radiographic findings are variable
  - Stage I: hilar adenopathy alone
  - Stage II: hilar adenopathy with parenchymal involvement
  - Stage III: parenchymal involvement alone
- Parenchymal involvement usually manifests as diffuse reticular infiltrates, but focal infiltrates, acinar shadows, nodules, and rare cavitation are seen
- Pleural effusion occurs in < 10% of patients

DIAGNOSTIC PROCEDURES

- Biopsy demonstrating noncaseating granulomas is required for diagnosis
- Easily accessible biopsy sites include lymph nodes, skin lesions, and salivary glands
- Transbronchial biopsy has a yield of 75–90%
- Bronchoalveolar lavage is usually characterized by an increase in lymphocytes with a high CD4/CD8 ratio; this may be used to follow disease activity, but not for diagnosis
- Some experts believe biopsy is unnecessary in stage I disease with a presentation highly suggestive of sarcoidosis

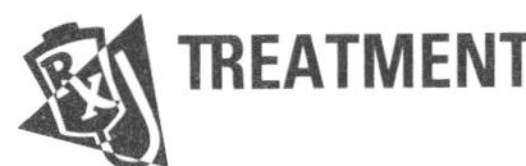

TREATMENT

MEDICATIONS

- Corticosteroids (oral prednisone, 0.5–1.0 mg/kg/day) are indicated for
  - Constitutional symptoms
  - Hypercalcemia
  - Iritis
  - Arthritis
  - Central nervous system involvement
  - Cardiac involvement
  - Hepatitis
  - Cutaneous lesions other than erythema nodosum
  - Symptomatic pulmonary lesions
- Long-term therapy is usually required over months to years
- Immunosuppressive drugs and cyclosporine have been tried when benefits of steroid therapy have been exhausted

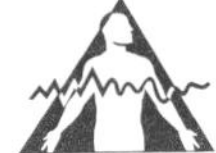

OUTCOME

FOLLOW-UP

- At a minimum, yearly physical examination, pulmonary function studies, chemistry panel, ophthalmologic evaluation, chest x-ray, and ECG

COMPLICATIONS

- Hemoptysis
- Pneumothorax
- Mycetoma formation in lung cavities
- Respiratory failure in advanced disease

PROGNOSIS

- 20% of patients with lung involvement suffer irreversible lung impairment, with progressive fibrosis, bronchiectasis, and cavitation
- Outlook is best for patients with stage I disease, worse with radiographic parenchymal involvement
- Erythema nodosum is associated with a good outcome
- Death from pulmonary insufficiency occurs in about 5% of patients

EVIDENCE

INFORMATION FOR PATIENTS

- American Lung Association
  - http://www.lungusa.org/site/pp.asp?c=dvLUK9O0E&b=35766
- National Institutes of Health
  - http://www.nlm.nih.gov/medlineplus/tutorials/sacroidosis.html
- National Heart, Lung, and Blood Institute
  - http://www.nhlbi.nih.gov/health/public/lung/other/sarcoidosis/index.htm

REFERENCE

- Baughman RP et al: Sarcoidosis. Lancet 2003;361:1111. [PMID:12672326]
- Paramothayan S et al: Corticosteroid therapy in pulmonary sarcoidosis: a systemic review. JAMA 2002;287:1301. [PMID:11886322]
- Statement on sarcoidosis. Joint Statement of the American Thoracic Society (ATS), the European Respiratory Society (ERS) and the World Association of Sarcoidosis and Other Granulomatous Disorders (WASOG) adopted by the ATS Board of Directors and by the ERS Executive Committee, February 1999. Am J Respir Crit Care Med 1999;160:736. [PMID:10430755]
- Thomas KW et al: Sarcoidosis. JAMA 2003;289:3300. [PMID:12824213]

Author(s)

Mark S. Chesnutt, MD

Thomas J. Prendergast, MD

Scabies

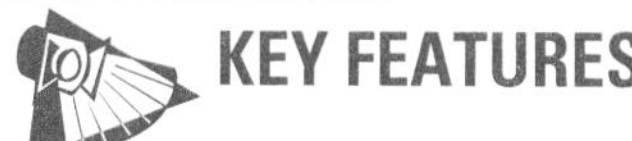

KEY FEATURES

ESSENTIALS OF DIAGNOSIS

- Generalized very severe itching
- Pruritic vesicles and pustules in "runs" or "galleries," especially on finger webs and the heels of the palms and in wrist creases
- Mites, ova, and brown dots of feces visible microscopically
- Red papules or nodules on the scrotum and on the penile glans and shaft are pathognomonic

GENERAL CONSIDERATIONS

- Caused by *Sarcoptes scabiei*
- Usually spares the head and neck (though these areas may be involved in the elderly, and in patients with AIDS)
- Usually acquired through the bedding of an infested individual or by other close contact

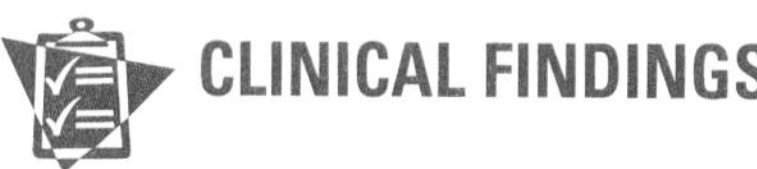

CLINICAL FINDINGS

SYMPTOMS AND SIGNS

- See Table 7
- Itching is almost always present and can be quite severe
- Lesions are more or less generalized excoriations with small pruritic vesicles, pustules, and "runs" or "burrows" in the web spaces and on the heels of the palms, wrists, elbows, and around the axillae
- Often, burrows are found only on the feet, as they have been scratched off in other locations
- The burrow appears as a short irregular mark, 2–3 mm long and the width of a hair
- Characteristic lesions may occur on the nipples in females and as pruritic papules on the scrotum or penis in males
- Pruritic papules may be seen over the buttocks

DIFFERENTIAL DIAGNOSIS

- Pediculosis (lice)
- Atopic dermatitis (eczema)
- Contact dermatitis
- Arthropod bites (insect bites)
- Urticaria
- Dermatitis herpetiformis

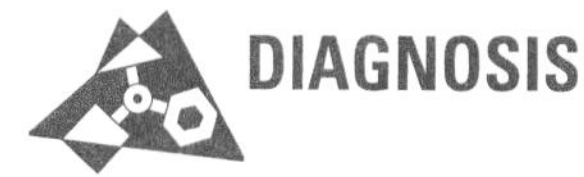

DIAGNOSIS

LABORATORY TESTS

- The diagnosis should be confirmed by microscopic demonstration of the organism, ova, or feces in a mounted specimen, best done on unexcoriated lesions from interdigital webs, wrists, elbows, or feet
- A bit of immersion oil is placed on the lesion and a No. 15 blade is used to scrape the lesion flat
- Diagnosis can also be confirmed in most cases with the burrow ink test: apply ink to the burrow and then do a very superficial shave biopsy by sawing off the burrow with a No. 15 blade, painlessly and bloodlessly; the mite, ova, and feces can be seen under the light microscope

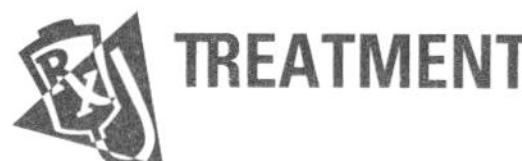

TREATMENT

MEDICATIONS

- Goal is to treat mites and control the dermatitis, which can last months after eradication of the mites, with mid-potency topical steroids (0.1% triamcinolone cream)
- Treatment consists of disinfestations; add systemic antibiotics for secondary pyoderma
- Permethrin 5% cream; treat with a single application for 8–12 h; may repeat in 1 week
- Crotamiton cream or lotion: an alternative, applied in the same way as permethrin but is used nightly for 4 nights; it is far less effective if used for only 48 h
- Benzyl benzoate: a lotion or emulsion in strengths from 20% to 35% and used as generalized applications (from collarbones down) overnight for two treatments 1 week apart; it is cosmetically acceptable, clean, and not overly irritating
- **Pregnant patients**: treat only if they have documented scabies; use permethrin 5% cream once for 12 h—or 5% or 6% sulfur in petrolatum applied nightly for 3 nights from the collarbones down
- **Treatment failures**: in immunocompetent hosts, most are due to incorrect use or incomplete treatment of the housing unit. Repeat treatment with permethrin once weekly for 2 weeks, with reeducation regarding the method and extent of application. Alternatively, ivermectin 200 μg/kg, single dose, is effective in about 75% of cases and in 95% of cases with two doses 2 weeks apart
- In immunosuppressed hosts and those with crusted (hyperkeratotic) scabies: multiple doses of ivermectin (every 2 weeks for two or three doses) plus topical therapy with permethrin once or twice weekly may be effective when topical treatment and oral therapy alone fail
- Persistent pruritic **postscabietic papules**: may be treated with mid- to high-potency steroids or with intralesional triamcinolone acetonide (2.5–5 mg/mL)

THERAPEUTIC PROCEDURES

- Bedding and clothing should be laundered or cleaned or set aside for 14 days in plastic bags
- Must treat all persons in a family or institutionalized group

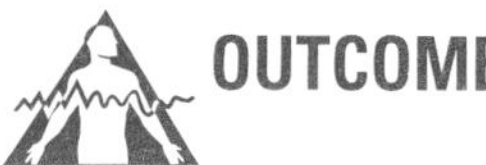

OUTCOME

WHEN TO REFER

- If there is a question about the diagnosis, if recommended therapy is ineffective, or if specialized treatment is necessary

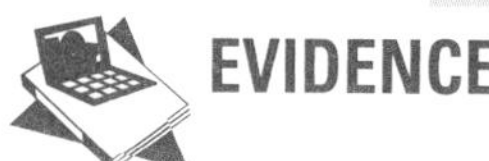

EVIDENCE

PRACTICE GUIDELINES

- Association for Genitourinary Medicine, Medical Society for the Study of Venereal Disease (London). 2002 national guideline on the management of scabies
  - http://www.guideline.gov/summary/summary.aspx?doc_id=3047&nbr=2273

WEB SITES

- American Academy of Dermatology
  - http://www.aad.org
- Centers for Disease Control and Prevention: Scabies Professional Information
  - http://www.dpd.cdc.gov/dpdx/HTML/Scabies.htm

INFORMATION FOR PATIENTS

- American Academy of Dermatology: Scabies
  - http://www.aad.org/public/Publications/pamphlets/Scabies.htm
  - http://www.niams.nih.gov/hi/topics/rosacea/rosacea.htm
- American Social Health Association: Scabies
  - http://www.ashastd.org/stdfaqs/scabies.html
- MedlinePlus: Scabies
  - http://www.nlm.nih.gov/medlineplus/ency/article/000830.htm

REFERENCES

- Chosidow O: Scabies and pediculosis. Lancet 2000;355:819. [PMID: 10711939]
- Gimenez Garcia R et al: Scabies in the elderly. J Eur Acad Dermatol Venereol 2004;18:105. [PMID: 14678549]

Author(s)

Timothy G. Berger, MD

Schistosomiasis

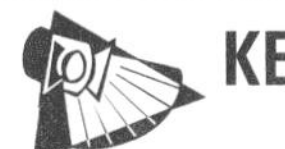

KEY FEATURES

ESSENTIALS OF DIAGNOSIS

- Exposure to infection in an endemic area

Acute phase

- Abrupt onset (2–6 weeks postexposure) of abdominal pain, weight loss, headache, fever, myalgia, diarrhea (sometimes bloody), dry cough, hepatomegaly, and eosinophilia

Chronic phase

- Either diarrhea, abdominal pain, blood in stool, hepatomegaly or hepatosplenomegaly, and bleeding from esophageal varices (*Schistosoma mansoni* or *Schistosoma japonicum* infection); or terminal hematuria, urinary frequency, and urethral and bladder pain (*Schistosoma haematobium* infection)
- Depending on species, characteristic eggs in feces, urine, or scrapings or biopsy of rectal or bladder mucosa

GENERAL CONSIDERATIONS

- The disease is caused mainly by three blood flukes (trematodes)
  - *S mansoni* causes intestinal schistosomiasis
    - Is widespread in Africa and occurs in the Arabian peninsula, South America, and the Caribbean
  - *S haematobium*
    - Causes vesical (urinary) schistosomiasis
    - Found throughout the Middle East and Africa
  - *S japonicum*
    - Causes Asiatic intestinal schistosomiasis, due to *S japonicum*
    - Important in China and the Philippines
- Except for the allergic response in the acute syndrome (see below), the disease is primarily due to delayed hypersensitivity
- The life span of the worms ranges from 5 to 30 years or more

DEMOGRAPHICS

- Infects more than 200 million persons worldwide, induces severe consequences in 20 million persons annually, resulting in over 200,000 deaths
- In the United States, an estimated 400,000 immigrants are infected, but transmission does not occur because appropriate snail intermediate hosts are absent

CLINICAL FINDINGS

SYMPTOMS AND SIGNS

- Many persons have light infections (< 100 eggs per gram of feces) and are asymptomatic
- 50–60% of people have symptoms and 5–10% have advanced organ damage
- Cercarial dermatitis produces a localized itchy erythematous or petechial rash to macules and papules that last up to 5 days

Acute schistosomiasis (Katayama fever)

- An allergic response to the developing schistosomes
- May occur with the three schistosomes (rare with *S haematobium*)
- The incubation period is 2–7 weeks; the severity of illness ranges from mild to (rarely) life-threatening
- Fever, malaise, urticaria, diarrhea (sometimes bloody), myalgia, dry cough
- Liver and spleen may be temporarily enlarged
- The patient becomes asymptomatic in 2–8 weeks

Chronic schistosomiasis

- This stage begins 6 months to several years after infection
- In *S mansoni* and *S japonicum* infections, findings include diarrhea, abdominal pain, irregular bowel movements, blood in the stool, a hard enlarged liver, and splenomegaly
- With subsequent slow progression over 5–15 years or longer, the following may appear: anorexia, weight loss, weakness, polypoid intestinal tumors, and features of portal and pulmonary hypertension
- Immune complex glomerulonephritis may occur
- In *S haematobium* infection, early symptoms of urinary tract disease are frequency and dysuria, followed by terminal hematuria and proteinuria

DIFFERENTIAL DIAGNOSIS

- Acute
  - Amebiasis
  - Bacterial dysentery, eg, *Shigella*, *Salmonella*
  - Viral hepatitis
  - Typhoid fever
  - Malaria
- Chronic
  - Typhoid fever
  - Visceral leishmaniasis
  - Lymphoma
  - Amebiasis
  - Portal hypertension due to other causes, eg, cirrhosis, portal vein thrombosis
  - Hematuria due to other causes, eg, urinary tract infections, renal cell carcinoma

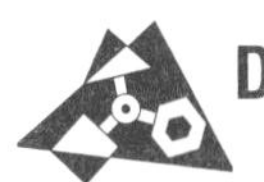

DIAGNOSIS

LABORATORY TESTS

- Screening is by testing for eggs (ova) and occult blood in feces and urine (the excretion of which may be irregular and require repeated testing), for protein and leukocytes in urine, and by serology
- Definitive diagnosis is by finding characteristic live eggs in excreta or mucosal biopsy
- In *S haematobium* infection, eggs may be found in the urine or, less frequently, in the stools. Eggs are sought in urine specimens collected between 9 AM and 2 PM or in 24-h collections. They are processed by membrane filtration (preferable) or by examination of the sediment
- In *S mansoni* and *S japonicum* infections, eggs may be found in stool specimens by direct examination, but concentration with a quantitative method (Kato-Katz) is often necessary; heavy infections are those with counts over 400 eggs per gram
- ELISA, immunoblot, and other tests may detect some egg-negative or ectopic infections
- Early in acute schistosomiasis, stool examination may be negative (examinations should be repeated for at least 6 months) but serological tests positive
- Anemia is common. Leukocytosis and marked eosinophilia, common during the acute stage, usually are absent in the chronic stage

IMAGING STUDIES

- In *S mansoni* and *S japonicum* infections, barium swallow, esophagoscopy, barium enema or colonoscopy, chest x-ray, or an ECG may be indicated. Ultrasound examination of the liver may show the pathognomonic pattern of periportal fibrosis and replaces the need for liver biopsy
- In advanced *S haematobium* disease, cystoscopy may show "sandy patches," ulcers, and areas of squamous metaplasia; lower abdominal plain films may show calcification of the bladder wall or ureters. Sonography is considered the imaging technique of choice but may fail to show the calcification. CT—which may demonstrate pathognomonic "turtle-

back" calcifications—intravenous pyelography, and retrograde cystography and pyelography may be useful

DIAGNOSTIC PROCEDURES

- If stool eggs are not found, biopsy may be necessary. Specimens should be examined as crush preparations between two glass slides and also examined histologically

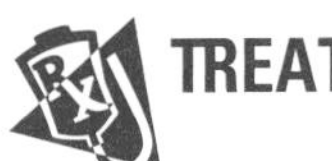

TREATMENT

MEDICATIONS

- Treatment should be given only if live ova are identified
- Praziquantel can be used to treat all species; alternative drugs of choice are oxamniquine for *S mansoni* and metrifonate for *S haematobium*
- The praziquantel dosage is 20 mg/kg—give twice in 1 day for *S haematobium* and *S mansoni* and three times in 1 day for *S japonicum* and *S mekongi*. The dosages should be given at 4- to 6-h intervals with water after a meal. The drug should not be used in pregnancy
- Oxamniquine is highly effective only in *S mansoni* infections. For strains in the western hemisphere and western Africa, a dose of 15 mg/kg is given once. Some recommend 40–60 mg/kg/day in two or three divided doses for 2–3 days in all of Africa and in the Arabian peninsula. When divided doses are needed, they are separated by 6–8 h. The drug is contraindicated in pregnancy
- Corticosteroids may be considered for (rarely) life-threatening acute schistosomiasis
- No specific treatment is indicated for bird cercarial dermatitis, except for topical applications to relieve itching

SURGERY

- In selected instances, surgery may be indicated for removal of polyps and for obstructive uropathy

THERAPEUTIC PROCEDURES

- For bleeding esophageal varices, sclerotherapy is the treatment of choice

OUTCOME

FOLLOW-UP

- After treatment, laboratory follow-up for continued passage of eggs is essential; start at 3 months and continue at intervals for 1 year; if found, viability should be determined, since dead eggs are passed for some months

COMPLICATIONS

- Portal hypertension with contracted liver, splenomegaly, pancytopenia, esophageal varices
- Pulmonary hypertension with cor pulmonale and edema due to right heart failure
- Large bowel stricture, granulomatous masses, colonic polyposis, and persistent *Salmonella* infection may occur
- Transverse myelitis, epilepsy, or optic neuritis may result from collateral circulation of eggs or ectopic worms
- Sequelae of *S haematobium* infection include bladder polyp formation, cystitis, chronic *Salmonella* infection, pyelitis, pyelonephritis, urolithiasis, hydronephrosis due to ureteral obstruction, renal failure, and death. Severe liver, lung, genital, or neurological disease is rare
- Bladder cancer has been associated with vesicular schistosomiasis

PROGNOSIS

- Cure rates with praziquantel > 85% are achieved at 6 months for *S haematobium*, *S mansoni*, and *S japonicum* infections, with marked reduction in egg counts (>90%) in those not cured
- In advanced disease with extensive involvement of the intestines, liver, bladder, or other organs, the outlook is poor even with treatment

WHEN TO REFER

- All patients with chronic schistosomiasis

WHEN TO ADMIT

- In areas where cysticercosis may coexist with a schistosomal infection being treated with praziquantel, treatment is best conducted in a hospital to monitor for death of cysticerci, which may be followed by neurological complications

PREVENTION

- Travelers to endemic areas should avoid swimming and other fresh water exposure. Use of topical agents to prevent cercarial penetration or oral prophylaxis has not been established

EVIDENCE

WEB SITES

- CDC—Division of Parasitic Diseases
  - http://www.cdc.gov/ncidod/dpd/parasites/schistosomiasis/default.htm
- Travelers' Health
  - http://www.cdc.gov/travel/diseases.htm#schisto

INFORMATION FOR PATIENTS

- Centers for Disease Control
  - http://www.cdc.gov/ncidod/dpd/parasites/schistosomiasis/factsht_schistosomiasis.htm
- National Institutes of Health
  - http://www.nlm.nih.gov/medlineplus/ency/article/001321.htm

REFERENCES

- Ghoneim MA: Bilharziasis of the genitourinary tract. BJU Int 2002;89(Suppl 1):22. [PMID: 11876729]
- Ross AG et al: Schistosomiasis. N Engl J Med 2002;346:1212. [PMID: 11961151]

Schizophrenia

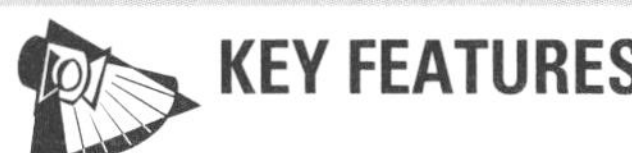

KEY FEATURES

ESSENTIALS OF DIAGNOSIS

- Massive disruption of thinking, mood, and overall behavior, as well as poor filtering of stimuli
- Schizophrenic disorders subdivided into types by prominent phenomena
  - **Disorganized (hebephrenic)**: incoherence and incongruous or silly affect
  - **Catatonic**: psychomotor disturbance or either excitement or rigidity
  - **Paranoid**: persecutory or grandiose delusions, and hallucinations
  - **Undifferentiated:** lack of symptoms specific enough to fit other types
  - **Residual**: for persons with a history of clear schizophrenia, but who presently exhibit only milder signs without overt psychosis

GENERAL CONSIDERATIONS

- Origin believed to have genetic, environmental, and neurotransmitter pathophysiologic components

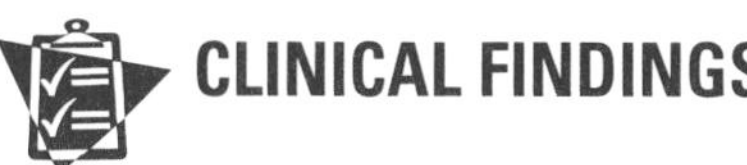

CLINICAL FINDINGS

SYMPTOMS AND SIGNS

- A history of a major disruption in the individual's life may precede gross psychotic deterioration
- Gradual decompensation usually predates the acute episode
- Symptoms of at least 6 months' duration
- **Positive** symptoms
  - Delusions are often paranoid, involving perceived threat from others
  - Hallucinations are typically auditory
  - Hypersensitivity to environmental stimuli, with feelings of enhanced sensory awareness
- **Negative** symptoms
  - Diminished sociability
  - Restricted affect
  - Impoverished speech
- **Appearance**: may be bizarre, though usually patients are just mildly unkempt
- **Motor activity**: generally reduced, although a broad spectrum is seen
- **Social function**: marked withdrawal, often with deterioration in personal care, disturbed interpersonal relationships
- **Speech**
  - Neologisms (made-up words or phrases)
  - Echolalia (repetition of others' words)
  - Verbigeration (repetition of senseless words or phrases)
- **Affect**: flat, occasionally inappropriate
- **Mood**: depression in most patients, less apparent during acute psychosis, may have rapidly alternating mood shifts irrespective of circumstances
- **Thought content**
  - Varies from paucity of ideas to rich delusions
  - Concrete thinking with inability to abstract
  - Inappropriate symbolism

DIFFERENTIAL DIAGNOSIS

- Schizophrenia should be distinguished from other psychoses
  - **Delusional disorders** are characterized by nonbizarre delusions with minimal impairment on daily life
  - **Schizoaffective disorders** fail to fit within the definitions of either schizophrenia or affective disorders
  - **Schizophreniform disorders** have a duration of less than 6 months, but more than 1 week
  - **Brief psychotic disorders** result from psychological stress, last less than 1 week, and have a much better prognosis
  - Late-life psychosis occurs after age 60 and is accompanied by cognitive impairment
  - **Atypical psychoses** are psychotic symptoms arising from a cause that may be apparent only later
  - Clues are precipitous onset and a good premorbid history
- Manic episodes
- Obsessive-compulsive disorder
- Psychotic depression
- Drug intoxication and abuse
- Thyroid, adrenal, and pituitary disorders
- Complex partial seizures and temporal lobe dysfunction may produce psychotic symptoms
- Drug toxicities, particularly overdoses of typical antipsychotics, can produce catatonia

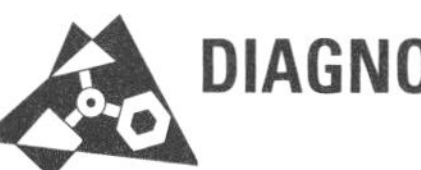

DIAGNOSIS

LABORATORY TESTS

- Tests to rule out metabolic and endocrine disorders, such as
  - Electrolytes, BUN, creatinine
  - Glucose, TSH; tests for endocrine disorders may be appropriate
- Toxicology screen

IMAGING STUDIES

- Ventricular enlargement and cortical atrophy on CT have been correlated with chronicity, cognitive impairment, and poor response to neuroleptics
- Decreased frontal lobe activity on positron emission tomography scan has been associated with negative symptoms
- MRI can exclude temporal lobe disorders

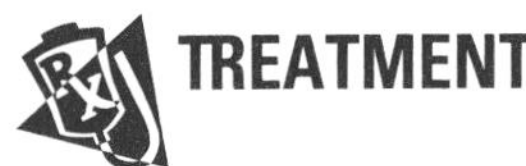

TREATMENT

MEDICATIONS

- See Tables 106 and 107
- Typical neuroleptic agents (phenothiazines, thioxanthenes, butyrophenones, dihydroindolones, dibenzoxazepines, and benzisoxazoles)
- Newer, atypical neuroleptics (clozapine, risperidone, olanzapine, quetiapine, ziprasidone, and aripiprazole)
  - Cause less tardive dyskinesia and extrapyramidal symptoms
  - Are more effective than typical agents on negative symptoms
- Antidepressant drugs may be used with antipsychotics if significant depression is present
- Resistant cases may require addition of lithium, carbamazepine, or valproate
- Addition of benzodiazepine can resolve catatonic symptoms and allow a lower neuroleptic dose

THERAPEUTIC PROCEDURES

- Social
  - Board and care homes with experienced staff can improve functioning and limit hospitalizations
  - Nonresidential self-help groups (Recovery, Inc.) should be used
  - Vocational rehabilitation and work agencies (Goodwill Industries, Inc.) can provide structured work situations
- Psychological
  - Need for psychotherapy varies markedly with patient status and history
  - Insight-oriented psychotherapy is often counterproductive
  - Cognitive-behavioral therapy with medication management may be efficacious
  - Family therapy may alleviate the patient's stress and assist relatives in coping
- Behavioral
  - Music from portable players with headphones can divert attention from auditory hallucinations

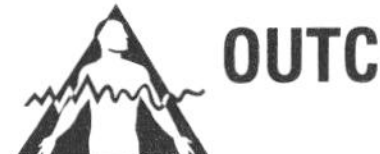

OUTCOME

FOLLOW-UP

- Clozapine
  - 1% risk of agranulocytosis
  - Weekly WBCs for 6 months, then every other week thereafter
  - Weekly WBCs for 1 month after discontinuation of clozapine
- Ziprasidone
  - Can cause QT prolongation
  - Pretreatment ECG and cardiac risk factor screen are necessary
- Quetiapine
  - Associated with cataracts
  - Ophthalmologic examination at initiation and biannually

COMPLICATIONS

- Neuroleptic malignant syndrome is uncommon but serious side effect of neuroleptics
- Tardive dyskinesia may occur after chronic use of neuroleptics
- Anticholinergic and adrenergic side effects are more frequent with low-potency neuroleptics
- Extrapyramidal symptoms are seen with high-potency neuroleptics
- Olanzapine has been associated with significant weight gain with case reports of type 2 diabetes

PROGNOSIS

- After removal of positive symptoms, prognosis is excellent in most patients
- Negative symptoms are more difficult to treat
- Prognosis is guarded when psychosis is associated with a history of serious drug abuse, owing to likely CNS damage
- Life expectancy is 20% shorter in schizophrenics, mostly because of higher mortality rates among young patients

WHEN TO ADMIT

- Gross disorganization
- Risk of self-harm or harm to others

EVIDENCE

PRACTICE GUIDELINES

- American Psychiatric Association: adult schizophrenia, 2004
  - http://www.guideline.gov/summary/summary.aspx?doc_id=5217
- American Academy of Child and Adolescent Psychiatry: children and adolescents with schizophrenia, 2000
  - http://www.guideline.gov/summary/summary.aspx?doc_id=3017

WEB SITES

- American Psychiatric Association
  - http://www.psych.org/
- Internet Mental Health
  - http://www.mentalhealth.com/
- National Institutes of Health—National Institute of Mental Health
  - http://www.nimh.nih.gov

INFORMATION FOR PATIENTS

- JAMA patient page: Schizophrenia. JAMA 2001;286:494. [PMID: 11484732]
- National Institute of Mental Health
  - http://www.nimh.nih.gov/healthinformation/schizophreniamenu.cfm

REFERENCES

- Eisendrath SJ, Chamberlain J: Psychiatry in the critical care unit. In: Current diagnosis and treatment in critical care, ed 2. Bongard FS, Sue DY (editors). Appleton & Lange, 2002
- Glassman AH et al: Antipsychotic drugs: prolonged QTc interval, torsade de pointes, and sudden death. Am J Psychiatry 2001;158:1774. [PMID:11691681]
- Kane JM et al: Efficacy and safety of aripiprazole and haloperidol versus placebo in patients with schizophrenia and schizoaffective disorder. J Clin Psychiatry 2002;63:763. [PMID:12363115]
- Rector NA et al: Cognitive behavioral therapy for schizophrenia: an empirical review. J Nerv Ment Dis 2001;189:278. [PMID:11379970]

Author(s)

Stuart J. Eisendrath, MD

Jonathan E. Lichtmacher, MD

Scleroderma (Systemic Sclerosis)

KEY FEATURES

ESSENTIALS OF DIAGNOSIS

- Diffuse thickening of skin, with telangiectasia and areas of increased pigmentation and depigmentation
- Raynaud's phenomenon in 90% of patients
- Systemic features of dysphagia, hypomotility of gastrointestinal tract, pulmonary fibrosis, and cardiac and renal involvement
- Positive test for antinuclear antibodies nearly universal

GENERAL CONSIDERATIONS

- A chronic disorder characterized by diffuse fibrosis of the skin and internal organs
- Two forms of systemic sclerosis are generally recognized: limited (80% of patients) and diffuse (20%)
- Microchimerism (long-term persisting cells from pregnancy) could be involved in the pathogenesis
- Patients presenting with systemic sclerosis or an eosinophilic fasciitis-like syndrome should be asked about tryptophan use, which is banned by the Food and Drug Administration

Eosinophilic fasciitis

- A rare disorder presenting with skin changes that resemble diffuse systemic sclerosis. The inflammatory abnormalities, however, are limited to the fascia rather than the dermis and epidermis.
- Unlike patients with systemic sclerosis, patients have peripheral blood eosinophilia, absence of Raynaud's phenomenon, a good response to prednisone, and an increased risk of developing aplastic anemia

DEMOGRAPHICS

- Symptoms usually appear in the third to sixth decades
- Women are affected about four times as frequently as men

CLINICAL FINDINGS

SYMPTOMS AND SIGNS

- Most frequently, skin involvement precedes visceral involvement
- Polyarthralgia and Raynaud's phenomenon (present in 90% of patients) are early manifestations
- With time the skin becomes thickened and hidebound, with loss of normal folds
- Telangiectasia, pigmentation, and depigmentation are characteristic
- Ulceration about the fingertips and subcutaneous calcification are seen
- Dysphagia from esophageal dysfunction (abnormalities in motility and later from fibrosis) is common
- Fibrosis and atrophy of the gastrointestinal tract cause hypomotility, and malabsorption results from bacterial overgrowth
- Diffuse pulmonary fibrosis and pulmonary vascular disease are reflected in low diffusing capacity and decreased lung compliance
- Cardiac abnormalities include pericarditis, heart block, myocardial fibrosis, and right heart failure secondary to pulmonary hypertension
- Systemic sclerosis renal crisis, resulting from obstruction of smaller renal blood vessels, indicates a grave prognosis

DIFFERENTIAL DIAGNOSIS

- Several conditions classified as "localized" sclerosis may mimic systemic morphea and limited systemic sclerosis. These disorders are generally limited to the skin (typically in a localized fashion) and are associated with excellent prognoses
- Eosinophilic fasciitis
- Eosinophilic-myalgia syndrome (due to tryptophan use)
- Overlap syndrome ("mixed connective tissue disease")
- Raynaud's disease
- Morphea
- Amyloidosis
- Graft-versus-host disease
- Cryoglobulinemia

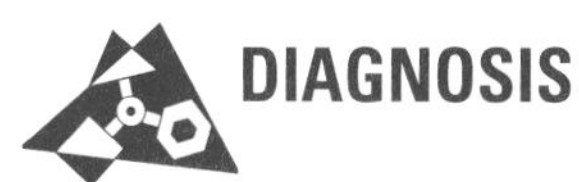

DIAGNOSIS

LABORATORY TESTS

- Antinuclear antibody tests are nearly always positive (Tables 76 and 82)
- The scleroderma antibody (SCL-70) directed against topoisomerase III is found in one-third of patients with diffuse systemic sclerosis and in 20% of those with CREST syndrome
- Anticentromere antibody is seen in 50% of those with CREST syndrome and in 1% of individuals with diffuse systemic sclerosis
- Elevation of the sedimentation rate is unusual
- Mild anemia is often present
- Proteinuria and cylindruria appear in association with renal involvement

Scleroderma (Systemic Sclerosis)

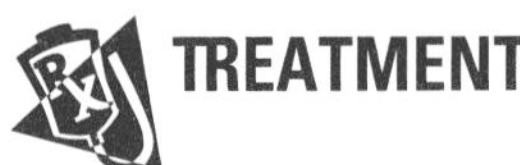

TREATMENT

MEDICATIONS

- Severe Raynaud's syndrome may respond to calcium channel blockers, eg, long-acting nifedipine, 30–120 mg/day, or to losartan, 50 mg/day
- Intravenous iloprost, a prostacyclin analog that causes vasodilation and platelet inhibition, is moderately effective in healing digital ulcers
- Intravenous prostaglandins (epoprostenol or PGE_2) or a subcutaneous prostacyclin analog (treprostinil) may be effective in pulmonary hypertension. An endothelin-1 antagonist, bosentan, improves symptoms and exercise tolerance in pulmonary hypertension
- Esophageal reflux can be reduced using antacids, H_2 blockers, and proton pump inhibitors (eg, omeprazole, 20–40 mg/day)
- Malabsorption due to bacterial overgrowth also responds to antibiotics, eg, tetracycline, 500 mg four times daily
- The hypertensive crises associated with systemic sclerosis renal crisis must be treated early and aggressively (in the hospital) with angiotensin-converting enzyme inhibitors, eg, captopril, 37.5–75 mg/day in three divided doses
- Prednisone has little or no role in the treatment of scleroderma
- Cyclophosphamide, a drug with many important side effects, may improve severe interstitial lung disease

SURGERY

- Digital sympathectomy may provide at least temporary relief in severe digital ischemia

THERAPEUTIC PROCEDURES

- Treatment is symptomatic and supportive

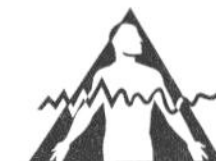

OUTCOME

COMPLICATIONS

- End-stage renal disease and often death from the malignant hypertension associated with scleroderma renal crisis
- Pulmonary hypertension
- Pulmonary fibrosis
- Profound gastrointestinal hypomotility and bacterial overgrowth
- Digital loss

PROGNOSIS

- Patients with CREST syndrome have a much better prognosis than those with diffuse disease, in large part because patients with limited disease do not develop renal failure or interstitial lung disease
- The 9-year survival rate in scleroderma averages approximately 40%
- The prognosis tends to be worse in those with diffuse scleroderma, in blacks, in males, and in older patients

WHEN TO REFER

- Patients should be managed in consultation with a rheumatologist

WHEN TO ADMIT

- Scleroderma renal crisis
- Advanced pulmonary hypertension

EVIDENCE

PRACTICE GUIDELINES

- Drake LA et al: Guidelines of care for scleroderma and sclerodermoid disorders. American Academy of Dermatology. J Am Acad Dermatol 1996;35:609.

WEB SITES

- American College of Rheumatology
  – http://www.rheumatology.org
- Scleroderma Foundation
  – http://www.scleroderma.org/

INFORMATION FOR PATIENTS

- American College of Rheumatology
  – http://www.rheumatology.org/public/factsheets/scler.asp
- National Institute of Arthritis and Musculoskeletal and Skin Diseases
  – http://www.niams.nih.gov/hi/topics/scleroderma/scleroderma.htm

REFERENCES

- Korn JH et al: Digital ulcers in systemic sclerosis: prevention by treatment with bosentan, an oral endothelin receptor antagonist. Arthritis Rheum 2004;50:3985. [PMID: 15593188]
- Rubin LJ et al: Bosentan therapy for pulmonary arterial hypertension. N Engl J Med 2002;346:896. [PMID: 11907289]
- Steen V et al: Predictors of isolated pulmonary hypertension in patients with systemic sclerosis and limited cutaneous involvement. Arthritis Rheum 2003;48:516. [PMID: 12571862]
- Steen VD: Scleroderma renal crisis. Rheum Dis Clin North Am 2003;29:315. [PMID: 12841297]
- Wigley FM: Clinical practice: Raynaud's phenomenon. N Engl J Med 2002;347:1001. [PMID: 12324557]

Author(s)

David B. Hellmann, MD, FACP
John H. Stone, MD, MPH

Sclerosing Cholangitis, Primary

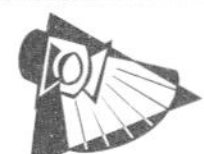

KEY FEATURES

ESSENTIALS OF DIAGNOSIS

- Males, aged 20–50 years old
- Often associated with ulcerative colitis
- Progressive jaundice, itching, and other features of cholestasis
- Diagnosis based on characteristic cholangiographic findings
- 10% risk of cholangiocarcinoma

GENERAL CONSIDERATIONS

- Characterized by a diffuse inflammation of the biliary tract leading to fibrosis and strictures of the biliary system
- Associated with the histocompatible antigens HLA-B8 and -DR3 or -DR4
- In patients with AIDS, sclerosing cholangitis may result from infections caused by cytomegalovirus (CMV), *Cryptosporidium*, or microsporum
- Occasional patients have clinical and histological features of both sclerosing cholangitis and autoimmune hepatitis. Even more rarely, an association with chronic pancreatitis (sclerosing pancreaticocholangitis) is seen, and this entity is often responsive to corticosteroids
- The diagnosis is difficult to make after biliary surgery or intrahepatic artery chemotherapy, which may result in bile duct injury
- Primary sclerosing cholangitis must be distinguished from idiopathic adulthood ductopenia, a rare disorder affecting young to middle-aged adults who manifest cholestasis resulting from loss of interlobular and septal bile ducts yet who have a normal cholangiogram

DEMOGRAPHICS

- The disease is most common in men aged 20–40 and is closely associated with ulcerative colitis (and occasionally Crohn's colitis), which is present in approximately two-thirds of patients; however, only 1–4% of patients with ulcerative colitis develop clinically significant sclerosing cholangitis
- As in ulcerative colitis, smoking is associated with a decreased risk of primary sclerosing cholangitis

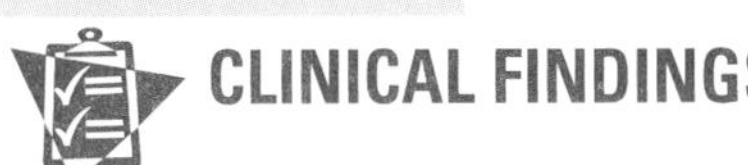

CLINICAL FINDINGS

SYMPTOMS AND SIGNS

- Progressive obstructive jaundice, frequently associated with malaise, pruritus, anorexia, and indigestion
- Occasional patients have clinical and histological features of both sclerosing cholangitis and autoimmune hepatitis

DIFFERENTIAL DIAGNOSIS

- Primary biliary cirrhosis
- Choledocholithiasis
- Cancer of pancreas or biliary tree
- Biliary stricture
- Drug-induced cholestasis, eg, chlorpromazine
- Inflammatory bowel disease complicated by cholestatic liver disease
- Idiopathic adulthood ductopenia
- *Clonorchis sinensis* (Chinese liver fluke)
- *Fasciola hepatica* (sheep liver fluke)
- Sclerosing cholangitis due to CMV, cryptosporidiosis, microsporidiosis (in AIDS)

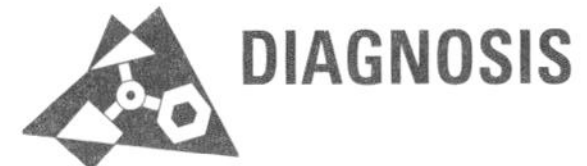

DIAGNOSIS

LABORATORY TESTS

- Patients may be diagnosed in the presymptomatic phase because of an elevated alkaline phosphatase level
- Antineutrophil cytoplasmic antibodies (ANCA), with fluorescent staining characteristics and target antigens distinct from those found in patients with Wegener's granulomatosis or vasculitis, are found in 70% of patients
- Serum antinuclear, anticardiolipin, and antithyroperoxidase antibodies and rheumatoid factor may be present

IMAGING STUDIES

- The diagnosis is generally made by endoscopic retrograde cholangiography (ERCP)
- Magnetic resonance cholangiography is increasingly being used as a noninvasive diagnostic approach but is less sensitive than ERCP for visualizing the intrahepatic ducts. Biliary obstruction by a stone or tumor should be excluded

DIAGNOSTIC PROCEDURES

- The disease may be confined to small intrahepatic bile ducts, in which case ERCP is normal and the diagnosis is suggested by liver biopsy
- Liver biopsy is needed for staging, which is based on the degree of inflammation and fibrosis

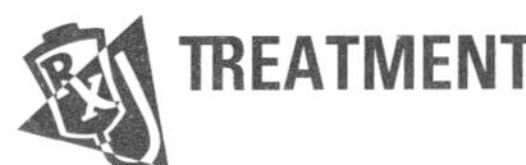

TREATMENT

MEDICATIONS

- Corticosteroids and broad-spectrum antimicrobial agents provide inconsistent results
- Episodes of acute bacterial cholangitis may be treated with ciprofloxacin
- Ursodeoxycholic acid in standard doses (10–15 mg/kg/day) may improve liver function test results but does not appear to alter the natural history. However, high-dose ursodeoxycholic acid (20 mg/kg/day) may reduce cholangiographic progression and liver fibrosis

SURGERY

- In patients without cirrhosis, surgical resection of a dominant bile duct stricture may lead to longer survival than endoscopic therapy by decreasing the subsequent risk of cholangiocarcinoma
- For patients with cirrhosis and clinical decompensation, liver transplantation is the procedure of choice

THERAPEUTIC PROCEDURES

- Careful endoscopic evaluation of the biliary tree may permit balloon dilation of localized strictures. If there is a major stricture, short-term placement of a stent may relieve symptoms and improve biochemical abnormalities with sustained improvement after the stent is removed
- Repeated balloon dilation of a recurrent dominant bile duct stricture may improve survival. However, long-term stenting may increase the rate of complications such as cholangitis

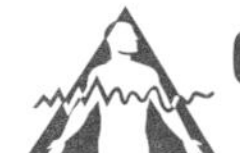

OUTCOME

COMPLICATIONS

- Complications of chronic cholestasis, such as osteoporosis and malabsorption of fat-soluble vitamins, may occur
- Cholangiocarcinoma
  - Occurs in at least 10% of cases
  - May be difficult to diagnose by cytological examination or biopsy because of false-negative results
  - A serum CA 19-9 level >100 units/mL is suggestive but not diagnostic of cholangiocarcinoma

PROGNOSIS

- Survival averages 10 years once symptoms appear
- Adverse prognostic markers
  - Older age, higher serum bilirubin and aspartate aminotransferase levels, lower albumin levels, and a history of variceal bleeding; variceal bleeding is also a risk factor for cholangiocarcinoma
- Actuarial survival rates with liver transplantation are as high as 85% at 3 years, but rates are much lower once cholangiocarcinoma has developed. Following transplantation, patients have an increased risk of nonanastomotic biliary strictures and—in those with ulcerative colitis—colon cancer
- Patients who are unable to undergo liver transplantation will ultimately require high-quality palliative care
- When the disease is confined to small intrahepatic bile ducts, the survival is longer and there is a lower rate of cholangiocarcinoma than with involvement of the large ducts

WHEN TO REFER

- All patients

PREVENTION

- In patients with ulcerative colitis, primary sclerosing cholangitis is an independent risk factor for the development of colorectal dysplasia and cancer, and strict adherence to a colonoscopic surveillance program is advisable

EVIDENCE

PRACTICE GUIDELINES

- Lee Y-M et al: Management of primary sclerosing cholangitis. Am J Gastroenterol 2002;97:528. PMID: 11922543

INFORMATION FOR PATIENTS

- National Digestive Diseases Information Clearinghouse
  - http://digestive.niddk.nih.gov/ddiseases/pubs/primarysclerosingcholangitis/index.htm
- National Institutes of Health
  - http://www.nlm.nih.gov/medlineplus/ency/article/000285.htm

REFERENCES

- Bjøro K et al: Liver transplantation for primary sclerosing cholangitis. J Hepatol 2004;40:570. [PMID: 15030971]
- Burak K et al: Incidence and risk factors for cholangiocarcinoma in primary sclerosing cholangitis. Am J Gastroenterol 2004;99:523. [PMID: 15056096]
- Talwalkar JA et al: Cost-minimization analysis of MRC versus ERCP for the diagnosis of primary sclerosing cholangitis. Hepatology 2004;40:39. [PMID: 15239084]

Author(s)

Lawrence S. Friedman, MD

Serum Sickness (Immune Complex Disease)

KEY FEATURES

ESSENTIALS OF DIAGNOSIS

- Fever, pruritus, and arthropathy
- Reaction is delayed in onset, usually 7–10 days, when specific IgG antibodies are generated against the allergen
- Immune complexes found circulating in serum or deposited in affected tissues

GENERAL CONSIDERATIONS

- Serum sickness reactions occur when immune complexes formed by the binding of drugs or heterologous serum to antibodies; these complexes deposit in the vascular endothelium and produce immune-mediated tissue injury
- The reaction occurs 7–10 days after exposure, when specific IgG antibodies are generated against the allergen
- The commonly affected organs include skin (urticaria, vasculitis), joints (arthritis), and kidney (nephritis)

CLINICAL FINDINGS

SYMPTOMS AND SIGNS

- Usually a self-limited illness, but can be a severe vasculitis
- Constitutional symptoms are common
- Fever
- Urticaria
- Arthritis
- Nephritis

DIFFERENTIAL DIAGNOSIS

- Infection
- Autoimmune hypersensitivity
- Vasculitis
- Systemic lupus erythematosus (SLE)
- Rheumatoid arthritis (RA)

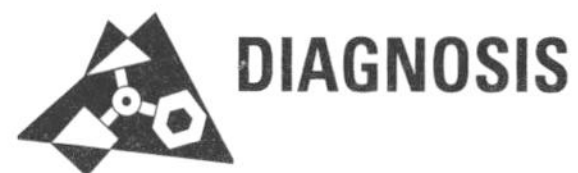

DIAGNOSIS

LABORATORY TESTS

- The specific IgG antibody may be present in sufficient quantity in serum to be detected by the precipitin-in-gel method; ELISA will detect antibodies present in lesser amounts
- Decreased C3, C4, or CH50 is nonspecific evidence of immune complex disease
- Immune complexes can be detected circulating in serum or deposited in affected tissues
- Increased erythrocyte sedimentation rate
- Red blood cell casts if nephritis is present

Seafood Poisoning p. 1149. Seborrheic Keratoses p. 1149. Sedative-Hypnotic Agent Overdose p. 1150.

Serum Sickness (Immune Complex Disease)

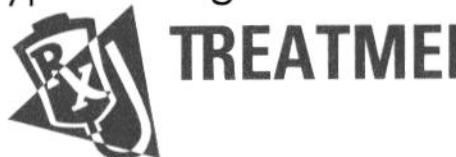

TREATMENT

MEDICATIONS

- Aspirin or nonsteroidal antiinflammatory drugs for fever and arthritis
- Antihistamines and topical steroids for dermatitis
- Systemic corticosteroids are used for systemic vasculitis manifesting as glomerulonephritis or neuropathy

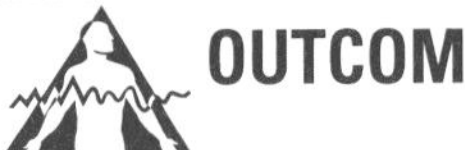

OUTCOME

PROGNOSIS

- Good to excellent if inciting antigen is identified and withdrawn (eg, drug, serum, etc)

WHEN TO REFER

- To an allergist for assistance in identifying inciting agent(s)
- To a rheumatologist if autoimmune disorder is suspected (eg, SLE, RA, or vasculitis)

PREVENTION

- Avoid known inciting agents

EVIDENCE

WEB SITE

- American Academy of Allergy, Asthma and Immunology
  - http://www.aaaai.org

INFORMATION FOR PATIENTS

- MedlinePlus: Serum Sickness
  - http://www.nlm.nih.gov/medlineplus/ency/article/000820.htm

REFERENCES

- Cuellar ML: Drug-induced vasculitis. Curr Rheumatol Rep 2002;4:55. [PMID: 11798983]
- Fiorentino DF: Cutaneous vasculitis. J Am Acad Dermatol 2003;48:311. [PMID: 12637912]
- Nigen S et al: Drug eruptions: approaching the diagnosis of drug-induced skin diseases. J Drugs Dermatol 2003;2:278. [PMID: 12848112]
- Venzor J: Urticarial vasculitis. Clin Rev Allergy Immunol 2002;23:201. [PMID: 12221865]

Author(s)

Jeffrey L. Kishiyama, MD
Daniel C. Adelman, MD

Sexual Dysfunction

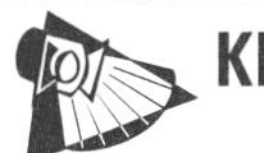

KEY FEATURES

ESSENTIALS OF DIAGNOSIS

- Large category of vasocongestive and orgasmic disorders
- Often involve problems of sexual adaptation, education, and technique

GENERAL CONSIDERATIONS

- Two most common conditions in men
  - Erectile dysfunction
  - Ejaculation disturbances
- Two most common conditions in women
  - Vaginismus
  - Frigidity

Erectile dysfunction

- The inability to achieve an erection adequate for satisfactory intercourse
- Causes can be psychological, physiologic, or both
- A history of occasional erections—especially nocturnal tumescence—can demonstrate a psychological origin

Ejaculation disturbances

- Ejaculation control is an acquired behavior that is minimal in adolescence and increases with experience
- Sexual ignorance, anxiety, guilt, depression, and relationship problems may interfere with learning control
- Interference with the sympathetic nerve distribution through surgery or trauma can be responsible

Vaginismus

- Conditioned response in which a spasm of the perineal muscles occurs when there is any stimulation of the area
- The desire is to avoid penetration

Frigidity

- Characterized by a general lack of sexual responsiveness
- Sexual activity varies from avoidance to an occasional orgasm
- Possible causes
  - Poor sexual techniques
  - Early traumatic sexual experiences
  - Marital problems
- Organic causes include
  - Conditions causing dyspareunia
  - Pelvic pathology
  - Mechanical obstruction
  - Neurologic deficits

CLINICAL FINDINGS

SYMPTOMS AND SIGNS

Erectile dysfunction

- Often mentioned only after direct questioning
- Patients sometimes use the term "impotence" to describe premature ejaculation

Ejaculation disturbances

- Patients may not relate symptoms without direct questions regarding their sex lives

Frigidity

- Difficulty in experiencing erotic sensation and lack of vasocongestive response
- Should be differentiated from orgasmic dysfunction, in which varying degrees of difficulty are experienced in achieving orgasm

DIFFERENTIAL DIAGNOSIS

- Depression or anxiety
- Underlying medical condition, eg, diabetes, peripheral vascular disease, hyperprolactinemia, hypogonadism
- Dyspareunia or chronic pelvic pain
- Drugs or substance use, eg, selective serotonin reuptake inhibitors (SSRIs), tricyclic antidepressants, alcohol

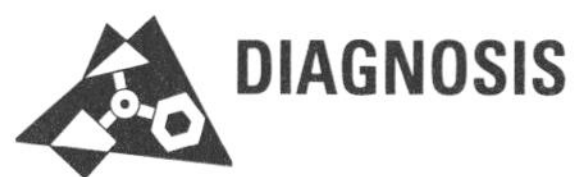

DIAGNOSIS

DIAGNOSTIC PROCEDURES

- Erectile dysfunction
  - Depression must be ruled out
  - Workup must differentiate between anatomic, endocrine, neurologic, and psychological causes
  - Even if an irreversible cause is identified, this knowledge may help the patient to accept the condition
- Other conditions
  - Clinical diagnosis

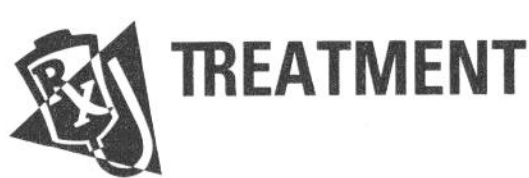

TREATMENT

MEDICATIONS

Erectile dysfunction

- Sildenafil (25–100 mg) vardenafil (2.5–20 mg), or tadalafil (5–20 mg) 1 hour before intercourse is useful
- Sildenafil, vardenafil, and tadalafil must not be used concurrently with nitrates owing to a risk of hypotension leading to sudden death

Ejaculation disturbances

- SSRIs have been effective because of their common effect in delaying ejaculation

THERAPEUTIC PROCEDURES

- Anxiety and guilt about parental injunctions against sex may contribute to sexual dysfunction

Erectile dysfunction

- The effect of this problem on relationships must be considered and addressed

Ejaculation disturbances

- Psychotherapy is best suited to cases in which interpersonal or intrapsychic problems predominate
- A combined behavioral-psychological approach is most effective

Vaginismus

- Responds well to desensitization with graduated Hegar dilators along with relaxation techniques
- Masters and Johnson have used behavioral approaches in all of the sexual dysfunctions, with concomitant supportive psychotherapy and with improvement of the communication patterns of the couple

Frigidity

- Organic causes (conditions causing dyspareunia, pelvic pathology, mechanical obstruction, and neurologic deficits) and contributing intrapersonal issues must be uncovered and addressed
- As with other psychosexual disorders, behavioral approaches with supportive psychotherapy and improved communication within couples can be effective

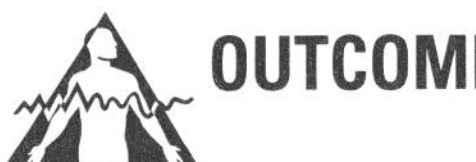

OUTCOME

PREVENTION

- The proximity of other people (eg, mother-in-law) in a household is frequently an inhibiting factor in sexual relationships; some social engineering may alleviate the problem

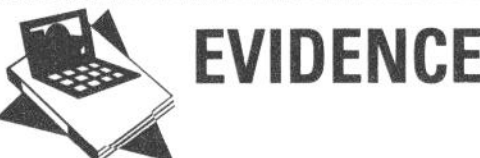

EVIDENCE

PRACTICE GUIDELINES

- American Academy of Family Physicians: Female Sexual Dysfunction: evaluation and treatment
  - http://www.aafp.org/afp/20000701/127.html
- National Guideline Clearinghouse: American Association of Clinical Endocrinologists: male sexual dysfunction, 2003
  - http://www.guideline.gov/summary/summary.aspx?doc_id=3725

WEB SITE

- American Psychiatric Association
  - http://www.psych.org/

INFORMATION FOR PATIENTS

- American Academy of Family Physicians
  - http://www.aafp.org/afp/20000701/141ph.html
- American College of Obstetricians and Gynecologists
  - http://www.medem.com/MedLB/article_detaillb.cfm?article_ID=ZZZ7P2WBT7C&sub_cat=2
- The Cleveland Clinic
  - http://www.clevelandclinicmeded.com/diseasemanagement/women/sex_dysfunction/sex_dysfunction.htm
- JAMA patient page: Male sexual dysfunction. JAMA 2004;291:3076. [PMID:15213218]
- JAMA patient page: Sexual dysfunction. JAMA 1999;281:584. [PMID:10022117]

REFERENCES

- Boyce EG et al: Sildenafil citrate, a therapeutic update. Clin Ther 2001;23:2. [PMID:11219477]
- Worthington JJ et al: Treatment of antidepressant-induced sexual dysfunction. Drugs Today 2003;39:887. [PMID:14702134]

Author(s)

Stuart J. Eisendrath, MD

Jonathan E. Lichtmacher, MD

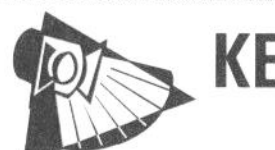

KEY FEATURES

GENERAL CONSIDERATIONS

- The most common sexually transmitted diseases (STDs) are
  - Gonorrhea
  - Syphilis
  - Condyloma acuminatum
  - Chlamydial genital infections
  - Herpesvirus genital infections
  - *Trichomonas* vaginitis
  - Chancroid
  - Granuloma inguinale
  - Scabies
  - Louse infestation
  - Bacterial vaginosis (among lesbians)
- Shigellosis, hepatitis A, B, and C, amebiasis, giardiasis, cryptosporidiosis, salmonellosis, and campylobacteriosis may also be transmitted by sexual (oral–anal) contact, especially in homosexual males
- Homosexual contact is a typical method of transmission of HIV, though bidirectional heterosexual transmission is occurring more commonly
- In most infections caused by sexually transmitted bacteria, spirochetes, chlamydiae, viruses, or protozoal agents, early lesions occur on genitalia or other sexually exposed mucous membranes; however, wide dissemination may occur, and involvement of nongenital tissues and organs may mimic many noninfectious disorders
- All STDs have subclinical or latent phases that play an important role in long-term persistence of the infection or in its transmission from infected (but largely asymptomatic) persons to other contacts

Sexual assault

- The risk of developing an STD following a sexual assault has not been established
- Victims of assault have a high baseline rate of infection
  - *Neisseria gonorrhoeae,* 6%
  - *Chlamydia trachomatis,* 10%
  - *Trichomonas vaginalis,* 15%
  - Bacterial vaginosis, 34%
- The risk of acquiring infection as a result of the assault is significant but is often lower than the preexisting rate
  - *N gonorrhoeae,* 6–12%
  - *C trachomatis,* 4–17%
  - *T vaginalis,* 12%
  - Syphilis, 0.5–3%
  - Bacterial vaginosis, 19%
- Although seroconversion to HIV has been reported following sexual assault when this was the only known risk, this risk is believed to be low. The likelihood of HIV transmission from anal or vaginal receptive intercourse when the source is known to be HIV positive is 1–3 per 1000
- Victims should be evaluated within 24 h after the assault

CLINICAL FINDINGS

SYMPTOMS AND SIGNS

- See individual diseases

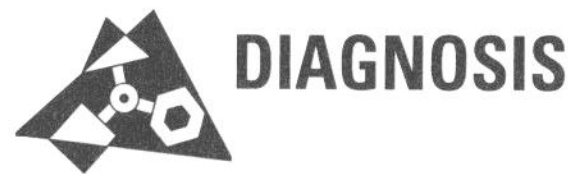

DIAGNOSIS

LABORATORY TESTS

- Simultaneous infection by several different agents is common
- Any person with an STD should be tested for syphilis; a repeat study should be done in 3 months if negative, since seroconversion is delayed after primary infection
- Laboratory examinations are of particular importance in the diagnosis of asymptomatic patients during the subclinical or latent phases of STDs

Sexual assault

- Victims should be evaluated within 24 h after the assault and cultures for *N gonorrhoeae and C trachomatis* (if culture is not available, nonculture tests, such as nucleic acid amplification tests, are acceptable)
- If the test is positive, it must be confirmed with a second test using a different target sequence
- Vaginal secretions are cultured and examined for *Trichomonas*
- If a discharge is present, if there is itching, or if secretions are malodorous, a wet mount should be examined for *Candida* and bacterial vaginosis
- A blood sample should be obtained for immediate serologic testing for syphilis, hepatitis B, and HIV

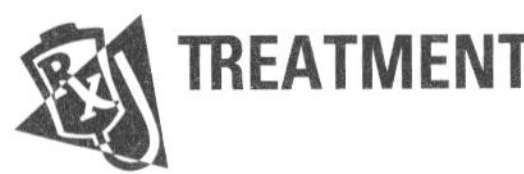

TREATMENT

MEDICATIONS

- The usefulness of presumptive therapy for victims of sexual assault is controversial
- If therapy is given, a reasonable regimen would be hepatitis B vaccination (without hepatitis B immune globulin, the first dose given at the initial evaluation and follow-up doses at 1–2 months and 4–6 months) and one dose of ceftriaxone, 125 mg IM, plus metronidazole, 2 g PO as a single dose, plus doxycycline, 100 mg PO BID for 7 days, or azithromycin, 1 g PO as a single dose
  - In premenopausal women, azithromycin should be used instead of doxycycline until the pregnancy status is determined
  - If the pregnancy test is positive, metronidazole should be given only after the first trimester
- Prophylactic postexposure treatment is recommended for 28 days if the individual seeks care within 72 hours of the assault and the source is known to be HIV infected
- If the status of the source is not known, and the victim presents within 72 hours of the assault, no firm recommendations can be made and the decision to treat is case-by-case
- If the patient seeks care > 72 hours after the assault, prophylaxis is not recommended

THERAPEUTIC PROCEDURES

- As a rule, sexual partners should be treated simultaneously to avoid prompt reinfection

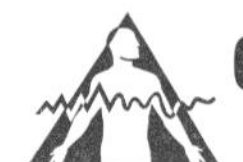

OUTCOME

FOLLOW-UP

- Follow-up examination for sexually transmitted disease after an assault should be repeated within 1–2 weeks, since concentrations of infecting organisms may not have been sufficient to produce a positive culture at the time of initial examination
- If prophylactic treatment was given, tests should be repeated only if the victim has symptoms
- If prophylaxis was not administered, the victim should be seen in 1 week so that any positive tests can be treated
- Follow-up serologic testing for syphilis and HIV infection should be performed in 6, 12, and 24 weeks if the initial tests are negative

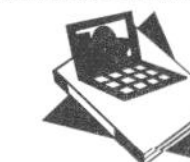

EVIDENCE

PRACTICE GUIDELINES

- Centers for Disease Control and Prevention: Sexually transmitted diseases treatment guidelines 2002. MMWR Recomm Rep 2002;51(RR-6):1. [PMID: 12184549]
- National Guideline Clearinghouse: Vaccine Preventable STDs. CDC, 2002.
  - http://www.guideline.gov/summary/summary.aspx?doc_id=3242

WEB SITE

- Centers for Disease Control and Prevention—National Center for STD, HIV, and TB Prevention, Division of Sexually Transmitted Diseases
  - http://www.cdc.gov/std/

INFORMATION FOR PATIENTS

- National Guideline Clearinghouse. STD guidelines. Centers for Disease Control, 2002.
  - http://www.guideline.gov/summary/summary.aspx?doc_id=3230
- National Institute of Allergy and Infectious Diseases
  - http://www.niaid.nih.gov/factsheets/stdinfo.htm
- American Academy of Family Physicians
  - http://familydoctor.org/165.xml
- Smith DK et al; US Department of Health and Human Services: Antiretroviral postexposure prophylaxis after sexual, injection-drug use, or other nonoccupational exposure to HIV in the United States. MMWR Recomm Rep 2005;54(RR-2):1. [PMID: 15660015]
- CDC National Prevention Information Network
  - http://www.cdcnpin.org/scripts/std/std.asp

REFERENCE

- Smith DK et al; US Department of Health and Human Services: Antiretroviral postexposure prophylaxis after sexual, injection-drug use, or other nonoccupational exposure to HIV in the United States. MMWR Recomm Rep 2005;54(RR-2):1. [PMID: 15660015]

Author(s)

Richard A. Jacobs, MD, PhD

Shigellosis

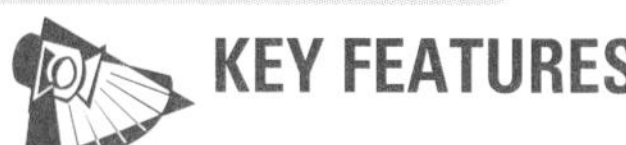

KEY FEATURES

ESSENTIALS OF DIAGNOSIS

- Diarrhea, often with blood and mucus
- Crampy abdominal pain, high fevers, and systemic toxicity
- White blood cells in stools; organism isolated on stool culture

GENERAL CONSIDERATIONS

- *Shigella* dysentery is a common disease, often self-limited and mild but occasionally serious
- Food-borne illness
- *Shigella sonnei* is the leading cause in the United States, followed by *Shigella flexneri*
- *Shigella dysenteriae* causes the most severe form of the illness
- There has been a rise in strains resistant to multiple antibiotics

DEMOGRAPHICS

- Residence in or travel to a foreign country
- Men who have sex with men at higher risk
- Exposure to contaminated food, especially in outbreak setting
- Approximately 450,000 cases (mostly due to *S sonnei*) occur in the United States each year
- In the developing world, *S flexneri* predominates

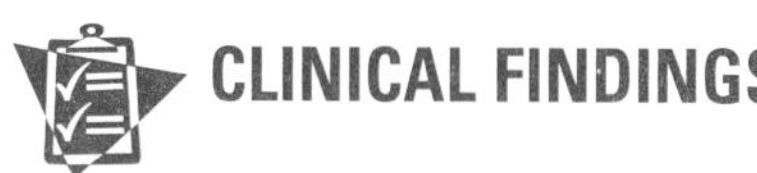

CLINICAL FINDINGS

SYMPTOMS AND SIGNS

- Table 131
- The illness usually starts abruptly, with diarrhea, lower abdominal cramps, and tenesmus
- The diarrheal stool often is mixed with blood and mucus
- Systemic symptoms are fever, chills, anorexia and malaise, and headache
- The abdomen is tender
- Temporary disaccharidase deficiency may follow the diarrhea

DIFFERENTIAL DIAGNOSIS

- Invasive diarrhea due to other bacteria
  - *Salmonella*
  - *Campylobacter*
  - Enteroinvasive *Escherichia coli*
  - *Yersinia enterocolitica*
- Amebic dysentery
- *Clostridium difficile* colitis
- Inflammatory bowel disease
- Viral gastroenteritis

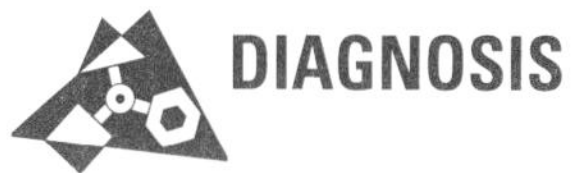

DIAGNOSIS

LABORATORY TESTS

- See Table 141
- The stool shows many leukocytes and red cells
- Stool culture is positive for shigellae in most cases, but blood cultures grow the organism in less than 5% of cases

DIAGNOSTIC PROCEDURES

- Sigmoidoscopic examination reveals an inflamed, engorged mucosa with punctate, sometimes large areas of ulceration

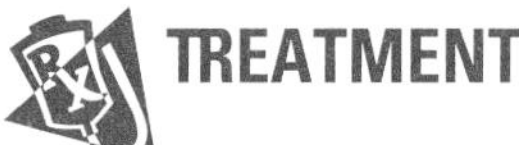

TREATMENT

MEDICATIONS

- Ciprofloxacin (contraindicated in pregnancy), 500 mg twice daily, or levofloxacin, 500 mg once daily for 3 days
- Trimethoprim-sulfamethoxazole, one double-strength tablet twice a day for 3 days (relegated to second-line therapy because of increasing drug resistance)
- Azithromycin, 500 mg on Day 1 then 250 mg daily for 4 days

THERAPEUTIC PROCEDURES

- Treatment of dehydration and hypotension is lifesaving in severe cases

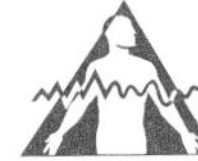

OUTCOME

COMPLICATIONS

- Temporary disaccharidase deficiency may follow the diarrhea
- Reactive arthritis (Reiter's) is an uncommon complication, usually occurring in HLA-B27 individuals infected by *Shigella*
- Hemolytic-uremic syndrome can occur after *S dysenteriae* type 1 infection

PROGNOSIS

- Complete recovery is the norm, although it may be several months before bowel habits are entirely normal

WHEN TO REFER

- If management consultation is needed

WHEN TO ADMIT

- Severe dehydration requiring parenteral fluid replacement

PREVENTION

- Wash hands with soap carefully and frequently, especially after going to the bathroom, after changing diapers, and before preparing foods or beverages
- Dispose of soiled diapers properly
- Disinfect diaper changing areas after using them
- Persons with diarrheal illness should not prepare food for others
- Travelers in the developing world should "boil it, cook it, peel it, or forget it"
- Avoid drinking pool water

EVIDENCE

PRACTICE GUIDELINES

- National Guideline Clearinghouse
  - http://www.guideline.gov/summary/summary.aspx?doc_id=2791

WEB SITE

- CDC—Division of Bacterial and Mycotic Diseases
  - http://www.cdc.gov/ncidod/dbmd/

INFORMATION FOR PATIENTS

- Centers for Disease Control and Prevention
  - http://www.cdc.gov/ncidod/dbmd/diseaseinfo/shigellosis_g.htm
- JAMA patient page: Preventing dehydration from diarrhea. JAMA 2001;185:362. [PMID: 11236756]
- JAMA patient page: Food-borne illnesses. JAMA 1999;281:1866. [PMID: 10340376]
- National Institutes of Health
  - http://www.nlm.nih.gov/medlineplus/ency/article/000295.htm

REFERENCES

- Ashkenazi S et al: Growing antimicrobial resistance of *Shigella* isolates. J Antimicrob Chemother 2003;51:427. [PMID: 12562716]
- Bhattacharya SK et al: An evaluation of current shigellosis treatment. Expert Opin Pharmacother 2003;4:1315. [PMID: 12877639]
- Thielman NM et al: Clinical practice. Acute infectious diarrhea. N Engl J Med 2004;350:38. [PMID: 14702426]

Author(s)

Henry F. Chambers, MD

Sickle Cell Anemia

KEY FEATURES

ESSENTIALS OF DIAGNOSIS

- Irreversibly sickled cells on peripheral blood smear
- Positive family history and lifelong personal history of hemolytic anemia
- Recurrent painful episodes
- Hemoglobin S is major hemoglobin seen on electrophoresis

GENERAL CONSIDERATIONS

- Autosomal recessive disorder in which abnormal hemoglobin leads to chronic hemolytic anemia with numerous clinical consequences
- Single DNA base change leads to amino acid substitution of valine for glutamine in sixth position on β-globin chain
- Abnormal tetramer designated hemoglobin S can form polymers that damage red blood cell (RBC) membrane
- Polymer formation and early membrane damage reversible, but with repeated sickling RBCs damaged beyond repair and become irreversibly sickled
- Sickling increased by increased RBC hemoglobin S concentration, RBC dehydration, acidosis, and hypoxemia
- Sickling retarded markedly by hemoglobin F; high hemoglobin F levels associated with more benign course
- Patients with heterozygous genotype (hemoglobin AS) have sickle cell trait
- Acute painful episodes as a result of vasoocclusion by sickled RBCs occur spontaneously or are provoked by infection, dehydration, or hypoxia

DEMOGRAPHICS

- Hemoglobin S gene carried in 8% of African-Americans
- Sickle cell anemia occurs in 1 birth in 400 in African-Americans
- Onset during first year of life, when hemoglobin F levels fall

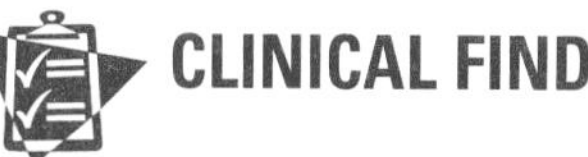

CLINICAL FINDINGS

SYMPTOMS AND SIGNS

- Chronic hemolytic anemia produces jaundice, pigment (calcium bilirubinate) gallstones, splenomegaly, and poorly healing ulcers over the lower tibia
- Anemia may be life threatening during hemolytic or aplastic crises
- Hemolytic crises result from splenic sequestration of sickled cells (primarily in childhood, before spleen has infarcted) or with coexistent disorders such as glucose-6-phosphate dehydrogenase deficiency
- Aplastic crises occur when bone marrow compensation is reduced by infection or folate deficiency
- Acute painful episodes, commonly in bones and chest, last hours to days and produce low-grade fever
- Acute vasoocclusion may cause priapism and strokes as a result of cavernous sinus thrombosis
- Repeated vasoocclusion affects heart (cardiomegaly, hyperdynamic precordium, systolic murmurs); liver; bone (ischemic necrosis, staphylococcal or salmonella osteomyelitis); spleen (infarction, asplenia); and kidney (infarction of renal medullary papillae, renal tubular concentrating defects, and gross hematuria)
- Retinopathy, blindness
- Increased susceptibility to infection as a result of hyposplenism, complement defects
- Hepatomegaly, nonpalpable spleen in adults
- Sickle cell trait: most often no symptoms or signs; acute vasoocclusion occurs only under extreme conditions
- May have episodes of gross hematuria or renal tubular defect causing inability to concentrate urine

DIFFERENTIAL DIAGNOSIS

- Other sickle cell syndromes: sickle cell trait, sickle thalassemia, or hemoglobin SC disease
- Osteomyelitis
- Hematuria from other cause
- Acute rheumatic fever
- Gaucher's disease (bone pain crises)

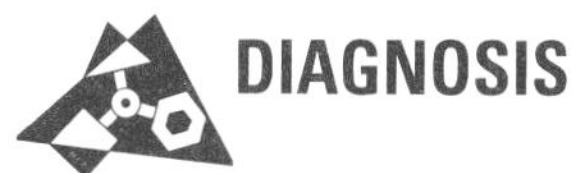

DIAGNOSIS

LABORATORY TESTS

- Serum indirect bilirubin, LDH, elevated; serum haptoglobin low
- Hematocrit usually 20–30%
- Reticulocyte count elevated
- Peripheral blood smear: irreversibly sickled cells comprise 5–50% of RBCs; reticulocytosis (10–25%); nucleated RBCs; Howell-Jolly bodies and target cells
- White blood cell count characteristically elevated to 12,000–15,000/μL; thrombocytosis may occur
- Screening test for sickle hemoglobin positive
- Hemoglobin electrophoresis confirms diagnosis
- Sickle cell anemia (homozygous S): hemoglobin S usually comprises 85–98% of hemoglobin and no hemoglobin A is present; hemoglobin F levels variably increased
- Sickle cell trait: complete blood cell count and peripheral blood smear normal; hemoglobin electrophoresis shows that hemoglobin S comprises ~40% of hemoglobin

IMAGING STUDIES

- Chest x-ray in acute chest syndrome
- Bone x-rays show characteristic abnormalities
- CT shows hepatomegaly and absence of spleen

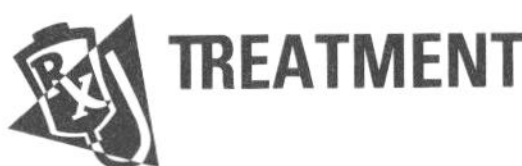

TREATMENT

MEDICATIONS

- Folic acid, 1 mg PO QD
- Hydroxyurea, 500–750 mg PO QD, increases hemoglobin F levels and reduces frequency of painful crises in patients whose quality of life is disrupted by frequent pain crises; long-term safety uncertain, concern exists about potential for secondary malignancies

THERAPEUTIC PROCEDURES

- Prenatal diagnosis and genetic counseling should be made available to those with personal or family history
- No specific treatment is available for sickle cell anemia
- Pneumococcal vaccination reduces incidence of infections
- Acute painful episodes: identify precipitating factors and treat infections if present; maintain good hydration, and administer oxygen if hypoxic
- Sickle cell trait: no treatment necessary; genetic counseling appropriate
- Transfusions for aplastic or hemolytic crises
- Exchange transfusion primarily indicated for treatment of intractable pain crises, priapism, and stroke
- Allogeneic bone marrow transplantation under investigation as possible curative option for severely affected young patients

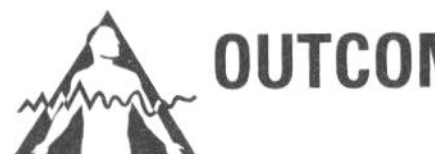

OUTCOME

COMPLICATIONS

- Sickle cell anemia becomes a chronic multisystem disease, with death from organ failure
- Acute chest syndrome

PROGNOSIS

- With improved supportive care, average life expectancy is now between ages 40 and 50

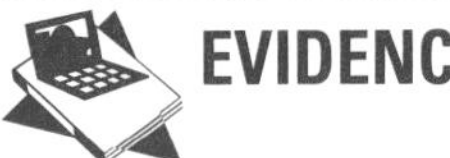

EVIDENCE

PRACTICE GUIDELINES

- Rees DC et al: Guidelines for the management of the acute painful crisis in sickle cell disease. Br J Haematol 2003;120:744. [PMID: 12614204]

WEB SITES

- Georgia Comprehensive Sickle Cell Center at Grady Health System
  - http://www.scinfo.org/
- National Library of Medicine Genetics Home Reference: Sickle Cell Anemia
  - http://ghr.nlm.nih.gov/condition=sicklecellanemia

INFORMATION FOR PATIENTS

- JAMA Patient Page: Sickle cell anemia. JAMA 1999;281:1768. [PMID: 10328078]
- National Heart, Lung, and Blood Institute: What Is Sickle Cell Anemia?
  - http://www.nhlbi.nih.gov/health/dci/Diseases/Sca/SCA_WhatIs.html
- Dolan DNA Learning Center: Sickle Cell Disease
  - http://www.yourgenesyourhealth.org/sickle/whatisit.htm
- Sickle Cell Disease Association of America: Frequently Asked Questions
  - http://www.sicklecelldisease.org/about_scd/faqs.phtml

REFERENCES

- Alexander N et al: Are there clinical phenotypes of homozygous sickle cell disease? Br J Haematol 2004; 126:606. [PMID: 15287956]
- Stuart MJ et al: Sickle-cell disease. Lancet 2004; 364:1343. [PMID: 15474138]
- Walters MC et al: Impact of bone marrow transplantation for symptomatic sickle cell disease: an interim report: multicenter investigation of bone marrow transplantation for sickle cell disease. Blood 2000;95:1918. [PMID: 10706855]

Author(s)

Charles A. Linker, MD

Sinusitis, Acute

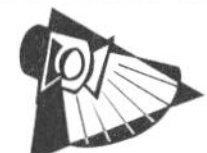

KEY FEATURES

ESSENTIALS OF DIAGNOSIS

- Pain is usually unilateral over the maxillary sinus or toothache-like
- Symptoms usually last for more than a week
- Change of secretions from mucoid to purulent green or yellow
- Occasional visible swelling or erythema over a sinus

GENERAL CONSIDERATIONS

- Diseases that swell the nasal mucous membrane, such as viral or allergic rhinitis, are usually the underlying cause
- Usually is a result of impaired mucociliary clearance and obstruction of the osteomeatal complex, resulting in the accumulation of mucous secretion in the sinus cavity that becomes secondarily infected by bacteria
- The typical pathogens are the same as those that cause acute otitis media: *Streptococcus pneumoniae*, other streptococci, *Haemophilus influenzae*, and, less commonly, *Staphylococcus aureus* and *Moraxella catarrhalis*
- About 25% of healthy asymptomatic individuals may, if sinus aspirates are cultured, harbor these bacteria
- Discolored nasal discharge and poor response to decongestants suggest sinusitis

DEMOGRAPHICS

- Uncommon compared with viral rhinitis, but still affects more than 14% of the population
- The prevalence of nosocomial sinusitis is as high as 40% in critically ill intubated patients

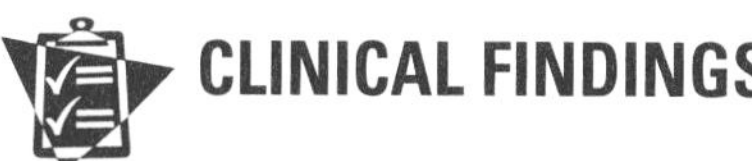

CLINICAL FINDINGS

SYMPTOMS AND SIGNS

- **Maxillary sinusitis**
  - Pain and pressure over the cheek
  - Pain may refer to the upper incisor and canine teeth
  - May result from dental infection, and tender teeth should be carefully examined for abscess
- **Ethmoid sinusitis**
  - Usually accompanied by maxillary sinusitis; the symptoms of maxillary sinusitis generally predominate
  - Pain and pressure over the high lateral wall of the nose that may radiate to the orbit
  - Periorbital cellulitis may be present
- **Sphenoid sinusitis**
  - Usually seen in the setting of pansinusitis
  - The patient may complain of a headache "in the middle of the head" and often points to the vertex
  - Sixth nerve palsy may occur as the abducens nerve courses just lateral to the sinus
- **Frontal sinusitis**
  - Usually pain and tenderness of the forehead
  - This is most easily elicited by palpation of the orbital roof just below the medial end of the eyebrow
  - Palpation here is more accurate than percussion of the supraorbital area or forehead

DIFFERENTIAL DIAGNOSIS

- Upper respiratory tract infection
- Viral rhinitis
- Allergic rhinitis
- Nasal polyposis
- Dental abscess
- Rhinocerebral mucormycosis
- Otitis media
- Pharyngitis
- Dacryocystitis
- Paranasal sinus cancer

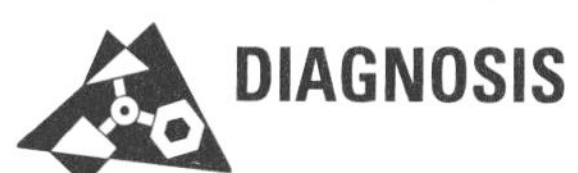

DIAGNOSIS

LABORATORY TESTS

- It is usually possible to make the diagnosis on clinical grounds alone

IMAGING STUDIES

- Routine radiographs are not cost-effective; they may be helpful when clinically based criteria are difficult to evaluate
  - Sinus x-rays can show soft tissue density without bone destruction
  - An air-fluid level may also be seen
- Coronal CT scans are reasonably sensitive, but not specific; sinus abnormalities can be seen in the majority of patients with an upper respiratory tract infection, whereas only 2% develop bacterial sinusitis
- Sinusitis is a clinical diagnosis for which CT may be helpful in confirming, denying, or monitoring

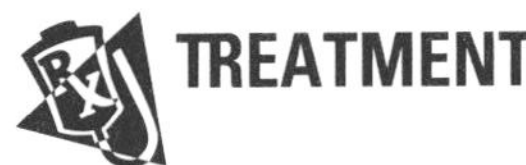

TREATMENT

MEDICATIONS

- Antibiotic use is the most cost-effective treatment
- For symptom improvement, use oral or nasal decongestants or both (eg, oral pseudoephedrine, 30–120 mg/dose, up to 240 mg/day; nasal oxymetazoline, 0.05%, or xylometazoline, 0.05–0.1%, one or two sprays in each nostril Q 6–8 h for up to 3 days
- Amoxicillin (500 mg PO three times a day), possibly with clavulanate (125 mg three times a day)
- Trimethoprim (TMP)-sulfamethoxazole (SMZ; 4 mg/kg TMP and 20 mg/kg SMZ PO twice daily; available as tablets with 80-mg or 160-mg TMP and 160-mg or 800-mg SMZ)
- Cephalexin (250–500 mg PO four times/day)
- Cefuroxime (250 mg PO twice daily)
- Cefaclor (250 mg PO three times/day)
- Cefixime (400 mg PO daily)
- Quinolones, such as ciprofloxacin (500 mg PO twice daily), levofloxacin (500 mg PO once daily), moxifloxacin (400 mg PO once daily), and sparfloxacin (200 mg PO once daily after an initial dose of 400 mg)
- Macrolides, such as azithromycin (500 mg PO once daily, possibly for only 3 days) or clarithromycin (500 mg PO twice daily for 14 days)

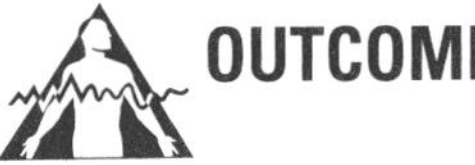

OUTCOME

COMPLICATIONS

- Mucocele; treatment is surgical
- Osteomyelitis requires prolonged antibiotics as well as removal of necrotic bone; the frontal sinus is most commonly affected, with bone involvement suggested by a tender puffy swelling of the forehead
- Cavernous sinus thrombosis
- Meningitis
- Epidural and intraparenchymal brain abscesses

PROGNOSIS

- Two thirds of untreated patients will improve symptomatically within 2 weeks

WHEN TO REFER

- Recurrent sinusitis or sinusitis that does not appear to respond clinically warrants evaluation by a specialist
- Any complication of sinusitis

EVIDENCE

PRACTICE GUIDELINES

- Institute for Clinical Systems Improvement: Acute Sinusitis in Adults, 2004.
  - http://www.icsi.org/knowledge/detail.asp?catID=29&itemID=148
- American College of Physicians: Principles of Appropriate Antibiotic Use for Acute Sinusitis in Adults, 2001.
  - http://www.guideline.gov/summary/summary.aspx?doc_id=2743&nbr=1969

WEB SITE

- Baylor College of Medicine Otolaryngology Resources on the Internet
  - http://www.bcm.tmc.edu/oto/othersa.html

INFORMATION FOR PATIENTS

- American Academy of Allergy, Asthma & Immunology: Sinusitis
  - http://www.aaaai.org/patients/resources/easy_reader/sinusitis.pdf
- American Academy of Family Physicians: Sinusitis
  - http://familydoctor.org/686.xml
- American Academy of Otolaryngology—Head and Neck Surgery: Doctor, What Is Sinusitis?
  - http://www.entnet.org/healthinfo/sinus/sinusitis.cfm
- National Institute of Allergy and Infectious Diseases: Sinusitis
  - http://www.niaid.nih.gov/factsheets/sinusitis.htm

REFERENCES

- Piccirillo JF: Clinical practice. Acute bacterial sinusitis. N Engl J Med 2004;351:902. [PMID: 15329428]
- Scheid EC et al: Acute bacterial rhinosinusitis in adults: part I. Evaluation. Am Fam Physician 2004;70:1685. [PMID: 15554486]
- Scheid EC et al: Acute bacterial rhinosinusitis in adults: part II. Treatment. Am Fam Physician 2004;70:1697. [PMID: 15554487]

Author(s)

Robert K. Jackler, MD
Michael J. Kaplan, MD

Sjögren's Syndrome

KEY FEATURES

ESSENTIALS OF DIAGNOSIS

- Dryness of eyes and dry mouth (sicca components); they occur alone or in association with rheumatoid arthritis or other connective tissue disease
- Rheumatoid factor and other autoantibodies common
- Increased incidence of lymphoma

GENERAL CONSIDERATIONS

- Chronic autoimmune dysfunction of exocrine glands in many areas of the body
- Dryness of the eyes, mouth, and other areas covered by mucous membranes
- Keratoconjunctivitis sicca results from inadequate tear production caused by lymphocyte and plasma cell infiltration of the lacrimal glands
- Frequently associated with a rheumatic disease, most often rheumatoid arthritis

Associated conditions

- Rheumatoid arthritis
- Systemic lupus erythematosus
- Primary biliary cirrhosis
- Scleroderma
- Polymyositis
- Hashimoto's thyroiditis
- Polyarteritis nodosa
- Idiopathic pulmonary fibrosis

DEMOGRAPHICS

- The disorder is predominantly a disease of women, in a ratio of 9:1
- Greatest incidence between age 40 and 60 years

CLINICAL FINDINGS

SYMPTOMS AND SIGNS

- Eyes
  - Ocular burning, itching, ropy secretions
  - "Grain of sand in the eye" sensation
- Parotid glands
  - Enlargement may be chronic or relapsing
  - Develops in one-third of patients
- Dryness of the mouth (xerostomia) leads to difficulty in swallowing dry foods (like crackers), to constant thirst for fluids, and to severe dental caries
- There may be loss of taste and smell
- Systemic manifestations
  - Dysphagia, pancreatitis
  - Pleuritis, obstructive lung disease (in the absence of smoking)
  - Neuropsychiatric dysfunction
  - Vasculitis
- Kidney
  - Renal tubular acidosis (type I, distal) occurs in 20% of patients
  - Chronic interstitial nephritis, which may result in impaired renal function, may be seen

DIFFERENTIAL DIAGNOSIS

- Sicca complex associated with other autoimmune disease, eg, sarcoidosis, rheumatoid arthritis, SLE, scleroderma
- Other causes of dry mouth or eyes, eg, anticholinergics, mumps, irradiation, seasonal allergies, irritation from smoking

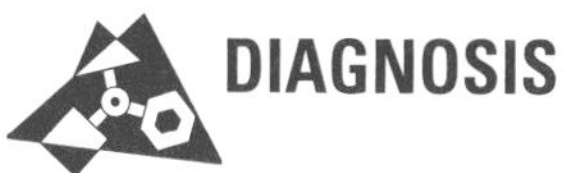

DIAGNOSIS

LABORATORY TESTS

- Rheumatoid factor is found in 70% of patients
- Antibodies against the cytoplasmic antigens SS-A and SS-B (also called Ro and La, respectively) are often present (Tables 76 and 82)
- When SS-A antibodies are present, extraglandular manifestations are far more common

DIAGNOSTIC PROCEDURES

- Lip biopsy is the only specific diagnostic technique and has minimal risk; if lymphoid foci are seen in accessory salivary glands, the diagnosis is confirmed
- Biopsy of the parotid gland should be reserved for patients with atypical presentations such as unilateral gland enlargement
- The Schirmer test, which measures the quantity of tears secreted

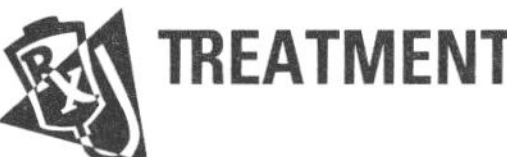

TREATMENT

MEDICATIONS

- Pilocarpine (5 mg four times daily) and the acetylcholine derivative cevimeline (30 mg three times daily) are helpful for severe xerostomia
- Atropinic drugs and decongestants decrease salivary secretions and should be avoided

THERAPEUTIC PROCEDURES

- Treatment is symptomatic and supportive
- Artificial tears applied frequently will relieve ocular symptoms and avert further desiccation
- Sipping water frequently or using sugar-free gums and hard candies usually relieves dry mouth symptoms
- A program of oral hygiene is essential to preserve dentition

OUTCOME

COMPLICATIONS

- A spectrum of lymphoproliferation ranging from benign to malignant may be found
- Malignant lymphomas and Waldenström's macroglobulinemia occur nearly 50 times more frequently than can be explained by chance alone in primary Sjögren's syndrome

PROGNOSIS

- Usually benign and consistent with a normal life span
- Prognosis is mainly influenced by the nature of the associated disease
- The patients (3–10% of the total Sjögren's population) at greatest risk of developing lymphoma have severe dryness, marked parotid gland enlargement, splenomegaly, vasculitis, peripheral neuropathy, anemia, and mixed monoclonal cryoglobulinemia

EVIDENCE

PRACTICE GUIDELINES

- Johns Hopkins University
  - http://www.hopkins-arthritis.som.jhmi.edu/edu/acr/acr.html#sjogrens

WEB SITE

- Sjögren's Syndrome Foundation
  - http://www.sjogrens.org

INFORMATION FOR PATIENTS

- National Institute of Arthritis and Musculoskeletal and Skin Diseases
  - http://www.niams.nih.gov/hi/topics/sjogrens/index.htm
- National Institute of Neurological Disorders and Stroke
  - http://www.ninds.nih.gov/health_and_medical/disorders/sjogrens_doc.htm

REFERENCES

- Garcia-Carrasco M et al: Primary Sjögren syndrome: clinical and immunologic disease patterns in a cohort of 400 patients. Medicine (Baltimore) 2002;81:270. [PMID: 12169882]
- Mariette X et al: Inefficacy of infliximab in primary Sjögren's syndrome: results of the randomized, controlled Trial of Remicade in Primary Sjögren's Syndrome (TRIPSS). Arthritis Rheum 2004;50:1270. [PMID: 15077311]
- Ono M et al: Therapeutic effect of cevimeline on dry eye in patients with Sjögren's syndrome: a randomized, double-blind clinical study. Am J Ophthalmol 2004;138:6. [PMID: 15234277]

Author(s)

David B. Hellmann, MD, FACP
John H. Stone, MD, MPH

Sleep Apnea, Obstructive

Skin Infections, Streptococcal p. 1151

KEY FEATURES

ESSENTIALS OF DIAGNOSIS

- Daytime somnolence or fatigue
- A history of loud snoring with witnessed apneic events
- Overnight polysomnography demonstrates apneic episodes with hypoxemia

GENERAL CONSIDERATIONS

- Upper airway obstruction results from a loss of pharyngeal muscle tone during sleep
- Patients with narrowed upper airways are predisposed to the condition
- Ingestion of alcohol or sedatives before sleep and nasal obstruction from any cause may precipitate or worsen the condition
- Cigarette smoking and hypothyroidism are risk factors

DEMOGRAPHICS

- Most patients are obese, middle-aged men

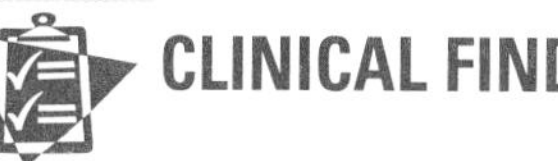

CLINICAL FINDINGS

SYMPTOMS AND SIGNS

- Patients complain of daytime somnolence or fatigue, morning sluggishness, or cognitive impairment
- Recent weight gain, headaches, and impotence may be present
- Bed partners usually report loud cyclical snoring and witnessed apneas with restlessness and thrashing movements during sleep
- Systemic hypertension is usually present
- Physical examination may show evidence of pulmonary hypertension with cor pulmonale
- Oropharyngeal narrowing due to excessive soft tissue may be seen
- A short, thick neck is common
- Bradydysrhythmias may occur during sleep
- Tachydysrhythmias may be seen once airflow is reestablished following an apneic episode

DIFFERENTIAL DIAGNOSIS

- Central sleep apnea
- Mixed sleep apnea
- Obesity-hypoventilation syndrome (Pickwickian syndrome)
- Narcolepsy
- Alcohol or sedative abuse
- Depression
- Hypothyroidism
- Seizure disorder

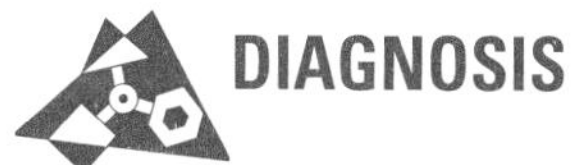

DIAGNOSIS

LABORATORY TESTS

- Erythrocytosis is common
- Thyroid-stimulating hormone should be checked

DIAGNOSTIC PROCEDURES

- Overnight polysomnography is essential to make the diagnosis
- Apneic episodes are defined as breath cessation for 10 seconds or more
- Hypopnea is defined as a decrement in airflow with a drop in oxyhemoglobin saturation of 4% or more
- An otolaryngologic examination should be performed
- Screening with home nocturnal pulse oximetry has a high negative predictive value if no desaturations are seen

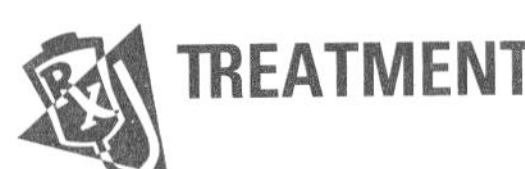

TREATMENT

MEDICATIONS

- Pharmacologic therapy is not successful

SURGERY

- Uvulopalatopharyngoplasty, the resection of pharyngeal tissue and removal of a portion of the soft palate and uvula, is helpful in approximately half of selected patients
- Nasal septoplasty is performed if gross nasal septal deformity is present
- Tracheostomy is the definitive therapy, but is reserved for life-threatening, refractory cases

THERAPEUTIC PROCEDURES

- Weight loss and avoidance of alcohol and hypnotic medications are initial steps
- 10–20% weight loss may be curative
- Nasal continuous positive airway pressure (CPAP) is curative in many patients
- Polysomnography is often necessary to determine the level of CPAP (usually 5–15 mm Hg) required
- Prosthetic devices inserted into the mouth to prevent pharyngeal occlusion can be modestly effective, but compliance is limiting

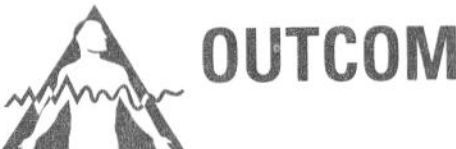

OUTCOME

COMPLICATIONS

- Cor pulmonale
- Life-threatening cardiac dysrhythmias
- Systemic hypertension

PROGNOSIS

- Only 75% of patients continue to use CPAP after 1 year

WHEN TO REFER

- For a sleep study

EVIDENCE

PRACTICE GUIDELINES

- National Guideline Clearinghouse
  - http://www.guideline.gov/summary/summary.aspx?doc_id=3181&nbr=2407&string=obstructive+sleep+apnea
- Littner M et al: Practice parameters for the use of laser-assisted uvulopalatoplasty: an update for 2000. Sleep 2001;24(5):603. [PMID:11480657]

INFORMATION FOR PATIENTS

- American Medical Association
  - http://www.medem.com/medlb/article_detaillb.cfm?article_ID=ZZZWT155MNC&sub_cat=593
- National Institute of Neurological Disorders and Stroke
  - http://www.ninds.nih.gov/disorders/sleep_apnea/sleep_apnea.htm

REFERENCES

- Bao G et al: Upper airway resistance syndrome—one decade later. Curr Op Pulm Med 2004;10:461. [PMID:15510051]
- Caples SM et al: Obstructive sleep apnea. Ann Intern Med 2005;142:187. [PMID:15684207]
- Flemons WW. Clinical practice. Obstructive sleep apnea. N Engl J Med 2002;347:498. [PMID:12181405]
- Shamsuzzaman AS et al: Obstructive sleep apnea: Implications for cardiac and vascular disease. JAMA 2003;290:1906. [PMID:14532320]
- Tishler PV et al: Incidence of sleep-disordered breathing in an urban adult population: the relative importance of risk factors in the development of sleep-disordered breathing. JAMA 2003;289:2230. [PMID:12734134]
- Yap WS et al: Central sleep apnea and hypoventilation syndrome. Curr Treat Options Neurol 2001;3:51. [PMID: 11123858]

Author(s)

Mark S. Chesnutt, MD

Thomas J. Prendergast, MD

Small Intestinal Neoplasms

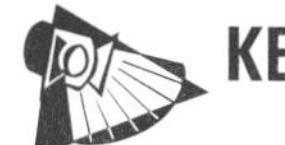

KEY FEATURES

ESSENTIALS OF DIAGNOSIS

- Acute gastrointestinal bleeding with hematochezia or melena or chronic gastrointestinal blood loss resulting in fatigue and iron deficiency anemia

GENERAL CONSIDERATIONS

- Benign and malignant tumors of the small intestine are rare
- Often no symptoms or signs
- Obstruction due to luminal narrowing or intussusception
- Benign tumors include single or multiple polyps, lipomas, benign gastrointestinal stromal tumors (GIST)
- Villous adenomas occur most commonly in the periampullary region of the duodenum and carry a high risk for invasive cancer
- Malignant small bowel tumors are extremely rare
- Adenocarcinoma occurs most commonly in the duodenum or proximal jejunum
- Ampullary carcinoma incidence is increased >200-fold in patients with familial adenomatous polyposis
- Nonampullary adenocarcinoma of the small intestine: 80% have metastasized at the time of diagnosis
- Lymphoma may arise primarily in the gastrointestinal tract or involve it secondarily in disseminated disease
- In the United States, primary lymphoma accounts for 5% of all lymphomas and 20% of small bowel malignancies
- Lymphoma occurs most commonly in the distal small intestine
- Majority are non-Hodgkin's intermediate or high-grade B cell lymphomas; T cell lymphomas occur in celiac sprue
- In the Middle East, lymphomas occur in immunoproliferative small intestinal disease
- Carcinoid tumors account for one-third of small intestinal tumors; >95% of gastrointestinal carcinoids occur in the rectum, appendix, or small intestine (especially ileum)
- Carcinoid tumors derive from neuroendocrine cells and secrete serotonin or its precursors
- Most are malignant, though many behave in an indolent fashion
- Even small carcinoid tumors may metastasize, usually by extension to the local lymph nodes and to the liver
- Carcinoid syndrome occurs in < 10% of patients and only in patients with hepatic metastasis; caused by tumor secretion of hormonal mediators
- Most malignant sarcomas arise from GIST; Kaposi's sarcoma is rare except in untreated AIDS

DEMOGRAPHICS

- Multiple small bowel polyps may suggest intestinal polyposis syndrome
- Hamartomas: Peutz-Jeghers syndrome, juvenile polyposis
- Adenomas or periampullary adenoma: familial adenomatous polyposis

CLINICAL FINDINGS

SYMPTOMS AND SIGNS

- Benign stromal tumors: most are asymptomatic, some may ulcerate and cause acute or chronic bleeding or obstruction
- Malignant small bowel tumors: anemia, bleeding, obstruction, or evidence of metastatic disease
- Nonampullary adenocarcinoma of the small intestine: obstruction, acute or chronic bleeding, or weight loss
- Ampullary carcinoma: jaundice due to bile duct obstruction or bleeding
- Primary lymphoma: abdominal pain, weight loss, nausea and vomiting, distention, anemia, and occult blood in the stool
- Carcinoid tumors: most asymptomatic; if symptomatic, usually with carcinoid syndrome with cramps, flushing, diarrhea, cyanosis, or bronchospasm, cardiac right-sided valvular lesions; intussusception with obstruction rare

DIFFERENTIAL DIAGNOSIS

- Crohn's disease

Benign polyps

- Mucosal polyps: adenomas, hamartomas, hyperplastic
- Lipoma
- Benign stromal tumor (leiomyoma)

Malignant lesions

- Adenocarcinoma
- Lymphoma (primary or secondary)
- Carcinoid
- Malignant stromal tumor (sarcoma)
- Kaposi's sarcoma

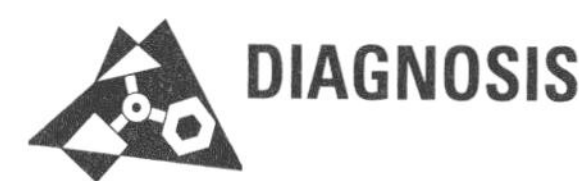

DIAGNOSIS

LABORATORY TESTS

- Alpha heavy chains in the serum in 70% of patients with lymphoma occurring in immunoproliferative small intestinal disease
- Hypoalbuminemia secondary to protein-losing enteropathy in lymphoma
- Urinary 5-hydroxyindoleacetic acid >10 mg/24 h and serum serotonin elevated in carcinoid tumors

IMAGING STUDIES

- Barium radiographic studies, either enteroclysis or a small bowel series, for diagnosis of small bowel tumors, primary lymphoma
- Chest and abdominal CT help to determine stage of primary lymphoma
- Video capsule imaging of small intestine
- Abdominal CT for carcinoid tumors, hepatic metastases
- Somatostatin receptor scintigraphy positive in >90% of hepatic metastases from carcinoid tumors
- Echocardiogram for carcinoid heart disease

DIAGNOSTIC PROCEDURES

- Enteroscopy to visualize and biopsy small intestinal tumors
- Endoscopic, percutaneous, or laparoscopic biopsy establishes the diagnosis of primary intestinal lymphoma
- Bone marrow biopsy, and, in some cases, lymphangiography for staging of primary lymphoma
- Proctoscopy: rectal carcinoids usually detected incidentally as submucosal nodules usually < 1 cm in size during proctoscopy
- Appendectomy: appendiceal carcinoids < 2 cm in size are identified in 0.3%

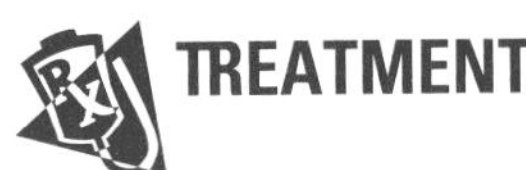

TREATMENT

MEDICATIONS

- Role of adjuvant chemotherapy in primary lymphoma is unclear
- Systemic chemotherapy with or without radiation therapy for primary lymphoma with extensive disease
- Octreotide, 150–500 μg SC three times daily, inhibits serotonin secretion, providing dramatic relief of symptoms in 90% of patients with carcinoid syndrome for a median period of 1 year

SURGERY

- Surgical or endoscopic excision of symptomatic benign tumors recommended
- Surgical excision of symptomatic benign stromal tumors if >3 cm
- Surgical resection of ampullary carcinoma is curative in up to 40%
- Resection of nonampullary adenocarcinoma for control of symptoms
- Resection of primary intestinal lymphoma for stage IE disease
- Surgical debulking for stage III or IV lymphoma
- Local excision of carcinoids of small intestine, appendix, rectum if < 2 cm in size and if evidence of lymphatic spread
- More extensive cancer resection operation is warranted for carcinoid tumors >2 cm in size since they are associated with metastasis in >20% of appendiceal and ~10% of rectal carcinoids
- Resection of hepatic metastases for refractory carcinoid syndrome, diarrhea

THERAPEUTIC PROCEDURES

- Hepatic artery occlusion and chemotherapy in hepatic metastases

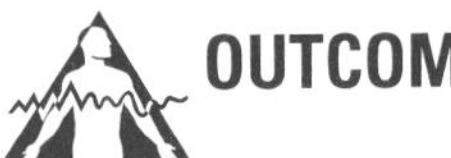

OUTCOME

FOLLOW-UP

- Periodic surveillance of periampullary region villous adenomas by endoscopic retrograde cholangiopancreatography or endoscopic ultrasound

COMPLICATIONS

- Cardiac right-sided valvular lesions are a late manifestation of metastatic carcinoid tumors

PROGNOSIS

- Carcinoid tumors: overall 5-year survival rate is 50%
- Carcinoid tumors: for disease confined to the small intestine, local excision cures >85%; for resectable disease with lymph node involvement, 5-year disease-free survival is 80%, but by 25 years, only 25% are disease free

EVIDENCE

PRACTICE GUIDELINES

- De Franco A et al: Imaging of small bowel tumors. Rays 2002;27:35. [PMID: 12696273]
- Kariv R et al: Malignant tumors of the small intestine—new insights into a rare disease. Isr Med Assoc J 2003;5:188. [PMID: 12725140]
- Miettinen M et al: Gastrointestinal stromal tumors (GISTs): definition, occurrence, pathology, differential diagnosis and molecular genetics. Pol J Pathol 2003;54:3. [PMID: 12817876]

WEB SITES

- MEDLINEplus—Small bowel resection
  - http://www.nlm.nih.gov/medlineplus/ency/article/002943.htm
- National Cancer Institute—Small intestine cancer
  - http://www.cancer.gov/cancerinfo/pdq/treatment/smallintestine/patient
- University of Alabama—Intestinal Neoplasms
  - http://cchs-dl.slis.ua.edu/clinical/oncology/gastrointestinal/instestinal.html

INFORMATION FOR PATIENTS

- Cleveland Clinic—Small intestine cancer
  - http://www.clevelandclinic.org/health/health-info/docs/1400/1446.asp?index=6225
- Columbia University of Physicians and Surgeons—Gastrointestinal cancers
  - http://cpmcnet.columbia.edu/texts/guide/hmg17_0010.html#17.35
- National Cancer Institute
  - http://www.cancer.gov/cancerinfo/pdq/treatment/smallintestine/patient

REFERENCES

- Bresman PS: Gastrointestinal lymphoma. Curr Treat Options Oncol 2003;4:21. [PMID: 12941202]
- Lograno R et al: Recent advances in cell biology, diagnosis, and therapy of gastrointestinal stromal tumor (GIST). Cancer Cell Biol 2004;3:251. [PMID: 14726714]
- Schnirer II et al: Carcinoid—a comprehensive review. Acta Oncol 2003;42:672. [PMID: 14690153]
- Torres M et al: Malignant tumors of the small intestine. J Clin Gastroenterol 2003;37:372. [PMID: 14564183]

Author(s)

Kenneth R. McQuaid, MD

Smallpox & Vaccinia

KEY FEATURES

ESSENTIALS OF DIAGNOSIS

- Prodromal high fever
- Eruption progressing from papules to vesicles to pustules, then crusts
- All lesions in the same stage
- Face and distal extremities (including palms and soles) favored

GENERAL CONSIDERATIONS

- Reintroduction of vaccination for first-responder and military population because of bioterrorist threat
- The incubation period for smallpox averages 12 days (7–17 days)
- Immunization with vaccinia is not recommended for persons with eczema, in whom widespread vaccinia (eczema vaccinatum) may result, with lesions resembling those of smallpox
- Exposure to a recently vaccinated person may lead to generalized disease in persons with certain skin diseases
- Prior vaccination does not prevent generalized vaccinia, but previously vaccinated individuals have milder disease
- Progression of the primary inoculation site to a large ulceration occurs in persons with systemic immune deficiency, with a possible fatal outcome

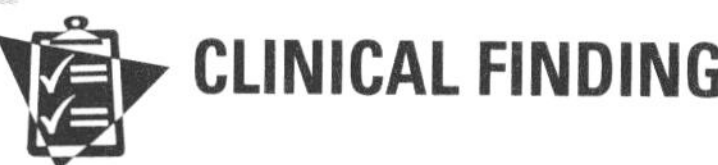

CLINICAL FINDINGS

SYMPTOMS AND SIGNS

- See Table 7

Smallpox

- **Prodrome:** abrupt onset of high fever, severe headaches, and backaches, with the infected person appearing quite ill
- **Infectious phase:** appearance of an enanthem, followed in 1–2 days by a skin eruption
  - Lesions begin as macules, progressing to papules, then pustules, and finally crusts over 14–18 days
  - The face is affected first, followed by the upper extremities, the lower extremities, and trunk, completely evolving over 1 week
  - Lesions are relatively monomorphous, especially in each anatomic region
- All lesions in same stage of development differentiates rash from varicella

Vaccinia

- Inoculation with vaccinia produces a papular lesion on day 2–3 that progresses to an umbilicated papule by day 4 and a pustular lesion by the end of the first week
- The lesion collapses centrally, and crusts, with the crust eventually detaching up to a month after the inoculation

DIFFERENTIAL DIAGNOSIS

- Generalized varicella zoster virus (VZV) infection
- Generalized herpes simplex virus (HSV)

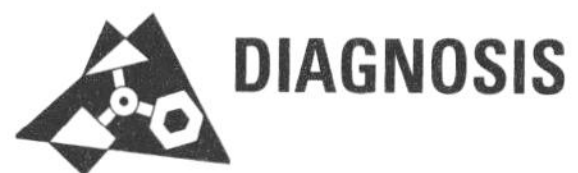

DIAGNOSIS

LABORATORY TESTS

- Direct fluorescent antibody testing for HSV and VZV are first-line diagnostic tests to differentiate VZV, HSV, vaccinia, and smallpox
- Smallpox is a clinical diagnosis but viral infection can be confirmed by electron microscopy, antigen detection, and PCR

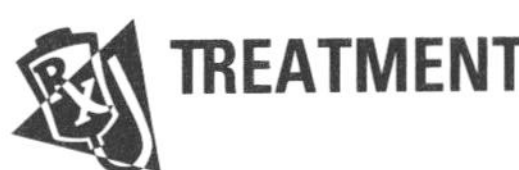

TREATMENT

MEDICATIONS

- No specific and proven antiviral therapy for vaccinia or smallpox
- Vaccinia immune globulin is used to treat eczema vaccinatum and progressive vaccinia
- Cidofovir may have some activity against these poxviruses

THERAPEUTIC PROCEDURES

- Strict respiratory and contact isolation crucial
- Patient should be immunized if in early stage of disease
- No antiviral therapy clearly effective
- Supportive care critical
- CDC should be contacted immediately in the event of suspected case(s)

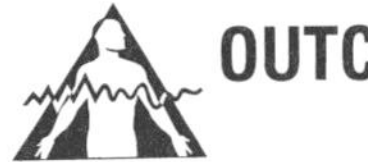

OUTCOME

COMPLICATIONS

- Serious complications in about 5/100,000 persons include encephalitis, progressive vaccinia, and eczema vaccinatum

PROGNOSIS

- Generalized vaccinia may be fatal

WHEN TO ADMIT

- Until the diagnosis is confirmed, strict isolation of the patient is indicated

PREVENTION

- U.S. vaccination campaign voluntary, focusing on first responders and military personnel

EVIDENCE

PRACTICE GUIDELINES

- Cono J et al; Centers for Disease Control and Prevention: Smallpox vaccination and adverse reactions. Guidance for clinicians, 2003
  - http://www.cdc.gov/mmwr/preview/mmwrhtml/rr5204a1.htm
- Rotz LD et al: Vaccinia (smallpox) vaccine: recommendations of the Advisory Committee on Immunization Practices, 2001
  - http://www.cdc.gov/mmwr/PDF/RR/RR5010.PDF
- Wharton et al: Recommendations for using smallpox vaccine in a pre-event vaccination program. Supplemental recommendations of the Advisory Committee on Immunization Practices and the Healthcare Infection Control Practices Advisory Committee, 2003
  - http://www.cdc.gov/mmwr/preview/mmwrhtml/rr5207a1.htm

WEB SITE

- Centers for Disease Control and Prevention
  - http://www.bt.cdc.gov/agent/smallpox/index.asp

INFORMATION FOR PATIENTS

- American Academy of Family Physicians: Smallpox Vaccine
  - http://familydoctor.org/740.xml
- Centers for Disease Control and Prevention: Smallpox Frequently Asked Questions
  - http://www.bt.cdc.gov/agent/smallpox/overview/faq.asp
- MedlinePlus: Smallpox Interactive Tutorial
  - http://www.nlm.nih.gov/medlineplus/tutorials/smallpox.html

REFERENCES

- Breman J et al: Diagnosis and management of smallpox. N Engl J Med 2002;346:1300. [PMID: 11923491]
- Mack T: A different view of smallpox and vaccination. N Engl J Med 2003;348:460. [PMID: 12496354]
- Sepkowitz K: How contagious is vaccinia? N Engl J Med 2003;348:439. [PMID: 12496351]

Author(s)

Timothy G. Berger, MD

Somatoform Disorders

KEY FEATURES

ESSENTIALS OF DIAGNOSIS

- Physical symptoms involve one or more organ systems
- Symptoms are not intentional
- Subjective complaints exceed objective findings
- Correlation exists between symptom development and psychosocial stress

GENERAL CONSIDERATIONS

- This diagnostic grouping includes **Conversion Disorder**, **Somatization Disorder**, **Pain Disorder Associated with Psychological Factors**, and **Hypochondriasis**
- It is difficult to discern whether the psychosocial distress seen in these conditions has caused or is the result of a chronic disease
- Vulnerability in an organ system and exposure to family members with somatization problems are thought to interact in the development of symptoms

DEMOGRAPHICS

- **Conversion disorder** is more common in lower socioeconomic classes and certain cultures
- **Somatization disorder** usually occurs before age 30 and is 10 times more common in women

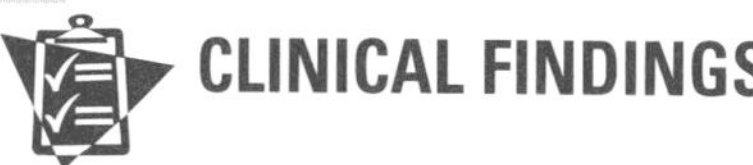

CLINICAL FINDINGS

SYMPTOMS AND SIGNS

- A precipitating emotional event often precedes somatic symptoms
- **Conversion disorder**
  - Psychic conflict is converted into physical symptoms
  - The somatic symptom is typically paralysis
  - The affected organ system may have symbolic meaning (eg, arm paralysis in marked anger)
- **Somatization disorder**
  - Multiple physical complaints are referable to several organ systems
  - Anxiety, panic disorder, and depression are often present
  - Preoccupation with medical and surgical issues often precludes other life activities
  - Patients have often undergone multiple surgeries and have evidence of longstanding symptoms
  - Multiple symptoms that frequently change and have eluded diagnosis by three or more physicians support this diagnosis
- **Pain disorder associated with psychological factors**
  - Patients have a long history of complaints of severe pain not consonant with anatomic and clinical signs
  - Exacerbations and remission of complaints correlate with psychogenic factors
- **Hypochondriasis**
  - Fear of disease and a preoccupation with the body
  - Patients exhibit perceptual amplification and heightened responsiveness
  - Family members who served as a role model for hypochondriacal behavior may be a clue to the diagnosis

DIFFERENTIAL DIAGNOSIS

- Depression must be considered in any patient with a condition judged to be somatoform
- Factitious disorders, which differ from this grouping in that symptom production is intentional
- Intoxication states

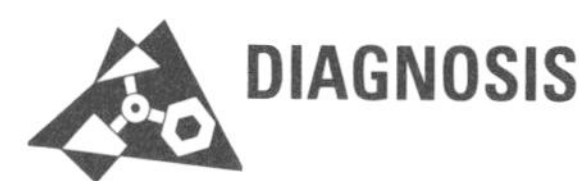

DIAGNOSIS

DIAGNOSTIC PROCEDURES

- In conversion disorder with pseudoseizures, video-EEG may be necessary to rule out epilepsy
- Since all somatoform disorders are diagnoses of exclusion, a workup sufficient to rule out physical illness is required

Smoke Inhalation p. 1152

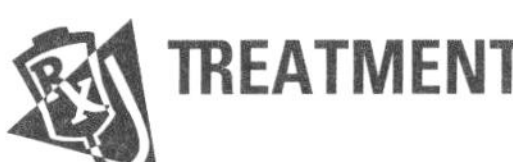

TREATMENT

MEDICATIONS

- Drugs should not be prescribed in place of frequent appointments

THERAPEUTIC PROCEDURES

- Behavioral
  - Biofeedback can be helpful in training patients to recognize symptoms and learn countermaneuvers that provide relief
- Psychological
  - Psychological intervention by the primary clinician should focus on pragmatic changes
  - Analytic approaches focused on exploration of early experiences often fail, since patients do not relate these to their current distress
  - Group therapy sometimes allows ventilation, improves coping, and focuses on interpersonal adjustment
  - Conversion disorder is sometimes helped by hypnosis or amobarbital interviews
- Social
  - Family members should attend appointments to learn how best to live with the patient
  - Peer support groups can encourage patients to accept and live with their problem
  - Communication with employers may be necessary to encourage long-term interest in the employee/patient

OUTCOME

FOLLOW-UP

- Regular appointments are helpful. These should be brief and not contingent on symptoms
- Care should be consolidated under a primary clinician, with consultants for evaluation only
- Ongoing reevaluation is important
- Somatoform disorders may coexist with physical illness, which can be overlooked

PROGNOSIS

- Intervention is most successful when instituted before chronicity develops

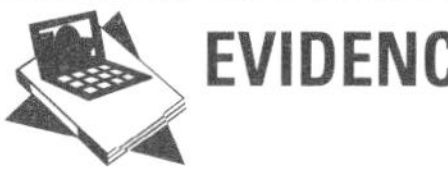

EVIDENCE

PRACTICE GUIDELINES

- American Academy of Family Physicians: Somatizing patients: Part I. Practical diagnosis
  - http://www.aafp.org/afp/20000215/1073.html
- American Academy of Family Physicians: Somatizing patients: Part II. Practical management
  - http://www.aafp.org/afp/20000301/1423.html
- American Academy of Family Physicians: In pursuit of perfection: A primary care physician's guide to body dysmorphic disorder
  - http://www.aafp.org/afp/991015ap/1738.html
- National Guideline Clearinghouse:VHA/DoD, 2004
  - http://www.guideline.gov/summary/summary.aspx?doc_id=3415

WEB SITES

- American Psychiatric Association
  - http://www.psych.org/
- Internet Mental Health
  - http://www.mentalhealth.com/

INFORMATION FOR PATIENTS

- American Academy of Family Physicians
  - http://familydoctor.org/162.xml
- American Academy of Family Physicians
  - http://www.aafp.org/afp/20000301/1431ph.html
- National Institutes of Health
  - http://www.nlm.nih.gov/medlineplus/ency/article/000922.htm

REFERENCES

- Eisendrath SJ: Factitious physical disorders. West J Med 1994;160:177. [PMID:8169474]
- Eisendrath SJ et al: Somatization disorders: effective management in primary care. J Musculoskel Med 1997;4:47.
- Yeung A: Somatoform disorders. West J Med 2001;176:253. [PMID:12208832]

Author(s)

Stuart J. Eisendrath, MD

Jonathan E. Lichtmacher, MD

Spasticity

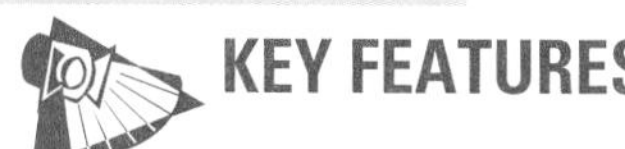

ESSENTIALS OF DIAGNOSIS

- The term "spasticity" is commonly used for an upper motor neuron deficit, but it properly refers to an increase in resistance to passive movement that affects different muscles to a different extent

GENERAL CONSIDERATIONS

- Spasticity is often a major complication of stroke, cerebral or spinal injury, static perinatal encephalopathy, and multiple sclerosis
- It may be exacerbated by decubitus ulcers, urinary or other infections, and nociceptive stimuli

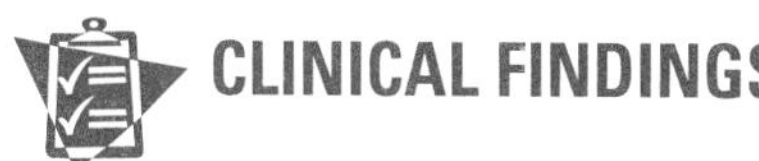

SYMPTOMS AND SIGNS

- A velocity-dependent increase in resistance to passive movement that affects different muscles to a different extent
- Not uniform in degree throughout the range of a particular movement
- Commonly associated with other features of pyramidal deficit

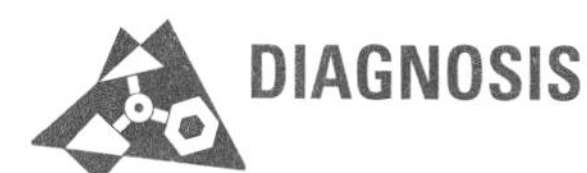

DIAGNOSTIC PROCEDURES

- Diagnosis made clinically

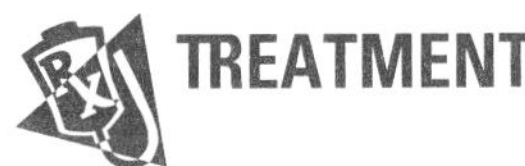

TREATMENT

MEDICATIONS

- Drug therapy is important, but it may increase functional disability when increased extensor tone is providing additional support for patients with weak legs
- Dantrolene
  - Weakens muscle contraction by interfering with the role of calcium
  - Best avoided in patients with poor respiratory function or severe myocardial disease
  - Begin with 25 mg QD, and build dose up by 25-mg increments every 3 days, depending on tolerance, to a maximum of 100 mg QID
  - Side effects: diarrhea, nausea, weakness, hepatic dysfunction (which may rarely be fatal, especially in women older than 35), drowsiness, lightheadedness, hallucinations
- Lioresal
  - An effective drug for treating spasticity of spinal origin and painful flexor (or extensor) spasms
  - Initial dose is 5 or 10 mg BID and then built up gradually
  - The maximum recommended daily dose is 80 mg
  - Side effects: gastrointestinal disturbances, lassitude, fatigue, sedation, unsteadiness, confusion, hallucinations
- Diazepam
  - May modify spasticity by its action on spinal interneurons and perhaps also by influencing supraspinal centers
  - Effective doses often cause intolerable drowsiness and vary with different patients
- Tizanidine is a centrally acting α_2-adrenergic agonist
  - As effective as these other agents but is probably better tolerated
  - The daily dose is built up gradually, usually to 8 mg taken three times daily
  - Side effects: sedation, lassitude, hypotension, dryness of the mouth
- Motor-point blocks by intramuscular phenol may reduce spasticity selectively in one or a few important muscles and may permit return of function in patients with incomplete myelopathies
- Intramuscular administration of botulinum toxin may also be helpful
- Intrathecal injection of phenol or absolute alcohol may be helpful in more severe cases, but greater selectivity can be achieved by nerve root or peripheral nerve neurolysis
  - These procedures should not be undertaken until the spasticity syndrome is fully evolved, ie, only after about 1 year or so, and only if long-term drug treatment either has not been helpful or carries a significant risk to the patient

SURGERY

- In patients with severe spasticity and limited use of the legs, a surgically implanted lioresal pump may provide significant relief and improve hygiene
- A number of surgical procedures, eg, adductor or heel cord tenotomy, may help in the management of spasticity and facilitate patient management
- Obturator neurectomy is helpful in patients with marked adductor spasms that interfere with personal hygiene or cause gait disturbances
- Posterior rhizotomy reduces spasticity, but its effect may be short-lived
- Anterior rhizotomy produces permanent wasting and weakness in the muscles that are denervated

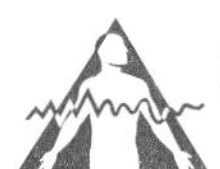

OUTCOME

WHEN TO REFER

- Refer early to a physical therapist

PREVENTION

- Physical therapy with appropriate stretching programs is important during rehabilitation after the development of an upper motor neuron lesion and in subsequent management of the patient
  - The aim is to prevent joint and muscle contractures and perhaps to modulate spasticity

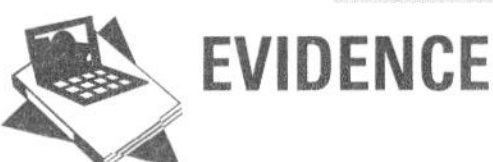

EVIDENCE

INFORMATION FOR PATIENTS

- National Institutes of Health
  - http://www.nlm.nih.gov/medlineplus/ency/article/003297.htm
- Worldwide Education and Awareness for Movement Disorders
  - http://www.wemove.org/spa/

REFERENCE

- Brashear A et al: Intramuscular injection of botulinum toxin for the treatment of wrist and finger spasticity after a stroke. N Engl J Med 2002;347:395. [PMID:12167681]

Author(s)

Michael J. Aminoff, DSc, MD, FRCP

Spherocytosis, Hereditary p. 1152.
Spinal Cord Compression, Malignant p. 1152.

Spinal Cord Tumors, Primary & Metastatic

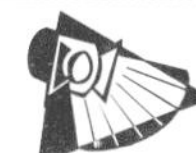

KEY FEATURES

ESSENTIALS OF DIAGNOSIS

- Pain, especially with extradural lesions
- Weakness, sensory disturbances, and reflex changes below the level of the lesion
- Bladder, bowel, and sexual dysfunction may occur

GENERAL CONSIDERATIONS

- Approximately 10% of spinal tumors are intramedullary
- Ependymoma is the most common type of intramedullary tumor; the remainder are other types of glioma
- Extramedullary tumors may be extradural or intradural in location
- Among the primary extramedullary tumors, neurofibromas and meningiomas are relatively common and benign and may be intra- or extradural
- Carcinomatous metastases, lymphomatous or leukemic deposits, and myeloma are usually extradural
- Common primary sites for metastases
  - Prostate
  - Breast
  - Lung
  - Kidney

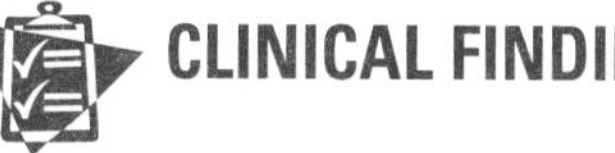

CLINICAL FINDINGS

SYMPTOMS AND SIGNS

- Tumors may lead to spinal cord dysfunction by
  - Direct compression
  - Ischemia secondary to arterial or venous obstruction
  - Invasive infiltration in the case of intramedullary lesions
- Symptoms usually develop insidiously
- Pain with extradural lesions
  - Characteristically aggravated by coughing or straining
  - May be radicular, localized to the back or felt diffusely in an extremity
  - May be accompanied by motor deficits, paresthesias, or numbness, especially in the legs
  - Often precedes specific neurologic symptoms in epidural metastases
- Sphincter disturbances may occur
- Localized spinal tenderness
- Segmental lower motor neuron deficit or dermatomal sensory changes (or both) may be found at the level of the lesion
- An upper motor neuron deficit and sensory disturbance are found below it

DIFFERENTIAL DIAGNOSIS

- Primary tumor, eg, ependymoma, meningioma, neurofibroma
- Lymphoma, leukemia, multiple myeloma
- Metastases, eg, cancer of the prostate, breast, lung, kidney
- Cervical or lumbar disk disease
- Multiple sclerosis
- Tuberculosis (Pott's disease)

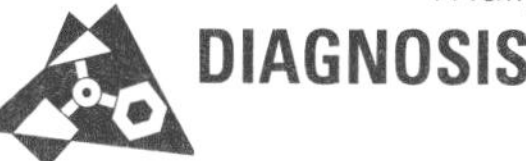

DIAGNOSIS

LABORATORY TESTS

- Cerebrospinal fluid removed at myelography
  - Is often xanthochromic
  - Contains a greatly increased protein concentration
  - Has normal cell content and glucose concentration

IMAGING STUDIES

- Findings on plain radiography are commonly abnormal with metastatic deposits
- MRI or CT myelography may be necessary to identify and localize the site of cord compression
- Indication to perform MRI or CT on an urgent basis
  - The combination of known tumor elsewhere in the body, back pain, and either abnormal plain films of the spine or neurologic signs of cord compression is an indication to perform MRI or CT on an urgent basis
- Some clinicians proceed to spinal MRI or myelography based solely on new back pain in a cancer patient
  - If a complete block is present at lumbar myelography, a cisternal myelogram is performed to determine the upper level of the block and the possibility of a block higher in the cord

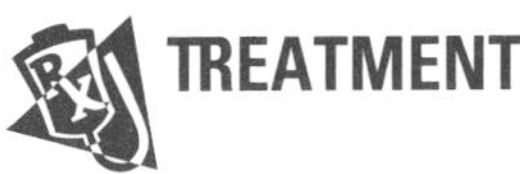

TREATMENT

MEDICATIONS

- Dexamethasone in high dosage (eg, 25 mg QID for 3 days, followed by rapid tapering of the dosage, depending on response) to reduce cord swelling and relieve pain

SURGERY

- Intramedullary tumors are treated by decompression and surgical excision (when feasible) and by irradiation
  - Prognosis depends on the cause and severity of cord compression before it is relieved
- Surgical decompression for epidural metastases is reserved for tumors that are unresponsive to irradiation or have previously been irradiated and for cases with an uncertain diagnosis

THERAPEUTIC PROCEDURES

- Epidural spinal metastases are treated with radiation, regardless of cell type
- Long-term outlook is poor, but radiation treatment may delay the onset of major disability

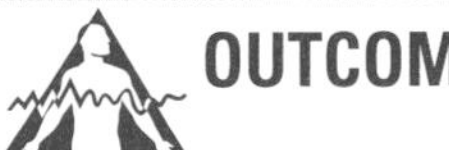

OUTCOME

PROGNOSIS

- Depends on the underlying lesion

WHEN TO ADMIT

- All patients

EVIDENCE

PRACTICE GUIDELINES

- American Society for Interventional and Therapeutic Neuroradiology: embolization of spinal arteriovenous fistulae, spinal arteriovenous malformations, and tumors of the spinal axis. Am J Neuroradiol 2001;22(8 Suppl):S28. [PMID: 11686072]
- National Guideline Clearinghouse
  - http://www.guideline.gov/summary/summary.aspx?doc_id=3639&nbr-2865&string=spinal+tumors

INFORMATION FOR PATIENTS

- American Cancer Society
  - http://www.cancer.org/docroot/cri/content/cri_2_4_4x_treatment_of_specific_types_of_brain_and_spinal_cord_tumors_3.asp?sitearea=cri
- National Institutes of Health
  - http://www.nlm.nih.gov/medlineplus/ency/article/001403.htm

REFERENCES

- Major PP: Efficacy of bisphosphonates in the management of skeletal complications of bone metastases and selection of clinical endpoints. Am J Clin Oncol 2002;25(6 Suppl 1):S10. [PMID:12562046]
- Shiff D: Spinal cord compression. Neurol Clin 2003;21:67. [PMID:12690645]
- Sundaresan N: Surgery for solitary metastases of the spine: rationale and results of treatment. Spine 2002;27:1802. [PMID:12195075]

Author(s)

Michael J. Aminoff, MD, DSc, FRCP

Spinal Cord Vascular Diseases

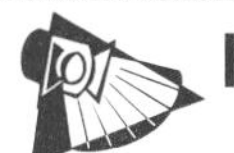

KEY FEATURES

ESSENTIALS OF DIAGNOSIS

- Sudden onset of back or limb pain and neurologic deficit in limbs
- Motor, sensory, or reflex changes in limbs depending on level of lesion
- Imaging studies distinguish between infarct and hematoma

GENERAL CONSIDERATIONS

Infarction of the spinal cord

- Rare and occurs only in the anterior spinal artery territory (which supplies the anterior two-thirds of the cord), because this artery is supplied by only a limited number of feeders
- Usually caused by interrupted flow in one or more of these feeders, eg, with aortic dissection, aortography, polyarteritis, or severe hypotension, or after surgical resection of the thoracic aorta
- Usually caudal because the anterior spinal artery receives numerous feeders in the cervical region

Epidural or subdural hemorrhage

- Occurs in association with bleeding disorders, anticoagulant drugs, trauma or lumbar puncture; epidural hemorrhage
- May also be related to a vascular malformation or tumor deposit

Arteriovenous malformation of the spinal cord

- Congenital lesions that present with spinal subarachnoid hemorrhage or myeloradiculopathy
- Most malformations are in the thoracolumbar region and are extramedullary
- Cervical arteriovenous malformations lead to symptoms and signs in the arms and are intramedullary

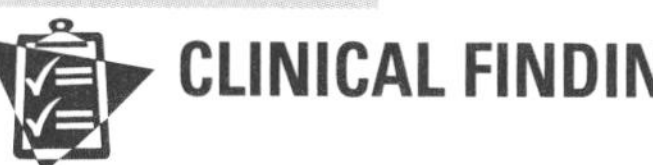

CLINICAL FINDINGS

SYMPTOMS AND SIGNS

Infarction of the spinal cord

- Acute onset of flaccid, areflexic paraplegia that evolves after a few days or weeks into a spastic paraplegia with extensor plantar responses
- Dissociated sensory loss, with impairment of appreciation of pain and temperature but preservation of vibration and position sense

Epidural or subdural hemorrhage

- Sudden severe back pain followed by an acute compressive myelopathy necessitating urgent CT or MRI and surgical evacuation

Arteriovenous malformation of the spinal cord

- Motor and sensory disturbances in the legs and sphincter disorders
- Pain in the legs or back often severe
- An upper, lower, or mixed motor deficit in the legs revealed on examination
- Sensory deficits also present and usually extensive, although occasionally confined to radicular distribution

DIFFERENTIAL DIAGNOSIS

- Primary tumor, eg, ependymoma, meningioma, neurofibroma
- Lymphoma, leukemia, multiple myeloma
- Metastases, eg, cancer of the prostate, breast, lung, kidney
- Cervical or lumbar disk disease
- Epidural abscess
- Multiple sclerosis
- Tuberculosis (Pott's disease)

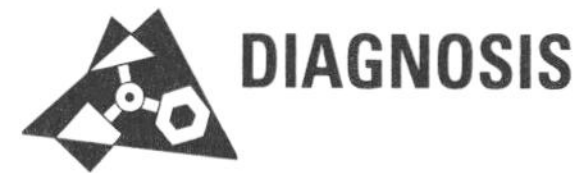

DIAGNOSIS

IMAGING STUDIES

- Urgent imaging (CR or MRI) is indicated for **epidural** or **subdural hemorrhage**
- **Arteriovenous malformation**
  - Myelography is a good screening test and (performed with the patient prone and supine) can show serpiginous filling defects due to enlarged vessels
  - Selective spinal arteriography confirms the diagnosis
  - Spinal MRI may not detect the disorder, and negative findings do not exclude the diagnosis

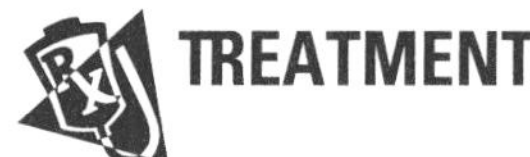

TREATMENT

SURGERY

- Epidural or subdural hemorrhage: urgent surgical evacuation is indicated
- Arteriovenous malformations of the spinal cord that are posterior to the cord can be treated by ligation of feeding vessels and excision of the fistulous anomaly or by embolization procedures

THERAPEUTIC PROCEDURES

- Infarction of the spinal cord: treatment is symptomatic

OUTCOME

PROGNOSIS

- Delay in treatment of an arteriovenous malformation of the spinal cord may lead to increased and irreversible disability or to death from recurrent subarachnoid hemorrhage

WHEN TO ADMIT

- All patients

EVIDENCE

PRACTICE GUIDELINES

- American Society for Interventional and Therapeutic Neuroradiology: embolization of spinal arteriovenous fistulae, spinal arteriovenous malformations, and tumors of the spinal axis. AJNR Am J Neuroradiol 2001;22(8 Suppl):S28. [PMID:11686072]

WEB SITE

- Neuromuscular Disease Center
  - http://www.neuro.wustl.edu/neuromuscular/

INFORMATION FOR PATIENTS

- National Institute of Neurological Diseases and Stroke
  - http://www.ninds.nih.gov/disorders/spinal_infarction/spinal_infarction.htm
  - http://www.ninds.nih.gov/disorders/avms/detail_avms.htm

REFERENCE

- Goodin DS: Neurological complications of aortic disease and surgery. In: Neurology and General Medicine, ed 3. Aminoff MJ (editor). Churchill Livingstone, 2001

Author(s)

Michael J. Aminoff, MD, DSc, FRCP

Spinal Trauma

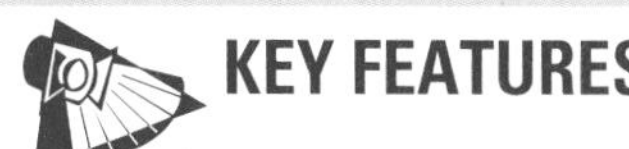

ESSENTIALS OF DIAGNOSIS

- History of trauma followed immediately or after a variable interval by an acute neurologic deficit
- Signs of myelopathy on examination

GENERAL CONSIDERATIONS

- Although spinal cord damage may result from whiplash injury, severe injury usually relates to fracture-dislocation causing compression or deformity of the cord either cervically or in the lower thoracic and upper lumbar regions
- Extreme hypotension following injury may also lead to cord infarction

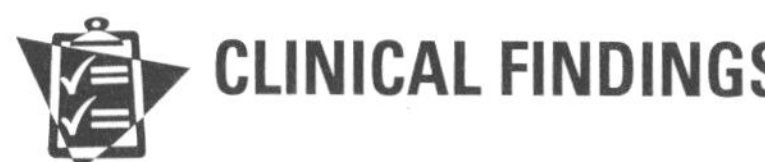

SYMPTOMS AND SIGNS

Total cord transection

- Immediate flaccid paralysis and loss of sensation below the level of the lesion
- Reflex activity is lost for a variable period; urinary and fecal retention
- As reflex function returns, spastic paraplegia or quadriplegia develops, with hyperreflexia and extensor plantar responses
- A flaccid atrophic (lower motor neuron) paralysis may be found depending on the segments of the cord affected
- The bladder and bowels regain some reflex function, permitting urine and feces to be expelled at intervals
- As spasticity increases, flexor or extensor spasms (or both) of the legs become troublesome, especially if the patient develops bed sores or a urinary tract infection
- Paraplegia with the legs in flexion or extension may eventually result

Lesser degrees of injury

- Mild limb weakness, distal sensory disturbance, or both
- Sphincter function may be impaired, urinary urgency and urgency incontinence being especially common
- A unilateral cord lesion leads to an ipsilateral motor disturbance with accompanying impairment of proprioception and contralateral loss of pain and temperature appreciation below the lesion (Brown-Séquard's syndrome)
- A central cord syndrome may lead to a lower motor neuron deficit and loss of pain and temperature appreciation, with sparing of posterior column functions
- A radicular deficit may occur at the level of the injury—or, if the cauda equina is involved, there may be evidence of disturbed function in several lumbosacral roots

DIFFERENTIAL DIAGNOSIS

- The history of the preceding trauma distinguishes the disorder from other causes of nontraumatic myelopathy

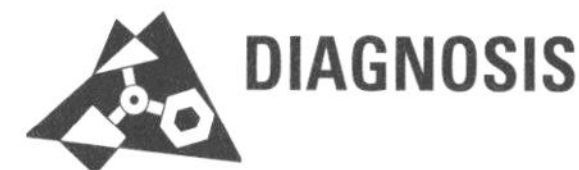

DIAGNOSTIC PROCEDURES

- Obtain history of trauma

Spinal Stenosis, Lumbar p. 1153

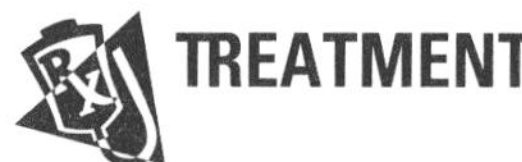

TREATMENT

MEDICATIONS

- Early treatment with high doses of corticosteroids (eg, methylprednisolone, 30 mg/kg by intravenous bolus, followed by 5.4 mg/kg/hour for 23 hours) can improve neurologic recovery if commenced within 8 hours after injury

SURGERY

- If there is cord compression, decompressive laminectomy and fusion

THERAPEUTIC PROCEDURES

- Immobilization
- Anatomic realignment of the spinal cord by traction and other orthopedic procedures is important

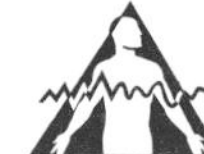

OUTCOME

FOLLOW-UP

- Subsequent care of the residual neurologic deficit—paraplegia or quadriplegia—requires treatment of spasticity and care of the skin, bladder, and bowels

COMPLICATIONS

- Decubiti
- Urinary tract infection
- Renal calculi
- Depression
- Pneumonia

WHEN TO ADMIT

- All patients (to a spinal trauma center, if available)

EVIDENCE

PRACTICE GUIDELINES

- National Guideline Clearinghouse
  - http://www.guideline.gov/summary/summary.aspx?doc_id=2964&nbr=2190&string=spinal+trauma
  - http://www.guideline.gov/summary/summary.aspx?doc_id=3564&nbr=2790&string=spinal+AND+trauma

INFORMATION FOR PATIENTS

- Mayo Clinic
  - http://www.mayoclinic.com/invoke.cfm?id=DS00460
- National Institute of Neurological Disorders and Stroke
  - http://www.ninds.nih.gov/disorders/sci/sci.htm

REFERENCES

- Gimenez y Robotta M et al: Strategies for regeneration and repair in spinal cord traumatic injury. Prog Brain Res 2002;137:191. [PMID:12440369]
- McDonald JW et al: Spinal-cord injury. Lancet 2002;359:417. [PMID: 11844532]

Author(s)

Michael J. Aminoff, DSc, MD, FRCP

Sporotrichosis p. 1153

Squamous Cell Carcinoma of the Skin

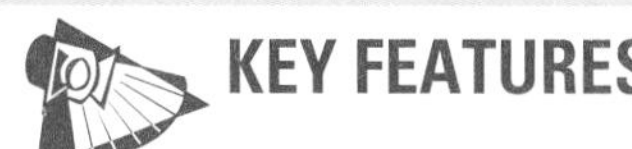

KEY FEATURES

ESSENTIALS OF DIAGNOSIS

- Nodule, ulcer, or patch usually on sun-exposed sites or in the genital area

GENERAL CONSIDERATIONS

- Squamous cell carcinoma (SCC) usually occurs subsequent to prolonged sun exposure on exposed parts in fair-skinned individuals who sunburn easily and tan poorly
- It may arise from an actinic keratosis

DEMOGRAPHICS

- SCC is about 20% as common as basal cell carcinoma

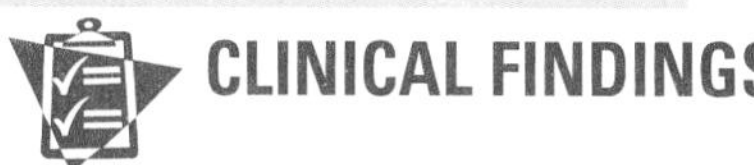

CLINICAL FINDINGS

SYMPTOMS AND SIGNS

- The lesions appear as small red, conical, hard nodules that occasionally ulcerate; they are not as distinctive as basal cell carcinomas and are more easily misdiagnosed clinically
- Since cutaneous SCC may metastasize, palpate draining nodes at affected area

DIFFERENTIAL DIAGNOSIS

- Actinic keratosis
- Basal cell carcinoma
- Seborrheic keratosis
- Warts
- Keratoacanthomas resemble squamous cell carcinoma histologically and for all practical purposes should be treated as though they were skin cancers

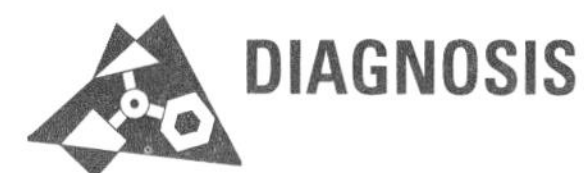

DIAGNOSIS

DIAGNOSTIC PROCEDURES

- The diagnosis is made by biopsy

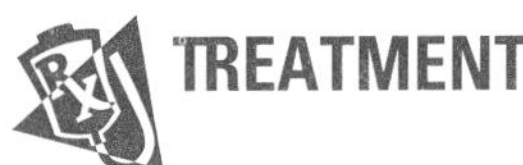

TREATMENT

SURGERY

- The preferred treatment of squamous cell carcinoma is excision
- Fresh tissue microscopically controlled excision (Mohs) is recommended for high-risk lesions (lips, temples, ears, nose) and for recurrent tumors

THERAPEUTIC PROCEDURES

- Electrodesiccation and curettage and x-ray radiation may be used for some lesions
- Some keratoacanthomas respond to intralesional injection of fluorouracil or methotrexate, but they must be excised if they do not

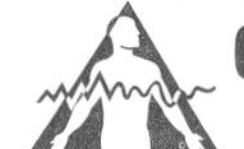

OUTCOME

FOLLOW-UP

- Follow-up must be more frequent and thorough than for basal cell carcinoma, starting at every 3 months, with careful examination of lymph nodes
- In addition, palpation of the lips is essential to detect hard or indurated areas that represent early squamous cell carcinoma; all such cases must be biopsied
- Multiple SCCs are very common on the sun-exposed skin of organ transplant patients because of the host's immunosuppressed state; the tumors begin to appear after 5 years of immunosuppression

COMPLICATIONS

- The frequency of metastasis is not precisely known, though metastatic spread is said to be less likely with SCC arising out of actinic keratoses than with those that arise de novo
- In actinically induced SCCs, rates of metastasis are estimated from retrospective studies to be 3–7%
- SCCs of the lip, oral cavity, tongue, and genitalia have much higher rates of metastasis and require special management

PROGNOSIS

- Tumor aggressiveness correlates with the size of the lesion, duration, location, origin, and degree of anaplasia
- Tumors of the scalp, eyelids, nose, ears, and lips invade subcutaneous tissues and have a greater risk of subclinical tumor extension

WHEN TO REFER

- If there is a question about the diagnosis, if recommended therapy is ineffective, or if specialized treatment is necessary

PREVENTION

- Sun protection and avoidance

EVIDENCE

PRACTICE GUIDELINES

- American Academy of Dermatology's Committee on Guidelines of Care for Cutaneous Squamous Cell Carcinoma
  - http://www.aad.org/professionals/pracmanage/guidelines/CutaneousSquamousCC.htm
- Miller SJ et al; NCCN Basal Cell and Squamous Cell Skin Cancer Practice Guidelines Panel. National Comprehensive Cancer Network: Basal Cell and Squamous Cell Skin Cancers v.1.2004
  - http://www.nccn.org/professionals/physician_gls/PDF/nmsc.pdf

WEB SITE

- National Cancer Institute: Skin Cancer Information for Patients and Health Professionals
  - http://www.cancer.gov/cancertopics/types/skin

INFORMATION FOR PATIENTS

- American Academy of Dermatology: Squamous Cell Carcinoma
  - http://www.aad.org/public/Publications/pamphlets/SquamousCellCarcinoma.htm
- American Cancer Society: Nonmelanoma Skin Cancer
  - http://www.cancer.org/docroot/CRI/CRI_2_3x.asp?rnav=cridg&dt=51
- MedlinePlus: Skin Cancer Interactive Tutorial
  - http://www.nlm.nih.gov/medlineplus/tutorials/skincancer.html

REFERENCES

- Fortina AB et al: Immunosuppressive level and other risk factors for basal cell carcinoma and squamous cell carcinoma in heart transplant recipients. Arch Dermatol 2004;140:1079.
- Garner KL et al: Basal and squamous cell carcinoma. Prim Care 2000;27:447. [PMID: 10815054]

Author(s)

Timothy G. Berger, MD

Status Epilepticus

Staphylococci Infections, Coagulase-Negative p. 1154

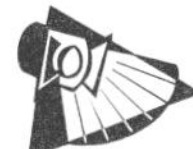

KEY FEATURES

ESSENTIALS OF DIAGNOSIS

- Occurrence of two or more convulsions with recovery of consciousness between attacks
- A fixed and enduring epileptic condition (for 30 minutes or more)

GENERAL CONSIDERATIONS

- Status epilepticus is a medical emergency
- Causes
  - Poor compliance with the anticonvulsant drug (most common)
  - Alcohol withdrawal
  - Intracranial infection or neoplasms
  - Stroke
  - Metabolic disorders
  - Drug overdose
- Mortality rate of convulsive status may be as high as 20%, with a high incidence of neurologic and mental sequelae
- Prognosis relates to the length of time between onset of status epilepticus and start of effective treatment

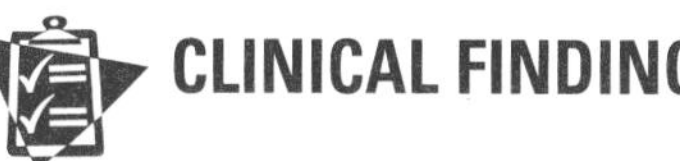

CLINICAL FINDINGS

SYMPTOMS AND SIGNS

- Two clinical subtypes: tonic-clonic convulsive status epilepticus and nonconvulsive status epilepticus
- Nonconvulsive status epilepticus is characterized by
  - Fluctuating abnormal mental status
  - Confusion
  - Impaired responsiveness
  - Automatism
  - Two subtypes: absence (petit mal) and complex partial status epilepticus

DIFFERENTIAL DIAGNOSIS

- Seizure due to hypoglycemia, electrolyte abnormality, alcohol withdrawal, cocaine, bacterial meningitis, herpes encephalitis, brain tumor, CNS vasculitis
- Syncope
- Cardiac arrhythmia
- Stroke or transient ischemic attack
- Pseudoseizure
- Panic attack
- Migraine
- Narcolepsy

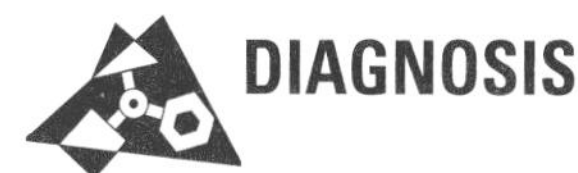

DIAGNOSIS

LABORATORY TESTS

- Electroencephalography (EEG) is essential in establishing the diagnosis of nonconvulsive status epilepticus and its two subtypes

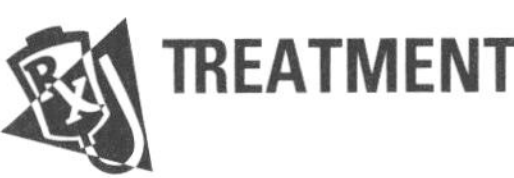

TREATMENT

MEDICATIONS

- See Table 98
- Initial treatment with IV lorazepam or diazepam is usually helpful regardless of the type of status epilepticus
- Phenytoin, phenobarbital, carbamazepine, and other drugs are also needed

Initial management

- Maintenance of the airway and 50% dextrose (25–50 mL) IV in case of hypoglycemia
- If seizures continue, give diazepam 10 mg IV over 2 minutes, and repeat after 10 minutes if necessary
  - Hypotension and respiratory depression may occur
- Alternatively, give lorazepam 4 mg IV bolus, repeat once after 10 minutes if necessary
  - Effective in halting seizures for a brief period but occasionally causes respiratory depression
- Also give phenytoin (18–20 mg/kg) IV at 50 mg/min for initiation of longer seizure control
  - The drug is best injected directly but can also be given in saline; it precipitates if injected into glucose-containing solutions
  - Because arrhythmias may develop during rapid administration of phenytoin, EKG monitoring is prudent
  - Phenytoin may cause hypotension, especially if diazepam has also been given
  - Phenytoin has been widely replaced by injectable fosphenytoin, which is rapidly and completely converted to phenytoin following IV administration
  - No dosing adjustments are necessary because fosphenytoin is expressed in terms of phenytoin equivalents (PE)
  - Fosphenytoin is less likely to cause reactions at the infusion site, can be given with all common IV solutions, and may be administered at a faster rate (150 mg PE/min). It is also more expensive

If seizures continue

- Phenobarbital is then given in a loading dose of 10–20 mg/kg IV by slow or intermittent injection (50 mg/min)
  - Respiratory depression and hypotension are common complications and should be anticipated
- If these measures fail, general anesthesia with ventilatory assistance and neuromuscular junction blockade may be required
- Alternatively, IV midazolam may control refractory status epilepticus
  - The suggested loading dose is 0.2 mg/kg, followed by 0.05–0.2 mg/kg/hour

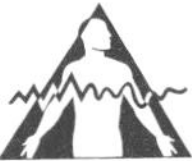

OUTCOME

FOLLOW-UP

- After status epilepticus is controlled, an oral drug program for the long-term management of seizures is started, and investigations into the cause of the disorder are pursued

WHEN TO REFER

- Many patients can benefit from the expertise of a neurologist

WHEN TO ADMIT

- All patients until seizure control is obtained

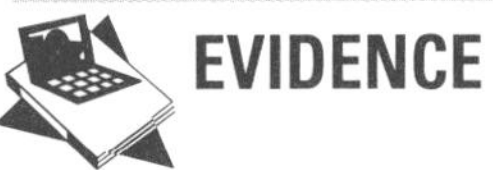

EVIDENCE

PRACTICE GUIDELINES

- National Guideline Clearinghouse
  - http://www.guideline.gov/summary/summary.aspx?doc_id=5091&nbr=3558&string=status+AND+epilepticus

INFORMATION FOR PATIENTS

- Epilepsy Foundation
  - http://www.epilepsyfoundation.org/answerplace/About-Epilepsy.cfm
- National Institute of Neurological Disorders and Stroke
  - http://www.ninds.nih.gov/disorders/epilepsy/epilepsy.htm

REFERENCES

- Alldredge BK et al: A comparison of lorazepam, diazepam, and placebo for the treatment of out-of-hospital status epilepticus. N Engl J Med 2001;345:631. [PMID:11547716]
- Benbadis SR et al: Advances in the treatment of epilepsy. Am Fam Physician 2001;64:91. [PMID:11456438]
- Kwan P et al: The mechanisms of action of commonly used antiepileptic drugs. Pharmacol Ther 2001;90:21. [PMID:11448723]
- Wu YW et al: Incidence and mortality of generalized convulsive status epilepticus in California. Neurology 2002;58:1070. [PMID:11940695]

Author(s)

Michael J. Aminoff, DSc, MD, FRCP

Stress & Adjustment Disorders

Still's Disease, Adult p. 1154. Storage Pool Disease p. 1154. Streptococcal, Group A Infections p. 1155.

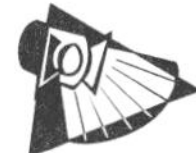

KEY FEATURES

ESSENTIALS OF DIAGNOSIS

- Anxiety or depression clearly secondary to an identifiable stress
- Subsequent symptoms of anxiety or depression commonly elicited by similar stress of lesser magnitude
- Alcohol and other drugs are commonly used in self-treatment

GENERAL CONSIDERATIONS

- Stress exists when the adaptive capacity of the individual is overwhelmed by events
- The event may be an insignificant one objectively considered
- Even favorable changes (eg, promotion and transfer) requiring adaptive behavior can produce stress
- For each individual, stress is subjectively defined, and the response to stress is a function of each person's personality and physiologic endowment
- The causes or sources of stress are different at different ages
  - Young adulthood
    1. Marriage or parent-child relationship
    2. Employment relationship
    3. Struggle to achieve financial stability
  - Middle years
    1. Changing spousal relationships
    2. Problems with aging parents
    3. Problems associated with having young adult offspring who themselves are encountering stressful situations
  - Old age
    1. Retirement
    2. Loss of physical capacity
    3. Major personal losses
    4. Thoughts of death
- Maladaptive behavior in response to stress is called adjustment disorder, with the major symptom specified (eg, "adjustment disorder with depressed mood")

CLINICAL FINDINGS

SYMPTOMS AND SIGNS

- Common subjective responses
  - Fear (of repetition of the stress-inducing event)
  - Rage (at frustration)
  - Guilt (over aggressive impulses)
  - Shame (over helplessness)
- Acute and reactivated stress manifestations
  - Restlessness
  - Irritability
  - Fatigue
  - Increased startle reaction
  - A feeling of tension
- Inability to concentrate, sleep disturbances (insomnia, bad dreams), and somatic preoccupations often lead to self-medication, most commonly with alcohol or other central nervous system depressants

DIFFERENTIAL DIAGNOSIS

- Anxiety disorders
- Affective disorders
- Personality disorders exacerbated by stress
- Somatic disorders with psychic overlay

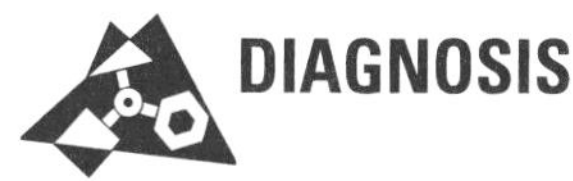

DIAGNOSIS

DIAGNOSTIC PROCEDURES

- Obtain history
- Identify precipitating sources of stress

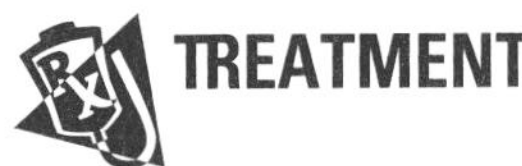

TREATMENT

MEDICATIONS

- Judicious use of sedatives (Table 105) (eg, lorazepam, 1–2 mg orally daily) for a limited time and as part of an overall treatment plan can provide relief

THERAPEUTIC PROCEDURES

- Behavioral
  - Stress reduction techniques include immediate symptom reduction (eg, rebreathing in a bag for hyperventilation) or early recognition and removal from a stress source before full-blown symptoms appear
  - It is often helpful for the patient to keep a daily log of stress precipitators, responses, and alleviators
  - Relaxation and exercise techniques are also helpful in reducing the reaction to stressful events
- Social
  - While it is not easy for the patient to make necessary changes (or they would have been made long ago), it is important for the clinician to establish the framework of the problem, since the patient's denial system may obscure the issues
  - Clarifying the problem allows the patient to begin viewing it within the proper context and facilitates the sometimes difficult decisions the patient eventually must make (eg, change of job or relocation of adult dependent offspring)
- Psychological
  - Prolonged in-depth psychotherapy is seldom necessary in cases of isolated stress response or adjustment disorder
  - Supportive psychotherapy with an emphasis on the here and now and strengthening of existing defenses is a helpful approach

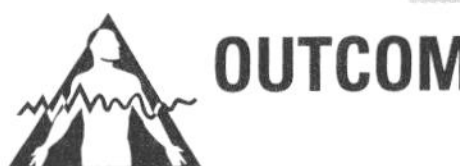

OUTCOME

PROGNOSIS

- A return to satisfactory function after a short period is part of the clinical picture of this syndrome
- Resolution may be delayed if others' responses to the patient's difficulties are thoughtlessly harmful or if the secondary gains outweigh the advantages of recovery
- The longer the symptoms persist, the worse the prognosis

EVIDENCE

PRACTICE GUIDELINES

- National Guideline Clearinghouse
  - http://www.guideline.gov/summary/summary.aspx?doc_id=1407

WEB SITES

- American Psychiatric Association
  - http://www.psych.org/
- Internet Mental Health
  - http://www.mentalhealth.com/

INFORMATION FOR PATIENTS

- American Academy of Family Physicians
  - http://familydoctor.org/healthfacts/167/
- American Academy of Family Physicians: Stress: Who Has Time for It? (for teens)
  - http://familydoctor.org/278.xml
- American Academy of Family Physicians: When You Are the Caregiver
  - http://www.aafp.org/afp/20001215/2621ph.html
- National Cancer Institute
  - http://www.cancer.gov/cancerinfo/pdq/supportivecare/adjustment/patient
- National Institutes of Health: Adjustment Disorders
  - http://www.nlm.nih.gov/medlineplus/ency/article/000932.htm

REFERENCES

- Ehlers A et al: Early psychological interventions for survivors of trauma: a review. Biol Psychiatry 2003;53:817. [PMID:12725974]
- Schoenfeld FB, Marmar CR, Neylan TC: Current concepts in pharmacotherapy for posttraumatic stress disorder. Psychiatr Serv 2004;55:519. [PMID:15128960]
- Vaiva G et al: Immediate treatment with propranolol decreases posttraumatic stress disorder two months after trauma. Biol Psychiatry 2003;54:947. Erratum in: Biol Psychiatry 2003;54:1471. [PMID:14573324]

Author(s)

Stuart J. Eisendrath, MD

Jonathan E. Lichtmacher, MD

Stroke, Intracerebral Hemorrhage

KEY FEATURES

ESSENTIALS OF DIAGNOSIS

- Hypertension is the usual cause
- Usually occurs suddenly and without warning, often during activity

GENERAL CONSIDERATIONS

Hypertensive intracerebral hemorrhage

- Spontaneous intracerebral hemorrhage in patients with no angiographic evidence of an associated vascular anomaly (eg, aneurysm or angioma) is usually due to hypertension
- Likely pathologic basis is microaneurysms that develop on perforating vessels 100–300 μm in diameter in hypertensive patients
- Occurs most frequently in the basal ganglia and less commonly in the pons, thalamus, cerebellum, and cerebral white matter
- Extension into the ventricular system or subarachnoid space may cause signs of meningeal irritation

Other causes

- May occur with hematologic and bleeding disorders (eg, leukemia, thrombocytopenia, hemophilia, or disseminated intravascular coagulation), anticoagulant therapy, liver disease, cerebral amyloid angiopathy, and primary or secondary brain tumors
- There is also an association with advancing age, male sex, and high alcohol intake
- Bleeding from an intracranial aneurysm or arteriovenous malformation is primarily into the subarachnoid space, but it may also be partly intraparenchymal
- In some cases, no specific cause for cerebral hemorrhage can be identified

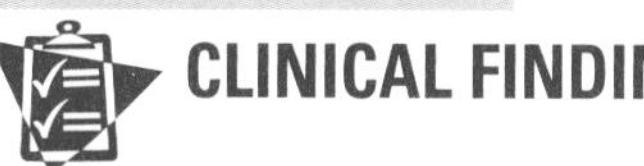

CLINICAL FINDINGS

SYMPTOMS AND SIGNS

Hemorrhage into the cerebral hemisphere

- Consciousness is initially lost or impaired in about 50% of patients
- Vomiting is frequent at the onset, and headache is sometimes present
- Focal symptoms and signs follow, depending on the site of the bleed
- With hypertensive hemorrhage, there is generally a rapidly evolving neurologic deficit with hemiplegia or hemiparesis
- A hemisensory disturbance occurs with more deeply placed lesions
- With lesions of the putamen, loss of conjugate lateral gaze may be present
- With thalamic hemorrhage, there may be a loss of upward gaze, downward or skew deviation of the eyes, lateral gaze palsies, and pupillary inequalities

Cerebellar hemorrhage

- Sudden onset of nausea and vomiting, disequilibrium, headache, and loss of consciousness that may terminate fatally within 48 hours
- Less commonly, the onset is gradual and episodic or slowly progressive, suggesting an expanding cerebellar lesion
- Onset and course can be intermediate
  - Lateral conjugate gaze palsies to the side of the lesion
  - Small reactive pupils
  - Contralateral hemiplegia; peripheral facial weakness
  - Ataxia of gait, limbs, or trunk
  - Periodic respiration
  - Or some combination of these findings

DIFFERENTIAL DIAGNOSIS

- Ischemic stroke
- Subarachnoid hemorrhage
- Space-occupying lesion, eg, brain tumor
- Subdural or epidural hemorrhage

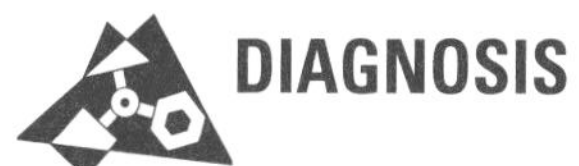

DIAGNOSIS

LABORATORY TESTS

- A complete blood cell count, platelet count, bleeding time, prothrombin and partial thromboplastin times, and liver and renal function tests may reveal a predisposing cause
- Lumbar puncture is contraindicated because it may cause herniation in patients with a large hematoma

IMAGING STUDIES

- CT scanning (without contrast) is important in confirming hemorrhage and for determining the size and site of the hematoma
- CT is superior to MRI for detecting intracranial hemorrhage of less than 48 hours' duration
- If the patient's condition permits further intervention, cerebral angiography may reveal an aneurysm or arteriovenous malformation

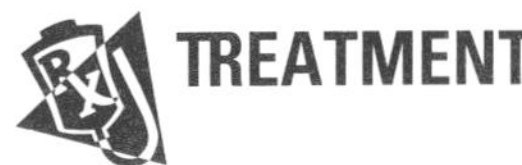

TREATMENT

SURGERY

- In cerebellar hemorrhage, prompt surgical evacuation of the hematoma is appropriate
- Decompression is helpful when a superficial hematoma in cerebral white matter is causing mass effect and herniation

THERAPEUTIC PROCEDURES

- In noncerebellar hemorrhage, neurologic management is generally conservative and supportive, either in cases of profound deficit with associated brainstem compression or more localized deficits
- The treatment of underlying structural lesions or bleeding disorders depends on their nature

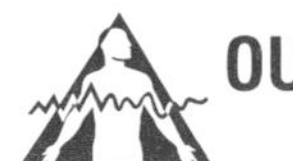

OUTCOME

PROGNOSIS

- Surgery for cerebellar hemorrhage may lead to complete resolution of the clinical deficit
- Untreated cerebellar hemorrhage can spontaneously deteriorate with a fatal outcome from brainstem herniation

WHEN TO ADMIT

- All patients

EVIDENCE

PRACTICE GUIDELINES

- American Academy of Neurology
  - http://www.aan.com/professionals/practice/pdfs/gl0097.pdf

INFORMATION FOR PATIENTS

- JAMA patient page: Hemorrhagic stroke. JAMA 2004;292:1916
- The Mayo Clinic
  - http://www.mayoclinic.com/invoke.cfm?id=DS00150
- National Institute of Neurological Disorders and Stroke
  - http://www.ninds.nih.gov/disorders/stroke/stroke.htm

REFERENCES

- Ariesen MJ et al: Risk factors for intracerebral hemorrhage in the general population: a systematic review. Stroke 2003;34:2065. [PMID:12843354]
- Hill MD et al: Rate of stroke recurrence in patients with primary intracerebral hemorrhage. Stroke 2000;31:123. [PMID:10625726]

Author(s)

Michael J. Aminoff, DSc, MD, FRCP

Stroke, Ischemic

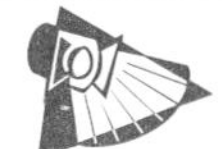

KEY FEATURES

ESSENTIALS OF DIAGNOSIS

- Thrombotic or embolic occlusion of a major vessel leads to cerebral infarction
- The resulting deficit depends on the particular vessel involved and the extent of any collateral circulation

GENERAL CONSIDERATIONS

- Strokes are traditionally subdivided into infarcts (thrombotic or embolic) and hemorrhages, but clinical distinction may not be possible
- A previous stroke is a risk factor for a subsequent stroke

DEMOGRAPHICS

- The third leading cause of death in the United States, despite a general decline in the incidence of stroke in the last 30 years

CLINICAL FINDINGS

SYMPTOMS AND SIGNS

- See Table 96
- Onset is usually abrupt, and there may then be very little progression except that due to brain swelling
- Examine the heart for murmur or arrhythmia and the carotid and subclavian arteries for bruits
- In hemiplegia of pontine origin, the eyes often deviate toward the paralyzed side
- In a hemispheric lesion, the eyes commonly deviate away from the hemiplegic side

Carotid circulation

- Ophthalmic artery occlusion
  - Symptomless in most
  - May produce amaurosis fugax—sudden and brief loss of vision in one eye
- Anterior cerebral artery occlusion distal to junction with anterior communicating artery
  - Weakness and cortical sensory loss in the contralateral leg and sometimes mild proximal arm weakness
  - May see contralateral grasp reflex, paratonic rigidity, and abulia (lack of initiative) or frank confusion
  - Urinary incontinence is common
- Middle cerebral artery occlusion
  - Contralateral hemiplegia, hemisensory loss, and homonymous hemianopia (ie, bilaterally symmetric loss of vision in half of the visual fields), with the eyes deviated to the side of the lesion
  - If the dominant hemisphere is involved, global aphasia is present
  - May be impossible to distinguish from occlusion of the internal carotid artery
  - May see considerable swelling of the hemisphere, leading to drowsiness, stupor, and coma
- Anterior main division occlusion of the middle cerebral artery
  - Expressive dysphasia, contralateral paralysis and loss of sensations in the arm, the face, and, to a lesser extent, the leg
- Posterior branch occlusion of the middle cerebral artery
  - Receptive (Wernicke's) aphasia and a homonymous visual field defect

Vertebrobasilar circulation

- Posterior cerebral artery occlusion may lead to
  - Thalamic syndrome of sensory loss
  - Ipsilateral facial, ninth and tenth cranial nerve lesions
  - Limb ataxia and numbness
  - Horner's syndrome, combined with contralateral sensory loss of the limb
- Occlusion of both vertebral arteries or the basilar artery
  - Coma with pinpoint pupils
  - Flaccid quadriplegia
  - Sensory loss
  - Variable cranial nerve abnormalities
- Partial basilar artery occlusion
  - Diplopia
  - Visual loss
  - Vertigo
  - Dysarthria
  - Ataxia
  - Weakness or sensory disturbances in some or all of the limbs
  - Discrete cranial nerve palsies
- Occlusion of any major cerebellar artery
  - Vertigo, nausea, vomiting, nystagmus, ipsilateral limb ataxia, and contralateral spinothalamic sensory loss in the limbs
  - Massive cerebellar infarction may lead to coma, tonsillar herniation, and death

DIFFERENTIAL DIAGNOSIS

- Hypoglycemia
- Transient ischemic attack
- Intracerebral hemorrhage or other mass lesion (eg, tumor)
- Focal seizure (Todd's paralysis)
- Migraine
- Peripheral causes of vertigo (Ménière's disease)

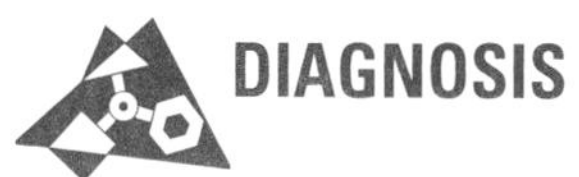

DIAGNOSIS

LABORATORY TESTS

- Complete blood cell count, sedimentation rate, blood glucose, and serologic tests for syphilis
- Antiphospholipid antibodies, serum lipids, and homocysteine
- ECG to help exclude a cardiac arrhythmia or recent myocardial infarction that might be a source of embolization
- Blood cultures if endocarditis is suspected

IMAGING STUDIES

- A CT scan of the head (without contrast) excludes cerebral hemorrhage, but may not distinguish between a cerebral infarct and a tumor
- CT scanning is preferable to MRI in the acute stage because it is quicker and hemorrhage is not easily detected by MRI in the first 48 hours
- In selected patients, carotid duplex studies, MRI and MR angiography, and conventional angiography may also be necessary
- Diffusion-weighted MRI is more sensitive than standard MRI in detecting cerebral ischemia
- Echocardiography if heart disease is suspected

DIAGNOSTIC PROCEDURES

- Holter monitoring if paroxysmal cardiac arrhythmia suspected

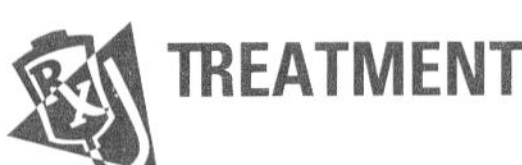

TREATMENT

MEDICATIONS

- Anticoagulants
  - If the CT shows no hemorrhage and there is a cardiac source of embolization, start intravenous heparin while warfarin is introduced for a target INR of 2–3 for the prothrombin time
  - Some physicians prefer to wait for 2 or 3 days before initiating anticoagulant treatment after the CT scan is repeated and there is no evidence of hemorrhagic transformation
- Thrombolytics
  - Intravenous thrombolytic therapy with recombinant tissue plasminogen activator (0.9 mg/kg to a maximum of 90 mg, with 10% given as a bolus over 1 minute and the remainder over 1 hour) is effective in reducing the neurologic deficit in selected patients who have no CT evidence of intracranial hemorrhage when administered within 3 hours after onset of ischemic stroke
  - Later administration has not been proved effective or safe
  - Contraindications include
    1. Recent hemorrhage
    2. Increased risk of hemorrhage (eg, treatment with anticoagulants), arterial puncture at a noncompressible site
    3. Systolic pressure above 185 mm Hg or diastolic pressure above 110 mm Hg

THERAPEUTIC PROCEDURES

- Early management consists of general supportive measures
- Avoid lowering the blood pressure of hypertensive patients within 2 weeks of stroke because ischemic areas may be further compromised—unless the systolic pressure exceeds 200 mm Hg, in which case it can be lowered gradually to 170–200 mm Hg and then, after 2 weeks, reduced further
- Physical therapy with early mobilization and active rehabilitation are important
- Occupational therapy may improve morale and motor skills
- Speech therapy may be beneficial in patients with expressive dysphasia or dysarthria

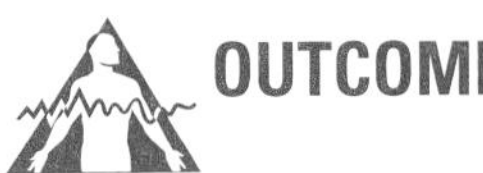

OUTCOME

PROGNOSIS

- The prognosis for survival after cerebral infarction is better than after cerebral or subarachnoid hemorrhage
- Loss of consciousness after a cerebral infarct implies a poorer prognosis than otherwise
- The extent of the infarct governs the potential for rehabilitation

PREVENTION

- Patients who have had a cerebral infarct are at risk for further strokes and for myocardial infarcts
- Statin therapy to lower serum lipid levels may reduce this risk
- Antiplatelet therapy with aspirin, 325 mg/day, reduces the recurrence rate by 30% among patients who have no cardiac cause for the stroke and who are not candidates for carotid endarterectomy
  - Nevertheless, the cumulative risk of recurrence of noncardioembolic stroke is still 3–7% annually
- A 2-year comparison did not show benefit of warfarin (INR 1.4–2.8) over aspirin (325 mg daily)
- Higher doses of warfarin should be avoided because they lead to an increased incidence of major bleeding

EVIDENCE

PRACTICE GUIDELINES

- Adams H et al: Guidelines for the early management of patients with ischemic stroke: 2005 guidelines update. A scientific statement from the Stroke Council of the American Heart Association/American Stroke Association. Stroke 2005;36:916. [PMID:15800252]
- Albers GW et al: Antithrombotic and thrombolytic therapy for ischemic stroke: the Seventh ACCP Conference on Antithrombotic and Thrombolytic Therapy. Chest 2004;126(3 Suppl):483S. [PMID:15383482]
- American Stroke Association/American Academy of Neurology Joint Report: Anticoagulants and antiplatelet agents in acute ischemic stroke. Stroke 2002;33:1934. [PMID:12105379]

WEB SITES

- Acute Cerebral Infarction Demonstration Case
  - http://www.brighamrad.harvard.edu/Cases/bwh/hcache/93/full.html
- Carotid Artery Stenosis Demonstration Case
  - http://www.brighamrad.harvard.edu/Cases/bwh/hcache/6/full.html

INFORMATION FOR PATIENTS

- UCSF Neurocritical Care and Stroke
  - http://www.ucsf.edu/stroke/patinfo.htm
- The Mayo Clinic
  - http://www.mayoclinic.com/invoke.cfm?id=DS00150

REFERENCES

- Albers GW et al: Intravenous tissue-type plasminogen activator for treatment of acute stroke: the Standard Treatment with Alteplase to Reverse Stroke (STARS) study. JAMA 2000;283:1145. [PMID:10703776]
- Bath P: Anticoagulants and antiplatelet agents in acute ischaemic stroke. Lancet Neurology 2002;1:405. [PMID:12849358]
- Caplan LR: Treatment of patients with stroke. Arch Neurol 2002;59:703. [PMID:12020249]
- Mohr JP et al: A comparison of warfarin and aspirin for the prevention of recurrent ischemic stroke. N Engl J Med 2001;345:1444. [PMID:11794192]
- Powers WJ: Oral anticoagulant therapy for the prevention of stroke. N Engl J Med 2001;345:1493. [PMID:11794201]
- Straus SE et al: New evidence for stroke prevention: scientific review. JAMA 2002;288:1388. [PMID:12234233]

Author(s)

Michael J. Aminoff, MD, DSc, FRCP

Strongyloidiasis

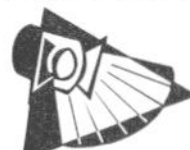

KEY FEATURES

ESSENTIALS OF DIAGNOSIS

- Pruritic dermatitis where larva penetrate
- Diarrhea, epigastric pain, nausea, malaise, weight loss
- Cough, transient pulmonary infiltrates
- Eosinophilia; characteristic larvae in stool specimens, duodenal aspirate, or sputum
- Hyperinfection syndrome: severe diarrhea, bronchopneumonia, ileus

GENERAL CONSIDERATIONS

- Infection is caused by *Strongyloides stercoralis* (2–2.5 × 30–50 mm)
- The primary host is humans
- The parasite maintains its life cycle both within humans and in soil. Infection occurs when filariform larvae in soil penetrate the skin, enter the bloodstream, and are carried to the lungs and ascend the bronchial tree to the glottis. The larvae are then swallowed and carried to the duodenum and upper jejunum, where they mature to the adult stage
- Recrudescence of a chronic asymptomatic infection may occur with immunosuppression; exacerbation may lead to the hyperinfection syndrome
- In the hyperinfection syndrome, autoinfection is greatly increased, resulting in a marked increase in the intestinal worm burden and in massive dissemination of filariform larvae to the lungs and most other tissues, where they can cause local inflammatory reactions and granuloma formation

DEMOGRAPHICS

- Endemic in tropical and subtropical regions; the prevalence is low, but in some areas disease rates exceed 25%
- Total world prevalence is 60 million
- In the United States, highest infection rates are found in immigrants from endemic areas, in parts of Appalachia (up to 4%), and in southeastern areas; Puerto Rico is also an endemic area
- Multiple infections in households are common, and prevalence may be high in mental institutions (2–4%)
- The infection is prevalent among immunosuppressed persons

CLINICAL FINDINGS

SYMPTOMS AND SIGNS

- Up to 30% are asymptomatic
- The time from larval penetration of the skin until their appearance in the feces is 3–4 weeks
- The acute syndrome is uncommon, in which cutaneous symptoms, usually of the feet, are followed by pulmonary and then intestinal symptoms
- Most present with chronic symptoms (continuous or with irregular exacerbations) that can persist for life due to autoinfection

Skin manifestations

- In acute infection, there may be focal edema, inflammation, petechiae, serpiginous or urticarial tracts, and intense itching
- In chronic infections, both stationary urticaria and larva currens occur, characterized by transient eruptions that migrate in serpiginous tracts

Intestinal manifestations

- Symptoms range from mild to severe, the most common being diarrhea, abdominal pain, and flatulence
- Anorexia, nausea, vomiting, and pruritus ani may be present; with increasing severity, fever and malaise may appear
- Diarrhea may alternate with constipation, and in severe cases the feces contain mucus and blood
- Malabsorption or a protein-losing enteropathy can result from a large worm burden

Pulmonary manifestations

- With migration of larvae through the lungs, symptoms may be limited to a dry cough and low-grade fever, dyspnea, wheezing, and hemoptysis may occur; asthma is rare
- Bronchopneumonia, bronchitis, pleural effusion, and miliary abscesses can develop; the cough may be productive of an odorless, mucopurulent sputum

Hyperinfection syndrome

- Intense dissemination of filariform larvae to the lungs and other tissues can result in pleural effusion, pericarditis and myocarditis, hepatic granulomas, cholecystitis, purpura, nephrotic syndrome, ulcerating lesions at all levels of the gastrointestinal tract, central nervous system involvement, paralytic ileus, perforation and peritonitis, gram-negative septicemia and meningitis (due to larval carriage of enterobacteria from the colon), cachexia, shock, and death

DIFFERENTIAL DIAGNOSIS

- Hookworm disease
- Ascariasis
- Giardiasis
- Amebiasis
- Acute eosinophilic pneumonia (Löffler's syndrome)
- Tropical pulmonary eosinophilia (*Wuchereria bancrofti, Brugia malayi*)
- Peptic ulcer disease
- Cutaneous larva migrans

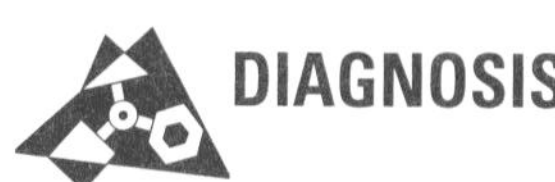

DIAGNOSIS

LABORATORY TESTS

Detection of eggs and larva

- Eggs are seldom found in feces
- Diagnosis requires finding the larval stages in feces or duodenal fluid. Four to six specimens, some unpreserved, should be collected at 2-day intervals or longer
- The sensitivity of direct microscopic examination of one specimen is about 30%; one-half of the specimens should be processed, unpreserved, in the Baermann concentration or agar plate culture methods, the sensitivities of which are high

Serological and hematological findings

- In chronic low-grade intestinal strongyloidiasis, the white blood cell count is often normal, with a slightly elevated percentage of eosinophils. However, with increasing larval migration, eosinophilia may reach 50% and leukocytosis 20,000/μL
- In immunocompromised patients, eosinophilia may not be seen and mild anemia may be present
- An ELISA is sensitive (84–95%) and specific (84–92%), as is Western blot, but cross-reactions can occur with the filaria and other helminthic infections. A positive test indicates current or past infection

Hyperinfection

- There may be hypoproteinemia, malabsorption, abnormal liver function, and extensive pulmonary opacities. Filariform larvae may appear in the urine. Eosinopenia is an unfavorable prognostic sign

IMAGING STUDIES

- Small bowel x-rays may show inflammation, prominent mucosal folds, bowel dilation, delayed emptying, or ulcerative duodenitis
- In chronic infections, the findings can resemble nontropical and tropical sprue,

or there may be narrowing, rigidity, and diminished peristalsis

- During pulmonary migration of larvae, chest films are normal or show fine miliary nodules or changing patches of pneumonitis, abscess, or effusion

DIAGNOSTIC PROCEDURES

- The diagnosis can sometimes be made by finding larvae in mucus obtained by the duodenal string test or by duodenal intubation and aspiration
- Duodenal biopsy is seldom indicated but will confirm the diagnosis in most. Rarely, larvae are found in sputum or bronchial washings during the pulmonary phase or in urine

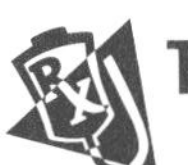

TREATMENT

MEDICATIONS

- Treatment should continue until the parasite is eradicated
- In concurrent infection with hookworm, strongyloidiasis, or ascariasis, eradicate the latter infections first

Ivermectin

- The drug of choice
- The dosage is 200 µg/kg PO; give a second dose within several days
- Cure rates range from 82% to 95%
- In the hyperinfection syndrome in immunocompromised patients, it may be necessary to prolong treatment or change to thiabendazole
- A parenteral formulation of ivermectin is available in some countries but is licensed only for veterinary use

Thiabendazole

- 25 mg/kg PO BID after meals (maximum, 1.5 g per dose) for 2–3 days. Repeat the course in 2 weeks
- A 5- to 7-day (or longer) course is needed for disseminated infections; side effects become severe
- Side effects, including headache, weakness, vomiting, vertigo, and decreased mental alertness, occur in 30% of patients and may be severe. Erythema multiforme and Stevens-Johnson syndrome can occur. The side effects can be decreased if the drug is taken after meals

Albendazole

- 400 mg PO BID for 3–7 days and repeated in 1 week; cure rates in several studies ranged from 38% to 95%
- Albendazole is less effective than ivermectin

OUTCOME

FOLLOW-UP

- Multiple stool examinations should be done at weekly intervals, preferably by the Baermann concentration method
- In selected instances, to control infections that cannot be eradicated, once-monthly treatments can be tried with a 1-day dose of ivermectin or 2-day course of thiabendazole

PROGNOSIS

- Favorable except in the hyperinfection syndrome and in infections associated with debilitating diseases

WHEN TO REFER

- Immunocompromised patients
- Disseminated disease

WHEN TO ADMIT

- Patients with the hyperinfection syndrome
- Severe pulmonary symptoms

EVIDENCE

PRACTICE GUIDELINES

- National Guideline Clearinghouse (imaging guidelines)
  - http://www.guideline.gov/summary/summary.aspx?doc_id=3258

INFORMATION FOR PATIENTS

- Centers for Disease Control and Prevention
  - http://www.dpd.cdc.gov/dpdx/HTML/Strongyloidiasis.htm
- National Institutes of Health
  - http://www.nlm.nih.gov/medlineplus/ency/article/000630.htm

REFERENCES

- Loutfy MR et al: Serology and eosinophil count in the diagnosis and management of strongyloidiasis in a non-endemic area. Am J Trop Med Hyg 2002;66:749. [PMID: 12224585]
- Zaha O et al: Efficacy of ivermectin for chronic strongyloidiasis: two single doses given 2 weeks apart. J Infect Chemother 2002;8:94. [PMID: 11957127]

Stupor & Coma

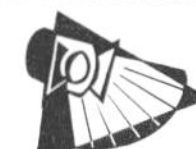

KEY FEATURES

ESSENTIALS OF DIAGNOSIS

- The stuporous patient is unresponsive except when subjected to repeated vigorous stimuli
- The comatose patient is unarousable and unable to respond to external events or inner needs, although reflex movements and posturing may be present

GENERAL CONSIDERATIONS

- Coma is a major complication of serious central nervous system disorders
- Abrupt onset of coma suggests subarachnoid hemorrhage, brainstem stroke, intracerebral hemorrhage, or acute herniation syndrome
- A slower onset and progression of coma occur with other structural or mass lesions
- A metabolic cause is likely with a preceding intoxicated state or agitated delirium
- **Intracranial causes**
  - Anoxic brain injury or head trauma
  - Ischemic stroke or intracerebral hemorrhage
  - Subarachnoid hemorrhage
  - Meningitis or encephalitis
  - Brainstem hemorrhage, infarct, or mass
  - Mass lesion causing brainstem compression
  - Subdural hematoma
  - Seizure
- **Metabolic causes**
  - Hypoglycemia
  - Diabetic ketoacidosis
  - Hyperglycemic hyperosmolar state
  - Drugs, eg, alcohol, opioids, sedatives, antidepressants, salicylates
  - Uremic or hepatic encephalopathy
  - Hypernatremia or hyponatremia
  - Hypercalcemia
  - Hypothermia
  - Heat stroke
  - Myxedema
  - Carbon monoxide poisoning

CLINICAL FINDINGS

SYMPTOMS AND SIGNS

- Response to painful stimuli
  - Purposive limb withdrawal from painful stimuli implies that sensory pathways from and motor pathways to the stimulated limb are functionally intact
  - Unilateral absence of responses to stimuli to both sides of the body implies a corticospinal lesion
  - Bilateral absence of responses suggests brainstem involvement, bilateral pyramidal tract lesions, or psychogenic unresponsiveness
  - Decorticate posturing with lesions of the internal capsule and rostral cerebral peduncle, decerebrate posturing with dysfunction or destruction of the midbrain and rostral pons
- Pupils
  - Hypothalamic disease processes may lead to unilateral Horner's syndrome
  - Bilateral diencephalic involvement or destructive pontine lesions leads to small but reactive pupils
  - Ipsilateral pupillary dilation with no response to light occurs with compression of the third cranial nerve, eg, with uncal herniation
  - The pupils are slightly smaller than normal but responsive to light in many metabolic encephalopathies
    1. They may be fixed and dilated following overdosage with atropine, scopolamine, or glutethimide
    2. They may be pinpoint (but responsive) with opiates
  - Pupillary dilation for several hours after cardiopulmonary arrest implies a poor prognosis
- Eye movements
  - Conjugate deviation of the eyes to the side suggests the presence of an ipsilateral hemispheric lesion or a contralateral pontine lesion
  - A mesencephaliclesion leads to downward conjugate deviation
  - Dysconjugate ocular deviation in coma implies a structural brainstem lesion (or preexisting strabismus)
- Oculomotor responses to passive head turning
  - In response to brisk rotation, flexion, and extension of the head, conscious patients with open eyes do not exhibit contraversive conjugate eye deviation (doll's-head eye response) unless there is voluntary visual fixation or bilateral frontal pathology
  - With cortical depression in lightly comatose patients, a brisk doll's-head eye response is seen
  - With brainstem lesions, this oculocephalic reflex becomes impaired or lost, depending on the lesion site
- Oculovestibular reflex
  - Tested by caloric stimulation using irrigation with ice water
  - In normal subjects, jerk nystagmus is elicited for about 2 or 3 minutes, with the slow component toward the irrigated ear
  - In unconscious patients with an intact brainstem, the fast component of the nystagmus disappears, so that the eyes tonically deviate toward the irrigated side for 2–3 minutes before returning to their original position
  - With impairment of brainstem function, the response is perverted and disappears
  - In metabolic coma, oculocephalic and oculovestibular reflex responses are preserved, at least initially
- Respiratory patterns
  - Cheyne-Stokes respiration may occur with bihemispheric or diencephalic disease or in metabolic disorders
  - Hyperventilation occurs with lesions of the brainstem tegmentum
  - Apneustic breathing (prominent end-inspiratory pauses) suggests damage at the pontine level
  - Atactic breathing (completely irregular pattern, with deep and shallow breaths occurring randomly): associated with lesions of the lower pons and medulla

DIFFERENTIAL DIAGNOSIS

- Brain death
- Persistent vegetative state
- Locked-in syndrome

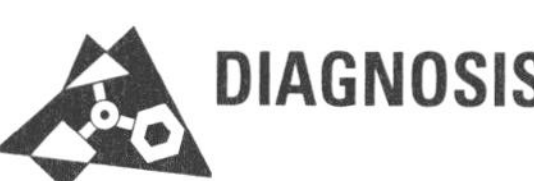

DIAGNOSIS

LABORATORY TESTS

- Serum glucose, electrolyte, and calcium levels
- Arterial blood gases
- Liver and renal function tests
- Toxicologic studies as indicated

IMAGING STUDIES

- CT scan to identify a structural lesion

DIAGNOSTIC PROCEDURES

- The diagnostic workup of the comatose patient must proceed concomitantly with management
- Lumbar puncture (if CT scan reveals no structural lesion) to exclude subarachnoid hemorrhage or meningitis

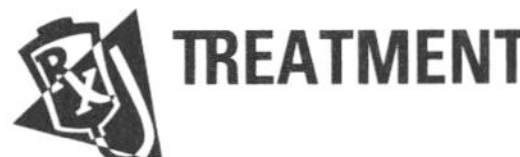

TREATMENT

MEDICATIONS

- Dextrose 50% (25 g), naloxone (0.4–1.2 mg), and thiamine (50 mg) are given intravenously

THERAPEUTIC PROCEDURES

- Treatment of coma depends on underlying cause
- Emergency measures
  - Supportive therapy for respiration or blood pressure is initiated
  - In hypothermia, all vital signs may be absent; all such patients should be rewarmed before the prognosis is assessed
  - The patient is positioned on one side with the neck partly extended, dentures removed, and secretions cleared by suction
  - If necessary, the patency of the airways is maintained with an oropharyngeal airway

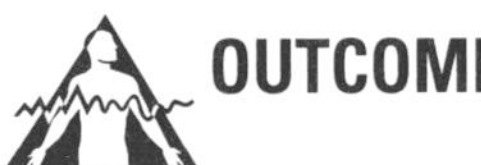

OUTCOME

WHEN TO ADMIT

- Admit all patients to an ICU

PROGNOSIS

- In coma because of cerebral ischemia and hypoxia, the absence of pupillary light reflexes at the time of initial examination implies little chance of regaining independence
- By contrast, preserved pupillary light responses, the development of spontaneous eye movements (roving, conjugate, or better), and extensor, flexor, or withdrawal responses to pain at this early stage imply a relatively good prognosis

EVIDENCE

INFORMATION FOR PATIENTS

- National Institute of Neurological Disorders and Stroke
  - http://www.ninds.nih.gov/disorders/coma/coma.htm

REFERENCE

- Booth CM et al: Is this patient dead, vegetative, or severely neurologically impaired? Assessing outcome for comatose survivors of cardiac arrest. JAMA 2004;291:870. [PMID:14970067]
- Laureys S et al: Brain function in coma, vegetative state, and related disorders. Lancet Neurol 2004;3:537. [PMID:15324722]
- Malik K, Hess DC: Evaluating the comatose patient. Rapid neurologic assessment is key to appropriate management. Postgrad Med 2002;111:38. [PMID:11868313]

Author(s)

Michael J. Aminoff, MD, DSc, FRCP

Subarachnoid Hemorrhage

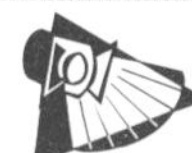

KEY FEATURES

ESSENTIALS OF DIAGNOSIS

- Sudden severe headache
- Signs of meningeal irritation usually present
- Obtundation or coma common
- Focal deficits frequently absent

GENERAL CONSIDERATIONS

- 5–10% of strokes are due to subarachnoid hemorrhage
- Hemorrhage is usually from rupture of an aneurysm or arteriovenous malformation
- No specific cause found in 20% of cases
- See Table 97

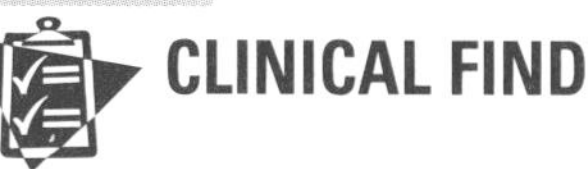

CLINICAL FINDINGS

SYMPTOMS AND SIGNS

- Sudden onset of headache with severity never experienced previously by the patient
- May be followed by nausea and vomiting and loss or impairment of consciousness (transient or progress to coma and death)
- Patient is often confused and irritable and may show other symptoms of an altered mental status
- Nuchal rigidity and other signs of meningeal irritation are seen, except in deeply comatose patients
- Focal neurologic deficits may be present and may suggest the site of the underlying lesion

DIFFERENTIAL DIAGNOSIS

- Meningitis
- Migraine
- Intracerebral hemorrhage
- Ischemic stroke

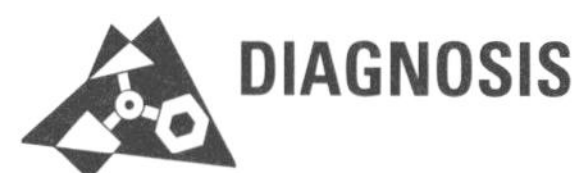

DIAGNOSIS

IMAGING STUDIES

- CT scan should be performed immediately to confirm that hemorrhage has occurred and to search for its source
- CT is faster and more sensitive in detecting hemorrhage in the first 24 hours than MRI
- Rarely, CT is normal in patients with suspected hemorrhage
  - If so, cerebrospinal fluid must be examined for blood or xanthochromia before the possibility of subarachnoid hemorrhage is discounted

DIAGNOSTIC PROCEDURES

- Cerebral arteriography helps to determine the source of bleeding
  - It is performed when the patient's condition has stabilized and surgery is feasible
- Bilateral carotid and vertebral arteriography are necessary because aneurysms are often multiple, while arteriovenous malformations may be supplied from several sources
- MR angiography may also permit visualization of vascular anomalies
  - Less sensitive than conventional arteriography

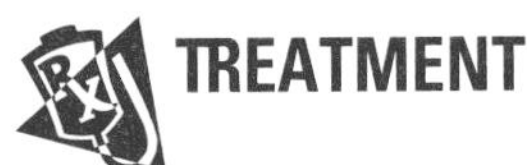

TREATMENT

MEDICATIONS

- Phenytoin to prevent seizures

SURGERY

- Causal lesion is treated surgically or by interventional radiology

THERAPEUTIC PROCEDURES

- Major aim is to prevent further hemorrhages
- Conscious patients
  - Confine to bed
  - Advise against exertion or straining
  - Treat symptomatically for headache and anxiety
  - Give laxatives or stool softeners
- Lower blood pressure gradually for severe hypertension, but not below a diastolic level of 90 mm Hg

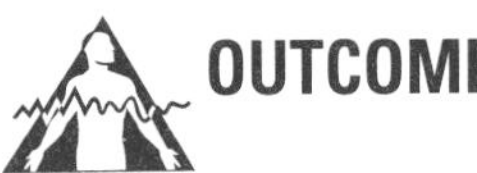

OUTCOME

PROGNOSIS

- Approxmately 20% of patients with aneurysms have further bleeding within 2 weeks and 40% within 6 months
- The greatest risk of further aneurysmal hemorrhage is within a few days of the initial bleed, thus early obliteration (within 2 days) is preferred

WHEN TO ADMIT

- All patients

PREVENTION

- See Intracranial Aneurysm

EVIDENCE

PRACTICE GUIDELINES

- American Society of Interventional and Therapeutic Neuroradiology. Mechanical and pharmacologic treatment of vasospasm. AJNR Am J Neuroradiol 2001;22(8 Suppl):S26. [PMID: 11686071]
- National Guideline Clearinghouse
  - http://www.guideline.gov/summary/summary.aspx?doc_id=3298&nbr=2524&string=subarachnoid+hemorrhage

WEB SITES

- CNS Pathology Index
  - http://medstat.med.utah.edu/WebPath/CNSHTML/CNSIDX.html
- 3-D Visualization of Brain Aneurysms
  - http://dpi.radiology.uiowa.edu/nlm/app/aneur/brain/aneur.html

INFORMATION FOR PATIENTS

- Brain Aneurysm Foundation
  - http://www.bafound.org/info/index.php
- National Institutes of Health
  - http://www.nlm.nih.gov/medlineplus/ency/article/000701.htm

REFERENCES

- Doerfler A et al: Endovascular treatment of cerebrovascular disease. Curr Opin Neurol 2004;17:481. [PMID:15247546]
- Molyneux A et al: International Subarachnoid Aneurysm Trial (ISAT) of neurosurgical clipping versus endovascular coiling in 2143 patients with ruptured intracranial aneurysms: a randomised trial. Lancet 2002;360:1267. [PMID:12414200]
- Polin RS et al: Efficacy of transluminal angioplasty for the management of symptomatic cerebral vasospasm following aneurysmal subarachnoid hemorrhage. J Neurosurg 2000;92:284. [PMID:10659016]
- Roos Y et al: Antifibrinolytic therapy for aneurysmal subarachnoid hemorrhage: a major update of a Cochrane review. Stroke 2003;34:2308. [PMID:12933970]
- Wiebers DO et al: Unruptured intracranial aneurysms: natural history, clinical outcome, and risks of surgical and endovascular treatment. Lancet 2003;362:103. [PMID:12867109]

Author(s)

Michael J. Aminoff, DSc, MD, FRCP

Superior Vena Cava Obstruction p. 1155.

Syndrome of Inappropriate Antidiuretic Hormone (SIADH)

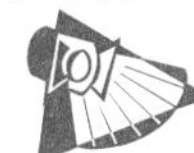

KEY FEATURES

ESSENTIALS OF DIAGNOSIS

- Serum sodium concentration less than 130 mEq/L
- Hypotonic, euvolemic hyponatremia

GENERAL CONSIDERATIONS

- Hyponatremia occurs from abnormal water balance rather than abnormal sodium balance
- Retention of electrolyte-free water because of impaired excretion and inappropriate antidiuretic hormone (ADH) excess results in hyponatremia and low serum osmolality
- Hospitalized patients treated with hypotonic fluid are at increased risk for hyponatremia
- Patterns of abnormal ADH secretion
  - Random secretion (eg, carcinomas)
  - Reset osmostat (eg, elderly, pulmonary diseases)
  - Leak of ADH (eg, basilar skull fractures)

Etiology

- **Central nervous system (CNS) disorders**
  - Head trauma
  - Stroke
  - Subarachnoid hemorrhage
  - Hydrocephalus
  - Brain tumor
  - Encephalitis
  - Guillain-Barré syndrome
  - Meningitis
  - Acute psychosis
  - Acute intermittent porphyria
- **Pulmonary lesions**
  - Tuberculosis
  - Bacterial pneumonia
  - Aspergillosis
  - Bronchiectasis
  - Neoplasms
  - Positive-pressure ventilation
- **Malignancies**
  - Bronchogenic carcinoma
  - Pancreatic carcinoma
  - Prostatic carcinoma
  - Renal cell carcinoma
  - Adenocarcinoma of colon
  - Thymoma
  - Osteosarcoma
  - Malignant lymphoma
  - Leukemia
- **Drugs: *Increased ADH production***
  - Antidepressants: tricyclics, monoamine oxidase inhibitors, selective serotonin reuptake inhibitors
  - Antineoplastics: cyclophosphamide, vincristine
  - Carbamazepine
  - Methylenedioxymethamphetamine (MDMA; Ecstasy)
  - Clofibrate
  - Neuroleptics: thiothixene, thioridazine, fluphenazine, haloperidol, trifluoperazine
- **Drugs: *Potentiated ADH action***
  - Carbamazepine
  - Chlorpropamide, tolbutamide
  - Cyclophosphamide
  - Nonsteroidal antiinflammatory drugs
  - Somatostatin and analogs
- **Others**
  - Postoperative
  - Pain
  - Stress
  - AIDS
  - Pregnancy (physiological)
  - Hypokalemia

DEMOGRAPHICS

- Most common cause of hyponatremia in hospitalized patients

CLINICAL FINDINGS

SYMPTOMS AND SIGNS

- Frequently asymptomatic
- Symptoms usually seen with serum sodium levels less than 120 mEq/L
- If symptomatic, primarily CNS symptoms of lethargy, weakness, confusion, delirium, and seizures
- Often symptoms are mistaken for primary neurological or metabolic disorders

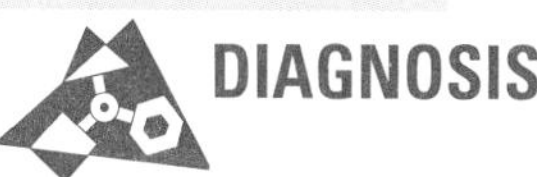

DIAGNOSIS

LABORATORY TESTS

- Decreased osmolality (< 280 mOsm/kg) with inappropriately increased urine osmolality (> 150 mOsm/kg)
- Low blood urea nitrogen (BUN) (< 10 mg/dL) and hypouricemia (< 4 mg/dL), which are not only dilutional but result from increased urea and uric acid clearances in response to the volume-expanded state
- A high BUN suggests a volume-contracted state, which excludes a diagnosis of SIADH

Syncope p. 1156.

Syndrome of Inappropriate Antidiuretic Hormone (SIADH)

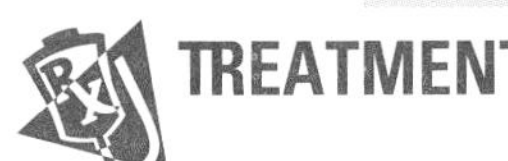

TREATMENT

MEDICATIONS

Symptomatic hyponatremia

- If CNS symptoms, hyponatremia should be rapidly treated at any level of serum sodium concentration
- Increase serum sodium concentration by ≤ 1–2 mEq/L/h and not > 25–30 mEq/L in first 2 days to prevent central pontine myelinolysis
- Rate should be reduced to 0.5–1 mEq/L/h as neurologic symptoms improve
- Initial goal: Achieve serum sodium concentration of 125–130 mEq/L, guarding against overcorrection
- Hypertonic (eg, 3%) saline plus furosemide (0.5–1 mg/kg IV) indicated for symptomatic hyponatremia
  - To determine how much 3% saline (513 mEq/L) to administer, obtain a spot urinary Na after a furosemide diuresis has begun
  - Excreted Na is replaced with 3% saline, empirically begun at 1–2 mL/kg/h, and then adjusted based on urinary output and urinary sodium (eg, after furosemide, urine volume may be 400 mL/h and sodium plus potassium excretion 100 mEq/L; excreted Na^+ is 40 mEq/h, which is replaced with 78 mL/h of 3% saline [40 mEq/h divided by 513 mEq/L])

Asymptomatic hyponatremia

- Correction rate: ≤ 0.5 mEq/L/h
  - Restrict water intake to 0.5–1 L/day
  - 0.9% saline with furosemide may be used when serum sodium < 120 mEq/L. Urinary sodium and potassium losses are replaced as above
  - Demeclocycline, 300–600 mg 2× daily, inhibits effect of ADH on distal tubule; is useful for patients who cannot adhere to water restriction or need additional therapy. Onset of action may be 1 week; concentrating may be permanently impaired. Therapy with demeclocycline in cirrhosis appears to increase renal failure risk
  - Selective vasopressin V2 antagonist
- Oral selective V2 antagonists may be available for treatment of SIADH in near future

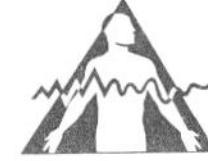

OUTCOME

FOLLOW-UP

- If symptomatic, measure plasma sodium ~Q 4 h and observe the patient closely

COMPLICATIONS

- Central pontine myelinolysis may occur from osmotically induced demyelination as a result of overly rapid correction of serum sodium (an increase of more than 1 mEq/L/h, or 25 mEq/L within the first day of therapy)
- Hypoxic-anoxic episodes during hyponatremia may contribute to the demyelination

PROGNOSIS

- Associated with underlying cause of SIADH
- Premenopausal women who develop hyponatremic encephalopathy from rapidly acquired hyponatremia (eg, postoperative hyponatremia) are about 25 times more likely than postmenopausal women to die or to suffer permanent brain damage

WHEN TO ADMIT

- Symptomatic hyponatremia
- Serum sodium < 120 mEq/L

EVIDENCE

WEB SITE

- Fall PJ: Hyponatremia and hypernatremia: A systematic approach to causes and their correction. Postgraduate Medicine Online, 2000
  - http://www.postgradmed.com/issues/2000/05_00/fall.htm

INFORMATION FOR PATIENTS

- American Association for Clinical Chemistry: Lab Tests Online: Sodium
  - http://labtestsonline.org/understanding/analytes/sodium/test.html
- Mayo Clinic: Low Blood Sodium in Older Adults
  - http://www.mayoclinic.com/invoke.cfm?id=AN00621
- MedlinePlus: ADH
  - http://www.nlm.nih.gov/medlineplus/ency/article/003702.htm
- MedlinePlus: Dilutional Hyponatremia (SIADH)
  - http://www.nlm.nih.gov/medlineplus/ency/article/000394.htm

REFERENCES

- Adrogue HJ et al: Hyponatremia. N Engl J Med 2000;342:1581. [PMID: 10824078]
- Cadnapaphornchai MA et al: Pathogenesis and management of hyponatremia. Am J Med 2000;109:688. [PMID: 11099692]
- Izzedine H et al: Angiotensin-converting enzyme inhibitor-induced syndrome of inappropriate secretion of antidiuretic hormone: case report and review of the literature. Clin Pharmacol Ther 2002;71:503. [PMID: 12087354]
- Oster JR et al: Hyponatremia, hypoosmolality, and hypotonicity: tables and fables. Arch Intern Med 1999;159:333. [PMID: 10030305]

Author(s)

Masafumi Fukagawa, MD, PhD
Kiyoshi Kurokawa, MD, MACP
Maxine A. Papadakis, MD

Syphilis

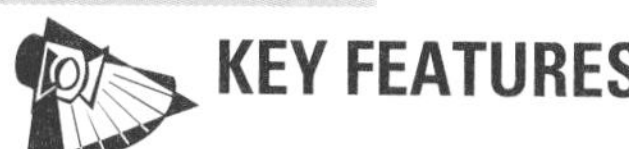

ESSENTIALS OF DIAGNOSIS

- Syphilis is a complex infectious disease caused by *Treponema pallidum*, a spirochete capable of infecting almost any organ or tissue in the body and causing protean clinical manifestations
- Transmission occurs most frequently during sexual contact (including oral sex); sites of inoculation are usually genital but may be extragenital

GENERAL CONSIDERATIONS

- The risk of syphilis after unprotected sex with an individual with early syphilis is ~30–50%
- Syphilis can be transferred from mother to fetus after the tenth week of pregnancy (congenital syphilis)
- Two major clinical stages: early (infectious) syphilis and late syphilis are separated by a symptom-free latent period. During early latency the infectious stage is liable to recur
- **Early (infectious) syphilis** includes
  - Primary lesions (chancre and regional lymphadenopathy)
  - Secondary lesions (commonly involving skin and mucous membranes, occasionally bone, central nervous system, or liver)
  - Relapsing lesions during early latency
  - Congenital lesions
- **Late syphilis** consists of the following:
  - So-called benign (gummatous) lesions involving skin, bones, and viscera
  - Cardiovascular disease (principally aortitis)
  - Central nervous system and ocular syndromes

DEMOGRAPHICS

- Between 1985 and 1990, there was a dramatic increase in infectious syphilis
- In 1998, a syphilis elimination program began targeting high-risk populations—women of childbearing age, sexually active teens, drug users, inmates of penal institutions, persons with multiple sexual partners or those who have sex with sex workers—and emphasizing screening, early treatment, contact tracing, and condom use
- A decrease in the number of primary and secondary cases was reported in 2001 (6103 cases) compared with 1998 (7035 cases)

CLINICAL FINDINGS

SYMPTOMS AND SIGNS

Primary

- Painless ulcer (chancre) on genitalia, perianal area, rectum, pharynx, tongue, lip, or elsewhere 2–6 weeks after exposure
- Nontender enlargement of regional lymph nodes

Secondary, early latent

- Generalized maculopapular skin rash
- Mucous membrane lesions, including patches and ulcers
- Weeping papules (condylomas) in moist skin areas
- Generalized nontender lymphadenopathy
- Fever
- Meningitis, hepatitis, osteitis, arthritis, iritis

Late latent ("hidden")

- No physical signs

Late (tertiary)

- Infiltrative tumors of skin, bones, liver (gummas)
- Aortitis, aneurysms, aortic regurgitation
- Central nervous system disorders, including meningovascular and degenerative changes, paresthesias, shooting pains, abnormal reflexes, dementia, or psychosis

DIFFERENTIAL DIAGNOSIS

- Primary syphilis (genital ulcer)
  - Herpes simplex virus
  - Chancroid
  - Granuloma inguinale
  - Lymphogranuloma venereum
  - Trauma
  - Neoplasm
- Secondary syphilis
  - Rash
  - Genital warts
- Tertiary syphilis
  - Other causes of aortic root disease
  - Other chronic meningitis

DIAGNOSIS

LABORATORY TESTS

- Serologic testing, microscopic detection of *T pallidum* in lesions, and other examinations (biopsies, lumbar puncture, x-rays) for evidence of tissue damage
- HIV test at the time of diagnosis

Nontreponemal antigen tests

- Most common are the VDRL and rapid plasma reagin (RPR)
- VDRL and RPR generally become positive 4–6 weeks after infection, or 1–3 weeks after a primary lesion. These serologic tests are not highly specific
- False-positive reactions are frequent in connective tissue diseases, infectious mononucleosis, malaria, HIV, febrile diseases, leprosy, injection drug use, infective endocarditis, old age, hepatitis C viral infection, and pregnancy
- False-negative results when very high antibody titers are present (the prozone phenomenon)
- RPR titers are often higher than VDRL titers and thus are not comparable
- Titers are used to assess adequacy of therapy

Treponemal antibody tests

- The fluorescent treponemal antibody absorption (FTA-ABS) helps determine whether a positive nontreponemal antigen test is indicative of syphilis or false-positive
- Because of its greater sensitivity, the FTA-ABS test is also of value when there is clinical evidence of syphilis but the nontreponemal serologic test is negative. The test is positive in most patients with primary syphilis and in virtually all with secondary syphilis
- The FTA-ABS test may revert to negative with adequate therapy
- False-positive FTA-ABS tests occur in systemic lupus erythematosus, Lyme disease, and hypergammaglobulinemia
- The *T pallidum* hemagglutination (TPHA) test and the particle agglutination test (TPPA) are comparable in sensitivity and specificity

DIAGNOSTIC PROCEDURES

- In primary and secondary syphilis, *T pallidum* may be shown by darkfield microscopic examination of fresh exudate from lesions or aspirated from regional lymph nodes
- Immunofluorescent staining for *T pallidum* of dried smears of fluid taken from early lesions may be helpful
- Cerebrospinal fluid (CSF) findings in neurosyphilis include elevation of total protein, lymphocytic pleocytosis, and a positive CSF VDRL
- CSF may, however, be completely normal
- CSF VDRL may be negative in 30–70% of cases of neurosyphilis
- CSF FTA-ABS is controversial

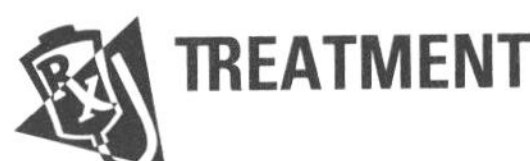

TREATMENT

MEDICATIONS

- For primary and secondary syphilis: benzathine penicillin G, 2.4 million units IM once
- For late latent syphilis or latent syphilis of unknown duration: benzathine penicillin G, 2.4 million units IM × 3 at 7 day intervals
- For neurosyphilis: aqueous penicillin G, 18–24 million units IV QD (3–4 million units Q 4 h or as a continuous infusion) for 10–14 days
- For patients allergic to penicillin, doxycycline, 100 mg PO BID for 14 days or tetracycline, 500 mg PO QID for 14 days, for infectious syphilis. In syphilis of more than 1-year duration or of unknown duration, treat for 28 days
- Preliminary data suggest azithromycin, 2 g PO once or ceftriaxone 1 g QD IM or IV for 8–10 days, is efficacious against infectious syphilis. Ceftriaxone, 2 g QD IM or IV for 10–14 days, can be used for neurosyphilis
- Patients with gonorrhea and exposure to syphilis should be treated with separate regimens effective against both diseases

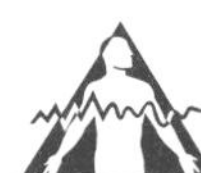

OUTCOME

FOLLOW-UP

- Syphilis patients must abstain from sexual activity until rendered noninfectious by antibiotic therapy
- Primary, secondary, early latent syphilis
  - Reexamine clinically and serologically at 6 and 12 months (at 3, 6, 9, 12, and 24 months if HIV infected)
  - If nontreponemal antibody titers fail to decrease 4-fold by 6 months, an HIV test should be repeated
  - A lumbar puncture should be considered
  - If careful follow-up cannot be ensured, treatment should be repeated with 2.4 million units of benzathine penicillin IM weekly for 3 weeks
- Latent syphilis
  - Repeat serologies at 6, 12, and 24 months
  - If titers increase 4-fold or if initially high titers (> 1:32) fail to decrease 4-fold by 12–24 months, an HIV test and lumbar puncture should be performed and retreatment given
- Neurosyphilis
  - Repeat lumbar puncture every 6 months
  - If CSF cell count has not decreased by 6 months or is not normal at 2 years, a second course of treatment is given

COMPLICATIONS

- The Jarisch-Herxheimer reaction, fever and aggravation of the clinical picture, may be prevented or modified by simultaneous administration of antipyretics or corticosteroids

PROGNOSIS

- Late syphilis may be highly destructive and permanently disabling and may lead to death.
- If left untreated, about one-third of people infected with syphilis will undergo spontaneous cure, about one-third will remain in the latent phase throughout life, and about one-third will develop serious late lesions

WHEN TO REFER

- If uncertain about interpretation of serologic tests, need for lumbar puncture, or optimal therapy, or if patient has severe penicillin allergy

WHEN TO ADMIT

- Admit for complications (stroke, meningoencephalitis, dementia, etc) or for careful observation for Jarisch-Herxheimer reaction

PREVENTION

- Avoidance of sexual contact
- Latex condoms
- Abortive penicillin therapy of procaine penicillin G 2.4 million units IM

EVIDENCE

PRACTICE GUIDELINES

- National Guideline Clearinghouse: 2002 national guidelines on the management of early syphilis. London: Association for Genitourinary Medicine (AGUM), Medical Society for the Study of Venereal Disease (MSSVD); 2002.
  - http://www.guideline.gov/summary/summary.aspx?doc_id=3036
  - http://www.guideline.gov/summary/summary.aspx?doc_id=3037
- National Guideline Clearinghouse: Screening for syphilis infection. United States Preventive Services Task Force, 2004.
  - http://www.guideline.gov/summary/summary.aspx?doc_id=5265
- National Guideline Clearinghouse: Diseases characterized by genital ulcers. Sexually transmitted diseases treatment guidelines. Centers for Disease Control and Prevention—MMWR Recomm Rep 2002;51(RR-6):11.
  - http://www.guideline.gov/summary/summary.aspx?doc_id=3233
- UK National Guidelines — Medical Society for the Study of Venereal Diseases — Late syphilis
  - http://www.mssvd.org.uk/PDF/CEG2001/late%20$%20final%20b%2031%2012%2002.pdf

WEB SITE

- Centers for Disease Control and Prevention—National Center for HIV, STD and TB Prevention—Division of Sexually Transmitted Diseases
  - http://www.cdc.gov/nchstp/dstd/SyphilisInfo.htm

INFORMATION FOR PATIENTS

- JAMA patient page: Syphilis. JAMA 2000;284:520. [PMID: 10939892]
- Centers for Disease Control and Prevention—Division of Sexually Transmitted Diseases
  - http://www.cdc.gov/std/Syphilis/STDFact-Syphilis.htm
- American Social Health Organization
  - http://www.ashastd.org/stdfaqs/syphilis.html

REFERENCES

- 2002 guidelines for treatment of sexually transmitted diseases. MMWR Recomm Rep 2002;51(RR-6):1. [PMID: 12184549]
- Hall CS et al: Managing syphilis in the HIV-infected patient. Curr Infect Dis Rep 2004;6:72. [PMID: 14733852]
- Marra CM et al: Normalization of cerebrospinal fluid abnormalities after neurosyphilis treatment: does HIV status matter? Clin Infect Dis 2004;38:1001. [PMID: 14745693]

Author(s)

Richard A. Jacobs, MD, PhD

Systemic Lupus Erythematosus

KEY FEATURES

ESSENTIALS OF DIAGNOSIS

- Occurs mainly in young women
- Rash over areas exposed to sunlight
- Joint symptoms in 90% of patients
- Multiple system involvement
- Depression of hemoglobin, white blood cells, platelets
- Antinuclear antibody with high titer to native DNA

GENERAL CONSIDERATIONS

- Systemic lupus erythematosus (SLE) is an inflammatory autoimmune disorder that affects multiple organ systems
- The clinical course is marked by spontaneous remission and relapses
- Four features of drug-induced lupus separate it from SLE
  - The sex ratio is nearly equal
  - Nephritis and central nervous system features are not ordinarily present
  - Hypocomplementemia and antibodies to native DNA are absent
  - The clinical features and most laboratory abnormalities often revert toward normal when the offending drug is withdrawn

DEMOGRAPHICS

- 85% of patients are women
- Occurs in 1:1000 white women but in 1:250 black women

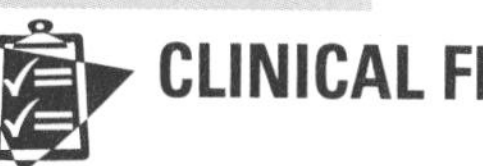

CLINICAL FINDINGS

SYMPTOMS AND SIGNS

- Fever, anorexia, malaise, and weight loss
- **Skin** lesions occur in most at some time; the characteristic "butterfly" rash affects fewer than 50%; alopecia is common
- **Raynaud's** phenomenon (20% of patients) often antedates other symptoms
- **Joint** symptoms, with or without active synovitis, occur in over 90% and are often the earliest manifestation. The arthritis is seldom deforming
- **Ocular:** conjunctivitis, photophobia, blurring of vision, and transient or permanent monocular blindness
- **Pulmonary**: pleurisy, pleural effusion, bronchopneumonia, pneumonitis, and restrictive lung disease
- **Cardiac:** pericarditis, myocarditis, arrhythmias. The typical verrucous endocarditis of Libman-Sacks is usually clinically silent but can produce acute or chronic valvular incompetence—most commonly mitral regurgitation—and can serve as a source of emboli
- **Mesenteric vasculitis** occasionally occurs and may resemble polyarteritis nodosa, including the presence of aneurysms in medium-sized blood vessels. Abdominal pain (particularly postprandial), ileus, peritonitis, and perforation may result
- **Neurological**: psychosis, organic brain syndrome, seizures, peripheral and cranial neuropathies, transverse myelitis, and strokes. Severe depression and psychosis may be exacerbated by the administration of large doses of corticosteroids
- **Glomerulonephritis:** several forms may occur, including mesangial, focal and diffuse proliferative, and membranous

DIFFERENTIAL DIAGNOSIS

- Drug-induced lupus (Table 80) (especially procainamide, hydralazine and isoniazid)
- Scleroderma
- Rheumatoid arthritis
- Inflammatory myopathy, especially dermatomyositis
- Rosacea
- Vasculitis, eg, polyarteritis nodosa
- Endocarditis
- Lyme disease

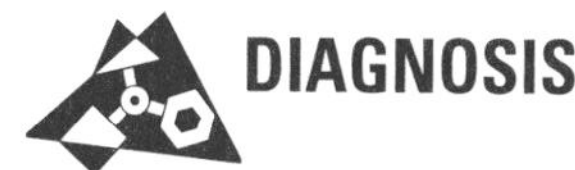

DIAGNOSIS

LABORATORY TESTS

- Production of many different autoantibodies (Tables 76, 82, and 83)
- Antinuclear antibody tests are sensitive but not specific for systemic lupus—ie, they are positive in most patients with lupus but are also positive in many patients with non-lupus conditions such as rheumatoid arthritis, hepatitis, and interstitial lung disease
- Antibodies to double-stranded DNA and to Sm are specific for SLE but not sensitive, since they are present in only 60% and 30% of patients, respectively
- Depressed serum complement—a finding suggestive of disease activity—often returns toward normal in remission
- Three types of antiphospholipid antibodies occur (Table 83)
  - The first causes the biological false-positive tests for syphilis
  - The second is lupus anticoagulant, a risk factor for venous and arterial thrombosis and miscarriage
  - The third is anticardiolipin antibody
- Abnormality of urinary sediment is almost always found in association with renal lesions. Red blood cells, with or without casts, and mild proteinuria are frequent

DIAGNOSTIC PROCEDURES

- The diagnosis can be made with reasonable probability if 4 of the 11 criteria set forth in Table 81 are met. These criteria should be viewed as rough guidelines that do not supplant clinical judgment in the diagnosis of SLE
- Renal biopsy is useful in deciding whether to treat with cyclophosphamide, and to rule out end-stage renal disease that may no longer benefit from treatment

Syringomyelia p. 1157

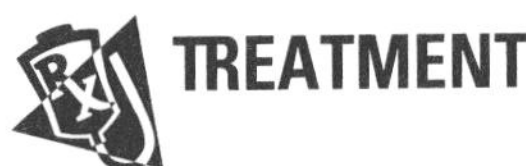

TREATMENT

MEDICATIONS

- Skin lesions often respond to the local administration of corticosteroids
- Minor joint symptoms can usually be alleviated by rest and nonsteroidal anti-inflammatory drugs (NSAIDs)
- Antimalarials (hydroxychloroquine) may be helpful in treating lupus rashes or joint symptoms that do not respond to NSAIDs
- Corticosteroids are required for the control of certain serious complications, such as thrombocytopenic purpura, hemolytic anemia, myocarditis, pericarditis, convulsions, and nephritis
- Immunosuppressive agents such as cyclophosphamide, chlorambucil, and azathioprine are used in cases resistant to corticosteroids. Cyclophosphamide improves renal survival. Overall patient survival, however, is no better than in the prednisone-treated group
- Systemic steroids are not usually given for minor arthritis, skin rash, leukopenia, or the anemia associated with chronic disease

THERAPEUTIC PROCEDURES

- Avoid sun exposure and use sunscreen

OUTCOME

COMPLICATIONS

- Thrombocytopenic purpura
- Hemolytic anemia
- Myocarditis
- Pericarditis
- Convulsions
- Nephritis

PROGNOSIS

- 10-year survival rate exceeds 85%
- In most patients, the illness pursues a relapsing and remitting course
- In some patients, the disease pursues a virulent course, leading to serious impairment of vital structures such as lung, heart, brain, or kidneys, and the disease may lead to death
- Accelerated atherosclerosis attributed, in part, to corticosteroid use, has been responsible for a rise in late deaths due to myocardial infarction

WHEN TO REFER

- Most patients should be followed in consultation with a rheumatologist and often a nephrologist

WHEN TO ADMIT

- Severe renal disease
- Pulmonary insufficiency
- Cardiac involvement
- Central nervous system disease
- Acute abdominal pain

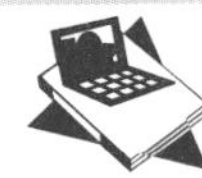

EVIDENCE

PRACTICE GUIDELINES

- Guidelines for referral and management of systemic lupus erythematosus in adults. American College of Rheumatology Ad Hoc Committee on Systemic Lupus Erythematosus Guidelines. Arthritis Rheum 1999;42:1785. [PMID: 10513791]
- National Guideline Clearinghouse
  - http://www.guideline.gov/summary/summary.aspx?doc_id=5675

WEB SITES

- Arthritis Foundation
  - http://www.arthritis.org
- Lupus Foundation of America
  - http://www.lupus.org

INFORMATION FOR PATIENTS

- National Institute of Arthritis and Musculoskeletal and Skin Diseases
  - http://www.niams.nih.gov/hi/topics/lupus/slehandout/index.htm

REFERENCES

- Asanuma Y et al: Premature coronary-artery atherosclerosis in systemic lupus erythematosus. N Engl J Med 2003;349:2407. [PMID: 14681506]
- Contreras G et al: Sequential therapies for proliferative lupus nephritis. N Engl J Med 2004;350:971. [PMID: 14999109]
- Mok CC: Cyclophosphamide for severe lupus nephritis: Where are we now? Arthritis Rheum 2004;50:3748. [PMID: 15593210]

Author(s)

David B. Hellmann, MD, FACP

John H. Stone, MD, MPH

Takayasu's Arteritis

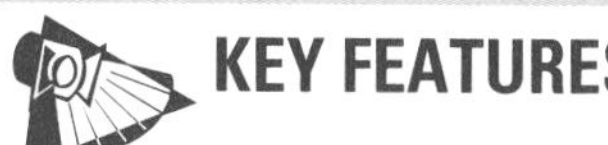

KEY FEATURES

ESSENTIALS OF DIAGNOSIS

- Polyarteritis with predilection for the branches of the aortic arch
- Segmental stenoses, occlusions, and aneurysms
- Elevated sedimentation rate

GENERAL CONSIDERATIONS

- A rare polyarteritis of unknown cause

DEMOGRAPHICS

- Predominantly affects Asian women age < 40

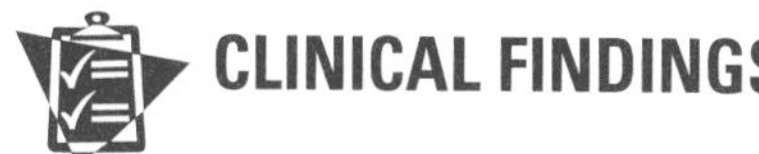

CLINICAL FINDINGS

SYMPTOMS AND SIGNS

- Clinical presentations depend on the stage of disease (early "inflammatory" or late "occlusive") and the vessels involved
- Early stages: fever, myalgias, arthralgias, and pain over the involved artery
- Later stages: syncope, dizziness, amaurosis fugax, stroke, angina, pulmonary hypertension, and claudication
- Hypertension in > 25% related to renal artery stenosis or aortic coarctation
- Vascular bruits, diminished peripheral pulses, or asymmetric blood pressure measurements

DIFFERENTIAL DIAGNOSIS

- Atheroocclusive disease
- Giant cell arteritis

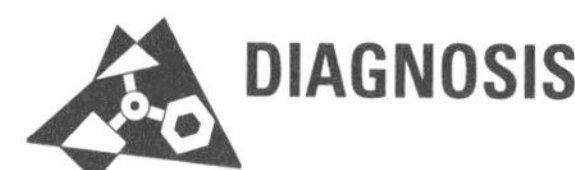

DIAGNOSIS

LABORATORY TESTS

- Leukocytosis
- Elevated sedimentation rate

IMAGING STUDIES

- Angiography shows combined occlusive and aneurysmal disease; the subclavian artery, descending thoracic aorta, renal artery, carotid artery, and mesenteric arteries are most commonly involved, but the ascending and abdominal aorta and the vertebral, coronary, pulmonary, iliac, and brachial arteries can also be affected
- MRA or CTA used for routine surveillance

Tachycardia, Paroxysmal Supraventricular p. 1157.
Tachycardia, Ventricular p. 1158.

Takayasu's Arteritis

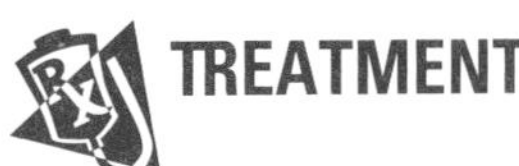

TREATMENT

MEDICATIONS

- Early, active stage: corticosteroids (eg, prednisone, 1 mg/kg PO QD)
- Cytotoxic agents may be added if steroids are ineffective

SURGERY

- Surgical or percutaneous intervention if disease indolent and clinical scenario warrants treatment
- Surgical indications are similar to those for arterial stenoses and aneurysms of other causes
- Percutaneous angioplasty or stenting can be done for short-segment stenoses, but there is a high recurrence rate

THERAPEUTIC PROCEDURES

- Histological examination of the resected artery shows nonspecific transmural inflammation or chronic fibrosis

OUTCOME

COMPLICATIONS

- Stroke
- Renal insufficiency
- Limb loss

PROGNOSIS

- Good if diagnosed and treated early

WHEN TO REFER

- Symptoms, signs, and diagnosis of Takayasu's arteritis

WHEN TO ADMIT

- Takayasu's arteritis with complication

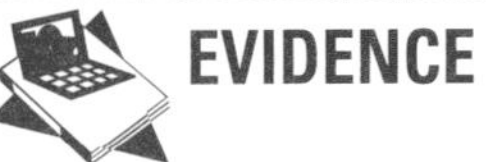

EVIDENCE

PRACTICE GUIDELINES

- Sabbadini MG et al: Takayasu's arteritis: therapeutic strategies. J Nephrol 2001;14:525. [PMID: 11783609]
- Weyand CM et al: Medium- and large-vessel vasculitis. N Engl J Med 2003;349:160. [PMID: 12853590]

INFORMATION FOR PATIENTS

- Cleveland Clinic: What You Need to Know About Takayasu Arteritis
  - http://www.clevelandclinic.org/health/health-info/docs/1700/1738.asp?index=7097
- Johns Hopkins Vasculitis Center: Types of Vasculitis: Takayasu Arteritis
  - http://vasculitis.med.jhu.edu/typesof/takayasu.html
- MedlinePlus: Vasculitis interactive tutorial
  - http://www.nlm.nih.gov/medlineplus/tutorials/vasculitis.html

REFERENCE

- Johnston SL et al: Takayasu arteritis: a review. J Clin Pathol 2002;55:481. [PMID: 12101189]

Author(s)

Louis M. Messina, MD

Tapeworm Infection, Beef

KEY FEATURES

ESSENTIALS OF DIAGNOSIS

- Generally asymptomatic
- Patients often discover segments of the tapeworm in clothing or stool

GENERAL CONSIDERATIONS

- Six tapeworms infect humans frequently
- The large tapeworms are *Taenia saginata* (the beef tapeworm, up to 25 m in length), *Taenia solium* (the pork tapeworm, 7 m), and *Diphyllobothrium latum* (the fish tapeworm, 10 m)
- A fourth large tapeworm, *T asiatica*, recently differentiated by DNA methods, has been found in China, the Koreas, Indonesia, and Southeast Asia. Although acquired by humans by ingestion of pig viscera, it apparently does not cause cysticercosis
- The small tapeworms are *Hymenolepis nana* (the dwarf tapeworm, 25–40 mm), *Hymenolepis diminuta* (the rodent tapeworm, 20–60 cm), and *Dipylidium caninum* (the dog tapeworm, 10–70 cm)
- Humans are the only definitive host of *T saginata* and *T solium*
- An adult tapeworm consists of a head (scolex), a neck, and a chain of individual segments (proglottids) in which eggs form in mature segments
- Humans are infected by eating raw or undercooked beef containing viable cysticerci, *Cysticercus bovis*. In human intestines, the cysticercus develops into an adult worm

DEMOGRAPHICS

- Four of the six tapeworms occur worldwide; the pork and fish tapeworms have more limited distribution
- The infection occurs in most countries with beef husbandry but is highly endemic in parts of the Far East, central and eastern Africa, and the central Asian area of the former Soviet Union
- Gravid segments of *T saginata* in the human intestine detach from the chain and are passed in feces to soil. When proglottids or eggs are ingested by grazing cattle or other domesticated bovines, the eggs hatch to release embryos that encyst in muscle as cysticerci

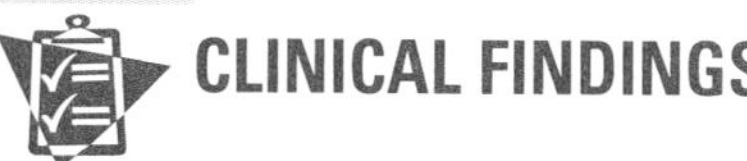

CLINICAL FINDINGS

SYMPTOMS AND SIGNS

- Large tapeworms are generally asymptomatic
- Occasionally, vague gastrointestinal symptoms (eg, nausea, diarrhea, abdominal pain) and systemic symptoms (eg, fatigue, hunger, dizziness) have been attributed to the infections
- Vomiting of proglottid segments or obstruction of the bile duct, pancreatic duct, or appendix is rare

DIFFERENTIAL DIAGNOSIS

- Pork, fish, dwarf, rodent, or dog tapeworms
- Chronic fatigue syndrome
- Chronic hepatitis
- Irritable bowel syndrome
- Amebiasis
- Ascariasis
- Enterobiasis (pinworm, mostly children)
- Hookworm disease
- Strongyloidiasis
- Celiac sprue or tropical sprue
- Pernicious anemia (*D latum*)

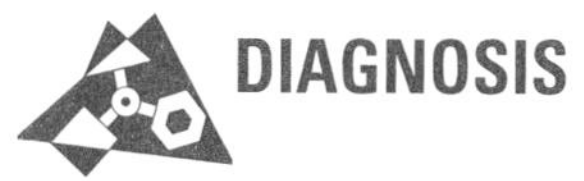

DIAGNOSIS

LABORATORY TESTS

- Serological tests are not available

DIAGNOSTIC PROCEDURES

- Infection is often discovered by the patient finding segments in stool, clothing, or bedding
- To determine the species, proglottid segments are either flattened between glass slides and examined microscopically for anatomic detail or differentiated by enzyme electrophoresis of glucose phosphate isomerase
- Eggs are infrequently present in stools, but the perianal cellophane tape test, as used to diagnose pinworm, is sometimes useful in detecting *T saginata* eggs. However, *Taenia* eggs look alike and do not permit species differentiation except by specialized methods

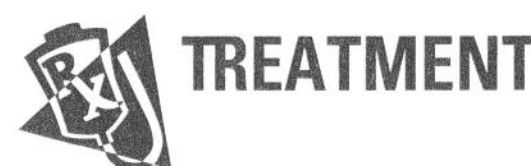

TREATMENT

MEDICATIONS

- Praziquantel in a single dose of 10 mg/kg achieves cure rates of about 99%. At this dose, side effects are minimal
- With a single dose of four tablets (2 g) of niclosamide (not available in the United States), cure rates over 90% can be anticipated. The drug is given in the morning before the patient has eaten. The tablets *must be chewed thoroughly* and swallowed with water. Eating may be resumed in 2 h. The drug usually produces no side effects
- Pre- and posttreatment purges are not used for either drug

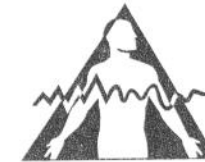

OUTCOME

FOLLOW-UP

- A disintegrating worm is usually passed within 24–48 h of treatment. Since efforts are not generally made to recover and identify the scolex, cure can be presumed only if regenerated segments have not reappeared 3–5 months later
- If it is preferred that parasitic cure be established immediately, the head (scolex) must be found in posttreatment stools; a laxative is given 2 h after treatment, and stools must be collected in a preservative for 24 h. To facilitate examination, toilet paper must be disposed of separately

PROGNOSIS

- Excellent with therapy

WHEN TO REFER

- For assistance in making the diagnosis
- Inability to clear the infection

PREVENTION

- *C bovis* is killed by cooking at 56°C or freezing at –10°C for 5 days. Pickling is not adequate

EVIDENCE

WEB SITE

- CDC—Division of Parasitic Diseases
  - http://www.cdc.gov/ncidod/dpd/parasites/taenia/default.htm
  - http://www.guideline.gov/summary/summary.aspx?doc_id=2707&nbr=1933&string=foodborne

INFORMATION FOR PATIENTS

- National Institutes of Health
  - http://www.nlm.nih.gov/medlineplus/ency/article/001391.htm
- The Mayo Clinic
  - http://www.mayoclinic.com/invoke.cfm?id=ID00002

REFERENCE

- Hoberg EP: Taenia tapeworms: their biology, evolution and socioeconomic significance. Microbes Infect 2002;4:859. [PMID: 12270733]

Tapeworm Infection, Dwarf

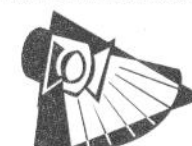

KEY FEATURES

ESSENTIALS OF DIAGNOSIS

- Infection may be asymptomatic
- Can cause nonspecific gastrointestinal symptoms of nausea, diarrhea, pain, and weight loss

GENERAL CONSIDERATIONS

- Six tapeworms infect humans frequently
- The large tapeworms are *Taenia saginata* (the beef tapeworm, up to 25 m in length), *Taenia solium* (the pork tapeworm, 7 m), and *Diphyllobothrium latum* (the fish tapeworm, 10 m)
- A fourth large tapeworm, *T asiatica*, recently differentiated by DNA methods, has been found in China, the Koreas, Indonesia, and Southeast Asia. Although acquired by humans by ingestion of pig viscera, it apparently does not cause cysticercosis
- The small tapeworms are *Hymenolepis nana* (the dwarf tapeworm, 25–40 mm), *Hymenolepis diminuta* (the rodent tapeworm, 20–60 cm), and *Dipylidium caninum* (the dog tapeworm, 10–70 cm)
- An adult tapeworm consists of a head (scolex), a neck, and a chain of individual segments (proglottids) in which eggs form in mature segments. The scolex is the attachment organ and generally lodges in the upper part of the small intestine
- Multiple infections are the rule for small tapeworms and may occur for *D latum*; however, it is rare for a person to harbor more than one or two of the taeniae

Dwarf tapeworm

- *H nana* is the most common cestode
- It can reach high prevalence, particularly in children, in regions of the world with poor fecal hygiene and in closed institutions worldwide
- Humans are the definitive host of *H nana*; rodent-adapted strains occur in rodents
- The life cycle is unusual in that both larval and adult stages are found in the human intestine, internal autoinfection can occur, and generally there is no intermediate host
- Transmission usually results from eggs transferred directly from human to human (the eggs are immediately infective) but sometimes involves fomites, water, or food or the swallowing of fleas

Rodent tapeworm

- *H diminuta* is a common parasite of rodents. Many arthropods (eg, rat fleas, beetles, and cockroaches) serve as intermediate hosts
- Humans—most commonly young children—are infected by accidentally swallowing the infected arthropods, usually in cereals or stored products

Dog tapeworm

- *D caninum* infection generally occurs in young children in close association with infected dogs or cats
- Transmission results from swallowing the infected intermediate hosts, ie, fleas or lice

CLINICAL FINDINGS

SYMPTOMS AND SIGNS

- Light infections are generally asymptomatic
- Heavy infections, particularly with *H nana*, may cause diarrhea, abdominal pain, anorexia, vomiting, weight loss, and irritability

DIFFERENTIAL DIAGNOSIS

- Chronic fatigue syndrome
- Chronic hepatitis
- Irritable bowel syndrome
- Amebiasis
- Ascariasis
- Enterobiasis (pinworm, mostly children)
- Hookworm disease
- Strongyloidiasis
- Celiac sprue or tropical sprue
- Pernicious anemia (*D latum*)

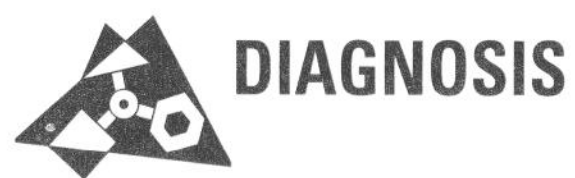

DIAGNOSIS

LABORATORY TESTS

- *H nana* and *H diminuta* infections are diagnosed by finding characteristic eggs in feces; proglottids are usually not seen
- *D caninum* infection is diagnosed by detection of proglottids (the size of melon seeds) in feces or after their active migration through the anus
- Serological tests are not available

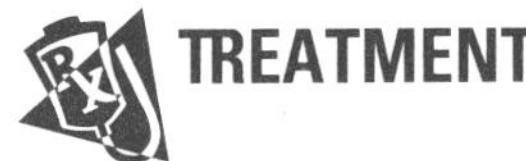

TREATMENT

MEDICATIONS

H nana

- Praziquantel, the drug of choice, produces 95% cure rates with a single 25-mg PO/kg dose
- Niclosamide (not available in the United States), the alternative drug, produces cure rates of 75% when given at a single dosage of four tablets (2 g) for 5–7 days; some workers repeat the course 5 days later. The drug is given in the morning before the patient has eaten. The tablets *must be chewed thoroughly* and swallowed with water. Eating may be resumed in 2 h. The drug usually produces no side effects

H diminuta and D caninum

- Treatment is with niclosamide or praziquantel in dosages as for *H nana*. Cure rates are not established

OUTCOME

WHEN TO REFER

- For persistent or progressive infection despite treatment

EVIDENCE

WEB SITE

- CDC—Division of Parasitic Diseases
  - http://www.cdc.gov/ncidod/dpd/parasites/taenia/default.htm

INFORMATION FOR PATIENTS

- Centers for Disease Control and Prevention
  - http://www.dpd.cdc.gov/dpdx/HTML/Taeniasis.htm
- National Institutes of Health
  - http://www.nlm.nih.gov/medlineplus/ency/article/001391.htm

REFERENCE

- Hoberg EP: Taenia tapeworms: their biology, evolution and socioeconomic significance. Microbes Infect 2002;4:859. [PMID: 12270733]

Tapeworm Infection, Fish

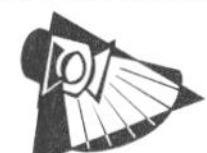

KEY FEATURES

ESSENTIALS OF DIAGNOSIS

- One of six tapeworms that commonly infect humans
- Infections are generally asymptomatic but occasionally there can be nonspecifc gastrointestinal discomfort
- Macrocytic megaloblastic anemia can develop

GENERAL CONSIDERATIONS

- Six tapeworms infect humans frequently. The large tapeworms are *Taenia saginata* (the beef tapeworm, up to 25 m in length), *Taenia solium* (the pork tapeworm, 7 m), and *Diphyllobothrium latum* (the fish tapeworm, 10 m)
- A fourth large tapeworm, *T asiatica*, recently differentiated by DNA methods, has been found in China, the Koreas, Indonesia, and Southeast Asia. Although acquired by humans by ingestion of pig viscera, it apparently does not cause cysticercosis
- The small tapeworms are *Hymenolepis nana* (the dwarf tapeworm, 25–40 mm), *Hymenolepis diminuta* (the rodent tapeworm, 20–60 cm), and *Dipylidium caninum* (the dog tapeworm, 10–70 cm)
- Four of the six tapeworms occur worldwide; the pork and fish tapeworms have more limited distribution
- An adult tapeworm consists of a head (scolex), a neck, and a chain of individual segments (proglottids) in which eggs form in mature segments. The scolex is the attachment organ and generally lodges in the upper part of the small intestine
- Multiple infections are the rule for small tapeworms and may occur for *D latum*; however, it is rare for a person to harbor more than one or two of the taeniae
- Eggs passed in human feces that reach fresh water are taken up first by crustaceans, which in turn are eaten by fish, both of which are intermediate hosts
- Human infection results from eating raw or inadequately cooked brackish or freshwater fish, including salmon
- Nonhuman reservoir hosts include dogs, bears, and other fish-eating mammals
- Some persons (mostly Scandinavian residents) who harbor the fish tapeworm develop a macrocytic megaloblastic anemia accompanied by thrombocytopenia and mild leukopenia. Gastric acidity is normal. The anemia is a result of the worm's competing with the host for vitamin B_{12}

DEMOGRAPHICS

- *D latum* is found in temperate and subarctic lake regions

CLINICAL FINDINGS

SYMPTOMS AND SIGNS

- Large tapeworm infections are generally asymptomatic
- Occasionally, vague gastrointestinal symptoms (eg, nausea, diarrhea, abdominal pain) and systemic symptoms (eg, fatigue, hunger, dizziness) have been attributed to the infections
- Vomiting of proglottid segments or obstruction of the bile duct, pancreatic duct, or appendix is rare
- If B_{12} deficiency develops, clinical findings are indistinguishable from those of pernicious anemia. They include glossitis, dyspnea, tachycardia, and neurological findings (numbness, paresthesias, disturbances of coordination, impairment of vibration and position sense, and dementia)

DIFFERENTIAL DIAGNOSIS

- Beef, pork, dwarf, rodent, or dog tapeworm
- Chronic fatigue syndrome
- Chronic hepatitis
- Irritable bowel syndrome
- Amebiasis
- Ascariasis
- Enterobiasis (pinworm, mostly children)
- Hookworm disease
- Strongyloidiasis
- Celiac sprue or tropical sprue
- Pernicious anemia (*D latum*)

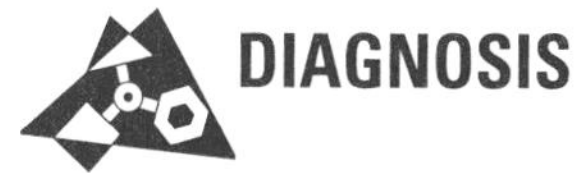

DIAGNOSIS

LABORATORY TESTS

- Diagnosed by finding characteristic operculated eggs in stool; repeat examinations and concentration may be necessary
- Proglottids are occasionally vomited or passed in feces; their internal morphology is diagnostic
- The presence of hydrochloric acid in the stomach differentiates tapeworm anemia from pernicious anemia; in both conditions, the Schilling test is abnormal

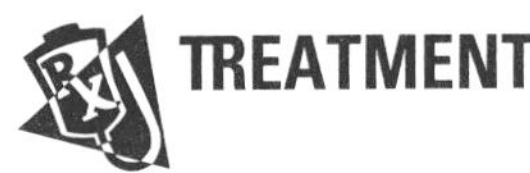

TREATMENT

MEDICATIONS

- Praziquantel in a single dose of 10 mg PO/kg achieves cure rates of about 99%. At this dose, side effects are minimal
- With a single dose of four tablets (2 g) of niclosamide (not available in the United States), cure rates over 90% can be anticipated. The drug is given in the morning before the patient has eaten. The tablets *must be chewed thoroughly* and swallowed with water. Eating may be resumed in 2 h. Niclosamide usually produces no side effects
- Pre- and posttreatment purges are not used for either drug
- The anemia and neurological manifestations respond to vitamin B_{12} as used in treatment of pernicious anemia

OUTCOME

FOLLOW-UP

- A disintegrating worm is usually passed within 24–48 h of treatment. Since efforts are not generally made to recover and identify the scolex, cure can be presumed only if regenerated segments have not reappeared 3–5 months later
- If it is preferred that parasitic cure be established immediately, the head (scolex) must be found in posttreatment stools; a laxative is given 2 h after treatment, and stools must be collected in a preservative for 24 h. To facilitate examination, toilet paper must be disposed of separately

WHEN TO REFER

- If confirmation of the diagnosis is needed or if symptoms are progressive despite therapy
- If there is difficulty distinguishing tapeworm-induced B_{12} deficiency from pernicious anemia

EVIDENCE

WEB SITE

- Centers for Disease Control and Prevention
  - http://www.cdc.gov/ncidod/dpd/parasites/taenia/default.htm

INFORMATION FOR PATIENTS

- National Institutes of Health
  - http://www.nlm.nih.gov/medlineplus/ency/article/001375.htm

REFERENCE

- Hoberg EP: Taenia tapeworms: their biology, evolution and socioeconomic significance. Microbes Infect 2002;4:859. [PMID: 12270733]

Tapeworm Infection, Pork

KEY FEATURES

ESSENTIALS OF DIAGNOSIS

- Generally asymptomatic
- Can cause nonspecific gastrointestinal symptoms of nausea, diarrhea, and pain

GENERAL CONSIDERATIONS

- Six tapeworms infect humans frequently
- The large tapeworms are *Taenia saginata* (the beef tapeworm, up to 25 m in length), *Taenia solium* (the pork tapeworm, 7 m), and *Diphyllobothrium latum* (the fish tapeworm, 10 m in length)
- A fourth large tapeworm, *T asiatica*, recently differentiated by DNA methods, has been found in China, the Koreas, Indonesia, and Southeast Asia. Although acquired by humans by ingestion of pig viscera, it apparently does not cause cysticercosis
- The small tapeworms are *Hymenolepis nana* (the dwarf tapeworm, 25–40 mm), *Hymenolepis diminuta* (the rodent tapeworm, 20–60 cm), and *Dipylidium caninum* (the dog tapeworm, 10–70 cm)
- Humans are the only definitive host of *T solium*
- An adult tapeworm consists of a head (scolex), a neck, and a chain of individual segments (proglottids) in which eggs form in mature segments
- Gravid segments of *T solium* in the human intestine detach themselves from the chain and are passed in feces to soil. When pigs ingest human feces containing proglottids and eggs, the eggs hatch to release embryos that encyst in muscle as cysticerci. Humans become infected when they eat undercooked pork containing viable *C cellulosae*. In the human intestines, the *Cysticercus* develops into an adult worm
- Humans are the intermediate host when they become infected with the larval (*Cysticercus*) stage by accidentally ingesting eggs in human feces; the eggs are immediately infectious (see *Cysticercosis*)
- Transmission of eggs may occur as a result of autoinfection (hand to mouth), direct person-to-person transfer, ingestion of food or drink contaminated by eggs, or (rarely) regurgitation of proglottids into the stomach

DEMOGRAPHICS

- The pork tapeworm is particularly prevalent in Mexico, Latin America, the Iberian Peninsula, the Slavic countries, Africa, Southeast Asia, India, and China
- In the United States and Canada, human infection is rare, usually encountered in persons infected abroad; cysticercosis in hogs is uncommon

CLINICAL FINDINGS

SYMPTOMS AND SIGNS

- Large tapeworms are generally asymptomatic
- Occasionally, vague gastrointestinal symptoms (eg, nausea, diarrhea, abdominal pain) and systemic symptoms (eg, fatigue, hunger, dizziness) have been attributed to the infections
- Vomiting of proglottid segments or obstruction of the bile duct, pancreatic duct, or appendix is rare

DIFFERENTIAL DIAGNOSIS

- Beef, fish, dwarf, rodent, and dog tapeworm
- Chronic fatigue syndrome
- Chronic hepatitis
- Irritable bowel syndrome
- Amebiasis
- Ascariasis
- Enterobiasis (pinworm, mostly children)
- Hookworm disease
- Strongyloidiasis
- Celiac sprue or tropical sprue
- Pernicious anemia (*D latum*)

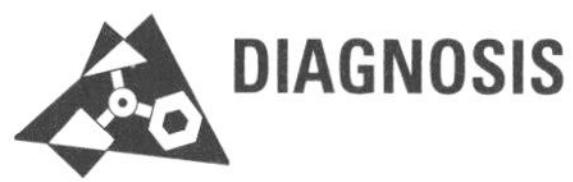

DIAGNOSIS

LABORATORY TESTS

- Infection is often discovered by the patient finding segments in stool, clothing, or bedding
- To determine the species, proglottid segments are either flattened between glass slides and examined microscopically for anatomic detail or differentiated by enzyme electrophoresis of glucose phosphate isomerase
- Serological tests are not available

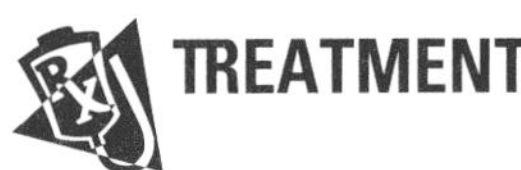

TREATMENT

MEDICATIONS

- Praziquantel in a single dose of 10 mg PO/kg achieves cure rates of about 99%. At this dose, side effects are minimal
- With a single dose of four tablets (2 g) of niclosamide (not available in the United States), cure rates of over 90% can be anticipated. The drug is given in the morning before the patient has eaten. The tablets *must be chewed thoroughly* and swallowed with water. Eating may be resumed in 2 h. The drug usually produces no side effects
- Neither drug kills eggs released from disintegrating segments; therefore, to avoid the theoretical possibility of cysticercosis from hatching eggs, give a moderate purgative 2–3 h after treatment to rapidly eliminate segments and eggs from the bowel. Instruct the patient about the need after defecation for careful washing of the hands and peranal area and for careful disposal of feces for 4 days after therapy
- A pretreatment purge is not used for either drug

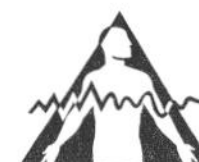

OUTCOME

FOLLOW-UP

- A disintegrating worm is usually passed within 24–48 h of treatment. Since efforts are not generally made to recover and identify the scolex, cure can be presumed only if regenerated segments have not reappeared 3–5 months later
- If it is preferred that parasitic cure be established immediately, the head (scolex) must be found in posttreatment stools; a laxative is given 2 h after treatment, and stools must be collected in a preservative for 24 h. To facilitate examination, toilet paper must be disposed of separately

COMPLICATIONS

- Cysticercosis occurs when humans are infected with the larval (*Cysticercus*) stage by accidentally ingesting eggs in human feces

WHEN TO REFER

- For persistent disease despite appropriate therapy

PREVENTION

- *C cellulosae* is killed by cooking at 65°C or freezing at –20°C for 12 h. Pickling is not adequate
- Because the prognosis is often poor in cerebral cysticercosis, *T solium* infections must be immediately eradicated

EVIDENCE

WEB SITE

- CDC—Division of Parasitic Diseases
  - http://www.cdc.gov/ncidod/dpd/parasites/taenia/default.htm

INFORMATION FOR PATIENTS

- Centers for Disease Control and Prevention
  - http://www.dpd.cdc.gov/dpdx/HTML/Taeniasis.htm
- National Institutes of Health
  - http://www.nlm.nih.gov/medlineplus/ency/article/001391.htm

REFERENCE

- Hoberg EP: Taenia tapeworms: their biology, evolution and socioeconomic significance. Microbes Infect 2002;4:859. [PMID: 12270733]

Testicular Cancer

Tardive Dyskinesia p. 1158

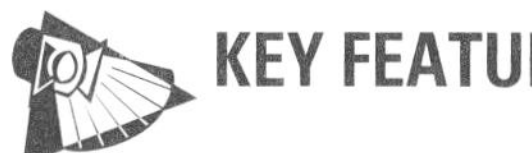

KEY FEATURES

ESSENTIALS OF DIAGNOSIS

- Most common neoplasm in men aged 20–35
- Typical presentation as a patient-identified painless nodule
- Orchiectomy necessary for diagnosis

GENERAL CONSIDERATIONS

- Rare, 2–3 new cases per 100,000 males in the United States each year
- 90–95% of all primary testicular tumors are germ cell tumors (seminoma and nonseminoma); remainder are nongerminal neoplasms (Leydig cell, Sertoli cell, gonadoblastoma)
- Lifetime probability of developing testicular cancer is 0.2% for an American white male
- Slightly more common on the right than on the left, bilateral in 1–2%
- Cause unknown
- History of unilateral or bilateral cryptorchism
- Risk of development of malignancy is highest for an intra-abdominal testis (1:20) and lower for an inguinal testis (1:80)
- Orchiopexy does not alter the malignant potential of the cryptorchid testis; it does facilitate examination and tumor detection
- 5–10% of these tumors occur in the contralateral, normally descended testis

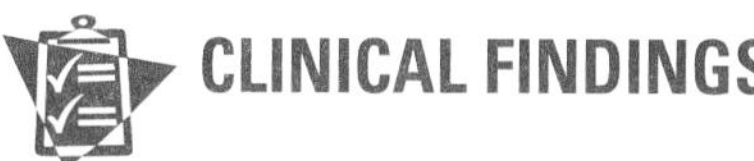

CLINICAL FINDINGS

SYMPTOMS AND SIGNS

- Most common symptom: painless enlargement of the testis
- Sensation of heaviness
- Acute testicular pain from intratesticular hemorrhage in ~10%
- Symptoms relating to metastatic disease, such as back pain (retroperitoneal metastases), cough (pulmonary metastases), or lower extremity edema (vena cava obstruction), in 10%
- Asymptomatic at presentation in 10%
- Physical examination: testicular mass or diffuse enlargement of the testis in the majority of cases
- Secondary hydroceles in 5–10%
- Supraclavicular adenopathy
- Retroperitoneal mass
- Gynecomastia in 5% of germ cell tumors

DIFFERENTIAL DIAGNOSIS

- Epidermoid cyst

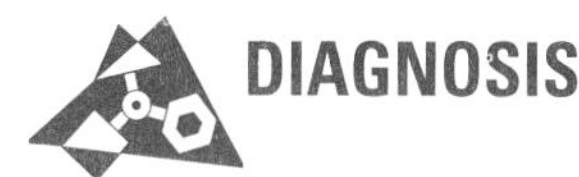

DIAGNOSIS

LABORATORY TESTS

- Human chorionic gonadotropin, α-fetoprotein, and lactate dehydrogenase
- Liver function tests

IMAGING STUDIES

- Scrotal ultrasound
- CT scanning of abdomen and pelvis

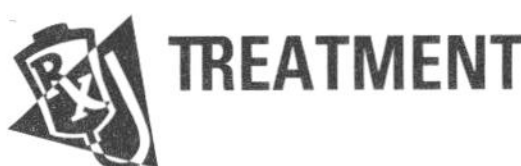

TREATMENT

SURGERY

- Radical orchiectomy by inguinal exploration with early vascular control of the spermatic cord structures
- Scrotal approaches and open testicular biopsies should be avoided

Seminomas

- Stage I and IIa (retroperitoneal disease < 10 cm in diameter) seminomas treated by radical orchiectomy and retroperitoneal irradiation have 5-year disease-free survival rates of 98% and 92–94%, respectively
- Stage IIb (> 10 cm retroperitoneal involvement) and stage III seminomas are treated with primary chemotherapy (etoposide and cisplatin or cisplatin, etoposide, and bleomycin)
- Among stage III patients, 95% will attain a complete response following orchiectomy and chemotherapy

Nonseminomas

- Up to 75% of stage A nonseminomas are cured by orchiectomy alone
- Modified retroperitoneal lymph node dissections have been designed to preserve the sympathetic innervation for ejaculation
- Selected patients who are reliable may be offered surveillance if:
  - Tumor is confined within the tunica albuginea
  - Tumor does not demonstrate vascular invasion
  - Tumor markers normalize after orchiectomy
  - Radiographic imaging (chest x-ray and CT) shows no evidence of disease
- Surveillance is done monthly for the first 2 years and bimonthly in year 3
  - Tumor markers at each visit
  - Chest x-ray and CT every 3–4 months
  - Majority of relapses occur within the first 8–10 months
  - With rare exceptions, patients who relapse can be cured by chemotherapy or surgery
  - The 5-year disease-free survival rate for stage A is 96% to 100%; for low-volume stage B disease, it is 90%
- Patients with bulky retroperitoneal disease (> 3 cm nodes) or metastases are treated with primary cisplatin-based combination chemotherapy following orchiectomy (etoposide and cisplatin or cisplatin, etoposide, and bleomycin)
- For a residual mass > 3 cm, retroperitoneal lymph node resection is mandatory
- If tumor markers fail to normalize following primary chemotherapy, salvage chemotherapy is required (cisplatin, etoposide, bleomycin, ifosfamide)

OUTCOME

PROGNOSIS

- Patients with bulky retroperitoneal or disseminated disease treated with primary chemotherapy followed by surgery have a 5-year disease-free survival rate of 55–80%

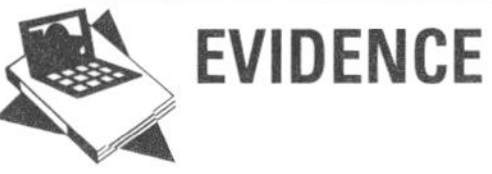

EVIDENCE

PRACTICE GUIDELINES

- Laguna MP et al: EAU guidelines on testicular cancer. Eur Urol 2001;40:102. [PMID: 11528185]
- Segal R et al: Surveillance programs for early stage non-seminomatous testicular cancer: a practice guideline. Can J Urol 2001;8:1184. [PMID: 11268306]

WEB SITES

- American Cancer Society—What is testicular cancer?
  - http://www.cancer.org/docroot/cri/content/cri_2_4_1x_what_is_testicular_cancer_41.asp?sitearea=cri
- National Cancer Institute—questions and answers about testicular cancer
  - http://cis.nci.nih.gov/fact/6_34.htm
- Testicular Cancer Resource Center
  - http://tcrc.acor.org/

INFORMATION FOR PATIENTS

- Mayo Clinic—Testicular cancer
  - http://www.mayoclinic.com/invoke.cfm?objectid=91B1CB36-2B25-4B93-8FB60CFCAC19B62D
- MedlinePlus—Testicular cancer
  - http://www.nlm.nih.gov/medlineplus/ency/article/001288.htm
- National Cancer Institute
  - http://cis.nci.nih.gov/fact/6_34.htm

REFERENCES

- Biggs ML et al: Differences in testis cancer survival by race and ethnicity: a population-based study, 1973–1999 (United States). Cancer Causes Control 2004;15:437. [PMID: 15286463]
- Bromen K et al: Testicular, other genital, and breast cancers in first-degree relatives of testicular cancer patients and controls. Cancer Epidemiol Biomarkers Prev 2004;13:1316. [PMID: 15298952]
- Oosterhof GO et al: Testicular tumours (nonseminomatous). BJU Int 2004;94:1196. [PMID: 15613163]

Author(s)

Marshall L. Stoller, MD

Peter R. Carroll, MD

Tetanus

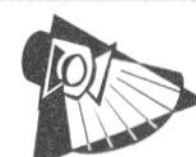

KEY FEATURES

ESSENTIALS OF DIAGNOSIS

- History of wound and possible contamination
- Jaw stiffness followed by spasms of jaw muscles (trismus)
- Stiffness of the neck and other muscles, dysphagia, irritability, hyperreflexia
- Finally, painful convulsions precipitated by minimal stimuli

GENERAL CONSIDERATIONS

- Caused by the neurotoxin tetanospasmin elaborated by *Clostridium tetani*
- Spores of this organism are ubiquitous in soil. When introduced into a wound, spores may germinate
- Tetanospasmin interferes with neurotransmission at spinal synapses of inhibitory neurons
- Minor stimuli result in uncontrolled spasms, and reflexes are exaggerated
- Most cases occur in unvaccinated individuals
- Persons at risk are the elderly, migrant workers, newborns, and injection drug users, who may acquire the disease through subcutaneous injections

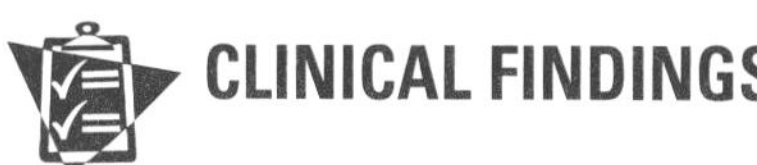

CLINICAL FINDINGS

SYMPTOMS AND SIGNS

- The first symptom may be pain and tingling at the site of inoculation, followed by spasticity of the muscles nearby
- Stiffness of the jaw, neck stiffness, dysphagia, and irritability are other early signs
- Hyperreflexia develops later, with spasms of the jaw muscles (trismus) or facial muscles and rigidity and spasm of the muscles of the abdomen, neck, and back
- Painful tonic convulsions precipitated by minor stimuli are common
- Spasms of the glottis and respiratory muscles may cause acute asphyxia
- The patient is awake and alert throughout the illness. The sensory examination is normal. The temperature is normal or only slightly elevated
- Urinary retention and constipation may result from spasm of the sphincters
- Respiratory arrest and cardiac failure are late, life-threatening events

DIFFERENTIAL DIAGNOSIS

- Meningitis
- Rabies
- Tetany due to hypocalcemia
- Strychnine poisoning
- Neuroleptic malignant syndrome
- Trismus due to peritonsillar abscess

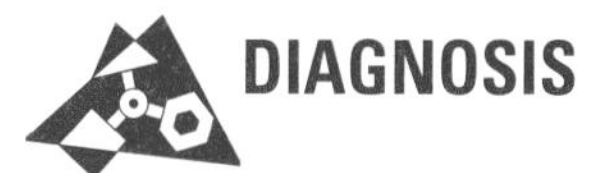

DIAGNOSIS

LABORATORY TESTS

- The diagnosis is made clinically

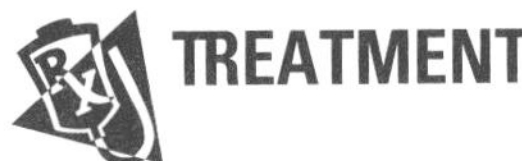

TREATMENT

MEDICATIONS

- Passive immunization should be used in nonimmunized individuals and those whose immunization status is uncertain whenever a wound is contaminated or likely to have devitalized tissue
- Tetanus immune globulin, 250 units, is given intramuscularly. Active immunization with tetanus toxoid should be started concurrently
- Table 133 provides a guide to prophylactic management
- Penicillin, 20 million units daily, is given to all patients—even those with mild illness—to eradicate toxin-producing organisms

THERAPEUTIC PROCEDURES

- Minimal stimuli can provoke spasms, so the patient should be placed at bed rest and monitored under the quietest conditions possible
- Sedation, paralysis with curare-like agents, and mechanical ventilation are often necessary to control tetanic spasms

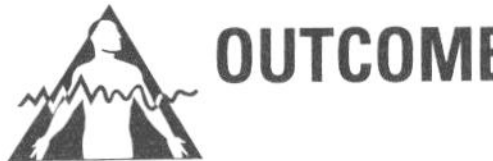

OUTCOME

COMPLICATIONS

- Respiratory arrest
- Pneumonia

PROGNOSIS

- High mortality rates are associated with a short incubation period, early onset of convulsions, and delay in treatment
- Contaminated lesions about the head and face are more dangerous than wounds on other parts of the body
- The overall mortality rate is about 40%, but this can be reduced with ventilator management

WHEN TO REFER

- For confirmation of the disease, refer to an infectious disease specialist
- For the specialized treatment of the neuromuscular symptoms, refer to a neurologist

WHEN TO ADMIT

- Any patient in whom there is clinical suspicion of the disease
- Intensive care unit may be needed

PREVENTION

- Tetanus is completely preventable by active immunization
- For primary immunization of adults, tetanus toxoid is administered as two doses 4–6 weeks apart, with a third dose 6–12 months later. Booster doses are given every 10 years or at the time of major injury if it occurs more than 5 years after a dose (Table 132)

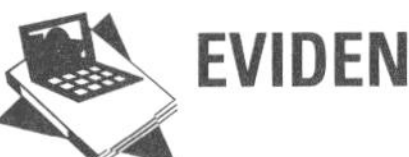

EVIDENCE

PRACTICE GUIDELINES

- National Guideline Clearinghouse: Immunization Guidelines
  - http://www.guideline.gov/summary/summary.aspx?doc_id=3180

WEB SITES

- CDC—National Immunization Program
  - http://www.cdc.gov/nip/publications/pink/tetanus.pdf
- Karolinska Institute—Directory of Bacterial Infections and Mycoses
  - http://www.mic.ki.se/Diseases/C01.html

INFORMATION FOR PATIENTS

- JAMA patient page: Immunizations. JAMA 1999;282:102.
- Mayo Clinic
  - http://www.mayoclinic.com/invoke.cfm?id=DS00227
- University of Utah Health Sciences Center
  - http://www.nfid.org/factsheets/tetanusadult.html

REFERENCES

- Attygalle D et al: New trends in the management of tetanus. Expert Rev Anti Infect Ther 2004;2:73. [PMID: 15482173]
- Hsu SS et al: Tetanus in the emergency department: a current review. J Emerg Med 2001;20:357. [PMID: 11348815]

Author(s)

Henry F. Chambers, MD

Thalassemia

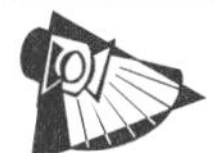

KEY FEATURES

ESSENTIALS OF DIAGNOSIS

- Microcytosis out of proportion to degree of anemia
- Positive family history or lifelong personal history of microcytic anemia
- Abnormal red blood cell (RBC) morphology with microcytes, acanthocytes, and target cells
- In β-thalassemia, elevated levels of hemoglobin A2 or F

GENERAL CONSIDERATIONS

- Hereditary disorders characterized by reduction in synthesis of globin chains (α or β), causing reduced hemoglobin synthesis and eventually hypochromic microcytic anemia
- Normal adult hemoglobin primarily hemoglobin A, a tetramer of two α-chains and two β-chains ($\alpha_2\beta_2$)
- α-Thalassemia syndromes determined by number of functional α-globin genes
  - Normal (four α-globin genes)
  - Silent carrier (three α-globin genes, normal hematocrit)
  - α-Thalassemia minor or trait [two α-globin genes, hematocrit 32–40%, mean cell volume (MCV) 60–75]
  - Hemoglobin H disease (one α-globin gene, hematocrit 22–32%, MCV 60-70)
  - Hydrops fetalis (0 α-globin genes)
- β-Thalassemia: Reduced β-globin chain synthesis results in relative increase in percentages of hemoglobins A2 and F compared with hemoglobin A, because β-like globins (γ and δ) substitute for missing β-chains
- With reduced β-chains, excess α-chains precipitate, causing hemolysis; bone marrow becomes hyperplastic, resulting in bony deformities, osteopenia, and pathological fractures

DEMOGRAPHICS

- α-Thalassemia occurs primarily in persons from southeast Asia and China and, less commonly, in blacks
- β-Thalassemia affects persons of Mediterranean origin (Italian, Greek) and to lesser extent Chinese, other Asians, and blacks

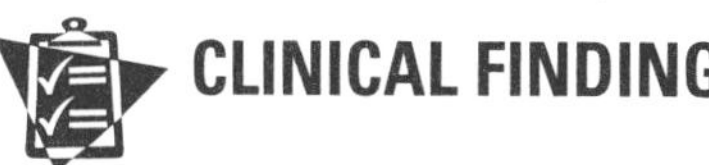

CLINICAL FINDINGS

SYMPTOMS AND SIGNS

- α-Thalassemia silent carriers: asymptomatic
- α-Thalassemia trait: clinically normal with mild microcytic anemia
- Hemoglobin H disease: chronic hemolytic anemia of variable severity, pallor, and splenomegaly
- Hydrops fetalis: fetal death
- Heterozygous for β-thalassemia (thalassemia minor): mild microcytic anemia
- Homozygous for mild β-thalassemia (thalassemia intermedia): chronic hemolytic anemia
- Homozygous for major β-thalassemia (thalassemia major): severe anemia requiring transfusion; growth failure; bony deformities (abnormal facial structure, pathological fractures); hepatosplenomegaly and jaundice

DIFFERENTIAL DIAGNOSIS

- Iron deficiency anemia (thalassemia has lower MCV, normal iron studies, more normal RBC count, more abnormal peripheral blood smear at modest levels of anemia)
- Other hemoglobinopathy (eg, sickle thalassemia, hemoglobin C disorders)
- Sideroblastic anemia
- Anemia of chronic disease

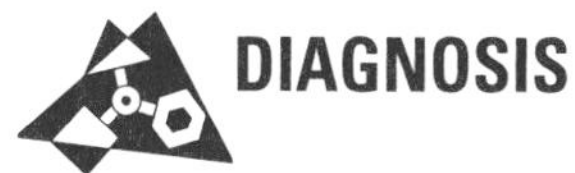

DIAGNOSIS

LABORATORY TESTS

α-Thalassemia trait

- Mild anemia (hematocrit 28-40%) with strikingly low MCV (60–75 fL)
- RBC count normal or increased
- Peripheral blood smear mildly abnormal: microcytes, hypochromia, occasional target cells, acanthocytes
- Reticulocyte count and iron studies normal
- Hemoglobin electrophoresis: no increase in percentage of hemoglobins A2 or F and no hemoglobin H (thus usually a diagnosis of exclusion)

Hemoglobin H disease

- Variably severe hemolytic anemia (hematocrit 22–32%) with remarkably low MCV (60–70 fL)
- Peripheral blood smear markedly abnormal: hypochromia, microcytosis, target cells, poikilocytosis
- Reticulocyte count elevated
- Hemoglobin electrophoresis: shows hemoglobin H comprises 10–40% of the hemoglobin

β-Thalassemia minor

- Mild anemia (hematocrit 28–40%) with MCV 55–75 fL
- RBC count normal or increased
- Peripheral blood smear mildly abnormal: hypochromia, microcytosis, target cells, basophilic stippling
- Reticulocyte count normal or slightly elevated
- Hemoglobin electrophoresis: elevated hemoglobin A2 to 4–8% and occasionally elevated hemoglobin F to 1–5%

β-Thalassemia major

- Severe anemia (hematocrit sometimes < 10% without transfusion)
- Peripheral blood smear bizarre: severe poikilocytosis, hypochromia, microcytosis, target cells, basophilic stippling, nucleated RBCs
- Hemoglobin electrophoresis: little or no hemoglobin A, variable amounts of hemoglobin A2, and major hemoglobin present is hemoglobin F

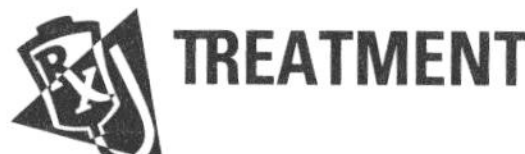

TREATMENT

MEDICATIONS

- Mild thalassemias (α-thalassemia trait or β-thalassemia minor) usually require no treatment and should be identified to avoid repeated evaluations for iron deficiency and inappropriate administration of supplemental iron
- α-Thalassemia trait and thalassemia intermedia may require transfusion during infection or other stress
- Hemoglobin H disease: folate supplementation; avoid medicinal iron and oxidative drugs such as sulfonamides
- Severe thalassemia: regular transfusions and folate supplementation

SURGERY

- Splenectomy indicated if hypersplenism causes marked increase in transfusion requirement

THERAPEUTIC PROCEDURES

- Prenatal diagnosis and genetic counseling should be offered
- Blood transfusions as above
- Allogeneic bone marrow transplantation for β-thalassemia major in children who have not yet experienced iron overload and chronic organ toxicity

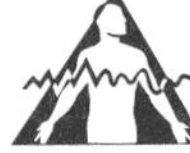

OUTCOME

COMPLICATIONS

- Bony deformities, osteopenia, and pathological fractures in β-thalassemia
- Complications of blood transfusions as below
- Splenomegaly may result from chronic hemolysis

PROGNOSIS

- Mild thalassemia (α-thalassemia trait or β-thalassemia minor): normal life expectancy
- Thalassemia intermedia: may develop transfusional iron overload; patients survive into adulthood but with hepatosplenomegaly and bony deformities
- β-Thalassemia major
  - Clinical course modified significantly by transfusion therapy, but transfusional iron overload causes heart failure, cirrhosis, and endocrinopathies, usually after > 100 units of transfusion
  - Death from cardiac failure usually occurs between ages 20 and 30
  - Long-term survival is > 80% in cases undergoing allogeneic bone marrow transplantation

PREVENTION

- Deferoxamine routinely given as iron-chelating agent to avoid or postpone hemosiderosis in transfusion-dependent patients; low-iron diet may also help

EVIDENCE

WEB SITES

- Children's Hospital Oakland: Thalassemia
  - http://www.thalassemia.com
- Cooley's Anemia Foundation
  - http://www.cooleysanemia.org
- Thalassemia Foundation of Canada: FAQ
  - http://www.thalassemia.ca/faq.html

INFORMATION FOR PATIENTS

- MedlinePlus: Thalassemia
  - http://www.nlm.nih.gov/medlineplus/ency/article/000587.htm
- National Heart, Lung, and Blood Institute: Thalassemia
  - http://www.nhlbi.nih.gov/health/dci/Diseases/Thalassemia/Thalassemia_WhatIs.html
- National Human Genome Research Institute: Learning About Thalassemia
  - http://www.genome.gov/page.cfm?pageID=10001221

REFERENCES

- Chaidos A et al: Treatment of beta-thalassemia patients with recombinant human erythropoietin: effect on transfusion requirements and soluble adhesion molecules. Acta Haematol 2004;111:189. [PMID: 15153710]
- Cunningham MJ et al: Complications of beta-thalassemia major in North America. Blood 2004;104:34. [PMID: 14988152]

Author(s)

Charles A. Linker, MD

Theophylline Toxicity p. 1159. Thiamin Deficiency p. 1159.

Thoracic Aortic Aneurysm

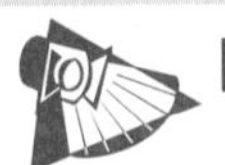

KEY FEATURES

GENERAL CONSIDERATIONS

- Aneurysms of the thoracic aorta account for < 10% of aortic aneurysms
- Causes: medial degeneration, chronic dissection, vasculitis, and collagen-vascular disease (Marfan's syndrome or Ehlers-Danlos syndrome), trauma, syphilis (rare)
- Type 1 extends from the left subclavian artery to the renal arteries, type 2 from the left subclavian artery to the iliac bifurcation, type 3 from the midthoracic to the infrarenal region, and type 4 from the diaphragmatic hiatus to the infrarenal region
- The prevalence of each type is roughly equal, but type 4 aneurysms have the lowest operative mortality (2–5%) and lowest risk of postoperative neurological deficits

CLINICAL FINDINGS

SYMPTOMS AND SIGNS

- Most are asymptomatic and discovered incidentally
- Substernal, back, or neck pain
- Dyspnea, stridor, or a brassy cough from pressure on the trachea
- Dysphagia from pressure on the esophagus
- Hoarseness from pressure on the left recurrent laryngeal nerve
- Neck and arm edema from external compression of the superior vena cava
- Aortic regurgitation murmur with aneurysms of the ascending aorta

DIFFERENTIAL DIAGNOSIS

- Lung neoplasm
- Thymoma
- Cyst
- Substernal goiter

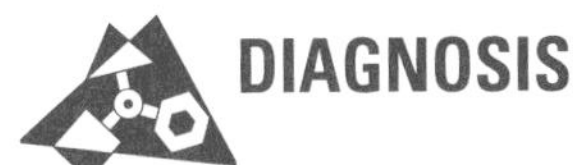

DIAGNOSIS

LABORATORY TESTS

- Preoperative evaluation: electrocardiogram, creatinine, complete blood count, and type and cross-match

IMAGING STUDIES

- CT scan and MRI/MRA
- Aortography: to assess involvement of the arch vessels, coronary arteries, and aortic valve

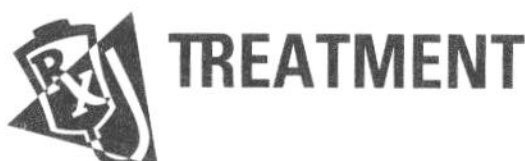

TREATMENT

MEDICATIONS

- Antihypertensives to control blood pressure
- β-Blockers to slow aneurysmal growth

SURGERY

- Indications for surgical treatment: new aortic insufficiency, presence of symptoms, rapid expansion, or size > 5 cm in good-risk surgical candidates
- Open surgical replacement with synthetic graft; sometimes requires left-sided heart bypass

THERAPEUTIC PROCEDURES

- Endovascular repair reduces cardiopulmonary risk, but the location of the aneurysm (proximity to arch vessels or spinal arteries) may preclude endovascular repair
- Endovascular treatment remains experimental

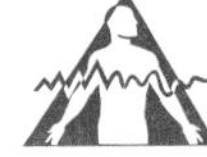

OUTCOME

FOLLOW-UP

- CT scan every 6–8 months

COMPLICATIONS

- Surgical complications
- Pulmonary complications
- Injury to recurrent laryngeal nerve, phrenic nerve, carotid and subclavian arteries
- Spinal cord paraplegia

PROGNOSIS

- Surgical morbidity and mortality are higher than with abdominal aortic aneurysms
- 30-day operative mortality is 8–20% with repair of type 1 and type 2 aneurysms
- 5-year survival for patients with unrepaired thoracic aneurysms > 6 cm is 20–25%

WHEN TO REFER

- Aneurysm diameter > 4.5 cm

WHEN TO ADMIT

- Symptomatic or ruptured aneurysm for elective repair when ≥ 6.0 cm

PREVENTION

- Cardiovascular risk factor assessment and modification
- Smoking cessation

EVIDENCE

PRACTICE GUIDELINES

- Eggebrecht H et al: Interventional management of aortic dissection. Herz 2002;27:539. [PMID: 12378400]

INFORMATION FOR PATIENTS

- Cleveland Clinic: Aneurysm
  - http://www.clevelandclinic.org/health/health-info/docs/3200/3209.asp?index=11143
- Mayo Clinic: Aortic Aneurysm
  - http://www.mayoclinic.com/invoke.cfm?objectid=FE3FE459-7D1E-405F-95E9339CD2E974B8
- MedlinePlus: Thoracic Aortic Aneurysm
  - http://www.nlm.nih.gov/medlineplus/ency/article/001119.htm

REFERENCES

- Chuter TAM et al: Multi-branched stent-graft for type III thoracoabdominal aortic aneurysm. J Vasc Interv Radiol 2001;12:391. [PMID: 11287522]
- Elefteriades JA: Natural history of thoracic aortic aneurysms: indications for surgery, and surgical versus nonsurgical risks. Ann Thorac Surg 2002;74:S1877. [PMID: 12440685]

Author(s)

Louis M. Messina, MD

Thoracic Outlet Syndrome

KEY FEATURES

ESSENTIALS OF DIAGNOSIS

- Subdivided into neurogenic, venous, and arterial types, depending on which structures are compressed in the interscalene triangle or costoclavicular space
- Neurogenic: most common (> 90%), often the most difficult to diagnose and treat; history of whiplash trauma or repetitive upper extremity activity, particularly overhead activity
- Venous: also called Paget-Schroetter syndrome or effort thrombosis; involves external compression of the subclavian vein by the first rib, anterior scalene muscle, clavicle, and costocoracoid ligament; often a history of repetitive upper arm exercises or clavicular fracture
- Arterial: least common; compression of the subclavian artery between the anterior and middle scalene muscles produces subclavian artery aneurysms, which result in digital ischemia caused by atheroemboli; arm claudication less common

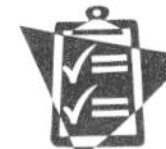

CLINICAL FINDINGS

SYMPTOMS AND SIGNS

Neurogenic

- Supraclavicular and anterior chest wall burning pain
- Segmental pain and paresthesias of the arm often in an ulnar nerve distribution
- Weakness of the intrinsic muscles of the hand
- Thenar or hypothenar muscle wasting (rare)
- Physical examination: supraclavicular tenderness, positive brachial plexus tension testing
- Positive Adson test
- Positive Roos test
- Positive Tinel sign
- Electrophysiological testing usually negative
- Presents as acute unilateral arm edema, axillary fullness, hand cyanosis, and enlarged shoulder and chest wall collateral veins
- Positive Wylie-Allen test, arm heaviness/tiredness with activity, digital ischemia or splinter hemorrhage secondary to emboli

DIFFERENTIAL DIAGNOSIS

- Other cause of brachial plexus neuropathy
- Neck disorder, eg, osteoarthritis, herniated disk, tumor
- Shoulder osteoarthritis
- Reflex sympathetic dystrophy
- Carpal tunnel syndrome

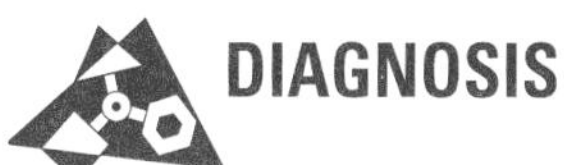

DIAGNOSIS

LABORATORY TESTS

- With thrombosis of vein, obtain plasma levels of antithrombin III, factor V Leiden, anticardiolipin antibody, fibrinogen, proteins C and S, lupus anticoagulant, homocysteine and prothrombin gene mutation

IMAGING STUDIES

- Neurogenic: chest film for cervical rib
- Venous: positional venography
- Arterial: angiography

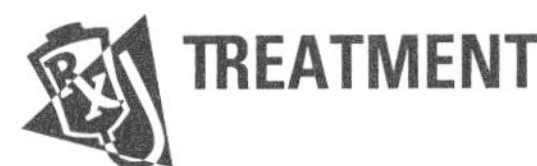

TREATMENT

MEDICATIONS

- Analgesics
- Muscle relaxants

SURGERY

Neurogenic

- Surgical resection of the hypertrophied anterior and middle scalene muscles, brachial plexus neurolysis, and resection of bony abnormalities in severe refractory cases
- Anterior scalene and first rib resection with venolysis; if axillary-subclavian vein thrombosis, preoperative thrombolysis followed immediately by surgery with intraoperative angioplasty of any residual venous stenosis, or surgical thrombectomy
- Removal of anterior and middle scalene muscles, resection of the aneurysm with polytetrafluoroethylene interposition graft

THERAPEUTIC PROCEDURES

Neurogenic

- Physical therapy: Edgelow Neurovascular Entrapment Self-Treatment (ENVEST) program
- Transcutaneous electrical nerve stimulation

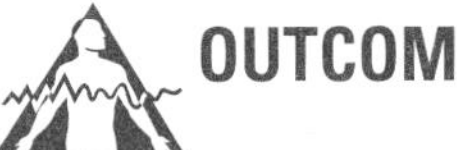

OUTCOME

COMPLICATIONS

- Loss of function
- Chronic venous stasis disease
- Ischemic ulceration

PROGNOSIS

- Neurogenic: after surgery symptoms return within 1 year in as many as 25% of patients
- Venous: prognosis is excellent with appropriate treatment

WHEN TO REFER

- Any suspected arterial or venous thoracic outlet syndrome
- Neurogenic thoracic outlet syndrome refractory to a dedicated course of medical treatment

WHEN TO ADMIT

- Acute venous occlusion
- Digital ischemia

PREVENTION

- Ergonomic workplace

EVIDENCE

PRACTICE GUIDELINES

- National Guideline Clearinghouse: Surgery for Thoracic Outlet Syndrome (TOS)
  - http://www.guideline.gov/summary/summary.aspx?doc_id=4211&nbr=3219&string=thoracic+AND+outlet+AND+syndrome
- Novak CB: Thoracic outlet syndrome. Clin Plast Surg 2003;30:175. [PMID: 12737351]

INFORMATION FOR PATIENTS

- American Academy of Orthopaedic Surgeons: Thoracic Outlet Syndrome
  - http://orthoinfo.aaos.org/fact/thr_report.cfm?Thread_ID=206&topcategory=Shoulder
- Cleveland Clinic: Thoracic Outlet Syndrome
  - http://www.clevelandclinic.org/health/health-info/docs/1300/1355.asp?index=6123
- Mayo Clinic: Thoracic Outlet Syndrome
  - http://www.mayoclinic.com/invoke.cfm?objectid=51E8E5FD-9ACA-4DAA-8DF2586D5F34C061
- MedlinePlus: Thoracic Outlet Syndrome
  - http://www.nlm.nih.gov/medlineplus/ency/article/001434.htm

REFERENCES

- Alexrod DA et al: Outcomes after surgery for thoracic outlet syndrome. J Vasc Surg 2001;33:1220. [PMID: 11389421]
- Pascarelli EF et al: Understanding work-related upper extremity disorders: clinical findings in 485 computer users, musicians, and others. J Occup Rehabil 2001;11:1. [PMID: 11706773]

Author(s)

Louis M. Messina, MD

Thromboangiitis Obliterans (Buerger's Disease)

KEY FEATURES

ESSENTIALS OF DIAGNOSIS

- An episodic and segmental inflammatory and thrombotic process of the peripheral arteries and veins
- Presents with claudication, rest pain
- Linked to tobacco use
- Episodic, with quiescent periods lasting weeks, months, or years

GENERAL CONSIDERATIONS

- Cause is unknown
- History of cold sensitivity or Raynaud's phenomenon
- Characterized by occlusion of distal arteries, producing claudication, rest pain, and tissue necrosis
- Associated with migratory superficial segmental thrombophlebitis; affected vein shows inflammatory infiltrate in the vessel wall, microabscesses, thrombus, or recanalization with perivascular fibrosis
- Clinical course is usually episodic, with acute exacerbations followed by remissions

DEMOGRAPHICS

- Most commonly occurs in men age < 40 who smoke, particularly those of eastern European or Asian background
- < 20% of affected patients are women

CLINICAL FINDINGS

SYMPTOMS AND SIGNS

- Intermittent claudication typically begins in the arch of the foot and progresses to the calf
- Rest pain and diminished sensation from ischemic neuropathy in > 70% of patients
- No pathognomonic signs
- Proximal pulses are normal; distal pulses are diminished or absent
- Affected digits may be pale, cyanotic, or erythematous
- Ulcers, typically located at the nail margins, in 75% of patients
- Allen test positive
- May have concomitant thrombophlebitis

DIFFERENTIAL DIAGNOSIS

- Limb ischemia resulting from emboli or atherosclerotic occlusive disease
- Autoimmune disorders: Raynaud's disease, polyarteritis nodosa, systemic lupus erythematosus, antiphospholipid antibody syndrome, Takayasu's arteritis
- Rare: ergotamine intoxication, cannabis arteritis, hypothenar hammer syndrome

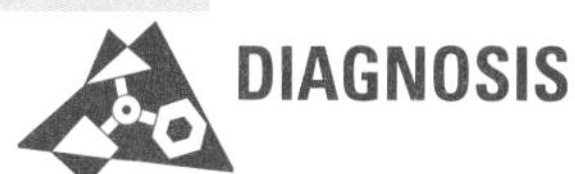

DIAGNOSIS

LABORATORY TESTS

- Obtain complete blood cell count, prothrombin time, partial thromboplastin time, sedimentation rate, antinuclear antibody, lupus anticoagulant, rheumatoid factor, anticentromere antibody, and antiphospholipid antibody

IMAGING STUDIES

- Angiography: involvement of distal arteries with sparing of proximal arteries, segmental appearance with skip areas, no vascular calcification, and extensive collateralization via tortuous "corkscrew" vessels
- Peripheral ultrasonography or angiography and echocardiography are done to exclude an embolic source

DIAGNOSTIC PROCEDURES

- Diagnosed by biopsy of affected vein

Thromboangiitis Obliterans (Buerger's Disease)

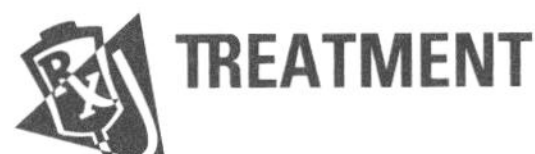

TREATMENT

MEDICATIONS

- Nonsteroidal antiinflammatory medications and opioids for pain control
- Aspirin, 325 mg PO QD, or other antiplatelet agents
- Calcium channel blockers
- Iloprost and vascular endothelial growth factor (VEGF) are investigational agents

SURGERY

- Sympathectomy is indicated for relief of intractable rest pain and healing of refractory ulcers, often in conjunction with digital amputation
- Amputation is reserved for patients with wet gangrene or severe rest pain

THERAPEUTIC PROCEDURES

- Smoking cessation, elimination of chewing tobacco and marijuana, and avoidance of nicotine replacement and exposure to second-hand smoke
- Local wound care: limited débridement, appropriate dressings, and IV antibiotics for cellulitis
- Moisturization of nonulcerated skin
- Lamb's wool between the toes, heel protectors, sheepskin-lined boots (Rooke boots)
- Supplemental oxygen by nasal cannula, hyperbaric oxygen

OUTCOME

COMPLICATIONS

- Gangrene
- Cellulitis
- Amputation/limb loss

PROGNOSIS

- Prognosis dependent on smoking cessation
- More than 90% of patients who quit smoking avoid amputation

WHEN TO REFER

- Refer patients with symptoms and signs of Buerger's disease to a vascular surgeon

WHEN TO ADMIT

- Limb-threatening ischemia

PREVENTION

- Tobacco cessation and nicotine avoidance

EVIDENCE

WEB SITE

- Johns Hopkins Vasculitis Center: Types of Vasculitis: Buerger's disease
  - http://vasculitis.med.jhu.edu/typesof/buergers.html

INFORMATION FOR PATIENTS

- Mayo Clinic: Buerger's Disease
  - http://www.mayoclinic.com/invoke.cfm?objectid=91D74792-B1CA-4B8C-97A6F3CCBAFA655F
- MedlinePlus: Thromboangiitis Obliterans
  - http://www.nlm.nih.gov/medlineplus/ency/article/000172.htm
- Merck Manual of Diagnosis and Therapy: Thromboangiitis Obliterans
  - http://www.merck.com/pubs/mmanual/section16/chapter212/212c.htm

REFERENCE

- Olin JW: Thromboangiitis obliterans (Buerger's disease). N Engl J Med 2000;343:864. [PMID: 10995867]

Author(s)

Louis M. Messina, MD

Thrombophlebitis, Superficial Veins

KEY FEATURES

ESSENTIALS OF DIAGNOSIS

- Induration, redness, and tenderness along a superficial vein
- Often a history of recent IV line or trauma
- No significant swelling of the extremity

GENERAL CONSIDERATIONS

- May occur spontaneously in patients with varicose veins, in pregnant or postpartum women, or with thromboangiitis obliterans or Behçet's disease
- May occur after trauma or after IV infusion
- Migratory superficial thrombophlebitis may occur in abdominal cancer such as carcinoma of the pancreas (Trousseau's syndrome)
- Long saphenous vein and its tributaries are most often involved
- Superficial thrombophlebitis is associated with occult deep vein thrombosis in ~20% of cases
- Pulmonary emboli are rare unless there is extension of clot into the deep veins

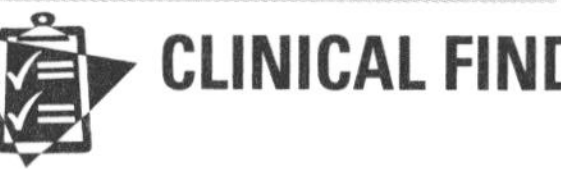

CLINICAL FINDINGS

SYMPTOMS AND SIGNS

- Dull pain in the region of the involved vein
- Induration, redness, and tenderness
- Dilated, thrombosed superficial veins
- No edema or deep calf tenderness
- Chills and high temperature suggest septic or suppurative phlebitis

DIFFERENTIAL DIAGNOSIS

- Deep vein thrombosis
- Cellulitis
- Lymphangitis
- Erythema nodosum
- Erythema induratum (associated with tuberculosis)
- Panniculitis

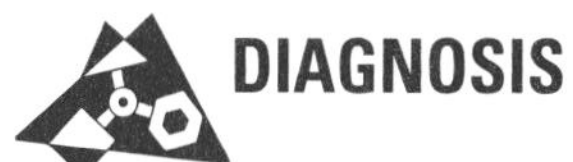

DIAGNOSIS

LABORATORY TESTS

- Blood culture: in septic thrombophlebitis, the causative organism is often *Staphylococcus* or a gram-negative rod
- Complete blood cell count

IMAGING STUDIES

- Ultrasonogram to rule out deep venous thrombosis and assess extent of superficial thrombosis

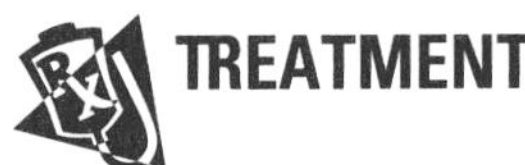

TREATMENT

MEDICATIONS

- Nonsteroidal antiinflammatory drugs
- Septic thrombophlebitis requires IV antibiotics for 7- to 10-day course
- Anticoagulation for rapidly progressing disease or extension into the deep system

SURGERY

- Excision of the involved vein indicated for symptoms that persist more than 2 weeks or for recurrent phlebitis
- Immediate excision of an infected vein if the patient becomes septic

THERAPEUTIC PROCEDURES

- Ambulation
- Warm compresses
- Limb elevation

OUTCOME

PROGNOSIS

- Course is generally benign and brief
- Prognosis depends on the underlying pathological process
- Phlebitis of a saphenous vein occasionally extends to the deep veins, which may cause chronic venous insufficiency, limb edema, and pulmonary emboli

WHEN TO REFER

- Suspected deep venous thrombosis
- Septic thrombophlebitis
- Recurrent thrombophlebitis
- Thrombophlebitis in suprageniculate greater saphenous vein

WHEN TO ADMIT

- Septic thrombophlebitis

EVIDENCE

PRACTICE GUIDELINES

- Kalodiki E et al: Superficial thrombophlebitis and low-molecular-weight heparins. Angiology 2002;53:659. [PMID: 12463618]
- Institute for Clinical Systems Improvement: Venous Thromboembolism, 2002
  - http://www.icsi.org/knowledge/detail.asp?catID=29&itemID=202

INFORMATION FOR PATIENTS

- Mayo Clinic: Thrombophlebitis
  - http://www.mayoclinic.com/invoke.cfm?id=DS00223
- MedlinePlus: Superficial Thrombophlebitis
  - http://www.nlm.nih.gov/medlineplus/ency/article/000199.htm
- Merck Manual of Medical Information: Superficial Thrombophlebitis
  - http://www.merck.com/mmhe/sec03/ch036/ch036c.html

REFERENCE

- Belcaro G et al: Superficial thrombophlebitis of the legs: a randomized, controlled, follow-up study. Angiology 1999;50:523. [PMID: 10431991]

Author(s)

Louis M. Messina, MD

Thrombotic Thrombocytopenic Purpura

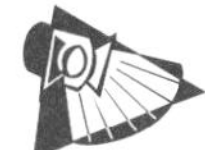

KEY FEATURES

ESSENTIALS OF DIAGNOSIS

- Thrombocytopenia
- Microangiopathic hemolytic anemia
- Normal coagulation tests
- Elevated serum lactate dehydrogenase (LDH)

GENERAL CONSIDERATIONS

- Uncommon syndrome characterized by microangiopathic hemolytic anemia, thrombocytopenia, noninfectious fever, neurological disorders, and renal insufficiency
- Markedly elevated serum LDH
- Pathogenesis appears to be deficiency of a von Willebrand factor–cleaving protease, in some cases resulting from antibody against the protease
- Occasionally precipitated by estrogen use, pregnancy, drugs, or infections (eg, HIV)

DEMOGRAPHICS

- Occurs primarily in young adults between ages 20 and 50
- Slight female predominance

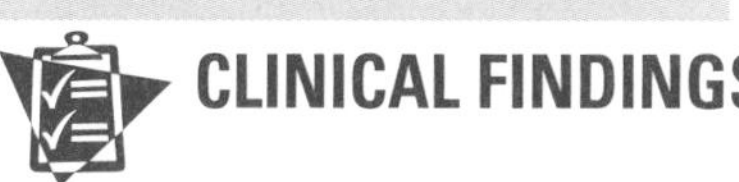

CLINICAL FINDINGS

SYMPTOMS AND SIGNS

- Fever may be present
- Pallor and symptoms of anemia
- Purpura, petechiae, and bleeding
- Neurological symptoms and signs, including headache, confusion, aphasia, and alterations in consciousness from lethargy to coma, may wax and wane over minutes; hemiparesis and seizures with more advanced disease
- Abdominal pain and tenderness resulting from pancreatitis

DIFFERENTIAL DIAGNOSIS

- Disseminated intravascular coagulation
- Hemolytic uremic syndrome
- Preeclampsia–eclampsia
- Meningitis
- Evan's syndrome (idiopathic thrombocytopenic purpura with autoimmune hemolytic anemia)

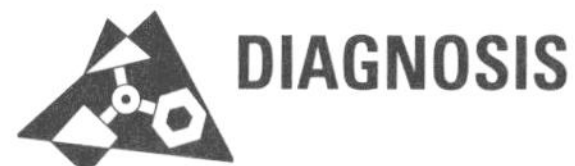

DIAGNOSIS

LABORATORY TESTS

- Peripheral smear shows microangiopathic changes with fragmented red blood cells (RBCs) (schistocytes, helmet cells, triangle forms)
- Anemia is universal and may be marked
- Usually marked reticulocytosis and occasional circulating nucleated RBCs
- Thrombocytopenia is invariably present and may be severe
- Increased indirect bilirubin and occasionally hemoglobinemia and hemoglobinuria from hemolysis; methemalbuminemia may impart brown color to plasma
- LDH markedly elevated in proportion to severity of hemolysis; Coombs test negative
- Coagulation tests (prothrombin time, partial thromboplastin time, fibrinogen) normal unless ischemic tissue damage causes secondary disseminated intravascular coagulation
- Elevated fibrin degradation products may be seen, as in other acutely ill patients
- Renal insufficiency, with abnormal urinalysis

DIAGNOSTIC PROCEDURES

- Pathologically, may see thrombi in capillaries and small arteries, with no evidence of inflammation

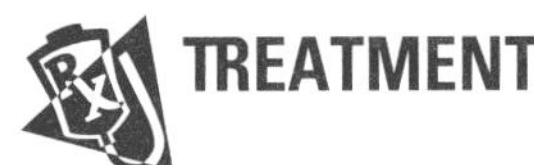

TREATMENT

MEDICATIONS

- Prednisone and antiplatelet agents (aspirin, 325 mg PO TID, and dipyridamole, 75 mg PO TID) have been used in addition to plasmapheresis, but their role is unclear
- Management of refractory patients who do not respond to plasmapheresis or have rapid recurrences is controversial
- Combination of splenectomy, corticosteroids, and dextran used with success
- Immunosuppression (eg, cyclophosphamide) also effective

SURGERY

- Splenectomy may be indicated for refractory disease
- Splenectomy during remission may prevent subsequent relapses

THERAPEUTIC PROCEDURES

- Emergent large-volume plasmapheresis is the treatment of choice for thrombotic thrombocytopenic purpura: 60–80 mL/kg of plasma removed and replaced with fresh-frozen plasma, continued daily until complete remission; optimal duration of plasmapheresis after remission unknown

OUTCOME

PROGNOSIS

- With plasmapheresis, formerly dismal prognosis has dramatically changed; 80–90% now recover completely
- Neurological abnormalities are usually reversed
- Most complete responses are durable, but 20% of cases are chronic and relapsing

EVIDENCE

PRACTICE GUIDELINES

- Allford SL et al: Guidelines on the diagnosis and management of the thrombotic microangiopathic haemolytic anaemias. Br J Haematol 2003;120:556. [PMID: 12588343]

INFORMATION FOR PATIENTS

- MedlinePlus: Thrombotic Thrombocytopenic Purpura
  - http://www.nlm.nih.gov/medlineplus/ency/article/000552.htm

REFERENCES

- Ahmad A et al: Rituximab for treatment of refractory/relapsing thrombotic thrombocytopenic purpura (TTP). Am J Hematol 2004;77:171. [PMID: 15389904]
- Knovich MA et al: Simplified assay for VWF cleaving protease (ADAMTS13) activity and inhibitor in plasma. Am J Hematol 2004;76:286. [PMID: 15224369]
- Zheng XL et al: Effect of plasma exchange on plasma ADAMTS13 metalloprotease activity, inhibitor level, and clinical outcome in patients with idiopathic and nonidiopathic thrombotic thrombocytopenic purpura. Blood 2004;103:4043. [PMID: 14982878]

Author(s)

Charles A. Linker, MD

Thyroid Cancer

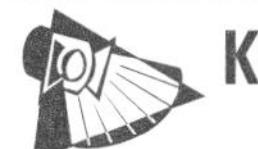

KEY FEATURES

ESSENTIALS OF DIAGNOSIS

- Painless swelling in region of thyroid
- Thyroid function tests usually normal
- Past history of head–neck radiation
- Positive thyroid fine needle aspiration biopsy

GENERAL CONSIDERATIONS

- Most thyroid cancers are microscopic and indolent. Larger ones require treatment

Papillary carcinoma

- Pure papillary or mixed papillary-follicular most common thyroid cancer (76%)
- Childhood head–neck radiation or nuclear fallout exposure imparts increased lifelong risk
- May be familial or associated with Cowden's disease or adenomatous polyposis coli
- Least aggressive thyroid malignancy, but spreads via thyroid lymphatics

Follicular carcinoma

- Second most common thyroid malignancy; generally more aggressive than papillary carcinoma
- Metastases commonly found in neck lymph nodes, bone, and lungs

Medullary thyroid carcinoma

- 4% of thyroid cancers
- One third sporadic, one third familial, one third associated with MEN type 2
- Early local metastases usually present, and late metastases may be in bones, lungs, adrenals, or liver
- Peptides (eg, serotonin) can cause symptoms and serve as tumor markers

Anaplastic thyroid carcinoma

- 1% of thyroid cancers
- Older patient with rapidly enlarging mass in multinodular goiter
- Most aggressive thyroid carcinoma; metastasizes early to surrounding lymph nodes and distant sites

Other thyroid malignancies

- 3% of thyroid cancers
- Lymphoma; metastatic bronchogenic, breast, and renal carcinomas, melanoma

CLINICAL FINDINGS

SYMPTOMS AND SIGNS

- Usually presents as palpable, firm, nontender nodule, but can arise from multinodular goiter
- Larger cancers can cause neck discomfort, dysphagia, or hoarseness
- ~3% present with metastasis to local lymph nodes and sometimes to distant sites such as bone or lung
- Metastatic differentiated carcinoma may secrete enough thyroxine to produce thyrotoxicosis
- Medullary carcinoma causes flushing, diarrhea, fatigue; ~5% develop Cushing's syndrome
- Anaplastic or longstanding tumors can produce hoarseness

DIFFERENTIAL DIAGNOSIS

- Benign thyroid nodule
- Subacute thyroiditis
- Benign multinodular goiter
- Lymphadenopathy due to other cause
- Metastasis from head and neck cancer
- Lymphoma

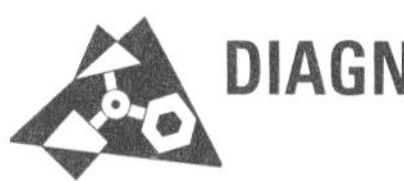

DIAGNOSIS

LABORATORY TESTS

- Serum thyroid-stimulating hormone (TSH), free tetraiodothyronine (T_4) generally normal unless concomitant thyroiditis; metastatic follicular carcinoma may secrete enough thyroxine to suppress TSH
- Serum thyroglobulin level high in most metastatic papillary and follicular tumors
  - Useful marker for recurrent or metastatic disease except if antithyroglobulin Ab present
  - Obtain serum thyroglobulin level preoperatively, postoperatively when hypothyroid (before ^{131}I therapy), and when euthyroid
- Serum calcitonin level frequently elevated in medullary thyroid carcinoma, but nonspecific test; obtain preoperatively and follow levels postoperatively as marker for recurrent or metastatic disease
- Serum carcinoembryonic antigen (CEA) levels usually elevated with medullary carcinoma; obtain preoperatively, repeat postoperatively as marker for recurrent or metastatic disease
- Genetic testing of siblings and children of patients with medullary carcinoma for *RET* protooncogene mutations, which occur in MEN-2 and familial medullary thyroid carcinoma

IMAGING STUDIES

- Radioiodine scanning not helpful preoperatively but useful postoperatively
- Preoperative neck ultrasound: in determining size and location of malignancy and neck metastases; especially useful if prior known metastases, persistent elevation in serum thyroglobulin, or detectable levels of antithyroglobulin antibodies
- Useful for postoperative surveillance for recurrence
- Chest x-ray or CT scan may demonstrate metastases, but iodinated contrast greatly reduces effectiveness of radioiodine scanning and therapy. Medullary carcinoma metastases in thyroid, nodes, and liver may calcify, but rarely do in lung
- Positive emission tomography (PET) scanning using
  - Useful in patients with elevated serum thyroglobulin (s/p thyroidectomy), especially with levels over 10 μg/mL and rising, who have normal whole-body RAI scan and unrevealing neck ultrasound
  - Can be combined with a CT scan
  - The resultant PET/CT fusion scan is 60% sensitive for detecting metastases not visible by other methods
  - Pretreatment with rhTSH can further increase sensitivity of ^{18}FDG-PET

DIAGNOSTIC PROCEDURES

- Fine-needle aspiration biopsy for clinically suspicious nodules

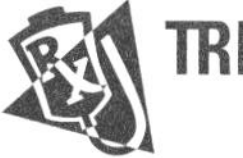

TREATMENT

MEDICATIONS

- Levothyroxine, 0.75–0.1 mg PO QD is begun immediately after thyroidectomy
  - Dosage adjusted using an ultrasensitive assay for serum TSH assay: suppress TSH below 0.1 mU/L for stage II disease and below 0.05 mU/L for stage III–IV disease
  - Patients receiving thyroxine suppression therapy, as a group, have slightly lower bone density than age-matched controls, but careful thyroxine suppression therapy has negligible effect on fracture risk
  - Determine bone densitometry periodically

SURGERY

- Surgical removal is treatment of choice for thyroid carcinomas
- Total or near-total thyroidectomy for most patients
- Subtotal thyroidectomy for adults aged < 45 with single tumor < 1 cm
- Surgical resection of metastases to brain (radiation or radioactive iodide therapy ineffective), and of bulky recurrent tumor in neck region
- Total thyroidectomy for medullary thyroid carcinoma; repeated neck dissections often required over time
- Prophylactic total thyroidectomy, ideally at age 6, in persons with *RET* protooncogene mutations
- Local resection, combined with radiation therapy, for anaplastic carcinoma

THERAPEUTIC PROCEDURES

- After thyroidectomy, patients with differentiated thyroid carcinomas receive radioiodine neck and whole-body scan after thyrotropin (rhTSH) administration or while hypothyroid
- Decision to treat with ^{131}I:
  - Patients with suspicious radioiodine uptake considered for ^{131}I therapy
  - Patients with stage 1 DTC, ^{131}I therapy does not improve survival, but does reduce local recurrence; ^{131}I given to those with a primary tumor over 1 cm diameter, tumor at the surgical margin, or lymph node involvement
- ^{131}I therapy cautions:
  - Pregnant women may not receive RAI therapy
  - Women are advised to avoid pregnancy for at least 4 months after therapy
  - Men have abnormal spermatozoa up to 6 months after therapy and must use contraceptive methods during that time
- External-beam radiation therapy for bone metastases

OUTCOME

FOLLOW-UP

- Monitor serum TSH, and adjust thyroxine dose (as above)
- Performing whole-body ^{131}I or ^{123}I scan at 2–4 months after total or near-total thyroidectomy will detect ~65% of metastases
- Perform another ^{131}I or ^{123}I whole-body scan ~6–12 months after the postoperative scan, and check serum thyroglobulin measurement while hypothyroid
- Monitor serum thyroglobulin levels
- Two successive whole-body scans negative for metastases are required for tentative diagnosis of remission
- Monitor serum calcitonin and CEA periodically after surgery for medullary carcinoma
- Surveillance of family of patients with medullary thyroid carcinoma

COMPLICATIONS

- Local or distant metastases, including occult lung metastases in 10–15%
- Medullary carcinomas may secrete serotonin and prostaglandins, producing flushing and diarrhea; or ACTH or corticotropin-releasing hormone, causing Cushing's syndrome. Coincident pheochromocytoma and hyperparathyroidism may occur in MEN-related cases
- Permanent hypothyroidism, possible hypoparathyroidism, and vocal cord palsy after radical neck surgery
- Immediate autotransplantation of incidentally resected parathyroids into neck muscles reduces postoperative hypoparathyroidism

PROGNOSIS

- For papillary (and follicular) carcinoma, generally excellent
- Palpable lymph node metastases in papillary thyroid cancer do not increase mortality, but do increase risk of local recurrence
- Prognosis worsened with follicular instead of papillary carcinoma, older age, male gender, bone or brain metastases, large pulmonary metastases, and lack of ^{131}I uptake into metastases
- Brain metastases (in 1%) reduce median survival to 12 months; prognosis improved by surgical resection
- Mortality increased twofold by 10 years and threefold by 25 years in patients not receiving ^{131}I ablation
- For medullary thyroid carcinoma, variable:
  - Overall 10-year survival rate 90% when confined to thyroid, 70% with metastases to cervical lymph nodes, and 20% with distant metastases
  - In MEN 2A, less aggressive tumors and in MEN 2B, more aggressive
  - Those staining heavily for calcitonin, usually less aggressive; prolonged survival despite extensive metastases
- For anaplastic thyroid carcinoma, poor

WHEN TO ADMIT

- Admit for thyroidectomy for at least 1 day postoperatively to monitor for late bleeding, airway problems, and tetany
- Admit for high-dose ^{131}I therapy

EVIDENCE

PRACTICE GUIDELINES

- AACE Medical Guidelines for Clinical Practice: 2001 thyroid carcinoma
  - http://www.aace.com/clin/guidelines/thyroid_carcinoma.pdf

WEB SITE

- American Thyroid Association
  - http://www.thyroid.org

INFORMATION FOR PATIENTS

- American Thyroid Association—Thyroid cancer
  - http://www.thyroid.org/patients/brochures/ThyroidCancer_brochure.pdf
- NIH Medline Plus Encyclopedia:
  - http://www.nlm.nih.gov/medlineplus/ency/article/001213.htm

REFERENCES

- Bal CS et al: Radioiodine dose for remnant ablation in differentiated thyroid carcinoma: a randomized trial of 509 patients. J Clin Endocrinol Metab 2004;89:1666. [PMID: 15070929]
- Clayman GL et al: Medullary thyroid cancer. Otolaryngol Clin North Am 2003;36:91. [PMID: 12803011]
- Fernandes JK et al: Overview of the management of differentiated thyroid cancer. Curr Treat Options Oncol 2005;6:47. [PMID: 15610714]
- Hamady ZZ et al: Surgical pathological second opinion in thyroid malignancy: impact on patients management and prognosis. Eur J Surg Oncol 2005;31:74. [PMID: 15642429]
- Lin JD et al: Papillary thyroid carcinomas with lung metastases. Thyroid 2004;14:1091. [PMID: 15650364]
- Machens A et al: Advances in the management of hereditary medullary thyroid cancer. J Intern Med 2005;257:50. [PMID: 15606376]
- Robbins RJ et al: Clinical review 156: recombinant human thyrotropin and thyroid cancer management. J Clin Endocrinol Metab 2003;88:1933. [PMID: 12727936]
- Sawka AM et al: A systematic review and metaanalysis of the effectiveness of radioactive iodine remnant ablation for well-differentiated thyroid cancer. J Clin Endocrinol Metab 2004;89:3668. [PMID: 15292285]

Author(s)

Paul A. Fitzgerald, MD

Thyroid Nodules & Multinodular Goiter

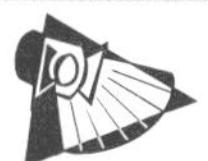

KEY FEATURES

ESSENTIALS OF DIAGNOSIS

- Single or multiple thyroid nodules commonly found with careful thyroid examinations
- Thyroid function tests mandatory
- Thyroid biopsy for single or dominant nodules or if history of head–neck radiation
- Ultrasound examination sometimes useful for biopsy and follow-up
- Clinical follow-up required

GENERAL CONSIDERATIONS

- Palpable enlargement of the thyroid (goiter) may be diffuse or nodular
- Most patients with goiter are euthyroid, but many have hypothyroidism or hyperthyroidism
- Causes of diffuse and multinodular goiters include
  - Benign multinodular goiter
  - Iodine deficiency
  - Pregnancy (in areas of iodine deficiency)
  - Graves' disease
  - Hashimoto's thyroiditis
  - Subacute thyroiditis, or infections
- Causes of solitary thyroid nodule include
  - Benign adenoma
  - Colloid nodule
  - Cys
  - Primary thyroid malignancy or (less frequently) metastatic neoplasm
- Risk of malignancy is higher
  - History of head-neck radiation in childhood
  - Family history of thyroid cancer
  - Personal history of another malignancy

DEMOGRAPHICS

- Goiter found in 4% of North American adults
- Incidence of goiter higher in iodine-deficient geographic areas (see Goiter, Endemic)

CLINICAL FINDINGS

SYMPTOMS AND SIGNS

- Most small thyroid nodules are asymptomatic and discovered incidentally on physical or radiologic examination
- Graves' disease, toxic multinodular goiter, hyperfunctioning nodules, and subacute thyroiditis can cause hyperthyroidism (eg, sweating, weight loss, anxiety, loose stools, heat intolerance, tachycardia, tremor)
- Hashimoto's thyroiditis may cause goiter and hypothyroidism (eg, fatigue, cold intolerance, constipation, weight gain, depression, dry skin, delayed return of deep tendon reflexes)
- Thyroid nodules or multinodular goiter can grow and cause cosmetic embarrassment, discomfort, hoarseness, or dysphagia. Large retrosternal multinodular goiters can cause dyspnea due to tracheal compression
- Malignancy is suggested by
  - Hoarsesness or vocal cord paralysis
  - Nodules in men or young women
  - Nodule that is solitary, firm, large, or adherent to trachea or strap muscles
  - Enlarged lymph nodes
  - Distant metastases
- Benign nodules are suggested by
  - Older women
  - Soft nodule
  - Multinodular goiter

DIFFERENTIAL DIAGNOSIS

- Benign multinodular goiter
- Iodine-deficient goiter
- Pregnancy (in areas of iodine deficiency)
- Graves' disease
- Hashimoto's thyroiditis
- Subacute (de Quervain's) thyroiditis
- Drugs causing hypothyroidism: lithium, amiodarone, propylthiouracil, methimazole, phenylbutazone, sulfonamides, interferon-α, iodide
- Infiltrating disease, eg, malignancy, sarcoidosis
- Suppurative thyroiditis
- Riedel's thyroiditis
- Nonthyroid neck mass, eg, lymphadenopathy, lymphoma, branchial cleft cyst

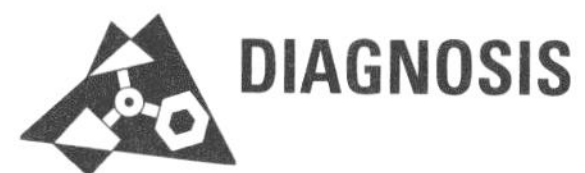

DIAGNOSIS

LABORATORY TESTS

- Obtain thyroid-stimulating hormone (TSH) (sensitive assay) and free thyroxine (FT_4) to exclude hypothyroidism or hyperthyroidism
- Antithyroperoxidase or antithyroglobulin antibodies usually very high in Hashimoto's thyroiditis; in patients with Hashimoto's thyroiditis, a palpable solitary thyroid nodule of ≥1 cm diameter has about an 8% chance of being malignant

IMAGING STUDIES

- Neck ultrasound indicated for most papalble thyroid nodules to accurately determine nodule size and consistency, to ascertain whether nodule is part of a multinodular goiter, and to follow nodule
- Solid nodules often malignant; cystic nodules usually benign
- Neck ultrasound preferred over CT and MRI because of accuracy
- Radioactive iodine (RAI; ^{123}I or ^{131}I) scans have limited usefulness in evaluation of thyroid nodules

DIAGNOSTIC PROCEDURES

- Fine-needle aspiration (FNA) biopsy of suspicious nodules (thyroiditis frequently coexists with malignancy); for cystic nodules, cytologic examination of centrifuged supernatant increases diagnostic yield
- FNA biopsy success is increased by ultrasound guidance
- Of thyroid FNA biopsies, ~70% are benign, 10% follicular neoplasm (suspicious cytology), 5% malignant, and 15% nondiagnostic. Among patients with follicular neoplasm (suspicious), ~20–40% harbor malignancy, with higher risk in young patients and if nodules fixed or >3 cm
- Cytology should be done on cystic fluid obtained at FNA
  - Cystic nodules yielding serous fluid are usually benign, those yielding bloody fluid have higher chance of malignancy
  - Repeat FNA biopsy if cytology nondiagnostic and nodule remains palpable
- Thyroid incidentalomas: nonpalpable small thyroid nodules are incidentally discovered by about 25–50% of scans of the neck (MRI, CT, ultrasound) done for other reasons.
  - Require ultrasound-guided FNA biopsy (USGFNAB) only if >1.5 cm or history of head-neck radiation in childhood

- Consider USGFNAB for nodules < 1.5 cm diameter if history of head–neck irradiation or a family history of thyroid cancer or a suspicious appearance on ultrasound (calcified, solitary, or irregular)
- Follow-up thyroid ultrasound in 3–4 months for nodules of borderline concern; growing lesions may be biopsied or resected

TREATMENT

MEDICATIONS

- Levothyroxine, 0.05–0.2 mg PO QD, if elevated TSH
- Consider "suppression" of nodules >2 cm with levothyroxine, 0.05–0.1 mg QD, if TSH elevated or normal. Avoid if baseline TSH is low suggesting autonomous thyroid hormone secretion, because levothyroxine will be ineffective and may cause thyrotoxicosis
  - Long-term suppression of TSH tends to keep nodules from enlarging and new nodules from developing, but few existing nodules actually shrink
  - Works best for younger patients
  - May increase risk for angina and arrhythmia in patients with cardiovascular disease
  - Causes small loss of bone density in many postmenopausal women not on estrogen replacement

SURGERY

- Surgical resection indicated for solitary nodule with history of head–neck radiation due to risk of malignancy
- Surgical resection of toxic adenoma cures hyperthyroidism
- Excision of multinodular goiters causing compressive symptoms

PROCEDURES

- Aspiration of cystic nodule with fluid sent for cytology. Multiple aspirations may be required because cysts tend to recur
- Regular clinical evaluation and thyroid palpation or ultrasound examinations in all patients; even patients with a "negative" FNAB require follow-up because the false-negative rate for FNAB is 4%
- Periodic bone densitometry in patients who are on levothyroxine suppression and at risk for osteoporosis

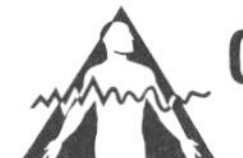

OUTCOME

FOLLOW-UP

- Regular periodic palpation of all thyroid nodules and rebiopsy if growth occurs
- Monitor patients on levothyroxine suppression for atrial arrhythmias and osteoporosis

PROGNOSIS

- Benign nodules usually persist or grow slowly and may involute. Malignant transformation is rare
- Prognosis of malignant nodules depends on histology (see Thyroid Cancer)
- Multinodular goiters tend to persist or grow slowly, even in iodine-deficient areas where iodine repletion usually does not shrink established goiters
- Patients with small incidentally discovered nonpalpable thyroid nodules are at very low risk for malignancy; nonpalpable thyroid nodules < 1 cm diameter are benign in 98.4% of cases; even those with malignancy have little morbidity and mortality

EVIDENCE

PRACTICE GUIDELINES

- AACE Practice Guidelines for Thyroid Nodule:
  - http://www.aace.com/clin/guidelines/thyroid_nodules.pdf

WEB SITE

- The American Thyroid Association
  - http://www.thyroid.org

INFORMATION FOR PATIENTS

- American Thyroid Association—Thyroid nodule
  - http://www.thyroid.org/patients/brochures/Nodules_brochure.pdf
- Mayo Clinic—Thyroid nodule
  - http://www.mayoclinic.com/invoke.cfm?objectid=6014E6CA-8B4E-49B0-ACA1FC378D888DAE

REFERENCES

- Day TA et al: Multinodular goiter. Otolaryngol Clin North Am 2003;36:35. [PMID:12803008]
- Hegedüs L: Clinical practice. The thyroid nodule. N Engl J Med 2004;351:1764. [PMID:15496625]
- Mackenzie EJ, Mortimer RH: Thyroid nodules and thyroid cancer. Med J Aust 2004;180:242. [PMID:14984346]
- Nam-Goong IS et al: Ultrasonography-guided fine-needle aspiration of thyroid incidentaloma: correlation with pathological findings. Clin Endocrinol (Oxf) 2004;60:21. [PMID:14678283]
- Sclabas GM et al: Fine-needle aspiration of the thyroid and correlation with histopathology in a contemporary series of 240 patients. Am J Surg 2003;186:702; discussion 709. [PMID:14672783]
- Yeh MW et al: False-negative fine-needle aspiration cytology results delay treatment and adversely affect outcome in patients with thyroid carcinoma. Thyroid 2004;14:207. [PMID:15072703]

Author(s)

Paul A. Fitzgerald, MD

Thyroiditis

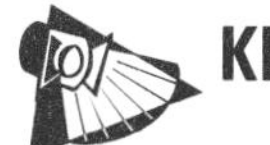

KEY FEATURES

ESSENTIALS OF DIAGNOSIS

- Swelling of thyroid gland, sometimes causing pressure symptoms in acute and subacute forms; painless enlargement or rubbery firmness in chronic form
- Thyroid function tests variable
- Serum antithyroperoxidase, antimicrosomal, antithyroglobulin antibody tests often positive

GENERAL CONSIDERATIONS

- Classification
  - Chronic lymphocytic (Hashimoto's) thyroiditis due to autoimmunity
  - Subacute thyroiditis (de Quervain's thyroiditis, granulomatous thyroiditis, and giant cell thyroiditis)
  - Suppurative thyroiditis
  - Riedel's thyroiditis
- Hashimoto's thyroiditis
  - Most common thyroid disorder in the United States
  - Frequency increased by dietary iodine supplementation; certain drugs (eg, amiodarone, interferon-α)
  - Associated with other autoimmune diseases, eg, diabetes mellitus, pernicious anemia, adrenal insufficiency (Schmidt's syndrome), other endocrine deficiencies (autoimmune polyglandular failure syndrome), inflammatory bowel disease, celiac disease; usually, concurrent with Graves' disease
- Postpartum thyroiditis is a form of autoimmune thyroiditis accompanied by transient hyperthyroidism followed by hypothyroidism
- Thyroiditis commonly occurs in patients with hepatitis C
- Suppurative thyroiditis is rare, caused by pyogenic organisms, usually during systemic infection
- Riedel's thyroiditis: rarest form

DEMOGRAPHICS

- Hashimoto's thyroiditis is often familial and is 6 times more common in women than men
- Subacute thyroiditis usually affects young and middle-aged women
- Riedel's thyroiditis usually affects middle-aged or elderly women
- Antithyroid antibodies are found in 3% of men and 13% of women
  - Women over age 60 years have a 25% incidence of having antithyroid antibodies
- Hashimoto's thyroiditis incidence varies by kindred and by race
  - In US adolescents and adults, antithyroid antibodies are found in 14.3% of whites, 10.9% of Mexican Americans, and 5.3% of African Americans

CLINICAL FINDINGS

SYMPTOMS AND SIGNS

Hashimoto's thyroiditis

- Thyroid gland usually diffusely enlarged, firm, and finely nodular. One lobe may be asymmetrically enlarged, raising concern for neoplasm
- Neck tightness; pain and tenderness not usually present
- Thyroiditis often progresses to hypothyroidism, which is usually permanent; uncommonly, thyroiditis causes transient thyrotoxicosis
- Rarely, a hypofunctioning gland may become hyperfunctioning with onset of coexistent Graves' disease
- Depression and chronic fatigue
- Mild dry mouth (xerostomia) or dry eyes (keratoconjunctivitis sicca) related to Sjögren's syndrome in ~33%
- Diplopia due to coexistent myasthenia gravis
- Manifestations of other autoimmune diseases listed above
- 40% of women and 20% of men exhibit focal thyroiditis at autopsy

Subacute thyroiditis

- Acute, usually painful, thyroid enlargement, with dysphagia. May have malaise or signs of thyrotoxicosis
- If no pain, called "silent thyroiditis"
- May persist for weeks or months

Suppurative thyroiditis

- Severe pain, tenderness, redness, and fluctuance around thyroid gland

Riedel's thyroiditis

- Usually causes hypothyroidism
- Enlargement often asymmetric; gland is stony hard and adherent to neck structures, causing dysphagia, dyspnea, pain, and hoarseness

DIFFERENTIAL DIAGNOSIS

- Benign multinodular goiter
- Iodine-deficient (endemic) goiter
- Graves' disease
- Thyroid cancer
- Other malignancies (eg, lymphoma)

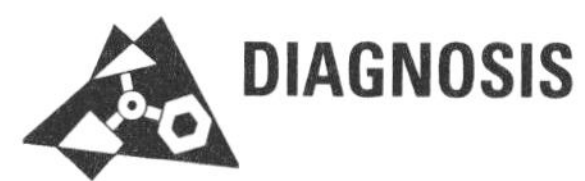

DIAGNOSIS

LABORATORY TESTS

- Thyroid-stimulating hormone (TSH) level is elevated if thyroiditis causes hypothyroidism, suppressed if it causes hyperthyroidism
- Serum-free tetraiodotyronine (T_4) usually elevated in acute and subacute thyroiditis with hyperthyroidism; normal or low in the chronic forms
- Hashimoto's thyroiditis: antithyroperoxidase levels increased in 95%; antithyroglobulin antibodies increased in 60% (very nonspecific)
- Thyroid autoantibodies also found in other types of thyroiditis, and mildly elevated titers found in 13% of asymptomatic women and 3% of asymptomatic men. Only 1% of the population has antibody titers >1:6400
- Subacute thyroiditis: erythrocyte sedimentation rate markedly elevated and antithyroid antibody titers low

IMAGING STUDIES

- Radioiodine uptake and scan usually not required; characteristically very low in initial, hyperthyroid phase of subacute thyroiditis, distinguishing thyroiditis from Graves' disease
- Radioiodine uptake may be high with an uneven scan in chronic thyroiditis, with enlargement of the gland, and low in Riedel's thyroiditis
- Ultrasound of thyroid helps distinguish thyroiditis from multinodular goiter or thyroid nodules that are suspicious for malignancy

DIAGNOSTIC PROCEDURES

- Biopsy may be required to distinguish asymmetric thyroiditis from carcinoma

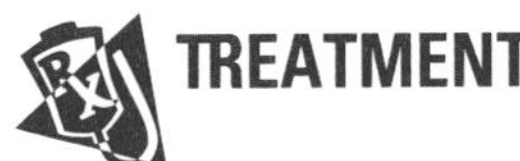

TREATMENT

MEDICATIONS

Hashimoto's thyroiditis

- Levothyroxine, 50–200 μg PO QD, if hypothyroidism or large goiter present
- In one study, selenium selenite (200 μg PO QD for 3 months) reduced serum antithyroperoxidase levels by 49% compared with 10% reduction with placebo
- If euthyroid (normal TSH) and minimal goiter, do not administer levothyroxine but follow patient until hypothyroidism develops

Subacute thyroiditis

- Aspirin is drug of choice, continue for several weeks
- Propranolol, 10–40 mg PO Q 6 h, for thyrotoxic symptoms
- Iodinated contrast agents promptly normalize triiodothyronine (T_3) levels and dramatically improve thyrotoxic symptoms. Sodium ipodate (Oragrafin, Biliv-ist) or iopanoic acid (Telepaque), 500 mg PO QD, until free T_4 normalizes
- Levothyroxine, 50–100 μg PO QD, if transient hypothyroidism is symptomatic

Suppurative thyroiditis

- Antibiotics

Riedel's thyroiditis

- Tamoxifen, 10 mg PO BID, usually induces partial to complete remissions within 3–6 months and must be continued for years
- Short-term glucocorticoid treatment for relief of pain and compression symptoms

SURGERY

- Suppurative thyroiditis requires surgical drainage when fluctuance is marked
- For Riedel's thyroiditis, surgery usually fails to permanently alleviate compression and is difficult due to dense fibrous adhesions

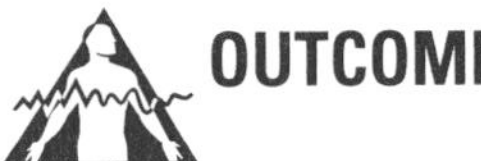

OUTCOME

FOLLOW-UP

- Euthyroid patients with Hashimoto's thyroiditis must be followed up long-term because hypothyroidism may develop years later

COMPLICATIONS

- Hashimoto's thyroiditis may lead to hypothyroidism or transient thyrotoxicosis
- Subacute and chronic thyroiditis can be complicated by dyspnea and, in Riedel's struma, vocal cord palsy from pressure on neck structures
- Riedel's thyroiditis usually occurs with other manifestations of multifocal systemic fibrosis syndrome, eg, retroperitoneal fibrosis, fibrosing mediastinitis
- Perimenopausal women with high antithyroperoxidase titers are at risk for depression independent of thyroid hormone levels
- Graves' disease may develop
- Carcinoma or lymphoma may be associated with chronic thyroiditis and must be considered if uneven painless enlargements continue despite treatment
- Hashimoto's thyroiditis may be associated with other autoimmune disorders

PROGNOSIS

- Hashimoto's thyroiditis has an excellent prognosis, because it either remains stable for years or progresses slowly to hypothyroidism, which is easily treated
- Subacute thyroiditis may smolder for months; spontaneous remissions and exacerbations are common
- Postpartum thyroiditis usually resolves with return to normal thyroid function

EVIDENCE

PRACTICE GUIDELINES

- Pearce EN et al: Thyroiditis. N Engl J Med 2003;348:2646. [PMID: 12826640]
- Slatosky J et al: Thyroiditis: differential diagnosis and management. Am Fam Physician 2000;61:1047. Erratum in Am Fam Physician 2000;62:318. [PMID: 10706157]

WEB SITES

- American Association of Clinical Endocrinologists
  - http://www.aace.com
- American Thyroid Association
  - http://www.thyroid.org

INFORMATION FOR PATIENTS

- American Thyroid Association
  - http://www.thyroid.org/patients/brochures/thyroiditis.pdf
- Mayo Clinic—Subacute thyroiditis
  - http://www.mayoclinic.com/invoke.cfm?objectid=7574A58E-05DE-4E78-9058AE99AB5C6829
- MEDLINEplus—Chronic thyroiditis
  - http://www.nlm.nih.gov/medlineplus/ency/article/000371.htm
- MEDLINEplus—Painless thyroiditis
  - http://www.nlm.nih.gov/medlineplus/ency/article/000388.htm
- MEDLINEplus—Subacute thyroiditis
  - http://www.nlm.nih.gov/medlineplus/ency/article/000375.htm

REFERENCES

- Dang AH et al: Lithium-associated thyroiditis. Endocr Pract 2002;8:232. [PMID: 12113638]
- Pearce EN et al: Thyroiditis. N Engl J Med 2003;348:2646. [PMID: 12826640]
- Stagnaro-Green A: Clinical review 152: postpartum thyroiditis. J Clin Endocrinol Metab 2002;87:4042. [PMID: 12213841]
- Su DH et al: Determining when to operate on patients with Hashimoto's thyroiditis with nodular lesions: the role of ultrasound-guided fine needle aspiration cytology. Acta Cytol 2004;48:622. [PMID: 15471253]

Author(s)

Paul A. Fitzgerald, MD

Tinea Corporis or Tinea Circinata

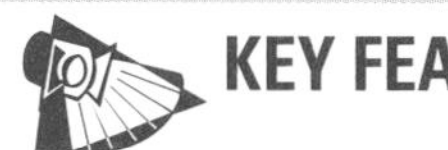

KEY FEATURES

ESSENTIALS OF DIAGNOSIS

- Ring-shaped lesions with an advancing scaly border and central clearing or scaly patches with a distinct border
- On exposed skin surfaces or the trunk
- Microscopic examination of scrapings or culture confirms the diagnosis

GENERAL CONSIDERATIONS

- The lesions are often on exposed areas of the body such as the face and arms
- All species of dermatophytes may cause this disease, but *Trichophyton rubrum* is the most common pathogen, usually representing extension onto the trunk or extremities of tinea cruris, pedis, or manuum
- Body ringworm usually responds promptly to conservative topical therapy or to griseofulvin by mouth within 4 weeks

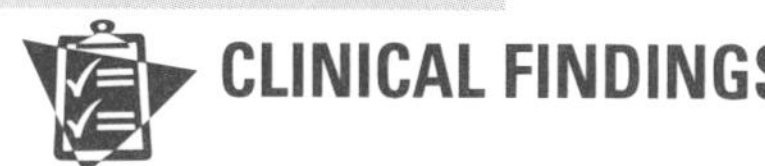

CLINICAL FINDINGS

SYMPTOMS AND SIGNS

- See Table 7
- Ring-shaped lesions with an advancing scaly border and central clearing or scaly patches with a distinct border
- Location: on exposed skin surfaces or the trunk
- Itching may be present
- A history of exposure to an infected cat may occasionally be obtained, usually indicating microsporum infection

DIFFERENTIAL DIAGNOSIS

- Psoriasis
- Impetigo
- Seborrheic dermatitis
- Secondary syphilis
- Pityriasis rosea
- Nummular eczema (discoid eczema, nummular dermatitis)
- Bacterial folliculitis

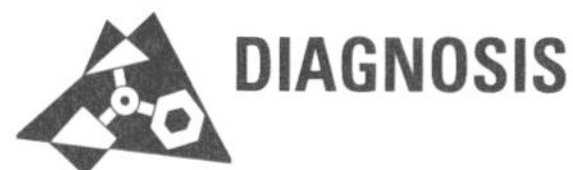

DIAGNOSIS

DIAGNOSTIC PROCEDURES

- Hyphae can be demonstrated by removing a peripheral scale and examining it microscopically using KOH
- The diagnosis may be confirmed by culture

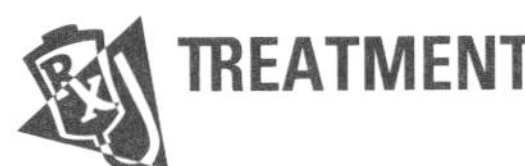

TREATMENT

MEDICATIONS

- See Table 6

Local measures

- Antifungal creams: miconazole, 2% cream; clotrimazole, 1% solution, cream, or lotion; ketoconazole, 2% cream; econazole, 1% cream or lotion; sulconazole, 1% cream; oxiconazole, 1% cream; ciclopirox, 1% cream; naftifine, 1% cream or gel; butenafine cream; and terbinafine, 1% cream
- Miconazole, clotrimazole, butenafine, and terbinafine are available OTC
- Allylamines (especially terbinafine and butenafine) require shorter courses and lead to the most rapid response and prolonged remissions
- In general, use of betamethasone-clotrimazole (Lotrisone) does not justify the expense

Systemic measures

- Griseofulvin (ultramicrosize), 250–500 mg PO twice daily, is used; typically, only 2–4 weeks of therapy are required
- Itraconazole as a single week-long pulse of 200 mg PO once daily is also effective in tinea corporis
- Terbinafine, 250 mg PO daily for 1 month, is an alternative

THERAPEUTIC PROCEDURES

- Treatment should be continued for 1–2 weeks after clinical clearing

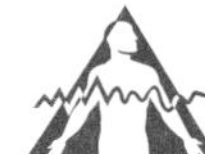

OUTCOME

PROGNOSIS

- Body ringworm usually responds promptly to conservative topical therapy or to griseofulvin by mouth within 4 weeks

WHEN TO REFER

- If there is a question about the diagnosis, if recommended therapy is ineffective, or if specialized treatment is necessary

EVIDENCE

WEB SITE

- American Academy of Dermatology: Superficial mycotic infections of the skin: Tinea corporis, tinea cruris, tinea faciei, tinea manuum, and tinea pedis
  - http://www.aad.org/professionals/pracmanage/guidelines/SupMycotic-TineaCorporis-Pedis.htm

INFORMATION FOR PATIENTS

- American Academy of Family Physicians: Tinea Infections: Athlete's Foot, Jock Itch and Ringworm
  - http://familydoctor.org/316.xml
- American Medical Association: Fungal Skin Infection
  - http://www.medem.com/search/article_display.cfm?path=TANQUERAYM_ContentItem&mstr=/M_ContentItem/ZZZ8W2QJU9C.html&soc=AMA&srch_typ=NAV_SERCH
- Mayo Clinic: Ringworm of the Body
  - http://www.mayoclinic.com/invoke.cfm?id=DS00489
- MedlinePlus: Tinea Corporis
  - http://www.nlm.nih.gov/medlineplus/ency/article/000877.htm

REFERENCES

- Crawford F et al: Topical treatments for fungal infections of the skin and nails of the foot. Cochrane Database Syst Rev 2000(2):CD001434. [PMID: 10796792]
- Gupta AK et al: Optimal management of fungal infections of the skin, hair, and nails. Am J Clin Dermatol 2004;5:225. [PMID: 15301570]
- Zuber TJ et al: Superficial fungal infection of the skin. Where and how it appears help determine therapy. Postgrad Med 2001;109:117. [PMID: 11198246]

Author(s)

Timothy G. Berger, MD

Tinea Cruris

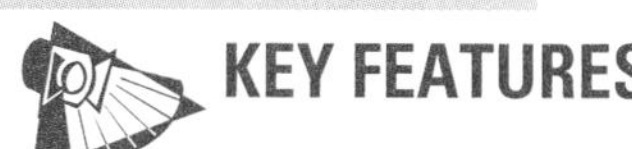

KEY FEATURES

ESSENTIALS OF DIAGNOSIS

- Marked itching in intertriginous areas, usually sparing the scrotum
- Peripherally spreading, sharply demarcated, centrally clearing erythematous lesions
- May have associated tinea infection of feet or toenails
- Laboratory examination with microscope or culture confirms diagnosis

GENERAL CONSIDERATIONS

- Must be distinguished from other lesions involving the intertriginous areas, such as candidiasis, seborrheic dermatitis, intertrigo, psoriasis of body folds ("inverse psoriasis"), erythrasma, and rarely tinea versicolor

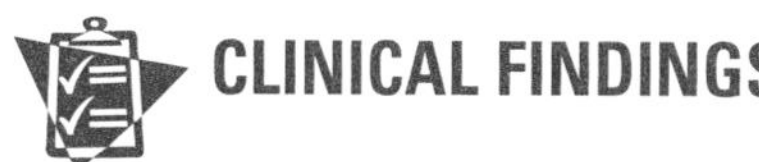

CLINICAL FINDINGS

SYMPTOMS AND SIGNS

- See Table 7
- Typical lesions are erythematous and sharply demarcated, with central clearing and active, spreading scaly peripheries
- Marked itching in intertriginous areas, usually sparing the scrotum
- May have associated tinea infection of feet or toenails
- The area may be hyperpigmented on resolution

DIFFERENTIAL DIAGNOSIS

- Erythrasma is best diagnosed with Wood's light—a brilliant coral-red fluorescence is seen
- Candidiasis
- Seborrheic dermatitis
- Intertrigo
- Psoriasis of body folds ("inverse psoriasis")
- Tinea versicolor (pityriasis versicolor)

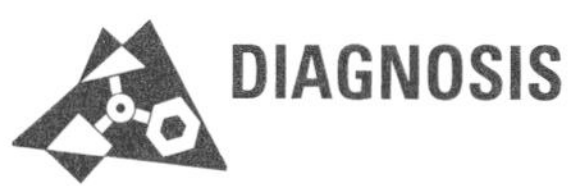

DIAGNOSIS

LABORATORY TESTS

- Hyphae can be demonstrated microscopically in potassium hydroxide preparations
- The organism may be cultured readily
- Tinea cruris must be distinguished from other lesions involving the intertriginous areas, such as candidiasis, seborrheic dermatitis, intertrigo, psoriasis of body folds ("inverse psoriasis"), erythrasma, and rarely tinea versicolor
- Candidiasis is generally bright red and marked by satellite papules and pustules outside of the main border of the lesion; *Candida* typically involves the scrotum
- Tinea versicolor can be diagnosed by the KOH preparation
- Seborrheic dermatitis also often involves the face, sternum, and axillae
- Intertrigo tends to be more red, less scaly, and present in obese individuals in moist body folds with less extension onto the thigh
- Inverse psoriasis is characterized by distinct plaques; other areas of typical psoriatic involvement should be checked, and the KOH examination will be negative

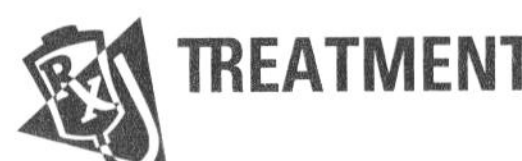

TREATMENT

MEDICATIONS

- See Table 6

General measures

- Drying powder [eg, miconazole nitrate (Zeasorb-AF])] should be dusted into the involved area in patients with excessive perspiration or occlusion of skin due to obesity

Local measures

- See preparations listed in *Tinea corporis*
- There is great variation in expense, with miconazole, clotrimazole, and terbinafine available OTC and usually at a lower price
- Terbinafine cream is curative in over 80% of cases after once-daily use for 7 days

Systemic measures

- Griseofulvin ultramicrosize is reserved for severe cases; give 250–500 mg orally twice daily for 1–2 weeks
- Itraconazole, 200 mg PO daily, or terbinafine, 250 mg PO daily, for 1 week, is also effective

THERAPEUTIC PROCEDURES

- Underwear should be loose fitting

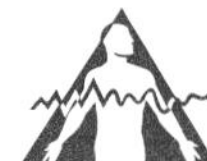

OUTCOME

WHEN TO REFER

- If there is a question about the diagnosis, if recommended therapy is ineffective, or if specialized treatment is necessary

EVIDENCE

WEB SITE

- American Academy of Dermatology: Superficial mycotic infections of the skin: Tinea corporis, tinea cruris, tinea faciei, tinea manuum, and tinea pedis
  - http://www.aad.org/professionals/pracmanage/guidelines/SupMycotic-TineaCorporis-Pedis.htm

INFORMATION FOR PATIENTS

- American Academy of Family Physicians: Tinea Infections: Athlete's Foot, Jock Itch and Ringworm
  - http://familydoctor.org/316.xml
- American Medical Association: Fungal Skin Infection
  - http://www.medem.com/search/article_display.cfm?path=TANQUERAYM_ContentItem&mstr=/M_ContentItem/ZZZ8W2QJU9C.html&soc=AMA&srch_typ=NAV_SERCH
- Mayo Clinic: Jock Itch
  - http://www.mayoclinic.com/invoke.cfm?objectid=0956F75F-3368-42AA-A0AA438D4694B2A7
- MedlinePlus: Jock Itch
  - http://www.nlm.nih.gov/medlineplus/ency/article/000876.htm

REFERENCES

- Crawford F et al: Topical treatments for fungal infections of the skin and nails of the foot. Cochrane Database Syst Rev 2000(2):CD001434. [PMID: 10796792]
- Gupta AK et al: Optimal management of fungal infections of the skin, hair, and nails. Am J Clin Dermatol 2004;5:225. [PMID: 15301570]
- Zuber TJ et al: Superficial fungal infection of the skin. Where and how it appears help determine therapy. Postgrad Med 2001;109:117. [PMID: 11198246]

Author(s)

Timothy G. Berger, MD

Tinea Manuum & Pedis

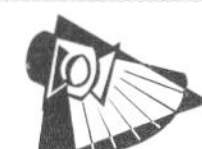

KEY FEATURES

ESSENTIALS OF DIAGNOSIS

- Most often presenting with asymptomatic scaling
- May progress to fissuring or maceration in toe web spaces
- Itching, burning, and stinging of interdigital webs, palms, and soles seen occasionally; deep vesicles in inflammatory cases
- The fungus is shown in skin scrapings examined microscopically or by culture of scrapings

GENERAL CONSIDERATIONS

- An extremely common acute or chronic dermatosis
- Certain individuals appear to be more susceptible than others
- Most infections are caused by *Trichophyton* species
- Interdigital tinea pedis is the most common cause of leg cellulitis in healthy individuals

CLINICAL FINDINGS

SYMPTOMS AND SIGNS

- See Table 7
- Most often presents with asymptomatic scaling that may progress to fissuring or maceration in toe web spaces
- Itching, burning, and stinging of interdigital webs, palms, and soles seen occasionally; deep vesicles in inflammatory cases
- Tinea pedis has several presentations that vary with the location
- On the sole and heel, may appear as chronic noninflammatory scaling, occasionally with thickening and cracking of the epidermis; this may extend over the sides of the feet in a "moccasin" distribution
- Often appears as a scaling or fissuring of the toe webs, perhaps with sodden maceration
- There may be grouped vesicles distributed anywhere on the soles or palms, generalized exfoliation of the skin of the soles, or nail involvement in the form of discoloration and thickening and crumbling of the nail plate

DIFFERENTIAL DIAGNOSIS

- Erythrasma
- Psoriasis
- Contact dermatitis
- Dyshidrosis (pomphylox)
- Scabies
- Pitted keratolysis
- Tinea pedis must be differentiated from other skin conditions involving the same areas, such as
  - Interdigital erythrasma (use Wood's light)
  - Psoriasis: repeated fungal cultures should be negative
- Contact dermatitis (from shoes) will often involve the dorsal surfaces and will respond to topical or systemic corticosteroids

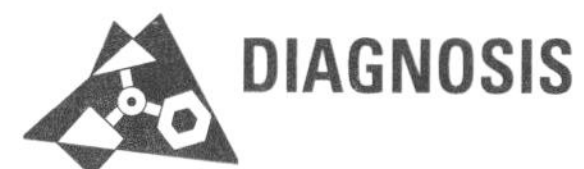

DIAGNOSIS

LABORATORY TESTS

- The KOH preparation is usually positive
- As the web spaces become more macerated, the KOH preparation and fungal culture are less often positive because bacterial species begin to dominate

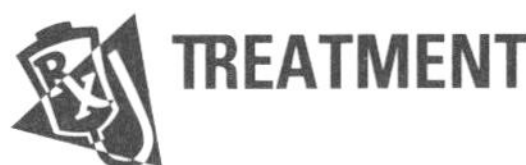

TREATMENT

MEDICATIONS

Local measures

- See Table 6
- Macerated stage—treat with aluminum subacetate solution soaks for 20 min twice daily
- Broad-spectrum antifungal creams and solutions (containing imidazoles or ciclopirox instead of tolnaftate and haloprogin) will help combat diphtheroids and other gram-positive organisms present at this stage and alone may be adequate therapy
- If topical imidazoles fail, try 1 week of once-daily allylamine treatment (terbinafine or butenafine)
- Dry and scaly stage—use any of the agents listed in *Tinea corporis*
- The addition of urea 10% lotion or cream (Carmol) under an occlusive dressing may increase the efficacy of topical treatments in thick ("moccasin") tinea of the soles

Systemic measures

- Griseofulvin should be used only for severe cases or those recalcitrant to topical therapy
- Itraconazole, 200 mg PO daily for 2 weeks or 400 mg daily for 1 week, or terbinafine, 250 mg PO daily for 2–4 weeks, may be used in refractory cases

THERAPEUTIC PROCEDURES

- Socks should be changed frequently, and absorbent nonsynthetic socks are preferred

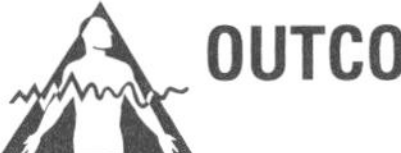

OUTCOME

FOLLOW-UP

- The use of powders containing antifungal agents (eg, Zeasorb-AF) or chronic use of antifungal creams may prevent recurrences, which occur commonly

WHEN TO REFER

- If there is a question about the diagnosis, if recommended therapy is ineffective, or if specialized treatment is necessary

PREVENTION

- The essential factor in prevention is personal hygiene
- Wear open-toed sandals if possible; use of rubber or wooden sandals in community showers and bathing places is often recommended
- Careful drying between the toes after showering is essential; a hair dryer used on low setting may be used

EVIDENCE

WEB SITES

- American Academy of Dermatology: Superficial mycotic infections of the skin: Tinea corporis, tinea cruris, tinea faciei, tinea manuum, and tinea pedis
  - http://www.aad.org/professionals/pracmanage/guidelines/SupMycotic-TineaCorporis-Pedis.htm
- MedlinePlus: Tinea Manuum Image
  - http://www.nlm.nih.gov/medlineplus/ency/imagepages/2531.htm

INFORMATION FOR PATIENTS

- American Academy of Family Physicians: Tinea Infections: Athlete's Foot, Jock Itch and Ringworm
  - http://familydoctor.org/316.xml
- Mayo Clinic: Athlete's Foot
  - http://www.mayoclinic.com/invoke.cfm?objectid=7469E5E7-F7D5-424F-A2552E60CC67C2FF
- MedlinePlus: Athlete's Foot
  - http://www.nlm.nih.gov/medlineplus/ency/article/000875.htm

REFERENCES

- Crawford F et al: Topical treatments for fungal infections of the skin and nails of the foot. Cochrane Database Syst Rev 2000(2):CD001434. [PMID: 10796792]
- Gupta AK et al: Optimal management of fungal infections of the skin, hair, and nails. Am J Clin Dermatol 2004;5:225. [PMID: 15301570]
- Roujeau JC et al: Chronic dermatomycoses of the foot as risk factors for acute bacterial cellulitis of the leg: a case-control study. Dermatology 2004;209:301. [PMID: 15539893]
- Zuber TJ et al: Superficial fungal infection of the skin. Where and how it appears help determine therapy. Postgrad Med 2001;109:117. [PMID: 11198246]

Author(s)

Timothy G. Berger, MD

Tinea Versicolor

KEY FEATURES

ESSENTIALS OF DIAGNOSIS

- Pale macules with fine scales that will not tan, or hyperpigmented macules
- Velvety, tan, pink, whitish, or brown macules that scale with scraping
- Central upper trunk the most frequent site
- Yeast and short hyphae observed on microscopic examination of scales

GENERAL CONSIDERATIONS

- Mild, superficial *Malassezia furfur* infection of the skin (usually of the trunk)
- Patients often first notice that involved areas will not tan, causing hypopigmentation
- High recurrence rate after treatment

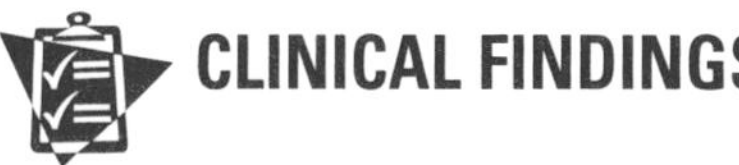

CLINICAL FINDINGS

SYMPTOMS AND SIGNS

- See Table 7
- Lesions are asymptomatic, with occasional itching
- The lesions are velvety, tan, pink, white, or brown macules that vary from 4–5 mm in diameter to large confluent areas
- The lesions initially do not look scaly, but scales may be readily obtained by scraping the area
- Lesions may appear on the trunk, upper arms, neck, face, and groin

DIFFERENTIAL DIAGNOSIS

- Seborrheic dermatitis
- Pityriasis rosea
- Postinflammatory pigmentary change (eg, acne, atopic dermatitis)
- Secondary syphilis
- Hansen's disease (leprosy)
- Vitiligo usually presents with periorificial lesions or lesions on the tips of the fingers; it (and not tinea versicolor) is characterized by total depigmentation, not just a lessening of pigmentation

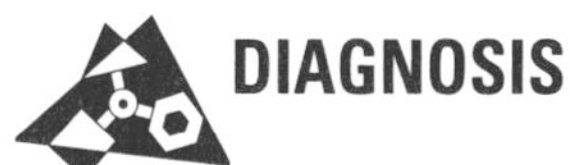

DIAGNOSIS

LABORATORY TESTS

- Large, blunt hyphae and thick-walled budding spores ("spaghetti and meatballs") may be seen under the 10× objective when skin scales have been cleared in 10% KOH
- Fungal culture is not useful

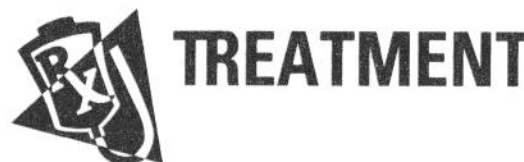

TREATMENT

MEDICATIONS

- See Table 6

Topical treatments

- Selenium sulfide lotion 2.5%, which may be applied from neck to waist daily and left on for 5–15 min for 7 days; this treatment is repeated weekly for a month and then monthly for maintenance
- Ketoconazole shampoo lathered on the chest and back and left on for 5 min may also be used weekly for maintenance
- Tinver lotion (contains sodium thiosulfate) is effective
- Sulfur-salicylic acid soap or shampoo (Sebulex) or zinc pyrithrone-containing shampoos used on a continuing basis may be effective prophylaxis

Systemic therapy

- Ketoconazole, 200 mg daily orally for 1 week or 400 mg as a single oral dose, results in short-term cure of 90% of cases; patients should be instructed not to shower for 8 to 12 h after taking ketoconazole, because it is delivered in sweat to the skin; the single dose may not work in more hot and humid areas

THERAPEUTIC PROCEDURES

- Stress to the patient that the raised and scaly aspects of the rash are being treated; the alterations in pigmentation may take months to fade or fill in
- Irritation and odor from these agents are common complaints from patients

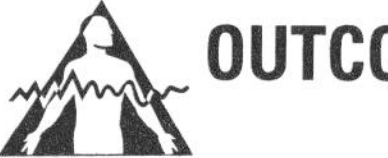

OUTCOME

COMPLICATIONS

- More protracted therapy with ketoconazole carries a small but finite risk of drug-induced hepatitis for a completely benign disease

PROGNOSIS

- Relapses are common: without maintenance therapy, recurrences will occur in over 80% of "cured" cases over the subsequent 2 years

WHEN TO REFER

- If there is a question about the diagnosis, if recommended therapy is ineffective, or if specialized treatment is necessary

EVIDENCE

WEB SITE

- American Academy of Dermatology
  - http://www.aad.org

INFORMATION FOR PATIENTS

- American Academy of Dermatology: Tinea Versicolor
  - http://www.aad.org/public/Publications/pamphlets/TineaVersicolor.htm
- American Medical Association: Fungal Skin Infection
  - http://www.medem.com/search/article_display.cfm?path=TANQUERAYM_ContentItem&mstr=/M_ContentItem/ZZZ8W2QJU9C.html&soc=AMA&srch_typ=NAV_SERCH
- Mayo Clinic: Tinea Versicolor
  - http://www.mayoclinic.com/invoke.cfm?objectid=D22A61A4-6AD5-4A4D-9DE869CA96BA739F
- MedlinePlus: Tinea Versicolor
  - http://www.nlm.nih.gov/medlineplus/ency/article/001465.htm

REFERENCES

- Crawford F et al: Topical treatments for fungal infections of the skin and nails of the foot. Cochrane Database Syst Rev 2000(2):CD001434. [PMID: 10796792]
- Gupta AK et al: Optimal management of fungal infections of the skin, hair, and nails. Am J Clin Dermatol 2004;5:225. [PMID: 15301570]
- Zuber TJ et al: Superficial fungal infection of the skin. Where and how it appears help determine therapy. Postgrad Med 2001;109:117. [PMID: 11198246]

Author(s)

Timothy G. Berger, MD

Tourette's Syndrome

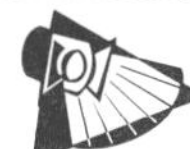

KEY FEATURES

ESSENTIALS OF DIAGNOSIS

- Multiple motor and phonic tics
- Symptoms begin before age 21 years
- Tics occur frequently for at least 1 year
- Tics vary in number, frequency, and nature over time

GENERAL CONSIDERATIONS

- The diagnosis of the disorder is often delayed for years, the tics being interpreted as psychiatric illness or some other form of abnormal movement
- Patients are thus often subjected to unnecessary treatment before the disorder is recognized

DEMOGRAPHICS

- Tics are noted first in childhood, generally between the ages of 2 and 15
- A family history is sometimes obtained
  - Inheritance has been attributed to an autosomal dominant gene with variable penetrance
  - Linkage to 18q22.1 has been noted in some instances

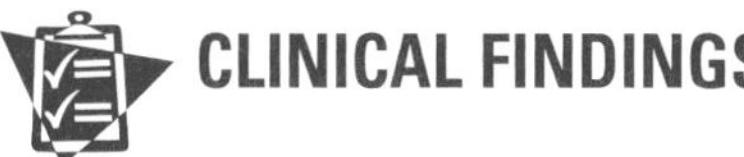

CLINICAL FINDINGS

SYMPTOMS AND SIGNS

- Motor tics
  - Initial manifestation in 80% of cases
  - Most commonly involve the face, head, shoulders, such as sniffing, blinking, frowning, shoulder shrugging, and head thrusting
- Phonic tics
  - Initial symptoms in 20% of cases
  - Commonly consist of grunts, barks, hisses, throat clearing, coughs, verbal utterances including coprolalia (obscene speech)
- All patients ultimately develop a combination of different motor and phonic tics
- Echolalia (repetition of the speech of others)
- Echopraxia (imitation of others' movements)
- Palilalia (repetition of words or phrases)
- Some tics may be self-mutilating in nature, such as
  - Nail-biting
  - Hair-pulling
  - Biting of the lips or tongue
- Obsessive-compulsive behaviors are commonly associated and may be more disabling than the tics themselves
- In addition to obsessive-compulsive behavior disorders, psychiatric disturbances may occur because of the associated cosmetic and social embarrassment

DIFFERENTIAL DIAGNOSIS

- Wilson's disease

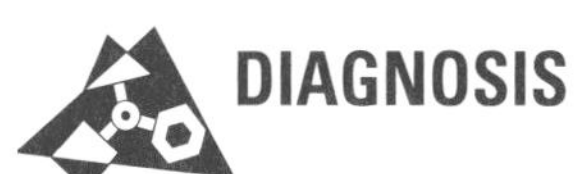

DIAGNOSIS

DIAGNOSTIC PROCEDURES

- Examination usually reveals no abnormalities other than the tics

Tinnitus p. 1159

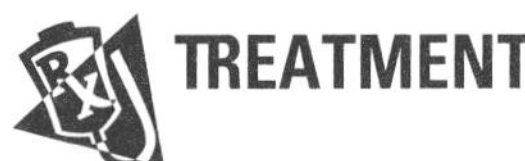

TREATMENT

MEDICATIONS

- Oral clonazepam (in a dose that depends on response and tolerance) or oral clonidine (2–5 μg/kg/day) may be helpful and prevents some of the long-term extrapyramidal side effects of haloperidol
- Haloperidol is started in a low daily dose (0.25 mg PO) that is gradually increased (by 0.25 mg every 4 or 5 days) until there is maximum benefit with a minimum of side effects or until side effects limit further increments
  - A total daily dose of between 2 and 8 mg is usually optimal, but higher doses are sometimes necessary
- Phenothiazines, such as fluphenazine (2–15 mg PO daily), have been used
  - Patients unresponsive to haloperidol are usually unresponsive to phenothiazines as well
- Pimozide is a dopamine-blocking drug related to haloperidol
  - May be helpful in patients who cannot tolerate or have not responded to haloperidol
  - Treatment is started with 1 mg PO daily, and the daily dose increased by 1–2 mg every 10 days
  - The average dose is between 7 and 16 mg daily
- Treatment with risperidone, calcium channel blockers, tetrabenazene, or clomipramine has yielded mixed results
- Injection of botulinum toxin type A at the site of the most distressing tics is sometimes worthwhile
- Bilateral high-frequency thalamic stimulation may help in otherwise intractable cases and is being studied

THERAPEUTIC PROCEDURES

- Treatment is symptomatic and may need to be continued indefinitely

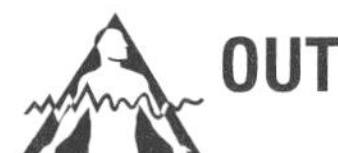

OUTCOME

PROGNOSIS

- The disorder is chronic, but the course may be punctuated by relapses and remissions

WHEN TO REFER

- When the diagnosis is uncertain
- For expertise in management, particularly when patients do not respond to conventional therapy

EVIDENCE

PRACTICE GUIDELINES

- Tourette Syndrome Association
  - http://www.tsa-usa.org/research/guidetodiagnosis.html

INFORMATION FOR PATIENTS

- Mayo Clinic
  - http://www.mayoclinic.com/invoke.cfm?id=DS00541
- National Institute of Neurological Disorders and Stroke
  - http://www.ninds.nih.gov/disorders/tourette/detail_tourette.htm
- Tourette Syndrome Association
  - http://www.tsa-usa.org/what_is/Faqs.html

REFERENCES

- Jankovic J: Tourette's syndrome. N Engl J Med 2001;345;1184. [PMID: 11642235]
- Leckman JF: Tourette's syndrome. Lancet 2002;360:1577. [PMID: 12443611]

Author(s)

Michael J. Aminoff, MD, DSc, FRCP

Toxoplasmosis in the Immunocompetent Patient

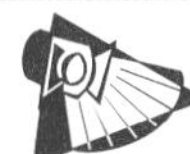

KEY FEATURES

ESSENTIALS OF DIAGNOSIS

Acute primary infection

- Fever, malaise, headache, lymphadenopathy (especially cervical), stiff neck, sore throat; occasionally, rash, hepatosplenomegaly, retinochoroiditis, confusion; in various combinations
- Positive serological tests with high and rising IgG and IgM
- Isolation of *Toxoplasma gondii* from blood or body fluids; tachyzoites in histological sections of tissue or cytological preparations of body fluids

GENERAL CONSIDERATIONS

- *T gondii*, an obligate intracellular protozoan, is found worldwide in humans and many species of animals and birds. The cat is the definitive host
- The parasite exists in three forms: the **trophozoite** (tachyzoite) (3 × 7 μm) is the rapidly proliferating form in tissues that causes acute disease. The **cyst**, containing viable bradyzoites, is the latent form that can persist indefinitely as a chronic infection, particularly in muscle and nerve tissue. The **oocyst** is the form passed only in the feces of the cat family. The oocysts, which contain infective sporozoites, are infectious within 12 h to several days after passage and can remain infective in moist soil for weeks or months
- Human infection results from ingestion of cysts in raw or undercooked meat; from ingestion of oocysts in contaminated food or water, by careless handling of contaminated cat litter, or from soil by soil-eating children; from transplacental transmission of trophozoites; or rarely, from direct inoculation of trophozoites, as in blood transfusion

DEMOGRAPHICS

- Antibody prevalence rates range from less than 5% in some parts of the world (absence of cats and minimal ingestion of meat) to 23% in the United States and over 80% in France

CLINICAL FINDINGS

SYMPTOMS AND SIGNS

- Over 80% of primary infections, including during pregnancy, are asymptomatic
- The incubation period for symptomatic persons is 1–2 weeks
- Generally, on recovery, both asymptomatic and symptomatic infections persist as chronic latent (cyst) infections

Primary infection in the immunocompetent host

- Most symptomatic infections are acute, mild, febrile multisystem illnesses that resemble infectious mononucleosis
- Lymphadenopathy, usually nontender, particularly of the head and neck, is most common
- Other features are malaise, myalgia, arthralgia, headache, sore throat, and maculopapular or urticarial rash
- Hepatosplenomegaly may occur
- Rarely, severe cases are complicated by pneumonitis, meningoencephalitis, hepatitis, myocarditis, polymyositis, and retinochloroditis
- Symptoms may fluctuate, but most patients recover spontaneously within a few weeks

Congenital infection

- Congenital transmission occurs only as a result of infection in a nonimmune (usually asymptomatic) woman during pregnancy

Retinochoroiditis

- Develops gradually weeks to years after congenital infection (generally bilateral) or as an acquired infection in a young child (generally unilateral)
- The inflammatory process may persist for weeks to months in focally necrotic retinal lesions
- Visual defects are accompanied by pain and photophobia
- Rarely, progression results in glaucoma and blindness

DIFFERENTIAL DIAGNOSIS

- Normal host
  - Infectious mononucleosis
  - Cytomegalovirus infection
  - Acute HIV infection
  - Lymphoma
  - Sarcoidosis
  - Tuberculosis
  - Cat-scratch disease
- Immunocompromised
  - CNS lymphoma or metastatic cancer
  - Bacterial brain abscess
  - Fungal brain abscess, eg, *Aspergillus*, histoplasma
  - Cryptococcoma
  - Tuberculoma
  - *Nocardia* brain abscess

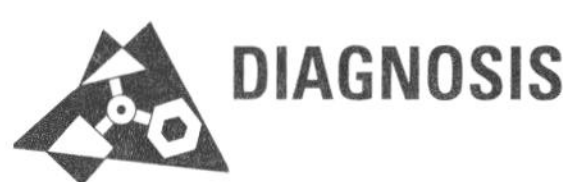

DIAGNOSIS

LABORATORY TESTS

- Diagnosis depends principally on serological tests
- Diagnosis is occasionally made from tissue (blood, bone marrow aspirates, cerebrospinal fluid sediment, sputum, and other tissues or body fluids or placental tissue) either by demonstration of trophozoites or characteristic histology, isolation of the organism in mice (more sensitive) or in tissue culture (more rapid, 3–6 days), or amplification of *T gondii* DNA by polymerase chain reaction (PCR)
- PCR has become particularly useful for testing amniotic fluid for congenital infection and testing immunocompromised patients for recrudescence

Serological tests

- Serological tests can be done on blood, cerebrospinal fluid, aqueous humor, and other body fluids
- Parallel testing of serial blood specimens collected 3–4 weeks apart is necesssary because a single high titer does not confirm the diagnosis
- The ELISA, immunosorbent, and immunofluorescent assay tests separate IgM and IgG antibody
- IgM antibody appears 1–2 weeks after start of infection, reaches a peak at 6–8 weeks, and then gradually declines over 18 months. As IgM antibody can persist for 5 years or longer, a positive finding does not necessarily represent recent infection; however, a negative finding does rule out acute infection
- False positive IgM tests are common and therefore should be confirmed
- IgG antibody appears within 1–2 weeks, peaks in 1–2 months, and may persist at high titers for years and at low levels for life. When positive, it reliably indicates present or past infection; when negative, it reliably rules out any infection
- IgA antibodies can be important in diagnosing acute infection because they rarely are found in chronic infection

Acute infection in immunocompetent patients

- Test initially for IgG antibody, which reliably establishes the presence or absence of infection

Toxic Shock Syndrome, *Staphylococcus aureus* p. 1160

Toxoplasmosis in the Immunocompetent Patient

- The diagnosis is established by seroconversion from negative to positive or by a fourfold rise in serological titers by any test
- A presumptive diagnosis is based on a single IgM titer of over 1:64 and a very high IgG titer (>1:1000). Confirmatory testing should always be done, preferably in a reference laboratory

Toxoplasmic retinochoroiditis

- This is usually associated with stable, usually low IgG titers and no IgM antibody. If IgG antibody in aqueous humor is higher than in the serum, the diagnosis is suspected
- Leukocyte counts are normal or reduced, often with lymphocytosis or monocytosis with rare atypical cells, but there is no heterophil antibody

IMAGING STUDIES

- Chest radiographs may show interstitial pneumonia

TREATMENT

MEDICATIONS

- The treatment of choice is pyrimethamine, 25–100 mg once daily, plus sulfadiazine, 1–1.5 g four times daily; continue this treatment for 3–4 weeks
- Folinic acid (leucovorin), 10–25 mg with each dose of pyrimethamine, should be given concurrently to avoid bone marrow suppression
- Patients should be screened for a history of sulfonamide sensitivity. To prevent crystal-induced nephrotoxicity, good urine output should be maintained; alkalinization with sodium bicarbonate may also be useful
- Pyrimethamine side effects include headache and gastrointestinal symptoms
- Clindamycin (600 mg four times daily) may be a useful alternative drug because it concentrates in the choroid
- Atovaquone (750 mg three or four times daily), dapsone, other macrolides, and immunotherapy are under evaluation
- The lymphadenopathic form of toxoplasmosis is usually not treated unless findings are severe or persist or there is overt visceral disease. If treatment is started, it should continue for 3–4 weeks and then be reassessed. Serological tests are not useful for evaluating the response to treatment
- Since most episodes of retinochoroiditis are self-limited, opinions vary on indications for and type of treatment

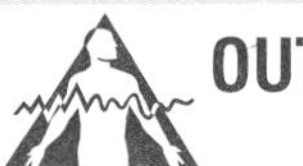

OUTCOME

FOLLOW-UP

- Platelet and white blood cell counts should be performed at least twice weekly while taking pyrimethamine

PROGNOSIS

- The outlook in immunocompetent adults is excellent and chronic asymptomatic infection is usually benign

WHEN TO REFER

- All patients with retinochoroiditis
- Progressive or unresponsive disease on therapy

WHEN TO ADMIT

- Stiff neck, confusion

PREVENTION

- Freezing of meat to –20°C for 2 days or heating to 60°C for 4 min kills cysts in tissues
- Hands, kitchen surfaces, and cooking utensils must be thoroughly cleaned after contact with raw meat
- Children's play areas should be protected from cat (and dog) feces. Indoor cats should be fed only dry, canned, or cooked meat. Litter boxes should be changed daily, as freshly deposited oocysts are not infective for 48 h

EVIDENCE

PRACTICE GUIDELINES

- National Guideline Clearinghouse
  - http://www.guideline.gov/summary/summary.aspx?doc_id=2277&nbr=1503&string=toxoplasmosis
  - http://www.guideline.gov/summary/summary.aspx?doc_id=3080&nbr=2306&string=toxoplasmosis

INFORMATION FOR PATIENTS

- Centers for Disease Control and Prevention
  - http://www.cdc.gov/ncidod/dpd/parasites/toxoplasmosis/factsht_toxoplasmosis.htm
- Center for the Evaluation of Risks to Human Reproduction
  - http://cerhr.niehs.nih.gov/genpub/topics/toxoplasmosis2-ccae.html

REFERENCES

- Derouin F: Anti-toxoplasmosis drugs. Curr Opin Investig Drugs 2001;2:1368. [PMID: 1890349]
- Kopecky D et al: Knowledge-based interpretation of toxoplasmosis serology test results including fuzzy temporal concepts—the Toxonet system. Medinfo 2001;10(Part 1):484. [PMID: 11604787]
- Luder CG et al: Toxoplasmosis: a persisting challenge. Trends Parasitol 2001;17:460. [PMID: 11587941]
- Montoya JG: Laboratory diagnosis of *Toxoplasma gondii* infection and toxoplasmosis. J Infect Dis 2002;185(Suppl 1):S73. [PMID: 11865443]

Toxoplasmosis in the Immunocompromised Patient

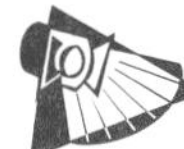

KEY FEATURES

ESSENTIALS OF DIAGNOSIS

- Central nervous system mass lesions; retinochoroiditis, pneumonitis, myocarditis less common
- Positive IgG titers moderately high; IgM antibody usually absent

GENERAL CONSIDERATIONS

- *Toxoplasma gondii*, an obligate intracellular protozoan, is found worldwide in humans and many species of animals and birds. The cat is the definitive host
- The parasite exists in three forms
  - The **trophozoite** (tachyzoite) (3 × 7 μm) is the rapidly proliferating form in tissues that causes acute disease
  - The **cyst**, containing viable bradyzoites, is the latent form that can persist indefinitely as a chronic infection, particularly in muscle and nerve tissue
  - The **oocyst** is the form passed only in the feces of the cat family. The oocysts, which contain infective sporozoites, are infectious within 12 h to several days after passage and can remain infective in moist soil for weeks or months
- Human infection results from ingestion of cysts in raw or undercooked meat; from ingestion of oocysts in contaminated food or water, by careless handling of contaminated cat litter, or from soil by soil-eating children; from transplacental transmission of trophozoites; or rarely, from direct inoculation of trophozoites, as in blood transfusion

DEMOGRAPHICS

- Antibody prevalence rates range from less than 5% in some parts of the world (absence of cats and minimal ingestion of meat) to 15–29% in the United States and over 80% in France

CLINICAL FINDINGS

SYMPTOMS AND SIGNS

- Over 80% of primary infections are asymptomatic
- The incubation period for symptomatic persons is 1–2 weeks
- Generally, on recovery, both asymptomatic and symptomatic infections persist as chronic latent (cyst) infections

Reactivated disease in the immunologically compromised host

- Occurs in patients with AIDS, cancer, or those given immunosuppressive drugs
- The infection may present in specific organs (brain, lungs, and eye most commonly, but also heart, skin, gastrointestinal tract, and liver) or as disseminated disease
- Between 30% and 50% of AIDS patients seropositive for past *Toxoplasma* infection will develop meningeal (uncommon), mass (single or multiple), or diffuse intracerebral *Toxoplasma* lesions, associated with clinical findings of fever, headache, altered mental status, seizures, and focal (or, infrequently, nonfocal) neurological deficits

DIFFERENTIAL DIAGNOSIS

- Normal host
  - Infectious mononucleosis
  - Cytomegalovirus infection
  - Acute HIV infection
  - Lymphoma
  - Sarcoidosis
  - Tuberculosis
  - Cat-scratch disease
- Immunocompromised
  - CNS lymphoma or metastatic cancer
  - Bacterial brain abscess
  - Fungal brain abscess, eg, *Aspergillus*, histoplasma
  - Cryptococcoma
  - Tuberculoma
  - *Nocardia* brain abscess

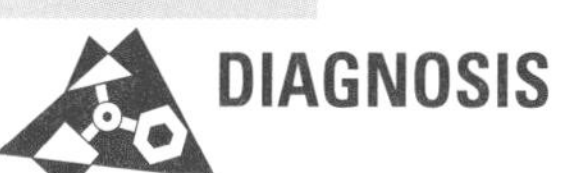

DIAGNOSIS

LABORATORY TESTS

- Diagnosis depends principally on serological tests
- Diagnosis is occasionally made from tissue (blood, bone marrow aspirates, cerebrospinal fluid sediment, sputum, and other tissues or body fluids or placental tissue) either by demonstration of trophozoites or characteristic histology, isolation of the organism in mice (more sensitive) or in tissue culture (more rapid, 3–6 days), or amplification of *T gondii* DNA by polymerase chain reaction

Serological tests

- Serological tests can be done on blood, cerebrospinal fluid, aqueous humor, and other body fluids
- Parallel testing of serial blood specimens collected 3–4 weeks apart is necesssary because a single high titer does not confirm the diagnosis
- The ELISA, immunosorbent, and immunofluorescent assay tests separate IgM and IgG antibody
- IgM antibody appears 1–2 weeks after start of infection, reaches a peak at 6–8 weeks, and then gradually declines over 18 months. As IgM antibody can persist for 5 years or longer, a positive finding does not necessarily represent recent infection; however, a negative finding does rule out acute infection
- False positive IgM tests are common and therefore should be confirmed
- IgG antibody appears within 1–2 weeks, peaks in 1–2 months, and may persist at high titers for years and at low levels for life. When positive, it reliably indicates present or past infection; when negative, it reliably rules out any infection
- IgA antibodies can be important in diagnosing acute infection because they rarely are found in chronic infection

Recrudescent infection in immunosuppressed patients

- Antibody titers cannot be depended on, since most patients have IgG titers that reflect past infection, significant rises are infrequent, and IgM antibody is rare
- Absence of IgG does not rule out the diagnosis of toxoplasmic retinochoroiditis or encephalitis
- The cerebrospinal fluid may show mild pleocytosis (predominantly lymphocytes and monocytes), elevated protein, and normal glucose

- In AIDS patients, *Toxoplasma* can sometimes be isolated from the blood or in cerebrospinal fluid (Wright-Giemsa stain or by PCR amplification)
- The diagnosis is presumed if the patient responds to empirical antibiotic treatment after a suggestive brain MRI is obtained

IMAGING STUDIES

- Chest radiographs may show interstitial pneumonia
- In HIV-infected persons, cerebral toxoplasmosis typically appears as multiple lesions with a predilection for the basal ganglion by MRI (the more sensitive test) or CT scan (typically: multiple, isodense or hypodense, ring-enhancing mass lesions)

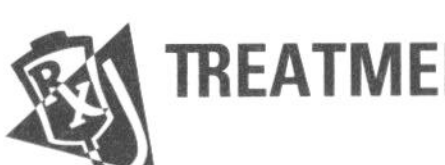

TREATMENT

MEDICATIONS

- Immunocompromised patients with active infection (primary or recrudescent) must be treated (Table 123)
- Therapy should continue for 4–6 weeks after cessation of symptoms—which may require up to a 6-month course, to be followed by drug prophylaxis as long as immunosuppression persists
- In HIV-infected persons, acute toxoplasmosis must be treated followed by continued prophylaxis; if there is positive IgG *Toxoplasma* serology but no symptoms, prophylaxis is desirable
- For prophylaxis, treat with trimethoprim-sulfamethoxazole (one double-strength tablet daily) or a combination of pyrimethamine, 25 mg orally once a week, plus dapsone, 100 mg orally daily

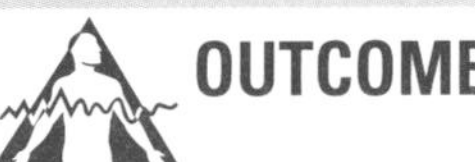

OUTCOME

PROGNOSIS

- In immunosuppressed patients, the disease is usually fatal if untreated; improvement occurs with early treatment, but recrudescence is common

WHEN TO REFER

- Refer to a clinician with expertise in this field

WHEN TO ADMIT

- Central nervous system symptoms
- Respiratory compromise

PREVENTION

- Freezing of meat to –20°C for 2 days or heating to 60°C for 4 min kills cysts in tissues
- Hands, kitchen surfaces, and cooking utensils must be thoroughly cleaned after contact with raw meat
- Children's play areas should be protected from cat (and dog) feces
- Indoor cats should be fed only dry, canned or cooked meet. Litter boxes should be changed daily, as freshly deposited oocysts are not infective for 48 h

EVIDENCE

PRACTICE GUIDELINES

- National Guideline Clearinghouse
  - http://www.guideline.gov/summary/summary.aspx?doc_id=3080
  - http://www.guideline.gov/summary/summary.aspx?.doc_id=3821

WEB SITE

- CDC—Division of Parasitic Diseases
  - http://www.cdc.gov/ncidod/dpd/parasites/toxoplasmosis/default.htm

INFORMATION FOR PATIENTS

- American Academy of Family Physicians
  - http://familydoctor.org/793.xml
- Centers for Disease Control
  - http://www.cdc.gov/ncidod/dpd/parasites/toxoplasmosis/factsht_toxoplasmosis.htm

REFERENCES

- Derouin F: Anti-toxoplasmosis drugs. Curr Opin Investig Drugs 2001;2:1368. [PMID: 11890349]
- Julander I et al: Polymerase chain reaction for diagnosis of cerebral toxoplasmosis in cerebrospinal fluid in HIV-positive patients. Scand J Infect Dis 2001;33:538. [PMID: 11515766]
- Kopecky D et al: Knowledge-based interpretation of toxoplasmosis serology test results including fuzzy temporal concepts—the Toxonet system. Medinfo 2001;10(Part 1):484. [PMID: 11604787]
- Montoya JG: Laboratory diagnosis of *Toxoplasma gondii* infection and toxoplasmosis. J Infect Dis 2002;185(Suppl 1):S73. [PMID: 11865443]

Transient Ischemic Attack

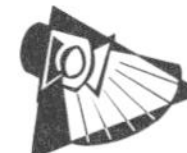

KEY FEATURES

ESSENTIALS OF DIAGNOSIS

- Acute, focal neurologic deficit
- Clinical deficit resolves completely within 24 hours

GENERAL CONSIDERATIONS

- Focal, ischemic, cerebral neurologic deficits that last for less than 24 hours (usually less than 1–2 hours)
- Embolization is an important etiology and may explain why separate attacks may affect different parts of the territory supplied by the same vessel
- Cardiac embolic sources
  - Rheumatic heart disease
  - Mitral valve disease
  - Cardiac arrhythmia
  - Infective endocarditis
  - Atrial myxoma
  - Mural thrombi after MI
  - Atrial septal defects and patent foramen ovale may permit emboli from the veins to reach the brain ("paradoxical emboli")
- Cerebrovascular sources
  - An ulcerated plaque on a major artery to the brain may be a source of emboli
  - In the anterior circulation, atherosclerotic changes occur most commonly near the carotid bifurcation extracranially and may cause a bruit
  - Other (less common) abnormalities of blood vessels that may cause transient ischemic attacks (TIAs)
    1. Fibromuscular dysplasia (particularly affects the cervical internal carotid artery)
    2. Atherosclerosis of the aortic arch
    3. Inflammatory arterial disorders such as giant cell arteritis, systemic lupus erythematosus, polyarteritis, and granulomatous angiitis
    4. Meningovascular syphilis
- Hypotension may reduce cerebral blood flow and rarely cause a TIA if a major extracranial artery to the brain is markedly stenosed
- The subclavian steal syndrome may lead to transient vertebrobasilar ischemia from stenosis or occlusion of one subclavian artery proximal to the source of the vertebral artery
- Hematologic causes
  - Polycythemia
  - Sickle cell disease
  - Hyperviscosity

DEMOGRAPHICS

- Proper treatment of TIAs can help prevent strokes
- About 30% of patients with stroke have a history of TIAs
- Risk of stroke is highest within one month after a TIA and then progressively declines
- Incidence of stroke is not related to the number or duration of individual TIAs but is increased in patients with hypertension or diabetes

CLINICAL FINDINGS

SYMPTOMS AND SIGNS

- Symptoms vary markedly among patients, but tend to be consistent in a given individual
- Onset abrupt, and recovery often occurs within a few minutes
- TIA in the carotid territory may manifest with
  - Weakness and heaviness of the contralateral arm, leg, or face, singly or in combination
  - Numbness or paresthesias may occur either as sole manifestation or with motor deficits
  - Dysphagia
  - Visual loss in the eye contralateral to affected limbs may occur
  - During an attack, examination may reveal flaccid weakness with pyramidal distribution, sensory changes, hyperreflexia or an extensor plantar response on the affected side, dysphasia, or any combination of these
  - A carotid bruit or cardiac abnormality may be present
- Vertebrobasilar TIA may manifest with
  - Vertigo
  - Ataxia
  - Diplopia
  - Dysarthria
  - Dimness or blurring of vision
  - Perioral numbness and paresthesias
  - Weakness or sensory complaints on one, both, or alternating sides of the body
  - Drop attacks due to bilateral leg weakness, without headache or loss of consciousness, may occur, in relation to head movements
  - Attacks may occur intermittently and stop spontaneously
- Findings in the subclavian steal syndrome may include
  - A bruit in the supraclavicular fossa,
  - Unequal radial pulses
  - A difference of 20 mm Hg or more between the systolic blood pressures in the arms

DIFFERENTIAL DIAGNOSIS

- Stroke
- Hypoglycemia
- Focal seizure (Todd's paralysis)
- Syncope
- Migraine
- Peripheral causes of vertigo (eg, Ménière's disease)

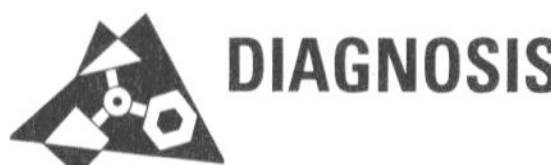

DIAGNOSIS

LABORATORY TESTS

- Complete blood cell count
- Fasting blood glucose and serum cholesterol and homocysteine
- Serologic test for syphilis
- Blood cultures if endocarditis is suspected

IMAGING STUDIES

- Chest x-ray
- CT scan of the head excludes cerebral hemorrhage or a rare tumor masquerading as a TIA
- Carotid duplex ultrasonography can detect significant stenosis of the internal carotid artery
- MR angiography may reveal stenotic lesions of large vessels
  - Less sensitive than conventional arteriography
- Patients with vertebrobasilar TIA are treated medically and are not subjected to arteriography unless there is clinical evidence of stenosis in carotid or subclavian arteries
- Echocardiography with bubble contrast is performed if a cardiac source is likely

DIAGNOSTIC PROCEDURES

- ECG
- Holter monitoring if a paroxysmal cardiac arrhythmia is suspected
- Assessment for hypertension, heart disease, hematologic disorders, diabetes mellitus, hyperlipidemia, and peripheral vascular disease

Tracheal Stenosis p. 1160

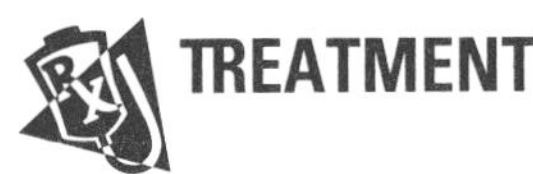

TREATMENT

MEDICATIONS

Embolization from the heart

- Anticoagulants should be started immediately unless contraindicated
- The fear of causing hemorrhage into an infarcted area is misplaced, since there is a far greater risk of further embolism to the cerebral circulation if treatment is withheld
- Use IV heparin (loading dose of 5000–10,000 units of standard molecular weight heparin, and maintenance infusion of 1000–2000 units/hour, depending on the partial thromboplastin time) while warfarin is introduced
- Warfarin is more effective than aspirin in reducing the incidence of cardioembolic events, but when contraindicated, aspirin (325 mg PO QD) may be used in nonrheumatic atrial fibrillation

Embolization from the cerebrovascular system

- In presumed or angiographically verified atherosclerotic changes in the extracranial or intracranial cerebrovascular circulation, antithrombotic medication is prescribed
- Treatment with aspirin, 325 mg PO QD, significantly reduces the frequency of TIA and stroke
- Dipyridamole added to aspirin does not offer any advantage over aspirin alone
- In patients intolerant of aspirin, clopidogrel may be used
- There is no convincing evidence that anticoagulant drugs are of value

SURGERY

- When there is a surgically accessible high-grade stenosis (70–99% in luminal diameter) on the side appropriate to carotid ischemic attacks and there is relatively little atherosclerosis elsewhere in the cerebrovascular system, carotid endarterectomy reduces the risk of ipsilateral carotid stroke, especially when TIAs are of recent onset (< 2 months)
- Surgery is not indicated for mild stenosis (< 30%); its benefits are unclear with severe stenosis plus diffuse intracranial atherosclerotic disease
- Surgical extracranial-intracranial arterial anastomosis is generally not helpful in TIAs associated with stenotic lesions of the distal internal carotid or the proximal middle cerebral arteries

THERAPEUTIC PROCEDURES

- Treatment is to prevent further TIAs and stroke
- Cigarette smoking should be stopped
- Cardiac sources of embolization, hypertension, diabetes, hyperlipidemia, arteritis, or hematologic disorders should be treated appropriately

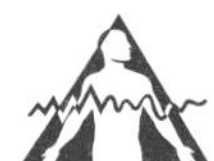

OUTCOME

PROGNOSIS

- In general, carotid TIAs are more likely than vertebrobasilar TIAs to be followed by stroke
- The stroke risk is greater
  - In patients older than 60 years
  - In diabetics
  - After TIAs that last longer than 10 minutes
  - With symptoms or signs of weakness, speech impairment, or gait disturbance

WHEN TO REFER

- If CT scan is normal, there is no cardiac source of embolization, and patient is a good operative risk, refer for possible endarterectomy

PREVENTION

- Anticoagulation of atrial fibrillation (except lone atrial fibrillation)
- Control of hypertension
- Control of lipids

EVIDENCE

PRACTICE GUIDELINES

- Adams RJ et al: Coronary risk evaluation in patients with transient ischemic attack and ischemic stroke: a scientific statement for healthcare professionals from the Stroke Council and the Council on Clinical Cardiology of the American Heart Association/American Stroke Association. Stroke 2003;34(9):2310. [PMID:12958318]
- Albers GW et al: Antithrombotic and thrombolytic therapy for ischemic stroke: the Seventh ACCP Conference on Antithrombotic and Thrombolytic Therapy. Chest 2004;126(3 Suppl):483S. [PMID:15383482]

WEB SITES

- Carotid Artery Stenosis Demonstration Case
  - http://www.brighamrad.harvard.edu/Cases/bwh/hcache/6/full.html
- Transient Ischemic Attacks
  - http://path.upmc.edu/cases/case114.html

INFORMATION FOR PATIENTS

- American Heart Association
  - http://www.americanheart.org/presenter.jhtml?identifier=4781
- Mayo Clinic
  - http://www.mayoclinic.com/invoke.cfm?id=DS00220
- National Institute of Neurological Disorders and Stroke
  - http://www.ninds.nih.gov/disorders/tia/tia.htm

REFERENCES

- Algra A et al: Oral anticoagulants versus antiplatelet therapy for preventing further vascular events after transient ischemic attack or minor stroke of presumed arterial origin. Stroke 2003;34:234. [PMID:12511782]
- Johnston SC et al: Transient ischemic attack. N Engl J Med 2002;347:1687. [PMID:12444184]

Author(s)

Michael J. Aminoff, MD, DSc, FRCP

Trichinosis

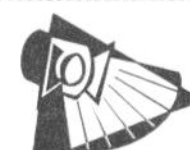

KEY FEATURES

ESSENTIALS OF DIAGNOSIS

- History of ingestion of raw or inadequately cooked pork, boar, or bear

First week

- Diarrhea, cramps, malaise

Second week to 1–2 months

- Muscle pain and tenderness, fever, periorbital and facial edema, conjunctivitis
- Eosinophilia and elevated serum enzymes; positive serological tests; larvae in muscle biopsy

GENERAL CONSIDERATIONS

- Caused worldwide by *Trichinella spiralis.* Four other species also identified
- Infection is usually acquired by eating viable encysted larvae in uncooked pork
- In some cases, the source of infection is the flesh of dogs (East Asia), horses (France), or wild animals, particularly bears, walruses, bush pigs, foxes, or cougars (United States)
- The adult worms (2–3.6 mm × 75–90 μm) survive for up to about 6 weeks
- In the natural cycle, larvae develop into adult worms in the intestines when a carnivore ingests parasitized muscle

DEMOGRAPHICS

- The disease is present wherever pork is eaten but is a greater problem in many temperate areas than in the tropics
- In the United States, there has been a marked reduction in prevalence in pigs (rates in commercial pork are 0–0.01%) and in incidence in humans; only about 10 human infections are reported yearly, 60% in association with eating wild game, mainly bear

CLINICAL FINDINGS

SYMPTOMS AND SIGNS

- The incubation period is 2–7 days (range: 12 h to 28 days)
- Findings range from asymptomatic to a mild short-lasting febrile illness to a severe multisystem illness that in rare cases is fatal

Intestinal stage

- When present, malaise, diarrhea, and abdominal cramps persist for 1–7 days; nausea and vomiting may occur
- Fever is rare

Muscle invasion stage

- This begins at the end of the first week and lasts about 6 weeks
- Findings include fever (low-grade to marked); muscle pain and tenderness, edema, and spasm; periorbital and facial edema; sweating; photophobia and conjunctivitis; weakness; pain on swallowing; dyspnea, coughing, and hoarseness; nail and subconjunctival hemorrhages; and rashes
- The most frequently parasitized muscles are the masseters, tongue, diaphragm, intercostal muscles, and extraocular, laryngeal, paravertebral, nuchal, deltoid, pectoral, gluteus, biceps, and gastrocnemius. Meningitis, encephalitis, myocarditis, bronchopneumonia, nephritis, and peripheral and cranial nerve disorders

Convalescent stage

- This generally begins in the second month but in severe infections may not begin before 3 months or longer
- Vague muscle pains for months
- Permanent muscular atrophy can occur

DIFFERENTIAL DIAGNOSIS

- Eosinophilia-myalgia syndrome
- Eosinophilic fasciitis
- Dermatomyositis
- Influenza
- Polyarteritis nodosa
- Viral gastroenteritis
- Polymyalgia rheumatica
- Fibromyalgia
- Sarcocystosis

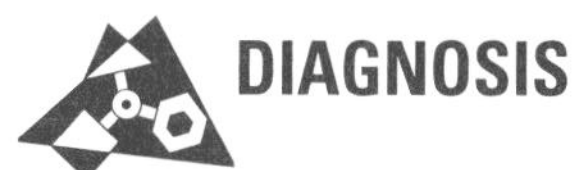

DIAGNOSIS

LABORATORY TESTS

- Elevated serum muscle enzymes (creatine kinase, lactate dehydrogenase, aspartate aminotransferase)
- There may be a marked hypergammaglobulinemia
- Absence of an elevated sedimentation rate is a useful diagnostic clue
- Leukocytosis and eosinophilia appear during the second week. The proportion of eosinophils rises to a maximum of 20–90% in the third or fourth week and then slowly declines to normal over the next few months
- Serological tests can detect most clinically manifest cases but are not sufficiently sensitive to detect low-level infections. Circulating antigen can be detected about 2 weeks after infection in heavily infected persons and in 3–4 weeks in light infections
- More than one antibody test should be used and then repeated to observe for seroconversion or for a rising titer. The bentonite flocculation (BF) test (positive titer, ≥1:5) is highly sensitive and is considered nearly 100% specific. It becomes positive in the third or fourth week, and reaches a maximum titer at about 2 months, and generally reverts to negative in 2–3 years. The immunofluorescence test (positive titer >16) is also highly sensitive, though less specific than the BF test; it may become positive in the second week. The IgM and IgG ELISAs also show high sensitivity and specificity
- Adult worms may be looked for in feces, though they are seldom found. In the second week, there are occasional larvae in blood, duodenal washings, and, rarely, in centrifuged spinal fluid

IMAGING STUDIES

- Chest films during the acute phase may show disseminated or localized infiltrates
- Late calcification of muscle cysts cannot be detected radiologically

DIAGNOSTIC PROCEDURES

- Confirmation of the diagnosis is by detection of larvae in muscle biopsies
- In the third to fourth weeks, biopsy of skeletal muscle (approximately 1 cm^3) may be definitive (particularly gastrocnemius and pectoralis), preferably at a site of swelling or tenderness or near tendinous insertions. Portions of the specimen should be examined micro-

scopically by compression between glass slides, by digestion, and by preparation of multiple histological sections. If the biopsy is done too early, larvae may not be detectable. Myositis even in the absence of larvae is a significant finding

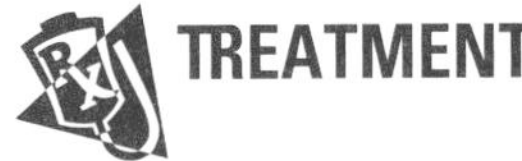

TREATMENT

MEDICATIONS

Intestinal phase

- Albendazole is the drug of choice in a dosage of 400 mg PO BID for 10 days
- Mebendazole is an alternative drug at a dosage of 200–300 mg PO TID for 3 days, followed by 400–500 mg PO TID for 10 days
- A third alternative drug is thiabendazole at a dosage of 25 mg/kg (maximum, 1.5 g per dose) twice daily after meals for 3–7 days; side effects, sometimes severe, are common
- Corticosteroids are contraindicated in the intestinal phase

Muscle invasion phase

- Severe infections require hospitalization and high doses of corticosteroids (40–60 mg/day for 1–2 days), followed by lower doses for several days or weeks to control symptoms. However, because corticosteroids may suppress the inflammatory response to adult worms, they should be used only when symptoms are severe
- Although specific drug treatment has not been shown to be effective in the muscle invasion stage, albendazole, mebendazole, or thiabendazole can be tried

THERAPEUTIC PROCEDURES

- Treatment is principally supportive, since in most cases recovery is spontaneous without sequelae

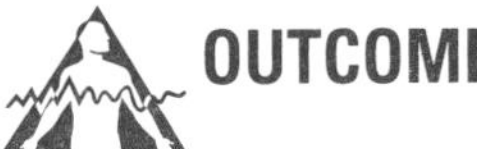

OUTCOME

FOLLOW-UP

- Antibody tests should be repeated to observe for seroconversion or for a rising titer

COMPLICATIONS

- Granulomatous pneumonitis
- Encephalitis
- Cardiac failure

PROGNOSIS

- Death is rare—sometimes within 2–3 weeks in overwhelming infections, more often in 4–8 weeks from a major complication such as cardiac failure or pneumonia

WHEN TO ADMIT

- Patients with severe muscle infections

PREVENTION

- The disease has been significantly reduced where public health measures prevent feeding of uncooked garbage to hogs and by animal inspections
- The primary safeguard is either adequate cooking of pork to 160°F (71°C) or freezing meat at –17°C for 20 days (longer if meat is over 15 cm thick). *T nativa* in game is often relatively resistant to freezing
- Low doses of gamma-irradiation are effective in killing larvae

EVIDENCE

PRACTICE GUIDELINES

- Gamble HR et al: International Commission on Trichinellosis: recommendations on methods for the control of *Trichinella* in domestic and wild animals intended for human consumption. Vet Parasitol 2000;93:393. PMID: 11099850

WEB SITE

- CDC—Division of Parasitic Diseases
  - http://www.cdc.gov/ncidod/dpd/parasites/trichinosis/default.htm

INFORMATION FOR PATIENTS

- Centers for Disease Control and Prevention
  - http://www.cdc.gov/ncidod/dpd/parasites/trichinosis/factsht_trichinosis.htm
- National Institutes of Health
  - http://www.nlm.nih.gov/medlineplus/ency/article/000631.htm

REFERENCES

- Bruschi F et al: New aspects of human trichinellosis: the impact of new *Trichinella* species. Postgrad Med J 2002;78:15. [PMID: 11796866]
- Kociecka W: Trichinellosis: human disease, diagnosis and treatment. Vet Parasitol 2000;93:365. [PMID: 11099848]
- Vojnikovic B et al: Severe trichinellosis cured with pulse doses of glucocorticoids. Coll Antropol 2001;25(Suppl):131. [PMID: 11817004]
- Watt G et al: Blinded, placebo-controlled trial of antiparasitic drugs for trichinosis myositis. J Infect Dis 2000;182:371. [PMID: 10882628]

Trichuriasis

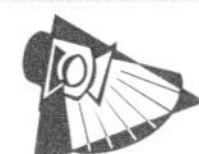

KEY FEATURES

ESSENTIALS OF DIAGNOSIS

- Light to moderate infections are generally asymptomatic
- Heavy infections can cause dysentery and blood loss in the stool
- The *Trichuris* dysentery syndrome is marked dysentery, anemia, rectal prolapse, clubbing of fingers, and growth stunting

GENERAL CONSIDERATIONS

- The slender worms, 30–50 mm in length, attach by means of their anterior whip-like end to the mucosa of the large intestine, particularly to the cecum
- Eggs are passed in the feces but require 2–4 weeks for larval development after reaching the soil before becoming infective; thus, person-to-person transmission is not possible
- Infections are acquired by ingestion of the infective egg. The larvae hatch in the small intestine and mature in the large bowel but do not migrate through the tissues

DEMOGRAPHICS

- *Trichuris trichiura* is a common intestinal parasite of humans throughout the world, particularly in the subtropics and tropics
- Persons of all ages are affected

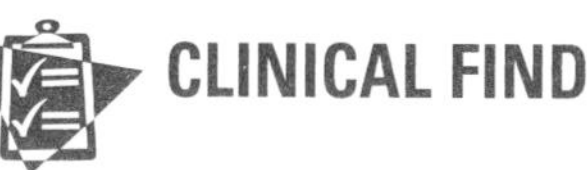

CLINICAL FINDINGS

SYMPTOMS AND SIGNS

- Light (fewer than 10,000 eggs per gram of feces) to moderate infections rarely cause symptoms
- Heavy infections (30,000 or more eggs per gram of feces) may be accompanied by abdominal cramps, tenesmus, diarrhea, distention, flatulence, and nausea and vomiting
- With persistent dysentery and blood loss into the stool, the *Trichuris* dysentery syndrome can appear, which is accompanied by anemia, rectal prolapse, clubbing of fingers, growth stunting, and possibly cognitive defects
- Adult worms are sometimes seen in stools
- Invasion of the appendix, with resulting appendicitis, is rare

DIFFERENTIAL DIAGNOSIS

- Lactase deficiency
- Giardiasis
- Tapeworm, eg, *Hymenolepis nana*
- Hookworm disease (with iron deficiency anemia)
- Strongyloidiasis
- Celiac sprue or tropical sprue

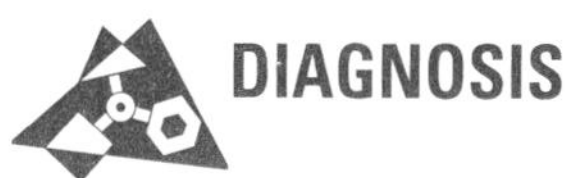

DIAGNOSIS

LABORATORY TESTS

- Diagnosis is by identification of characteristic eggs and, sometimes, adult worms in stools
- Eosinophilia (5–20%) is common with all but light infections
- Charcot-Leyden crystals may be seen in stool
- Severe iron deficiency anemia may be present with heavy infections

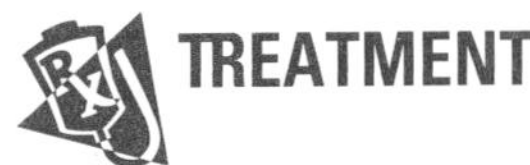

TREATMENT

MEDICATIONS

- Patients with asymptomatic light infections do not require treatment
- For those with heavier or symptomatic infections, give mebendazole or albendazole. Thiabendazole should *not* be used because it is not effective and because it is potentially toxic
- Iron replacement may be needed for anemia

Albendazole

- A single oral dose of 400 mg has resulted in cure rates of 33–90%, with marked reduction in egg counts in those not cured
- Daily treatment for 3 days improves cure rates
- Albendazole should not be used in pregnancy

Mebendazole

- Oral dosage of 100 mg twice daily before or after meals for 3 days results in cure rates of 60–80%, with marked reduction in ovum counts in the remaining patients
- There may be an advantage for the tablets to be chewed before swallowing
- In mild disease, a 500-mg oral dose may be sufficient, whereas in severe trichuriasis a longer course of treatment (up to 6 days) or a repeat course will often be necessary
- Gastrointestinal side effects from the drug are rare
- The drug is contraindicated in pregnancy

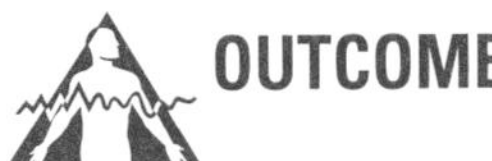

OUTCOME

PROGNOSIS

- The prognosis is excellent with treatment

EVIDENCE

WEB SITE

- CDC—Division of Parasitic Diseases
  - http://www.cdc.gov/ncidod/dpd/parasites/whipworm/default.htm

INFORMATION FOR PATIENTS

- Centers for Disease Control and Prevention
  - http://www.dpd.cdc.gov/dpdx/HTML/Trichuriasis.htm
- National Institutes of Health
  - http://www.nlm.nih.gov/medlineplus/ency/article/001364.htm

REFERENCES

- Crompton DW et al: Nutritional impact of intestinal helminthiasis during the human life cycle. Annu Rev Nutr 2002;22:35. [PMID: 12055337]
- Pedersen S et al: Whipworm-nutrition interaction. Trends Parasitol 2001;17(10):470. [PMID: 11642259]

Trigeminal Neuralgia

KEY FEATURES

ESSENTIALS OF DIAGNOSIS

- Brief episodes of stabbing facial pain
- Pain is in the territory of the second and third division of the trigeminal nerve
- Pain exacerbated by touch

GENERAL CONSIDERATIONS

- Trigeminal neuralgia (tic douloureux) is most common in middle and later life
- It affects women more frequently than men

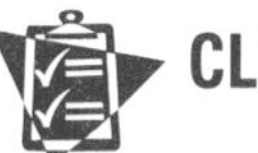

CLINICAL FINDINGS

SYMPTOMS AND SIGNS

- Momentary episodes of sudden lancinating facial pain
- Commonly arises near one side of the mouth and shoots toward the ear, eye, or nostril on that side
- The pain may be triggered by touch, movement, drafts, and eating. To prevent further attacks, many patients try to hold the face still
- Symptoms remain confined to the distribution of the trigeminal nerve (usually the second or third division) on one side only
- Neurologic examination shows no abnormality unless trigeminal neuralgia is symptomatic of some underlying lesion, such as multiple sclerosis or a brainstem neoplasm

DIFFERENTIAL DIAGNOSIS

- Atypical facial pain
  - Especially common in middle-aged women
  - Generally a constant burning pain that may have a restricted distribution at onset but soon spreads to the rest of the face on the affected side and sometimes involves the other side of the face, the neck, and the back of the head as well
- Temporomandibular joint dysfunction
  - Occurs with malocclusion, abnormal bite, or faulty dentures
  - May cause tenderness of the masticatory muscles
  - An association between pain onset and jaw movement
  - Diagnosis requires dental examination and x-rays
- Giant cell arteritis—may have pain on mastication
- Sinusitis and ear infections
- Glaucoma
- Multiple sclerosis
- Brainstem tumor
- Dental caries or abscess
- Otitis media
- Glossopharyngeal neuralgia
- Postherpetic neuralgia

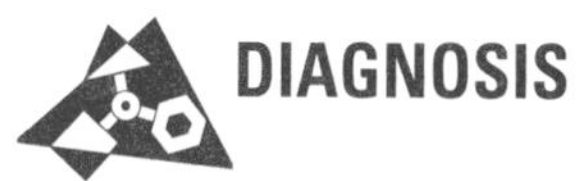

DIAGNOSIS

IMAGING STUDIES

- CT scans and cerebral MRIs are normal in patients with classic trigeminal neuralgia but should nevertheless be performed to exclude structural causes

DIAGNOSTIC PROCEDURES

- The characteristic features of the pain in trigeminal neuralgia usually distinguish it from other causes of facial pain
- In a young patient presenting with trigeminal neuralgia, multiple sclerosis must be suspected even if there are no other neurologic signs
  - In such a patient, findings on evoked potential testing, head MRI, and examination of cerebrospinal fluid may be corroborative

Tricyclic Antidepressant Overdose p. 1161.

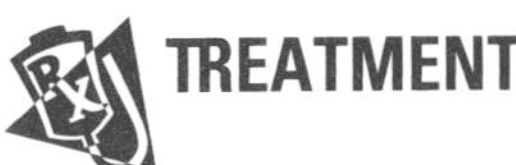

TREATMENT

MEDICATIONS

- Oxcarbazepine or carbamazepine is most helpful (monitor blood cell counts and liver function tests)
- Phenytoin is second choice (Table 98)
- Baclofen (10–20 mg PO three or four times daily) may be helpful, alone or in combination with carbamazepine or phenytoin
- Gabapentin up to 2400 mg PO/day is given in divided doses may relieve pain in patients refractory to conventional therapy and those with multiple sclerosis

SURGERY

- Surgical exploration, radiofrequency rhizotomy, and gamma radiosurgery should be reserved for specialized centers

OUTCOME

PROGNOSIS

- Spontaneous remissions for several months or longer may occur
- Progression of the disorder
  - Episodes of pain become more frequent
  - Remissions become shorter and less common
  - A dull ache may persist between the episodes of stabbing pain

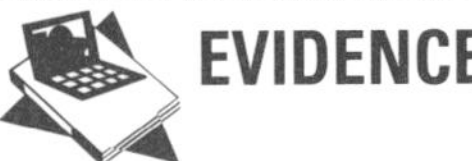

EVIDENCE

PRACTICE GUIDELINES

- National Guideline Clearinghouse
  - http://www.guideline.gov/summary/summary.aspx?doc_id=4671&nbr=3405&string=trigeminal+AND+neuralgia
  - http://www.guideline.gov/summary/summary.aspx?doc_id=4111&nbr=3156&string=trigeminal+AND+neuralgia

INFORMATION FOR PATIENTS

- The Mayo Clinic
  - http://www.mayoclinic.com/invoke.cfm?id=DS00446
- National Institute of Neurological Disorders and Stroke
  - http://www.ninds.nih.gov/disorders/trigemin/trigemin.htm

REFERENCES

- Kondziolka DE et al: Stereotactic radiosurgery for the treatment of trigeminal neuralgia. Clin J Pain 2002;18;42. [PMID: 11803302]
- Liu JK, Apfelbaum RI: Treatment of trigeminal neuralgia. Neurosurg Clin North Am 2004;15:319. [PMID: 15246340]
- Rozen TD: Trigeminal neuralgia and glossopharyngeal neuralgia. Neurol Clin 2004;22:185. [PMID: 15062534]
- Sindrup SH et al: Pharmacotherapy of trigeminal neuralgia. Clin J Pain 2002;18;22. [PMID: 11803299]

Author(s)

Michael J. Aminoff, DSc, MD, FRCP

Trypanosomiasis, African (*T b gambiense*)

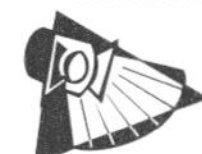

KEY FEATURES

ESSENTIALS OF DIAGNOSIS

- History of exposure to tsetse flies with bite lesion usually absent
- Hemolymphatic stage symptoms usually absent
- Trypanosomes in blood or lymph node aspirates; positive serology

Meningoencephalitic stage

- Insomnia
- Motor and sensory disorders, abnormal reflexes
- Somnolence to coma
- Trypanosomes and increased white blood cells and protein in cerebrospinal fluid

GENERAL CONSIDERATIONS

- Caused by *Trypanosoma brucei gambiense* [see also Trypanosomiasis, African (*T b rhodesiense*)]. Both are hemoflagellates
- The organisms are transmitted by bites of tsetse flies (glossina species), which inhabit shaded areas along rivers
- Humans are the principal mammalian host; it is uncertain if there is an animal reservoir, but domestic animals can be infected
- Trypanosomes ingested in a blood meal undergo a developmental period of 18–35 days in the fly; when the fly feeds again on a new mammalian host, the infective stage is injected

DEMOGRAPHICS

- Found in moist sub-Saharan savanna and riverine forests of west and central Africa up to the eastern Rift Valley
- About 50,000 deaths occur yearly
- Of new infections yearly, approximately 100,000 are Gambian but only several hundred are Rhodesian

CLINICAL FINDINGS

SYMPTOMS AND SIGNS

- Generally a long asymptomatic period in which chancres are rare and the hemolymphatic stage may be absent or may go unnoticed
- When symptoms do manifest after weeks to years, they are often initially mild and ignored by the patient

The hemolymphatic (early) stage

- Fever, headache, joint pains, and malaise may recur at irregular intervals corresponding to waves of parasitemia
- Between febrile episodes there are symptom-free periods
- Transient rashes may appear, often pruritic and papular or circinate
- Examination may reveal mild enlargement of the liver and spleen

The meningoencephalitic (late) stage

- This stage appears only months after infection
- With progression, death occurs within several years
- Insomnia, anorexia, personality changes, apathy, and headaches are early findings
- A variety of motor or tonus disorders may develop, including tremors, seizures, disturbances of speech, gait, and reflexes; somnolence appears late
- Sensory involvement includes hyperaesthesia and pruritis
- The patient becomes severely emaciated and, finally, comatose
- Death often results from secondary infection

DIFFERENTIAL DIAGNOSIS

- *Trypanosoma brucei rhodesiense* infection
- Malaria
- Influenza and pneumonia
- Tuberculosis
- Infectious mononucleosis
- Leukemia or lymphoma
- HIV
- Arbovirus encephalitis
- Wilson's disease
- Psychosis due to other causes, eg, neurosyphilis

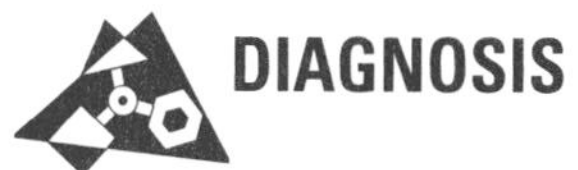

DIAGNOSIS

LABORATORY TESTS

- Anemia, increased sedimentation rate, thrombocytopenia, and increased serum globulin are common
- Eosinophilia is not seen
- Detection in blood is very difficult in Gambian infection (unlike Rhodesian infection)
- Definitive diagnosis requires identifying motile organisms in wet films and after Giemsa or Wright's staining of thin and thick blood films; or aspirates of bite lesions, lymph nodes, or bone marrow; or of cerebrospinal fluid
- Because the number of trypanosomes in blood fluctuates (they may be undetectable 3 of 5 days but are more common during febrile periods), multiple anticoagulated specimens should be examined daily for as long as 15 days
- Other diagnostic tests with blood are intraperitoneal inoculation of rodents (sensitive but effective only for *T b rhodesiense*), culture, Millipore filtration, and DEAE-cellulose anion exchange centrifugation

Cerebrospinal fluid

- Cerebrospinal fluid is clear and shows an increase in pressure, lymphocytes, and protein
- Large eosinophilic plasma cells (Mott cells) are rarely seen but are considered pathognomic
- With progression of the disease, the parasite is more likely to be found in cerebrospinal fluid than in blood or lymph nodes
- To detect the organism, the fluid should be examined within 20 min (to avoid parasitic lysis) and centrifuged twice (doubles sensitivity), inoculated into an experimental animal, and cultured

Antibody detection assays

- Several antibody detection assays are used epidemiologically and for case finding for Gambian infections
- False-positive results can be due to animal trypanosomes that are noninfectious to humans
- A field-adapted card agglutination test (sensitivity about 96%, specificity high) detects circulating and cerebrospinal fluid antigen. Positive results of these antigen and antibody tests should be followed by parasitic confirmatory testing
- Circulating IgM antibody becomes positive about 12 days after infection; its titers may fluctuate or be undetectable during brief periods of excess antigen,

and a negative test does not rule out infection
- In late central nervous system disease, though both circulating antibody and parasitemia may fall below detectable levels, serological tests of the cerebrospinal fluid (including IgM) may prove useful

IMAGING STUDIES

- MRI and CT scans are nonspecific

DIAGNOSTIC PROCEDURES

- If present, only soft lymph nodes should be selected for aspiration (25-gauge needle); after the node is gently kneaded, the aspirate is examined immediately for motile organisms
- Electroencephalograms are nonspecific

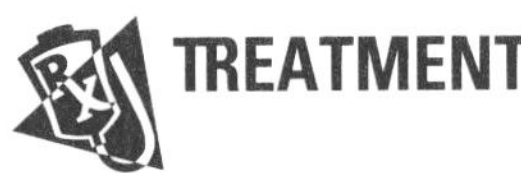

TREATMENT

MEDICATIONS

- Because all of the drugs used (except eflornithine) are highly toxic (mortality during drug treatment can reach 5–10%), specific detection of the organism rather than immunoassays is a prerequisite for treatment

The hemolymphatic stage

- The drug of choice is intravenous suramin [100–200 mg (test dose), then 1 g on Days 1, 3, 7, 14, and 21]
- Suramin side effects include vomiting, pruritis, paresthesias, and peripheral neuropathy
- Alternative drugs of choice are intravenous eflornithine (400 mg/kg/day in four divided doses for 14 days, followed by 300 mg/kg/day orally for 3–4 weeks; cure rate 97%) or pentamidine (4 mg/kg/day intramuscularly for 7–10 days; cure rate 93%)

The meningoencephalitic stage

- In central nervous system involvement, use melarsoprol and eflornithine, rather than suramin and pentamidine, which do not adequately cross the blood-brain barrier
- Drug of choice is intravenous melarsoprol, 2–3.6 mg/kg/day for 3 days; after 1 week, 3.6 mg/kg/d for 3 days; repeat after 10–21 days. Relapse rates for infections, formerly low (5–8%), have markedly increased
- Melarsoprol causes a reactive encephalopathy in up to 10% of patients; this complication has a 50% mortality rate and may be prevented by corticosteroids
- Alternative treatments are eflornithine (as above) or intravenous tryparsamide, 30 mg/kg (maximum: 2 g) every 5 days for 12 injections, plus intravenous suramin, 100–200 mg (test dose), followed by 10 mg/kg every 5 days for 12 injections; the treatment may be repeated in 1 month
- Systemic eflornithine is highly effective and associated with only mild toxicity in early and late *T b gambiense* infections
- Eflornithine is expensive, and its continued availability (from WHO) is uncertain. In the United States, eflornithine has been approved for topical use to remove facial hair; suramin and melarsoprol are available only from the CDC Drug Service, Centers for Disease Control and Prevention, Atlanta, GA

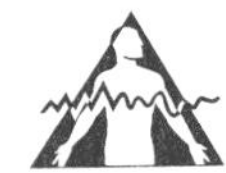

OUTCOME

FOLLOW-UP

- Proper follow-up to ensure detection of the encephalitic stage requires initial cerebrospinal fluid examination, repeat studies at intervals during treatment, 3 months after treatment, and then at 6-month intervals for 2 years

PROGNOSIS

- Most patients—even those with advanced disease—recover following treatment
- Relapses are uncommon (about 2%)
- When therapy is started late, irreversible brain damage or death is common
- Most persons will die if untreated

WHEN TO REFER

- Diagnosis and treatment are best done by a specialist

WHEN TO ADMIT

- All patients who are in a presumed or confirmed meningoencephalitic stage

PREVENTION

- Individual prevention should include wearing long sleeves and trousers, avoiding dark-colored clothing, and using mosquito nets while sleeping. Repellents have no effect
- Pentamidine is used in chemoprophylaxis (controversial). One intramuscular injection (4 mg/kg, maximum 300 mg) protects for 3–6 months. It may suppress early symptoms, resulting in late recognition of the disease. The drug is toxic and should be used only for persons at high risk (ie, those with constant, heavy exposure to tsetse flies in areas with known transmission of Gambian disease)
- Performing serological tests every 6 months during exposure and for 3 years afterward is the safest method for detecting the disease at an early stage

EVIDENCE

WEB SITE

- CDC—Division of Parasitic Diseases
  - http://www.cdc.gov/ncidod/dpd/parasites/trypanosomiasis/default.htm

INFORMATION FOR PATIENTS

- Centers for Disease Control and Prevention
  - http://www.cdc.gov/ncidod/dpd/parasites/trypanosomiasis/factsht_wa_trypanosomiasis.htm
- National Institutes of Health
  - http://www.nlm.nih.gov/medlineplus/ency/article/001362.htm

REFERENCES

- Burchmore RJ et al: Chemotherapy of human African trypanosomiasis. Curr Pharm Des 2002;8:256. [PMID: 11860365]
- Legros D et al: Treatment of human African trypanosomiasis—present situation and needs for research and development. Lancet Infect Dis 2002;2:437. [PMID: 12127356]
- Lejon V et al: Stage determination and follow-up in sleeping sickness. Med Trop (Mars) 2001;61:355. [PMID: 11803826]

Trypanosomiasis, African (*T b rhodesiense*)

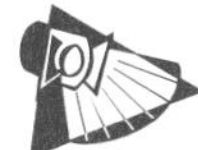

KEY FEATURES

ESSENTIALS OF DIAGNOSIS

- History of exposure to tsetse flies

Hemolymphatic stage

- Irregular fevers, headaches, joint pains, malaise, pruritus, papular skin rash, edemas
- Posterior cervical or generalized lymphadenopathy; hepatosplenomegaly
- Anemia, weight loss
- Trypanosomes in blood or lymph node aspirates; positive serology

Meningoencephalitic stage

- Insomnia, motor and sensory disorders, abnormal reflexes, somnolence to coma
- Trypanosomes and increased white blood cells and protein in cerebrospinal fluid

GENERAL CONSIDERATIONS

- Caused by *Trypanosoma brucei rhodesiense* and *Trypanosoma brucei gambiense* [see Trypanosomiasis, African (*T b gambiense*)], both hemoflagellates
- The organisms are transmitted by bites of tsetse flies (glossina species), which inhabit shaded areas along rivers
- Trypanosomes ingested in a blood meal undergo a developmental period of 18–35 days in the fly; when the fly feeds again on a new mammalian host, the infective stage is injected

DEMOGRAPHICS

- *T b rhodesiense* occurs to the east of the Rift Valley in the savannah of east and southeast Africa and along the shores of Lake Victoria
- *T b rhodesiense* infection is primarily a zoonosis of game animals; humans are infected sporadically
- About 50,000 deaths occur yearly
- Of new infections yearly, approximately 100,000 are Gambian but only several hundred are Rhodesian
- Among visitors to the East African game parks, infections are rare, with about one case a year appearing in the United States

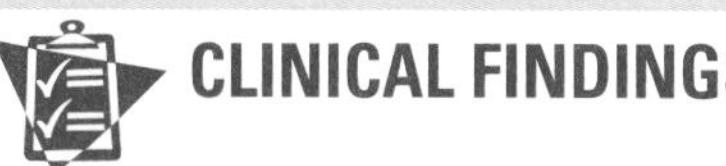

CLINICAL FINDINGS

SYMPTOMS AND SIGNS

- Infections go through the following three stages, which are virulent, and untreated patients die within weeks to a year

The trypanosomal chancre

- There is is a local pruritic, painful inflammatory reaction (3–10 cm) with regional lymphadenopathy that appears about 48 h after the tsetse fly bite and lasts 2–4 weeks

The hemolymphatic (early) stage

- High fever, severe headache, joint pains, and malaise recur at irregular intervals
- Between febrile episodes symptom-free periods may last up to 2 weeks
- Transient rashes may appear, often pruritic and papular or circinate
- Examination reveals mild enlargement of the liver and spleen, and edema (peripheral, pleural, ascites, etc)
- Nodes of the posterior cervical group (Winterbottom's sign) may be enlarged
- With progression of the disease, there is weight loss and debilitation
- Myocardial involvement may appear early, and the patient may succumb to myocarditis before meningoencephalitic signs appear

The meningoencephalitic (late) stage

- This stage appears within a few weeks or months of onset
- Insomnia, anorexia, personality changes, apathy, and headaches are early findings
- A variety of motor or tonus disorders may develop, including tremors, seizures, disturbances of speech, gait, and reflexes; somnolence appears late
- Sensory involvement includes hyperaesthesia and pruritis
- The patient becomes severely emaciated and, finally, comatose. Death often results from secondary infection

DIFFERENTIAL DIAGNOSIS

- *Trypanosoma brucei gambiense* infection
- Influenza and pneumonia
- Tuberculosis
- Malaria
- Infectious mononucleosis
- Leukemia or lymphoma
- HIV
- Arbovirus encephalitis
- Wilson's disease
- Psychosis due to other causes, eg, neurosyphilis

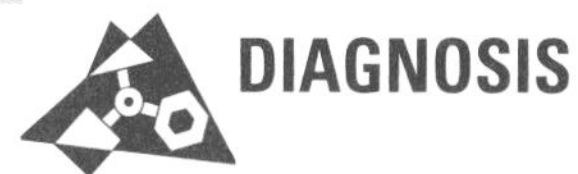

DIAGNOSIS

LABORATORY TESTS

- Anemia, increased sedimentation rate, and thrombocytopenia are common. Eosinophilia is not seen
- Detection in blood is usually possible in Rhodesian infection (but very difficult in Gambian infection)
- Definitive diagnosis requires identifying motile organisms in wet films and after Giemsa or Wright staining of thin and thick blood films; of aspirates of bite lesions, lymph nodes, or bone marrow; or of cerebrospinal fluid. Because the number of trypanosomes in blood fluctuates (they may be undetectable 3 out of 5 days but are more common during febrile periods), multiple anticoagulated specimens should be examined daily for as many as 15 days using 10–15 mL for centrifugation; the trypanosomes are concentrated in the buffy coat
- Other diagnostic tests with blood are intraperitoneal inoculation of rodents, culture, Millipore filtration, and DEAE-cellulose anion-exchange centrifugation
- Cerebrospinal fluid is clear and shows an increase in pressure, lymphocytes, and protein. Large eosinophilic plasma cells (Mott cells) are rarely seen but are considered pathognomic
- With progression of the disease, the parasite is more likely to be found in cerebrospinal fluid than in blood or lymph nodes. To detect the organism, the fluid should be examined within 20 min (to avoid parasitic lysis) and centrifuged twice (doubles sensitivity), inoculated into an experimental animal, and cultured
- Several antibody detection assays are available. False-positive results can be due to animal trypanosomes that are noninfectious to humans. A field-adapted card agglutination test (sensitivity about 96%, specificity high) detects circulating and cerebrospinal fluid antigen. Positive results of these antigen and antibody tests should be followed by parasitic confirmatory testing
- Circulating IgM antibody becomes positive about 12 days after infection; its titers may fluctuate or be undetectable during brief periods of excess antigen, and a negative test does not rule out infection
- In late central nervous system disease, though both circulating antibody and parasitemia may fall below detectable levels, serological tests of the cerebrospinal fluid (including IgM) may prove useful

IMAGING STUDIES

- MRI and CT scans are nonspecific

DIAGNOSTIC PROCEDURES

- Only soft lymph nodes should be selected for aspiration (25-gauge needle); after the node is gently kneaded, the aspirate is examined immediately for motile organisms
- Electroencephalograms are nonspecific

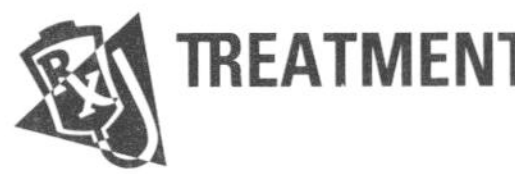

TREATMENT

MEDICATIONS

- Because all of the drugs used (except eflornithine) are highly toxic (mortality during drug treatment can reach 5–10%), specific detection of the organism rather than immunoassays is a prerequisite for treatment

Early disease, the hemolymphatic stage

- The drug of choice is intravenous suramin [100–200 mg (test dose), then 1 g on Days 1, 3, 7, 14, and 21]
- Suramin side effects include vomiting, pruritis, paresthesias, and peripheral neuropathy
- Alternative drug of choice is pentamidine (4 mg/kg/day intramuscularly for 7–10 days; cure rate 93%)

Late disease with central nervous system involvement

- In central nervous system involvement, use melarsoprol, rather than suramin and pentamidine, which do not adequately cross the blood-brain barrier
- Drug of choice is intravenous melarsoprol, 2–3.6 mg/kg/day for 3 days; after 1 week, 3.6 mg/kg/d for 3 days; repeat after 10–21 days
- Melarsoprol causes a reactive encephalopathy in up to 10% of patients; this complication has a 50% mortality rate and may be prevented by corticosteroids
- Systemic eflornithine should not be used, as its efficacy is inconsistent
- Suramin and melarsoprol are available only from the CDC Drug Service, Centers for Disease Control and Prevention, Atlanta, GA

OUTCOME

FOLLOW-UP

- Proper follow-up to ensure detection of the encephalitic stage requires initial cerebrospinal fluid examination, repeat studies at intervals during treatment, 3 months after treatment, and then at 6-month intervals for 2 years

PROGNOSIS

- Most patients—even those with advanced disease—recover following treatment. Relapses are uncommon (about 2%)
- When therapy is started late, irreversible brain damage or death is common
- Most persons with African trypanosomiasis will die if untreated

WHEN TO REFER

- Diagnosis and treatment are best done by a specialist

WHEN TO ADMIT

- All patients with suspected or confirmed meningoencephalitic disease

PREVENTION

- Individual prevention in endemic areas should include wearing long sleeves and trousers, avoiding dark-colored clothing, and using mosquito nets while sleeping. Repellents have no effect
- Pentamidine should not be used in chemoprophylaxis

EVIDENCE

WEB SITE

- CDC—Division of Parasitic Diseases
  - http://www.cdc.gov/ncidod/dpd/parasites/trypanosomiasis/default.htm

INFORMATION FOR PATIENTS

- Centers for Disease Control and Prevention
  - http://www.cdc.gov/ncidod/dpd/parasites/trypanosomiasis/factsht_ea_trypanosomiasis.htm
- National Institutes of Health
  - http://www.nlm.nih.gov/medlineplus/ency/article/001362.htm

REFERENCES

- Burchmore RJ et al: Chemotherapy of human African trypanosomiasis. Curr Pharm Des 2002;8:256. [PMID: 11860365]
- Legros D et al: Treatment of human African trypanosomiasis—present situation and needs for research and development. Lancet Infect Dis 2002;2:437. [PMID: 12127356]
- Lejon V et al: Stage determination and follow-up in sleeping sickness. Med Trop (Mars) 2001;61:355. [PMID: 11803826]

Trypanosomiasis, American (Chagas' Disease)

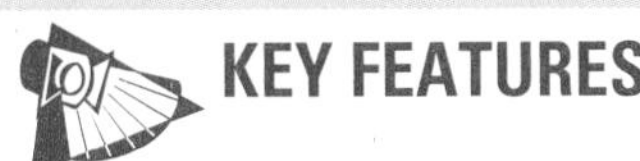

KEY FEATURES

ESSENTIALS OF DIAGNOSIS

Acute stage

- Inflammatory lesion at site of inoculation; prolonged fever, tachycardia, hepatosplenomegaly, lymphadenopathy, myocarditis
- Parasites in peripheral blood, positive serological tests

Chronic stage

- Heart failure with cardiac arrhythmias
- In some regions, dysphagia, severe constipation, and radiological evidence of megaesophagus or megacolon
- Positive xenodiagnosis or hemoculture, positive serological tests; abnormal ECG

GENERAL CONSIDERATIONS

- Caused by *Trypanosoma cruzi*, a protozoan parasite of humans and wild and domestic animals found in wild animals and in humans from southern South America to southern United States
- The disease is often acquired in childhood; the proportion of infected persons increases with age
- In many countries in South America, Chagas' disease is the most important cause of heart disease
- The organism has a predilection for myocardium, smooth muscle, and central nervous system glial cells

DEMOGRAPHICS

- An estimated 13 million people are infected, mostly in rural areas, resulting in about 45,000 deaths yearly from cardiac disease
- In the United States, less than 10 instances of local transmission have been confirmed
- A large number of immigrants to the United States from endemic areas of Latin America (particularly Central America) are infected (estimated 50,000–100,000)
- A few infections following blood transfusion have been reported

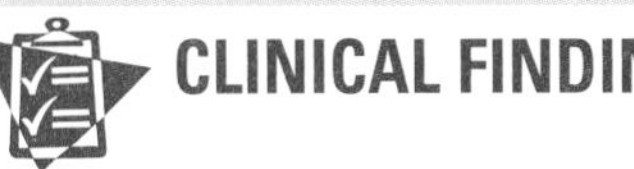

CLINICAL FINDINGS

SYMPTOMS AND SIGNS

- Up to 70% of infected persons remain asymptomatic despite lifelong infection

Acute stage

- Seen principally in children
- Lasts 2–4 months and leads to death in up to 10% of cases
- The earliest findings are at the site of inoculation either in the eye—Romaña's sign (unilateral bipalpebral edema, conjunctivitis, local lymphadenopathy)—or in the skin—a chagoma (furuncle-like lesion with local lymphadenopathy)
- Subsequent findings include fever, malaise, headache, hepatosplenomegaly, and generalized lymphadenopathy
- Acute myocarditis may lead to biventricular failure, but arrhythmias are rare
- Meningoencephalitis is limited to young children and is often fatal

Latent stage (indeterminate phase)

- This asymptomatic stage may last 10–30 years but the serological tests and sometimes parasitological examination confirm the presence of the infection

Chronic stage

- Usually manifested by cardiac disease in the third and fourth decades of life, with arrhythmias, congestive heart failure (often with prominent right-sided findings), ventricular aneurysms, and systemic or pulmonary embolization originating from mural thrombi. Valvular lesions are absent. Sudden cardiac arrest in young adults may occur from ventricular fibrillation
- Megacolon and megaesophagus occur in some areas of Chile, Argentina, and Brazil; findings include dysphagia, regurgitation, constipation, sigmoid volvulus, bacterial overgrowth in the small intestine, and parotid gland hypertrophy. Megasyndromes can also affect the urinary tract
- In immunosuppressed persons—including infrequently in AIDS patients and transplant recipients—latent Chagas' disease may reactivate. Common findings are cardiomyopathy and brain lesions indistinguishable from cerebral toxoplasmosis

DIFFERENTIAL DIAGNOSIS

- Acute stage: malaria, rheumatic fever, African trypanosomiasis
- Myocarditis due to other causes, eg, coxsackievirus, Rocky Mountain spotted fever, toxoplasmosis, drugs
- Arrhythmia or congestive heart failure due to other causes, eg, sick sinus syndrome, coronary artery disease
- Toxic megacolon due to inflammatory bowel disease or *Clostridium difficile*-associated colitis
- Idiopathic achalasia

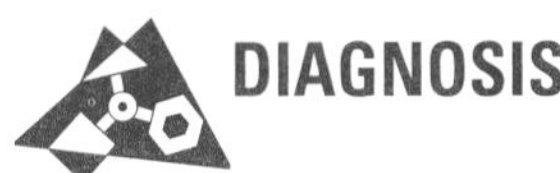

DIAGNOSIS

LABORATORY TESTS

- Laboratory tests will identify most acute and congenital cases and up to 40% of chronic ones
- In the **acute phase**, the organism may be found as motile trypanosomes in anticoagulated blood; as Giemsa-stained trypanosomes in anticoagulated blood used to prepare thin and thick or buffy coat films; or by blood culture or animal inoculation. Occasionally, amastigotes can be found in tissue aspirates or biopsies of chagomas or lymph nodes by direct examination, staining, or culture
- In the **chronic phase**, the organism is rarely found directly, but may be detected by culture, animal inoculation, or xenodiagnosis. The latter consists of permitting uninfected laboratory-reared bugs of the local major vector to feed on the patients and then examining their intestinal contents for trypanosomes
- In **both acute and chronic** infection, blood should also be cultured using appropriate media and inoculated into laboratory mice or rats 3–10 days old
- *Trypanosoma rangeli*, a nonpathogenic blood trypanosome also found in humans in Central America and northern South America, must not be mistaken for *T cruzi* trypomastogotes
- Several highly sensitive IgG serological tests (hemagglutination inhibition, complement fixation, ELISA, Western blot, immunofluorescence, others) are available. However, up to three of these tests should be done because false negative (including some cases of depressed immune response) and false positive tests are common. The latter may occur in other infections, including leishmaniasis, malaria, syphilis, and *T rangeli* infection, and in autoimmune diseases. For ELISA and immunofluorescent tests, sensitivity is 93–98% and specificity (excluding leishmaniasis) is 99%
- IgM antibodies are elevated early in the acute stage but are replaced by IgG antibodies as the disease progresses. Maximum titers are reached in 3–4 months; thereafter, titers can remain positive at a

low level for life. In chronic infections, when circulating organisms are difficult to find, the polymerase chain reaction and recombinant DNA methods often assess effectiveness of chemotherapy (clearance of parasites), whereas the serological tests do not

IMAGING STUDIES

- Right bundle branch block and arrhythmias are the most significant electrocardiographic abnormalities
- In certain regions of South America, radiological examination may show megaesophagus, megacolon, or cardiac enlargement with characteristic apical aneurysms

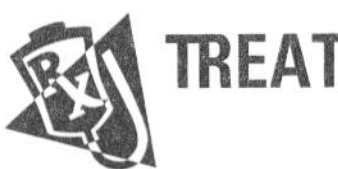

TREATMENT

MEDICATIONS

- Treatment is inadequate because the two drugs used, nifurtimox and benznidazole, often cause severe side effects, must be used for a long period, and are ineffective in chronic infection
- Treatment is indicated in acute infection (regardless of the time since infection) but not in latent infection and is controversial in the chronic stage
- Nifurtimox is given orally in daily doses of 8–10 mg/kg in four divided doses after meals for 90–120 days. It generally produces gastrointestinal complaints, weight loss, tremors, and peripheral neuropathy. Hallucinations, pulmonary infiltrates, and convulsions are rare. In the United States, nifurtimox is available only from the Parasitic Disease Drug Service, Centers for Disease Control, Atlanta, GA
- Benznidazole—not available in the United States—is given at a dosage of 5 mg/kg/day for 60 days. Its side effects include granulocytopenia, rash, and peripheral neuropathy. The drug is better tolerated by children
- In the chronic stage, digoxin is not well tolerated. The most effective antiarrhythmic drug is amiodarone. Cardiac pacemakers are used for atrioventricular block. Amiodarone and angiotensin-converting enzyme inhibitors may result in better survival in selected patients

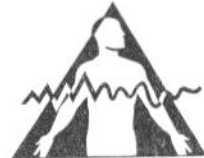

OUTCOME

COMPLICATIONS

- Chronic disease complications, including cardiac disease and sudden cardiac arrest
- Megacolon and megaesophagus, constipation, sigmoid volvulus, and parotid gland hypertrophy. Megasyndromes can also affect the urinary tract

PROGNOSIS

- Adults with chronic heart disease may die of the disease
- The use of nifurtimox and benznidazole reduces the duration and severity of infection, but cure is achieved in only about 70% of patients. In the chronic phase, although parasitemia may disappear in up to 70% of patients, treatment does not alter the serological reaction, cardiac function, or progression of the disease

WHEN TO REFER

- All patients should be referred to an infectious disease specialist
- Refer to a cardiologist for either acute or chronic cardiac disease
- Refer to a gastroenterologist for any megasyndromes

PREVENTION

- In South America, a major eradication program based on improved housing, use of residual pyrethroid insecticides, and screening of blood donors has achieved striking reductions in infections in children
- In endemic areas, blood should not be used for transfusion unless at least two serological tests are negative; otherwise, blood can be treated with gentian violet to kill the parasites
- Immigrants from endemic areas should be tested

EVIDENCE

WEB SITE

- CDC—Division of Parasitic Diseases
  - http://www.cdc.gov/ncidod/dpd/parasites/chagasdisease/default.htm

INFORMATION FOR PATIENTS

- Centers for Disease Control and Prevention
  - http://www.cdc.gov/ncidod/dpd/parasites/chagasdisease/factsht_chagas_disease.htm
- National Institutes of Health
  - http://www.nlm.nih.gov/medlineplus/ency/article/001372.htm

REFERENCES

- Umezawa ES et al: Chagas' disease. Lancet 2002;359:627. [PMID: 11867143]
- Urbina JA: Specific treatment of Chagas disease: current status and new developments. Curr Opin Infect Dis 2001;14(6):733. [PMID: 11964893]

Tuberculosis, Bones & Joints

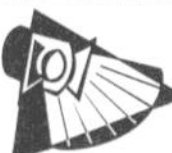

KEY FEATURES

ESSENTIALS OF DIAGNOSIS

- In most cases, a single site of bone or joint is infected
- Spine—especially lower thoracic—or knee are the most common sites
- Chest x-ray abnormal in less than half

GENERAL CONSIDERATIONS

- Infection of the musculoskeletal system is caused by hematogenous spread from a primary lesion in the respiratory tract
- It may occur shortly after primary infection or may be seen years later as a disease reactivation
- Tuberculosis of the thoracic or lumbar spine (Pott's disease) usually occurs in the absence of extraspinal infection
- Tuberculosis of peripheral joints is almost always monarticular, with the knee the most common site

DEMOGRAPHICS

- A disease of children, the elderly, or those with HIV infection

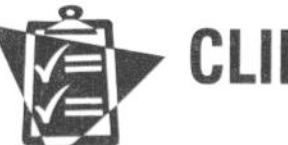

CLINICAL FINDINGS

SYMPTOMS AND SIGNS

- Onset is generally insidious without systemic symptoms
- Pain may be mild at onset, is usually worse at night, and may be accompanied by stiffness
- As the disease process progresses, limitation of joint motion becomes prominent because of muscle contractures and joint destruction
- Symptoms of pulmonary tuberculosis may also be present
- Local findings during the early stages may be limited to tenderness, soft tissue swelling, joint effusion, and increase in skin temperature about the involved area
- Abscess formation with spontaneous drainage externally leads to sinus formation
- Progressive destruction of bone in the spine may cause a gibbus deformity

DIFFERENTIAL DIAGNOSIS

- All subacute and chronic infections (bacterial, fungal) of bone
- Gonococcal arthritis
- Mycotic bone infection
- Pyogenic osteomyelitis or septic arthritis
- Rheumatoid arthritis
- Sporotrichosis
- Metastatic cancer
- Osseous dysplasia

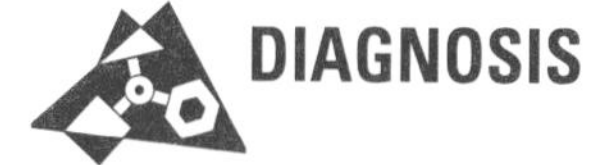

DIAGNOSIS

LABORATORY TESTS

- Recovery of the acid-fast organism from joint fluid, pus, or tissue specimens

IMAGING STUDIES

- The earliest changes are soft tissue swelling and distention of the joint capsule by the effusion
- Subsequently, bone atrophy causes thinning of the trabecular pattern, narrowing of the cortex, and enlargement of the medullary canal
- As joint disease progresses, destruction of cartilage, both in the spine and in peripheral joints, is manifested by narrowing of the joint cleft and focal erosion of the articular surface, especially at the margins
- With spinal tuberculosis, CT scanning is helpful in demonstrating paraspinal soft tissue extensions of the infection (eg, psoas abscess, epidural extension)

DIAGNOSTIC PROCEDURES

- Biopsy of the bony lesion, synovium, or a regional lymph node may demonstrate the characteristic histopathological picture of caseating necrosis and giant cells

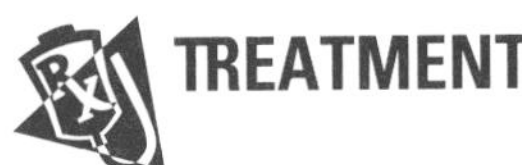

TREATMENT

MEDICATIONS

- See *Tuberculosis*
- Four oral drugs: isoniazid, 300 mg/day; rifampin, 600 mg/day; pyrazinamide, 25 mg/kg/day; and ethambutol, 15 mg/kg/day
- If the isolate is sensitive to isoniazid and rifampin, the ethambutol can be stopped, with the pyrazinamide maintained for 2 months. Isoniazid and rifampin are continued for at least 6 months

SURGERY

- Surgical debridement is indicated for recurrent joint effusions and other indicators of poor clinical response to antituberculous medications

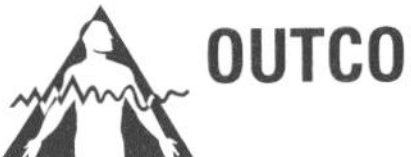

OUTCOME

COMPLICATIONS

- Destruction of bones or joints may occur in a few weeks or months if adequate treatment is not provided
- Deformity due to joint destruction, abscess formation with spread into adjacent soft tissues, and sinus formation are common

EVIDENCE

PRACTICE GUIDELINES

- Centers for Disease Control and Prevention
  - http://www.cdc.gov/mmwr/preview/mmwrhtml/rr5211a1.htm
- Infectious Diseases Society of America
  - http://www.journals.uchicago.edu/CID/journal/issues/v31n3/000549/000549.web.pdf
- National Guideline Clearinghouse
  - http://www.guideline.gov/summary/summary.aspx?doc_id=2663

INFORMATION FOR PATIENTS

- National Institutes of Health
  - http://www.nlm.nih.gov/medlineplus/ency/article/000417.htm

REFERENCE

- Wardle N et al: Orthopaedic manifestations of tuberculosis. Hosp Med 2004;65:228. [PMID: 15127678]

Author(s)

David B. Hellmann, MD, FACP
John H. Stone, MD, MPH

Tuberculosis in HIV

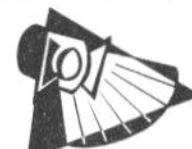

KEY FEATURES

ESSENTIALS OF DIAGNOSIS

- Fatigue, weight loss, fever, night sweats, and cough
- Pulmonary infiltrates on chest radiograph, most often apical
- Positive tuberculin skin test reaction (most cases)
- Acid-fast bacilli on smear of sputum or sputum culture positive for *Mycobacterium tuberculosis* (MTB)

GENERAL CONSIDERATIONS

- Latent tuberculosis infection (LTBI) occurs when bacilli are contained within granulomata, the typical response to infection in immunocompetent persons
  - Nontransmissible, but may become active disease if a host's immune function becomes impaired
  - Reactivation occurs within 2 years in up to 50% of HIV+ patients
- Nonadherence is a major cause of treatment failure, disease transmission, and development of drug resistance

DEMOGRAPHICS

- HIV increases the risk of reactivation disease
- Risk factors for drug resistance include
  - Immigration from a region with drug-resistant tuberculosis
  - Close contact with a patient infected with drug-resistant tuberculosis
  - Unsuccessful prior therapy
  - Patient noncompliance

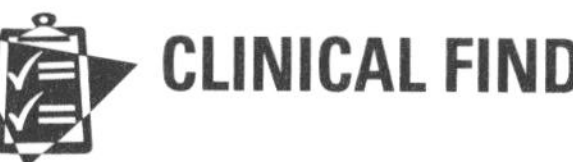

CLINICAL FINDINGS

SYMPTOMS AND SIGNS

- Cough is the most common symptom
- Blood-streaked sputum is common, frank hemoptysis is rare
- Slowly progressive constitutional symptoms
  - Malaise
  - Anorexia
  - Weight loss
  - Fever
  - Night sweats
- Patients appear chronically ill and malnourished
- Chest examination is nonspecific; posttussive apical rales are classic
- Extrapulmonary disease is especially common, often with lymphadenitis or miliary disease
- Atypical presentations are common

DIFFERENTIAL DIAGNOSIS

- Pneumonia or lung abscess
- Lung cancer
- Lymphoma
- *Mycobacterium avium* complex (or other nontuberculous mycobacteria)
- Sarcoidosis
- Fungal infection, eg, histoplasmosis
- Endocarditis
- Nocardiosis

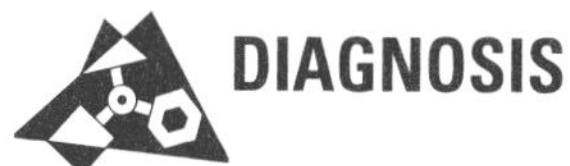

DIAGNOSIS

LABORATORY TESTS

- Tuberculin skin test (Table 22)
- Definitive diagnosis depends on recovery of *M tuberculosis* from cultures or identification with DNA or RNA amplification techniques
- Three consecutive first AM sputum samples are advised
- Cultures on solid media to identify *M tuberculosis* may require 12 weeks; liquid medium culture systems can identify growth in several days
- DNA fingerprinting with restriction fragment-length polymorphism analysis can identify individual strains
- Pleural fluid cultures for tuberculosis are positive in only 25% of effusions

IMAGING STUDIES

- In early HIV disease, radiographic features resemble those of patients who do not have HIV disease
- Atypical radiographic features are seen in late HIV infection
  - Lower lung
  - Diffuse or miliary infiltrates
  - Pleural effusions
  - Hilar and lymph node involvement

DIAGNOSTIC PROCEDURES

- Sputum induction is required for patients unable to voluntarily produce a sample
- Bronchoscopy may be considered in smear-negative patients in whom there is a high suspicion of disease

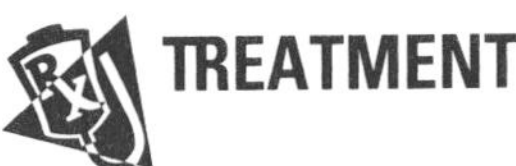

TREATMENT

MEDICATIONS

- See Tables 23 and 24
- Patients with HIV disease and tuberculosis respond best when the HIV infection is treated concurrently; in some cases, prolonged antituberculous therapy may be warranted
- Multiple drugs to which the organism is susceptible are used
- At least two new drugs are added when treatment failure is suspected
- When a twice- or thrice-weekly regimen is used, dosages are increased (Table 24)
- Treatment is similar to treatment of tuberculosis in HIV-negative patients, with the following additional considerations
  - Directly observed therapy (DOT) is indicated for all HIV+ patients
  - Longer duration of therapy
  - Awareness of drug interactions between rifampin or rifabutin and protease inhibitors or nonnucleoside reverse transcriptase inhibitors used to treat HIV
  - Pyridoxine (10–50 mg PO QD) should be given to all HIV+ patients on isoniazid to reduce nervous system side effects
- **Extrapulmonary disease**
  - In most cases, regimens effective for pulmonary disease are adequate
  - Nine months of therapy for miliary, meningeal, bone, or joint involvement
  - Corticosteroids reduce complications of tuberculous pericarditis and meningitis

SURGERY

- Early debridement and drainage are recommended for skeletal involvement

THERAPEUTIC PROCEDURES

- Needle biopsy of the pleura reveals granulomatous inflammation in 60% of patients with tuberculous pleural effusions
- Culture of three pleural biopsy specimens combined with microscopic examination increases the diagnostic yield to 90%
- Complete blood cell count, lung function tests, blood urea nitrogen, and creatinine should be checked at baseline
- Visual acuity and red-green color vision testing before initiating ethambutol
- Audiometry prior to streptomycin therapy
- Routine monitoring for evidence of drug toxicity is not recommended

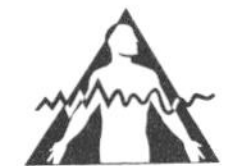

OUTCOME

FOLLOW-UP

- Monthly visits are recommended for outpatients
- Monthly sputum smears and cultures should be done until documented negative
- Patients with negative sputum after 2 months of therapy should have smear and culture repeated at the end of therapy
- Patients with multidrug-resistant tuberculosis (MDRTB) should have sputum smear and culture monthly throughout therapy
- Chest x-ray is recommended on conclusion of successful therapy
- Patients whose cultures do not turn negative or have persistent symptoms after 3 months of therapy should be evaluated for MDRTB

COMPLICATIONS

- Development of drug resistance

WHEN TO REFER

- All cases of drug-resistant TB
- All cases of TB in HIV+ patients
- DOT is recommended for all patients with MDRTB and those receiving twice- or thrice-weekly therapy

WHEN TO ADMIT

- Patients who are incapable of self-care or likely to expose susceptible individuals to tuberculosis
- Hospitalization is not necessary for initial therapy in most patients
- Hospitalized patients require isolation in an appropriately ventilated room until three sputums from different days are negative for MTB organisms

PREVENTION

- Despite a negative purified protein derivative (PPD) skin test, HIV+ patients who are close contacts of patients with active MTB should receive 12 months of preventive therapy (see Tuberculosis, Latent Infection)
- HIV+ patients with positive PPD skin tests but without active MTB should be treated (see Tuberculosis, Latent Infection)
- All suspected and confirmed cases of MTB should be reported to local and state public health authorities

EVIDENCE

PRACTICE GUIDELINES

- Long R et al: Canadian Tuberculosis Committee of the Centre for Infectious Disease Prevention and Control, Population and Public Health Branch, Health Canada. Recommendations for screening and prevention of tuberculosis in patients with HIV and for screening for HIV in patients with tuberculosis and their contacts. CMAJ 2003;169:789. [PMID:14557318]
- National Guideline Clearinghouse
  - http://www.guideline.gov/summary/summary.aspx?doc_id=3080&nbr=2306&string=tuberculosis+and+hiv

INFORMATION FOR PATIENTS

- Centers for Disease Control and Prevention
  - http://www.cdc.gov/hiv/pubs/brochure/oi_tb.htm

REFERENCE

- American Thoracic Society/Centers for Disease Control and Prevention/Infectious Diseases Society of America: Treatment of tuberculosis. Am J Respir Crit Care Med 2003;167:603. [PMID: 12588714]
- Zunla A et al: Impact of HIV infection on tuberculosis. Postgrad Med J 2000;76:259. [PMID: 10775277]

Author(s)

Mark S. Chesnutt, MD

Thomas J. Prendergast, MD

Tuberculosis, Latent Infection

Tuberculosis, Intestinal p. 1161

KEY FEATURES

ESSENTIALS OF DIAGNOSIS

- A positive tuberculin skin test
- No evidence of active infection with tuberculosis
- A history (knowingly or not) of exposure to *Mycobacterium tuberculosis* (MTB)

GENERAL CONSIDERATIONS

- Targeted skin testing is used to identify persons at high risk for tuberculosis (TB) and who would benefit from treatment of latent tuberculosis infection (LTBI)
- LTBI describes patients who have been infected with *M tuberculosis*, but do not have active disease
- Individuals with LTBI have contained, but not eradicated infection
- The importance of identifying and treating LTBI is to prevent reactivation disease
- LTBI is nontransmissible, but may become active disease if a host's immune function becomes impaired
- Without preventive therapy, 10% of patients with LTBI will have reactivation during their lifetime, with 50% of cases occurring within 2 years of primary infection
- Reactivation occurs within 2 years in up to 50% of HIV+ patients with LTBI
- 2–10 weeks are required for primary infection to manifest an immune response to skin testing
- Persons who have received bacillus Calmette-Guérin (BCG) may have a positive purified protein derivative (PPD) tuberculin test for the rest of their lives

CLINICAL FINDINGS

SYMPTOMS AND SIGNS

- Patients are asymptomatic
- The disease is uncovered by screening with the tuberculin skin test
- Any pulmonary or constitutional symptoms should prompt an evaluation for active disease prior to prophylactic treatment

DIFFERENTIAL DIAGNOSIS

- Vaccine BCG

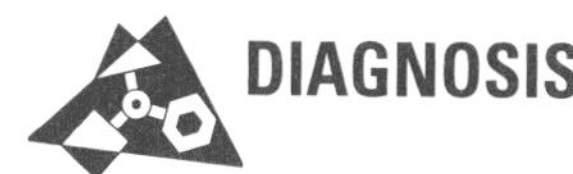

DIAGNOSIS

LABORATORY TESTS

- All patients with risk factors should be tested for HIV

IMAGING STUDIES

- Chest x-ray is required to rule out active pulmonary tuberculosis

DIAGNOSTIC PROCEDURES

- The Mantoux test is the preferred skin test (Table 22)
  - 0.1 mL of PPD containing 5 tuberculin units is injected intradermally on the volar forearm
  - Transverse width in millimeters of induration at 48–72 hours is measured
- False-positive tuberculin skin test reactions occur in patients previously vaccinated against MTB with BCG
- Prior vaccination with BCG does not alter the interpretation of the tuberculin skin test
- False-negative tests may result from
  - Improper technique
  - Concurrent infections
  - Malnutrition
  - Advanced age
  - Immunosuppression of any kind
  - Fulminant MTB infection
- Because of waning immunity, some patients with LTBI may have a negative skin test many years after exposure
- Two-step testing or "boosting"
  - Performed to reduce the likelihood that a boosted reaction will later be misinterpreted as a recent infection in individuals who will be tested repeatedly (health care workers)
  - A second test is performed 1–3 weeks after a negative test
  - If negative, the patient is uninfected or anergic; if positive, a "boosted reaction" is likely
- Anergy testing is not recommended to distinguish a true-negative test from anergy

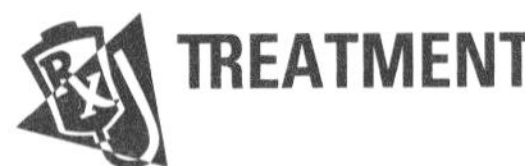

TREATMENT

MEDICATIONS

- Treatment substantially reduces the risk that infection will progress to active disease
- Patients suspected of having active disease should be treated with multidrug regimens until the diagnosis is confirmed or excluded
- Exposed persons who are skin-test–negative and HIV-negative may be observed without treatment or treated for 6 months
- Isoniazid (INH)
  - 9 months oral treatment (=270 doses within 12 months)
  - 300 mg QD or 15 mg/kg twice weekly
  - Coadministration of pyridoxine, 10–50 mg PO QD, for patients at risk of INH neuropathy (diabetes, uremia, malnutrition, alcoholism, HIV infection, pregnancy, seizure disorder)
  - INH plus pyridoxine is appropriate for pregnant or lactating women
- Rifampin/pyrazinamide (RIF/PZA)
  - 2 months (=60 doses within 3 months)
  - 10 mg/kg PO QD RIF to maximum of 600 mg/day and 15–20 mg/day PZA to maximum of 2 g/day
- Rifampin
  - 4-month oral regimen (=120 doses over 4 months)
  - Used for patients who cannot receive INH or PZA
- Contacts of persons with INH-resistant, RIF-sensitive MTB should receive RIF/PZA or RIF regimens
- Contacts of persons with multidrug-resistant TB (MDRTB) should receive two drugs to which the organism is sensitive
- HIV+ contacts should be treated for 12 months

THERAPEUTIC PROCEDURES

- It is not necessary to routinely monitor liver function tests unless there are abnormalities at baseline or clinical reasons to obtain the measurements

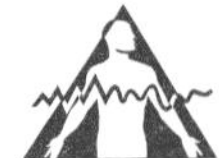

OUTCOME

FOLLOW-UP

- All contacts of persons with MDRTB should be monitored for 2 years regardless of treatment
- Patients being treated for LTBI should be seen monthly to evaluate for evidence of active TB, hepatitis, and adherence to treatment

COMPLICATIONS

- Development of active TB
- Drug toxicity

PROGNOSIS

- Almost all properly treated patients with TB can be cured
- Relapse rates are < 5% with current regimens
- Treatment failure is most commonly due to nonadherence

WHEN TO REFER

- HIV+ patients receiving antiretroviral therapy should be referred to TB and HIV experts if they are to receive rifampin therapy

PREVENTION

- Close contacts of patients with active TB should be retested 10–12 weeks after a negative test
- Despite a negative skin test, close contacts of patients with TB should consider treatment if they are immunosuppressed

EVIDENCE

PRACTICE GUIDELINES

- Centers for Disease Control and Prevention; American Thoracic Society. Update: adverse event data and revised American Thoracic Society/CDC recommendations against the use of rifampin and pyrazinamide for treatment of latent tuberculosis infection—United States, 2003. MMWR Morb Mortal Wkly Rep 2003;52(31):735
- Neff M et al: ATS, CDC, and IDSA update recommendations on the treatment of tuberculosis. Am Fam Physician 2003;68(9):1854,1857,1861. [PMID:14620606]

INFORMATION FOR PATIENTS

- Centers for Disease Control and Prevention
  - http://www.cdc.gov/nchstp/tb/faqs/qa.htm
- National Institute of Allergy and Infectious Disease
  - http://www.niaid.nih.gov/factsheets/tb.htm

REFERENCES

- American Thoracic Society and The Centers for Disease Control and Prevention: Diagnostic standards and classification of tuberculosis in adults and children. Am J Respir Crit Care Med 2000;161(4 Part 1):1376. [PMID: 10764337]
- American Thoracic Society and The Centers for Disease Control and Prevention: Targeted tuberculin testing and treatment of latent tuberculosis infection. Am J Respir Crit Care Med 2000;161(4 Part 2):S221. [PMID: 10764341]
- American Thoracic Society/Centers for Disease Control and Prevention/Infectious Diseases Society of America: treatment of tuberculosis. Am J Respir Crit Care Med 2003;167:603. [PMID: 12588714]

Author(s)

Mark S. Chesnutt, MD
Thomas J. Prendergast, MD

Tuberculosis, Pulmonary

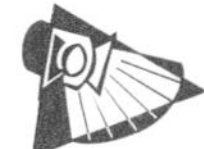

KEY FEATURES

ESSENTIALS OF DIAGNOSIS

- Cough and constitutional symptoms
- Pulmonary infiltrates on chest radiograph, most often apical
- Positive tuberculin skin test reaction (most cases)
- Acid-fast bacilli on smear of sputum or sputum culture positive for *Mycobacterium tuberculosis* (MTB)

GENERAL CONSIDERATIONS

- **Primary infection**
  - Occurs with inhalation of airborne droplets containing viable tubercle bacilli and subsequent lymphangitic and hematogenous spread before immunity develops
  - Up to one-third of new urban cases are from primary infection acquired by person-to-person transmission
- **Progressive primary tuberculosis**
  - Occurs in 5% of cases, with pulmonary and constitutional symptoms
- **Latent tuberculosis infection** (LTBI)
  - Occurs when bacilli are contained within granulomata
  - Nontransmissible, but may become active disease if a host's immune function becomes impaired
- Resistance to one or more drugs is seen in 15% of tuberculosis patients in the United States and is increasing
- Nonadherence is a major cause of treatment failure, disease transmission, and development of drug resistance

DEMOGRAPHICS

- Infects 20–40% of the world population annually (3 million deaths)
- Occurs disproportionately among malnourished, homeless, and marginally housed individuals
- Increased risks of reactivation
  - Gastrectomy
  - Silicosis
  - Diabetes mellitus
  - HIV
  - Immunosuppressive drugs
- Risk factors for drug resistance
  - Immigration from regions with drug-resistant tuberculosis
  - Close contact with patients infected with drug-resistant tuberculosis
  - Unsuccessful prior therapy
  - Patient noncompliance with treatment

CLINICAL FINDINGS

SYMPTOMS AND SIGNS

- Cough is the most common symptom
- Blood-streaked sputum is common, frank hemoptysis is rare
- Slowly progressive constitutional symptoms include malaise, anorexia, weight loss, fever, and night sweats
- Patients appear chronically ill
- Chest examination is nonspecific; posttussive apical rales are classic
- Atypical presentations are becoming more common, usually among the elderly and HIV+ patients

DIFFERENTIAL DIAGNOSIS

- Pneumonia or lung abscess
- Lung cancer or lymphoma
- *Myobacterium avium* complex (or other nontuberculous mycobacteria)
- Sarcoidosis
- Fungal infection, eg, histoplasmosis
- Endocarditis
- Silicosis or asbestosis
- Nocardiosis

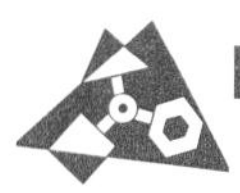

DIAGNOSIS

LABORATORY TESTS

- Tuberculin skin test (Table 22)
- Definitive diagnosis is *M tuberculosis* on culture or identification with DNA or RNA amplification techniques
- Three consecutive first AM sputum samples are advised
- Cultures on solid media may require 12 weeks; liquid medium culture systems can identify growth in several days
- DNA fingerprinting with restriction fragment-length polymorphism analysis can identify individual strains
- Pleural fluid cultures are positive in only 25% of tuberculous effusions

IMAGING STUDIES

Chest x-ray

- Primary disease
  - There may be homogeneous infiltrates, hilar and paratracheal lymph node enlargement, and/or segmental atelectasis
  - Cavitation may be seen with progressive disease
- Reactivation disease
  - There may be fibrocavitary apical disease, nodules, and infiltrates, usually in apical or posterior segments of upper lobes, but in other locations in 30% of cases
  - More commonly in elderly patients
- Miliary pattern (diffuse small nodular densities) reflects hematologic or lymphangitic spread
- Ghon (calcified primary focus) and Ranke (calcified primary focus with calcified hilar lymph node) complexes represent healed primary infection

DIAGNOSTIC PROCEDURES

- Sputum induction is required for patients unable to voluntarily produce a sample
- Bronchoscopy may be considered in smear-negative patients in whom there is a high suspicion of disease
- Needle biopsy of the pleura reveals granulomatous inflammation in 60% of tuberculous pleural effusions; culture of three pleural biopsy specimens combined with microscopic examination increases the diagnostic yield to 90%

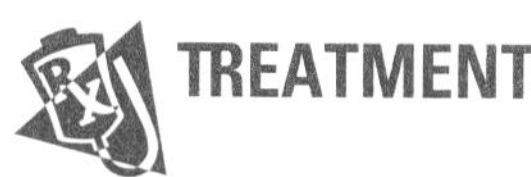

TREATMENT

MEDICATIONS

- See dosages in Table 24
- Multiple drugs to which the organism is susceptible are used; at least two new drugs are added when treatment failure is suspected; when a twice- or thrice-weekly regimen is used, dosages are increased (Tables 23 and 24)
- Coadminister pyridoxine, 10–50 mg/day, for patients at risk of isoniazid neuropathy (diabetes, uremia, malnutrition, alcoholism, HIV infection, pregnancy, seizure disorder)

HIV patients

- 6-month rather than 9-month regimen
- Daily isoniazid (INH), rifampin (RIF), and pyrazinamide (PZA) for 2 months
- Ethambutol (EMB) or streptomycin added where prevalence of INH resistance is 4% or higher
- If isolate is RIF- and INH-sensitive, continue these two drugs for 4 months
- Therapy is continued for at least 3 months beyond documentation of sputum cultures negative for MTB
- Directly observed therapy (DOT) regimens
  - INH/RIF/PZA plus EMB or streptomycin daily for 2 months, then INH/RIF 2–3 times/week for 4 months if susceptibility is demonstrated

- INH/RIF/PZA plus EMB or streptomycin daily for 2 weeks, then 2 times/week for 6 weeks, then INH/RIF 2 times/week for 4 months if susceptibility is demonstrated
- INH/RIF/PZA plus EMB or streptomycin 3 times/week for 6 months

Drug-resistant TB

- MTB resistant only to INH can be treated with 6 months of RIF/PZA plus EMB or streptomycin or 12 months of RIF/EMB
- Treatment requires individualized daily treatment with DOT under an experienced clinician
- Most strains have at least INH or RIF resistance and require three drugs to which susceptibility is proven
- The three-drug regimen is continued until negative cultures are documented; a two-drug regimen is continued for another 12–24 months

Pregnant or lactating women

- INH, RIF, and EMB, with EMB excluded if INH resistance is unlikely
- The teratogenicity of PZA is unknown and streptomycin is contraindicated owing to a risk of congenital deafness
- Pyridoxine should be given with INH
- Breastfeeding is not contraindicated

Extrapulmonary disease

- In most cases, regimens effective for pulmonary disease are adequate
- 9 months of therapy for miliary, meningeal, bone, or joint involvement
- Corticosteroids reduce complications of tuberculous pericarditis and meningitis

SURGERY

- Early debridement and drainage are recommended for skeletal involvement

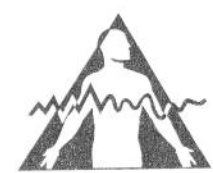

OUTCOME

FOLLOW-UP

- Complete blood cell counts, lung function tests, and renal function should be checked at baseline
- Visual acuity and red-green color vision testing before initiating EMB and audiometry prior to streptomycin use
- Routine monitoring for evidence of drug toxicity should be considered
- Monthly visits with monthly sputum smears and cultures until documented negative
- If sputum is negative after 2 months of therapy, repeat smear and culture at the end of therapy
- Patients with multidrug-resistant tuberculosis (MDRTB) should have sputum smear and culture monthly throughout therapy
- Chest x-ray is recommended on conclusion of successful therapy
- Patients whose cultures do not turn negative or have persistent symptoms after 3 months of therapy should be evaluated for MDRTB

COMPLICATIONS

- Development of drug resistance

PROGNOSIS

- Without therapy, 10% of patients with LTBI will have reactivation during their lifetime, with 50% of cases occurring within 2 years of primary infection
- Almost all properly treated patients with tuberculosis can be cured; relapse rates are less than 5% with current regimens
- The main cause of treatment failure is nonadherence to therapy

WHEN TO REFER

- All cases of drug-resistant TB
- DOT is recommended with MDRTB and those receiving twice- or thrice-weekly therapy

WHEN TO ADMIT

- Patients who are incapable of self-care or likely to expose susceptible individuals to tuberculosis
- Hospitalization is not necessary for initial therapy in most patients
- Hospitalized patients require isolation in an appropriately ventilated room until three sputums from different days are negative for MTB organisms

PREVENTION

- Vaccine bacillus Calmette-Guérin (BCG)
- BCG not recommended in the United States because of its variable effectiveness, the low prevalence of TB infection, and the interference of the vaccine with determination of LTBI
- All suspected and confirmed cases of MTB should be reported to local and state public health authorities

EVIDENCE

PRACTICE GUIDELINES

- American Thoracic Society, Centers for Disease Control and Prevention, Infectious Diseases Society of America: Treatment of tuberculosis. Am J Respir Crit Care Med 2003;167:603. [PMID:12588714]

WEB SITE

- CDC's Division of Tuberculosis Elimination
  - http://www.cdc.gov/nchstp/tb/

INFORMATION FOR PATIENTS

- National Institute of Allergy and Infectious Disease
  - http://www.niaid.nih.gov/publications/pubTB/TBEnglish06.pdf

REFERENCES

- Diagnostic Standards and Classification of Tuberculosis in Adults and Children. American Thoracic Society and Centers for Disease Control and Prevention. Am J Respir Crit Care Med 2000;161(4 Part 1):1376. [PMID:10764337]
- Frieden TR et al: Tuberculosis. Lancet 2003;362:887. [PMID:13678977]
- Jasmer RM et al: Clinical practice. Latent tuberculosis infection. N Engl J Med 2002;347:1860. [PMID:12466511]
- Small PM et al: Management of tuberculosis in the United States. N Engl J Med 2001;345:189. [PMID:11463015]
- Treatment of tuberculosis. MMWR 2003;52(RR11):1
  - http://www.cdc.gov/mmwr/preview/mmwrhtml/rr5211a1.htm)]

Author(s)

Mark S. Chesnutt, MD
Thomas J. Prendergast, MD

Tuberculous Meningitis

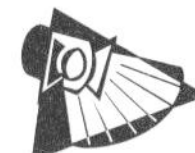

KEY FEATURES

ESSENTIALS OF DIAGNOSIS

- Gradual onset of listlessness, irritability, and anorexia
- Headache, vomiting, and seizures common
- Cranial nerve abnormalities typical
- Tuberculous focus may be evident elsewhere
- Cerebrospinal fluid shows several hundred lymphocytes per microliter, low glucose, and high protein

GENERAL CONSIDERATIONS

- Caused by rupture of a meningeal tuberculoma resulting from earlier hematogenous seeding of tubercle bacillus from a pulmonary focus, or may be a consequence of miliary spread

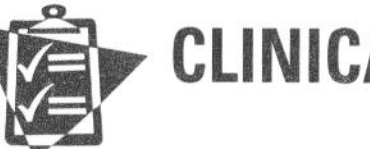

CLINICAL FINDINGS

SYMPTOMS AND SIGNS

- The onset is usually gradual, with listlessness, irritability, anorexia, and fever, followed by headache, vomiting, convulsions, and coma
- In older patients, headache and behavioral changes are prominent early symptoms. Nuchal rigidity and cranial nerve palsies occur as the meningitis progresses
- Evidence of active tuberculosis elsewhere or a history of prior tuberculosis is present in up to 75% of patients
- The tuberculin skin test is usually (not always) positive

DIFFERENTIAL DIAGNOSIS

- May be confused with any other type of meningitis, but the gradual onset, the predominantly lymphocytic pleocytosis of the spinal fluid, and evidence of tuberculosis elsewhere often point to the diagnosis
- Chronic lymphocytic meningitis due to fungi (cryptococcus, coccidioides, histoplasma), brucellosis, leptospirosis, syphilis, Lyme disease, HIV infection, neurocysticercosis
- Carcinomatous meningitis
- Sarcoidosis
- Subdural hematoma

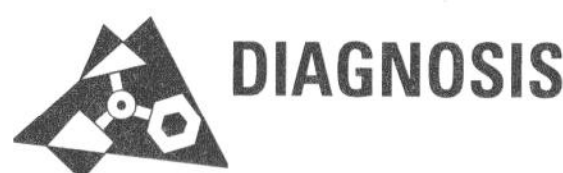

DIAGNOSIS

LABORATORY TESTS

- The spinal fluid is frequently yellowish, with increased pressure, 100–500 cells/μL (predominantly lymphocytes, though neutrophils may be present early during infection), increased protein, and decreased glucose (Table 130)
- Acid-fast stains of cerebrospinal fluid usually are negative, and cultures also may be negative in 15–25% of cases

IMAGING STUDIES

- Chest x-ray often reveals abnormalities compatible with tuberculosis but may be normal

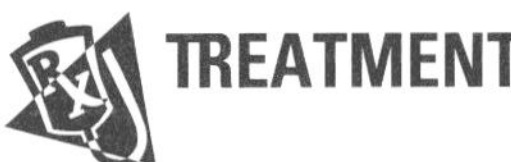

TREATMENT

MEDICATIONS

- Presumptive diagnosis followed by early, empirical antituberculous therapy is essential for survival and to minimize sequelae
- Even if cultures are not positive, a full course of therapy is warranted if the clinical setting is suggestive of tuberculous meningitis
- Regimens that are effective for pulmonary tuberculosis (but adminstered for 12 months) are effective also for tuberculous meningitis (Table 24)
- Rifampin, isoniazid, and pyrazinamide all penetrate into cerebrospinal fluid well
- The penetration of ethambutol is more variable, but therapeutic concentrations can be achieved, and the drug has been successfully used for meningitis
- Some authorities recommend the addition of corticosteroids for patients with focal deficits or altered mental status. Dexamethasone, 0.15 mg/kg four times daily for 1–2 weeks, then discontinued in a tapering regimen over 4 weeks, may be used

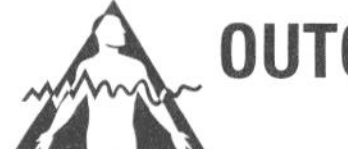

OUTCOME

COMPLICATIONS

- Result from inflammatory exudate primarily involving the basilar meninges and arteries
  - Chronic brain syndrome
  - Seizure disorders
  - Cranial nerve palsies
  - Stroke
  - Obstructive hydrocephalus

PROGNOSIS

- High morbidity and mortality associated with stupor, coma, focal neurological deficits

WHEN TO REFER

- Consultation with a physician experienced in the treatment of tuberculosis is recommended

WHEN TO ADMIT

- Recommended for all suspected cases for initial evaluation and treatment

EVIDENCE

PRACTICE GUIDELINES

- Tuberculous Meningitis
  - http://www.guideline.gov/summary/summary.aspx?doc_id=4670

WEB SITE

- eMedicine
  - http://www.emedicine.com/NEURO/topic385.htm

INFORMATION FOR PATIENTS

- JAMA patient page: Lumbar puncture. JAMA 2002;288:2056.
- JAMA patient page: Meningitis. JAMA 1999;281:1560.
- National Institutes of Health
  - http://www.nlm.nih.gov/medlineplus/ency/article/000650.htm

REFERENCES

- Bidstrup C et al: Tuberculous meningitis in a country with a low incidence of tuberculosis: still a serious disease and a diagnostic challenge. Scand J Infect Dis 2002;34:811. [PMID: 12578148]
- Johansen IS et al: Improved sensitivity of nucleic acid amplification for rapid diagnosis of tuberculous meningitis. J Clin Microbiol 2004;42:3036. [PMID: 15243056]
- Thwaites GE et al: Diagnosis of adult tuberculous meningitis by use of clinical and laboratory features. Lancet 2002;360:1287. [PMID: 12414204]

Author(s)

Henry F. Chambers, MD

Tubular Necrosis, Acute

KEY FEATURES

ESSENTIALS OF DIAGNOSIS

- Acute renal failure
- Fractional excretion of sodium (FE_{Na}) > 1% if oliguric
- Urine sediment with pigmented granular casts and renal tubular epithelial cells

GENERAL CONSIDERATIONS

- Acute renal failure as a result of tubular damage
- Accounts for 85% of intrinsic acute renal failure
- Two major causes are ischemia and nephrotoxin exposure
- Ischemic acute renal failure occurs in prolonged hypotension or hypoxemia such as with dehydration, shock, and sepsis and after major surgical procedures
- Nephrotoxin exposure includes both exogenous and endogenous toxins

Exogenous nephrotoxins

- Aminoglycosides
- Vancomycin, acyclovir
- Radiographic contrast media
- Antineoplastics, such as cisplatin and organic solvents, and heavy metals (mercury, cadmium, and arsenic)

Endogenous nephrotoxins

- Myoglobinuria as a consequence of rhabdomyolysis
- Hemoglobinuria, massive intravascular hemolysis
- Hyperuricemia
- Bence Jones protein, paraproteins

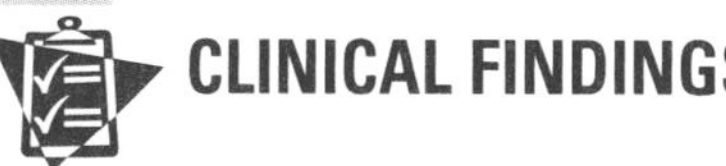

CLINICAL FINDINGS

SYMPTOMS AND SIGNS

- See Renal Failure, Acute

DIFFERENTIAL DIAGNOSIS

- Prerenal azotemia (eg, dehydration)
- Postrenal azotemia (benign prostatic hyperplasia)
- Other renal causes of acute renal failure
  - Acute glomerulonephritis: immune complex (eg, IgA nephropathy), pauci-immune (eg, Wegener's granulomatosis), antiglomerular basement membrane disease
  - Acute interstitial nephritis: drugs (eg, β-lactams), infections (eg, *Streptococcus*), immune (eg, systemic lupus erythematosus)

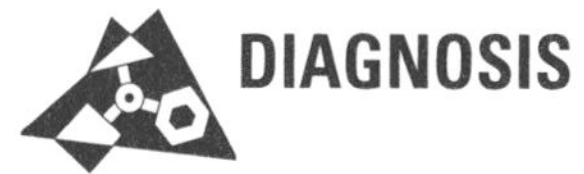

DIAGNOSIS

LABORATORY TESTS

- Serum creatinine (Cr) and blood urea nitrogen (BUN) elevated
- BUN–creatinine ratio < 20:1 in acute tubular necrosis
- Hyperkalemia
- Anion gap metabolic acidosis
- Hyperphosphatemia
- Urinalysis: Urine may be brown with pigmented granular casts or "muddy brown" casts; renal tubular epithelial cells and epithelial cell casts
- FE_{Na} = clearance of Na^+/GFR = clearance of Na^+/creatinine clearance = (urine Na^+/plasma Na^+)/(urine Cr/plasma Cr) × 100
- FE_{Na} high (>1%) in acute tubular necrosis

IMAGING STUDIES

- Renal ultrasonography

DIAGNOSTIC PROCEDURES

- Renal biopsy is rarely indicated

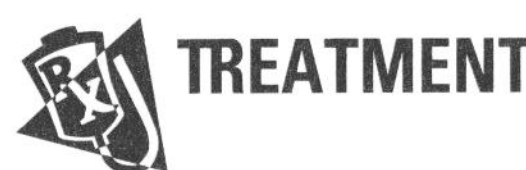

TREATMENT

MEDICATIONS

- Stop offending agent and correct ischemia
- Loop diuretics in moderation, with or without thiazide, for volume maintenance
- Phosphate-binding agents
  - Aluminum hydroxide, 500 mg PO TID with meals
  - Calcium carbonate, 500–1500 mg PO TID with meals
  - Calcium acetate, 667 mg 2–4 tabs PO TID with meals
  - Sevelamer, 800–1600 mg PO TID with meals

THERAPEUTIC PROCEDURES

- Dietary protein restriction of 0.6 g/kg/day in certain settings
- Nutritional support
- Avoid volume overload
- Avoid hyperkalemia
- Avoid magnesium-containing antacids and laxatives
- Hemodialysis, peritoneal dialysis: indications include
  - Uremic symptoms such as pericarditis, encephalopathy, or coagulopathy
  - Fluid overload unresponsive to diuresis
  - Refractory hyperkalemia
  - Severe metabolic acidosis (pH < 7.20)
  - Neurological symptoms such as seizures or neuropathy

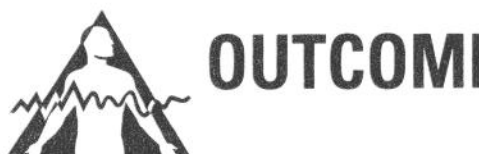

OUTCOME

COMPLICATIONS

- Loop diuretics in large doses may cause deafness

PROGNOSIS

- Nonoliguric acute tubular necrosis has a better outcome
- Mortality from acute renal failure is 20–50% in medical illness and up to 70% in a surgical setting
- Increased mortality with advanced age, severe underlying disease, and multisystem organ failure
- Leading causes of death are infections, fluid and electrolyte disturbances, and worsening of underlying disease

WHEN TO REFER

- Rapidly rising BUN/Cr

WHEN TO ADMIT

- Decompensation from acute renal failure; volume overload; hyperkalemia; uremic symptoms

PREVENTION

- Monitor patients closely with rising serum creatinine after radiographic contrast media

EVIDENCE

WEB SITE

- National Kidney and Urologic Diseases Information Clearinghouse
  - http://kidney.niddk.nih.gov/

INFORMATION FOR PATIENTS

- Mayo Clinic: Kidney Failure
  - http://www.mayoclinic.com/invoke.cfm?id=DS00280
- MedlinePlus: Acute Tubular Necrosis
  - http://www.nlm.nih.gov/medlineplus/ency/article/000512.htm
- MedlinePlus: Kidney Failure Interactive Tutorial
  - http://www.nlm.nih.gov/medlineplus/tutorials/kidneyfailure/htm/index.htm

REFERENCES

- Albright RC Jr: Acute renal failure: a practical update. Mayo Clin Proc 2001;76:67. [PMID: 11155415]
- Murphy SW et al: Contrast nephropathy. J Am Soc Nephrol 2000;11:177. [PMID: 10616853]
- Nissenson AR: Acute renal failure: definition and pathogenesis. Kidney Int 1998;66(Suppl):S7. [PMID: 9573567]
- Perazella MA: Crystal-induced acute renal failure. Am J Med 1999;106:459. [PMID: 10225250]
- Vanholder R et al: Rhabdomyolysis. J Am Soc Nephrol 2000;11:1553. [PMID: 10906171]

Author(s)

Suzanne Watnick, MD

Gail Morrison, MD

Tularemia

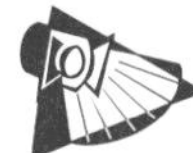

KEY FEATURES

ESSENTIALS OF DIAGNOSIS

- History of contact with rabbits, other rodents, and biting arthropods (eg, ticks in summer) in endemic area
- Fever, headache, nausea, and prostration
- Papule progressing to ulcer at site of inoculation
- Enlarged regional lymph nodes
- Serological tests or culture of ulcer, lymph node aspirate, or blood confirm the diagnosis

GENERAL CONSIDERATIONS

- An infection of wild rodents—particularly rabbits and muskrats—with *Francisella (Pasteurella) tularensis*
- Usually acquired by contact with animal tissues (eg, trapping muskrats, skinning rabbits), from ticks, or from biting flies
- Risk factors for pneumonic tularemia include lawn-mowing and brush-cutting, underscoring the potential for probable aerosol transmission of the organism
- The incubation period is 2–10 days
- *F tularensis* has been classified as a high-priority agent for potential bioterrorism use because of its virulence and relative ease of dissemination

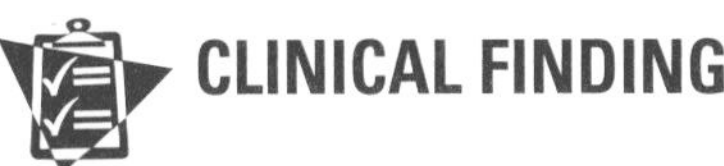

CLINICAL FINDINGS

SYMPTOMS AND SIGNS

- Infection often produces a local lesion and widespread organ involvement but may be entirely asymptomatic
- Fever, headache, and nausea begin suddenly
- A local lesion—a papule at the site of inoculation—develops and soon ulcerates
- The local lesion may be on the skin of an extremity or in the eye
- Regional lymph nodes may become enlarged and tender and may suppurate
- Pneumonia may develop from hematogenous spread of the organism or may be primary after inhalation of infected aerosols, which are responsible for human-to-human transmission
- Following ingestion of infected meat or water, an enteric form may be manifested by gastrointestinal symptoms, stupor, and delirium
- Hematogenous spread may produce meningitis, perisplenitis, pericarditis, pneumonia, and osteomyelitis
- In any type of involvement, the spleen may be enlarged and tender and there may be nonspecific rashes, myalgias, and prostration

DIFFERENTIAL DIAGNOSIS

- Anthrax
- Cat-scratch disease
- Infectious mononucleosis
- Plague
- Typhoid fever
- Lymphoma
- Rickettsial disease, eg, epidemic typhus, Q fever
- Rat-bite fever
- Meningococcemia
- Sporotrichosis
- Herpes simplex virus conjunctivitis

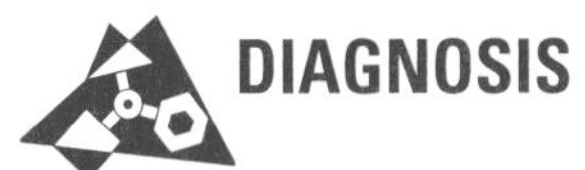

DIAGNOSIS

LABORATORY TESTS

- Culturing the organism from blood or infected tissue requires special media. For this reason and because cultures of *F tularensis* may be hazardous to laboratory personnel, the diagnosis is usually made serologically
- A positive agglutination test (>1:80) develops within 2 weeks and may persist for several years
- Culture of ulcer, lymph node aspirate, or blood confirms the diagnosis

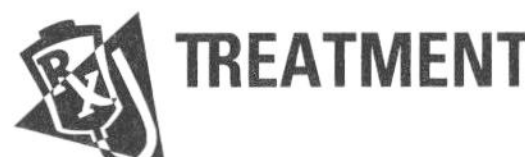

TREATMENT

MEDICATIONS

- Streptomycin, 7.5–10 mg/kg intramuscularly or intravenously every 12 h for 7–10 days
- Chloramphenicol, 50–100 mg/kg/day, is indicated for meningitis

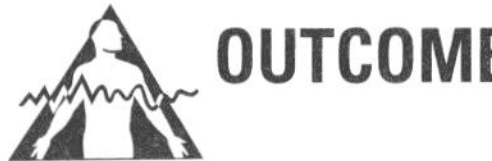

OUTCOME

COMPLICATIONS

- Hematogenous spread may produce meningitis, perisplenitis, pericarditis, pneumonia, and osteomyelitis

WHEN TO REFER

- Early referral to an infectious disease specialist may aid in management

WHEN TO ADMIT

- Serious cases
- Any complications from hematogenous spread

EVIDENCE

PRACTICE GUIDELINES

- National Guideline Clearinghouse
  - http://www.guideline.gov/summary/summary.aspx?doc_id=2981

WEB SITES

- CDC—Emergency Preparedness and Response
  - http://www.bt.cdc.gov/agent/tularemia/index.asp
- Karolinska Institute—Directory of Bacterial Infections and Mycoses
  - http://www.mic.ki.se/Diseases/C01.html

INFORMATION FOR PATIENTS

- National Institute of Allergy and Infectious Diseases
  - http://www.niaid.nih.gov/factsheets/tularemia.htm
- National Institutes of Health
  - http://www.nlm.nih.gov/medlineplus/ency/article/000856.htm

REFERENCES

- Centers for Disease Control and Prevention (CDC): Tularemia associated with a hamster bite—Colorado, 2004. MMWR Morb Mortal Wkly Rep 2005;53:1202. [PMID: 15635290]
- Feldman KA et al: An outbreak of primary pneumonic tularemia on Martha's Vineyard. N Engl J Med 2001;345:1601. [PMID: 11757506]

Author(s)

Henry F. Chambers, MD

Typhoid Fever

Turner's Syndrome (Gonadal Dysgenesis) p. 1162

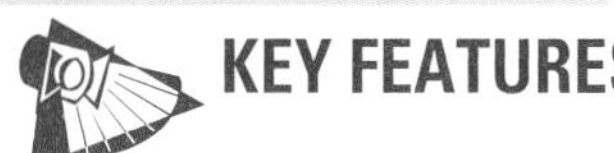

KEY FEATURES

ESSENTIALS OF DIAGNOSIS

- Gradual onset of malaise, headache, sore throat, cough, and either diarrhea or constipation
- Rose spots, relative bradycardia, splenomegaly, and abdominal distention and tenderness
- Leukopenia; blood, stool, and urine culture positive for *Salmonella*

GENERAL CONSIDERATIONS

- The term "typhoid fever" applies when *Salmonella enterica* subspecies *enterica* serotype typhi is the cause of enteric fever accompanied by bacteremia
- Enteric fever generally refers to a typhoidal type illness caused by serotypes other than typhi
- Infection is transmitted by consumption of contaminated food or drink
- Infection begins when organisms cross the intestinal mucosa. Bacteremia occurs, and the infection then localizes principally in the lymphoid tissue of the small intestine (particularly within 60 cm of the ileocecal valve). Peyer's patches become inflamed and may ulcerate, with involvement greatest during the third week of disease
- The incubation period is 5–14 days

DEMOGRAPHICS

- 400 cases per year in the United States, mostly among travelers
- An estimated 21 million cases of typhoid fever and 200,000 deaths occur worldwide

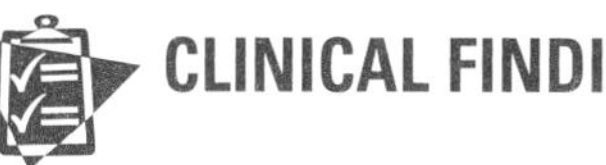

CLINICAL FINDINGS

SYMPTOMS AND SIGNS

Prodromal stage

- Increasing malaise, headache, cough, and sore throat
- Often with abdominal pain and constipation, while the fever ascends in a stepwise fashion
- During the early prodrome, physical findings are few
- There may be marked constipation

Later stage

- After about 7–10 days, the fever reaches a plateau and the patient is much more ill, appearing exhausted and often prostrated
- Marked constipation may develop into "pea soup" diarrhea
- Splenomegaly, abdominal distention and tenderness, relative bradycardia, dicrotic pulse, and occasionally meningismus appear
- The rash (rose spots) commonly appears during the second week of disease. The individual spot, found principally on the trunk, is a pink papule 2–3 mm in diameter that fades on pressure. It disappears in 3–4 days

DIFFERENTIAL DIAGNOSIS

- Brucellosis
- Tuberculosis
- Infective endocarditis
- Q fever and other rickettsial infections
- Other causes of acute diarrhea
- Viral hepatitis
- Lymphoma
- Adult Still's disease
- Malaria

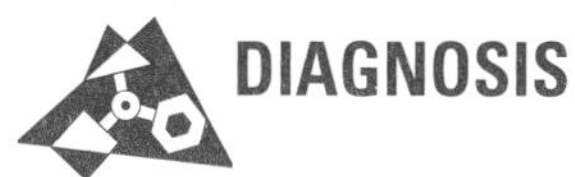

DIAGNOSIS

LABORATORY TESTS

- Best diagnosed by isolation of the organism from blood culture, which is positive in the first week of illness in 80% of patients who have not taken antibiotics
- Cultures of bone marrow occasionally are positive when blood cultures are not
- Stool culture is not reliable because it may be positive in gastroenteritis without typhoid fever

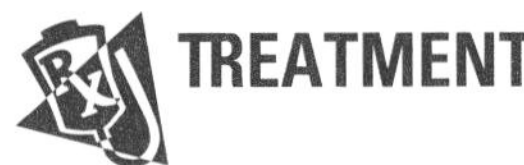

TREATMENT

MEDICATIONS

- Ciprofloxacin, 500 mg orally twice daily or 400 mg intravenously twice daily for 5–7 days
- Ceftriaxone, 2 g intravenously once daily for 10–14 days
- Azithromycin, 1 g orally for 5 days
- Dexamethasone (3 mg/kg over 30 min intravenously, then 1 mg/kg every 6 h for 8 doses) reduces mortality in patients with severe typhoid fever (eg, those with delirium, coma, shock)
- Many strains are resistant to ampicillin and chloramphenicol; resistance to trimethoprim-sulfamethoxazole is increasing

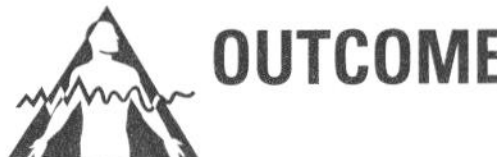

OUTCOME

FOLLOW-UP

- Follow-up examination, with blood cultures for fever, as relapse can occur

COMPLICATIONS

- Complications occur in about 30% of untreated cases and account for 75% of all deaths
- Intestinal hemorrhage, manifested by a sudden drop in temperature and signs of shock followed by dark or fresh blood in the stool, or intestinal perforation, accompanied by abdominal pain and tenderness, is most likely to occur during the third week

PROGNOSIS

- Mortality rate is about 2% in treated cases
- With complications, the prognosis is poor
- Relapses occur in 5–10% of cases; these are treated the same as primary infection
- A residual carrier state frequently persists in spite of chemotherapy

WHEN TO REFER

- Report to the public health department to trace contacts or carriers
- Refer early to an infectious disease specialist

WHEN TO ADMIT

- For intravenous antibiotics or supportive care

PREVENTION

- Immunization is not always effective but should be provided for household contacts of a typhoid carrier, for travelers to endemic areas, and during epidemic outbreaks
- A multiple-dose oral vaccine and a single-dose parenteral vaccine are available
- Adequate waste disposal and protection of food and water supplies from contamination are important public health measures to prevent salmonellosis
- Carriers must not be permitted to work as food handlers

EVIDENCE

PRACTICE GUIDELINES

- National Guideline Clearinghouse: Immunization Information
  - http://www.guideline.gov/summary/summary.aspx?doc_id=3180

WEB SITES

- CDC—Division of Bacterial and Mycotic Diseases
  - http://www.cdc.gov/ncidod/dbmd/
- Karolinska Institute—Directory of Bacterial Infections and Mycoses
  - http://www.mic.ki.se/Diseases/C01.html

INFORMATION FOR PATIENTS

- Centers for Disease Control and Prevention
  - http://www.cdc.gov/ncidod/dbmd/diseaseinfo/typhoidfever_g.htm
- National Institutes of Health
  - http://www.nlm.nih.gov/medlineplus/ency/article/001332.htm

REFERENCES

- Parry CM et al: Typhoid fever. N Engl J Med 2002;347:1770. [PMID: 12456854]
- Steinberg EB et al: Typhoid fever in travelers: who should be targeted for prevention? Clin Infect Dis 2004;39:186. [PMID: 15307027]

Author(s)

Henry F. Chambers, MD

Typhus, Endemic p. 1162. Typhus, Epidemic Louse-Borne p. 1163.
Typhus, Scrub p. 1163.

Ulcerative Colitis

KEY FEATURES

ESSENTIALS OF DIAGNOSIS

- Bloody diarrhea
- Lower abdominal cramps and fecal urgency
- Anemia, low serum albumin
- Negative stool cultures
- Sigmoidoscopy is key to diagnosis

GENERAL CONSIDERATIONS

- Idiopathic inflammatory condition that involves the mucosal surface of the colon, resulting in diffuse friability and erosions with bleeding
- In 50% of cases, disease is confined to the rectosigmoid region (proctosigmoiditis); 30% extend to the splenic flexure (left-sided colitis); <20% extend more proximally (extensive colitis)
- Most affected patients experience periods of symptomatic flare-ups and remissions

DEMOGRAPHICS

- More common in nonsmokers and former smokers, severity may worsen in patients who stop smoking
- Appendectomy at age <20 reduces risk

CLINICAL FINDINGS

SYMPTOMS AND SIGNS

- Bloody diarrhea
- Cramps, abdominal pain
- Fecal urgency and tenesmus
- Abdominal tenderness, rebound tenderness
- Bright red blood on digital rectal examination
- Diarrhea infrequent
- Rectal bleeding and mucus intermittent
- Fecal urgency and tenesmus
- Left lower quadrant cramps, relieved by defecation
- No significant abdominal tenderness
- Diarrhea more severe with frequent bleeding
- Abdominal pain and tenderness
- Mild fever

Severe disease

- >6–10 bloody bowel movements per day
- Signs of hypovolemia and impaired nutrition
- Abdominal pain and tenderness

Fulminant disease

- Rapid progression of symptoms and signs of severe toxicity (hypovolemia, hemorrhage requiring transfusion, and abdominal distention with tenderness) over 1–2 weeks in fulminant colitis

Toxic megacolon

- Colonic dilation of >6 cm on plain films with signs of toxicity, occurring in < 2%, heightens risk of perforation

Extracolonic manifestations

- Occur in 25% of cases
- Erythema nodosum, pyoderma gangrenosum
- Episcleritis
- Thromboembolic events
- Oligoarticular, nondeforming arthritis
- Sclerosing cholangitis, with risk of cholangiocarcinoma

DIFFERENTIAL DIAGNOSIS

- Infectious colitis: *Salmonella, Shigella, Campylobacter,* amebiasis, *Clostridium difficile,* enteroinvasive *Escherichia coli*
- Ischemic colitis
- Crohn's disease
- Diverticular disease
- Colon cancer
- Antibiotic-associated diarrhea or pseudomembranous colitis
- Infectious proctitis: gonorrhea, chlamydia, herpes, syphilis
- Radiation colitis or proctitis
- Cytomegalovirus colitis in AIDS

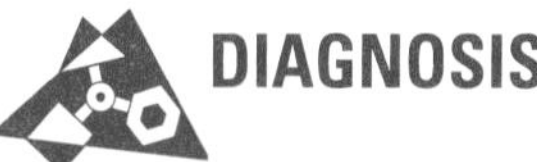

DIAGNOSIS

LABORATORY TESTS

- Obtain hematocrit, erythrocyte sedimentation rate, and serum albumin
- Anemia in moderate to severe disease
- Hypoalbuminemia in moderate to severe disease
- Antineutrophil cytoplasmic antibodies with perinuclear staining (p-ANCA) in 50–70%; sometimes useful to distinguish from Crohn's disease in patients with indeterminate colitis
- Stools for bacterial (including *C difficile*) culture, ova and parasites

IMAGING STUDIES

- Plain abdominal radiographs
- Barium enema is of little utility and may precipitate toxic megacolon

DIAGNOSTIC PROCEDURES

- Sigmoidoscopy establishes diagnosis
- Colonoscopy should not be performed in patients with severe disease because of the risk of perforation, but after improvement colonoscopy is recommended to determine extent of disease, and for cancer surveillance

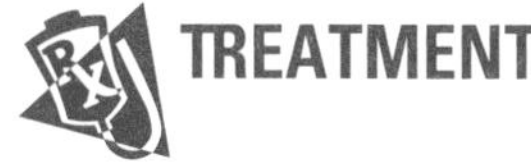

TREATMENT

MEDICATIONS

Mild to moderate colitis

- Mesalamine, 800 mg PO TID (Asacol) or 1 g PO QID (Pentasa), balsalazide, 2.25 g PO TID, or sulfasalazine, 500 mg PO BID and increased gradually over 1–2 weeks to 2 g PO BID; 50–75% improve
- Folic acid, 1 mg PO QD, should be given to all patients taking sulfasalazine
- Corticosteroid therapy to patients who fail to improve after 2–3 weeks
- Hydrocortisone foam or enemas (80–100 mg BID), or prednisone, 20–30 mg BID, tapering after 2 weeks by no more than 5 mg/week, slower tapering after 15 mg/day
- Antidiarrheal agents (eg, loperamide, 2 mg, diphenoxylate with atropine, 1 tablet, or tincture of opium, 8–15 drops up

to four times daily), but should not be given in the acute phase of illness

Distal colitis

- Mesalamine suppository, 500 mg PR BID for proctitis, and as an enema 4 g PR QHS for proctosigmoiditis, for 3–12 weeks; 75% of patients improve
- Hydrocortisone suppository or foam for proctitis and hydrocortisone enema (80–100 mg) for proctosigmoiditis; less effective

Severe colitis

- Corticosteroid therapy improves 50–75%
- Methylprednisolone, 48–64 mg, or hydrocortisone 300 mg, in 3 divided doses
- Hydrocortisone enema, 100 mg BID as a drip over 30 min
- Immunosuppressive agents: cyclosporine, 4 mg/kg/day IV, improves 60–75% of patients with severe colitis that is not improving after 7–10 days of intravenous steroids

Fulminant colitis and toxic megacolon

- Broad-spectrum antibiotics targeting anaerobes and gram-negative bacteria
- Mercaptopurine or azathioprine long-term therapy for patients with severe steroid-resistant colitis

Maintenance therapy

- Sulfasalazine, 1–1.5 g PO BID; olsalazine, 500 mg PO BID; and mesalamine, 800 mg PO TID (Asacol) or 500 mg PO QID (Pentasa) reduce relapse rate from 75% to < 33%
- For distal colitis: mesalamine suppositories (500 mg PO QD) or oral mesalamine, balsalazide, or sulfasalazine reduce the relapse rate from 80–90% to < 20% within 1 year

Refractory disease

- Mercaptopurine or azathioprine
- Infliximab (5 mg/kg); efficacy unproven in controlled trials

SURGERY

- Total proctocolectomy with ileostomy (standard ileostomy, continent ileostomy, or ileoanal anastomosis) required in 25% of patients
- Indications for surgery include patients with severe disease (eg, severe hemorrhage) who fail to improve after 7–10 days of corticosteroid or cyclosporine therapy; perforation; refractory disease requiring chronic steroids to control symptoms; fulminant colitis or toxic megacolon that worsens or fails to improve within 48–72 h; dysplasia or carcinoma on surveillance colonoscopic biopsies

THERAPEUTIC PROCEDURES

Mild to moderate colitis

- Regular diet
- Limit intake of caffeine and gas-producing vegetables
- Fiber supplements (eg, psyllium, 3.4 g PO BID; methylcellulose, 2 g PO BID; bran powder, 1 tbsp PO BID)

Severe colitis

- Discontinue all oral intake
- Avoid opioid and anticholinergic agents
- Restore circulating volume with fluids and blood
- Correct electrolyte abnormalities

Fulminant colitis and toxic megacolon

- Nasogastric suction, roll patients from side to side and onto the abdomen
- Serial examinations and abdominal plain films to look for worsening dilation

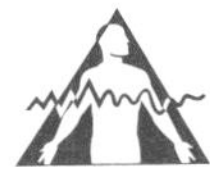

OUTCOME

COMPLICATIONS

- Toxic megacolon
- Colon cancer
- Sclerosing cholangitis with risk of cholangiocarcinoma

PROGNOSIS

- Lifelong disease characterized by exacerbations and remissions
- In most patients, disease is readily controlled by medical therapy without need for surgery
- Majority never require hospitalization
- Surgery results in complete cure of the disease

WHEN TO REFER

- Patients with severe or refractory disease requiring immunomodulatory therapy

WHEN TO ADMIT

- Hospitalize patients with severe colitis

PREVENTION

- Colon cancer occurs in ~0.5–1% per year of patients who have had colitis for >10 years
- Colonoscopy with multiple random mucosal biopsies recommended every 1–2 years in patients with extensive colitis, beginning 8–10 years after diagnosis
- Folic acid, 1 mg PO QD, decreases risk of colon cancer

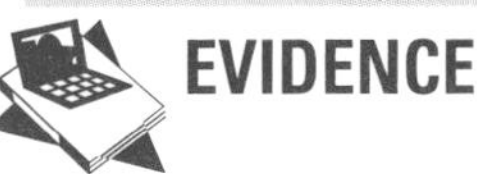

EVIDENCE

PRACTICE GUIDELINES

- Bebb JR et al: Systematic review: how effective are the usual treatments for ulcerative colitis? Aliment Pharmacol Ther 2004;20:143. [PMID: 15362049]
- Kornbluth A et al: Ulcerative colitis practice guidelines in adults (update): American College of Gastroenterology, Practice Parameters Committee. Am J Gastroenterol 2004;99:1371. [PMID: 15233681]

WEB SITES

- Crohn's & Colitis Foundation of America
  - www.ccfa.org/research/info/aboutuc (also contains patient information)
- National Digestive Diseases Information Clearinghouse—Ulcerative Colitis
  - http://digestive.niddk.nih.gov/ddiseases/pubs/colitis/index.htm
- WebPath Gastrointestinal Pathology Index
  - http://medstat.med.utah.edu/WebPath/GIHTML/GIIDX.html

INFORMATION FOR PATIENTS

- Mayo Clinic
  - http://www.mayoclinic.com/invoke.cfm?id=DS00104
- National Digestive Diseases Information Clearinghouse
  - http://digestive.niddk.nih.gov/ddiseases/pubs/colitis/

REFERENCES

- Gan SI et al: A new look at toxic megacolon: an update and review of incidence, etiology, pathogenesis, and management. Am J Gastroenterol 2003;98:2363. [PMID: 14638335]
- Hanauer S: Medical therapy for ulcerative colitis 2004. Gastroenterology 2004;126:1582. [PMID: 15168369]
- Rizello F et al: Review article: medical therapy of severe ulcerative colitis. Aliment Pharmacol Ther 2003;17(Suppl 2):7. [PMID: 12786606]
- Vecchi M et al: Review article: diagnosis, monitoring and treatment of distal colitis. Aliment Pharmacol Ther 2003;17(Suppl 2):2. [PMID: 12786605]

Author(s)

Kenneth R. McQuaid, MD

Urinary Incontinence

KEY FEATURES

GENERAL CONSIDERATIONS

- Urinary incontinence is the involuntary loss of urine
- Urinary continence depends on both bladder and sphincteric mechanisms; dysfunction of either component may result in incontinence
- Most common in older patients
- Prevalence 5–15% in the community, > 50% in long-term care facilities

Classification

- **Total incontinence**: uncontrolled loss of urine at all times and in all positions. Results when sphincteric efficiency is lost (previous surgery, nerve damage, cancerous infiltration) or when an abnormal connection between the urinary tract and the skin exists that bypasses the urinary sphincter (vesicovaginal or ureterovaginal fistulas)
- **Stress incontinence:** loss of urine associated with activities that increase intra-abdominal pressure (coughing, sneezing, lifting, exercising), though not in the supine position, results from urethral sphincteric insufficiency due to laxity of the pelvic floor musculature—in multiparous women or after pelvic surgery
- **Urge incontinence:** loss of urine that is preceded by a strong, unexpected urge to void, unrelated to position or activity, results from detrusor hyperreflexia or sphincter dysfunction due to inflammatory conditions or neurogenic disorders of the bladder
- **Overflow incontinence:** loss of urine in patients with chronic urinary retention results from the chronically distended bladder receiving an additional increment of urine, so that intravesical pressure just exceeds the outlet resistance, allowing a small amount of urine to dribble out

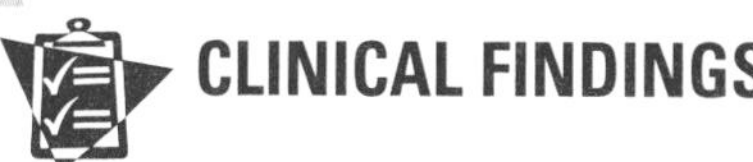

CLINICAL FINDINGS

SYMPTOMS AND SIGNS

- History permits subclassification into one of the four categories of incontinence
- Physical examination is done to exclude fistula in cases of total incontinence, neurological abnormalities (spasticity, flaccidity, rectal sphincter tone, bulbocavernosus reflex) in cases of urge incontinence, or distended bladder in cases of overflow incontinence

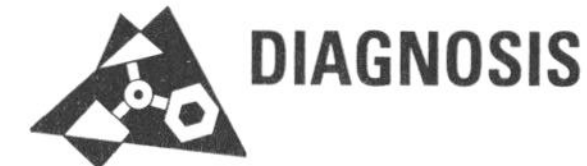

DIAGNOSIS

LABORATORY TESTS

- Urinalysis and urine culture to exclude urinary tract infection.
- Serum creatinine to exclude renal dysfunction
- Cystograms to demonstrate fistula sites and descensus of the bladder neck (descent of bladder neck more than 1.5 cm on straining view) in cases of stress incontinence
- Urethral catheterization or ultrasonography to assess postvoid residual urine volume

DIAGNOSTIC PROCEDURES

- History, supplemented with a voiding diary

Special tests

- Urodynamic evaluation can assess both bladder and sphincteric function and is indicated
  - In patients with moderate to severe incontinence
  - When neurological disease is suspected
  - When infection and neoplasm have been excluded in urge incontinence
- Cystometry to assess bladder capacity, accommodation, sensation, voluntary control, contractility, and response to pharmacological intervention
  - Normal adult bladder capacity = 350–500 mL
  - Decreased capacity occurs in incontinence, infections, interstitial cystitis, radiation damage, upper motor neuron lesions, and postoperative changes
  - Increased bladder capacity occurs with chronic urinary tract obstruction, lower motor neuron lesions, and sensory neuropathies
- Urethral profilometry, electromyography, or combined video studies to assess sphincteric function

Urinary Incontinence

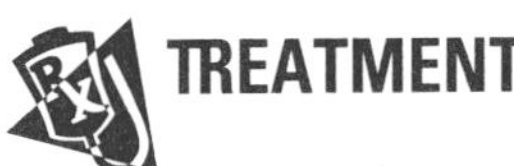

TREATMENT

MEDICATIONS

- Urge incontinence: anticholinergic medications (oxybutynin, 5–15 mg/day, or tolterodine, 2–4 mg/day) or tricyclic antidepressants (imipramine, 25–75 mg PO at bedtime)

SURGERY

- Total incontinence
  - Congenital defects and acquired lesions require surgical correction
  - Sphincter injuries following prostatectomy may be managed by surgical reconstruction with a sling or artificial urinary sphincter
- Stress incontinence
  - Bladder neck descends below the midportion of the pubic symphysis
  - Surgical treatment centers on placing the bladder neck into an appropriate anatomic location, allowing increased intra-abdominal pressure to be transmitted to the bladder and bladder neck

THERAPEUTIC PROCEDURES

- Overflow incontinence
  - Placement of a urethral catheter in the acute setting
  - Further treatment must address the underlying disease

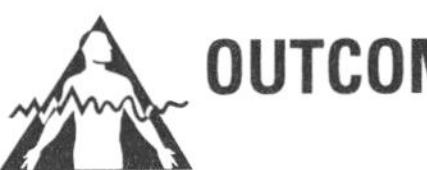

OUTCOME

PROGNOSIS

- Surgery is usually corrective for stress incontinence

EVIDENCE

PRACTICE GUIDELINES

- Urinary incontinence. American Medical Directors Association, 2001
  - http://www.guidelines.gov/summary/summary.aspx?doc_id=1812&nbr=1038&string=urinary+incontinence

INFORMATION FOR PATIENTS

- American Academy of Family Physicians—Urinary incontinence: embarrassing but treatable
  - http://familydoctor.org/healthfacts/189/
- National Institute on Aging
  - http://www.niapublications.org/engagepages/urinary.asp
- National Kidney and Urologic Diseases Information Clearinghouse
  - http://kidney.niddk.nih.gov/kudiseases/pubs/uiwomen/index.htm

REFERENCES

- Davila GW et al: Current treatment options for female urinary incontinence—a review. Int J Fertil Women's Med 2004;49:102. [PMID: 15303311]
- Foldspang A et al: Risk of postpartum urinary incontinence associated with pregnancy and mode of delivery. Acta Obstet Gynecol Scand 2004;83:923. [PMID: 15453887]
- Hannestad YS et al: Familial risk of urinary incontinence in women: population based cross sectional study. BMJ 2004;329:889. [PMID: 15485965]
- Parkkinen A et al: Physiotherapy for female stress urinary incontinence: individual therapy at the outpatient clinic versus home-based pelvic floor training: a 5-year follow-up study. Neurourol Urodyn 2004;23:643. [PMID: 15382186]
- Rohr G et al: Reproducibility and validity of simple questions to identify urinary incontinence in elderly women. Acta Obstet Gynecol Scand 2004;83:969. [PMID: 15453896]

Author(s)

Marshall, L. Stoller, MD
Peter R. Carroll, MD

Urinary Incontinence in Elderly

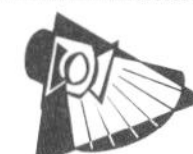

KEY FEATURES

ESSENTIALS OF DIAGNOSIS

- Delirium is the most common cause of transient or potentially reversible incontinence
- Detrusor overactivity (urge incontinence) is the most common cause of established incontinence

GENERAL CONSIDERATIONS

Transient causes (the mnemonic "DIAPPERS")

- Delirium (most common cause in hospitalized patients)
- Infection (symptomatic urinary tract infection)
- Atrophic urethritis and vaginitis
- Pharmaceuticals (eg, potent diuretics, anticholinergics, psychotropics, opioid analgesics, α-blockers [in women], α-agonists [in men], and calcium channel blockers)
- Psychological factors (severe depression with psychomotor retardation)
- Excess urinary output (diuretics, excess fluid intake, hyperglycemia and peripheral edema and its associated nocturia)
- Restricted mobility (see Immobility in Elderly)
- Stool impaction

Established causes

- Detrusor overactivity (urge incontinence)
  - Uninhibited bladder contractions that cause leakage
  - Most common cause of established geriatric incontinence, accounting for two-thirds of cases; usually idiopathic
- Urethral incompetence (stress incontinence)
- Urethral obstruction
- Detrusor underactivity (overflow incontinence)

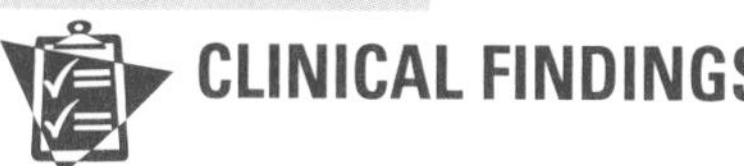

CLINICAL FINDINGS

SYMPTOMS AND SIGNS

- Atrophic urethritis and vaginitis
  - Vaginal mucosal friability, erosions, telangiectasia, petechiae, or erythema
- Detrusor overactivity (urge incontinence)
  - Women complain of urinary leakage after the onset of an intense urge to urinate that cannot be forestalled
- Urethral incompetence (stress incontinence)
  - Urinary loss occurs with laughing, coughing, or lifting heavy objects
- Urethral obstruction
  - Dribbling incontinence after voiding
  - Urge incontinence due to detrusor overactivity (which coexists in two-thirds of cases), or overflow incontinence due to urinary retention
- Detrusor underactivity (overflow incontinence)
  - Urinary frequency, nocturia, and frequent leakage of small amounts

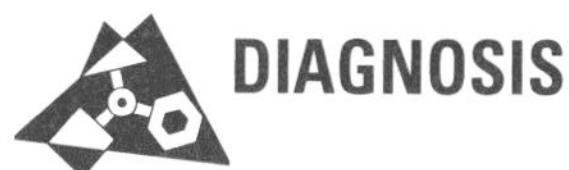

DIAGNOSIS

LABORATORY TESTS

- Review medications
- Check urinalysis for infection
- Consider tests for hyperglycemia, hypercalcemia, diabetes insipidus

IMAGING STUDIES

- Ultrasonography can determine postvoid residual
- Renal ultrasound to exclude hydronephrosis in men whose postvoid residual exceeds 150 mL, particularly if the incontinence developed suddenly
- In older men for whom surgery is planned, urodynamic confirmation of obstruction is strongly advised

DIAGNOSTIC PROCEDURES

- To test for **stress incontinence**, have the patient relax her perineum and cough vigorously (a single cough) while standing with a full bladder
  - Instantaneous leakage indicates stress incontinence if urinary retention has been excluded by postvoid residual determination using ultrasound
  - A delay of several seconds or persistent leakage suggests the problem is caused by an uninhibited bladder contraction induced by coughing
- Because **detrusor overactivity** may be due to bladder stones or tumor, the abrupt onset of otherwise unexplained urge incontinence—especially if accompanied by perineal or suprapubic discomfort or sterile hematuria—should be investigated by cystoscopy and cytologic examination of the urine
- An elevated postvoid residual (generally over 450 mL) distinguishes detrusor underactivity from detrusor overactivity and stress incontinence, but only urodynamic testing differentiates it from urethral obstruction in men

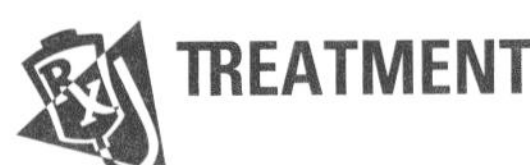

TREATMENT

MEDICATIONS

Transient causes

- Discontinue all anticholinergic agents or substitute with less anticholinergic effects (eg, sertraline instead of desipramine)

Established causes

- Detrusor overactivity: oxybutynin (2.5–5 mg PO TID or QID), long-acting oxybutynin (5–15 mg PO QD), or tolterodine (1–2 mg PO BID) may reduce episodes of incontinence; watch for delirium, dry mouth, or urinary retention
- Urethral incompetence (stress incontinence): topical or oral estrogens may be helpful if atrophic vaginitis with urethral irritation is present
- Urethral obstruction: for prostatic obstruction without retention, treatment with α-blocking agents (eg, terazosin, 1–10 mg PO QD; prazosin, 1–5 mg PO BID; tamsulosin, 0.4–0.8 mg QD) may relieve symptoms
- Detrusor underactivity: antibiotics (only for symptomatic upper urinary tract infection or as prophylaxis against recurrent symptomatic infections with intermittent catheterization)
- Detrusor overactivity
  - The cornerstone is behavioral therapy
  - Patients are instructed to void every 1–2 h while awake (increased by 30 min until the interval is 4–5 h)
  - Pelvic floor exercises, behavioral approaches, and biofeedback can be extremely helpful
  - In refractory cases, where intermittent catheterization is feasible, the physician may choose to induce urinary retention with a bladder relaxant and have the patient empty the bladder three or four times daily
- Urethral incompetence (stress incontinence)
  - Pelvic muscle and pelvic floor exercises are effective for mild to moderate stress incontinence; they can be combined with biofeedback, electrical stimulation, or vaginal cones
  - A pessary or a tampon (for women with exercise-associated stress incontinence)
- Urethral obstruction
  - For the nonoperative candidate, use an intermittent or indwelling catheter
- Detrusor underactivity
  - Augmented voiding techniques (eg, double voiding, suprapubic pressure)
  - Intermittent or indwelling catheterization

SURGERY

- Although a last resort, surgery is the most effective treatment for stress incontinence, resulting in a cure rate of 75–85% even in older women
- Surgical decompression is the most effective treatment for urethral obstruction, especially in the setting of urinary retention

OUTCOME

COMPLICATIONS

- The most important complication is restriction of social activity
- In immobile patients, incontinence increases the risk for pressure ulcers

PROGNOSIS

- Some incontinence resolves spontaneously
- In most patients, treatment of exacerbating factors, and pharmacologic and nonpharmacologic treatments can substantially reduce the severity

WHEN TO REFER

- Refer to a multidisciplinary incontinence clinic or geriatrician if there is no response to first-line measures

PREVENTION

- Weight loss may be beneficial especially for stress incontinence

EVIDENCE

PRACTICE GUIDELINES

- Urinary incontinence in adults: acute and chronic management. Clinical Practice Guideline, No. 2, 1996 update. United States Department of Health and Human Services. Public Health Service, AHCPR. Publication No. 96-0682.
- National Guidelines Clearinghouse
  - Continence for Women. Association of Women's Health, Obstetric and Neonatal Nurses, 2000
  - Urinary Incontinence. The John A. Hartford Foundation Institute for Geriatric Nursing, 2003.
- http://www.guideline.gov/summary/summary.aspx?doc_id=3507

WEB SITE

- MedlinePlus: Urinary Incontinence
  - http://www.nlm.nih.gov/medlineplus/urinaryincontinence.html

INFORMATION FOR PATIENTS

- American Academy of Family Physicians
  - http://familydoctor.org/189.xml
- JAMA patient page: incontinence. JAMA 1998;280:2054. [PMID: 9863861]
- Parmet S et al: JAMA patient page. Stress incontinence. JAMA 2003;290:426. [PMID: 12865384]

REFERENCE

- Burgio KL: Behavioral vs drug treatment for urge urinary incontinence in older women: a randomized, controlled trial. JAMA 1998;280:1995. [PMID: 9863850]

Author(s)

Helen Chen, MD

C. Bree Johnston, MD

Urinary Stone Disease

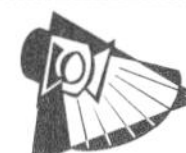

KEY FEATURES

GENERAL CONSIDERATIONS

- 240,000–720,000 Americans per year
- Males > females (3:1)
- Initial presentation predominates in the third and fourth decades
- Incidence is greatest during hot summer months
- Geographic factors (high humidity and elevated temperatures); diet (sodium and protein intake, excess intake of oxalate and purines); fluid intake; and genetic factors (cystinuria; distal renal tubular acidosis) contribute to urinary stone formation
- Five major types of urinary stones: calcium oxalate, calcium phosphate, struvite, uric acid, and cystine
- Most urinary stones contain calcium (85%) and are radiopaque; uric acid stones are radiolucent
- **Hypercalciuric calcium nephrolithiasis** (>250 mg/24 h) can be caused by absorptive, resorptive, and renal disorders (Table 89)
  - **Absorptive hypercalciuria** is secondary to increased absorption of calcium at the level of the small bowel, predominantly in the jejunum, and can be further subdivided into types I, II, and III. **Type I absorptive hypercalciuria** is independent of calcium intake. There is increased urinary calcium on a regular or even a calcium-restricted diet. **Type II absorptive hypercalciuria** is diet dependent. **Type III absorptive hypercalciuria** is secondary to a renal phosphate leak, which results in increased vitamin D synthesis and secondarily increased small bowel absorption of calcium
  - Resorptive hypercalciuria is secondary to hyperparathyroidism. Hypercalcemia, hypophosphatemia, hypercalciuria, and an elevated serum parathyroid hormone level are found
  - Renal hypercalciuria occurs when the renal tubules are unable to efficiently reabsorb filtered calcium, and hypercalciuria and secondary hyperparathyroidism result
- **Hyperuricosuric calcium nephrolithiasis** is secondary to dietary excesses or uric acid metabolic defects
- **Hyperoxaluric calcium nephrolithiasis** is usually due to primary intestinal disorders, including chronic diarrhea, inflammatory bowel disease, or steatorrhea
- **Hypocitraturic calcium nephrolithiasis** is secondary to disorders associated with metabolic acidosis including chronic diarrhea, type I (distal) renal tubular acidosis, and chronic hydrochlorothiazide treatment
- **Uric acid calculi:** contributing factors include low urinary pH, myeloproliferative disorders, malignancy with increased uric acid production, abrupt and dramatic weight loss, and uricosuric medications
- **Struvite calculi** (magnesium-ammonium-phosphate, "staghorn" calculi) occur with recurrent urinary tract infections with urease-producing organisms, including *Proteus*, *Pseudomonas*, *Providencia*, and, less commonly, *Klebsiella*, staphylococci, and *Mycoplasma*; urine pH ≥ 7.2
- **Cystine calculi**
- Inherited disorder with recurrent stone disease

CLINICAL FINDINGS

SYMPTOMS AND SIGNS

- Colicky pain in the flank, usually severe
- Nausea and vomiting
- Patients constantly moving—in sharp contrast to those with an acute abdomen
- Pain episodic and radiates anteriorly over the abdomen
- With stone in the ureter, pain may be referred into the ipsilateral testis or labium
- With stone at the ureterovesical junction, marked urinary urgency and frequency
- Stone size does not correlate with severity of symptoms

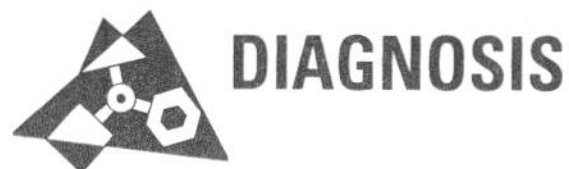

DIAGNOSIS

LABORATORY TESTS

- Urinalysis: microscopic or gross (~10%) hematuria. Absence of microhematuria does not exclude urinary stones
- Urinary pH: persistent urinary pH < 5.0 is suggestive of uric acid or cystine stones; persistent pH ≥ 7.2 is suggestive of a struvite stone

Metabolic evaluation

- Stone analysis on recovered stones
- Uncomplicated first-time stone formers: serum calcium, phosphate, electrolytes, and uric acid
- Recurrent stone formers or patients with a family history of stone disease: 24-h urine collection on a random diet for volume, urinary pH, and calcium, uric acid, oxalate, phosphate, and citrate excretion
- To subcategorize patients, if necessary: a second 24-h urine collection on a restricted calcium (400 mg/day) and sodium (100 mEq/day) diet
- Serum parathyroid hormone

IMAGING STUDIES

- Spiral CT sensitivity exceeds that of ultrasound or intravenous urography
- Plain film of the abdomen and renal ultrasound will diagnose most stones
- Plain film of the abdomen: radiopaque stones
- Abdominal ultrasonography: stones at the ureterovesical junction can be imaged if patient has a full bladder

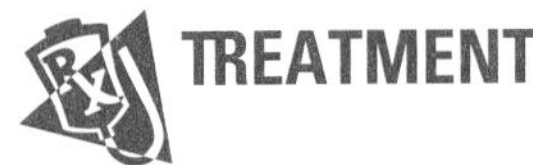

TREATMENT

MEDICATIONS

- **Type I absorptive hypercalciuria:** cellulose phosphate, 10–15 g in 3 divided doses given with meals to decrease bowel absorption of calcium. Follow-up metabolic surveillance every 6–8 months to exclude hypomagnesemia, secondary hyperoxaluria, and recurrent calculi. Thiazide therapy can decrease renal calcium excretion
- **Type II absorptive hypercalciuria:** decrease calcium intake by 50% (to approximately 400 mg QD). There is no specific medical therapy
- **Type III absorptive hypercalciuria:** orthophosphates (250 mg TID) to inhibit vitamin D synthesis
- **Renal hypercalciuria:** thiazides (effective long-term)
- **Hyperuricosuric calcium nephrolithiasis:** dietary purine restrictions or allopurinol, 300 mg PO QD (or both)
- **Hyperoxaluric calcium nephrolithiasis:** measures to curtail the diarrhea or steatorrhea, oral calcium supplements with meals, and encouraging increased fluid intake
- **Hypocitraturic calcium nephrolithiasis:** potassium citrate, 20 mEq PO TID
- **Uric acid calculi:** potassium citrate, 20 mEq PO TID, to increase urinary pH above 6.2. Patients should monitor their urinary alkalinization with Nitrazine pH paper. If hyperuricemia is present, allopurinol, 300 mg PO QD
- **Struvite calculi:** after stone extraction consider suppressive antibiotics. Acetohydroxamic acid, an effective urease inhibitor, is poorly tolerated
- **Cystine calculi:** difficult to manage medically. Prevention by increased fluid intake, alkalinization of the urine above pH 7.5 (monitored with Nitrazine pH paper), penicillamine and tiopronin

SURGERY

- **Resorptive hypercalciuria:** surgical resection of the parathyroid adenoma
- **Infection with ureteral obstruction:** a medical emergency requiring both prompt drainage by a ureteral catheter or a percutaneous nephrostomy tube, and antibiotics
- **Ureteral stones:** stones < 6 mm in diameter will usually pass spontaneously. Conservative observation with appropriate pain medications for up to 6 weeks
  - Therapeutic intervention required if spontaneous passage does not occur
  - Indications for earlier intervention include severe pain unresponsive to medications, fever, persistent nausea and vomiting requiring intravenous hydration
  - Distal ureteral stones—either ureteroscopic stone extraction or in situ extracorporeal shock wave lithotripsy (ESWL)
  - Proximal and midureteral stones can be treated with ESWL or ureteroscopic extraction, and a double-J ureteral stent to ensure adequate drainage
- **Renal stones:** conservative observation for patients presenting without pain, urinary tract infections, or obstruction. Intervention if calculi become symptomatic or grow in size. For renal stones < 2.5 cm, treat by ESWL. For stones in the inferior calix or those >3 cm, treat by percutaneous nephrolithotomy. Perioperative antibiotics as indicated by preoperative urine cultures

THERAPEUTIC PROCEDURES

- Forced intravenous fluid diuresis is not productive and exacerbates pain

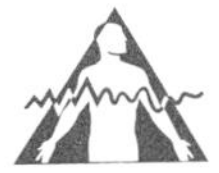

OUTCOME

PREVENTION

- Increased fluid intake to void 1.5–2.0 L/day to reduce stone recurrence. Patients are encouraged to ingest fluids during meals, 2 h after each meal, prior to going to sleep in the evening, and during the night
- Reduce sodium intake
- Reduce animal protein intake during individual meals

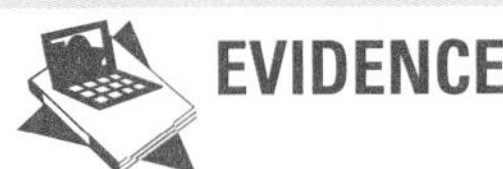

EVIDENCE

PRACTICE GUIDELINES

- National Guideline Clearinghouse
  - http://www.guideline.gov/summary/summary.aspx?doc_id=3266&nbr=2492&string=urinary+AND+stones
- Sandhu C et al: Urinary tract stones–Part II: current status of treatment. Clin Radiol 2003;58:422. [PMID: 12788311]

INFORMATION FOR PATIENTS

- Cleveland Clinic—Kidney Stones
  - http://www.clevelandclinic.org/health/health-info/docs/0000/0046.asp?index=4349
- Mayo Clinic—Kidney Stones
  - http://www.mayoclinic.com/invoke.cfm?id=DS00282
- NIH Medline Plus—Kidney Stone Tutorial
  - http://www.nlm.nih.gov/medlineplus/tutorials/kidneystones.html

REFERENCES

- Meschi T et al: Body weight, diet and water intake in preventing stone disease. Urol Int 2004;72(Suppl 1):29. [PMID: 15133330]
- Stoller ML et al: The primary stone event: a new hypothesis involving a vascular etiology. J Urol 2004;171:1920. [PMID: 15076312]
- Teichman JM: Clinical practice. Acute renal colic from ureteral calculus. N Engl J Med 2004;350:684. [PMID: 14960744]

Author(s)

Marshall L. Stoller, MD

Peter R. Carroll, MD

Urticaria & Angioedema

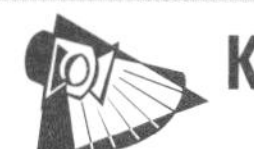

KEY FEATURES

ESSENTIALS OF DIAGNOSIS

- Eruptions of evanescent wheals or hives
- Itching is usually intense but may on rare occasions be absent
- Special forms of urticaria have special features (dermographism; cholinergic, solar, or cold urticaria)
- Most incidents are acute and self-limited over a period of 1–2 weeks
- Chronic urticaria (episodes lasting >6 weeks) may have an autoimmune basis

GENERAL CONSIDERATIONS

- The most common causes of acute urticaria are foods, viral infections, and medications
- **Nonallergic** causes of urticaria
  - Drugs, eg, atropine, pilocarpine, morphine, and codeine
  - Arthropod bites, eg, insect bites and bee stings
  - Physical factors such as heat, cold, sunlight, and pressure
  - Neurogenic factors such as in cholinergic urticaria induced by exercise, excitement, hot showers
- **Allergic** causes of urticaria
  - Penicillins, aspirin, and other medications
  - Inhalants, eg, feathers and animal danders
  - Ingestion of shellfish, tomatoes, or strawberries
  - Injections of sera and vaccines; external contactants, eg, various chemicals and cosmetics
  - Infections such as hepatitis
- Chronic urticaria (episodes lasting >6 weeks) may have an autoimmune basis; the cause is often not found
- Autoimmune thyroid disease may coexist, but treatment of the thyroid disease does not improve the urticaria
- Physical forms of urticaria have special features (dermographism; cholinergic, solar, or cold urticaria)

DEMOGRAPHICS

- Chronic uritcaria is most common in young adult women

CLINICAL FINDINGS

SYMPTOMS AND SIGNS

- See Table 7
- Lesions are itchy red swellings of a few millimeters to many centimeters
- The morphology of the lesions may vary over a period of minutes to hours
- Individual lesions in true urticaria last less than 24 h, and often only 2–4 h
- Angioedema is involvement of deeper vessels, with swelling of the lips, eyelids, palms, soles, and genitalia in association with more typical lesions
- Angioedema is no more likely than urticaria to be associated with systemic complications such as laryngeal edema or hypotension
- In cholinergic urticaria, triggered by a rise in core body temperature (hot showers, exercise), wheals are 2–3 mm in diameter with a large surrounding red flare
- Vasculitis
- Erythema multiforme
- Contact dermatitis (eg, poison oak or ivy)
- Cellulitis

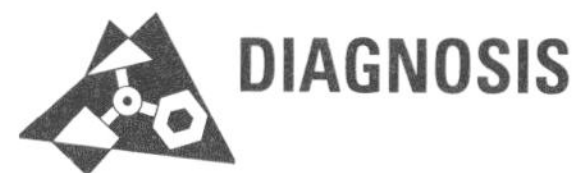

DIAGNOSIS

LABORATORY TESTS

- Laboratory studies are not likely to be helpful in the evaluation of acute or chronic urticaria unless there are suggestive findings in the history and physical examination
- Quantitative immunoglobulins, cryoglobulins, cryofibrinogens, and antinuclear antibodies are often sought in urticaria but are rarely found
- Liver tests may be elevated, since a serum sickness-like prodrome, with urticaria, may be associated with acute hepatitis B infection

DIAGNOSTIC PROCEDURES

- In patients with individual slightly purpuric lesions that persist past 24 h, a skin biopsy may help exclude urticarial vasculitis

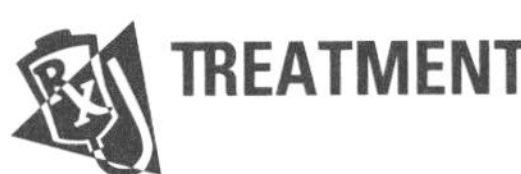

TREATMENT

MEDICATIONS

- H_1 antihistamines
  - Hydroxyzine, 10 mg PO twice daily to 25 mg three times daily to even 100 mg three times daily, may be very useful if tolerated; giving hydroxyzine as one dose of 50–75 mg at night may reduce sedation and other side effects
  - Cyproheptadine, 4 mg PO four times daily, may be useful for cold urticaria
- Add "nonsedating" or less sedating antihistamines if the generic sedating antihistamines are not effective
  - Fexofenadine is given in a dosage of 60 mg PO twice a day
  - Loratadine in a dosage of 10 mg PO/day is similar to the other H_1 antihistamines in effectiveness
  - Cetirizine, a metabolite of hydroxyzine, may be sedating (13% of patients) and is given in a dosage of 10 mg PO/day
  - Doxepin (a tricyclic antidepressant), 25 mg PO three times daily, or, more commonly, 25–75 mg at bedtime, can be very effective in chronic urticaria; it has anticholinergic side effects
- H_2 antihistamines in combination with H_1 blockers may be helpful in patients with symptomatic dermatographism
- Adjuvants
  - Calcium channel blockers (used for at least 4 weeks)
  - Terbutaline, 1.25–2.5 mg three times daily
  - Colchicine, 0.6 mg PO twice daily
  - Danazol
  - Warfarin
  - Systemic steroids in a dose of about 40 mg daily will usually suppress acute and chronic urticaria; however, the use of corticosteroids is rarely indicated
  - Topical treatment is rarely rewarding

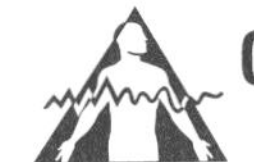

OUTCOME

PROGNOSIS

- Acute urticaria usually lasts only a few days to 6 weeks
- 50% of patients whose urticaria persists for more than 6 weeks will have it for years

WHEN TO REFER

- If there is a question about the diagnosis, if recommended therapy is ineffective, or if specialized treatment is necessary

EVIDENCE

PRACTICE GUIDELINES

- The diagnosis and management of urticaria: a practice parameter: part I: acute urticaria/angioedema: part II: chronic urticaria/angioedema. Joint Task Force on Practice Parameters, 2000
  - http://www.guideline.gov/summary/summary.aspx?doc_id=3622&nbr=2848
- Grattan C et al: British Association of Dermatologists. Management and diagnostic guidelines for urticaria and angioedema. Br J Dermatol 2001;144:708. [PMID: 11298527]

WEB SITE

- American Academy of Dermatology
  - http://www.aad.org

INFORMATION FOR PATIENTS

- American Academy of Allergy, Asthma & Immunology: Allergic Skin Conditions
  - http://www.aaaai.org/patients/publicedmat/tips/allergicskinconditions.stm
- American Academy of Dermatology: Urticaria—Hives
  - http://www.aad.org/public/Publications/pamphlets/Urticaria-Hives.htm
- Mayo Clinic: Hives and Angioedema
  - http://www.mayoclinic.com/invoke.cfm?id=DS00313

REFERENCES

- Black AK et al: Antihistamines in urticaria and angioedema. Clin Allergy Immunol 2002;17:249. [PMID: 12113219]
- Caproni M et al: Chronic idiopathic and chronic autoimmune urticaria: clinical and immunopathological features of 68 subjects. Acta Dermatol Venereol 2004;84:288. [PMID: 15339073]
- Gaig P et al: Epidemiology of urticaria in Spain. J Invest Allergol Clin Immunol 2004;14:214. [PMID: 15552715]
- Grattan CE et al: Chronic urticaria. J Am Acad Dermatol 2002;46:657. [PMID: 12004303]
- Kaplan AP: Diagnostic tests for urticaria and angioedema. Clin Allergy Immunol 2000;15:111. [PMID: 10943290]

Author(s)

Timothy G. Berger, MD

Vaginal Bleeding, Abnormal Premenopausal

Urticaria, Cold p. 1164.
Uterine Prolapse p. 1165.

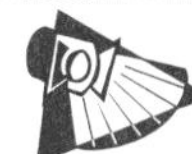

KEY FEATURES

ESSENTIALS OF DIAGNOSIS

- Blood loss of over 80 mL per cycle
- Excessive bleeding, often with the passage of clots, may occur at regular menstrual intervals (**menorrhagia**) or irregular intervals (**dysfunctional uterine bleeding**)
- Etiology most commonly involves dysfunctional uterine bleeding on a hormonal basis

GENERAL CONSIDERATIONS

- Average normal menstrual bleeding lasts 4 days (range, 2–7 days), with a mean blood loss of 40 mL
- Bleeding cycles less than 21 days apart are likely anovular
- Blood loss of over 80 mL per cycle is abnormal and frequently produces anemia
- **Ovulation bleeding**, a single episode of spotting between regular menses, is quite common. Heavier or irregular intermenstrual bleeding warrants investigation
- **Anovulatory bleeding** (dysfunctional uterine bleeding) is usually caused by overgrowth of endometrium due to estrogen stimulation without adequate progesterone to stabilize growth

DEMOGRAPHICS

- Anovulation associated with high estrogen levels commonly occurs in teenagers, in women aged late 30s to late 40s, and in extremely obese women or those with polycystic ovary syndrome

CLINICAL FINDINGS

SYMPTOMS AND SIGNS

- Obtain
  - A careful description of the duration and amount of flow, related pain, and relationship to the last menstrual period (LMP). The presence of blood clots or the degree of inconvenience caused by the bleeding may be more useful indicators
  - A history of pertinent illnesses or weight change
  - A history of all medications taken in the past month
  - A history of coagulation disorders in the patient or family members
- Perform a careful pelvic examination to look for pregnancy, uterine myomas, adnexal masses, or infection

DIFFERENTIAL DIAGNOSIS

- Ovulation bleeding (spotting episode between menses)
- Anovulatory cycle (dysfunctional uterine bleeding)
- Polycystic ovary syndrome (type of anovulatory cycle)
- Pregnancy
- Ectopic pregnancy
- Spontaneous abortion
- Uterine leiomyomas (fibroids)
- Endometrial polyp
- Cervicitis or pelvic inflammatory disease
- Adenomyosis (uterine endometriosis)
- Cervical cancer
- Cervical polyp
- Endometrial hyperplasia
- Endometrial cancer
- Hypothyroidism
- Hyperprolactinemia
- Diabetes mellitus
- Bleeding disorder, eg, von Willebrand's disease

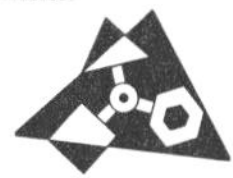

DIAGNOSIS

LABORATORY TESTS

- Cervical smears as needed for cytological and culture studies
- Complete blood cell count, sedimentation rate, and glucose levels
- Pregnancy test
- Thyroid function and blood clotting should be considered
- Tests for ovulation in cyclic menorrhagia include
  - Basal body temperature records
  - Serum progesterone measured 1 week before the expected onset of menses
  - Analysis of an endometrial biopsy specimen for secretory activity shortly before the onset of menstruation

IMAGING STUDIES

- Ultrasound can evaluate endometrial thickness or diagnose intrauterine or ectopic pregnancy or adnexal masses
- Endovaginal ultrasound with saline infusion sonohysterography can diagnose endometrial polyps or subserous myomas
- MRI can definitively diagnose submucous myomas and adenomyosis

DIAGNOSTIC PROCEDURES

- In women over age 35, perform endometrial sampling to rule out endometrial hyperplasia or carcinoma prior to initiation of hormonal therapy for dysfunctional uterine bleeding
- If cancer of the cervix is suspected, colposcopically directed biopsies and endocervical curettage are indicated as first steps
- Hysteroscopy can visualize endometrial polyps, submucous myomas, and exophytic endometrial cancers. It is useful immediately before D&C

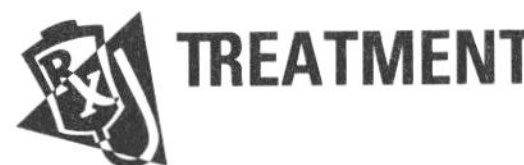

TREATMENT

MEDICATIONS

- **Dysfunctional uterine bleeding**
  - Give medroxyprogesterone acetate, 10 mg PO/day, or norethindrone acetate, 5 mg PO/day, for 10–14 days starting on day 15 of the cycle, following which withdrawal bleeding (medical curettage) occurs
  - Repeat treatment for several cycles and reinstitute if amenorrhea or dysfunctional bleeding recurs
  - In women who are bleeding actively, any combination oral contraceptive can be given four times daily for 1 or 2 days followed by two pills daily through day 5 and then one pill daily through day 20; after withdrawal bleeding occurs, pills are taken in the usual dosage for three cycles
- **Heavy bleeding**
  - For intractable heavy bleeding, danazol, 200 mg PO four times daily, is sometimes used to create an atrophic endometrium
  - Alternatively, a gonadotropin-releasing hormone agonist such as depot leuprolide, 3.75 mg IM monthly, or nafarelin, 0.2–0.4 mg intranasally twice daily, can be used for up to 6 months to create a temporary cessation of menstruation by ovarian suppression
  - IV conjugated estrogens, 25 mg Q 4 h for three or four doses, can be used, followed by oral conjugated estrogens, 2.5 mg daily, or ethinyl estradiol, 20 μg daily, for 3 weeks, with the addition of medroxyprogesterone acetate, 10 mg daily for the last 10 days of treatment, or a combination oral contraceptive daily for 3 weeks. This will thicken the endometrium and control the bleeding
- **Menorrhagia**
  - Nonsteroidal antiinflammatory drugs in the usual antiinflammatory doses will often reduce blood loss in menorrhagia—even that associated with an intrauterine device
  - Prolonged use of a progestin, as in a minipill, in injectable contraceptives, or in the therapy of endometriosis, can also lead to intermittent bleeding, sometimes severe. In this instance, the endometrium is atrophic and fragile. If bleeding occurs, it should be treated with estrogen as follows: ethinyl estradiol, 20 μg/day for 7 days, or conjugated estrogens, 1.25 mg/day for 7 days

THERAPEUTIC PROCEDURES

- Discuss stressful situations that may contribute to anovulation, such as prolonged emotional turmoil or excessive use of drugs or alcohol
- If the abnormal bleeding is not controlled by hormonal treatment, a D&C is necessary to check for incomplete abortion, polyps, submucous myomas, or endometrial cancer
- D&C is usually not necessary in women under age 40
- Endometrial ablation through the hysteroscope with laser photocoagulation or electrocautery is an option; this technique is designed to reduce or prevent any future menstrual flow

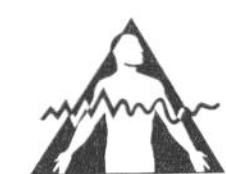

OUTCOME

FOLLOW-UP

- Monitor for the development of iron-deficiency anemia

WHEN TO REFER

- Refer if bleeding does not stop with first-line therapy or if expertise is needed with a procedure

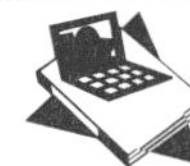

EVIDENCE

PRACTICE GUIDELINES

- American College of Obstetricians and Gynecologists (ACOG). Management of anovulatory bleeding, 2000
  - http://www.guideline.gov/summary/summary.aspx?doc_id=3964&nbr=3102
- Brigham and Women's Hospital. Common gynecologic problems: a guide to diagnosis and treatment, 2002
  - http://www.guideline.gov/summary/summary.aspx?doc_id=3486&nbr=2712

INFORMATION FOR PATIENTS

- American Academy of Family Physicians: Abnormal Uterine Bleeding
  - http://familydoctor.org/470.xml
- Mayo Clinic: Vaginal Bleeding
  - http://www.mayoclinic.com/invoke.cfm?id=HO00159
- MedlinePlus: Vaginal Bleeding Between Periods
  - http://www.nlm.nih.gov/medlineplus/ency/article/003156.htm
- MedlinePlus: Dysfunctional Uterine Bleeding
  - http://www.nlm.nih.gov/medlineplus/ency/article/000903.htm

REFERENCES

- Dubinsky TJ: Value of sonography in the diagnosis of abnormal vaginal bleeding. J Clin Ultrasound 2004;32:348. [PMID: 15293302]
- Hurskainen R et al: Levonorgestrel-releasing intrauterine system in the treatment of heavy menstrual bleeding. Curr Opin Obstet Gynecol 2004;16:487. [PMID: 15534445]

Author(s)

H. Trent MacKay, MD, MPH

Vaginal Bleeding, Postmenopausal

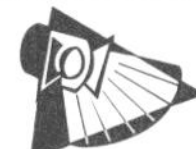

KEY FEATURES

ESSENTIALS OF DIAGNOSIS

- Vaginal bleeding that occurs 6 months or more following cessation of menstrual function
- Bleeding is usually painless
- Bleeding may be a single episode of spotting or profuse bleeding for days or months

GENERAL CONSIDERATIONS

- The most common causes are
  - Atrophic endometrium
  - Endometrial proliferation or hyperplasia
  - Endometrial or cervical cancer
  - Administration of estrogens without added progestin
- Risk factors
  - Obesity
  - Nulliparity
  - Diabetes
  - History of anovulation
  - Tamoxifen therapy

CLINICAL FINDINGS

SYMPTOMS AND SIGNS

- Uterine bleeding is usually painless, but pain will be present if the cervix is stenotic, if bleeding is severe and rapid, or if infection or torsion or extrusion of a tumor is present
- The vulva and vagina should be inspected for areas of bleeding, ulcers, or neoplasms

DIFFERENTIAL DIAGNOSIS

- Atrophic endometrium
- Endometrial hyperplasia or proliferation
- Endometrial cancer
- Atrophic vaginitis
- Perimenopausal bleeding
- Endometrial polyp
- Unopposed exogenous estrogen
- Cervical cancer
- Uterine leiomyomas (fibroids)
- Trauma
- Bleeding disorder
- Cervical polyp
- Cervical ulcer
- Vaginal cancer
- Vulvar cancer

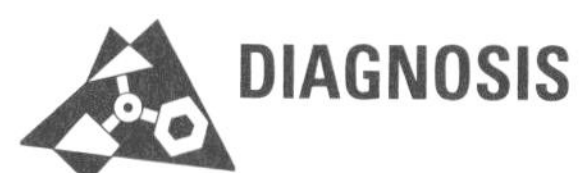

DIAGNOSIS

LABORATORY TESTS

- A cytologic smear of the cervix and vaginal pool should be taken

IMAGING STUDIES

- Transvaginal sonography should be used to measure endometrial thickness
- A measurement of 5 mm or less indicates a low likelihood of hyperplasia or endometrial cancer, although up to 4% of endometrial cancers may be missed with sonography

DIAGNOSTIC PROCEDURES

- If the endometrial thickness by transvaginal sonography is > 5 mm, endocervical curettage and endometrial aspiration should be performed, preferably in conjunction with hysteroscopy

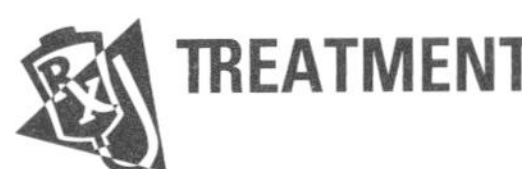

TREATMENT

MEDICATIONS

- Treat simple endometrial hyperplasia with cyclic progestin therapy (medroxyprogesterone acetate, 10 mg PO/day, or norethindrone acetate, 5 mg PO/day) for 21 days of each month for 3 months
- A repeat D&C or endometrial biopsy should be performed, and if tissues are normal and estrogen replacement therapy is reinstituted, a progestin should be prescribed in a cyclic or continuous regimen

SURGERY

- Aspiration curettage (with polypectomy if indicated) will frequently be curative
- If endometrial hyperplasia with atypical cells or carcinoma of the endometrium is found, hysterectomy is necessary

OUTCOME

FOLLOW-UP

- Annual visit for pelvic examination and transvaginal sonography

COMPLICATIONS

- Endometrial cancer
- Complex hyperplasia with atypia has a high risk of becoming adenocarcinoma of the endometrium and requires hysterectomy

WHEN TO REFER

- Refer for hysteroscopy by gynecologist

PREVENTION

- Avoidance of unopposed estrogen therapy
- Weight reduction
- Simple endometrial hyperplasia responds well to medical therapy

EVIDENCE

PRACTICE GUIDELINES

- Scottish Intercollegiate Guidelines Network. Investigation of post-menopausal bleeding. A national clinical guideline. 2002.
  - http://www.guideline.gov/summary/summary.aspx?doc_id=3456&nbr=2682
- American Cancer Society guidelines on testing for early endometrial cancer detection-update 2001.
  - http://www.guideline.gov/summary/summary.aspx?doc_id=2749&nbr=1975

INFORMATION FOR PATIENTS

- American Academy of Family Physicians: Abnormal Uterine Bleeding
  - http://familydoctor.org/470.xml
- American College of Obstetricians and Gynecologists: Endometrial Hyperplasia
  - http://www.medem.com/MedLB/article_detaillb.cfm?article_ID=ZZZ7Z2GWQMC&sub_cat=9
- American College of Surgeons: About D&C for Uterine Bleeding Problems
  - http://www.facs.org/public_info/operation/dncbleed.pdf
- American College of Surgeons: Hysteroscopy
  - http://www.medem.com/medlb/article_detaillb.cfm?article_ID=ZZZNOLS2RWC&sub_cat=9
- Mayo Clinic: Vaginal Bleeding
  - http://www.mayoclinic.com/invoke.cfm?id=HO00159

REFERENCE

- Tabor A et al: Endometrial thickness as a test for endometrial cancer in women with postmenopausal vaginal bleeding. Obstet Gynecol 2002;99:663. [PMID: 12039131]

Author(s)

H. Trent MacKay, MD, MPH

Vaginitis

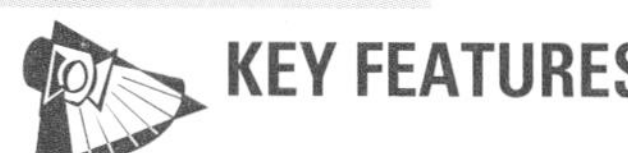

KEY FEATURES

ESSENTIALS OF DIAGNOSIS

- Vaginal irritation, pruritus, pain, or unusual discharge

GENERAL CONSIDERATIONS

- Inflammation and infection of the vagina are common
- Results from a variety of pathogens, allergic reactions to vaginal contraceptives or other products, or the friction of coitus
- The normal vaginal pH is 4.5 or less, and *Lactobacillus* is the predominant organism
- At the time of the midcycle estrogen surge, clear, elastic, mucoid secretions from the cervical os are often profuse
- In the luteal phase and during pregnancy, vaginal secretions are thicker, white, and sometimes adherent to the vaginal walls
- These normal secretions can be confused with vaginitis by concerned women

Candida albicans

- Pregnancy, diabetes, and use of broad-spectrum antibiotics or corticosteroids predispose to *Candida* infections
- Heat, moisture, and occlusive clothing also contribute to the risk

Trichomonas vaginalis

- This protozoal flagellate infects the vagina, Skene's ducts, and lower urinary tract in women and the lower genitourinary tract in men
- It is transmitted through coitus

Bacterial vaginosis

- This condition is considered to be a polymicrobial (overgrowth of *Gardnerella* and other anaerobes) and is not sexually transmitted

Condylomata acuminata (genital warts)

- Caused by various types of the human papillomavirus
- Sexually transmitted
- Pregnancy and immunosuppression favor growth

CLINICAL FINDINGS

SYMPTOMS AND SIGNS

- Take a careful history
  - Onset of the last menstrual period
  - Recent sexual activity
  - Use of contraceptives, tampons, or douches
  - Vaginal burning, pain, pruritus
  - Profuse or malodorous discharge
- The physical examination: careful inspection of the vulva and speculum examination of the vagina and cervix

Candida albicans

- Pruritus
- Vulvovaginal erythema
- White curd-like discharge that is not malodorous

Trichomonas vaginalis

- Pruritus and a malodorous frothy, yellow-green discharge
- Diffuse vaginal erythema and red macular lesions on the cervix in severe cases

Bacterial vaginosis

- Increased malodorous discharge without obvious vulvitis or vaginitis
- Discharge is grayish, frothy

Condylomata acuminata

- Warty growths on the vulva, perianal area, vaginal walls, or cervix
- Vulvar lesions: obviously wart-like
- Fissures may be at the fourchette
- Vaginal lesions may show diffuse hypertrophy or a cobblestone appearance
- These lesions may be related to dysplasia and cervical cancer

DIFFERENTIAL DIAGNOSIS

- Normal vaginal discharge
- Bacterial vaginosis
- *Trichomonas* vaginitis
- *Candida* vulvovaginitis
- Atrophic vaginitis
- Genital warts (condyloma acuminata)
- Friction from intercourse
- Reaction to douches, tampons, condoms, soap

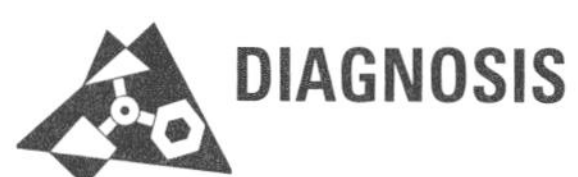

DIAGNOSIS

LABORATORY TESTS

- The cervix is cultured for *Gonococcus* or *Chlamydia* if applicable
- The vaginal pH is frequently > 4.5 in infections due to trichomonads (pH of 5.0–5.5) and bacterial vaginosis
- Examine a specimen of vaginal discharge microscopically
  - In a drop of 0.9% saline solution (wet mount) to search for motile organisms with flagella (trichomonads) and epithelial cells covered with bacteria to such an extent that cell borders are obscured (clue cells)
  - In a drop of 10% potassium hydroxide to search for the filaments and spores of *Candida* and an amine-like "fishy" odor of *Trichomonas*
- Cultures with Nickerson's medium may be used if *Candida* is suspected but not demonstrated
- Vaginal cultures are generally not useful in diagnosis

DIAGNOSTIC PROCEDURES

- Vulvar or cervical lesions of condylomata acuminata may be visible by colposcopy only after pretreatment with 4% acetic acid, when they appear whitish, with prominent papillae

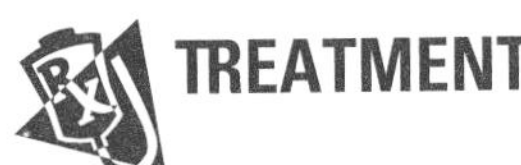

TREATMENT

MEDICATIONS

Candida albicans

- Women with uncomplicated vulvovaginal candidiasis will usually respond to a 1- to 3-day regimen of a topical azole
- Women with complicated infection (including four or more episodes in 1 year, severe signs and symptoms, nonalbicans species, uncontrolled diabetes, HIV infection, corticosteroid treatment, or pregnancy) should receive 7–14 days of a topical regimen or two doses of fluconazole 3 days apart. (Pregnant women should use only topical azoles.)
- Three-day regimens
  - Butoconazole (2% cream, 5 g)
  - Clotrimazole (two 100-mg vaginal tablets)
  - Terconazole (0.8% cream, 5 g, or 80 mg suppository)
  - Miconazole (200-mg vaginal suppository) once daily
- Seven-day regimens
  - Clotrimazole (1% cream or 100-mg vaginal tablet)
  - Miconazole (2% cream, 5 g, or 100-mg vaginal suppository)
  - Terconazole (0.4% cream, 5 g) once daily
- Single-dose regimens
  - Clotrimazole (500-mg tablet)
  - Tioconazole ointment (6.5%, 5 g)
  - Fluconazole, 150 mg PO
- Fourteen-day regimens
  - Nystatin (100,000-unit vaginal tablet once daily)
  - Boric acid capsules (600-mg gelatin capsule inserted vaginally, daily)
- Recurrent candidal vulvovaginitis: ketoconazole, 100 mg PO once daily for up to 6 months

Trichomonas vaginalis

- Recommend treatment of both partners
  - Metronidazole, 2 g PO, single dose
  - For treatment failure in the absence of reexposure, retreat with metronidazole, 500 mg twice a day for 7 days
  - If this is not effective, metronidazole susceptibility testing can be arranged with the Centers for Disease Control and Prevention

Bacterial vaginosis

- Metronidazole, 500 mg PO twice daily for 7 days
- Clindamycin vaginal cream (2%, 5 g), once daily for 7 days
- Metronidazole gel (0.75%, 5 g), twice daily for 5 days
- Metronidazole, 2 g PO as a single dose
- Clindamycin, 300 mg PO twice daily for 7 days

Condylomata acuminata

- For vulvar warts
  - Podophyllum resin 25% in tincture of benzoin (do not use during pregnancy or on bleeding lesions). Wash off after 2–4 h
  - 80–90% trichloroacetic or bichloroacetic acid. Apply carefully to avoid the surrounding skin
- Freezing with liquid nitrogen
- Patient-applied regimens include podofilox 0.5% solution or gel and imiquimod 5% cream
- Vaginal warts may be treated with cryotherapy with liquid nitrogen, trichloroacetic acid, or podophyllum resin
- Interferon is not recommended for routine use

THERAPEUTIC PROCEDURES

- Routine examination of sex partners is not necessary for the management of genital warts. However, partners may wish to be examined for detection and treatment of genital warts and other sexually transmitted diseases

Condylomata acuminata

- Vulvar warts: freezing with cryoprobe and electrocautery
- Vaginal warts: extensive warts may require treatment with CO_2 laser under anesthesia

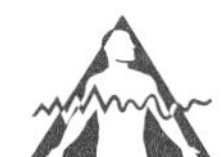

OUTCOME

FOLLOW-UP

- Examination for pelvic infection

EVIDENCE

PRACTICE GUIDELINES

- Centers for Disease Control and Prevention. Sexually Transmitted Diseases Treatment Guidelines—2002
  - http://www.cdc.gov/mmwr/preview/mmwrhtml/rr5106a1.htm

INFORMATION FOR PATIENTS

- American Social Health Association: Vaginitis
  - http://www.ashastd.org/stdfaqs/vaginitis.html
- National Institute of Allergy and Infectious Diseases: Vaginitis Due to Vaginal Infections
  - http://www.niaid.nih.gov/factsheets/stdvag.htm
- National Institute of Child Health & Human Development: Vaginitis
  - http://www.nichd.nih.gov/publications/pubs/vagtoc.htm
- MedlinePlus: Sexually Transmitted Diseases Interactive Tutorial
  - http://www.nlm.nih.gov/medlineplus/tutorials/sexuallytransmitteddiseases.html

REFERENCES

- Anderson MR et al: Evaluation of vaginal complaints. JAMA 2004;291:1368. [PMID: 15026404]
- Holmes KK et al: Effectiveness of condoms in preventing sexually transmitted infections. Bull World Health Organ 2004;82:454. [PMID: 15356939]
- Sexually transmitted disease treatment guidelines 2002. Centers for Disease Control and Prevention. MMWR Recomm Rep 2002;51(RR-6):1. [PMID: 12184549]

Author(s)

H. Trent MacKay, MD, MPH

Varicella & Herpes Zoster

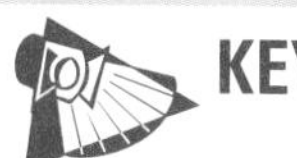

KEY FEATURES

ESSENTIALS OF DIAGNOSIS

- Fever and malaise before visible skin lesions (varicella)
- Pain before onset of skin lesions in a dermatome (herpes zoster)
- Typical incubation period of 2–3 weeks between exposure and clinical onset

GENERAL CONSIDERATIONS

- Chickenpox is spread by inhalation of infective droplets or by contact with skin lesions

DEMOGRAPHICS

- Disease manifestations include chickenpox (varicella), which occurs typically in children, and shingles (zoster), which occurs more commonly in elderly or immunocompromised individuals

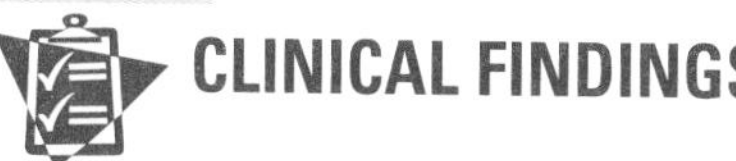

CLINICAL FINDINGS

SYMPTOMS AND SIGNS

Varicella (chickenpox)

- Fever and malaise mild in children, marked in adults
- Vesicular eruptions often first involve oropharynx
- Rash involves face, scalp, and trunk and then moves out to the extremities
- Lesions erupt over 1–5 days so all stages of eruption present simultaneously
- Vesicles and pustules are superficial, elliptical, with slightly serrated borders
- Multinucleated giant cells on Tzanck smear of materials from vesicle bases

Herpes zoster (shingles)

- Pain is often severe and precedes the lesions
- Lesions follow any nerve route distribution (thoracic and lumbar most common)
- Vesicular skin lesions resemble varicella
- Lesions on tip of nose indicate potential ophthalmic involvement
- Facial palsy, vertigo, tinnitus, deafness, or external ear lesions suggest geniculate ganglion involvement

DIFFERENTIAL DIAGNOSIS

Varicella (chickenpox)

- Herpes simplex (cold or fever sore; genital herpes)
- Herpes zoster (shingles)
- Contact dermatitis
- Scabies
- Atopic dermatitis (eczema) (acute)
- Miliaria (heat rash)
- Photodermatitis
- Smallpox
- Rickettsialpox
- Hand, foot, and mouth disease

Herpes zoster (shingles)

- Contact dermatitis (eg, poison oak or ivy)
- Herpes simplex
- Varicella (chickenpox)
- Erysipelas
- Prodromal pain mimics angina, peptic ulcer, appendicitis, biliary or renal colic

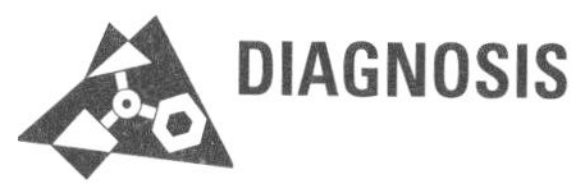

DIAGNOSIS

LABORATORY TESTS

- Leukopenia often present in varicella
- Zoster symptoms and signs often highly characteristic, not requiring further diagnostic testing
- When diagnosis remains in doubt, direct fluorescent antibody (DFA) testing, viral culture, and polymerase chain reaction (PCR) testing can be helpful

DIAGNOSTIC FINDINGS

- Most patients with a history of exposure and clinical symptoms and signs of varicella do not need further diagnostic testing

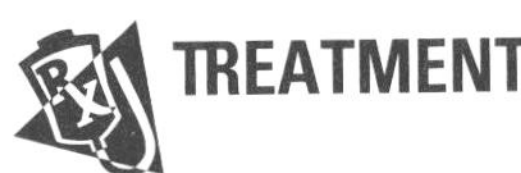

TREATMENT

MEDICATIONS

- Acyclovir or related drugs can reduce the duration and severity of chickenpox or zoster infection, especially when started early, but is seldom needed in immunocompetent patients
- Acyclovir may reduce the likelihood and/or severity of postherpetic neuralgia
- Acyclovir usually indicated in immunocompromised patients with systemic varicella infection
- Foscarnet may be useful in acyclovir-resistant varicella, especially in patients taking long-term acyclovir therapy
- Prevention: varicella immunoglobulin is effective in preventing chickenpox in exposed individuals
- Vaccination, with live, attenuated virus, is 85% effective at preventing disease and 95% effective at preventing serious complications
- Adults should receive a second vaccine dose 1–2 months after the first dose
- Postherpetic neuralgia: initial treatment with acyclovir and corticosteroids may reduce the incidence and severity
- Once established, pain may be treated with tricyclic antidepressants, lidocaine patches, and antiepileptics such as carbamazepine and gabapentin

THERAPEUTIC PROCEDURES

- Isolate patients with active vesicles or pneumonia from seronegative patients

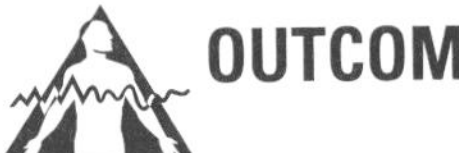

OUTCOME

COMPLICATIONS

Varicella (chickenpox)

- Interstitial pneumonia more common in adults than children
- Ischemic strokes, though uncommon, may be due to an associated vasculitis
- Hepatitis occurs in 0.1%
- Encephalitis, characterized by ataxia, nystagmus, and even death, is rare (0.025%)
- Reye's syndrome may occur in conjunction with aspirin use, usually in children
- Congenital malformations occur with first-trimester infections

Herpes zoster (shingles)

- Skin lesions beyond the dermatome, visceral lesions, and encephalitis occur in immunocompromised individuals
- Postherpetic neuralgia occurs in 60–70% of elderly patients; corticosteroids are controversial but may be of some benefit when tapered over 21 days for prevention of postherpetic neuralgia

PROGNOSIS

- Total duration of varicella from onset of symptoms to disappearance of crusts usually ≤ 2 weeks
- Zoster symptoms and lesions usually resolve within 6 weeks

WHEN TO REFER

- Refer patients with synchronous progression of the lesions, which raises the concern for smallpox, to local health department and infectious disease experts for confirmation

WHEN TO ADMIT

- Consider hospitalization for signs of visceral involvement, especially pulmonary involvement. Varicella pneumonia can be lethal, especially in adults and in immunocompromised patients

EVIDENCE

PRACTICE GUIDELINES

- General recommendations on immunization: recommendations of the Advisory Committee on Immunization Practices (ACIP) and the American Academy of Family Physicians (AAFP). American Academy of Family Physicians; Centers for Disease Control and Prevention, 2002
  - http://www.guideline.gov/summary/summary.aspx?doc_id=3180&nbr=2406&string=varicella+and+treatment

WEB SITE

- National Institute of Allergy and Infectious Diseases, National Institutes of Health
  - http://www.niaid.nih.gov/

INFORMATION FOR PATIENTS

- NIAID Facts About Shingles (Varicella-Zoster Virus)
  - http://www.niaid.nih.gov/factsheets/shinglesfs.htm
- Web MD varicella
  - http://my.webmd.com/content/healthwise/129/32072

REFERENCES

- Ampofo K et al: Persistence of immunity to live attenuated varicella vaccine in healthy adults. Clin Infect Dis 2002;34:774. [PMID: 11830801]
- Gnann JW Jr et al: Herpes zoster. N Engl J Med 2002;347:340. [PMID: 12151472]
- Hall S et al: Second varicella infections: are they more common than previously thought? Pediatrics 2002;109:1068. [PMID: 12042544]

Author(s)

Wayne X. Shandera, MD

Ana Moran, MD

Varicose Veins

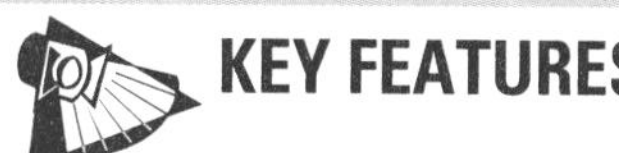

KEY FEATURES

ESSENTIALS OF DIAGNOSIS

- Dilated, tortuous superficial veins in the lower extremities
- May be asymptomatic or associated with fatigue, aching discomfort, thrombosis, bleeding, or localized pain
- Edema, pigmentation, and ulceration suggest concomitant venous stasis disease

GENERAL CONSIDERATIONS

- Abnormally dilated veins in the legs produced by venous reflux and valvular incompetence
- Long saphenous vein and its tributaries most commonly involved; short saphenous vein may also be affected
- Primary varicosities: inherited vein wall or valve defect
- Secondary varicosities: valve damage after thrombophlebitis, trauma, deep venous thrombosis, arteriovenous fistula, pregnancy, or pelvic tumor
- With long-standing disease, the skin may develop secondary changes such as fibrosis, chronic edema, and skin pigmentation and atrophy
- Risk factors: female gender, pregnancy, family history, prolonged standing, and history of phlebitis

DEMOGRAPHICS

- Occur in 15% of adults
- Increased frequency after pregnancy

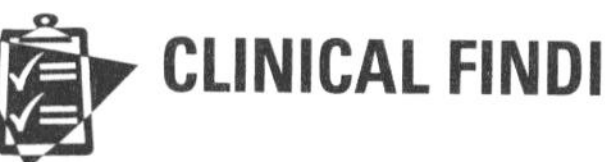

CLINICAL FINDINGS

SYMPTOMS AND SIGNS

- Dull, aching heaviness and fatigue, worsened by standing
- Itching from eczematoid dermatitis
- Dilated, tortuous, elongated veins, visible when the patient is standing
- Smaller, flat, blue-green reticular veins, telangiectasias, and spider veins
- Signs of chronic venous insufficiency: brownish pigmentation and thinning of the skin above the ankle, edema, fibrosis, scaling dermatitis, and ulceration

DIFFERENTIAL DIAGNOSIS

- Klippel-Trenaunay syndrome: varicose veins, limb hypertrophy, and a cutaneous birthmark (portwine stain or venous malformation)

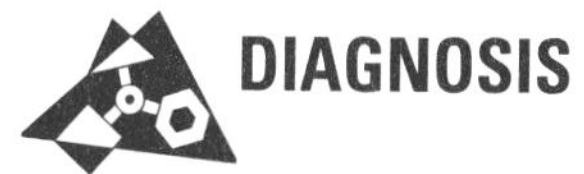

DIAGNOSIS

IMAGING STUDIES

- Duplex ultrasonography detects location of incompetent valves; helpful preoperatively

DIAGNOSTIC PROCEDURES

- Brodie-Trendelenburg test positive

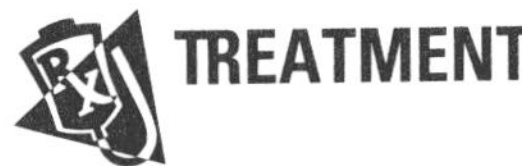

TREATMENT

SURGERY

- Indications: disabling pain, recurrent superficial thrombophlebitis, erosion of the overlying skin with bleeding, and manifestations of chronic venous insufficiency (particularly ulceration)
- Varicose vein excision (stab avulsion) combined with high ligation of the saphenofemoral junction or ligation of perforator branches
- Stripping of the entire saphenous system rarely required

THERAPEUTIC PROCEDURES

- Periodic leg elevation
- Regular exercise
- Knee-high or thigh-high elastic graduated (20–30 mm Hg) compression stockings
- Compression bandages (Ace wrap or Unna boot) when complicated by ulceration
- Compression sclerotherapy: injection of 23.4% hypertonic saline or 2.5% sodium morrhuate and compression stockings

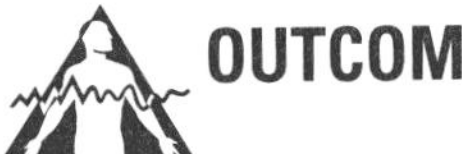

OUTCOME

COMPLICATIONS

- Ulceration, bleeding, chronic stasis dermatitis, superficial venous thrombosis, and thrombophlebitis

PROGNOSIS

- Recurrence rate is ~10%
- Even after adequate treatment, secondary tissue changes may not regress

PREVENTION

- Continued use of compression stockings, leg elevation, and exercise

EVIDENCE

INFORMATION FOR PATIENTS

- Cleveland Clinic: Varicose Veins
  - http://www.clevelandclinic.org/health/health-info/docs/3200/3218.asp?index=11201
- MedlinePlus: Varicose Veins
  - http://www.nlm.nih.gov/medlineplus/ency/article/001109.htm
- MedlinePlus: Varicose Veins interactive tutorial
  - http://www.nlm.nih.gov/medlineplus/tutorials/varicoseveins.html

REFERENCES

- Belcaro G et al: Endovascular sclerotherapy, surgery, and surgery plus sclerotherapy in superficial venous incompetence: a randomized, 10-year follow-up trial—final results. Angiology 2000;51:529. [PMID: 10917577]
- Bradbury A et al: The relationship between lower limb symptoms and superficial and deep venous reflux on duplex ultrasonography: The Edinburgh Vein Study. J Vasc Surg 2000;32:921. [PMID: 11054224]

Author(s)

Louis M. Messina, MD

Vascular Disease, Peripheral

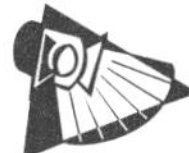

KEY FEATURES

ESSENTIALS OF DIAGNOSIS

- Peripheral vascular disease (PVD) is a common cause of disability
- A predictor of cardiovascular morbidity and mortality
- Leg pain occurs reproducibly after walking a fixed distance
- Forefoot pain with limb elevation

GENERAL CONSIDERATIONS

- Type 1 disease affects about 10–15% of patients with PVD and is limited to the aorta and common iliac arteries
- Type 2 disease (~25% of patients) involves the aorta and common iliac and external iliac arteries
- Type 3 disease (~60–70% of patients) involves the aorta and iliac, femoral, popliteal, and tibial arteries
- High incidence of coexisting cerebrovascular and coronary artery disease
- ~30% have severe triple-vessel coronary artery disease

DEMOGRAPHICS

- Risk factors for type 1 disease: younger men and middle-aged women who are heavy smokers or who have hyperlipidemia
- Risk factors for type 2 and type 3 disease: older age, male gender, diabetes, hypertension, hypercholesterolemia

CLINICAL FINDINGS

SYMPTOMS AND SIGNS

- Claudication, rest pain, ulceration, gangrene
- Male erectile dysfunction with occlusive disease of iliac arteries
- Leriche's syndrome: bilateral hip and buttock claudication, erectile dysfunction, absent femoral pulses
- Claudication is pain, numbness, or weakness in calves, thighs, or buttocks from walking, relieved with rest
- Ischemic rest pain occurs across dorsum of foot with elevation and is relieved with dependency; implies severe arterial insufficiency, impending limb loss
- Absent or weak femoral pulse or presence of iliac or femoral bruit suggests inflow disease
- Normal femoral pulse but diminished or absent popliteal pulse indicates superficial femoral artery stenosis or occlusion
- Normal femoral and popliteal pulses but nonpalpable dorsalis pedis or posterior tibial pulse indicate tibial disease
- Ratio of ankle to brachial systolic blood pressures (ankle-brachial index [ABI]) useful in gauging arterial insufficiency
- Normal ABI is 1.0
- Claudication occurs at ABI < 0.8
- Rest pain and nonhealing ulcers occur at ABI < 0.4
- Toe-brachial index can be used in diabetic or renal failure patients when tibial arteries are calcified and noncompressible
- Penile-brachial index (PBI) can be used when vasogenic impotence is suspected; PBI < 0.6 suggests significant arterial disease
- Index measurements monitor progression of disease and assess effect of therapeutic intervention
- Atrophy of skin, subcutaneous tissues, and muscles, elevation pallor, dependent rubor, hair loss, and coolness of the skin indicate advanced ischemia
- Ulcers over pressure points

DIFFERENTIAL DIAGNOSIS

- Musculoskeletal disorder
- Lumbar spinal stenosis or nerve root compression (neurogenic or pseudoclaudication)
- Venous disease
- Peripheral neuropathy
- Nocturnal leg cramps
- Arterial embolism
- Thromboangiitis obliterans (Buerger's disease)
- Polyarteritis nodosa
- For popliteal artery occlusion with unilateral claudication in young, healthy person, consider popliteal artery entrapment, trauma, compression by Baker's cyst, popliteal adventitial cystic disease
- Reflex sympathetic dystrophy
- Raynaud's disease

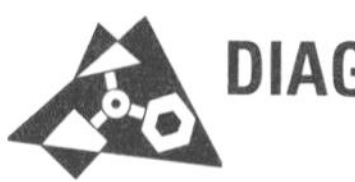

DIAGNOSIS

IMAGING STUDIES

- Radiographs of the lower leg and foot to rule out osteomyelitis underlying an infected ulcer or to identify calcification of potential runoff vessels
- Duplex ultrasonogram used for diagnosis and in routine follow-up of infrainguinal bypass grafts to screen for graft stenoses
- Gadolinium-enhanced MRA in patients with severe renal insufficiency or contrast allergy
- Angiography indicated for percutaneous endovascular treatment or in preparation for surgical intervention

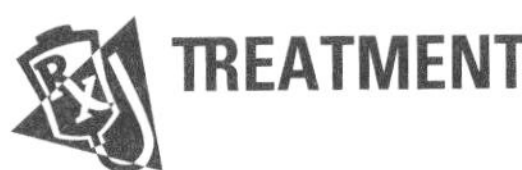

TREATMENT

MEDICATIONS

- Pentoxifylline, 400 mg PO TID; unclear efficacy
- Cilostazol, 100 mg PO BID; side effects: headache, dizziness in ~20%; contraindicated in heart failure
- Propionyl-L-carnitine, 1000 mg PO BID
- Ginkgo biloba extract, 120 mg PO QD; may increase risk of bleeding
- Aspirin, 81 mg PO QD
- Clopidogrel, 75 mg PO QD, or warfarin, dosed to maintain INR of 2.0–3.0; reserved for patients with unreconstructable disease and postoperative patients with higher risk of graft thrombosis because of hypercoagulable state, suboptimal conduit, poor distal runoff
- Sildenafil, 25–50 mg 30 min to 4 h before sexual activity for male erectile dysfunction

SURGERY

- Local wound care and débridement for ulcers
- Percutaneous or open surgery considered for low-risk patients with short-distance claudication that impairs ability to work or perform activities of daily living or with rest pain or gangrene
- Medical management optimized preoperatively
- Consider stress testing or coronary angiography preoperatively

Open surgery

- Aortobifemoral bypass grafting with bifurcated polytetrafluoroethylene or Dacron graft anastomosed end to end with infrarenal abdominal aorta and end to side to each common femoral artery has 10-year patency rate of 80%
- Axillary-femoral or femoral-femoral bypass graft for high-risk patients has lower 10-year patency rate of 50%
- Autogenous greater saphenous vein as bypass conduit for infrainguinal occlusive disease; 5-year patency rate of 75–80%
- Thomboendarterectomy is alternative to bypass for short-segment lesions in larger arteries in type 1 disease
- Long-segment closed superficial femoral artery endarterectomy combined with distal stenting is alternative to femoral popliteal bypass in high-risk surgical patients with suboptimal veins
- Lumbar sympathectomy is reserved for symptomatic patients with unreconstructable disease
- Iliac artery revascularization male erectile dysfunction

THERAPEUTIC PROCEDURES

- Blood pressure control, tobacco cessation, and lipid-lowering medications
- Initiation of daily exercise program

Endovascular techniques

- Stent angioplasty of common iliac artery stenoses with self-expanding (Wall) stents or balloon-expandable (Palmaz) stents has 3-year patency rate of 70–80%
- Angiography or stenting of distal lesions (external iliac or infrainguinal arteries) is not as successful: 3-year primary patency rate of 55–60%; lesions most amenable to this treatment are discrete, short-segment (< 5 cm), concentric lesions in noncalcified large-diameter vessels

OUTCOME

FOLLOW-UP

- Serial pulse examination and ABIs
- Duplex ultrasound surveillance is advised at 6-month intervals to detect stenotic, or "threatened," grafts before they progress to occlusion

COMPLICATIONS

- Operative complications for open aortic surgery: myocardial infarction or arrhythmia, renal insufficiency, bowel ischemia, impotence or retrograde ejaculation, and blue toe syndrome
- Late complications: graft thrombosis, graft infection, and aortoduodenal fistula
- Angiogram complications: hematoma, pseudoaneurysm, arteriovenous fistula, retroperitoneal hemorrhage, arterial occlusion, dissection or rupture, distal emboli, contrast nephropathy
- Operative mortality is 2–5% for open aortic surgery and 1–3% for infrainguinal bypass

PROGNOSIS

- Of patients with claudication, 25% will eventually develop ischemic rest pain or ulceration, 10% will require amputation; 5-year survival of 50%
- 5-year patency rate for infrainguinal saphenous vein grafts is 60–80%

WHEN TO REFER

- Lifestyle-limiting short-distance claudication
- Rest pain
- Ischemic ulceration

WHEN TO ADMIT

- Limb-threatening ischemia

EVIDENCE

PRACTICE GUIDELINES

- National Guideline Clearinghouse
  - http://www.guideline.gov/summary/summary.aspx?doc_id=5393&nbr=3696&string=arterial+AND+disease

INFORMATION FOR PATIENTS

- American Heart Association: Peripheral Vascular Disease
  - http://www.americanheart.org/presenter.jhtml?identifier=4692
- JAMA Patient Page: Peripheral arterial disease. JAMA 2001;286:1406.
- MedlinePlus: Arteriosclerosis of the Extremities
  - http://www.nlm.nih.gov/medlineplus/ency/article/000170.htm

REFERENCES

- Hiatt WR: Medical treatment of peripheral arterial disease and claudication. N Engl J Med 2001;344:1608. [PMID: 11372014]
- Muradin GSR et al: Balloon dilation and stent implantation for treatment of femoropopliteal arterial disease: meta-analysis. Radiology 2001;221:137. [PMID: 11568332]

Author(s)

Louis M. Messina, MD

Venous Insufficiency, Chronic

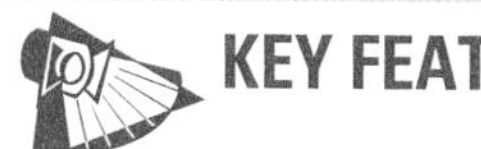

KEY FEATURES

ESSENTIALS OF DIAGNOSIS

- History of varicose veins, phlebitis, or leg injury
- Early sign: ankle edema
- Late signs: varicosities, pigmentation, stasis dermatitis, and induration from fibrosis of the subcutaneous tissue and skin, and ulceration

GENERAL CONSIDERATIONS

- Causes: deep venous thrombosis (most common), leg trauma, varicose veins, obstruction of the pelvic veins, or congenital or acquired arteriovenous fistula or venous anomaly

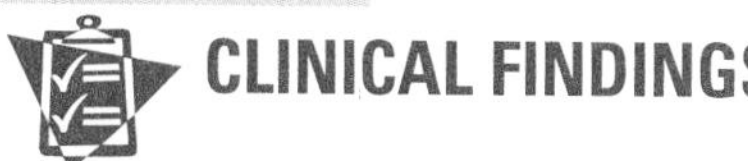

CLINICAL FINDINGS

SYMPTOMS AND SIGNS

- Progressive edema of the leg with dull aching discomfort
- Varicosities often present
- Stasis dermatitis, brownish pigmentation, brawny induration, and ulceration
- Thin, shiny, atrophic, and cyanotic skin
- Cellulitis
- Weeping dermatitis
- Venous stasis ulcers

DIFFERENTIAL DIAGNOSIS

- Congestive heart failure
- Chronic renal disease, nephrotic syndrome
- Cirrhosis
- Hypoalbuminemia
- Lymphedema
- Other causes of chronic leg ulcers, eg, autoimmune diseases (Felty's syndrome), arterial insufficiency, sickle cell anemia, erythema induratum, and fungal infections

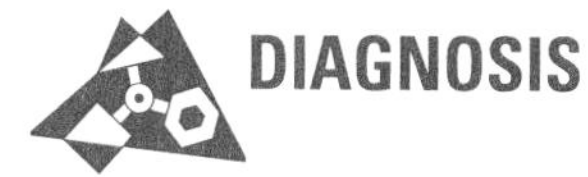

DIAGNOSIS

LABORATORY TESTS

- Electrolytes, albumin, complete blood cell count

IMAGING STUDIES

- Venous ultrasonogram to rule out deep venous thrombosis

Vasculitis, Cryoglobulinemic p. 1165. Vegetative State, Persistent p. 1165.

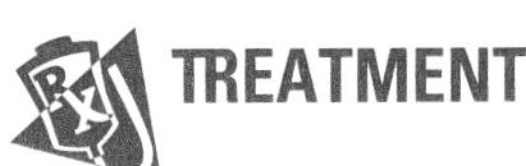

TREATMENT

MEDICATIONS

- Unna boot, semipermeable hydrophilic foam dressing, or calcium alginate dressing for weepy ulcers
- Systemic antibiotics and topical antifungal agents (eg, clotrimazole 1% cream or miconazole 2% cream) for active infection
- Zinc oxide ointment with ichthammol, 3%, QD or BID for chronic dermatitis

SURGERY

- Wide débridement and skin grafting in combination with open or endoscopic ligation of incompetent saphenous and perforating veins
- Venous reconstructive surgery is rarely indicated

THERAPEUTIC PROCEDURES

Acute care

- Bed rest with leg elevation and wet saline compresses for acute weeping dermatitis
- Deep venous thrombosis prophylaxis and external compression

Chronic care

- Intermittent periodic elevation of the legs during the day and elevation of the legs at night (kept above the level of the heart with pillows under the mattress); avoidance of long periods of sitting or standing; knee- or thigh-high graduated compression stockings (20–30 mm Hg); regular exercise
- Wet-to-dry normal saline, hydrogel, silvadine, or Promogran dressings plus Ace wrap compression, or an Unna boot or Wound VAC for venous ulcerations

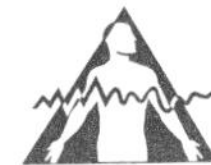

OUTCOME

COMPLICATIONS

- Cellulitis
- Limb loss

PROGNOSIS

- Recurrent venous stasis ulcers and progressive stasis changes of the skin are not uncommon

WHEN TO REFER

- Nonhealing wound
- Progression of venous stasis disease

WHEN TO ADMIT

- Sepsis
- Refractory cellulitis
- Threatened limb loss

PREVENTION

- Early and aggressive management of acute deep venous thrombosis
- Surgical treatment (eg, sclerosis or stripping) of varicose veins

EVIDENCE

PRACTICE GUIDELINES

- Buller HR et al: Antithrombotic therapy for venous thromboembolic disease: the Seventh ACCP Conference on Antithrombotic and Thrombolytic Therapy. Chest 2004;126(Suppl):401S. [PMID: 15383479]

INFORMATION FOR PATIENTS

- MedlinePlus: Venous Insufficiency
  - http://www.nlm.nih.gov/medlineplus/ency/article/000203.htm
- National Lymphedema Network: When It's Not Lymphedema
  - http://www.lymphnet.org/lymphlink1099.html
- Penn State College of Medicine: Chronic Venous Insufficiency
  - http://www.hmc.psu.edu/healthinfo/c/chronicvenous.htm

REFERENCE

- Mohr DN et al: The venous stasis syndrome after deep venous thrombosis or pulmonary embolism: a population-based study. Mayo Clin Proc 2000;75:1249. [PMID: 11126832]

Author(s)

Louis M. Messina, MD

Venous Stasis Ulcers

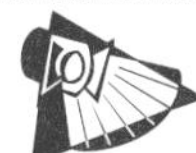

KEY FEATURES

ESSENTIALS OF DIAGNOSIS

- Past history of varicosities, thrombophlebitis, or postphlebitic syndrome
- Irregular ulceration, often on the medial aspect of the lower legs above the malleolus
- Edema of the legs, varicosities, hyperpigmentation, and red and scaly areas (stasis dermatitis) and scars from old ulcers support the diagnosis

GENERAL CONSIDERATIONS

- Patients at risk may have a history of venous insufficiency, either with obvious varicosities or with a past history of thrombophlebitis, or with immobility of the calf muscle group (paraplegics, etc)
- Red, pruritic patches of stasis dermatitis often precede ulceration
- Because venous insufficiency is the most common cause of lower leg ulceration, testing of venous competence is a required part of the evaluation even when no changes of venous insufficiency are present

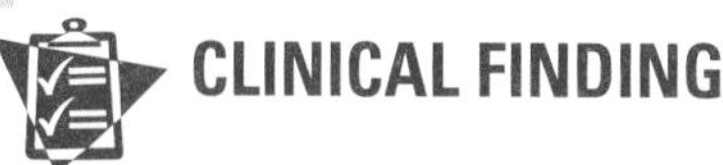

CLINICAL FINDINGS

SYMPTOMS AND SIGNS

- Classically, chronic edema is followed by a dermatitis, which is often pruritic; these changes are followed by hyperpigmentation, skin breakdown, and eventually sclerosis of the skin of the lower leg
- The ulcer base may be clean, but it may have a yellow fibrin eschar that often requires surgical treatment
- Ulceration is often on the *medial* aspect of the lower legs above the malleolus
- Edema of the legs, varicosities, hyperpigmentation, and red and scaly areas (stasis dermatitis) and scars from old ulcers support the diagnosis
- Ulcers that appear on the feet, toes, or above the knees are atypical for venous stasis—consider other diagnoses

DIFFERENTIAL DIAGNOSIS

- Arterial insufficiency (arterial ulcer)
- Bacterial pyoderma (eg, infected wound or bite)
- Trauma
- Diabetic ulcer
- Pressure ulcer
- Vasculitis
- Pyoderma gangrenosum
- Skin cancer
- Infection (eg, mycobacterial, fungal, tertiary syphilis, leishmaniasis, amebiasis)
- Sickle cell anemia
- Embolic disease (including cholesterol emboli)
- Cryoglobulinemia
- Calciphylaxis

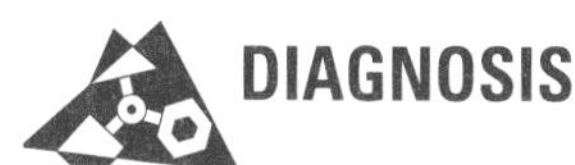

DIAGNOSIS

LABORATORY TESTS

- Thorough evaluation of the patient's vascular system (including measurement of the ankle-brachial index) is essential

IMAGING STUDIES

- Doppler ultrasound is usually sufficient (except in the diabetic) to elucidate the cause of most vascular cases of lower leg ulceration

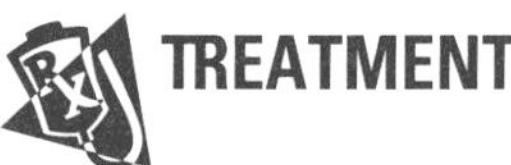

TREATMENT

MEDICATIONS

Cleaning of the ulcer

- The patient is instructed to clean the base with saline or cleansers such as Safclens or Cara-klenz daily
- Once the base is clean
  - The ulcer is treated with metronidazole gel to reduce bacterial growth and odor
  - Any red dermatitic skin is treated with a medium- to high-potency steroid ointment
  - The ulcer is then covered with an occlusive hydroactive dressing (Duoderm or Cutinova) or a polyurethane foam (Allevyn) followed by an Unna zinc paste boot, changed weekly

Systemic therapy

- Pentoxifylline, 400 mg three times daily, administered with compression accelerates healing
- Zinc supplementation is occasionally beneficial in patients with low serum zinc levels
- If cellulitis accompanies the ulcer, systemic antibiotics are recommended

SURGERY

- A curette or small scissors can be used to remove the yellow fibrin eschar, under local anesthesia if the areas are very tender
- Grafting for severe or nonhealing ulcers
  - Full- or split-thickness grafts often do not take, and pinch grafts (small shaves of skin laid onto the bed) may be more effective
  - Cultured epidermal cell grafts—or Apligraf, a bilayered skin construct—may accelerate wound healing, but they are very expensive

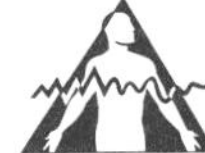

OUTCOME

PROGNOSIS

- The ulcer should begin to heal within weeks, and healing should be complete within 2–3 months

WHEN TO REFER

- If there is a question about the diagnosis, if recommended therapy is ineffective, or if specialized treatment is necessary

PREVENTION

- Elevation of an edematous leg above the heart for more than 2 h two times a day
- Compression stockings to reduce edema
  - Compression should achieve a pressure of 30 mm Hg below the knee and 40 mm Hg at the ankle
  - The stockings should not be used in patients with arterial insufficiency with an ankle-brachial pressure index less than 0.7
  - Pneumatic sequential compression devices may be of great benefit

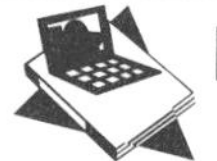

EVIDENCE

PRACTICE GUIDELINES

- Registered Nurses Association of Ontario. Assessment and management of venous leg ulcers, 2004
  - http://www.guideline.gov/summary/summary.aspx?doc_id=5309&nbr=3632
- Smith & Nephew Ltd. Grace P, editor. Guidelines for the management of leg ulcers in Ireland, 2002
  - http://www.guideline.gov/summary/summary.aspx?doc_id=3616&nbr=2842

WEB SITE

- American Academy of Dermatology
  - http://www.aad.org

INFORMATION FOR PATIENTS

- Mayo Clinic: Venostasis
  - http://www.mayoclinic.com/invoke.cfm?id=AN00628
- MedlinePlus: Stasis Dermatitis
  - http://www.nlm.nih.gov/medlineplus/ency/article/000834.htm
- MedlinePlus: Varicose Veins
  - http://www.nlm.nih.gov/medlineplus/ency/article/001109.htm
- Radiological Society of North America: Venous Ultrasound
  - http://www.radiologyinfo.org/content/ultrasound-venous.htm

REFERENCES

- de Araujo T et al: Managing the patient with venous ulcers. Ann Intern Med 2003;138:326. [PMID: 12585831]
- McMullin GM: Improving the treatment of leg ulcers. Med J Aust 2001;175:375. [PMID: 11700817]

Author(s)

Timothy G. Berger, MD

Vertigo

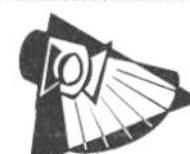

KEY FEATURES

ESSENTIALS OF DIAGNOSIS

- Either a sensation of motion when there is no motion or an exaggerated sense of motion in response to a given bodily movement
- Cardinal symptom of vestibular disease
- Must differentiate peripheral from central causes of vestibular dysfunction

GENERAL CONSIDERATIONS

- Causes of vestibular disorders can be determined based on the duration of symptoms (seconds, hours, days, months) and whether auditory symptoms are present (Table 11)
- Vertigo can occur as a side effect of anticonvulsants (eg, phenytoin), antibiotics (eg, aminoglycosides, doxycycline, metronidazole), hypnotics (eg, diazepam), analgesics (eg, aspirin), and tranquilizing drugs and alcohol

Endolymphatic hydrops (Ménière's disease)

- Results from distension of the endolymphatic compartment of the inner ear; the primary lesion appears to be in the endolymphatic sac, which filters and excretes endolymph
- Although a precise cause of hydrops cannot usually be established, two causes are syphilis and head trauma
- Episodic vertigo resembling Ménière's disease but without accompanying auditory symptoms is known as recurrent vestibulopathy
  - The pathogenic mechanism of this symptom complex is usually unknown, although a few patients suffer from a variant of migraine and others develop the classic syndrome of endolymphatic hydrops

CLINICAL FINDINGS

SYMPTOMS AND SIGNS

- See Table 11
- Perform Romberg test; evaluate gait; observe for nystagmus

Peripheral vestibulopathy

- Vertigo usually sudden; may be so severe that patient is unable to walk or stand; frequently accompanied by nausea and vomiting
- Tinnitus and hearing loss may accompany; support otologic origin
- **Nystagmus** usually horizontal with rotary component; fast phase usually beats away from diseased side
- Visual fixation tends to inhibit nystagmus except in very acute peripheral lesions or with CNS disease
- Positioning nystagmus can be induced with **Nylen-Bárány** and **Fukada tests**, which are of limited use when patient able to visually fixate; may be overcome by observing in the dark using electronystagmographic recording
- **Nylen-Bárány test:** Patient is in sitting position with head turned to right and is quickly lowered to supine position with head extending over the edge of table and placed 30° lower than the body; watch for nystagmus for 30 s. Repeat with head turned to left; perform maneuver without turning head
- **Fukuda test:** Patient walks in place with eyes closed; is useful for detecting subtle defects. Positive response observed when patient rotates, usually toward side of diseased labyrinth
- **Positional vertigo**: Symptoms usually develop seconds after head movement (latency period) and subside in 10–60 s; constant repetition of positional change leads to habituation
- Central lesions: no latent period, fatigability, or habituation of symptoms and signs
- **Ménière's syndrome:** episodic vertigo, usually for 1–8 h; low-frequency sensorineural hearing loss, often fluctuating; tinnitus, usually low tone and "blowing" in quality; aural pressure sensation. Symptoms wax and wane as endolymphatic pressure rises and falls. Caloric testing reveals loss/impairment of thermally induced nystagmus on involved side
- **Labyrinthitis:** acute onset of continuous, usually severe vertigo lasting several days to a week, hearing loss, tinnitus. During recovery (several weeks) rapid head movements may cause transient vertigo. Hearing may return to normal or be permanently impaired in involved ear

Central vestibulopathy

- Vertigo tends to develop gradually, often progressively more severe and debilitating
- Nystagmus not always present but can occur in any direction and may be dissociated in both eyes; it is often nonfatigable, vertical rather than horizontal, without latency, unsuppressed by visual fixation

DIFFERENTIAL DIAGNOSIS

- Imbalance
- Light-headedness
- Syncope

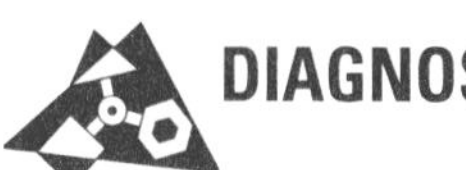

DIAGNOSIS

LABORATORY TESTS

- Electronystagmography is useful in differentiating central from peripheral causes of vertigo

IMAGING STUDIES

- The evaluation of central audiovestibular dysfunction usually requires MRI of the brain

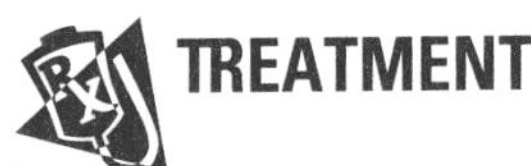

TREATMENT

MEDICATIONS

- Most common drug classes used (antihistamines, anticholinergics, sedative-hypnotics) reserved for patients with prominent nausea and vomiting; are best tapered and halted when symptoms resolve (in 1–2 weeks)
- In **acute severe vertigo**, vestibular suppressants (eg, diazepam, 2.5–5 mg SL, PO, or IV) may abate attack
- Relief from nausea and vomiting usually requires antiemetic delivered IM or by rectal suppository
- **Less severe vertigo** may be alleviated with antihistamines (eg, meclizine, 25 mg PO, or cyclizine or dimenhydrinate, 25–50 mg PO Q 6 h)
- Scopolamine (0.5 mg/day transdermal) beneficial in recurrent vertigo; side effects (dry mouth, blurred vision, urinary obstruction) often limit use (1/2 or even 1/4 patch may help without side effects)
- Drug combination may help if single drug fails
- In **Ménière's disease**, treatment is intended to lower endolymphatic pressure; low-salt diet (< 2 g sodium daily), at times supplemented by hydrochlorothiazide, 50–100 mg PO daily, adequately controls symptoms in most
- Prednisone used for clusters refractory to diuretics, low-salt diet, vestibular suppressants

SURGERY

- Surgical remedies reserved for those who remain substantially disabled despite prolonged, varied trial of medical therapy and exercises
- Selective section of the vestibular portion of the CN VIII brings relief of vertigo in > 90% of such patients
- Surgical removal of semicircular canals (labyrinthectomy) also highly effective; is appropriate only for patients with little or no hearing in involved ear

THERAPEUTIC PROCEDURES

- Bed rest may reduce severity of acute vertigo
- In **chronic or recurrent vertigo**, physical activity should be encouraged once nausea and vomiting resolve
- In general, patients should repeatedly perform maneuvers that provoke vertigo—up to the point of nausea or fatigue—to habituate them
- Patients refractory to conventional therapy may benefit from formal rehabilitation program under guidance of physical therapist
- Head maneuvers may help in managing **positioning vertigo;** these are as effective as vestibular habituation exercises and less time consuming
- Some refractory patients will benefit from selective chemical destruction of the vestibular hair cell population by infusion of ototoxins (eg, gentamicin) transtympanically into middle ear; 80–90% of Ménière's syndrome patients relieved of severe vertigo

OUTCOME

WHEN TO REFER

- Audiological evaluation, caloric stimulation, electronystagmography, CT scan or MRI, and brainstem auditory evoked potential studies are indicated in patients with persistent vertigo or when CNS disease is suspected
- For patients with recalcitrant vertigo or clusters of attacks, specialty referral may be useful

EVIDENCE

PRACTICE GUIDELINES

- Cesarani A et al: The treatment of acute vertigo. Neurol Sci 2004;25(Suppl 1):S26. [PMID: 15045617]

WEB SITE

- Baylor College of Mediine Otolaryngology Resources on the Internet
  - http://www.bcm.tmc.edu/oto/othersa.html

INFORMATION FOR PATIENTS

- American Hearing Research Foundation: Benign Paroxysmal Positional Vertigo (BPPV)
  - http://www.american-hearing.org/name/bppv.html
- MedlinePlus: Vertigo-Associated Disorders
  - http://www.nlm.nih.gov/medlineplus/ency/article/001432.htm
- National Institute on Deafness and Other Communication Disorders: Balance Disorders
  - http://www.nidcd.nih.gov/health/balance/balance_disorders.asp
- National Institute on Deafness and Other Communication Disorders: Ménière's Disease
  - http://www.nidcd.nih.gov/health/balance/meniere.asp
- Vestibular Disorders Association: Vestibular Disorders: An Overview
  - http://www.vestibular.org/overview.html

REFERENCES

- Angeli SI et al: Systematic approach to benign paroxysmal positional vertigo in the elderly. Otolaryngol Head Neck Surg 2003;128:719. [PMID: 12748567]
- Brandt T et al: General vestibular testing. Clin Neurophysiol 2005;116:406. [PMID: 15661119]
- Guilemany JM et al: Clinical and epidemiological study of vertigo at an outpatient clinic. Acta Otolaryngol 2004;124:49. [PMID: 14977078]
- Lempert T et al: Episodic vertigo. Curr Opin Neurol 2005;18:5. [PMID: 15655395]

Author(s)

Robert K. Jackler, MD
Michael J. Kaplan, MD

Visceral Artery Insufficiency

Vestibular Schwannoma (Acoustic Neuroma) p. 1167.
Vibrio Infections p. 1167.
Visceral Artery Aneurysms p. 1167.

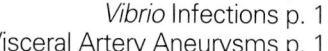

KEY FEATURES

ESSENTIALS OF DIAGNOSIS

- Chronic intestinal ischemia: epigastric or periumbilical pain, bloating or diarrhea, and food avoidance (diagnosis of exclusion)
- Acute intestinal ischemia: severe epigastric and periumbilical abdominal pain and a high leukocyte count

GENERAL CONSIDERATIONS

- Chronic intestinal ischemia results from atherosclerotic occlusive lesions at the origins of the superior mesenteric, celiac, and inferior mesenteric arteries
- Acute intestinal ischemia may result from embolic occlusion of a visceral branch of the abdominal aorta, generally in patients with mitral valvular disease, atrial fibrillation, or left ventricular mural thrombus; thrombosis of an atherosclerotic mesenteric vessel; or low-flow or shock state resulting from cardiac failure or arterial spasm induced by ergot or cocaine intoxication; or postcoarctectomy syndrome
- Emboli are responsible for almost half of cases
- Celiac axis compression syndrome: stenosis of the celiac artery caused by external compression of the arcuate ligament may cause chronic mesenteric ischemia
- Mesenteric vein occlusion causes 5–15% of cases of acute mesenteric ischemia
- Risk factors for mesenteric vein occlusion: hypercoagulable state (malignancy; protein C, protein S, or antithrombin III deficiency; presence of anticardiolipin or antiphospholipid antibody; polycythemia vera), intraabdominal sepsis, previous splenectomy or portal angiography or sclerotherapy, portal hypertension, and cirrhosis

DEMOGRAPHICS

- Almost 30% of patients with peripheral vascular disease have asymptomatic occlusive disease of the mesenteric arteries

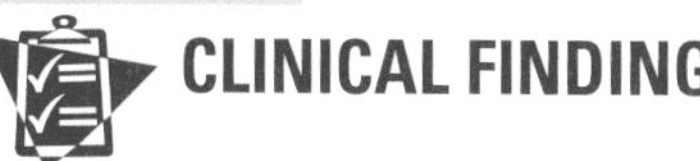

CLINICAL FINDINGS

SYMPTOMS AND SIGNS

- Chronic mesenteric ischemia: epigastric or periumbilical postprandial pain, often accompanied by bloating or diarrhea, and, at later stages, food avoidance (sitophobia), resulting in weight loss
- Acute mesenteric ischemia: sudden onset of severe epigastric and periumbilical abdominal pain, acidosis and hypotension, with minimal appreciable findings on abdominal examination except abdominal distension
- Ischemic colitis: bouts of crampy lower abdominal pain and mild—often bloody—diarrhea

DIFFERENTIAL DIAGNOSIS

- Peptic ulcer disease
- Gastroesophageal reflux
- Bowel obstruction
- Pancreatitis
- Irritable bowel syndrome
- Malignancy

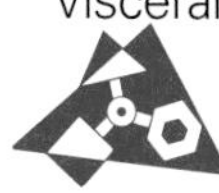

DIAGNOSIS

LABORATORY TESTS

- Obtain complete blood cell count and electrolytes
- Arterial blood gas if suspect acidosis
- Hypercoagulable workup may be indicated for mesenteric vein thrombosis

IMAGING STUDIES

- Visceral angiography indicated in any person older than 45 who appears chronically ill, with risk factors for arterial occlusive disease and no other identifiable cause for abdominal symptoms
- Mesenteric artery thrombosis from atherooclusive disease causes occlusion at the origin of the vessel
- Emboli most often lodge within the superior mesenteric artery at the first jejunal branch
- With shock or arterial spasm, vessels are pruned but patent
- Mesenteric vein occlusion: contrast-enhanced abdominal CT scan or arterial portography

DIAGNOSTIC PROCEDURES

- Ischemic colitis: colonoscopy reveals segmental inflammatory changes, most prominent in the watershed areas of the rectosigmoid junction and splenic flexure

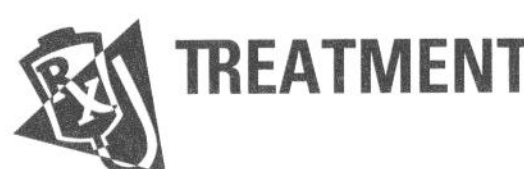

TREATMENT

MEDICATIONS

- Long-term anticoagulation for mesenteric vein thrombosis
- Broad-spectrum antibiotics for acute mesenteric ischemia
- Catheter-directed thrombolytics (alteplase, 0.5–1 mg/h) for thrombotic disease or vasodilators (papaverine, 30–60 mg/h) for nonocclusive disease
- Perioperative nutritional supplementation

SURGERY

- Surgical or endovascular management is directed toward restoration of anterograde visceral arterial flow
- Chronic mesenteric ischemia: transaortic endarterectomy and mesenteric artery bypass
  - A 5–9% mortality rate and a 10–25% recurrence rate at long-term follow-up
  - A higher recurrence rate with stenting of short-segment lesions; these patients require routine angiographic follow-up
- Acute mesenteric ischemia: emergent laparotomy indicated for patients with embolic disease, acidosis, hemodynamic instability, or severe or progressive abdominal pain
  - Surgical options include thomboembolectomy or bypass and resection of any nonviable bowel
  - Second-look operation if any bowel is of questionable viability
- Celiac axis compression syndrome: division of the arcuate ligament yields variable postoperative results
- Ischemic colitis: conservative management is usually adequate; surgery indicated for progressive symptoms or stricture formation

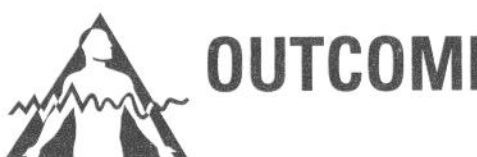

OUTCOME

COMPLICATIONS

- Bowel infarction
- Intraabdominal sepsis

PROGNOSIS

- Mortality approaches 80% in acute bowel infarction

WHEN TO REFER

- Symptoms and signs of acute or chronic mesenteric ischemia

WHEN TO ADMIT

- Acute mesenteric ischemia

EVIDENCE

PRACTICE GUIDELINES

- Moneta GL: Screening for mesenteric vascular insufficiency and follow-up of mesenteric artery bypass procedures. Semin Vasc Surg 2001;14:186. [PMID: 11561279]
- Trompeter M et al: Non-occlusive mesenteric ischemia: etiology, diagnosis, and interventional therapy. Eur Radiol 2002;12:1179. Dec 21. [PMID: 11976865]

INFORMATION FOR PATIENTS

- Albany Medical Center: Acute Mesenteric Ischemia
  - http://www.amc.edu/Vascular/vas_visceral_info.htm#Acute
- Mayo Clinic: Intestinal Ischemia
  - http://www.mayoclinic.com/invoke.cfm?objectid=61253DCD-5CF2-4204-83572DEB6DD0CB89
- MedlinePlus: Mesenteric Artery Ischemia
  - http://www.nlm.nih.gov/medlineplus/ency/article/001156.htm

REFERENCES

- Kasirajan K et al: Chronic mesenteric ischemia: Open surgery versus percutaneous angioplasty and stenting. J Vasc Surg 2001;33:63. [PMID: 11137925]
- Klotz S et al: Diagnosis and treatment of nonocclusive mesenteric ischemia after open heart surgery. Ann Thorac Surg 2001;72:1583. [PMID: 11722048]

Author(s)

Louis M. Messina, MD
Lawrence M. Tierney, Jr., MD

Vitamin B_{12} Deficiency

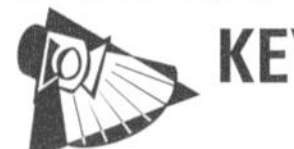

KEY FEATURES

ESSENTIALS OF DIAGNOSIS

- Macrocytic anemia
- Macroovalocytes and hypersegmented neutrophils on peripheral blood smear
- Serum vitamin B_{12} level < 100 pg/mL

GENERAL CONSIDERATIONS

- All vitamin B_{12} is absorbed from diet (foods of animal origin)
- After ingestion, vitamin B_{12} binds to intrinsic factor, a protein secreted by gastric parietal cells
- Vitamin B_{12}-intrinsic factor complex is absorbed in terminal ileum by cells with specific receptors for the complex; it is then transported through plasma and stored in the liver
- Liver stores are sufficient such that vitamin B_{12} deficiency develops only > 3 years after vitamin B_{12} absorption ceases
- Causes of vitamin B
  - Decreased intrinsic factor production: pernicious anemia (most common cause), gastrectomy
  - Dietary deficiency (only in vegans)
  - Competition for B_{12} in gut: blind loop syndrome, fish tapeworm (rare)
  - Decreased ileal B_{12} absorption: surgical resection, Crohn's disease, metformin
  - Pancreatic insufficiency
  - *Helicobacter pylori* infection
  - Transcobalamin II deficiency (rare)
- Pernicious anemia is associated with atrophic gastritis and other autoimmune diseases, eg, immunoglobulin A (IgA) deficiency, polyglandular endocrine failure syndromes

DEMOGRAPHICS

- Pernicious anemia is hereditary, though rare clinically before age 35

CLINICAL FINDINGS

SYMPTOMS AND SIGNS

- Megaloblastic anemia, which may be severe
- Pallor and mild icterus
- Glossitis and vague gastrointestinal disturbances (eg, anorexia, diarrhea)
- Neurological manifestations: peripheral neuropathy usually occurs first; then subacute combined degeneration of the spinal cord affecting posterior columns, causing difficulty with position and vibration sensation and balance; then, in advanced cases, central nervous system, causing dementia or other neuropsychiatric changes
- Decreased vibration and position sensation
- Neurological manifestations occasionally precede hematological changes; patients with suspicious neurological symptoms and signs should be evaluated for vitamin B_{12} deficiency despite normal mean cell volume (MCV) and absence of anemia

DIFFERENTIAL DIAGNOSIS

- Folic acid deficiency (other cause of megaloblastic anemia)
- Myelodysplastic syndrome (other cause of macrocytic anemia with abnormal morphology)
- Other cause of peripheral neuropathy, ataxia, or dementia

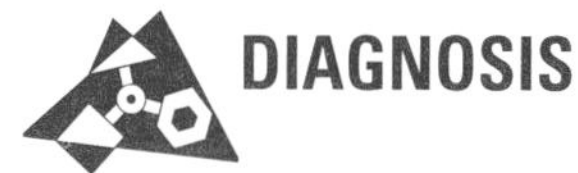

DIAGNOSIS

LABORATORY TESTS

- Anemia of variable severity; hematocrit may be as low as 10–15%
- MCV strikingly elevated: 110–140 fL; may be normal if coexistent thalassemia or iron deficiency
- Serum vitamin B_{12} level low, usually < 100 pg/mL (normal 150–350 pg/mL), establishes diagnosis
- Serum methylmalonic acid or homocysteine level elevations can confirm diagnosis when serum vitamin B_{12} level is borderline
- Peripheral blood smear: macro-ovalocytes characteristic; hypersegmented neutrophils with mean lobe count > 4, or ≥ 1 six-lobed neutrophils; anisocytosis and poikilocytosis
- Reticulocyte count reduced
- Pancytopenia present in severe cases
- Serum lactate dehydrogenase (LDH) elevated and indirect bilirubin modestly increased

DIAGNOSTIC PROCEDURES

- Schilling test used to document decreased absorption of oral vitamin B_{12} characteristic of pernicious anemia
- Vitamin B_{12}, 1000 μg given IM to saturate transport proteins, then radiolabeled vitamin B_{12} given PO, and 24-h urine collected to determine how much vitamin B_{12} is absorbed and excreted; abnormal excretion of < 3% occurs with impaired absorption of oral vitamin B_{12}
- In second stage of Schilling test (done 2 months after vitamin B_{12} replacement), radiolabeled vitamin B_{12} is given with intrinsic factor; in pernicious anemia, low absorption should normalize
- Bone marrow morphology is characteristic: marked erythroid hyperplasia, megaloblastic changes in erythroid series, and giant metamyelocytes in myeloid series

Vitamin A Deficiency p. 1168. Vitamin B_6 Deficiency p. 1168.

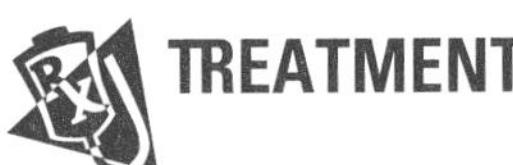

TREATMENT

MEDICATIONS

- Vitamin B_{12}, 100 µg IM QD for 1 week, then every week for 1 month, then every month for life, for pernicious anemia
- Oral cobalamin, 1000 µg PO QD, may be tried instead of parenteral therapy but must be continued indefinitely
- Antibiotics if vitamin B_{12} deficiency is caused by bacterial overgrowth in a blind loop
- Pancreatic enzymes if deficiency is due to pancreatic insufficiency
- Anthelmintic agent if deficiency is due to fish tapeworm
- **Note**: Large doses of folic acid may produce hematological responses in cases of vitamin B_{12} deficiency but allow neurological damage to progress

OUTCOME

FOLLOW-UP

- Pernicous anemia is a lifelong disorder; if patients discontinue monthly therapy, the vitamin deficiency will recur
- Brisk reticulocytosis occurs 5–7 days after therapy, and the hematological picture normalizes in 2 months
- Follow serum vitamin B_{12} level

COMPLICATIONS

- Nervous system complications include subacute combined degeneration of the spinal cord, psychosis, and dementia
- Atrophic gastritis in pernicious anemia is associated with increased risk of gastric carcinoma
- Hypokalemia may complicate the first several days of parenteral vitamin B_{12} therapy in pernicious anemia, particularly if anemia is severe

PROGNOSIS

- Patients with pernicious anemia respond to parenteral vitamin B_{12} therapy with immediate improvement in sense of well-being
- Nervous system manifestations are reversible if they are of relatively short duration (< 6 months) but may be permanent if treatment is not initiated promptly

EVIDENCE

WEB SITE

- National Institutes of Health, Office of Dietary Supplements: Vitamin B_{12}
  - http://ods.od.nih.gov/factsheets/vitaminb12.asp

INFORMATION FOR PATIENTS

- American Academy of Family Physicians: Vitamin B-12
  - http://familydoctor.org/765.xml
- Mayo Clinic: Vitamin Deficiency Anemia
  - http://www.mayoclinic.com/invoke.cfm?id=DS00325
- MedlinePlus: Pernicious Anemia
  - http://www.nlm.nih.gov/medlineplus/ency/article/000569.htm
- MedlinePlus: Vitamin B_{12}
  - http://www.nlm.nih.gov/medlineplus/druginfo/uspdi/202596.html

REFERENCES

- Andres E et al: Vitamin B_{12} (cobalamin) deficiency in elderly patients. CMAJ 2004;171:251. [PMID: 15289425]
- Bolaman Z et al: Oral versus intramuscular cobalamin treatment in megaloblastic anemia: a single-center, prospective, randomized, open-label study. Clin Ther 2003; 25:3124. [PMID: 14749150]

Author(s)

Charles A. Linker, MD

von Willebrand's Disease

Vitamin C Deficiency p. 1168. Vitamin E Deficiency p. 1169.
Vitamin K Deficiency p. 1169. Vocal Cord Dysfunction p. 1169.

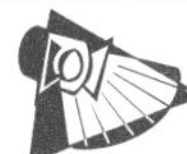

KEY FEATURES

ESSENTIALS OF DIAGNOSIS

- Family history with autosomal dominant pattern of inheritance
- Bleeding time prolonged, either at baseline or after challenge with aspirin
- Factor VIII antigen or ristocetin cofactor levels reduced
- Factor VIII coagulant activity levels reduced in some patients

GENERAL CONSIDERATIONS

- Most common congenital disorder of hemostasis
- Autosomal dominant transmission
- Characterized by deficient or defective von Willebrand factor (vWF), a protein that mediates platelet adhesion
- Platelets adhere to subendothelium via vWF, which binds to platelet receptor composed of glycoprotein Ib (missing in Bernard-Soulier syndrome)
- Platelet aggregation normal in von Willebrand's disease
- vWF has separate function protecting from degradation factor VIII coagulant protein (factor VIII:C, deficient in hemophilia A); may thus secondarily cause coagulation disturbance because of deficient factor VIII:C levels, but coagulopathy is rarely severe
- Subtypes of von Willebrand's disease
  - Type I (80% of cases): quantitative decrease in vWF
  - Type IIa: qualitative abnormality prevents multimer formation; only small multimers present that cannot mediate platelet adhesion
  - Type IIb: qualitative abnormality causes rapid clearance of functional large multimeric forms
  - Type III: rare autosomal recessive disorder in which vWF nearly absent
  - Pseudo-von Willebrand disease: rare disorder in which platelets bind large vWF multimers with excessive avidity, causing their clearance from plasma

DEMOGRAPHICS

- Common disorder affecting both men and women

CLINICAL FINDINGS

SYMPTOMS AND SIGNS

- Mild bleeding in most cases
- Rarely as severe as hemophilia, and spontaneous hemarthroses do not occur
- Mucosal bleeding usually (epistaxis, gingival bleeding, menorrhagia), but gastrointestinal bleeding may occur
- Incisional bleeding usually occurs after surgery or dental extractions
- Bleeding tendency is exacerbated by aspirin
- Bleeding tendency decreases during pregnancy or estrogen use

DIFFERENTIAL DIAGNOSIS

- Other qualitative platelet disorders, eg, uremia, aspirin use, Glanzmann's thrombasthenia
- Thrombocytopenia
- Hemophilia
- Waldenström's macroglobulinemia

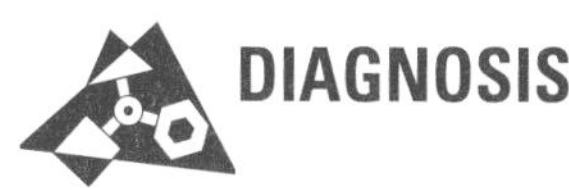

DIAGNOSIS

LABORATORY TESTS

- Platelet number and morphology normal
- Bleeding time usually (not always) prolonged; measure whenever diagnosis is considered because it correlates most closely with clinical bleeding
- When bleeding time is normal in von Willebrand's disease, it will be prolonged markedly by aspirin; normal persons prolong their bleeding time to a minor extent with aspirin but rarely out of the normal range
- In the most common form of von Willebrand's disease (type I), vWF plasma levels are reduced, as measured by factor VIII antigen or by ristocetin cofactor activity
- When factor VIII antigen is reduced, may also see a decrease in factor VIII coagulant (factor VIII:C) levels; when factor VIII:C levels < 25%, partial thromboplastin time is prolonged
- Platelet aggregation studies with standard agonists (ADP, collagen, thrombin) are normal, but platelet aggregation in response to ristocetin may be subnormal
- In difficult cases, it may be helpful to perform a direct assay of the multimeric composition of vWF

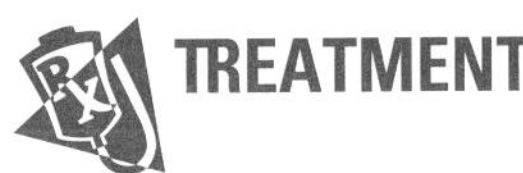

TREATMENT

MEDICATIONS

- Desmopressin, 0.3 μg/kg IV × 1, is useful for mild type I von Willebrand's disease
  - vWF levels usually rise 2- to 3-fold in 30–90 min, apparently via release of stored vWF from endothelial cells
  - Can be given only every 24 h as stores of vWF become depleted
- Desmopressin is not effective in type IIa von Willebrand's disease, in which no endothelial stores are present
- Desmopressin may be harmful in type IIb, leading to thrombocytopenia and increased bleeding
- Factor VIII concentrate, eg, Humate-P (Armour), 20–50 U/kg depending on disease severity, is treatment of choice if factor replacement is required; some (not all) of these products contain functional vWF and they do not transmit HIV or hepatitis
- ε-Aminocaproic acid (EACA; Amicar) is useful as adjunctive therapy during dental procedures; after either cryoprecipitate or desmopressin, 4 g PO Q 4 h to reduce the likelihood of bleeding

THERAPEUTIC PROCEDURES

- In mild bleeding disorder, no treatment is routinely given other than aspirin avoidance
- In preparation for surgical or dental procedures, measure bleeding time as the best indicator of bleeding likelihood; prophylactic therapy may be reasonably withheld if the procedure is minor and bleeding time is normal

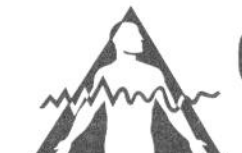

OUTCOME

PROGNOSIS

- Prognosis is excellent
- In most cases, bleeding disorder is mild
- In more serious cases, replacement therapy is effective

EVIDENCE

PRACTICE GUIDELINES

- Laffan M et al: The diagnosis of von Willebrand disease: a guideline from the UK Haemophilia Centre Doctors' Organization.Haemophilia 2004;10:199. [PMID: 15086318]
- Pasi KJ et al: Management of von Willebrand disease: a guideline from the UK Haemophilia Centre Doctors' Organization. Haemophilia 2004;10:218. [PMID: 15086319]

WEB SITE

- National Hemophilia Foundation
  - http://www.hemophilia.org

INFORMATION FOR PATIENTS

- National Heart, Lung, and Blood Institute: von Willebrand Disease
  - http://www.nhlbi.nih.gov/health/dci/Diseases/vWD/vWD_WhatIs.html
- National Hemophilia Foundation: von Willebrand Disease
  - http://www.hemophilia.org/bdi/bdi_types3.htm
- MedlinePlus: von Willebrand's Disease
  - http://www.nlm.nih.gov/medlineplus/ency/article/000544.htm

REFERENCES

- Federici AB et al: Biologic response to desmopressin in patients with severe type 1 and type 2 von Willebrand disease: results of a multicenter European study. Blood 2004;103:2032. [PMID: 14630825]
- Laffan M et al: The diagnosis of von Willebrand disease: a guideline from the UK Haemophilia Centre Doctors' Organization. Haemophilia 2004;10:199. [PMID: 15086318]

Author(s)

Charles A. Linker, MD

Vulvar Cancer

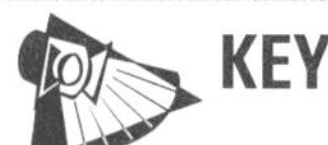

KEY FEATURES

ESSENTIALS OF DIAGNOSIS

- History of genital warts
- History of prolonged vulvar irritation, with pruritus, local discomfort, or slight bloody discharge
- Early lesions may suggest or include nonneoplastic epithelial disorders
- Late lesions appear as a mass, an exophytic growth, or a firm, ulcerated area in the vulva
- Biopsy is necessary to make the diagnosis

GENERAL CONSIDERATIONS

- The vast majority of cancers of the vulva are squamous lesions; basal cell carcinomas are also found
- Several subtypes (particularly 16, 18, and 31) of the human papillomavirus have been identified in some but not all vulvar cancers
- As with squamous cell lesions of the cervix, a grading system of vulvar intraepithelial neoplasia (VIN) from mild dysplasia to carcinoma in situ has been established

DEMOGRAPHICS

- Usually occurs in women over 50 years of age
- The likelihood that a superimposed vulvar cancer will develop in a woman with a nonneoplastic epithelial disorder (vulvar dystrophy) ranges from 1% to 5%

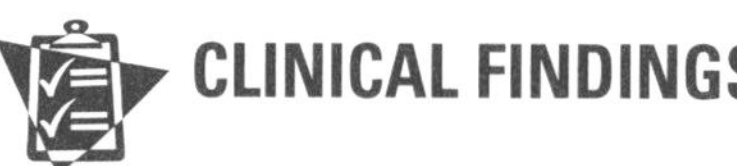

CLINICAL FINDINGS

SYMPTOMS AND SIGNS

- Early lesions may suggest or include nonneoplastic epithelial disorders
- Late lesions appear as a mass, an exophytic growth, or a firm, ulcerated area in the vulva

DIFFERENTIAL DIAGNOSIS

- Chronic granulomatous lesions (eg, lymphogranuloma venereum, syphilis), condylomas, hidradenoma, or neurofibroma
- Genital warts (condyloma acuminata)
- Lichen sclerosus
- Lichen planus
- Ulcer: herpes simplex virus, chancroid, syphilis, granuloma inguinale, lymphogranuloma venereum, Behçet's syndrome
- Hidradenitis suppurativa
- Vulvar intraepithelial neoplasia
- Psoriasis
- Paget's disease
- Papillary hidradenoma
- Bartholin's cyst or abscess

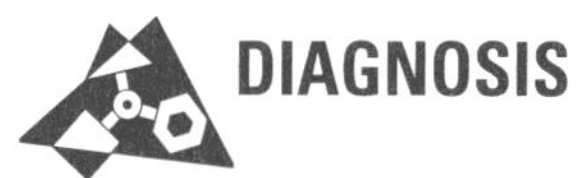

DIAGNOSIS

LABORATORY TESTS

- Pathologic examination of biopsies of lesion(s)

IMAGING STUDIES

- Preoperative colposcopy of vulva, vagina, and cervix
- Pelvic CT scan to rule out lymphadenopathy

DIAGNOSTIC PROCEDURES

- Biopsy is essential for the diagnosis and should be performed with any localized atypical vulvar lesion, including white patches
- Multiple skin-punch specimens can be taken in the office under local anesthesia, with care to include tissue from the edges of each lesion sampled
- Lichen sclerosus and other associated leukoplakic changes in the skin should be biopsied

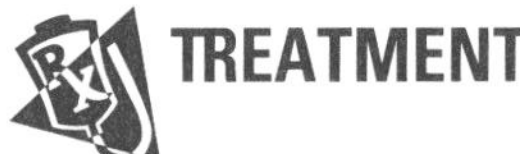

TREATMENT

MEDICATIONS

- A 7:3 combination of betamethasone and crotamiton is particularly effective for itching
- After an initial response, fluorinated steroids should be replaced with hydrocortisone because of their skin atrophying effect
- For lichen sclerosus, apply clobetasol propionate cream 0.05% twice daily for 2–3 weeks, then once daily until symptoms resolve. Application one to three times a week can be used for long-term maintenance therapy

SURGERY

- **In situ carcinoma**
  - In situ squamous cell carcinoma of the vulva and small, invasive basal cell carcinoma of the vulva should be excised with a wide margin
  - If the squamous carcinoma in situ is extensive or multicentric, laser therapy or superficial surgical removal of vulvar skin may be required. In this way, the clitoris and uninvolved portions of the vulva may be spared. Skin grafting may be necessary, but mutilating vulvectomy is avoided
- **Invasive carcinoma**
  - Invasive carcinoma confined to the vulva without evidence of spread to adjacent organs or to the regional lymph nodes will necessitate radical vulvectomy and inguinal lymphadenectomy if the patient is able to withstand surgery
  - Debilitated patients may be candidates for palliative irradiation only

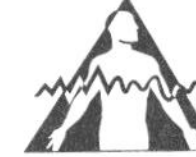

OUTCOME

FOLLOW-UP

- Examination every 3 months for 2 years postoperatively, then every 6 months for an additional 3 years

COMPLICATIONS

- Depends on extent of surgery
- Wound infection
- Wound breakdown
- Lymphedema may occur as a late complication in up to 30%

PROGNOSIS

- Basal cell carcinomas very seldom metastasize, and carcinoma in situ by definition has not metastasized. With adequate excision, the prognosis for both lesions is excellent
- Patients with invasive vulvar carcinoma 3 cm in diameter or less without inguinal lymph node metastases who can sustain radical surgery have about a 90% chance of a 5-year survival. If the lesion is > 3 cm and has metastasized, the likelihood of 5-year survival is less than 25%

WHEN TO REFER

- All patients with invasive vulvar carcinoma should be referred to a gynecologic oncologist

PREVENTION

- Careful examination of the vulva for premalignant lesions at all gynecologic examinations

EVIDENCE

PRACTICE GUIDELINES

- Benedet JL et al: FIGO staging classifications and clinical practice guidelines in the management of gynecologic cancers. FIGO Committee on Gynecologic Oncology. Int J Gynaecol Obstet 2000;70:209. [PMID: 11041682]

WEB SITE

- National Cancer Institute: Vulvar Cancer Information for Patients and Health Professionals
  - http://www.cancer.gov/cancertopics/types/vulvar/

INFORMATION FOR PATIENTS

- American Academy of Family Physicians: Vulvar Cancer
  - http://familydoctor.org/753.xml
- American Cancer Society: Vulvar Cancer
  - http://www.cancer.org/docroot/CRI/CRI_2_3x.asp?rnav=cridg&dt=45
- MedlinePlus: Cancer—vulva
  - http://www.nlm.nih.gov/medlineplus/ency/article/000902.htm

REFERENCES

- Cardosi RJ et al: Diagnosis and management of vulvar and vaginal intraepithelial neoplasia. Obstet Gynecol Clin North Am 2001;28:685. [PMID: 11766145]
- Hopkins MP et al: Carcinoma of the vulva. Obstet Gynecol Clin North Am 2001;28:791. [PMID: 11766152]

Author(s)

H. Trent MacKay, MD, MPH

Waldenström's Macroglobulinemia

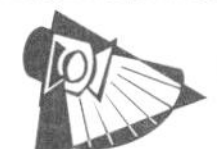

KEY FEATURES

ESSENTIALS OF DIAGNOSIS

- Symptoms nonspecific: splenomegaly common on examination
- Monoclonal immunoglobulin M (IgM) paraprotein
- Infiltration of bone marrow by plasmacytic lymphocytes
- Absence of lytic bone disease

GENERAL CONSIDERATIONS

- Malignant disease of B cells that appear to be hybrid of lymphocytes and plasma cells
- Cells characteristically secrete IgM paraprotein, and this macroglobulin causes many clinical manifestations

DEMOGRAPHICS

- Occurs mainly in patients aged 60–79

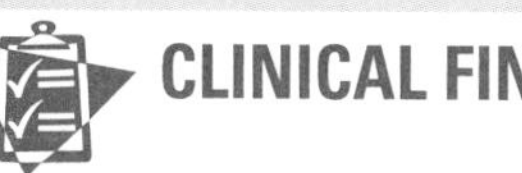

CLINICAL FINDINGS

SYMPTOMS AND SIGNS

- Insidious fatigue related to anemia
- Mucosal or gastrointestinal bleeding related to engorged blood vessels and platelet dysfunction with hyperviscosity syndrome (usually when viscosity > 4 times that of water)
- Nausea, vertigo, or visual disturbances; or alterations in consciousness from mild lethargy to stupor and coma with hyperviscosity syndrome
- Symptoms of cold agglutinin disease or peripheral neuropathy from IgM paraprotein
- Hepatosplenomegaly or lymphadenopathy may be present
- Retinal vein engorgement
- Purpura may be present
- Bone tenderness absent

DIFFERENTIAL DIAGNOSIS

- Monoclonal gammopathy of uncertain significance
- Multiple myeloma
- Chronic lymphocytic leukemia
- Lymphoma

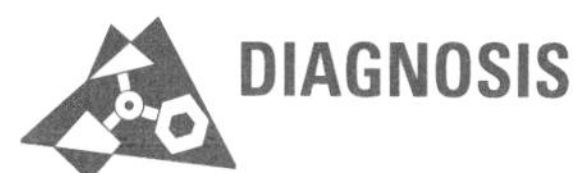

DIAGNOSIS

LABORATORY TESTS

- Anemia nearly universal, and rouleau formation common
- White blood cell and platelet count usually normal
- Peripheral blood smear: abnormal plasmacytic lymphocytes usually in small numbers
- Serum protein electrophoresis (SPEP) demonstrates monoclonal IgM spike in β- or γ-globulin region
- Serum viscosity usually increased above normal (> 1.4–1.8 times viscosity of water)
- No strict correlation between paraprotein concentration and serum viscosity
- Coombs, cold agglutinin, or cryoglobulin tests may be positive because of IgM paraprotein
- If macroglobulinemia is suspected but SPEP shows only hypogammaglobulinemia, repeat SPEP while maintaining blood at 37°C, because paraprotein may precipitate at room temperature
- No evidence of renal failure

IMAGING STUDIES

- Bone x-rays: normal

DIAGNOSTIC PROCEDURES

- Bone marrow aspiration and biopsy: characteristic infiltration by the plasmacytic lymphocytes

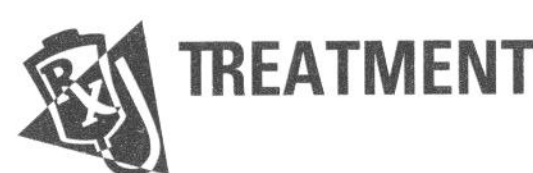

TREATMENT

MEDICATIONS

- Chemotherapy with:
  - Chlorambucil, cyclophosphamide, or fludarabine
  - Cladribine
  - Rituximab (monoclonal antibody)

THERAPEUTIC PROCEDURES

- Emergent plasmapheresis for marked hyperviscosity syndrome (stupor or coma)
- Plasmapheresis alone periodically for some patients
- Autologous stem cell transplantation in younger patients with more aggressive disease

OUTCOME

PROGNOSIS

- Median survival rate is 3–5 years; some patients may survive 10 years or longer

EVIDENCE

PRACTICE GUIDELINES

- Gertz MA et al: Treatment recommendations in Waldenström's macroglobulinemia: consensus panel recommendations from the Second International Workshop on Waldenström's Macroglobulinemia. Semin Oncol 2003;30:121. [PMID: 12720120]
- Kyle RA et al: Prognostic markers and criteria to initiate therapy in Waldenström's macroglobulinemia: consensus panel recommendations from the Second International Workshop on Waldenström's Macroglobulinemia. Semin Oncol 2003;30:116. [PMID: 12720119]

WEB SITE

- International Waldenström's Macroglobulinemia Foundation
  - http://www.iwmf.com/

INFORMATION FOR PATIENTS

- American Cancer Society: Detailed Guide: Waldenström's Macroglobulinemia
  - http://www.cancer.org/docroot/CRI/CRI_2_3x.asp?rnav=cridg YOURMOMMAdt=76
- MedlinePlus: Macroglobulinemia of Waldenström
  - http://www.nlm.nih.gov/medlineplus/ency/article/000588.htm
- National Cancer Institute: Waldenström's Macroglobulinemia Facts
  - http://cis.nci.nih.gov/fact/6_4.htm
- Research Fund for Waldenström's: What Is Waldenström's Macroglobulinemia?
  - http://www.waldenstromsresearch.org/whatis.htm

REFERENCES

- Johnson SA et al: Waldenström's macroglobulinaemia. Blood Rev 2002;16:175. [PMID: 12163003]
- Kyle RA et al: Long-term follow-up of IgM monoclonal gammopathy of undetermined significance. Blood 2003;102:3759. [PMID: 12881316]
- Munshi NC et al: Role for high-dose therapy with autologous hematopoietic stem cell support in Waldenström's macroglobulinemia. Semin Oncol 2003;30:282. [PMID: 12720153]

Author(s)

Charles A. Linker, MD

Warts

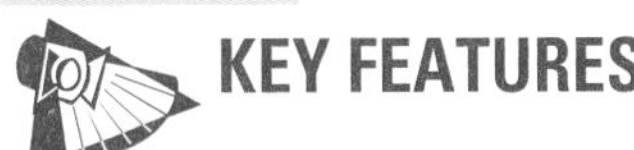

KEY FEATURES

ESSENTIALS OF DIAGNOSIS

- Verrucous papules anywhere on the skin or mucous membranes, usually no larger than 1 cm in diameter
- Prolonged incubation period (average 2–18 months); spontaneous "cures" are frequent (50%)
- "Recurrences" (new lesions) are frequent

GENERAL CONSIDERATIONS

- Caused by human papillomaviruses (HPVs)
- Especially in genital warts, simultaneous infection with numerous wart types is common
- Genital HPVs are divided into low-risk and high-risk types depending on the likelihood of their association with cervical and anal cancer

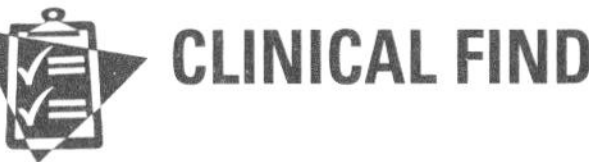

CLINICAL FINDINGS

SYMPTOMS AND SIGNS

- There are usually no symptoms
- Tenderness on pressure occurs with plantar warts; itching occurs with anogenital warts
- Occasionally a wart will produce mechanical obstruction (eg, nostril, ear canal, urethra)
- Warts vary widely in shape, size, and appearance
- Flat warts are most evident under oblique illumination
- Subungual warts may be dry, fissured, and hyperkeratotic and may resemble hangnails or other nonspecific changes
- Plantar warts resemble plantar corns or calluses

DIFFERENTIAL DIAGNOSIS

- Nongenital warts
  - Actinic keratosis
  - Squamous cell carcinoma
  - Molluscum contagiosum
  - Seborrheic keratosis
  - Skin tag (acrochordon)
  - Nevus
  - Verrucous zoster (in AIDS)
- Genital warts *(*condyloma acuminata)
  - Secondary syphilis (condyloma lata)
  - Psoriasis
  - Seborrheic keratosis
  - Molluscum contagiosum
  - Bowenoid papulosis and squamous cell carcinoma
  - Lichen planus
  - Pearly penile papules
  - Skin tag (acrochordon)

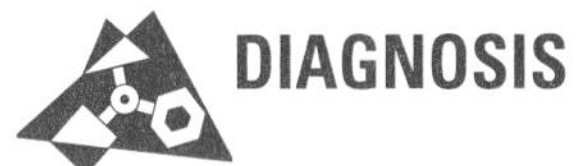

DIAGNOSIS

LABORATORY TESTS

- Clinical diagnosis

DIAGNOSTIC PROCEDURES

- Biopsy may be necessary for definitive diagnosis

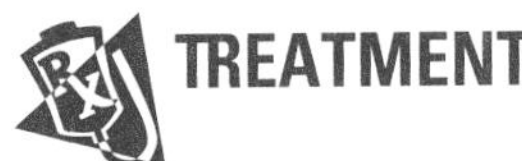

TREATMENT

MEDICATIONS

Liquid nitrogen

- Apply to achieve a thaw time of 20–45 s; two freeze-thaw cycles are used every 2–4 weeks for several visits
- Scarring will occur if used incorrectly
- May cause permanent depigmentation in darkly pigmented individuals
- It is useful on dry penile warts and on filiform warts on the face and body

Keratolytic agents and occlusion

- Any of the following salicylic acid products may be used against common warts or plantar warts: Occlusal, Trans-Ver-Sal, and Duofilm
- Plantar warts may be treated by applying a 40% salicylic acid plaster (Mediplast) after paring; the plaster may be left on for 5–6 days, then removed, the lesion pared down, and another plaster applied; it may take months to eradicate
- Chronic occlusion alone with water-impermeable tape (duct tape, adhesive tape) for months may be effective

Podophyllum resin

- Paint each anogenital wart carefully (protecting normal skin) every 2–3 weeks with 25% podophyllum resin (podophyllin) in compound tincture of benzoin
- Avoid use in pregnancy
- The purified active component of the resin, podofilox, is available for use at home twice daily three consecutive days a week for cycles of 4–6 weeks; it is less irritating and more effective than podophyllum resin
- May need multiple cycles of treatment

Imiquimod

- A 5% cream of this local interferon inducer can clear external genital warts, particularly in women
- Treatment is once daily on 3 alternate days per week; response may take up to 12 weeks; recurrences may occur
- There is less risk in pregnancy than with podophyllum resin and it appears to be the "patient-administered" treatment of choice in women
- In men, the more rapid response, lower cost, and similar efficacy make podophyllotoxin the initial treatment of choice, with imiquimod used for recurrences or refractory cases
- May be used to treat superficial flat warts

Other agents

- Bleomycin diluted to 1 unit/mL injected into plantar and common warts; do not use on digital warts because of the potential complications of Raynaud's phenomenon, nail loss, and terminal digital necrosis
- Cimetidine, 35–50 mg/kg daily, for younger patients with common warts
- Apply aquaric acid dibutylester 0.2–2% directly to the warts from once weekly to five times weekly to induce a mild contact dermatitis; most warts clear over 10–20 weeks
- Injection of candida antigen may be used in the same way

Retinoids

- Tretinoin (Retin-A) cream or gel applied topically twice daily may be effective for facial or beard flat warts
- Extensive warts may remit after 4–8 weeks of oral retinoids

THERAPEUTIC PROCEDURES

Operative removal

- For genital warts, snip biopsy (scissors) removal followed by light electrocautery is more effective than cryotherapy but does scar

Laser therapy

- The CO_2 laser effectively treats recurrent warts, periungual warts, plantar warts, and condylomata acuminata
- It leaves open wounds that must fill in with granulation tissue over 4–6 weeks and is best reserved for warts resistant to other modalities
- Soaking warts in hot (42.2°C) water for 10–30 min daily for 6 weeks can result in dramatic involution

OUTCOME

PROGNOSIS

- Development of new lesions is common
- Warts may disappear spontaneously or may be unresponsive to treatment

WHEN TO REFER

- If there is a question about the diagnosis, if recommended therapy is ineffective, or if specialized treatment is necessary

PREVENTION

- The use of condoms may reduce transmission of genital warts
- A person with flat warts should be educated about the infectivity of warts and advised not to scratch the areas
- Using an electric shaver may prevent autoinoculation

EVIDENCE

PRACTICE GUIDELINES

- Centers for Disease Control and Prevention. Human papillomavirus infection. Sexually transmitted diseases treatment guidelines 2002
  - http://www.guideline.gov/summary/summary.aspx?doc_id=3240&nbr=2466

WEB SITE

- American Academy of Dermatology
  - http://www.aad.org

INFORMATION FOR PATIENTS

- American Academy of Dermatology: Warts
  - http://www.aad.org/public/Publications/pamphlets/Warts.htm
- American Academy of Family Physicians: Warts
  - http://familydoctor.org/209.xml
- MedlinePlus: Warts
  - http://www.nlm.nih.gov/medlineplus/ency/article/000885.htm

REFERENCES

- Focht DR 3rd et al: The efficacy of duct tape vs cryotherapy in the treatment of verruca vulgaris (the common wart). Arch Pediatr Adolesc Med 2002;156:971. [PMID: 12361440]
- Gibbs S: Local treatments for cutaneous warts: systematic review. BMJ 2002;325:461. [PMID: 12202325]
- Wiley DJ: External genital warts: diagnosis, treatment and prevention. Clin Infect Dis 2002;35(Suppl 2):S210. [PMID: 12353208]

Author(s)

Timothy G. Berger, MD

Wegener's Granulomatosis

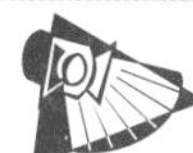

KEY FEATURES

ESSENTIALS OF DIAGNOSIS

- Triad of upper respiratory tract disease, lower respiratory disease, and glomerulonephritis
- Suspect this diagnosis whenever mundane respiratory systems (eg, nasal congestion, sinusitis) are refractory to usual treatment
- Pathology defined by the triad of small vessel vasculitis, granulomatous inflammation, and necrosis
- Cytoplasmic antineutophil cytoplasmic antibody (c-ANCA) pattern of immunofluorescence has moderate sensitivity and excellent specificity if confirmed by an enzyme immunoassay for antibodies to proteinase-3
- 10% of patients have a perinuclear (p)-ANCA pattern on immunofluorescence testing for ANCA, caused by antibodies to myeloperoxidase
- Renal disease often rapidly progressive

GENERAL CONSIDERATIONS

- The disease presents as vasculitis of small arteries, arterioles, and capillaries, necrotizing granulomatous lesions of both upper and lower respiratory tract, and glomerulonephritis

DEMOGRAPHICS

- Annual incidence of 10 per million
- Occurs most commonly in the fourth and fifth decades of life
- Affects men and women with equal frequency

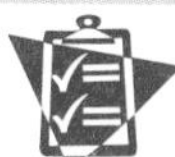

CLINICAL FINDINGS

SYMPTOMS AND SIGNS

- Usually develops over 4–12 months
- Fever, malaise, and weight loss
- 90% of patients present with upper or lower respiratory tract symptoms or both
- Upper respiratory tract symptoms can include
  - Nasal congestion, sinusitis
  - Otitis media, mastoiditis
  - Inflammation of the gums
  - Stridor due to subglottic stenosis
- Physical examination can be remarkable for congestion, crusting, ulceration, bleeding, and even perforation of the nasal mucosa
- The lung is affected initially in 40% and eventually in 80%, with symptoms including cough, dyspnea, and hemoptysis
- Renal involvement (75%) may be subclinical until renal insufficiency is advanced
- Other early symptoms can include
  - Unilateral proptosis (from pseudotumor)
  - Red eye from scleritis
  - Arthritis
  - Purpura
  - Dysesthesia due to neuropathy
  - Destruction of the nasal cartilage with "saddle nose" deformity occurs late
- Patients are at high risk for venous thrombotic events (deep venous thrombosis, pulmonary embolus)

DIFFERENTIAL DIAGNOSIS

- Polyarteritis nodosa
- Microscopic polyangiitis
- Churg-Strauss syndrome
- Chronic sinusitis
- Goodpasture's disease
- Systemic lupus erythematosus
- Sarcoidosis

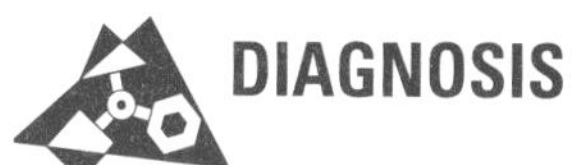

DIAGNOSIS

LABORATORY TESTS

- Cytoplasmic pattern of immunofluorescence (c-ANCA)
  - Caused by antibodies to proteinase-3, a constituent of neutrophil granules
  - Has a high specificity (> 90%)
  - In the setting of active disease, the sensitivity of c-ANCA is also reasonably high (= 70%)
- The p-ANCA pattern
  - Caused by antibodies to myeloperoxidase and is much less specific than c-ANCA
  - Approximately 10–25% of patients with classic Wegener's granulomatosis have p-ANCA
- The urinary sediment in the renal disease invariably contains red cells, with or without white cells, and red cell casts

IMAGING STUDIES

- Chest CT is more sensitive than chest x-ray for infiltrates, nodules, masses, and cavities

PROCEDURES

- ANCA testing does not eliminate the need in most cases for confirmation of the diagnosis by tissue biopsy
- The full range of pathologic changes is usually evident only on thoracoscopic lung biopsy. Histologic features include vasculitis, granulomatous inflammation, geographic necrosis, and acute and chronic inflammation
- Renal biopsy discloses a segmental necrotizing glomerulonephritis with multiple crescents (characteristic but not diagnostic)

Weakness & Paralysis p. 1170

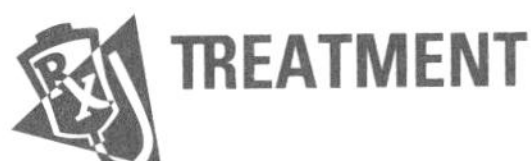

TREATMENT

MEDICATIONS

- Prednisone and oral cyclophosphamide
- Methotrexate, 20–25 mg/week, is a reasonable substitute for oral cyclophosphamide in patients who do not have immediately life-threatening disease

THERAPEUTIC PROCEDURES

- Early treatment is crucial in preventing renal failure and may be lifesaving

OUTCOME

FOLLOW-UP

- Complete blood cell count every 2 weeks for patients on daily cyclophosphamide

COMPLICATIONS

Permanent disease-related complications

- Suffered by 85% of patients
- End-stage renal disease
- Decreased hearing
- Visual impairment
- Subglottic stenosis
- Saddle-nose deformity

Permanent treatment-related complications

- Suffered by 40% of patients
- Multitudinous effects of corticosteroids
- Cyclophosphamide
  - Bone marrow hypoplasia
  - Secondary malignancy (bladder, leukemia)
  - Hemorrhagic cystitis
  - Infertility

PROGNOSIS

- Without treatment it is invariably fatal, most patients surviving < 1 year after diagnosis
- Remissions have been induced in up to 75% of patients treated with cyclophosphamide and prednisone, though half of these patients eventually suffer disease recurrences

WHEN TO REFER

- All patients should be monitored by a rheumatologist. Other subspecialty consultations may be appropriate

WHEN TO ADMIT

- Alveolar hemorrhage
- Rapidly progressive glomerulonephritis

EVIDENCE

WEB SITE

- http://vasculitis.med.jhu.edu

REFERENCES

- Regan MJ et al: Treatment of Wegener's granulomatosis. Rheum Dis Clin North Am 2001;27:863. [PMID: 11723769]
- Stone JH; The Wegener's Granulomatis Etanercept Trial Research Group: Limited versus severe Wegener's granulomatosis: baseline data on patients in the Wegener's granulomatosis etanercept trial. Arthritis Rheum 2003;48:2299. [PMID: 12905485]

Author(s)

David B. Hellmann, MD, FACP
John H. Stone, MD, MPH

Weight Loss, Involuntary

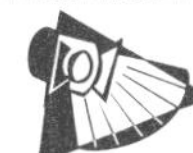

KEY FEATURES

ESSENTIALS OF DIAGNOSIS

- Decreased caloric intake
- Fever
- Change in bowel habits
- Secondary confirmation (eg, changes in clothing size)
- Substance abuse
- History of age-appropriate cancer screening

GENERAL CONSIDERATIONS

- Body weight is determined by a person's caloric intake, absorptive capacity, metabolic rate, and energy losses
- Involuntary weight loss is clinically significant when it exceeds 5% or more of usual body weight over a 6- to 12-month period
- Often indicates serious physical or psychological illness
- Most common causes are cancer (~30% of cases), gastrointestinal disorders (~15%), and dementia or depression (~15%)
- In approximately 15–25% of cases, no cause for the weight loss can be found

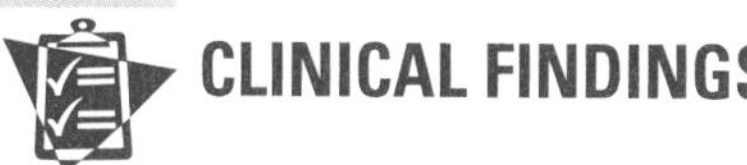

CLINICAL FINDINGS

SYMPTOMS AND SIGNS

- History should include medication profile and 24-h diet recall
- Night sweats, cough, breast mass, constipation, hematochezia, bone pain suggest cancer
- Nausea, vomiting, diarrhea, abdominal pain suggest gastrointestinal disease
- Anhedonia, sleep disorder, suicidal ideation, recent psychosocial stressors suggest depression
- Memory loss, wandering, isolation suggest dementia
- Physical examination for evidence of cancer

DIFFERENTIAL DIAGNOSIS

Medical

- Malignancy
- Gastrointestinal disorders, eg, malabsorption, pancreatic insufficiency, peptic ulcer
- Hyperthyroidism
- Chronic heart, lung, or renal disease
- Uncontrolled diabetes mellitus
- Mesenteric ischemia (ischemic bowel)
- Dysphagia
- Anorexia due to azotemia
- Hypercalcemia
- Tuberculosis
- Subacute bacterial endocarditis

Psychosocial

- Depression
- Dementia
- Alcoholism
- Anorexia nervosa
- Loss of teeth, poor denture fit
- Social isolation
- Poverty
- Inability to shop or prepare food

Drug-related

- Nonsteroidal anti-inflammatory drugs
- Antiepileptics
- Digoxin
- Selective serotonin reuptake inhibitors

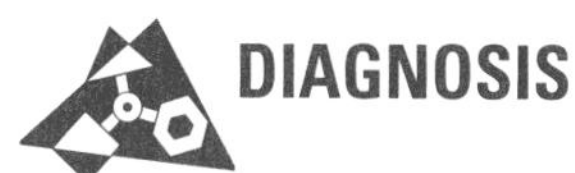

DIAGNOSIS

LABORATORY TESTS

- Obtain complete blood cell count
- Serologic tests
- Serum thyroid-stimulating hormone
- Urinalysis
- Fecal occult blood tests

IMAGING STUDIES

- Chest x-ray
- Abdominal CT scan or upper gastrointestinal series, or both
- When these tests are normal, more definitive gastrointestinal investigation (eg, tests for malabsorption; endoscopy) and cancer screening (eg, Pap smear, mammography, prostate-specific antigen)

DIAGNOSTIC PROCEDURES

- If initial diagnostic work-up is unrevealing, follow-up is preferable to further diagnostic testing

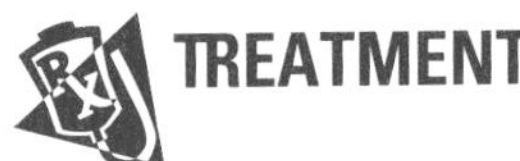

TREATMENT

MEDICATIONS

- Appetite stimulants (mild to moderate effectiveness): corticosteroids, progestational agents, dronabinol, and serotonin antagonists
- Anabolic agents: growth hormone and testosterone derivatives
- Anticatabolic agents: omega-3 fatty acids, pentoxifylline, hydrazine sulfate, and thalidomide

THERAPEUTIC PROCEDURES

- Treatment of the underlying disorder
- Consultation with dietician
- Caloric supplementation to achieve intake of 30–40 kcal/kg/day
- Oral feeding is preferred, but temporary nasojejunal tube, or permanent cutaneous gastric or jejunal tube may be necessary

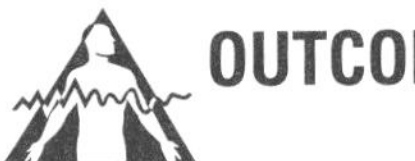

OUTCOME

PROGNOSIS

- Rapid unintentional weight loss is predictive of morbidity and mortality
- Mortality rates at 2-year follow-up
  - 8% for unexplained involuntary weight loss
  - 19% for weight loss due to nonmalignant disease
  - 79% for weight loss due to malignant disease

EVIDENCE

PRACTICE GUIDELINES

- American Academy of Family Physicians, American Dietetic Association, Nutrition Screening Initiative: Nutrition Management for Older Adults (Specific Guidelines for Cancer, COPD, CHF, CHD, Dementia, Diabetes Mellitus, Hypertension, Osteoporosis), 2002.
  - http://www.aafp.org/x16705.xml
- American Medical Directors Association: Altered Nutritional Status, 2001.
  - http://www.guideline.gov/summary/summary.aspx?doc_id=3304&nbr=2530

INFORMATION FOR PATIENTS

- Mayo Clinic: When you have no appetite: Tips to get the nutrition you need
  - http://www.mayoclinic.com/invoke.cfm?id=HQ01134
- Mayo Clinic: Illness and appetite: What to do when nothing tastes right
  - http://www.mayoclinic.com/invoke.cfm?objectid=C596EDA8-DEBC-444F-B01153A818A2C304&MOTT=HQ01134
- MedlinePlus: Unintentional Weight Loss
  - http://www.nlm.nih.gov/medlineplus/ency/article/003107.htm
- National Institutes of Health: The Widespread Effects of Depression
  - http://www.nih.gov/news/WordonHealth/apr2003/depression.htm

REFERENCES

- Gazewood JD et al: Diagnosis and management of weight loss in the elderly. J Fam Pract 1998;47:19. [PMID: 9673603]
- Lankisch P et al: Unintentional weight loss: diagnosis and prognosis. The first prospective follow-up study from a secondary referral centre. J Intern Med 2001;249:41. [PMID: 11168783]
- Poehlman ET et al: Energy expenditure, energy intake, and weight loss in Alzheimer disease. Am J Clin Nutr 2000;71:650S. [PMID: 10681274]

Author(s)

Ralph Gonzales, MD

Weight Loss & Malnutrition in Elderly

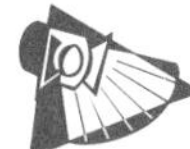

KEY FEATURES

ESSENTIALS OF DIAGNOSIS

- Unintended weight loss exceeding 5% in 1 month or 10% in 6 months
- Failure to thrive

GENERAL CONSIDERATIONS

- Undernutrition affects substantial numbers of elderly persons and often precedes hospitalization for "failure to thrive"
- "Failure to thrive"
  - A syndrome lacking a consensus definition but generally represents a constellation of weight loss, weakness, and progressive functional decline
  - The label is typically applied when some triggering event—loss of social support, a bout of depression or pneumonia, the addition of a new medication—pulls a struggling elderly person below the threshold of successful independent living
- Poor fitting dentures or oral health problems may contribute to nutritional problems, particularly in those with dementia
- Medications may alter taste or appetite
- Total caloric needs are reduced by about 30% in the elderly, but protein needs may be increased
- Risk factors for malnutrition include
  - Chronic disease
  - Functional and cognitive impairment
  - Depression

CLINICAL FINDINGS

SYMPTOMS AND SIGNS

- A 10% loss of weight suggests severe malnutrition
- A loss of 5% suggests moderate malnutrition
- Subcutaneous tissue loss can be best evaluated in the subscapular, suprailiac, and triceps skinfolds
- A body mass index under 22 should raise concern about significant malnutrition

DIFFERENTIAL DIAGNOSIS

Medical

- Chronic heart, lung disease
- Dementia
- Oral problems (eg, poor denture fit)
- Dysphagia
- Dysgeusia
- Mesenteric ischemia
- Cancer
- Diabetes
- Hyperthyroidism
- Malabsorption

Psychosocial

- Alcoholism/substance use
- Depression/dementia
- Social isolation
- Limited funds
- Problems with shopping or food preparation
- Inadequate assistance with feeding

Drug-related

- Nonsteroidal anti-inflammatory drugs
- Antiepileptics
- Digoxin
- Selective serotonin reuptake inhibitors
- Anticholinergics

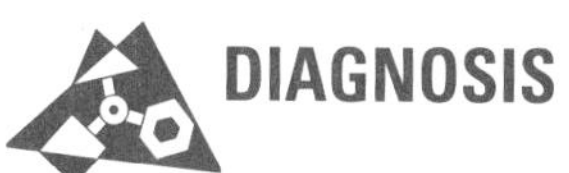

DIAGNOSIS

LABORATORY TESTS

- Laboratory studies are intended to uncover an occult metabolic or neoplastic cause
- Useful laboratory studies include complete blood cell count, serum chemistries (including glucose, TSH, creatinine, calcium), urinalysis

IMAGING STUDIES

- Chest x-ray
- Further imaging (eg, mammography, colonoscopy) as dictated by the clinical presentation

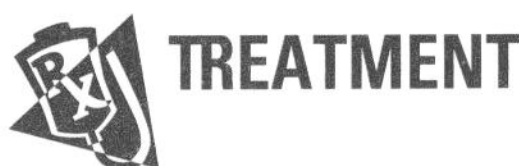

TREATMENT

THERAPEUTIC PROCEDURES

- Aim for a caloric intake of about 25 kcal/kg, based on ideal body weight
- Nutritional supplements may lead to weight gain; use of instant breakfast powder in whole milk (for those who can tolerate dairy products) is a less costly alternative
- For those who have lost the ability to feed themselves, assiduous hand feeding may allow maintenance of weight
- Artificial nutrition and hydration ("tube feeding") is an alternative, but it deprives the patient of the taste and texture of food as well as the social milieu typically associated with mealtime
- If the patient makes repeated attempts to pull out the tube during a trial of artificial nutrition, the treatment burden becomes substantial, and the utility of tube feeding should be reconsidered
- Megestrol acetate has not been shown to increase body mass in the elderly
- Treatment of depression with mirtazapine has been associated with modest weight gain

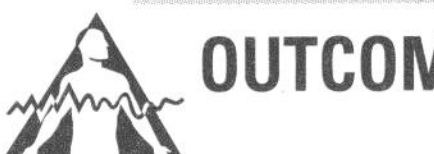

OUTCOME

FOLLOW-UP

- Patients with malnutrition are at higher risk for death, functional decline, and nursing home placement

COMPLICATIONS

- Hospitalized patients with malnutrition are more likely to experience multiple life-threatening complications

PROGNOSIS

- Though commonly used, there is no evidence that tube feeding prolongs life in patients with end-stage dementia

WHEN TO REFER

- Early involvement of a nutritionist may be helpful
- Consider dental or denture evaluation

WHEN TO ADMIT

- Malnutrition is rarely an indication for admission in and of itself
- The threshold for admission should be lower when a malnourished patient presents with an acute illness such as pneumonia

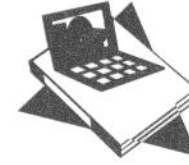

EVIDENCE

PRACTICE GUIDELINES

- American Academy of Family Physicians
  - http://www.aafp.org/afp/20020215/640.html
- National Guidelines Clearinghouse: American Medical Directors Association, 2001
  - http://www.guideline.gov/summary/summary.aspx?doc_id=3304

WEB SITES

- Administration on Aging
  - http://www.aoa.dhhs.gov
- American Geriatrics Society
  - http://www.americangeriatrics.org
- Merck Manual of Geriatrics
  - http://www.merck.com/mrkshared/mm_geriatrics/home.jsp

INFORMATION FOR PATIENTS

- Federal nutrition.gov
  - http://www.info.gov.hk/elderly/english/healthinfo/selfhelptips/common-e.htm
- JAMA patient page: healthy diet. JAMA 2000;283:2198. [PMID: 10791513]
- Mayo Clinic
  - http://www.mayoclinic.com/invoke.cfm?id=HA00019
- National Institute on Aging
  - http://www.niapublications.org/engagepages/nutrition.asp

REFERENCES

- Covinsky KE: The relationship between clinical assessments of nutritional status and adverse outcomes in older hospitalized medical patients. J Am Geriatr Soc 1999;47:532. [PMID: 10323645]
- Finucane TE: Tube feeding in patients with advanced dementia: a review of the evidence. JAMA 1999;282:1365. [PMID: 10527184]
- Robertson RG et al: Geriatric failure to thrive. Am Fam Physician 2004;70:343. [PMID: 15391093]

Author(s)

Helen Chen, MD

C. Bree Johnston, MD

Whipple's Disease

KEY FEATURES

ESSENTIALS OF DIAGNOSIS

- Multisystem disease
- Fever, lymphadenopathy, arthralgias
- Malabsorption
- Duodenal biopsy with PAS-positive macrophages with characteristic bacillus

GENERAL CONSIDERATIONS

- Rare multisystem illness caused by infection with the bacillus *Tropheryma whippelei*
- Source of infection is unknown; no cases of human-to-human spread have been documented

DEMOGRAPHICS

- May occur at any age but most commonly affects white men in the fourth to sixth decades

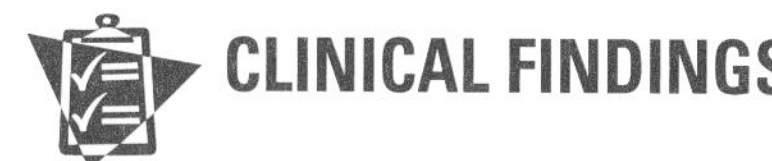

CLINICAL FINDINGS

SYMPTOMS AND SIGNS

- Clinical manifestations are protean
- Arthralgias or a migratory, nondeforming arthritis in 80%
- Gastrointestinal symptoms in 75% include abdominal pain, diarrhea, and variable malabsorption with distention, flatulence, and steatorrhea
- Weight loss in almost all patients
- Protein-losing enteropathy with hypoalbuminemia and edema
- Intermittent low-grade fever in >50%
- Chronic cough
- Generalized lymphadenopathy
- Myocardial involvement: congestive heart failure or valvular regurgitation
- Ocular: uveitis, vitreitis, keratitis, retinitis, and retinal hemorrhages
- CNS involvement in ~10%: dementia, lethargy, coma, seizures, myoclonus, or hypothalamic signs
- Cranial nerve findings: ophthalmoplegia or nystagmus
- Physical examination
  - Low-grade fever
  - Hypotension (late)
  - Lymphadenopathy in 50%
  - Heart murmurs
  - Peripheral joint inflammation, swelling
  - Neurological findings
  - Hyperpigmentation on sun-exposed areas in up to 40%

DIFFERENTIAL DIAGNOSIS

- Malabsorption due to other cause, eg, celiac or tropical sprue
- Inflammatory bowel disease
- Sarcoidosis
- Reactive arthritis (Reiter's syndrome)
- Systemic vasculitis
- Infective endocarditis
- Intestinal lymphoma
- Familial Mediterranean fever
- Behçet's syndrome
- Intestinal *Mycobacterium-avium intracellulare* (in AIDS)

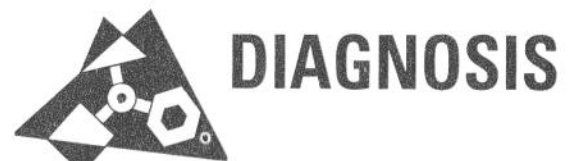

DIAGNOSIS

LABORATORY TESTS

- PCR confirms diagnosis by demonstrating the presence of 16S ribosomal RNA of *T whippelei* in blood, cerebrospinal fluid, vitreous fluid, synovial fluid, or cardiac valves; sensitivity of 97%, specificity of 100%

DIAGNOSTIC PROCEDURES

- Endoscopic biopsy of the duodenum demonstrates infiltration of the lamina propria with PAS-positive macrophages that contain gram-positive, non–acid-fast bacilli, and dilatation of the lacteals
- Biopsy of other involved organs or lymph nodes for histological evaluation of the involved tissues may be necessary

Wernicke's Encephalopathy p. 1170

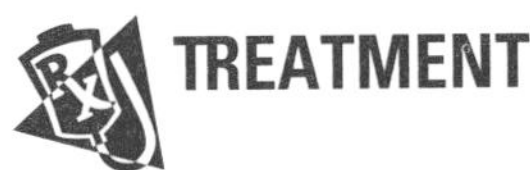

TREATMENT

MEDICATIONS

- Trimethoprim-sulfamethoxazole (1 double-strength tablet PO BID for 1 year) is recommended as first-line therapy
- Alternatives: ceftriaxone or fluoroquinolones

THERAPEUTIC PROCEDURES

- Prolonged treatment for at least 1 year is required
- After antibiotic treatment, repeat biopsies for PCR; negative results predict a low likelihood of clinical relapse

OUTCOME

FOLLOW-UP

- Patients must be followed closely after treatment for recurrence

COMPLICATIONS

- Some neurological signs may be permanent

PROGNOSIS

- Antibiotic therapy results in a dramatic clinical improvement within several weeks
- Complete response within 1–3 months
- Relapse may occur in up to one-third of patients after discontinuation of treatment
- If untreated, the disease is fatal

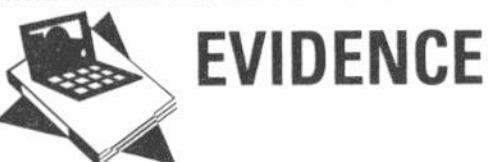

EVIDENCE

INFORMATION FOR PATIENTS

- Cleveland Clinic—Whipple's disease
  - http://www.clevelandclinic.org/health/health-info/docs/1200/1236.asp?index=5958
- Medical College of Wisconsin—Whipple's disease
  - http://healthlink.mcw.edu/article/930591431.html
- National Digestive Diseases Information Clearinghouse
  - http://digestive.niddk.nih.gov/ddiseases/pubs/whipple/index.htm
- National Institute of Neurological Disorders and Stroke
  - http://www.ninds.nih.gov/disorders/whipples/whipples.htm

REFERENCE

- Bai JC: Whipple's disease. Clin Gastroenterol Hepatol 2004;2:849. [PMID: 15476147]

Author(s)

Kenneth R. McQuaid, MD

Wilson's Disease

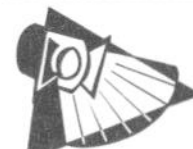

KEY FEATURES

ESSENTIALS OF DIAGNOSIS

- Characterized by excessive deposition of copper in the liver and brain
- Rare autosomal recessive disorder that usually occurs between the first and third decades
- Serum ceruloplasmin, the plasma copper-carrying protein, is low. Urinary excretion of copper is high

GENERAL CONSIDERATIONS

- The genetic defect, localized to chromosome 13, affects a copper-transporting adenosine triphosphatase (ATP7B) in the liver and leads to oxidative damage of hepatic mitochondria
- Over 200 different mutations in the Wilson disease gene have been identified, making genetic diagnosis impractical; most patients are compound heterozygotes (ie, carry two different mutations)
- The major physiological aberration is excessive absorption of copper from the small intestine and decreased excretion of copper by the liver, resulting in increased tissue deposition, especially in the liver, brain, cornea, and kidney

DEMOGRAPHICS

- Adolescents and young adults

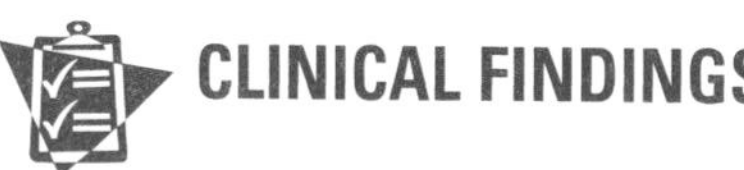

CLINICAL FINDINGS

SYMPTOMS AND SIGNS

- Consider the diagnosis in any child or young adult with the following
  - Hepatitis, splenomegaly with hypersplenism, portal hypertension
  - Hemolytic anemia
  - Neurological or psychiatric abnormalities
  - Chronic or fulminant hepatitis
- Hepatic involvement may range from elevated liver tests (although the alkaline phosphatase may be low) to cirrhosis and portal hypertension
- Neurological manifestations
  - Related to basal ganglia dysfunction
  - Resting, postural, or kinetic tremor
  - Dystonia of the bulbar musculature with resulting dysarthria and dysphagia
- Psychiatric features include behavioral and personality changes and emotional lability
- **Kayser-Fleischer ring**
  - Pathognomonic sign
  - Brownish or gray-green pigmented granular deposits in Descemet's membrane in the cornea close to the endothelial surface
  - Usually most marked at the superior and inferior poles of the cornea
  - It can frequently be seen with the naked eye and almost invariably by slit lamp examination
  - It may be absent in patients with hepatic manifestations only but is usually present in those with neuropsychiatric disease

DIFFERENTIAL DIAGNOSIS

- Acute hepatitis
- Cholestasis
- Acute hepatic failure
- Chronic hepatitis
- Cirrhosis
- Hepatomegaly
- Other cause of hepatitis, fulminant hepatic failure, or cirrhosis, eg, viral, toxins, hemochromatosis
- Tremor due to other causes, eg, Parkinson's disease, essential tremor
- Dementia due to other causes, eg, Huntington's disease
- Behavior change due to other medical illness, eg, neurosyphilis, brain tumor

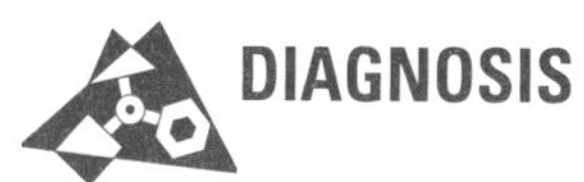

DIAGNOSIS

LABORATORY TESTS

- Increased urinary copper excretion (>100 μg/24 h) or low serum ceruloplasmin levels (<20 μg/dL), and elevated hepatic copper concentration (>250 μg/g of dry liver). However, increased urinary copper and low serum ceruloplasmin levels are not specific for Wilson's disease
- In equivocal cases (when the serum ceruloplasmin level is normal), the diagnosis may require demonstration of low radiolabeled copper incorporation into ceruloplasmin or urinary copper determination after a penicillamine challenge

DIAGNOSTIC PROCEDURES

- Liver biopsy may show acute or chronic hepatitis or cirrhosis and is used to quantify hepatic copper

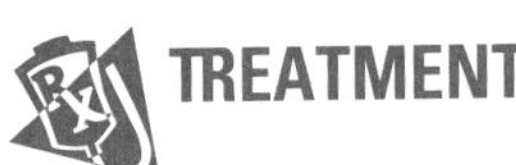

TREATMENT

MEDICATIONS

- Oral penicillamine (0.75–2 g/day in divided doses) is the drug of choice, enhancing urinary excretion of chelated copper. Add pyridoxine, 25–50 mg/week, since penicillamine is an antimetabolite of this vitamin
- If penicillamine treatment cannot be tolerated because of gastrointestinal, hypersensitivity, or autoimmune reactions, consider the use of trientine, 250–500 mg three times a day
- Oral zinc acetate, 50 mg three times a day, interferes with intestinal absorption of copper, promotes fecal copper excretion, and may be used as maintenance therapy after decoppering with a chelating agent or as first-line therapy in presymptomatic or pregnant patients
- Ammonium tetrathiomolybdate complexes copper in the intestinal tract and has shown promise as initial therapy for neurological Wilson's disease
- Treatment should continue indefinitely
- Once the serum nonceruloplasmin copper level is within the normal range, the dose of chelating agent can be reduced to the minimum necessary for maintaining that level

SURGERY

- Liver transplantation is indicated for fulminant hepatitis (often after plasma exchange as a stabilizing measure), end-stage cirrhosis, and, in selected cases, intractable neurological disease

THERAPEUTIC PROCEDURES

- Early treatment to remove excess copper is essential before it can produce neurological or hepatic damage
- Early in the treatment phase, restrict dietary copper (shellfish, organ foods, and legumes)

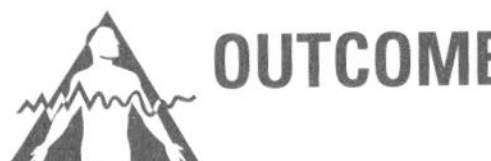

OUTCOME

FOLLOW-UP

- Serum nonceruloplasmin copper
- Urine copper

COMPLICATIONS

- Fulminant hepatitis and cirrhosis
- Renal calculi, the Fanconi defect, renal tubular acidosis, hypoparathyroidism, and hemolytic anemia may occur

PROGNOSIS

- The prognosis is good if effective treatment occurs before liver or brain damage
- The disease may stabilize with treatment in cirrhosis

PREVENTION

- Family members, especially siblings, require screening with serum ceruloplasmin, liver function tests, and slit lamp examination

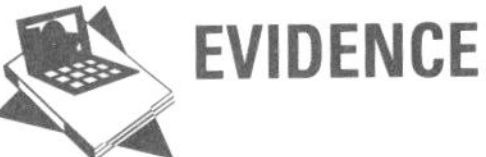

EVIDENCE

PRACTICE GUIDELINES

- National Guideline Clearinghouse
  - http://www.guideline.gov/summary/summary.aspx?ss=15&doc_id=3865&nbr=3075&string=Wilson's%20AND%20Disease
- Roberts EA et al: A practice guideline on Wilson disease. Hepatology 2003;37:1475. [PMID: 12774027]

WEB SITES

- Hepatic Ultrasound Images
  - http://www.sono.nino.ru/english/hepar_en.html
- Online Mendelian Inheritance in Man
  - http://www3.ncbi.nlm.nih.gov/entrez/dispomim.cgi?id=277900
- Pathology Index
  - http://www-medlib.med.utah.edu/WebPath/LIVEHTML/LIVERIDX.html

INFORMATION FOR PATIENTS

- Mayo Clinic
  - http://www.mayoclinic.com/invoke.cfm?id=DS00411
- National Digestive Diseases Information Clearinghouse
  - http://digestive.niddk.nih.gov/ddiseases/pubs/wilson/index.htm
- National Institute of Neurological Disorders and Stroke
  - http://www.ninds.nih.gov/health_and_medical/disorders/wilsons_doc.htm

REFERENCE

- Ferenci P: Review article: diagnosis and current therapy of Wilson's disease. Aliment Pharmacol Ther 2004;19:157. [PMID: 14723607]

Author(s)

Lawrence S. Friedman, MD

Zollinger-Ellison Syndrome

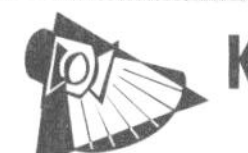

KEY FEATURES

ESSENTIALS OF DIAGNOSIS

- Peptic ulcer disease, severe and atypical
- Gastric acid hypersecretion
- Diarrhea common, relieved by nasogastric suction
- Most cases are sporadic; 25% with multiple endocrine neoplasia (MEN) type 1

GENERAL CONSIDERATIONS

- Caused by gastrin-secreting gut neuroendocrine tumors (gastrinomas), which result in hypergastrinemia and acid hypersecretion
- Gastrinomas cause < 1% of peptic ulcers
- Primary gastrinomas may arise in the pancreas (25%), duodenal wall (45%), lymph nodes (5–15%), or other locations (20%)
- Most gastrinomas are solitary or multifocal nodules that are potentially resectable; 25% are small multicentric gastrinomas associated with MEN 1 that are more difficult to resect
- Gastrinomas are malignant in less than two-thirds; one-third have already metastasized to the liver at initial presentation
- Screening for Zollinger-Ellison syndrome with fasting gastrin levels indicated for patients with ulcers refractory to standard therapies, giant ulcers (>2 cm), ulcers located distal to the duodenal bulb, multiple duodenal ulcers, frequent ulcer recurrences, ulcers associated with diarrhea, ulcers occurring after ulcer surgery, ulcers with complications, ulcers with hypercalcemia or a family history of ulcers, and ulcers not related to *Helicobacter pylori* or nonsteroidal antiinflammatory drugs (NSAIDs)

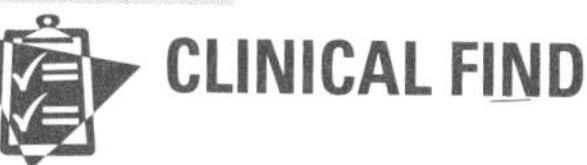

CLINICAL FINDINGS

SYMPTOMS AND SIGNS

- Peptic ulcers in >90%, usually solitary and in proximal duodenal bulb, but may be multiple or in distal duodenum
- Isolated gastric ulcers do not occur
- Gastroesophageal reflux symptoms
- Diarrhea, steatorrhea, and weight loss (in ~33%) secondary to pancreatic enzyme inactivation

DIFFERENTIAL DIAGNOSIS

- Peptic ulcer disease due to other cause, eg, NSAIDs, *H pylori*
- Gastroesophageal reflux disease, esophagitis, gastritis, pancreatitis, or cholecystitis
- Diarrhea due to other cause
- Other gut neuroendocrine tumor: carcinoid, insulinoma, VIPoma, glucagonoma, somatostatinoma
- Hypergastrinemia due to other cause: atrophic gastritis, gastric outlet obstruction, pernicious anemia, chronic renal failure

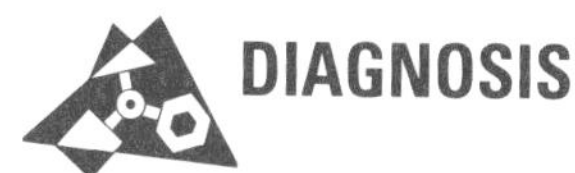

DIAGNOSIS

LABORATORY TESTS

- Fasting serum gastrin concentration increased (>150 pg/mL) in patients not taking H_2 receptor antagonists for 24 h or proton pump inhibitor for 6 days
- Obtain serum calcium, parathyroid hormone, prolactin, leutinizing hormone, follicle-stimulating hormone, and growth hormone level in all patients with Zollinger-Ellison syndrome to exclude MEN 1
- Gastric pH of >3.0 implies hypochlorhydria and excludes gastrinoma

IMAGING STUDIES

- CT, MRI, and transabdominal ultrasound have sensitivity of < 50–70% for hepatic metastases and 35% for primary tumors
- Somatostatin receptor scintigraphy (SRS) with SPECT has high sensitivity (>80%) for detecting hepatic metastases, as well as primary tumors
- Endoscopic ultrasonography (EUS) is indicated in patients with negative SRS, has sensitivity of >90% for tumors of the pancreatic head and ~50% for tumors in the duodenal wall or adjacent lymph nodes
- Combination of SRS and EUS can localize >90% of primary gastrinomas preoperatively

DIAGNOSTIC PROCEDURES

- Secretin stimulation test distinguishes Zollinger-Ellison syndrome from other causes of hypergastrinemia
- Secretin, 2 units/kg IV, produces a rise in serum gastrin of >200 pg/mL within 2–30 min in 85% of patients with gastrinoma

Yellow Fever p. 1170

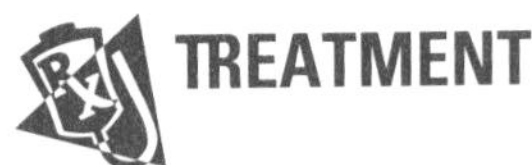

TREATMENT

MEDICATIONS

- Proton pump inhibitors (omeprazole, rabeprazole, pantoprazole, esomeprazole, or lansoprazole), 40–120 mg/day, titrated to achieve a basal acid output of <10 mEq/h for metastatic disease

SURGERY

- Primary resection of gastrinoma at laparotomy for localized disease
- Preoperative studies and intraoperative palpation and sonography allow successful localization and resection in the majority of cases
- Surgical resection of isolated hepatic metastases

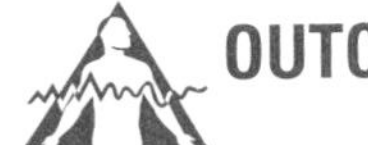

OUTCOME

COMPLICATIONS

- In patients with unresectable disease, complications of gastric acid hypersecretion can be prevented in almost all cases by sufficient doses of proton pump inhibitors
- Treatment options for metastatic disease include interferon, octreotide, combination therapy, and chemoembolization

PROGNOSIS

- 15-year survival of patients without liver metastases at initial presentation is >80%
- 10-year survival of patients with hepatic metastases is 30%

WHEN TO REFER

- All patients with Zollinger-Ellison syndrome should be referred to a gastrointestinal surgeon with expertise in evaluation and management

EVIDENCE

PRACTICE GUIDELINES

- Gibril F et al: Zollinger-Ellison syndrome revisited: diagnosis, biologic markers, associated inherited disorders, and acid hypersecretion. Curr Gastroenterol Rep 2004;6:454. [PMID: 15527675]
- Quan C et al: Management of peptic ulcer disease not related to *Helicobacter pylori* or NSAIDs. Am J Gastroenterol 2002;97:2950. [PMID: 12492176]

WEB SITES

- MEDLINEplus—Zollinger-Ellison syndrome
  - http://www.nlm.nih.gov/medlineplus/ency/article/000325.htm
- National Digestive Diseases Information Clearinghouse—Zollinger-Ellison syndrome
  - http://digestive.niddk.nih.gov/ddiseases/pubs/zollinger/index.htm

INFORMATION FOR PATIENTS

- Cleveland Clinic—Zollinger-Ellison syndrome
  - http://www.clevelandclinic.org/health/health-info/docs/1200/1238.asp?index=5956
- Florida State University College of Medicine—Zollinger-Ellison Syndrome
  - http://fsumed-dl.slis.ua.edu/clinical/gastroenterology/upper/stomach disorders/zollinger.html
- Mayo Clinic—Zollinger-Ellison syndrome
  - http://www.mayoclinic.com/invoke.cfm?objectid=00895C9E-1914-4475-86F645783A952DE7

REFERENCE

- Norton J et al: Resolved and unresolved controversies in the surgical management of patients with Zollinger-Ellison syndrome. Ann Surg 2004;240:757. [PMID: 15492556]

Author(s)

Kenneth R. McQuaid, MD

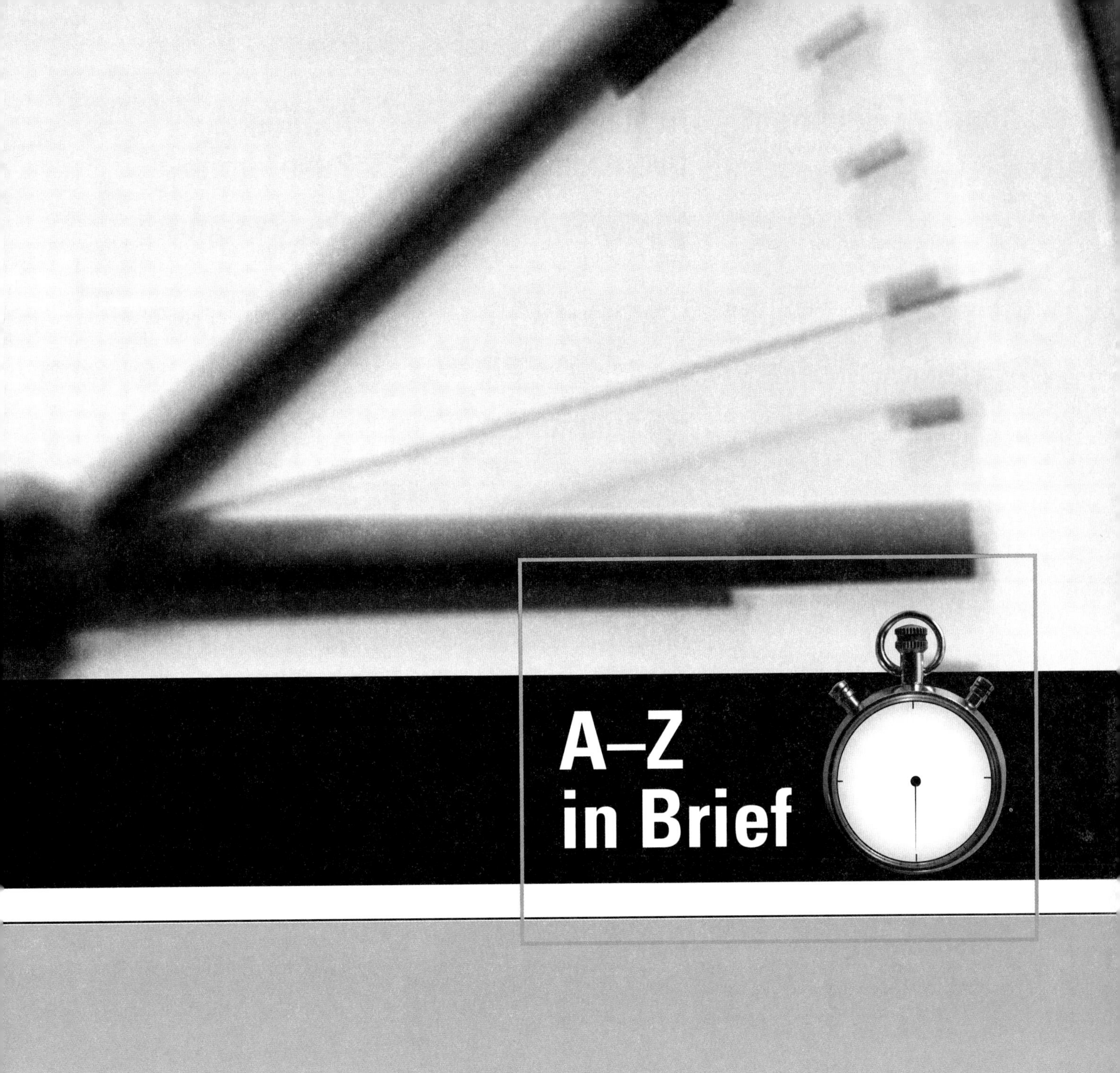

A–Z in Brief

Abortion, Recurrent

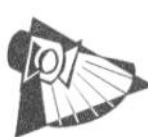

KEY FEATURES

- Defined as loss of three or more previable (< 500 g) pregnancies in succession
- Women with three previous unexplained losses have a 70–80% chance of carrying a subsequent pregnancy to viability

CLINICAL FINDINGS

- Occurs in 0.4–0.8% of all pregnancies
- Clinical findings are similar to those in spontaneous abortion

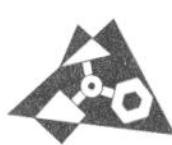

DIAGNOSIS

- Preconception therapy aims to detect maternal or paternal defects contributing to abortion; these are found in about 50% of couples
- Polycystic ovaries, thyroid abnormalities, and diabetes should be ruled out
- Hypercoagulable states should be ruled out
- Endometrial tissue should be examined to determine the adequacy of its response to hormones in the postovulatory phase
- Hysteroscopy or hysterography can exclude uterine abnormalities
- Chromosomal analysis of partners identifies balanced translocations in 5% of couples

TREATMENT

- Early prenatal care and frequent office visits are routine
- Complete bed rest is justified only for bleeding or pain
- Empiric sex steroid therapy is contraindicated

Author(s)

William R. Crombleholme, MD

Acetaminophen Overdose

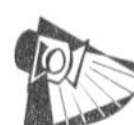

KEY FEATURES

- Toxic dose: > 200 mg/kg or 7 g (acute) or > 4–6 g/day (chronic)
- Nausea, vomiting early after acute ingestion
- Hepatic necrosis evident after 24–36 h
- Fulminant hepatic failure can occur

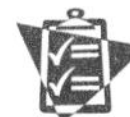

CLINICAL FINDINGS

- Early: nausea and vomiting
- After 24 h: elevated transaminases, evidence of hepatic dysfunction and fulminant hepatic failure
- Massive overdose can cause coma, hypotension, metabolic acidosis

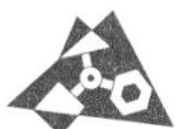

DIAGNOSIS

- Elevated serum acetaminophen level (> 150 mg/L at 4 h or 75 mg/L at 8 h)
- Chronic excessive dosing may produce only moderately elevated levels
- Elevated hepatic transaminases, prothrombin time/INR, bilirubin
- Metabolic acidosis, encephalopathy indicate poor prognosis

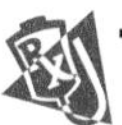

TREATMENT

- Oral activated charcoal 60–100 g mixed in aqueous slurry (if given within 2–3 h of acute ingestion)
- Oral *N*-acetylcysteine (NAC), 140 mg/kg loading dose, followed by 70 mg/kg Q 4 h
- Traditional US oral regimen: 72 h
- UK/Europe: IV NAC for 20 h (IV formulation Acetadote™ now approved in USA)
- Alternate oral treatment end point: may stop NAC if no evident liver injury at 36 h after ingestion
- Fulminant liver failure may require emergency liver transplantation

Author(s)

Kent R. Olson, MD

Acidosis, Respiratory

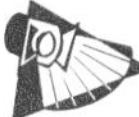

KEY FEATURES

- Respiratory acidosis results from decreased alveolar ventilation and subsequent hypercapnia. The clinician must be mindful of readily reversible causes, such as from opioids
- Acute compensation is an increase in serum HCO_3^- of 1 mEq/L per 10 mm Hg increase in Pco_2, and for chronic respiratory acidosis (after 6–12 h), an increase in serum HCO_3^- of 3.5 mEq/L per 10 mm Hg increase in Pco_2
- When chronic respiratory acidosis is corrected suddenly, there is a 2- to 3-day lag in renal bicarbonate excretion, resulting in posthypercapnic metabolic alkalosis

CLINICAL FINDINGS

- Acutely, somnolence, confusion, myoclonus, asterixis
- Increased intracranial pressure (papilledema, pseudotumor cerebri)
- Coma from CO_2 narcosis

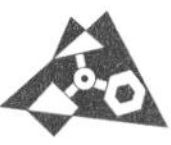

DIAGNOSIS

- Low arterial pH, increased Pco_2
- In the chronic state, HCO_3^- may be elevated along with hypochloremia from NH_4^+ and Cl^- renal loss (Table 85)

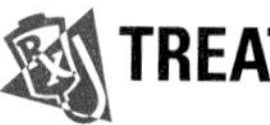

TREATMENT

- Administer naloxone, 0.04–2 mg IV, for possible drug overdose
- For all forms of respiratory acidosis, treatment is to improve ventilation

Author(s)

Masafumi Fukagawa, MD, PhD, FJSIM
Kiyoshi Kurokawa, MD, MACP
Maxine A. Papadakis, MD

Acrocyanosis

KEY FEATURES

- An uncommon vasospastic disorder characterized by persistent cyanosis of the hands and feet and, to a lesser degree, the forearms and legs
- Associated with arteriolar vasoconstriction combined with dilation of the subcapillary venous plexus of the skin
- Worse in cold weather; does not completely disappear during warm
- Occurs primarily in women, most common in the teens and 20s; may improve with advancing age or during pregnancy

CLINICAL FINDINGS

- Symmetric coldness, sweating, slight edema, cyanotic discoloration of the hands or feet
- Peripheral pulses are normal
- Pain, trophic lesions, and disability do not occur

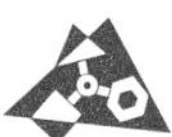

DIAGNOSIS

- Characteristic clinical picture

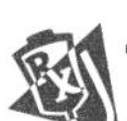

TREATMENT

- Avoidance of cold exposure

Author(s)

Louis M. Messina, MD

Actinic Keratosis

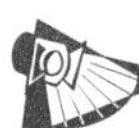

KEY FEATURES

- Actinic keratoses are considered premalignant, but only 1:1000 lesions/year progresses to become squamous cell carcinoma

CLINICAL FINDINGS

- Actinic keratoses are small (0.2–1 cm) patches—flesh-colored, pink, or slightly hyperpigmented—that feel like sandpaper and are tender when the finger is drawn over them
- They occur on sun-exposed parts of the body in persons of fair complexion

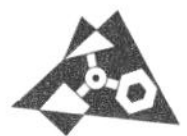

DIAGNOSIS

- Clinical
- Differential diagnosis includes squamous cell carcinoma, Bowen's disease (squamous cell carcinoma in situ), nonpigmented seborrheic keratosis, psoriasis, seborrheic dermatitis, seborrheic keratosis, Paget's disease. See differential diagnosis for *Scaly lesions*

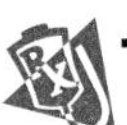

TREATMENT

- Liquid nitrogen is a rapid, effective method of eradication. The lesions crust and disappear in 10–14 days
- An alternative treatment is the use of 1–5% fluorouracil cream.
  - This agent may be rubbed into the lesions morning and night until they become red and sore, crusted, and eroded (usually 2–3 weeks), and then it is stopped
  - Alternatively, 5-fluorouracil 0.5% cream once daily for 4–6 weeks

Author(s)

Timothy G. Berger, MD

Adenovirus Infections

KEY FEATURES

- More than 40 types, which produce a variety of clinical syndromes
- Usually self-limited except in immunosuppressed hosts

CLINICAL FINDINGS

- Common cold
- Nonstreptococcal exudative pharyngitis
- Lower respiratory tract infections
- Epidemic keratoconjunctivitis
- Hemorrhagic cystitis
- Acute gastroenteritis
- Disseminated disease in transplant recipients

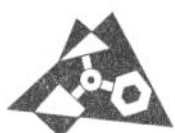

DIAGNOSIS

- Can be cultured from appropriate specimens when definitive diagnosis is desired

TREATMENT

- Disease usually self-limited
- Immunocompromised patients often treated with ribavirin, although efficacy unclear
- Vaccine against certain strains used in military personnel to prevent outbreaks

Author(s)

Wayne X. Shandera, MD

Ana Moran, MD

Alkalosis, Respiratory

KEY FEATURES

- Acute respiratory alkalosis symptoms are related to decreased cerebral blood flow
- Causes include the following:
  - Hyperventilation syndrome
  - Hypoxia, including severe anemia
  - CNS-mediated disorders (anxiety hyperventilation, cerebrovascular accident, infection, trauma, tumor, pharmacological and hormonal stimulation [salicylates, nicotine, xanthines], pregnancy [progesterone], hepatic failure, septicemia, recovery from metabolic acidosis, heat exposure)
  - Pulmonary disease
  - Mechanical overventilation

CLINICAL FINDINGS

- Acutely, light-headedness, anxiety, paresthesias, numbness about the mouth, and a tingling sensation in the hands and feet
- Tetany in severe alkalosis from a fall in ionized calcium
- In chronic cases, findings are those of the responsible condition

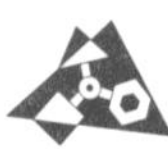

DIAGNOSIS

- Elevated arterial blood pH, with low Pco_2
- Serum bicarbonate is decreased in chronic respiratory alkalosis. Although serum HCO_3^- is frequently below 15 mEq/L in metabolic acidosis, it is unusual to see such a low level in respiratory alkalosis, and its presence implies a superimposed (noncompensatory) metabolic acidosis

TREATMENT

- Treatment is directed toward the underlying cause
- In acute hyperventilation syndrome from anxiety, rebreathing into a paper bag increases Pco_2. Sedation may be necessary if the process persists
- Rapid correction of chronic respiratory alkalosis may result in metabolic acidosis as Pco_2 is increased in the setting of previous compensatory decrease in HCO_3^-

Author(s)

Masafumi Fukagawa, MD, PhD, FJSIM
Kiyoshi Kurokawa, MD, MACP
Maxine A. Papadakis, MD

Alkaptonuria

KEY FEATURES

- Alkaptonuria is caused by a recessively inherited deficiency of the enzyme homogentisic acid oxidase
- Homogentisic acid accumulates slowly in cartilage throughout the body, leading to degenerative joint disease of the spine and peripheral joints

CLINICAL FINDINGS

- Back pain; difficult to distinguish from ankylosing spondylitis
- On radiograph, sacroiliac joints are not fused
- Examination shows slight darkish-blue color below the skin in areas overlying cartilage, such as in the ears, called "ochronosis"
- In some patients, more severe hyperpigmentation in the sclera, conjunctiva, and cornea
- Accumulation of metabolites in heart valves can lead to aortic or mitral stenosis
- Predisposition to coronary artery disease

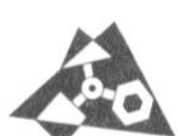

DIAGNOSIS

- Homogentisic acid is present in large amounts in the urine, which turns black spontaneously on exposure to air
- Quantitative analysis of homogentisic acid in urine or plasma

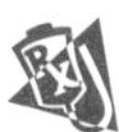

TREATMENT

- Nonsteroidal antiinflammatory drugs for arthritis
- Replacement of defective heart valves and joints
- Although the syndrome causes considerable morbidity, life expectancy is reduced only modestly

Author(s)

Reed E. Pyeritz, MD, PhD

Allergic Bronchopulmonary Aspergillosis (ABPA)

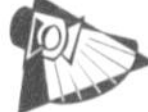

KEY FEATURES

- Also known as allergic bronchopulmonary mycosis
- A bronchopulmonary hypersensitivity disorder caused by allergy to fungal antigens
- Seen in atopic asthmatics aged 20–40 years, usually in response to *Aspergillus* species

CLINICAL FINDINGS

- Symptoms
  - Dyspnea
  - Wheezing
  - Cough
  - Brown-flecked sputum
- Relapses after therapy common
- Complications
  - Bronchiectasis
  - Hemoptysis
  - Pulmonary fibrosis

DIAGNOSIS

- Primary criteria
  1. History of asthma
  2. Peripheral eosinophilia
  3. Immediate skin reactivity
  4. Precipitating antibodies to *Aspergillus* antigen
  5. Elevated serum IgE
  6. Pulmonary infiltrates
  7. Central bronchiectasis
- Secondary criteria
  - *Aspergillus* in sputum
  - History of brown-flecked sputum
  - Delayed skin reactivity to *Aspergillus* antigen
- Presence of primary criteria 1–6 makes diagnosis almost certain

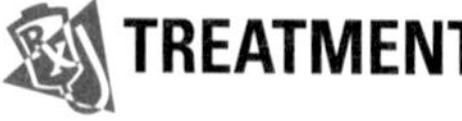

TREATMENT

- Prednisone, 0.5–1 mg/kg/day for at least 2 months, then careful tapering
- Itraconazole, 200 mg QD to BID, may be added for steroid-dependent patients
- Bronchodilators are helpful

Author(s)

Mark S. Chesnutt, MD
Thomas J. Prendergast, MD

Amenorrhea, Primary

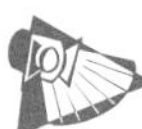

KEY FEATURES

- Menarche ordinarily occurs between 11 and 15 years (average in US, 12.7 years)
- Primary amenorrhea is failure of any menses to appear
- Evaluation is recommended at age 14 if no menarche or breast development or if height in lowest 3%; recommended at age 16 if no menarche
- Causes of primary amenorrhea:
  - Hypothalamic-pituitary (low-normal FSH): idiopathic delayed puberty; pituitary tumor; hypothalamic amenorrhea (eg, stress, weight change, exercise); anorexia nervosa; hypothyroidism; Cushing's syndrome; GnRH or gonadotropin deficiency (eg, Kallmann's syndrome or craniopharyngioma)
  - Hyperandrogenism (low-normal FSH): adrenal tumor or adrenal hyperplasia; polycystic ovary syndrome; ovarian tumor; exogenous androgenic steroids
  - Ovarian causes (high FSH): gonadal dysgenesis (Turner's syndrome); autoimmune ovarian failure; ovarian enzyme deficiencies (rare)
  - Pseudohermaphroditism (high LH): testosterone synthesis defect, complete androgen resistance (testicular feminization)
  - Anatomic defect (normal FSH): vaginal agenesis, absent uterus, atrophic endometrium, imperforate hymen
  - Pregnancy (high hCG)

CLINICAL FINDINGS

- Nausea, amenorrhea, breast engorgement, and weight gain suggest pregnancy
- Headaches or visual field abnormalities suggest pituitary or hypothalamic tumor
- Obesity and short stature suggest Cushing's syndrome
- Hirsutism, virilization, and acne suggest excessive testosterone
- Short stature suggests growth hormone or thyroid hormone deficiency
- Short stature and gonadal dysgenesis indicate Turner's syndrome
- Tall stature suggests eunuchoidism or gigantism
- Anosmia suggests Kallmann's syndrome
- Perform external pelvic and rectal examination to assess for hymenal patency and presence of a uterus

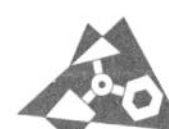

DIAGNOSIS

- Serum FSH, LH, prolactin, testosterone, TSH, free T_4, and pregnancy test
- Serum electrolytes
- Further hormone evaluation if patient is virilized or hypertensive
- Obtain MRI of hypothalamus and pituitary if low-normal FSH and LH, especially if high prolactin
- Karyotyping

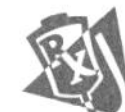

TREATMENT

- Treatment directed at underlying cause
- Hormone replacement therapy for females with permanent hypogonadism
- See *Amenorrhea, Secondary & Menopause*

Author(s)

Paul A. Fitzgerald, MD

Anaerobic Infections, Bacteremia & Endocarditis

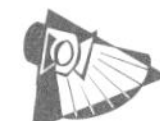

KEY FEATURES

- Anaerobic bacteremia usually originates from the GI tract, the oropharynx, decubitus ulcers, or the female genital tract. Endocarditis resulting from anaerobic and microaerophilic streptococci and bacteroides (rare) originates from the same sites

CLINICAL FINDINGS

- Related to site of original and metastatic infection

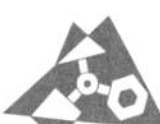

DIAGNOSIS

- Culture of blood and affected tissues

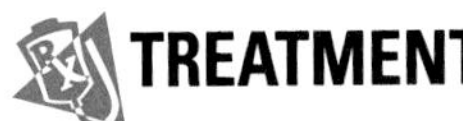

TREATMENT

- Most cases of anaerobic or microaerophilic streptococcal endocarditis can be effectively treated with 12–20 million units of penicillin G daily for 4–6 weeks, but optimal therapy for other types of anaerobic bacterial endocarditis must rely on laboratory guidance
- Metronidazole, 500 mg IV Q 8 h, should be used if *Bacteroides* sp is identified

Author(s)

Henry F. Chambers, MD

Anaerobic Infections, Central Nervous System

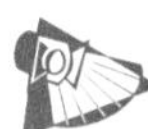

KEY FEATURES

- Common cause of brain abscess, subdural empyema, or septic CNS thrombophlebitis
- The organisms reach CNS by direct extension from sinusitis, otitis, or mastoiditis or by hematogenous spread from chronic lung infections

CLINICAL FINDINGS

- Various neurological deficits

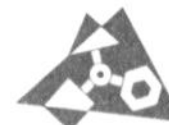

DIAGNOSIS

- CT scan
- Culture of infected tissue

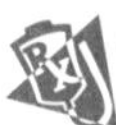

TREATMENT

- Antimicrobial therapy (eg, penicillin, 20 million units IV, in combination with metronidazole, 500–750 mg IV Q 8 h) is an important adjunct to surgical drainage
- Duration of antibiotic therapy is 6–8 weeks
- Some small multiple brain abscesses can be treated with antibiotics alone without surgical drainage

Author(s)

Henry F. Chambers, MD

Anaerobic Infections, Chest

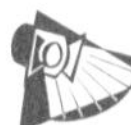

KEY FEATURES

- Frequently occur in the setting of poor oral hygiene and periodontal disease, aspiration of saliva (which contains 108 anaerobic organisms per milliliter in addition to aerobes)
- May lead to necrotizing pneumonia, lung abscess, and empyema
- Polymicrobial infection is the rule. Anaerobes—particularly *Prevotella melaninogenica,* fusobacteria, and peptostreptococci—are frequently isolated etiological agents

CLINICAL FINDINGS

- Fever, productive cough, night sweats, weight loss
- Poor dentition (frequently)

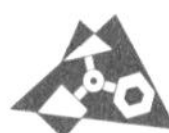

DIAGNOSIS

- Pleural fluid culture
- Chest x-ray film
- CT scan

TREATMENT

- Clindamycin, 600 mg IV once, followed by 300 mg PO Q 6–8 h, is the treatment of choice
- Penicillin, 2 million units IV Q 4 h, followed by amoxicillin, 750–1000 mg PO Q 12 h, is a reasonable alternative
- These infections respond slowly; a duration of 3–4 weeks or more of antimicrobial therapy is typical

Author(s)

Henry F. Chambers, MD

Anaerobic Infections, Intra-Abdominal

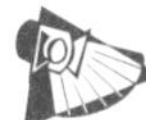

KEY FEATURES

- In the colon, there are up to 10^{11} anaerobes per gram of content, predominantly *Bacteroides fragilis*, clostridia, and peptostreptococci
- These organisms play a central role in most intra-abdominal abscesses (diverticulitis, appendicitis, or perirectal abscess) and may also participate in hepatic abscess and cholecystitis
- The bacteriology of these infections includes anaerobes as well as enteric gram-negative rods and, on occasion, enterococci

CLINICAL FINDINGS

- Related to infected organ

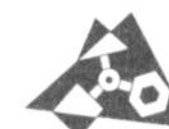

DIAGNOSIS

- Exam, laboratory tests, and CT scan

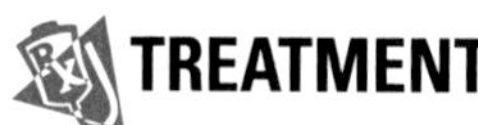

TREATMENT

- Therapy should be directed both against anaerobes and gram-negative aerobes
- Antibiotics that are reliably active against *B fragilis* include metronidazole, chloramphenicol, imipenem, ampicillin-sulbactam, ticarcillin-clavulanic acid, piperacillin-tazobactam
- Table 140 summarizes the antibiotic regimens for management of moderate to moderately severe infections (eg, patient hemodynamically stable, good surgical drainage possible or established, low APACHE score, no multiple-organ failure) and severe infections (eg, major peritoneal soilage, large or multiple abscesses, patient hemodynamically unstable), particularly if drug-resistant organisms are suspected

Author(s)

Henry F. Chambers, MD

Anaerobic Infections, Skin & Soft Tissue

 KEY FEATURES

- Usually occur after trauma, with inadequate blood supply, in association with diabetes, or after surgery and are most common in areas contaminated by oral or fecal flora
- Several terms (eg, bacterial synergistic gangrene, synergistic necrotizing cellulitis, necrotizing fasciitis, nonclostridial crepitant cellulitis) have been used to classify these infections. Although there are some differences in microbiology among them, their differentiation on clinical grounds alone is difficult
- All are mixed infections caused by aerobic and anaerobic organisms

 CLINICAL FINDINGS

- There may be progressive tissue necrosis and a putrid odor

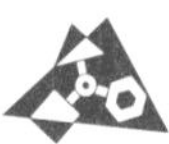 DIAGNOSIS

- Surgical exploration

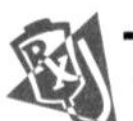 TREATMENT

- Broad-spectrum antibiotics active against both anaerobes and gram-positive and gram-negative aerobes (eg, piperacillin-tazobactam or vancomycin plus metronidazole plus gentamicin or tobramycin) should be instituted empirically and modified by culture results (Tables 127, 128, and 140)
- Require aggressive surgical débridement of necrotic tissue for cure

Author(s)

Henry F. Chambers, MD

Anaerobic Infections, Upper Respiratory Tract

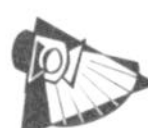 KEY FEATURES

- *Prevotella melaninogenica* and anaerobic spirochetes are commonly involved in periodontal infections
- These organisms, fusobacteria, and peptostreptococci may cause chronic sinusitis, peritonsillar abscess, chronic otitis media, and mastoiditis

 CLINICAL FINDINGS

- Related to infected organ

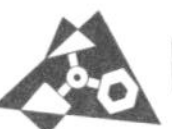 DIAGNOSIS

- Culture
- CT scan

 TREATMENT

- Tables 127 and 128
- Oral anaerobic organisms have been uniformly susceptible to penicillin, but there has been a trend of increasing penicillin resistance, usually resulting from β-lactamase production
- Penicillin, 1–2 million units IV Q 4 h (if parenteral therapy is required) or 0.5 g orally QID for less severe infections, or clindamycin, 600 mg IV Q 8 h or 300 mg PO Q 6 h), can be used
- Indolent, established infections (eg, mastoiditis or osteomyelitis) may require prolonged courses of therapy (eg, 4–6 weeks or longer)

Author(s)

Henry F. Chambers, MD

Anal Cancer

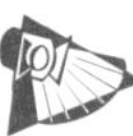 KEY FEATURES

- Carcinoma of the anus is relatively rare: only 1–2% of all cancers of the large intestine and anus
- Squamous cancers (keratinizing, transitional cell, and cloacogenic; 80%); adenocarcinomas, 20%
- Increased incidence among
  - People practicing receptive anal intercourse
  - Those with a history of other sexually transmitted diseases
  - Those with HIV infection
- Human papillomavirus (HPV) infection in >80%
- Increased risk in combined HIV and HPV infection

 CLINICAL FINDINGS

- Anal bleeding
- Pain
- Local tumor

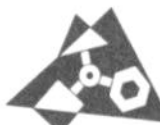 DIAGNOSIS

- Anoscopy and biopsy for diagnosis
- MRI and endoluminal ultrasonogram for staging

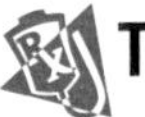 TREATMENT

- Local excision for small superficial lesions of the perianal skin
- Combined-modality therapy for tumors invading the sphincter or rectum: external radiation with simultaneous chemotherapy (fluorouracil and either mitomycin or cisplatin)
- Local control achieved in 80% of patients
- Radical surgery (abdominoperineal resection) for patients who fail chemotherapy and radiation therapy
- 5-year survival rate
  - 60–70% for localized (stages I–III) disease
  - >25% for metastatic (stage IV) disease

Author(s)

Kenneth R. McQuaid, MD

Anal Fissures

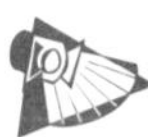

KEY FEATURES

- Linear or rocket-shaped ulcers, usually < 5 mm
- Most commonly in the posterior midline; 10% anteriorly
- Arise from trauma during defecation

CLINICAL FINDINGS

- Severe, tearing pain during defecation followed by throbbing discomfort
- May lead to constipation because of fear of recurrent pain
- Mild associated hematochezia
- Chronic fissures fibrosis and a skin tag at the outermost edge (sentinel pile)

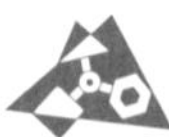

DIAGNOSIS

- Diagnosis confirmed by visual inspection of the anal verge while gently separating the buttocks
- Digital and anoscopic examinations may cause severe pain and may not be possible

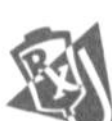

TREATMENT

- Fiber supplements
- Sitz baths
- Hydrocortisone 1% ointment
- Topical nitroglycerin 0.2–0.5% ointment applied by cotton swab to the anus and anal canal BID for 6–8 weeks heals up to 80% of patients with chronic anal fissure
- Botulinum toxin (20 units) injection into the anal sphincter heals 90% of chronic fissures
- Partial lateral internal sphincterotomy is effective for chronic or recurrent fissures but may be complicated by minor fecal incontinence

Author(s)

Kenneth R. McQuaid, MD

Anemia, Hemolytic

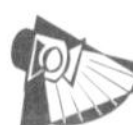

KEY FEATURES

- Anemia only when RBC survival very short or bone marrow ability to compensate impaired
- RBC production failure causes hematocrit to fall ~3% points/week; if faster, suspect blood loss, hemolysis
- **Coombs positive hemolytic anemia** may be autoimmune or related to drugs, infection, lymphoproliferative disease, Rh or ABO incompatibility
- **Coombs negative hemolytic anemia** may be intrinsic RBC disease
  - Abnormal hemoglobin: sickle cell disease, thalassemia, methemoglobinemia
  - Membrane defect: hereditary spherocytosis, hereditary elliptocytosis, paroxysmal nocturnal hemoglobinuria
  - Enzyme defect: G6PD deficiency, pyruvate kinase deficiency
- **Coombs negative hemolytic anemia** may be extrinsic
  - Microangiopathic hemolytic anemia: TPP, HUS, DIC, prosthetic valve hemolysis, metastatic adenocarcinoma, vasculitis, malignant hypertension, HELLP syndrome
  - Splenic sequestration
  - *Plasmodium, Clostridium, Borrelia* infection
  - Burns

CLINICAL FINDINGS

- Symptoms of anemia
- Jaundice, pigment gallstones, cholecystitis in chronic cases
- Palpable spleen

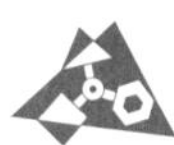

DIAGNOSIS

- Serum haptoglobin may be low
- Reticulocytosis present unless second disorder (infection, folate deficiency) superimposed on hemolysis
- Transient hemoglobinemia with intravascular hemolysis
- Hemoglobinuria when capacity for reabsorption of hemoglobin by renal tubular cells exceeded
- Urine hemosiderin test positive; indicates prior intravascular hemolysis
- Hemoglobinemia and methemalbuminemia if severe intravascular hemolysis
- Indirect bilirubin elevated, total bilirubin elevated to ≥4 mg/dL
- Serum LDH levels elevated in microangiopathic hemolysis; may be elevated in other hemolytic anemias

TREATMENT

- Treat underlying cause
- Folic acid, 1 mg PO QD
- Transfusions possible

Author(s)

Charles A. Linker, MD

Anemia of Chronic Disease

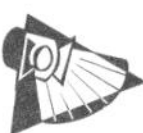

KEY FEATURES

- Many chronic systemic diseases associated with mild or moderate anemia (eg, chronic infection or inflammation, cancer, liver disease)
- Anemia of chronic renal failure has different pathophysiology (reduced erythropoietin); is usually more severe
- Largely caused by sequestration of iron within reticuloendothelial system
- Decreased dietary intake of folate or iron common in ill patients, causing coexistent folate or iron deficiency
- Many also have ongoing GI bleeding
- Hemodialysis patients regularly lose iron and folate during dialysis

CLINICAL FINDINGS

- Symptoms of anemia, which is usually modest
- Suspect diagnosis in patients with known chronic diseases

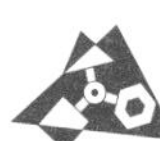

DIAGNOSIS

- Hematocrit usually > 25% (except in renal failure); if < 25%, evaluate for coexistent iron deficiency or folic acid deficiency
- Mean corpuscular volume usually normal or slightly low
- Red blood cell morphology nondiagnostic; reticulocyte count neither strikingly reduced nor increased
- Low serum iron, low transferrin saturation
- Normal or increased serum ferritin; serum ferritin < 30 μg/L suggests coexistent iron deficiency
- Normal or increased bone marrow iron stores

TREATMENT

- In most cases, no treatment necessary
- Purified recombinant erythropoietin (eg, 30,000 units SC every week) effective for anemia of renal failure, AIDS, cancer, rheumatoid arthritis
- In renal failure, optimal response to erythropoietin requires adequate dialysis
- Erythropoietin very expensive; used only when patient is transfusion-dependent or when quality of life clearly improved by hematological response

Author(s)

Charles A. Linker, MD

Anemia, Sideroblastic

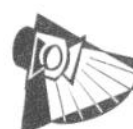

KEY FEATURES

- Heterogeneous group of disorders in which reduced hemoglobin synthesis occurs because of failure to incorporate heme into protoporphyrin to form hemoglobin
- Iron accumulates, particularly in mitochondria
- Sometimes represents stage in evolution of a generalized bone marrow disorder (myelodysplasia) that may terminate in acute leukemia
- Other causes include chronic alcoholism and lead poisoning

CLINICAL FINDINGS

- Symptoms of anemia; no other specific clinical features

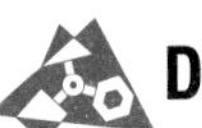

DIAGNOSIS

- Anemia usually moderate, hematocrit 20–30%
- Mean corpuscular volume usually normal or slightly increased, but occasionally low, leading to confusion with iron deficiency
- Peripheral blood smear characteristically shows dimorphic population of RBCs: 1 normal and 1 hypochromic
- Coarse basophilic stippling of RBCs and serum lead level elevated in lead poisoning
- Bone marrow iron stain shows generalized increase in iron stores and ringed sideroblasts (RBCs with iron deposits encircling the nucleus) and marked erythroid hyperplasia (resulting from ineffective erythropoiesis)
- Serum iron and transferrin saturation high

TREATMENT

- Occasionally, transfusion required for severe anemia
- Erythropoietin therapy not usually effective

Author(s)

Charles A. Linker, MD

Angina Pectoris, Unstable

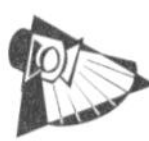

KEY FEATURES

- Accelerating or "crescendo" pattern of angina pectoris (see Angina pectoris)
- Worse prognosis than stable angina because more likely to progress to myocardial infarction
- Unstable new-onset angina, if exertional and responsive to rest and medication, is not associated with poor prognosis

CLINICAL FINDINGS

- Angina occurs at rest or with less exertion than previously
- Lasts longer
- Is less responsive to medication

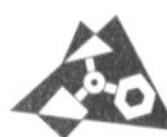

DIAGNOSIS

- Most patients with unstable angina manifest ECG changes during pain: ST-segment depression, T wave flattening, or inversion
- ST-segment elevation is more ominous and has to be considered and treated as myocardial infarction until proved otherwise
- Possible left ventricular dysfunction during pain and for a period afterward
- See Angina pectoris for other symptoms and signs

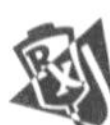

TREATMENT

- Hospitalization, bed rest, telemetry, and supplemental oxygen
- Rule out myocardial infarction with 3 serial cardiac enzymes (troponin I, troponin T, and CK-MB) Q 6–8 h and follow-up ECGs
- Cardiology consultation
- Benzodiazepine sedation if anxiety is present
- **Aspirin** (first-line therapy): 325 mg immediately, and then once daily
- **Heparin** (first-line therapy) if symptoms onset within the past 24 hours, stuttering, or unremitting
- **Low-molecular-weight heparin** (eg, enoxaparin 1 mg/kg subcutaneously Q 12 h), slightly superior to IV heparin
- **Clopidogrel:** 300 mg loading dose, then 75 mg/day, sometimes added
- **Nitroglycerin** (first-line therapy): sublingual, oral, or topical initially, but continuous drip if pain persists or recurs
  - Continuous BP monitoring required
  - Start at 10 μg/min, titrate up to 1 μg/kg/min over 30–60 minutes, increasing to higher doses if needed
- **Opioids,** for unrelieved pain or pulmonary congestion
- **β-blockers** (first-line therapy) oral or intravenous for more rapid effect
  - For example, metoprolol 5-mg doses × 3 at 5-min intervals, unless overt heart failure
  - Titrate up for goal heart rate of 60/min as tolerated by BP
- Reduce systolic BP to 100–120 mm Hg with nitroglycerin and β-blockers, except in patients with history of severe hypertension
- Early exercise or pharmacologic stress testing or coronary arteriography
- If continued pain despite above medications, fluctuating ST-segment depression, or positive cardiac enzymes, consider GIIb/IIIa receptor blockers (eg, tirofiban, 0.4 mg/kg/min for 30 min, then 0.1 μg/kg/min) pending emergent arteriography
- Thrombolytics have no role in unstable angina without ST-segment elevation

Author(s)

Thomas M. Bashore, MD

Christopher B. Granger, MD

Angiostrongyliasis Costaricensis

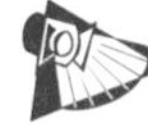

KEY FEATURES

- The helminth causes an eosinophilic ileocolitis
- Has been identified in humans (predominantly children) in Mexico, Central America, Venezuela, Brazil, and United States
- The known geographic range of the parasite in rodents (the definitive host) extends from northern South America to Texas
- Infection occurs from ingestion of the larvae in the intermediate host (slugs, snails) or from food contaminated by larvae in slug or snail mucus
- In humans, the larvae mature in the mesenteric vessels

CLINICAL FINDINGS

- The inflammatory response to adult worms, larvae, and eggs can be severe, resulting in a marked eosinophilic granulomatous reaction and vasculitis and ischemic necrosis of the intestine
- Most cases involve the ileocecal region, appendix, ascending colon, regional nodes
- Findings include fever, right lower quadrant abdominal pain and a mass, leukocytosis, and eosinophilia
- Some patients have relapsing symptoms that can continue for months
- Bowel complications include perforation, bleeding, incomplete or complete obstruction, and infarction. The intra-abdominal mass can mimic tumor

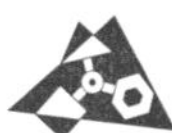

DIAGNOSIS

- Neither eggs or larvae are passed in stool; diagnosis is made by agglutination serologic test

TREATMENT

- There is no specific treatment; albendazole, thiabendazole, or mebendazole can be tried
- Operative treatment is frequently necessary

Angiitis of the CNS, Primary

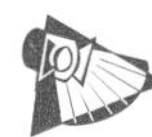

KEY FEATURES

- Small and medium-sized vasculitis limited to the brain and spinal cord

CLINICAL FINDINGS

- Biopsy-proved cases have predominated in men who present with a history of weeks to months of headaches, encephalopathy, and multifocal strokes
- Systemic symptoms and signs are absent

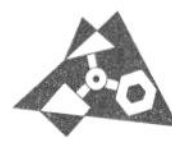

DIAGNOSIS

- MRI of the brain is almost always abnormal
- Spinal fluid often reveals a mild lymphocytosis and a modest increase in protein level
- Angiograms classically reveal a "string of beads" pattern produced by alternating segments of arterial narrowing and dilation
- However, neither MRI nor angiogram appearance is specific for vasculitis
- Definitive diagnosis requires a compatible clinical picture; exclusion of infection, neoplasm, or metabolic disorder or drug exposure (eg, cocaine) that can mimic primary angiitis of the central nervous system; and a positive brain biopsy
- Many patients who fit this clinical profile (stroke, headache, but no encephalopathy) and have disease diagnosed by angiography (but not biopsy) probably have vasospasm rather than true vasculitis
- Routine laboratory tests are usually normal

TREATMENT

- Usually improve with prednisone therapy
- May require cyclophosphamide

Author(s)

David B. Hellmann, MD, FACP
John H. Stone, MD, MPH

Ankle Sprains

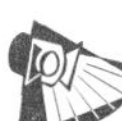

KEY FEATURES

- Most involve the lateral ligament complex, particularly the anterior talofibular ligament

CLINICAL FINDINGS

- Varus sprains include a spectrum of severity, ranging from slight loss of function to prompt swelling, prominent pain, and inability to bear weight
- Tenderness and marked swelling are typically present
- Hemorrhage from torn ligaments and damaged peroneal muscle tendons may cause substantial ecchymosis

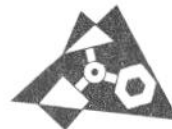

DIAGNOSIS

- Stability of the anterior talofibular and calcaneofibular ligaments should be assessed with the "anterior drawer" sign: With the foot held in slight plantar flexion, the examiner cups the patient's heel with one hand and the patient's shin with the other. The examiner then applies gentle anterior force in the plane of the patient's foot. Excessive anterior motion of the foot constitutes a positive test (grade III sprain). (Grades I and II correspond to mild to moderate injuries)
- Plain x-rays exclude bony injury

TREATMENT

- RICE (*r*est, *i*ce, *c*ompression, *e*levation)
- Early application of a compression dressing is essential to control swelling and provide stability to the joint
- Weight bearing should be minimal, with liberal use of crutches
- Patients should be informed that symptoms from lateral ankle sprains may take weeks or months to resolve, and that this period will be prolonged by premature attempts to bear weight on the injured ankle
- Surgical repairs of ruptured lateral ligaments provide excellent outcomes but are usually necessary only in cases of chronically unstable joints

Author(s)

David B. Hellmann, MD, FACP
John H. Stone, MD, MPH

Anorectal Infections

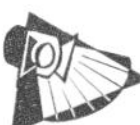

KEY FEATURES

- Proctitis is inflammation of the distal 15 cm of rectum
  - Most cases are sexually transmitted, especially by anal-receptive intercourse
  - Causes include
    - *Neisseria gonorrhoeae*
    - *Treponema pallidum* (syphilis)
    - *Chlamydia trachomatis*, herpes simplex virus type 2 (HSV-2)
    - Human papillomavirus (HPV)
- Venereal warts (condylomata acuminata) are caused by HPV occur in up to 50% of homosexual men
- Proctocolitis is inflammation that extends above the rectum to the sigmoid colon or more proximally
  - Causes: *Campylobacter, Entamoeba histolytica*, *Shigella*, and enteroinvasive *Escherichia coli*

CLINICAL FINDINGS

- Proctitis
  - Anorectal discomfort
  - Tenesmus
  - Constipation
  - Discharge
- Gonorrhea proctitis
  - Itching
  - Burning
  - Tenesmus
  - Mucopurulent discharge
- Complications of untreated gonorrheal infections
  - Strictures
  - Fissures
  - Fistulas
  - Perirectal abscesses
- Anal syphilis: asymptomatic, chancre, or proctitis
- In primary syphilis, chancre may mimic a fissure, fistula, or ulcer; in secondary syphilis, condylomata lata, foul-smelling mucous discharge, and inguinal lymphadenopathy
- *C trachomatis* causes proctitis similar to gonorrhea or lymphogranuloma venereum, proctocolitis with fever and bloody diarrhea, painful perianal ulcerations, anorectal strictures and fistulas, and inguinal lymphadenopathy (buboes)
- HSV-2 proctitis
  - Severe pain, itching, constipation, tenesmus, urinary retention, and radicular pain

– Small vesicles or ulcers in the perianal area or anal canal
- Venereal warts are noted on the perianal skin and within the anal canal; otherwise asymptomatic
- Higher rate of HPV progression to high-grade dysplasia or anal cancer in HIV-positive individuals

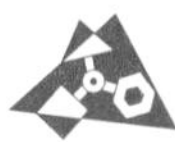

DIAGNOSIS

- Gonorrhea proctitis: blind swab of the anal canal has sensitivity of < 60%
- Gram's stain and culture from the rectum during anoscopy, cultures from the urethra and pharynx in men, and cultures from the cervix in women
- Anal syphilis: dark-field microscopy of scrapings from the chancre or condylomata
- Serum VDRL positive in 75% of primary and 99% of secondary cases
- Culture of rectal discharge or rectal biopsy for *C trachomatis* has sensitivity of >80%
- Sigmoidoscopy in HSV-2 shows vesicular or ulcerative lesions in the distal rectum
- Diagnosis by viral culture or HSV-2 antigen detection assays of vesicular fluid

TREATMENT

- Cefixime, 400 mg PO once, ceftriaxone 250 mg IM once, or ciprofloxacin, 500 mg PO once, for *N gonorrhoeae*
- Doxycycline, 100 mg PO BID for 10 days, or ofloxacin, 300 mg PO BID for 21 days, for *C trachomatis*
- Benzathine penicillin G, 2.4 million units IM once, or doxycycline, 100 mg PO BID for 2 weeks, for *T pallidum*
- Acyclovir, 400 mg PO 5 times daily for 5–10 days, for HSV-2
  - Chronic acyclovir suppressive therapy for patients with AIDS and recurrent relapses
- Podophyllum resin applied topically for small perianal warts from HPV; CO_2 laser surgery or cryosurgery for anal lesions; higher relapse rate after therapy in HIV-positive individuals
- Examine and treat patient's sexual partners
- Surveillance anoscopy every 3–6 months in HIV-positive individuals

Author(s)

Kenneth R. McQuaid, MD

Antiarrhythmic Agent Overdose

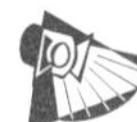

KEY FEATURES

- Quinidine, disopyramide, and procainamide are class Ia antiarrhythmic agents, and flecainide is a class Ic agent

CLINICAL FINDINGS

- Arrhythmias, syncope, hypotension

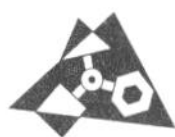

DIAGNOSIS

- Blood levels of quinidine and procainamide (and active metabolite NAPA) are generally available from hospital lab
- ECG monitoring for QRS and QT interval prolongation
  - Widening of the QRS complex (> 100–120 ms)
  - With type Ia drugs, a lengthened QT interval and atypical or polymorphous ventricular tachycardia (torsades de pointes) may occur

TREATMENT

- Administer activated charcoal, 60–100 g PO or via gastric tube, mixed in aqueous slurry for ingestions within 1 h; do not use for comatose or convulsing patients unless they are endotracheally intubated
- Consider gastric lavage for recent (1 h) large ingestions
- Consider whole bowel irrigation for ingestion of sustained-release formulations
- Perform continuous cardiac monitoring
- Treat cardiotoxicity (hypotension, QRS interval widening) with IV boluses of sodium bicarbonate, 50–100 mEq
- Torsades de pointes ventricular tachycardia may be treated with IV magnesium or overdrive pacing

Author(s)

Kent R. Olson, MD

Antipsychotic Agent Overdose

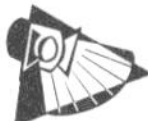

KEY FEATURES

- Chlorpromazine and related drugs used as antiemetics, antipsychotic agents, and potentiators of analgesic and hypnotic drugs

CLINICAL FINDINGS

- Drowsiness, orthostatic hypotension, especially with α-blocking agents
- Large overdose: obtundation, miosis, severe hypotension, tachycardia, convulsions, coma
- Prolongation of QRS and/or QT interval and ventricular arrhythmias may occur (particularly with thioridazine and haloperidol)
- With therapeutic or toxic doses, a parkinsonian-like extrapyramidal dystonic reaction, with spasmodic contractions of the face and neck muscles, extensor rigidity of the back muscles, carpopedal spasm, and motor restlessness, can occur
- Severe rigidity, hyperthermia, and metabolic acidosis (neuroleptic malignant syndrome) may occasionally occur and are life threatening

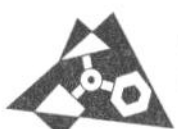

DIAGNOSIS

- Clinical

TREATMENT

- Activated charcoal 60–100 g (in aqueous slurry) PO or via gastric tube. Do not use for comatose or convulsing patients unless they are endotracheally intubated
- Consider gastric lavage for large ingestions
- Treat hypotension with fluids and pressor agents; hypotension and cardiac arrhythmias and widened QRS intervals (thioridazine) may respond to IV NaHCO3 as used for tricyclic antidepressants
- Treat hyperthermia, maintain cardiac monitoring
- For extrapyramidal signs, give diphenhydramine, 0.5–1 mg/kg IV, or benztropine mesylate, 0.01–0.02 mg/kg IM; continue with PO doses for 1–2 days

- Bromocriptine, 2.5–7.5 mg/day PO, may treat neuroleptic malignant syndrome
- Dantrolene, 2–5 mg/kg IV, can lessen muscle contractions

Author(s)

Kent R. Olson, MD

Aortic Regurgitation

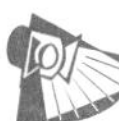

KEY FEATURES

- Nonrheumatic causes are more common than rheumatic heart disease
- Nonrheumatic causes include bicuspid valves, infective endocarditis, hypertension, cystic medial necrosis, Marfan's syndrome, aortic dissection, ankylosing spondylitis, Reiter's syndrome, and syphilis

CLINICAL FINDINGS

- High-pitched, decrescendo diastolic murmur along the left sternal border
- Hyperactive, enlarged left ventricle
- Wide pulse pressure with peripheral signs
- Usually slowly progressive and asymptomatic until middle age, although onset may sometimes be rapid, as in infective endocarditis or myocardial infarction
- Exertional dyspnea and fatigue are the most frequent symptoms, but paroxysmal nocturnal dyspnea and pulmonary edema may also occur
- May present with left-sided failure or chest pain
- Coronary artery disease and syncope are less common than in aortic stenosis

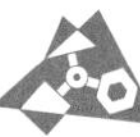

DIAGNOSIS

- ECG: left ventricular hypertrophy
- CXR: left ventricular and sometimes aortic dilation
- Echo-Doppler confirms the diagnosis and estimates severity
- Serial assessments of left ventricular size and function are critical in determining the timing of valve replacement
- CT or MRI can estimate aortic root size and exclude ascending aneurysm
- Cardiac catheterization can help quantify severity and preoperatively to evaluate the coronary and aortic root anatomy

TREATMENT

- Surgery is often urgently required in rapid-onset regurgitation (even with active infection)
- Vasodilators (eg, hydralazine, nifedipine, and angiotensin-converting enzyme inhibitors) may be used to reduce severity of regurgitation
- In chronic cases, vasodilators can postpone surgery in asymptomatic patients
- Surgery is usually indicated once aortic regurgitation causes symptoms
- Surgery is also indicated for those who have an ejection fraction < 55% or increasing end-systolic left ventricular volume
- Operative mortality is usually 3–5%

Author(s)

Thomas M. Bashore, MD

Christoper B. Granger, MD

Aortic Stenosis

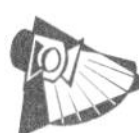

KEY FEATURES

- Two common scenarios: congenital bicuspid valve or acquired valvular degeneration caused by progressive valvular calcification (sclerosis precedes stenosis)
- Increasingly common with age
- In developed countries, most common valve lesion requiring surgery
- Much more frequent in men, smokers, and patients with hypercholesterolemia and hypertension

CLINICAL FINDINGS

- Delayed and diminished carotid pulses
- Soft, absent, or paradoxically split S_2
- Harsh systolic murmur, sometimes with thrill along left sternal border, often radiating to the neck; may be louder at apex in older patients
- With bicuspid valve, usually asymptomatic until middle or old age
- Left ventricular hypertrophy progresses over time
- Patients may present with left ventricular failure, angina pectoris, or syncope
- Syncope, typically exertional, may be due to stimulation of reflex baroreceptors or to arrhythmias (usually ventricular tachycardia, sometimes sinus bradycardia)

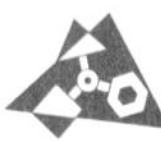

DIAGNOSIS

- ECG: usually shows left ventricular hypertrophy
- CXR fluoroscopy: calcified valve
- Echo-Doppler is usually diagnostic and can estimate the aortic valve gradient
- Cardiac catheterization provides confirmatory data, assesses hemodynamics, and excludes concomitant coronary artery disease
- Stenosis must be distinguished from supravalvular and outflow obstruction of the left ventricular infundibulum

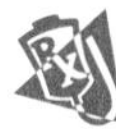

TREATMENT

- After onset of heart failure, angina, or syncope, the mortality rate without surgery is 50% within 3 yr
- Aortic valve replacement (in middle age or older) or Ross procedure (in younger age) is indicated for all symptomatic patients, and those with left ventricular dysfunction or peak gradient > 64 mm Hg
- Surgical mortality rate is 2–5%, higher (10%) with age > 75, substantially higher with left ventricular dysfunction, severe coronary disease, or prior myocardial infarction
- Balloon valvuloplasty in adolescents

Author(s)

Thomas M. Bashore, MD

Christopher B. Granger, MD

Aphthous Ulcer

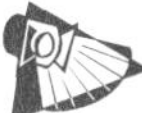

KEY FEATURES

- Canker sore or ulcerative stomatitis
- Large or persistent areas of ulcerative stomatitis may be secondary to erythema multiforme or drug allergies, acute herpes simplex, pemphigus, pemphigoid, bullous lichen planus, Behçet's disease, or inflammatory bowel disease
- Cause remains uncertain, although an association with human herpesvirus 6 has been suggested

CLINICAL FINDINGS

- Very common and easy to recognize
- Found on nonkeratinized mucosa (eg, buccal and labial mucosa and not gingiva or palate)
- May be single or multiple, are usually recurrent, and appear as small (usually 1–2 mm but sometimes 1–2 cm), round painful ulcerations with yellow-gray fibrinoid centers surrounded by red halos
- The painful stage lasts 7–10 days; healing is completed in 1–3 weeks

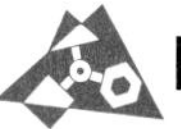

DIAGNOSIS

- Based on clinical appearance
- Squamous cell carcinoma may occasionally present in this fashion. When the diagnosis is not clear, incisional biopsy is indicated

TREATMENT

- Topical steroids (triamcinolone acetonide, 0.1%, or fluocinonide ointment, 0.05%) in an adhesive base (Orabase-Plain) provide symptomatic relief
- Other topical therapies are diclofenac 3% in hyaluronan 2.5%, doxymycine-cyanoacrylate, mouthwashes containing the enzymes amyloglucosidase and glucose oxidase, and amlexanox 5% oral paste
- A 1-week tapering course of prednisone (40–60 mg PO daily) can be used

Author(s)

Robert K. Jackler, MD

Michael J. Kaplan, MD

Arbovirus Encephalitides

KEY FEATURES

- Arthropod-borne viruses
- St. Louis and California encephalitides common in United States
- West Nile encephalitis identified in 1999; now present in much of United States
- Disease in United States tends to occur in outbreaks during periods of mosquito proliferation

CLINICAL FINDINGS

- Age-dependent; residual neurologic deficits more likely in the elderly
- Fevers, sore throat, stiff neck, nausea, vomiting, lethargy, coma
- Signs of meningeal irritation, tremors, cranial nerve palsies are common
- CSF: elevated protein, elevated opening pressure and lymphocytosis
- Motor weakness common in West Nile infection

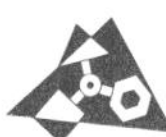

DIAGNOSIS

- Clinical symptoms, with history of mosquito or other vector exposure
- Lymphocytopenia
- Polymerase chain reaction assays may be diagnostic
- West Nile: serum and CSF IgM ELISA confirm the diagnosis

TREATMENT

- Vigorous supportive measures
- Prevention: mosquito control measures

Author(s)

Wayne X. Shandera, MD

Ana Moran, MD

Arsenic Poisoning

KEY FEATURES

- Found in some pesticides and industrial chemicals

CLINICAL FINDINGS

- Symptoms usually appear within 1 h after ingestion but may be delayed as long as 12 h
- Abdominal pain, vomiting, watery diarrhea, and skeletal muscle cramps
- Profound dehydration and shock may occur
- In chronic poisoning, symptoms can be vague but often include those of peripheral sensory neuropathy

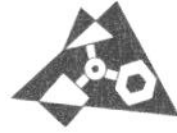

DIAGNOSIS

- Urinary arsenic levels may be falsely elevated after certain meals (eg, seafood) that contain large quantities of relatively nontoxic organic arsenic

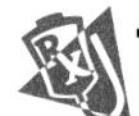

TREATMENT

EMERGENCY MEASURES

- Perform gastric lavage and administer 60–100 g of activated charcoal mixed in aqueous slurry

ANTIDOTE

- For symptomatic patients or those with massive overdose, give dimercaprol injection (BAL), 10% solution in oil, 3–5 mg/kg IM Q 4–6 h for 2 days. The side effects include nausea, vomiting, headache, and hypertension
- Follow dimercaprol with oral penicillamine, 100 mg/kg/day in 4 divided doses (maximum, 2 g/day), or succimer (DMSA), 10 mg/kg Q 8 h for 1 week
- Consult a medical toxicologist or regional poison control center for advice regarding chelation

Author(s)

Kent R. Olson, MD

Arthritis & Inflammatory Bowel Diseases

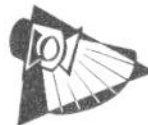

KEY FEATURES

- 20% of patients with inflammatory bowel disease have arthritis
- Second most common extraintestinal manifestation (after anemia)

CLINICAL FINDINGS

- Two distinct forms of arthritis occur
  - Peripheral arthritis—usually a nondeforming asymmetric oligoarthritis of large joints—in which the activity of the joint disease parallels that of the bowel disease
  - Spondylitis that is indistinguishable by symptoms or x-ray film from ankylosing spondylitis and follows a course independent of the bowel disease. About 50% of these patients are HLA-B27-positive
- About two-thirds of patients with Whipple's disease experience arthralgia or arthritis, most often an episodic, large-joint polyarthritis. The arthritis usually precedes gastrointestinal manifestations by years and resolves as the diarrhea develops

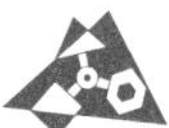

DIAGNOSIS

- Clinical
- Differential diagnosis includes reactive arthritis (Reiter's syndrome), ankylosing spondylitis, psoriatic arthritis, Whipple's disease

TREATMENT

- Controlling the intestinal inflammation usually eliminates the peripheral arthritis
- Spondylitis often requires NSAIDs, which need to be used cautiously because they may activate the bowel disease in a few patients

Author(s)

David B. Hellmann, MD, FACP

John H. Stone, MD, MPH

Arthritis in Sarcoidosis

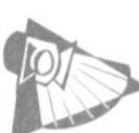

KEY FEATURES

- May occur early (within 6 months of onset of symptoms) or late
- Often associated with erythema nodosum
- Rarely deforming

CLINICAL FINDINGS

- Early arthritis
  - Usually begins in one or both ankles and can additively involve knees, wrists, and hands
  - Strongly associated with erythema nodosum and often produces more periarticular swelling than frank joint swelling
  - Axial skeleton spared
  - Commonly self-limited, resolving after several weeks or months and rarely resulting in chronic arthritis, joint destruction, or significant deformity
- Late arthritis is less severe and less widespread
- Dactylitis (sausage digit) may occur in association with overlying cutaneous sarcoidosis
- Often associated with erythema nodosum

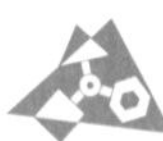

DIAGNOSIS

- Contingent on demonstration of other extraarticular manifestations of sarcoidosis and biopsy evidence of noncaseating granulomas
- In chronic arthritis, radiographs show typical changes in the bones of the extremities with intact cortex and cystic changes

TREATMENT

- Usually symptomatic and supportive
- A short course of corticosteroids may be effective in severe and progressive joint disease
- Colchicine may be of value

Author(s)

David B. Hellmann, MD, FACP

John H. Stone, MD, MPH

Arthritis, Viral

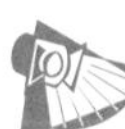

KEY FEATURES

- Arthritis may be a manifestation of many viral infections
- Generally mild and of short duration, terminating without lasting ill effects

CLINICAL FINDINGS

- Mumps arthritis may occur in the absence of parotitis
- Rubella arthritis, which occurs more commonly in adults than in children, may appear immediately before, during, or soon after the disappearance of the rash. Its usual polyarticular and symmetric distribution mimics that of rheumatoid arthritis
- In adults, polyarthritis may follow infection with human parvovirus B19
- Transient polyarthritis may be associated with type B hepatitis and typically occurs before the onset of jaundice; it may occur in anicteric hepatitis as well
- Hepatitis C infection may be associated with chronic polyarthralgia or polyarthritis that mimics rheumatoid arthritis

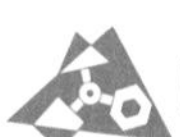

DIAGNOSIS

- Viral serologies

TREATMENT

- NSAIDs are the mainstay of treatment for most forms of viral arthritis
- Symptoms secondary to hepatitis C virus may respond to interferon-α if the virological response is good

Author(s)

David B. Hellmann, MD, FACP

John H. Stone, MD, MPH

Asbestosis

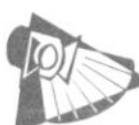

KEY FEATURES

- A nodular interstitial fibrosis occurring in workers chronically exposed to asbestos fibers
- Cigarette smoking increases the prevalence of pleural and parenchymal changes and markedly increases the incidence of lung carcinoma

CLINICAL FINDINGS

- Inexorably progressive dyspnea, inspiratory crackles
- Clubbing and cyanosis present in some patients
- Lower lungs involved more than upper lungs
- Pulmonary function tests show restrictive dysfunction and reduced diffusing capacity

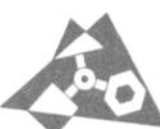

DIAGNOSIS

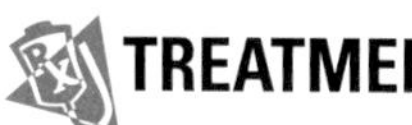

- Radiographic features
  - Interstitial fibrosis
  - Thickened pleura
  - Calcified pleural plaques on lateral chest walls and diaphragm
- High-resolution CT— the best imaging method

TREATMENT

- No specific treatment

Author(s)

Mark S. Chesnutt, MD

Thomas J. Prendergast, MD

Ascites, Malignant

KEY FEATURES

- Two-thirds of cases are due to peritoneal carcinomatosis from
  - Adenocarcinomas of the ovary
  - Uterus
  - Pancreas
  - Stomach
  - Colon
  - Lung
  - Breast
- One-third of cases are due to lymphatic obstruction or portal hypertension from
  - Hepatocellular carcinoma
  - Diffuse hepatic metastases

CLINICAL FINDINGS

- Nonspecific abdominal discomfort and weight loss
- Increased abdominal girth
- Nausea or vomiting caused by partial or complete intestinal obstruction

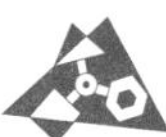

DIAGNOSIS

- Abdominal CT
  - Useful to demonstrate primary malignancy or hepatic metastases
  - Seldom confirms diagnosis of peritoneal carcinomatosis
- Paracentesis demonstrates
  - Low serum ascites–albumin gradient (< 1.1 mg/dL)
  - Increased total protein (>2.5 g/dL)
  - Elevated WBC (often both neutrophils and mononuclear cells but with a lymphocyte predominance)
- Ascitic fluid cytology is positive in 95%
- Laparoscopy is diagnostic in patients with negative cytology

TREATMENT

- Diuretics not useful in controlling ascites
- Periodic large-volume paracentesis for symptomatic relief
- Intraperitoneal chemotherapy sometimes used
- Prognosis is extremely poor: only 10% survival at 6 months
- Ovarian cancer is an exception; with surgical debulking and intraperitoneal chemotherapy, long-term survival is possible

Author(s)

Kenneth R. McQuaid, MD

Aspiration of Gastric Contents, Acute

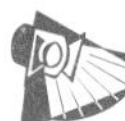

KEY FEATURES

- Also known as Mendelson's syndrome
- One of the most common causes of ARDS
- Severity depends on the characteristics and amount of gastric contents; more severe injury is caused by more acidic pH

CLINICAL FINDINGS

- Abrupt onset of respiratory distress with cough, wheezing, and fever
- Hypoxemia and bibasilar crackles may be noted immediately
- Chest x-ray demonstrates infiltrates in dependent lung zones within hours
- Fever and leukocytosis occur even with no bacterial superinfection
- Secondary pulmonary infection occurs in 25% of patients, usually after 2–3 days
- Hypotension secondary to alveolar injury and intravascular volume depletion is common

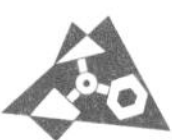

DIAGNOSIS

- History of aspiration or condition known to predispose to it
- Sudden onset of respiratory distress with hypoxia and typical radiographic features
- Exclusion of other cardiopulmonary conditions causing hypoxia and infiltrates

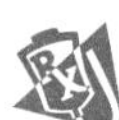

TREATMENT

- Acute treatment
  - Airway protection and supplemental oxygen
  - Ventilatory support as needed
- No evidence supports routine use of corticosteroids or prophylactic antibiotics

Author(s)

Mark S. Chesnutt, MD

Thomas J. Prendergast, MD

Aspiration of Gastric Contents, Chronic

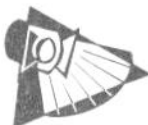

KEY FEATURES

- May result from primary disorders of the larynx or esophagus

CLINICAL FINDINGS

- Chronic cough
- Nocturnal asthma or symptoms
- Interstitial lung disease
- Bronchiectasis
- Recurrent lung infections

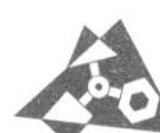

DIAGNOSIS

- Ambulatory monitoring of esophageal pH detects pathologic reflux
- Esophagogastroscopy and barium swallow may be necessary to rule out esophageal disease
- Swallowing evaluation by a speech pathologist

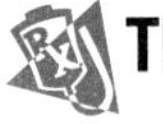

TREATMENT

- Elevation of the head of the bed
- Cessation of smoking
- Weight reduction
- Avoidance of caffeinated products and alcohol
- Acid-suppressive therapy (eg, proton pump inhibitors; see *Gastroesophageal Reflux Disease*)
- Metoclopramide may be helpful in some patients
- Nissen fundoplication for pathologic reflux despite medical therapy
- Speech–swallowing therapy

Author(s)

Mark S. Chesnutt, MD

Thomas J. Prendergast, MD

Asthma, Occupational

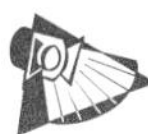 KEY FEATURES

- Estimated 2–5% of all asthma cases are related to occupation

 CLINICAL FINDINGS

- Dyspnea, wheezing, and cough, which correlate with the workplace
- Patients will often report feeling better in the evenings or during weekends and vacations

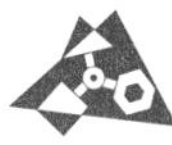 DIAGNOSIS

- Requires a high index of suspicion and a careful history of work exposures
- Spirometry before and after exposure to the implicated substance
- Peak flow measurements at and outside of the workplace
- Bronchial provocation testing is helpful in some cases

 TREATMENT

- Bronchodilators
- Avoidance of further exposure to the offending agent

Author(s)

Mark S. Chesnutt, MD

Thomas J. Prendergast, MD

Atrial Flutter

 KEY FEATURES

- Ectopic impulse formation occurs at atrial rates of 250–350/min, with transmission of every second, third, or fourth impulse through the AV node to the ventricles
- Atrial flutter is less common than fibrillation
- Occurs most often in chronic obstructive pulmonary disease (COPD) and less commonly with rheumatic or coronary heart disease, congestive heart failure, atrial septal defect, or surgically repaired congenital heart disease
- Ventricular rate control is attempted as in atrial fibrillation but is much more difficult to achieve
- Risk of systemic embolization is slightly increased

 CLINICAL FINDINGS

- Regular pulse with heart rate between 250–350 bpm
- Symptoms include anxiety, shortness of breath, light-headedness
- Physical findings of COPD

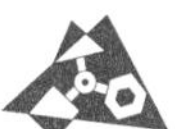 DIAGNOSIS

- ECG: characteristic atrial flutter waves transmitted in a regular 2:1, 3:1, or 4:1 pattern to the ventricles

TREATMENT

- Initially, digoxin, a β-blocker, or a calcium channel blocker (Table 40) is used for rate control; conversion to sinus rhythm may result
- If not, ibutilide converts atrial flutter to sinus rhythm in ~50–70% of patients within 60–90 min
- Electrical cardioversion (25–50 J) is effective in ~90% of patients
- Precardioversion anticoagulation is not necessary for atrial flutter of < 48 h duration except in the setting of mitral valve disease
- Anticoagulation is prudent in chronic atrial flutter, particularly because transient periods of atrial fibrillation are common in these patients
- In chronic atrial flutter, rate control is often difficult; amiodarone is the drug of choice
- In patients in whom drug therapy is refractory, consider radiofrequency ablation of a possible atypical reentry circuit

Author(s)

Thomas M. Bashore, MD

Christopher B. Granger, MD

Atrial Septal Defect

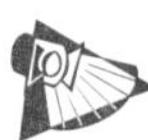

KEY FEATURES

- Three forms
  - Persistent ostium secundum (mid-septum) (80% of cases)
  - Persistent ostium primum (low septum)
  - Sinus venosus defect (upper septum)
- Oxygenated blood from higher-pressure left atrium passes into right atrium, increasing right ventricular output and pulmonary blood flow
- Prolonged high flow through pulmonary circulation often leads to pulmonary hypertension
- Right-to-left shunting and cyanosis (Eisenmenger's syndrome) in 15%
- Patent foramen ovale (present in 20–30% of adults) is responsible for most paradoxical emboli

CLINICAL FINDINGS

- Most small or moderate ASDs are asymptomatic
- Large shunts can produce exertional dyspnea or cardiac failure, usually after the fourth decade
- Moderately loud systolic ejection murmur in the second and third interspaces; S_2 widely split, does not vary with breathing
- Prominent right ventricular and pulmonary artery pulsations

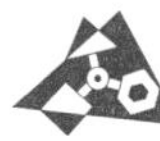

DIAGNOSIS

- ECG: incomplete or complete RBBB, right axis deviation, RVH
- Chest x-ray: large pulmonary arteries, increased pulmonary vascularity, enlarged right atrium and ventricle
- Echocardiography usually diagnostic
  - Saline bubble contrast and Doppler flow can demonstrate shunting
  - Transesophageal echo has superior sensitivity for small shunts and patent foramen ovale
- Cardiac catheterization can show increase in oxygen saturation between venae cava and right ventricle, quantify shunt, and measure pulmonary vascular resistance

TREATMENT

- Small shunts do not require surgery
- Large shunts generally require surgery
- Surgery contraindicated in Eisenmenger's syndrome
- Percutaneous closure devices now available

Author(s)

Thomas M. Bashore, MD

Christopher B. Granger, MD

Atropine and Anticholinergic Poisoning

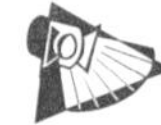

KEY FEATURES

- Atropine, scopolamine, belladonna, diphenoxylate with atropine, *Datura stramonium, Hyoscyamus niger,* some mushrooms, tricyclic antidepressants, and antihistamines are antimuscarinic agents with variable CNS effects

CLINICAL FINDINGS

- Dryness of the mouth, thirst, difficulty swallowing, blurring of vision
- Dilated pupils, flushed skin, tachycardia, fever, delirium, myoclonus, ileus, flushed appearance
- Antidepressants and antihistamines may induce convulsions
- Diphenhydramine commonly causes delirium, tachycardia, and seizures; massive overdose may mimic tricyclic antidepressant poisoning
- Terfenadine and astemizole cause QT interval prolongation and torsades de pointes and were removed from US market

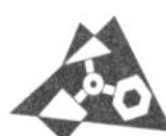

DIAGNOSIS

- Clinical or diagnosis by serum level

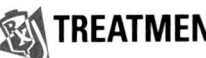

TREATMENT

Emergency and supportive measures

- Administer activated charcoal 60–100 g mixed in aqueous slurry PO or via gastric tube. Do not use for comatose or convulsing patients unless they are endotracheally intubated

Specific treatment

- For pure atropine or related anticholinergic syndrome, if symptoms are severe (eg, hyperthermia or excessively rapid tachycardia), give physostigmine salicylate, 0.5–1 mg IV slowly over 5 min, with ECG monitoring, until symptoms are controlled
- Bradyarrhythmias and convulsions are a hazard with physostigmine administration, and it should **not** be used in patients with tricyclic antidepressant overdose

Author(s)

Kent R. Olson, MD

Avascular Necrosis of Bone

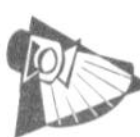

KEY FEATURES

- A complication of
  - Corticosteroid use
  - Trauma
  - Systemic lupus erythematosus (SLE)
  - Pancreatitis
  - Alcoholism
  - Gout
  - Sickle cell disease
  - Infiltrative diseases (eg, Gaucher's disease)
- Most commonly affected sites are the proximal and distal femoral heads
- The natural history is usually progression of the bony infarction to cortical collapse, resulting in significant joint dysfunction

CLINICAL FINDINGS

- Hip or knee pain
- Many patients with hip disease first present with pain referred to the knee; however, internal rotation of the hip—not movement of the knee—is painful

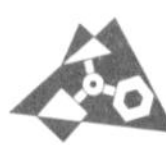

DIAGNOSIS

- Initially, radiographs are often normal; MRI, CT scan, and bone scan are all more sensitive techniques
- Differential diagnosis
  - Osteoarthritis or rheumatoid arthritis
  - Fracture
  - Joint pain resulting from other cause

TREATMENT

- Avoidance of weight bearing on the affected joint for at least several weeks
- Surgical core decompression is controversial
- Total hip replacement is the usual outcome for all patients who are suitable candidates

Author(s)

David B. Hellmann, MD, FACP

John H. Stone, MD, MPH

Bacteremia, Salmonella

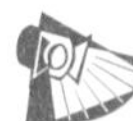

KEY FEATURES

- This complication tends to occur in immunocompromised persons and is seen in HIV-infected individuals, who typically have bacteremia without an obvious source

CLINICAL FINDINGS

- May be manifested by prolonged or recurrent fevers or local infection in bone, joints, pleura, pericardium, lungs, or other sites
- Mycotic abdominal aortic aneurysms may also be a complication

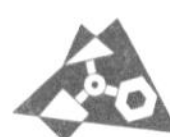

DIAGNOSIS

- Serotypes other than *Salmonella typhi* usually are isolated in culture

TREATMENT

- Treatment is the same as for typhoid fever (see enteric or typhoid fever) plus drainage of any abscesses
- In HIV-infected patients, relapse is common, and lifelong suppressive therapy may be needed
- Ciprofloxacin, 500 mg BID, is effective both for therapy of acute infection and for suppression of recurrence

Author(s)

Henry F. Chambers, MD

Bacteremia, Staphylococcal

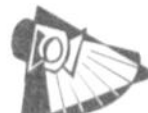

KEY FEATURES

- Although staphylococcal bacteremia commonly arises from skin lesions or IV catheters, whenever *Staphylococcus aureus* is recovered from blood cultures, the possibility of endocarditis, osteomyelitis, or other metastatic deep infections must be considered

CLINICAL FINDINGS

- There may be symptoms and signs related to source of infection

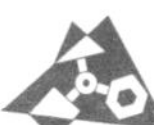

DIAGNOSIS

- Transesophageal echocardiography is a sensitive and cost-effective method for excluding underlying endocarditis and should be considered for patients for whom the pretest probability of endocarditis is 5% or higher and perhaps for all patients with unexplained *S aureus* bacteremia

TREATMENT

- The appropriate duration of therapy for uncomplicated bacteremia arising from a removable source (eg, IV device) or drainable focus (eg, skin abscess) has not been well defined, but a 10- to 14-day course of therapy appears to be the minimum
- Nafcillin or oxacillin, 1.5 g IV Q 4–6 h, cefazolin, 500–1000 mg Q 8 h, or vancomycin, 1000 mg Q 12 h, is recommended for uncomplicated staphylococcal bacteremia
- Vancomycin, which is less efficacious than β-lactams, should be reserved for treatment of methicillin-resistant strains or for infection in patients with serious penicillin allergy
- Resistance to vancomycin remains rare and should not affect the choice of empiric therapy
- Cases of vancomycin treatment failures in which the staphylococcal isolate exhibits a vancomycin MIC ≥ 4 μg/mL should be reported to the Centers for Disease Control and Prevention to help track this potentially serious and emerging problem

Author(s)

Henry F. Chambers, MD

Bacterial Overgrowth, Small Intestine

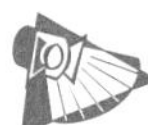

KEY FEATURES

- Overgrowth of bacteria in normally sterile segments of small bowel; may result in malabsorption of fat with steatorrhea
- Causes include
  - Gastric achlorhydria
  - Anatomic abnormalities of the small intestine with stagnation (afferent limb of Billroth II gastrojejunostomy, small intestine diverticula, obstruction, blind loop, radiation enteritis)
  - Small intestine motility disorders (scleroderma, diabetic enteropathy, chronic intestinal pseudo-obstruction)
  - Gastrocolic or coloenteric fistula (Crohn's disease, malignancy, surgical resection)
  - Miscellaneous disorders (AIDS, chronic pancreatitis)

CLINICAL FINDINGS

- Many patients are asymptomatic
- Abdominal distention, weight loss, and steatorrhea
- Watery diarrhea

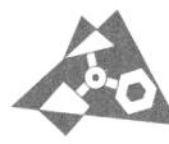

DIAGNOSIS

- Qualitative or quantitative fecal fat assessment abnormal
- D-xylose absorption abnormal
- Aspirate and culture of proximal jejunal secretion demonstrate $>10^5$ organisms/mL
- ^{13}C- or ^{14}C-xylose breath test or glucose breath test
- Megaloblastic anemia secondary to vitamin B_{12} deficiency
- Schilling test abnormal in phases I and II (without and with intrinsic factor) but normalizes after a course of antibiotics
- Small bowel barium radiography: helpful to document conditions predisposing to intestinal stasis
- Empirical antibiotic trial can be used as a diagnostic and therapeutic maneuver

TREATMENT

- Correct the anatomic defect when possible
- Ciprofloxacin, 500 mg PO BID, norfloxacin, 400 mg PO BID, amoxicillin clavulanate, 875 mg PO BID, or combination of metronidazole, 250 mg PO TID, and trimethoprim-sulfamethoxazole 160/800 mg PO BID, or cephalexin, 250 mg PO QID, for 1–2 weeks
- If symptoms recur off antibiotics, cyclic therapy (eg, 1 week of 4) may be sufficient
- Avoid continuous antibiotics to prevent bacterial antibiotic resistance
- Octreotide in small doses may be of benefit

Author(s)

Kenneth R. McQuaid, MD

Balantidiasis

KEY FEATURES

- *Balantidium coli* is a large intestinal protozoan found worldwide but particularly in the tropics
- Pigs are the reservoir host, but the agent is found in other animals and insects
- The disease is rare in humans, occurring as an acute or chronic infection (sporadic or in outbreaks) resulting from ingestion of cysts passed in stools of humans or swine
- In properly treated mild to moderate symptomatic cases, the prognosis is good
- In spite of treatment, fatalities have occurred in severe infections as a result of intestinal perforation or hemorrhage

CLINICAL FINDINGS

- Many infections are asymptomatic and need not be treated
- Chronic recurrent diarrhea, alternating with constipation, is most common, but mild diarrhea to severe dysentery with bloody mucoid stools, tenesmus, and colic may occur
- Rarely, instances of infection in the lung, liver, and vagina can occur

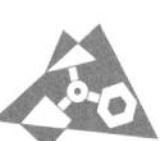

DIAGNOSIS

- Identify trophozoites in liquid stools, cysts in formed stools, or the trophozoite in scrapings or biopsy of ulcers of the large bowel. Specimens must be examined rapidly or placed in preservative

TREATMENT

- The treatment of choice is tetracycline hydrochloride, 500 mg PO QID for 10 days. The alternative drug is iodoquinol (diiodohydroxyquin), 650 mg PO TID for 21 days
- Occasional success has also been reported with metronidazole (750 mg PO TID for 5 days) or paromomycin PO (25–30 mg/kg [base] in 3 divided doses for 5–10 days)

Bartholin's Duct Cyst and Abscess

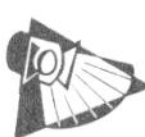

KEY FEATURES

- Trauma or infection may cause obstruction of the gland; drainage of secretions is prevented, leading to pain, swelling, and abscess formation
- The infection usually resolves and pain disappears, but stenosis of the duct outlet with distention often persists
- Reinfection causes recurrent tenderness and further enlargement of the duct

CLINICAL FINDINGS

- Periodic painful swelling on either side of the introitus and dyspareunia
- A fluctuant swelling 1–4 cm in diameter in the inferior portion of either labium minus is a sign of occlusion of Bartholin's duct
- Tenderness is evidence of active infection

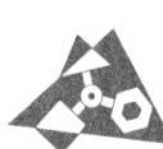

DIAGNOSIS

- Pus or secretions from the gland should be cultured for gonococci, chlamydiae, and other pathogens

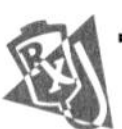

TREATMENT

- Treat according to culture results
- Frequent warm soaks may be helpful
- If an abscess develops, aspiration or incision and drainage are the simplest forms of therapy, but the problem may recur
- Marsupialization (in the absence of an abscess), incision and drainage with the insertion of an indwelling Word catheter, or laser treatment will establish a new duct opening. Antibiotics are unnecessary unless cellulitis is present
- An asymptomatic cyst does not require therapy

Author(s)

H. Trent MacKay, MD, MPH

Behçet's Syndrome

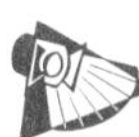

KEY FEATURES

- Causes recurrent attacks of oral aphthous ulcers, genital ulcers, uveitis, and skin lesions
- Onset usually in young adults, aged 25–35 yr
- Blindness, CNS abnormalities, and thrombosis or rupture of large vessels are the most serious complications

CLINICAL FINDINGS

- Recurrent oral and genital ulcers
- Eye abnormalities include
  - Keratitis
  - Retinal vasculitis
  - Anterior uveitis (often with hypopyon, or pus in the anterior chamber)
- Seronegative arthritis occurs in about two-thirds of patients, most commonly affecting the knees and ankles
- CNS abnormalities include
  - Cranial nerve palsies
  - Convulsions
  - Encephalitis
  - Mental disturbances
  - Spinal cord lesions
- Clinical course may be chronic but is often characterized by remissions and exacerbations

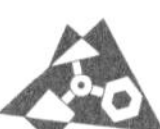

DIAGNOSIS

- Clinical diagnosis
- CNS lesions may mimic multiple sclerosis radiologically
- Differential diagnosis
  - Inflammatory bowel disease
  - Systemic lupus erythematosus
  - Recurrent aphthous ulcers
  - Herpes simplex infection
  - Ankylosing spondylitis
  - Reactive arthritis (Reiter's syndrome)
  - Syphilis
  - Sarcoidosis
  - HIV infection

TREATMENT

- Corticosteroids, azathioprine, chlorambucil, pentoxifylline, and cyclosporine have been used with beneficial results

Author(s)

David B. Hellmann, MD, FACP
John H. Stone, MD, MPH

Bernard-Soulier Syndrome

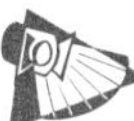

KEY FEATURES

- Rare autosomal recessive disorder
- Platelets cannot adhere to subendothelium because of lack of receptors (composed of glycoprotein Ib) for von Willebrand factor

CLINICAL FINDINGS

- Often severe mucosal and postoperative bleeding

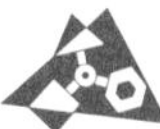

DIAGNOSIS

- Thrombocytopenia may be present
- Bleeding time markedly prolonged
- Platelet aggregation normal in response to standard agonists (collagen, adenosine 5'-diphosphate, thrombin), but platelets fail to aggregate in response to ristocetin
- Normal plasma von Willebrand factor level

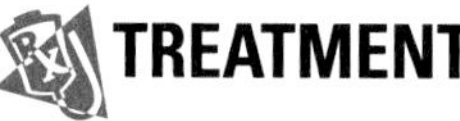

TREATMENT

- Platelet transfusion when necessary

Author(s)

Charles A. Linker, MD

Berylliosis

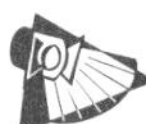

KEY FEATURES

- An acute or chronic pulmonary disorder related to beryllium exposure
- Exposure occurs in machining and handling of beryllium products and alloys; beryllium miners are *not* at risk

CLINICAL FINDINGS

- Acute berylliosis is a toxic, ulcerative tracheobronchitis and chemical pneumonitis after intense, severe exposure
- Chronic berylliosis is a more common, systemic disease resembling sarcoidosis

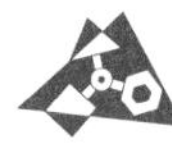

DIAGNOSIS

- The beryllium lymphocyte proliferation test is a useful diagnostic test

TREATMENT

- Avoid exposure to beryllium
- Corticosteroids are often prescribed despite lack of proven efficacy

Author(s)

Mark S. Chesnutt, MD
Thomas J. Prendergast, MD

Beta-Blocker Overdose

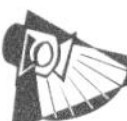

KEY FEATURES

- The most toxic β-blocker is propranolol, which competitively blocks β_1- and β_2- adrenoceptors and also has direct membrane-depressant and CNS effects

CLINICAL FINDINGS

- Hypotension and bradycardia are common with mild or moderate intoxication
- Cardiac depression from more severe poisoning is often unresponsive to conventional β-adrenergic stimulants such as dopamine and norepinephrine
- With propranolol and other lipid-soluble drugs, seizures and coma may occur

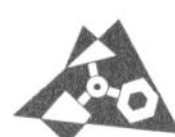

DIAGNOSIS

- Diagnosis is clinical
- Routine toxicology screening does not usually include β-blockers

TREATMENT

- Initially, treat bradycardia or heart block with atropine, 0.5–2 mg IV, isoproterenol, 2–20 μg/min by IV infusion, titrated to desired heart rate
- If the above measures are not successful in reversing bradycardia and hypotension, give glucagon, 5–10 mg IV, followed by infusion of 1–5 mg/h
- Administer activated charcoal, 60–100 g PO or via gastric tube, mixed in aqueous slurry; repeated doses may be given

Author(s)

Kent R. Olson, MD

Biliary Stricture

KEY FEATURES

- Results from surgical anastomosis or injury in about 95% of cases
- Cholangitis is the most common complication
- Significant hepatocellular disease resulting from secondary biliary cirrhosis is inevitable if not treated

CLINICAL FINDINGS

- Ductal injury may not be recognized in the immediate postoperative period
- With complete occlusion, jaundice develops rapidly; more often, a tear is accidentally made in the duct, with excessive or prolonged bile loss from the surgical drains as the earliest manifestation
- Typically, episodes of pain, fever, chills, and jaundice occur within a few weeks to months after cholecystectomy
- Right upper quadrant abdominal tenderness. There may be jaundice during an attack of cholangitis and right upper quadrant abdominal tenderness

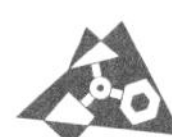

DIAGNOSIS

- Serum alkaline phosphatase is usually elevated. Hyperbilirubinemia is variable, fluctuating in the range of 5–10 mg/dL during exacerbations. Blood cultures may be positive during an episode of cholangitis
- Surgical exploration may be needed to differentiate from cholangiocarcinoma

TREATMENT

- Endoscopic retrograde cholangiopancreatography or percutaneous transhepatic cholangiography can demonstrate the stricture, permit biopsy, and allow dilation and multiple stent placement
- Endoscopic ultrasonography, intraductal ultrasonography, and cholangioscopy may help exclude malignancy
- Operative treatment frequently necessitates performance of an end-to-end ductal repair, choledochojejunostomy, or hepaticojejunostomy to reestablish bile flow into the intestine

Author(s)

Lawrence S. Friedman, MD

Bites, Snake

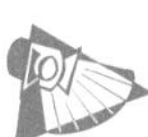

KEY FEATURES

- Venom may be neurotoxic (coral snake) or cytolytic (rattlesnakes, other pit vipers)
- Neurotoxins cause respiratory paralysis; cytolytic venoms cause tissue digestion and hemolysis with destruction of endothelial lining of blood vessels

CLINICAL FINDINGS

- Manifestations of rattlesnake envenomation: local pain, redness, swelling, extravasation of blood
- Perioral tingling, metallic taste, nausea, vomiting, hypotension, ptosis, coagulopathy, dysphagia, diplopia, and respiratory arrest can occur
- Coagulopathy common and includes prolonged PT and thrombocytopenia (sometimes severe)

TREATMENT

- Immobilize patient and bitten area in neutral position
- Avoid manipulation of area
- Do not apply ice or tourniquet
- Incision and suction of bite by unskilled persons probably not useful
- Transport patient to medical facility
- **Pit viper (eg, rattlesnake)** envenomation
  - For local signs (eg, swelling, pain, ecchymosis) but no systemic symptoms, 4–6 vials of crotalid antivenin (CroFab) by slow IV drip in 250–500 mL saline; repeat doses of 2 vials Q 6 h for up to 18 h
  - For more serious envenomation with marked local effects and systemic toxicity (eg, hypotension, coagulopathy), higher doses and additional vials may be required. Monitor vital signs and blood coagulation profile. Type and cross-match blood
  - Adequacy of venom neutralization indicated by improvement in symptoms and signs and slowed swelling rate
- **Elapid (coral snake)** envenomation
  - 1–2 vials of specific antivenom as soon as possible; call regional poison control center to locate antisera

Author(s)

Kent R. Olson, MD

Bites, Spider & Scorpion

CLINICAL FINDINGS

- Toxin of most species of spiders in the US causes only local pain, redness, swelling
- Venomous black widow spiders (*Latrodectus mactans*) cause generalized muscular pains, muscle spasms, rigidity
- Brown recluse spider (*Loxosceles reclusa*) causes progressive local necrosis as well as hemolytic reactions (rare)
- Stings by most scorpions in US cause only local pain; stings by the more toxic *Centruroides* species (found in southwestern US) may cause muscle cramps, twitching and jerking, and occasionally hypertension, convulsions, and pulmonary edema

TREATMENT

Black widow spider bites

- Relieve pain with parenteral narcotics or muscle relaxants (eg, methocarbamol, 15 mg/kg)
- Calcium gluconate 10%, 0.1–0.2 mL/kg IV, may relieve muscle rigidity
- Antivenin is available; because of concerns about acute hypersensitivity reactions it is often reserved for very young or elderly patients and those who do not respond to the above measures
- Horse serum sensitivity testing required (instruction and testing materials are in the antivenin kit)

Brown recluse spider bites

- No universally accepted management; some authorities recommend early excision of the bite site, whereas others use oral corticosteroids
- Anecdotal reports claim success with dapsone and colchicine

Scorpion stings

- For *Centruroides* stings, some toxicologists use a specific antivenom developed in Arizona, but this is neither FDA approved nor widely available

Author(s)

Kent R. Olson, MD

Blastomycosis

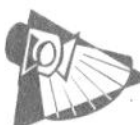

KEY FEATURES

- Most often in men infected during outdoor activities
- Geographically limited to south central and midwestern US and Canada
- A few cases found in Mexico and Africa

CLINICAL FINDINGS

- Pulmonary infection most common with cough, fever, dyspnea, chest pain; may be asymptomatic
- May resolve or progress, with bloody and purulent sputum, pleurisy, fever, chills, weight loss, prostration
- When disseminated, lesions mostly affect skin, bones, urogenital system
- Verrucous cutaneous lesions with abrupt downward sloping border. Border extends slowly, leaving central atrophic scar. Left untreated, may mimic skin cancer
- Bone lesions often in ribs and vertebrae
- Epididymitis, prostatitis, and other involvement of the male urogenital system
- CNS involvement uncommon
- In HIV-infected persons, disease may progress rapidly; dissemination common

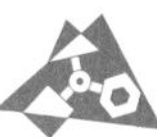

DIAGNOSIS

- Leukocytosis and anemia
- Chest x-ray or CT scan: pulmonary infiltrates and enlarged regional lymph nodes
- Bone x-ray: both destructive and proliferative lesions
- Serologic tests available but not sensitive or specific enough for definitive diagnosis
- Clinical specimen: organism is a thick-walled cell 5–20 μm in diameter; may have single broad-based bud. *Blastomyces* grows readily on culture

TREATMENT

- Itraconazole, 100–200 mg PO QD for at least 2–3 mo, for non–life-threatening, non-CNS disease, response rate of > 80%
- Amphotericin B, 0.3–0.6 mg/kg/day IV for total dose of 1.5–2.5 g, for CNS disease or treatment failures
- Monitor patients several years for relapse

Author(s)

Samuel A. Shelburne, MD

Richard J. Hamill, MD

Bone & Joint Mycotic Infections

KEY FEATURES

- **Candidal osteomyelitis**
  - Occurs in malnourished patients undergoing prolonged hospitalization for cancer, neutropenia, trauma, complicated abdominal surgical procedures, or injection drug use
  - Infected IV catheters frequently serve as a hematogenous source
- **Coccidioidomycosis**
  - Usually secondary to a primary pulmonary infection
  - Arthralgia with periarticular swelling, especially in the knees and ankles, occurring as a nonspecific manifestation of systemic coccidioidomycosis, should be distinguished from actual bone or joint infection
  - Osseous lesions commonly occur in cancellous bone of the vertebrae or near the ends of long bones at tendinous insertions; these lesions are initially osteolytic and thus may mimic metastatic tumor or myeloma

CLINICAL FINDINGS

- Joint and bone pain and swelling

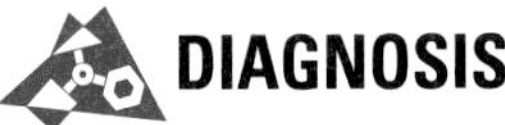

DIAGNOSIS

- Culture studies of synovial fluid
- **Coccidioidomycosis**
  - Recovery of *Coccidioides immitis* from the lesion or histologic examination of tissue obtained by open biopsy
  - Rising titers of complement-fixing antibodies also provide evidence of the disseminated nature of the disease

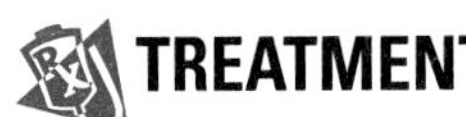

TREATMENT

- **Candidal:** fluconazole, 200 mg PO BID, is probably as effective as amphotericin
- **Coccidioidomycosis**
  - Itraconazole, 200 mg BID for 6–12 mo
  - May require operative excision of infected bone and soft tissue
  - Amputation may be the only solution for stubbornly progressive infections

Author(s)

David B. Hellmann, MD, FACP

John H. Stone, MD, MPH

Bone Tumors & Tumor-Like Lesions

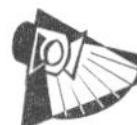

KEY FEATURES

- Persistent pain, swelling, or tenderness of a skeletal part
- Pathologic ("spontaneous") fractures
- Suspicious areas of bony enlargement, deformity, radiodensity, or radiolucency on x-ray
- Histologic evidence of bone neoplasm on biopsy specimen
- Primary tumors of bone are relatively uncommon in comparison with secondary or metastatic neoplasms
- Osteosarcoma, the most common malignancy of bone, typically occurs in adolescents

CLINICAL FINDINGS

- Osteosarcoma may present as pain or swelling in a bone or joint (especially in or around the knee)
- When the symptoms appear following a sports-related injury, accurate diagnosis may be delayed

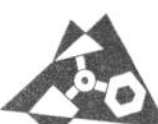

DIAGNOSIS

- Biopsy (which is not always definitive)
- Differential diagnosis
  - Benign developmental skeletal abnormalities
  - Metastatic neoplastic disease
  - Infections (eg, osteomyelitis)
  - Posttraumatic bone lesions
  - Metabolic disease of bone
  - Osteoid osteomas
  - Osteosarcoma
  - Fibrosarcomas
  - Enchondromas
  - Chondromyxoid fibromas
  - Chondrosarcomas
  - Giant cell tumors (osteoclastomas)
  - Chondroblastomas
  - Ewing's sarcoma

TREATMENT

- Chemotherapy for some
- Osteosarcomas: treated by resection and chemotherapy; 5-year survival rate of 60%
- Osteoid osteomas (seen in children and adolescents) should be surgically removed
- Tumors derived from cartilage treated with appropriate curettement or surgery have good prognosis
- Ewing's sarcoma (affects children, adolescents, and young adults), has a 50% mortality rate in spite of chemotherapy, irradiation, and surgery

Author(s)

David B. Hellmann, MD, FACP

John H. Stone, MD, MPH

Bradycardias

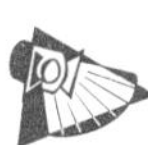

KEY FEATURES

- Bradycardia most commonly results from impaired sinus node function or from conduction abnormalities, which can occur between sinus node and atrium, within atrioventricular (AV) node or intraventricular conduction pathways
- Sick sinus syndrome (SSS) occurs most commonly in the elderly and is often caused by drugs (digitalis, calcium channel blockers, β-blockers, sympatholytic agents, antiarrhythmics) and less often by sarcoidosis, amyloidosis, Chagas' disease, and various cardiomyopathies
- AV block subtypes:
  - First-degree and second-degree Mobitz type I block occur with: (1) heightened vagal tone in normal individuals; (2) drugs that block the AV node, often in individuals with organic heart disease; and (3) ischemia, infarction, inflammatory processes, fibrosis, calcification, or infiltration
  - Second-degree Mobitz type II block occurs with organic heart disease involving the infranodal conduction system
  - Third-degree (complete) block occurs with lesions distal to the His bundle; associated with bilateral bundle branch block

CLINICAL FINDINGS

- **SSS, first- and second-degree block**
  - Most patients are asymptomatic
  - Rarely, patients experience syncope, dizziness, confusion, palpitations, heart failure, or angina pectoris
  - Symptoms are nonspecific and thus must coincide temporally with arrhythmias
- **Third-degree block**
  - Patients may be asymptomatic or may complain of weakness, dyspnea, or abrupt syncope if heart rate < 35/min
  - Slow ventricular rate, usually < 50/min, that does not increase with exercise
  - S_1 varies in intensity
  - Wide pulse pressure and changing systolic BP level
  - Cannon venous pulsations in the neck

DIAGNOSIS

- SSS: ECG shows sinus arrest, sinoatrial exit block (a pause equal to a multiple of the underlying PP interval or progressive shortening of the PP interval before a pause), or persistent sinus bradycardia
- Prolonged ambulatory Holter monitoring or event recorder may be required to document correspondence of bradycardia with symptoms
- AV block
  - First-degree: PR interval > 0.21 s with all atrial impulses conducted
  - Second-degree: intermittent blocked beats
  - Mobitz type I second-degree: progressive lengthening of PR interval and shortening of RR interval before the blocked beat
  - Mobitz type II second-degree: intermittent nonconducted atrial beats are not preceded by a lengthening PR interval
  - Third-degree (complete): ventricular rate usually < 50/min, wide QRS, and no supraventricular impulses being conducted to the ventricles
  - Narrow QRS complexes suggest nodal block
  - Wide QRS complexes suggest infranodal block
- Electrophysiological studies may be necessary for accurate localization

TREATMENT

- Discontinue offending drugs
- SSS: oral theophylline sometimes effective, especially for sinus bradycardia
- Most symptomatic patients require permanent (preferably dual-chamber) pacemaker implantation
- First-degree and Mobitz type I block: discontinue offending drugs; other therapy is not usually needed
- Mobitz type II block: prophylactic ventricular pacemaker implantation is usually required because of risk of progression to third-degree block
- Third-degree block: permanent pacemaker implantation; temporary pacing if permanent pacing is delayed

Author(s)

Thomas M. Bashore, MD

Christopher B. Granger, MD

Brain Death

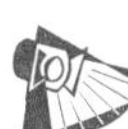

KEY FEATURES

- Irreversible coma without any brainstem reflexes, including the pupillary, corneal, oculovestibular, oculocephalic, oropharyngeal, and respiratory reflexes, and should have been in this condition for at least 6 h

CLINICAL FINDINGS

- Coma (irreversible)
- No response to external stimulation
- No brainstem reflexes
- No spontaneous respirations and no respirations during apnea test

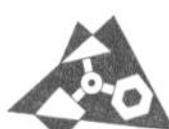

DIAGNOSIS

- The apnea test (presence or absence of spontaneous respiratory activity at a Paco$_2$ of at least 60 mm Hg) serves to determine whether the patient is capable of respiratory activity
- An isoelectric electroencephalogram recorded according to the recommendations of the American Electroencephalographic Society is especially helpful in confirming the diagnosis
- Alternatively, the demonstration of an absent cerebral circulation by intravenous radioisotope cerebral angiography or four-vessel contrast cerebral angiography can be confirmatory

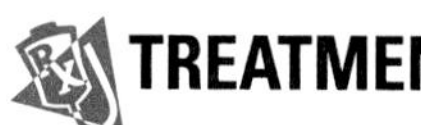

TREATMENT

- Palliative care

Author(s)

Michael J. Aminoff, MD, DSc, FRCP

Brain Mass, AIDS

KEY FEATURES

- AIDS patients may present with primary cerebral lymphoma, cerebral toxoplasmosis, or cryptococcal meningitis
- Progressive multifocal leukoencephalopathy (PML) or cytomegalovirus meningoencephalitis can occasionally have similar clinical presentations and overlapping MRI findings

CLINICAL FINDINGS

- Disturbances in cognition or consciousness
- Focal motor or sensory deficits
- Aphasia
- Seizures
- Cranial neuropathies

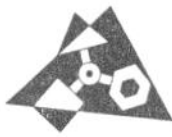

DIAGNOSIS

- Neither CT nor MRI findings distinguish primary cerebral lymphoma from toxoplasmosis
- Serologic tests for toxoplasmosis are unreliable in AIDS patients; therefore, empiric treatment helps in diagnosis
- CT scans are usually normal in cryptococcal meningitis
- Diagnosis of cryptococcal meningitis is made with positive cerebrospinal fluid India ink staining in 75–80% of cases and cryptococcal antigen tests in 95% of cases

TREATMENT

- See Non-Hodgkin's Lymphoma, Toxoplasmosis, Cryptococcal meningitis

Author(s)

Michael J. Aminoff, MD, DSc, FRCP

Brain Metastases

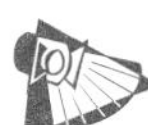

KEY FEATURES

- The most common source of intracranial metastasis is cancer of the lung followed by cancer of the breast, kidney, and gastrointestinal tract
- 10–15% of brain metastases are of unknown primary source
- Most common metastatic carcinomas to the leptomeninges are breast, lymphomas, and leukemia

CLINICAL FINDINGS

- Intracranial metastases and primary cerebral neoplasms present similarly
- Leptomeningeal metastases cause multifocal neurologic deficits from infiltration of nerve roots, direct invasion of the brain or spinal cord, or obstructive hydrocephalus. Cranial nerve palsies are common

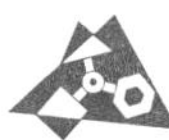

DIAGNOSIS

- Laboratory and radiology studies are the same as for primary neoplasms
- Lumbar puncture is needed only if carcinomatous meningitis is suspected; elevated cerebrospinal fluid pressure, pleocytosis, increased protein levels, and decreased glucose concentration are seen. Malignant cells may be found
- In leptomeningeal metastases, CT scans show contrast enhancement in the basal cisterns or hydrocephalus without any evidence of mass lesions
  - Gadolinium-enhanced MRI frequently shows leptomeningeal involvement
  - Myelography may show deposits on multiple nerve roots

TREATMENT

- A single cerebral metastasis may be irradiated, followed by surgical excision in some cases
- Leptomeningeal metastases receive irradiation and intrathecal methotrexate. Prognosis is poor, with only about a 10% 1-yr survival. Palliative care is important

Author(s)

Michael J. Aminoff, MD, DSc, FRCP

Breast Abscess

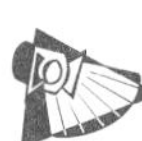

KEY FEATURES

- In lactating women, common during nursing; infection is generally caused by *Staphylococcus aureus*
- In nonlactating young or middle-aged women, subareolar abscesses are rare
- In the nonlactating breast, consider inflammatory carcinoma

CLINICAL FINDINGS

- Redness, tenderness, and induration in the breast

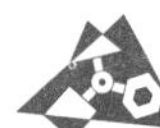

DIAGNOSIS

- In lactating women, diagnosis is generally clinical
- In nonlactating women, incision and biopsy of indurated breast tissue are indicated to rule out malignancy
- Differential diagnosis
  - Breast cancer, especially inflammatory or Paget's disease of the breast
  - Local irritation or trauma
  - Fat necrosis
  - Fibroadenoma

TREATMENT

- **Lactating women**
  - In early stages, continue nursing and treat with antibiotics: dicloxacillin or oxacillin, 250 mg PO QID for 7–10 days
  - If mass develops with local or systemic signs of infection, discontinue nursing and refer for surgical drainage
- **Nonlactating women**
  - If abscess can be percutaneously drained and completely resolves, patient may be monitored conservatively
  - However, an abscess will tend to recur after aspiration unless area is explored during a quiescent interval with excision of the involved ducts
  - Biopsy is generally required to rule out malignancy

Author(s)

Armando E. Giuliano, MD

Breast Augmentation Disorders

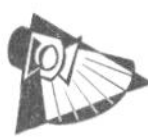 KEY FEATURES

- At least 4 million American women have had breast implants
- No increase in autoimmune disease associated with implants
- No increased risk of breast cancer associated with implants, but cancer can develop in implant patients

 CLINICAL FINDINGS

- Capsule contraction or scarring around the implant occurs in 15–25% of patients, leading to a firmness and distortion of the breast that can be painful
- Implant rupture may occur in as many as 5–10% of women, and bleeding of gel through the capsule is even more common

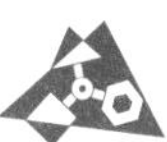 DIAGNOSIS

- Breast cancer may be more difficult to diagnose because mammography is less able to detect early lesions if implants are present

 TREATMENT

- Women should consider removal of implants if they have significant pain or symptoms of autoimmune illness
- If a cancer develops, it should be treated in the same manner as in women without implants
- Radiotherapy of the augmented breast often results in marked capsular contracture

Author(s)

Armando E. Giuliano, MD

Breast Cancer, Male

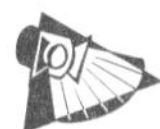 KEY FEATURES

- Rare
- Average age, 60 yr
- Poorer prognosis than for female breast cancer (even stage I)
- Blood-borne metastases are usually present
- Hormonal influences likely play an important role

 CLINICAL FINDINGS

- Painless lump beneath the areola, usually found after age 50
- Nipple discharge, retraction, or ulceration
- Gynecomastia not uncommonly precedes or accompanies male breast cancer
- Examination usually shows a hard, ill-defined, nontender mass beneath the nipple or areola
- Cancer staging is the same in men as in women

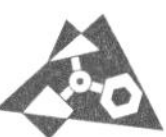 DIAGNOSIS

- Biopsy is required to confirm diagnosis
- Differential diagnosis
  - Gynecomastia
  - Metastatic cancer from another site (eg, prostate)
  - Fatty breast enlargement of obesity

 TREATMENT

- Modified radical mastectomy in operable patients
- Irradiation for localized, symptomatic metastases to skin, lymph nodes, or skeleton
- Adjuvant chemotherapy is used for the same indications as in female breast cancer
- Tamoxifen, 20 mg PO QD, for advanced-stage male breast cancer
- Castration produces regression in 60–70%, with average duration of remission of 30 mo and life prolongation; also relieves bone pain from metastases
- Medical adrenalectomy with aminoglutethimide, 250 mg PO QID, for relapse or resistant disease
- Estrogen therapy (diethylstilbestrol, 5 mg PO TID), or aromatase inhibitors may be effective as secondary hormonal manipulation after medical adrenalectomy
- 5- and 10-yr survival rates
  - Stage I: 58% and 38%, respectively
  - Stage II: 38% and 10%, respectively
  - All stages: 36% and 17%, respectively

Author(s)

Armando E. Giuliano, MD

Breast Fat Necrosis

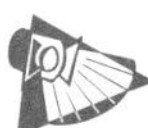

KEY FEATURES

- Rare
- Thought to be caused by trauma, but history of trauma present in only about half of patients
- Common after segmental resection, radiation therapy, or postmastectomy flap reconstruction of the breast

CLINICAL FINDINGS

- Breast mass
- Often associated with skin or nipple retraction
- Indistinguishable from cancer by examination
- Occasionally, ecchymosis present

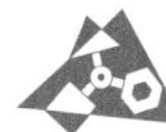

DIAGNOSIS

- Needle biopsy often adequate for diagnosis
- Occasionally, mass must be excised to exclude carcinoma
- Differential diagnosis
  - Breast cancer
  - Fibroadenoma
  - Breast abscess
  - Fibrocystic disease or cyst
  - Paget's disease of the breast

TREATMENT

- If untreated, mass effect gradually disappears

Author(s)

Armando E. Giuliano, MD

Breast Fibroadenoma

KEY FEATURES

- Common benign neoplasm
- Most frequent in young women
- Occurs somewhat more frequently and at an earlier age in black women
- Multiple fibroadenomas in 10–15% of affected patients

CLINICAL FINDINGS

- Round or ovoid, rubbery, discrete, relatively mobile, nontender mass, 1–5 cm in diameter
- Usually discovered incidentally
- Rarely occurs after menopause unless patient is receiving hormone replacement therapy

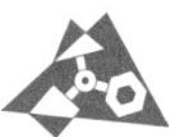

DIAGNOSIS

- Breast ultrasonography useful in differentiating cystic from solid mass
- Needle biopsy or fine-needle aspiration generally adequate for diagnosis
- Excision with pathological examination if diagnosis remains uncertain
- Differential diagnosis
  - Fibrocystic disease or cyst
  - Breast cancer
  - Lipoma
  - Phyllodes tumor
  - Breast abscess
  - Intraductal papilloma
  - Fat necrosis

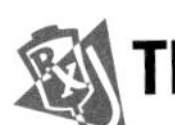

TREATMENT

- No treatment necessary

Author(s)

Armando E. Giuliano, MD

Bronchial Obstruction

KEY FEATURES

- May be caused by retained secretions, aspiration of foreign bodies (eg, peanut, hot dog), bronchogenic carcinoma, extrinsic compression, or metastatic tumors
- Recurrent pneumonia in the same location or slow resolution (>3 months) of a pneumonia suggests obstruction

CLINICAL FINDINGS

- Dyspnea, cough, wheezing, and pulmonary infection may occur
- Prolonged expiration and localized wheezing may be found
- Complete obstruction of a main stem bronchus may manifest with
  - Asymmetric chest expansion
  - Mediastinal shift
  - Absent breath sounds
  - Dullness to percussion
- X-ray films may show
  - Atelectasis
  - Postobstructive infiltrates
  - Air trapping
- CT scan may demonstrate the nature and exact location of obstruction

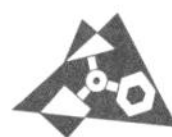

DIAGNOSIS

- Bronchoscopy is required for definitive diagnosis

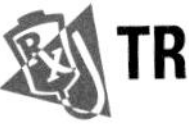

TREATMENT

- Treatment of infection, if present
- Definitive treatment depends on the cause of the obstruction

Author(s)

Mark S. Chesnutt, MD

Thomas J. Prendergast, MD

Bulimia Nervosa

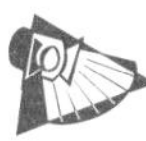

KEY FEATURES

- Uncontrolled episodes of binge eating at least twice weekly for 3 months
- Recurrent inappropriate compensation to prevent weight gain, such as self-induced vomiting, laxatives, diuretics, fasting, or excessive exercise
- Overconcern with weight and body shape
- Occurs predominantly in young, white, middle- and upper-class women

CLINICAL FINDINGS

- Consuming large quantities of easily ingested high-calorie foods, usually in secrecy, followed by vomiting, cathartics, or diuretics accompanied by feelings of guilt or depression
- Body weight fluctuates but generally within 20% of desirable weight
- Menstruation is usually preserved

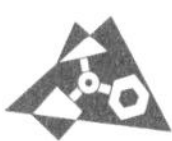

DIAGNOSIS

- History and identification of behavioral features
- Differential diagnosis
  - Anorexia nervosa
  - Depression
  - Obsessive-compulsive disorder
  - Personality disorder
  - Substance abuse

TREATMENT

- Antidepressant medications such as fluoxetine hydrochloride and other selective serotonin reuptake inhibitors
- Psychotherapy (individual, group, family)

Author(s)

Robert B. Baron, MD, MS

Bursitis

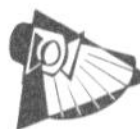

KEY FEATURES

- Inflammation from trauma, infection, or arthritis (eg, gout, rheumatoid arthritis, or osteoarthritis)
- Subdeltoid, olecranon, ischial, trochanteric, semimembranous-gastrocnemius (Baker's cyst), and prepatellar bursae are common locations

CLINICAL FINDINGS

- More likely than arthritis to begin abruptly and be tender and swollen
- Active and passive range of motion is usually much more limited in arthritis than in bursitis

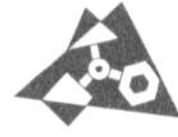

DIAGNOSIS

- Acute swelling and redness calls for aspiration to rule out infection
- A bursal fluid white blood cell count of greater than 1000/μL indicates inflammation from infection, rheumatoid arthritis, or gout
- In septic bursitis, the white cell count averages over 50,000/μL; most cases are caused by *Staphylococcus aureus*
- Chronic, stable olecranon bursa swelling without erythema or other signs of inflammation is unlikely to be infected and does not require aspiration
- A bursa can become symptomatic when it ruptures (eg, Baker's cyst, which, on rupture, can cause calf pain and swelling that mimic thrombophlebitis)
- Treatment of a ruptured cyst includes rest, leg elevation, and injection of triamcinolone, 20–40 mg, into the knee (which communicates with the cyst)

TREATMENT

- Traumatic bursitis responds to local heat, rest, immobilization, NSAIDs, and local corticosteroid injections
- Bursectomy is indicated only when there are repeated infections
- Avoid repetitive minor trauma to the olecranon bursa by not resting the elbow on a hard surface or by wearing an elbow pad

Author(s)

David B. Hellmann, MD, FACP

John H. Stone, MD, MPH

Calcium Channel Blocker Overdose

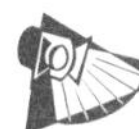

KEY FEATURES

- All calcium channel blockers (including verapamil, diltiazem, nifedipine, nicardipine, amlodipine, felodipine, isradipine, nisoldipine, nimodipine) share the ability to cause arteriolar vasodilation and depression of cardiac contractility after acute overdose

CLINICAL FINDINGS

- Bradycardia, AV nodal block, hypotension, or a combination
- With severe poisoning, cardiac arrest may occur

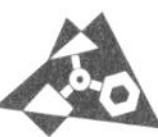

DIAGNOSIS

- Clinical
- Junctional bradycardia is a common finding with even moderate verapamil poisoning

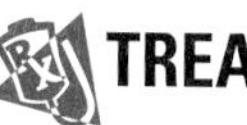

TREATMENT

- Administer activated charcoal 60–100 g mixed in aqueous slurry PO or via gastric tube. Do not use for comatose or convulsing patients unless they are endotracheally intubated
- In addition, perform whole-bowel irrigation as soon as possible if a sustained-release product has been ingested
- Treat hypotension and bradycardia with calcium chloride IV
  - Start with calcium chloride 10%, 10 mL, or calcium gluconate, 20 mL. Repeat the dose Q 3–5 min
  - The optimum (or maximum) dose has not been established, but there are reports of success after as much as 10–12 g of calcium chloride
  - Calcium is most useful in reversing negative inotropic effects and is less effective for AV nodal blockade and bradycardia
- Epinephrine infusion, 1–4 μg/min initially, and glucagon, 5–10 mg IV, have also been given with variable success
- A transcutaneous or internal cardiac pacemaker may be needed

Author(s)

Kent R. Olson, MD

Calluses & Corns, Feet & Toes

KEY FEATURES

- Callosities and corns are caused by pressure and friction resulting from faulty weight bearing, orthopedic deformities, improperly fitting shoes, neuropathies

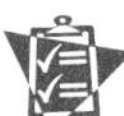

CLINICAL FINDINGS

- Tenderness on pressure and "after-pain" are the only symptoms
- The hyperkeratotic well-localized overgrowths always occur at pressure points
- Fingerprint lines are preserved over the surface (not so in warts)
- On paring, a glassy core is found (differentiating these disorders from plantar warts, which have multiple capillary bleeding points or black dots when pared)
- A soft corn often occurs laterally on the proximal portion of the fourth toe as a result of pressure against the bony structure of the interphalangeal joint of the fifth toe

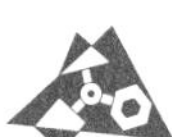

DIAGNOSIS

- Clinical

TREATMENT

- Treatment consists of correcting mechanical abnormalities that cause friction and pressure
- Shoes must be properly fitted and orthopedic deformities corrected
- Callosities may be removed by careful paring of the callus after a warm-water soak or with keratolytic agents as found in various brands of corn pads
- Plantar hyperkeratosis of the heels can be treated successfully using 20% urea (Ureacin 20), urea/lactic acid combinations (Ulactin), or 12% lactic acid (Lac-Hydrin) nightly and a pumice stone after soaking in water

Author(s)

Timothy G. Berger, MD

Campylobacter Infections

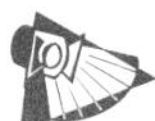

KEY FEATURES

- Microaerophilic, motile, gram-negative rods
- Two species infect humans
  - *Campylobacter jejuni*, an important cause of diarrheal disease
  - *Campylobacter fetus* subsp *fetus*, typically causes systemic infection and not diarrhea
- Dairy cattle and poultry are important reservoirs

CLINICAL FINDINGS

- *Campylobacter* gastroenteritis
  - Fever
  - Abdominal pain
  - Diarrhea characterized by loose, watery, or bloody stools
  - Disease is self-limited, but its duration can be shortened with antimicrobial therapy
- *C fetus*
  - Causes systemic infections that can be fatal, including primary bacteremia, endocarditis, meningitis, and focal abscesses
  - Infrequently causes gastroenteritis
  - Infected patients are often elderly, debilitated, or immunocompromised
  - Closely related species, collectively termed "*Campylobacter*-like organisms," cause bacteremia in HIV-infected individuals

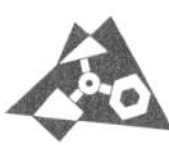

DIAGNOSIS

- Blood culture
- Stool culture

TREATMENT

- Both erythromycin, 250–500 mg QID for 5–7 days, and ciprofloxacin, 500 mg BID for 3–5 days, are effective regimens
- *C fetus*: Systemic infections respond to therapy with gentamicin, chloramphenicol, ceftriaxone, or ciprofloxacin. Ceftriaxone or chloramphenicol should be used to treat infections of the central nervous system because of their ability to penetrate the blood–brain barrier

Author(s)

Henry F. Chambers, MD

Cancer, Infectious Complications

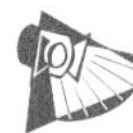

KEY FEATURES

- Increased susceptibility to bacterial, opportunistic infection
- Caused by impaired host defense mechanisms or myelosuppressive/immunosuppressive chemotherapy effects
- ≥ 50% of infections in neutropenic patients endogenous
- Incidence of bacteremia rises with WBC count < 1000/μL, granulocytes < 200/μL
- Common infections
  - *Enterobacteriaceae*
  - *Pseudomonas*
  - *Staphylococcus*
  - *Streptococcus*
  - *Corynebacterium*
  - *C difficile*
- Increased infection risk with prolonged neutropenia or post-bone marrow transplantation (BMT)
  - Fungal
  - Parasitic
  - Viral

CLINICAL FINDINGS

- Fever in neutropenia (not always in patients on corticosteroids)
- Shaking chills, hypotension, breathing difficulties

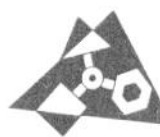

DIAGNOSIS

- CBC with differential
- Urinalysis
- CXR
- Urine, blood cultures
- Symptom-directed evaluation

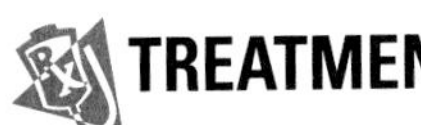

TREATMENT

Prophylaxis

- PO antibiotics in low risk, levofloxacin in higher risk
- IVIG with B-cell malignancies (chronic lymphocytic leukemia, multiple myeloma, BMT), acute infections
- G-CSF and GM-CSF
  - Reduce duration of neutropenia and frequency/severity of infection after myelosuppressive chemotherapy or BMT for nonmyeloid malignancies
  - For prophylaxis and/or treatment

Therapy

- Treat immediately before cultures positive
- Initial monotherapy with 3rd-generation cephalosporin or combination β-lactam
- Add vancomycin or amphotericin B based on clinical suspicion, culture results, prolonged fever in absence of positive cultures
- For persistent fevers or clinical deterioration, change gram-negative coverage to broader spectrum agent (eg, imipenem/meropenem)
- If *Stenotrophomonas* suspected, add TMP-SMX

Author(s)

Hope Rugo, MD

Candidiasis, Oral

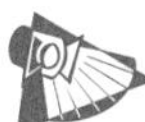

KEY FEATURES

- Commonly encountered among denture wearers, in patients in debilitated states, in persons with diabetes or anemia, in those undergoing chemotherapy or local irradiation, or in persons taking corticosteroids or broad-spectrum antibiotics
- Often heralds HIV infection
- Angular cheilitis is a symptom, although it can be seen in nutritional deficiencies

CLINICAL FINDINGS

- Painful creamy-white curd-like patches
- White patches can be easily rubbed off by a tongue depressor, unlike leukoplakia or lichen planus, revealing an underlying irregular erythema

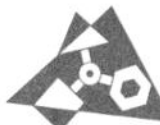

DIAGNOSIS

- Clinical
- A wet preparation using potassium hydroxide will reveal spores and may show nonseptate mycelia
- Biopsy will show intraepithelial pseudomycelia of *Candida albicans*

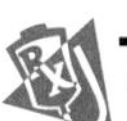

TREATMENT

- Medications
  - Fluconazole (100 mg daily for 7–14 days)
  - Ketoconazole (200–400 mg with breakfast [requires acidic gastric environment for absorption] for 7–14 days)
  - Clotrimazole troches (10 mg dissolved orally 5 times daily)
  - Nystatin vaginal troches (100,000 units dissolved PO 5 times daily) or mouth rinses (500,000 units [5 mL of 100,000 units/mL] held in the mouth before swallowing TID)
- Shorter duration therapy with fluconazole is effective
- In HIV infection, longer courses may be needed, and itraconazole (200 mg PO daily) may be indicated in fluconazole-refractory cases
- 0.12% chlorhexidine or half-strength hydrogen peroxide mouth rinses may provide local relief
- Nystatin powder (100,000 units/g) applied to dentures 3 or 4 times daily for several weeks may help denture wearers

Author(s)

Robert K. Jackler, MD
Michael J. Kaplan, MD

Carbon Monoxide Poisoning

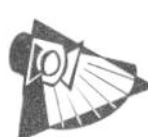

KEY FEATURES

- Avidly binds to hemoglobin, which results in reduced oxygen-carrying capacity and altered delivery of oxygen to cells

CLINICAL FINDINGS

- At low carbon monoxide levels (carboxyhemoglobin < 25%) there may be headache, dizziness, nausea
- With higher levels, confusion, dyspnea, and syncope may occur
- Hypotension, coma, and seizures are common with levels > 50–60%
- Survivors of acute severe poisoning may develop permanent neurological deficits

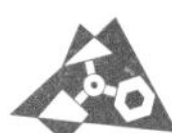

DIAGNOSIS

- Suspect in the setting of severe headache or acutely altered mental status, especially if multiple victims
- Diagnosis depends on specific measurement of the arterial or venous carboxyhemoglobin saturation, although the level may have declined if high-flow oxygen therapy has already been administered
- Routine arterial blood gas testing and pulse oximetry are not useful because they may give falsely normal oxyhemoglobin saturation levels

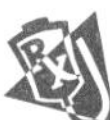

TREATMENT

- Remove victim from exposure
- Administer 100% oxygen by tight-fitting high-flow reservoir face mask or endotracheal tube
- Hyperbaric oxygen can provide 100% oxygen under higher than atmospheric pressures, further shortening the half-life; it may be useful if readily available for patients with coma or seizures and in pregnant women

Author(s)

Kent R. Olson, MD

Carcinoid Syndrome, Malignant

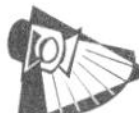

KEY FEATURES

- Uncommon
- Caused by tumors of argentaffin cells such as carcinoid tumors of the small bowel metastatic to the liver; less commonly, primary carcinoid tumors of lung or stomach
- Related syndromes occur in patients with pancreatic tumors
- Caused by release of vasoactive substances: serotonin, histamine, catecholamines, prostaglandins, vasoactive intestinal peptide

CLINICAL FINDINGS

- Facial flushing, telangiectasias
- Abdominal cramps and diarrhea
- Bronchospasm
- Edema of the head and neck (especially with bronchial carcinoid)
- Cardiac valvular lesions (tricuspid or pulmonary stenosis or regurgitation)

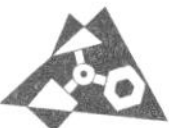

DIAGNOSIS

- 24-h urine 5-hydroxyindoleacetic acid (5-HIAA) is increased to > 25 mg/day

TREATMENT

- Prednisone, 15–30 mg/day
- Hydration and diphenoxylate with atropine for diarrhea
- Octreotide acetate, 100–600 μg/day SC in 2–4 divided doses, is the most effective agent for reducing symptoms and levels of urinary 5-HIAA
- Surgical resection of localized carcinoid tumors
- Cyproheptadine, 4 mg PO TID, or methysergide maleate, 2 mg PO TID (up to 16 mg) for severe diarrhea
- Cimetidine and phenothiazines also helpful
- Chemotherapy is moderately effective in metastatic disease

Author(s)

Hope Rugo, MD

Carcinoid Tumors, Bronchial

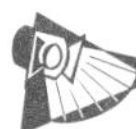

KEY FEATURES

- Diagnosis includes carcinoid and bronchial gland tumors, which are low-grade malignancies
- Most patients are younger than 60 years
- Men and women are affected equally
- Tumors grow slowly and rarely metastasize

CLINICAL FINDINGS

- Common symptoms
  - Hemoptysis
  - Cough
  - Focal wheezing
  - Recurrent pneumonia
- Carcinoid syndrome is rare
- Bronchoscopy may reveal a pink or purple tumor in a central airway
- Complications involve bleeding and airway obstruction rather than tumor invasion or spread

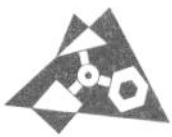

DIAGNOSIS

- Biopsy may be complicated by significant bleeding
- CT is useful to localize lesions and follow their growth over time
- Octreotide scintigraphy may aid in tumor localization

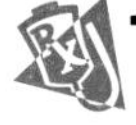

TREATMENT

- Surgical excision is necessary in some cases
- Prognosis is generally favorable
- Most bronchial carcinoid tumors are resistant to radiation or chemotherapy

Author(s)

Mark S. Chesnutt, MD

Thomas J. Prendergast, MD

Carcinoid Tumors, Gastric

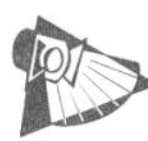

KEY FEATURES

- Gastric carcinoids are rare tumors, accounting for < 1% of gastric neoplasms
- Occur sporadically (20%) or secondary to chronic hypergastrinemia (80%)
- Most sporadic carcinoids
  - Solitary
  - >2 cm in size
  - Have strong propensity for metastatic spread and carcinoid syndrome
- Carcinoids secondary to chronic hypergastrinemia
  - Occur in association either with pernicious anemia (75%) or Zollinger-Ellison syndrome with multiple endocrine neoplasia type I (5%)
  - They tend to be multicentric, are < 1 cm in size, and have a low potential for metastatic spread and carcinoid syndrome
- Metastatic gastric carcinoid causes elevated serum levels of 5-hydroxytryptophan (unlike metastatic small intestinal carcinoid, which causes elevated levels of serotonin or 5-hydroxyindoleacetic acid)

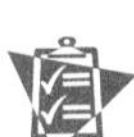

CLINICAL FINDINGS

- Most are asymptomatic and are detected incidentally during endoscopy
- Gastric carcinoids may ulcerate, causing occult GI bleeding and anemia
- Metastatic gastric carcinoids may present with atypical carcinoid syndrome manifested by flushing and diarrhea

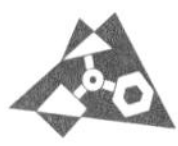

DIAGNOSIS

- Endoscopy demonstrates solitary or multiple nodules, which may be umbilicated or ulcerated
- Diagnosis is confirmed by biopsy showing small, round cells proved to be neuroendocrine cells by silver and immunohistochemical stains
- Staging includes abdominal CT scan and nuclear somatostatin receptor scintography

TREATMENT

- Small lesions are treated with endoscopic resection followed by periodic endoscopic surveillance
- Alternatively, antrectomy reduces serum gastrin levels and may lead to regression in patients with multiple lesions
- Large or multiple carcinoids are treated with surgical tumor resection
- Symptomatic metastatic disease is treated with resection, if possible
  - Somatostatin analog therapy (octreotide) or hepatic arterial chemoembolization is sometimes useful

Author(s)

Kenneth R. McQuaid, MD

Cardiomyopathy, Hypertrophic

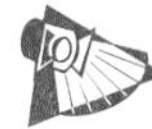

KEY FEATURES

- Myocardial hypertrophy impinging on the left ventricular (LV) cavity, narrowing the LV outflow tract during systole, can cause dynamic obstruction
- Obstruction is worsened by sympathetic stimulation, digoxin, postextrasystolic beats, Valsalva's maneuver, peripheral vasodilator drugs
- Inherited form has autosomal dominant inheritance and usually presents in early adulthood
- Acquired form presents as diastolic dysfunction in elderly patients with a long history of hypertension
- Atrial fibrillation is a long-term consequence and a poor prognostic sign
- Ventricular arrhythmias are common
- Sudden death may occur, often in athletes after extraordinary exertion

CLINICAL FINDINGS

- Often presents with dyspnea, chest pain, or syncope (typically postexertional)
- Physical examination: prominent "a" wave in jugular pulse, bisferiens carotid pulse, sustained or triple apical impulse, and loud S_4
- Loud systolic murmur along left sternal border that increases with upright posture or Valsalva's maneuver and decreases with squatting; mitral regurgitation is frequently present

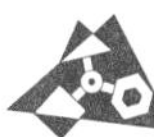

DIAGNOSIS

- Chest x-ray: often unimpressive
- ECG: LV hypertrophy and, occasionally, septal Q waves in the absence of myocardial infarction
- Echo-Doppler: ventricular hypertrophy, which may be asymmetric; usually normal or enhanced contractility and signs of dynamic obstruction; systolic anterior motion of mitral valve if outflow tract obstruction; can confirm outflow tract gradient and diastolic filling abnormalities

TREATMENT

- β-blockers (Table 47) indicated in symptomatic individuals, especially

when dynamic outflow obstruction is noted on echocardiogram
- Calcium channel blockers, especially verapamil (Table 49), or disopyramide also effective
- Diuretics (Table 46) for high diastolic and pulmonary capillary wedge pressures
- Nonsurgical septal ablation by injection of alcohol into septal branches of the left coronary artery
- Implantable defibrillator for malignant ventricular arrhythmias or unexplained syncope
- Attempt cardioversion of atrial fibrillation
- Endocarditis prophylaxis

Author(s)

Thomas M. Bashore, MD
Christopher B. Granger, MD

Cardiomyopathy, Peripartum

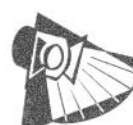 KEY FEATURES

- Defined as heart failure during pregnancy or in the first 6 mo postpartum in a woman with no other cause
- Incidence from 1:4000 to 1:1000, higher in Africa; at risk are older women, mothers with twins, and patients with pregnancy-induced hypertension
- Cause unknown
- Mortality is 6% at 5 yr in patients with cardiomegaly 6 mo from symptom onset, with 50% recurrence rate in subsequent pregnancy and a 19% mortality rate

 CLINICAL FINDINGS

- Congestive heart failure
- Sinus tachycardia and atrial or ventricular arrhythmias
- Death may result from a fatal arrhythmia or embolism

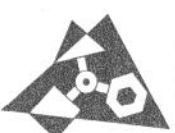 DIAGNOSIS

- Clinical presentation with echocardiographic findings of dilated cardiomyopathy and exclusion of other causes

 TREATMENT

- Treat as for other causes of congestive heart failure (see Congestive Heart Failure)

Author(s)

William R. Crombleholme, MD

Cardiomyopathy, Primary Dilated

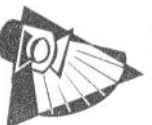 KEY FEATURES

- Left ventricular (LV) dilation and systolic dysfunction (ejection fraction < 50%)
- Symptoms and signs of congestive heart failure (most commonly dyspnea)
- Causes
  - Chronic alcohol abuse
  - Unrecognized myocarditis
  - Chronic tachycardia
  - Amyloidosis
  - Sarcoidosis
  - Hemochromatosis
  - Arrhythmogenic right ventricular (RV) dysplasia
  - Uhl's disease
- Often no cause can be identified
- Not associated with ischemic heart disease, hypertension, valvular disease, or congenital defects

 CLINICAL FINDINGS

- Heart failure usually develops gradually, but initial presentation may be severe biventricular failure
- Physical examination
  - Low blood pressure
  - Rales
  - Edema
  - Cardiomegaly
  - Elevated jugular venous pressure, S_3 and S_4 gallops
  - Murmurs of mitral and tricuspid regurgitation
- Arterial and pulmonary emboli
- Annual mortality rate of 11–13%

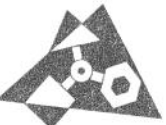 DIAGNOSIS

- ECG: low QRS voltage, sinus tachycardia, LBBB, ventricular or atrial arrhythmias
- Chest x-ray film: cardiomegaly, pulmonary venous congestion, pleural effusions
- Echo-Doppler
  - LV dilatation, thinning, and global dysfunction
  - Can exclude valvular or other lesions
- Exercise or pharmacologic stress myocardial perfusion imaging may suggest underlying coronary disease

- Cardiac MRI helpful in infiltrative diseases

 TREATMENT

- Few cases are amenable to specific therapy
- Discontinue alcohol use
- Treat thyroid dysfunction, acromegaly, pheochromocytoma
- Immunosuppressive therapy is not indicated
- Treat congestive heart failure (see *Congestive heart failure*)
- Long-term anticoagulation for emboli
- Consider biventricular pacing (resynchronization) and implantable cardioverter-defibrillator

Author(s)

Thomas M. Bashore, MD

Christopher B. Granger, MD

Carotid Artery Aneurysm

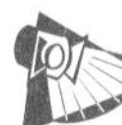 KEY FEATURES

- Much more common in the intracerebral than the cervical portion of carotid arteries
- Most often, cervical aneurysms arise in the common carotid artery, are fusiform, and are associated with atherosclerosis
- Traumatic aneurysms can be related to healing of an internal carotid dissection or to penetrating trauma
- Mycotic aneurysms can be caused by staphylococcal, *Escherichia coli*, or tuberculous infections
- Other causes: vasculitides, Behçet's disease, Takayasu's disease, fibromuscular dysplasia, and segmental arterial mediolysis

 CLINICAL FINDINGS

- Pulsatile mass in the neck
- Neck pain
- Cranial nerve dysfunction
- Transient ischemic attack or stroke

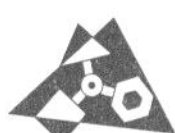 DIAGNOSIS

- Diagnosis confirmed by angiography

 TREATMENT

- Surgery indicated for aneurysms resulting from penetrating trauma, aneurysms associated with neurological deficit, mycotic aneurysms, enlarging aneurysms, and aneurysms > 2 cm diameter
- Primary repair of the artery indicated for most penetrating injuries
- Carotid resection and interposition grafting or simple carotid ligation indicated for most other aneurysms

Author(s)

Louis M. Messina, MD

Carotid Body Tumor

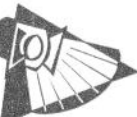 KEY FEATURES

- Carotid body tumors are also called paraganglionomas or chemodectomas
- Rare
- Usually present as painless neck masses
- Most are slow growing and benign, but lymph node metastases have been reported

 CLINICAL FINDINGS

- If untreated, they are locally invasive; a large tumor may cause vagus or hypoglossal nerve deficit from mass effect or may encircle the internal carotid artery to the skull base

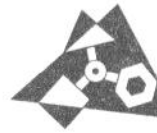 DIAGNOSIS

- Biopsy is contraindicated; diagnosis is made by angiography or MRA
- The tumor is hypervascular, splays the internal and external carotid arteries, and produces angiographic tumor blush in the center of a widened carotid bifurcation

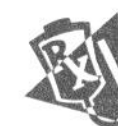 TREATMENT

- Preoperative angiography is performed for tumor embolization and test occlusion of the internal carotid artery for tumors > 4 cm diameter
- Resection of large tumors is complicated by cranial nerve injury in 40%
- Excellent prognosis after complete resection; survival is equal to that of age-matched controls and long-term recurrence of only 6%

Author(s)

Louis M. Messina, MD

Carotid Dissection

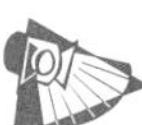

KEY FEATURES

- A false channel in the wall of the carotid artery produced by a tear in the intima
- May be spontaneous or traumatic (shearing of the internal carotid artery between the C2 and C3 transverse processes during deceleration injuries)

CLINICAL FINDINGS

- Classic triad of symptoms: unilateral neck pain or headache, stroke or transient ischemic attack, and incomplete Horner's syndrome (miosis and ptosis without anhidrosis)

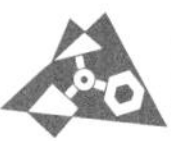

DIAGNOSIS

- Diagnosis confirmed at angiography or CT angiography
- Noncontrast CT of the head to confirm no intracranial hemorrhage

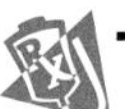

TREATMENT

- Primary treatment is heparin followed by warfarin anticoagulation (to an INR of 2.0–3.0)
- With such treatment, 60–85% of carotid dissections will recannulate in 3–6 mo with complete or near-complete neurological recovery
- Recurrent dissection occurs in ~3% at 3 years and ~12% at 10 years
- Recurrent dissection most often involves a different cervical vessel, which justifies use of long-term aspirin
- Surgery (usually carotid interposition) or carotid stenting is indicated for ongoing symptoms with residual stenosis or aneurysm

Author(s)

Louis M. Messina, MD

Carpal Tunnel Syndrome

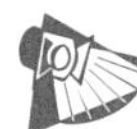

KEY FEATURES

- An entrapment neuropathy from compression of the median nerve in the carpal tunnel, particularly from synovitis of the tendon sheaths or carpal joints and recent or poorly healed fractures
- Most often afflicts those who perform repetitive hand movements
- Associated with pregnancy, rheumatoid arthritis, myxedema, amyloidosis, sarcoidosis, leukemia (tissue infiltration), acromegaly, and hyperparathyroidism

CLINICAL FINDINGS

- Pain, burning, or tingling in the distribution of the median nerve
- Aching pain may radiate proximally into the forearm and occasionally to the shoulder
- Pain is exacerbated by manual activity, particularly by extremes of volar flexion or dorsiflexion of wrist
- Impairment of sensation in the median nerve distribution may be demonstrable
- Tinel's or Phalen's sign may be positive. (Tinel's sign is shock-like pain on volar wrist percussion; Phalen's sign is pain in the distribution of the median nerve when both wrists are flexed 90° with the dorsal aspects of the hands held in apposition for 1 min)
- Muscle weakness or atrophy, especially of the thenar eminence, appears later than sensory disturbances

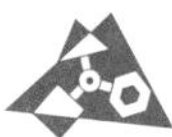

DIAGNOSIS

- Electromyography and determinations of segmental sensory and motor conduction delay

TREATMENT

- Change of manual activity (or ergonomic improvements); splinting of the hand and forearm at night
- NSAIDs and/or injection of corticosteroid by an experienced operator into the carpal tunnel
- Operative division of the volar carpal ligament gives lasting relief from pain

Author(s)

David B. Hellmann, MD, FACP

John H. Stone, MD, MPH

Cat Scratch Disease

KEY FEATURES

- Cat scratch disease is an acute infection of children and young adults caused by *Bartonella henselae*
- It is transmitted from cats to humans as the result of a scratch or bite
- Disseminated forms of the disease—bacillary angiomatosis and peliosis hepatis—occur in HIV-infected persons

CLINICAL FINDINGS

- A papule or ulcer will develop at the inoculation site within a few days in one-third of patients
- Fever, headache, and malaise occur 1–3 weeks later
- The regional lymph nodes become enlarged, often tender, and may suppurate
- Lymphadenopathy resembles that resulting from neoplasm, tuberculosis, lymphogranuloma venereum, and bacterial lymphadenitis
- Encephalitis occurs rarely

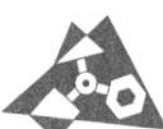

DIAGNOSIS

- Clinical
- Special cultures for *Bartonella,* serology, or excisional biopsy, although rarely necessary, confirm the diagnosis
- The biopsy reveals necrotizing lymphadenitis and is itself not specific for cat scratch disease

TREATMENT

- Cat scratch disease is usually self-limited, requiring no specific therapy
- Bacillary angiomatosis and endocarditis respond to treatment with a macrolide (eg, azithromycin, 500 mg QD) or doxycycline, 100 mg BID for 4–8 weeks

Author(s)

Henry F. Chambers, MD

Cataract

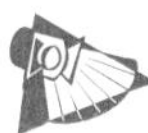

KEY FEATURES

- Cataract means lens opacity
- Cataracts usually occur bilaterally
- Senile (age-related) cataract is the most common type
- Most persons older than 60 have some degree of lens opacity
- Other causes include congenital infections, diabetes mellitus, chronic corticosteroid use, uveitis, and ocular trauma

CLINICAL FINDINGS

- Usually gradually progressive visual impairment

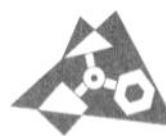

DIAGNOSIS

- Ophthalmoscopy, particularly with a dilated pupil, shows opacities in the red reflex
- As the cataract progresses, retinal visualization becomes increasingly difficult

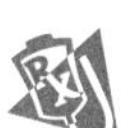

TREATMENT

- When visual impairment significantly affects daily activities, surgical therapy is usually warranted
- Treatment involves surgical removal and insertion of an intraocular lens of appropriate refractive power

Author(s)

Paul Riordan-Eva, FRCOphth

Cerumen Impaction

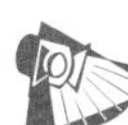

KEY FEATURES

- Cerumen is a protective secretion produced by the outer portion of the ear canal
- In most individuals, the ear canal is self-cleansing
- In most cases, cerumen impaction is self-induced through ill-advised attempts at cleaning the ear

CLINICAL FINDINGS

- Fullness in ear
- Conductive hearing loss when accumulation blocks the canal

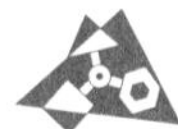

DIAGNOSIS

- Made by otoscopic inspection

TREATMENT

- Recommended hygiene consists of cleaning the external opening with a washcloth over the index finger without entering the canal itself
- May be relieved with detergent ear drops (eg, 3% hydrogen peroxide; 6.5% carbamide peroxide), mechanical removal, suction, or irrigation
- Irrigation is performed with water at body temperature to avoid a vestibular caloric response, which could produce nystagmus and nausea. The stream should be directed at the ear canal wall adjacent to the cerumen plug
- Irrigation should be performed only when the tympanic membrane is known to be intact
- Use of jet irrigators designed for cleaning teeth (eg, WaterPik) for wax removal should be avoided because they may result in tympanic membrane perforations
- After irrigation, the ear canal should be thoroughly dried (eg, by instilling isopropyl alcohol or using a hair blow-dryer on low-power setting) to reduce the likelihood of inducing external otitis
- Specialty referral for cleaning under microscopic guidance is indicated when the impaction has not responded to routine measures or if the patient has a history of chronic otitis media or tympanic membrane perforation

Author(s)

Robert K. Jackler, MD

Michael J. Kaplan, MD

Cervical Polyps

KEY FEATURES

- Commonly occur after menarche and are occasionally noted in postmenopausal women
- The cause is not known, but inflammation may play an etiologic role
- Must be differentiated from polypoid neoplastic disease of the endometrium, small submucous pedunculated myomas, and endometrial polyps
- Cervical polyps rarely contain malignant foci

CLINICAL FINDINGS

- Discharge and abnormal vaginal bleeding
- Abnormal bleeding should not be ascribed to a cervical polyp without sampling the endocervix and endometrium

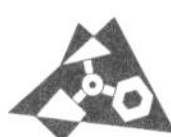

DIAGNOSIS

- The polyps are visible in the cervical os on speculum examination

TREATMENT

- Cervical polyps can generally be removed in the office by avulsion with a uterine packing forceps or ring forceps
- If the cervix is soft, patulous, or definitely dilated and the polyp is large, surgical D&C is required (especially if the pedicle is not readily visible)
- Because of the possibility of endometrial disease, cervical polypectomy should be accompanied by endometrial sampling, and all tissue removed should be submitted for microscopic examination

Author(s)

H. Trent MacKay, MD, MPH

Cervicitis

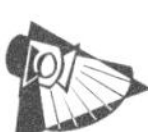

KEY FEATURES

- Infection of the cervix must be distinguished from physiologic ectopy of columnar epithelium, which is common in young women
- Infection may result from a sexually transmitted pathogen such as *Neisseria gonorrhoeae, Chlamydia,* or herpesvirus
- In most cases, none of these organisms can be isolated

CLINICAL FINDINGS

- Mucopurulent cervicitis is characterized by a red edematous cervix with a purulent yellow discharge
- Herpesvirus presents with vesicles and ulcers on the cervix during a primary herpetic infection

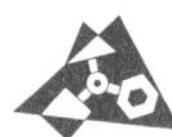

DIAGNOSIS

- Mucopurulent cervicitis is an insensitive predictor of either gonorrheal or chlamydial infection and in addition has a low positive predictive value

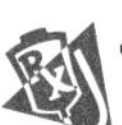

TREATMENT

- Treatment should be based on microbiologic testing
- Presumptive antibiotic treatment is not indicated unless there is a high prevalence of either *N gonorrhoeae* or *Chlamydia* in the population or if the patient is unlikely to return for treatment
- Three months after treatment, approximately 20% of women will have persistent or recurrent mucopus in the cervix, not explained by relapse or reinfection

Author(s)

H. Trent MacKay, MD, MPH

Chancroid

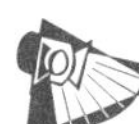

KEY FEATURES

- A sexually transmitted disease caused by the gram-negative bacillus *Haemophilus ducreyi*
- Incubation period is 3–5 days

CLINICAL FINDINGS

- Initial lesion at the site of inoculation is a vesicopustule that breaks down to form a painful, soft ulcer with a necrotic base, surrounding erythema, and undermined edges
- Multiple lesions, started by autoinoculation, and inguinal adenitis often develop
- The adenitis is usually unilateral and consists of tender, matted nodes of moderate size with overlying erythema. These may become fluctuant and rupture spontaneously
- With lymph node involvement, fever, chills, and malaise may develop
- Balanitis and phimosis are frequent complications in men
- Women may have no external signs of infection

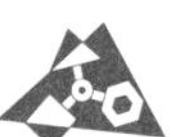

DIAGNOSIS

- Culturing a swab of the lesion onto special medium

TREATMENT

- A single dose of either azithromycin, 1 g PO, or ceftriaxone, 250 mg IM, is effective treatment
- Effective multiple-dose regimens are amoxicillin-potassium clavulanate, 500/125 mg, PO TID for 7 days; erythromycin, 500 mg PO QID for 7 days; or ciprofloxacin, 500 mg PO BID for 3 days

Author(s)

Henry F. Chambers, MD

Cholecystectomy, Pre- & Post- Syndrome

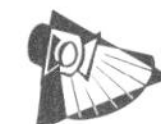

KEY FEATURES

PRECHOLECYSTECTOMY

- In a few patients (mostly women) with biliary colic, conventional radiographic studies of the upper gastrointestinal tract and gallbladder, including cholangiography, are unremarkable
  - However, emptying of the gallbladder is markedly reduced on gallbladder scintigraphy after injection of cholecystokinin
  - This may occur from fibrotic stenosis, adhesions or kinking of the cystic duct, ampullary spasm, or biliary dyskinesia

POSTCHOLECYSTECTOMY

- After cholecystectomy, some continue to complain about right upper quadrant pain, flatulence, and fatty food intolerance
- Choledocholithiasis or common duct stricture should be ruled out as a cause of persistent symptoms
- Pain has been associated with dilation of the cystic duct remnant, neuroma formation in the ductal wall, foreign body granuloma, or traction on the common duct by a long cystic duct

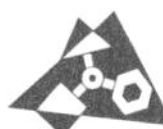

DIAGNOSIS

- Abdominal or endoscopic ultrasonography or retrograde cholangiography may exclude biliary tract disease
- Biliary manometry may document elevated baseline sphincter of Oddi pressures typical of sphincter dysfunction
- Biliary scintigraphy and magnetic resonance cholangiopancreatography following IV secretin shows promise as a screening test for sphincter dysfunction

TREATMENT

- Cholecystectomy is usually curative for precholecystectomy symptoms
- Endoscopic sphincterotomy can relieve symptoms of postcholecystectomy syndrome associated with a dilated common bile duct and elevated liver tests or elevated sphincter pressure on manometry

Author(s)

Lawrence S. Friedman, MD

Chromoblastomycosis

KEY FEATURES

- A chronic, principally tropical cutaneous infection
- Usually affects young men who are agricultural workers and are infected by traumatic inoculation or due to contact with soil
- Caused by several species of closely related black molds (*Fonsecaea* species and *Phialophora* species)

CLINICAL FINDINGS

- Cutaneous lesions usually occur on a lower extremity and begin as a papule or ulcer
- Over months to years, papules enlarge to become vegetating, papillomatous, verrucous, elevated nodules
- Satellite lesions may appear along lymphatics
- Secondary bacterial infection may occur
- Elephantiasis may result

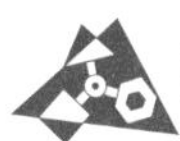

DIAGNOSIS

- Potassium hydroxide preparations of pus or skin scrapings are helpful, showing brown, thick-walled, spherical, sometimes septate cells
- The type of reproduction found in culture determines the species
- *Fonsecaea pedrosoi* is the pathogen in most cases

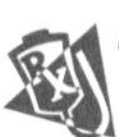

TREATMENT

- Itraconazole, 200–400 mg PO QD for 6–18 mo, achieves response rate of 65%
- Addition of flucytosine to itraconazole may improve response rates
- Cryosurgery alone for smaller lesions
- Surgical excision of involved areas increases cure rates with extent of infection being major determinant of successful outcome
- Terbinafine may be equivalent to itraconazole but clinical experience is lacking

Author(s)

Samuel A. Shelburne, MD

Richard J. Hamill, MD

Churg-Strauss Syndrome

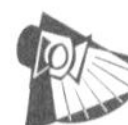

KEY FEATURES

- Idiopathic vasculitis of small and medium-sized arteries seen in patients with symptoms of asthma
- Affects multiple organ systems, most commonly skin and lung, but heart, GI tract, and peripheral nerve involvement may also be affected

CLINICAL FINDINGS

- Marked peripheral eosinophilia
- Chest x-ray findings range from transient infiltrates to pulmonary nodules

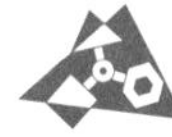

DIAGNOSIS

- Tissue biopsy demonstrating eosinophilic vasculitis is required to confirm the diagnosis and exclude other causes

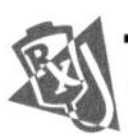

TREATMENT

- Combination therapy with corticosteroids (prednisone, 1 mg/kg/day, tapering over 3–6 months) and cyclophosphamide (1–2 mg/kg/day, tapered 1 year after remission is achieved)

Author(s)

Mark S. Chesnutt, MD

Thomas J. Prendergast, MD

Clonidine Overdose

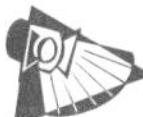

KEY FEATURES

- Symptoms usually resolve in 24 h
- Deaths are rare
- Similar symptoms may occur after ingestion of topical nasal decongestants chemically similar to clonidine (oxymetazoline, tetrahydrozoline, α-naphazoline, brimonidine)

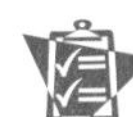

CLINICAL FINDINGS

- Bradycardia, hypotension, miosis, respiratory depression, and coma are caused by central α_2-adrenergic effects
- Hypertension occasionally occurs as a result of peripheral α_1-adrenergic effects

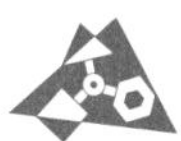

DIAGNOSIS

- Clinical

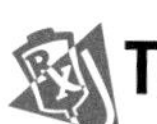

TREATMENT

- Symptomatic treatment is usually sufficient
  - Maintain blood pressure with IV fluids
  - Dopamine can also be used
  - Atropine is usually effective for bradycardia
- Administer activated charcoal, 60–100 g PO or via gastric tube, mixed in aqueous slurry; do not use for comatose or convulsing patients unless it can be given by gastric tube and the airway is protected by a cuffed endotracheal tube
- There is no specific antidote
  - Tolazoline should not be used for clonidine overdose because its effects are unpredictable
  - Naloxone has had anectodal success

Author(s)

Kent R. Olson, MD

Clostridial Myonecrosis

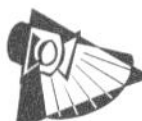 KEY FEATURES

- Sudden onset of pain and edema in wound
- Systemic toxicity
- Presence of gas in infected tissue
- Gram-positive rods on Gram stain or culture

 CLINICAL FINDINGS

- Hypotension and tachycardia
- Painful, edematous wound with surrounding pale skin
- Foul-smelling brown, blood-tinged discharge

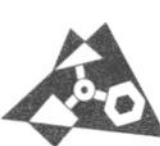 DIAGNOSIS

- Gram stain shows paucity of white blood cells and gram-positive rods
- Anaerobic culture grows *Clostridium* spp

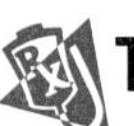 TREATMENT

- Surgical débridement with radical excision as necessary
- Penicillin, 2 million units Q 3 h (other antimicrobials active against anaerobes are also effective)
- Anecdotally, hyperbarbic oxygen may be beneficial in conjunction with surgery and antimicrobial therapy

Author(s)

Henry F. Chambers, MD

Coagulopathy of Liver Disease

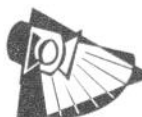 KEY FEATURES

- All coagulation factors except factor VIII synthesized in liver
- With hepatic insufficiency, vitamin K–dependent factors (factors II, VII, IX, X) and factor V are first to be affected
- Because of rapid turnover (half-life 6 h), factor VII level declines first
- Decreased fibrinogen synthesis does not occur unless liver disease is severe
- Liver disease also increases fibrinolysis because liver synthesizes α_2-antiplasmin (main inhibitor of fibrinolysis)
- Biliary tract disease may lead to vitamin K malabsorption
- Congestive splenomegaly may cause thrombocytopenia

 CLINICAL FINDINGS

- Bleeding at any site from coagulopathy
- Oozing at venipuncture sites from excessive fibrinolysis
- Clinical signs of liver disease
- No response to vitamin K
- Disseminated intravascular coagulation (DIC) may occur in end-stage liver disease

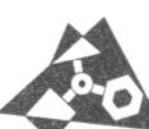 DIAGNOSIS

- PT more prolonged than PTT
- Early in course of liver disease, only PT affected
- Platelet count may be reduced by low levels of thrombopoietin, hypersplenism, bone marrow suppression by alcohol, folic acid deficiency
- Fibrinogen levels and thrombin time normal unless dysfibrinogenemia present
- Peripheral blood smear may show target cells

 TREATMENT

- Long-term treatment with factor replacement usually ineffective
- Fresh-frozen plasma is treatment of choice, but volume overload limits ability to maintain hemostatic factor levels
- Factor IX concentrates contraindicated because of tendency to cause DIC
- Platelet transfusion may help if thrombocytopenia present, but platelet recovery usually disappointing because of hypersplenism

Author(s)

Charles A. Linker, MD

Coal Worker's Pneumoconiosis

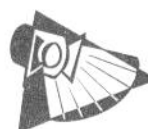

KEY FEATURES

- An occupational pulmonary disease resulting from macrophages ingesting inhaled coal dust
- Cigarette smoking may have an additive detrimental effect on ventilatory function

CLINICAL FINDINGS

- Simple coal worker's pneumoconiosis is usually asymptomatic
- Pulmonary function tests may be normal
- Complicated disease, "progressive massive fibrosis," resembles complicated silicosis, with conglomeration and contraction in upper lung zones

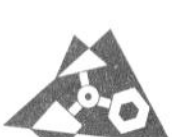

DIAGNOSIS

- Chest x-ray shows diffuse small opacities prominent in upper lungs

TREATMENT

- No therapy has demonstrated efficacy in controlled trials
- As with many other progressive inflammatory disorders of the lung, steroids have been tried

Author(s)

Mark S. Chesnutt, MD

Thomas J. Prendergast, MD

Coarctation of the Aorta

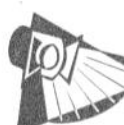

KEY FEATURES

- Narrowing of the aortic arch distal to the origin of the left subclavian artery
- Collateral circulation through intercostal arteries and branches of subclavian arteries
- Cause of secondary hypertension
- Bicuspid aortic valve in 50%

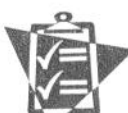

CLINICAL FINDINGS

- Usually no symptoms until hypertension produces left ventricular (LV) failure or cerebral hemorrhage (sometimes associated with congenital cerebral aneurysms)
- Strong arterial pulsations in the neck and suprasternal notch
- Hypertension in the arms, but blood pressure is normal or low in the legs
- Delayed or weak femoral pulsations
- Harsh systolic murmur heard in the back

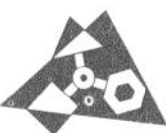

DIAGNOSIS

- ECG: left ventricular hypertrophy (LVH)
- Chest x-ray: scalloping of the ribs as a result of enlarged collateral intercostal arteries
- Echo-Doppler is diagnostic and can estimate severity of obstruction
- MRI or CT provides excellent visualization of coarctation area
- Cardiac catheterization: measurement of gradient across stenosis

TREATMENT

- Up to age 20: all coarctations should be resected
- Younger than age 40: surgery advisable if refractory hypertension or significant LVH
- Surgical mortality rate is 1–4%
- Older than age 50: considerable surgical mortality
- Percutaneous stenting is the procedure of choice, but balloon angioplasty is also done
- Most untreated patients younger than 50 die of complications, LV failure, or cerebral hemorrhage
- About 25% of corrected patients remain hypertensive

Author(s)

Thomas M. Bashore, MD

Christopher B. Granger, MD

Cold Agglutinin Disease

KEY FEATURES

- Acquired hemolytic anemia caused by IgM autoantibodies against RBCs, which characteristically do not react with cells at 37°C but only at lower temperatures
- Because blood temperature rarely falls below 20°C, only antibodies active at higher temperatures than this produce clinical effects
- In cooler parts of the circulation (fingers, nose, ears), IgM binds to RBC and fixes complement. When RBC returns to warmer temperature, IgM antibody dissociates, leaving complement on the cell. Lysis rarely occurs, but C3b present on RBC recognized by Kupffer cells in liver, resulting in RBC sequestration
- Most cases of chronic cold agglutinin disease idiopathic
- Occurs in *Mycoplasma* pneumonia, infectious mononucleosis, Waldenström's macroglobulinemia

CLINICAL FINDINGS

- Mottled or numb fingers or toes on exposure to cold
- Hemolytic anemia, rarely severe
- Hemoglobinuria with exposure to cold

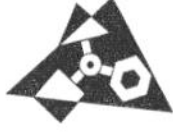

DIAGNOSIS

- Mild anemia, with reticulocytosis and spherocytes
- Direct Coombs test positive for complement only
- Occasionally (in low-titer cold agglutinin disease), only the more sensitive micro-Coombs test is positive

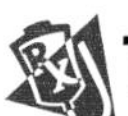

TREATMENT

- Mild disease: Avoid exposure to cold
- Severe disease: alkylating agents (eg, cyclophosphamide) or immunosuppressive agents (eg, cyclosporine)
- Splenectomy and prednisone usually ineffective
- High-dose IVIG (2 g/kg) may be effective temporarily
- Rituximab, 375 mg/m^2 IV every week for 4 weeks, may be effective

Author(s)

Charles A. Linker, MD

Colitis, Microscopic

KEY FEATURES

- Chronic watery diarrhea with normal-appearing mucosa at endoscopy
- Much more common in women, especially in the fifth to sixth decades
- Associated with chronic NSAID use in up to half; idiopathic in the remainder

CLINICAL FINDINGS

- Chronic or recurrent diarrhea
- May remit spontaneously after many years

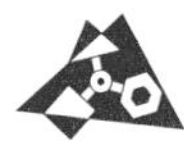

DIAGNOSIS

- Sigmoidoscopy or colonoscopy with biopsy
- Histologic evaluation of mucosal biopsies shows lymphocytic inflammation in the lamina propria

TREATMENT

- Bulking agents or antidiarrheal agents (loperamide, cholestyramine) for mild disease
- Bismuth subsalicylate (2 tablets QID) for 2 months may be effective
- 5-Aminosalicylates (sulfasalazine, mesalamine) are of unproved benefit
- Delayed-release budesonide (Entocort) 9 mg PO QD for 6–8 weeks has demonstrated efficacy in controlled studies

Author(s)

Kenneth R. McQuaid, MD

Colorectal Cancer, Hereditary Nonpolyposis

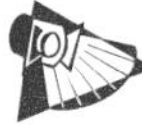

KEY FEATURES

- Markedly increased risk of colorectal cancer and other cancers, including endometrial, ovarian, renal or vesical, hepatobiliary, gastric, small intestine
- Accounts for up to 5% of all colorectal cancers
- Autosomal dominant
- Caused by a defect in one of several genes: *hMLH1, hMSH2, hMSH6, pPMS1,* and *hPMS2*
- Associated with a 70–80% lifetime risk of colorectal carcinoma and a >30% lifetime risk of endometrial cancer
- Develops at an earlier age (mean, 44 years) than sporadic colorectal cancers, and >66% arise proximal to the splenic flexure
- Associated with markedly improved survival compared with sporadic colorectal cancers

CLINICAL FINDINGS

- Few colonic adenomas; adenomas flat, and more often contain villous features or high-grade dysplasia
- Metachronous cancers within 10 years occur in up to 45% of patients

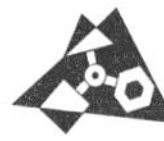

DIAGNOSIS

- Obtain thorough family history of cancer
- Offer genetic testing to patients whose families fulfill the Amsterdam criteria
  - ≥3 first-degree family members with corectal cancer (or 1 of the other associated cancers)
  - Colon cancer involving at least 2 generations
  - ≥1 colon cancer diagnosed before age 50
- Consider genetic testing
  - For individuals with colorectal cancer or endometrial cancer diagnosed before age 50 (especially if right-sided, undifferentiated, or signet ring) or adenoma before age 40
  - For those with colorectal cancer who have a first-degree relative with colorectal cancer or extracolonic cancer diagnosed before age 50

- For those with a personal history of 2 HNPCC-associated cancers
- Test tumor tissues of affected individuals or family members for microsatellite instability
  - Absence of microsatellite instability virtually excludes diagnosis of HNPCC

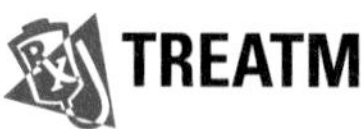

TREATMENT

- If genetic testing documents HNPCC gene mutation, screen affected relatives with colonoscopy every 1–2 years beginning at age 25 (or 5 years younger than the earliest diagnosed family cancer)
- In families that fulfill the Amsterdam criteria or that have tumors with proved microsatellite instability but do not have a documented gene mutation, recommend colonoscopic screening for all family members
- Subtotal colectomy with ileorectal anastomosis if cancer is found (followed by annual surveillance of the rectal stump)
- Endometrial aspiration or transvaginal ultrasound screening for endometrial cancer in women beginning at age 25–35
- Prophylactic hysterectomy and oophorectomy considered in women of post–child-bearing age

Author(s)

Kenneth R. McQuaid, MD

Connective Tissue Disease, Mixed

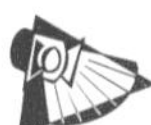

KEY FEATURES

- Features of more than one rheumatic disease; overlap connective tissue disease is the preferred designation for patients having features of different rheumatic diseases
- Patients with overlapping features of systemic lupus erythematosus (SLE), systemic sclerosis, and polymyositis
  - Initially, these patients were thought to have a distinct entity (mixed connective tissue disease) defined by a specific autoantibody to ribonuclear protein (RNP)
  - With time, in many patients, the manifestations evolve to one predominant disease, such as scleroderma, and many patients with antibodies to RNP have clear-cut SLE

CLINICAL FINDINGS

- Characteristics of multiple rheumatic diseases

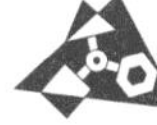

DIAGNOSIS

- Clinical
- Differential diagnosis
  - SLE
  - Scleroderma
  - Polymyositis
  - Sjögren's syndrome
  - Rheumatoid arthritis
  - Eosinophilic fasciitis
  - Graft-versus-host disease

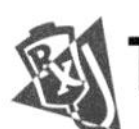

TREATMENT

- Symptom directed
- SLE, systemic sclerosis, or polymyositis features are treated the same way as the diseases

Author(s)

David B. Hellmann, MD, FACP

John H. Stone, MD, MPH

Contraception, Emergency

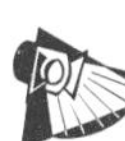

KEY FEATURES

- Information on clinics or individual clinicians providing emergency contraception in the United States may be obtained by calling 1-888-668-2528

TREATMENT

MEDICATION

- The following methods should be started within 72 h after unprotected coitus:
  - Levonorgestrel, 0.75 mg given in two doses 12 h apart (available in the US prepackaged as Plan B); has a 1% failure rate and is associated with less nausea and vomiting than the following combination regimen
  - Ethinyl estradiol, 50 μg, with 0.5 mg norgestrel (available in the US prepackaged as Preven), given in a regimen of two tablets initially followed by two tablets 12 h later
  - A comparable regimen includes four pills 12 h apart of Lo/Ovral, Nordette, or Levlen or the same regimen with the yellow pills of Triphasil or Tri-Levlen. The failure rate is approximately 3%, and antinausea medication should be provided
  - Ethinyl estradiol, 2.5 mg BID for 5 days. This regimen is as efficacious as the others but is associated with a higher likelihood of nausea, vomiting, and breast tenderness
  - Mifepristone, 10 mg as a single dose, has the same failure rate as the levonorgestrel regimen, with minimal side effects, and appears to be effective given up to 120 h after unprotected intercourse. It is not currently available at this dose in the US

INTRAUTERINE DEVICES

- Copper-bearing intrauterine devices (IUDs) inserted within 5 days after one episode of unprotected midcycle coitus will prevent pregnancy
- The disadvantage of this method is possible infection, especially in rape cases
- The advantage is ongoing contraceptive protection if this is desired in a patient for whom the IUD is a suitable choice

Author(s)

H. Trent MacKay, MD, MPH

Contraception, Periodic Abstinence

KEY FEATURES

- **Periodic abstinence during fertile periods**
  - Most effective when intercourse restricted to postovular phase of cycle or barrier method used at other times
  - Women should identify fertile periods (see Infertility, Female)
- **"Symptothermal" natural family planning**
  - Patient-observed increase in clear elastic cervical mucus, brief abdominal midcycle discomfort ("mittelschmerz")
  - Unprotected intercourse is avoided from shortly after the menstrual period until 48 h after ovulation, as identified by a sustained rise in temperature and the disappearance of clear elastic mucus
- In the **calendar method,** after the length of the menstrual cycle has been observed for at least 8 mo, the following calculations are made
  - The first fertile day is determined by subtracting 18 days from the shortest cycle
  - The last fertile day is determined by subtracting 11 days from the longest cycle
- **Basal body temperature method** shows the safe time for intercourse after ovulation has passed
  - Take temperature immediately upon awakening, before any activity
  - A slight drop in temperature often occurs 12–24 h before ovulation, and a rise of about 0.4°C occurs 1–2 days after ovulation
  - The risk of pregnancy increases starting 5 days before the day of ovulation, peaks on the day of ovulation, and then rapidly decreases to zero by the day after ovulation
- **The Standard Days Method** uses a set of beads to remind the couple to avoid intercourse during days 8 through 19 of the cycle. Typical use failure rate may be about 12%

Author(s)

H. Trent MacKay, MD, MPH

Contraception, Sterilization

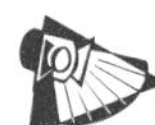

KEY FEATURES

- In the United States, sterilization is the most popular method of birth control for couples who want no more children
- Vasectomy is a safe, simple procedure in which the vas deferens is severed and sealed through a scrotal incision under local anesthesia
- Female sterilization is performed via laparoscopic bipolar electrocoagulation or plastic ring application on the uterine tubes or via minilaparotomy with tubal resection
- The cumulative 10-year failure rate for all methods combined is 1.85%, varying from 0.75% for postpartum partial salpingectomy and laparoscopic unipolar coagulation to 3.65% for spring clips
- Essure is approved by the Food and Drug Administration. The method involves the placement of an expanding microcoil of titanium into the proximal uterine tube under hysteroscopic guidance. The efficacy rate at 1 year is 99.8%

Author(s)

H. Trent MacKay, MD, MPH

Cor Pulmonale

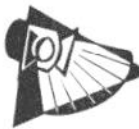

KEY FEATURES

- Right ventricular (RV) hypertrophy and failure from hypoxia-associated lung disease or pulmonary vascular disease
- Most common cause: chronic obstructive pulmonary disease (COPD)
- Less frequent causes
  - Pneumoconiosis
  - Pulmonary fibrosis
  - Kyphoscoliosis
  - Primary pulmonary hypertension
  - Repeated pulmonary embolization
  - Sleep apnea (Pickwickian syndrome)

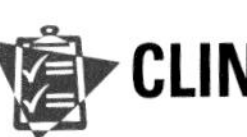

CLINICAL FINDINGS

- Predominant symptoms—intensified with RV failure—are related to the underlying pulmonary disorder
  - Chronic productive cough
  - Exertional dyspnea
  - Wheezing
  - Easy fatigability
  - Weakness
- Other possible findings
  - Dependent edema
  - Right upper quadrant pain (hepatic congestion)
  - Cyanosis
  - Clubbing
  - Distended neck veins
  - RV heave
  - Gallop
- Polycythemia is often present
- Arterial oxygen saturation often < 85%

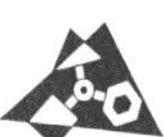

DIAGNOSIS

- Symptoms and signs of COPD with elevated jugular venous pressure, parasternal lift, edema, hepatomegaly, ascites
- ECG
  - Tall, peaked P waves (P pulmonale), right axis deviation, and RV hypertrophy
  - Q waves in leads II, III, and aVF may mimic myocardial infarction
  - Frequent, nonspecific supraventricular arrhythmias
- Chest x-ray film
  - Enlarged right ventricle and pulmonary artery
  - Possible signs of pulmonary parenchymal disease
- Pulmonary function tests to confirm underlying lung disease

- Echocardiogram or angiography to exclude primary left ventricular failure as a cause of right-sided heart failure
- Multi-slice CT scan to exclude pulmonary emboli

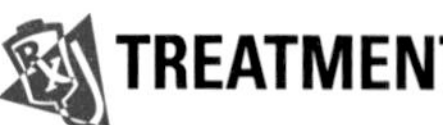

TREATMENT

- Treat underlying lung disease
- Oxygen, salt and fluid restriction, and diuretics, often in combination
- Compensated cor pulmonale has the same prognosis as the underlying lung disease
- Average life expectancy is 2–5 yr when congestive signs appear, but survival is significantly longer when uncomplicated emphysema is the cause

Author(s)

Thomas M. Bashore, MD

Christopher B. Granger, MD

Coxsackievirus Infections

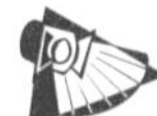

KEY FEATURES

- Named after a town in northern New York State, the coxsackievirus causes several clinical syndromes
- More than 50 serotypes and 2 major subgroups: A and B
- Enterovirus occurs most often during the summer months

CLINICAL FINDINGS

- Herpangina (subtype A): sudden-onset fevers, headaches, myalgias, and petechiae on the soft palate that become shallow ulcers. Resolves in 3 days
- Epidemic pleurodynia (Bornholm disease, subtype B): pleuritic chest pain, systemic symptoms, including headache, malaise, pharyngitis
- Aseptic meningitis (subtypes A and B): fever, headache, stiff neck, and CSF lymphocytosis. Encephalitis and transverse myelitis may occur
- Acute pericarditis (subtype B): positional, pleuritic chest pain, fevers and myalgias. Clinical and echocardiographic signs of pericarditis
- Hand-foot-and-mouth disease (subtype A): stomatitis and vesicular rash on hands and feet
- Hepatitis, renal disease, and myocarditis are also caused by coxsackievirus infections

DIAGNOSIS

- Clinical diagnosis
- No reliable laboratory abnormality
- Neutralizing antibodies appear during convalescence

TREATMENT

- Supportive measures
- In severe cases, immunoglobulin treatment is sometimes used (anecdotal evidence)

Author(s)

Wayne X. Shandera, MD

Ana Moran, MD

Cyanide Poisoning

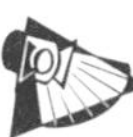

KEY FEATURES

- In gaseous form, hydrogen cyanide is an important component of fire smoke
- Cyanide-generating glycosides also found in the pits of apricots and other related plants
- Cyanide is generated by breakdown of nitroprusside; poisoning can result from rapid high-dose infusions
- Also formed by metabolism of acetonitrile, found in some over-the-counter fingernail glue removers
- Cyanide is rapidly absorbed by inhalation, skin absorption, ingestion

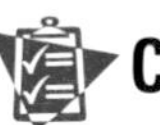

CLINICAL FINDINGS

- Onset of toxicity is nearly instantaneous after inhalation but may be delayed for minutes to hours after ingestion of cyanide salts or cyanogenic plants or chemicals
- Effects include headache, dizziness, nausea, abdominal pain, and anxiety followed by confusion, syncope, shock, seizures, coma, and death
- "Bitter almond" odor may be detected on the victim's breath or in vomitus, although this is not a reliable finding

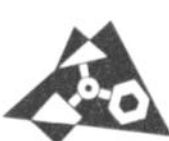

DIAGNOSIS

- The venous oxygen saturation may be elevated (> 90%) in severe poisonings because tissues have failed to take up arterial oxygen
- Obtain blood cyanide levels (not usually readily available)

TREATMENT

- Remove the victim from exposure, taking care to avoid exposure to rescuers
- Administer activated charcoal 60–100 g mixed in aqueous slurry PO or via gastric tube. Do not use for comatose or convulsing patients unless they are endotracheally intubated.
- At the scene, induce emesis if charcoal is not immediately available
- Stop or slow the nitroprusside infusion rate for suspected cyanide toxicity
- In the US, there are prepackaged cyanide antidotes (Table 146)

Author(s)

Kent R. Olson, MD

Cytomegalovirus (CMV) Infection

KEY FEATURES

- Most CMV infections asymptomatic
- Age-related rise in seroprevalence
- Acute acquired CMV infection is similar to infectious mononucleosis, except unusual to develop pharyngeal symptoms
- Most CMV-related diseases occur in immunocompromised, especially HIV infected, persons
  - CMV retinitis
  - Gastrointestinal (GI) and hepatobiliary disease
  - Pulmonary disease
  - Neurologic disease
- Major pathogen in transplant recipients by both direct infection and reactivation of latent infection, increasing rates of transplant rejection

CLINICAL FINDINGS

- CMV inclusion disease, with CNS and hepatic malfunction, occurs in infants born to acutely infected mothers
- CMV retinitis, with neovascular and proliferative retinal lesions, occurs primarily in advanced AIDS
- GI and hepatobiliary CMV, with esophagitis, small bowel inflammation, colitis, or cholangiopathy, occurs in AIDS or with high-dose chemotherapy
- Pneumonitis occurs in transplant recipients and HIV-infected patients
- Neurologic manifestations include polyneuropathy, transverse myelitis, encephalitis

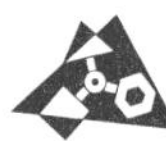

DIAGNOSIS

- Characteristic clinical symptoms in immunosuppressed patients
- Tzanck smear, CMV antibodies, and polymerase chain reaction (PCR) helpful in the proper clinical context
- Tissue biopsy showing characteristic histology used to document invasive disease

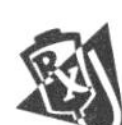

TREATMENT

- Acute, severe infections: IV ganciclovir, valganciclovir, foscarnet, and cidofovir
- Improvement of immunosuppression especially important in AIDS and transplant patients
- Prophylactic therapy: IV ganciclovir, oral valganciclovir or high-dose valacyclovir
- Antigen or PCR tests often used in transplant patients to guide preemptive therapy
- Prevention: no CMV vaccine currently available
- Use CMV-negative blood products in immunosuppressed patients

Author(s)
Wayne X. Shandera, MD
Ana Moran, MD

Dengue

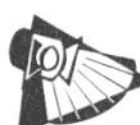

KEY FEATURES

- Extremely common togavirus infection transmitted by the bite of the *Aedes* mosquito
- Incubation period is typically 7–10 days (can be longer)
- Found throughout the tropics
- In United States, occurs in southern Texas and Puerto Rico

CLINICAL FINDINGS

- Usually nonspecific; self-limited febrile illness that typically lasts 3–7 days followed by a remission
- Severe dengue associated with fevers, terrible body aches ("breakbone"), pharyngitis, hemorrhage, and shock
- Rash is very common in the remission period or early in a second febrile phase
- Rash has maculopapular, petechial, or other morphology, appears first on the hands and feet and spreads to the arms, legs, trunk, and neck, usually sparing the face
- Death seen in cases of dengue hemorrhagic fever and dengue shock syndrome

DIAGNOSIS

- Consider diagnosis in travelers recently returned from endemic areas
- Leukopenia is characteristic
- Thrombocytopenia is common in the hemorrhagic form of the disease
- Rapid serological testing is available

TREATMENT

- No specific antiviral therapy
- Supportive measures, including analgesics (avoid aspirin) and hydration
- Prevention: a vaccine has been developed but is not yet available commercially
- Mosquito control measures

Author(s)
Wayne X. Shandera, MD
Ana Moran, MD

Dermatitis Herpetiformis

 KEY FEATURES

- Highest prevalence in Scandinavia
- Is associated with HLA antigens -B8, -DR3, and -DQ2
- Associated with gluten-sensitive enteropathy, but in the great majority it is subclinical
- Ingestion of gluten plays a role in the exacerbation of skin lesions

 CLINICAL FINDINGS

- Uncommon disease manifested by pruritic papules, vesicles, and papulovesicles mainly on the elbows, knees, buttocks, posterior neck, scalp
- Patients with dermatitis herpetiformis are at increased risk for gastrointestinal lymphoma, and this risk is reduced by a gluten-free diet

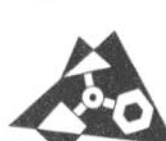 DIAGNOSIS

- Diagnosis is made by light microscopy, which demonstrates neutrophils at the dermal papillary tips
- Direct immunofluorescence studies show granular deposits of IgA along the dermal papillae
- Circulating antiendomysium antibodies and antibodies to tissue transglutaminase are present in 70% of cases
- Differential diagnosis includes weeping or encrusted lesions (crusted lesions), impetigo, contact dermatitis (acute)
- Any vesicular dermatitis can become crusted

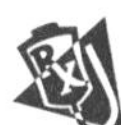 TREATMENT

- Strict long-term avoidance of dietary gluten has been shown to decrease the dose of dapsone (usually 100–200 mg/day) required to control the disease and may even eliminate the need for drug treatment

Author(s)

Timothy G. Berger, MD

Dermatitis, Seborrheic

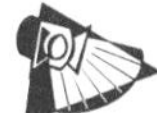 KEY FEATURES

- May represent an inflammatory reaction to *Malassezia furfur* yeasts
- The tendency is to lifelong recurrences, with outbreaks lasting weeks, months, or years

 CLINICAL FINDINGS

- Greasy scales and underlying erythema
- Scalp, central face, presternal, interscapular areas, umbilicus, and body folds
- They occur on sun-exposed parts of the body in persons of fair complexion
- See Table 7
- Differential diagnosis
  - Psoriasis
  - Atopic dermatitis (eczema)
  - Tinea capitis
  - Contact dermatitis
  - Tinea versicolor
  - Pityriasis rosea

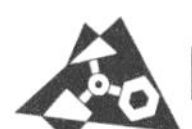 DIAGNOSIS

- Clinical

 TREATMENT

Scalp

- Shampoos that contain zinc pyrithione or selenium daily
- These may be alternated with ketoconazole shampoo (1% or 2%) used twice weekly
- Tar shampoos
- Topical corticosteroid solutions or lotions twice daily

Facial

- A mild corticosteroid (hydrocortisone 1%, alclometasone, desonide) used intermittently and not near the eyes
- Add ketoconazole (Nizoral) 2% cream BID If control is not obtained with intermittent topical corticosteroid use
- Topical tacrolimus (Protopic) and pimecrolimus (Elidel) are steroid-sparing alternatives
  - Only use when other agents are ineffective
  - Use in a limited area for a brief time
  - Avoid these agents for patients with known immunosuppression, HIV infection, bone marrow and organ transplantation, lymphoma, at high risk for lymphoma, and those with a prior history of lymphoma

Nonhairy/Intertriginous areas

- 1% or 2.5% hydrocortisone, desonide, or alclometasone dipropionate cream twice weekly for maintenance
- Ketoconazole cream may be added
- Tacrolimus or pimecrolimus

Author(s)

Timothy G. Berger, MD

Diverticulosis

KEY FEATURES

- Incidence increases with age in Western societies
  - 5% at age < 40
  - 30% at age 60
  - 50% at age >80
- Uncommon in developing countries
- Most are asymptomatic, discovered incidentally at sigmoidoscopy or colonoscopy or on barium enema
- Causes
  - Diet deficient in fiber
  - Abnormal motility
  - Hereditary factors
  - Ehlers-Danlos syndrome
  - Marfan's syndrome
  - Scleroderma

CLINICAL FINDINGS

- Nonspecific complaints
  - Chronic constipation
  - Abdominal pain
  - Fluctuating bowel habits
- Physical examination usually normal
  - May reveal mild left lower quadrant tenderness
- Complications occur in 33%, including lower GI bleeding and diverticulitis

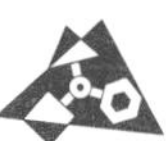

DIAGNOSIS

- Routine laboratory studies normal
- Barium enema best demonstrates diverticula
- Colonoscopy

TREATMENT

- High-fiber diet or fiber supplements (bran powder, psyllium or methylcellulose 1–2 tbsp PO BID)

Author(s)

Kenneth R. McQuaid, MD

Down Syndrome

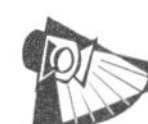

KEY FEATURES

- Caused by simple trisomy for chromosome 21 or unbalanced translocations involving the long arm of chromosome 21
- Risk of an affected fetus increases exponentially with age of mother at conception and begins a marked rise after age 35
- At maternal age 45, risk is 1 in 40

CLINICAL FINDINGS

- Usually diagnosed at birth
- Typical facial features
- Hypotonia
- Single palmar crease
- Serious problems at birth or early in childhood, including duodenal atresia, congenital heart disease (especially atrioventricular canal defects), and leukemia
- Mental retardation, although intelligence varies across a wide spectrum
- Alzheimer-like dementia in the fourth or fifth decade
- Affected patients who survive childhood have a reduced life expectancy

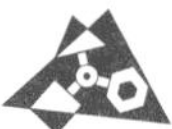

DIAGNOSIS

- Cytogenetic analysis
- Most affected individuals have simple trisomy for chromosome 21
- Others have unbalanced translocations, usually resulting from a parent with a balanced translocation, incurring a substantial risk of Down syndrome in future offspring
- Can be detected in the early second trimester through screening maternal serum for alpha-fetoprotein and certain hormones (triple screen) and by observation of increased nuchal skin thickness on fetal ultrasonogram

TREATMENT

- No treatment is effective for the mental impairment
- Congenital heart disease, duodenal atresia, and acute leukemia, if present, are treated by standard approaches
- Genetic counseling is essential for parents of a newly diagnosed child
- Prenatal diagnosis should be offered for subsequent pregnancies

Author(s)

Reed E. Pyeritz, MD, PhD

Dupuytren's Contracture

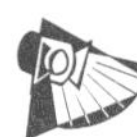

KEY FEATURES

- Hyperplasia of the palmar fascia and related structures, with nodule formation and contracture
- Cause is unknown
- Occurs primarily in white men older than 50 yr. The incidence is higher among alcoholics and patients with chronic systemic disorders (especially cirrhosis)
- Also associated with systemic fibrosing syndrome, which includes Peyronie's disease, mediastinal and retroperitoneal fibrosis, and Riedel's struma

CLINICAL FINDINGS

- Slowly progressive chronic disease
- Nodular or cord-like thickening of one or both hands, with the fourth and fifth fingers most commonly affected
- Tightness of the involved digits, with inability to satisfactorily extend the fingers
- The contracture is well tolerated because it exaggerates the normal position of function of the hand, although resulting cosmetic problems may be unappealing

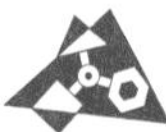

DIAGNOSIS

- Clinical findings outlined above

TREATMENT

- If the palmar nodule is growing rapidly, injections of triamcinolone into the nodule may be of benefit
- Surgical intervention is indicated in patients with significant flexion contractures, depending on the location, but recurrence is not uncommon

Author(s)

David B. Hellmann, MD, FACP

John H. Stone, MD, MPH

Effusions, Malignant, Pleural, Pericardial, & Peritoneal

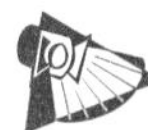

KEY FEATURES

- Half of undiagnosed effusions in patients not known to have cancer are malignant
- Occur in pleural, pericardial, and peritoneal spaces
- Caused by direct neoplastic involvement of serous surface or obstruction of lymphatic drainage

CLINICAL FINDINGS

- Chest pain
- Shortness of breath
- Cough
- Hypotension
- Muffled heart sounds
- Abdominal distention

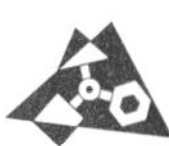

DIAGNOSIS

- Thoracentesis, pericardiocentesis, or paracentesis; send fluid for cytology, cell count and differential, protein content, lactate dehydrogenase level
- Malignant effusions are generally bloody; chylous effusions occur with thoracic duct obstruction or enlarged mediastinal lymph nodes in lymphoma
- If pleural cytology is negative on two occasions but suspicion of tumor high, thoracoscopic pleural biopsy may be helpful
- Differential diagnosis: congestive heart failure, pulmonary embolism, trauma, infections
- Effusions are a complication of some chemotherapeutic agents

TREATMENT

- Treatment of underlying malignancy is often ineffective in relieving effusions
- Pleural: Diuretics are used to minimize reexpansion pulmonary edema after thoracentesis
- Thoracentesis alone controls fewer than 10% of pleural effusions but may be useful in conjunction with systemic chemotherapy
- Closed water-seal drainage with a chest tube for 3–4 days, followed by chemosclerosis with talc or mitoxantrone, if necessary
- Pleuroperitoneal shunting occasionally helpful, but patient must pump shunt 100 times 5 times/day
- Pleurectomy is effective but has a high complication rate, and is rarely indicated
- Pericardial: Pericardial window or stripping achieves good control (also useful for constrictive pericarditis after radiation therapy)
- Peritoneal: Diuretics are used in initial treatment of small to moderate effusions and as adjunctive treatment after large-volume paracentesis

Author(s)

Hope Rugo, MD

Ehrlichiosis

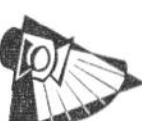

KEY FEATURES

- Tick-borne gram-negative obligate intracellular bacteria
- Two main clinical entities: human granulocytic ehrlichiosis (typically *Ehrlichia phagocytophila*) and human monocytic ehrlichiosis (typically *E chaffeensis*)
- Bacteria form morulae, intracytoplasmic aggregates within leukocytes
- In the United States, mainly found in mid-Atlantic, southeastern, and central states
- May see coinfection with other tick-borne illnesses (eg, Lyme disease)

CLINICAL FINDINGS

- Prodrome of malaise, rigors, and nausea, followed by fever, headache, and rash
- Respiratory failure, renal failure, and encephalopathy may ensue in severe cases

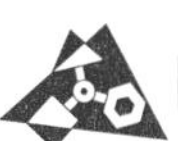

DIAGNOSIS

- Leukopenia, lymphopenia, thrombocytopenia, and elevated liver function tests common
- May see morulae in cytoplasm of leukocytes
- PCR from whole blood useful
- Indirect fluorescent antibody test available from CDC

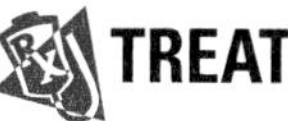

TREATMENT

- Doxycycline is treatment of choice, usually given for 7–10 days
- Attention to tick removal and acquisition is mainstay of prevention

Author(s)

Wayne X. Shandera, MD

Ana Moran, MD

Enterococcal Infections

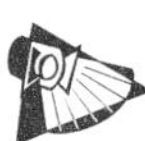

KEY FEATURES

- Two species—*Enterococcus faecalis* and *Enterococcus faecium*—are responsible for most human enterococcal infections

CLINICAL FINDINGS

- Wound infections
- Urinary tract infection
- Bacteremia
- Endocarditis
- Meningitis

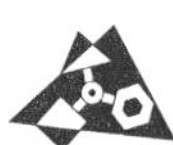

DIAGNOSIS

- Cultures of affected fluids or tissue

TREATMENT

- Most enterococcal infections can still be treated with penicillin, 3 million units Q 4 h; ampicillin (which is slightly more active than penicillin in vitro), 2 g Q 6 h; or vancomycin, 1 g Q 12 h
- Because these antibiotics are not bactericidal for enterococci, gentamicin, 1 mg/kg Q 8 h, is added for treatment of endocarditis or other serious infection
- Quinupristin/dalfopristin and linezolid are FDA approved for treatment of infections caused by vancomycin-resistant strains of enterococci
- Quinupristin/dalfopristin is not active against strains of *E faecalis* and should be used only for infections caused by *E faecium*. Linezolid, an oxazolidinone, is active against both *E faecalis* and *E faecium*

Author(s)

Henry F. Chambers, MD

Enteropathy, Protein-Losing

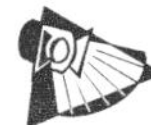

KEY FEATURES

- Defined as excessive loss of serum proteins into GI tract
- Essential diagnostic features
  - Hypoalbuminemia
  - Elevated fecal α_1-antitrypsin level
- Causes include
  - Mucosal disease with ulceration
  - Lymphatic obstruction
  - Idiopathic change in permeability of mucosal capillaries

CLINICAL FINDINGS

- Hypoalbuminemia
- Edema
- Lymphocytopenia (< 1000/μL), hypoglobulinemia, hypocholesterolemia in lymphatic obstruction

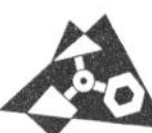

DIAGNOSIS

- Obtain lymphocyte count, serum albumin, protein electrophoresis, cholesterol, ANA, and C3 levels
- Gut α_1-antitrypsin clearance (24-h volume of feces × stool concentration of α_1-antitrypsin/serum α_1-antitrypsin concentration) of >13 mL/24 h is diagnostic
- Stool samples of ova and parasites
- Stool qualitative fecal fat determination
- Upper endoscopy with small bowel biopsy
- Small bowel barium series
- Barium enema or colonoscopy
- CT scan of the abdomen
- Lymphangiography (rarely needed)
- Laparotomy with full-thickness intestinal biopsy

TREATMENT

- Treat underlying disease
- Low-fat diets supplemented with medium-chain triglycerides for cases caused by lymphatic obstruction
- Octreotide may benefit some patients

Author(s)

Kenneth R. McQuaid, MD

Eosinophilia-Myalgia Syndrome

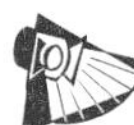

KEY FEATURES

- The eosinophilia-myalgia syndrome was first noted in patients who ingested tryptophan until it was banned by the US Food and Drug Administration

CLINICAL FINDINGS

- Begins weeks to months after beginning ingestion of tryptophan
- A syndrome of severe generalized myalgias and cutaneous abnormalities ranging from hives to generalized swelling and induration of the arms and legs develops
- Other common clinical manifestations include pulmonary symptoms, fever, myopathy, lymphadenopathy, and ascending polyneuropathy
- Death, especially from neurologic involvement, can occur

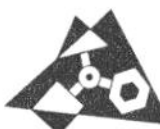

DIAGNOSIS

- Peripheral eosinophilia (> 1000/μL) is characteristic
- Mild elevations of aldolase with normal creatine kinase levels and, frequently, positive ANA tests
- Full-thickness biopsies may reveal features of systemic sclerosis, evidence of fasciitis or myositis, or small-vessel vasculitis

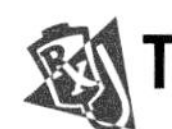

TREATMENT

- Although some patients improve after discontinuing tryptophan, others progress and require corticosteroid therapy, which is not always effective

Author(s)

David B. Hellmann, MD, FACP

John H. Stone, MD, MPH

Epicondylitis, Lateral & Medial

 KEY FEATURES

- Better known by their sports associations: tennis elbow and golf elbow, respectively
- The conditions are caused by overuse
- Pain results from minor tears in the tendons of the forearm's extensor and flexor muscles

 CLINICAL FINDINGS

- Pain and point tenderness at the site of tendon insertion
- Grasping and squeezing, in such tasks as shaking hands or opening jars, are impaired and cause pain. The pain may be reproduced by extension **(lateral epicondylitis)** or flexion **(medial epicondylitis)** of the wrist against pressure

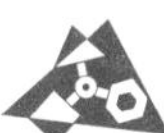 DIAGNOSIS

- Clinical

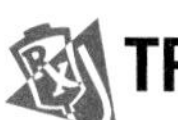 TREATMENT

- The use of "counterforce" straps (bands worn distal to the elbow, over the bulk of the forearm musculature), intended to decrease the forces transmitted to the elbow during activity, are inadequate substitutes for rest
- Symptoms that persist after 2 weeks of conservative therapy usually respond to infiltration of triamcinolone, 10–20 mg, mixed with 1% lidocaine, 1–2 mL, around the involved epicondyle

Author(s)

David B. Hellmann, MD, FACP

John H. Stone, MD, MPH

Epididymitis, Acute

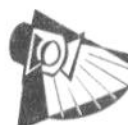 KEY FEATURES

- Painful enlargement of the epididymis, relieved by scrotal elevation
- Fever and irritative voiding symptoms are common
- In advanced cases, infection can spread to the testis and entire scrotal contents tender to palpation
- **Sexually transmitted form**: typically in men under age 40, associated with urethritis, and caused by *Chlamydia trachomatis* or *Neisseria gonorrhoeae*
- **Nonsexually transmitted form**: in older men, associated with urinary tract infections and prostatitis, and caused by gram-negative rods

 CLINICAL FINDINGS

- Symptoms can follow acute physical strain, trauma, or sexual activity
- Associated symptoms of urethritis and urethral discharge or cystitis (irritative voiding symptoms)
- Pain in the scrotum may radiate along the spermatic cord
- Fever and scrotal swelling
- Differential diagnosis
  - Tumors of the testis
  - Testicular torsion

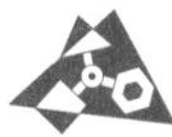 DIAGNOSIS

- Complete blood count: leukocytosis and left shift
- In **sexually transmitted** variety, Gram stain of urethral discharge: white cells and gram-negative intracellular diplococci (*N gonorrhoeae*) or white cells without visible organisms (nongonococcal urethritis, *C trachomatis*)
- In **nonsexually transmitted** variety, urinalysis: pyuria, bacteriuria, hematuria; urine cultures may reveal pathogen

 TREATMENT

- **Sexually transmitted** variety: antibiotics for 21 days, treat sexual partner also
- **Nonsexually transmitted** variety: antibiotics for 21–28 days
- Evaluate urinary tract to identify underlying disease
- Bed rest with scrotal elevation
- Prompt treatment usually results in a favorable outcome
- Delayed or inadequate treatment may result in epididymoorchitis, decreased fertility, abscess formation

Author(s)

Marshall L. Stoller, MD

Peter R. Carroll, MD

Epiglottitis

KEY FEATURES

- Suspect epiglottitis (or, more correctly, supraglottitis) when a patient complains of
  - Rapidly developing sore throat
  - Odynophagia (pain on swallowing) which is disproportional to apparently minimal oropharyngeal findings on examination
- May be viral or bacterial in origin

CLINICAL FINDINGS

- Swollen, erythematous epiglottis on laryngoscopy

DIAGNOSIS

- Unlike in children, indirect laryngoscopy is generally safe

TREATMENT

- Hospitalization and initial admission to intensive care unit
- IV antibiotics (eg, ceftizoxime, 1–2 g IV Q 8–12 h; or cefuroxime, 750–1500 mg IV Q 8 h)
- Dexamethasone, usually 4–10 mg as initial bolus and then 4 mg IV Q 6 h, and observation of the airway
- Corticosteroids may be tapered as signs and symptoms resolve. Similarly, substitution of oral antibiotics may be appropriate to complete a 10-day course
- When epiglottitis is recognized early in the adult, it is usually possible to avoid intubation
- Indications for intubation are dyspnea or rapid pace of sore throat (where progression to airway compromise may occur before the effects of corticosteroids and antibiotics take hold)
- If the patient is not intubated, monitor oxygen saturation with continuous pulse oximetry

Author(s)

Robert K. Jackler, MD

Michael J. Kaplan, MD

Erythromelalgia

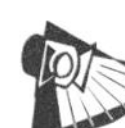

KEY FEATURES

- Paroxysmal bilateral vasodilatory disorder of unknown cause
- Idiopathic (primary) erythromelalgia occurs in otherwise healthy persons
- Affects men and women equally
- Secondary erythromelalgia occurs in patients with polycythemia vera, hypertension, gout, and neurological diseases

CLINICAL FINDINGS

- Erythema, warmth, and bilateral burning pain that lasts minutes to hours, at first involving circumscribed areas on the balls of the feet or palms and often progressing to involve the entire extremity
- Symptoms occur in response to vasodilation produced by exercise or heat (eg, at night when the extremities are warmed under bedclothes)
- Relief may be obtained by cooling and elevating the affected extremity

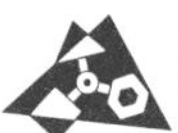

DIAGNOSIS

- No findings between attacks
- During attacks, skin temperature and arterial pulsations are increased, and involved areas are warm, erythematous, and sweaty

TREATMENT

Primary erythromelalgia

- Avoid warm environments
- Aspirin, 650 mg Q 4–6 h
- β-blockers, epidural corticosteroid injections, and lidocaine patches

Secondary erythromelalgia

- Treatment of the primary disease process

Author(s)

Louis M. Messina, MD

Esophageal Diverticula

KEY FEATURES

- Zenker's diverticulum is a protrusion of pharyngeal mucosa at the pharyngoesophageal junction between the inferior pharyngeal constrictor and the cricopharyngeus
- Esophageal diverticula occur in the mid or distal esophagus secondary to motility disorders (diffuse esophageal spasm, achalasia) or may develop above esophageal strictures

CLINICAL FINDINGS

- Zenker's diverticulum
  - Dysphagia and regurgitation
  - Oropharyngeal dysphagia with coughing or throat discomfort
- As the diverticulum enlarges and retains food, any of the following may occur
  - Halitosis
  - Spontaneous regurgitation of undigested food
  - Nocturnal choking
  - Gurgling in the throat
  - Protrusion in the neck may occur
- Complications include
  - Aspiration pneumonia
  - Bronchiectasis
  - Lung abscess
- Esophageal diverticula: seldom symptomatic
- Risk of perforation at endoscopy

DIAGNOSIS

- Barium esophagogram

TREATMENT

- Treatment directed at the underlying disorder
- Small asymptomatic diverticula may be observed
- Symptomatic upper esophageal myotomy and surgical diverticulectomy lead to improvement in >90%

Author(s)

Kenneth R. McQuaid, MD

Esophageal Injury, Caustic

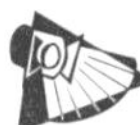

KEY FEATURES

- Follows accidental or deliberate (suicidal) ingestion of alkali (drain cleaners, etc) or acid

CLINICAL FINDINGS

- Severe burning and chest pain, gagging, dysphagia, and drooling
- Aspiration results in stridor and wheezing

DIAGNOSIS

- Examine circulatory status
- Assess airway patency, including laryngoscopy
- Chest and abdominal radiographs
- Endoscopy

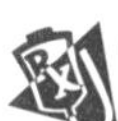

TREATMENT

- Supportive treatment, IV fluids, analgesics
- Nasogastric lavage and oral antidotes should *not* be administered
- Endoscopy within the first 24 hours to assess extent and severity of mucosal damage
- Patients with mild damage (edema, erythema, exudates, or superficial ulcers)
  - Recover quickly
  - Have low risk of stricture
  - May be advanced from liquids to regular diet over 24–48 hours
- Patients with severe injury (deep or circumferential ulcers or necrosis)
  - Have a high risk (up to 65%) of acute perforation with mediastinitis or peritonitis, bleeding, stricture, or esophageal-tracheal fistulas
  - Must be kept fasting and monitored closely for signs of deterioration that warrant emergency surgery
- Surgery: esophagectomy and colonic or jejunal interposition, nasoenteric feeding tube
- Neither steroids nor antibiotics are recommended
- Strictures develop in up to 70% of patients with serious esophageal injury weeks to months after initial injury, requiring recurrent dilations
- Esophageal squamous carcinoma occurs in 2–3%, warranting endoscopic surveillance 15–20 years after the caustic ingestion

Author(s)

Kenneth R. McQuaid, MD

Esophageal Webs & Rings

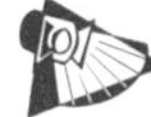

KEY FEATURES

- Esophageal webs are thin, diaphragm-like membranes of squamous mucosa typically in the mid or upper esophagus
  - May be multiple in congenital graft-versus-host disease, pemphigoid, epidermolysis bullosa, pemphigus vulgaris
  - Web plus iron deficiency anemia is known as Plummer-Vinson syndrome
- Esophageal rings are smooth, circumferential, thin (< 4 mm) mucosal structures in the distal esophagus at the squamocolumnar junction
  - Are associated with hiatal hernia
  - May be related to gastroesophageal reflux disease

CLINICAL FINDINGS

- Solid-food dysphagia, characteristically intermittent and not progressive, with rings <13 mm in diameter

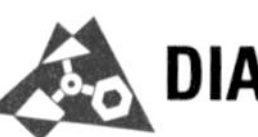

DIAGNOSIS

- Barium esophagogram with full esophageal distention
- Endoscopy less sensitive for detection of subtle webs and rings

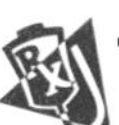

TREATMENT

- Passage of a large (>16-mm diameter) bougie dilator to disrupt the web or ring
- Single dilation, repeat dilations, graduated dilation for ringed esophagus
- Proton pump inhibitor chronic therapy for patients who have heartburn or who require repeated dilation

Author(s)

Kenneth R. McQuaid, MD

Esophagitis, Pill-Induced

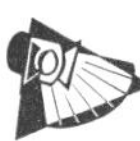 KEY FEATURES

- Various medications may injure the esophagus through direct, prolonged mucosal contact
- Most commonly implicated
  - Alendronate
  - Clindamycin
  - Doxycycline
  - Iron
  - NSAIDs
  - Potassium chloride pills
  - Quinidine
  - Risedronate
  - Tetracycline
  - Trimethoprim-sulfamethoxazole
  - Vitamin C
  - Zalcitabine
  - Zidovudine
- Injury is most likely to occur if pills are swallowed without water or while supine
- Hospitalized or bed-bound patients are at greater risk

 CLINICAL FINDINGS

- Severe retrosternal chest pain
- Odynophagia
- Dysphagia

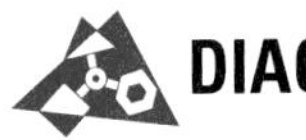 DIAGNOSIS

- Endoscopy reveals one or several discrete, shallow or deep ulcers
- Severe esophagitis with stricture, hemorrhage, or perforation

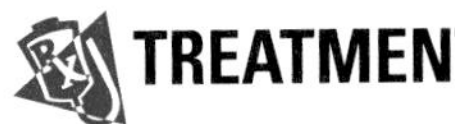 TREATMENT

- Prevention by instructing patients to take pills with 4 oz water and to remain upright for 30 minutes after ingestion
- Known offending agents should not be given to patients with esophageal dysmotility, dysphagia, or strictures

Author(s)

Kenneth R. McQuaid, MD

Factitious Disorder

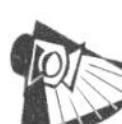 KEY FINDINGS

- Self-induced symptoms or false physical and laboratory findings in an attempt to deceive clinicians
- Unlike the somatoform disorders, symptom production is intentional
- No apparent external motivation for the deceptive behaviors other than achieving the sick role
- In Munchausen syndrome, the deception is carried out by the patient
- In Munchausen by proxy, a parent creates an illness in a child so that the parent can maintain a relationship with clinicians
- Patients are frequently connected in some way to the health professions and often are migratory

 CLINICAL FINDINGS

- Deceptions may involve
  - Fever
  - Self-mutilation
  - Hemorrhage
  - Hypoglycemia
  - Seizures
  - Many other symptoms
  - False physical and/or laboratory findings
- Presentations are often dramatic and exaggerated, but the duplicity may also be complex and difficult to recognize

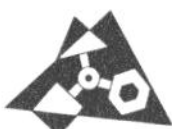 DIAGNOSIS

- Determining that physical or laboratory findings are false

TREATMENT

- Early psychiatric consultation is indicated
- Two main treatment strategies
  - Conjoint confrontation of the patient by both the primary clinician and the psychiatrist
    - ▫ The patient's disorder is portrayed as a cry for help, and psychiatric treatment is recommended
  - Avoidance of direct confrontation and attempt to provide a face-saving way to relinquish the symptom without overt disclosure of the disorder's origin

Author(s)

Stuart J. Eisendrath, MD

Jonathan E. Lichtmacher, MD

Familial Mediterranean Fever

 KEY FEATURES

- Episodic bouts of acute peritonitis associated with serositis involving the joints and pleura
- Rare autosomal recessive disorder
- Almost exclusively affects people of Mediterranean ancestry, especially Sephardic Jews, Armenians, Turks, and Arabs
- Unknown pathogenesis
- Patients lack a protease in serosal fluids that normally inactivates interleukin-8 and complement factor 5A

 CLINICAL FINDINGS

- Symptom onset before the age of 20
- Fever
- Severe abdominal pain and abdominal tenderness with guarding or rebound tenderness
- Joint pain, inflammation
- Pleuritic chest pain, pleural effusion
- Secondary amyloidosis (renal, hepatic) occurs in 25% of cases and can lead to death

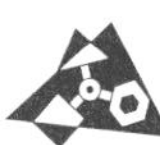 DIAGNOSIS

- Usually a clinical diagnosis
- Gene responsible for familial Mediterranean fever (*MEFV*) has been identified
- Diagnosis can be established by genetic testing

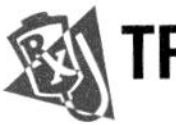 TREATMENT

- Patients may undergo unnecessary exploratory laparotomy
- Untreated, attacks resolve within 24–48 hours
- Colchicine, 0.6 mg PO BID–TID
  - Decreases the frequency and severity of attacks
  - Can prevent or arrest amyloidosis

Author(s)

Kenneth R. McQuaid, MD

Fascioliasis

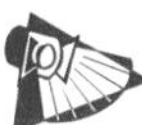

KEY FEATURES

- Infection results from ingestion of encysted metacercariae on watercress or other aquatic vegetables or in water
- Eggs of worm infect snails; snails subsequently infect vegetation
- Most prevalent in sheep-raising countries, particularly where raw salads are eaten

CLINICAL FINDINGS

- Tender, enlarged liver, fever, leukocytosis, and marked eosinophilia (to 90%) seen in acute illness
- Right upper quadrant pain, headache, anorexia and vomiting, myalgia, urticaria, and other allergic reactions
- Jaundice, cachexia, and prostration may appear in severe illness
- Chronic latent phase may be asymptomatic or characterized by hepatomegaly and other findings
- In chronic obstructive phase, clinical picture similar to sclerosing cholangitis, biliary cirrhosis, or choledocholithiasis

DIAGNOSIS

- Diagnosis established by detecting eggs in feces; sometimes eggs only found in biliary drainage
- Ultrasonography and endoscopic retrograde cholangiopancreatography (ERCP) may show parasites in gallbladder
- Eosinophilia is characteristic, and hypergammaglobulinemia and abnormal liver function tests may be present
- ELISA is highly sensitive and specific in detection of antibody and antigen, particularly in acute infections

TREATMENT

- Triclabendazole (Novartis Agribusiness in US) is the drug of choice; 10 mg/kg given once with food achieves a cure rate of 80%. In severe infection, 20 mg/kg in divided doses for 1 day is sometimes recommended. Treatment may need to be repeated
- Bithionol (given as for paragonimiasis) is the alternative drug of choice
- In biliary obstruction due to *Fasciola,* endoscopic biliary sphincterotomy with extraction of the flukes has been effective and safe

Fasciolopsiasis

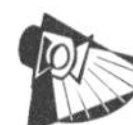

KEY FEATURES

- *Fasciolopsis buski* is a common parasite of humans and pigs in central and southern Asia
- When eggs shed in stools reach water, they hatch to produce free-swimming larvae that penetrate and develop in the flesh of snails. Cercariae escape from snails and infect various water plants, which are then eaten by humans (water chestnuts, bamboo shoots)

CLINICAL FINDINGS

- After an incubation period of 2–3 mo, manifestations of gastrointestinal irritation appear in all but light infections
- In severe infections, there may be nausea, upper abdominal pain, diarrhea, sometimes alternating with constipation
- Ascites and edema of the face and lower extremities may occur late as well as intestinal obstruction, ileus, and cachexia

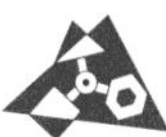

DIAGNOSIS

- Diagnosis depends on finding characteristic eggs or, occasionally, flukes in the stools
- Leukocytosis with moderate eosinophilia is common
- No serologic test is available
- The adult worms live for 6 mo; absence from the endemic area for a longer period makes the diagnosis unlikely

TREATMENT

- The drug of first choice is praziquantel, 25 mg/kg 3 times in 1 day only
- The alternative drug is niclosamide (not available in US), given every other day for 3 doses. Taken in the morning before eating, the tablets must be chewed thoroughly and swallowed with water. Resume eating in 2 h
- In light infections—even without treatment—the prognosis is good; generally, spontaneous cure occurs within 1 yr

Fatty Liver of Pregnancy, Acute

KEY FEATURES

- Acute hepatic failure in the third trimester of pregnancy
- Mortality of 20–30% with early delivery
- Etiology unknown in most cases
- 20% linked to fetal LCHAD deficiency
- Fatty engorgement of hepatocytes seen on CT of liver and on biopsy
- Incidence of 1:14,000 deliveries

CLINICAL FINDINGS

- Gradual onset of flu-like symptoms
- Progression to abdominal pain, jaundice, encephalopathy, disseminated intravascular coagulation, and death
- Signs of hepatic failure are present on examination
- All etiologies of fulminant hepatic failure should be considered, but transaminase levels are lower (< 500 U/mL) in acute fatty liver of pregnancy

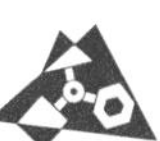

DIAGNOSIS

- Marked elevation of alkaline phosphatase
- Only moderate alanine aminotransferase and aspartate aminotransferase elevations
- Prothrombin time and bilirubin are elevated
- Leukocytosis with thrombocytopenia
- Hypoglycemia may be extreme
- Levels of toxins known to cause liver failure should be measured

TREATMENT

- Supportive care includes administration of glucose, platelets, and fresh frozen plasma as needed
- Diagnosis mandates immediate delivery, preferably vaginally
- Low protein diet
- Resolution of encephalopathy occurs over days
- Recurrence rates are unclear

Author(s)

William R. Crombleholme, MD

Fecal Incontinence

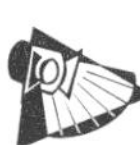

KEY FEATURES

- Occurs in up to 10% of the elderly
- Minor incontinence is slight soilage of undergarments that tends to occur after bowel movements or with straining or coughing
- Causes
  - Local anal problems such as hemorrhoids and skin tags
  - Ulcerative proctitis
  - Chronic diarrheal conditions
  - Irritable bowel syndrome
- Major incontinence is complete uncontrolled loss of stool
- Causes
  - Significant sphincteric or neurologic damage resulting from obstetric trauma (especially forceps delivery, episiotomy, or pudendal nerve damage)
  - Prolapse
  - Prior anal surgery
  - Physical trauma
  - Aging
  - Diabetes mellitus
  - Dementia
  - Multiple sclerosis
  - Spinal cord injury
  - Cauda equina syndrome

CLINICAL FINDINGS

- Incontinence of stool, minor or major

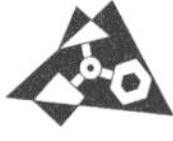

DIAGNOSIS

- Confirm an intact anocutaneous reflex by stimulation of perianal skin
- Digital examination during relaxation and squeezing to assess resting tone and external sphincter function and to exclude fecal impaction
- Anoscopy to assess for prolapse of rectal mucosal hemorrhoids
- Proctosigmoidoscopy to exclude rectal neoplasm or proctitis
- Anal ultrasonography to assess integrity of sphincter
- Anal manometry and surface electromyography to assess rectal sensation, resting and voluntary squeeze pressures, and innervation

TREATMENT

- Minor incontinence
  - Fiber supplements
  - Bulking agents
  - Loose application of a cotton ball near the anal opening
  - Kegel perineal strengthening exercises
- Major incontinence
  - Antidiarrheal drugs (eg, loperamide, 2 mg before meals and prophylactically before social engagements, shopping trips, etc)
  - Scheduled toilet use after glycerin suppositories or tap water enemas
- Provide elderly more time and assistance to reach toilet
- Prevent stool impaction and "overflow" incontinence
- Biofeedback training with anal sphincter exercises for patients with reduced sensation or poor voluntary squeeze pressures
- Surgical intervention in patients who have failed medical therapy, especially patients with traumatic disruption of sphincters

Author(s)

Kenneth R. McQuaid, MD

Femoral Aneurysm

KEY FEATURES

- True aneurysms of the femoral artery are less common than popliteal or aortic aneurysms or femoral pseudoaneurysms
- Causes
  - Injury produced by IV drug abuse
  - Femoral artery puncture for angiography
  - Pevious surgery
  - Femoral catheter insertion

CLINICAL FINDINGS

- Pulsatile groin mass
- Symptoms resulting from arterial thrombosis, peripheral embolization, or compression of adjacent structures with resultant venous thrombosis or neuropathy
  - Rupture is rare
- Arterial thrombosis leads to amputation in up to 30% of patients

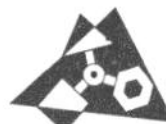

DIAGNOSIS

- Ultrasonography
- Conventional angiography

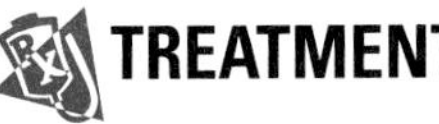

TREATMENT

True Aneurysms

- Incidence of complications is lower than with popliteal aneurysms
- Patients with combined disease undergo repair of aortoiliac and popliteal aneurysms before repair of the femoral aneurysm

Pseudoaneurysms

- Uninfected, small (< 5 cm) traumatic pseudoaneurysms
  - Can be treated by ultrasonogram-guided compression of the aneurysm neck or by thrombin injection
  - 90% reported success rate
- If compression not successful, open repair is required
- Open repair is also advised for any pseudoaneurysm after femoral bypass surgery
- Mycotic aneurysms should be widely débrided with proximal and distal ligation or interposition grafting using autologous vein

Author(s)

Louis M. Messina, MD

Femoral Neuropathy

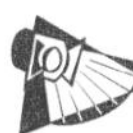

KEY FEATURES

- May occur in diabetics or from compression by retroperitoneal neoplasms or hematomas; may also result from pressure from the inguinal ligament when the thighs are markedly flexed and abducted, as in the lithotomy position
- The neuropathy may be asymptomatic, resolve rapidly and spontaneously, or become progressively more disabling

CLINICAL FINDINGS

- Weakness of the quadriceps muscle
- Sensory impairment over the anteromedian aspect of the thigh and sometimes also of the leg to the medial malleolus
- Depressed or absent knee jerk

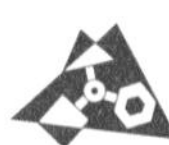

DIAGNOSIS

- Electromyography and nerve conduction velocities are often indispensable for accurate localization of the focal lesion

TREATMENT

- Improvement may occur if any compression is relieved

Author(s)

Michael J. Aminoff, MD, DSc, FRCP

Fibromuscular Dysplasia

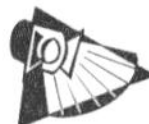

KEY FEATURES

- Nonatherosclerotic, noninflammatory disease of unknown cause characterized by segmental irregularity of small and medium-sized muscular arteries
- Occurs predominantly in women aged 30–50 years
- Family history of disease often present
- Most frequently involved vessels are the renal, carotid, and common iliac arteries
- Four recognized histological types: medial fibrodysplasia (> 80%), intimal fibroplasia, medial hyperplasia, and perimedial dysplasia

CLINICAL FINDINGS

- Renovascular hypertension
- Renal insufficiency
- Transient ischemic attacks
- Claudication
- Intracranial aneurysms present in as many as half of patients with internal carotid fibromuscular dysplasia

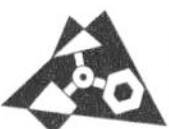

DIAGNOSIS

- Angiography: "string of beads" pattern of disease

TREATMENT

- Aspirin, 325 mg PO QD
- Percutaneous angioplasty for symptomatic patients
- Stents offer no any advantage over angioplasty alone
- More complex lesions require interposition grafting

Author(s)

Louis M. Messina, MD

Fibromyalgia

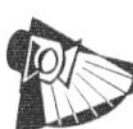

KEY FEATURES

- One of the most common rheumatic syndromes in ambulatory medicine
- Although many of the clinical features of the two conditions overlap, musculoskeletal pain predominates in fibromyalgia and lassitude dominates chronic fatigue syndrome
- Cause is unknown

CLINICAL FINDINGS

- Chronic aching pain and stiffness, often involving the entire body but with prominence of pain around neck, shoulders, low back, and hips
- Fatigue, sleep disorders, subjective numbness, chronic headaches, and irritable bowel symptoms are common
- Physical examination is normal except for "trigger points" of pain produced by palpation of various areas such as the trapezius, the medial fat pad of the knee, and the lateral epicondyle of the elbow

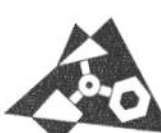

DIAGNOSIS

- Diagnosis of exclusion
- Thyroid function tests are useful because hypothyroidism can produce a secondary fibromyalgia syndrome
- Polymyositis produces weakness rather than pain
- Polymyalgia rheumatica produces shoulder and girdle pain, is associated with an elevated sedimentation rate and anemia, and occurs after age 50

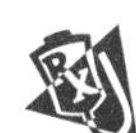

TREATMENT

- Patients can be comforted that they have a syndrome treatable by specific, though imperfect, therapies and that the course is not progressive
- Amitriptyline, fluoxetine, chlorpromazine, or cyclobenzaprine reduce symptoms in some patients
- Amitriptyline is initiated at a dosage of 10 mg at bedtime and gradually increased to 40–50 mg depending on efficacy and toxicity
- Exercise programs are also beneficial
- Opioids, NSAIDs, and corticosteroids are ineffective

Author(s)

David B. Hellmann, MD, FACP

John H. Stone, MD, MPH

Focal Segmental Glomerular Sclerosis

KEY FEATURES

- Idiopathic or secondary to heroin use, morbid obesity, HIV infection

CLINICAL FINDINGS

- Nephrotic syndrome
- Microscopic hematuria in 80%
- Hypertension
- Decreased renal function at diagnosis in 25–50%

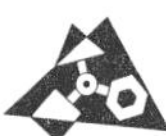

DIAGNOSIS

- Renal biopsy:
  - Light microscopy shows focal segmental glomerular sclerosis;
  - Immunofluorescence shows IgM and C3;
  - Electron microscopy shows fusion of epithelial foot processes

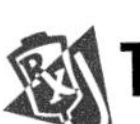

TREATMENT

- Nephrology consultation
- Prednisone, 1–1.5 mg/kg/day PO for 2–3 mo followed by a slow steroid taper
- Remission in > 50% of patients, most within 5–9 mo
- Cytotoxic drug therapy produces remission in < 20% of those refractory to steroids

Author(s)

Suzanne Watnick, MD

Gail Morrison, MD

Folic Acid Deficiency

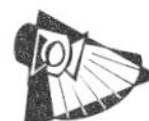

KEY FEATURES

- Folic acid present in most fruits and vegetables (especially citrus fruits and green leafy vegetables)
- Daily requirements of 50–100 μg/day usually met in the diet
- Total body stores of folate enough to supply requirements for 2–3 mo
- Most common cause of folate deficiency is inadequate dietary intake, which occurs in alcoholics, anorectic patients, persons who do not eat fresh fruits and vegetables, and those who overcook food
- Other causes: decreased absorption (tropical sprue, drugs, eg, phenytoin, sulfasalazine, trimethoprim-sulfamethoxazole); increased requirement (chronic hemolytic anemia, pregnancy, exfoliative skin disease); loss (dialysis); and inhibition of reduction to active form (methotrexate)

CLINICAL FINDINGS

- Megaloblastic anemia, which may be severe
- Glossitis and vague GI disturbances (eg, anorexia, diarrhea)
- No neurological abnormalities, unlike vitamin B_{12} deficiency

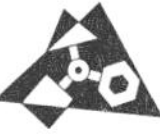

DIAGNOSIS

- Megaloblastic anemia identical to that in vitamin B_{12} deficiency (eg, macro-ovalocytes, hypersegmented neutrophils (see Vitamin B_{12} deficiency)
- Red blood cell folate level < 150 ng/mL
- Serum vitamin B_{12} level normal
- Distinguish from anemia of liver disease (macrocytic anemia with target cells but no megaloblastic changes)

TREATMENT

- Folic acid, 1 mg PO QD, for patients with folate deficiency or increased folate requirements
- Rapid improvement in sense of well-being, reticulocytosis in 5–7 days, and total correction of hematological abnormalities within 2 months

Author(s)

Charles A. Linker, MD

Fragile X Mental Retardation

KEY FEATURES

- Fragile X mental retardation accounts for more cases of retardation in males than any condition except Down syndrome
- Inherited as an X-linked condition
- About 1 in 2000 males is affected

CLINICAL FINDINGS

- Affected males show macro-orchidism (enlarged testes) after puberty, large ears and a prominent jaw, high-pitched voice, and mental retardation. Some show evidence of a mild connective tissue defect, with joint hypermobility and mitral valve prolapse
- Affected (heterozygous) women show no physical signs other than early menopause, but they may have learning difficulties or frank retardation
- Premutation carriers (men and women with 55–200 CGG repeats) may develop ataxia and tremor as older adults

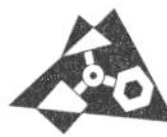

DIAGNOSIS

- Cytogenetic studies demonstrate a small gap, or fragile site, near the tip of the long arm of the X chromosome
- Fragile site is due to expansion of a trinucleotide repeat (CGG) near a gene called *FMR1*
- One *FMR1* allele with ≥ 200 repeats results in mental retardation in virtually all men and about 60% of women
- Clinical DNA diagnosis for the number of CCG repeats can be performed for any male or female who has unexplained mental retardation
- Prenatal DNA diagnosis can be performed

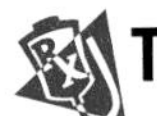

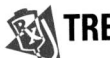

TREATMENT

- None

Author(s)

Reed E. Pyeritz, MD, PhD

Galactorrhea

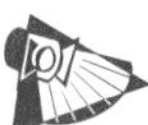

KEY FEATURES

- Lactation that occurs without breast-feeding
- Usual cause: hyperprolactinemia from either overproduction of prolactin by pituitary adenoma or loss of prolactin inhibition by dopamine
- Nipple stimulation and nipple rings can increase prolactin
- Idiopathic (benign) galactorrhea
  - Many parous women can express a small amount of breast milk
  - Prolactin level is normal
- Normal breast milk may vary in color, but bloody discharge raises suspicion of cancer

CLINICAL FINDINGS

- Unilateral or bilateral milky nipple discharge
- Oligomenorrhea, amenorrhea, or infertility
- Pituitary prolactinomas may co-secrete growth hormone, causing acromegaly
- Large pituitary tumors may cause
  - Headaches
  - Visual field defects
  - Pituitary insufficiency (hypogonadism, hypothyroidism, adrenal insufficiency, growth hormone deficiency)

DIAGNOSIS

- Evaluation required for galactorrhea if:
  - Significant in amount
  - In a nulliparous woman
  - Associated with amenorrhea, headache, visual field abnormalities, or other symptoms implying endocrinopathy
- Serum prolactin level is elevated (Table 110)
- Urine or serum hCG is elevated if pregnancy causes galactorrhea
- TSH high if hypothyroidism causes hyperprolactinemia
- MRI of the pituitary and hypothalamus indicated for nonpregnant patients
  - If prolactin is persistently elevated (>200 ng/dL) with no discernible cause
  - If patient has headaches or visual field defects

TREATMENT

- Reassure if prolactin is normal or if parous woman
- Correct underlying cause of elevated prolactin (Table 110)
- Discontinue potentially offending medications, and recheck in a few weeks
- Cabergoline or bromocriptine can reduce galactorrhea regardless of cause
- Treat prolactinoma using medication, surgery, or radiation (see *Hyperprolactinemia*)

Author(s)

Paul A. Fitzgerald, MD

Gamma Hydroxybutyrate Overdose

KEY FEATURES

- A popular drug of abuse and for sexual assault; consumed as a liquid or powder added to a drink
- Other related chemicals with similar effects include butanediol and gamma-butyrolactone (GBL)
- A prolonged withdrawal syndrome has been described in some heavy chronic users

CLINICAL FINDINGS

- Symptoms after ingestion include drowsiness and lethargy followed by coma with respiratory depression
- Muscle twitching and seizures are sometimes observed
- Recovery is usually rapid, with patients awakening within a few hours

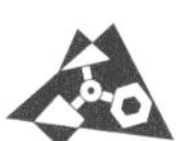

DIAGNOSIS

- Urine GHB analysis can be obtained from National Medical Labs and some forensic labs

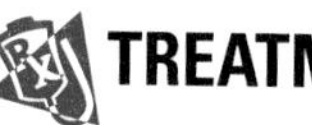

TREATMENT

- Administer activated charcoal, 60–100 g PO or via gastric tube, mixed in aqueous slurry for recent ingestions
- Do not use for comatose patients unless it can be given by gastric tube and the airway is first protected by a cuffed endotracheal tube
- There is no specific treatment
- GHB withdrawal syndrome may require very large doses of benzodiazepines over several days

Author(s)

Kent R. Olson, MD

Gastritis, Atrophic

KEY FEATURES

- An autoimmune disorder involving the fundic glands
- Results in achlorhydria and vitamin B_{12} malabsorption
- Fundic histology shows severe gland atrophy and intestinal metaplasia
- Inflammation and autoimmune destruction of the parietal cells lead to loss of intrinsic factor

CLINICAL FINDINGS

- Hypergastrinemia may induce hyperplasia of gastric enterochromaffin-like cells, development of small, multicentric carcinoid tumors in 5%
- Risk of adenocarcinoma is increased threefold
  - Prevalence 1–3%

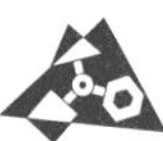

DIAGNOSIS

- Endoscopy with biopsy
- Achlorhydria leads to pronounced hypergastrinemia (>1000 pg/mL)
- Parietal cell antibodies present in 90%
- Low serum vitamin B_{12} level
- Megaloblastic (macrocytic) anemia

TREATMENT

- One-time endoscopic screening for adenocarcinoma or carcinoids recommended
- Patients with dysplasia or small carcinoids require periodic endoscopic surveillance
- Vitamin B_{12} 1000 mg SC every month if B_{12} deficiency documented

Author(s)

Kenneth R. McQuaid, MD

Gastroenteritis, *Escherichia coli*

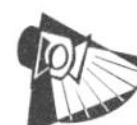

KEY FEATURES

- *E coli* causes gastroenteritis by organism growth in the gut with toxin production
- Enterotoxin causes hypersecretion in the small intestine

CLINICAL FINDINGS

- Table 131
- **Enterotoxigenic** *E coli*
  - Elaborates either a heat-stable or a heat-labile toxin that mediates diarrhea, including traveler's diarrhea
- **Enteroinvasive** *E coli*
  - Invades cells, causing bloody diarrhea and dysentery similar to infection with *Shigella* species
- **Enterohemorrhagic** *E coli*
  - Produces two Shiga-like toxins that mediate nonbloody diarrhea, hemorrhagic colitis, hemolytic uremic syndrome, and thrombotic thrombocytopenic purpura
  - Serotype O157:H7 is responsible for most cases in the United States
  - Elderly individuals and young children are most severely affected; hemolytic uremic syndrome is more common in the latter group

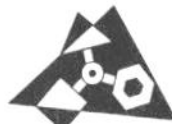

DIAGNOSIS

- *E coli* O157:H7 is not identified by routine stool cultures. Isolation requires identification of sorbitol-negative colonies of *E coli* on sorbitol-MacConkey agar followed by serologic testing to confirm serotype

TREATMENT

- Antimicrobial therapy does not alter the course of the disease and may increase the risk of hemolytic uremic syndrome. Treatment is primarily supportive

Author(s)

Henry F. Chambers, MD

Gastroenteritis, *Salmonella*

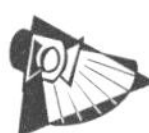

KEY FEATURES

- The most common form of salmonellosis is acute enterocolitis
- Numerous *Salmonella* serotypes may cause enterocolitis
- The incubation period is 8–48 h after ingestion of contaminated food or liquid

CLINICAL FINDINGS

- Fever (often with chills), nausea and vomiting, cramping abdominal pain, and diarrhea, which may be grossly bloody, lasting 3–5 days
- Usually self-limited, but bacteremia with localization in joints or bones may occur, especially in patients with sickle cell disease

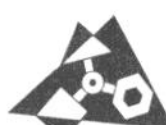

DIAGNOSIS

- Culturing the organism from the stool

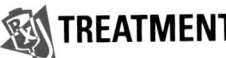

TREATMENT

- Mild to moderate disease can be treated symptomatically
- For severe diarrhea, either ciprofloxacin, 500 mg BID for 3 days, or levofloxacin, 500 mg once daily for 3 days, is effective; trimethoprim-sulfamethoxazole DS BID for 3 days is an effective alternative

Author(s)

Henry F. Chambers, MD

Gastroenteritis, Viral

KEY FEATURES

- Viruses are major cause of infectious diarrhea
- Include rotaviruses, Norwalk and Norwalk-like caliciviruses, and enteric adenoviruses

CLINICAL FINDINGS

- Gastroenteritis usually includes both vomiting and nonbloody diarrhea
- Often occurs in an epidemic fashion in closed environments (eg, cruise ships, schools)

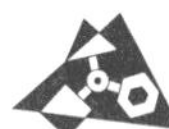

DIAGNOSIS

- Generally restricted to outbreak investigations
- ELISA and PCR assays of stool

TREATMENT

- Supportive care with fluid and electrolyte replacement
- Environmental sanitation key to containing and preventing outbreaks
- Rotavirus vaccination suspended for fear it caused intussusception in infants (although data are controversial)

Author(s)

Wayne X. Shandera, MD

Ana Moran, MD

Gastrointestinal Bleeding, Occult

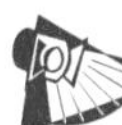

KEY FEATURES

- Presence of a positive fecal occult blood test (FOBT) or iron deficiency anemia in an adult with no visible fecal blood loss
- 1–2.5% of patients in screening programs have a positive FOBT
- 2% of men and 5% of women have iron deficiency anemia
- In premenopausal women
  - Most common cause is menstrual and pregnancy-associated iron loss
  - GI blood loss in 10%
  - No cause determined in 30–50%
- In men and postmenopausal women
  - Blood loss in the colon in 15–30%
  - In the upper GI tract in 35–55%
  - Malignancy in 10%
- Most common causes: neoplasms; vascular abnormalities (vascular ectasias, portal hypertensive gastropathy); acid-peptic lesions; infections (nematodes [especially hookworm], tuberculosis); medications (especially NSAIDs or aspirin); inflammatory bowel disorder or malabsorption (celiac sprue)

CLINICAL FINDINGS

- Positive FOBT
- Iron deficiency anemia

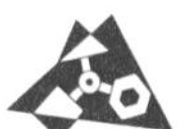

DIAGNOSIS

- Colonoscopy with or without upper endoscopy is indicated
  - For all adults older than 40–45 with positive FOBTs or iron deficiency anemia
  - For premenopausal women and younger men with GI symptoms
  - For those with family history of GI cancer
  - For those with anemia disproportionate to the estimated menstrual blood loss
- Unless upper GI tract symptoms are present, colonoscopy should be done first
- Upper endoscopy indicated in patients with upper GI tract symptoms or iron deficiency anemia after nondiagnostic colonoscopy
- Small bowel enteroscopy, small bowel series or enteroclysis, video capsule device if persistent unexplained chronic GI blood loss or anemia that responds poorly to iron supplementation. Rarely, angiography or intraoperative endoscopy is indicated

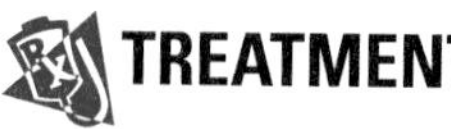

TREATMENT

- Colonoscopy, upper endoscopy, and small bowel enteroscopy allow detection of biopsy or exclusion of benign and malignant neoplasms or endoscopic cautery of vascular ectasias

Author(s)

Kenneth R. McQuaid, MD

Gastroparesis

KEY FEATURES

- Chronic condition characterized by intermittent, waxing and waning symptoms of nausea, bloating, early satiety, and vomiting in the absence of any mechanical lesions
- Caused by endocrine disorders (diabetes mellitus, hypothyroidism, cortisol deficiency), postsurgical (vagotomy, partial gastric resection, fundoplication, gastric bypass, Whipple procedure), neurologic (Parkinson's disease, muscular and myotonic dystrophy, autonomic dysfunction, multiple sclerosis, postpolio syndrome, porphyria), rheumatologic (progressive systemic sclerosis), infections (postviral, Chagas' disease), amyloidosis, paraneoplastic syndromes, medications, and anorexia nervosa
- Cause may not always be identified

CLINICAL FINDINGS

- Manifestations of gastroparesis may be chronic or intermittent
- Early satiety, bloating, nausea, and postprandial vomiting (1–3 hours after meals)

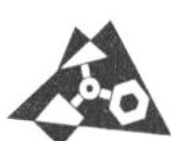

DIAGNOSIS

- Plain-film radiography shows dilatation of the esophagus and stomach
- Endoscopy or barium radiography (upper GI series) excludes mechanical obstruction
- Gastric scintigraphy with a low-fat solid meal assesses gastric emptying
- Gastric retention of 60% after 2 hours or more than 10% after 4 hours is abnormal

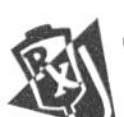

TREATMENT

- No specific therapy
- Acute exacerbations: Nasogastric suction and IV fluids, correction of electrolyte disturbance
- Chronic treatment: Small, frequent meals low in fiber, milk, gas-forming foods, and fat
- Jejunal feeding via external feeding tube or jejunostomy if oral feeding cannot meet nutritional needs
- Parenteral nutrition seldom required unless there is a diffuse gastric and intestinal motility disorder
- Avoid opioids, anticholinergics
- In diabetics, maintain glucose levels < 200 mg/dL
- Metoclopramide, 5–20 mg PO QID or 5–10 mg IV or SC before meals, and erythromycin, 125–250 mg PO BID or 3 mg/kg IV Q 8 h
- Tegaserod, 6–12 mg BID, enhances gastric emptying; however, its role in gastroparesis requires further study
- Gastric decompression: Patients with severe gastroparesis may require placement of a percutaneous endoscopic gastrostomy (PEG) to decompress the stomach
- Gastric pacing with internally implanted neurostimulators

Author(s)

Kenneth R. McQuaid, MD

Gaucher's Disease

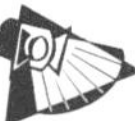

KEY FEATURES

- Gaucher's disease is caused by a deficiency of β-glucocerebrosidase, which leads to an accumulation of sphingolipid within phagocytic cells throughout the body
- Inherited as an autosomal recessive
- Most common in people of Ashkenazi Jewish ancestry
- Over 200 mutations have been found to cause Gaucher's disease
- Two uncommon forms of Gaucher's disease, types II and III, involve neurological accumulation of sphingolipid and neurological problems
- Type II is of infantile onset and has a poor prognosis

CLINICAL FINDINGS

- Episodes of bone pain
- Anemia and thrombocytopenia are common, due primarily to hypersplenism and marrow infiltration with Gaucher cells
- Cortical erosions of bones, especially vertebrae and femur, due to local infarctions

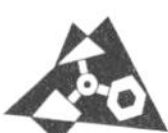

DIAGNOSIS

- Bone marrow aspirates reveal typical Gaucher cells, which have an eccentric nucleus and periodic acid–Schiff–positive inclusions, along with wrinkled cytoplasm and inclusion bodies of a fibrillar type
- Serum acid phosphatase elevated
- Deficient glucocerebrosidase activity in leukocytes

TREATMENT

- Supportive treatment of bone pain; avoid risks for fractures
- Splenectomy for thrombocytopenia
- Enzyme replacement therapy
- Imiglucerase, a recombinant form of the enzyme glucocerebrosidase, 30 units/kg/mo IV, reduces total body stores of glycolipid and improves orthopedic and hematological, but not neurological, manifestations
- During enzyme therapy, monitor platelet count in blood, and the size of the liver and spleen on MRI
- An initial skeletal survey will detect occult bone involvement; new onset of bone pain requires evaluation for possible fracture

Author(s)

Reed E. Pyeritz, MD, PhD

Gender Identity Disorder

KEY FEATURES

- Gender identity reflects a biological self-image and is usually well developed by age 3 or 4 years of age
- Gender dysphoria occurs when a sexual identity is developed that is opposite the biological identity

CLINICAL FINDINGS

- Transsexuals assume a fixed role of attitudes, feelings, fantasies, and choices typical of the opposite sex
  - They typically lack interest in their genitals as evidence of their gender or as a focus for erotic behavior
- A desire for sex change starts early and may culminate in assumption of a feminine lifestyle, hormonal treatment, and use of surgical procedures such as castration and vaginoplasty

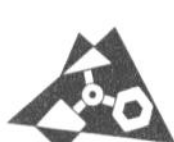

DIAGNOSIS

- Clinical
- Aversion and operant condition are frequently tried but only occasionally result in a behavioral change
- Genital reconstructive surgeries are sometimes performed, but many patients are screened out by trial periods living as the intended sex

Author(s)

Stuart J. Eisendrath, MD

Jonathan E. Lichtmacher, MD

Genital Prolapse

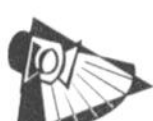

KEY FEATURES

- Cystocele, rectocele, and enterocele are vaginal hernias commonly seen in multiparous women
- Cystocele is a hernia of the bladder wall into the vagina, causing a soft anterior fullness
- Cystocele may be accompanied by urethrocele, which is not a hernia but a sagging of the urethra after its detachment from the pubic symphysis during childbirth
- Rectocele is a herniation of the terminal rectum into the posterior vagina, causing a collapsible pouch-like fullness
- Enterocele is a vaginal vault hernia containing small intestine, usually in the posterior vagina and resulting from a deepening of the pouch of Douglas
- Enterocele may also accompany uterine prolapse or follow hysterectomy, when weakened vault supports or a deep unobliterated cul-de-sac containing intestine protrudes into the vagina
- All three types of hernia may occur in combination

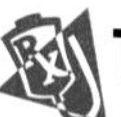

TREATMENT

- Supportive measures include a high-fiber diet. Weight reduction in obese patients and limitation of straining and lifting are helpful
- Pessaries may reduce cystocele, rectocele, or enterocele temporarily and are helpful in women who do not wish surgery or are chronically ill
- The only cure for symptomatic cystocele, rectocele, or enterocele is corrective surgery. The prognosis after an uncomplicated procedure is good

Author(s)

H. Trent MacKay, MD, MPH

Gingivitis, Necrotizing Ulcerative

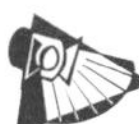

KEY FEATURES

- Trench mouth, Vincent's infection
- Often caused by an infection of both spirochetes and fusiform bacilli
- Is common in young adults under stress (classically at examination time)
- Underlying systemic diseases may also predispose to this disorder

CLINICAL FINDINGS

- Painful acute gingival inflammation and necrosis, often with bleeding
- Halitosis
- Fever
- Cervical lymphadenopathy

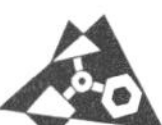

DIAGNOSIS

- Clinical
- Culture

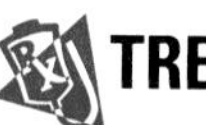

TREATMENT

- Warm half-strength peroxide rinses and oral penicillin (250 mg TID daily for 10 days) may help
- Dental gingival curettage may prove necessary

Author(s)

Robert K. Jackler, MD

Michael J. Kaplan, MD

Glanzmann's Thrombasthenia

KEY FEATURES

- Rare autosomal recessive disorder in which platelets are unable to aggregate because of lack of receptors (containing glycoproteins IIb and IIIa) for fibrinogen, which form bridges between platelets during aggregation

CLINICAL FINDINGS

- Mucosal (epistaxis, gingival) bleeding, menorrhagia, and postoperative bleeding. Variable severity but may be severe

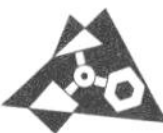

DIAGNOSIS

- Platelet numbers and morphology normal, but bleeding time markedly prolonged. Platelets fail to aggregate in response to typical agonists (adenosine 5'-diphosphate, collagen, thrombin) but aggregate normally in response to ristocetin

TREATMENT

- Platelet transfusions when necessary, but limited by tendency of patients to develop multiple alloantibodies

Author(s)

Charles A. Linker, MD

Glaucoma, Acute Angle-Closure

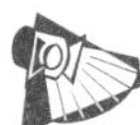

KEY FEATURES

- Primary acute angle-closure glaucoma occurs in eyes with narrow anterior chamber angles, such as in the elderly, hyperopes, and Asians
- May be precipitated by pupillary dilation from sitting in the dark, from stress, rarely by pharmacologic mydriasis for ophthalmologic examination, or from medications with anticholinergic or sympathomimetic activity
- Secondary acute angle-closure glaucoma occurs in uveitis

CLINICAL FINDINGS

- Extreme ocular pain
- Blurred vision, typically with halos around lights
- Nausea and vomiting
- The eye is red and the cornea is cloudy, usually with a moderately dilated, nonreactive pupil

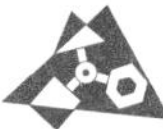

DIAGNOSIS

- Markedly elevated intraocular pressure with shallow anterior chamber in both eyes

TREATMENT

- Immediate evaluation and treatment by an ophthalmologist are essential
- IV and oral acetazolamide and topical agents to lower intraocular pressure
- Topical pilocarpine is used after intraocular pressure is reduced to reverse the angle closure
- Definitive treatment is generally laser peripheral iridotomy, which is usually performed prophylactically on the fellow eye, or surgical peripheral iridectomy

Author(s)

Paul Riordan-Eva, FRCOphth

Glaucoma, Chronic Open-Angle

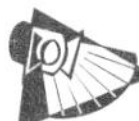

KEY FEATURES

- Usually bilateral optic neuropathy characterized by optic disk cupping and progressive visual field loss, generally associated with elevated intraocular pressure
- Primary open-angle glaucoma: intraocular pressure is elevated because of abnormal drainage of aqueous; generally more severe in African-Americans
- Chronic angle-closure glaucoma: intraocular pressure is elevated as a result of obstruction to aqueous flow; more common in Asians
- Secondary open-angle glaucoma: occurs after ocular trauma, in uveitis, and with chronic topical or systemic corticosteroid therapy
- Normal-tension glaucoma: intraocular pressure not elevated
- Ocular hypertension: elevated intraocular pressure without optic disk cupping or visual field loss

CLINICAL FINDINGS

- Asymptomatic until severe visual loss has developed
- Visual fields progressively constrict, but central vision (acuity) remains good until late

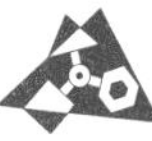

DIAGNOSIS

- Screening by measurement of intraocular pressure, optic disk examination, and visual field testing are essential to early diagnosis
- All persons older than 40 should undergo measurement of intraocular pressure and ophthalmoscopy every 2–5 y
- In diabetics and those with a family history of glaucoma, annual examinations are indicated

TREATMENT

- See Table 10
- Topical prostaglandin analogs and β-adrenergic blocking agents are the most commonly used agents to reduce intraocular pressure
- Other topical agents include α-adrenergic agonists, carbonic anhydrase inhibitors, and cholinergic agonists

- Surgical therapy, such as trabeculectomy or laser trabeculoplasty, may be undertaken if medical therapy is inadequate

Author(s)

Paul Riordan-Eva, FRCOphth

Glomerulonephritis, Cryoglobulin-Associated

KEY FEATURES

- Essential (mixed) cryoglobulinemia is a disorder associated with cold-precipitable immunoglobulins (cryoglobulins)
- Glomerular disease occurs from the precipitation of cryoglobulins in glomerular capillaries
- Causes include underlying bacterial, fungal, and viral infections (eg, hepatitis B and C)

CLINICAL FINDINGS

- Necrotizing skin lesions in dependent areas
- Arthralgias
- Fever
- Hepatosplenomegaly

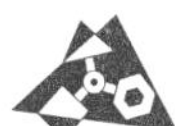

DIAGNOSIS

- Serum complement levels are low
- Renal biopsy: rapidly progressive glomerulonephritis with crescents

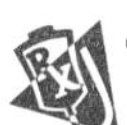

TREATMENT

- Aggressive treatment of the underlying infection
- Pulse corticosteroids, plasma exchange, and cytotoxic agents
- α-Interferon for hepatitis C–related cryoglobulinemia of benefit in subset of patients

Author(s)

Suzanne Watnick, MD

Gail Morrison, MD

Glomerulonephritis, Membranoproliferative

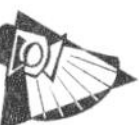

KEY FEATURES

- Idiopathic or secondary to immune complex or paraprotein deposition and thrombotic microangiopathic glomerulonephritides
- Presents with nephritic or nephrotic features
- Most patients are older than 30 years
- Two major subgroups: type I and type II; type II less common than type I

CLINICAL FINDINGS

Type I

- History of recent upper respiratory tract infection in ~33%
- Nephrotic syndrome

Type II

- Glomerulonephritis findings

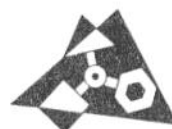

DIAGNOSIS

Type I

- Serum complement levels are low
- Renal biopsy: light microscopy shows glomerular basement membrane is thickened by immune complex deposition, abnormal mesangial cell proliferation, "splitting" appearance to the capillary wall; immunofluorescence shows IgG, IgM, and granular deposits of C3, C1q, and C4

Type II

- Renal biopsy: light microscopy findings similar to type I, but electron microscopy shows dense deposit of homogeneous material replacing part of the glomerular basement membrane
- C3 nephritic factor, a circulating IgG antibody, found in serum

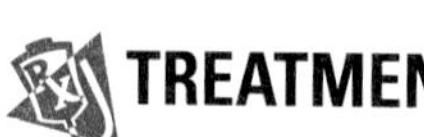

TREATMENT

- Treatment is controversial
- Corticosteroid therapy
- Antiplatelet drugs: aspirin, 500–975 mg/day, plus dipyridamole, 225 mg/day
- In the past, 50% of patients progressed to end-stage renal disease in 10 years;

fewer now with introduction of more aggressive therapy
- Prognosis less favorable with type II disease, early renal insufficiency, hypertension, and persistent nephrotic syndrome
- Renal transplantation, but both types may recur thereafter

Author(s)

Suzanne Watnick, MD

Gail Morrison, MD

Glomerulonephritis, Pauci-Immune

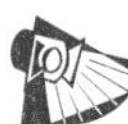

KEY FEATURES

- Pauci-immune glomerular lesions are seen with small-vessel vasculitides, Wegener's granulomatosis, microscopic polyangiitis, and Churg–Strauss syndrome
- Antineutrophil cytoplasmic antibody–associated glomerulonephritis can also present as a primary renal lesion

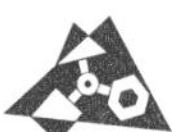

CLINICAL FINDINGS

- Fever, malaise, weight loss
- Hematuria
- Proteinuria
- Purpura
- Mononeuritis multiplex
- In Wegener's, 90% have upper or lower respiratory tract lesions that bleed

DIAGNOSIS

- A cytoplasmic pattern of ANCA (c-ANCA) is specific for antiproteinase 3 antibodies, whereas a perinuclear pattern (p-ANCA) is specific for antimyeloperoxidase antibodies
- Renal biopsy: necrotizing lesions and crescents signify a rapidly progressive glomerulonephritis

TREATMENT

- Institute treatment early; prognosis depends mainly on extent of glomerular involvement before treatment is started
- High-dose corticosteroids (methylprednisolone, 1–2 g/day for 3 days, followed by prednisone, 1 mg/kg for 1 mo, with a slow taper over the next 6 mo) and cytotoxic agents (cyclophosphamide, 1.5–2 mg/kg PO for 3 mo, tapered over 1 year)
- Monitor ANCA levels to help determine efficacy of treatment

Author(s)

Suzanne Watnick, MD

Gail Morrison, MD

Glomerulonephritis, Postinfectious

KEY FEATURES

- Causes include infection from nephritogenic group A β-hemolytic streptococci, especially type 12; bacteremia (eg, *Staphylococcus aureus* sepsis); infective endocarditis; shunt infections; hepatitis B, cytomegalovirus infection, infectious mononucleosis, coccidioidomycosis, malaria, and toxoplasmosis

CLINICAL FINDINGS

- Oliguria
- Edema
- Hypertension, variable

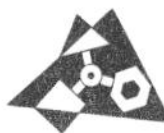

DIAGNOSIS

- Serum complement levels are low
- Antistreptolysin O (ASO) titers sometimes high
- Urinalysis: cola-colored urine, with red blood cells, red cell casts, and proteinuria
- 24-h urine protein < 3.5 g/day
- Renal biopsy
  - Light microscopy shows diffuse proliferative glomerulonephritis
  - Immunofluorescence shows IgG and C3 in a granular pattern in the mesangium and along the capillary basement membrane
  - Electron microscopy shows large, dense subepithelial deposits or "humps"

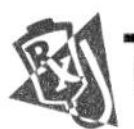

TREATMENT

- Supportive measures
- Antibiotics, as indicated for infection
- Antihypertensive mediations
- Salt and water restriction
- Diuretics

Author(s)

Suzanne Watnick, MD

Gail Morrison, MD

Glossitis & Glossodynia

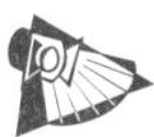

KEY FEATURES

- **Glossitis**
  - Inflammation of the tongue with loss of filiform papillae leads to glossitis
  - May be secondary to nutritional deficiencies (eg, niacin, riboflavin, iron, or vitamin E), drug reactions, dehydration, irritants, and possibly autoimmune reactions or psoriasis
- **Glossodynia**
  - Burning and pain of the tongue; it may occur with or without glossitis
  - It has been associated with diabetes, drugs (eg, diuretics), tobacco, xerostomia, and candidiasis as well as the causes of glossitis
  - Periodontal disease is not a factor

CLINICAL FINDINGS

- Rarely painful
- Glossitis: red, smooth-surfaced tongue

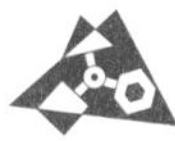

DIAGNOSIS

- Clinical

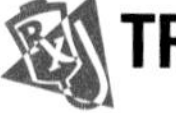

TREATMENT

- **Glossitis**
  - If the primary cause cannot be treated, consider empiric nutritional replacement therapy
- **Glossodynia**
  - Reassurance that there is no infection or tumor
  - Anxiolytic medications and evaluation of possible psychological status may be useful
  - Treating possible underlying causes, changing chronic medications to alternative ones, and smoking cessation may resolve symptoms
  - Consider an empiric trial of gabapentin for symptom control

Author(s)

Robert K. Jackler, MD

Michael J. Kaplan, MD

Glossopharyngeal Neuralgia

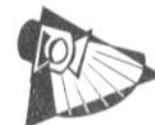

KEY FEATURES

- An uncommon disorder with throat pain similar in quality to that in trigeminal neuralgia

CLINICAL FINDINGS

- Pain occurs in the throat, about the tonsillar fossa, and sometimes deep in the ear and at the back of the tongue
- The pain may be precipitated by swallowing, chewing, talking, or yawning and is sometimes accompanied by syncope

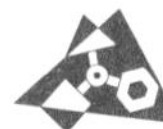

DIAGNOSIS

- In most instances, no underlying structural abnormality is present
- Microvascular compression of glossopharyngeal nerve may be underlying pathogenesis
- Multiple sclerosis or other brainstem lesions are sometimes responsible

TREATMENT

- Oxcarbazepine or carbamazepine is the treatment of choice and should be tried before any surgical procedures are considered
- Microvascular decompression is generally preferred over destructive surgical procedures such as partial rhizotomy in medically refractory, idiopathic cases and is often effective without causing severe complications

Author(s)

Michael J. Aminoff, MD, DSc, FRCP

Glucose-6-Phosphate Dehydrogenase Deficiency

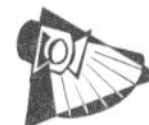

KEY FEATURES

- Hereditary enzyme defect causing episodic hemolytic anemia because of decreased ability of RBCs to deal with oxidative stresses
- Hemoglobin may become oxidized, forming precipitants called Heinz bodies, which cause membrane damage, leading to removal of RBCs by spleen
- X-linked recessive disorder affecting 10–15% of black American males, who have a variant G6PD with 15% of normal enzyme activity; in addition, enzyme activity declines rapidly as RBC ages past 40 days
- Mediterranean variants have extremely low enzyme activity
- Female carriers are affected only when unusually high percentage of cells producing normal enzyme are inactivated (rare)

CLINICAL FINDINGS

- Usually healthy, without chronic hemolytic anemia or splenomegaly
- Hemolysis occurs with oxidative stress resulting from either infection or exposure to certain drugs
- Common drugs initiating hemolysis: dapsone, primaquine, quinidine, quinine, sulfonamides, and nitrofurantoin
- Hemolytic episode self-limited, even with continued use of offending drug, because older RBCs (with low G6PD activity) removed and replaced with young RBCs (with adequate G6PD activity)
- Chronic hemolytic anemia in severe G6PD deficiency (eg, Mediterranean variants)

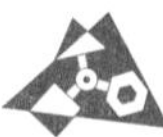

DIAGNOSIS

- Coombs test is negative
- Blood is normal between hemolytic episodes
- Reticulocytosis and increased indirect bilirubin during hemolytic episodes
- G6PD enzyme assays low, especially in severe cases of G6PD deficiency

- G6PD enzyme assays may be misleadingly normal if performed shortly after hemolytic episode when enzyme-deficient RBCs have been removed
- RBC smear, although not diagnostic, may reveal "bite" cell
- Heinz bodies may be seen on peripheral blood smear with crystal violet stain

TREATMENT

- Avoid known oxidant drugs
- Otherwise, no treatment necessary

Author(s)

Charles A. Linker, MD

Gnathostomiasis

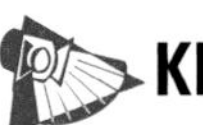

KEY FEATURES

- Infection is usually caused by the larval stage of the nematode *Gnathostoma spinigerum*
- Infection is most common in southeast Asia, China, India, Ecuador, Israel, East Africa, and Mexico, where the infection is most commonly associated with eating raw fresh-water fish, especially sushi, sashimi, and ceviche

CLINICAL FINDINGS

- Within **24–48 h**, larval migration through the intestine can cause acute epigastric pain, vomiting, urticaria, and eosinophilia. The worm then migrates to subcutaneous and other tissues, causing pruritic subcutaneous swelling up to 25 cm across, occasionally accompanied by stabbing pain
- Over **weeks to years**, the swelling may remain constant or move continuously
- Occasionally the worm becomes visible under the skin
- Internal organs and the eye (with eventual blindness) may also be invaded
- Spontaneous pneumothorax, leukorrhea, hematemesis, hematuria, hemoptysis, coughing, edema of the pharynx, spinal cord invasion, eosinophilic meningoencephalitis, or subarachnoid hemorrhage can occur

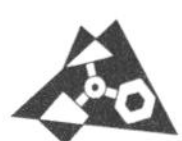

DIAGNOSIS

- Diagnosis can be made by surgical removal of the worm when it appears close to the skin
- Marked eosinophilia is common, except for central nervous system involvement
- Serodiagnosis by immunoblot assay or ELISA is promising

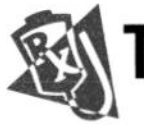

TREATMENT

- Ivermectin, 200 μg/kg PO daily for 2 days, or albendazole, 400 mg PO twice daily for 21 days; larval death appears to occur slowly, and cure rates may reach 95%
- Courses of prednisolone provide temporary relief of symptoms

Goodpasture's Syndrome, Renal

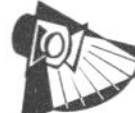

KEY FEATURES

- Clinical constellation of glomerulonephritis and pulmonary hemorrhage
- Injury mediated by antiglomerular basement membrane (anti-GBM) antibodies
- Up to one third of patients with anti-GBM glomerulonephritis have no evidence of lung injury
- 10–15% of patients with rapidly progressive acute glomerulonephritis have anti-GBM
- Incidence in males ~6 times that in females
- Occurs most commonly in the second and third decades
- Associated with influenza A infection, hydrocarbon solvent exposure, and HLA-DR2 and -B7 antigens

CLINICAL FINDINGS

- Upper respiratory tract infection precedes onset in 20–60% of cases
- Hemoptysis, dyspnea, and possible respiratory failure
- Hypertension
- Edema

DIAGNOSIS

- Complement levels are normal
- Sputum contains hemosiderin-laden macrophages
- Chest x-rays show shifting pulmonary infiltrates
- Diffusion capacity of carbon monoxide is markedly increased
- Circulating anti-GBM antibodies positive in > 90%
- Renal biopsy is diagnostic

TREATMENT

- Combination of plasma exchange therapy to remove circulating antibodies and administration of immunosuppressive drugs to prevent formation of new antibodies
- Corticosteroids: pulse doses of prednisone or methylprednisolone, 1–2 g/day for 3 days, then 1 mg/kg/day
- Cyclophosphamide, 2–3 mg/kg/day

- Plasmapheresis, performed daily for up to 2 weeks
- Prognosis poor in patients with oliguria and a serum creatinine > 6–7 mg/dL

Author(s)

Suzanne Watnick, MD

Gail Morrison, MD

Granuloma Inguinale

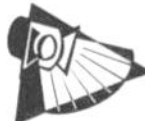

KEY FEATURES

- A chronic, relapsing granulomatous anogenital infection caused by *Calymmatobacterium (Donovania) granulomatis*
- The incubation period is 8 days to 12 weeks

CLINICAL FINDINGS

- Onset is insidious
- Lesions occur on the skin or mucous membranes of the genitalia or perineal area
- Lesions are relatively painless, infiltrated nodules that soon slough. A shallow, sharply demarcated ulcer forms, with a beefy-red friable base of granulation tissue. The lesion spreads by contiguity. The advancing border has a characteristic rolled edge of granulation tissue
- Superinfection with spirochete-fusiform organisms is common. The ulcer then becomes purulent, painful, foul smelling, and extremely difficult to treat

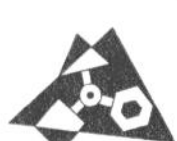

DIAGNOSIS

- Culture

TREATMENT

- Doxycycline, 100 mg PO BID for 21 days
- Trimethoprim-sulfamethoxazole DS (160 mg/800 mg) PO BID, azithromycin, 1 g PO once weekly for 3 weeks

Author(s)

Henry F. Chambers, MD

Haemophilus Infections

KEY FEATURES

- Cause sinusitis, otitis, bronchitis, epiglottitis, pneumonitis, cellulitis, arthritis, meningitis, and endocarditis
- Alcoholism, smoking, chronic lung disease, advanced age, and HIV infection are important risk factors

CLINICAL FINDINGS

- Typical **bacterial pneumonia**, with purulent sputum containing a predominance of gram-negative, pleomorphic rods
- **Epiglottitis** is characterized by an abrupt onset of fever, drooling, and inability to handle secretions
  - Often a severe sore throat despite an unimpressive examination of the pharynx
  - Stridor and respiratory distress result from laryngeal obstruction
- **Meningitis** with sinusitis or otitis

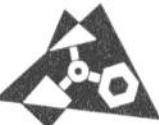

DIAGNOSIS

- Culture: *Haemophilus* species frequently colonize the upper respiratory tract; in the absence of positive pleural fluid or blood cultures, distinguishing pneumonia from colonization or from bacterial bronchitis is difficult
- Epiglottitis: The diagnosis is best made by direct visualization of the cherry-red, swollen epiglottis at laryngoscopy

TREATMENT

- For sinusitis, otitis, or respiratory tract infection, use oral amoxicillin, 750 mg, or amoxicillin, 875 mg, with clavulanate, 125 mg, BID for 10–14 days
- For penicillin allergy, use cefuroxime axetil, 250 mg BID, or trimethoprim-sulfamethoxazole, 800/160 mg PO BID for 10 days
- In the seriously ill patient, use cefuroxime, 750 mg Q 8 h, or ceftriaxone, 1 g/day, pending organism susceptibilities
- *H influenzae* meningitis (Table 128)

Author(s)

Henry F. Chambers, MD

Headache, Cluster

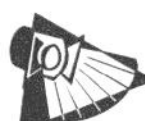

KEY FEATURES

- Affects mainly middle-aged men
- May relate to a vascular headache or a disturbance of a serotonergic mechanism
- There is often no family history of headache or migraine

CLINICAL FINDINGS

- Severe unilateral periorbital pain occurring daily for several weeks
  - Often accompanied by ipsilateral nasal congestion, rhinorrhea, redness of the eye, lacrimation, or Horner's syndrome
- Episodes often occur at night and last for less than 2 h
- Precipitants of an attack
  - Alcohol
  - Stress
  - Glare
  - Specific foods
- Spontaneous remission occurs, and the patient remains well for weeks or months before another bout occurs
- Typical attacks may occur without remission. This variant is chronic cluster headache

TREATMENT

- Sumatriptan 6 mg SC, dihydroergotamine (1–2 mg SC), or inhalation of 100% oxygen (7 L/min for 15 min) may be effective
- Butorphanol tartrate nasal spray, 1 mg (1 spray in 1 nostril), repeated after 60–90 min if necessary, may help
- For prophylaxis, give ergotamine tartrate as rectal suppositories (0.5–1 mg HS or BID), PO (2 mg QD), or by SC injection (0.25 mg TID for 5 days per week)
- Other potentially helpful prophylactic agents include valproate, cyproheptadine, lithium carbonate (monitored by plasma lithium determination), prednisone (20–40 mg daily or on alternate days for 2 weeks, followed by gradual withdrawal), and verapamil (240–480 mg daily)

Author(s)

Michael J. Aminoff, MD, DSc, FRCP

Headache, Tension

KEY FEATURES

- Constant daily headaches that are often vise-like or tight in quality
- May be exacerbated by emotional stress, fatigue, noise, or glare
- Patients also frequently complain of poor concentration and other vague nonspecific symptoms

CLINICAL FINDINGS

- The headaches are usually generalized
- May be most intense about the neck or back of the head
- Are not associated with focal neurologic symptoms

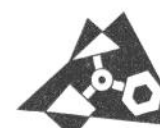

DIAGNOSIS

- Diagnosis is made after exclusion of other causes of headache (see individual diagnoses, eg, *Sinusitis, Acute*)

TREATMENT

- When treatment with simple analgesics is not effective, a trial of antimigrainous agents (see *Headache, Migraine*) is worthwhile
- Techniques to induce relaxation are also useful and include massage, hot baths, and biofeedback
- Exploration of underlying causes of chronic anxiety is often rewarding
- Anecdotal reports of beneficial responses to local injection of botulinum toxin type A have been published

Author(s)

Michael J. Aminoff, MD, DSc, FRCP

Heavy Chain Disease

KEY FEATURES

- A rare gammopathy with excess production of a homogeneous α, γ, or μ heavy chain

CLINICAL FINDINGS

- Clinical presentation is more typical of lymphoma than multiple myeloma
- γ chain disease presents as a lymphoproliferative disorder with autoimmune features
- α chain disease is frequently associated with severe diarrhea and infiltration of the lamina propria of the small intestine with abnormal plasma cells
- μ chain disease is associated with chronic lymphocytic leukemia

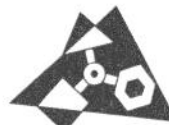

DIAGNOSIS

- Immunofluorescence staining of biopsy tissue with anti-heavy chain antibodies

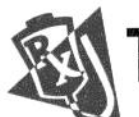

TREATMENT

- Treat with chemotherapy as for a lymphoproliferative disorder
- If μ chain disease, treat underlying chronic lymphocytic leukemia
- Referral to medical oncologist is advised

Author(s)

Jeffrey L. Kishiyama, MD

Daniel C. Adelman, MD

Hemoglobinuria, Paroxysmal Nocturnal

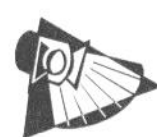

KEY FEATURES

- Acquired clonal stem cell disorder causing abnormal sensitivity of RBC membrane to lysis by complement
- Defect involves increased binding of C3b and increased vulnerability to lysis by complement
- Suspect diagnosis in confusing cases of hemolytic anemia or pancytopenia

CLINICAL FINDINGS

- Hemoglobinuria (reddish-brown urine), particularly in first morning urine
- Anemia
- Increased susceptibility to thrombosis, especially of mesenteric and hepatic veins
- May progress to aplastic anemia, myelodysplasia, or acute myelogenous leukemia

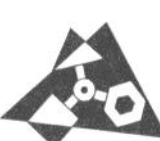

DIAGNOSIS

- Sucrose hemolysis test is best screening test
- Anemia of variable severity
- Reticulocytosis may or may not be present
- Blood smear abnormalities (eg, macro-ovalocytes) are nondiagnostic
- Urine hemosiderin test useful (indicates episodic intravascular hemolysis)
- Serum lactate dehydrogenase characteristically elevated
- Iron deficiency common because of chronic iron loss from hemoglobinuria
- WBC and platelet count may be low
- Bone marrow morphology variable; may show generalized hypoplasia or erythroid hyperplasia
- Flow cytometric assays may confirm diagnosis by demonstrating absence of CD59

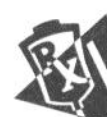

TREATMENT

- Iron replacement often indicated for iron deficiency; may improve anemia but also may cause transient increase in hemolysis
- Prednisone, including alternate-day regimens, may be effective in decreasing hemolysis
- Allogeneic bone marrow transplantation for severe cases and cases of transformation to myelodysplasia

Author(s)

Charles A. Linker, MD

Hemolytic Disease in Newborn

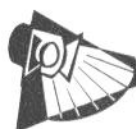

KEY FEATURES

- Anti-Rho(D) antibody is responsible for most severe instances
- Occurs when a Rho(D)-negative woman carries a Rho(D)-positive fetus and develops antibodies against Rho(D)
- The antibody developed against Rho(D) persists and poses a threat of hemolytic disease in subsequent Rho(D)-positive fetuses
- Passive immunization of Rho(D)-negative mothers after delivery destroys fetal Rho(D)-positive cells and prevents formation of antibodies, which would cause disease in subsequent Rho(D)-positive gestations

CLINICAL FINDINGS

- Routine antibody screen is positive

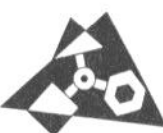

DIAGNOSIS

- Because hemolytic disease may occur in association with Rh subgroups or other red blood cell antigens, atypical antibodies should be assessed at 28 weeks in all pregnancies

TREATMENT

- Rho(D) immunoglobulin (Ig) is given to the mother within 72 h after delivery to prevent future erythroblastosis
- Additional protection is afforded by the routine administration of the Ig at week 28; the passive antibody titer is too low to harm the Rho(D)-positive fetus
- Rho(D) Ig should also be given after abortion, ectopic pregnancy, abruptio placenta, other antepartum bleeding, or amniocentesis or chorionic villus sampling

Author(s)

William R. Crombleholme, MD

Hemolytic Transfusion Reactions

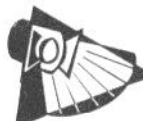

KEY FEATURES

- Severe reactions usually involve mismatches in ABO system resulting from clerical errors and mislabeled specimens
- Hemolysis is rapid and intravascular; most reactions occur in surgical patients under anesthesia
- Severity depends on RBC dose
- Less severe reactions caused by minor antigen systems
- Hemolysis is slower and extravascular and may be delayed for 5–10 days after transfusion
- Duffy, Kidd, Kell, and C and E loci of Rh system are antigens most commonly involved
- Most transfusion reactions are not hemolytic but related to antigens present on WBCs

CLINICAL FINDINGS

- Fever, chills, backache, headache
- Apprehension, dyspnea, hypotension, vascular collapse
- Disseminated intravascular coagulation (DIC)
- Renal failure from acute tubular necrosis
- Generalized bleeding and oliguria in patients under general anesthesia

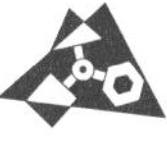

DIAGNOSIS

- Hematocrit fails to rise as expected
- Renal failure
- DIC (low fibrinogen, elevated fibrin degradation products, thrombocytopenia, prolonged PT)
- Hemoglobinemia (plasma pink and hemoglobinuria)
- Indirect bilirubin rises
- Offending alloantibody detectable in patient's serum

TREATMENT

- Stop transfusion immediately
- Check identification of recipient and blood
- Return donor transfusion bag with pilot tube to blood bank with fresh sample of

recipient's blood for retyping and repeat of cross-match
- Centrifuge sample of anticoagulated blood from recipient; if free hemoglobin present, hydrate patient vigorously to prevent acute tubular necrosis. Forced diuresis with mannitol may help prevent renal damage

Author(s)

Charles A. Linker, MD

Hemoptysis

KEY FEATURES

- Expectoration of blood originating below the vocal cords
- Massive hemoptysis
  - >200–600 mL of blood/24 hours
  - Hemodynamic or airway compromise
- Causes can be classified anatomically
  - Airway (bronchitis, bronchiectasis, malignancy)
  - Pulmonary vasculature (congestive heart failure, mitral stenosis, pulmonary emboli, arteriovenous malformation [AVM])
  - Parenchymal (pneumonia, crack use, autoimmune diseases, or iatrogenesis)

CLINICAL FINDINGS

- Blood-tinged sputum to frank blood
- Dyspnea may be mild or severe

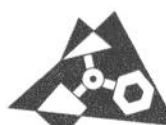

DIAGNOSIS

- Chest x-ray may demonstrate the cause
- High-resolution CT of the chest can diagnose bronchiectasis and AVM as well as many malignancies
- Bronchoscopy is indicated when there is a suspicion of malignancy or a normal chest x-ray

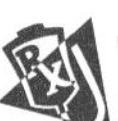

TREATMENT

- In massive hemoptysis, airway protection and circulatory support are first steps
- Patients should be placed in decubitus position with affected lung down
- Rigid bronchoscopy and surgical consultation are necessary in uncontrollable hemorrhage
- Bronchoscopy and angiography can localize lesions
- Embolization is initially effective in 85% of cases, although 20% rebleed in 1 year

Author(s)

Mark S. Chesnutt, MD

Thomas J. Prendergast, MD

Hemorrhagic Fever & Hantavirus

KEY FEATURES

- Diverse group of illnesses associated with animal contact (eg, ticks, mosquitoes, rodents)
- Most prominent in tropics but have worldwide distribution
- Often named for area where they occur (eg, Omsk hemorrhagic fever)
- Includes Ebola, Lassa, Marburg fever, and hantavirus pulmonary syndrome (Sin Nombre virus)

CLINICAL FINDINGS

- Usually present with high fever, leukopenia, altered mental status; hemorrhagic diathesis not a feature of hantavirus
- Marked toxicity and death may occur; acute respiratory distress syndrome may develop as a manifestation of hantavirus pulmonary syndrome

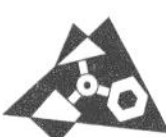

DIAGNOSIS

- Usually made by serologic testing in proper clinical setting
- Polymerase chain reaction testing becoming more widely available

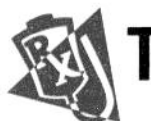

TREATMENT

- Supportive care key
- Patients must be isolated
- Hantavirus and Lassa fever infections treated with ribavarin
- Prevention by reducing the likelihood of vector contact (eg, rodents for Sin Nombre)

Author(s)

Wayne X. Shandera, MD

Ana Moran, MD

Henoch-Schönlein Purpura

 KEY FEATURES

- The most common systemic vasculitis in children
- Occurs in adults as well

 CLINICAL FINDINGS

- Purpuric skin lesions typically located on the lower extremities; may also be seen on the hands, arms, trunk, and buttocks
- Joint symptoms are present in most patients; the knees and ankles are most commonly involved
- Abdominal pain secondary to vasculitis of the intestinal tract is often associated with gastrointestinal bleeding
- Hematuria signals the presence of a glomerular lesion that is usually reversible, although it occasionally may progress to renal insufficiency

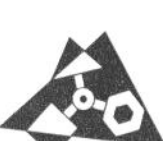 DIAGNOSIS

- Skin biopsy can demonstrate leukocytoclastic vasculitis with IgA deposition
- Kidney biopsy reveals segmental glomerulonephritis with crescents and mesangial deposition of IgA
- Differential diagnosis
  - Immune thrombocytopenic purpura
  - Meningococcemia
  - Rocky Mountain spotted fever
  - Rheumatoid arthritis (including juvenile form)
  - Polyarteritis nodosa
  - Endocarditis
  - Cryoglobulinemia

 TREATMENT

- Usually self-limited, lasting 1–6 weeks, and subsiding without sequelae if renal involvement is not severe
- Chronic courses with persistent or intermittent skin disease are more likely to occur in adults than children
- The efficacy of treatment is not well established

Author(s)

David B. Hellmann, MD, FACP

John H. Stone, MD, MPH

Hepatitis D (Delta)

 KEY FEATURES

- Hepatitis D virus (HDV) causes hepatitis only in the presence of hepatitis B surface antigen (HBsAg); it is cleared when the latter is cleared
- May coinfect with hepatitis B virus (HBV) or may superinfect a person with chronic hepatitis B, usually by percutaneous exposure
- New cases of hepatitis D are infrequent; cases seen today are usually those infected years ago who survived the impact of hepatitis D and now have inactive cirrhosis

 CLINICAL FINDINGS

- When acute hepatitis D is coincident with acute HBV infection, the infection is generally similar in severity to acute hepatitis B alone
- In chronic hepatitis B, superinfection by HDV appears to carry a worse short-term prognosis, often resulting in fulminant hepatitis or severe chronic hepatitis that progresses rapidly to cirrhosis
- Patients with longstanding chronic hepatitis D and B often have inactive cirrhosis

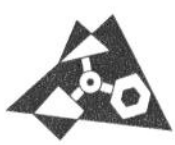 DIAGNOSIS

- Diagnosis is made by detecting antibodies to hepatitis D antigen (anti-HDV) or, where available, HDV RNA in serum

TREATMENT

- Interferon alfa-2a, 9 million units three times a week for 48 weeks, leads to clearance of HDV RNA in 50% of patients; relapse common after discontinuing drug
- Three-fold increased risk of hepatocellular carcinoma
- Hospitalization is necessary for patients with intractable nausea and vomiting who need parenteral fluids
- Encephalopathy or severe coagulopathy indicates impending acute hepatic failure; hospitalization is mandatory
- Hepatitis D is best prevented by preventing hepatitis B (eg, with HBV vaccine—see Hepatitis B, Acute)

Author(s)

Lawrence S. Friedman, MD

Hepatopathy, Ischemic

 KEY FEATURES

- Caused by an acute fall in cardiac output resulting from, for example, acute myocardial infarction or arrhythmia
- Usually in a patient with passive congestion of the liver

 CLINICAL FINDINGS

- Clinical hypotension may be absent
- The precipitating event can be arterial hypoxemia resulting from respiratory failure
- In severe cases, encephalopathy may develop
- The mortality rate resulting from the underlying disease is high; however, in patients who recover, the aminotransferase levels return to normal quickly, usually within 1 week, in contrast to viral hepatitis
- Hepatojugular reflux is present, and with tricuspid regurgitation the liver may be pulsatile
- Ascites may be out of proportion to peripheral edema

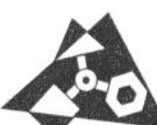 DIAGNOSIS

- The hallmark is a rapid, striking elevation of serum aminotransferase levels (often > 5000 units/L); an early rapid rise in the serum lactate dehydrogenase level is also typical, but elevations of serum alkaline phosphatase and bilirubin are usually mild. The prothrombin time may be prolonged
- In passive congestion of the liver caused by right-sided heart failure, the serum bilirubin level may be elevated, occasionally as high as 40 mg/dL, resulting partly from hypoxia of perivenular hepatocytes. Serum alkaline phosphatase levels are normal or slightly elevated
- Ascites generally has a high serum ascites-albumin gradient (> 1.1) and a protein content of more than 2.5 g/dL

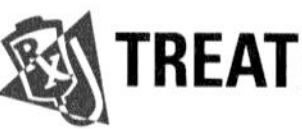

- Supportive. Treat underlying cardiac disease

Author(s)

Lawrence S. Friedman, MD

Hepatopulmonary Syndrome

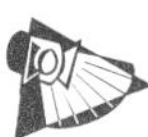

KEY FEATURES

- Characteristic triad
  - Chronic liver disease
  - Increased alveolar-arterial gradient at room air
  - Intrapulmonary vascular dilations or arteriovenous communications that result in a right-to-left intrapulmonary shunt

CLINICAL FINDINGS

- Dyspnea and arterial deoxygenation in the upright position (orthodeoxia) and relieved by recumbency
- The diagnosis should be suspected in a cirrhotic patient with a pulse oximetry level ≤92%

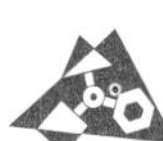

DIAGNOSIS

- Contrast-enhanced echocardiography is a sensitive screening test for detecting pulmonary vascular dilations, whereas macroaggregated albumin lung perfusion scanning is more specific and is used to confirm the diagnosis
- High-resolution CT may be useful for detecting dilated pulmonary vessels that may be amenable to embolization

TREATMENT

- Medical therapy has been disappointing; however, IV methylene blue may improve oxygenation by inhibiting nitric oxide-induced vasodilation
- The syndrome may reverse with liver transplantation; postoperative mortality is increased when the preoperative arterial oxygen tension is ≤50 mm Hg or with substantial intrapulmonary shunting
- Liver transplantation is contraindicated in moderate to severe pulmonary hypertension (mean pulmonary pressure >35 mm Hg), although treatment with epoprostenol or basentan may reduce pulmonary hypertension and thereby facilitate liver transplantation
- TIPS may provide palliation in patients with hepatopulmonary syndrome awaiting transplantation

Author(s)

Lawrence S. Friedman, MD

Hepatorenal Syndrome

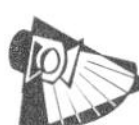

KEY FEATURES

- Diagnosed when other causes of renal disease have been excluded in the setting of end-stage liver disease

CLINICAL FINDINGS

- In **type I** hepatorenal syndrome, the serum creatinine doubles to a level >2.5 mg/dL or the creatinine clearance halves to < 20 mL/min in fewer than 2 weeks
- **Type II** hepatorenal syndrome is chronic and slowly progressive
- The cause is unknown, but the pathogenesis involves intense renal vasoconstriction. Histologically, the kidneys are normal

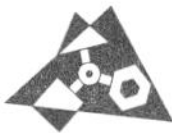

DIAGNOSIS

- Azotemia, hyponatremia, oliguria, unremarkable urinary sediment, no proteinuria
- 24-h urinary sodium < 10 mEq
- Renal function fails to improve after IV infusion of 1.5 L of isotonic saline

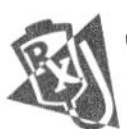

TREATMENT

- Improvement may follow IV infusion of the long-acting vasoconstrictor ornipressin and albumin (but with a high rate of ischemic side effects), ornipressin and dopamine, terlipressin (a long-acting vasopressin analog) and albumin, norepinephrine and albumin, or octreotide, midodrine, an α-adrenergic drug, and albumin
- Survival benefit has occurred with the molecular adsorbent recirculating system (MARS), a modified dialysis method that selectively removes albumin-bound substances
- Improvement may also follow TIPS placement
- Mortality is high without liver transplantation; death is due to complicating infection or hemorrhage

Author(s)

Lawrence S. Friedman, MD

Hiccups

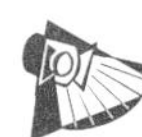

KEY FEATURES

- Usually benign and self-limited but may be persistent and a sign of serious underlying illness
- Causes of self-limited hiccups
  - Gastric distention
  - Sudden temperature changes
  - Alcohol ingestion
  - Emotion
- Causes of recurrent or persistent hiccups
  1. CNS: neoplasms, infections, cerebrovascular accident, trauma
  2. Metabolic: uremia, hypocapnia (hyperventilation)
  3. Irritation of the vagus or phrenic nerve
     - Head, neck: foreign body in ear, goiter, neoplasms
     - Thorax: pneumonia, empyema, neoplasms, myocardial infarction, pericarditis, aneurysm, esophageal obstruction, reflux esophagitis
     - Abdomen: subphrenic abscess, hepatomegaly, hepatitis, cholecystitis, gastric distention, gastric neoplasm, pancreatitis, pancreatic malignancy
  4. Surgical: general anesthesia, postoperative
  5. Psychogenic and idiopathic

CLINICAL FINDINGS

- Detailed neurologic examination

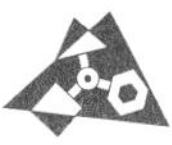

DIAGNOSIS

- Serum creatinine, liver enzymes
- Chest radiograph, chest fluoroscopy
- CT of the head, chest, abdomen
- Echocardiography
- Bronchoscopy
- Upper endoscopy

TREATMENT

Acute hiccups

- Irritation of the nasopharynx by tongue traction, lifting the uvula with a spoon, catheter stimulation of the nasopharynx, or eating 1 tsp dry granulated sugar
- Interruption of the respiratory cycle by breath holding, Valsalva's maneuver, sneezing, gasping, or rebreathing into a bag
- Stimulation of the vagus nerve by carotid massage
- Irritation of the diaphragm by holding knees to chest or by continuous posi-

tive airway pressure during mechanical ventilation
- Relief of gastric distention by belching or insertion of an NG tube

Chronic hiccups

- Chlorpromazine, 25–50 mg PO or IM TID–QID
- Anticonvulsants (phenytoin, carbamazepine), benzodiazepines (lorazepam, diazepam), metoclopramide, baclofen, and occasionally general anesthesia

Author(s)

Kenneth R. McQuaid, MD

Homocystinuria

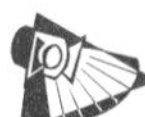

KEY FEATURES

- Caused by cystathionine β-synthase deficiency, which results in extreme elevations of plasma and urinary homocysteine levels
- Autosomal recessive pattern of inheritance

CLINICAL FINDINGS

- Similar to Marfan's syndrome in body habitus and ectopia lentis
- Mental retardation often present
- Cardiovascular events caused by repeated arterial or venous thromboses
- Life expectancy is reduced, especially in untreated and pyridoxine-unresponsive patients
- Myocardial infarction, stroke, and pulmonary embolism are most common causes of death

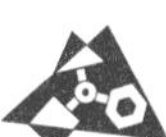

DIAGNOSIS

- Diagnosis suspected in patients in the second and third decades of life who have repeated arterial or venous thromboses and no other risk factors
- DNA analysis can detect mutations in the cystathionine β-synthase gene
- Amino acid analysis of plasma is helpful diagnostic test: elevated plasma methionine levels

TREATMENT

- In ~50% of cases, β-synthase deficiency improves biochemically and clinically with pharmacological doses of pyridoxine and folate
- Treatment from infancy can prevent retardation and the other clinical problems
- Pyridoxine nonresponders must be treated with dietary reduction in methionine and supplementation of cysteine
- Vitamin betaine useful in reducing plasma methionine levels
- Anticoagulation for documented venous thrombosis
- Prophylactic use of warfarin not recommended

Author(s)

Reed E. Pyeritz, MD, PhD

Human T-Cell Lymphotrophic Virus (HTLV)

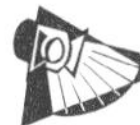

KEY FEATURES

- Retroviruses, types I and II
- HTLV-1 are the causative agents of adult T cell leukemia/lymphoma (ATL) and HTLV-associated myelopathy (HAM)
- Endemic in Caribbean, southern Japan, sub-Saharan Africa, and southeastern United States

CLINICAL FINDINGS

- ATL presents with diffuse lymphadenopathy, skin lesions, hypercalcemia, and lytic bone lesions
- HAM characterized by progressive motor weakness, spastic paraparesis, and sensory disturbances
- HTLV predisposes to usual AIDS-associated opportunistic infections

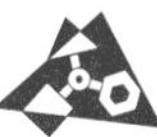

DIAGNOSIS

- Serologic testing for HTLV antibodies
- HTLV-associated ATL confirmed by proviral DNA integration

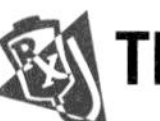

TREATMENT

- ATL treated like other non-Hodgkin's lymphomas
- HAM treated with corticosteroids
- No benefit to antiretroviral therapy
- Blood supply is now screened for HTLV-1 because transfusion is a recognized mode of transmission

Author(s)

Wayne X. Shandera, MD

Ana Moran, MD

Hypercalcemia, Malignant

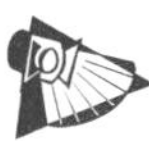

KEY FEATURES

- Occurs in 10–20% of patients with cancer
- Less frequent now with routine use of bisphosphonates for metastatic bone disease
- Common causes include cancers of breast, lung, kidney, and head and neck and multiple myeloma and lymphoma
- Most result from bony metastases, but 20% are unrelated to bony lesions
- Parathyroid hormone–related protein identified in two thirds of patients with malignant hypercalcemia

CLINICAL FINDINGS

- Nausea and vomiting
- Constipation
- Polyuria
- Muscular weakness and hyporeflexia
- Confusion, psychosis, tremor, lethargy

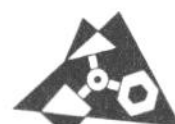

DIAGNOSIS

- Serum calcium increased
- ECG: shortening of the QT interval
- Renal insufficiency
- Be sure to adjust serum calcium level for low albumin or check ionized calcium level

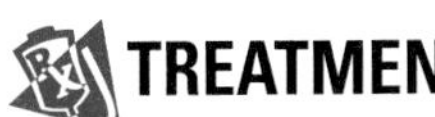

TREATMENT

- Emergency treatment: hydration (3–4 L/day of 0.9% saline) followed by furosemide, 10–40 mg IV. Aggressive hydration is critical
- Definitive treatment: bisphosphonate (eg, zoledronic acid), 4 mg IV over 15 min with adequate hydration, normalizes serum calcium in < 3 days in 80–100%
- Gallium nitrate, 100–200 mg/m^2/day continuous IV infusion for 5 days
- Calcitonin, 4–8 IU/kg IM, SC, or intranasally Q 12 h, in conjunction with bisphosphonates
- Chemotherapy and prednisone effective in reducing serum calcium in lymphoid cancers
- Do not replace phosphate when calcium–phosphate product is high

Author(s)

Hope Rugo, MD

Hyperemesis Gravidarum

KEY FEATURES

- Persistent severe vomiting during pregnancy

CLINICAL FINDINGS

- Weight loss
- Dehydration
- Starvation ketosis
- Hypochloremic alkalosis
- Hypokalemia
- Mild elevation in liver enzymes

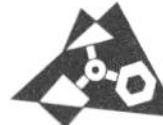

DIAGNOSIS

- TSH and free T_4 should be checked because thyroid dysfunction can be associated

TREATMENT

- Hospitalization with NPO and IV fluids and vitamins PRN
- Total parenteral nutrition is rarely necessary
- As soon as possible, start a dry diet with 6 small daily feedings and clear liquids 1 h after meals
- Prochlorperazine rectal suppositories may be useful
- Once stabilized, patients may remain at home, even if IV fluids are required
- To limit the risk of teratogenicity, drug use in the first half of pregnancy should be limited to those of major importance to life and health (Tables 71, 74)

Author(s)

William R. Crombleholme, MD

Hypermagnesemia

KEY FEATURES

- Almost always the result of renal insufficiency and excessive magnesium intake (eg, antacids, laxatives, IV administration)
- Suppresses secretion of parathyroid hormone with consequent hypocalcemia

CLINICAL FINDINGS

- Muscle weakness
- Decreased deep tendon reflexes
- Mental obtundation
- Confusion
- Weakness, even flaccid paralysis
- Hypotension
- There may be respiratory muscle paralysis or cardiac arrest

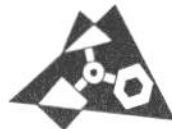

DIAGNOSIS

- In the common setting of renal failure, elevated BUN, serum creatinine, phosphate, and uric acid; serum K^+ may be elevated
- Serum Ca^{2+} is often low
- ECG may show increased PR interval, broadened QRS complexes, and peaked T waves, probably related to associated hyperkalemia

TREATMENT

- Treatment is directed toward therapy of renal insufficiency
- Calcium antagonizes Mg^{2+} and may be given IV as calcium chloride, 500 mg or more at a rate of 100 mg (4.5 mmol)/min
- Hemodialysis or peritoneal dialysis may be indicated

Author(s)

Masafumi Fukagawa, MD, PhD, FJSIM
Kiyoshi Kurokawa, MD, MACP
Maxine A. Papadakis, MD

Hyperphosphatemia

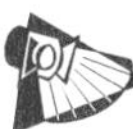 KEY FEATURES

- Chronic renal insufficiency from decreased excretion of phosphorus and decreased renal hydroxylation of 25-OH-vitamin D to 1,25-OH_2-vitamin D is the most common cause
- Hyperphosphatemia in chronic renal failure leads to secondary hyperparathyroidism and renal osteodystrophy
- A serum calcium X serum phosphorus product > 70 markedly increases the risk of nephrocalcinosis and soft tissue calcification

 CLINICAL FINDINGS

- Clinical symptoms are those of the underlying disorders (eg, chronic renal failure, hypoparathyroidism)

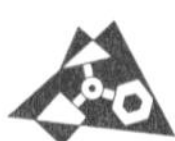 DIAGNOSIS

- Other blood chemistry values are those of the underlying disease (renal failure, hypoparathyroidism)

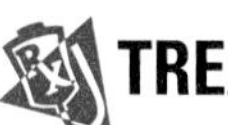 TREATMENT

- Treatment is that of the underlying disease and of associated hypocalcemia if present
- In acute and chronic renal failure, dialysis will reduce serum phosphate
- Phosphate absorption can be reduced by calcium carbonate, 0.5–1.5 g TID with meals (500-mg tablets) (preferred to aluminum hydroxide because of concerns about aluminum toxicity)
- Another phosphate binder is sevelamer hydrochloride titrated to target phosphorus levels using 800–1600 mg three times daily with meals (400- to 800-mg tablets and 403-mg capsules); does not contain calcium or aluminum and may be especially useful in hypercalcemia or uremia

Author(s)

Masafumi Fukagawa, MD, PhD, FJSIM
Kiyoshi Kurokawa, MD, MACP
Maxine A. Papadakis, MD

Hypersomnia

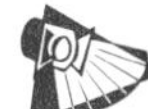 KEY FEATURES

- Classification
  - **Sleep apnea**
    - See Obstructive Sleep Apnea
  - **Narcolepsy**
    - See Narcolepsy
  - **Kleine-Levin syndrome**
    - Occurs mostly in young men
    - Associated with antecedent neurologic insults
  - **Nocturnal myoclonus**

 CLINICAL FINDINGS

- **Kleine-Levin syndrome**
  - Hypersomnic attacks lasting up to 2 days and occurring 3–4 times/year
  - Awakening is accompanied by hyperphagia, hypersexuality, irritability, confusion
  - Usually remits after age 40
- **Nocturnal myoclonus**
  - Periodic lower leg movements occur during sleep
  - Subsequent daytime sleepiness, anxiety, depression, cognitive impairment

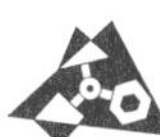 DIAGNOSIS

- Clinical or during a sleep study

TREATMENT

- **Kleine-Levin syndrome**
  - No treatment is known
- **Nocturnal myoclonus**
  - Clonazepam can be used with variable results
  - Dopaminergic agents (bromocriptine, carbodopa/levodopa) can be useful in some

Author(s)

Stuart J. Eisendrath, MD
Jonathan E. Lichtmacher, MD

Hyperthermia

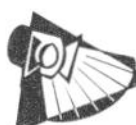 KEY FEATURES

- A rapidly life-threatening complication
- May be due to poisoning by amphetamines (especially ecstasy), atropine and other anticholinergic drugs, cocaine, dinitrophenol and pentachlorophenol, phencyclidine, salicylates, strychnine, tricyclic antidepressants, other agents
- Overdose of serotonin reuptake inhibitors (eg, fluoxetine, paroxetine, sertraline) or use in a patient taking monoamine oxidase inhibitor may cause agitation, hyperactivity, hyperthermia (**serotonin syndrome**)
- Haloperidol and other antipsychotic agents can cause rigidity and hyperthermia (**neuroleptic malignant syndrome**)
- **Malignant hyperthermia** is associated with general anesthetic agents (rare)

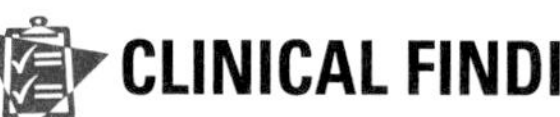 CLINICAL FINDINGS

- Severe hyperthermia (temperature > 40–41°C) may rapidly cause brain damage and multiorgan failure

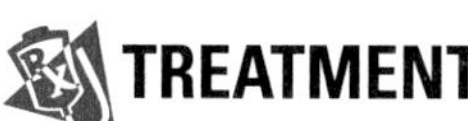 TREATMENT

- Remove clothing; spray with tepid water; fan patient
- If rectal temperature not normal in 30–60 min or there is significant muscle rigidity or hyperactivity, induce neuromuscular paralysis with nondepolarizing neuromuscular blocker (pancuronium, vecuronium)
- Once paralyzed, patient must be intubated and mechanically ventilated
- With seizures, absence of visible muscular convulsive movements may give false impression that brain seizure activity has ceased; this must be confirmed by EEG
- Dantrolene, 2–5 mg/kg IV, may be effective for muscle rigidity unresponsive to neuromuscular blockade (ie, **malignant hyperthermia**)
- Bromocriptine, 2.5–7.5 mg PO daily, for **neuroleptic malignant syndrome**
- Cyproheptadine, 4 mg PO Q h for 3–4 doses, for **serotonin syndrome**

Author(s)

Kent R. Olson, MD

Hyperuricemia

KEY FEATURES

- Complication of rapidly proliferating malignancies as well as treatment-associated tumor lysis of hematological malignancies
- May be worsened by thiazide diuretic use
- Rapid increase in serum uric acid can result in acute urate nephropathy caused by uric acid crystallization in the distal tubules, collecting ducts, and renal parenchyma
- To prevent urate nephropathy, serum uric acid must be reduced before chemotherapy

CLINICAL FINDINGS

- Acute renal failure
- Gouty arthritis (generally only with history of gout)

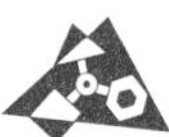

DIAGNOSIS

- At-risk patients should have BID measurements of serum uric acid, phosphate, calcium, and creatinine for the first 2–3 days after initiation of chemotherapy
- Serum uric acid concentration > 15 mg/dL imposes a high risk of uric acid nephropathy

TREATMENT

Prophylaxis

- Allopurinol, 600 mg PO 12–24 h before chemotherapy followed by 300 mg PO QD; higher doses (900–1200 mg/day) are used when severe hyperuricemia is anticipated
- IV dosing when oral not tolerated
- Maintain adequate hydration
- Alkalinize urine with sodium bicarbonate, 6–8 g PO QD, or by infusion of 1 L of D_5W with 2–3 ampules of sodium bicarbonate; goal urine pH = 7.0

Emergency treatment

- Hydration with 2–4 L of fluid per day
- Alkalinization of the urine as above
- Allopurinol, 900–1200 mg/day
- In severe cases, emergency hemodialysis

Author(s)

Hope Rugo, MD

Hyperventilation Syndromes

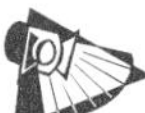

KEY FEATURES

- Hyperventilation is an increase in alveolar ventilation leading to hypocapnia
- Causes include
  - Pregnanc
  - Hypoxemia
  - Obstructive and infiltrative lung disease
  - Sepsis
  - Liver failure
  - Fever
  - Pain
- "Central neurogenic hyperventilation" describes monotonous, sustained deep breathing seen in comatose patients with brain stem injury

CLINICAL FINDINGS

- Acute hyperventilation
  - Hyperpnea
  - Paresthesias
  - Carpopedal spasm
  - Tetany
  - Anxiety
- Chronic hyperventilation presents nonspecifically
  - Fatigue
  - Dyspnea
  - Anxiety
  - Palpitations
  - Dizziness

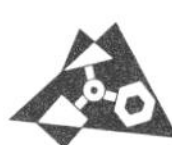

DIAGNOSIS

- Symptoms must be reproduced during voluntary hyperventilation

TREATMENT

- When organic causes have been excluded, rebreathing expired gas from a paper bag decreases respiratory alkalemia and its symptoms
- Anxiolytics may be helpful

Author(s)

Mark S. Chesnutt, MD

Thomas J. Prendergast, MD

Hypoventilation, Primary Alveolar

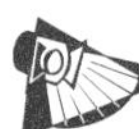

KEY FEATURES

- A rare syndrome ("Ondine's curse") of unknown cause
- Characterized by inadequate alveolar ventilation despite normal airways, lungs, chest wall, respiratory muscles, and neurologic function
- Patients are usually nonobese males in their 40s and 50s

CLINICAL FINDINGS

- Lethargy, headache, and somnolence
- Dyspnea is not present
- Erythrocytosis may be present

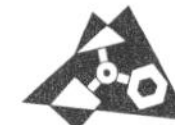

DIAGNOSIS

- Arterial blood gas values show hypoxemia and hypercapnia, which improve with voluntary hyperventilation

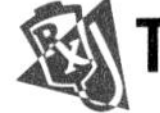

TREATMENT

- Ventilatory stimulants are not effective
- Mechanical augmentation of ventilation via phrenic nerve stimulation, rocking bed, or ventilators may be helpful
- Supplemental oxygen should be given, with the caveat that nocturnal oxygen be given only if sleep study demonstrates that it is effective and safe

Author(s)

Mark S. Chesnutt, MD

Thomas J. Prendergast, MD

Immunoglobulin A Deficiency, Selective

KEY FEATURES

- The most common primary immunodeficiency disorder, estimated to affect 1 in 500 individuals

CLINICAL FINDINGS

- Most patients are asymptomatic
- Frequent and recurrent infections such as sinusitis, otitis, and bronchitis
- Can be associated with IgG subclass deficiency
- Increased atopic and autoimmune diseases
- Most severe consequence is serum sickness or anaphylaxis that develops after the infusion of IgA-containing plasma products (when the patient has anti-IgA antibodies)

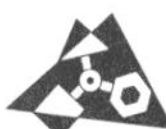

DIAGNOSIS

- The absence of serum IgA with normal levels of total serum IgG and IgM

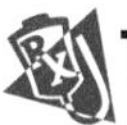

TREATMENT

- Treatment with commercial immune globulin is ineffective because IgA is present only in trace quantities in these preparations
- Antibiotics as needed for infections

Author(s)

Jeffrey L. Kishiyama, MD
Daniel C. Adelman, MD

Impetigo

KEY FEATURES

- A contagious and autoinoculable infection of the skin caused by staphylococci or rarely streptococci (or both)

CLINICAL FINDINGS

- See Table 7
- The lesions consist of macules, vesicles, bullae, pustules, and honey-colored gummy crusts that when removed leave denuded red areas
- The face and other exposed parts are most often involved
- Ecthyma is a deeper form of impetigo caused by staphylococci or streptococci, with ulceration and scarring; it occurs frequently on the legs and other covered areas

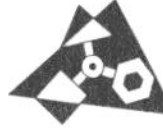

DIAGNOSIS

- Culture confirms the diagnosis
- Differential diagnosis
  - Contact dermatitis (acute)
  - Herpes simplex

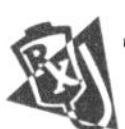

TREATMENT

- Cephalexin, 250 mg PO QID daily
- Doxycycline 100 mg PO BID can be used for penicillin allergy and methicillin-resistant *S aureus*
- Recurrent impetigo, which is due to nasal carriage of *S aureus*, is treated with rifampin, 600 mg PO QD, or intranasal mupirocin ointment twice daily for 5 days
- Refer if questionable diagnosis or if therapy is ineffective

Author(s)

Timothy G. Berger, MD

Infertility, Assisted Reproductive Technologies

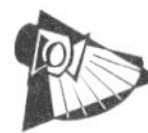

KEY FEATURES

- Couples who have not responded to traditional infertility treatments may benefit from in vitro fertilization (IVF), gamete intrafallopian transfer (GIFT), and zygote intrafallopian transfer (ZIFT)
- Age is an important determinant of success: For couples younger than 35, the average rate of live birth is 37% per cycle, whereas the rate for women older than 42 is 4%. More than one-third of pregnancies have been multiple

CLINICAL FINDINGS

- See Infertility, Female

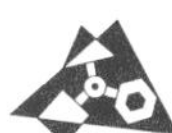

DIAGNOSIS

- See Infertility, Female

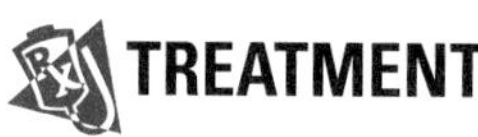

TREATMENT

- All procedures involve ovarian stimulation to produce multiple oocytes, oocyte retrieval by transvaginal sector scan-guided needle aspiration, and handling of the oocytes outside the body
- With IVF, the eggs are fertilized in vitro and the embryos transferred to the uterine fundus. Extra embryos may be cryopreserved for subsequent cycles
- GIFT involves the placement of sperm and eggs in the uterine tube by laparoscopy or minilaparotomy and is more invasive than IVF
- GIFT is not appropriate for women with severe tubal diseases and is less successful than IVF with male factor infertility because fertilization cannot be documented
- With ZIFT, fertilization occurs in vitro, and the early development of the embryo occurs in the uterine tube after transfer by laparoscopy or minilaparotomy
- Intracytoplasmic sperm injection allows fertilization with a single sperm, which is helpful in the setting of severe oligospermia or obstructive azoospermia

Author(s)

H. Trent MacKay, MD, MPH

Interstitial Lung Disease, Respiratory Bronchiolitis-Associated

KEY FEATURES

- Presentation similar to usual interstitial pneumonitis (UIP) but in younger patients
- Patients are invariably heavy smokers
- Prognosis is better than in UIP; median survival >10 years

CLINICAL FINDINGS

- Age 40–45 years
- Insidious dry cough with exertional dyspnea over months to years
- Diffuse, fine, late inspiratory crackles on exam

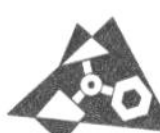

DIAGNOSIS

- Pulmonary function test shows restriction with decreased DLCO, usually less severe than that seen in UIP
- Biopsy shows increased numbers of macrophages localized within the peribronchiolar space; alveolar architecture is preserved, honeycomb change and fibrosis are minimal

TREATMENT

- Spontaneous remission in up to 20% of patients
- Smoking cessation is crucial
- Corticosteroids are thought to be effective, although no randomized trial supports this

Author(s)

Mark S. Chesnutt, MD

Thomas J. Prendergast, MD

Intertrigo

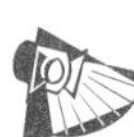

KEY FEATURES

- Caused by the macerating effect of heat, moisture, friction
- Especially likely to occur in obese persons and in humid climates

CLINICAL FINDINGS

- Symptoms are itching, stinging, burning
- Body folds develop fissures, erythema, and sodden epidermis, with superficial denudation
- Candidiasis may complicate intertrigo

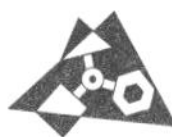

DIAGNOSIS

- KOH prep and Wood's light to rule out *Candida,* tinea, and erythrasma
- Differential diagnosis
  - Candidiasis
  - Tinea cruris (jock itch)
  - Psoriasis of body folds ("inverse psoriasis")
  - Erythrasma
  - Cellulitis
  - Seborrheic dermatitis
  - Tinea versicolor (pityriasis versicolor; rarely)
  - Scratching resulting from pediculosis (lice)
  - Contact dermatitis

TREATMENT

- Maintain hygiene in the area, and keep it dry
- Compresses may be useful acutely
- Hydrocortisone 1% and an imidazole cream or nystatin cream are effective
- Recurrences are common

Author(s)

Timothy G. Berger, MD

Iron Poisoning

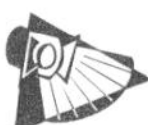

KEY FEATURES

- Most children's preparations contain 12–15 mg of elemental iron per dose vs. 60–90 mg for most adult-strength preparations
- Iron is corrosive to GI tract and has depressant effects on myocardium and on peripheral vascular resistance

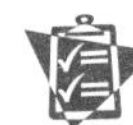

CLINICAL FINDINGS

- Ingestion of < 30 mg/kg of elemental iron usually produces only mild GI upset
- Ingestion of > 40–60 mg/kg may cause vomiting, hematemesis, diarrhea, hypotension, and metabolic acidosis
- Death may occur from massive fluid losses and bleeding, metabolic acidosis, peritonitis from intestinal perforation, fulminant hepatic failure

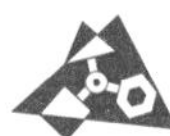

DIAGNOSIS

- Serum iron levels > 350–500 μg/dL are potentially toxic; levels > 1000 μg/dL usually associated with severe poisoning
- Plain abdominal x-ray film may reveal radiopaque tablets

TREATMENT

- Treat hypotension aggressively with IV crystalloid solutions (0.9% saline or lactated Ringer's solution)
- Perform whole-bowel irrigation to remove unabsorbed pills, particularly when intact tablets are visible on abdominal x-ray film
- Administer balanced polyethylene glycol-electrolyte solution (CoLyte, GoLYTELY) into the stomach via gastric tube at 1–2 L/h until rectal effluent is clear
- Activated charcoal not effective
- For symptomatic toxicity, and particularly with markedly elevated serum iron levels (eg, > 800–1000 μg/dL), administer 10–15 mg/kg/h of deferoxamine by constant IV infusion; higher doses (up to 40–50 mg/kg/h) have been used in massive poisonings. Prolonged infusion (> 36–48 h) has been associated with acute respiratory distress syndrome

Author(s)

Kent R. Olson, MD

Isoniazid Poisoning

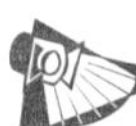

KEY FEATURES

- Acute ingestion of as little as 1.5–2 g can cause toxicity, and severe poisoning is likely to occur after ingestion of more than 80–100 mg/kg
- May cause hepatitis with chronic use

CLINICAL FINDINGS

- Confusion, slurred speech, and seizures may occur abruptly after acute overdose
- Severe lactic acidosis—disproportional to the severity of seizures—is probably due to inhibited metabolism of lactate

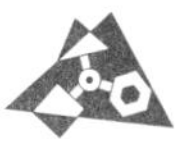

DIAGNOSIS

- Diagnosis is based on a history of ingestion and the presence of severe acidosis associated with seizures
- Isoniazid is not usually included in routine toxicological screening, and serum levels are not readily available

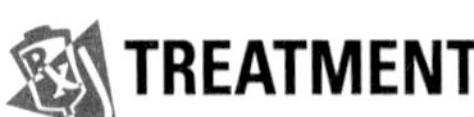

TREATMENT

- Seizures may require higher than usual doses of benzodiazepines (eg, lorazepam, 3–5 mg IV)
- Pyridoxine (vitamin B_6) is a specific antagonist of the acute toxic effects and is usually successful in controlling seizures that do not respond to benzodiazepines. Give 5 g IV over 1–2 min or, if the amount ingested is known, a gram-for-gram equivalent amount of pyridoxine
- Administer activated charcoal, 60–100 g PO or via gastric tube, mixed in aqueous slurry; do not use for comatose or convulsing patients unless it can be given by gastric tube and the airway is protected by a cuffed endotracheal tube

Author(s)

Kent R. Olson, MD

Kawasaki Syndrome

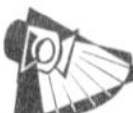

KEY FEATURES

- Mucocutaneous lymph node syndrome
- Usually affects children younger than 10, at times in an epidemic fashion
- No clear infectious cause identified

CLINICAL FINDINGS

- Fever universal
- Bilateral nonexudative conjunctivitis
- Mucous membrane involvement
- Polymorphous rash
- Cervical lymphadenopathy

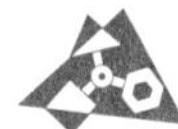

DIAGNOSIS

- Clinical based on combination of above findings
- Potential for arteritis of coronary vessels leading to myocardial infarction

TREATMENT

- High-dose aspirin
- IV immunoglobulin
- Warfarin for coronary artery aneurysms
- Corticosteroids for refractory disease
- Interventional catheter treatment, including stent implantation

Author(s)

Wayne X. Shandera, MD

Ana Moran, MD

Klinefelter's Syndrome

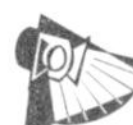

KEY FEATURES

- Males with 1 extra X chromosome (XXY)

CLINICAL FINDINGS

- Boys are normal in appearance before puberty; after puberty, they have disproportionately long legs and arms, a female escutcheon, gynecomastia, and small testes
- Infertility resulting from azoospermia; the seminiferous tubules are hyalinized
- Mental retardation is somewhat more common than in the general population, and many have learning problems
- Higher risk of breast cancer
- Heightened risk of diabetes mellitus

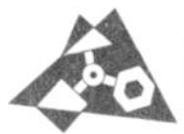

DIAGNOSIS

- Cytogenetic analysis

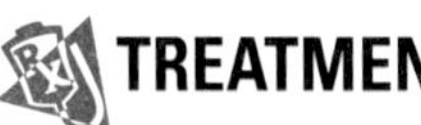

TREATMENT

- Testosterone administration is advisable after puberty but will not restore fertility
- Intracytoplasmic sperm injection is possible using sperm obtained by testicular extraction

Author(s)

Reed E. Pyeritz, MD, PhD

Knee, Overuse Syndromes

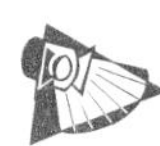

KEY FEATURES

- Runners, particularly those who overtrain, fail to stretch before running, or do not attain the proper level of conditioning before starting a running program, may develop a variety of painful overuse syndromes of the knee
- Most of these conditions are forms of tendinitis or bursitis that can be diagnosed on examination
- The most common conditions include anserine bursitis, iliotibial band syndrome, and popliteal and patellar tendinitis

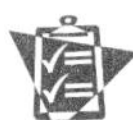

CLINICAL FINDINGS

- Symptoms worsen with continued running
- Anserine bursitis results in pain medial and inferior to the knee joint over the medial tibia
- The iliotibial band syndrome results in pain on the lateral side of the knee
- Patellar tendinitis, a cause of anterior knee discomfort, typically occurs at the tendon's insertion into the patella rather than at its more inferior insertion

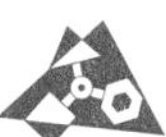

DIAGNOSIS

- Confirm the diagnoses by palpating the relevant sites around the knee
- Not associated with joint effusions or other signs of synovitis

TREATMENT

- Rest and abstention from the associated physical activities for a period of days to weeks are essential
- Once the acute pain has subsided, a program of gentle stretching (particularly before resuming exercise) may prevent recurrence
- Corticosteroid with lidocaine injections may be useful when intense discomfort is present, but caution must be used when injecting corticosteroids into the region of a tendon since rupture may occur

Author(s)

David B. Hellmann, MD, FACP
John H. Stone, MD, MPH

Labor, Preterm

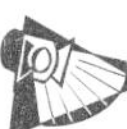

KEY FEATURES

- Labor beginning before 37th week of pregnancy
- Responsible for 85% of neonatal illnesses and deaths

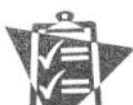

CLINICAL FINDINGS

- Risk factors
  - History of preterm labor
  - Premature rupture of membranes
  - Urinary tract infection
  - Diethylstilbestrol exposure
  - Multiple gestation
  - Abdominal or cervical surgery
  - Cervical length of < 25 mm by second-trimester ultrasonogram

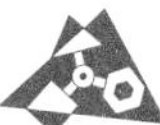

DIAGNOSIS

- Fetal fibronectin measurement in cervicovaginal specimens can differentiate true from false labor
- A level < 50 ng/mL has a negative predictive value of 93–97% for delivery in 7–14 days among women with a history of preterm delivery currently having contractions

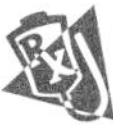

TREATMENT

- Low rates of preterm delivery are associated with successful education of patients in identifying regular, frequent contractions
- Magnesium sulfate IV, 4–6-g bolus followed by infusion of 2–3 g/h titrated to blood levels of 6–8 mg/dL
- Terbutaline (2.5 μg/min IV titrated to a maximum 20 μg/min or 2.5–5 mg PO Q 2–4 h) relaxes the myometrium via B_2-receptor activation
- Nifedipine, 10–20 mg PO Q 4–6 h

Author(s)

William R. Crombleholme, MD

Lactase Deficiency

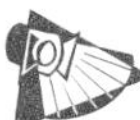

KEY FEATURES

- Partial to complete lactose intolerance affects ~50 million people in the United States
- Occurs in 90% of Asian Americans, 70% of African Americans, 95% of Native Americans, 50% of Mexican Americans, 60% of Jewish Americans, 25% of Caucasian adults
- Also occurs secondary to Crohn's disease, sprue, viral gastroenteritis, giardiasis, short bowel syndrome, malnutrition

CLINICAL FINDINGS

- Bloating, abdominal cramps, and flatulence 1–3 hours after ingesting milk products
- Diarrhea

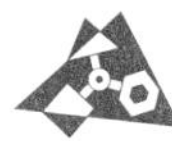

DIAGNOSIS

- Diarrheal specimens have an increased osmotic gap and pH < 6.0
- Hydrogen breath test: After ingestion of 50 g lactose, a rise in breath hydrogen of >20 ppm within 90 minutes is a positive test
- Empirical trial of a lactose-free diet for 2 weeks, leading to resolution of symptoms
- Differential diagnosis: inflammatory bowel disease, mucosal malabsorptive disorders, irritable bowel syndrome, pancreatic insufficiency

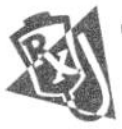

TREATMENT

- Eliminate or restrict milk products
- Spread dairy product intake throughout the day
- Use lactase enzyme supplements (eg, nonprescription formulation [LactAid]) when ingesting dairy products
- Calcium supplementation

Author(s)

Kenneth R. McQuaid, MD

Larva Migrans, Cutaneous

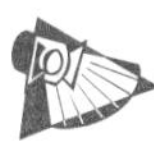

KEY FEATURES

- Caused by larvae of the dog and cat hookworms, *Ancylostoma braziliense* and *Ancylostoma caninum*
- Prevalent throughout the tropics and subtropics, including southeastern US
- Moist sandy soil (eg, beaches, children's sand piles) contaminated by dog or cat feces is a common site of infection

CLINICAL FINDINGS

- At the site of larval entry, particularly on the hands or feet, up to several hundred minute, intensely pruritic erythematous papules appear
- Two to 3 days later, serpiginous eruptions appear as the larvae migrate at a rate of several millimeters a day
- The process may continue for weeks; the lesions may become severely pruritic, vesiculate, encrusted, or secondarily infected
- Without treatment, the larvae eventually die and are absorbed

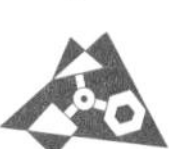

DIAGNOSIS

- Clinical and the frequent eosinophilia
- Biopsy is usually not indicated

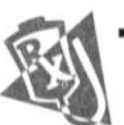

TREATMENT

- Mild transient cases may not require treatment
- For mild cases, use thiabendazole, applied topically TID for 5 or more days as a 15% cream, which can be formulated in a hygroscopic base using crushed 500-mg tablets
- For more severe cases, oral treatment is indicated. Give ivermectin, 200 μg/kg for 1 or 2 days, and albendazole, 400 mg BID for 3–5 days or 400 mg daily for 7 days
- Thiabendazole, given PO as for strongyloidiasis, is less satisfactory because of its toxicity
- Antihistamines can help control pruritus
- Antibiotic (ointment or oral) may be necessary to treat secondary infections

Lead Poisoning

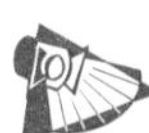

KEY FEATURES

- Toxicity is usually from subacute or chronic exposure to contaminated dust or fumes
- Acute ingestion of lead fishing weights or curtain weights can cause poisoning

CLINICAL FINDINGS

- Abdominal pain, constipation, headache, irritability
- Coma and convulsions in severe poisoning
- Chronic intoxication can cause learning disorders (in children) and motor neuropathy (eg, wristdrop)

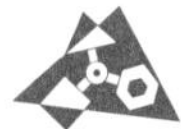

DIAGNOSIS

- Blood lead level
- Microcytic anemia with basophilic stippling and elevated free erythrocyte protoporphyrin may be seen
- Can be misdiagnosed as porphyria

TREATMENT

- For recent ingestion, give activated charcoal, 60–100 g PO or via gastric tube, mixed in aqueous slurry
- If a large lead object remains visible on stomach x-ray film, repeated cathartics, whole-bowel irrigation, endoscopy, or surgical removal may be necessary
- Consult a medical toxicologist or regional poison control center for advice about chelation. For severe intoxication (encephalopathy or levels > 70–100 μg/dL), give edetate calcium disodium (EDTA), 1500 mg/m^2/kg/day (~50 mg/kg/day) in 4–6 divided doses or as a continuous IV infusion
- Dimercaprol, 4–5 mg/kg IM Q 4 h for 5 days, can be added
- Less severe symptoms with blood lead levels between 55 and 69 μg/dL may be treated with EDTA alone in dosages as above
- Succimer (dimercaptosuccinic acid), 10 mg/kg PO Q 8 h for 5 days, then Q 12 h for 2 weeks

Author(s)

Kent R. Olson, MD

Leishmaniasis, Mucocutaneous

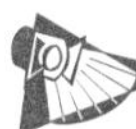

KEY FEATURES

- Caused by the leishmania (viannia) group of organisms; most common is *Leishmania (V) brasiliensis* in Central and South America

CLINICAL FINDINGS

- The **initial lesion**, single or multiple, is on exposed skin; at first it is papular, then nodular, and later may ulcerate or become wart-like or papillomatous. Local healing follows, with scarring within several months to a year
- **Subsequent** nasooral involvement occurs in a few patients. It may appear concurrently with the initial lesion, shortly after healing, or after many years. Extensive destruction of the soft tissues and cartilage of the nose, oral cavity, and lips may follow and may extend to the larynx and pharynx
- Secondary bacterial infection is common
- Fever, keratitis, lymphangitis, weight loss, and anemia may be present

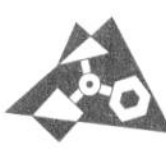

DIAGNOSIS

- Diagnosis by detecting amastigotes in scrapings, biopsy impressions, or aspirated tissue fluid is difficult
- The organism grows with difficulty in culture or in hamster inoculation
- The skin test can be useful
- Standard serological tests are often not useful; a direct agglutination for IgM antibodies may become positive in 4–6 weeks and subsequently an IgG test may become positive, but at low titer

TREATMENT

- See *Leishmaniasis*
- Failure rates are high in severe disease even when a full course (28 days) of sodium stibogluconate is used. If repeated and extended antimony treatment fails, amphotericin B desoxycholate or pentamidine is used
- Corticosteroids may control inflammation from release of antigens

Listeriosis

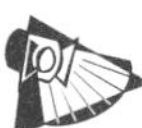

KEY FEATURES

- *Listeria monocytogenes* is a motile, gram-positive rod that is a facultative intracellular organism
- Most cases of infections are sporadic, but outbreaks have been traced to eating contaminated food, especially unpasteurized dairy products

CLINICAL FINDINGS

- Five types of infection are recognized
  - Infection during pregnancy, usually in the last trimester, produces a mild febrile illness without an apparent primary focus. This is a relatively benign disease that may resolve without therapy
  - Granulomatosis infantisepticum is a neonatal infection characterized by disseminated abscesses and granulomas and a high mortality rate
  - Bacteremia with or without sepsis syndrome is an infection of neonates or immunocompromised adults. The presentation is that of a febrile illness without a recognized source
  - Meningitis affects infants younger than 2 mo and adults, ranking third and fourth, respectively, among the common causes of bacterial meningitis. Adults with meningitis are usually immunocompromised, and cases have been associated with HIV infection
  - Focal infections, including adenitis, brain abscess, endocarditis, osteomyelitis, and arthritis, occur rarely

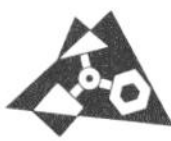

DIAGNOSIS

- Table 130
- In meningitis, cerebrospinal fluid shows a neutrophilic pleocytosis

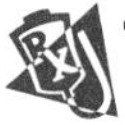

TREATMENT

- Tables 127 and 129
- The drug of choice is probably ampicillin, 8–12 g/day IV in 4–6 divided doses (the higher dose is recommended in cases of meningitis)
- Trimethoprim-sulfamethoxazole is an effective alternative

Author(s)

Henry F. Chambers, MD

Lithium Toxicity

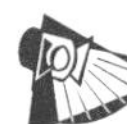

KEY FEATURES

- Occurs at serum lithium levels >2 mEq/L
- Sodium loss (from diarrhea, diuretics, perspiration) results in elevated lithium levels
- Toxicity is more severe in the elderly

CLINICAL FINDINGS

- Diarrhea, vomiting
- Tremors, marked weakness, confusion
- Dysarthria, ataxia, vertigo, choreoathetosis, hyperreflexia
- Myoclonus, seizures, opisthotonos, coma

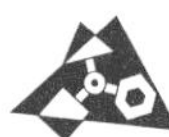

DIAGNOSIS

- Serum lithium levels confirm the diagnosis

TREATMENT

- Induced emesis and gastric lavage for massive ingestions or levels >2.5 mEq/L
- Osmotic or saline diuresis in patients with normal renal function
- Urinary alkalinization with sodium bicarbonate or acetazolamide

Author(s)

Stuart J. Eisendrath, MD

Jonathan E. Lichtmacher, MD

Livedo Reticularis

KEY FEATURES

- An uncommon vasospastic disorder of unknown cause that results in a painless, mottled discoloration on large areas of the extremities in a fishnet pattern with reticulated cyanotic areas surrounding a paler central core
- Occurs in men and women of all ages
- In most instances, entirely benign
- Infrequently associated with an occult malignancy, polyarteritis nodosa, atherosclerotic microemboli, or antiphospholipid antibody syndrome

CLINICAL FINDINGS

- Arteriolar vasoconstriction with capillary and venous dilation
- Most apparent on the thighs
- Can occur on the forearms or lower abdomen
- Most pronounced in cold weather
- Paresthesias, coldness, or numbness in a few patients
- Peripheral pulses are normal
- Affected regions may be cool
- Skin ulceration is rare

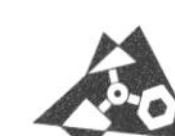

DIAGNOSIS

- Clinical diagnosis

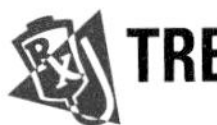

TREATMENT

- Protection from exposure to cold
- Vasodilators seldom indicated
- If ulcerations or gangrene, exclude an underlying systemic disease

Author(s)

Louis M. Messina, MD

Liver Neoplasms, Benign

KEY FEATURES

- The most common benign hepatic neoplasm is the **cavernous hemangioma**, often found incidentally on ultrasonography; hormonal therapy may cause these lesions to enlarge
- Two benign lesions occur in women. **Focal nodular hyperplasia** occurs at all ages. **Liver cell adenoma**, most common in the third and fourth decades of life, is usually caused by oral contraceptives

CLINICAL FINDINGS

- Focal nodular hyperplasia is often asymptomatic. Liver cell adenoma usually presents with acute abdominal pain because of necrosis of the tumor with hemorrhage. The only physical finding in both lesions is a palpable abdominal mass in a few cases

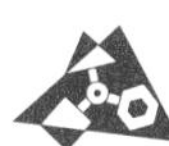

DIAGNOSIS

- Cavernous hemangioma must be differentiated from other liver lesions, usually by MRI. Rarely, fine-needle biopsy is needed
- Focal nodular hyperplasia appears as a hypervascular mass, occasionally with a central hypodense "stellate" scar on CT
- Liver cell adenoma is a hypovascular tumor and is a cold defect on liver scan
- In focal nodular hyperplasia and liver cell adenoma, the liver function is usually normal. Arterial-phase helical CT and MRI can distinguish an adenoma from focal nodular hyperplasia in 80–90% of cases

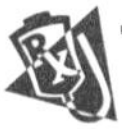

TREATMENT

- Cavernous hemangiomas rarely require treatment. Regression of benign hepatic tumors may follow cessation of oral contraceptives. Treatment of focal nodular hyperplasia is resection only in the symptomatic patient. The prognosis is excellent
- Liver cell adenoma often undergoes necrosis and rupture; resection is advised, even in asymptomatic persons

Author(s)

Lawrence S. Friedman, MD

Locked-In Syndrome

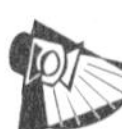

KEY FEATURES

- Acute destructive lesions (eg, infarction, hemorrhage, demyelination, encephalitis) involving the ventral pons and sparing the tegmentum
- Patient is mute and quadriparetic but conscious
- Such a patient can mistakenly be regarded as comatose
- Physicians should recognize that "locked-in" individuals are fully aware of their surroundings

CLINICAL FINDINGS

- Mute, quadriplegic patient
- Conscious state
- Patient is capable of blinking and of voluntary eye movement in the vertical plane
- Preserved pupillary responses to light

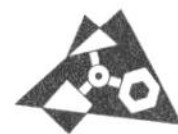

DIAGNOSIS

- Brain imaging with CT or MRI scan
- Obtain the expertise of a clinician familiar with this disorder to aid in the diagnosis

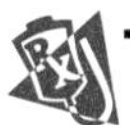

TREATMENT

- The prognosis is variable, but recovery has occasionally been reported, in some cases including resumption of independent daily life, although this may take up to 2 or 3 yr

Author(s)

Michael J. Aminoff, MD, DSc, FRCP

LSD & Hallucinogens

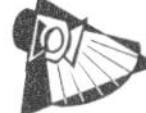

KEY FEATURES

- The mechanism of toxicity and the clinical effects vary for each substance

CLINICAL FINDINGS

- **Anticholinergic delirium**
  - Dilated pupils, flushed skin, dry mucous membranes, tachycardia, and urinary retention
- **LSD**
  - Marked visual hallucinations and perceptual distortion, widely dilated pupils, and mild tachycardia
- **Phencyclidine (PCP)**
  - Can produce fluctuating delirium and coma, often with vertical and horizontal nystagmus
- **Toluene** and other hydrocarbon solvents (eg, butane, trichloroethylene, "chemo")
  - Euphoria, delirium, and fatal dysrhythmias

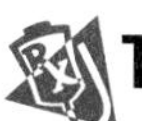

TREATMENT

- For recent ingestions, administer activated charcoal, 60–100 g PO or via gastric tube, mixed in aqueous slurry
- Treat anticholinergic delirium with physostigmine salicylate, 0.5–1 mg IV slowly over 5 min, with ECG monitoring, until symptoms are controlled. Bradyarrhythmias and convulsions can occur with physostigmine use, and it should be avoided in tricyclic antidepressant overdose
- Treat dysphoria, agitation, or psychosis from LSD or mescaline with lorazepam, 1–2 mg PO or IV, or haloperidol, 2–5 mg
- Monitor patients who have sniffed solvents for cardiac dysrhythmias; β-blockers (eg, propranolol, 1–5 mg IV, or esmolol, 250–500 μg/kg IV, then 50 μg/kg/min by infusion) may be used

Author(s)

Kent R. Olson, MD

Lupus Anticoagulant

KEY FEATURES

- IgM or IgG antibody that produces prolonged PTT by binding to phospholipid used in PTT assay
- A laboratory artifact that does not cause clinical bleeding
- Occurs in 5–10% of patients with systemic lupus erythematosus; more common in patients without underlying disorder and in patients taking phenothiazines

CLINICAL FINDINGS

- No bleeding unless a second disorder is present (eg, thrombocytopenia, hypoprothrombinemia, prolonged bleeding time)
- Increased risk of thrombosis and recurrent spontaneous abortions

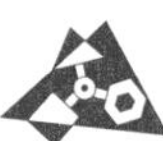

DIAGNOSIS

- PTT prolonged, fails to correct when patient's plasma is mixed in 1:1 dilution with normal plasma because lupus anticoagulant acts as inhibitor
- PT normal or slightly prolonged
- Serum fibrinogen level and thrombin time normal
- Russell viper venom test is a sensitive assay designed to demonstrate presence of lupus anticoagulant
- False-positive VDRL test for syphilis
- A related autoantibody, anticardiolipin, can be detected by separate assays
- Factor VIIIc level, measured when acquired factor VIII inhibitor suspected, is normal in patients with lupus anticoagulant

TREATMENT

- No specific treatment necessary
- Prednisone usually rapidly eliminates lupus anticoagulant, but it is unclear whether it affects thrombotic tendency
- Anticoagulation in standard doses for patients with thromboses
- Because of artificially prolonged PTT, heparin therapy is difficult to monitor; thus, low-molecular-weight heparin may be preferred
- Warfarin dose needs to be increased if baseline PT prolonged

Author(s)

Charles A. Linker, MD

Lymphocytic Choriomeningitis

KEY FEATURES

- Arenavirus infection of CNS
- Main reservoir is house mouse, but other domestic animals may harbor virus
- Virus spread from animal to human by infected oronasal secretions, urine, or feces
- Person-to-person spread rare

CLINICAL FINDINGS

- Symptoms are biphasic with a prodromal phase followed by a meningeal phase
- Fever, malaise, headache, and cough are common in prodromal phase
- Neck and back stiffness with a positive Kernig's sign are common in the meningeal phase
- Obstructive hydrocephalus is rare but serious complication

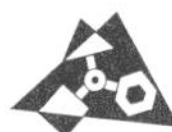

DIAGNOSIS

- Leukocytosis or leukopenia
- Cerebrospinal fluid lymphocytic pleocytosis common
- Cerebrospinal fluid PCR for lymphocytic choriomeningitis virus is available, although rarely used
- Complement-fixing antibodies appear during second week of infection and may aid in diagnosis

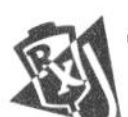

TREATMENT

- No specific antiviral therapy
- Supportive measures

Author(s)

Wayne X. Shandera, MD
Ana Moran, MD

Lymphogranuloma Venereum

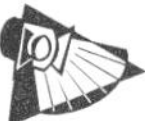

KEY FEATURES

- An acute and chronic sexually transmitted disease
- Caused by *Chlamydia trachomatis* types L1–L3

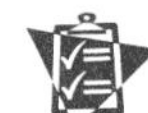

CLINICAL FINDINGS

- In **men**
  - The initial vesicular or ulcerative lesion (on the external genitalia) is evanescent and often goes unnoticed
  - Inguinal buboes appear 1–4 weeks after exposure, are often bilateral, and have a tendency to fuse, soften, and break down to form multiple draining sinuses, with extensive scarring
- In **women**
  - The genital lymph drainage is to the perirectal glands
  - Early anorectal manifestations are proctitis with tenesmus and bloody purulent discharge
  - Late manifestations are chronic cicatrizing inflammation of the rectal and perirectal tissue. These changes lead to obstipation and rectal stricture and, occasionally, rectovaginal and perianal fistulas. They are also seen in homosexual men

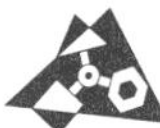

DIAGNOSIS

- The complement fixation test may be positive, but cross-reaction with other chlamydiae occurs
- Specific immunofluorescence tests for IgM are more specific for acute infection

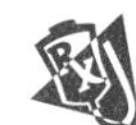

TREATMENT

- Doxycycline, 0.1 g PO BID for 21 days; erythromycin, 500 mg PO QID; or trimethoprim-sulfamethoxazole, 160/800 mg PO BID for 21 days

Author(s)

Henry F. Chambers, MD

Lymphoma, Gastric

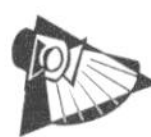 KEY FEATURES

- Second most common gastric malignancy, 3–6% of gastric cancers
- More than 95% are non-Hodgkin's B-cell lymphomas
- May be primary (gastric mucosal lymphoma) or secondary (in patients with nodal lymphomas)
- ~60% of primary gastric lymphomas are mucosa-associated lymphoid tissue (MALT)
- B cells of nodal origin may be distinguished from B cells derived from MALT (CD19- and CD20-positive)
- Infection with *Helicobacter pylori* is an important risk factor for primary gastric lymphoma
- >85% of low-grade primary gastric lymphomas and 40% of high-grade lymphomas are associated with *H pylori*

 CLINICAL FINDINGS

- Abdominal pain
- Weight loss
- Upper GI bleeding

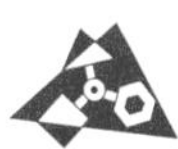 DIAGNOSIS

- Endoscopy with biopsy useful in diagnosis
- Abdominal and chest CT and endoscopic ultrasonography useful in staging

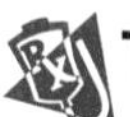 TREATMENT

- Primary low-grade gastric lymphomas are usually localized to the stomach wall (stage IE) or adjacent lymph nodes (stage IIE) and have an excellent prognosis
- Nodal lymphomas with secondary gastric involvement are usually at an advanced stage and thus seldom curable
- Complete lymphoma regression occurs in 75% of cases of stage IE low-grade lymphoma after successful *H pylori* eradication
- Patients with stage IE or IIE low-grade lymphomas who are not infected with *H pylori* or fail to respond to eradication therapy can be treated successfully with surgical resection, local radiation therapy, or combination therapy
- Stage IEE or IIEE high-grade lymphomas are treated with resection and CHOP chemotherapy (cyclophosphamide, hydroxydaunomycin, Oncovin, prednisone)
- Stage III or IV primary lymphomas are treated with combination chemotherapy; surgical resection is no longer recommended
- Long-term survival of primary gastric lymphoma for stage I is >85% and for stage II 35–65%

Author(s)

Kenneth R. McQuaid, MD

Macular Degeneration, Age-Related

 KEY FEATURES

- Age-related macular degeneration is the leading cause of permanent visual loss in the elderly
- Exact cause is unknown but a precursor is the development of macular drusen
- Two subtypes: atrophic and exudative

 CLINICAL FINDINGS

- Loss of central vision
- Atrophic subtype is characterized by progressive, bilateral visual loss of moderate severity resulting from atrophy and degeneration of the outer retina
- Exudative subtype is characterized by rapid and severe unilateral visual loss, with a high risk of subsequent involvement of the fellow eye
- Older patients developing sudden central visual loss, particularly paracentral distortion or scotoma with preservation of central acuity, should be referred urgently to an ophthalmologist for assessment

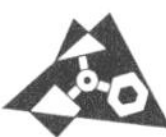 DIAGNOSIS

- On ophthalmoscopic examination, various abnormalities are visualized in the macula
- Fundal photography after IV fluorescein (fluorescein angiography) is often required

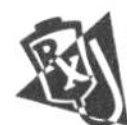 TREATMENT

- No specific treatment is available for atrophic macular degeneration, but patients often benefit from low vision aids
- Retinal laser photocoagulation, including photodynamic therapy, or retinal surgery may be beneficial in exudative disease

Author(s)

Paul Riordan-Eva, FRCOphth

Measles

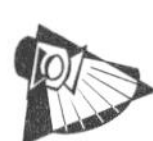

KEY FEATURES

- Transmitted by inhalation of infected respiratory droplets
- Estimated 1 million deaths annually worldwide, mainly from gastroenteritis
- Declining US incidence because of widespread vaccine use

CLINICAL FINDINGS

- Initial prodrome of malaise and fever; rash 3–4 days later
- Fever persists through the early rash
- Koplik's spots, tiny "table crystals" on mucous membranes, are pathognomonic and appear 2 days before rash
- Rash begins as pin-sized papules on face and behind ears, spreading to trunk and then extremities
- Pulmonary involvement occurs in up to 5% of cases and is most common cause of death
- Encephalitis in up to 0.1% of cases
- Subacute sclerosing panencephalitis (SSPE) is a rare, late CNS complication, largely among rural boys

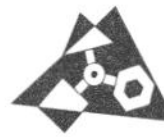

DIAGNOSIS

- Often difficult to differentiate clinical symptoms from other viral illnesses
- Koplik's spots clinch the diagnosis
- History of exposure to patients with measles helpful but not always present
- Leukopenia usually present
- Lymphocyte count < 2000/μL associated with poor prognosis
- Fourfold rise in measles antibody titer is diagnostic

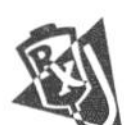

TREATMENT

- Supportive measures
- High-dose vitamin A recommended in children
- Antibiotics for bacterial pneumonia superinfection
- Prevention: measles vaccination of children and young adults
- Postexposure prophylaxis: Live virus vaccine may be effective in prevention up to 5 days postexposure in susceptible individuals
- Pregnant women and immunocompromised individuals should avoid vaccination, although HIV-infected adults can be safely vaccinated

Author(s)

Wayne X. Shandera, MD

Ana Moran, MD

Meniscus Tears, Medial

KEY FEATURES

- The most common knee injuries encountered in primary care; tears result from twisting on the knee joint while the foot is weight bearing

CLINICAL FINDINGS

- There is usually a tearing or popping sensation followed by severe pain
- In contrast to ligamentous injuries, in which hemorrhage causes immediate swelling, effusions from meniscal injuries accumulate over hours and are typically worse the day after the injury
- Several days after resolution (full or partial), there may be joint locking or instability, recurrent swelling with activity, and pain

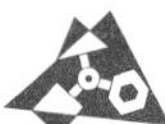

DIAGNOSIS

- Joint effusion is usually present
- Tenderness may be localized to the medial joint line, and range of motion in the knee may be restricted
- In the absence of an acutely painful knee, perform a McMurray's test: With the patient supine with the hip and knee in full flexion, place one hand on the involved knee and the other on the ipsilateral foot. As the foot is externally rotated, extend the patient's knee. The presence of a "snap" (palpable or audible) suggests a medial meniscus lesion
- MRI confirms the diagnosis if plain films exclude other conditions

TREATMENT

- Initial management is elevation, a compression dressing, and ice
- Weight bearing should be minimized for the first few days but may be resumed slowly thereafter
- Quadriceps-strengthening exercises by a physical therapist
- Surgery is reserved for patients with symptoms that recur on resumption of normal activities or for patients with irreducible locking caused by mechanical problems

Author(s)

David B. Hellmann, MD, FACP

John H. Stone, MD, MPH

Meralgia Paresthetica

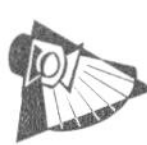

KEY FEATURES

- The lateral femoral cutaneous nerve, a sensory nerve arising from the L2 and L3 roots, may be compressed or stretched in obese or diabetic patients and during pregnancy
- Hyperextension of the hip or increased lumbar lordosis—as during pregnancy—leads to nerve compression by the posterior fascicle of the ligament. However, entrapment of the nerve at any point along its course may cause similar symptoms, and several other anatomic variations predispose the nerve to damage when it is stretched

CLINICAL FINDINGS

- Pain, paresthesia, or numbness occurs about the outer aspect of the thigh, usually unilaterally, and is sometimes relieved by sitting

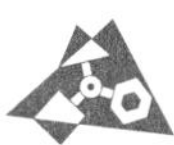

DIAGNOSIS

- Examination shows no abnormalities except in severe cases when cutaneous sensation is impaired in the affected area

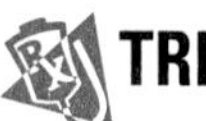

TREATMENT

- Symptoms are usually mild and commonly settle spontaneously
- Hydrocortisone injections medial to the anterosuperior iliac spine often relieve symptoms temporarily, whereas nerve decompression by transposition may provide more lasting relief

Author(s)

Michael J. Aminoff, MD, DSc, FRCP

Mercury Poisoning

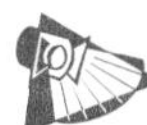

KEY FEATURES

- Acute mercury poisoning usually occurs by ingestion of inorganic mercuric salts or inhalation of metallic mercury vapor

CLINICAL FINDINGS

- Mercury salts: metallic taste, salivation, thirst, a burning sensation in the throat, discoloration and edema of oral mucous membranes, abdominal pain, vomiting, bloody diarrhea, and shock. Direct nephrotoxicity causes acute renal failure
- Inhalation of high concentrations of metallic mercury vapor may cause acute fulminant chemical pneumonia
- Chronic mercury poisoning causes weakness, ataxia, intention tremors, irritability, and depression
- Exposure to alkyl (organic) mercury derivatives from contaminated fish or fungicides used on seeds has caused ataxia, tremors, convulsions, and catastrophic birth defects

TREATMENT

Acute poisoning

- There is no effective specific treatment for mercury vapor pneumonitis
- For acute ingestion of mercuric salts
  - Remove ingestion by gastric lavage, and administer activated charcoal 60–100 g in aqueous slurry PO or via gastric tube
  - Administer chelation therapy with BAL (British Anti-Lewisite) or DMSA (succimer)
  - Contact a poison control center or medical toxicologist for assistance

Chronic poisoning

- Remove from exposure
- Neurological toxicity is not considered reversible with chelation, although some recommend a trial of succimer

Author(s)

Kent R. Olson, MD

Mesothelioma, Peritoneal

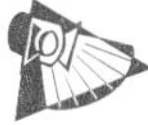

KEY FEATURES

- Rare malignancy of peritoneum, pleura
- History of asbestos exposure in >70%

CLINICAL FINDINGS

- Abdominal pain or bowel obstruction
- Increased abdominal girth, with small to moderate ascites

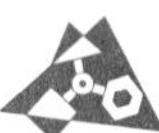

DIAGNOSIS

- Chest radiograph shows pulmonary asbestosis in >50%
- Ascitic fluid is hemorrhagic, with low serum-ascites albumin gradient
- Ascitic fluid cytology is often negative
- Abdominal CT reveals sheet-like masses involving the mesentery and omentum
- Diagnosis at laparotomy or laparoscopy

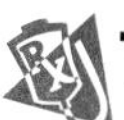

TREATMENT

- Prognosis is extremely poor, but long-term survivors have been described who received a combination of radiation therapy and systemic or intraperitoneal chemotherapy

Author(s)

Kenneth R. McQuaid, MD

Methanol and Ethylene Glycol Poisoning

KEY FEATURES

- The toxicity of both agents is caused by metabolism to toxic organic acids—methanol to formic acid, ethylene glycol to glycolic and oxalic acids

CLINICAL FINDINGS

- Shortly after ingestion of either agent, patients usually appear drunk
- After several hours, there is tachypnea, confusion, convulsions, and coma
- Methanol intoxication frequently causes visual disturbances, whereas ethylene glycol often produces oxalate crystalluria and renal failure

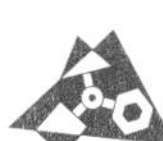

DIAGNOSIS

- Initially, the serum osmolality (and osmolar gap) is usually increased. After several hours, there is a severe anion gap metabolic acidosis
- Ethylene glycol often produces oxalate crystalluria
- Alcoholic ketoacidosis also can cause a combined anion gap acidosis and osmolar gap

TREATMENT

- Empty stomach by gastric lavage and administer activated charcoal if ingestion is within 60 min (however, charcoal is not very effective)
- Administer ethanol or fomepizole to block metabolism of methanol and ethylene glycol to their toxic metabolites; contact a regional poison control center for indications and dosing
- For significant toxicity (manifested by severe metabolic acidosis, altered mental status, serum methanol, or ethylene glycol level > 50 mg/dL or osmolar gap > 10 mOsm/L), perform hemodialysis as soon as possible

Author(s)

Kent R. Olson, MD

Methemoglobinemia

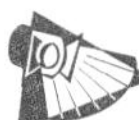

KEY FEATURES

- Agents include benzocaine, aniline, nitrites, nitrogen oxide gases, nitrobenzene, dapsone, phenazopyridine, and many other oxidants
- Dapsone has a long half-life and may produce prolonged or recurrent methemoglobinemia

CLINICAL FINDINGS

- Dizziness, nausea, headache, dyspnea, confusion, seizures, coma
- Severity of symptoms depends on the percentage of hemoglobin oxidized to methemoglobin
  - Severe poisoning is usually present when methemoglobin fractions are > 40–50%
  - Even at low levels (15–20%), victims appear cyanotic because of the chocolate-brown color of methemoglobin

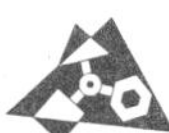

DIAGNOSIS

- Po_2 results are normal on arterial blood gas determinations; pulse oximetry gives inaccurate oxygen saturation measurements
- Severe metabolic acidosis
- Hemolysis may occur, especially in patients with glucose-6-phosphate dehydrogenase deficiency

TREATMENT

- Administer high-flow oxygen
- Administer activated charcoal, 60–100 g PO or via gastric tube, mixed in aqueous slurry for ingestions within 1 h; repeat-dose activated charcoal may enhance dapsone elimination
- For symptomatic patients, administer methylene blue, 1–2 mg/kg (0.1–0.2 mL/kg of 1% solution) IV
  - The dose may be repeated once in 15–20 min if necessary
  - Patients with glucose-6-phosphate dehydrogenase deficiency may not respond to methylene blue

Author(s)

Kent R. Olson, MD

Minimal Change Disease

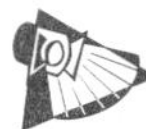

KEY FEATURES

- Most common in children; occurs occasionally in adults
- Equal distribution between men and women

CLINICAL FINDINGS

- Nephrotic syndrome

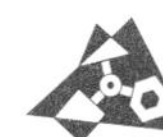

DIAGNOSIS

- Renal biopsy
  - Light microscopy and immunofluorescence: no changes
  - Electron microscopy: characteristic fusion of epithelial foot processes

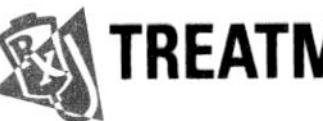

TREATMENT

- Prednisone, 1 mg/kg/day for up to 16 weeks, continued for several weeks after complete remission of proteinuria
- Cyclophosphamide or chlorambucil for patients with steroid resistance or relapses
- Progression to end-stage renal disease is rare but more common in adults
- Complications most often related to prolonged steroid use

Author(s)

Suzanne Watnick, MD

Gail Morrison, MD

Mitral Regurgitation

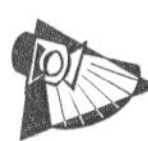

KEY FEATURES

- Mitral regurgitation results from displacement of papillary muscles (dilated cardiomyopathy), excessive length of chordae or myxomatous degeneration of leaflets (mitral prolapse), or noncontraction of annulus (annular calcification)
- Places a volume load on heart (increased preload), but reduces afterload, resulting in enlarged left ventricle (LV) and initial increase in ejection fraction (EF)
- Over time, LV weakens and EF drops

CLINICAL FINDINGS

- Pansystolic murmur at the apex, radiating into the axilla
- Often associated with an S_3
- Hyperdynamic LV impulse
- Brisk carotid upstroke
- May be asymptomatic for many years (or life)
- When regurgitation develops acutely, left atrial pressure rises abruptly, leading to pulmonary edema if severe
- When regurgitation progresses more slowly, exertional dyspnea and fatigue worsen gradually over many years
- Left atrial enlargement may lead to atrial fibrillation and systemic embolization
- Predisposition to infective endocarditis

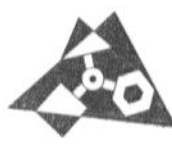

DIAGNOSIS

- ECG: left atrial abnormality or atrial fibrillation and LV hypertrophy
- Chest x-ray film: left atrial and ventricular enlargement
- Echo-Doppler confirms the diagnosis and estimates severity
- Transesophageal echocardiography may reveal the cause and identify candidates for valvular repair
- Coronary angiography is often indicated (especially after age 45) to determine the presence of coronary artery disease before valve surgery

TREATMENT

- Antibiotic prophylaxis for dental and other procedures
- ACE inhibitor therapy to reduce afterload
- Acute mitral regurgitation resulting from endocarditis, myocardial infarction, and ruptured chordae tendineae often requires emergency surgery
- Chronic regurgitation usually requires surgery when symptoms develop
- Because irreversible deterioration of LV function may occur before the onset of symptoms, surgery is indicated in asymptomatic patients with a declining EF (< 60%) or marked LV dilation
- Surgical valve repair using the thoracoscopic approach can avoid the complications of prosthetic valves
- Novel percutaneous approaches to mitral valve repair include transseptal stitching of leaflets (Alfieri procedure) and coronary sinus crimping to reduce annular size

Author(s)

Thomas M. Bashore, MD

Christopher B. Granger, MD

Mitral Stenosis

KEY FEATURES

- Underlying rheumatic heart disease in almost all patients (although history of rheumatic fever is often absent)

CLINICAL FINDINGS

- Localized mid-diastolic, low-pitch murmur whose duration varies with the severity of stenosis and heart rate
- A sharp opening snap is widely distributed over the chest
- Low-pitched rumble at apex with patient in left decubitus position, increased by brief exercise
- Moderate stenosis (valve area 1.8–1.3 cm^2): exertional dyspnea and fatigue common, especially with tachycardia
- Severe stenosis (valve area < 1.0 cm^2): pulmonary congestion at rest, with dyspnea, fatigue, right-sided heart failure, orthopnea, paroxysmal nocturnal dyspnea, and occasional hemoptysis
- Sudden increase in heart rate may precipitate pulmonary edema
- Paroxysmal or chronic atrial fibrillation develops in ~50–80%, may precipitate dyspnea or pulmonary edema

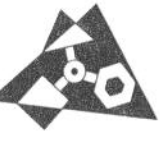

DIAGNOSIS

- ECG typically shows left atrial abnormality and, often, atrial fibrillation
- Echo-Doppler confirms diagnosis and quantifies severity by assigning 1–4 points to each of 4 observed parameters, with 1 being the least involvement and 4 the greatest
  - Mitral leaflet thickening
  - Mitral leaflet mobility
  - Submitral scarring
  - Commissural calcium
- Cardiac catheterization to detect valve, coronary, or myocardial disease, usually done only after a decision to intervene has been made

TREATMENT

- Control heart rate
- Attempt conversion of atrial fibrillation
- Once atrial fibrillation occurs, provide lifelong anticoagulation with warfarin, even if sinus rhythm is restored
- Intervention to relieve stenosis indicated for symptoms (eg, pulmonary edema,

decline in exercise capacity) or evidence of pulmonary hypertension

- Percutaneous balloon valvuloplasty when there is minimal mitral regurgitation
- Surgical valve replacement in combined stenosis and regurgitation or when the mitral valve is significantly distorted and calcified
- Operative mortality rate is ~1–3%

Author(s)

Thomas M. Bashore, MD

Christopher B. Granger, MD

Mitral Valve Prolapse

KEY FEATURES

- Usually asymptomatic
- When symptomatic, symptoms include nonspecific chest pain, dyspnea, fatigue, and ventricular or supraventricular arrhythmias
- Most patients are female, many are thin, and some have minor chest wall deformities
- The significance of mitral valve prolapse (MVP) is disputed because it is diagnosed frequently in healthy young women (up to 10%)
- In occasional patients, MVP is not benign
- Infective endocarditis may occur, chiefly in patients with murmurs

CLINICAL FINDINGS

- One or more characteristic midsystolic clicks, often but not always followed by a late systolic murmur
- Findings are accentuated in the standing position
- A single midsystolic click is usually benign
- The late or pansystolic murmur may presage significant mitral regurgitation, often resulting from rupture of chordae tendineae

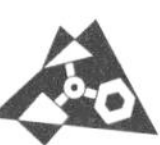

DIAGNOSIS

- The diagnosis is primarily clinical but can be confirmed by echo-Doppler
- Echocardiography: Marked thickening or redundancy of the valve is associated with a higher incidence of complications

TREATMENT

- Usually, no treatment is indicated
- In asymptomatic patients, serial clinical examinations to rule out progression to mitral regurgitation
- In patients with murmurs, antibiotic prophylaxis before dental work and other procedures
- β-Blockers for supraventricular arrhythmias
- A cardioverter-defibrillator for symptomatic ventricular tachycardia
- If regurgitation evolves, treat as indicated for mitral regurgitation (see Mitral Regurgitation)

Author(s)

Thomas M. Bashore, MD

Christopher B. Granger, MD

Molluscum Contagiosum

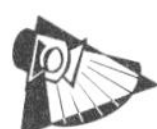

KEY FEATURES

- Caused by a poxvirus
- The lesions are autoinoculable and spread by wet skin-to-skin contact
- In sexually active individuals, lesions may be confined to the penis, pubis, and inner thighs and are considered a sexually transmitted disease
- Common in AIDS, usually with a helper T cell count < 100/μL. AIDS patients tend to develop extensive lesions over the face and neck as well as in the genital area
- Lesions are difficult to eradicate in AIDS unless immunity improves, in which case spontaneous clearing may occur

CLINICAL FINDINGS

- Presents as single or multiple rounded, dome-shaped, waxy papules 2–5 mm in diameter that are umbilicated
- Lesions at first are firm, solid, and flesh colored but on reaching maturity become softened, whitish, or pearly gray and may suppurate
- The principal sites are the face, lower abdomen, and genitals
- Individual lesions persist for ~2 mo

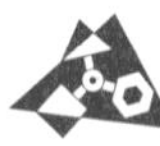

DIAGNOSIS

- Clinical; based on the distinctive central umbilication of the dome-shaped lesion
- Differential diagnosis
  - Warts
  - Varicella (chickenpox)
  - Basal cell carcinoma
  - Lichen planus
  - Smallpox
  - Cutaneous cryptococcosis (in AIDS)

TREATMENT

- The best treatment is by curettage or applications of liquid nitrogen as for warts but more briefly
- When lesions are frozen, the central umbilication often becomes more apparent
- Light electrosurgery with a fine needle is also effective

Author(s)

Timothy G. Berger, MD

Monoamine Oxidase Inhibitor Overdose

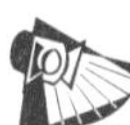

KEY FEATURES

- Ingestion of tyramine-containing foods (eg, aged cheese and red wines) or any sympathomimetic drug may cause a severe hypertensive reaction
- Severe or fatal hyperthermia (serotonin syndrome) may occur when monoamine oxidase (MAO) inhibitors are given with meperidine, fluoxetine, paroxetine, fluvoxamine, venlafaxine, tryptophan, dextromethorphan, moclobemide, or other serotonin-enhancing drugs
- The serotonin syndrome can also occur with selective serotonin reuptake inhibitors (SSRIs) in large doses or in combination with other SSRIs, even in the absence of an MAO inhibitor or meperidine

CLINICAL FINDINGS

- Acute overdose: agitation, hypertension, and tachycardia followed in several hours by hypotension, convulsions, and hyperthermia
- Food or drug hypertensive reaction: hypertension, tachycardia, headache, possible intracranial hemorrhage
- Serotonin syndrome: agitation, confusion, muscle hyperactivity, hyperthermia

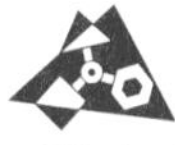

DIAGNOSIS

- Clinical

TREATMENT

- Acute ingestion: Administer activated charcoal, 60–100 g PO or via gastric tube, mixed in aqueous slurry if ingestion is within 1 h
- Treat severe hypertension with nitroprusside, phentolamine, or other rapid-acting vasodilators
- Treat hypotension with fluids and positioning, but avoid use of pressor agents if possible
- Observe patients for at least 24 h because hyperthermia may be delayed (see Hyperthermia)
- Cyproheptadine, 4 mg PO (or by gastric tube) Q h for 3 or 4 doses, can be effective

Author(s)

Kent R. Olson, MD

Monoclonal Gammopathy of Uncertain Significance (MGUS)

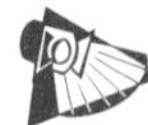

KEY FEATURES

- Stable quantity of M protein in the serum without symptoms or signs of multiple myeloma, macroglobulinemia, amyloidosis, or lymphoma
- MGUS increases with age and is seen in 3% in persons 70 years of age or older
- Lymphoid malignancies, amyloidosis, or multiple myeloma will develop in as many as one-third of patients with apparently benign monoclonal gammopathies
- Risk of developing a malignant disorder is 12% at 10 years, 25% at 20 years, and 30% at 25 years

CLINICAL FINDINGS

- Asymptomatic
- No lymphadenopathy, splenomegaly, or bony lesions of multiple myeloma

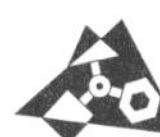

DIAGNOSIS

- Monoclonal spike on serum protein electrophoresis, confirmed by immunoelectrophoresis to be a homogeneous immunoglobulin with either κ or γ light chains
- Parameters that suggest a favorable prognosis include
  - Concentrations of homogeneous immunoglobulin less than 2 g/dL
  - No increase in concentration of the immunoglobulin from the time of diagnosis
  - No decrease in the concentration of normal immunoglobulins
  - Absence of a homogeneous light chain in the urine, and normal hematocrit and serum albumin

TREATMENT

- No specific treatment
- Monitor periodically for changes in serum M proteins, urinary Bence-Jones proteins, evidence of renal failure, ane-

mia, hypercalcemia, lytic bone lesions, or bone marrow plasmacytoses

Author(s)

Jeffrey L. Kishiyama, MD
Daniel C. Adelman, MD

Mononucleosis

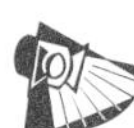 KEY FEATURES

- Acute infection can occur at any age but most common in 10–35 year olds
- Epstein-Barr virus (EBV) is the causative agent; similar syndromes are caused by cytomegalovirus (CMV), acute HIV infection, and toxoplasmosis
- EBV shows a strong serologic association with HIV-related lymphomas, nasopharyngeal carcinoma, Burkitt's lymphoma, oral hairy leukoplakia, and posttransplant lymphoproliferative disorder

 CLINICAL FINDINGS

- Fever, sore throat common
- Lymphadenopathy very common
- Splenomegaly (50%)
- Maculopapular rash uncommon (15%) except in patients receiving ampicillin (90%)
- Exudative pharyngitis common
- Hepatitis, mononeuropathy, aseptic meningitis, hemolytic anemia uncommon
- Secondary bacterial infections of the throat
- Splenic rupture is rare but dramatic
- Nonspecific ECG changes (5%)

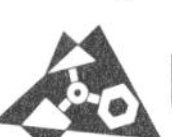 DIAGNOSIS

- Combination of sore throat, fever, fatigue, adenopathy, and splenomegaly suggests the diagnosis
- Chronicity of pharyngitis makes infectious mononucleosis more likely than bacterial pharyngitis
- Granulocytopenia with lymphocytosis, especially large, atypical lymphocytes
- Hemolytic anemia and thrombocytopenia
- Heterophil antibody and Monospot tests usually positive
- Antibody (IgM) titers to early antigens including viral capsid antigen can be useful early in disease

TREATMENT

- 95% of patients recover without antiviral therapy
- Acyclovir and other antiviral drugs are without verified clinical benefit
- Chronic EBV syndromes are increasingly recognized, especially in the immunodeficient (Duncan's syndrome)

Author(s)

Wayne X. Shandera, MD
Ana Moran, MD

Moraxella catarrhalis Infection

 KEY FEATURES

- An infection caused by a gram-negative aerobic coccus, *Moraxella catarrhalis,* that is morphologically and biochemically similar to *Neisseria*

 CLINICAL FINDINGS

- Sinusitis, bronchitis, otitis, and pneumonia
- Bacteremia and meningitis have also been reported in immunocompromised patients

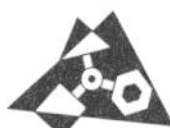 DIAGNOSIS

- Culture
- The organism frequently colonizes the respiratory tract, and differentiation of colonization from infection can be difficult
- If *M catarrhalis* is the predominant isolate, therapy should be directed against it

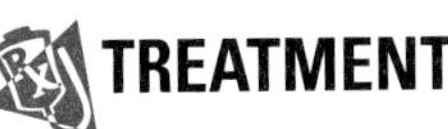

- Amoxicillin-clavulanate, ampicillin-sulbactam, trimethoprim-sulfamethoxazole, ciprofloxacin, and second- and third-generation cephalosporins
- Treatment is similar to that for *Haemophilus* infections (see Haemophilus Infections)
- Typically produces β-lactamase and, therefore, is usually resistant to ampicillin and amoxicillin

Author(s)

Henry F. Chambers, MD

Mucormycosis

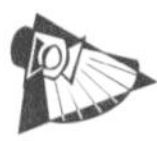 KEY FEATURES

- The term "mucormycosis" (zygomycosis, phycomycosis) applies to opportunistic infections caused by members of the genera *Rhizopus, Mucor, Absidia,* and *Cunninghamella*
- Predisposing conditions include diabetic ketoacidosis, chronic renal failure, use of corticosteroids or cytotoxic drugs

 CLINICAL FINDINGS

- Invasive disease of sinuses, orbits, lungs
- In acidotic diabetic patients, black necrotic lesions of nose or sinuses or new cranial nerve abnormalities
- Cerebral invasion may ensue in the absence of therapy
- Widely disseminated disease more common after aggressive chemotherapy

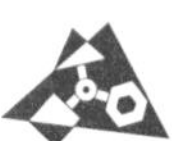 DIAGNOSIS

- Cultures frequently negative
- Biopsy almost always required for diagnosis. Histology demonstrates organisms in tissues as broad, branching nonseptate hyphae

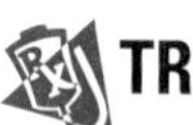 TREATMENT

- High-dose amphotericin B, 1–1.5 mg/kg/day IV, for prolonged period
- Control of diabetes and other underlying conditions is essential
- Extensive repeated surgical débridement of necrotic, nonperfused tissue
- Even with timely treatment, mortality is 30–50% for localized disease and higher for disseminated disease

Author(s)

Samuel A. Shelburne, MD

Richard J. Hamill, MD

Mumps

 KEY FEATURES

- Spread by respiratory droplets
- Produces inflammation of salivary glands (eg, parotitis) and occasionally orchitis and meningitis

 CLINICAL FINDINGS

- Parotid tenderness and overlying facial edema common
- Fever and malaise variable
- Orchitis 7–10 days after parotitis; rarely leads to sterility
- Meningitis third most common manifestation
- Other complications include pancreatitis, oophoritis, thyroiditis, neuritis, hepatitis, myocarditis, encephalitis

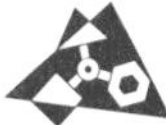 DIAGNOSIS

- Symptom onset occurs 14–21 days postexposure
- Painful, swollen parotid and other salivary glands
- Orchitis, pancreatitis, or meningitis in setting of parotitis is usually diagnostic
- Lymphocytosis and elevated serum amylase are common
- Serologic testing may be useful but not commonly done
- Serum neutralization titers best for determining immunity

 TREATMENT

- Supportive measures
- Febrile patients should be kept on bed rest and isolated while there is parotid swelling
- Orchitis can be managed with scrotal support and ice packs
- Prevention: mumps live virus vaccine is safe and highly effective
- Vaccine should be avoided in pregnant women and immunocompromised individuals
- Vaccine probably safe in adults with asymptomatic HIV infection

Author(s)

Wayne X. Shandera, MD

Ana Moran, MD

Muscle Cramps

 KEY FEATURES

- Muscle cramps are usually caused by sports or occupational muscle injury
  - Idiopathic (most common)
  - Electrolyte disorders (hypocalcemia, hypokalemia, hyponatremia, hypoglycemia, hyperkalemia, hypermagnasemia, alkalosis)
  - Systemic diseases (diabetes mellitus, Parkinson's disease, CNS or spinal cord lesions, spinal stenosis, peripheral neuropathy, hemodialysis, peripheral vascular disease, hyperthyroidism or hypothyroidism)
  - Pregnancy
  - Peripheral vascular disease (exertional claudication)
  - HMGCoA reductase inhibitor (statin)-related ause myalgia; serum CK levels may be elevated in the presence of rhabdomyolysis
  - Vitamin D deficiency (bone pain)
  - Drugs: cisplatin, vincristine, cholinesterase inhibitors, bisphosphonates, chemotherapy (eg, imatinib)
  - Acute arsenic intoxication can cause muscle cramps along with dysphagia, nausea, vomiting, and thirst
  - Dermatomyositis and polymyositis can cause diffuse muscle pain; CK levels are elevated
  - Diffuse muscle tenderness, especially with "trigger points" and normal serum CK levels may indicate fibromyalgia
  - Hemodialysis

CLINICAL FINDINGS

- Muscle cramping, often nocturnal
- Physical exam usually normal or shows signs of associated conditions listed above
- Exertional claudication and reduced pedal pulses suggest lower extremity arterial occlusive disease

 DIAGNOSIS

- Obtain serum calcium, potassium, sodium, glucose, magnesium levels
- Consider magnesium deficiency in tetany unresponsive to calcium
- If leg cramps during walking, consider serum TSH and Doppler ankle–brachial index evaluation for peripheral vascular disease

- Serum CK level is elevated in enzyme deficiencies, such as McArdle's disease and carnitine palmitoyltransferase II deficiency

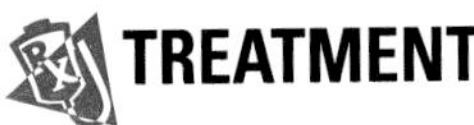

TREATMENT

- Correct electrolyte disorders
- Gabapentin, 600–1200 mg/day divided PO BID–TID, for recurrent, severe, or prolonged muscle cramping. May cause leukopenia or CNS effects
- Quinine only for severe nocturnal cramping. May cause arrhythmias, dizziness, hemolytic-uremic syndrome, and agranulocytosis
- Calcium or magnesium citrate supplementation for pregnancy-associated leg cramps
- Pentoxifylline, cilostazol, angioplasty, or arterial bypass for claudication (see *Vascular Disease, Peripheral*)
- Botulinum toxin injections for recurrent cervicofacial dystonias, laryngeal dystonias, and hand cramps

Author(s)

Paul A. Fitzgerald, MD

Muscular Dystrophies

KEY FEATURES

- Inherited myopathic disorders are characterized by progressive muscle weakness and wasting
- They are subdivided by mode of inheritance, age at onset, and clinical features (Table 102)
- A genetic defect on the short arm of the X chromosome occurs in Duchenne dystrophy. The affected gene codes for the protein dystrophin, which is almost absent from the diseased muscles
- Dystrophin levels are generally normal in the Becker variety, but the protein is qualitatively altered
- Duchenne muscular dystrophy is detectable in pregnancy

CLINICAL FINDINGS

- Muscle weakness, often in a characteristic distribution
- Age at onset and inheritance pattern depend on specific dystrophy
- Duchenne dystrophy
  - Pseudohypertrophy of muscles often occurs at some stage
  - Intellectual retardation is common
  - Skeletal deformities, muscle contractures, and cardiac involvement may be present

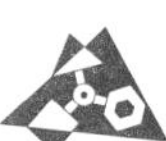

DIAGNOSIS

- The serum creatine kinase level is increased, especially in the Duchenne and Becker varieties, and mildly increased in limb-girdle dystrophy
- Electromyography may confirm myopathic weakness rather than neurogenic
- Histopathologic examination of muscle biopsy specimen can distinguish between various muscle diseases

TREATMENT

- No specific treatment for the muscular dystrophies
- Is important to encourage patients to lead as normal lives as possible
- Prolonged bed rest must be avoided because inactivity often leads to worsening of the underlying muscle disease
- Physical therapy and orthopedic procedures may help counteract deformities or contractures

Author(s)

Michael J. Aminoff, MD, DSc, FRCP

Myasthenic Syndrome

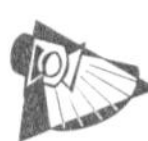

KEY FEATURES

- Clinical similarity to myasthenia gravis, but myasthenic syndrome occurs mainly as a paraneoplastic syndrome (Table 156)
- There is defective release of acetylcholine in response to a nerve impulse, leading to weakness, especially of the proximal muscles of the limbs
- May be associated with small cell lung carcinoma, sometimes developing before the tumor is diagnosed, and occasionally occurs with certain autoimmune diseases

CLINICAL FINDINGS

- Variable weakness, typically improving with activity
- Dysautonomic symptoms may also be present
- A history of malignant disease may be obtained
- Unlike myasthenia gravis, power steadily increases with sustained contraction

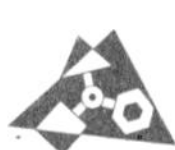

DIAGNOSIS

- Electrophysiologic diagnosis: the muscle response to stimulation of its motor nerve increases remarkably if the nerve is stimulated repetitively at high rates, even in muscles that are not clinically weak

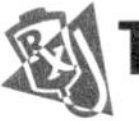

TREATMENT

- Plasmapheresis and immunosuppressive drug therapy (prednisone and azathioprine), in addition to therapy directed at a tumor
- Prednisone is usually initiated in a daily dose of 60–80 mg and azathioprine in a daily dose of 2 mg/kg
- Guanidine hydrochloride (25–50 mg/kg/day in divided doses) is occasionally helpful in seriously disabled patients, but adverse effects of the drug include marrow suppression
- The response to treatment with anticholinesterase drugs such as pyridostigmine or neostigmine, either alone or in combination with guanidine, is variable

Author(s)

Michael J. Aminoff, MD, DSc, FRCP

Mycetoma

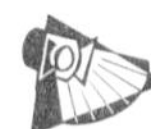

KEY FEATURES

- Mycetoma is a chronic local, slowly progressive, destructive infection
- Begins in subcutaneous tissues, frequently after localized trauma, and spreads to contiguous structures
- Maduromycosis is mycetoma caused by true fungi
- Actinomycetoma is mycetoma caused by *Nocardia* and *Actinomadura*

CLINICAL FINDINGS

- Lesion begins as a papule, nodule, or abscess that, over months to years, forms multiple abscesses and sinus tracts ramifying deep into the tissue
- Secondary bacterial infection may occur in large open ulcers

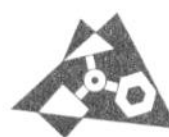

DIAGNOSIS

- X-ray films may show destructive changes in underlying bone
- Tissue Gram's stain reveals large hyphae with maduromycosis and fine branching hyphae with actinomycetoma
- Species is often identifiable by the color of characteristic grains within infected tissues

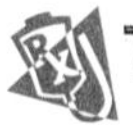

TREATMENT

- For maduromycosis: ketoconazole or itraconazole for months
- For actinomycetoma: trimethoprim-sulfamethoxazole, 160/800 mg PO BID, or dapsone, 100 mg PO BID after meals, for months. Streptomycin, 14 mg/kg/d IM, may be useful during first month of therapy
- Oral medications must be continued for several months after clinical cure to prevent relapse
- Débridement assists healing
- Prognosis of maduromycosis is poor, although prolonged ketoconazole or itraconazole therapy combined with surgical debridement yields a response rate of 70%. Amputation is necessary in far-advanced cases
- Prognosis of actinomycetoma is good because it usually responds to sulfonamides and sulfones, especially if treated early

Author(s)

Samuel A. Shelburne, MD

Richard J. Hamill, MD

Myocarditis, Acute

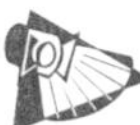

KEY FEATURES

- Focal or diffuse inflammation of the myocardium
- Primary causes: acute viral infection or postviral immune response
- Secondary causes
  - Nonviral pathogens, such as bacterial, rickettsial, spirochetal, fungal, or parasitic
  - Toxins, drugs (especially cocaine)
  - Immunologic disorders (eg, systemic lupus erythematosus)
- Many cases resolve spontaneously
- In other cases, cardiac function deteriorates progressively and may lead to dilated cardiomyopathy

CLINICAL FINDINGS

- Onset: several days to a few weeks after onset of an acute febrile illness or respiratory infection
- Congestive heart failure, gradual or abrupt and fulminant
- Symptoms: chest pain (pleuritic or nonspecific), dyspnea
- Physical examination: tachycardia, gallop rhythm, edema, or conduction defect
- Emboli due to procoagulant effect of cytokines, decreased myocardial contractility, and blood pooling

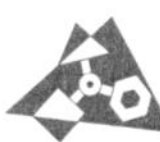

DIAGNOSIS

- Elevated white blood count, erythrocyte sedimentation rate, troponin I (in 33%), CK-MB (in 10%)
- ECG: sinus tachycardia, ventricular ectopy, nonspecific repolarization changes, or intraventricular conduction delay; occasionally, ST-T changes may mimic acute myocardial infarction
- Chest x-ray film: nonspecific, cardiomegaly is common, pulmonary venous hypertension, even pulmonary edema
- Echocardiogram: cardiomegaly and contractile dysfunction
- Myocardial biopsy, although not sensitive, may reveal a characteristic inflammatory pattern

TREATMENT

- Specific antimicrobial therapy for any identified infectious agent

- Immunosuppressive therapy for acute (< 6 mo) myocarditis only if myocardial biopsy suggests ongoing inflammation
- Otherwise, treat heart failure and arrhythmias
- Evaluation for cardiac transplantation

Author(s)

Thomas M. Bashore, MD

Christopher B. Granger, MD

Myoclonus

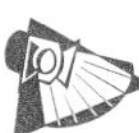 KEY FEATURES

- Myoclonic jerks are sudden, shock-like muscle contractions
- Occasional myoclonic jerks may occur in anyone, especially when drifting into sleep
- General or multifocal myoclonus: common in patients with idiopathic epilepsy and certain hereditary disorders
- Generalized myoclonic jerking may accompany metabolic encephalopathies, result from levodopa therapy, occur in alcohol or drug withdrawal states, or follow anoxic brain damage
- It is common in subacute sclerosing panencephalitis and Creutzfeldt-Jakob disease

 CLINICAL FINDINGS

- Myoclonus can be focal or generalized and can occur spontaneously or in response to certain stimuli (eg, noise)

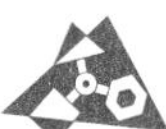 DIAGNOSIS

- Clinical
- An electroencephalogram is often helpful in clarifying an epileptic basis, and CT or MRI scan may reveal the causal lesion

 TREATMENT

- May respond to certain anticonvulsant drugs, especially valproic acid, or to one of the benzodiazepines, particularly clonazepam (Table 98)
- It may also respond to piracetam (up to 16.8 g daily)
- Myoclonus after anoxic brain damage is often responsive to oxitriptan and sometimes to clonazepam
- Oxitriptan is given in gradually increasing doses up to 1–1.5 mg daily
- In patients with segmental myoclonus, a localized lesion (spinal or cerebral) should be searched for and treated appropriately

Author(s)

Michael J. Aminoff, MD, DSc, FRCP

Myotonic Dystrophy

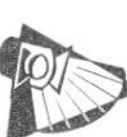 KEY FEATURES

- A slowly progressive, dominantly inherited myopathic disorder
- Usually manifests itself in the third or fourth decade but occasionally appears early in childhood
- The genetic defect has been localized to the long arm of chromosome 19

 CLINICAL FINDINGS

- Complaints of muscle stiffness
- Marked delay occurs before affected muscles can relax after a contraction; this can often be demonstrated clinically by delayed relaxation of the hand after sustained grip or by percussion of the belly of a muscle
- Weakness and wasting of the facial, sternocleidomastoid, and distal limb muscles
- Cataracts, frontal baldness, testicular atrophy, diabetes mellitus, cardiac abnormalities, and intellectual changes

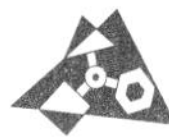 DIAGNOSIS

- Electromyographic sampling of affected muscles reveals myotonic discharges in addition to changes suggestive of myopathy

 TREATMENT

- Phenytoin, 100 mg PO TID; quinine sulfate, 300–400 mg PO TID; or procainamide, 0.5–1 g PO QID; phenytoin is preferred because the other drugs may have undesirable effects on cardiac conduction
- Tocainide and mexiletine have also been used
- Neither the weakness nor the course of the disorder is influenced by treatment

Author(s)

Michael J. Aminoff, MD, DSc, FRCP

Narcolepsy

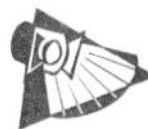 KEY FEATURES

- A disorder of excessive sleepiness, manifesting in "sleep attacks"
- Disorder begins in early adult life
- Affects both sexes equally
- Severity levels off at ~30 years of age

 CLINICAL FINDINGS

- Tetrad of symptoms
  - Sudden, brief sleep attacks during any type of activity
  - Cataplexy, a loss of specific or generalized muscle tone
  - Sleep paralysis: a flaccidity of muscles with full consciousness while falling or waking from sleep
  - Hypnagogic hallucinations, preceding sleep or occurring during a sleep attack

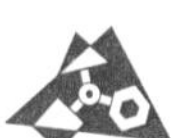 DIAGNOSIS

- Sleep study
  - Attacks are characterized by abrupt transition into REM sleep, a necessary criterion for diagnosis

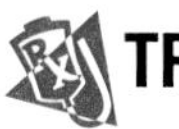 TREATMENT

- Dextroamphetamine, 10 mg PO Q AM
- Modafinil, 200 mg PO Q AM
  - Mechanism of action is unknown, but risk of abuse is thought to be lower than with stimulants
- Imipramine, 75–100 mg PO QD, is effective in treatment of cataplexy but not narcolepsy

Author(s)

Stuart J. Eisendrath, MD

Jonathan E. Lichtmacher, MD

Nasal Trauma

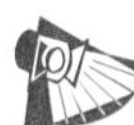 KEY FEATURES

- The nasal pyramid is the most frequently fractured bone in the body
- Epistaxis and pain are common, as are soft tissue hematomas ("black eye")
- Septal hematomas may become infected; *Staphylococcus aureus* is the predominant organism
- Persistent functional or cosmetic defects may be repaired by delayed reconstructive nasal surgery

 CLINICAL FINDINGS

- Fracture is suggested by crepitance or palpably mobile bony segments
- Intranasal examination should be performed in all cases to rule out septal hematoma, which appears as a widening of the anterior septum, visible just posterior to the columella. The septal cartilage receives its only nutrition from its closely adherent mucoperichondrium
- It is important to ensure that there is no palpable step-off of the infraorbital rim, which would indicate the presence of a zygomatic complex fracture

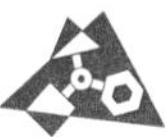 DIAGNOSIS

- Radiologic confirmation may be helpful but is not necessary in uncomplicated nasal fractures

 TREATMENT

- Treatment is aimed at maintaining long-term nasal airway patency and nasal aesthetics
- Closed reduction, using topical 4% cocaine and locally injected 1% lidocaine, should be attempted within 1 week of injury
- In the presence of marked nasal swelling, it is best to wait several days for the edema to subside before undertaking reduction
- An untreated subperichondrial hematoma will result in loss of the nasal cartilage with resultant saddle-nose deformity

Author(s)

Robert K. Jackler, MD

Michael J. Kaplan, MD

Nausea & Vomiting of Pregnancy

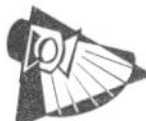 KEY FEATURES

- "Morning sickness"
- Up to 75% of women complain of nausea and vomiting during early pregnancy
- Vast majority of symptomatic patients note nausea throughout the day
- Symptoms are particularly common with multiple pregnancy and hydatidiform mole
- High estrogen levels are believed to be responsible
- Exerts no adverse effects on the pregnancy and does not presage complications

 CLINICAL FINDINGS

- Morning or evening nausea and vomiting usually begin soon after the first missed period and ceases after the fifth month
- Persistent, severe vomiting is hyperemesis gravidarum, a distinct entity (see Hyperemesis Gravidarum)

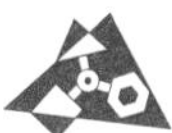 DIAGNOSIS

- Clinical

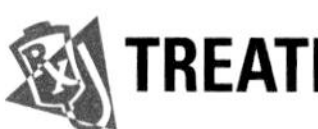 TREATMENT

- Reassurance and dietary advice are adequate in most cases
- Vitamin B_6, 50–100 mg PO QD, is nontoxic and may help some patients
- To limit the risk of teratogenicity, drug use in the first half of pregnancy should be limited to those of major importance to life and health (Tables 71 and 74)

Author(s)

William R. Crombleholme, MD

Nephritis, Interstitial

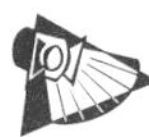

KEY FEATURES

- Interstitial inflammatory response with edema and possible tubular cell damage, responsible for ~10–15% of cases of intrinsic renal failure
- Causes of **acute** interstitial nephritis
  - Drugs (> 70% of cases), including penicillins, cephalosporins, sulfonamides, erythromycin, tetracycline, vancomycin, thiazides, furosemide, nonsteroidal anti-inflammatory drugs, rifampin, phenytoin, allopurinol, cimetidine
  - Infectious diseases, including streptococcal infections, leptospirosis, cytomegalovirus, Epstein-Barr virus, histoplasmosis, Rocky Mountain spotted fever, *Mycoplasma, Toxoplasma*
  - Immunologic disorders, including systemic lupus erythematosus, Sjögren's syndrome, sarcoidosis, cryoglobulinemia
  - Idiopathic
- Causes of **chronic** interstitial nephritis
  - Obstructive uropathy
  - Vesicoureteral reflux (reflux nephropathy)
  - Analgesic nephropathy
  - Heavy metals (lead, cadmium, mercury, bismuth)
  - Multiple myeloma
  - Gout

CLINICAL FINDINGS

- Fever (> 80%)
- Transient maculopapular rash (25–50%)
- Arthralgias

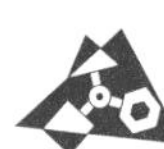

DIAGNOSIS

- Peripheral blood eosinophilia (80%)
- Acute renal insufficiency
- Pyuria (including eosinophiluria), white blood cell casts, and hematuria (95%)
- Proteinuria usually modest
- Differential diagnosis
  - Acute tubular necrosis
  - Acute glomerulonephritis
  - Prerenal azotemia
  - Chronic glomerulopathy (eg, diabetes)
  - Hypertensive nephrosclerosis
  - Obstructive uropathy

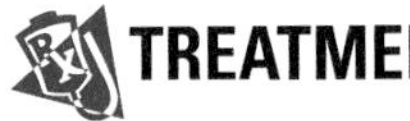

TREATMENT

- Supportive measures
- Removal of inciting agent
- Prednisone, 1–2 mg/kg/day for 1–2 weeks, followed by a prednisone taper if renal failure persists after removal of the inciting agent
- Prognosis good; recovery occurs over weeks to months
- Dialysis may be necessary in up to 33%
- Patients rarely progress to end-stage renal disease
- Prognosis worse in those with prolonged courses of oliguric failure and advanced age

Author(s)

Suzanne Watnick, MD

Gail Morrison, MD

Nephritis, Lupus

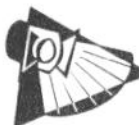

KEY FEATURES

- Renal involvement is common in systemic lupus erythematosus (SLE), occurring in 35–90% of SLE patients

CLINICAL FINDINGS

- Urinalysis: hematuria and proteinuria

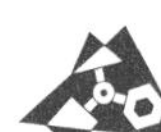

DIAGNOSIS

- Renal biopsy shows 1 of 5 histological patterns: type I, normal; type II, mesangial proliferative; type III, focal and segmental proliferative; type IV, diffuse proliferative; type V, membranous nephropathy

TREATMENT

- No treatment required for types I and II
- Immunosuppressive therapy with corticosteroids and cytotoxic agents for extensive type III lesions and all type IV lesions
- Indications for treatment of type V disease are unclear
- Corticosteroids: methylprednisolone, 1 g IV QD for 3 days, followed by prednisone, 60 mg PO QD for 4–6 weeks
- Cytotoxic agents: cyclophosphamide, IV every month for 6 doses and then every 3 mo for 6 doses
- Cyclosporine useful
- Mycophenolate mofetil may be helpful
- Monitoring serum creatinine, dsDNA antibodies, C3, C4, and CH50, urinary protein, and sediment can be useful during treatment
- Renal transplantation, but recurrent renal disease occurs in 8% of cases

Author(s)

Suzanne Watnick, MD

Gail Morrison, MD

Nephropathy, Diabetic

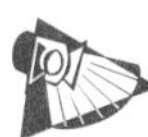

KEY FEATURES

- Most common cause of end-stage renal disease in US
- Type 1 diabetes mellitus imposes a 30–40% risk of nephropathy after 20 years
- Type 2 imposes a 15–20% risk after 20 years
- Males, African-Americans, and Native Americans are at higher risk

CLINICAL FINDINGS

- Diabetic retinopathy is often present
- Microalbuminuria develops within 10–15 years after onset of diabetes and progresses over the next 3–7 years to overt proteinuria

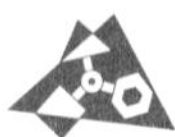

DIAGNOSIS

- Increase in GFR at onset
- With the development of macroalbuminuria, GFR returns to normal and then to subnormal as nephropathy progresses
- Renal biopsy: most common lesion is diffuse glomerulosclerosis, but nodular glomerulosclerosis (Kimmelstiel-Wilson nodules) is pathognomonic

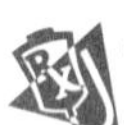

TREATMENT

- Strict glycemic control and treatment of hypertension slow progression of diabetic nephropathy
- ACE inhibitors and angiotensin II receptor antagonists lower the rate of progression to clinical proteinuria and overt renal failure

Author(s)

Suzanne Watnick, MD

Gail Morrison, MD

Nephropathy, Immunoglobulin A

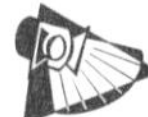

KEY FEATURES

- Primary renal disease of IgA deposition in the glomerular mesangium
- Inciting cause unknown
- Associated with hepatic cirrhosis, celiac disease, and HIV and cytomegalovirus infections
- Most common form of acute glomerulonephritis in US
- Usually occurs in children and young adults
- Males affected 2–3 times more often than females

CLINICAL FINDINGS

- Gross hematuria, frequently associated with an upper respiratory tract infection (50%), GI symptoms (10%), or flu-like illness (15%)
- Urine becomes red or cola-colored 1–2 days after illness onset
- Asymptomatic microscopic hematuria may be found incidentally
- Hypertension
- Nephrotic syndrome possible

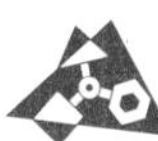

DIAGNOSIS

- Persistent microscopic hematuria and proteinuria
- Serum creatinine and blood urea nitrogen sometimes elevated
- Serum IgA level is increased in ≤ 50% of patients
- Serum complement levels usually normal
- Renal biopsy: light microscopy shows focal glomerulonephritis with and proliferation of mesangial cells; immunofluorescence shows diffuse mesangial IgA, IgG, and C3 deposits
- Skin biopsy: granular deposits of IgA in dermal capillaries

TREATMENT

- ~33% of patients experience spontaneous remission
- Chronic microscopic hematuria and stable serum creatinine in 50–60%; progressive renal insufficiency in 40–50%
- Prognosis worse if proteinuria > 1 g/day
- Angiotensin-converting enzyme inhibitors or angiotensin II receptor-blocking drugs to reduce blood pressure and proteinuria (Table 48)
- Methylprednisolone, 1 g/day IV for 3 days during months 1, 3, and 5, plus prednisone, 0.5 mg/kg QOD for 6 mo in nephrotic patients with glomerular filtration rate 60–70 mL/min
- Fish oil, 2–5 g/day, debatable
- Renal transplantation

Author(s)

Suzanne Watnick, MD

Gail Morrison, MD

Nephropathy, Membranous

KEY FEATURES

- Most common cause of primary nephrotic syndrome in adults
- Caused by immune complex deposition in the subepithelial portion of glomerular capillary walls
- Associated with infections such as hepatitis B, endocarditis, syphilis; autoimmune disease such as systemic lupus erythematosus, mixed connective tissue disease, thyroiditis; carcinoma; certain drugs such as gold, penicillamine, captopril
- Occurs most commonly in adults in the fifth and sixth decades

CLINICAL FINDINGS

- Nephrotic syndrome

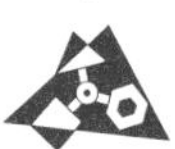

DIAGNOSIS

- Renal biopsy: light microscopy: increased capillary wall thickness; immunofluorescence: IgG and C3 along capillary loops; electron microscopy: discontinuous dense deposits along the subepithelial surface of the basement membrane

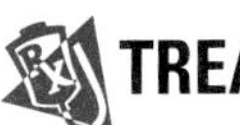

TREATMENT

- Treatment is controversial
- Patients with proteinuria of < 4 g/day: close monitoring, low-salt diet, strict blood pressure control, and ACE inhibitor
- Patients with proteinuria of 4–8 g/day and normal renal function: consider immunosuppressive regimens with corticosteroids and chlorambucil or cyclophosphamide (or cyclosporine) for 6 mo
- Patients with proteinuria of > 8 g/day and possible renal dysfunction: consider cyclosporine as a first-line immunosuppressant or corticosteroids with a cytotoxic agent
- Renal transplantation

Author(s)

Suzanne Watnick, MD

Gail Morrison, MD

Nephrotic Syndrome

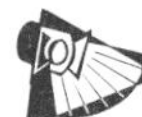

KEY FEATURES

- In adults, most commonly idiopathic
- Associated with diabetes mellitus, amyloidosis, or systemic lupus erythematosus in 33%

CLINICAL FINDINGS

- Peripheral edema with serum albumin < 3 g/dL
- Edema can become generalized
- Dyspnea caused by pulmonary edema, pleural effusions, and diaphragmatic compromise with ascites
- Abdominal distention from ascites
- Increased susceptibility to infection because of urinary loss of immunoglobulins and complement
- Hypercoagulable state, with renal vein thrombosis and venous thromboemboli, particularly in membranous nephropathy

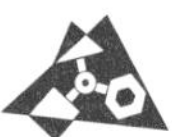

DIAGNOSIS

- Urinalysis: proteinuria; few cellular elements or casts
- Oval fat bodies appear as "grape clusters" under light microscopy and "Maltese crosses" under polarized light
- Serum albumin < 3 g/dL, serum protein < 6 g/dL
- Hyperlipidemia
- Elevated erythrocyte sedimentation rate
- Send serum complement levels, serum and urine protein electrophoresis, ANA, and serologic tests for hepatitis as indicated
- Renal biopsy indicated in adults with new-onset idiopathic nephrotic syndrome if a primary renal disease is suspected
- Renal biopsy useful for prognosis and treatment decisions
- Four most common lesions: minimal change disease, focal glomerular sclerosis, membranous nephropathy, and membranoproliferative glomerulonephritis (Table 93)

TREATMENT

- Protein intake should replace total daily urinary protein losses
- Salt and water restriction for edema
- Loop and thiazide diuretics in combination
- Antilipidemic agents
- Corticosteroids, cytotoxic agents as indicated for primary renal lesion
- Warfarin in patients with thrombosis for at least 3–6 mo

Author(s)

Suzanne Watnick, MD

Gail Morrison, MD

Neurogenic Arthropathy (Charcot's Joint)

KEY FEATURES

- Joint destruction resulting from loss or diminution of proprioception, pain, and temperature perception
- As normal muscle tone and protective reflexes are lost, secondary degenerative joint disease ensues
- Traditionally associated with tabes dorsalis; more frequently seen in diabetic neuropathy, syringomyelia, spinal cord injury, pernicious anemia, leprosy, and peripheral nerve injury

CLINICAL FINDINGS

- An enlarged, boggy, painless joint with extensive cartilage erosion, osteophyte formation, and multiple loose-joint bodies

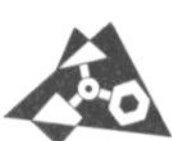

DIAGNOSIS

- Radiographic changes may be degenerative or hypertrophic in the same patient
- Differential diagnosis
  - Repeated trauma (causing degenerative joint disease)
  - Rheumatoid arthritis
  - Chronic hemarthrosis (bleed)
  - Chondrocalcinosis (eg, pseudogout, hemochromatosis, Wilson's disease)

TREATMENT

- Directed against the primary disease
- Mechanical devices are used to assist in weight bearing and prevention of further trauma
- In some instances, amputation becomes unavoidable

Author(s)

David B. Hellmann, MD, FACP

John H. Stone, MD, MPH

Neuroleptic Malignant Syndrome

KEY FEATURES

- A catatonia-like state manifested by
  - Extrapyramidal signs
  - Blood pressure changes
  - Altered consciousness
  - Hyperpyrexia
- Uncommon complication of neuroleptic treatment
- Comorbid affective disorder as well as concomitant lithium use may increase risk
- In most cases, occurs within 2 weeks of starting neuroleptic agent

CLINICAL FINDINGS

- Muscle rigidity, involuntary movements, confusion, dysarthria, dysphagia
- Pallor, cardiovascular instability, pulmonary congestion, diaphoresis
- Can result in stupor, coma, death

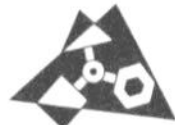

DIAGNOSIS

- Elevated creatinine kinase and leukocytosis with left shift in 50% of cases

TREATMENT

- Control of fever and IV fluid support
- Bromocriptine, 2.5–10 mg TID, and amantadine, 100–200 mg BID, are useful
- Dantrolene, 50 mg IV PRN to maximum of 10 mg/kg/day, can alleviate rigidity
- ECT has been used in resistant cases
- Clozapine has been used safely in patients with a history of NMS

Author(s)

Stuart J. Eisendrath, MD

Jonathan E. Lichtmacher, MD

Nevi, Congenital

KEY FEATURES

- In contrast to the common nevi that appear after birth, congenital nevi by definition are present at birth
- The management of small congenital nevi—less than a few centimeters in diameter—is controversial. The majority will never become malignant, but some experts believe that the risk of melanoma in these lesions may be somewhat increased

CLINICAL FINDINGS

- Most nevi are small and look like ordinary pigmented acquired nevi
- Giant congenital nevi may be quite large and involve the trunk, upper back, or shoulders
- The surface of the lesion may be smooth or irregular
- Color may range from pale tan to brown-black
- May be associated with an overgrowth of hair

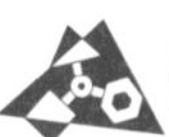

DIAGNOSIS

- Clinical or by biopsy

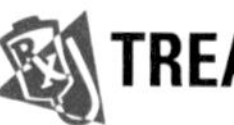

TREATMENT

- Because 1% of whites are born with these lesions, management should be conservative and excision advised only for lesions in cosmetically nonsensitive areas where the patient cannot easily see the lesion and note any suspicious changes
- Excision should be considered for congenital nevi whose contour (bumpiness, nodularity) or color (different shades) makes it difficult for examiners to note early signs of malignant change
- Giant congenital melanocytic nevi (> 5% body surface area) are at greater risk for development of melanoma, and surgical removal in stages is often recommended

Author(s)

Timothy G. Berger, MD

Nevi, Dysplastic or Atypical

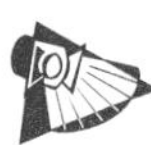

KEY FEATURES

- The term "atypical nevus" or "atypical mole" has supplanted "dysplastic nevus"
- It is estimated that 5–10% of the US population have 1 or more atypical nevi
- There is an increased risk of melanoma in the following populations
  - Patients with 50 or more nevi with 1 or more atypical moles and 1 mole at least 8 mm or larger
  - Patients with a few to many definitely atypical moles. These patients deserve education and regular (usually every 6–12 mo) follow-up
  - Kindreds with familial melanoma (numerous atypical nevi and a strong family history) deserve even closer attention because the risk of developing single or even multiple melanomas in these individuals approaches 50% by age 50

CLINICAL FINDINGS

- The moles are large (> 5 mm in diameter), with an ill-defined, irregular border and irregularly distributed pigmentation

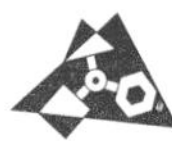

DIAGNOSIS

- The diagnosis is made clinically and not histologically

TREATMENT

- Moles should be removed only if they are suspected to be melanomas

Author(s)

Timothy G. Berger, MD

Niacin Deficiency

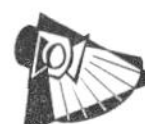

KEY FEATURES

- Most commonly results from alcoholism and nutrient–drug interactions
- Can also occur in inborn errors of metabolism
- Manifestations are nonspecific

CLINICAL FINDINGS

- Common complaints include anorexia, weakness, irritability, mouth soreness, glossitis, stomatitis, weight loss
- More advanced deficiency results in the classic triad of pellagra: dermatitis, diarrhea, dementia
- Advanced pellagra can result in death

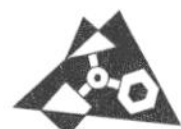

DIAGNOSIS

- Diagnosis of pellagra is made clinically
- Measure niacin metabolites, particularly *N*-methylnicotinamide, in the urine
- Serum and red blood cell nicotinamide adenine dinucleotide and nicotinamide adenine dinucleotide phosphate levels are low

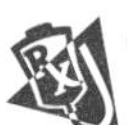

TREATMENT

- Niacin, usually given as nicotinamide, 10–150 mg PO QD

Author(s)

Robert B. Baron, MD, MS

Nipple Discharge

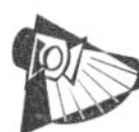

KEY FEATURES

- The most common causes of nipple discharge in the nonlactating breast, in order of decreasing frequency, are:
  - Duct ectasia
  - Intraductal papilloma
  - Carcinoma
- Factors to be assessed by history and physical examination:
  - Nature of discharge (serous, bloody, or other)
  - Discharge associated with a mass
  - Unilateral or bilateral discharge
  - Single or multiple duct discharge
  - Discharge is spontaneous (persistent or intermittent) or must be expressed
  - Discharge is produced by pressure at a single site or by general pressure on breast
  - Relationship of discharge to menses
  - Premenopausal or postmenopausal patient
  - Patient taking oral contraceptives or estrogen

CLINICAL FINDINGS

- Unilateral, spontaneous serous or serosanguineous discharge from a single duct usually caused by intraductal papilloma or, rarely, intraductal cancer
- Bloody discharge is worrisome for malignancy
- In premenopausal women, spontaneous brown or green discharge, from multiple ducts, unilaterally or bilaterally, most marked just before menstruation, is often due to fibrocystic condition
- In the nonlactating breast, milky discharge from multiple ducts occurs as a result of hyperprolactinemia in certain endocrine syndromes, from certain drugs (antipsychotics), or from fibrocystic condition
- A clear, serous, or milky discharge from single or multiple ducts can occur on oral contraceptives or estrogen replacement therapy or can be due to fibrocystic condition. The discharge is more evident just before menstruation and disappears on stopping the medication
- Purulent discharge may originate in a subareolar abscess

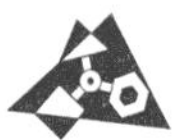

DIAGNOSIS

- If unilateral discharge present from single duct, involved duct can be identified by pressure at different sites around nipple at margin of areola

- Cytological examination of discharge may identify malignant cells, but if negative, does not rule out cancer
- Check serum prolactin and thyroid-stimulating hormone levels if discharge is milky
- Mammography may be helpful if localization of lesion is not possible
- Differential diagnosis
  - Galactorrhea (eg, pregnancy, postpartum, hyperprolactinemia)
  - Mammary duct ectasia
  - Intraductal papilloma
  - Breast cancer
  - Oral contraceptives or estrogen replacement therapy
  - Fibrocystic condition
  - Subareolar abscess

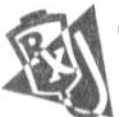

TREATMENT

- Any mass or, in the case of duct ectasia or intraductal papilloma, any involved duct should be excised
- Abscesses require drainage or removal along with the related lactiferous sinus
- When localization is not possible, no mass is palpable, and discharge is nonbloody, the patient should be reexamined every 6 mo for 1 yr, and mammography performed

Author(s)

Armando E. Giuliano, MD

Nocardiosis

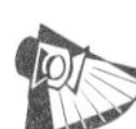

KEY FEATURES

- *Nocardia asteroides*, an aerobic filamentous soil bacterium, causes pulmonary and systemic nocardiosis
- Bronchopulmonary abnormalities (eg, alveolar proteinosis) predispose to colonization, but infection is unusual unless the patient is also receiving systemic corticosteroids or is otherwise immunosuppressed
- Central nervous system involvement commonly accompanies pulmonary infection

CLINICAL FINDINGS

- Pulmonary involvement usually begins with malaise, loss of weight, fever, and night sweats
- Cough and production of purulent sputum are the chief complaints
- Dissemination may involve any organ
  - Brain abscesses and subcutaneous nodules are most frequent
  - Dissemination is seen exclusively in immunocompromised patients

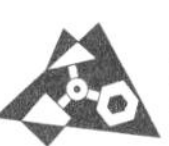

DIAGNOSIS

- *N asteroides* is a branching, filamentous gram-positive bacterium that is weakly acid-fast
- Identification is made by culture
- Chest x-ray may show infiltrates accompanied by pleural effusion. The lesions may penetrate through the chest wall and invade the ribs

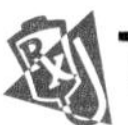

TREATMENT

- IV trimethoprim-sulfamethoxazole is initially administered at a dosage of 5–10 mg/kg/day (trimethoprim) and continued with trimethoprim-sulfamethoxazole PO, one double-strength tablet BID
- Surgical procedures such as drainage and resection may be needed as adjunctive therapy
- Response may be slow, and therapy must be continued for at least 6 mo
- The prognosis in systemic nocardiosis is poor when therapy is delayed

Author(s)

Henry F. Chambers, MD

Obesity-Hypoventilation Syndrome

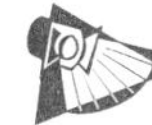

KEY FEATURES

- Massive obesity and alveolar hypoventilation while awake
- Hypoventilation resulting from blunted ventilatory drive and increased mechanical load imposed on the chest
- Obstructive sleep apnea in most

CLINICAL FINDINGS

- Obesity
- Lethargy, headache, hypersomnolence
- Loud snoring if accompanied by obstructive sleep apnea
- Dyspnea often absent
- Signs of cyanosis and cor pulmonale may be found
- Many patients have polycythemia

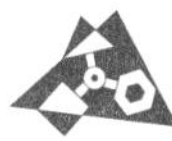

DIAGNOSIS

- Arterial blood gas measurements confirm daytime hypoxemia and hypercapnia, which improve with voluntary hyperventilation
- Nocturnal sleep study helpful to evaluate for obstructive sleep apnea

TREATMENT

- Mainly consists of weight loss
- Noninvasive positive-pressure ventilation is helpful in some patients
- Respiratory stimulants (medroxyprogesterone acetate, 10–20 mg Q 8 h, theophylline, acetazolamide) may help
- If present, obstructive sleep apnea must be treated aggressively
- Treatment of comorbid conditions

Author(s)

Mark S. Chesnutt, MD

Thomas J. Prendergast, MD

Opioid Poisoning

KEY FEATURES

- Widely varying potencies and durations of action (eg, some illicit fentanyl derivatives are 2000 times more potent than morphine)

CLINICAL FINDINGS

- Heroin's duration of action usually 3–5 h; methadone, 48–72 h
- Euphoria, drowsiness, and constricted pupils can occur with mild intoxication
- Severe intoxication may cause hypotension, bradycardia, hypothermia, coma, pulmonary edema, respiratory arrest
- Death usually from apnea or pulmonary aspiration
- Propoxyphene may cause seizures and prolong QRS interval. Tramadol, dextromethorphan, and meperidine also occasionally cause seizures. Meperidine metabolite normeperidine can cause seizures, particularly with repeated use in renal insufficiency
- Skin-popping, especially with "black tar" heroin, associated with wound botulism

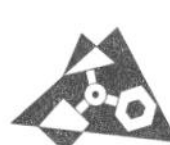

DIAGNOSIS

- Routine urine toxicology screening usually positive for patients with heroin, morphine, codeine overdose
- Toxicology screening may be falsely negative if opioid is methadone, fentanyl, oxycodone

TREATMENT

- Activated charcoal, 60–100 g PO or via gastric tube, mixed in aqueous slurry if ingestion within 1 h; not for comatose or convulsing patients unless airway protected by cuffed endotracheal tube
- Naloxone, 0.4–2 mg IV; repeat to maintain airway reflexes and spontaneous breathing. Effect duration: ~2–3 h; repeated doses may be necessary for intoxication by methadone or other long-acting drugs. Large doses (10–20 mg) possible for propoxyphene, codeine, fentanyl derivatives. Continuous observation for at least 3 h after the last naloxone dose is mandatory

Author(s)

Kent R. Olson, MD

Osmolar Gap

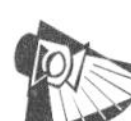

KEY FEATURES

- Alcohol quickly equilibrates between intracellular and extracellular water, adding 22 mOsm/L for every 1000 mg/L
- When measured osmolality exceeds that calculated from values of serum Na^+ and glucose and blood urea nitrogen, consider ethanol intoxication as an explanation of the discrepancy (osmolar gap)
- Toxic alcohol ingestion, particularly methanol or ethylene glycol, can produce an osmolar gap with an anion gap metabolic acidosis. However, the combination of anion gap metabolic acidosis and an osmolar gap exceeding 10 mOsm/kg is not specific for toxic alcohol ingestion
- Nearly half of patients with alcoholic ketoacidosis or lactic acidosis have similar findings, caused in part by elevations of endogenous glycerol, acetone, and acetone metabolites

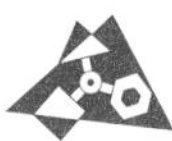

DIAGNOSIS

- The following substances can produce an osmolar gap:
  - Methanol
  - Ethylene glycol
  - Isopropyl alcohol
  - Ethanol toxicity
  - Acetone
  - Propylene glycol
  - Severe alcoholic or diabetic ketoacidosis
  - Lactic acidosis

Author(s)

Masafumi Fukagawa, MD, PhD, FJSIM
Kiyoshi Kurokawa, MD, MACP
Maxine A. Papadakis, MD

Osteomyelitis, *Staphylococcus aureus*

KEY FEATURES

- *S aureus* is the cause of approximately 60% of all cases of osteomyelitis
- Osteomyelitis may occur by direct inoculation (eg, from an open fracture or as a result of surgery), by extension from a contiguous focus of infection or open wound or, more commonly, by hematogenous spread

CLINICAL FINDINGS

- Acute, abrupt local symptoms and systemic toxicity; or insidious onset of vague pain over the site of infection, progressing to local tenderness
- Fever is absent in one-third of cases

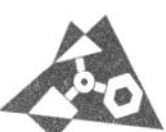

DIAGNOSIS

- Isolation of *S aureus* from the blood (60%), bone, or a contiguous focus of a patient with signs and symptoms of focal bone infection
- Bone biopsy and culture should be considered if blood cultures are sterile
- Bone scan and gallium scan can identify the site of bone infection
- Spinal infection (unlike malignancy) traverses the disk space to involve the contiguous vertebral body
- MRI is slightly less sensitive than bone scan but has a specificity of 90%. MRI is indicated when epidural abscess is suspected in association with vertebral osteomyelitis

TREATMENT

- Duration is 4–6 weeks or longer
- Parenteral regimens are advised during the acute phase:
  - Nafcillin or oxacillin, 9–12 g/day in 6 divided doses, is the drug of choice
  - Cefazolin, 1 g Q 6–8 h
- Vancomycin, 1 g Q 12 h, may be used for penicillin-allergic patients
- Oral regimens are dicloxacillin or cephalexin, 1 g Q 6 h, plus rifampin, 300 mg BID (prevents late relapse and is advised)

Author(s)

Henry F. Chambers, MD

Panbronchiolitis, Diffuse

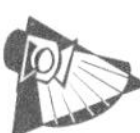

KEY FEATURES

- Idiopathic disorder of respiratory bronchioles
- Diagnosed frequently in Japan; underrecognized in the United States
- Slightly more prevalent in men, usually presenting between ages 30 and 70 years
- Approximately 66% of patients are nonsmokers
- May progress to diffuse bronchiectasis and respiratory failure

CLINICAL FINDINGS

- Marked dyspnea, cough, and sputum production
- Wheezing may occur
- Crackles and rhonchi are noted
- Most patients have history of chronic pansinusitis

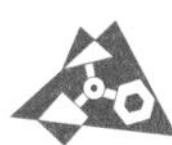

DIAGNOSIS

- Pulmonary function tests reveal obstructive airflow abnormalities
- Chest x-ray shows a distinct pattern of diffuse small nodular shadows and hyperinflation
- Open-lung biopsy is necessary for diagnosis

TREATMENT

- Chronic low-dose macrolide antibiotics (eg, erythromycin, 200–600 mg/day for 2–6 months)
- β_2-agonists or ipratropium bromide
- Treatment of sinus disease
- Corticosteroids have been used despite lack of evidence supporting their efficacy
- Treatment of bronchial infections is aided by sputum analysis

Author(s)

Mark S. Chesnutt, MD

Thomas J. Prendergast, MD

Paracoccidioidomycosis

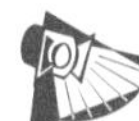

KEY FEATURES

- *Paracoccidioides brasiliensis* is a dimorphic fungus with limited geographic distribution to Mexico, Central and South America
- Long asymptomatic periods enable persons to travel far from endemic area before symptoms occur
- Primary infection is probably acquired through inhalation

CLINICAL FINDINGS

- Paracoccidioidomycosis is similar to other endemic fungi, beginning with a primary pulmonary infection is often asymptomatic or mild and self-limited
- Subacute paracoccidioidomycosis affects children and adolescents with dissemination from pulmonary focus leading to fever, malaise, hepatosplenomegaly
- Chronic symptomatic paracoccidioidomycosis in adults may occur several years after exposure, usually with pulmonary involvement and ulceration of oronasopharynx
- Extensive coalescent ulcerations may result in destruction of the epiglottis, vocal cords, uvula; extensive ulcerations of the upper gastrointestinal tract may prevent caloric intake leading to cachexia
- Extension to lips and face may occur; skin lesions are variable in appearance and may have necrotic central crater with hard hyperkeratotic borders
- Papules ulcerate and enlarge peripherally and deeper into subcutaneous tissue
- Lymph node enlargement, eventually ulcerating and forming draining sinuses
- Hepatosplenomegaly and central nervous system involvement
- Cough indicates pulmonary involvement, but symptoms may be mild despite marked radiographic findings
- Differential diagnosis includes mucocutaneous leishmaniasis and syphilis

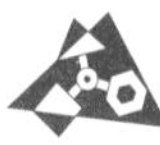

DIAGNOSIS

- Routine laboratory tests are nonspecific, but serologic tests are useful
- Immunodiffusion serologic tests positive in 98% of progressive cases
- Complement fixation titers correlate with severity of disease and fall with effective therapy
- Diagnosis is confirmed by finding *P brasiliensis* as spherical cells with many buds arising from it in sputum, pus, or tissue specimens
- Histologic stains are often more sensitive since organism grows slowly and erratically in culture

TREATMENT

- Itraconazole, 100–200 mg/day PO, for at least 6 months is treatment of choice
- Response is usually seen within the first month, with effective control within 2–6 months
- Relapse may occur following intraconazole therapy
- Patients need to be monitored for several years following completion of therapy
- Sulfonamides and amphotericin B can be used in patients who cannot tolerate itraconazole

Author(s)

Samuel A. Shelburne, MD

Richard J. Hamill, MD

Paralysis, Periodic

KEY FEATURES

- Episodes of flaccid weakness or paralysis occur, sometimes in association with abnormalities of the plasma potassium level
- May have a familial (dominant inheritance) basis
- The hypokalemic variety is commonly associated with hyperthyroidism in young Asian men
- The familial hyperkalemic periodic paralysis may have a defect in the sodium channel gene on the long arm of chromosome 17

CLINICAL FINDINGS

- **Hypokalemic periodic paralysis**
  - Attacks tend to occur on awakening, after exercise, or after a heavy meal and may last for several days
  - Strength is normal between attacks
- **Hyperkalemic periodic paralysis:** attacks also tend to occur after exercise but usually last for < 1 h
- **Normokalemic periodic paralysis:** similar clinically to the hyperkalemic variety, but the plasma potassium level remains normal during attacks

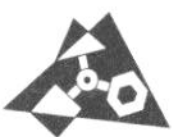

DIAGNOSIS

- Clinical and plasma potassium

TREATMENT

- **Hypokalemic periodic paralysis**
  - Patients should avoid excessive exertion
  - A low-carbohydrate, low-salt diet may help prevent attacks, as may acetazolamide, 250–750 mg PO QD
  - An ongoing attack may be aborted by potassium chloride given PO or by IV drip, provided the ECG can be monitored and renal function is satisfactory
  - Treatment of associated hyperthyroidism prevents recurrences
- **Hyperkalemic periodic paralysis**
  - Attacks may be terminated by IV calcium gluconate (1–2 g) or by IV diuretics (furosemide, 20–40 mg), glucose, or glucose and insulin
  - Daily acetazolamide or chlorothiazide may prevent recurrences
- **Normokalemic periodic paralysis:** treatment is with acetazolamide

Author(s)

Michael J. Aminoff, MD, DSc, FRCP

Paraneoplastic Syndromes

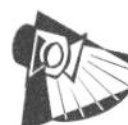

KEY FEATURES

- Occur in ≤ 15% of patients with cancer
- Small cell lung cancer is most common tumor association
- Can occur despite relatively limited neoplastic growth
- May provide an early clue to presence of certain types of cancer
- Course usually parallels course of the cancer: Effective cancer treatment should be accompanied by resolution of the syndrome; conversely, recurrence of the cancer is sometimes heralded by return of syndrome
- Metabolic or toxic effects of the syndrome (eg, hypercalcemia, hyponatremia) may be a more urgent hazard to life than the underlying cancer
- Caused by:
  - Tumor product such as ectopic hormone production (serotonin in carcinoid syndrome, PTH-related peptide in hypercalcemia, ACTH in Cushing's syndrome, ADH in the syndrome of inappropriate antidiuretic hormone secretion [SIADH])
  - Destruction of normal tissues by tumor products (local secretion of cytokines leading to hypercalcemia)
  - Unknown mechanisms such as circulating immune complexes stimulated by the tumor or unidentified tumor products (eg, certain neurologic syndromes or osteoarthropathy resulting from bronchogenic carcinoma)

CLINICAL FINDINGS

- Hypercalcemia, hyponatremia
- Cushing's syndrome, SIADH
- Neuropathy, encephalitis, cerebellar degeneration
- Dermatomyositis, Sweet's syndrome
- Polycythemia, thrombocytosis
- Renal disease
- Diarrhea
- Arthropathy

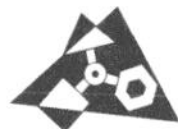

DIAGNOSIS

- See Table 156

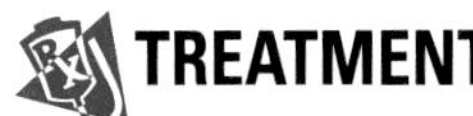

TREATMENT

- Treatment of underlying malignancy
- Bisphosphonates, corticosteroids (depending on tumor type) for hypercalcemia
- Symptomatic measures

Author(s)

Hope Rugo, MD

Paraphilias

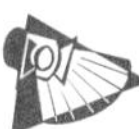

KEY FEATURES

- Atypical objects or orientations for sexual excitement
- Stimuli can vary from common objects such as a woman's shoe, a child, instruments of torture, or aggressive acts
- Disorders are differentiated by the object or activity used to achieve arousal

CLINICAL FINDINGS

- Exhibitionism is the achievement of arousal by exposing genitalia to strangers
- Transvestism consists of recurrent cross-dressing in a heterosexual man often in masturbation foreplay
- Voyeurism involves attaining arousal watching sexual activities or disrobing of an unknowing person
- Pedophilia is the use of a child to achieve sexual arousal and often gratification
- Incest involves a sexual relationship with a person—usually a child—in the immediate family
- Sexual sadism involves inflicting pain upon the sexual object as a means of arousal
- Sexual masochism is from erotic pleasure being achieved by being humiliated, enslaved, or physically bound or restrained
- Necrophilia is sexual intercourse with a dead body or use of parts of a corpse for sexual excitation

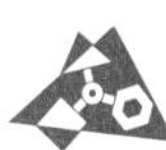

DIAGNOSIS

- Is based on clinical history and often court-ordered evaluations

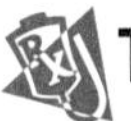

TREATMENT

- Behavioral therapy
- Gonadotropin antagonists
- Medroxyprogesterone acetate
- Selective serotonin reuptake inhibitors (eg, fluoxetine)

Author(s)

Stuart J. Eisendrath, MD

Jonathan E. Lichtmacher, MD

Paraquat Poisoning

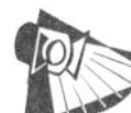

KEY FEATURES

- Used as a herbicide

CLINICAL FINDINGS

- Concentrated solutions are highly corrosive to oropharynx, esophagus, and stomach
- Fatal dose after absorption may be as small as 4 mg/kg
- If ingestion of paraquat is not rapidly fatal because of its corrosive effects, the herbicide may cause progressive pulmonary fibrosis, with death ensuing after 2–3 weeks

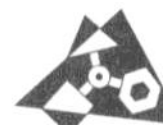

DIAGNOSIS

- Clinical
- Serum paraquat levels can be obtained through Syngenta (1-800-327-8633)
- Paraquat levels associated with a high likelihood of death: 2 mg/L at 4 h, 0.9 mg/L at 6 h, and 0.1 mg/L at 24 h after ingestion

TREATMENT

- Administer 60 g of activated charcoal PO or by gastric tube. Results of charcoal hemoperfusion, 8 h/day for 2–3 weeks, are equivocal
- Supplemental oxygen should be withheld unless the Po_2 is < 70 mm Hg because oxygen may contribute to the pulmonary damage

Author(s)

Kent R. Olson, MD

Parasomnias

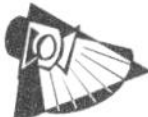

KEY FEATURES

MOST COMMON DISORDERS

Sleep terror

- Distinct from sleep panic attacks
- Usually seen in preadolescent boys, although it may occur in adults

Nightmares

- Occur during REM sleep, unlike sleep terror, which occurs in stage 3 or 4

Sleepwalking

- Includes ambulation or other intricate behaviors while asleep
- Episodes can occur during stage 3 or 4 or REM sleep
- Causative factors include medical conditions and drugs of abuse

Enuresis

- Involuntary micturition during sleep occurring in a patient who usually has control
- Most common 3–4 hours after bedtime, but not limited to a specific stage of sleep

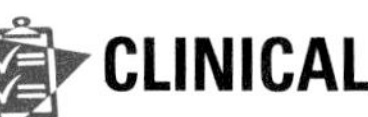

CLINICAL FINDINGS

- Sleep terror
  - Fear, sweating, tachycardia, and confusion for several minutes
  - Abrupt, terrifying arousal in sleep
  - Amnesia for the event
- Enuresis
  - Confusion during the event and amnesia after it are common

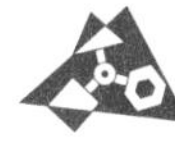

DIAGNOSIS

- Sleep walking is confirmed by a sleep study

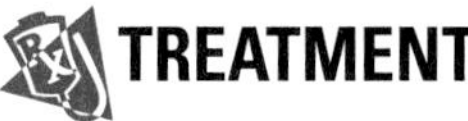

TREATMENT

Sleep terror and nightmares

- Benzodiazepines (diazepam, 5–20 mg QHS, suppresses stage 3 and 4 sleep)

Enuresis

- Desmopressin nasal spray is increasingly the treatment of choice
- Alternatively, imipramine, 50–100 mg QHS
- Behavioral approaches (eg, bells that ring when a pad is wet) have been successful

Author(s)

Stuart J. Eisendrath, MD

Jonathan E. Lichtmacher, MD

Parvovirus

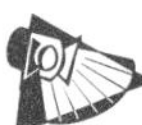

KEY FEATURES

- Widespread infection (by age 15 years, approximately 50% of children have detectable IgG). Causes several syndromes

CLINICAL FINDINGS

- In children, an exanthematous illness ("fifth disease," erythema infectiosum) is characterized by a fiery red "slapped cheek" appearance, circumoral pallor, and a subsequent lacy, maculopapular, evanescent rash on the trunk and limbs. Malaise, headache, and pruritus (especially in palms and soles) occur, but little fever
- In immunosuppressed patients—including those with HIV infection, posttransplantation, or hematologic conditions such as sickle cell disease—transient aplastic crisis and pure red blood cell aplasia may occur
- Middle-aged persons (especially women) develop a limited symmetric polyarthritis that mimics systemic lupus erythematosus and rheumatoid arthritis, preferentially involving the proximal interphalangeal joints of the hands and the wrists and knees
- Arthralgias are uncommon in children. Rashes, especially facial, are uncommon in adults. In pregnancy, fetal loss and hydrops fetalis are reported sequelae

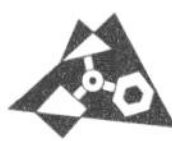

DIAGNOSIS

- Clinical diagnosis (Table 126) may be confirmed by an elevated titer of IgM anti-parvovirus antibodies in serum or with polymerase chain reaction

TREATMENT

- In healthy persons, treatment is symptomatic
  - Nonsteroidal anti-inflammatory drugs for arthalgias
  - Transfusions as needed for transient aplastic crises
- In immunosuppressed patients, intravenous immunoglobulin reduces degree of anemia

Author(s)

Wayne X. Shandera, MD

Ana Moran, MD

Patellofemoral Syndrome

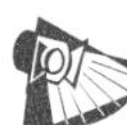

KEY FEATURES

- Anterior knee pain
- A variety of injuries or anatomic abnormalities predispose patients to irregular patellar movements, leading to the patellofemoral syndrome
- Predisposing conditions include
  - Imbalance of quadriceps strength
  - Patella alta
  - Recurrent patellar subluxation
  - Direct trauma to the patella
  - Meniscal injuries

CLINICAL FINDINGS

- Pain is in the front of the knee, around or underneath the patella
- Because of the flexion load, patients may have difficulty going up or down staircases
- May have crepitus, joint locking, or sensations of joint instability

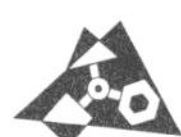

DIAGNOSIS

- The history is generally more useful than the physical examination in establishing the diagnosis, but a significant number of patients have characteristic physical findings
- When the knee is held in slight flexion, gentle pressure against the patella as the patient contracts the quadriceps muscles may reproduce the symptoms. In some cases, with the knee extended and the quadriceps relaxed, the typical pain may be reproduced by digital pressure under the medial or lateral border of the patella, with side-to-side movement of the bone

TREATMENT

- Avoidance of flexion loads and strengthening of the quadriceps

Author(s)

David B. Hellmann, MD, FACP

John H. Stone, MD, MPH

Patent Ductus Arteriosus

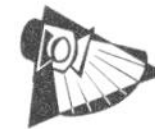

KEY FEATURES

- Embryonic ductus arteriosus fails to close, resulting in continuous (systolic and diastolic) shunt of blood from aorta to left pulmonary artery (PA)
- Usually located near the origin of the left subclavian artery
- Effect of persistent left-to-right shunt on PA pressure depends on size of ductus
- Small or moderate size patent ductus usually asymptomatic until middle age
- Large patent ductus causes pulmonary hypertension, and Eisenmenger's syndrome may result

CLINICAL FINDINGS

- Symptoms only if left ventricular (LV) failure or pulmonary hypertension develops
- Heart typically normal size or slightly enlarged
- Hyperdynamic apical impulse
- Wide pulse pressure and low diastolic pressure
- Continuous rough "machinery" murmur
- Thrill common
- Advanced disease: cyanotic lower legs (especially toes) in contrast to normally pink fingers

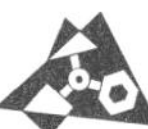

DIAGNOSIS

- ECG: Normal tracing or LV hypertrophy
- Chest x-ray film
  - Normal-sized heart or LV and left atrial enlargement
  - Prominent PA, aorta, and left atrium
- Echo-Doppler is helpful, but lesion best visualized by MRI, CT, or contrast angiography
- Cardiac catheterization can assess ductus and shunt size and direction and PA pressure

TREATMENT

- Large shunts: high mortality early in life
- Smaller shunts: compatible with long survival; congestive heart failure most common complication

- Antibiotic prophylaxis mandatory to prevent endocarditis
- Surgical ligation or if ductus size is small enough, transcatheter closure using either coils or occluder devices
- Ductus closure usually attempted unless pulmonary hypertension and right-to-left shunting is present

Author(s)

Thomas M. Bashore, MD

Christopher B. Granger, MD

Penicillium marneffei Infection

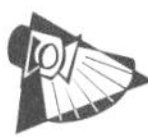

KEY FEATURES

- *Penicillium marneffei* is a dimorphic fungus, endemic in southeast Asia
- Causes systemic infection in both immunocompetent and immunocompromised persons
- Disseminated infections occur in advanced AIDS, including in travelers returning from southeast Asia

CLINICAL FINDINGS

- Fever
- Lymphadenopathy, hepatosplenomegaly
- Generalized umbilicated papular rash
- Cough
- Diarrhea

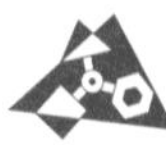

DIAGNOSIS

- Identification of the organism on smears, histopathological specimens, or culture; the fungus produces a characteristic red pigment in culture
- Best sites for isolation include skin, blood, bone marrow, respiratory tract, lymph nodes

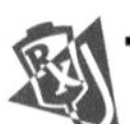

TREATMENT

- Itraconazole, 400 mg PO QD for 8 weeks, for mild to moderate infection
- Amphotericin B, 0.5–0.7 mg/kg/day, for severe disease
- Because relapse rate after successful treatment is 30%, use maintenance therapy with itraconazole, 200–400 mg PO QD

Author(s)

Samuel A. Shelburne, MD

Richard J. Hamill, MD

Perianal Abscess & Fistula

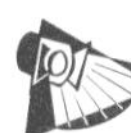

KEY FEATURES

- Infection of anal glands located at the base of the anal crypts at the dentate line, leading to abscess formation
- Causes include anal fissure and Crohn's disease
- Fistula in ano arises in an anal crypt and is usually preceded by an anal abscess
- Causes of fistulas that connect to the rectum include Crohn's disease, lymphogranuloma venereum, rectal tuberculosis, cancer

CLINICAL FINDINGS

- Perianal abscess: throbbing, continuous perianal pain
- Erythema, fluctuance, and swelling in the perianal region on external exam
- Swelling in the ischiorectal fossa on digital rectal exam
- Fistula in ano: purulent discharge itching, tenderness, and pain

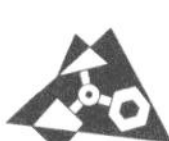

DIAGNOSIS

- Anorectal exam, anoscopy
- Fistulogram

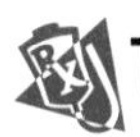

TREATMENT

- Perianal abscess treated by local surgical incision under anesthesia, ischiorectal abscess by drainage in the operating room
- Fistula in ano is treated by surgical excision under anesthesia
- Fistulas caused by Crohn's disease are frequently asymptomatic and may be treated initially with antibiotics (metronidazole, 250 mg PO TID, or ciprofloxacin, 500 mg PO BID)
- Patients with persistent or recurrent symptoms due to Crohn's disease are treated with immunomodulators (6-mercaptopurine, 1–1.5 mg/kg/day) or the anti-TNF antibody infliximab (5 mg/kg IV at 2 and 6 weeks)

Author(s)

Kenneth R. McQuaid, MD

Pericardial Effusion

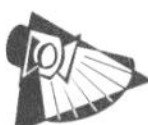

KEY FEATURES

- Can develop from any form of pericarditis
- Slow development of large effusions may produce no hemodynamic effects
- Rapid appearance of smaller effusions can cause cardiac tamponade (elevated intrapericardial pressure that restricts venous return and ventricular filling), leading to shock and death

CLINICAL FINDINGS

- Pain in acute inflammatory pericarditis; neoplastic and uremic effusions are often painless
- Dyspnea and cough, especially with tamponade
- Other symptoms reflect primary disease
- Pericardial friction rub may be present (even with large effusions)
- Pulsus paradoxus (> 10 mm Hg decline in systolic pressure during inspiration)
- Tachycardia, tachypnea, narrow pulse pressure, and preserved systolic pressure are characteristic of tamponade
- Elevation of central venous pressure, edema, or ascites in chronic processes

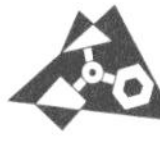

DIAGNOSIS

- ECG: often reveals nonspecific T wave changes and low QRS voltage. Electrical alternans is pathognomonic but uncommon
- CXR: normal or enlarged cardiac silhouette with a globular configuration
- Echocardiography is the primary mode of diagnosis and can distinguish effusion from congestive heart failure
- Diagnostic pericardiocentesis or biopsy is often indicated for microbiologic and cytologic studies

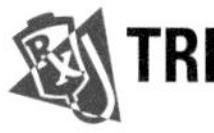

TREATMENT

- Small effusions can be followed clinically and by echocardiogram
- Urgent pericardiocentesis is required for tamponade
- Partial pericardiectomy may be required for recurrent effusion in neoplastic disease and uremia
- Additional therapy (eg, dialysis) for the primary disease

Author(s)

Thomas M. Bashore, MD

Christopher B. Granger, MD

Pericarditis, Acute

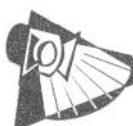 KEY FEATURES

- Acute inflammation of the pericardium
- Causes
  - Infections
  - Autoimmune diseases
  - Uremia
  - Neoplasms
  - Radiation
  - Drug toxicity
  - Hemopericardium
  - Postcardiac surgery
  - Contiguous inflammatory processes of the heart or lung (eg, myocardial infarction [MI], Dressler's syndrome, idiopathic)
- Viral infections are the most common cause; acute pericarditis often follows upper respiratory tract infection
- Males, usually younger than age 50, are most commonly affected

 CLINICAL FINDINGS

- Often associated with pleuritic chest pain, relieved by sitting, that radiates to the neck, shoulders, back, or epigastrium
- Dyspnea and fever
- Pericardial friction rub with or without evidence of pericardial effusion or constriction
- Pericardial involvement
- Bacterial pericarditis: rare; patients appear toxic and are often critically ill
- Neoplastic pericarditis: often painless, hemodynamic compromise
- Dressler's syndrome (post-MI pericarditis)
  - Occurs within days to 3 months post-MI
  - Usually self-limited
  - Treated with aspirin, nonsteroidal anti-inflammatory drugs (NSAIDs), or corticosteroids

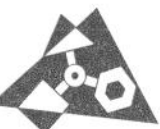 DIAGNOSIS

- Usually clinical
- Leukocytosis
- ECG
  - Generalized ST-T wave changes, characteristic progression beginning with diffuse ST elevations, followed by a return to baseline, then T wave inversions
  - PR depression indicates atrial injury
- Chest x-ray film
  - Frequently normal
  - Cardiac enlargement if pericardial effusion
  - Signs of related pulmonary disease
- Echocardiogram
  - Often normal in inflammatory pericarditis
  - Otherwise, can demonstrate pericardial effusion, tamponade
- Rising titers in paired sera may confirm viral infection
- Cardiac enzymes slightly elevated if a myocarditic component
- Cytology of pericardial effusion or pericardial biopsy
- MRI and CT scan can visualize adjacent tumor when present

 TREATMENT

- Treat underlying causes (eg, antibiotics for bacterial infection, dialysis for uremia)
- Symptomatic treatment with NSAIDs or aspirin for pain
- Corticosteroids for unresponsive cases and Dressler's syndrome
- Symptoms usually subside in several days to weeks
- Constrictive pericarditis develops rarely but may require pericardial resection
- Partial pericardiectomy for tamponade
- Drainage of malignant effusion, instillation of chemotherapeutic agents or tetracycline to prevent recurrence
- Pericardial windows are rarely effective

Author(s)

Thomas M. Bashore, MD

Christopher B. Granger, MD

Pericarditis, Constrictive

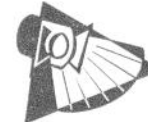 KEY FEATURES

- Generally caused by inflammation leading to a thickened, fibrotic, adherent pericardium that restricts diastolic filling and produces chronically elevated venous pressures
- Most common causes: radiation therapy, cardiac surgery, viral pericarditis
- Less common causes: tuberculosis, histoplasmosis

 CLINICAL FINDINGS

- Slowly progressive dyspnea, fatigue, and weakness
- Chronic edema, hepatic congestion, and ascites out of proportion to degree of peripheral edema
- Elevated jugular venous pressure with a rapid *y* descent
- Increased jugular venous pressure during inspiration (Kussmaul's sign)
- Pericardial knock in early diastole
- Atrial fibrillation is common
- Pulsus paradoxus is unusual

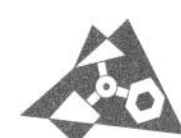 DIAGNOSIS

- Chest x-ray film
  - Normal heart size or cardiomegaly
  - Pericardial calcification is common and best seen on lateral view
- Echocardiography: thick pericardium and small chambers
- CT and MRI may be more sensitive than echocardiography; septal "bounce" reflects rapid early filling
- Exclude restrictive cardiomyopathy and cardiac tamponade

 TREATMENT

- Diuretic agents (Table 46)
- Complete surgical pericardiectomy is usually required in symptomatic patients but carries relatively high mortality rate (up to 15%)

Author(s)

Thomas M. Bashore, MD

Christopher B. Granger, MD

Peritonitis, Tuberculous

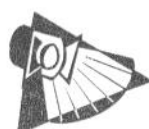

KEY FEATURES

- Tuberculous involvement of the peritoneum
- Accounts for < 2% of all causes of ascites in the United States
- Incidence higher among those with HIV disease, urban poor, nursing home residents, and immigrants from underdeveloped countries
- In the United States, half have underlying cirrhosis and ascites from portal hypertension

CLINICAL FINDINGS

- Low-grade fever
- Abdominal pain
- Anorexia, weight loss
- Abdominal swelling, clinically apparent ascites
- Abdominal examination shows doughy consistency

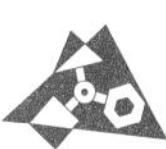

DIAGNOSIS

- Tuberculin skin tests positive in half (Table 22)
- Chest radiographs abnormal in >70%
- Active pulmonary tuberculosis disease in < 25%
- Ultrasound examination shows ascites in >90%
- Ascitic fluid total protein >3.5 g/dL, lactate dehydrogenase >90 units/L, or mononuclear cell-predominant leukocytosis >500/μL; each has a sensitivity of 70–80% but limited specificity
- Ascitic fluid smears for acid-fast bacilli are usually negative; cultures are positive in only 20%
- Ascitic fluid cultures of high-volume paracentesis fluid have increased sensitivity of ~85%
- Ascitic fluid adenosine deaminase activity has limited predictive value in cirrhotic ascites
- Laparoscopy establishes diagnosis
- Characteristic peritoneal nodules are visible in >90%
- Peritoneal biopsy reveals granulomas
- Peritoneal biopsy cultures are positive in < 66% and require at least 4–6 weeks

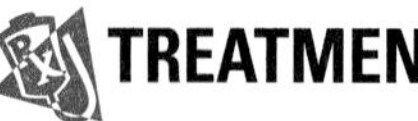

TREATMENT

- Tuberculosis, initial treatment (Table 24)
- Antituberculous drugs characteristics (Table 23)

Author(s)

Kenneth R. McQuaid, MD

Pesticide Poisoning

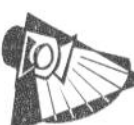

KEY FEATURES

- Includes organophosphates and carbamates
- Inhibit the enzyme acetylcholinesterase and increase acetylcholine activity at nicotinic and muscarinic receptors and in CNS
- Most are absorbed through intact skin
- Most chemical warfare "nerve agents" are organophosphates

CLINICAL FINDINGS

- Abdominal cramps, diarrhea, vomiting, excessive salivation, sweating, seizures, lacrimation, constricted pupils, wheezing, bronchorrhea, skeletal muscle weakness, respiratory arrest
- Initial tachycardia is usually followed by bradycardia
- Symptoms may persist or recur for days, especially with highly lipid-soluble agents such as fenthion or dimethoate

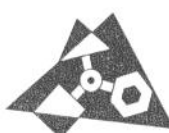

DIAGNOSIS

- Serum and red blood cell cholinesterase activity is usually at least 50% below baseline with severe intoxication

TREATMENT

- Administer activated charcoal 60–100 g PO in aqueous slurry recent ingestions
- If the agent is on the victim's skin or hair, wash with soap or shampoo and water. Care providers must avoid skin exposure by wearing gloves and waterproof aprons
- Administer atropine, 2 mg IV, and give repeated doses as needed (may need several hundred milligrams) to dry bronchial secretions and decrease wheezing
- Administer pralidoxime, 1–2 g IV, as soon as possible, and give a continuous infusion (200–400 mg/h) as long as there is any evidence of acetylcholine excess. Pralidoxime is of questionable benefit for carbamate poisoning

Author(s)

Kent R. Olson, MD

Petroleum Distillate Poisoning

KEY FEATURES

- Toxicity may occur from inhalation of the vapor or as a result of pulmonary aspiration of the liquid during or after ingestion

CLINICAL FINDINGS

- Table 147
- Aspiration pneumonitis
- With some hydrocarbons, severe systemic poisoning after oral ingestion
- Systemic intoxication can also occur by inhalation
- Vertigo, muscular incoordination, irregular pulse, myoclonus, and seizures occur with serious poisoning and may be due to hypoxemia or systemic effects of the agents
- Chlorinated and fluorinated hydrocarbons (eg, trichloroethylene, freons) and many other hydrocarbons can cause ventricular arrhythmias because of increased sensitivity of the myocardium to the effects of endogenous catecholamines

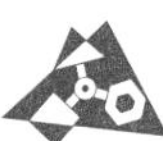

DIAGNOSIS

- Coughing or choking immediately after ingestion suggests pulmonary aspiration
- Chest X-ray findings may be delayed for several hours

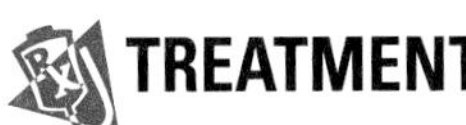

TREATMENT

- Table 147
- Move the patient to fresh air
- Administration of activated charcoal (60–100 g mixed in aqueous slurry PO or via gastric tube) may be helpful if the preparation contains toxic solutes (eg, an insecticide) or is an aromatic or halogenated product
- Observe the victim for 6–8 h for signs of aspiration pneumonitis
- Corticosteroids are not recommended
- If fever occurs, give a specific antibiotic only after identification of the bacterial pathogens
- Because of the risk of arrhythmias, use bronchodilators only with caution in patients with chlorinated or fluorinated solvent intoxication

Author(s)

Kent R. Olson, MD

Plantar Fasciitis

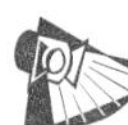

KEY FEATURES

- The most common cause of foot pain in outpatient medicine
- Results from constant strain on the plantar fascia at its insertion into the medial tubercle of the calcaneus
- The majority of cases occur in patients with no associated disease. Most occur from excessive standing and improper footwear

CLINICAL FINDINGS

- Severe pain on the bottoms of the feet in the morning—the first steps out of bed in particular—but the pain subsides after a few minutes of ambulation

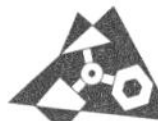

DIAGNOSIS

- Pain with palpation over the plantar fascia's insertion on the medial heel
- Radiographs have no role in the diagnosis of this condition; heel spurs frequently exist in patients without plantar fasciitis, and most symptomatic patients do not have heel spurs
- Differential diagnosis
  - Enthesopathy resulting from seronegative spondyloarthropathy
  - Achilles tendinitis
  - Metatarsal stress fracture
  - Genital herpes (referred pain from sacral ganglion)
  - Retrocalcaneal bursitis

TREATMENT

- An interval of days without prolonged standing and the use of arch supports
- NSAIDs may provide some relief
- In severe cases, a corticosteroid with lidocaine injection (small volume—no more than a total of 1.5 mL) directly into the most tender area on the sole of the foot is helpful

Author(s)

David B. Hellmann, MD, FACP
John H. Stone, MD, MPH

Pleuritis

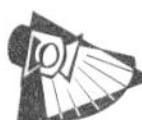

KEY FEATURES

- Irritation of the parietal pleura causes the pain associated with pleuritis

CLINICAL FINDINGS

- Pain
  - Localized, sharp, and fleeting
  - Worsened by cough, sneeze, movement, or deep breathing
- Shoulder pain may be referred when there is irritation of the central portion of the ipsilateral diaphragmatic pleura

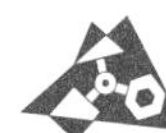

DIAGNOSIS

- The setting in which pain occurs can often narrow the broad list of potential causes
- In young, healthy individuals, pleuritis is usually due to a viral respiratory infection
- Pleural effusion, pleural thickening, or pneumothorax require additional diagnostic and therapeutic measures

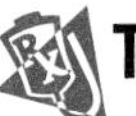

TREATMENT

- Treatment is directed at the underlying disease
- NSAIDs (indomethacin, 25 mg BID–TID) may help pain relief
- Codeine (30–60 mg TID) may control cough
- Intercostal nerve blocks are occasionally helpful

Author(s)

Mark S. Chesnutt, MD
Thomas J. Prendergast, MD

Plexopathies

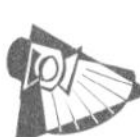

KEY FEATURES

- **Brachial plexus neuropathy** may be idiopathic, follow trauma, or result from congenital anomalies, neoplastic involvement, or injury by various physical agents; rarely, may be familial
- **Cervical rib syndrome** is the compression of the C8 and T1 roots or the lower trunk of the brachial plexus by a cervical rib or band arising from the seventh cervical vertebra
- **Lumbosacral plexus** lesions may develop in association with diabetes, cancer, or bleeding disorders, after injury, or occasionally without known cause

CLINICAL FINDINGS

- **Brachial plexus neuropathy**: Initially, severe pain about the shoulder, then, within days, weakness, reflex changes, and sensory changes, especially involving C5 and C6. Symptoms usually unilateral but may be bilateral. Wasting of affected muscles can be profound
- **Cervical rib syndrome**: weakness and wasting of intrinsic hand muscles, especially those in the thenar eminence. Pain and numbness is in the medial two fingers and the ulnar border of the hand and forearm. Compression of the subclavian artery may also occur
- **Lumbosacral plexus lesions**: pain and weakness, more so than sensory symptoms; symptoms depends on the level of neurologic involvement

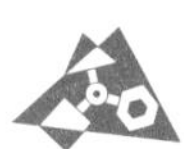

DIAGNOSIS

- X-ray films can show a cervical rib or a large transverse process of the seventh cervical vertebra; normal findings do not exclude the possibility of a cervical band. Adson's test for diagnosing compression of the subclavian artery is a diminished or obliterated radial pulse when the seated patient inhales deeply and turns the head to one side or the other
- Electrodiagnostic evaluation helps localize a lesion and is important for differential diagnosis

TREATMENT

- Symptomatic or surgical excision of the rib or band in cervical rib syndrome
- Physical therapy is especially important in idiopathic cases
- Treat underlying cause

Author(s)

Michael J. Aminoff, MD, DSc, FRCP

Pneumonia, Chlamydial

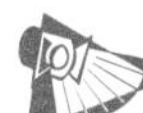

KEY FEATURES

- *Chlamydia pneumoniae* causes pneumonia and bronchitis
- *C pneumoniae* causes approximately 10% of community-acquired pneumonias
- *C pneumoniae* is second only to *Mycoplasma* as an agent of atypical pneumonia
- *C pneumoniae* has been associated seroepidemiologically with coronary artery disease

CLINICAL FINDINGS

- The clinical presentation is that of an atypical pneumonia

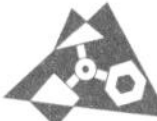

DIAGNOSIS

- Microimmunofluorescence or complement fixation test of acute and convalescent sera

TREATMENT

- Doxycycline, 100 mg BID for 10–14 days
- Azithromycin, 500 mg once on day 1, then 250 mg QD for 4 days more
- Levofloxacin, 500 mg QD for 10–14 days

Author(s)

Henry F. Chambers, MD

Pneumonia, Eosinophilic

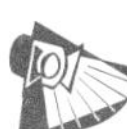

KEY FEATURES

- One of a diverse group of eosinophilic pulmonary syndromes

CLINICAL FINDINGS

- Fever, night sweats, weight loss, and dyspnea
- Pulmonary infiltrates on chest x-ray are invariably peripheral
- Peripheral eosinophilia

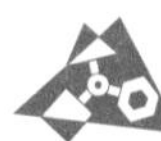

DIAGNOSIS

- Chest x-ray with peripheral airspace and interstitial infiltrates
- Peripheral eosinophilia
- Bronchoalveolar lavage to document eosinophils in the lung and exclude other causes
- Lung biopsy may be required

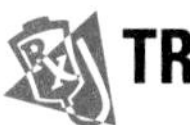

TREATMENT

- Oral prednisone (1 mg/kg/day) for 1–2 weeks and tapered over many months usually results in dramatic improvement
- Most patients require 10–15 mg prednisone every other day for 1 year or longer to prevent relapses

Author(s)

Mark S. Chesnutt, MD

Thomas J. Prendergast, MD

Pneumonia, Usual Interstitial

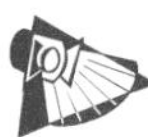

KEY FEATURES

- Clinical presentation is similar to that of other idiopathic fibrosing interstitial pneumonias
- Median survival is approximately 3 years

CLINICAL FINDINGS

- Age 55–60 with slight male predominance
- Insidious dry cough with months to years of exertional dyspnea
- Clubbing is present at diagnosis in 25–50%
- Pulmonary function tests: restriction and decreased diffusion capacity
- ANA and RF are positive in 25% of patients without documented collagen vascular disease

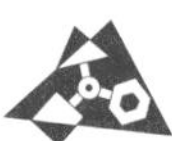

DIAGNOSIS

- Chest x-ray findings: decreased lung volumes with linear or reticular bibasilar or subpleural opacities
- HRCT shows minimal ground-glass and variable honeycomb change
- Normal chest x-ray findings in 2–10% at diagnosis
- Biopsy shows nonuniform distribution of fibrosis, with loss of type I pneumocytes and proliferation of alveolar type II cells
- Usual interstitial pneumonia can be diagnosed with 90% confidence in patients older than 65 with classic features, avoiding biopsy

TREATMENT

- No randomized study has demonstrated a benefit to any treatment
- Response to corticosteroids and cytotoxic agents is 15% at best

Author(s)

Mark S. Chesnutt, MD

Thomas J. Prendergast, MD

Pneumonitis, Acute Interstitial

KEY FEATURES

- Known clinically as Hamman-Rich syndrome

CLINICAL FINDINGS

- Wide age range, including many young patients
- Acute onset of dyspnea followed by rapid development of respiratory failure
- Preceding viral syndrome is reported by 50% of patients
- Clinical course is indistinguishable from idiopathic ARDS

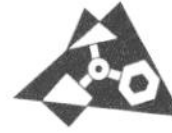

DIAGNOSIS

- X-ray film shows diffuse bilateral airspace consolidation
- Areas of ground-glass attenuation are seen on HRCT
- Biopsy resembles the organizing phase of diffuse alveolar damage, with fibrosis and minimal collagen deposition
- Pathologically similar to usual interstitial pneumonitis but more homogeneous, and honeycombing is typically absent

TREATMENT

- Supportive care including mechanical ventilation is critical
- Benefit of specific therapies is unclear
- 50–90% of patients die within 2 months
- Course is not progressive if patient survives
- Lung function may be permanently impaired in survivors

Author(s)

Mark S. Chesnutt, MD

Thomas J. Prendergast, MD

Pneumonitis, Nonspecific Interstitial

KEY FEATURES

- Clinical presentation and features are similar to usual interstitial pneumonia (UIP) but with distinct pathologic findings and better prognosis
- The median survival is >10 years

CLINICAL FINDINGS

- Age 45–55 with slight female predominance
- Onset of dyspnea and cough over months; otherwise, presentation is similar to that of UIP

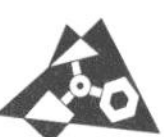

DIAGNOSIS

- Radiographically, may be indistinguishable from UIP
- The most typical HRCT finding is bilateral areas of ground-glass attenuation and fibrosis with rare honeycombing
- Biopsy shows varying degrees of patchy inflammation and fibrosis, which are uniform in time. Honeycombing is scant
- See Tables 28 and 29

TREATMENT

- Corticosteroids are thought to be effective, but no prospective clinical studies have been published
- Prognosis is good overall, but it depends on the degree of fibrosis at diagnosis

Author(s)

Mark S. Chesnutt, MD

Thomas J. Prendergast, MD

Pneumonitis, Radiation

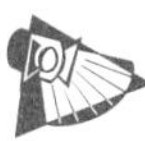

KEY FEATURES

- Usually presents 2–3 months after completion of radiation therapy
- Radiographic findings correlate poorly with symptoms
- Resolution typically occurs after 2–3 weeks; death from ARDS is unusual

CLINICAL FINDINGS

- Insidious onset of dyspnea, dry cough, chest fullness or pain, weakness, and fever
- Inspiratory crackles may be heard
- In severe disease, respiratory distress and cyanosis may be present
- Leukocytosis and elevated ESR are common

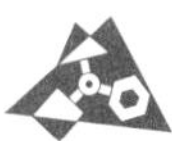

DIAGNOSIS

- Chest x-ray usually shows alveolar or nodular infiltrate limited to the irradiated area; air bronchograms are common
- Pulmonary function tests: reduced volumes, compliance, and diffusion capacity
- Hypoxemia

TREATMENT

- Aspirin, cough suppression, and bed rest
- Corticosteroids have not been proved effective, but prednisone (1 mg/kg/day PO) is usually given for 1 week, reduced to 20–40 mg/day for several weeks before a slow taper

Author(s)

Mark S. Chesnutt, MD

Thomas J. Prendergast, MD

Poliomyelitis

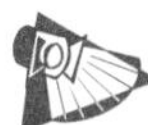

KEY FEATURES

- Enteroviral infection (three serotypes) of lower motor neurons
- Infection transmitted by fecal-oral route
- Rare in the developed world
- Targeted for global eradication by the World Health Organization

CLINICAL FINDINGS

- Fever, headache, stiff neck
- Lower motor neuron lesions lead to weakness, decreased deep tendon reflexes, muscle wasting
- 95% of infected patients are asymptomatic; the remainder have 1 of 3 grades:
  - Minor (abortive) polio: fever, headache, diarrhea, sore throat
  - Nonparalytic polio: fever, headache, meningitis, and muscle spasms without paralysis
  - Paralytic polio (rare, 0.1%): Paralysis occurs any time during febrile period. Can be further subdivided into spinal polio, in which paralysis mainly affects muscles innervated by spinal nerves, and bulbar polio, which affects muscles supplied by the cranial nerves

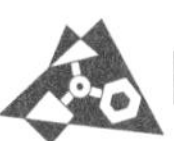

DIAGNOSIS

- Diagnosis rarely made; majority of patients are asymptomatic
- CSF lymphocytosis
- Characteristic clinical symptoms and viral recovery from stools or neutralizing antibodies clinch the diagnosis

TREATMENT

- Supportive measures, including bed rest and careful monitoring for bulbar symptoms
- Prevention: inactive parenteral vaccine has replaced oral vaccine in developed world
- Adults not at high risk are not routinely vaccinated
- To avoid precipitation of paralysis, IM injections should be avoided for 1 mo after vaccination

Author(s)

Wayne X. Shandera, MD

Ana Moran, MD

Polychondritis, Relapsing

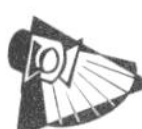

KEY FEATURES

- Inflammatory destructive lesions of cartilaginous structures, principally the ears, nose, trachea, larynx, and chest wall cartilage
- Associated conditions include
  - Systemic lupus erythematosus
  - Rheumatoid arthritis
  - Hashimoto's thyroiditis
  - Cancer (especially multiple myeloma)

CLINICAL FINDINGS

- The cartilage is painful, swollen, and tender during an attack
- Subsequently becomes atrophic, resulting in permanent deformity
- Noncartilaginous manifestations of the disease include fever, episcleritis, uveitis, deafness, aortic insufficiency, and rarely glomerulonephritis
- In 85% of patients, a migratory, asymmetric, and seronegative arthropathy occurs, affecting both large and small joints and the costochondral junctions

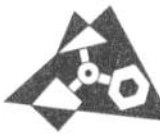

DIAGNOSIS

- Clinical
- Differential diagnosis
  - Other causes of ear deformity (skin cancer, cauliflower ear [cartilage dissolution posttrauma], chondritis or perichondritis, chondrodermatitis nodularis helicis)
  - Other causes of nose deformity (syphilis, rhinophyma [rosacea], Hansen's disease [leprosy], Wegener's granulomatosis)

TREATMENT

- Prednisone, 0.5–1 mg/kg/day, is often effective
- Dapsone, 100–200 mg/day, may also be effective, sparing the need for long-term high-dose corticosteroid treatment

Author(s)

David B. Hellmann, MD, FACP

John H. Stone, MD, MPH

Polycystic Kidney Disease

KEY FEATURES

- Common hereditary disease, affecting 1:1000 to 1:400 individuals in US
- 50% develop end-stage renal disease by age 60
- 10% of dialysis patients
- Variable penetrance
- At least 2 genes in disorder: *ADPKD1* on the short arm of chromosome 16 (86% of patients) and *ADPKD2* on chromosome 4
- Family history positive in 75%

CLINICAL FINDINGS

- Abdominal or flank pain caused by infection, bleeding into cysts, nephrolithiasis, rupture of cyst, urinary tract infection, renal cell carcinoma
- Fever caused by infection
- Nephrolithiasis, primarily calcium oxalate stones, in up to 20%
- Hypertension in 50%
- Abdominal mass
- Arterial aneurysms in the circle of Willis in 10–15%
- Mitral valve prolapse in up to 25%
- Aortic aneurysms
- Aortic valve abnormalities

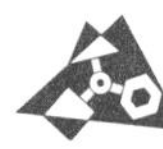

DIAGNOSIS

- Renal ultrasonogram: diagnostic depending on age and number of cysts
- Urinalysis: may be normal because cysts do not communicate directly with the urinary tract, but blood cultures may be positive
- CT scan: infected cyst has increased wall thickness
- Cerebral arteriography screening: not recommended unless family history of aneurysms or patient undergoing elective surgery prone to cause hypertension

TREATMENT

- Cyst rupture
  - Bed rest
  - Analgesics, not nonsteroidal anti-inflammatory drugs
- Cyst pain: decompression
- Cyst infection:
  - Antibiotics: fluoroquinolones, trimethoprim-sulfamethoxazole, and chloramphenicol IV for 2 weeks followed by long-term PO therapy
- Hydration (2–3 L/day)
- Antihypertensive agents, but diuretics used cautiously because effect on renal cyst formation is unknown

Author(s)

Suzanne Watnick, MD

Gail Morrison, MD

Polyneuropathy, Chronic Inflammatory

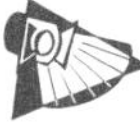

KEY FEATURES

- Clinically similar to Guillain-Barré syndrome but with relapsing or progressive course over months or years
- In the relapsing form, partial recovery may occur after relapses, or no recovery between exacerbations
- Remission may occur spontaneously, but frequently is progression to severe functional disability
- Usually ascending, symmetric weakness
- Paresthesias more variable

CLINICAL FINDINGS

- A symmetric sensory, motor, or mixed deficit, which may be most marked distally or proximally
- See Guillain-Barré Syndrome

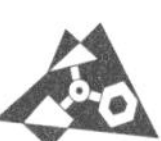

DIAGNOSIS

- Electrodiagnostic studies: marked slowing of motor and sensory conduction and focal conduction block. Signs of partial denervation may be present owing to secondary axonal degeneration
- Nerve biopsy may show chronic perivascular inflammatory infiltrates in endoneurium and epineurium without accompanying evidence of vasculitis, but normal nerve biopsy or the presence of nonspecific abnormalities does not exclude the diagnosis

TREATMENT

- Prednisone, 60 mg PO QD for 2–3 mo
- If no response has occurred despite 3 mo of treatment, a higher dose may be tried. In responsive cases, the dose is gradually tapered, but most patients become corticosteroid dependent, often requiring prednisone, 20 mg on alternate days, on a long-term basis
- Patients unresponsive to corticosteroids may benefit from a cytotoxic drug such as azathioprine
- Short-term benefit with plasmapheresis may occur

- High-dose intravenous immunoglobulin treatment (eg, 400 mg/kg/day) may produce clinical improvement lasting for weeks to months

Author(s)

Michael J. Aminoff, MD, DSc, FRCP

Pompholyx (Dyshidrotic Eczema)

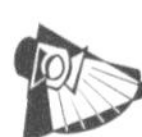 KEY FEATURES

- "Tapioca" vesicles of 1–2 mm on the palms, soles, and sides of fingers, associated with pruritus
- Scaling and fissuring may follow drying of the blisters
- Patients often have an atopic background and report flares with stress
- Patients with widespread dermatitis due to any cause may develop pompholyx-like eruptions as a part of an autoeczematization response

 CLINICAL FINDINGS

- Table 7

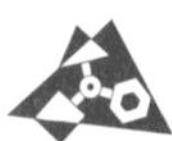 DIAGNOSIS

- KOH examination will reveal hyphae in cases of bullous tinea, which may be confused with pompholyx
- Differential diagnosis
  - Vesicular tinea
  - Contact dermatitis
  - Tinea pedis with dermatophytid reaction of palms
  - Scabies
  - Use of nonsteroidal anti-inflammatory drugs

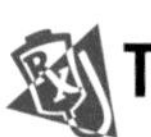 TREATMENT

- See Table 6
- Systemic corticosteroids should be avoided in this chronic condition
- A high-potency topical corticosteroid used early in the attack may help abort the flare and ameliorate pruritus
- PUVA
- Avoid anything that irritates the skin; patients should wear cotton gloves inside vinyl gloves when doing dishes or other wet chores, use long-handled brushes instead of sponges, and use a hand cream after washing the hands

Author(s)

Timothy G. Berger, MD

Popliteal Aneurysm

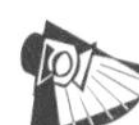 KEY FEATURES

- 85% of all peripheral artery aneurysms

 CLINICAL FINDINGS

- Symptoms caused by arterial thrombosis, peripheral embolization, or compression of adjacent structures with resultant venous thrombosis or neuropathy; rarely caused by rupture
- Arterial thrombosis leads to amputation in up to 30% of patients

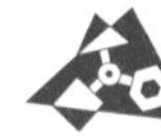 DIAGNOSIS

- Ultrasonogram diagnostic to measure the diameter of the aneurysm and rule out aortic abdominal aneurysms
- MRA or conventional arteriography required before operative repair

 TREATMENT

- Surgery recommended for all asymptomatic aneurysms > 2 cm and all symptomatic aneurysms regardless of size
- Catheter-directed thrombolysis can be attempted if no patent distal vessels for bypass
- Saphenous vein bypass graft with proximal and distal ligation of the aneurysm if patent outflow vessel is identified for bypass
- Resection of the aneurysm in addition to grafting is required for large aneurysms producing popliteal vein or nerve compression

Author(s)

Louis M. Messina, MD

Popliteal Artery Occlusion

 KEY FEATURES

- Causes atheroocclusive disease; popliteal aneurysm thrombosis, entrapment syndrome, adventitial cystic disease; trauma; extrinsic compression by Baker's cyst

Popliteal entrapment syndrome

- From anatomic anomalies, leading to arterial compression in popliteal space
- 4 types: abnormal course of popliteal artery, medial insertion of gastrocnemius muscle medial head, and abnormal accessory slip of gastrocnemius or popliteus muscles

Popliteal adventitial disease

- Formation of cysts in popliteal artery wall; arterial lumen compressed, causing stenosis, occlusion
- Affects healthy men 40–50 yr

 CLINICAL FINDINGS

- Absent popliteal pulses with ABI < 1.0
- Claudication, rest pain
- Bilateral disease
- Claudication symptoms may be atypical

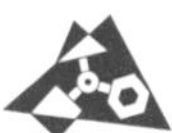 DIAGNOSIS

- MRA, positional angiography
- Bilateral multifocal lesions: atheroocclusive disease
- With entrapment, patent artery impinged with passive dorsiflexion or active plantar flexion of ankle
- Ultrasonography to diagnose large adventitial and Baker's cysts
- Most adventitial cysts are small, appear as thickening of popliteal artery wall on MRA
- Conventional angiogram for knee dislocation and abnormal pulse exam or ABI

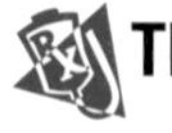 TREATMENT

- Angioplasty for short-segment atheroocclusive disease
- Bypass surgery for severe arterial insufficiency secondary to atheroocclusive disease
- Entrapment: surgical transection of abnormal muscle or short-segment bypass with greater or lesser saphenous vein if artery occluded

- Ultrasonogram-guided aspiration of adventitial cysts, which frequently recur
- Interposition bypass graft curative

Author(s)

Louis M. Messina, MD

Porphyria Cutanea Tarda

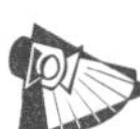 KEY FEATURES

- Noninflammatory blisters on sun-exposed sites, especially the dorsal hands
- Hypertrichosis, skin fragility
- Associated liver disease
- Elevated urine porphyrins
- The disease is associated with ingestion of certain medications (eg, estrogens), and liver disease from alcoholism or hepatitis C

 CLINICAL FINDINGS

- Table 7

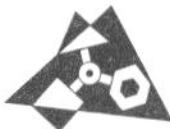 DIAGNOSIS

- Urinary uroporphyrins are elevated two- to five-fold above coproporphyrins
- There may be abnormal liver function tests, evidence of hepatitis C infection, increased liver iron stores, and hemochromatosis gene mutations
- Differential diagnosis
  - Pseudoporphyria: dialysis, medications (tetracycline, nonsteroidal anti-inflammatory drugs)
  - Contact dermatitis
  - Scabies

TREATMENT

- Phlebotomy without oral iron supplementation at a rate of 1 unit every 2–4 weeks will gradually lead to improvement
- 200 mg of hydroxychloroquine twice weekly will increase the excretion of porphyrins, improving the skin disease
- Stopping all triggering medications and stopping alcohol consumption may lead to improvement
- Most patients improve with treatment
- Sunscreens are ineffective, and barrier sun protection with clothing is required for prevention

Author(s)

Timothy G. Berger, MD

Postherpetic Neuralgia

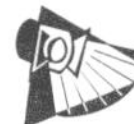 KEY FEATURES

- Past history of herpes zoster (shingles)
- Occurrence of pain for months or years in the same dermatomal distribution as was affected by the herpes zoster
- The zoster vaccine markedly reduces morbidity from herpes zoster and post-herpetic neuralgia among older adults

 CLINICAL FINDINGS

- Severe pain, sometimes burning or tingling and quite disabling, occurs in areas of prior shingles

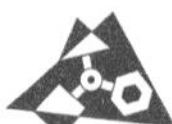 DIAGNOSIS

- A history of shingles and the presence of cutaneous scarring resulting from shingles aid in the diagnosis

 TREATMENT

- Management of the established complication is essentially medical
- If simple analgesics fail to help, a trial of a tricyclic drug (eg, amitriptyline, up to 100–150 mg/day) in conjunction with a phenothiazine (eg, perphenazine, 2–8 mg/day) is often effective
- Other patients respond to carbamazepine (up to 1200 mg/day), phenytoin (300 mg/day), or gabapentin (up to 3600 mg/day)
- Topical application of capsaicin cream (eg, Zostrix, 0.025%) or 5% lidocaine may also be helpful

Author(s)

Michael J. Aminoff, MD, DSc, FRCP

Pregnancy, Third-Trimester Bleeding

 KEY FEATURES

- Vaginal bleeding occurs in 5–10% of women in late pregnancy

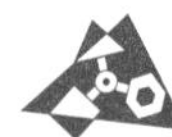 CLINICAL FINDINGS

- Painless vaginal bleeding is characteristic of placenta previa
- Strong uterine contractions, continuous pain, and tenderness are more often associated with abruptio placentae

DIAGNOSIS

- Placental causes must be differentiated from nonplacental causes
- Complete blood count should be ordered, with blood typed and cross-matched
- Coagulation studies may be indicated
- Ultrasonography can determine placental location
- Speculum and digital pelvic exams are avoided until placenta previa is excluded
- Amniocentesis may be performed to assess for fetal lung maturity in patients < 36 weeks' gestational age

 TREATMENT

- Approach should be conservative and expectant unless fetal distress or risk of severe maternal hemorrhage occurs
- Patients should be hospitalized and placed on bed rest with fetal monitoring
- Hospitalization and bed rest are continued if the patient is < 36 weeks' gestation
- Home management may be considered in selected patients
- Betamethasone, 12 mg IM × 2 12–24 h apart, is indicated if fetal lung immaturity is present

Author(s)

William R. Crombleholme, MD

Pregnancy, Thyroid Disease

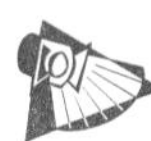

KEY FEATURES

- **Thyrotoxicosis**
  - May result in fetal anomalies, late abortion, or preterm labor and fetal hyperthyroidism with goiter
  - Thyroid storm in late pregnancy or labor is a life-threatening emergency
  - Keep free T_4 in the high-normal range during pregnancy
- **Recurrent postpartum thyroiditis**
  - A hyperthyroid state of 1–3-mo duration followed by hypothyroidism
  - Occurs 3–6 mo after delivery
  - Spontaneous recovery occurs in 90% after 3–6 mo
- **Maternal hypothyroidism**
  - Even subclinical elevation of TSH may impact neuropsychological fetal development
  - Check TSH level at the first prenatal visit in suspected hypothyroidism

CLINICAL FINDINGS

- Presentation is similar to that of the nonpregnant state. In first trimester persistent nausea, vomiting, and weight loss could be misdiagnosed as hyperemesis gravidarum

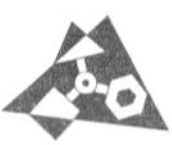

DIAGNOSIS

- Total T_4 and total T_3 normally elevated in pregnancy; free T_4 and free T_3 unchanged. Suppressed TSH can occur in up to 10% of normal pregnancy
- Thyroperoxidase antibodies and thyroglobulin antibodies are present in recurrent postpartum thyroiditis

TREATMENT

- Treat thyrotoxicosis with propylthiouracil. The initial dose is 100–150 mg PO TID QD. A maintenance dose of 100 mg/day minimizes the chance of fetal hypothyroidism
- Treat maternal hypothyroidism with T_4 to maintain normal TSH

Author(s)

William R. Crombleholme, MD

Prion Diseases

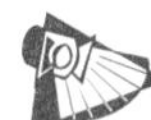

KEY FEATURES

- Proteinaceous infectious particles
- Transmissible agents that cause conversion of brain protein to abnormal isoform
- Cause disease in both humans (Creutzfeldt-Jakob) and animals (scrapie)
- Disease in human has sporadic, familial, iatrogenic, and new-variant forms

CLINICAL FINDINGS

- Classic Creutzfeldt-Jakob disease (CJD) occurs in late middle age
- Rapidly progressive dementia, myoclonic fasciculations, and ataxia
- New variant form occurs in younger individuals and is associated with consumption of infected beef
- New variant with longer duration, more psychiatric and cerebellar symptoms versus classic form

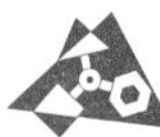

DIAGNOSIS

- Combination of clinical findings, characteristic EEG, and MRI
- CSF can be analyzed for tau and 14-3-3 protein

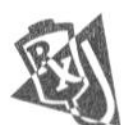

TREATMENT

- No specific therapy available
- Disinfection of neurosurgical equipment key for prevention of iatrogenic transmission

Author(s)

Wayne X. Shandera, MD

Ana Moran, MD

Prostatitis, Chronic Bacterial

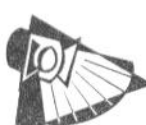

KEY FEATURES

- Irritative voiding symptoms
- Perineal or suprapubic discomfort, often dull and poorly localized
- Positive expressed prostatic secretions and culture
- Although chronic bacterial prostatitis may evolve from acute bacterial prostatitis, many men have no history of acute infection
- Most common: gram-negative rods
- Less common: *Enterococcus*

CLINICAL FINDINGS

- Variable; some patients are asymptomatic; most have irritative voiding symptoms, low back and perineal pain
- Many report a history of urinary tract infections
- Physical examination often unremarkable; prostate may feel normal, boggy, or indurated

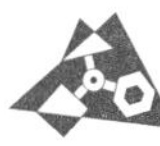

DIAGNOSIS

- Culture secretions or postprostatic massage urine specimen
- Urinalysis: normal unless a secondary cystitis is present
- Expressed prostatic secretions: > 10 leukocytes/hpf, especially lipid-laden macrophages
- Differential diagnosis
  - Chronic urethritis
  - Cystitis
  - Perianal disease

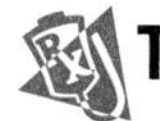

TREATMENT

- Anti-inflammatory agents (indomethacin, ibuprofen)
- Quinolones, trimethoprim-sulfamethoxazole, carbenicillin, erythromycin, or cephalexin, for 6–12 weeks
- Regimens
  - Ciprofloxacin, 250–500 mg PO Q 12 h for 1–3 months
  - Ofloxacin, 200–400 mg PO Q 12 h for 1–3 months
  - Trimethoprim-sulfamethoxazole, 160/800 mg PO Q 12 h for 1–3 months (increasing resistance noted [up to 20%])
- Hot sitz baths

- Relax pelvic floor with micturition
- Difficult to cure
- Symptoms and recurrent urinary tract infections can be controlled by suppressive antibiotic therapy

Author(s)

Marshall L. Stoller, MD

Peter R. Carroll, MD

Prostatodynia

KEY FEATURES

- Prostatodynia is a noninflammatory disorder that affects young and middle-aged men and has variable causes, including voiding dysfunction and over facilitated pelvic floor musculature

CLINICAL FINDINGS

- Variable, no history of urinary tract infections; hesitancy and interruption of flow; lifelong history of voiding difficulty
- Physical examination is unremarkable, except increased anal sphincter tone and periprostatic tenderness may be observed

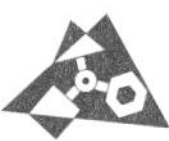

DIAGNOSIS

- Urinalysis: normal
- Expressed prostatic secretions: normal numbers of leukocytes
- Urodynamic testing: dysfunctional voiding (detrusor contraction without urethral relaxation, high urethral pressures, spasms of the urinary sphincter); indicated in patients failing empiric trials of α-blockers or anticholinergics
- Differential diagnosis
  - Acute cystitis, other prostatitis syndromes
  - Acute bacterial prostatitis
  - Chronic bacterial prostatitis
  - Nonbacterial prostatitis

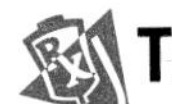

TREATMENT

- α-Blocking agents: terazosin, 1–10 mg PO QD; or doxazosin, 1–8 mg PO QD
- Anticholinergics
- Diazepam
- Biofeedback techniques
- Sitz baths
- Prognosis is variable depending on the specific cause

Author(s)

Marshall L. Stoller, MD

Peter R. Carroll, MD

Pruritus

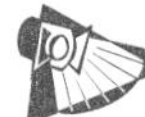

KEY FEATURES

- Causes of generalized pruritus
  - Dry skin—whether naturally occurring and aggravated by climatic conditions or arising from disease states
  - Scabies, dermatitis herpetiformis, atopic dermatitis, pruritus vulvae et ani, miliaria, insect bites, pediculosis, contact dermatitis, drug reactions, urticaria, urticarial eruptions of pregnancy, psoriasis, lichen planus, lichen simplex chronicus, exfoliative dermatitis, folliculitis, bullous pemphigoid, fiberglass dermatitis
- Persistent pruritus not explained by cutaneous disease should prompt a staged workup for systemic causes
- Other causes: endocrine disorders such as hypo- or hyperthyroidism, psychiatric disturbances, lymphoma, leukemia, iron deficiency anemia, certain neurological disorders

CLINICAL FINDINGS

- Bilirubin may be normal in patients with hepatic pruritus, and the severity of the liver disease may not correlate with the degree of itching
- Burning or itching involving the face, scalp, and genitalia may be manifestations of primary depression and is treatable with drugs such as tricyclics (amitriptyline, imipramine, doxepin), SSRIs, and other antidepressants

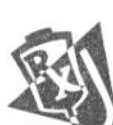

TREATMENT

- Naltrexone and nalmefene relieve the pruritus of liver disease
- Uremia in conjunction with hemodialysis and the pruritus of obstructive biliary disease may be helped by phototherapy with ultraviolet B or PUVA
- Idiopathic pruritus and pruritus accompanying serious internal disease may not respond to any type of therapy
- Pruritus accompanying specific skin disease will subside when the disease is controlled

Author(s)

Timothy G. Berger, MD

Pseudoallergic Reactions

KEY FEATURES

- Resemble immediate hypersensitivity reactions but are not mediated by allergen-IgE interaction; instead, direct mast cell activation occurs
- Examples of pseudoallergic or "anaphylactoid" reactions are the "red man syndrome" from rapid infusion of vancomycin, direct mast cell activation by opioids, and radiocontrast reactions
- If a patient has had an anaphylactoid reaction to conventional radiocontrast media, the risk for a second reaction on reexposure may be as high as 30%
- Unlike IgE-mediated reactions, these can often be prevented by prophylactic medical regimens

CLINICAL FINDINGS

- Mimics allergic reactions, from urticaria/angioedema to anaphylaxis

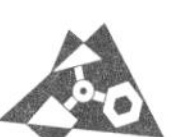

DIAGNOSIS

- Clinical

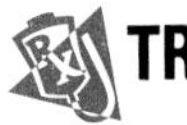

TREATMENT

- Slow (vancomycin infusion) or stop (radiocontrast) exposure
- Antihistamines, bronchodilators, and steroids
- Prevention: low-osmolality contrast preparations
- Prevention: prophylactic administration of prednisone (50 mg PO Q 6 h beginning 18 h before contrast) and diphenhydramine (25–50 mg IM 60 min before the contrast)
- The use of the lower-osmolality radiocontrast media in combination with the pretreatment regimen decreases the incidence of reactions to less than 1%

Author(s)

Jeffrey L. Kishiyama, MD

Daniel C. Adelman, MD

Pseudogout & Chondrocalcinosis

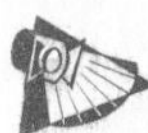

KEY FEATURES

- Also known as calcium pyrophosphate dihydrate deposition disease (CPPD)
- Chondrocalcinosis is the presence of calcium-containing salts in articular cartilage
- May be familial and is associated with hemochromatosis, hyperparathyroidism, ochronosis, diabetes mellitus, true gout, hypothyroidism, Wilson's disease
- Usually seen in individuals 60 yr and older
- Pseudogout attacks of the knee especially common 1–2 days after general surgery

CLINICAL FINDINGS

- CPPD can be asymptomatic, cause recurrent, acute attacks of monoarthritis (pseudogout), or result in chronic arthritis resembling either osteoarthritis or rheumatoid arthritis
- Pseudogout, like gout, frequently develops 24–48 h after major surgery
- CPPD with osteoarthritic changes of second and third metacarpophalangeals suggests hemochromatosis

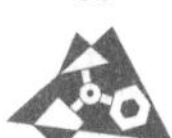

DIAGNOSIS

- Identification of calcium pyrophosphate crystals in joint aspirates is diagnostic
- Rhomboid-shaped pseudogout crystals are blue when parallel and yellow when perpendicular to the axis of the compensator with polarized light microscopy. Needle-shaped gout crystals give the opposite color pattern
- X-ray examination shows not only calcification (usually symmetric) of cartilaginous structures but also signs of osteoarthritis
- Normal serum urate levels

TREATMENT

- Treatment is directed at the primary disease, if present
- NSAIDs are used for acute episodes. Colchicine is sometimes used for prophylaxis but is generally ineffective for acute episodes
- Intra-articular injection of triamcinolone, 10–40 mg

Author(s)

David B. Hellmann, MD, FACP

John H. Stone, MD, MPH

Pulmonary Alveolar Proteinosis

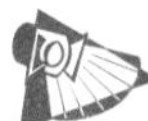

KEY FEATURES

- Phospholipid accumulation within alveolar spaces
- May be primary (idiopathic) or secondary to immune deficiency, hematologic malignancies, or inhalation of mineral dusts, or may occur after lung infections

CLINICAL FINDINGS

- Progressive dyspnea
- Chest x-ray shows bilateral pulmonary infiltrates suggestive of edema
- Spontaneous remission occurs in some; others develop progressive respiratory insufficiency
- Pulmonary infection with *Nocardia* or fungi may occur

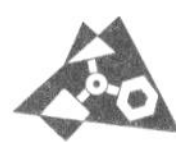

DIAGNOSIS

- Based on characteristic findings on alveolar lavage, a milky appearance, and periodic acid–Schiff–positive lipoproteinaceous material, with typical clinical and radiographic features
- Biopsy is necessary in some cases

TREATMENT

- Therapy consists of periodic whole-lung lavage

Author(s)

Mark S. Chesnutt, MD

Thomas J. Prendergast, MD

Pulmonary Edema, Acute

KEY FINDINGS

- Acute onset or worsening of dyspnea at rest
- Tachycardia, diaphoresis, cyanosis
- Pulmonary rales, rhonchi, expiratory wheezes
- CXR shows interstitial and alveolar edema with or without cardiomegaly
- Arterial hypoxemia
- Cardiac causes include acute myocardial infarction (MI) or ischemia, congestive heart failure (CHF), valvular regurgitation, and mitral stenosis
- Noncardiac causes include IV narcotics, increased intracerebral pressure, high altitude, sepsis, medications, inhaled toxins, transfusion reactions, shock, and disseminated intravascular coagulation

CLINICAL FINDINGS

- Severe dyspnea; pink, frothy sputum; diaphoresis; and cyanosis
- Rales, wheezing, or rhonchi in all lung fields
- Sudden onset in acute exacerbations of CHF or acute MI

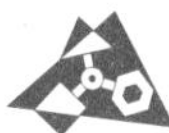

DIAGNOSIS

- Characteristic clinical findings
- CXR: pulmonary vascular congestion, increased interstitial markings, and butterfly pattern of alveolar edema; heart enlarged or normal in size
- Echocardiography: assesses ejection fraction, atrial pressure
- Pulmonary capillary wedge pressure: always elevated (usually > 25 mm Hg) in cardiogenic pulmonary edema, normal or even low in noncardiogenic pulmonary edema

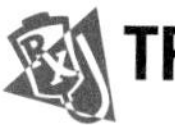

TREATMENT

- Place patient in a sitting position with legs dangling over the side of the bed
- Give oxygen by mask for Pa_{O_2} < 60 mm Hg
- Noninvasive pressure support ventilation or endotracheal intubation and mechanical ventilation for respiratory distress
- Morphine, 4–8 mg IV or SC, repeated PRN after 2–4 h (avoid in patients with narcotic-induced and neurogenic pulmonary edema)

- Diuretic IV (Table 46)
- Nitroglycerin SL, PO, or IV
- Inhaled β-adrenergic agonists or IV aminophylline for bronchospasm
- Parenteral vasodilator (eg, nitroprusside IV) for elevated arterial pressure
- Positive inotropic agents in low-output states, hypotension

Author(s)

Thomas M. Bashore, MD

Christopher B. Granger, MD

Pulmonary Hemosiderosis, Idiopathic

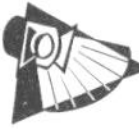 KEY FEATURES

- Recurrent pulmonary hemorrhage with hemoptysis
- Usually in children or young adults
- No known underlying cause
- Multiple episodes can result in interstitial fibrosis and pulmonary failure

 CLINICAL FINDINGS

- Hemoptysis, recurrent
- Dyspnea
- Alveolar infiltrates on chest x-ray
- Anemia, often iron deficient

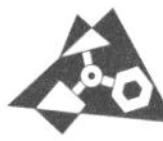 DIAGNOSIS

- Exclusion of other causes of alveolar hemorrhage
- Hemoptysis, dyspnea, cough
- Chest radiograph opacities
- Iron-deficiency anemia
- Hemosiderin-laden macrophages on bronchoalveolar lavage and lung biopsy specimens

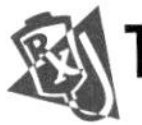 TREATMENT

- Corticosteroids may be useful for acute episodes

Author(s)

Mark S. Chesnutt, MD

Thomas J. Prendergast, MD

Pulmonary Hypertension, Primary

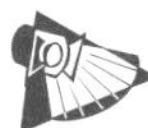 KEY FEATURES

- Elevated pulmonary vascular resistance and hypertension in the absence of other cardiac or pulmonary disease
- Pathological findings: diffuse narrowing of pulmonary arterioles
- The diet pills fenfluramine, dexfenfluramine, and phentermine may cause a picture indistinguishable from primary pulmonary hypertension

 CLINICAL FINDINGS

- Clinical findings are similar to pulmonary hypertension from other causes
- Characteristically occurs in young women
- Weakness and fatigue from right-sided heart failure, low cardiac output
- Edema, ascites, peripheral cyanosis, and effort-related syncope as right-sided heart failure advances

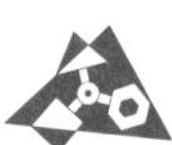 DIAGNOSIS

- ECG: right ventricular and atrial hypertrophy
- CXR: enlarged right ventricle, enlarged main pulmonary arteries with reduced peripheral branches
- Echocardiography, lung scanning, and (if necessary) pulmonary angiography are essential to exclude secondary causes

TREATMENT

- Death usually occurs in 2–8 yr
- Long-term anticoagulation is recommended by some experts
- Vasodilator drugs are controversial because of possible life-threatening systemic hypotension
- Nifedipine and diltiazem (Table 50) may be effective but only in early disease
- Epoprostenol (a potent pulmonary vasodilator) by continuous IV infusion may slow (but not halt) symptom progression in advanced disease
- Nitric oxide by inhalation is sometimes given for nonresponders to epoprostenol
- Bosentan (an oral endothelin antagonist) may become the treatment of choice for all stages of disease
- Heart–lung transplantation is definitive treatment

Author(s)

Thomas Bashore, MD

Christopher B. Granger, MD

Pulmonary Radiation Fibrosis

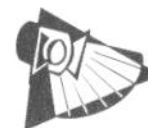 KEY FEATURES

- Typically seen in patients who receive a full course of radiation therapy for breast or lung cancer
- Pulmonary fibrosis develops after a 6- to 12-week period of well-being
- Fibrosis may occur without preceding pneumonitis

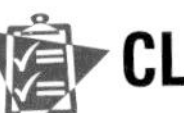 CLINICAL FINDINGS

- Most patients are asymptomatic; slowly progressive dyspnea may occur
- Cor pulmonale and chronic respiratory failure are rare

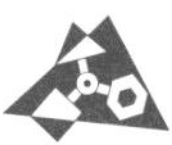 DIAGNOSIS

- Radiographic findings
  - Obliteration of normal lung markings
  - Dense interstitial and pleural fibrosis
  - Reduced lung volumes
  - Tenting of the diaphragm
  - Sharp delineation of radiation margins

 TREATMENT

- No specific therapy is effective; corticosteroids are of no value

Author(s)

Mark S. Chesnutt, MD

Thomas J. Prendergast, MD

Pulmonary Stenosis

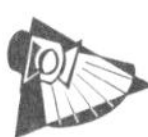

KEY FEATURES

- Increased resistance to right ventricular (RV) outflow, increased RV pressure, decreased pulmonary blood flow
- Often associated with other cardiac lesions
- Without shunting, arterial saturation normal, but severe stenosis causes peripheral cyanosis through decreased cardiac output
- Clubbing and polycythemia occur only with right-to-left shunting from patent foramen ovale or atrial septal defect

CLINICAL FINDINGS

- Mild: asymptomatic
- Moderate: asymptomatic early, with symptoms of dyspnea, syncope, and chest pain evolving in adulthood
- Severe: right-sided congestive heart failure and sudden death in the 20s and 30s
- Palpable parasternal lift
- Loud, harsh systolic ejection murmur and thrill in second left interspace, radiating to left shoulder
- P_2 delayed and soft or absent; ejection click, decreases with inspiration

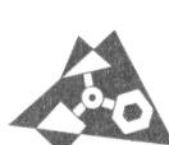

DIAGNOSIS

- ECG
  - Right axis deviation or RV hypertrophy
  - Peaked P waves
- Chest x-ray film
  - Heart size normal
  - RV and right atrium prominent
  - Pulmonary artery dilatation
- Echo-Doppler
  - Diagnostic
  - Can determine gradient across valve
  - Find subvalvular obstruction

TREATMENT

- Treatment indicated for symptomatic patients and those with RV hypertrophy and elevated pulmonary artery gradients > 50 mm Hg
- Treatment of choice: percutaneous balloon valvuloplasty
- Surgical commissurotomy or if valve is dysplastic, pulmonic valve replacement
- Surgery has excellent long-term results but a 2–4% operative mortality rate

Author(s)

Thomas M. Bashore, MD

Christopher B. Granger, MD

Pulmonary Veno-Occlusive Disease

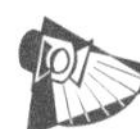

KEY FEATURES

- A rare cause of postcapillary pulmonary hypertension
- Occurs in children and young adults
- Characterized by progressive fibrotic occlusion of pulmonary veins and venules with secondary hypertensive changes in the pulmonary arteriolar bed

CLINICAL FINDINGS

- Difficult to recognize in early stages
- Progressive dyspnea
- Fatigue, exertional syncope
- Cardiac exam findings consistent with elevated right-sided pressures (see *Pulmonary Hypertension, Primary*)

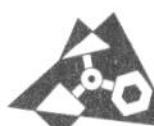

DIAGNOSIS

- Chest x-ray shows prominent symmetric interstitial markings, Kerley B lines, dilated pulmonary arteries, and normal left atrium and ventricle
- Premortem diagnosis is difficult but can be made with open-lung biopsy

TREATMENT

- No effective therapy; most patients die within 2 years

Author(s)

Mark S. Chesnutt, MD

Thomas J. Prendergast, MD

Q Fever

KEY FEATURES

- Caused by *Coxiella burnetii*, a rickettsia that infects cows, goats, and sheep
- Transmission to humans occurs by inhalation of dry feces, milk, or dust contaminated by them
- Typical incubation period is 7–21 days

CLINICAL FINDINGS

- Febrile illness with headache, myalgias, nonproductive cough
- Pneumonitis and granulomatous hepatitis commonly seen
- Endocarditis, usually of the aortic valve, can occur in chronic *Coxiella* infections
- Clinical course is variable, from acute to chronic and relapsing

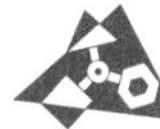

DIAGNOSIS

- Elevated liver enzymes
- Leukocytosis
- A rise in the complement-fixing antibody titer is diagnostic
- A serum enzyme-linked immunoassay is also available and helpful

TREATMENT

- Prevention: a vaccine is being developed for high-risk people who handle livestock or are laboratory workers
- Doxycycline and related medications are effective at treating most manifestations of the disease
- Endocarditis usually requires addition of a second agent, a sulfa, rifampin, or a fluoroquinolone, and therapy is usually needed for long periods, sometimes years
- In endocarditis, the rate of clinical failure with antibiotics is high, and surgical value replacement is often necessary

Author(s)

Wayne X. Shandera, MD

Ana Moran, MD

Rabies

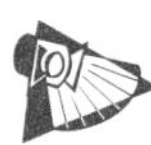

KEY FEATURES

- A rhabdovirus infection causing encephalitis, transmitted by infected saliva after an animal bite
- Bats, raccoons, skunks, foxes, and coyotes are most common vectors in the United States
- Human cases rare in the United States
- Incubation period of 3–7 weeks, proportional to distance from wound to CNS
- Usually fatal unless patients receive postexposure prophylaxis

CLINICAL FINDINGS

- Prodrome includes pain at site of bite, fever, nausea
- CNS symptoms begin about 10 days later with encephalitis or paralysis
- Encephalitis: delirium and extremely painful laryngeal spasms that lead to hydrophobia
- Paralysis: less common; ascending paralysis resembles Guillain-Barré syndrome
- Both encephalitic and paralytic forms progress to coma, autonomic dysfunction, death

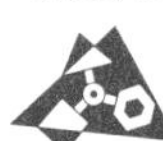

DIAGNOSIS

- History of animal bite, initial viral prodrome followed by CNS symptoms suggests diagnosis
- Diagnosis is confirmed with fluorescent antibody testing of the sacrificed animal brain
- Skin biopsy from the patient's posterior neck has ~80% sensitivity; PCR may play a role in future diagnosis

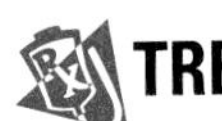

TREATMENT

- Animal bite wounds should not be sutured; local wound cleansing, debridement, and flushes are useful
- Treatment includes both passive antibody and vaccination
- When the disease is under serious consideration, use of postexposure immunization should be based on clinical guidelines, and on recommendations of local health officials
- Prevention: immunization of household dogs and avoidance of animals associated with rabies (bats, foxes, raccoons, skunks)

Author(s)

Wayne X. Shandera, MD

Ana Moran, MD

Radial Neuropathy

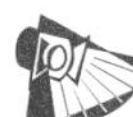

KEY FEATURES

- Radial nerve is particularly liable to compression or injury in the axilla (eg, by crutches or by pressure when the arm hangs over the back of a chair)
- The neuropathy may be asymptomatic, resolve rapidly and spontaneously, or become progressively more disabling

CLINICAL FINDINGS

- Percussion of the nerve at the site of the lesion may lead to paresthesias in its distal distribution
- Leads to weakness or paralysis of muscles supplied by the nerve, including the triceps, except in cases involving injury near the spiral groove in which the triceps is spared (Saturday night palsy)
- Sensory changes may also occur in a small area on the back of the hand between the thumb and index finger
- If injured at or above the elbow, its purely motor posterior interosseous branch, supplying the extensors of the wrist and fingers, may be involved immediately below the elbow, but there is sparing of the extensor carpi radialis longus, so that the wrist can still be extended
- The superficial radial nerve may be compressed by handcuffs or a tight watch strap

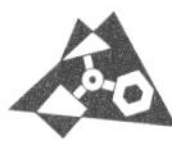

DIAGNOSIS

- Electromyography and nerve conduction studies help localize the focal lesion

TREATMENT

- If acute compression is the cause, then no treatment is needed in most cases
- If repetitive mechanical trauma is responsible, this is avoided by occupational adjustment

Author(s)

Michael J. Aminoff, MD, DSc, FRCP

Rash, Heat

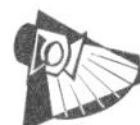

KEY FEATURES

- Burning
- Itching
- Superficial aggregated small vesicles, papules, or pustules on covered areas of the skin, usually the trunk
- More common in hot, moist climates

CLINICAL FINDINGS

- Table 7

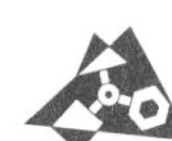

DIAGNOSIS

- Clinical
- Differential diagnosis
  - Folliculitis
  - Drug eruption

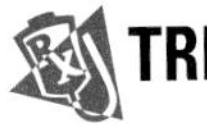

TREATMENT

- See Table 6
- Triamcinolone acetonide, 0.1% lotion or cream applied two to four times daily
- Can cause hyperthermia
- Refer if recommended therapy is ineffective

Author(s)

Timothy G. Berger, MD

Rat-Bite Fever

KEY FEATURES

- Rat-bite fever is an uncommon acute infectious disease caused by *Spirillum minus*. It is transmitted to humans by the bite of a rat
- Inhabitants of rat-infested slum dwellings and laboratory workers are at greatest risk

CLINICAL FINDINGS

- Rat bite heals promptly, but 1 to several weeks later the site becomes swollen, indurated, and painful; assumes a dusky purplish hue; and may ulcerate. Regional lymphangitis and lymphadenitis
- Fever, chills, malaise, myalgia, arthralgia, and headache
- Splenomegaly
- A sparse, dusky-red maculopapular rash on the trunk and extremities
- Arthritis
- After a few days, symptoms subside, only to reappear again in a few more days
- Relapsing fever for 3–4 days alternating with afebrile periods lasting 3–9 days; may persist for weeks

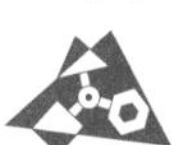

DIAGNOSIS

- Leukocytosis
- Nontreponemal test for syphilis often falsely positive
- Organism may be identified in dark-field examination of the ulcer exudate or an aspirated lymph node
- Differential diagnosis
  - Streptobacillary fever
  - Tularemia
  - Rickettsial disease (eg, Rocky Mountain spotted fever, epidemic typhus)
  - Ehrlichiosis
  - *Pasteurella multocida* infection
  - Relapsing fever

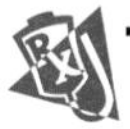

TREATMENT

- Procaine penicillin G, 600,000 units IM Q 12 h, or tetracycline hydrochloride, 0.5 g PO Q 6 h, for 10–14 days
- The usual mortality rate of about 10% can be markedly reduced by prompt diagnosis and antimicrobial treatment

Author(s)

Richard A. Jacobs, MD, PhD

Relapsing Fever

KEY FEATURES

- Caused by *Borrelia recurrentis*
- Endemic in many parts of the world
- Both tick-borne and louse-borne disease occur
- For tick-borne disease, main reservoir is rodents, which serve as the source of infection for ticks
- In the US, infected ticks are found throughout the west, especially in mountainous areas
- Clinical cases are uncommon in humans
- Tick-borne relapsing fever is not transmitted from person to person
- In louse-borne disease, when an infected person harbors lice, the lice become infected with *Borrelia*
- Large epidemics may occur

CLINICAL FINDINGS

- Abrupt onset of fever, chills, tachycardia, nausea and vomiting, arthralgia, and severe headache
- Hepatomegaly and splenomegaly, rashes
- Delirium, neurological and psychological abnormalities
- The attack terminates, usually abruptly, after 3–10 days
- After an interval of 1–2 weeks, relapse occurs, and 3–10 relapses may occur before recovery

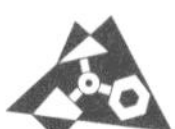

DIAGNOSIS

- During episodes of fever, large spirochetes can be seen in blood smears stained with Wright's or Giemsa stain. Organisms can be cultured in special media
- Anti-*Borrelia* antibodies develop during the illness
- The Weil-Felix test for rickettsioses, nontreponemal serologic tests for syphilis, and indirect fluorescent antibody and Western blot tests for *Borrelia burgdorferi* may be falsely positive
- Cerebrospinal fluid abnormalities occur in patients with meningeal involvement
- Mild anemia and thrombocytopenia are common
- Differential diagnosis: malaria, leptospirosis, meningococcemia, typhoid fever, yellow fever, epidemic typhus, rat-bite fever

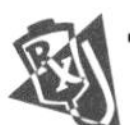

TREATMENT

- For louse-borne relapsing fever: tetracycline or erythromycin, 0.5 g PO once, or procaine penicillin G, 400,000–600,000 units IM once
- For tick-borne relapsing fever: tetracycline or erythromycin, 0.5 g PO QID for 5–10 days
- Jarisch-Herxheimer reactions occur commonly and may be life-threatening. Treatment with aspirin—but not hydrocortisone—may ameliorate this reaction.
- With treatment, the initial attack is shortened and relapses are largely prevented
- Overall mortality rate is ~5%
- Fatalities most common in old, debilitated, or very young patients
- Prevention of relapsing fever is by prevention of tick bites and delousing procedures

Author(s)

Richard A. Jacobs, MD, PhD

Renal Artery Aneurysm

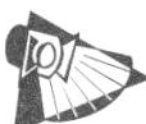 KEY FEATURES

- Incidence: ~1% of adults
- Many affected patients are asymptomatic
- Causes: medial degeneration, trauma, and injury after renal biopsy or percutaneous nephrolithostomy

 CLINICAL FINDINGS

- Most are asymptomatic
- Rupture is initial presentation in 5%
  - Hematuria/flank pain
  - Hypertension
  - Renal insufficiency

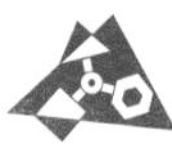 DIAGNOSIS

- CT scan
- Conventional angiography indicated if planning intervention

 TREATMENT

- Indications for treatment
  - Size > 2 cm
  - Local symptoms
  - Renovascular hypertension
  - Distal embolization
  - Growth on serial imaging
  - Occurrence in women of childbearing age
- Surgical treatment
  - Excision with interposition grafting
  - Infrequently, ex vivo reconstruction if aneurysm extends into branch vessels
- Interposition grafting of main renal arteries > 5 mm in diameter yields 5-year primary patency rate of ~70%
- Stent grafts for saccular aneurysms of main renal artery
- Endovascular embolization with microcoils for interlobar artery aneurysms

Author(s)

Louis M. Messina, MD

Respiratory Syncytial Virus

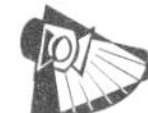 KEY FEATURES

- Annual outbreaks of pneumonia, bronchiolitis, and tracheobronchitis in the very young
- Premature infants with bronchopulmonary dysplasia are at highest risk
- Other risk factors
  - Male gender
  - Age < 6 months
  - Day care exposure
- Upper respiratory tract infection and tracheobronchitis in older children or adults

 CLINICAL FINDINGS

- Annual epidemics occur in winter and spring
- Average incubation period is 5 days. Inoculation may occur through the nose or the eyes
- In RSV bronchiolitis, proliferation and necrosis of bronchiolar epithelium develop, producing
  - Obstruction from sloughed epithelium and increased mucus secretion
  - Low-grade fever, tachypnea, and wheezes
  - Hyperinflated lungs, decreased gas exchange, and increased work of breathing
- Otitis media is a frequent complication, often with concomitant *Streptococcus pneumoniae* infection

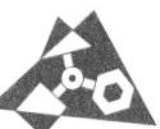 DIAGNOSIS

- Culture of nasopharyngeal secretions remains standard for diagnosis
- Rapid diagnosis possible by viral antigen identification in nasal washings using an ELISA or immunofluorescent assay

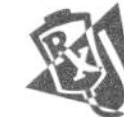 TREATMENT

- Hydration, humidification of inspired air, and ventilatory support as needed
- In non-high risk populations, although bronchodilating agents, ribavirin, and corticosteroids are widely used, evidence is lacking to support their effectiveness
- In immunocompromised adults, hyperimmune RSV immunoglobulin G (1500 mg/kg) is effective in combination with ribavirin
- Monoclonal RSV antibody, palivizumab, at 15 mg/kg, can be given prophylactically, parenterally at 15 mg/kg monthly for 6 months during the season of high transmission, to infants with high risk factors such as prematurity, bronchopulmonary dysplasia, and congenital heart disease

Author(s)

Wayne X. Shandera, MD

Ana Moran, MD

Retinal Detachment

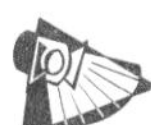

KEY FEATURES

- Retinal detachment is most commonly secondary to development of a tear in the retina, which is usually spontaneous but may be secondary to trauma
- Spontaneous detachment most common in patients age > 50
- Cataract extraction and myopia are the two most common predisposing conditions

CLINICAL FINDINGS

- Blurred vision in the involved eye, becoming progressively worse
- Often described as "a curtain coming down over the eye"
- Central vision remains intact until the macula becomes detached
- May be associated with "flashes" and "floaters"
- No pain or redness

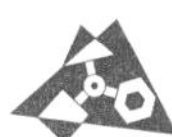

DIAGNOSIS

- On ophthalmoscopic examination, the retina may be seen hanging like a gray cloud

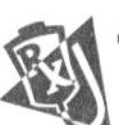

TREATMENT

- Immediate referral to ophthalmologist is critical
- During transportation, patient's head should be positioned so that the detached portion of the retina will fall back with the aid of gravity
- Surgical therapy involves closing the retinal tears by creating a permanent adhesion between the neurosensory retina, retinal pigment epithelium, and choroid
- Indentation of the sclera with a silicone sponge or buckle, drainage of subretinal fluid, surgical removal of the vitreous (vitrectomy), or injection of an expansile gas into the vitreous cavity may be required. (Expansile gas within the eye, which may persist for weeks, is a contraindication to air travel, mountaineering at high altitude, and nitrous oxide anesthesia.)
- About 80% of uncomplicated cases are cured with one operation, 15% need further surgical therapy, and 5% never reattach

Author(s)

Paul Riordan-Eva, FRCOphth

Rheumatic Manifestations of Cancer

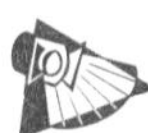

KEY FEATURES

- Patients with malignancy-associated **dermatomyositis** tend to be older and have the type of cancer anticipated by their age and gender profiles
- **Hypertrophic pulmonary osteoarthropathy** should be suspected in middle-aged or older patients with polyarthritis that mimics rheumatoid arthritis but is associated with new-onset clubbing and periosteal new bone formation
- **Palmar fasciitis** is characterized by bilateral palmar swelling and finger contraction and may be the first indication of cancer, particularly ovarian carcinoma
- Acute leukemia can produce joint pains that are disproportionately severe in comparison to the minimal swelling and heat that are present. **Leukemic arthritis** complicates about 5% of cases
- Rheumatic manifestations of myelodysplastic syndromes include cutaneous vasculitis, lupus-like syndromes, neuropathy, and episodic intense arthritis
- **Erythromelalgia**, a painful warmth and redness of the extremities that (unlike Raynaud's disease) improves with cold exposure or with elevation of the extremity, is often associated with myeloproliferative diseases

CLINICAL FINDINGS

- Rheumatic symptoms tend to improve or resolve with treatment of the cancer, but may return with cancer recurrence

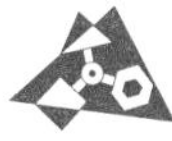

DIAGNOSIS

- Malignancy workups should focus on screening tests appropriate to patient's age (eg, colonoscopy in patients older than 50 yr). "Fishing expeditions" are not indicated

TREATMENT

- Corticosteroids are often helpful for arthritic symptoms
- Erythromelalgia may respond to ASA, 325 mg QD or BID

Author(s)

David B. Hellmann, MD, FACP

John H. Stone, MD, MPH

Rheumatic Manifestations of HIV

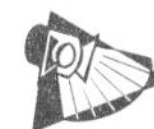

KEY FEATURES

- Infection with HIV virus has been associated with various rheumatic disorders, most commonly arthralgias or Reiter's syndrome. More rare are the occurence of myositis, psoriatic arthritis, Sjögren's syndrome, or vasculitis
- It is possible that these disorders stem directly from HIV infection itself or from the many other infections that occur in immunodeficient patients
- The rheumatic syndromes may follow the diagnosis of AIDS or may precede it by several months

CLINICAL FINDINGS

- Arthralgias
- Some rheumatic manifestations (eg, the arthritis of Reiter's syndrome or the cutaneous findings in psoriasis) tend to be accentuated in patients with HIV

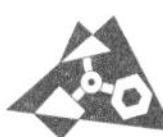

DIAGNOSIS

- Same criteria as for non-HIV–infected patients

TREATMENT

- Many patients respond to nonsteroidal anti-inflammatory drugs, although a few are unresponsive and develop progressive deformities
- Immunosuppressive agents must be used with great caution. However, with the use of highly active antiretroviral therapy (HAART), the paradoxic use of immunosuppression in HIV patients with inflammatory disease is sometimes required

Author(s)

David B. Hellmann, MD, FACP

John H. Stone, MD, MPH

Rheumatism, Palindromic

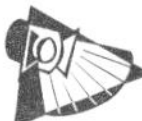 KEY FEATURES

- Frequent recurring attacks at irregular intervals of acutely inflamed joints
- In some patients, palindromic rheumatism is a prodrome of rheumatoid arthritis

 CLINICAL FINDINGS

- Periarticular pain with swelling
- Attacks cease within several hours to several days
- Knee and fingers are most commonly affected, but any peripheral joint may be involved
- Systemic manifestations other than fever do not occur
- Although hundreds of attacks may take place over a period of years, there is no permanent articular damage

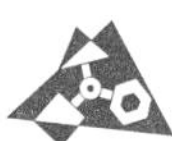 DIAGNOSIS

- Clinical
- Laboratory findings are usually normal

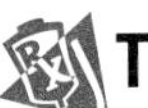 TREATMENT

- Nonsteroidal anti-inflammatory drugs are usually all that is required during the attacks
- Hydroxychloroquine may be of value in preventing recurrences

Author(s)

David B. Hellmann, MD, FACP

John H. Stone, MD, MPH

Riboflavin Deficiency

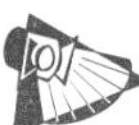 KEY FEATURES

- Almost always occurs in combination with deficiencies of other vitamins
- Caused by dietary inadequacy, interactions with a variety of medications, alcoholism, and other causes of protein-calorie undernutrition

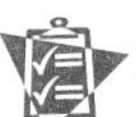 CLINICAL FINDINGS

- Cheilosis, angular stomatitis, glossitis
- Seborrheic dermatitis
- Weakness
- Corneal vascularization
- Anemia

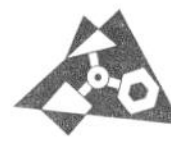 DIAGNOSIS

- Measure serum levels of the riboflavin-dependent enzyme erythrocyte glutathione reductase. Activity coefficients > 1.2–1.3 suggest riboflavin deficiency
- Less commonly measured: urinary riboflavin excretion and serum levels of plasma and red blood cell flavins

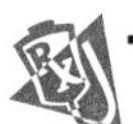 TREATMENT

- Riboflavin, 5–15 mg PO QD, until clinical findings are resolved

Author(s)

Robert B. Baron, MD, MS

Right Middle Lobe Syndrome

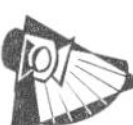 KEY FEATURES

- Recurrent or persistent atelectasis of the right middle lobe
- Related to the relatively long length and narrow diameter of the right middle lobe bronchus and the oval opening to the lobe
- Important to exclude obstructing lesion such as bronchogenic carcinoma

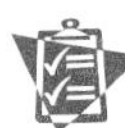 CLINICAL FINDINGS

- Radiographic finding of recurrent atelectasis of right middle lobe
- Recurrent or slowly resolving pneumonia

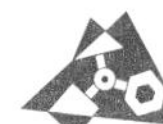 DIAGNOSIS

- CT scan or bronchoscopy is often necessary to rule out obstructing tumor
- Foreign body aspiration or other benign causes of atelectasis must be excluded

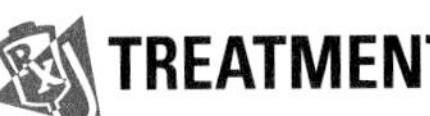

- Treatment is of the underlying condition

Author(s)

Mark S. Chesnutt, MD

Thomas J. Prendergast, MD

Rocky Mountain Spotted Fever

KEY FEATURES

- Caused by *Rickettsia rickettsii*, a parasite of ticks, transmitted by tick bites
- Most cases occur in the middle and southern Atlantic seaboard and the central Mississippi River valley
- Most cases occur in late spring and summer
- Typical incubation period is 2–14 days (median, 7 days)

CLINICAL FINDINGS

- Initial symptoms include fevers, chills, headache, nausea and vomiting
- Cough and pneumonitis often occur early in the disease
- Rash (not always found) begins as a faint macule that progresses to large maculopapules and often petechiae
- Rash begins on the wrists and ankles, characteristically involves palms and soles, and spreads to arms, legs, and trunk
- About 3–5% of recognized cases in the United States are fatal

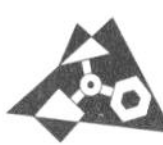

DIAGNOSIS

- Thrombocytopenia
- Hyponatremia
- Hepatitis
- CSF low glucose
- Immunohistological staining for *R rickettsii* in skin biopsy specimens and serological testing are the keys to a definitive diagnosis

TREATMENT

- Doxycycline or chloramphenicol are usually highly effective
- Prevention: protective clothing and avoiding tick bites

Author(s)

Wayne X. Shandera, MD

Ana Moran, MD

Rotator Cuff Injuries

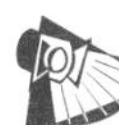

KEY FEATURES

- The majority of shoulder problems stem from disorders of the rotator cuff
- Rotator cuff tendinitis, subacromial bursitis, partial and complete rotator cuff tears, and calcific tendinitis frequently cause similar symptoms

CLINICAL FINDINGS

- Nonspecific localized shoulder pain
- Locking sensations occur with motion (particularly abduction) of the shoulder
- Maximum tenderness is usually noted over the supraspinatus insertion
- Range of motion pain is worst between 60° and 120° of abduction, the site of greatest impingement of the rotator cuff tissues between the humerus and coracoacromial arch
- With rotator cuff tears, there may be an inability to abduct or flex the shoulder depending on the site of the tear, although full range of motion may be maintained by the shoulder's accessory rotator muscles
- Complete tears usually have positive "drop" signs: inability to sustain passive abduction of the arm to 90°

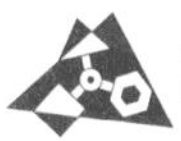

DIAGNOSIS

- Clinical features; MRI may be of use

TREATMENT

- Rest and abstention from inciting activities, along with NSAIDs
- For symptoms that persist after 2 weeks of conservative therapy, injection of 1 mL triamcinolone (40 mg/mL) with 2–3 mL of lidocaine hydrochloride (1–2%) may help. The procedure, along with continued rest, may be repeated after 2–3 weeks
- Physical therapy is valuable if the patient fails to maintain the shoulder's normal range of motion
- Aside from patients with complete rotator cuff tears, only those who fail to improve after months of conservative therapy are candidates for operation

Author(s)

David B. Hellmann, MD, FACP

John H. Stone, MD, MPH

Rubella

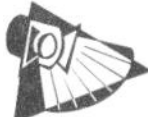

KEY FEATURES

- Spread by respiratory droplets
- Rare disease in United States
- Nonspecific features makes it difficult to distinguish from other viral infections

CLINICAL FINDINGS

- Mild fever, malaise, and arthralgias, which are more common in women
- Cervical, postauricular lymphadenopathy common
- Fine, pink rash lasts 3 days in each area
- Rash typically starts on the face and spreads to trunk and extremities
- Exposure during pregnancy can lead to fetal infection and death
- Postinfectious encephalopathy is rare, few long-term sequelae
- Congenital rubella associated with CNS, cutaneous, ophthalmic (cataracts), otic (deafness), and cardiac disease

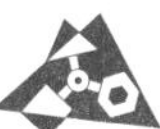

DIAGNOSIS

- Exposure 14–21 days before symptom onset
- Leukopenia common
- Diagnosis established by clinical findings and rise in serum rubella antibody titers

TREATMENT

- Symptomatic treatment and supportive measures
- Prevention: live attenuated virus is safe and highly effective
- Women should be immunized when not pregnant

Author(s)

Wayne X. Shandera, MD

Ana Moran, MD

Sciatic Nerve Palsy

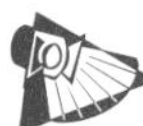

KEY FEATURES

- Misplaced deep intramuscular injections are probably the most common cause
- Trauma to the buttock, hip, or thigh may also be responsible
- The resulting clinical deficit depends on whether the whole nerve or only certain fibers have been affected
- In general, the peroneal fibers of the sciatic nerve are more susceptible to damage than those destined for the tibial nerve
- The common peroneal nerve itself may be compressed or injured in the region of the head and neck of the fibula (eg, by sitting with crossed legs or wearing high boots)

CLINICAL FINDINGS

- There is weakness of dorsiflexion and eversion of the foot, accompanied by numbness or blunted sensation of the anterolateral aspect of the calf and dorsum of the foot

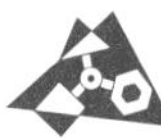

DIAGNOSIS

- Suggested clinically and may be confirmed by electromyography
- A sciatic nerve lesion may be difficult to distinguish from peroneal neuropathy unless there is electromyographic evidence of involvement of the short head of the biceps femoris muscle

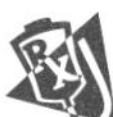

TREATMENT

- Unless trauma has interrupted the continuity of the nerve, treatment is supportive
- Avoid pressure on the nerve

Author(s)

Michael J. Aminoff, MD, DSc, FRCP

Seafood Poisoning

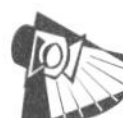

KEY FEATURES

- In the majority of cases, the seafood has a normal appearance and taste (scombroid may have a peppery taste)

CLINICAL FINDINGS

- A variety of intoxications may occur, including scombroid, ciguatera, paralytic shellfish, and puffer fish poisoning (Table 148)
- Abrupt respiratory arrest may occur with acute paralytic shellfish and puffer fish poisoning

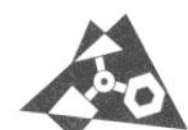

DIAGNOSIS

- Table 148

TREATMENT

- Observe patients for at least 4–6 h
- Replace fluid and electrolyte losses from gastroenteritis with IV saline or other crystalloid solution
- For recent ingestions, administer activated charcoal, 60–100 g PO or via gastric tube, mixed in aqueous slurry; do not use for comatose or convulsing patients unless it can be given by gastric tube and the airway is first protected by a cuffed endotracheal tube
- There is no specific antidote for paralytic shellfish or puffer fish poisoning
- Ciguatera: Acute neurological symptoms may respond to mannitol, 1 g/kg IV (anecdotal)
- Scombroid: Antihistamines such as diphenhydramine, 25–50 mg IV, and the H_2 blocker cimetidine, 300 mg IV, are usually effective. For severe reactions, also give epinephrine, 0.3–0.5 mL of a 1:1000 solution SC

Author(s)

Kent R. Olson, MD

Seborrheic Keratoses

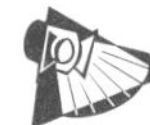

KEY FEATURES

- Seborrheic keratoses are common, especially in the elderly and may be mistaken for melanomas or other types of cutaneous neoplasms

CLINICAL FINDINGS

- Seborrheic keratoses are benign plaques, beige to brown or even black, 3–20 mm in diameter, with a velvety or warty surface
- They appear to be stuck or pasted onto the skin

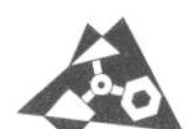

DIAGNOSIS

- Clinical

TREATMENT

- Although they may be frozen with liquid nitrogen or curetted if they itch or are inflamed, no treatment is needed

Author(s)

Timothy G. Berger, MD

Sedative-Hypnotic Agent Overdose

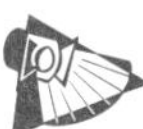

KEY FEATURES

- Sedative-hypnotics depress the CNS reticular activating system, cerebral cortex, and cerebellum

CLINICAL FINDINGS

- **Mild intoxication** produces euphoria, slurred speech, ataxia, and even hypoglycemia
- With **severe intoxication**, stupor, coma, bradycardia, hypotension, hypothermia, and respiratory arrest may occur
- Death is usually from respiratory arrest or pulmonary aspiration of gastric contents
- Massively intoxicated patients may appear dead, with no reflex responses or even electroencephalographic activity

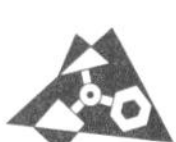

DIAGNOSIS

- Ethanol serum levels > 300 mg/dL (0.3 g/dL; 65 mmol/L) usually produce coma in a novice user, but regular users may remain awake at much higher levels
- Phenobarbital levels > 80–100 mg/L usually cause coma

TREATMENT

- Administer activated charcoal, 60–100 g PO or via gastric tube, mixed in aqueous slurry if given within 1 h of ingestion; do not use for comatose patients unless it can be given by gastric tube and the patient is intubated endotracheally
- Hemodialysis may be necessary for severe phenobarbital intoxication but not for most other drugs in this group
- Flumazenil is a specific benzodiazepine antagonist and has no effect on other sedative-hypnotic agents. Give flumazenil, IV 0.2 mg over 30–60 s, repeated in 0.5-mg increments as needed up to a total dose of 3–5 mg. Caution: It may induce seizures in patients with preexisting seizures, benzodiazepine addiction, or concomitant overdose with tricyclic antidepressants

Author(s)

Kent R. Olson, MD

Severe Acute Respiratory Syndrome (SARS)

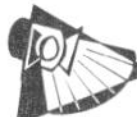

KEY FEATURES

- Travel to endemic area within 10 days before symptom onset, including mainland China, Hong Kong, Singapore, Taiwan, Vietnam, and Toronto
- Persistent fever, dry cough, dyspnea in most cases
- Mortality: as high as 10% in clinically diagnosed cases

CLINICAL FINDINGS

- SARS is an atypical pneumonia that affects all age groups
- The incubation period is 2–7 days; it can be spread to contacts of affected patients for 10 days. Mean time from onset of clinical symptoms to hospital admission is 3–5 days
- In all clinical cases, persistent fever is present; chills/rigor, cough, shortness of breath, rales, and rhonchi are the rule
- Many patients report headache, myalgias, and sore throat
- Watery diarrhea occurs in some patients late in the course of the illness
- Elderly patients may report malaise and delirium, without fever

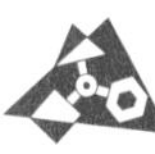

DIAGNOSIS

- Serologic tests are available, but seroconversion may not occur until 3 weeks after the onset of symptoms
- Detection rates for the virus using conventional RT-PCR are low in the first 7 days of illness. Positivity rates on urine, nasopharyngeal aspirate, and stool specimens are 42%, 68%, and 97%, respectively, on day 14 of illness
- Case definitions
  - **Suspected case** is defined as a person with fever > 38°C, cough or difficultly in breathing, and close contact with a suspected case or recent travel to endemic area
  - **Probable case** is defined as a suspected case with radiographic changes of pneumonia or acute respiratory distress syndrome; or a suspected case positive for the virus in one of more laboratory assays; or a suspected case with necropsy evidence of acute respiratory distress syndrome of unknown cause

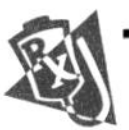

TREATMENT

- No specific treatment
- Supportive therapy is mainstay
- Benefit of ribavirin in treating SARS is controversial. Limited data suggest that doses of 2 g/day may be effective and not produce adverse reactions
- High-dose pulse methylprednisolone during the clinical progression phase (with development of radiologic evidence of pneumonia and hypoxemia) may be associated with more favorable clinical improvement

Author(s)

Wayne X. Shandera, MD

Ana Moran, MD

Short Bowel Syndrome

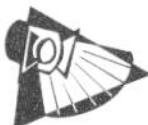

KEY FEATURES

- Malabsorptive condition following removal of significant portions of the small intestine
- Causes: Crohn's disease, mesenteric infarction, radiation enteritis, trauma
- Type and degree of malabsorption depend on length and site of resection and degree of adaptation of remaining bowel

CLINICAL FINDINGS

- Terminal ileal resection: watery diarrhea, malabsorption of bile salts and vitamin B_{12}, low serum vitamin B_{12} levels, abnormal Schilling test, steatorrhea and malabsorption of fat-soluble vitamins, cholesterol gallstones, calcium oxalate kidney stones
- Extensive (>40–50%) small bowel resection: short bowel syndrome, characterized by weight loss and diarrhea, folate, iron, or calcium malabsorption

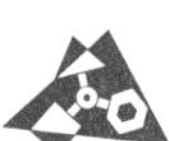

DIAGNOSIS

- Clinical diagnosis based on presence of diarrhea and malabsorption with prior bowel resection

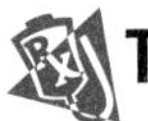

TREATMENT

TERMINAL ILEAL RESECTION

- Vitamin B_{12} injections IM monthly
- If watery diarrhea, bile salt binding resins (eg, cholestyramine, 2–4 g PO TID with meals)
- If steatorrhea, low-fat diet and vitamins, medium-chain triglycerides
- Calcium supplements to bind oxalate

EXTENSIVE SMALL BOWEL RESECTION

- If the colon is preserved, 100 cm of proximal jejunum may be sufficient to maintain adequate oral nutrition with a low-fat, high–complex-carbohydrate diet
- If the colon has been removed, at least 200 cm of proximal jejunum is typically required to maintain oral nutrition
- Parenteral vitamin supplementation
- Monitor levels of zinc and magnesium
- Antidiarrheal agents (eg, loperamide, 2–4 mg PO TID)
- Octreotide
- H_2 receptor antagonists to reduce acid hypersecretion
- TPN required if < 100–200 cm of proximal jejunum intact
- TPN has an estimated annual mortality rate of 2–5% resulting from TPN-induced liver disease, sepsis, loss of venous access
- Small intestinal transplantation

Author(s)

Kenneth R. McQuaid, MD

Silicosis

KEY FEATURES

- Extensive or prolonged inhalation of free silica results in small, rounded opacities (silicotic nodules) throughout the lung

CLINICAL FINDINGS

- Calcification of peripheral hilar lymph nodes ("eggshell" calcification) strongly suggests silicosis
- Incidence of pulmonary tuberculosis is increased in patients with silicosis

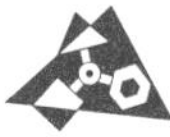

DIAGNOSIS

- Simple silicosis is usually asymptomatic without effect on pulmonary function tests
- Complicated silicosis presents with large conglomerate densities in the upper lung; dyspnea with restrictive and obstructive dysfunction is common

TREATMENT

- All patients require a tuberculin skin test and current chest x-ray
- Patients with suspected old pulmonary tuberculosis should be treated with multidrug regimens

Author(s)

Mark S. Chesnutt, MD
Thomas J. Prendergast, MD

Skin Infections, Streptococcal

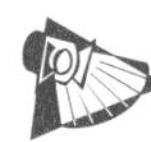

KEY FEATURES

- Group A β-hemolytic streptococci are not normal skin flora
- Usually result from colonization of normal skin by contact with other infected individuals or by preceding streptococcal respiratory infection

CLINICAL FINDINGS

- Impetigo is a focal, vesicular, pustular lesion with a thick, amber-colored crust that has a "stuck-on" appearance
- Erysipelas is a painful superficial cellulitis that frequently involves the face. It is indurated, slightly elevated, and well demarcated from the surrounding normal skin

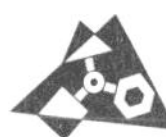

DIAGNOSIS

- Cultures obtained from a wound or pustule are likely to grow group A β-hemolytic streptococci
- Blood cultures are occasionally positive

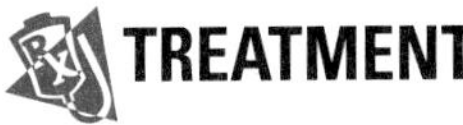

TREATMENT

- Parenteral antibiotics are indicated for patients with facial erysipelas or evidence of systemic infection
  - Penicillin, 2 million units IV Q 4 h, is the drug of choice
  - Cefazolin, 500 mg IV or IM Q 8 h is an alternative
- Initial therapy for severely ill patients or those who have risk factors for staphylococcal infection (eg, injection drug use, wound infection, diabetes) should include a drug, such as nafcillin, 1.5 g IV Q 6 h, that is also active against *Staphylococcus aureus*
- Patients who do not require parenteral therapy may be treated with amoxicillin, 750 mg twice daily for 7–10 days
- Relatively high prevalence of resistance among strains makes macrolides a less attractive alternative for penicillin-allergic patients

Author(s)

Henry F. Chambers, MD

Smoke Inhalation

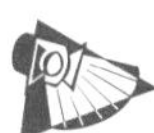

KEY FEATURES

- 33% of patients treated for burn injuries also have pulmonary injury from smoke inhalation
- Injury occurs as a result of impaired oxygenation, thermal injury to the upper airway, and chemical injury to the lung

CLINICAL FINDINGS

- Pulmonary edema, increased upper airway secretions, stridor, and respiratory failure may be present
- ARDS may develop 1–2 days after exposure
- Sloughing of the airway mucosa may occur in 2–3 days, leading to airway obstruction, atelectasis, and worsening hypoxemia
- Bacterial colonization and pneumonia are common 5–7 days after exposure

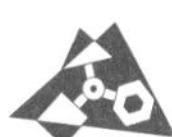

DIAGNOSIS

- Typically, a history of smoke exposure is easily obtained or presumed
- Examination of the upper airway with a laryngoscope or bronchoscope is superior to physical exam
- Arterial blood gases are necessary to evaluate oxygenation and rule out carbon monoxide poisoning

TREATMENT

- Supplemental oxygen, humidified air, bronchodilators, and suctioning of mucosal debris and secretions
- Positive end-expiratory pressure has been advocated when there is pulmonary edema
- Corticosteroids are unhelpful and may be harmful
- Monitoring for bacterial infection is important, but prophylactic antibiotics are not recommended

Author(s)

Mark S. Chesnutt, MD

Thomas J. Prendergast, MD

Spherocytosis, Hereditary

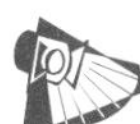

KEY FEATURES

- Disorder of RBC membrane, leading to chronic hemolytic anemia
- Autosomal dominant disease of variable severity
- Membrane defect is in spectrin, an RBC skeleton protein, resulting in decreased surface–volume ratio and a spherical RBC shape, which is less deformable
- Hemolysis occurs because of trapping of RBCs within the spleen

CLINICAL FINDINGS

- Often diagnosed in childhood, but milder cases discovered incidentally late in life. Family history often positive
- Anemia may or may not be present because bone marrow may be able to compensate for shortened RBC survival
- Severe anemia (aplastic crisis) may occur with folic acid deficiency or infection
- Jaundice and pigment (calcium bilirubinate) gallstones and cholecystitis in chronic hemolysis
- Palpable spleen

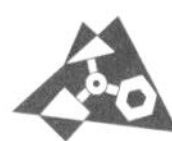

DIAGNOSIS

- Microcytic, hyperchromic anemia of variable severity; hematocrit may be normal
- Increased mean corpuscular hemoglobin concentration, often > 36 g/dL
- Reticulocytosis present
- Peripheral blood smear shows small percentage of spherocytes, small cells that have lost their central pallor
- Indirect bilirubin often increased
- Coombs test negative
- Increased osmotic fragility (abnormally vulnerable to swelling induced by hypotonic media), although nonspecific

TREATMENT

- Folic acid, 1 mg PO QD
- Splenectomy, which eliminates site of hemolysis
- Splenectomy may not be necessary in very mild cases discovered late in adult life

Author(s)

Charles A. Linker, MD

Spinal Cord Compression, Malignant

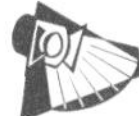

KEY FEATURES

- Oncological emergency
- Complication of metastatic solid tumor, lymphoma, or myeloma
- Carcinomatous meningitis (leptomeningeal disease) occurs in 3–8% of all cancers

CLINICAL FINDINGS

- Back pain (in > 80%) aggravated by lying down, weight bearing, sneezing, coughing
- Progressive weakness of the lower extremities
- Sensory loss (usually in the lower extremities)
- Less commonly, chest or abdominal pain, signs of nerve root compression
- Late findings: bowel and bladder dysfunction
- Carcinomatous meningitis: sequential cranial nerve abnormalities, stroke, hydrocephalus

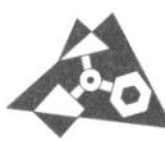

DIAGNOSIS

- MRI with and without contrast
- Bone radiographs and bone scans can detect vertebral metastases but do not assess spinal cord or nerve root compromise
- Carcinomatous meningitis diagnosed by gadolinium-enhanced MRI scans showing enhancement of the meninges or by CSF cytology showing malignant cells

TREATMENT

- Emergency surgery yields superior neurological outcomes for lesions involving a single vertebra with extension to only 1 superior or inferior vertebra compared with radiation alone with surgery for nonresponse
- Other indications for emergency surgery include spinal cord compression without a diagnosis of malignancy, already maximal doses of radiation to involved area, or progressive neurological deficits during radiation
- Radiation therapy either as primary therapy or after surgery

- Cyber knife for previously radiated sites
- High-dose corticosteroids (eg, dexamethasone, 10–100 mg IV) as soon as possible followed by lower dose (eg, dexamethasone, 4–6 mg Q 6 h IV PO) throughout course of radiation
- Chemotherapy for lymphomas and multiple myeloma in conjunction with or after radiation
- Carcinomatous meningitis treated with radiation, usually whole brain and spinal cord, or intrathecal chemotherapy, most commonly methotrexate and cytarabine

Author(s)

Hope Rugo, MD

Spinal Stenosis, Lumbar

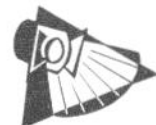

KEY FEATURES

- May be congenital or, more commonly, acquired
- Narrowing of the spinal canal most frequently results from enlarging osteophytes at the facet joints, hypertrophy of the ligamentum flavum, and protrusion or bulging of intervertebral disks
- Exactly how spinal stenosis results in pain is not defined
- Most patients with lumbar spinal stenosis are older than 60 yr

CLINICAL FINDINGS

- When low back pain is the chief symptom, it is bilateral and often diffuse over the buttocks
- Gradual onset of pain, weakness, or unsteadiness in both legs precipitated by walking or prolonged standing and relieved by sitting
- The onset of symptoms with standing by itself, the location of the maximal discomfort to the thighs, and the preservation of pedal pulses help distinguish the "pseudoclaudication" of spinal stenosis from true claudication caused by vascular insufficiency
- May have fewer symptoms walking uphill than down

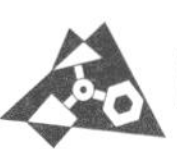

DIAGNOSIS

- MRI
- Differential diagnosis
  - Claudication (arterial insufficiency)
  - Disk herniation
  - Lumbar facet joint degenerative arthritis
  - Sacroiliitis (eg, ankylosing spondylitis, epidural abscess or tumor, piriformis syndrome)

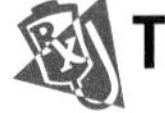

TREATMENT

- Weight loss and exercises aimed at reducing lumbar lordosis, which aggravates symptoms of spinal stenosis
- When disabling symptoms persist, decompressive laminectomy can provide at least short-term relief in about 80% of patients

Author(s)

David B. Hellmann, MD, FACP

John H. Stone, MD, MPH

Sporotrichosis

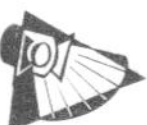

KEY FEATURES

- Sporotrichosis is a chronic fungal infection caused by *Sporothrix schenckii*
- Found worldwide; most patients have had contact with soil, sphagnum moss, or decaying wood
- Infection occurs via skin inoculation, usually on the hand, arm, or foot, especially during gardening
- Disseminated sporotrichosis is rare in immunocompetent patients but occurs in immunocompromised patients, especially those with AIDS and alcohol abuse

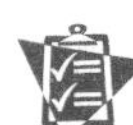

CLINICAL FINDINGS

- Begins with a hard, nontender subcutaneous nodule, which later adheres to overlying skin and ulcerates
- Within days to weeks, similar nodules develop along lymphatics draining the area, and these may ulcerate. The lymphatics become indurated and are easily palpated
- Disseminated sporotrichosis presents with widespread cutaneous, lung, bone, joint, and central nervous system involvement

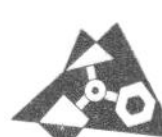

DIAGNOSIS

- Cultures are needed to establish the diagnosis
- Antibody tests may be useful in disseminated disease, especially meningitis

TREATMENT

- Itraconazole, 200–400 mg PO QD, for several months for localized lymphocutaneous disease and mild cases of disseminated disease
- Saturated solution of potassium iodide, 5 drops TID, increasing to 40–50 drops TID, or terbinafine, 500 mg PO twice daily, for several months, are alternatives for localized disease
- Amphotericin B, 1–2 g IV, for meningeal and disseminated disease
- Joint involvement may require arthrodesis
- Lymphocutaneous sporotrichosis has a good prognosis; pulmonary, joint, and disseminated sporotrichosis respond less favorably

Author(s)

Samuel A. Shelburne, MD

Richard J. Hamill, MD

Staphylococci Infections, Coagulase-Negative

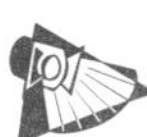

KEY FEATURES

- An important cause of infections of intravascular and prosthetic devices and of wound infection after cardiothoracic surgery
- Less virulent than *Staphylococcus aureus*, and infections tend to be more indolent
- Normal flora of human skin

CLINICAL FINDINGS

- Often associated with a foreign body
- Fever, a new murmur, instability of the prosthesis, and signs of embolization are evidence of prosthetic valve infection

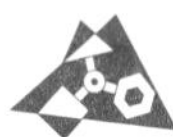

DIAGNOSIS

- Infection (vs isolation as a contaminant) is more likely if the patient has a foreign body or an intravascular device in place
- Infection is more likely if the same strain is isolated from 2 or more blood cultures and from the foreign body site
- Contamination is more likely when a single blood culture is positive or if more than 1 strain is isolated from blood cultures. Antimicrobial susceptibility and speciation can help determine whether multiple strains have been isolated.

TREATMENT

- Remove the foreign body or intravascular device when possible
  - Sometimes treatment with antibiotics is preferable
  - Surgical management may become necessary
- Vancomycin, 1 g IV Q 12 h, is the treatment of choice
- Duration of therapy is not established for infections caused by foreign devices, which may be eliminated by simply removing the infected device
- Treat bone or a prosthetic valve infection for 6 weeks
- Vancomycin plus rifampin, 300 mg PO BID, and gentamicin, 1 mg/kg IV Q 8 h, is recommended for prosthetic valve endocarditis caused by methicillin-resistant strains

Author(s)

Henry F. Chambers, MD

Still's Disease, Adult

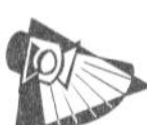

KEY FEATURES

- A variant of rheumatoid arthritis
- High spiking fevers are much more prominent, especially at the outset, than in rheumatoid arthritis

CLINICAL FINDINGS

- The fever is dramatic, often spiking to 40°C, associated with sweats and chills, and then plunging to several degrees below normal
- An evanescent salmon-colored nonpruritic rash, chiefly on the chest and abdomen, is a characteristic feature but is easily missed because it often appears only with the fever spike
- Sore throat
- Lymphadenopathy
- Joint symptoms are mild or absent in the beginning, but a destructive arthritis, especially of the wrists, may develop months later
- Anemia and leukocytosis, with white blood cell counts sometimes exceeding 40,000/μL, are the rule
- About one-third of patients have recurrent episodes

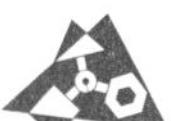

DIAGNOSIS

- A diagnosis of exclusion (of other causes of fever and arthritis)
- Strongly suggested by the fever pattern, sore throat, and classic rash

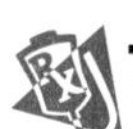

TREATMENT

- About half of the patients respond to high-dose aspirin (eg, 1 g TID) or other nonsteroidal anti-inflammatory drugs
- About half require prednisone, sometimes in doses > 60 mg/day

Author(s)

David B. Hellmann, MD, FACP
John H. Stone, MD, MPH

Storage Pool Disease

KEY FEATURES

- Group of mild bleeding disorders characterized by defective secretion of platelet granule contents (especially adenosine 5'-diphosphate) that stimulate platelet aggregation

CLINICAL FINDINGS

- Mild increase in bruising and postoperative bleeding

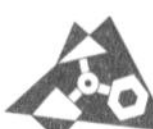

DIAGNOSIS

- Platelets normal in number and morphology
- Bleeding time slightly prolonged, especially after aspirin
- Variable abnormalities in platelet aggregation studies

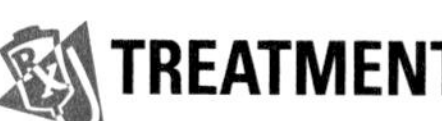

TREATMENT

- Most patients do not require treatment
- Avoid aspirin
- Platelet transfusions transiently correct bleeding tendency
- Desmopressin, 0.3 μg/kg IV Q 24 h, may be helpful

Author(s)

Charles A. Linker, MD

Streptococcal, Group A Infections

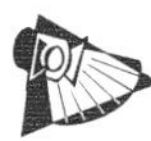

KEY FEATURES

- Arthritis, pneumonia, empyema, endocarditis, and necrotizing fasciitis are relatively uncommon infections that may be caused by group A streptococci

CLINICAL FINDINGS

- Arthritis generally occurs in association with cellulitis
- Pneumonia and empyema often are characterized by extensive tissue destruction and an aggressive, rapidly progressive clinical course
- Endocarditis (rare) should be suspected when bacteremia accompanies pneumonia, particularly if the patient uses injection drugs; the tricuspid valve is most commonly involved
- Necrotizing fasciitis is a rapidly spreading infection involving the fascia of deep muscle. The clinical findings at presentation range from severe cellulitis to systemic toxicity and severe pain
- Any streptococcal infection, especially necrotizing fasciitis, can be associated with streptococcal toxic shock syndrome, characterized by invasion of skin or soft tissues, acute respiratory distress syndrome, and renal failure

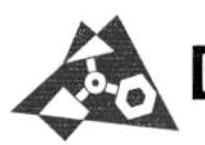

DIAGNOSIS

- Culture of affected site or blood

TREATMENT

- Arthritis: IV penicillin G, 2 million units Q 4 h, and frequent percutaneous needle aspiration
- Pneumonia/empyema: high-dose penicillin and chest tube drainage for treatment of the empyema
- Endocarditis: 4 million units of penicillin G Q 4 h for 4 weeks
- Necrotizing fasciitis: Early, extensive débridement is essential for survival
- Toxic shock syndrome: IV penicillin; consider the addition of clindamycin (600 mg IV Q 8 h to halt toxin production) and IV immune globulin

Author(s)

Henry F. Chambers, MD

Stroke, Lacunar

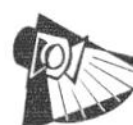

KEY FEATURES

- Small lesions (usually < 5 mm in diameter)
  - Occur in the distribution of short, penetrating arteries in the basal ganglia, pons, cerebellum, anterior limb of the internal capsule, and, less commonly, the deep cerebral white matter
- Risk factors include poorly controlled hypertension and diabetes
- Generally have a good prognosis, with partial or complete resolution often occurring over 4–6 weeks

CLINICAL FINDINGS

- There are several clinical syndromes
  - Contralateral pure motor or pure sensory deficit
  - Ipsilateral ataxia with crural paresis
  - Dysarthria with clumsiness of the hand
- Deficits may progress over 24–36 h before stabilizing

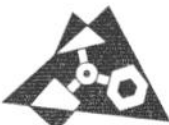

DIAGNOSIS

- Sometimes visible on CT scans as small, punched-out, hypodense areas, but in other patients no abnormality is seen
- In some instances, patients with a clinical syndrome suggestive of lacunar infarction are found to have a severe hemispheric infarct on CT scanning

TREATMENT

- Treat hypertension or diabetes
- Avoid tobacco use
- Anticoagulation is not indicated
- Aspirin, 325 mg PO QD, is of uncertain benefit

Author(s)

Michael J. Aminoff, MD, DSc, FRCP

Superior Vena Cava Obstruction

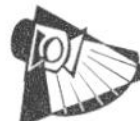

KEY FEATURES

- A rare disorder caused by partial or complete obstruction of the superior vena cava
- Most frequent causes
  - Superior mediastinal tumors (eg, adenocarcinoma of the lung, lymphoma, thyroid carcinoma, thymoma, teratoma, synovial cell carcinoma, angiosarcoma)
  - Chronic fibrotic mediastinitis, either idiopathic or secondary to tuberculosis, histoplasmosis, pyogenic infections, or drugs (eg, methysergide)
  - Thrombophlebitis secondary to indwelling central venous catheters or pacemaker wires
  - Aneurysm of the aortic arch
  - Constrictive pericarditis

CLINICAL FINDINGS

- Swelling of the neck and face
- Headache
- Dizziness, stupor, syncope
- Visual disturbances
- Bending over or lying down accentuates symptoms
- Dilated anterior chest wall veins and/or collateral veins
- Facial flushing
- Brawny edema and cyanosis of the face and arms
- Cerebral and laryngeal edema

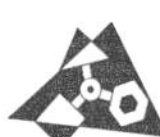

DIAGNOSIS

- Usually suggested by the history and physical examination
- Duplex ultrasonogram offers limited view of central veins
- CT scan or MRA
- Contrast venography is reserved for patients undergoing surgical or endoscopic treatment

TREATMENT

- Malignant tumors: endovascular stenting, chemotherapy, or external beam radiation
- Mediastinal fibrosis or constrictive pericarditis: surgical excision of the fibrous tissue or pericardial sac

- Thrombophlebitis: removal of central venous catheter, head elevation, and short-course warfarin anticoagulation or thrombolysis, and venous angioplasty or venous bypass

Author(s)

Louis M. Messina, MD

Syncope

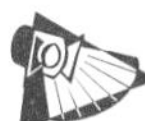

KEY FEATURES

- Transient (few seconds to a few minutes) loss of consciousness and postural tone
- Abrupt onset
- Caused by inadequate cerebral blood flow
- Often leads to injury
- Prompt recovery without resuscitative measures
- Causes include cardiac, vascular, and neurological processes
- Most common in the elderly
- More likely in those with heart disease, older men, and young women prone to vasovagal episodes
- 30% of adults will experience ≥ 1 syncopal episode
- Accounts for ~3% of ER visits

CLINICAL FINDINGS

VASOVAGAL SYNCOPE

- Caused by excessive vagal tone or impaired reflex control of the peripheral circulation
- "Common faint" occurs most often
- Often initiated by stressful, painful, or claustrophobic experiences
- Nausea, diaphoresis, tachycardia, and pallor are common premonitory symptoms
- Other varieties: carotid sinus hypersensitivity, postmicturition, or cough syncope

ORTHOSTATIC (POSTURAL) SYNCOPE

- Caused by impaired vasoconstrictive response to assuming upright posture, leading to abrupt decrease in venous return
- Occurs in those with advanced age; diabetes or other cause of autonomic neuropathy; blood loss or hypovolemia; and vasodilator, diuretic, or adrenergic-blocker drug therapy

CARDIOGENIC SYNCOPE

- Caused by rhythm disturbances (sick sinus syndrome, atrioventricular block, tachyarrhythmias) or mechanical causes (eg, aortic stenosis, pulmonary stenosis, hypertrophic obstructive cardiomyopathy, pulmonary hypertension, atrial myxoma)
- Episodes are often exertional

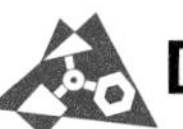

DIAGNOSIS

- Initial evaluation yields a specific cause in only 50% of cases
- Physical examination: orthostatic changes in blood pressure and pulse, carotid sinus massage, and cardiac exam
- Resting ECG: arrhythmias, accessory pathways, infarction, hypertrophy, and other abnormalities
- Do tilt-table testing before invasive studies unless clinical and ambulatory ECG evaluation suggests a cardiac cause

VASOVAGAL SYNCOPE

- Characteristic history
- Carotid sinus massage under carefully monitored conditions or tilt-table testing may be diagnostic

ORTHOSTATIC SYNCOPE

- > 20 mm Hg decline in blood pressure immediately on standing
- Tilt-table testing and Valsalva's maneuver are diagnostic

CARDIOGENIC SYNCOPE

- Echocardiography to rule out mechanical causes
- If rhythm disturbance suspected, ambulatory ECG monitoring indicated. May need to repeat several times, up to 3 days
- Event recorder and transtelephone ECG monitoring indicated for more intermittent presyncopal episodes
- Electrophysiological studies indicated for recurrent episodes and nondiagnostic ambulatory ECGs

TREATMENT

VASOMOTOR SYNCOPE

- Lying down or avoiding the inciting stimuli
- β-blockers may be helpful
- Permanent pacing for those with bradycardic responses to syncope

ORTHOSTATIC SYNCOPE

- Discontinue offending drugs; stand up slowly; fludrocortisone rarely

CARDIOGENIC SYNCOPE

- Treat the underlying disorder

Author(s)

Thomas M. Bashore, MD

Christopher B. Granger, MD

Syringomyelia

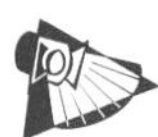

KEY FEATURES

- Destruction of gray and white matter adjacent to the central canal of the cervical spinal cord leads to cavitation and fluid collection within the cord
- Associated with Arnold-Chiari malformation, sometimes with accompanying meningomyelocele
- Cord cavitation may also occur with cord injury or neoplasm at any level of the cord

CLINICAL FINDINGS

- Cervical lesions: segmental atrophy, areflexia, and loss of pain and temperature appreciation in a "cape" distribution owing to the destruction of fibers crossing in front of the central canal. Often there is thoracic kyphoscoliosis
- A pyramidal and sensory deficit may be present in the legs
- Upward extension of the cavitation (syringobulbia) leads to dysfunction of the lower brainstem and thus to bulbar palsy, nystagmus, and sensory loss over one or both sides of the face

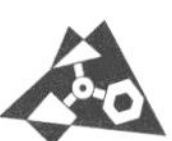

DIAGNOSIS

- X-ray films of the skull and cervical spine may show skeletal abnormalities. CT scans show caudal displacement of the fourth ventricle in Arnold-Chiari malformation. MRI or positive-contrast myelography may demonstrate the malformation itself
- Focal cord enlargement is found at myelography or by MRI in patients with cavitation related to past injury or intramedullary neoplasms

TREATMENT

- Treatment of Arnold-Chiari malformation with associated syringomyelia is by suboccipital craniectomy and upper cervical laminectomy, with the aim of decompressing the malformation at the foramen magnum
- In cavitation associated with intramedullary tumor, treatment is surgical, but radiation therapy may be necessary if complete removal is not possible
- Posttraumatic syringomyelia is also treated surgically if it leads to increasing neurologic deficits or to intolerable pain

Author(s)

Michael J. Aminoff, MD, DSc, FRCP

Tachycardia, Paroxysmal Supraventricular

KEY FEATURES

- Most common paroxysmal tachycardia
- Often occurs in patients without structural heart disease
- Attacks begin and end abruptly and may last a few seconds to several hours or longer
- In the absence of heart disease, serious effects are rare
- Usually caused by atrioventricular (AV) nodal reentry tachycardia
- One third of cases caused by an AV accessory pathway

CLINICAL FINDINGS

- Heart rate is 140–240 bpm (usually 160–220 bpm) and perfectly regular (despite exercise or change in position)
- Patients may be asymptomatic except for awareness of rapid heartbeat
- Some patients have mild chest pain or shortness of breath, especially when episodes are prolonged, even in the absence of associated cardiac abnormalities
- May result from digitalis toxicity, when it is commonly associated with AV block

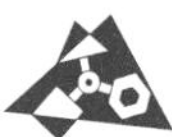

DIAGNOSIS

- ECG or telemetry
  - Perfectly regular rhythm with heart rate between 140–240 bpm (usually 160–220 bpm)
  - P wave usually differs in contour from sinus beats
  - Accessory pathways (eg, Wolff-Parkinson-White syndrome) are often associated with a short PR interval and sometimes with an early delta wave at the onset of a wide, slurred QRS complex

TREATMENT

- Attack should be terminated quickly if the patient has congestive heart failure, syncope, or angina or underlying cardiac or coronary disease
- Mechanical measures should be attempted first:
  - Valsalva's maneuver, stretching the arms and body, lowering the head between the knees, coughing, and breath holding
  - Carotid sinus massage unilaterally for 10–20 s (do not perform if patient has carotid bruits or a history of transient ischemic attacks)
- If mechanical measures fail, give adenosine (initial 6 mg IV bolus; then, if no response after 1–2 min, a second 12-mg IV bolus, followed by a third if necessary; Table 40
- Alternative agents for narrow-complex supraventricular tachycardias include IV calcium channel blockers (diltiazem, verapamil), β-blockers (esmolol), and digoxin (Table 40)
- Do not use digoxin, verapamil, or β-blockers if premature supraventricular tachycardia is associated with a known or suspected accessory pathway
- For patients who are hemodynamically unstable or if adenosine and verapamil are contraindicated or ineffective, synchronized electrical cardioversion (beginning at 100 J) is almost always successful
- Avoid electrical cardioversion if digitalis toxicity is suspected or documented
- Radiofrequency ablation for patients with recurrent symptomatic reentry supraventricular tachycardia, whether from dual pathways within the AV node or accessory pathways
- **Medications as preventive measure**
  - Oral digoxin is the usual first choice for narrow-complex supraventricular tachycardias
  - Verapamil, alone or in combination with digitalis, is a second choice
  - β-blockers are also effective (Table 40)
  - Use sotalol or amiodarone in patients with structural heart disease
- For wide-complex supraventricular tachycardias without atrial fibrillation or flutter (generally resulting from accessory pathways), use a combination of agents to increase refractoriness in the bypass tract (class Ia or Ic antiarrhythmic agents) and in the AV node (verapamil, digoxin, and β-blockers). Class III agents are also sometimes used (Table 40)

Author(s)

Thomas M. Bashore, MD

Christopher B. Granger, MD

Tachycardia, Ventricular

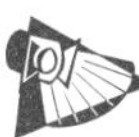

KEY FEATURES

- Defined as 3 or more consecutive ventricular premature beats
- Usually, rate is 160–240/min and moderately regular
- Either nonsustained (< 30 s) or sustained (> 30 s)
- Nonsustained ventricular tachycardia without underlying heart disease does not imply a poor prognosis
- Sustained ventricular tachycardia usually occurs with cardiac disease and carries an unfavorable prognosis
- When there is significant left ventricular dysfunction, sudden death is common

CLINICAL FINDINGS

- Causes include acute myocardial infarction, dilated cardiomyopathy, coronary artery disease, hypertrophic cardiomyopathy, mitral valve prolapse, myocarditis, and other forms of myocardial disease
- May be asymptomatic or associated with syncope or milder symptoms of impaired cerebral perfusion

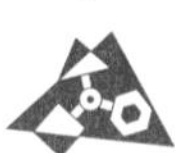

DIAGNOSIS

- ECG: runs of ≥ 3 ventricular beats
- Distinguishing between ventricular tachycardia and aberrant conduction of supraventricular tachycardia may be difficult
- Torsades de pointes, a form of ventricular tachycardia in which QRS morphology twists around the baseline, has a poor prognosis and may occur with hypokalemia, hypomagnesemia, or drugs that prolong the QT interval

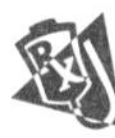

TREATMENT

- Empiric magnesium sulfate 1 g IV
- Nonsustained ventricular tachycardias with structural heart disease
  - β-blockers reduce the incidence of sudden death by 40–50%
  - Avoid other antiarrhythmic agents (except, possibly, amiodarone)
- Acute sustained ventricular tachycardia
  - In unstable patients (hypotension, heart failure, or myocardial ischemia), immediate synchronized DC cardioversion with 100–360 J
  - In stable patients, lidocaine 1 mg/kg IV bolus; procainamide or amiodarone are alternative, second-line agents (Table 40)
- Recurrent symptomatic or sustained ventricular tachycardia: implantable cardioverter-defibrillator device
- In patients with preserved left ventricular function: amiodarone, optimally in combination with a β-blocker
- Electrophysiological studies may help identify candidates for radiofrequency ablation of a tachycardia focus

Author(s)

Thomas M. Bashore, MD
Christopher B. Granger, MD

Tardive Dyskinesia

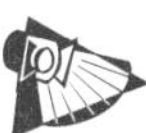

KEY FEATURES

- A syndrome of involuntary stereotyped movements of the face, mouth, tongue, trunk, limbs
- Occurs after months or (typically) years of treatment in 20–35% of neuroleptic agent users
- Predisposing factors
  - Older age
  - Cigarette smoking
  - Diabetes
- Atypical antipsychotics appear to be lower risk
- Symptoms do not necessarily worsen and may improve even when neuroleptics are continued

CLINICAL FINDINGS

- Early signs
  - Fine worm-like tongue movements
  - Difficulty sticking out the tongue
  - Facial tics
  - Increased blink frequency
  - Jaw movements
- Late signs
  - Lip smacking
  - Chewing motions
  - Disturbed gag reflex
  - Puffing of the cheeks
  - Respiratory distress
  - Disturbed speech
  - Choreoathetoid movements

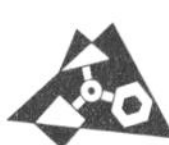

DIAGNOSIS

- Differentiate early signs of TD from reversible side effects of medicines such as tricyclic antidepressants and antiparkinsonism agents

TREATMENT

- Emphasis should be on prevention by using lowest effective dose
- Stop anticholinergic drugs and gradually discontinue neuroleptic dose
- Benzodiazepines, buspirone, phosphatidylcholine, clonidine, calcium channel blockers, vitamin E, and propranolol are of limited usefulness in treating symptoms

Author(s)

Stuart J. Eisendrath, MD
Jonathan E. Lichtmacher, MD

Theophylline Toxicity

 KEY FEATURES

- The usual serum half-life of theophylline is 4–6 h, but this may increase to > 20 h after overdose

 CLINICAL FINDINGS

- Mild intoxication causes nausea, vomiting, tachycardia, tremulousness
- Ventricular and supraventricular tachyarrhythmias, hypotension, and seizures occur in severe intoxication (serum levels > 100 mg/L)
- Status epilepticus is common and often intractable to usual anticonvulsants
- Symptoms may be delayed for hours after acute ingestion, especially if a sustained-release preparation was taken
- Serious toxicity may develop at lower levels (ie, 40–60 mg/L) with chronic intoxication

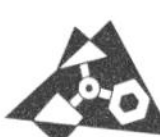 DIAGNOSIS

- Serum theophylline concentration
- Hypokalemia, hyperglycemia, and metabolic acidosis are common after acute overdose

 TREATMENT

- After acute ingestion, administer activated charcoal
- Repeated doses of activated charcoal may enhance gut decontamination and elimination by "gut dialysis"
- Whole-bowel irrigation should be considered for large ingestions involving sustained-release preparations
- Hemodialysis is indicated for status epilepticus or markedly elevated serum theophylline levels (eg, > 100 mg/L after acute overdose or possibly for levels > 60 mg/L with chronic intoxication)
- Treat seizures with benzodiazepines (lorazepam, 2–3 mg IV, or diazepam, 5–10 mg IV) or phenobarbital, 10–15 mg/kg IV. Phenytoin is not effective
- Hypotension and tachycardia may respond to β-blocker therapy even in low doses: Administer esmolol, 25–50 μg/kg/min by IV infusion, or propranolol, 0.5–1 mg IV

Author(s)

Kent R. Olson, MD

Thiamin Deficiency

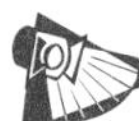 KEY FEATURES

- Most common cause: alcoholism
- Other causes: malabsorption, dialysis, chronic protein-calorie undernutrition
- In patients with marginal thiamin stores, symptoms and signs can be precipitated by IV dextrose solutions

 CLINICAL FINDINGS

- Early manifestations include anorexia, muscle cramps, paresthesias, and irritability
- Advanced deficiency chiefly affects cardiovascular system (wet beriberi) or nervous system (dry beriberi)
- Wet beriberi
  - Occurs with severe physical exertion and high carbohydrate intake
  - Characterized by marked peripheral vasodilation resulting in high-output heart failure with dyspnea, tachycardia, cardiomegaly, pulmonary and peripheral edema, and warm extremities
- Dry beriberi
  - Occurs with inactivity and low-calorie intake
  - Involves both peripheral and central nervous systems
  - Peripheral nerve involvement includes symmetric motor and sensory neuropathy with pain, paresthesias, and loss of reflexes in legs more than the arms
  - Central nervous system involvement includes Wernicke-Korsakoff syndrome

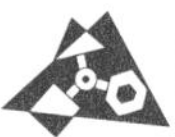 DIAGNOSIS

- Clinical response to empiric thiamine therapy
- Biochemical tests: erythrocyte transketolase activity and urinary thiamin excretion coefficient > 15–20% suggest thiamin deficiency

TREATMENT

- Thiamine, 50–100 mg IV or IM QD for the first few days, followed by 5–10 mg PO QD
- Therapeutic doses of other water-soluble vitamins
- Treatment results in complete resolution of symptoms and signs in 50% of patients (half immediately and half over days); the remaining 50% obtain only partial resolution or no benefit

Author(s)

Robert B. Baron, MD, MS

Tinnitus

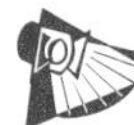 KEY FEATURES

- Tinnitus is the perception of abnormal ear or head noises
- Intermittent periods of mild, high-pitched tinnitus lasting for several minutes are common in normal-hearing persons
- Persistent tinnitus usually indicates the presence of sensory hearing loss
- When severe and persistent, tinnitus may interfere with sleep and the ability to concentrate, resulting in considerable psychological distress

 CLINICAL FINDINGS

- Pulsatile tinnitus is often described by the patient as listening to one's own heartbeat
  - Should be distinguished from tonal tinnitus
  - Although often caused by conductive hearing loss, this symptom may indicate a vascular abnormality, such as glomus tumor, carotid vaso-occlusive disease, arteriovenous malformation, or aneurysm
- A staccato "clicking" tinnitus may result from middle-ear muscle spasm, sometimes associated with palatal myoclonus. The patient typically perceives a rapid series of popping noises, lasting seconds to a few minutes, accompanied by a fluttering feeling in the ear

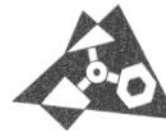 DIAGNOSIS

- MR angiography should be considered in cases in which vascular abnormality is suspected

TREATMENT

- The most important treatment is avoidance of exposure to excessive noise, ototoxic agents, and other factors that may cause cochlear damage
- Masking the tinnitus with music or through amplification of normal sounds with a hearing aid may bring relief
- Oral antidepressants (eg, oral nortriptyline at an initial dosage of 50 mg at bedtime) often impact tinnitus-induced sleep disorder and depression

Author(s)

Robert K. Jackler, MD

Michael J. Kaplan, MD

Toxic Shock Syndrome, *Staphylococcus aureus*

KEY FEATURES

- Strains of staphylococci may produce toxins that can cause four important entities
  - Scalded skin syndrome, typically in children, or bullous impetigo in adults
  - Necrotizing pneumonitis in children
  - Toxic shock syndrome (TSS)
  - Enterotoxin food poisoning
- Most cases (≥ 90%) of TSS have been reported in women of childbearing age, especially common within 5 days of the onset of a menstrual period in women who have used tampons
- Nonmenstrual cases of TSS are now about as common as menstrual cases. Organisms from various sites, including the nasopharynx, bones, vagina, and rectum, or wounds have all been associated with the illness

CLINICAL FINDINGS

- Abrupt onset of fever, vomiting, and watery diarrhea
- A diffuse macular erythematous rash and nonpurulent conjunctivitis are common, and desquamation, especially of the palms and soles, is typical during recovery

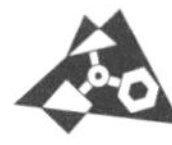

DIAGNOSIS

- Blood cultures are negative because symptoms are due to the effects of the toxin and not to the invasive properties of the organism

TREATMENT

- Rapid rehydration, antistaphylococcal drugs, management of renal or cardiac failure, and removal of sources of toxin, (eg, removal of tampon, drainage of abscess)

Author(s)

Henry F. Chambers, MD

Tracheal Stenosis

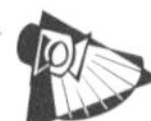

KEY FEATURES

- As an acquired disorder, usually results from previous tracheotomy or endotracheal intubation
- Idiopathic cases occur, mostly in women
- Complications include recurrent pulmonary infection and respiratory failure

CLINICAL FINDINGS

- Dyspnea, cough, and inability to clear pulmonary secretions occurring weeks to months after tracheal cannulation or intubation

DIAGNOSIS

- Wheezing, a palpable tracheal thrill, or harsh breath sounds may be detected, but often not until tracheal diameter is decreased by 50%
- Diagnosis is confirmed by plain films or CT of the trachea

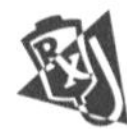

TREATMENT

- Surgical reconstruction, endotracheal stent placement, or laser photoresection

Author(s)

Mark S. Chesnutt, MD

Thomas J. Prendergast, MD

Tremor, Essential

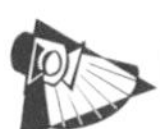

KEY FEATURES

- The cause is uncertain, but it is sometimes inherited in an autosomal dominant manner
- Tremor may begin at any age and is enhanced by emotional stress

CLINICAL FINDINGS

- Postural tremor usually involves one or both hands, the head, or the hands and head, whereas the legs tend to be spared
- Speech may also be affected if the laryngeal muscles are involved
- Examination reveals no other abnormalities
- Ingestion of a small quantity of alcohol commonly provides remarkable but short-lived relief by an unknown mechanism
- Although the tremor may become more conspicuous with time, it generally leads to little disability, and treatment is often unnecessary
- Occasionally, it interferes with manual skills and leads to impairment of handwriting

TREATMENT

- Propranolol, either intermittently or indefinitely, 60–240 mg PO QD
- Primidone may be helpful, but patients are often very sensitive to it. They are, therefore, started on 50 mg PO QD, and the daily dose is increased by 50 mg every 2 weeks depending on the response; a maintenance dose of 125 mg TID is commonly effective
- Occasional patients do not respond to these measures but are helped by alprazolam (up to 3 mg daily in divided doses), clozapine (30–50 mg twice daily), mirtazapine (15 or 30 mg at night), or topiramate (up to 400 mg daily titrated over 6–8 weeks)
- Disabling tremor unresponsive to medical treatment may be helped by unilateral or bilateral high-frequency thalamic stimulation

Author(s)

Michael J. Aminoff, MD, DSc, FRCP

Trench Fever

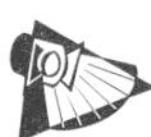 KEY FEATURES

- A self-limited, louse-borne relapsing febrile disease caused by *Bartonella quintana*
- Epidemic infection in louse-infested troops and civilians during wars; endemic in scattered geographic areas (eg, Central America)
- An urban equivalent of trench fever has been described among the homeless
- Humans acquire infection when infected lice feces enter sites of skin breakdown

 CLINICAL FINDINGS

- Onset of symptoms is abrupt, and fever lasts 3–5 days with relapses
- The patient complains of weakness and severe pain behind the eyes and typically in the back and legs
- Lymphadenopathy, splenomegaly, and a transient maculopapular rash may appear
- Subclinical infection is frequent, and a carrier state is recognized
- The differential diagnosis includes other febrile, self-limited states such as dengue, leptospirosis, malaria, relapsing fever, and typhus

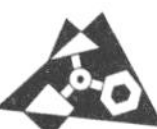 DIAGNOSIS

- Blood cultures: *B quintana* will grow in standard BACTEC media, but growth may require incubation for 4–6 weeks
- Positive serology with a compatible clinical syndrome: either documented seroconversion or high titer of antibody (≥ 1:1600) in single ELISA or immunofluorescence test

 TREATMENT

- Doxycycline, 100 mg PO BID, or azithromycin, 500 mg PO, for 4–6 weeks for uncomplicated bacteremia, although recovery can occur in the absence of therapy
- Patients with endocarditis should be treated for 4–6 mo, with addition of a third-generation cephalosporin or aminoglycoside for the first 3 weeks

Author(s)

Henry F. Chambers, MD

Tricyclic Antidepressant Overdose

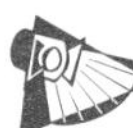 KEY FEATURES

- Tricyclic antidepressants (TCAs) contain both anticholinergic and cardiac depressant properties (quinidine-like sodium channel blockade)
- Newer antidepressants such as trazodone, fluoxetine, paroxetine, sertraline, bupropion, venlafaxine, and fluvoxamine are not chemically related to the TCAs and do not generally produce cardiotoxic effects. However, they may cause seizures and serotonin syndrome (see Monoamine Oxidase Inhibitor Overdose) in overdoses

 CLINICAL FINDINGS

- Severe symptoms may occur abruptly within 30–60 min after acute overdose
- Anticholinergic effects include dilated pupils, tachycardia, dry mouth, flushed skin, muscle twitching, decreased peristalsis
- Quinidine-like cardiotoxic effects include QRS interval widening (> 0.12 s), ventricular arrhythmias, atrioventricular block, and hypotension
- Seizures and coma are common with severe intoxication
- Life-threatening hyperthermia may result from status epilepticus and anticholinergic-induced impairment of sweating

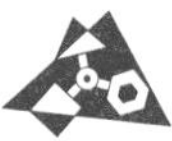 DIAGNOSIS

- QRS interval correlates with the severity of intoxication more reliably than the serum drug level

TREATMENT

- Observe patients for at least 6 h, and admit if there are anticholinergic effects or signs of cardiotoxicity
- Administer activated charcoal 60–100 g mixed in aqueous slurry PO or via gastric tube
- Consider gastric lavage after recent large ingestions
- Treat cardiotoxic effects with boluses of sodium bicarbonate (50–100 mEq IV). Maintain the pH between 7.45 and 7.50. Alkalinization does not promote excretion of tricyclics

Author(s)

Kent R. Olson, MD

Tuberculosis, Intestinal

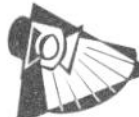 KEY FEATURES

- Common in developing nations; rare in the United States
- Incidence in the United States rising in immigrant groups and patients with AIDS
- Caused by *Mycobacterium tuberculosis* and *M bovis*

 CLINICAL FINDINGS

- Active pulmonary tuberculosis in < 50%
- Most common involvement is ileocecal
- Chronic abdominal pain, obstructive symptoms, weight loss, diarrhea
- Abdominal mass palpable
- Complications include
  - Intestinal obstruction
  - Hemorrhage
  - Fistula formation

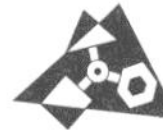 DIAGNOSIS

- PPD skin test may be negative, especially in weight loss or AIDS
- Barium enema, small bowel follow-through
- Colonoscopy
- Differential diagnosis: Crohn's disease, carcinoma, intestinal amebiasis
- Definitive diagnosis by either endoscopic or surgical biopsy revealing acid-fast bacilli and caseating granuloma or by positive cultures
- Detection of tubercle bacilli in biopsy specimens by PCR

 TREATMENT

- Tuberculosis, initial treatment (Table 24)
- Antituberculous drugs characteristics (Table 23)

Author(s)

Kenneth R. McQuaid, MD

Turner's Syndrome (Gonadal Dysgenesis)

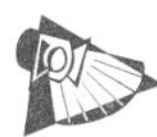

KEY FEATURES

- Chromosomal disorder associated with primary hypogonadism, short stature, other phenotypic anomalies
- Common cause of primary amenorrhea and early ovarian failure
- Patients with classic syndrome lack one X chromosome (45,XO karyotype)
- Incidence: about 1:10,000 female newborns
- < 3% survive to term
- Diagnosis suspected: at birth, small newborns, often with lymphedema; in childhood, short stature

CLINICAL FINDINGS

- Features variable and may be subtle if mosaicism
- Short stature, hypogonadism, webbed neck, high-arched palate, short fourth metacarpals, wide-spaced nipples, recurrent otitis media, hypertension, renal abnormalities, coarctation of aorta
- Hypogonadism presents as delayed adolescence (80%) or early ovarian failure (20%)
- Prone to:
  - Keloid formation after ear piercing or surgery
  - Hypothyroidism, diabetes mellitus, dyslipidemia, hypertension, and osteoporosis

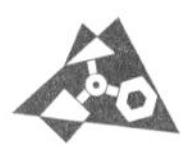

DIAGNOSIS

- Serum FSH and LH levels elevated
- Karyotype shows 45,XO (or X chromosome abnormalities, or mosaicism)
- Serum growth hormone and IGF-I levels normal
- Yearly physical examinations and periodic thyroid, lipid, and glucose testing recommended
- Echocardiogram by age 16 years

TREATMENT

- Growth hormone, 0.1 unit/kg/day SC, plus androgen (eg, oxandrolone) for ≥4 years before epiphyseal fusion increases final height by ~10 cm over mean predicted height of 144.2 cm
- Estrogen therapy after age 12 (eg, conjugated estrogens, 0.3 mg PO on days 1–21/month)
- Estrogen plus progestin hormone replacement therapy after growth stops
- Life expectancy reduced

Author(s)

Paul A. Fitzgerald, MD

Typhus, Endemic

KEY FEATURES

- Caused by *Rickettsia typhi* (ubiquitous)
- Transmitted from rats (*R typhi*) to humans by fleas
- Less severe disease than epidemic typhus

CLINICAL FINDINGS

- Gradual onset of malaise, cough, fever, and headache
- Maculopapular rash concentrated on trunk with rapid fading

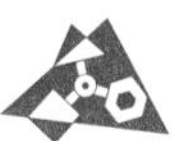

DIAGNOSIS

- Thrombocytopenia and elevated liver function tests common
- Antibody testing establishes diagnosis

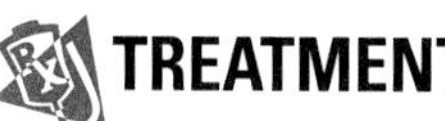

TREATMENT

- Tetracycline, doxycyline, choramphenicol given until more than 3 full days of defervescence

Author(s)

Wayne X. Shandera, MD

Samuel Shelburne, MD

Typhus, Epidemic Louse-Borne

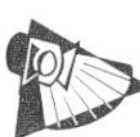

KEY FEATURES

- Infection with *Rickettsia prowazekii,* parasite of the body louse
- Transmission favored by famine, crowded living conditions, war
- Recrudescent typhus (Brill's disease) can occur years after initial exposure
- Ubiquitous, with rare US cases associated with flying squirrels or travel

CLINICAL FINDINGS

- Prodrome of malaise, cough, and headache followed by acute onset of fever, chills, and prostration
- Conjunctivitis, splenomegaly, and macular rash that starts in the axilla common

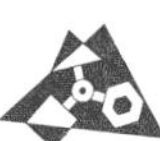

DIAGNOSIS

- Diffuse symptoms with abrupt onset of fever, chills, and prostration
- Macular rash does not appear in all cases
- Antibodies usually appear within 1 week of symptom onset (IgM for acute disease, IgG for Brill's disease)

TREATMENT

- Tetracycline and chloramphenicol effective when given for 4–10 days

Author(s)

Wayne X. Shandera, MD

Ana Moran, MD

Typhus, Scrub

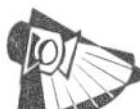

KEY FEATURES

- Caused by *Orienta tsutsugamushi,* a parasite of rodents, and transmitted by mites
- Mites live on vegetation, but bite humans who contact infested vegetation
- Occurs most commonly in Southeast Asia, western Pacific, and Australia
- Typical incubation period is 7–21 days

CLINICAL FINDINGS

- Malaise, chills, severe headache, backache
- Site of the bite turns from a papule to a flat black eschar with enlarged regional lymph nodes
- Gradual onset of fever with an accompanying macular rash
- Pneumonitis, myocarditis, encephalitis, granulomatous hepatitis, and GI hemorrhage are late complications

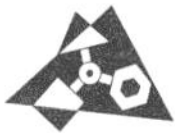

DIAGNOSIS

- Fluorescein-labeled antirickettsial assays or enzyme-linked immunoassays are available to make the diagnosis
- PCR is an increasingly used and very sensitive way to confirm the diagnosis

TREATMENT

- Doxycycline or chloramphenicol for 3–7 days
- Mortality rate for untreated patients may be as high as 30%
- Prevention: long-acting miticides and insecticides

Author(s)

Wayne X. Shandera, MD

Ana Moran, MD

Ulnar Neuropathy

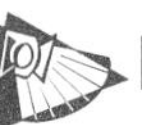

KEY FEATURES

- Commonly in the elbow where the nerve runs behind the medial epicondyle and descends into the cubital tunnel
- In the condylar groove, the ulnar nerve is exposed to pressure or trauma. Moreover, any increase in the carrying angle of the elbow, whether congenital, degenerative, or traumatic, may cause excessive stretching of the nerve when the elbow is flexed
- May also result from thickening or distortion of the anatomic structures forming the cubital tunnel, and the resulting symptoms may be aggravated by flexion of the elbow because the tunnel is then narrowed by tightening of its roof or inward bulging of its floor
- May also develop at the wrist or in the palm of the hand, usually owing to repetitive trauma or to compression from ganglia or benign tumors

CLINICAL FINDINGS

- Sensory changes in the medial $1\frac{1}{2}$ digits and along the medial border of the hand
- Weakness of the ulnar-innervated muscles in the forearm and hand, with lesions at the elbow
- With a cubital tunnel lesion there may be relative sparing of the flexor carpi ulnaris muscle
- Lesions at the wrist or palm cause weakness, sensory deficits, or both, restricted to the hand

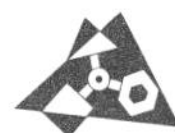

DIAGNOSIS

- Electrophysiologic evaluation using nerve stimulation techniques allows precise localization of the lesion

TREATMENT

- If repetitive mechanical trauma is responsible, this is avoided by occupational adjustment or job retraining
- If conservative measures are unsuccessful in relieving symptoms and preventing further progression, surgical treatment may be necessary. This consists of nerve transposition if the lesion is in the condylar groove or a release procedure if it is in the cubital tunnel

Author(s)

Michael J. Aminoff, MD, DSc, FRCP

Ureter & Renal Pelvis Cancer

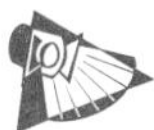 KEY FEATURES

- Most cancers of the ureter and renal pelvis are transitional cell carcinomas
- Rare; occur more commonly in smokers, those with Balkan nephropathy, those exposed to Thorotrast (a contrast agent with radioactive thorium in use until the 1960s), and those with a long history of analgesic abuse

 CLINICAL FINDINGS

- Gross or microscopic hematuria in most
- Flank pain secondary to bleeding and obstruction less common

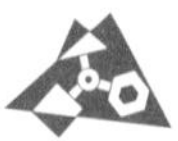 DIAGNOSIS

- Urinary cytology: often positive
- IV pyelography and abdominal CT: intraluminal filling defect, unilateral nonvisualization of the collecting system, and hydronephrosis
- Differential diagnosis
  - Calculi
  - Blood clots
  - Papillary necrosis
  - Inflammatory or infectious lesions

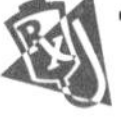 TREATMENT

- Treatment is based on the site, size, depth of penetration, and number of tumors present
- Most are excised with laparoscopic or open nephroureterectomy (renal pelvic and upper ureteral lesions) or segmental excision of the ureter (distal ureteral lesions)
- Direct biopsy, fulguration, or resection is sometimes possible using a ureteroscope
- Endoscopic resection indicated in patients with limited renal function and in the management of focal, low-grade, upper tract cancers

Author(s)

Marshall L. Stoller, MD

Peter R. Carroll, MD, FACS

Urethritis & Cervicitis, Chlamydial

 KEY FEATURES

- *Chlamydia trachomatis* immunotypes D–K are isolated in about 50% of cases of nongonococcal urethritis and cervicitis by appropriate techniques
- Coinfection with gonococci is common
- Postgonococcal (ie, chlamydial) urethritis may persist after successful treatment of the gonococcus

 CLINICAL FINDINGS

- Urethritis and occasionally epididymitis, prostatitis, or proctitis
- Females may be asymptomatic or may have signs and symptoms of cervicitis, salpingitis, or pelvic inflammatory disease

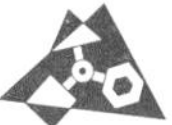 DIAGNOSIS

- The urethral or cervical discharge tends to be less painful and less purulent in chlamydial versus gonococcal infection
- Direct immunofluorescence assay, ELISA, and a DNA probe test, although less sensitive than culture, are sometimes used to confirm the diagnosis and for screening
- Ligase chain reaction (LCR) test
  - Has superior sensitivity compared with all other methods
  - Has excellent specificity, approaching 100%
  - Can be performed on urine
  - Will likely replace all other methods for diagnosis of chlamydial urethritis and cervicitis

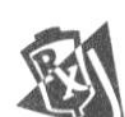 TREATMENT

- Sexual partners of infected patients should also be treated
- Therapy often must be given presumptively
- A single oral 1-g dose of azithromycin is effective for uncomplicated urethritis and cervicitis and has the advantage of improved patient compliance and minimal toxicity
- Doxycycline, 100 mg BID for 7 days

Author(s)

Henry F. Chambers, MD

Urticaria, Cold

 KEY FEATURES

- Can be familial (autosomal dominant) or acquired
- Urticaria may develop on even limited exposure to cold (eg, wind, freezer compartments)
- Most cases of acquired cold urticaria are idiopathic but can be associated with medication (eg, griseofulvin), infection, cryoglobulinemia, or syphilis

 CLINICAL FINDINGS

- Usually occurs only on exposed areas but in markedly sensitive individuals can be generalized and fatal
- Immersion in cold water may result in severe systemic reactions, including shock; histamine release occurs

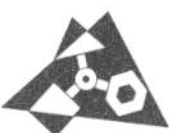 DIAGNOSIS

- Apply ice cube to the forearm skin for 5 min, remove, and observe the area for 10 min. As the skin rewarms, an urticarial wheal appears at the site and may be accompanied by itching

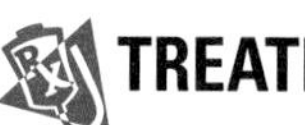 TREATMENT

- Cyproheptadine, 16–32 mg/day in divided doses

Author(s)

Richard Cohen, MD, MPH

Uterine Prolapse

KEY FEATURES

- Most commonly occurs as a delayed result of childbirth injury to the pelvic floor (particularly the transverse cervical and uterosacral ligaments)
  - Unrepaired obstetric lacerations of the levator musculature and perineal body augment the weakness
  - Attenuation of the pelvic structures with aging can worsen the prolapse
- In **slight prolapse,** the uterus descends only partway down the vagina
- In **moderate prolapse,** the corpus descends to the introitus and the cervix protrudes slightly beyond
- In **marked prolapse (procidentia),** the entire cervix and uterus protrude beyond the introitus and the vagina is inverted
- Inability to walk comfortably because of protrusion or discomfort from the presence of a vaginal mass is an indication that surgical treatment should be considered

TREATMENT

- The type of surgery depends on extent of prolapse and the desire for menstruation, pregnancy, and coitus
- The simplest, most effective procedure is vaginal hysterectomy with appropriate repair of the cystocele and rectocele
- If pregnancy is desired, a partial resection of the cervix with plication of the cardinal ligaments can be attempted
- For older women who do not desire coitus, partial obliteration of the vagina is surgically simple and effective
- A well-fitted vaginal pessary (eg, inflatable doughnut type, Gellhorn pessary) may give relief if surgery is not an option

Author(s)

H. Trent MacKay, MD, MPH

Vasculitis, Cryoglobulinemic

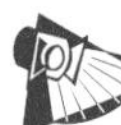

KEY FEATURES

- **Type I** cryoglobulins (monoclonal proteins that lack rheumatoid factor activity) are more commonly seen in lymphoproliferative disease and usually cause hyperviscosity syndromes rather than vasculitis
- **Type II** (monoclonal antibody with rheumatoid factor activity) and **type III** (polyclonal antibody with rheumatoid factor activity) cryoglobulins cause vasculitis and are associated with hepatitis C and connective tissue diseases (eg, Sjögren's syndrome)

CLINICAL FINDINGS

- Palpable purpura
- Peripheral neuropathy
- Abnormal liver function tests
- Abdominal pain
- Pulmonary disease

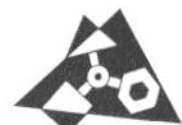

DIAGNOSIS

- Compatible clinical picture and a positive serum test for cryoglobulins
- Differential diagnosis includes other causes of palpable purpura and peripheral neuropathy (eg, polyarteritis nodosa, rheumatoid arthritis, sarcoidosis)
- Associated conditions
  - Hepatitis C or B
  - Lymphoproliferative disorders (eg, multiple myeloma, Waldenström's macroglobulinemia, chronic lymphocytic leukemia)
  - Sjögren's syndrome, systemic lupus erythematosus

TREATMENT

- Because 90% of cryoglobulinemia cases are associated with hepatitis C infections, the optimal approach to treatment is viral suppression with interferon-alpha with or without ribavirin
- Because immunosuppressive agents may facilitate viral replication, corticosteroids, cyclophosphamide, and other agents should be reserved for organ-threatening complications

Author(s)

David B. Hellmann, MD, FACP

John H. Stone, MD, MPH

Vegetative State, Persistent

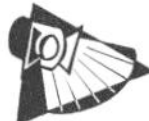

KEY FEATURES

- Patients with severe bilateral hemispheric disease may show some improvement from an initially comatose state, so that, after a variable interval, they appear to be awake but display no movement
- This persistent vegetative state has been variously referred to as akinetic mutism, apallic state, or coma vigil
- Most patients in a persistent vegetative state will die in months or years, but partial recovery has occasionally occurred and in rare instances has been sufficient to permit communication or even independent living

CLINICAL FINDINGS

- Patients appear to be awake with open eyelids but lie motionless
- No evidence of awareness or higher mental activity
- Simulate coma
- Unresponsive

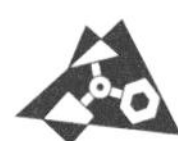

DIAGNOSIS

- Obtain the expertise of a clinician familiar with this syndrome to aid in the diagnosis

Author(s)

Michael J. Aminoff, MD, DSc, FRCP

Venous Thrombosis, Intracranial

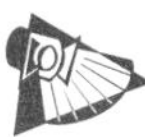 KEY FEATURES

- May occur in association with intracranial or maxillofacial infections, hypercoagulable states, polycythemia, sickle cell disease, and cyanotic congenital heart disease and in pregnancy or during the puerperium

 CLINICAL FINDINGS

- Headache, focal or generalized convulsions, drowsiness, confusion, increased intracranial pressure, focal neurological deficits, and less commonly meningeal irritation

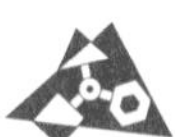 DIAGNOSIS

- Confirmed by CT scanning and MRI, MR venography, or angiography

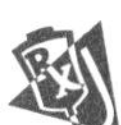 TREATMENT

- Anticonvulsant drugs if seizures have occurred
- Antiedema agents (eg, dexamethasone, 4 mg QID and continued as necessary) to reduce intracranial pressure
- Anticoagulation with dose-adjusted IV heparin followed by oral anticoagulation for 6 mo reduces morbidity and mortality of venous sinus thrombosis
- In cases refractory to heparin, endovascular techniques including catheter-directed thrombolytic therapy (urokinase) and thrombectomy are sometimes helpful

Author(s)

Michael J. Aminoff, MD, DSc, FRCP

Ventricular Septal Defect

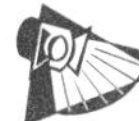 KEY FEATURES

- Opening in membranous (most) or muscular (rest) portion of interventricular septum, permitting blood in high-pressure left ventricle to shunt into low-pressure right ventricle
- Presentation in adults depends on size of shunt and presence or absence of associated pulmonic stenosis
- Small to moderate shunts are often asymptomatic
- Moderate shunts may lead to pulmonary vascular disease and right-sided failure
- Shunt reversal occurs in ~25% of cases, producing Eisenmenger's syndrome

 CLINICAL FINDINGS

- Small shunts: loud, harsh holosystolic murmur in third and fourth left interspaces along the sternum and, occasionally, mid-diastolic flow murmur
- Systolic thrill common
- Large shunts: right ventricular volume and pressure overload may cause pulmonary hypertension and cyanosis

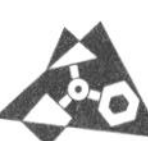 DIAGNOSIS

- ECG: left and/or right ventricular hypertrophy if shunt is reversed
- CXR: increased pulmonary vascularity
- Echo-Doppler is diagnostic and can assess magnitude of shunt and pulmonary artery pressure
- Cardiac CT and MRI can visualize defect and other anatomic abnormalities
- Cardiac catheterization usually reserved for those with at least moderate shunting and can measure pulmonary vascular resistance and degree of pulmonary hypertension

 TREATMENT

- Endocarditis occurs more often with smaller shunts; antibiotic prophylaxis is mandatory
- Small shunts do not require closure in asymptomatic patients
- Large shunts should be surgically or percutaneously repaired
- Surgical mortality is 2–3%, but ≥ 50% if pulmonary hypertension is present
- Surgery is contraindicated in Eisenmenger's syndrome
- Percutaneous closure devices are now available

Author(s)

Thomas M. Bashore, MD

Christopher B. Granger, MD

Vestibular Schwannoma (Acoustic Neuroma)

KEY FEATURES

- Eighth nerve schwannomas are among the most common of intracranial tumors
- The lesions arise within the internal auditory canal and gradually grow to involve the cerebellopontine angle, eventually compressing the pons and resulting in hydrocephalus
- Any individual with a unilateral or asymmetric sensorineural hearing loss should be evaluated for an intracranial mass lesion
- Other lesions of the cerebellopontine angle such as meningioma and epidermoids may have similar audiovestibular manifestations

CLINICAL FINDINGS

- Typical auditory symptoms are unilateral hearing loss with deterioration of speech discrimination exceeding that predicted by the degree of pure-tone loss
- Nonclassic presentations, such as sudden unilateral hearing loss, are fairly common
- Vestibular dysfunction more often takes the form of continuous dysequilibrium than episodic vertigo

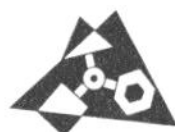

DIAGNOSIS

- Diagnosis is made by enhanced MRI, although auditory evoked responses may have a role in screening

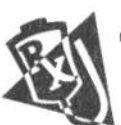

TREATMENT

- Microsurgical excision is most often indicated, although small tumors in older individuals may be managed with stereotactic radiotherapy or simply followed with serial imaging studies

Author(s)

Robert K. Jackler, MD

Michael J. Kaplan, MD

Vibrio Infections

KEY FEATURES

- Vibrios other than *Vibrio cholerae* that cause human disease are *V parahaemolyticus, V vulnificus,* and *V alginolyticus*
- Infection is acquired by exposure to organisms in raw or undercooked crustaceans or shellfish and warm (> 20°C) ocean waters and estuaries
- Oysters are implicated in up to 90% of food-related cases

CLINICAL FINDINGS

- *V parahaemolyticus* causes acute watery diarrhea with fever, typically within 24 h after ingestion of contaminated shellfish. The disease is self-limited, and antimicrobial therapy is usually not necessary
- *V vulnificus* and *V alginolyticus,* neither of which cause diarrhea, cause cellulitis and primary bacteremia after ingestion of contaminated shellfish or exposure to seawater
  - Cellulitis with or without sepsis may occur with bulla formation, necrosis, and extensive soft tissue destruction, at times requiring débridement and amputation
  - The infection can progress rapidly and be severe in immunocompromised individuals, especially those with cirrhosis, with death rates of 50%

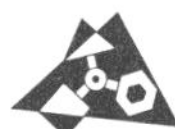

DIAGNOSIS

- Culture

TREATMENT

- Doxycycline, 100 mg PO BID for 7–10 days, is the drug of choice for cellulitis or bacteremia; fluoroquinolones and third-generation cephalosporins are also effective
- *V vulnificus* may be susceptible to penicillin, ampicillin, cephalosporins, chloramphenicol, aminoglycosides, and fluoroquinolones
- *V parahaemolyticus* and *V alginolyticus* are resistant to penicillin and ampicillin, but susceptibilities otherwise are similar to *V vulnificus*

Author(s)

Henry F. Chambers, MD

Visceral Artery Aneurysms

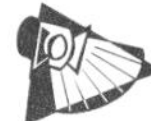

KEY FEATURES

- Hepatic artery aneurysms are the most common
- Splenic artery aneurysms ~30%
- Superior mesenteric, celiac, gastric, and gastroepiploic artery aneurysms each represent about 5% of visceral aneurysms
- Aneurysms of mesenteric branch vessels are rare and often associated with connective tissue disease or vasculitis
- Historically, almost 10% mortality rate, resulting from rupture
- Causes of hepatic artery aneurysm: medial degeneration, injury during cholangiography, hepatic biopsy, blunt abdominal trauma
- Causes of splenic artery aneurysm: medial fibroplasia, portal hypertension, splenomegaly, pregnancy, amphetamine use, local inflammation
- Causes of superior mesenteric artery aneurysm: infective endocarditis, septic emboli, atherosclerosis
- Causes of celiac artery aneurysm: atherosclerosis

CLINICAL FINDINGS

- Usually asymptomatic
- If ruptured, patient presents with hypotension and abdominal pain

DIAGNOSIS

- High-resolution CT scanning has increased detection of incidental mesenteric aneurysms

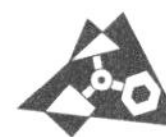

TREATMENT

- Asymptomatic splenic aneurysms < 2 cm rarely rupture
- No treatment unless patient is pregnant
- For symptomatic aneurysms and aneurysms > 2 cm, surgical aneurysmectomy or aneurysmorrhaphy with ligation of branches or endovascular (embolization) management

Author(s)

Louis M. Messina, MD

Vitamin A Deficiency

KEY FEATURES

- One of the most common vitamin deficiency syndromes in developing countries
- Most common cause of blindness in developing countries
- In the US, occurs most commonly in the elderly and urban poor or from fat malabsorption syndromes or mineral oil laxative abuse

CLINICAL FINDINGS

- Night blindness (early)
- Dryness (xerosis) of conjunctivae and small white patches on the conjunctivae (Bitot's spots) (early)
- Ulceration and necrosis of the cornea (keratomalacia), perforation, endophthalmitis, and blindness (late)
- Xerosis and hyperkeratinization of the skin
- Loss of taste

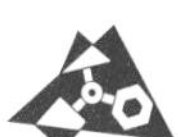

DIAGNOSIS

- Abnormalities of dark adaptation
- Serum vitamin A levels below normal range of 30–65 mg/dL

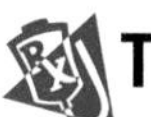

TREATMENT

- Early deficiency: vitamin A 30,000 IU PO QD for 1 week
- Advanced deficiency: vitamin A 20,000 units/kg PO QD for at least 5 days

Author(s)

Robert B. Baron, MD, MS

Vitamin B_6 Deficiency

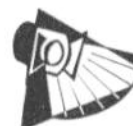

KEY FEATURES

- Vitamin B_6 deficiency most commonly occurs as a result of alcoholism or a variety of medications, especially isoniazid, cycloserine, penicillamine, and oral contraceptives
- Can also occur in a number of inborn errors of metabolism

CLINICAL FINDINGS

- Mouth soreness, glossitis, cheilosis, weakness, irritability
- Severe deficiency can result in peripheral neuropathy, anemia, seizures

DIAGNOSIS

- Serum pyridoxal phosphate levels are below normal levels of > 50 ng/mL

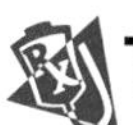

TREATMENT

- Vitamin B_6, 10–20 mg PO QD, is usually adequate
- Patients taking medications that interfere with pyridoxine metabolism may need doses as high as 100 mg/day. Patients with inborn errors of metabolism require up to 600 mg/day
- Prophylaxis with vitamin B_6 should be routinely given to patients receiving medications (such as isoniazid) that interfere with pyridoxine metabolism and to elderly, urban poor, or alcoholic patients

Author(s)

Robert B. Baron, MD, MS

Vitamin C Deficiency

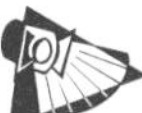

KEY FEATURES

- Vitamin C deficiency is most commonly due to dietary inadequacy among urban poor, elderly, and chronic alcoholics and to chronic illnesses such as cancer and chronic renal failure

CLINICAL FINDINGS

- Early: nonspecific malaise and weakness
- Late: scurvy
- Early scurvy is characterized by perifollicular hyperkeratotic papules, petechiae and purpura, splinter hemorrhages, bleeding gums, hemarthroses, and subperiosteal hemorrhages
- Late scurvy is characterized by edema, oliguria, neuropathy, intracerebral hemorrhage, and death
- Anemia is common
- Wound healing is impaired

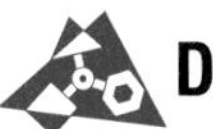

DIAGNOSIS

- Characteristic skin lesions
- Atraumatic hemarthrosis
- Plasma ascorbic acid levels low, typically < 0.1 mg/dL

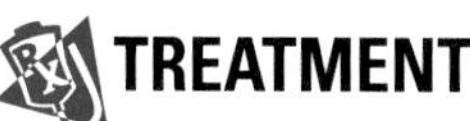

TREATMENT

- Ascorbic acid (vitamin C), 300–1000 mg PO QD

Author(s)

Robert B. Baron, MD, MS

Vitamin E Deficiency

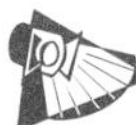

KEY FEATURES

- Most commonly results from severe malabsorption (eg, cystic fibrosis), abetalipoproteinemia (genetic disorder), and chronic cholestatic liver disease (including biliary atresia)

CLINICAL FINDINGS

- Areflexia, disturbances of gait, decreased proprioception and vibration, and ophthalmoplegia

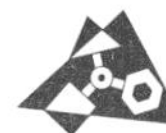

DIAGNOSIS

- Plasma vitamin E level below normal range of 0.5–0.7 mg/dL

TREATMENT

- Vitamin E supplementation, although optimum therapeutic dose has not been clearly defined

Author(s)

Robert B. Baron, MD, MS

Vitamin K Deficiency

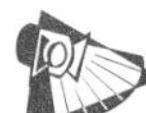

KEY FEATURES

- Vitamin K plays role in coagulation as a cofactor for the posttranslational carboxylation of factors II, VII, IX, and X. These modified factors are better able to participate in activation of factors X and II. Without this carboxylation, hemostasis is impaired
- Vitamin K is supplied exogenously in diet (primarily in leafy vegetables) and endogenously from synthesis by intestinal bacteria
- May be due to poor diet, malabsorption, and broad-spectrum antibiotics that suppress colonic flora
- Body stores of vitamin K are small; deficiency may develop in 1 week

CLINICAL FINDINGS

- No specific clinical features
- Bleeding may occur at any site

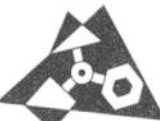

DIAGNOSIS

- PT prolonged to greater extent than PTT
- Only PT prolonged with mild vitamin K deficiency; fibrinogen level, thrombin time, and platelet count not affected
- Response to vitamin K therapy distinguishes it from hepatic coagulopathy
- Surreptitious warfarin use causes laboratory features indistinguishable from vitamin K deficiency

TREATMENT

- Vitamin K, 15 mg SC once, completely corrects laboratory abnormalities in 12–24 h
- Prognosis excellent; vitamin K deficiency is completely corrected with replacement

Author(s)

Charles A. Linker, MD

Vocal Cord Dysfunction

KEY FEATURES

- A syndrome of acute and chronic upper airway obstruction characterized by paradoxical vocal cord adduction

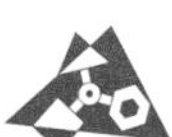

CLINICAL FINDINGS

- May present as dyspnea and wheezing and be confused with asthma
- Symptoms do not respond to a bronchodilator

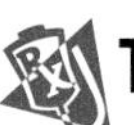

DIAGNOSIS

- Direct visualization of adduction of the vocal cords with both inspiration and expiration is diagnostic
- Spirometry shows evidence of upper airway obstruction but is normal immediately after an attack
- Bronchial provocation test normal

TREATMENT

- Speech therapy

Author(s)

Mark S. Chesnutt, MD

Thomas J. Prendergast, MD

Weakness & Paralysis

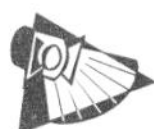

KEY FEATURES

- Loss of muscle power may result from
  - Central disease involving the upper or lower motor neurons
  - Peripheral disease involving the roots, plexus, or peripheral nerves
  - Disorders of neuromuscular transmission
  - Primary disorders of muscle

CLINICAL FINDINGS

- Weakness resulting from **upper motor neuron lesions** is characterized by selective involvement of certain muscle groups and is associated with spasticity, increased tendon reflexes, and extensor plantar responses
- **Lower motor neuron lesions** lead to muscle wasting as well as weakness, with flaccidity and loss of tendon reflexes, but no change in the plantar responses unless the neurons subserving them are directly involved
  - Fasciculations may be evident over affected muscles only in lower motor neuron or more peripheral neuropathic lesions
- In distinguishing between a **root, plexus, or peripheral nerve lesion,** the distribution of the motor deficit and of any sensory changes is of particular importance
- In **disturbances of neuromuscular transmission,** weakness is patchy in distribution, often fluctuates over short periods of time, and is not associated with sensory changes
- In **myopathic disorders,** weakness is usually most marked proximally in the limbs, is not associated with sensory loss or sphincter disturbance, and is not accompanied by muscle wasting or loss of tendon reflexes, at least not until an advanced stage

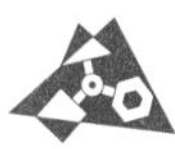

DIAGNOSIS

- See individual disorders

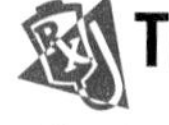

TREATMENT

- See individual disorders

Author(s)

Michael J. Aminoff, MD, DSc, FRCP

Wernicke's Encephalopathy

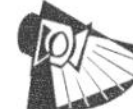

KEY FEATURES

- Caused by thiamin deficiency
- In United States, occurs most commonly in alcoholic patients
- It may also occur in patients with AIDS, in patients with hyperemesis gravidarum, or after surgery for morbid obesity

CLINICAL FINDINGS

- Triad of confusion, ataxia, and nystagmus leading to ophthalmoplegia (lateral rectus muscle weakness, conjugate gaze palsies)
- Peripheral neuropathy may be present

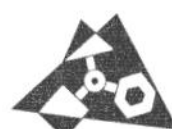

DIAGNOSIS

- The diagnosis is confirmed by the response to treatment within 1 or 2 days, which must not be delayed while laboratory confirmation is obtained

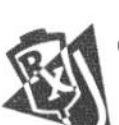

TREATMENT

- In suspected cases, thiamin 50 mg, is given IV immediately and then IM on a daily basis until a satisfactory diet can be ensured
- IV glucose given before thiamin may precipitate the syndrome or worsen the symptoms

Author(s)

Michael J. Aminoff, MD, DSc, FRCP

Yellow Fever

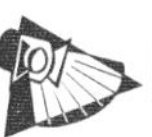

KEY FEATURES

- Zoonotic viral infection transmitted by the bite of the *Aedes* mosquito
- Found in South America and sub-Saharan Africa (not Asia)
- Incubation period is typically 3–6 days
- Adults and children equally susceptible

CLINICAL FINDINGS

- Mild form (85%): fevers, malaise, retro-orbital pain, nausea, photophobia, bradycardia
- Severe form (15%): begins with the same symptoms as the mild form of the disease; then, after initial remission of symptoms, a toxic phase ensues with fever, bradycardia, hypotension, jaundice, delirium, hemorrhage

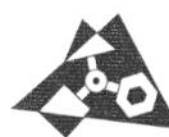

DIAGNOSIS

- Leukopenia often but not always present
- Abnormal liver function tests, including prolonged PT
- Proteinuria, often in large quantities
- Serologic diagnosis with rapid enzyme immunoassay

TREATMENT

- Supportive measures, including analgesia and hydration
- No specific antiviral therapy
- Prevention: a highly effective and safe vaccine is available and should be used when living or traveling to endemic areas
- Prevention: mosquito control measures

Author(s)

Wayne X. Shandera, MD

Ana Moran, MD

Reference Tables

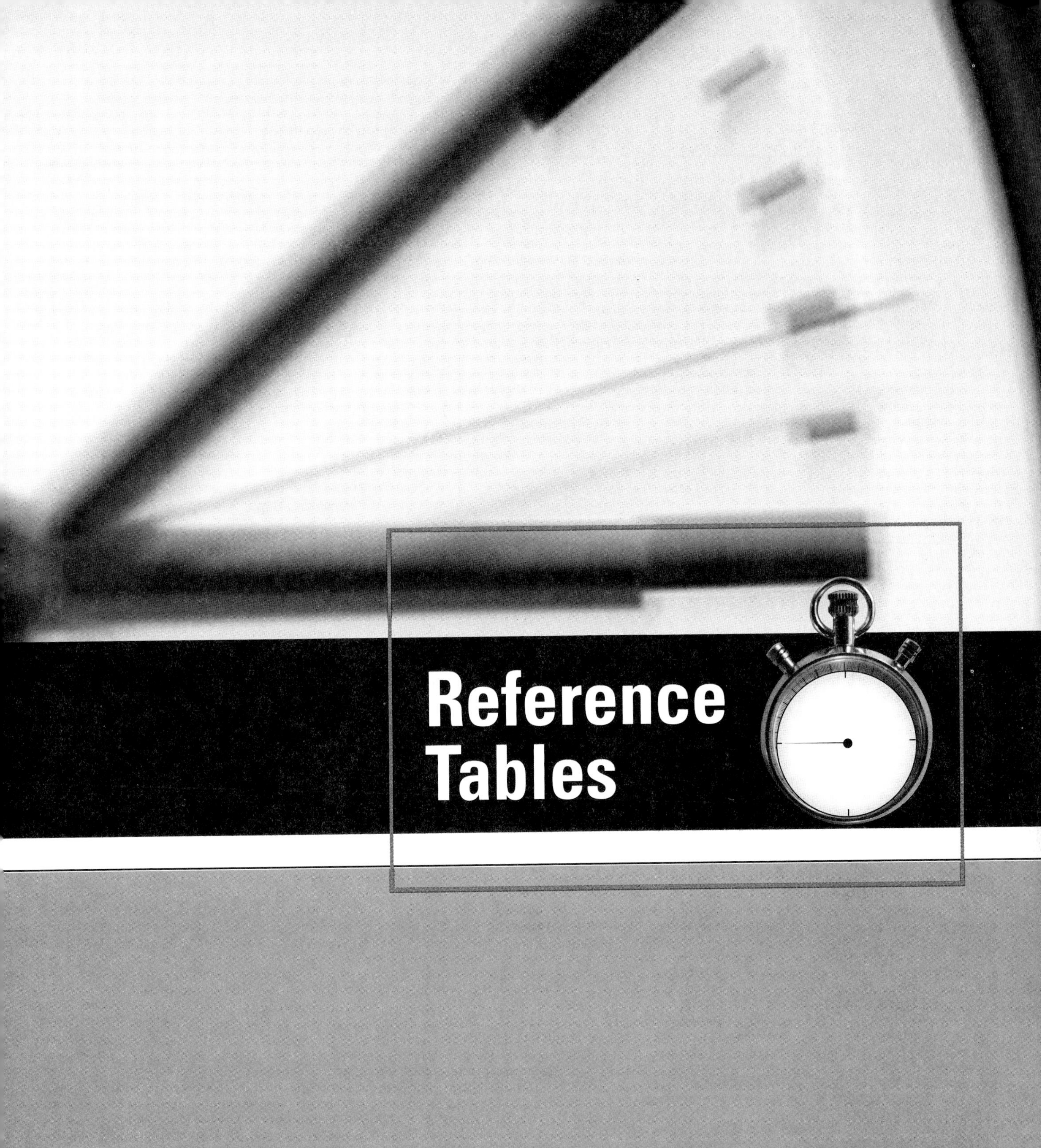

Table 1. Acetaminophen, COX-2 inhibitors, and useful nonsteroidal anti-inflammatory drugs.

Drug	Usual Dose for Adults ≥ 50 kg	Usual Dose for Adults < 50 kg[1]	Cost per Unit	Cost for 30 Days[2]	Comments[3]
Acetaminophen[4] (Tylenol, Datril, etc)	650 mg q4h or 975 mg q6h	10–15 mg/kg q4h (oral); 15–20 mg/kg q4h (rectal)	\$0.02/325 mg (oral) OTC; \$0.45/650 mg (rectal) OTC	\$7.20 (oral); \$81.00 (rectal)	Not an NSAID because it lacks peripheral anti-inflammatory effects. Equivalent to aspirin as analgesic and antipyretic agent.
Aspirin[5]	650 mg q4h or 975 mg q6h	10–15 mg/kg q4h (oral); 15–20 mg/kg q4h (rectal)	\$0.02/325 mg OTC; \$0.26/600 mg (rectal) OTC	\$7.20 (oral); \$46.80 (rectal)	Available also in enteric-coated form that is more expensive and more slowly absorbed but better tolerated.
Celecoxib[4] (Celebrex)	200 mg qd (osteoarthritis); 100–200 mg bid (rheumatoid arthritis)	100 mg qd–bid	\$1.91/100 mg; \$3.14/200 mg	\$94.20 OA; \$188.40 RA	Cyclooxygenase-2 inhibitor. No antiplatelet effects. Lower doses for elderly who weigh < 50 kg. Lower incidence of endoscopic gastrointestinal ulceration. Not known if true lower incidence of gastrointestinal bleeding. Possible link to cardiovascular toxicity. Celecoxib is contraindicated in sulfonamide allergy.
Choline magnesium salicylate[6] (Trilasate, others)	1000–1500 mg tid	25 mg/kg tid	\$0.57/500 mg	\$153.90	Salicylates cause less gastrointestinal distress and renal impairment than NSAIDs but are probably less effective in pain management than NSAIDs.
Diclofenac (Voltaren, Cataflam, others)	50–75 mg bid–tid		\$0.86/50 mg; \$1.04/75 mg	\$77.40; \$93.60	May impose higher risk of hepatotoxicity. Low incidence of gastrointestinal side effects. Enteric-coated product; slow onset.
Diclofenac Sustained Release (Voltaren-XR, others)	100–200 mg qd		\$2.81/100 mg	\$168.60	
Diflunisal[7] (Dolobid, others)	500 mg q12h		\$1.29/500 mg	\$77.40	Fluorinated acetylsalicylic acid derivative.
Etodolac (Lodine, others)	200–400 mg q6–8h		\$1.26/300 mg	\$151.20	Perhaps less gastrointestinal toxicity.
Fenoprofen calcium (Nalfon, others)	300–600 mg q6h		\$0.51/300 mg or 600 mg	\$61.20	Perhaps more side effects than others, including tubulointerstitial nephritis.
Flurbiprofen (Ansaid)	50–100 mg tid–qid		\$0.79/50 mg; \$1.19/100 mg	\$94.80; \$142.80	Adverse gastrointestinal effects may be more common among elderly.
Ibuprofen (Motrin, Advil, Rufen, others)	400–800 mg q6h	10 mg/kg q6–8h	\$0.28/600 mg Rx; \$0.05/200 mg OTC	\$33.60; \$9.00	Relatively well tolerated. Less gastrointestinal toxicity.
Indomethacin (Indocin, Indometh, others)	25–50 mg bid–qid		\$0.38/25 mg; \$0.64/50 mg	\$45.60; \$76.80	Higher incidence of dose-related toxic effects, especially gastrointestinal and bone marrow effects.
Ketoprofen (Orudis, Oruvail, others)	25–75 mg q6–8h (max 300 mg/d)		\$0.96/50 mg Rx; \$1.07/75 mg Rx; \$0.09/12.5 mg OTC	\$172.80; \$128.40; \$16.20	Lower doses for elderly.
Ketorolac tromethamine (Toradol)	10 mg q4–6h to a maximum of 40 mg/d PO		\$0.93/10 mg	Not recommended	Short-term use (< 5 days) only; otherwise, increased risk of gastrointestinal side effects.

(*continued*)

Table 1. Acetaminophen, COX-2 inhibitors, and useful nonsteroidal anti-inflammatory drugs. (continued)

Drug	Usual Dose for Adults ≥ 50 kg	Usual Dose for Adults < 50 kg[1]	Cost per Unit	Cost for 30 Days[2]	Comments[3]
Ketorolac tromethamine[8] (Toradol)	60 mg IM or 30 mg IV initially, then 30 mg q6h IM or IV		$3.89/30 mg	Not recom-mended	Intramuscular or intravenous NSAID as alternative to opioid. Lower doses for elderly. Short-term use (< 5 days) only.
Magnesium salicyl-ate (various)	650 mg q4h		$0.17/325 mg OTC	$40.80	
Meclofenamate sodium[9] (Meclomen)	50–100 mg q6h		$3.40/100 mg	$408.00	Diarrhea more common.
Mefenamic acid (Ponstel)	250 mg q6h		$2.28/250 mg	$273.60	
Nabumetone (Relafen)	500–1000 mg once daily (max dose 2000 mg/d)		$1.30/500 mg; $1.53/750 mg	$91.80	May be less ulcerogenic than ibuprofen, but overall side effects may not be less.
Naproxen (Naprosyn, Anaprox, Aleve [OTC], others)	250–500 mg q6–8h	5 mg/kg q8h	$1.16/500 mg Rx; $0.09/220 mg OTC	$104.40; $8.10 OTC	Generally well tolerated. Lower doses for elderly.
Oxaprozin (Day-pro, others)	600–1200 mg once daily		$1.51/600 mg	$90.60	Similar to ibuprofen. May cause rash, pruritus, pho-tosensitivity.
Piroxicam (Feldene, others)	20 mg daily		$2.64/20 mg	$79.20	Single daily dose convenient. Long half-life. May cause higher rate of gastrointestinal bleeding and dermatologic side effects. High adverse drug reac-tion rate in the elderly.
Sodium salicylate	325–650 mg q3–4h		$0.08/650 mg OTC	$19.20	
Sulindac (Clinoril, others)	150–200 mg bid		$0.98/150 mg; $1.21/200 mg	$58.80; $72.60	May cause higher rate of gastrointestinal bleeding. May have less nephrotoxic potential.
Tolmetin (Tolectin)	200–600 mg qid		$0.65/200 mg; $1.62/600 mg	$78.00; $194.40	Perhaps more side effects than others, including anaphylactic reactions.

Modified from Jacox AK et al: *Management of Cancer Pain: Quick Reference Guide for Clinicians No. 9.* AHCPR Publication No. 94-0593. Rockville, MD: Agency for Health Care Policy and Research, Public Health Service, U.S. Department of Health and Human Services. March 1994.

[1]Acetaminophen and NSAID dosages for adults weighing less than 50 kg should be adjusted for weight.

[2]Average wholesale price (AWP, for AB-rated generic when available) for quantity listed. Source: *Red Book* Update, Vol. 24, No. 4, April 2005. AWP may not accurately represent the actual pharmacy cost because wide contractual variations exist among institutions.

[3]The adverse effects of headache, tinnitus, dizziness, confusion, rashes, anorexia, nausea, vomiting, gastrointestinal bleeding, diarrhea, nephrotoxicity, visual disturbances, etc, can occur with any of these drugs. Tolerance and efficacy are subject to great individual variations among patients. Note: All NSAIDs can increase serum lithium levels.

[4]Acetaminophen and celecoxib lack the antiplatelet activities of other NSAIDs.

[5]May inhibit platelet aggregation for 1 week or more and may cause bleeding.

[6]May have minimal antiplatelet activity.

[7]Administration with antacids may decrease absorption.

[8]Has the same gastrointestinal toxicities as oral NSAIDs.

[9]Coombs-positive autoimmune hemolytic anemia has been associated with prolonged use.

OTC = over-the-counter; Rx = prescription; OA = osteoarthritis; RA = rheumatoid arthritis.

Table 2. Useful opioid agonist analgesics.

Drug	Approximate Equianalgesic Dose[1]		Usual Starting Dose				Potential Advantages	Potential Disadvantages
			Adults ≥ 50 kg Body Weight		Adults < 50 kg Body Weight			
	Oral	Parenteral	Oral	Parenteral	Oral	Parenteral		
OPIOID AGONISTS[2]								
Fentanyl	Not available	0.1 (100 mcg) q1h	Not available	50–100 mcg IV/IM q1h or 0.5–1.5 mcg/kg/h IV infusion	Not available	0.5–1 mcg/kg IV q1–4h or 1–2 mcg/kg IV x1, then 0.5–1 mcg/kg/h infusion	Possibly less neuroexcitatory effects, including in renal failure. Oral transmucosal formulation also available.	
Fentanyl Transdermal	Not available orally but can use "2:1 Rule[2]" for transdermal formulation	Not available	Not available orally but 25 mcg patch q72h	Not available	Not available orally but 25 mcg patch q72h	Not available	Stable medication blood levels	Not for use in opioid-naïve patients
Hydromorphone[3] (Dilaudid)	7.5 mg q3–4h	1.5 mg q3–4h	6 mg q3–4h; $0.37/2 mg	1.5 mg q3–4h; $1.06/2 mg	0.06 mg/q3–4h	0.015 mg/kg q3–4h	Similar to morphine. Available in injectable high-potency preparation, rectal suppository.	Short duration. (Extended release formulation (Palladone) recently approved by the FDA, limited availability.)
Hydromorphone (Palladone, extended release hydromorphone)	12 mg q24h	Not available	12 mg q24h; $7.70/12 mg	Not available	Not available	Not available		
Levorphanol (Levo-Dromoran)	4 mg q6–8h	2 mg q6–8h	4 mg q6–8h; $1.07/2 mg	2 mg q6–8h; $3.96/2 mg	0.04 mg/kg q6–8h	0.02 mg q6–8h	Longer-acting than morphine sulfate.	
Meperidine[4] (Demerol)	300 mg q2–3h; normal dose 50–150 mg q3–4h	100 mg q3h; $0.69/50 mg	Not recommended; $0.69/50 mg	100 mg q3h; $0.98/100 mg	Not recommended	0.75 mg/kg q2–3h	May be useful for acute pain if the patient is intolerant to morphine.	Short duration. Metabolite in high concentrations may cause seizures.
Methadone (Dolophine, others)	20 mg q6–8h	10 mg q6–8h	20 mg q6–8h; $0.15/10 mg	10 mg q6–8h; $3.75/10 mg	0.2 mg/kg q6–8h	0.1 mg/kg q6–8h	Somewhat longer-acting than morphine. Useful in cases of intolerance to morphine.	Analgesic duration shorter than plasma duration. May accumulate, requiring close monitoring during first weeks of treatment. Equianalgesic ratios vary with dose.
Morphine[3] Immediate release (Roxanol)	30 mg q3–4h (repeat around- the-clock dosing); 60 mg q3–4h (single or intermittent dosing)	10 mg q3–4h	30 mg q3–4h; $0.18/15 mg	10 mg q3–4h; $0.76/10 mg	0.3 mg/kg q3–4h	0.1 mg/kg q3–4h	Standard of comparison; multiple dosage forms available.	No unique problems when compared with other opioids.

(continued)

Table 2. Useful opioid agonist analgesics. (continued)

Drug	Approximate Equianalgesic Dose[1]		Usual Starting Dose				Potential Advantages	Potential Disadvantages
			Adults ≥ 50 kg Body Weight		Adults < 50 kg Body Weight			
	Oral	Parenteral	Oral	Parenteral	Oral	Parenteral		
Morphine Controlled-release[3] (MS Contin, Oramorph)	90–120 mg q12h	Not available	90–120 mg q12h; $1.89/30 mg	Not available	Not available	Not available		
Morphine Extended release (Kadian, Avinza)	180–240 mg q24h	Not available	20–30 mg q24h; $2.65/30 mg	Not available	Not available	Not available	Once-daily dosing	
Oxycodone (Roxicodone, OxyIR)	30 mg q3–4h	Not available	10 mg q3–4h; $0.35/5 mg	Not available	0.2 mg/kg q3–4h	Not available	Similar to morphine.	
Oxycodone Controlled release (Oxycontin)	40 mg q12h	Not available	20–40 mg q12h; $3.12/20 mg					
Oxymorphone[5] (Numorphan)	Not available	1 mg q3–4h	Not available	1 mg q3–4h; $3.26/1 mg			Active metabolite of oxycodone	
COMBINATION OPIOID-NSAID PREPARATIONS								
Codeine[6,7] (with aspirin or acetaminophen)[8]	180–200 mg q3–4h; normal dose, 15–60 mg q4–6h	130 mg q3–4h	60 mg q4–6h; $0.64/60 mg	60 mg q2h (IM/SC); $1.06/60 mg	0.5–1 mg/kg q3–4h	Not recommended	Similar to morphine.	Closely monitor for efficacy as patients vary in their ability to convert the prodrug codeine to morphine
Hydrocodone[5] (in Lorcet, Lortab, Vicodin, others)[8]	30 mg q3–4h	Not available	10 mg q3–4h; $0.32/5 mg	Not available	0.2 mg/kg q3–4h	Not available		Combination with acetaminophen limits dosage titration.
Oxycodone[6] (in Percocet, Percodan, Tylox, others)[8]	30 mg q3–4h	Not available	10 mg q3–4h; $0.31/5 mg	Not available	0.2 mg/kg q3–4h	Not available	Similar to morphine.	Combination with acetaminophen and aspirin limits dosage titration.

Modified from Jacox AK et al: *Management of Cancer Pain: Quick Reference Guide for Clinicians No. 9.* AHCPR Publication No. 94–0593. Rockville, MD. Agency for Health Care Policy and Research, Public Health Service, U.S. Department of Health and Human Services. March 1994. Reproduced in part from Hosp Formul 1994;29(8 Part 2):586. (Erstad BL: A rational approach to the management of acute pain states.) Copyright by Advanstar Communications, Inc.

[1]Published tables vary in the suggested doses that are equianalgesic to morphine. Clinical response is the criterion that must be applied for each patient; titration to clinical efficacy is necessary. Because there is not complete cross-tolerance among these drugs, it is usually necessary to use a lower than equianalgesic dose initially when changing drugs and to retitrate to response.

[2]Dosing of transdermal fentanyl can be based on the "2:1 Rule"—the approximate equianalgesic dose of transdermal fentanyl in mcg/h is half the 24 hour mg dose of oral morphine.

[3]***Caution:*** For morphine, hydromorphone, and oxymorphone, rectal administration is an alternative route for patients unable to take oral medications. Equianalgesic doses may differ from oral and parenteral doses. A short-acting opioid should normally be used for initial therapy.

[4]Not recommended for chronic pain. Doses listed are for brief therapy of acute pain only. Switch to another opioid for long-term therapy.

[5]***Caution:*** Recommended doses do not apply for adult patients with renal or hepatic insufficiency or other conditions affecting drug metabolism.

[6]***Caution:*** Doses of aspirin and acetaminophen in combination products must also be adjusted to the patient's body weight (Table 5–6).

[7]***Caution:*** Doses of codeine above 60 mg often are not appropriate because of diminishing incremental analgesia with increasing doses but continually increasing nausea, constipation, and other side effects.

[8]***Caution:*** Monitor total acetaminophen dose carefully, including any OTC use. Total acetaminophen dose maximum 4 g/d. If liver impairment or heavy alcohol use, maximum is 2 g/d.

Note: Average wholesale price (AWP, generic when available) for quantity listed. Source: *Red Book* Update, Vol. 24, No. 4, April 2005. AWP may not accurately represent the actual pharmacy because wide contractual variations exist among institutions.

Patient Name ______________ Date ________
Source: Pt ________ Other ________

HISTORY ITEMS	ABNORMAL	ACTION	RESULT AND COMMENTS
"Have you had any falls in the last year?"	Yes	Gait assessment Further exam, home evaluation and PT Osteoporosis and injury risk assessment	________
"Do you have trouble with stairs, lighting, bathroom hazards, or other home hazards?"	Yes to any	Home evaluation or PT	________
"Do you have a problem with urine leaks or accidents?"	Yes	Rule out transient (DIAPPERS) History (stress, urge), exam, PVR	________
"Over the past month, have you often been bothered by feeling sad, depressed, or hopeless?"	Yes to either	GDS or other depression assessment	________
"During the past month, have you often been bothered by little interest or pleasure in doing things?"	Yes to either		
Do you ever feel unsafe where you live?	Yes	Explore further, social work, APS	________
Does anyone threaten you or hurt you?	Yes		
Is pain a problem for you?	Yes	Evaluate ________	

Do you have any problems with any of the following areas? Who assists? Do you use any devices? (for "yes" answers, consider causes, social services, and home eval/PT/OT)

Doing strenuous activities like fast walking/bicycling?	________
Cooking?	________
Shopping?	________
Doing heavy housework like washing windows?	________
Doing laundry?	________
Getting to a place beyond walking distance by driving or taking a bus?	________
Managing finances?	________
Getting out of bed/transfer?	________
Dressing?	________
Toilet?	________
Eating?	________
Walking?	________
Bathing (sponge bath, tub, or shower)?	________

Review medications that the patient brought in Also ask about herbs, vitamins, supplements, and nonprescription medications	Confusion about medications > 5 medications Doesn't bring in	Consider simplification Medi-set or other aid Consider home visit	________
PHYSICAL EXAM ITEMS (The next few items may be performed by nursing staff in some settings)			
Weight/BMI And ask "have you lost weight?" If so, how much?	BMI < 21 Loss of 5% since last visit Or 10% over 1 year	Alert provider or nutrition evaluation Consider medical, dental, social causes	________
Jaeger Card or Snellen eye chart Test each eye (with glasses)	Can't read 20/40	Alert provider or refer	________
Whisper short sentences at 6–12 inches (out of visual view) OR audioscopy	Unable to hear Retest/refer	Cerumen check Hearing handicap inventory	________
Name three objects/re-ask in 5 minutes Clock draw test	Misses any or unable	MMSE	________
"Rise from the chair (do not use arms to get up), walk 10 feet, turn, walk back to the chair and sit down"	Observed problem or unable in < 10 seconds	Further gait and neurologic exam Home evaluation and PT	________
"Touch the back of your head with your hands" "Pick up the pencil"	Unable to do either	Further exam Consider OT	________

(Remember to ask about the 3 items!)

Other areas of concern: caregiver stress, alcohol use, social isolation, exercise, driving, advance directives and health care wishes.

Table 3. Simple geriatric screen. PT = physical therapy; DIAPPERS = delirium, infection, atrophic urethritis or vaginitis, pharmaceuticals, psychological factors, excess urinary output, restricted mobility, stool impaction; PVR = postvoid residual; GDS = Geriatric Depression Screen; APS = Adult Protective Services; OT = occupational therapy; BMI = body mass index; MMSE = Mini-Mental State Exam. (Modified from Lachs M et al: A simple procedure for general screening for functional disability in elderly patients. Ann Intern Med 1990;112:699 and Moore AA et al: Screening for common problems in ambulatory elderly: clinical confirmation of a screening instrument. Am J Med 1996;100:438.)

COMPLETE IF INDICATED CLINICALLY
(Ask general question and then ask specific questions to the right.)

Orientation *(Score 1 for each correct; max = 10)*

Where are you?
- Name this place (building or hospital)
- What floor are you on now?
- What state are you in?
- What country are you in?
- (If not in a country, score correct if city is correct.)
- What city are you in (or near) now?

What is the date today?
- What year is it?
- What season is it?
- What month is it?
- What is the day of the week?
- What is the date today?

Registration *(Score 1 for each object correctly repeated; max = 3)*

Name three objects (ball, flag, and tree) and have the patient repeat them.
(Say objects at about 1 word per second. If patient misses object, ask patient to repeat them after you until he/she learns them. Stop at 6 repeats.)

Attention and calculation *(Score 1 for each correct to 65; max = 5)*

Subtract 7s from 100 in a serial fashion to 65
(Alternatively, subtract serial 3s from 20 or spell WORLD backwards.)

Recall *(Score 1 for each object recalled; max = 3)*

Do you recall the names of the three objects?

Language (max = 8)

Ask the patient to provide names of a watch and pen as you show them to him/her
(Score 1 for each object correct; max = 2)

Repeat "No ifs, ands, or buts."
(Only one trial. Score 1 if correct; max = 1)

Give the patient a piece of plain blank paper and say, "Take the paper in your right hand (1), fold it in half (2), and put it on the floor (3)."
(Score 1 for each part done correctly; max = 3)

Ask the patient to read and perform the following task written on paper: Close your eyes.
(Score 1 if patient closes eyes; max = 1)

Ask the patient to write a sentence on a piece of paper.
(Score total of 1 if sentence has a subject, object and verb; max = 1)

Construction

Ask patient to copy the two interlocking pentagons.
(Score total of 1, if all 10 angles are present and the two angles intersect. Ignore tremor and rotation; max = 1)

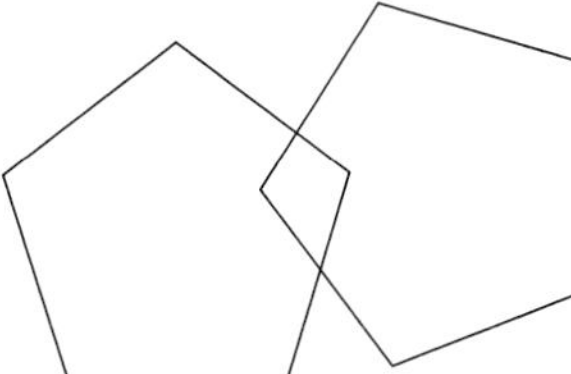

Total Score *(Maximum = 30, likely organic < 27)*

Figure 1. Mini-mental State Exam. (Adapted from Folstein MF et al: Mini-mental state: a practical method for grading the cognitive state of patients for the clinician. J Psychiatr Res 1975;12:189.)

Table 4. Yesavage's Geriatric Depression Scale (short form).

1. Are you basically satisfied with your life? (no)
2. Have you dropped many of your activities and interests? (yes)
3. Do you feel that your life is empty? (yes)
4. Do you often get bored? (yes)
5. Are you in good spirits most of the time? (no)
6. Are you afraid that something bad is going to happen to you? (yes)
7. Do you feel happy most of the time? (no)
8. Do you often feel helpless? (yes)
9. Do you prefer to stay home at night, rather than go out and do new things? (yes)
10. Do you feel that you have more problems with memory than most? (yes)
11. Do you feel it is wonderful to be alive now? (no)
12. Do you feel pretty worthless the way you are now? (yes)
13. Do you feel full of energy? (no)
14. Do you feel that your situation is hopeless? (yes)
15. Do you think that most persons are better off than you are? (yes)

Score one point for each response that matches the yes or no answer after the question.

Key: Scores: 3 ± 2 = normal; 7 ± 3 = mildly depressed; 12 ± 2 = very depressed.

Table 5. Fall risk factors and targeted interventions.

Risk Factor	Targeted Intervention
Postural hypotension (> 20 mm Hg drop in systolic blood pressure, or systolic blood pressure < 90 mm Hg)	Behavioral recommendations, such as hand clenching, elevation of head of bed; discontinuation or substitution of high-risk medications
Use of benzodiazepine or sedative-hypnotic agent	Education about sleep hygiene; discontinuation or substitution of medications
Use of three prescription medications	Review of medications
Environmental hazards	Appropriate changes; installation of safety equipment (eg, grab bars)
Gait impairment	Gait training, assistive devices, balance or strengthening exercises
Impairment in transfer or balance	Balance exercises, training in transfers, environmental alterations (eg, grab bars)
Impairment in leg or arm muscle strength or limb range of motion	Exercise with resistance bands or putty, with graduated increases in resistance

Table 6. Useful topical dermatologic therapeutic agents.

Agent	Formulations, Strengths, and Prices[1]	Apply	Potency Class	Common Indications	Comments
Corticosteroids					
Hydrocortisone acetate	Cream 1%: $3.60/30 g Ointment 1%: $3.72/30 g Lotion 1%: $20.20/120 mL	bid	Low	Seborrheic dermatitis. Pruritus ani. Intertrigo.	Not the same as hydrocortisone butyrate or valerate! Not for poison oak! OTC lotion (Aquinil HC). OTC solution (Scalpicin, T Scalp).
	Cream 2.5%: $8.95/30 g	bid	Low	As for 1% hydrocortisone.	Perhaps better for pruritus ani. Not clearly better than 1%. More expensive. Not OTC.
Alclometasone dipropionate (Aclovate)	Cream 0.05%: $20.42/15 g Ointment 0.05%: $42.60/45 g	bid	Low	As for hydrocortisone.	More efficacious than hydrocortisone. Perhaps causes less atrophy.
Desonide	Cream 0.05%: $15.45/15 g Ointment 0.05%: $40.15/60 g Lotion 0.05%: $32.83/60 mL	bid	Low	As for hydrocortisone. For lesions on face or body folds resistant to hydrocortisone.	More efficacious than hydrocortisone. Can cause rosacea or atrophy. Not fluorinated.
Prednicarbate (Dermatop)	Emollient cream 0.1%: $21.83/15 g Ointment 0.1%: $21.65/15 g	bid	Medium	As for triamcinolone.	May cause less atrophy. No generic formulations. Preservative-free.
Triamcinolone acetonide	Cream 0.1%: $3.60/15 g Ointment 0.1%: $3.60/15 g Lotion 0.1%: $42.44/60 mL	bid	Medium	Eczema on extensor areas. Used for psoriasis with tar. Seborrheic dermatitis and psoriasis on scalp.	Caution in body folds, face. Economical in 0.5-lb and 1-lb sizes for treatment of large body surfaces. Economical as solution for scalp.
	Cream 0.025%: $3.00/15 g Ointment 0.025%: $5.25/80 g	bid	Medium	As for 0.1% strength.	Possibly less efficacy and few advantages over 0.1% formulation.
Fluocinolone acetonide	Cream 0.025%: $3.05/15 g Ointment 0.025%: $4.20/15 g	bid	Medium	As for triamcinolone.	
	Solution 0.01%: $11.00/60 mL	bid	Medium	As for triamcinolone solution.	
Mometasone furoate (Elocon)	Cream 0.1%: $29.41/15 g Ointment 0.1%: $24.30/15 g Lotion 0.1%: $60.91/60 mL	qd	Medium	As for triamcinolone.	Often used inappropriately on the face or in children. Not fluorinated.
Diflorasone diacetate	Cream 0.05%: $36.78/15 g Ointment 0.05%: $51.86/30 g	bid	High	Nummular dermatitis. Allergic contact dermatitis. Lichen simplex chronicus.	
Amcinonide (Cyclocort)	Cream 0.1%: $20.58/15 g Ointment 0.1%: $30.68/30 g	bid	High	As for betamethasone.	

(continued)

Table 6. Useful topical dermatologic therapeutic agents. (continued)

Agent	Formulations, Strengths, and Prices[1]	Apply	Potency Class	Common Indications	Comments
Fluocinonide (Lidex)	Cream 0.05%: $10.61/15 g Gel 0.05%: $21.01/15 g Ointment 0.05%: $21.25/15 g Solution 0.05%: $27.27/60 mL	bid	High	As for betamethasone. Gel useful for poison oak.	Economical generics. Lidex cream can cause stinging on eczema. Lidex emollient cream preferred.
Betamethasone dipropionate (Diprolene)	Cream 0.05%: $7.80/15 g Ointment 0.05%: $9.40/15 g Lotion 0.05%: $30.49/60 mL	bid	Ultra-high	For lesions resistant to high-potency steroids. Lichen planus. Insect bites.	Economical generics available.
Clobetasol propionate (Temovate)	Cream 0.05%: $24.71/15 g Ointment 0.05%: $24.71/15 g Lotion 0.05%: $53.10/50 mL	bid	Ultra-high	As for betamethasone dipropionate.	Somewhat more potent than diflorasone. Limited to 2 continuous weeks of use. Limited to 50 g or less per week. Cream may cause stinging; use "emollient cream" formulation. Generic available.
Halobetasol propionate (Ultravate)	Cream 0.05%: $34.75/15 g Ointment 0.05%: $34.75/15 g	bid	Ultra-high	As for clobetasol.	Same restrictions as clobetasol. Cream does not cause stinging. Compatible with calcipotriene (Dovonex).
Flurandrenolide (Cordran)	Tape: $47.31/80″ × 3″ roll Lotion 0.05%: $45.42/60 mL	q12h	Ultra-high	Lichen simplex chronicus.	Protects the skin and prevents scratching.
Nonsteroidal anti-inflammatory agents					
Tacrolimus[2] (Protopic)	Ointment 0.1%: $67.82/30 g Ointment 0.03%: $63.46/30 g	bid	N/A	Atopic dermatitis.	Steroid substitute not causing atrophy or striae. Burns in ≥ 40% of patients with eczema.
Pimecrolimus[2] (Elidel)	Cream 1%: $56.53/30 g	bid	N/A	Atopic dermatitis.	Steroid substitute not causing atrophy or striae.
Antibiotics (for acne)					
Clindamycin phosphate	Solution 1%: $12.09/30 mL Gel 1%: $38.13/30 mL Lotion 1%: $53.06/60 mL Pledget 1%: $50.25/60	bid	N/A	Mild papular acne.	Lotion is less drying for patients with sensitive skin.
Erythromycin	Solution 2%: $7.53/60 mL Gel 2%: $24.73/30 g Pledget 2%: $26.07/60	bid	N/A	As for clindamycin.	Many different manufacturers. Economical.
Erythromycin/ Benzoyl peroxide (Benzamycin)	Gel: $68.60/23.3 g Gel: $128.00/46.6 g	bid	N/A	As for clindamycin. Can help treat comedonal acne.	No generics. More expensive. More effective than other topical antibiotics. Main jar requires refrigeration.
Clindamycin/ Benzoyl peroxide (Benzeclin)	Gel: $64.97/25 g Gel: $122.84/50 g	bid		As for benzamycin.	No generic. More effective than either agent alone.

(*continued*)

Table 6. Useful topical dermatologic therapeutic agents. (continued)

Agent	Formulations, Strengths, and Prices[1]	Apply	Potency Class	Common Indications	Comments
Antibiotics (for impetigo)					
Mupirocin (Bactroban)	Ointment 2%: $42.75/22 g Cream 2%: $34.39/15 g	tid	N/A	Impetigo, folliculitis.	Because of cost, use limited to tiny areas of impetigo. Used in the nose twice daily for 5 days to reduce staphylococcal carriage.
Antifungals					
Clotrimazole	Cream 1%: $5.29/15 g OTC Solution 1%: $5.69/10 mL	bid	N/A	Dermatophyte and candida infections.	Available OTC. Inexpensive generic cream available.
Miconazole	Cream 2%: $2.36/30 g OTC	bid	N/A	As for clotrimazole.	As for clotrimazole.
Other imidazoles					
Econazole (Spectazole)	Cream 1%: $19.27/15 g	qd	N/A	As for clotrimazole.	No generic. Somewhat more effective than clotrimazole and miconazole.
Ketoconazole	Cream 2%: $16.85/15 g	qd	N/A	As for clotrimazole.	No generic. Somewhat more effective than clotrimazole and miconazole.
Oxiconazole (Oxistat)	Cream 1%: $23.66/15 g Lotion 1%: $39.83/30 mL	bid	N/A		
Sulconazole (Exelderm)	Cream 1%: $12.56/15 g Solution 1%: $27.05/30 mL	bid	N/A	As for clotrimazole.	No generic. Somewhat more effective than clotrimazole and miconazole.
Other antifungals					
Butenafine (Mentax)	Cream 1%: $40.27/15 g	qd	N/A	Dermatophytes.	Fast response; high cure rate; expensive. Available OTC.
Ciclopirox (Loprox) (Penlac)	Cream 0.77%: $47.13/30 g Lotion 0.77%: $96.15/60 mL Solution 8%: $137.46/6.6 mL	bid	N/A	As for clotrimazole.	No generic. Somewhat more effective than clotrimazole and miconazole.
Naftifine (Naftin)	Cream 1%: $44.16/30 g Gel 1%: $71.01/60 mL	qd	N/A	Dermatophytes.	No generic. Somewhat more effective than clotrimazole and miconazole.
Terbinafine (Lamisil)	Cream 1%: $6.79/12 g OTC	qd	N/A	Dermatophytes.	Fast clinical response. OTC.
Antipruritics					
Camphor/menthol	Compounded lotion (0.5% of each)	bid–tid	N/A	Mild eczema, xerosis, mild contact dermatitis.	
Pramoxine hydrochloride (Prax)	Lotion 1%: $13.33/120 mL	qid	N/A	Dry skin, varicella, mild eczema, pruritus ani.	OTC formulations (Prax, Aveeno Anti-Itch Cream or Lotion; Itch-X Gel). By prescription mixed with 1% or 2% hydrocortisone.
Doxepin (Zonalon)	Cream 5%: $64.19/30 g	qid	N/A	Topical antipruritic, best used in combination with appropriate topical steroid to enhance efficacy.	Can cause sedation.

(continued)

Table 6. Useful topical dermatologic therapeutic agents. (continued)

Agent	Formulations, Strengths, and Prices[1]	Apply	Potency Class	Common Indications	Comments
Emollients					
Aveeno	Cream, lotion, others	qd–tid	N/A	Xerosis, eczema.	Choice is most often based on personal preference by patient.
Aqua glycolic	Cream, lotion, shampoo, others	qd–tid	N/A	Xerosis, ichthyosis, keratosis pilaris. Mild facial wrinkles. Mild acne or seborrheic dermatitis.	Contains 8% glycolic acid. Available from other makers, eg, Alpha Hydrox, or generic 8% glycolic acid lotion. May cause stinging on eczematous skin.
Aquaphor	Ointment: $7.50/50 g	qd–tid	N/A	Xerosis, eczema. For protection of area in pruritus ani.	Not as greasy as petrolatum.
Carmol	Lotion 10%: $8.80/180 mL Cream 20%: $8.75/90 g	bid	N/A	Xerosis.	Contains urea as humectant. Nongreasy hydrating agent (10%); debrides keratin (20%).
Complex 15	Lotion: $6.48/240 mL Cream: $4.82/75 g	qd–tid	N/A	Xerosis. Lotion or cream recommended for split or dry nails.	Active ingredient is a phospholipid.
DML	Cream, lotion, facial moisturizer: $6.30/240 mL	qd–tid	N/A	As for Complex 15.	Face cream has sunscreen.
Eucerin	Cream: $5.10/120 g Lotion: $5.10/240 mL	qd–tid	N/A	Xerosis, eczema.	Many formulations made. Eucerin Plus contains alphahydroxy acid and may cause stinging on eczematous skin. Facial moisturizer has SPF 25 sunscreen.
Lac-Hydrin-Five	Lotion: $10.12/240 mL OTC	bid	N/A	Xerosis, ichthyosis, keratosis pilaris.	Rx product is 12%.
Lubriderm	Lotion: $5.03/300 mL	qd–tid	N/A	Xerosis, eczema.	Unscented usually preferred.
Neutrogena	Cream, lotion, facial moisturizer: $7.39/240 mL	qd–tid	N/A	Xerosis, eczema.	Face cream has titanium-based sunscreen.
SBR Lipocream	Cream: $7.43/30 g	qd-tid	N/A	Xerosis, eczema.	Less greasy but effective moisturizer.
Triceram Cream	Cream: $30.00/3.4-oz tube	bid	N/A	Xerosis, eczema.	Contains ceramide; anti-inflammatory and nongreasy moisturizer.
U-Lactin	Lotion: $7.13/240 mL	qd	N/A	Hyperkeratotic heels.	Moisturizes and removes keratin.

[1]Average wholesale price (AWP, for AB-rated generic when available) for quantity listed. AWP may not accurately represent the actual pharmacy cost because wide contractual variations exist among institutions. Source: *Red Book Update*, Vol. 24, No. 4, May 2005.

[2]Topical tacrolimus and pimecrolimus should only be used when other topical treatments are ineffective. Treatment duration should be limited to an area and be as brief as possible. Treatment with these agents should be avoided in persons with known immunosuppression, HIV infection, bone marrow and organ transplantation, lymphoma, at high risk for lymphoma, and those with a prior history of lymphoma.

OTC = over-the-counter; N/A = not applicable.

Table 7. Morphologic categorization of skin lesions and diseases.

Pigmented	Freckle, lentigo, seborrheic keratosis, nevus, blue nevus, halo nevus, dysplastic nevus, melanoma
Scaly	Psoriasis, dermatitis (atopic, stasis, seborrheic, chronic allergic contact or irritant contact), xerosis (dry skin), lichen simplex chronicus, tinea, tinea versicolor, secondary syphilis, pityriasis rosea, discoid lupus erythematosus, exfoliative dermatitis, actinic keratoses, Bowen's disease, Paget's disease, intertrigo
Vesicular	Herpes simplex, varicella, herpes zoster, dyshidrosis (vesicular dermatitis of palms and soles), vesicular tinea, dermatophytid, dermatitis herpetiformis, miliaria, scabies, photosensitivity
Weepy or encrusted	Impetigo, acute contact allergic dermatitis, any vesicular dermatitis
Pustular	Acne vulgaris, acne rosacea, folliculitis, candidiasis, miliaria, any vesicular dermatitis
Figurate ("shaped") erythema	Urticaria, erythema multiforme, erythema migrans, cellulitis, erysipelas, erysipeloid, arthropod bites
Bullous	Impetigo, blistering dactylitis, pemphigus, pemphigoid, porphyria cutanea tarda, drug eruptions, erythema multiforme, toxic epidermal necrolysis
Papular	Hyperkeratotic: warts, corns, seborrheic keratoses Purple-violet: lichen planus, drug eruptions, Kaposi's sarcoma Flesh-colored, umbilicated: molluscum contagiosum Pearly: basal cell carcinoma, intradermal nevi Small, red, inflammatory: acne, miliaria, candidiasis, scabies, folliculitis
Pruritus[1]	Xerosis, scabies, pediculosis, bites, systemic causes, anogenital pruritus
Nodular, cystic	Erythema nodosum, furuncle, cystic acne, follicular (epidermal) inclusion cyst
Photodermatitis (photodistributed rashes)	Drug, polymorphic light eruption, lupus erythematosus
Morbilliform	Drug, viral infection, secondary syphilis
Erosive	Any vesicular dermatitis, impetigo, aphthae, lichen planus, erythema multiforme
Ulcerated	Decubiti, herpes simplex, skin cancers, parasitic infections, syphilis (chancre), chancroid, vasculitis, stasis, arterial disease

[1]Not a morphologic class but included because it is one of the most common dermatologic presentations.

Table 8. Skin reactions due to systemic drugs.

Reaction	Appearance	Distribution and Comments	Common Offenders
Toxic erythema	Morbilliform, maculopapular, exanthematous reactions.	The most common skin reaction to drugs. Often more pronounced on the trunk than on the extremities. In previously exposed patients, the rash may start in 2–3 days. In the first course of treatment, the eruption often appears about the seventh to ninth days. Fever may be present.	Antibiotics (especially ampicillin and trimethoprim-sulfamethoxazole), sulfonamides and related compounds (including thiazide diuretics, furosemide, and sulfonylurea hypoglycemic agents), and barbiturates.
Erythema multiforme major	Target-like lesions. Bullae may occur. Mucosal involvement.	Mainly on the extensor aspects of the limbs.	Sulfonamides, penicillamine, barbiturates, and NSAIDs.
Erythema nodosum	Inflammatory cutaneous nodules.	Usually limited to the extensor aspects of the legs. May be accompanied by fever, arthralgias, and pain.	Oral contraceptives.
Allergic vasculitis	Inflammatory changes may present as urticaria that lasts over 24 hours, hemorrhagic papules ("palpable purpura"), vesicles, bullae, or necrotic ulcers.	Most severe on the legs.	Sulfonamides, indomethacin, phenytoin, allopurinol, and ibuprofen.
Purpura	Itchy, petechial macular rash.	Dependent areas. Results most typically from thrombocytopenia.	Thiazides, sulfonamides, sulfonylureas, barbiturates, quinine, and sulindac.
Eczema	Similar to contact dermatitis.	A rare reaction in patients previously sensitized by external exposure who are given the same or a related substance systemically.	Penicillin, neomycin, phenothiazines, and local anesthetics.
Exfoliative dermatitis and erythroderma	Red and scaly.	Entire skin surface.	Allopurinol, sulfonamides, isoniazid, gold, or carbamazepine.
Photosensitivity: increased sensitivity to light, often of ultraviolet A wavelengths, but may be due to UVB or visible light as well	Sunburn, vesicles, papules in photodistributed pattern.	Exposed skin of the face, the neck, and the backs of the hands and, in women, the lower legs. Exaggerated response to ultraviolet light.	Sulfonamides and sulfonamide-related compounds (thiazide diuretics, furosemide, sulfonylureas), tetracyclines, phenothiazines, sulindac, amiodarone, and NSAIDs.
Drug-related lupus erythematosus	May present with a photosensitive rash accompanied by fever, polyarthritis, myalgia, and serositis.	Less severe than systemic lupus erythematosus, sparing the kidneys and central nervous system. Recovery often follows drug withdrawal.	Hydralazine, procainamide; less often, isoniazid, phenytoin, lisinopril, hydrochlorothiazide; diltiazem; may cause subacute lupus erythematosus.

(continued)

Table 8. Skin reactions due to systemic drugs. (continued)

Reaction	Appearance	Distribution and Comments	Common Offenders
Lichenoid and lichen planus–like eruptions	Pruritic, erythematous to violaceous polygonal papules that coalesce or expand to form plaques.	May be in photo- or nonphotodistributed pattern.	Bismuth, carbamazepine, chlordiazepoxide, chloroquine, chlorpropamide, dapsone, ethambutol, furosemide, gold salts, hydroxychloroquine, methyldopa, penicillamine, phenothiazines, propranolol, quinidine, quinine, quinacrine, streptomycin, sulfonylureas, tetracyclines, thiazides, and triprolidine.
Fixed drug eruptions	Single or multiple demarcated, round, erythematous plaques that often become hyperpigmented.	Recur at the same site when the drug is repeated. Hyperpigmentation, if present, remains after healing.	Numerous drugs, including antimicrobials, analgesics, barbiturates, cardiovascular drugs, heavy metals, antiparasitic agents, antihistamines, phenolphthalein, ibuprofen, and naproxen.
Toxic epidermal necrolysis	Large sheets of erythema, followed by separation, which looks like scalded skin.	Rare.	In adults, the eruption has occurred after administration of many classes of drugs, particularly anticonvulsants, antibiotics, sulfonamides, and NSAIDs.
Urticaria	Red, itchy wheals that vary in size from < 1 cm to many centimeters. May be accompanied by angioedema.	Chronic urticaria is rarely caused by drugs.	Acute urticaria: penicillins, NSAIDs, sulfonamides, opiates, and salicylates. Angioedema is common in patients receiving ACE inhibitors.
Pruritus	Itchy skin without rash.		Pruritus ani may be due to overgrowth of candida after systemic antibiotic treatment. NSAIDs may cause pruritus without a rash.
Hair loss		Hair loss most often involves the scalp, but other sites may be affected.	A predictable side effect of cytotoxic agents and oral contraceptives. Diffuse hair loss also occurs unpredictably with a wide variety of other drugs, including anticoagulants, antithyroid drugs, newer antimicrobials, cholesterol-lowering agents, heavy metals, corticosteroids, androgens, NSAIDs, retinoids (isotretinoin, etretinate), and β-blockers.
Pigmentary changes	Flat hyperpigmented areas.	Forehead and cheeks (chloasma, melasma). The most common pigmentary disorder associated with drug ingestion. Improvement is slow despite stopping the drug.	Oral contraceptives are the usual cause.
	Blue-gray discoloration.	Light-exposed areas.	Chlorpromazine and related phenothiazines.
	Brown or blue-gray pigmentation.	Generalized.	Heavy metals (silver, gold, bismuth, and arsenic). Arsenic, silver, and bismuth are not used therapeutically, but patients who receive gold for rheumatoid arthritis may show this reaction.
	Yellow color.	Generalized.	Usually quinacrine.

(continued)

Table 8. Skin reactions due to systemic drugs. (continued)

Reaction	Appearance	Distribution and Comments	Common Offenders
Pigmentary changes (continued)	Blue-black patches on the shins.		Minocycline, chloroquine.
	Blue-black pigmentation of the nails and palate and depigmentation of the hair.		Chloroquine.
	Slate-gray color.	Primarily in photoexposed areas.	Amiodarone.
	Brown discoloration of the nails.	Especially in more darkly pigmented patients.	Zidovudine (azidothymidine; AZT), hydroxyurea.
Psoriasiform eruptions	Scaly red plaques.	May be located on trunk and extremities. Palms and soles may be hyperkeratotic. May cause psoriasiform eruption or worsen psoriasis.	Chloroquine, lithium, β-blockers, and quinacrine.
Pityriasis rosea–like eruptions	Oval, red, slightly raised patches with central scale.	Mainly on the trunk.	Barbiturates, bismuth, captopril, clonidine, gold salts, methopromazine, metoprolol, metronidazole, and tripelennamine.

NSAIDs = nonsteroidal anti-inflammatory drugs; ACE = angiotensin-converting enzyme.

Table 9. The inflamed eye: Differential diagnosis of common causes.

	Acute Conjunctivitis	Acute Uveitis	Acute Glaucoma[1]	Corneal Trauma or Infection
Incidence	Extremely common	Common	Uncommon	Common
Discharge	Moderate to copious	None	None	Watery or purulent
Vision	No effect on vision	Often blurred	Markedly blurred	Usually blurred
Pain	Mild	Moderate	Severe	Moderate to severe
Conjunctival injection	Diffuse; more toward fornices	Mainly circumcorneal	Mainly circumcorneal	Mainly circumcorneal
Cornea	Clear	Usually clear	Steamy	Clarity change related to cause
Pupil size	Normal	Small	Moderately dilated and fixed	Normal
Pupillary light response	Normal	Poor	None	Normal
Intraocular pressure	Normal	Commonly low but may be elevated	Elevated	Normal
Smear	Causative organisms	No organisms	No organisms	Organisms found only in corneal ulcers due to infection

[1]Angle-closure glaucoma.

Table 10. Topical ophthalmic agents.

Agent	Representative Cost/Size [1]	Sig	Indications
AGENTS FOR GLAUCOMA AND OCULAR HYPERTENSION			
Sympathomimetics			
Apraclonidine HCl 0.5% solution (Iopidine)	$66.48/5 mL	1 drop three times daily	Reduction of intraocular pressure. Expensive. Reserve for treatment of resistant cases.
Apraclonidine HCl 1% solution (Iopidine)	$11.03/unit dose 0.1 mL	1 drop 1 hour before and immediately after anterior segment laser surgery	To control or prevent elevations of intraocular pressure after laser trabeculoplasty or iridotomy.
Brimonidine tartrate 0.2% solution (Alphagan)	$32.65/5 mL	1 drop two or three times daily	Reduction of intraocular pressure.
Dipivefrin HCl 0.1% solution (Propine)[2]	$14.07/5 mL	1 drop every 12 hours	Open-angle glaucoma.
Epinephrine HCl 0.25%, 0.5% (Epifrin), 1%, and 2% solution (various)[3]	1%: $49.69/15 mL 2%: $54.36/15 mL	1 drop twice daily	
β-Adrenergic blocking agents			
Betaxolol HCl 0.5% solution and 0.25% suspension (Betoptic S)[4]	0.5%: $44.56/10 mL 0.25%: $78.24/10 mL	1 drop twice daily	Reduction of intraocular pressure.
Carteolol HCl 1% solution (Ocupress)[5]	$37.07/10 mL	1 drop twice daily	
Levobunolol HCl 0.25% and 0.5% solution (Betagan)[5]	0.5%: $32.25/10 mL	1 drop once or twice daily	
Metipranolol HCl 0.3% solution (OptiPranolol)[5]	$26.85/10 mL	1 drop twice daily	
Timolol 0.25% and 0.5% solution (Betimol)[5]	0.5%: $42.84/10 mL	1 drop once or twice daily	
Timolol maleate 0.25% and 0.5% solution (Timoptic) and 0.25% and 0.5% gel (Timoptic-XE)[5]	0.5% solution: $32.29/10 mL 0.5% gel: $32.30/5 mL	1 drop once or twice daily	
Miotics			
Pilocarpine HCl (various)[6] 1–4%, 6%, 8%, and 10%	2%: $11.80/15 mL	1 drop three or four times daily	Reduction of intraocular pressure, treatment of acute or chronic angle-closure glaucoma, and pupillary constriction.
Pilocarpine HCl 4% gel (Pilopine HS)	$42.00/4 g	Apply 0.5-inch ribbon in lower conjunctival sac at bedtime	
Carbonic anhydrase inhibitors			
Dorzolamide HCl 2% solution (Trusopt)	$55.88/10 mL	1 drop three times daily	Reduction of intraocular pressure.
Brinzolamide 1% suspension (Azopt)	$67.80/10 mL	1 drop three times daily	
Prostaglandin analogs			
Bimatoprost 0.03% solution (Lumigan)	$66.45/2.5 mL	1 drop once daily at night	
Latanoprost 0.005% solution (Xalatan)	$58.84/2.5 mL	1 drop once or twice daily at night	
Travoprost 0.004% solution (Travatan)	$59.70/2.5 mL	1 drop once daily at night	Reduction of intraocular pressure.

(continued)

Table 10. Topical ophthalmic agents. (continued)

Agent	Representative Cost/Size [1]	Sig	Indications
Prostaglandin analogs (continued)			
Unoprostone 0.15% solution (Rescula)	$51.50/5 mL	1 drop twice daily	
Combined preparations			
Xalacom (latanoprost 0.005% and timolol 0.5%)	Not available in the United States	1 drop daily in the morning	Reduction of intraocular pressure.
Cosopt (dorzolamide 2% and timolol 0.5%)	$53.51/5 mL	1 drop twice daily	Reduction of intraocular pressure.
		ANTI-INFLAMMATORY AGENTS	
Nonsteroidal anti-inflammatory agents[7]			
Diclofenac sodium 0.1% solution (Voltaren)	$67.61/5 mL	1 drop to operated eye four times daily beginning 24 hours after cataract surgery and continuing through first 2 postoperative weeks	Treatment of postoperative inflammation following cataract extraction and laser corneal surgery.
Flurbiprofen sodium 0.03% solution (various)	$8.73/2.5 mL	1 drop every half hour beginning 2 hours before surgery; 1 drop to operated eye four times daily beginning 24 hours after cataract surgery	Inhibition of intraoperative miosis. Treatment of cystoid macular edema and inflammation after cataract surgery.
Ketorolac tromethamine 0.5% solution (Acular)	$71.53/5 mL	1 drop four times daily	Relief of ocular itching due to seasonal allergic conjunctivitis.
Corticosteroids[8]			
Dexamethasone sodium phosphate 0.1% solution (various)	$17.31/5 mL	1 or 2 drops as often as indicated by severity; use every hour during the day and every 2 hours during the night in severe inflammation; taper off as inflammation decreases	Treatment of steroid-responsive inflammatory conditions of anterior segment.
Dexamethasone sodium phosphate 0.05% ointment (various)	$6.34/3.5 g	Apply thin coating on lower conjunctival sac three or four times daily	
Fluorometholone 0.1% suspension (various)[9]	$26.16/10 mL	1 or 2 drops as often as indicated by severity; use every hour during the day and every 2 hours during the night in severe inflammation; taper off as inflammation decreases	
Fluorometholone 0.25% suspension (FML Forte)[9]	$37.60/10 mL		
Fluorometholone 0.1% ointment (FML S.O.P.)	$34.00/3.5 g	Apply thin coating on lower conjunctival sac three or four times daily	
Medrysone 1% suspension (HMS)	$33.24/10 mL	1 or 2 drops as often as indicated by severity of inflammation; use every hour during the day and every 2 hours during the night in severe inflammation; taper off as inflammation decreases	
Prednisolone acetate 0.12% suspension (Pred Mild)	$36.14/10 mL		
Prednisolone acetate 0.125% suspension (various)	$36.96/10 mL		
Prednisolone sodium phosphate 0.125% solution (various)	$27.29/10 mL		

(*continued*)

Table 10. Topical ophthalmic agents. (continued)

Agent	Representative Cost/Size [1]	Sig	Indications
Corticosteroids[8] (continued)			
Prednisolone acetate 1% suspension (various)	$23.10/10 mL	1 or 2 drops as often as indicated by severity of inflammation; use every hour during the day and every 2 hours during the night in severe inflammation; taper off as inflammation decreases	Treatment of steroid-responsive inflammatory conditions of anterior segment.
Prednisolone sodium phosphate 1% solution (various)	$24.06/10 mL		
Rimexolone 1% suspension (Vexol)	$49.32/10 mL		
Mast cell stabilizers			
Cromolyn sodium 4% solution (Crolom)	$37.20/10 mL	1 drop four to six times daily	Allergic conjunctivitis.
Ketotifen fumarate 0.025% solution (Zaditor)	$66.80/5 mL	1 drop two to four times daily	Allergic conjunctivitis.
Lodoxamide tromethamine 0.1% solution (Alomide)	$69.12/10 mL	1 or 2 drops four times daily (up to 3 months)	Allergic conjunctivitis and vernal keratoconjunctivitis.
Nedocromil sodium 2% solution (Alocril)	$79.85/5 mL	1 drop twice daily	Allergic conjunctivitis.
Olopatadine hydrochloride 0.1% solution (Patanol)	$74.16/5 mL	1 drop twice daily	Allergic conjunctivitis.
ANTIBIOTIC OINTMENTS AND SOLUTIONS			
Bacitracin 500 units/g ointment (various)[10]	$4.75/3.5 g	Refer to package insert (instructions vary)	Infections involving lid, conjunctiva, or cornea.
Chloramphenicol 1% (10 mg/g) ointment (Ocu-chlor)[11]	$1.65/3.5 g		As above, with both gram-positive and gram-negative coverage.
Ciprofloxacin HCl (Ciloxan)	0.3% solution: $50.46/5 mL 0.3% ointment: $50.46/3.5 g		
Erythromycin 0.5% ointment (various)[12]	$5.62/3.5 g		
Gatifloxacin 0.3% solution (Zymar)	$56.42/5 mL		
Gentamicin sulfate 0.3% solution (various)	$8.17/5 mL		
Gentamicin sulfate 0.3% ointment (various)	$19.67/3.5 g		
Moxifloxacin sulfate 0.5% solution (Vigamox)	$51.24/3 mL		
Norfloxacin 0.3% solution (Chibroxin)	Not available in the United States		
Ofloxacin 0.3% solution (Ocuflox)	$50.81/5 mL		
Polymyxin B sulfate 500,000 units, powder for solution (Polymyxin B Sulfate Sterile)[13]	$12.60/500,000 units		
Tobramycin 0.3% solution (various) Tobramycin 0.3% ointment (Tobrex)	$15.00/5 mL $53.88/3.5 g	Refer to package insert (instructions vary)	As above, with both gram-positive and gram-negative coverage.

(continued)

Table 10. Topical ophthalmic agents. (continued)

Agent	Representative Cost/Size [1]	Sig	Indications
		SULFONAMIDES	
Sulfacetamide sodium 10% solution (various)	$5.08/15 mL	1 or 2 drops every 1–3 hours	Conjunctivitis, corneal ulcer, and other superficial ocular infections due to susceptible microorganisms.
Sulfacetamide sodium 10% ointment (various)	$8.10/3.5 g	Apply small amount (0.5 inch) into lower conjunctivitis sac once to four times daily and at bedtime	Conjunctivitis, corneal ulcer, and other superficial ocular infections due to susceptible microorganisms.
Note: Many combination products containing antibiotics, antibiotics and steroids, or sulfonamides and steroids are available as solutions, suspensions, or ointments.			
		TOPICAL ANTIFUNGAL AGENTS	
Natamycin 5% suspension (Natacyn)	$147.36/15 mL	1 drop every 1–2 hours	Fungal blepharitis, conjunctivitis, and keratitis caused by susceptible organisms. Drug of choice for *Fusarium solani* keratitis.
		TOPICAL ANTIVIRAL AGENTS	
Ganciclovir 4.5 mg surgical insert (Vitrasert)	$5000.00 each	1 implant every 5–8 months	Treatment of cytomegalovirus retinitis in patients with AIDS.
Trifluridine 1% solution (Viroptic)	$104.95/7.5 mL	1 drop onto cornea every 2 hours while awake for a maximum daily dose of 9 drops until resolution occurs; then an additional 7 days of 1 drop every 4 hours while awake (minimum five times daily)	Primary keratoconjunctivitis and recurrent epithelial keratitis due to herpes simplex virus types 1 or 2.[14]
		TOPICAL ANTIHISTAMINICS[15]	
Levocabastine HCl 0.05% ophthalmic solution (Livostin)	$81.29/10 mL	1 drop four times daily (up to 2 weeks)	Allergic conjunctivitis; temporary relief of seasonal allergic conjunctivitis.
Emedastine difumarate 0.05% solution (Emadine)	$54.60/5 mL	1 drop four times daily	Allergic conjunctivitis.

[1]Average wholesale price (AWP, for AB-rated generic when available) for quantity listed. Source: *Red Book,* Update, Vol. 24, April 2005. AWP may not accurately represent the actual pharmacy cost because wide contractual variations exist among institutions.

[2]Macular edema occurs in 30% of patients.

[3]May (rarely) increase blood pressure. ***Caution:*** Avoid in patients with sulfite hypersensitivity (some brands contain sulfite).

[4]Cardioselective (β_1) β-blocker.

[5]Nonselective (β_1 and β_2) β-blocker. Monitor all patients for systemic side effects, particularly exacerbation of asthma.

[6]Decreased night vision, headaches possible.

[7]Cross-sensitivity to aspirin and other nonsteroidal anti-inflammatory drugs.

[8]Long-term use may increase intraocular pressure or cause cataracts.

[9]May be less likely to elevate intraocular pressure.

[10]Little efficacy against gram-negative organisms (except *Neisseria*).

[11]Aplastic anemia has been reported with prolonged ophthalmic use. Use only in serious infections for which less toxic drugs are ineffective or contraindicated.

[12]Also indicated for prophylaxis of ophthalmia neonatorum due to *N gonorrhoeae* or *C trachomatis.* Increasing resistance of *S pneumoniae* and *P aeruginosa* has been noted.

[13]No gram-positive coverage.

[14]Recurrences are common and call for additional 7-day treatment.

[15]Antihistamines (topical) are potential sensitizers and may produce local reactions.

Table 11. Common vestibular disorders: Differential diagnosis based on classic presentations.

Duration of Typical Vertiginous Episodes	Auditory Symptoms Present	Auditory Symptoms Absent
Seconds	Perilymphatic fistula	Positioning vertigo (cupulolithiasis), vertebrobasilar insufficiency, cervical vertigo
Hours	Endolymphatic hydrops (Meniere's syndrome, syphilis)	Recurrent vestibulopathy, vestibular migraine
Days	Labyrinthitis, labyrinthine concussion	Vestibular neuronitis
Months	Acoustic neuroma, ototoxicity	Multiple sclerosis, cerebellar degeneration

Table 12. Classification of severity of chronic stable asthma.

	Symptoms	Nighttime Symptoms	Lung Function
Mild intermittent	Symptoms ≤ 2 times a week Asymptomatic and normal PEF between exacerbations Exacerbations brief (few hours to few days); intensity may vary	≤ 2 times a month	FEV_1 or PEF ≥ 80% predicted PEF variability ≤ 20%
Mild persistent	Symptoms > 2 times a week but < 1 time a day Exacerbations may affect activity	> 2 times a month	FEV_1 or PEF > 80% predicted PEF variability 20–30%
Moderate persistent	Daily symptoms Daily use of inhaled short-acting β_2-agonist Exacerbations affect activity Exacerbations ≥ 2 times a week; may last days	> 1 time a week	FEV_1 or PEF > 60% to < 80% predicted PEF variability > 30%
Severe persistent	Continual symptoms Limited physical activity Frequent exacerbations	Frequent	FEV_1 or PEF ≤ 60% predicted PEF variability > 30%

Adapted from National Asthma Education and Prevention Program. Expert Panel Report 2: Guidelines for the Diagnosis and Management of Asthma. National Institutes of Health Pub. No. 97-4051. Bethesda, MD, 1997.

Key: PEF = peak expiratory flow; FEV_1 = forced expiratory volume in the first second.

Table 13. Classification of severity of asthma exacerbations.

	Mild	Moderate	Severe	Impending Respiratory Failure
Symptoms				
Breathlessness	With activity	With talking	At rest	At rest
Speech	Sentences	Phrases	Words	Mute
Signs				
Body position	Able to recline	Prefers sitting	Unable to recline	Unable to recline
Respiratory rate	Increased	Increased	Often > 30/min	> 30/min
Use of accessory respiratory muscles	Usually not	Commonly	Usually	Paradoxical thoracoabdominal movement
Breath sounds	Moderate wheezing at mid- to end-expiration	Loud wheezes throughout expiration	Loud inspiratory and expiratory wheezes	Little air movement without wheezes
Heart rate (beats/min)	< 100	100–120	> 120	Relative bradycardia
Pulsus paradoxus (mm Hg)	< 10	10–25	Often > 25	Often absent
Mental status	May be agitated	Usually agitated	Usually agitated	Confused or drowsy
Functional assessment				
PEF (% predicted or personal best)	> 80	50–80	< 50 or response to therapy lasts < 2 hours	< 50
Sa_{O_2} (%, room air)	> 95	91–95	< 91	< 91
Pa_{O_2} (mm Hg, room air)	Normal	> 60	< 60	< 60
Pa_{CO_2} (mm Hg)	< 42	< 42	≥ 42	≥ 42

Adapted from National Asthma Education and Prevention Program. Expert Panel Report 2: Guidelines for the Diagnosis and Management of Asthma. National Institutes of Health Pub. No. 97-4051. Bethesda, MD, 1997.
PEF = peak expiratory flow.

Table 14. Stepwise approach for managing asthma.[1]

	Long-Term Control	Quick Relief	Education
Step 1: Mild intermittent	No daily medication needed.	Short-acting bronchodilator: **inhaled β_2-agonists** as needed for symptoms. Intensity of treatment will depend on severity of exacerbation. Use of short-acting **inhaled β_2-agonists** > 2 times a week may indicate the need for long-term control therapy.	Teach basic facts about asthma Teach inhaler/inhalation chamber technique Discuss roles of medications Develop self-management and action plans Discuss appropriate environmental control measures
Step 2: Mild persistent	One daily medication: **Anti-inflammatory:** either **inhaled corticosteroid** (low doses) or **cromolyn** or **nedocromil** Less desirable alternatives: sustained-release **theophylline** or **leukotriene modifier**	Step 1 actions plus: Use of short-acting **inhaled β_2-agonists** on a daily basis, or increasing use, indicates the need for additional long-term control therapy.	Step 1 actions plus: Teach self-monitoring Refer to group education if available Review and update self-management plan
Step 3: Moderate persistent	Daily medication: Either **Anti-inflammatory: inhaled corticosteroid** (medium dose) or **Inhaled corticosteroid** (low-medium dose) and a **long-acting bronchodilator** (long-acting **inhaled β_2-agonist,** sustained-release **theophylline** or long-acting **β_2-agonist tablets**) If needed: **Anti-inflammatory: inhaled corticosteroid** (medium-high dose) and **Long-acting bronchodilator** (long-acting **inhaled β_2-agonist,** sustained-release **theophylline** or long-acting **β_2-agonist tablets**)	As for step 2.	Step 1 actions plus: Teach self-monitoring Refer to group education if available Review and update self-management plan
Step 4: Severe persistent	Daily medication: **Anti-inflammatory: inhaled corticosteroid** (high dose) and **Long-acting bronchodilator** (long-acting **inhaled β_2-agonist,** sustained release **theophylline** or long-acting **inhaled β_2-agonist tablets**) and **Corticosteroid tablets or syrup** (1–2 mg/kg/d, generally not to exceed 60 mg/d)	As for step 2.	Step 2 and 3 actions plus: Refer to individual education, counseling

Step down: Review treatment every 1–6 months; a gradual stepwise reduction in treatment may be possible.
Step up: If asthma control is not maintained, consider step up to next treatment level after reviewing medication technique, adherence, and environmental control.

Modified from National Asthma Education and Prevention Program. Expert Panel Report 2: Guidelines for the Diagnosis and Management of Asthma. National Institutes of Health Pub. No. 97-4051. Bethesda, MD, 1997.

[1]Preferred treatments are in bold text; however, specific medication plans should be tailored to individual patients.

Table 15. Long-term control medications for asthma.[1]

Drug	Important Formulations	Usual Adult Dosage	Cost[2]	Comments
Inhaled corticosteroids[3]				
Beclomethasone dipropionate (QVAR)	40 mcg/puff	Two or three puffs BID	\$56.90/7.30 g	Chlorofluorocarbon-free; hydrofluoralkane propellant
	80 mcg/puff	One to two puffs BID	\$71.70/7.30 g	
Budesonide (Pulmicort Turbuhaler)	Dry powder delivery system: 200 mcg/puff; 200 puffs/inhaler	One inhalation twice a day	\$158.15/inhaler	Dry powder
Flunisolide (AeroBid)	MDI: 250 mcg/puff; 100 puffs/inhaler	Two to four puffs twice a day	\$77.57/7 g	Chlorofluorocarbon propellant
Fluticasone (Flovent)	MDI: 44, 110, or 220 mcg/puff; 120 puffs/inhaler	Two or three puffs (of 110 mcg) twice a day	\$91.79/13 g (110 μg)	Chlorofluorocarbon propellant
Fluticasone (Flovent Rotadisk)	Dry powder delivery system: 44, 88, 220 mcg/blister; 4 blisters/Rotadisk, 15 Rotadisks per tube	One or two puffs (of 88 mcg) twice a day	\$61.70/60 88-μg disks	Dry powder
Triamcinolone acetonide (Azmacort)	MDI: 100 mcg/puff; 240 puffs/inhaler	Two or three puffs four times a day, or four to six puffs twice daily	\$75.60/20 g	Chlorofluorocarbon propellant
Systemic corticosteroids				
Methylprednisolone (many)	Tablets: 4 mg	5–60 mg daily to every other day as needed	\$0.54/4 mg	
Prednisolone (many)	Tablets: 5 mg	5–60 mg daily to every other day as needed	\$0.04/5 mg	
Prednisone (many)	Tablets: 1, 2.5, 5, 10, 20, 50 mg	5–60 mg daily to every other day as needed	\$0.04/5 mg	
Combination inhaled corticosteroid and long-acting β_2-agonist				
Fluticasone and salmeterol (Advair Diskus)	Dry powder delivery system: 100, 250, or 500 mcg fluticasone per dose and 50 mcg salmeterol per dose	One puff twice a day of 250/50; cannot use more than one puff twice a day due to salmeterol component	\$162.05/60 250/50 disks	Dry powder
Cromolyn (Intal)	MDI: 800 mcg per puff: 200 puffs/inhaler	2–4 puffs 4 times a day	\$92.94/14.2 g	Chlorofluorocarbon propellant
	Nebulizer solution: 20 mg/2 mL ampule	20 mg (2 mL) four times a day	\$0.82/2 mL	Administer with powered nebulizer

Nedocromil (Tilade)	MDI: 1.75 mg/puff; 112 puffs/inhaler	Two puffs four times a day	$69.86/16.2 g	Chlorofluorocarbon propellant
Long-acting β_2 agonists[4]				
Salmeterol (Serevent Diskus)	Dry powder: 50 mcg/blister; 60 blisters per pack	One blister every 12 hours	$100.16/60	Dry powder
Formoterol (Foradil Aerolizer)	Dry powder: 12 mcg/capsule; 60 capsules/Aerolizer	One capsule every 12 hours	$79.83/60	Dry powder
Sustained-release albuterol (Proventil Repetab)	Sustained-release tablet, 4 mg	One tablet every 12 hours	$1.24/4 mg	Usually reserved for nocturnal symptoms not improved with other therapies
Theophylline (many)	Sustained-release tablets and capsules	Initially 10 mg/kg/d up to 300 mg maximum; then 200–600 mg every 8–24 hours	$0.33/200 mg	Maintenance dose guided by serum drug level. Absorption and dosing vary with brand
Leukotriene modifiers				
Montelukast (Singulair)	Tablet, 10 mg	One tablet each evening	$3.15/10 mg $94.96/mo	
Zafirlukast (Accolate)	Tablet, 20 mg	One tablet twice a day	$1.33/20 mg $79.91/mo	Administration with meals decreases bioavailability; take at least 1 hour before or 2 hours after meals
Zileuton (Zyflo)	Tablet, 600 mg	One tablet four times a day	$0.85/600 mg $102.14/mo	Monitor hepatic enzymes

[1]Only drugs available in the United States are listed.
[2]Average wholesale price (AWP, for AB-rated generic when available) for quantity listed. Source: *Red Book*, Update, Vol. 24, No. 4. April 2005. AWP may not accurately represent actual pharmacy cost because wide contractual variations exist among institutions.
[3]Dosing should be individualized. See text.
[4]Not for acute relief of symptoms.
MDI = metered-dose inhaler.

Table 16. Quick-relief medications for asthma.[1]

Drug	Important Formulations	Usual Adult Dosage	Cost[2]	Comments
Short-acting Inhaled β_2-agonists				
Albuterol (Proventil, Ventolin)	MDI: 90 mcg/puff, 200 puffs/canister	Two puffs 5 minutes before exercise Two puffs every 4–6 hours as needed	$29.79/17 g	Preferred formulation in most cases. Chlorofluorocarbon propellant.
	Nebulizer solutions: 5 mg/mL (0.5%)	1.25–5 mg (0.25–1 mL) in 2–3 mL of normal saline every 4–8 hours as needed	$14.99/20 mL	Administer with powered nebulizer. More frequent dosing is acceptable for acute or severe exacerbations.
	Unit dose: 0.083%, 3 mL	One dose every 4–8 hours as needed	$1.22/unit	May mix with cromolyn or ipratropium nebulizer solutions.
	Tablets: 2 mg, 4 mg	2–4 mg orally every 6–8 hours	$31.14/100 2-mg tablets	Extended-release 4-mg tablet (Proventil Repetab) available for use every 12 hours.
Albuterol HFA (Proventil HFA)	MDI: 90 mcg/puff, 200 puffs/canister	Two puffs 5 minutes before exercise Two puffs every 4–6 hours as needed	$42.20/6.7 g	Nonchlorofluorocarbon propellant.
Pirbuterol (Maxair Autoinhaler)	MDI 200 mcg/puff, 400 puffs/canister	Two puffs every 4–6 hours as needed	$87.96/14 g	Breath-activated MDI system. Chlorofluorocarbon propellant.
Terbutaline (Brethine)	Tablets: 2.5 mg, 5 mg	2.5–5 mg orally three times a day	$62.21/100 5-mg tablets	Tremor, nervousness, palpitations common; therefore not recommended.
	Injection solution, 1 mg/mL	0.25 mg (0.25 mL) subcutaneously; may be repeated once in 30 minutes	$32.48/1 mg	Onset of action 30 minutes. Not limited to β_2-agonist effects.
Anticholinergics				
Ipratropium bromide (Atrovent)	MDI: 18 mcg/puff, 200 puffs/canister	Two to four puffs every 6 hours	$66.85/14 g	Chlorofluorocarbon propellant.
	Unit dose nebulizer solution, 0.2 mg/mL (0.02%), 2.5 mL (0.5 mg)	0.25–0.5 mg (1–2 mL) every 6 hours	$1.66/unit	
Systemic corticosteroids				
Methylprednisolone (many)	Tablets: 4 mg	40–60 mg/d as single dose or in two divided doses for 3–10 days	$11.00/4-mg dose-pack	
Methylprednisolone sodium succinate (many)	Intravenous injection solution vials: 40, 125, 500 mg	0.5–1 mg/kg every 6 hours	$3.58/125-mg vial	
Prednisolone (many)	Tablets: 5 mg Syrup: 15 mg/5 mL	40–60 mg/d as single dose or in two divided doses for 3–10 days	$0.04/5-mg tablet $6.21/240 mL syrup	
Prednisone (many)	Tablets: 1, 2.5, 5, 10, 20, 50 mg	40–60 mg/d as single dose or in two divided doses for 3–10 days	$0.04/5 mg	

[1]Only drugs available in the United States are listed.
[2]Average wholesale price (AWP, for AB-rated generic when available) for quantity listed. Source: *Red Book,* Update, Vol. 24., No. 4, April 2005. AWP may not accurately represent the actual pharmacy cost because wide contractual variations exist among institutions.
MDI = metered-dose inhaler.

Table 17. Patterns of disease in advanced COPD.

	Type A: Pink Puffer (Emphysema Predominant)	Type B: Blue Bloater (Bronchitis Predominant)
History and physical examination	Major complaint is dyspnea, often severe, usually presenting after age 50. Cough is rare, with scant clear, mucoid sputum. Patients are thin, with recent weight loss common. They appear uncomfortable, with evident use of accessory muscles of respiration. Chest is very quiet without adventitious sounds. No peripheral edema.	Major complaint is chronic cough, productive of mucopurulent sputum, with frequent exacerbations due to chest infections. Often presents in late 30s and 40s. Dyspnea usually mild, though patients may note limitations to exercise. Patients frequently overweight and cyanotic but seem comfortable at rest. Peripheral edema is common. Chest is noisy, with rhonchi invariably present; wheezes are common.
Laboratory studies	Hemoglobin usually normal (12–15 g/dL). Pa_{O_2} normal to slightly reduced (65–75 mm Hg) but Sa_{O_2} normal at rest. Pa_{CO_2} normal to slightly reduced (35–40 mm Hg). Chest radiograph shows hyperinflation with flattened diaphragms. Vascular markings are diminished, particularly at the apices.	Hemoglobin usually elevated (15–18 g/dL). Pa_{O_2} reduced (45–60 mm Hg) and Pa_{CO_2} slightly to markedly elevated (50–60 mm Hg). Chest radiograph shows increased interstitial markings ("dirty lungs"), especially at bases. Diaphragms are not flattened.
Pulmonary function tests	Airflow obstruction ubiquitous. Total lung capacity increased, sometimes markedly so. DL_{CO} reduced. Static lung compliance increased.	Airflow obstruction ubiquitous. Total lung capacity generally normal but may be slightly increased. DL_{CO} normal. Static lung compliance normal.
Special evaluations		
$\dot{V}/\dot{Q}$ matching	Increased ventilation to high $\dot{V}/\dot{Q}$ areas, ie, high dead space ventilation.	Increased perfusion to low $\dot{V}/\dot{Q}$ areas.
Hemodynamics	Cardiac output normal to slightly low. Pulmonary artery pressures mildly elevated and increase with exercise.	Cardiac output normal. Pulmonary artery pressures elevated, sometimes markedly so, and worsen with exercise.
Nocturnal ventilation	Mild to moderate degree of oxygen desaturation not usually associated with obstructive sleep apnea.	Severe oxygen desaturation, frequently associated with obstructive sleep apnea.
Exercise ventilation	Increased minute ventilation for level of oxygen consumption. Pa_{O_2} tends to fall, Pa_{CO_2} rises slightly.	Decreased minute ventilation for level of oxygen consumption. Pa_{O_2} may rise; Pa_{CO_2} may rise signficantly.

DL_{CO} = single-breath diffusing capacity for carbon monoxide; $\dot{V}/\dot{Q}$ = ventilation-perfusion.

Table 18. Home oxygen therapy: requirements for Medicare coverage.[1]

Group I (any of the following):

1. $PaO_2 \leq 55$ mm Hg or $SaO_2 \leq 88\%$ taken at rest breathing room air, while awake.
2. During sleep (prescription for nocturnal oxygen use only):
   a. $PaO_2 \leq 55$ mm Hg or $SaO_2 \leq 88\%$ for a patient whose awake, resting, room air PaO_2 is ≥ 56 mm Hg or $SaO_2 \geq 89\%$,

   or

   b. Decrease in $PaO_2 > 10$ mm Hg or decrease in $SaO_2 > 5\%$ associated with symptoms or signs reasonably attributed to hypoxemia (eg, impaired cognitive processes, nocturnal restlessness, insomnia).
3. During exercise (prescription for oxygen use only during exercise):
   a. $PaO_2 \leq 55$ mg Hg or $SaO_2 \leq 88\%$ taken during exercise for a patient whose awake, resting, room air PaO_2 is ≥ 56 mm Hg or $SaO_2 \geq 89\%$,

   and

   b. There is evidence that the use of supplemental oxygen during exercise improves the hypoxemia that was demonstrated during exercise while breathing room air.

Group II[2]:

$PaO_2 = 56–59$ mm Hg or $SaO_2 = 89\%$ if there is evidence of any of the following:

1. Dependent edema suggesting congestive heart failure.
2. P pulmonale on ECG (P wave > 3 mm in standard leads II, III, or aVF).
3. Hematocrit > 56%.

[1]Health Care Financing Administration, 1989.

[2]Patients in this group must have a second oxygen test 3 months after the initial oxygen set-up.

Table 19. Characteristics and treatment of selected pneumonias.

Organism; Appearance on Smear of Sputum	Clinical Setting	Complications	Laboratory Studies	Antimicrobial Therapy[1,2]
Streptococcus pneumoniae (pneumococcus). Gram-positive diplococci.	Chronic cardiopulmonary disease; follows upper respiratory tract infection	Bacteremia, meningitis, endocarditis, pericarditis, empyema	Gram stain and culture of sputum, blood, pleural fluid	Preferred[3]: Penicillin G, amoxicillin. Alternative: Macrolides, cephalosporins, doxycycline, fluoroquinolones, clindamycin, vancomycin, TMP-SMZ, linezolid.
Haemophilus influenzae. Pleomorphic gram-negative coccobacilli.	Chronic cardiopulmonary disease; follows upper respiratory tract infection	Empyema, endocarditis	Gram stain and culture of sputum, blood, pleural fluid	Preferred[3]: Cefotaxime, ceftriaxone, cefuroxime, doxycycline, azithromycin, TMP-SMZ. Alternative: Fluoroquinolones, clarithromycin.
Staphylococcus aureus. Plump gram-positive cocci in clumps.	Residence in chronic care facility, nosocomial, influenza epidemics; cystic fibrosis, bronchiectasis, injection drug use	Empyema, cavitation	Gram stain and culture of sputum, blood, pleural fluid	For methicillin-susceptible strains: Preferred: A penicillinase-resistant penicillin with or without rifampin, or gentamicin. Alternative: A cephalosporin; clindamycin, TMP-SMZ, vancomycin, a fluoroquinolone. For methicillin-resistant strains: Vancomycin with or without gentamicin or rifampin, linezolid.
Klebsiella pneumoniae. Plump gram-negative encapsulated rods.	Alcohol abuse, diabetes mellitus; nosocomial.	Cavitation, empyema	Gram stain and culture of sputum, blood, pleural fluid	Preferred: Third-generation cephalosporin. For severe infections, add an aminoglycoside. Alternative: Aztreonam, imipenem, meropenem, β-lactam/β-lactamase inhibitor, an aminoglycoside, or a fluoroquinolone.
Escherichia coli. Gram-negative rods.	Nosocomial; rarely, community-acquired	Empyema	Gram stain and culture of sputum, blood, pleural fluid	Same as for *Klebsiella pneumoniae*.
Pseudomonas aeruginosa. Gram-negative rods.	Nosocomial; cystic fibrosis, bronchiectasis	Cavitation	Gram stain and culture of sputum, blood	Preferred: An antipseudomonal β-lactam plus an aminoglycoside. Alternative: Ciprofloxacin plus an aminoglycoside or an antipseudomonal β-lactam.
Anaerobes. Mixed flora.	Aspiration, poor dental hygiene	Necrotizing pneumonia, abscess, empyema	Culture of pleural fluid or of material obtained by transtracheal or transthoracic aspiration	Preferred: Clindamycin, β-lactam/β-lactamase inhibitor, imipenem.

(*continued*)

Table 19. Characteristics and treatment of selected pneumonias. (continued)

Organism; Appearance on Smear of Sputum	Clinical Setting	Complications	Laboratory Studies	Antimicrobial Therapy[1,2]
Mycoplasma pneumoniae. PMNs and monocytes; no bacteria.	Young adults; summer and fall	Skin rashes, bullous myringitis; hemolytic anemia	PCR. Culture.[4] Complement fixation titer.[5] Cold agglutinin serum titers are not helpful as they lack sensitivity and specificity.	Preferred: Doxycycline or erythromycin. Alternative: Clarithromycin; azithromycin, or a fluoroquinolone.
Legionella species. Few PMNs; no bacteria.	Summer and fall; exposure to contaminated construction site, water source, air conditioner; community-acquired or nosocomial	Empyema, cavitation, endocarditis, pericarditis	Direct immunofluorescent examination or PCR of sputum or tissue; culture of sputum or tissue.[4] Urinary antigen assay for *L pneumophila* serogroup 1.	Preferred: A macrolide with or without rifampin; a fluoroquinolone. Alternative: Doxycycline with or without rifampin, TMP-SMZ.
Chlamydia pneumoniae. Nonspecific.	Clinically similar to *M pneumoniae*, but prodromal symptoms last longer (up to 2 weeks). Sore throat with hoarseness common. Mild pneumonia in teenagers and young adults.	Reinfection in older adults with underlying COPD or heart failure may be severe or even fatal	Isolation of the organism is very difficult. Serologic studies include microimmunofluorescence with TWAR antigen. PCR at selected laboratories.	Preferred: Doxycycline. Alternative: Erythromycin, clarithromycin, azithromycin, or a fluoroquinolone.
Moraxella catarrhalis. Gram-negative diplococci.	Preexisting lung disease; elderly; corticosteroid or immunosuppressive therapy	Rarely, pleural effusions and bacteremia	Gram stain and culture of sputum, blood, pleural fluid	Preferred: A second- or third-generation cephalosporin; a fluoroquinolone. Alternative: TMP-SMZ, amoxicillin-clavulanic acid, or a macrolide.
Pneumocystis jiroveci. Nonspecific.	AIDS, immunosuppressive or cytotoxic drug therapy, cancer	Pneumothorax, respiratory failure, ARDS, death	Methenamine silver, Giemsa, or DFA stains of sputum or bronchoalveolar lavage fluid	Preferred: TMP-SMZ or pentamidine isethionate plus prednisone. Alternative: Dapsone plus trimethoprim; clindamycin plus primaquine; trimetrexate plus folinic acid.

[1]Antimicrobial sensitivities should guide therapy when available. (Modified from: The choice of antibacterial drugs. Med Lett Drugs Ther 2004;43:69, and from Bartlett JG et al: Practice guidelines for the management of community-acquired pneumonia in adults. Clin Infect Dis 2000;31:347.)
[2]For additional antimicrobial therapy information, see Infectious Disease: Antimicrobial Therapy: Tables 37–1 (drugs of choice), 37–5 and 37–7 (doses per day), and 37–4, 37–8, and 37–9 (pharmacology and dosage adjustment for renal dysfunction).
[3]Consider penicillin resistance when choosing therapy. See text.
[4]Selective media are required.
[5]Fourfold rise in titer is diagnostic.
Key: TMP-SMZ = trimethoprim-sulfamethoxazole; PCR = polymerase chain reaction; COPD = chronic obstructive pulmonary disease; ARDS = acute respiratory distress syndrome.

Table 20. Scoring system for risk class assignment for PORT prediction rule.

Patient Characteristic	Points Assigned[1]
Demographic factor	
Age: men	Number of years
Age: women	Number of years minus 10
Nursing home resident	10
Comorbid illnesses	
Neoplastic disease[2]	30
Liver disease[3]	20
Congestive heart failure[4]	10
Cerebrovascular disease[5]	10
Renal disease[6]	10
Physical examination finding	
Altered mental status[7]	20
Respiratory rate ≥ 30 breaths/min	20
Systolic blood pressure < 90 mm Hg	20
Temperature ≤ 35°C or ≥ 40°C	15
Pulse ≥ 125 beats/min	10
Laboratory or radiographic finding	
Arterial pH < 7.35	30
Blood urea nitrogen ≥ 30 mg/dL	20
Sodium < 130 mEq/L	20
Glucose > 250 mg/dL	10
Hematocrit < 30%	10
Arterial Po_2 < 60 mm Hg	10
Pleural effusion	10

Modified and reproduced, with permission, from Fine MJ et al: A prediction rule to identify low-risk patients with community-acquired pneumonia. N Engl J Med 1997;336:243.

[1]A total point score for a given patient is obtained by summing the patient's age in years (age minus 10 for women) and the points for each applicable characteristic.

[2]Any cancer except basal or squamous cell of the skin that was active at the time of presentation or diagnosed within 1 year before presentation.

[3]Clinical or histologic diagnosis of cirrhosis or another form of chronic liver disease.

[4]Systolic or diastolic dysfunction documented by history, physical examination and chest radiograph, echocardiogram, MUGA scan, or left ventriculogram.

[5]Clinical diagnosis of stroke or transient ischemic attack or stroke documented by MRI or CT scan.

[6]History of chronic renal disease or abnormal blood urea nitrogen and creatinine concentration documented in the medical record.

[7]Disorientation (to person, place, or time, not known to be chronic), stupor, or coma.

Table 21. PORT risk class 30-day mortality rates and recommendations for site of care.

Number of Points	Risk Class	Mortality at 30 days (%)	Recommended Site of Care
Absence of predictors	I	0.1–0.4	Outpatient
≤ 70	II	0.6–0.7	Outpatient
71–90	III	0.9–2.8	Outpatient or brief inpatient
91–130	IV	8.2–9.3	Inpatient
≥ 130	V	27.0–31.1	Inpatient

Data from Fine MJ et al: A prediction rule to identify low-risk patients with community-acquired pneumonia. N Engl J Med 1997;336:243.

Table 22. Classification of positive tuberculin skin test reactions.[1]

Reaction Size	Group
≥ 5 mm	1. HIV-positive persons. 2. Recent contacts of individuals with active tuberculosis. 3. Persons with fibrotic changes on chest x-rays suggestive of prior tuberculosis. 4. Patients with organ transplants and other immunosuppressed patients (receiving the equivalent of > 15 mg/d of prednisone for 1 month or more).
≥ 10 mm	1. Recent immigrants (< 5 years) from countries with a high prevalence of tuberculosis (eg, Asia, Africa, Latin America). 2. HIV-negative injection drug users. 3. Mycobacteriology laboratory personnel. 4. Residents of and employees[2] in the following high-risk congregate settings: correctional institutions; nursing homes and other long-term facilities for the elderly; hospitals and other health care facilities; residential facilities for AIDS patients; and homeless shelters. 5. Persons with the following medical conditions that increase the risk of tuberculosis: gastrectomy, ≥ 10% below ideal body weight, jejunoileal bypass, diabetes mellitus, silicosis, chronic renal failure, some hematologic disorders, (eg leukemias, lymphomas), and other specific malignancies (eg, carcinoma of the head or neck and lung). 6. Children < 4 years of age or infants, children, and adolescents exposed to adults at high risk.
≥ 15 mm	1. Persons with no risk factors for tuberculosis.

Adapted from: Screening for tuberculosis and tuberculosis infection in high-risk populations: recommendations of the Advisory Council for the Elimination of Tuberculosis. MMWR Morb Mortal Wkly Rep 1995;44(RR-11):19.

[1]A tuberculin skin test reaction is considered positive if the transverse diameter of the *indurated* area reaches the size required for the specific group. All other reactions are considered negative.

[2]For persons who are otherwise at low risk and are tested at entry into employment, a reaction of > 15 mm induration is considered positive.

Table 23. Characteristics of antituberculous drugs.[1]

Drug	Most Common Side Effects	Tests for Side Effects	Drug Interactions	Remarks
Isoniazid	Peripheral neuropathy, hepatitis, rash, mild CNS effects.	AST and ALT; neurologic examination.	Phenytoin (synergistic); disulfiram.	Bactericidal to both extracellular and intracellular organisms. Pyridoxine, 10 mg orally daily as prophylaxis for neuritis; 50–100 mg orally daily as treatment.
Rifampin	Hepatitis, fever, rash, flu-like illness, gastrointestinal upset, bleeding problems, renal failure.	CBC, platelets, AST and ALT.	Rifampin inhibits the effect of oral contraceptives, quinidine, corticosteroids, warfarin, methadone, digoxin, oral hypoglycemics; aminosalicyclic acid may interfere with absorption of rifampin. Significant interactions with protease inhibitors and nonnucleoside reverse transcriptase inhibitors.	Bactericidal to all populations of organisms. Colors urine and other body secretions orange. Discoloring of contact lenses.
Pyrazinamide	Hyperuricemia, hepatotoxicity, rash, gastrointestinal upset, joint aches.	Uric acid, AST, ALT.	Rare.	Bactericidal to intracellular organisms.
Ethambutol	Optic neuritis (reversible with discontinuance of drug; rare at 15 mg/kg); rash.	Red-green color discrimination and visual acuity (difficult to test in children under 3 years of age).	Rare.	Bacteriostatic to both intracellular and extracellular organisms. Mainly used to inhibit development of resistant mutants. Use with caution in renal disease or when ophthalmologic testing is not feasible.
Streptomycin	Eighth nerve damage, nephrotoxicity.	Vestibular function (audiograms); BUN and creatinine.	Neuromuscular blocking agents may be potentiated and cause prolonged paralysis.	Bactericidal to extracellular organisms. Use with caution in older patients or those with renal disease.

[1]See also Chapter 37.

Key: AST = aspartate aminotransferase; ALT = alanine aminotransferase; CBC = complete blood count; BUN = blood urea nitrogen.

Table 24. Recommended dosages for the initial treatment of tuberculosis.

Drugs	Daily	Cost[1]	Twice a Week[2]	Cost[1]/wk	Three Times a Week[2]	Cost[1]/wk
Isoniazid	5 mg/kg Max: 300 mg/dose	$0.13/300 mg	15 mg/kg Max: 900 mg/dose	$0.78	15 mg/kg Max: 900 mg/dose	$1.17
Rifampin	10 mg/kg Max: 600 mg/dose	$3.80/600 mg	10 mg/kg Max: 600 mg/dose	$7.60	10 mg/kg Max: 600 mg/dose	$11.40
Pyrazinamide	15–30 mg/kg Max: 2 g/dose	$4.40/2 g	50–70 mg/kg Max: 4 g/dose	$17.60	50–70 mg/kg Max: 3 g/dose	$19.80
Ethambutol	5–25 mg/kg Max: 2.5 g/dose	$11.36/2.5 g	50 mg/kg Max: 2.5 g/dose	$22.72	25–30 mg/kg Max: 2.5 g/dose	$34.08
Streptomycin	15 mg/kg Max: 1 g/dose	$9.75/1 g	25–30 mg/kg Max: 1.5 g/dose	$39.00	25–30 mg/kg Max: 1.5 g/dose	$58.50

[1]Average wholesale price (AWP, for AB-rated generic when available) for quantity listed. Source: *Red Book*, Update, Vol. 24, No. 4, April 2005. AWP may not accurately represent the actual pharmacy cost because wide contractual variations exist among institutions.
[2]All intermittent dosing regimens should be used with directly observed therapy.

Table 25. TNM staging for lung cancer.

Stage	T	N	M	Description
0	Tis			Carcinoma in situ
IA IB	T1 T2	N0 N0	M0 M0	Limited local disease without nodal or distant metastases
IIA IIB	T1 T2 T3	N1 N1 N0	M0 M0 M0	Limited local disease with ipsilateral hilar or peribronchial nodal involvement but not distant metastases *or* Locally invasive disease without nodal or distant metastases
IIIA	T3 T1–3	N1 N2	M0 M0	Locally invasive disease with ipsilateral or peribronchial nodal involvement but not distant metastases *or* Limited or locally invasive disease with ipsilateral mediastinal or subcarinal nodal involvement but not distant metastases
IIIB	Any T T4	N3 Any N	M0 M0	Any primary with contralateral mediastinal or hilar nodes, or ipsilateral scalene or supraclavicular nodes *or* Unresectable local invasion with any degree of adenopathy but no distant metatases; malignant pleural effusion
IV	Any T	Any N	M1	Distant metastases
Primary Tumor (T)				
TX	Primary tumor cannot be assessed; or tumor proved by the presence of malignant cells in sputum or bronchial washings but not visualized by imaging or bronchoscopy.			
T0	No evidence of primary tumor.			
Tis	Carcinoma in situ.			
T1	A tumor ≤ 3 cm in greatest dimension, surrounded by lung or visceral pleura, and without evidence of invasion proximal to a lobar bronchus at bronchoscopy.			
T2	A tumor > 3.0 cm in greatest dimension, or a tumor of any size that either involves a main bronchus (but is ≥ 2 cm distal to the carina), invades the visceral pleura, or has associated atelectasis or obstructive pneumonitis extending to the hilar region. Any associated atelectasis or obstructive pneumonitis must involve less than an entire lung.			
T3	A tumor of any size with direct extension into the chest wall (including superior sulcus tumors), the diaphragm, the mediastinal pleura, or the parietal pericardium; or a tumor in the main bronchus < 2 cm distal to the carina without involving the carina; or associated atelectasis or obstructive pneumonitis of the entire lung.			
T4	A tumor of any size with invasion of the mediastinum, heart, great vessels, trachea, esophagus, vertebral body, or carina; or with a malignant pleural or pericardial effusion; or with satellite tumor nodules within the ipsilateral lobe of the lung containing the primary tumor.			
Regional Lymph Nodes (N)				
NX	Regional lymph nodes cannot be assessed.			
N0	No demonstrable metastasis to regional lymph nodes.			
N1	Metastasis to lymph nodes in the peribronchial or the ipsilateral hilar region, or both, including direct extension.			
N2	Metastasis to ipsilateral mediastinal lymph nodes and/or subcarinal lymph nodes.			
N3	Metastasis to contralateral mediastinal lymph nodes, contralateral hilar lymph nodes, ipsilateral or contralateral scalene or supraclavicular lymph nodes.			
Distant Metastases (M)				
MX	Presence of distant metastasis cannot be assessed.			
M0	No (known) distant metastasis.			
M1	Distant metastasis present.			

Adapted from Mountain CF: Revisions in the international system for staging lung cancer. Chest 1997;111:1710.

Table 26. Approach to staging of patients with lung cancer.

Part A: Recommended tests for all patients
- Complete blood count
- Electrolytes, calcium, alkaline phosphatase, albumin, AST, ALT, total bilirubin, creatinine
- Chest radiograph
- CT of chest through the adrenal glands[1,2]
- Pathologic confirmation of malignancy[3]

Part B: Recommended tests for selected but not all patients

Test	Indication
CT with contrast of liver or liver ultrasound	Elevated liver function tests; abnormal non-contrast-enhanced CT of liver or abnormal clinical evaluation
CT with contrast of brain or MRI of brain	CNS symptoms or abnormal clinical evaluation
Whole body ^{18}F-fluoro-deoyx-D-glucose positron emission tomography scan (FDG-PET)	To evaluate the mediastinum in patients who are candidates for surgery
Radionuclide bone scan	Elevated alkaline phosphatase (bony fraction), elevated calcium, bone pain, or abnormal clinical evaluation
Pulmonary function tests	If lung resection or thoracic radiotherapy planned
Quantitative radionuclide perfusion lung scan or exercise testing to evaluate maximum oxygen consumption	Patients with borderline resectability due to limited cardiovascular status

Modified and reproduced, with permission, from: Pretreatment evaluation of non-small cell lung cancer. Consensus Statement of the American Thoracic Society and the European Respiratory Society. Am J Respir Crit Care Med 1997;156:320.

[1]May not be necessary if patient has obvious M1 disease on chest x-ray or physical examination.

[2]Intravenous iodine contrast enhancement is not essential but is recommended in probable mediastinal invasion.

[3]While optimal in most cases, tissue diagnosis may not be necessary prior to surgery in some cases where the lesion is enlarging or the patient will undergo surgical resection regardless of the outcome of a biopsy.

Table 27. Approximate survival rates following treatment for lung cancer.

Non-Small Cell Lung Cancer: Mean 5-Year Survival Following Resection		
Stage	**Clinical Staging**	**Surgical Staging**
IA (T1N0M0)	60%	74%
IB (T2N0M0)	38%	61%
IIA (T1N1M0)	34%	55%
IIB (T2N1M0, T3N0M0)	23%	39%
IIIA	9–13%	22%
IIIB[1]	3–7%	
IV[1]	1%	
Small Cell Lung Cancer: Survival Following Chemotherapy		
	Mean 2-Year	
Stage	**Survival**	**Median Survival**
Limited	15–20%	14–20 months
Extensive	< 3%	8–13 months

Data from multiple sources. Modified and reproduced, with permission, from Reif MS et al: Evidence-based medicine in the treatment of non-small cell cancer. Clin Chest Med 2000;21:107.

[1]Independent of therapy, generally not surgical patients.

Table 28. Differential diagnosis of interstitial lung disease.

Drug-related
- Antiarrhythmic agents (amiodarone)
- Antibacterial agents (nitrofurantoin, sulfonamides)
- Antineoplastic agents (bleomycin, cyclophosphamide, methotrexate, nitrosoureas)
- Antirheumatic agents (gold salts, penicillamine)
- Phenytoin

Environmental and occupational (inhalation exposures)
- Dust, inorganic (asbestos, silica, hard metals, beryllium)
- Dust, organic (thermophilic actinomycetes, avian antigens, aspergillus species)
- Gases, fumes, and vapors (chlorine, isocyanates, paraquat, sulfur dioxide)
- Ionizing radiation
- Talc (injection drug users)

Infections
- Fungus, disseminated (*Coccidioides immitis, Blastomyces dermatitidis, Histoplasma capsulatum*)
- Mycobacteria, disseminated
- *Pneumocystis jiroveci*
- Viruses

Primary pulmonary disorders
- Cryptogenic organizing pneumonitis (COP)
- Idiopathic fibrosing interstitial pneumonia: Acute interstitial pneumonitis, desquamative interstitial pneumonitis, nonspecific interstitial pneumonitis, usual interstitial pneumonitis, respiratory bronchiolitis-associated interstitial lung disease
- Pulmonary alveolar proteinosis

Systemic disorders
- Acute respiratory distress syndrome
- Amyloidosis
- Ankylosing spondylitis
- Autoimmune disease: Dermatomyositis, polymyositis, rheumatoid arthritis, systemic sclerosis (scleroderma), systemic lupus erythematosus
- Chronic eosinophilic pneumonia
- Goodpasture's syndrome
- Idiopathic pulmonary hemosiderosis
- Inflammatory bowel disease
- Langerhans cell histiocytosis (eosinophilic granuloma)
- Lymphangitic spread of cancer (lymphangitic carcinomatosis)
- Lymphangioleiomyomatosis
- Pulmonary edema
- Pulmonary venous hypertension, chronic
- Sarcoidosis
- Wegener's granulomatosis

Table 29. Idiopathic fibrosing interstitial pneumonias.

Name and Clinical Presentation	Histopathology	Radiographic Pattern	Response to Therapy and Prognosis
Usual interstitial pneumonia (UIP) Age 55–60, slight male predominance. Insidious dry cough and dyspnea lasting months to years. Clubbing present at diagnosis in 25–50%. Diffuse fine late inspiratory crackles on lung auscultation. Restrictive ventilatory defect and reduced diffusing capacity on pulmonary function tests. ANA and RF positive in 25% in the absence of documented collagen-vascular disease.	Patchy, temporally and geographically nonuniform distribution of fibrosis, honeycomb change, and normal lung. Type I pneumocytes are lost, and there is proliferation of alveolar type II cells. "Fibroblast foci" of actively proliferating fibroblasts and myofibroblasts. Inflammation is generally mild and consists of small lymphocytes. Intra-alveolar macrophage accumulation is present but is not a prominent feature.	Diminished lung volume. Increased linear or reticular bibasilar and subpleural opacities. Unilateral disease is rare. High-resolution CT scanning shows minimal ground-glass and variable honeycomb change. Areas of normal lung may be adjacent to areas of advanced fibrosis. Between 2% and 10% have normal chest radiographs and high-resolution CT scans on diagnosis.	No randomized study has demonstrated improved survival compared with untreated patients. Inexorably progressive. Response to corticosteroids and cytotoxic agents at best 15%, and these probably represent misclassification of histopathology. Median survival approximately 3 years, depending on stage at presentation. Current interest in antifibrotic agents.
Respiratory bronchiolitis-associated interstitial lung disease (RB-ILD)[1] Age 40–45. Presentation similar to that of UIP though in younger patients. Similar results on pulmonary function tests, but less severe abnormalities. Patients with respiratory bronchiolitis are invariably heavy smokers.	Increased numbers of macrophages evenly dispersed within the alveolar spaces. Rare fibroblast foci, little fibrosis, minimal honeycomb change. In RB-ILD the accumulation of macrophages is localized within the peribronchiolar air spaces; in DIP,[1] it is diffuse. Alveolar architecture is preserved.	May be indistinguishable from UIP. More often presents with a nodular or reticulonodular pattern. Honeycombing rare. High-resolution CT more likely to reveal diffuse ground-glass opacities and upper lobe emphysema.	Spontaneous remission occurs in up to 20% of patients, so natural history unclear. Smoking cessation is essential. Prognosis clearly better than that of UIP: median survival greater than 10 years. Corticosteroids thought to be effective, but there are no randomized clinical trials to support this view.
Acute interstitial pneumonitis (AIP) Clinically known as Hamman-Rich syndrome. Wide age range, many young patients. Acute onset of dyspnea followed by rapid development of respiratory failure. Half of patients report a viral syndrome preceding lung disease. Clinical course indistinguishable from that of idiopathic ARDS.	Pathologic changes reflect acute response to injury within days to weeks. Resembles organizing phase of diffuse alveolar damage. Fibrosis and minimal collagen deposition. May appear similar to UIP but more homogeneous and there is no honeycomb change—though this may appear if the process persists for more than a month in a patient on mechanical ventilation.	Diffuse bilateral airspace consolidation with areas of ground-glass attenuation on high-resolution CT scan.	Supportive care (mechanical ventilation) critical but effect of specific therapies unclear. High initial mortality: Fifty to 90 percent die within 2 months after diagnosis. Not progressive if patient survives. Lung function may return to normal or may be permanently impaired.
Nonspecific interstitial pneumonitis (NSIP) Age 45–55. Slight female predominance. Similar to UIP but onset of cough and dyspnea over months, not years.	Nonspecific in that histopathology does not fit into better-established categories. Varying degrees of inflammation and fibrosis, patchy in distribution but uniform in time, suggesting response to single injury. Most have lymphocytic and plasma cell inflammation without fibrosis. Honeycombing present but scant. Some have advocated division into cellular and fibrotic subtypes.	May be indistinguishable from UIP. Most typical picture is bilateral areas of ground-glass attenuation and fibrosis on high-resolution CT. Honeycombing is rare.	Treatment thought to be effective, but no prospective clinical studies have been published. Prognosis overall good but depends on the extent of fibrosis at diagnosis. Median survival greater than 10 years.

(*continued*)

Table 29. Idiopathic fibrosing interstitial pneumonias. (continued)

Name and Clinical Presentation	Histopathology	Radiographic Pattern	Response to Therapy and Prognosis
Cryptogenic organizing pneumonitis (formerly bronchiolitis obliterans organizing pneumonia [BOOP]) Typically age 50–60 but wide variation. Abrupt onset, frequently weeks to a few months following a flu-like illness. Dyspnea and dry cough prominent, but constitiutional symptoms are common: fatigue, fever, and weight loss. Pulmonary function tests usually show restriction, but up to 25% show concomitant obstruction.	Included in the idiopathic interstitial pneumonias on clinical grounds. Buds of loose connective tissue (Masson bodies) and inflammatory cells fill alveoli and distal bronchioles.	Lung volumes normal. Chest radiograph typically shows interstitial and parenchymal disease with discrete, peripheral alveolar and ground-glass infiltrates. Nodular opacities common. High-resolution CT shows subpleural consolidation and bronchial wall thickening and dilation.	Rapid response to corticosteroids in two-thirds of patients. Long-term prognosis generally good for those who respond. Relapses are common.

[1]Includes desquamative interstitial pneumonia (DIP).
Key: ANA = antinuclear antibody; RF = rheumatoid factor; UIP = usual interstitial pneumonia; ARDS = acute respiratory distress syndrome.

Table 30. Frequency of specific symptoms and signs in patients at risk for pulmonary thromboembolism.

	UPET[1] PE+ (n = 327)	PIOPED[2] PE+ (n = 117)	PIOPED[2] PE– (n = 248)
Symptoms			
Dyspnea	84%	73%	72%
Respirophasic chest pain	74%	66%	59%
Cough	53%	37%	36%
Leg pain	nr	26%	24%
Hemoptysis	30%	13%	8%
Palpitations	nr	10%	18%
Wheezing	nr	9%	11%
Anginal pain	14%	4%	6%
Signs			
Respiratory rate ≥ 16 UPET, ≥ 20 PIOPED	92%	70%	68%
Crackles (rales)	58%	51%	40%[3]
Heart rate ≥ 100/min	44%	30%	24%
Fourth heart sound (S_4)	nr	24%	13%[3]
Accentuated pulmonary component of second heart sound (S_2P)	53%	23%	13%[3]
T ≥ 37.5 °C UPET, ≥ 38.5 °C PIOPED	43%	7%	12%
Homans' sign	nr	4%	2%
Pleural friction rub	nr	3%	2%
Third heart sound (S_3)	nr	3%	4%
Cyanosis	19%	1%	2%

[1]Data from the Urokinase-Streptokinase Pulmonary Embolism Trial, as reported in Bell WR, Simon TL, DeMets DL: The clinical features of submassive and massive pulmonary emboli. Am J Med 1977;62:355.
[2]Data from patients enrolled in the PIOPED study, as reported in Stein PD et al: Clinical, laboratory, roentgenographic, and electrocardiographic findings in patients with acute pulmonary embolism and no preexisting cardiac or pulmonary disease. Chest 1991;100:598.
[3]$P < .05$ comparing patients in the PIOPED study.
PE+ = confirmed diagnosis of pulmonary embolism; PE– = diagnosis of pulmonary embolism ruled out; nr = not reported.

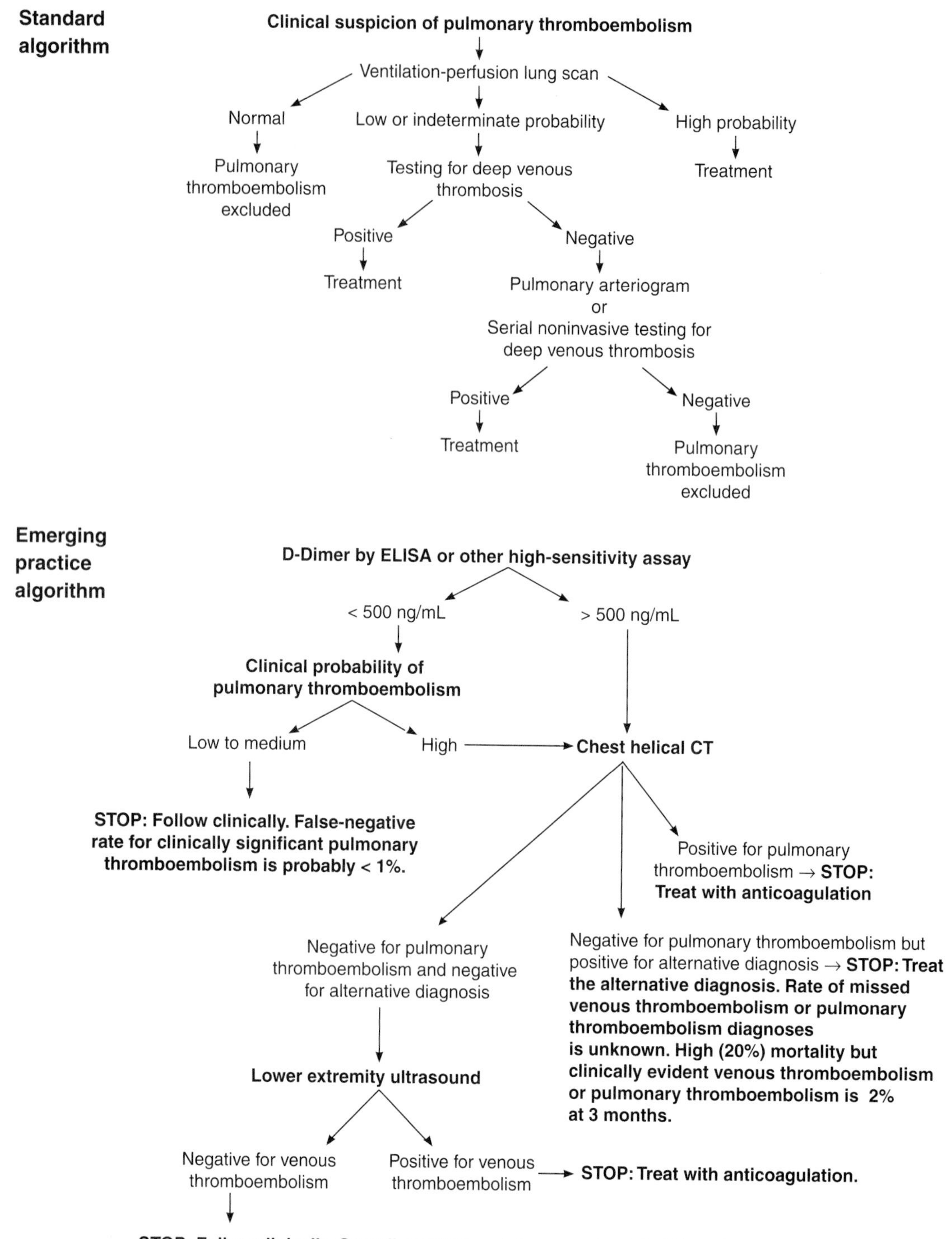

Figure 2. Two simple algorithms to guide evaluation of suspected venous thromboembolism. The standard algorithm is based on the results of ventilation-perfusion lung scanning using PIOPED data. Management of patients with ventilation-perfusion lung scans of low and indeterminate probability must always be guided by clinical judgment based upon cumulative clinical information and the degree of suspicion of pulmonary thromboembolism. The second algorithm uses D-dimer, helical CT, and venous ultrasonography to describe an evidence-based, efficient evaluation that reflects emerging practice. This second algorithm is not based on the experience of the standard ventilation-perfusion approach but anticipates a shift toward use of helical CT as the primary diagnostic test in pulmonary thromboembolism.

Table 31. Selected methods for the prevention of venous thromboembolism.

Risk Group	Recommendations for Prophylaxis
Surgical patients	
General surgery	
Low-risk: Minor procedures, age under 40, and no clinical risk factors	Early ambulation
Moderate risk: Minor procedures with additional thrombosis risk factors; age 40–60, and no other clinical risk factors; or major operations with age under 40 without additional clinical risk factors	ES, or LDUH, or LMWH, or IPC; plus early ambulation if possible
Higher risk: Major operation, over age 40 or with additional risk factors	LDUH, or LMWH, or IPC
Higher risk plus increased risk of bleeding	ES or IPC
Very high risk: Multiple risk factors	LDUH, or higher-dose LMWH, plus ES or IPC
Selected very high risk	Consider ADPW, INR 2.0–3.0, or postdischarge LMWH
Orthopedic surgery	
Elective total hip replacement surgery	Subcutaneous LMWH, or ADPW, or adjusted-dose heparin started preoperatively; plus IPC or ES
Elective total knee replacement surgery	LMWH, or ADPW, or IPC
Hip fracture surgery	LMWH or ADPW
Neurosurgery	
Intracranial neurosurgery	IPC with or without ES; LDUH and postoperative LMWH are acceptable alternatives; IPC or ES plus LDUH or LMWH may be more effective than either modality alone in high-risk patients.
Acute spinal cord injury	LMWH; IPC and ES may have additional benefit when used with LMWH. In the rehabilitation phase, conversion to full-dose warfarin may provide ongoing protection.
Trauma	
With an identifiable risk factor for thromboembolism	LMWH; IPC or ES if there is a contraindication to LMWH; consider duplex ultrasound screening in very high risk patients; IVC filter insertion if proximal DVT is identified and anticoagulation is contraindicated.
Medical patients	
Acute myocardial infarction	Subcutaneous LDUH, or full-dose heparin; if heparin is contraindicated, IPC and ES may provide some protection.
Ischemic stroke with impaired mobility	LMWH or LDUH or danaparoid; IPC or ES if anticoagulants are contraindicated
General medical patients with clinical risk factors; especially patients with cancer, congestive heart failure, or severe pulmonary disease	Low-dose LMWH, or LDUH
Cancer patients with indwelling central venous catheters	Warfarin, 1 mg/d, or LMWH

Recommendations assembled from Geerts WH et al: Prevention of venous thromboembolism. Chest 2001;119(Suppl):132.
ADPW = adjusted-dose perioperative warfarin: begin 5–10 mg the day of or the day following surgery; adjust dose to INR 2.0–3.0.
DVT = deep venous thrombosis.
ES = elastic stockings.
IPC = intermittent pneumatic compression.
IVC = inferior vena cava.
LDUH = low-dose unfractionated heparin: 5000 units subcutaneously every 8–12 hours starting 1–2 hours before surgery.
LMWH = low-molecular-weight heparin. See Table 9–24 for dosing regimens.

Table 32. Selected low-molecular-weight heparin and heparinoid regimens to prevent venous thromboembolism.

Risk Group	Drug	Subcutaneous Dose[1]	Administration Regimen	Cost[2]
General surgery, moderate risk	Dalteparin (Fragmin)	2500 units	1–2 h preop and qd postop	$17.22/dose
	Enoxaparin (Lovenox)	20 mg	1–2 h preop and qd postop	$21.41/dose
	Nadroparin (Fraxiparin)	2850 units	2–4 h preop and qd postop	No price available: Not available in USA
	Tinzaparin (Innohep)	3500 units	2 h preop and qd postop	$28.22/dose
General surgery, high risk	Dalteparin (Fragmin)	5000 units	8–12 preop and qd postop	$27.95/dose
	Danaparoid (Orgaran)	750 units	1–4 h preop and q12 h postop	No price available: Not available in USA
	Enoxaparin (Lovenox)	40 mg	1–2 h preop and qd postop	$28.54/dose
	Enoxaparin (Lovenox)	30 mg	q12 h starting 8–12 h postop	$21.41/dose
Orthopedic surgery	Dalteparin (Fragmin)	5000 units	8–12 h preop and qd starting 12–24 h postop	$27.95/dose
	Dalteparin (Fragmin)	2500 units	6–8 h postop then 5000 units qd	$17.22/dose
	Danaparoid (Orgaran)	750 units	1–4 preop and q12 h postop	No price available: Not available in USA
	Enoxaparin (Lovenox)	30 mg	q12 h starting 12–24 h postop	$21.41/dose
	Enoxaparin (Lovenox)	40 mg	qd starting 10–12 h preop	$28.54/dose
	Nadroparin (Fraxiparin)	38 units/kg	12 h preop, 12 h postop, and qd on postop days 1, 2, 3; then increase to 57 units/kg qd	No price available: Not available in USA
	Tinzaparin (Innohep)	75 units/kg	qd starting 12–24 h postop	$36.29/dose (60 kg pt).
	Tinzaparin (Innohep)	4500 units	12 h preop and qd postop	$36.29/dose
Major trauma	Enoxaparin (Lovenox)	30 mg	q12h starting 12–36 h postinjury if hemostatically stable	$21.41/dose
Acute spinal cord injury	Enoxaparin (Lovenox)	30 mg	q12h	$21.41/dose
Medical conditions	Dalteparin (Fragmin)	2500 units	qd	$17.22/dose
	Danaparoid (Orgaran)	750 units	q12h	No price available: Not available in USA
	Enoxaparin (Lovenox)	40 mg	qd	$28.54/dose
	Nadroparin (Fraxiparin)	2850 units	qd	No price available: Not available in USA

Modified and reproduced with permission, from Geerts WH et al: Prevention of venous thromboembolism. Chest 2001;119:132S.
[1]Dose expressed in anti-Xa units; for enoxaparin, 1 mg = 100 anti-Xa units.
[2]Average wholesale price (AWP, for AB-rated generic when available) for quantity listed. Source: *Red Book* Update, Vol. 24, No. 4, April 2005. AWP may not accurately represent the actual pharmacy cost because wide contractual variations exist among institutions.
Preop = preoperatively; Postop = postoperatively; qd = once daily.

Table 33. Intravenous heparin dosing based on body weight.

Initial dosing

1. Load with 80 units/kg IV, then
2. Initiate a maintenance infusion at 18 units/kg/h
3. Check activated partial thromboplastin time (aPTT) in 6 hours

Dose adjustment schedule based on aPTT results

< 35 s (< 1.2 × control)	Rebolus with 80 units/kg; increase infusion by 4 units/kg/h
35–45 s (1.2–1.5 × control)	Rebolus with 40 units/kg; increase infusion by 2 units/kg/h
46–70 s (1.5–2.3 × control)	No change
71–90 s (2.3–3 × control)	Decrease infusion rate by 2 units/kg/h
> 90 s (> 3 × control)	Stop infusion for 1 hour, then decrease infusion by 3 units/kg/h

Repeat aPTT every 6 hours for the first 24 hours. If the aPTT is 46–70 s after 24 hours, then recheck once daily every morning. If the aPTT is outside this therapeutic range at 24 hours, continue checking every 6 hours until it is 46–70 s. Once it has been in the therapeutic range on two consecutive measurements after 24 hours, check once daily every morning.

Adapted from Raschke RA et al: The weight-based heparin dosing nomogram compared with a "standard care" nomogram. Ann Intern Med 1993;119:874.

Table 34. Selected low-molecular-weight heparin anticoagulation regimens.

Drug	Suggested Treatment Dose [1] (Subcutaneous)
Dalteparin	200 units/kg once daily (not to exceed 18,000 units/dose)
Enoxaparin	1.5 mg/kg once daily (single dose not to exceed 180 mg)
Nadroparin	86 units/kg twice daily for 10 days, or 171 units/kg once daily (single dose not to exceed 17,000 units)
Tinzaparin	175 units/kg once daily

Modified and reproduced with permission, from Hyers TM et al: Antithrombotic therapy for venous thromboembolic disease. Chest 2001;119(Suppl):176S.

[1]Dose expressed in anti-Xa units; for enoxaparin, 1 mg = 100 anti-Xa units.

Table 35. Selected causes of hypersensitivity pneumonitis.

Disease	Antigen	Source
Farmer's lung	*Micropolyspora faeni, Thermoactinomyces vulgaris*	Moldy hay
"Humidifier" lung	Thermophilic actinomycetes	Contaminated humidifiers, heating systems, or air conditioners
Bird fancier's lung ("pigeon-breeder's disease")	Avian proteins	Bird serum and excreta
Bagassosis	*Thermoactinomyces sacchari* and *T vulgaris*	Moldy sugar cane fiber (bagasse)
Sequoiosis	Graphium, aureobasidium, and other fungi	Moldy redwood sawdust
Maple bark stripper's disease	*Cryptostroma (Coniosporium) corticale*	Rotting maple tree logs or bark
Mushroom picker's disease	Same as farmer's lung	Moldy compost
Suberosis	*Penicillium frequentans*	Moldy cork dust
Detergent worker's lung	*Bacillus subtilis* enzyme	Enzyme additives

Table 36. Causes of pleural fluid transudates and exudates.

Transudates	Exudates
Congestive heart failure (≈90% of cases)	Pneumonia (parapneumonic effusion)
Cirrhosis with ascites	Cancer
Nephrotic syndrome	Pulmonary embolism
Peritoneal dialysis	Bacterial infection
Myxedema	Tuberculosis
Acute atelectasis	Connective tissue disease
Constrictive pericarditis	Viral infection
Superior vena cava obstruction	Fungal infection
Pulmonary embolism	Rickettsial infection
	Parasitic infection
	Asbestos
	Meigs' syndrome
	Pancreatic disease
	Uremia
	Chronic atelectasis
	Trapped lung
	Chylothorax
	Sarcoidosis
	Drug reaction
	Post-myocardial infarction syndrome

Table 37. Characteristics of important exudative pleural effusions.

Etiology or Type of Effusion	Gross Appearance	White Blood Cell Count (cells/mcL)	Red Blood Cell Count (cells/mcL)	Glucose	Comments
Malignant effusion	Turbid to bloody; occasionally serous	1000 to < 100,000 M	100 to several hundred thousand	Equal to serum levels; < 60 mg/dL in 15% of cases	Eosinophilia uncommon; positive results on cytologic examination
Uncomplicated parapneumonic effusion	Clear to turbid	5000–25,000 P	< 5000	Equal to serum levels	Tube thoracostomy unnecessary
Empyema	Turbid to purulent	25,000–100,000 P	< 5000	Less than serum levels; often very low	Drainage necessary; putrid odor suggests anaerobic infection
Tuberculosis	Serous to serosanguineous	5000–10,000 M	< 10,000	Equal to serum levels; occasionally < 60 mg/dL	Protein > 4.0 g/dL and may exceed 5 g/dL; eosinophils (> 10%) or mesothelial cells (> 5%) make diagnosis unlikely
Rheumatoid effusion	Turbid; greenish yellow	1000–20,000 M or P	< 1000	< 40 mg/dL	Secondary empyema common; high LDH, low complement, high rheumatoid factor, cholesterol crystals are characteristic
Pulmonary infarction	Serous to grossly bloody	1000–50,000 M or P	100 to > 100,000	Equal to serum levels	Variable findings; no pathognomonic features
Esophageal rupture	Turbid to purulent; red-brown	< 5000 to > 50,000 P	1000–10,000	Usually low	High amylase level (salivary origin); pneumothorax in 25% of cases; effusion usually on left side; pH < 6.0 strongly suggests diagnosis
Pancreatitis	Turbid to serosanguineous	1000–50,000 P	1000–10,000	Equal to serum levels	Usually left-sided; high amylase level

Key: M = mononuclear cell predominance; P = polymorphonuclear leukocyte predominance; LDH = lactate dehydrogenase.

Table 38. Selected disorders associated with ARDS.

Systemic Insults	Pulmonary Insults
Trauma	Aspiration of gastric contents
Sepsis	Embolism of thrombus, fat, air, or amniotic fluid
Pancreatitis	Miliary tuberculosis
Shock	Diffuse pneumonia (eg, SARS)
Multiple transfusions	Acute eosinophilic pneumonia
Disseminated intravascular coagulation	Cryptogenic organizing pneumonitis
Burns	Upper airway obstruction
Drugs and drug overdose	Free-base cocaine smoking
Opioids	Near-drowning
Aspirin	Toxic gas inhalation
Phenothiazines	Upper airway obstruction
Tricyclic andtidepressants	Nitrogen dioxide
Amiodarone	Chlorine
Chemotherapeutic agents	Sulfur dioxide
Nitrofurantoin	Ammonia
Protamine	Smoke
Thrombotic thrombocytopenic purpura	Oxygen toxicity
Cardiopulmonary bypass	Lung contusion
Head injury	Radiation exposure
Paraquat	High-altitude exposure
	Lung reexpansion or reperfusion

ARDS = acute respiratory distress syndrome; SARS = severe acute respiratory syndrome.

Table 39. Thrombolytic therapy for acute myocardial infarction.

	Streptokinase	Alteplase; Tissue Plasminogen Activator (t-PA)	Reteplase	Tenecteplase (TNK-t-PA)
Source	Group C streptococcus	Recombinant DNA	Recombinant DNA	Recombinant DNA
Half-life	20 minutes	5 minutes	15 minutes	20 minutes
Usual dose	1.5 million units	100 mg	20 units	40 mg
Administration	750,000 units over 20 minutes followed by 750,000 units over 40 minutes	Initial bolus of 15 mg, followed by 50 mg infused over the next 30 minutes and 35 mg over the following 60 minutes	10 units as a bolus over 2 minutes, repeated after 30 minutes	Single weight-adjusted bolus, 0.5 mg/kg
Anticoagulation after infusion	Aspirin, 325 mg daily; there is no evidence that adjunctive heparin improves outcome following streptokinase	Aspirin, 325 mg daily; heparin, 5000 units as bolus, followed by 1000 units per hour infusion, subsequently adjusted to maintain PTT 1.5–2 times control	Aspirin, 325 mg; heparin as with t-PA	Aspirin, 325 mg daily
Clot selectivity	Low	High	High	High
Fibrinogenolysis	+++	+	+	+
Bleeding	+	+	+	+
Hypotension	+++	+	+	+
Allergic reactions	++	0	0	+
Reocclusion	5–20%	10–30%	—	5–20%
Approximate cost[1]	$562.50	$3404.78	$2872.50	$2917.48

PTT = partial thromboplastin time.
[1]Average wholesale price (AWP, for AB-rated generic when available) for quantity listed. Source: *Red Book* Update, Vol. 24, No. 4, April 2005. AWP may not accurately represent the actual pharmacy cost because wide contractual variations exist among institutions.

Table 40. Antiarrhythmic drugs.

Agent	Intravenous Dosage	Oral Dosage	Therapeutic Plasma Level	Route of Elimination	Side Effects
Class Ia: Action: Sodium channel blockers: Depress phase 0 depolarization; slow conduction; prolong repolarization. **Indications:** Supraventricular tachycardia, ventricular tachycardia, prevention of ventricular fibrillation, symptomatic ventricular premature beats.					
Quinidine	6–10 mg/kg (intramuscularly or intravenously) over 20 min (rarely used parenterally)	200–400 mg every 4–6 h or every 8 h (long-acting)	2–5 mg/mL	Hepatic	GI, ↓LVF, ↑Dig
Procainamide	100 mg/1–3 min to 500–1000 mg; maintain at 2–6 mg/min	50 mg/kg/d in divided doses every 3–4 h or every 6 h (long-acting)	4–10 mg/mL; NAPA (active metabolite), 10–20 μg/mL	Renal	SLE, hypersensitivity, ↓LVF
Disopyramide		100–200 mg every 6–8 h	2–8 mg/mL	Renal	Urinary retention, dry mouth, markedly ↓LVF
Moricizine		200–300 mg every 8 h	***Note:*** Active metabolites	Hepatic	Dizziness, nausea, headache, ↓theophylline level, ↓LVF
Class Ib: Action: Shorten repolarization. **Indications:** Ventricular tachycardia, prevention of ventricular fibrillation, symptomatic ventricular beats.					
Lidocaine	1–2 mg/kg at 50 mg/min; maintain at 1–4 mg/min		1–5 mg/mL	Hepatic	CNS, GI
Mexiletine		100–300 mg every 6–12 h; maximum: 1200 mg/d	0.5–2 mg/mL	Hepatic	CNS, GI, leukopenia
Phenytoin	50 mg/5 min to 1000 mg (12 mg/kg); maintain at 200–400 mg/d	200–400 mg every 12–24 h	5–20 mg/mL	Hepatic	CNS, GI
Class Ic: Action: Depress phase 0 repolarization; slow conduction. *Propafenone* is a weak calcium channel blocker and β-blocker and prolongs action potential and refractoriness. **Indications:** Life-threatening ventricular tachycardia or fibrillation, refractory supraventricular tachycardia.					
Flecainide		100–200 mg twice daily	0.2–1 mg/mL	Hepatic	CNS, GI, ↓↓LVF, incessant VT, sudden death
Propafenone		150–300 mg every 8–12 h	***Note:*** Active metabolites	Hepatic	CNS, GI, ↓↓LVF, ↑Dig
Class II: Action: β-blocker, slows AV conduction. ***Note:*** Other β-blockers may also have antiarrhythmic effects but are not yet approved for this indication in the United States. **Indications:** Supraventricular tachycardia; may prevent ventricular fibrillation.					
Esmolol	500 mg/kg over 1–2 min; maintain at 25–200 mg/kg/min	Other β-blockers may be used concomitantly	0.15–2 mg/mL	Hepatic	↓LVF, bronchospasm
Propranolol	1–5 mg at 1 mg/min	40–320 mg in 1–4 doses daily (depending on preparation)	Not established	Hepatic	↓LVF, bradycardia, AV block, bronchospasm
Metoprolol	2.5–5 mg	50–200 mg daily	Not established	Hepatic	↓LVF, bradycardia, AV block

(continued)

Table 40. Antiarrhythmic drugs. (continued)

Agent	Intravenous Dosage	Oral Dosage	Therapeutic Plasma Level	Route of Elimination	Side Effects
Class III: Action: Prolong action potential. **Indications:** *Amiodarone:* refractory ventricular tachycardia, supraventricular tachycardia, prevention of ventricular tachycardia, atrial fibrillation, ventricular fibrillation; *dofetilide:* atrial fibrillation and flutter; *sotalol:* ventricular tachycardia, atrial fibrillation; *bretylium:* ventricular fibrillation, ventricular tachycardia; *ibutilide:* conversion of atrial fibrillation and flutter.					
Amiodarone	150 mg infused rapidly, followed by 1-mg/min infusion for 6 h (360 mg) and then 0.5 mg/min; additional 150 mg as needed	800–1600 mg/d for 7–21 days; maintain at 100–400 mg/d (higher doses may be needed)	1–5 mg/mL	Hepatic	Pulmonary fibrosis, hypothyroidism, hyperthyroidism, corneal and skin deposits, hepatitis, ↑Dig, neurotoxicity, GI
Sotalol		80–160 mg every 12 h (higher doses may be used for life-threatening arrhythmias)		Renal (dosing interval should be extended if creatinine clearance is < 60 mL/min)	Early incidence of torsade de pointes, ↓LVF, bradycardia, fatigue (and other side effects associated with β-blockers)
Dofetilide		500 mg twice daily		Renal (dose must be reduced with renal dysfunction)	Torsade de pointes in 3%; interaction with cytochrome P-450 inhibitors
Ibutilide	1 mg over 10 min, followed by a second infusion of 0.5–1 mg over 10 min			Hepatic and renal	Torsade de pointes in up to 5% of patients within 3 h after administration; patients must be monitored with defibrillator nearby
Bretylium	5–10 mg/kg over 5–10 min; maintain at 0.5–2 mg/min; maximum: 30 mg/kg		0.5–1.5 mg/mL	Renal	Hypotension, nausea
Class IV: Action: Slow calcium channel blockers. **Indications:** Supraventricular tachycardia.					
Verapamil	10–20 mg over 2–20 min; maintain at 5 mg/kg/min	80–120 mg every 6–8 h; 240–360 mg once daily with sustained-release preparation	0.1–0.15 mg/mL	Hepatic	↓LVF, constipation, ↑Dig, hypotension
Diltiazem	0.25 mg/kg over 2 min; second 0.35-mg/kg bolus after 15 min if response is inadequate; infusion rate, 5–15 mg/h	180–360 mg daily in 1–3 doses depending on preparation (oral forms not approved for arrhythmias)		Hepatic metabolism, renal excretion	Hypotension, ↓LVF
Adenosine	6 mg rapidly followed by 12 mg after 1–2 min if needed; use half these doses if administered via central line.			Adenosine receptor stimulation, metabolized in blood	Transient flushing, dyspnea, chest pain, AV block, sinus bradycardia; effect ↓ by theophylline, ↑ by dipyridamole
Digoxin	0.5 mg over 20 min followed by increment of 0.25 or 0.125 mg to 1–1.5 mg over 24 h	1–1.5 mg over 24–36 h in 3 or 4 doses; maintenance, 0.125–0.5 mg/d	0.7–2 mg/mL	Renal	AV block, arrhythmias, GI, visual changes

AV = atrioventricular; CNS = central nervous system; ↑Dig = elevation of serum digoxin level; GI = gastrointestinal (nausea, vomiting, diarrhea); ↓LVF = reduced left ventricular function; NAPA = *N*-acetylprocainamide; SLE = systemic lupus erythematosus; VT = ventricular tachycardia.

Table 41. Lifestyle modifications to manage hypertension.[1]

Modification	Recommendation	Approximate Systolic BP Reduction, Range
Weight reduction	Maintain normal body weight (BMI, 18.5–24.9)	5–20 mm Hg/10-kg weight loss
Adopt DASH eating plan	Consume a diet rich in fruits, vegetables, and low-fat dairy products with a reduced content of saturated fat and total fat	8–14 mm Hg
Dietary sodium reduction	Reduce dietary sodium intake to no more than 100 mEq/L (2.4 g sodium or 6 g sodium chloride)	2–8 mm Hg
Physical activity	Engage in regular aerobic physical activity such as brisk walking (at least 30 minutes per day, most days of the week)	4–9 mm Hg
Moderation of alcohol consumption	Limit consumption to no more than two drinks per day (1 oz or 30 mL ethanol [eg, 24 oz beer, 10 oz wine, or 3 oz 80-proof whiskey]) in most men and no more than one drink per day in women and lighter-weight persons	2–4 mm Hg

From Chobanian AV et al: The Seventh Report of the Joint National Committee on Prevention, Detection, Evaluation, and Treatment of High Blood Pressure: the JNC 7 report. JAMA 2003;289:2560.

BMI = body mass index calculated as weight in kilograms divided by the square of height in meters; BP = blood pressure; DASH = Dietary Approaches to Stop Hypertension.

[1]For overall cardiovascular risk reduction, stop smoking. The effects of implementing these modifications are dose and time dependent and could be higher for some individuals.

Table 42. Classification and management of blood pressure for adults aged 18 years or older.

BP Classification	Systolic BP, mm Hg[1]		Diastolic BP, mm Hg[1]	Management		
				Lifestyle Modification	Initial Drug Therapy	
					Without Compelling Indication	With Compelling Indications[2]
Normal	< 120	and	< 80	Encourage		
Prehypertension	120–139	or	80–89	Yes	No antihypertensive drug indicated	Drugs for the compelling indications[3]
Stage 1 hypertension	140–159	or	90–99	Yes	Thiazide-type diuretics for most; may consider ACE inhibitor, ARB, β-blocker, CCB, or combination	Drug(s) for the compelling indications Other antihypertensive drugs (diuretics, ACE inhibitor, ARB, β-blocker, CCB) as needed
Stage 2 hypertension	≥ 160	or	≥ 100	Yes	Two-drug combination for most (usually thiazide-type diuretic and ACE inhibitor or ARB or β-blocker or CCB)[4]	Drug(s) for the compelling indications Other antihypertensive drugs (diuretics, ACE inhibitor, ARB, β-blocker, CCB) as needed

From Chobanian AV et al: The Seventh Report of the Joint National Committee on Prevention, Detection, Evaluation, and Treatment of High Blood Pressure: the JNC 7 report. JAMA 2003;289:2560.

ACE = angiotensin-converting enzyme; ARB = angiotensin receptor blocker; BP = blood pressure; CCB = calcium channel blocker.

[1]Treatment determined by highest BP category.

[2]See Table 11–10.

[3]Treat patients with chronic kidney disease or diabetes to BP goal of less than 130/80 mm Hg.

[4]Initial combined therapy should be used cautiously in those at risk for orthostatic hypotension.

Table 43. Identifiable causes of hypertension.

Sleep apnea
Drug-induced or drug-related (see Table 11–11)
Chronic kidney disease
Primary aldosteronism
Renovascular disease
Chronic steroid therapy and Cushing's syndrome
Pheochromocytoma
Coarctation of the aorta
Thyroid or parathyroid disease

From Chobanian AV et al: The Seventh Report of the Joint National Committee on Prevention, Detection, Evaluation, and Treatment of High Blood Pressure: the JNC 7 report. JAMA 2003;289:2560.

Table 44. Causes of resistant hypertension.

Improper blood pressure measurement
Volume overload and pseudotolerance
Excess sodium intake
Volume retention from kidney disease
Inadequate diuretic therapy
Drug-induced or other causes
Nonadherence
Inadequate doses
Inappropriate combinations
Nonsteroidal anti-inflammatory drugs; cyclooxygenase-2 inhibitors
Cocaine, amphetamines, other illicit drugs
Sympathomimetics (decongestants, anorectics)
Oral contraceptives
Adrenal steroids
Cyclosporine and tacrolimus
Erythropoietin
Licorice (including some chewing tobacco)
Selected over-the-counter dietary supplements and medicines (eg, ephedra, ma haung, bitter orange)
Associated conditions
Obesity
Excess alcohol intake
Identifiable causes of hypertension (see Table 11–3)

From Chobanian AV et al: The Seventh Report of the Joint National Committee on Prevention, Detection, Evaluation, and Treatment of High Blood Pressure: the JNC 7 report. JAMA 2003;289:2560.

Table 45. Clinical trial and guideline basis for compelling indications for individual drug classes.

High-Risk Conditions with Compelling Indication[1]	Recommended Drugs						Clinical Trial Basis[2]
	Diuretic	β-Blocker	ACE Inhibitor	ARB	CCB	Aldosterone Antagonist	
Heart failure	•	•	•	•		•	ACC/AHA Heart Failure Guideline, MERIT-HF, COPERNICUS, CIBIS, SOLVD, AIRE, TRACE, ValHEFT, RALES
Post-myocardial infarction		•	•			•	ACC/AHA Post-MI Guideline, BHAT, SAVE, Capricorn, EPHESUS
High coronary disease risk	•	•	•		•		ALLHAT, HOPE, ANBP2, LIFE, CONVINCE
Diabetes	•	•	•	•	•		NKF-ADA Guideline, UKPDS, ALLHAT
Chronic kidney disease			•	•			NKF Guideline, Captopril Trial, RENAAL, IDNT, REIN, AASK
Recurrent stroke prevention	•		•				PROGRESS

From Chobanian AV et al: The Seventh Report of the Joint National Committee on Prevention, Detection, Evaluation, and Treatment of High Blood Pressure: the JNC 7 report. JAMA 2003;289:2560.

AASK = African American Study of Kidney Disease and Hypertension; ACC/AHA = American College of Cardiology/American Heart Association; ACE = angiotensin converting enzyme; AIRE = Acute Infarction Ramipril Efficacy; ALLHAT = Antihypertensive and Lipid-Lowering Treatment to Prevent Heart Attack Trial; ANBP2 = Second Australian National Blood Pressure Study; ARB = angiotensin receptor blocker; BHAT = β-Blocker Heart Attack Trial; CCB = calcium channel blocker; CIBIS = Cardiac Insufficiency Bisoprolol Study; CONVINCE = Controlled Onset Verapamil Investigation of Cardiovascular End Points; COPERNICUS = Carvedilol Prospective Randomized Cumulative Survival Study; EPHESUS = Eplerenone Post-Acute Myocardial Infarction Heart Failure Efficacy and Survival Study; HOPE = Heart Outcomes Prevention Evaluation Study; IDNT = Irbesartan Diabetic Nephropathy Trial; LIFE = Losartan Intervention For Endpoint Reduction in Hypertension Study; MERIT-HF = Metoprolol CR/XL Randomized Intervention Trial in Congestive Heart Failure; NKF-ADA = National Kidney Foundation–American Diabetes Association; PROGRESS = Perindopril Protection Against Recurrent Stroke Study; RALES = Randomized Aldactone Evaluation Study: REIN, Ramipril Efficacy in Nephropathy Study; RENAAL, Reduction of Endpoints in Non-Insulin-Dependent Diabetes Mellitus with the Angiotensin II Antagonist Losartan Study; SAVE = Survival and Ventricular Enlargement Study; SOLVD = Studies of Left Ventricular Dysfunction; TRACE = Trandolapril Cardiac Evaluation Study; UKPDS = United Kingdom Prospective Diabetes Study; ValHEFT = Valsartan Heart Failure Trial.

[1]Compelling indications for antihypertensive drugs are based on benefits from outcome studies or existing clinical guidelines; the compelling indication is managed in parallel with the blood pressure.

[2]Conditions for which clinical trials demonstrate benefit of specific classes of antihypertensive drugs.

Table 46. Antihypertensive drugs: diuretics.

Drug	Proprietary Name	Initial Dosage	Dosage Range	Cost per Unit	Cost of 30 Days Treatment[1] (Average Dosage)	Adverse Effects	Comments
THIAZIDES AND RELATED DIURETICS							
Hydrochlorothiazide	Esidrix, Hydro-Diuril	12.5 or 25 mg once daily	12.5–50 mg once daily	$0.08/25 mg	$2.40	↓ K^+, ↓ Mg^{2+}, ↑ Ca^{2+}, ↓ Na^+, ↑ uric acid, ↑ glucose, ↑ LDL cholesterol, ↑ triglycerides; rash, erectile dysfunction.	Low dosages effective in many patients without associated metabolic abnormalities; metolazone more effective with concurrent renal insufficiency; indapamide does not alter serum lipid levels.
Chlorthalidone	Hygroton, Thaliton	12.5 or 25 mg once daily	12.5–50 mg once daily	$0.23/25 mg	$6.90		
Metolazone	Zaroxolyn	1.25 or 2.5 mg once daily	1.25–5 mg once daily	$1.48/5 mg	$44.40		
	Mykrox	0.5 mg once daily	0.5–1 mg once daily	$1.24/0.5 mg	$37.20		
Indapamide	Lozol	2.5 mg once daily	2.5–5 mg once daily	$0.83/2.5 mg	$24.90		
LOOP DIURETICS							
Furosemide	Lasix	20 mg twice daily	40–320 mg in 2 or 3 doses	$0.16/40 mg	$9.60	Same as thiazides, but higher risk of excessive diuresis and electrolyte imbalance. Increases calcium excretion.	**Furosemide:** Short duration of action a disadvantage; should be reserved for patients with renal insufficiency or fluid retention. Poor antihypertensive. **Torsemide:** Effective blood pressure medication at low dosage.
Ethacrynic acid	Edecrin	50 mg once daily	50–100 mg once or twice dily	$0.75/50 mg	$45.00		
Bumetanide	Bumex	0.25 mg twice daily	0.5–10 mg in 2 or 3 doses	$0.45/1 mg	$27.00		
Torsemide	Demadex	2.5 mg once daily	5–10 mg once daily	$0.70/10 mg	$21.00		
ALDOSTERONE RECEPTOR BLOCKERS							
Spironolactone	Aldactone	12.5 or 25 mg once daily	12.5–100 mg once daily	$0.46/25 mg	$13.80	Hyperkalemia, metabolic acidosis, gynecomastia.	Can be useful add-on therapy in patients with refractory hypertension.
Amiloride	Midamor	5 mg once daily	5–10 mg once daily	$0.47/5 mg	$14.10		
Eplerenone	Inspra	25 mg once daily	25–100 mg once daily	$3.60/25 mg	$108.00		

(continued)

Table 46. Antihypertensive drugs: diuretics. (continued)

Drug	Proprietary Name	Initial Dosage	Dosage Range	Cost per Unit	Cost of 30 Days Treatment[1] (Average Dosage)	Adverse Effects	Comments
COMBINATION PRODUCTS							
Hydrochlorothiazide and triamterene	Dyazide (25/50 mg); Maxzide (25/37.5 mg)	1 tab once daily	1 or 2 tabs once daily	$0.36	$10.80	Same as thiazides plus GI disturbances, hyperkalemia rather than hypokalemia, headache; triamterene can cause kidney stones and renal dysfunction; spironolactone causes gynecomastia. Hyperkalemia can occur if this combination is used in patients with renal failure or those taking ACE inhibitors.	Use should be limited to patients with demonstrable need for a potassium-sparing agent.
Hydrochlorothiazide and amiloride	Moduretic (50/5 mg)	1/2 tab once daily	1 or 2 tabs once daily	$0.42	$12.60		
Hydrochlorothiazide and spironolactone	Aldactazide (25/25 mg)	1 tab once daily	1 or 2 tabs once daily	$0.50	$15.00		

LDL = low-density lipoprotein; GI = gastrointestinal; ACE = angiotensin-converting enzyme.

[1]Average wholesale price (AWP, for AB-rated generic when available) for quantity listed. Source: *Red Book* Update, Vol. 24, No. 4, April 2005. AWP may not accurately represent the actual pharmacy cost because wide contractual variations exist among institutions.

Table 47. Antihypertensive drugs: β-adrenergic blocking agents.

Drug	Proprietary Name	Initial Dosage	Dosage Range	Cost per Unit	Cost of 30 Days Treatment (Based on Average Dosage)[1]	Special Properties					Comments[5]
						β_1 Selectivity[2]	ISA[3]	MSA[4]	Lipid Solubility	Renal vs Hepatic Elimination	
Acebutolol	Sectral	200 mg once daily	200–1200 mg in 1 or 2 doses	$1.34/400 mg	$ 40.20	+	+	+	+	H > R	Positive ANA; rare LE syndrome; also indicated for arrhythmias. Doses > 800 mg have β_1 and β_2 effects.
Atenolol	Tenormin	25 mg once daily	25–200 mg once daily	$0.83/50 mg	$24.90	+	0	0	0	R	Also indicated for angina pectoris and post-MI. Doses > 100 mg have β_1 and β_2 effects.
Betaxolol	Kerlone	10 mg once daily	10–40 mg once daily	$1.10/10 mg	$33.00	+	0	0	+	H > R	
Bisoprolol and hydrochlorothiazide	Ziac	5 mg/6.25 mg	2.5–10 mg plus 6.25 mg	$1.14/2.5/6.25 mg	$34.20	+	0	0	0	R = H	Low-dose combination approved for initial therapy. Bisoprolol also effective for heart failure.
Carteolol	Cartrol	2.5 mg once daily	2.5–10 mg once daily	$1.36/5 mg	$40.80	0	+	0	+	R > H	
Carvedilol	Coreg	6.25 mg	12.5–100 mg in 2 doses	$1.83/25 mg	$109.80 (25 mg twice a day)	0	0	0	+++	H > R	α:β-Blocking activity 1:9; may cause orthostatic symptoms; effective for congestive heart failure.
Labetalol	Normodyne, Trandate	100 mg twice daily	200–1200 mg in 2 doses	$0.71/200 mg	$42.60	0	0/+	0	++	H	α:β-Blocking activity 1:3; more orthostatic hypotension, fever, hepatotoxicity.

(continued)

Table 47. Antihypertensive drugs: β-adrenergic blocking agents.[1] (continued)

Drug	Proprietary Name	Initial Dosage	Dosage Range	Cost per Unit	Cost of 30 Days Treatment (Based on Average Dosage)[2]	Special Properties					Comments[5]
						β_1 Selectivity[3]	ISA[4]	MSA[5]	Lipid Solubility	Renal vs Hepatic Elimination	
Metoprolol	Lopressor	50 mg in 1 or 2 doses	50–200 mg in 1 or 2 doses	$0.55/50 mg	$33.00	+	0	+	+++	H	Also indicated for angina pectoris and post-MI. Approved for heart failure. Doses > 100 mg have β_1 and β_2 effects.
	Toprol XL (SR preparation)	50 mg once daily	50–200 mg once daily	$1.28/100 mg	$38.40						
Nadolol	Corgard	20 mg once daily	20–160 mg once daily	$1.05/40 mg	$31.50	0	0	0	0	R	
Penbutolol	Levatol	20 mg once daily	20–80 mg once daily	$1.80/20 mg	$54.00	0	+	0	++	R > H	
Pindolol	Visken	5 mg twice daily	10–60 mg in 2 doses	$0.70/5 mg	$42.00	0	++	+	+	H > R	In adults, 35% renal clearance.
Propranolol	Inderal	20 mg twice daily	40–320 mg in 2 doses	$0.51/40 mg	$30.60	0	0	++	+++	H	Once-daily SR preparation also available. Also indicated for angina pectoris and post-MI.
Timolol	Blocadren	5 mg twice daily	10–40 mg in 2 doses	$0.38/10 mg	$ 22.80	0	0	0	++	H > R	Also indicated for post-MI. 80% hepatic clearance.

ISA = intrinsic sympathomimetic activity; MSA = membrane-stabilizing activity; ANA = antinuclear antibody; LE = lupus erythematosus; MI = myocardial infarction; SR = sustained release; 0 = no effect; +, ++, +++ = some, moderate, most effect.

[1]Average wholesale price (AWP, for AB-rated generic when available) for quantity listed. Source: *Red Book* Update, Vol. 25, No. 4, April 2005. AWP may not accurately represent the actual pharmacy cost because wide contractual variations exist among institutions.

[2]Agents with β_1 selectivity are less likely to precipitate bronchospasm and decreased peripheral blood flow *in low doses*, but selectivity is only relative.

[3]Agents with ISA cause less resting bradycardia and lipid changes.

[4]MSA generally occurs at concentrations greater than those necessary for β-adrenergic blockade. The clinical importance of MSA by β-blockers has not been defined.

[5]Adverse effects of all β-blockers: bronchospasm, fatigue, sleep disturbance and nightmares, bradycardia and atrioventricular block, worsening of congestive heart failure, cold extremities, gastrointestinal disturbances, impotence, ↑triglycerides, ↓HDL cholesterol, rare blood dyscrasias.

Table 48. Antihypertensive drugs: ACE inhibitors and angiotensin II receptor blockers.

Drug	Proprietary Name	Initial Dosage	Dosage Range	Cost per Unit	Cost of 30 Days Treatment (Average Dosage)[1]	Adverse Effects	Comments
ACE INHIBITORS							
Benazepril	Lotensin	10 mg once daily	5–40 mg in 1 or 2 doses	$1.05/20 mg	$31.50	Cough, hypotension, dizziness, renal dysfunction, hyperkalemia, angioedema; taste alteration and rash (may be more frequent with captopril); rarely, proteinuria, blood dyscrasia. Contraindicated in pregnancy.	More fosinopril is excreted by the liver in patients with renal dysfunction (dose reduction may or may not be necessary). Captopril and lisinopril are active without metabolism. Captopril, enalapril, lisinopril, and quinapril are approved for congestive heart failure.
Captopril	Capoten	25 mg twice daily	50–300 mg in 2 or 3 doses	$0.65/25 mg	$39.00		
Enalapril	Vasotec	5 mg once daily	5–40 mg in 1 or 2 doses	$1.52/20 mg	$45.60		
Fosinopril	Monopril	10 mg once daily	10–80 mg in 1 or 2 doses	$1.19/20 mg	$35.70		
Lisinopril	Prinivil, Zestril	5–10 mg once daily	5–40 mg once daily	$1.06/20 mg	$31.80		
Moexipril	Univasc	7.5 mg once daily	7.5–30 mg in 1 or 2 doses	$1.33/ 7.5 mg	$39.90		
Perindopril	Aceon	4 mg once daily	4–16 mg in 1 or 2 doses	$2.07/8 mg	$62.10		
Quinapril	Accupril	10 mg once daily	10–80 mg in 1 or 2 doses	$1.23/20 mg	$36.90		
Ramipril	Altace	2.5 mg once daily	2.5–20 mg in 1 or 2 doses	$1.59/5 mg	$47.70		
Trandolapril	Mavik	1 mg once daily	1–8 mg once daily	$1.15/4 mg	$34.50		
ANGIOTENSIN II RECEPTOR BLOCKERS							
Candesartan cilexitil	Atacand	16 mg once daily	8–32 mg once daily	$1.63/16 mg	$48.95	Hyperkalemia, renal dysfunction, rare angioedema. Combinations have additional side effects. Contraindicated in pregnancy.	Losartan has a very flat dose-response curve. Valsartan and irbesartan have wider dose-response ranges and longer durations of action. Addition of low-dose diuretic (separately or as combination pills) increases the response.
Candesartan cilexitil/ HCTZ	Atacand HCT	16 mg/ 12.5 mg once daily	8–32 mg of candesartan once daily	$2.21/16 mg/12.5 mg	$66.25		
Eprosartan	Teveten	600 mg once daily	400–800 mg in 1–2 doses	$1.44/ 600 mg	$43.20		
Eprosartan/ HCTZ	Teveten HCT	600 mg/ 12.5 mg once daily	600 mg/12.5 mg or 600 mg/25 mg once daily	$1.44/ 600 mg/ 12.5 mg	$43.20		
Irbesartan	Avapro	150 mg once daily	150–300 mg once daily	$1.69/ 150 mg	$50.76		
Irbesartan and hydrochlorothiazide	Avalide	150 mg/ 12.5 mg once daily	150–300 mg irbesartan daily	$2.09/ 150 mg	$62.58		
Losartan	Cozaar	50 mg once daily	25–100 mg in 1 or 2 doses	$1.67/50 mg	$50.10		

(*continued*)

Table 48. Antihypertensive drugs: ACE inhibitors and angiotensin II receptor blockers.[1] (continued)

Drug	Proprietary Name	Initial Dosage	Dosage Range	Cost per Unit	Cost of 30 Days Treatment (Average Dosage)[1]	Adverse Effects	Comments
ANGIOTENSIN II RECEPTOR BLOCKERS (continued)							
Losartan and hydrochlorothiazide	Hyzaar	50 mg/12.5 mg once daily	One or 2 tablets once daily	$1.67/50 mg/12.5 mg/tablet	$50.10	Hyperkalemia, renal dysfunction, rare angioedema. Combinations have additional side effects. Contraindicated in pregnancy.	Losartan has a very flat dose-response curve. Valsartan and irbesartan have wider dose-response ranges and longer durations of action. Addition of low-dose diuretic (separately or as combination pills) increases the response.
Olmesartan	Benicar	20 mg once daily	20–40 mg daily	$1.61/20 mg	$48.24		
Olmesartan and HCTZ	Benicar HCT	20 mg/12.5 mg daily	20–40 mg olmesartan daily	$1.62/20 mg/12.5 mg	$48.60		
Telmisartan	Micardis	40 mg once daily	20–80 mg once daily	$1.74/40 mg	$52.33		
Telmisartan and HCTZ	Micardis HCT	40 mg/12.5 mg once daily	20–80 mg telmisartan daily	$1.87/40 mg/12.5 mg	$56.06		
Valsartan	Diovan	80 mg once daily	80–320 mg once daily	$1.92/160 mg	$57.72		
Valsartan and HCTZ	Diovan HCT	80 mg/12.5 mg once daily	80–320 mg valsartan daily	$2.09/160 mg/12.5 mg	$62.82		

ACE = angiotensin-converting enzyme; HCTZ = hydrochlorothiazide.
[1]Average wholesale price (AWP, for AB-rated generic when available) for quantity listed. Source: *Red Book* Update, Vol. 24, No. 4, April 2005. AWP may not accurately represent the actual pharmacy cost because wide contractual variations exist among institutions.

Table 49. Antihypertensive drugs: calcium channel blocking agents.

Drug	Proprietary Name	Initial Dosage	Dosage Range	Cost of 30 Days Treatment (Average Dosage)[1]	Special Properties: Peripheral Vasodilation	Special Properties: Cardiac Automaticity and Conduction	Special Properties: Contractility	Adverse Effects	Comments
NONDIHYDROPYRIDINE AGENTS									
Diltiazem	Cardizem SR	90 mg twice daily	180–360 mg in 2 doses	$67.20 (120 mg twice daily)	++	↓↓	↓↓	Edema, headache, bradycardia, GI disturbances, dizziness, AV block, congestive heart failure, urinary frequency.	Also approved for angina.
	Cardizem CD; Cartia XT	180 mg daily	180–360 mg daily	$53.27 (240 mg daily)					
	Dilacor XR	180 or 240 mg daily	180–480 mg daily	$34.50 (240 mg daily)					
	Tiazac SA	240 mg daily	180–540 mg daily	$62.74 (240 mg daily)					
Verapamil	Calan SR Isoptin SR Verelan	180 mg daily	180–480 mg in 1 or 2 doses	$46.80	++	↓↓↓	↓↓↓	Same as diltiazem but more likely to cause constipation and congestive heart failure.	Also approved for angina and arrhythmias.
	Covera HS			$66.00 (240 mg daily)					
DIHYDROPYRIDINES									
Amlodipine	Norvasc	5 mg daily	5–20 mg daily	$68.55 (10 mg daily)	+++	↓/0	↓/0	Edema, dizziness, palpitations, flushing, headache, hypotension, tachycardia, GI disturbances, urinary frequency, worsening of congestive heart failure (may be less common with felodipine, amlodipine).	Amlodipine, nicardipine, and nifedipine also approved for angina.
Felodipine	Plendil	5 mg daily	5–20 mg daily	$72.30 (10 mg daily)	+++	↓/0	↓/0		
Isradipine	DynaCirc	2.5 mg twice daily	2.5–5 mg twice daily	$133.50 (5 mg twice daily)	+++	↓/0	↓		
	DynaCirc CR	5 mg daily	5–10 mg daily	$95.40 (10 mg daily)					
Nicardipine	Cardene	20 mg three times daily	20–40 mg three times daily	$41.20 (20 mg three times daily)	+++	↓/0	↓		
	Cardene SR	30 mg twice daily	30–60 mg twice daily	$57.02 (30 mg twice daily)					
Nifedipine	Adalat CC	30 mg daily	30–120 mg daily	$82.80 (60 mg daily)	+++	↓	↓↓		
	Procardia XL	30 mg daily	30–120 mg daily	$68.70 (60 mg daily)					
Nisoldipine	Sular	20 mg/d	20–60 mg/d	$51.90 (40 mg daily)	+++	↓/0	↓		

GI = gastrointestinal; AV = atrioventricular.

[1]Average wholesale price (AWP, for AB-rated generic when available) for quantity listed. Source: *Red Book* Update, Vol. .24, No. 4, April 2005. AWP may not accurately represent the actual pharmacy cost because wide contractual variations exist among institutions.

Table 50. α-Adrenoceptor blocking agents, sympatholytics, and vasodilators.

Drug	Proprietary Name	Initial Dosage	Dosage Range	Cost per Unit	Cost of 30 Days Treatment (Average Dosage)[1]	Adverse Effects	Comments
α-ADRENOCEPTOR BLOCKERS							
Prazosin	Minipress	1 mg hs	2–20 mg in 2 or 3 doses	$0.78/5 mg	$46.80 (5 mg twice daily)	Syncope with first dose; postural hypotension, dizziness, palpitations, headache, weakness, drowsiness, sexual dysfunction, anticholinergic effects, urinary incontinence; first-dose effects may be less with doxazosin.	May ↑ HDL and ↓ LDL cholesterol. May provide short-term relief of obstructive prostatic symptoms. Less effective in preventing cardiovascular events than diuretics.
Terazosin	Hytrin	1 mg hs	1–20 mg in 1 or 2 doses	$1.60/1, 2, 5, 10 mg	$48.00 (5 mg daily)		
Doxazosin	Cardura	1 mg hs	1–16 mg daily	$0.97/4 mg	$29.10 (4 mg daily)		
CENTRAL SYMPATHOLYTICS							
Clonidine	Catapres	0.1 mg twice daily	0.2–0.6 mg in 2 doses	$0.22/0.1 mg	$13.20 (0.1 mg twice daily)	Sedation, dry mouth, sexual dysfunction, headache, bradyarrhythmias; side effects may be less with guanfacine. Contact dermatitis with clonidine patch. Methyldopa also causes hepatitis, hemolytic anemia, fever.	"Rebound" hypertension may occur even after gradual withdrawal. Methyldopa should be avoided in favor of safer agents.
	Catapres TTS	0.1 mg/d patch weekly	0.1–0.3 mg/d patch weekly	$26.73/0.2 mg	$106.92 (0.2 mg weekly)		
Guanabenz	Wytensin	4 mg twice daily	8–64 mg in 2 doses	$0.98/4 mg	$58.80 (4 mg twice daily)		
Guanfacine	Tenex	1 mg once daily	1–3 mg daily	$0.87/1 mg	$26.10 (1 mg daily)		
Methyldopa	Aldomet	250 mg twice daily	500–2000 mg in 2 doses	$0.63/500 mg	$37.80 (500 mg twice daily)		
PERIPHERAL NEURONAL ANTAGONISTS							
Reserpine	Serpasil	0.05 mg once daily	0.05–0.25 mg daily	$0.32/0.1 mg	$9.60 (0.1 mg daily)	Depression (less likely at low dosages, ie, < 0.25 mg), night terrors, nasal stuffiness, drowsiness, peptic disease, gastrointestinal disturbances, bradycardia.	
DIRECT VASODILATORS							
Hydralazine	Apresoline	25 mg twice daily	50–300 mg in 2–4 doses	$0.05/25 mg	$3.00 (25 mg twice daily)	GI disturbances, tachycardia, headache, nasal congestion, rash, LE-like syndrome.	May worsen or precipitate angina.
Minoxidil	Loniten	5 mg once daily	5–40 mg qd	$1.29/10 mg	$38.70 (10 mg qd)	Tachycardia, fluid retention, headache, hirsutism, pericardial effusion, thrombocytopenia.	Should be used in combination with β-blocker and diuretic.

GI = gastrointestinal; LE = lupus erythematosus.

[1]Average wholesale price (AWP, for AB-rated generic when available) for quantity listed. Source: *Red Book* Update, Vol. 24, No. 4, April 2005. AWP may not accurately represent the actual pharmacy cost because wide contractual variations exist among institutions.

Table 51. Drugs for hypertensive emergencies and urgencies.

Agent	Action	Dosage	Onset	Duration	Adverse Effects	Comments
PARENTERAL AGENTS (INTRAVENOUSLY UNLESS NOTED)						
Nitroprusside (Nipride)	Vasodilator	0.25–10 mcg/kg/min	Seconds	3–5 minutes	GI, CNS; thiocyanate and cyanide toxicity, especially with renal and hepatic insufficiency; hypotension.	Most effective and easily titratable treatment. Use with β-blocker in aortic dissection.
Nitroglycerin	Vasodilator	0.25–5 mcg/kg/min	2–5 minutes	3–5 minutes	Headache, nausea, hypotension, bradycardia.	Tolerance may develop. Useful primarily with myocardial ischemia.
Labetalol (Normodyne, Trandate)	β- and α-Blocker	20–40 mg every 10 minutes to 300 mg; 2 mg/min infusion	5–10 minutes	3–6 hours	GI, hypotension, bronchospasm, bradycardia, heart block.	Avoid in congestive heart failure, asthma. May be continued orally.
Esmolol (Brevibloc)	β-Blocker	Loading dose 500 mcg/kg over 1 minute; maintenance, 25–200 mcg/kg/min	1–2 minutes	10–30 minutes	Bradycardia, nausea.	Avoid in congestive heart failure, asthma. Weak antihypertensive.
Fenoldopam (Corlopam)	Dopamine receptor agonist	0.1–1.6 mcg/kg/min	4–5 minutes	< 10 minutes	Reflex tachycardia, hypotension, ↑ intraocular pressure.	May protect renal function.
Nicardipine (Cardene)	Calcium channel blocker	5 mg/h; may increase by 1–2.5 mg/h every 15 minutes to 15 mg/h	1–5 minutes	3–6 hours	Hypotension, tachycardia, headache.	May precipitate myocardial ischemia.
Enalaprilat (Vasotec)	ACE inhibitor	1.25 mg every 6 hours	15 minutes	6 hours or more	Excessive hypotension.	Additive with diuretics; may be continued orally.
Furosemide (Lasix)	Diuretic	10–80 mg	15 minutes	4 hours	Hypokalemia, hypotension.	Adjunct to vasodilator.
Hydralazine (Apresoline)	Vasodilator	5–20 mg intravenously or intramuscularly (less desirable); may repeat after 20 minutes	10–30 minutes	2–6 hours	Tachycardia, headache, GI.	Avoid in coronary artery disease, dissection. Rarely used except in pregnancy.
Diazoxide (Hyperstat)	Vasodilator	50–150 mg repeated at intervals of 5–15 minutes, or 15–30 mg/min by intravenous infusion to a maximum of 600 mg	1–2 minutes	4–24 hours	Excessive hypotension, tachycardia, myocardial ischemia, headache, nausea, vomiting, hyperglycemia. Necrosis with extravasation.	Avoid in coronary artery disease and dissection. Use with β-blocker and diuretic. Mostly obsolete.
Trimethaphan (Arfonad)	Ganglionic blocker	0.5–5 mg/min	1–3 minutes	10 minutes	Hypotension, ileus, urinary retention, respiratory arrest. Liberates histamine; use caution in allergic individuals.	Useful in aortic dissection. Otherwise rarely used.

(*continued*)

Table 51. Drugs for hypertensive emergencies and urgencies. (continued)

Agent	Action	Dosage	Onset	Duration	Adverse Effects	Comments
			ORAL AGENTS			
Nifedipine (Adalat, Procardia)	Calcium channel blocker	10 mg initially; may be repeated after 30 minutes	15 minutes	2–6 hours	Excessive hypotension, tachycardia, headache, angina, myocardial infarction, stroke.	Response unpredictable.
Clonidine (Catapres)	Central sympatholytic	0.1–0.2 mg initially; then 0.1 mg every hour to 0.8 mg	30–60 minutes	6–8 hours	Sedation.	Rebound may occur.
Captopril (Capoten)	ACE inhibitor	12.5–25 mg	15–30 minutes	4–6 hours	Excessive hypotension.	

GI = gastrointestinal; CNS = central nervous system; ACE = angiotensin-converting enzyme.

Table 52. Causes of nausea and vomiting.

Visceral afferent stimulation	**Infections** **Mechanical obstruction** Gastric outlet obstruction: peptic ulcer disease, malignancy, gastric volvulus Small intestinal obstruction: adhesions, hernias, volvulus, Crohn's disease, carcinomatosis **Dysmotility** Gastroparesis: diabetic, medications, postviral, postvagotomy Small intestine: scleroderma, amyloidosis, chronic intestinal pseudo-obstruction, familial myoneuropathies **Peritoneal irritation** Peritonitis: perforated viscus, appendicitis, spontaneous bacterial peritonitis Viral gastroenteritis: Norwalk agent, rotavirus "Food poisoning": toxins from *Bacillus cereus*, *Staphylococcus aureus*, *Clostridium perfringens* Hepatitis A or B Acute systemic infections **Hepatobiliary or pancreatic disorders** Acute pancreatitis Cholecystitis or choledocholithiasis **Topical gastrointestinal irritants** Alcohol, NSAIDs, oral antibiotics **Postoperative** **Other** Cardiac disease: acute myocardial infarction, congestive heart failure Urologic disease: stones, pyelonephritis
CNS disorders	**Vestibular disorders** Labyrinthitis, Meniere's syndrome, motion sickness, migraine **Increased intracranial pressure** CNS tumors, subdural or subarachnoid hemorrhage **Migraine** **Infections** Meningitis, encephalitis **Psychogenic** Anticipatory vomiting, bulimia, psychiatric disorders
Irritation of chemoreceptor trigger zone	**Antitumor chemotherapy** **Drugs and medications** Calcium channel blockers Opioids Anticonvulsants Antiparkinsonism drugs β-Blockers, antiarrhythmics, digoxin Nicotine **Radiation therapy** **Systemic disorders** Diabetic ketoacidosis Uremia Adrenocortical crisis Parathyroid disease Hypothyroidism Pregnancy Paraneoplastic syndrome

NSAIDs = nonsteroidal anti-inflammatory drugs; CNS = central nervous system.

Table 53. Common antiemetic dosing regimens.

	Dosage	Route
Serotonin 5-HT$_3$ antagonists		
Ondansetron	8 mg or 0.15 mg/kg once daily	IV
	8 mg twice daily	PO
Granisetron	1 mg or 0.01 mg/kg once daily	IV
	2 mg once daily	PO
Dolasetron	100 mg or 1.8 mg/kg once daily	IV
	100–200 mg once daily	PO
Corticosteroids		
Dexamethasone	8–20 mg once daily	IV
	4–20 mg once or twice daily	PO
Methylprednisolone	40–100 mg once daily	IV
Dopamine receptor antagonists		
Metoclopramide	10–30 mg or 0.5 mg/kg every 6–8 hours	IV
	10–20 mg every 6–8 hours	PO
Prochlorperazine	5–20 mg every 4–6 hours	PO, IM, IV
	25 mg suppository every 6 hours	PR
Promethazine	25 mg every 4–6 hours	PO, PR, IM
Trimethobenzamide	250 mg every 6–8 hours	PO
	200 mg every 6–8 hours	IM, PR
Sedatives		
Diazepam	2–5 mg every 4–6 hours	PO, IV
Lorazepam	1–2 mg every 4–6 hours	PO, IV

IV = intravenously; PO = orally; IM = intramuscularly; PR = per rectum.

Table 54. Causes of ascites.

NORMAL PERITONEUM
Portal hypertension (SAAG ≥ 1.1 g/dL)
1. Hepatic congestion[1]
Congestive heart failure
Constrictive pericarditis
Tricuspid insufficiency
Budd-Chiari syndrome
Veno-occlusive disease
2. Liver disease[2]
Cirrhosis
Alcoholic hepatitis
Fulminant hepatic failure
Massive hepatic metastases
Hepatic fibrosis
Acute fatty liver of pregnancy
3. Portal vein occlusion
Hypoalbuminemia (SAAG < 1.1 g/dL)
Nephrotic syndrome
Protein-losing enteropathy
Severe malnutrition with anasarca
Miscellaneous conditions (SAAG < 1.1 g/dL)
Chylous ascites
Pancreatic ascites
Bile ascites
Nephrogenic ascites
Urine ascites
Myxedema (SAAG ≥ 1.1 g/dL)
Ovarian disease
DISEASED PERITONEUM (SAAG < 1.1 g/dL)[2]
Infections
Bacterial peritonitis
Tuberculous peritonitis
Fungal peritonitis
HIV-associated peritonitis
Malignant conditions
Peritoneal carcinomatosis
Primary mesothelioma
Pseudomyxoma peritonei
Massive hepatic metastases
Hepatocellular carcinoma
Other conditions
Familial Mediterranean fever
Vasculitis
Granulomatous peritonitis
Eosinophilic peritonitis

[1]Hepatic congestion usually associated with SAAG ≥ 1.1 g/dL and ascitic fluid total protein > 2.5 g/dL.
[2]There may be cases of "mixed ascites" in which portal hypertensive ascites is complicated by a secondary process such as infection. In these cases, the SAAG is ≥ 1.1 g/dL.
SAAG = serum-ascites albumin gradient.

Table 55. Treatment options for peptic ulcer disease.

Active *Helicobacter pylori*–associated ulcer

1. Treat with anti-*H pylori* regimen for 10–14 days. Treatment options:

   Proton pump inhibitor twice daily[1]
   Clarithromycin 500 mg twice daily
   Amoxicillin 1 g twice daily (or metronidazole 500 mg twice daily, if penicillin allergic)

   Proton pump inhibitor twice daily[1]
   Bismuth subsalicylate two tablets four times daily
   Tetracycline 500 mg four times daily
   Metronidazole 250 mg four times daily

   Ranitidine bismuth citrate 400 mg twice daily (not available in the United States)
   Clarithromycin 500 mg twice daily
   Amoxicillin 1 g or tetracycline 500 mg or metronidazole 500 mg twice daily

   (Proton pump inhibitors administered before meals. Avoid metronidazole regimens in areas of known high resistance or in patients who have failed a course of treatment that included metronidazole.)
2. After completion of 10–14-day course of *H pylori* eradication therapy, continue treatment with proton pump inhibitor[1] once daily or H_2-receptor antagonist (as below) for 4–8 weeks to promote healing.

Active ulcer not attributable to *H pylori*

1. Consider other causes: NSAIDs, Zollinger-Ellison syndrome, gastric malignancy. Treatment options:
   Proton pump inhibitors[1]:
   Uncomplicated duodenal ulcer: treat for 4 weeks
   Uncomplicated gastric ulcer: treat for 8 weeks
   H_2-receptor antagonists:
   Uncomplicated duodenal ulcer: cimetidine 800 mg, ranitidine or nizatidine 300 mg, famotidine 40 mg, once daily at bedtime for 6 weeks
   Uncomplicated gastric ulcer: cimetidine 400 mg, ranitidine or nizatidine 150 mg, famotidine 20 mg, twice daily for 8 weeks
   Complicated ulcers: proton pump inhibitors are the preferred drugs

Prevention of ulcer relapse

1. NSAID-induced ulcer: prophylactic therapy for high-risk patients (prior ulcer disease or ulcer complications, use of corticosteroids or anticoagulants, age > 70 years with serious comorbid illnesses).
   Treatment options:

   Proton pump inhibitor once daily
   COX-2 selective NSAID (celecoxib)
   (In special circumstances: misoprostol 200 mcg 3–4 times daily)
2. Long-term "maintenance" therapy indicated in patients with recurrent ulcers who either are *H pylori*-negative or who have failed attempts at eradication therapy: once-daily proton pump inhibitor[1] or H_2-receptor antagonist at bedtime (cimetidine 400–800 mg, nizatidine or ranitidine 150–300 mg, famotidine 20–40 mg)

[1]Proton pump inhibitors: omeprazole 20 mg, rabeprazole 20 mg, lansoprazole 30 mg, pantoprazole 40 mg, esomeprazole 40 mg.
All proton pump inhibitors are given twice daily except esomeprazole (once daily).
NSAIDs = nonsteroidal anti-inflammatory drugs; COX-2 = cyclooxygenase-2.

Table 56. Staging of colorectal cancer.

Joint Committee Classification	TNM			Dukes Class[1]
Stage 0				
Carcinoma in situ	Tis	N0	M0	
Stage I				
Tumor invades submucosa	T1	N0	M0	Dukes A
Tumor invades muscularis propria	T2	N0	M0	Dukes B_1
Stage II				
Tumor invades into subserosa or into nonperitonealized pericolic or perirectal tissues	T3	N0	M0	Dukes B_1 or B_2
Tumor perforates the visceral peritoneum or directly invades other organs or structures	T4	N0	M0	Dukes B_2
Stage III				
Any degree of bowel wall perforation with lymph node metastasis				
One to three pericolic or perirectal lymph nodes involved	Any T	N1	M0	Dukes C_1
Four or more pericolic or perirectal lymph nodes involved	Any T	N2	M0	Dukes C_2
Metastasis to lymph nodes along a vascular trunk	Any T	N3	M0	
Stage IV				
Presence of distant metastasis	Any T	Any N	M1	Dukes D

[1]Gastrointestinal Tumor Study Group modification of Dukes classification.

Table 57. Recommendations for colorectal cancer screening.[1]

Average-risk individuals ≥ 50 years old[2]

- Annual fecal occult blood testing
- Flexible sigmoidoscopy every 5 years
- Annual fecal occult blood testing *and* flexible sigmoidoscopy every 5 years
- Colonoscopy every 10 years
- Barium enema every 5 years

Individuals with a family history of a first-degree member with colorectal neoplasia[3]

- Single first-degree relative with colorectal cancer diagnosed at age ≥ **60 years:** Begin screening at age 40. Screening guidelines same as average-risk individual; however, preferred method is colonoscopy every 10 years.
- Single first-degree relative with colorectal cancer diagnosed at age **< 60 years,** or multiple first-degree relatives: Begin screening at age 40 or at age 10 years younger than age at diagnosis of the youngest affected relative, whichever is first in time. Recommended screening: colonoscopy every 5 years.

[1]For recommendations for families with inherited polyposis syndromes or hereditary nonpolyposis colon cancer, see separate section.
[2]Colorectal cancer screening and surveillance: clinical guidelines and rationale. Gastroenterology 2003;124:544.
[3]Screening Recommendations of American College of Gastroenterology. Am J Gastroenterol 2000;95:868.

Table 58. Classification of jaundice.

Type of Hyperbilirubinemia	Location and Cause
Unconjugated hyperbilirubinemia (predominant indirect-reacting bilirubin)	Increased bilirubin production (eg, hemolytic anemias, hemolytic reactions, hematoma, pulmonary infarction) Impaired bilirubin uptake and storage (eg, posthepatitis hyperbilirubinemia, Gilbert's syndrome, Crigler-Najjar syndrome, drug reactions)
Conjugated hyperbilirubinemia (predominant direct-reacting bilirubin)	**HEREDITARY CHOLESTATIC SYNDROMES** Faulty excretion of bilirubin conjugates (eg, Dubin-Johnson syndrome, Rotor's syndrome) or mutation in genes coding for bile salt transport proteins (eg, progressive familial intrahepatic cholestasis syndromes and benign recurrent intrahepatic cholestasis) **HEPATOCELLULAR DYSFUNCTION** Biliary epithelial damage (eg, hepatitis, hepatic cirrhosis) Intrahepatic cholestasis (eg, certain drugs, biliary cirrhosis, sepsis, postoperative jaundice) Hepatocellular damage or intrahepatic cholestasis resulting from miscellaneous causes (eg, spirochetal infections, infectious mononucleosis, cholangitis, sarcoidosis, lymphomas, industrial toxins) **BILIARY OBSTRUCTION** Choledocholithiasis, biliary atresia, carcinoma of biliary duct, sclerosing cholangitis, choledochal cyst, external pressure on common duct, pancreatitis, pancreatic neoplasms

Table 59. Hyperbilirubinemic disorders.

	Nature of Defect	Type of Hyperbilirubinemia	Clinical and Pathologic Characteristics
Gilbert's syndrome	Glucuronyl transferase deficiency	Unconjugated (indirect) bilirubin	Benign, asymptomatic hereditary jaundice. Hyperbilirubinemia increased by 24- to 36-hour fast. No treatment required. Prognosis excellent.
Dubin-Johnson syndrome[1]	Faulty excretory function of hepatocytes	Conjugated (direct) bilirubin	Benign, asymptomatic hereditary jaundice. Gallbladder does not visualize on oral cholecystography. Liver darkly pigmented on gross examination. Biopsy shows centrilobular brown pigment. Prognosis excellent.
Rotor's syndrome			Similar to Dubin-Johnson syndrome, but liver is not pigmented and the gallbladder is visualized on oral cholecystography. Prognosis excellent.
Benign recurrent intrahepatic cholestasis[2]	Cholestasis, often on a familial basis	Unconjugated plus conjugated (total) bilirubin	Episodic attacks of jaundice, itching, and malaise. Onset in early life and may persist for a lifetime. Alkaline phosphatase increased. Cholestasis found on liver biopsy. (Biopsy is normal during remission.) Prognosis excellent.
Recurrent jaundice of pregnancy			Benign cholestatic jaundice of unknown cause, usually occurring in the third trimester of pregnancy. Itching, gastrointestinal symptoms, and abnormal liver excretory function tests. Cholestasis noted on liver biopsy. Prognosis excellent, but recurrence with subsequent pregnancies or use of birth control pills is characteristic.

[1]The Dubin-Johnson syndrome is caused by a point mutation in the gene coding for an organic anion transporter in bile canaliculi on chromosome 10q23–24.
[2]Mutations in genes which control hepatocellular transport systems that are involved in the formation of bile and inherited as autosomal recessive traits are on chromosomes 18q21–22, 2q24, and 7q21 in families with progressive familial intrahepatic cholestasis. Gene mutations on chromosome 18q21–22 alter a P-type ATPase expressed in the small intestine and liver and others on chromosome 2q24 alter the bile acid export pump and cause benign recurrent intrahepatic cholestasis.

Table 60. Liver function tests: Normal values and changes in two types of jaundice.

Tests	Normal Values	Hepatocellular Jaundice	Uncomplicated Obstructive Jaundice
Bilirubin			
Direct	0.1–0.3 mg/dL	Increased	Increased
Indirect	0.2–0.7 mg/dL	Increased	Increased
Urine bilirubin	None	Increased	Increased
Serum albumin/total protein	Albumin, 3.5–5.5 g/dL	Albumin decreased Total protein, 6.5–8.4 g/dL	Unchanged
Alkaline phosphatase	30–115 units/L	Increased (+)	Increased (++++)
Prothrombin time	INR of 1.0–1.4. After vitamin K, 10% increase in 24 hours	Prolonged if damage severe and does not respond to parenteral vitamin K	Prolonged if obstruction marked, but responds to parenteral vitamin K
ALT, AST	ALT, 5–35 units/L; AST, 5–40 units/L	Increased in hepatocellular damage, viral hepatitis	Minimally increased

INR = international normalized ratio; ALT = alanine aminotransferase; AST = aspartate aminotransferase.

Table 61. Common serologic patterns in hepatitis B virus infection and their interpretation.

HBsAg	Anti-HBs	Anti-HBc	HBeAg	Anti-HBe	Interpretation
+	–	IgM	+	–	Acute hepatitis B
+	–	IgG[1]	+	–	Chronic hepatitis B with active viral replication
+	–	IgG	–	+	Chronic hepatitis B with low viral replication
+	+	IgG	+ or –	+ or –	Chronic hepatitis B with heterotypic anti-HBs (about 10% of cases)
–	–	IgM	+ or –	–	Acute hepatitis B
–	+	IgG	–	+ or –	Recovery from hepatitis B (immunity)
–	+	–	–	–	Vaccination (immunity)
–	–	IgG	–	–	False-positive; less commonly, infection in remote past

[1]Low levels of IgM anti-HBc may also be detected.

Table 62. Modified Child-Turcotte-Pugh classification for cirrhosis.

Parameter	Numerical Score		
	1	2	3
Ascites	None	Slight	Moderate to severe
Encephalopathy	None	Slight to moderate	Moderate to severe
Bilirubin (mg/dL)	< 2.0	2–3	> 3.0
Albumin (g/dL)	> 3.5	2.8–3.5	< 2.8
Prothrombin time (seconds increased)	1–3	4–6	> 6.0

Total numerical score	Child-Turcotte-Pugh class
5–6	A
7–9	B
10–15	C

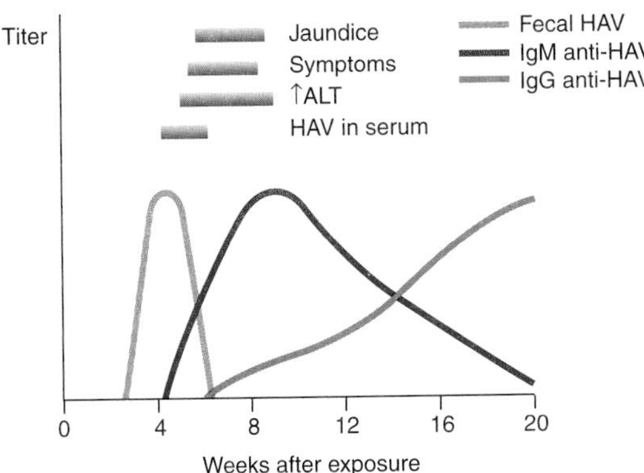

Figure 3. **The typical course of acute type A hepatitis. (HAV, hepatitis A virus; anti-HAV, antibody to hepatitis A virus; ALT, alanine aminotransferase.)** (Reprinted from Koff RS: Acute viral hepatitis. In: *Handbook of Liver Disease*. Friedman LS, Keeffe EB [editors], 2nd ed. © 2004, with permission from Elsevier.)

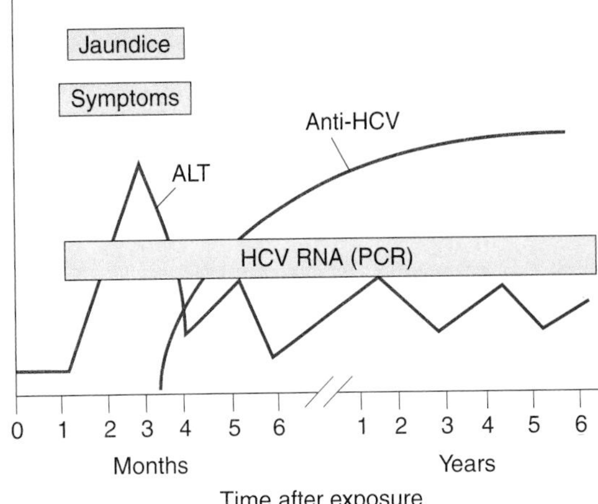

Figure 4. **The typical course of acute and chronic hepatitis C.** (ALT, alanine aminotransferase; Anti-HCV, antibody to hepatitis C virus by enzyme immunoassay; HCV RNA [PCR], hepatitis C viral RNA by polymerase chain reaction.)

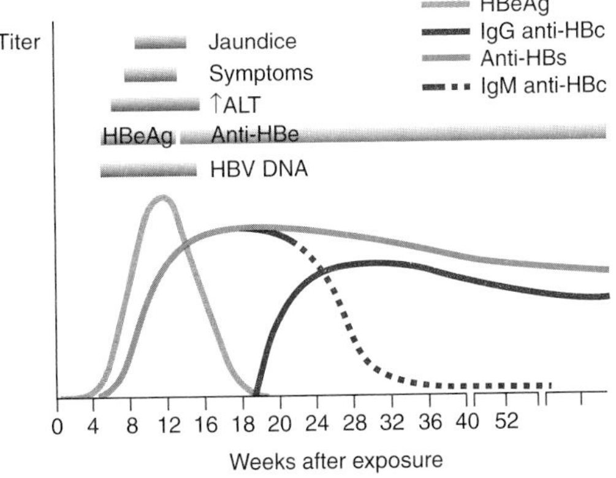

Figure 5. **The typical course of acute type B hepatitis. (HBsAg, hepatitis B surface antigen; anti-HBs, antibody to HBsAg; HBeAg, hepatitis Be antigen; anti-HBe, antibody to HBeAg; anti-HBc, antibody to hepatitis B core antigen; ALT, alanine aminotransferase.)** (Reprinted from Koff RS: Acute viral hepatitis. In: *Handbook of Liver Disease*. Friedman LS, Keeffe EB [editors], 2nd ed. © 2004, with permission from Elsevier.)

Table 63. Diseases of the biliary tract.

	Clinical Features	Laboratory Features	Diagnosis	Treatment
Gallstones	Asymptomatic	Normal	Ultrasound	None
Gallstones	Biliary pain	Normal	Ultrasound	Laparoscopic cholecystectomy
Cholesterolosis of gallbladder	Usually asymptomatic	Normal	Oral cholecystography	None
Adenomyomatosis	May cause biliary pain	Normal	Oral cholecystography	Laparoscopic cholecystectomy if symptomatic
Porcelain gallbladder	Usually asymptomatic, high risk of gallbladder cancer	Normal	X-ray or CT	Laparoscopic cholecystectomy
Acute cholecystitis	Epigastric or right upper quadrant pain, nausea, vomiting, fever, Murphy's sign	Leukocytosis	Ultrasound, HIDA scan	Antibiotics, laparoscopic cholecystectomy
Chronic cholecystitis	Biliary pain, constant epigastric or right upper quadrant pain, nausea	Normal	Ultrasound (stones), oral cholecystography (nonfunctioning gallbladder)	Laparoscopic cholecystectomy
Choledocholithiasis	Asymptomatic or biliary pain, jaundice, fever; gallstone pancreatitis	Cholestatic liver function tests; leukocytosis and positive blood cultures in cholangitis; elevated amylase and lipase in pancreatitis	Ultrasound (dilated ducts), MRCP, ERCP	Endoscopic sphincterotomy and stone extraction; antibiotics for cholangitis

HIDA = hepatic iminodiacetic acid; MRCP = magnetic resonance cholangiopancreatography; ERCP = endoscopic retrograde cholangiopancreatography.

Table 64. Severity index for acute pancreatitis.

CT Grade	Points	Necrosis %	Necrosis Additional Points	Severity Index	Mortality Rate (%)
A Normal pancreas	0	0	0	0	0
B Pancreatic enlargement	1	0	0	1	0
C Pancreatic inflammation and/or peripancreatic fat	2	< 30	2	4	0
D Single peripancreatic fluid collection	3	30–50	4	7	
E Two or more fluid collections or retroperitoneal air	4	> 50	6	10	> 17

Adapted from Balthazar EJ: Acute pancreatitis: assessment of severity with clinical and CT evaluation. Radiology 2002;223:603.

Table 65. Classification systems for Papanicolaou smears.

Numerical	Dysplasia	CIN	Bethesda System
1	Benign	Benign	Normal
2	Benign with inflammation	Benign with inflammation	Normal, ASC-US
3	Mild dysplasia	CIN I	Low-grade SIL
3	Moderate dysplasia	CIN II	High-grade SIL
3	Severe dysplasia	CIN III	High-grade SIL
4	Carcinoma in situ	CIN III	High-grade SIL
5	Invasive cancer	Invasive cancer	Invasive cancer

CIN = cervical intraepithelial neoplasia; ASC-US = atypical squamous cells of undetermined significance; SIL = squamous intraepithelial lesion.

Table 66. FIGO staging of cancer of the cervix.

Preinvasive carcinoma	
Stage 0	Carcinoma in situ.
Invasive carcinoma	
Stage I	Carcinoma strictly confined to the cervix.
IA	Invasive cancer diagnosed only by microscopy. All gross lesions, even with superficial invasion, are stage IB.
	IA1 Measured invasion of stroma no greater than 3 mm in depth and no wider than 7 mm.
	IA2 Measured invasion of stroma greater than 3 mm in depth and no greater than 5 mm in depth and no wider than 7 mm.
IB	Clinical lesions confined to the cervix or preclinical lesions greater than 1A.
	IB1 Clinical lesions no greater than 4 cm.
	IB2 Clinical lesions greater than 4 cm.
Stage II	Carcinoma extends beyond the cervix but has not extended to the pelvic wall. The carcinoma involves the vagina but not as far as the lower third.
IIA	No obvious parametrial involvement.
IIB	Obvious parametrial involvement.
Stage III	Carcinoma has extended either to the lower third of the vagina or to the pelvic sidewall. All cases of hydronephrosis.
IIIA	Involvement of lower third of vagina. No extension to pelvic sidewall.
IIIB	Extension onto the pelvic wall and/or hydronephrosis or nonfunctioning kidney.
Stage IV	Carcinoma extended beyond the true pelvis or clinically involving the mucosa of the bladder or rectum.
IVA	Spread of growth to adjacent organs.
IVB	Spread of growth to distant organs.

Table 67. Ovarian functional and neoplastic tumors.

Tumor	Incidence	Size	Consistency	Menstrual Irregularities	Endocrine Effects	Potential for Malignancy	Special Remarks
Follicle cysts	Rare in childhood; frequent in menstrual years; never in post-menopausal years.	< 6 cm, often bilateral.	Moderate	Occasional	Occasional anovulation with persistently proliferative endometrium	None	Usually disappear spontaneously within 2–3 months.
Corpus luteum cysts	Occasional, in menstrual years.	4–6 cm, unilateral.	Moderate	Occasional delayed period	Prolonged secretory phase	None	Functional cysts. Intraperitoneal bleeding occasionally.
Theca lutein cysts	Occurs with hydatidiform mole, choriocarcinoma; also with gonadotropin or clomiphene therapy.	To 4–5 cm, multiple, bilateral. (Ovaries may be ≥ 20 cm in diameter.)	Tense	Amenorrhea	hCG elevated as a result of trophoblastic proliferation	None	Functional cysts. Hematoperitoneum or torsion of ovary may occur. Surgery is to be avoided.
Inflammatory (tubo-ovarian abscess)	Concomitant with acute salpingitis.	To 15–20 cm, often bilateral.	Variable, painful	Menometrorrhagia	Anovulation usual	None	Unilateral removal indicated if possible.
Endometriotic cysts	Never in preadolescent or postmenopausal years. Most common in women aged 20–40 years.	To 10–12 cm, occasionally bilateral.	Moderate to softened	Rare	None	Very rare	Associated pelvic endometriosis. Medical treatment or conservative surgery recommended.
Teratoid tumors:							
Benign teratomas (dermoid cysts)	Childhood to post-menopause.	< 15 cm; 15% are bilateral.	Moderate to softened	None	None	Rare	Torsion can occur. Partial oophorectomy recommended.
Malignant teratomas	< 1% of ovarian tumors. Usually in infants and young adults.	> 20 cm, unilateral.	Irregularly firm	None	Occasionally, hCG elevated	All	Surgery alone may be curative.
Cystadenoma, cystadenocarcinoma	Common in reproductive years.	Serous: < 25 cm, 33% bilateral; mucinous: up to 1 cm, 10% bilateral.	Moderate to softened	None	None	> 50% for serous, about 5% for mucinous	Peritoneal implants often occur with serous, rarely with mucinous. If mucinous tumor is ruptured, pseudomyxoma peritonei may occur.

Endometrioid carcinoma	15% of ovarian carcinomas.	Moderate, 13% bilateral.	Firm	None	None	All	Adenocarcinoma of endometrium coexists in 15–30% of cases.
Fibroma	< 5% of ovarian tumors.	Usually < 15 cm.	Very firm	None	None	Rare	Ascites in 20% (rarely, pleural fluid).
Arrhenoblastoma	Rare. Average age 30 years or more.	Often small (< 10 cm), unilateral.	Firm to softened	Amenorrhea	Androgens elevated	< 20%	Recurrences are moderately sensitive to irradiation.
Theca cell tumor (thecoma)	Uncommon.	< 10 cm, unilateral.	Firm	Occasional irregularity	Estrogens or androgens elevated	< 1%	
Granulosa cell tumor	Uncommon. Usually in prepubertal girls or women older than 50 years.	May be very small.	Firm to softened	Menometrorrhagia	Estrogens elevated	15–20%	Recurrences are moderately sensitive to irradiation.
Dysgerminoma	About 1–2% of ovarian tumors.	< 30 cm, bilateral in 33%.	Moderate to softened	None	—	All	Very radiosensitive.
Brenner tumor	About 1% of ovarian tumors.	< 30 cm, unilateral.	Firm	None	—	Very rare	> 50% occur in postmenopausal years.
Secondary ovarian tumors	10% of fatal malignant disease in women.	Varies; often bilateral.	Firm to softened	Occasional	Very rare (thyroid, adrenocortical origin)	All	Bowel or breast metastases to ovary common.

Table 68. Commonly used low-dose oral contraceptives.

Name	Progestin	Estrogen (Ethinyl Estradiol)	Cost per Month[1]
		COMBINATION	
Alesse	0.1 mg levonorgestrel	20 mcg	$35.32
Loestrin 1/20 Microgestin 1/20	1 mg norethindrone acetate	20 mcg	$35.84 $28.66
Mircette	0.15 mg desogestrel	20 mcg	$37.54
Loestrin 1.5/30 Microgestin 1.5/30	1.5 mg norethindrone acetate	30 mcg	$50.33 $28.94
Lo-Ovral Low-ogestrel	0.3 mg dl-norgestrel	30 mcg	$37.54 $30.52
Nordette Levlen Levora	0.15 mg levonorgestrel	30 mcg	$31.93 $36.50 $30.93
Ortho-Cept Desogen	0.15 mg desogestrel	30 mcg	$48.33 $34.02
Yasmin	3 mg drospirenone	30 mcg	$41.46
Brevicon Modicon Necon 0.5/35	0.5 mg norethindrone	35 mcg	$39.48 $47.97 $32.14
Demulen 1/35 Zovia 1/35E	1 mg ethynodiol diacetate	35 mcg	$37.07 $29.88
Norinyl 1/35 Ortho-Novum 1/35 Necon 1/35	1 mg norethindrone	35 mcg	$46.19 $48.33 $29.49
Ortho-Cyclen	0.25 mg norgestimate	35 mcg	$41.97
Ovcon 35	0.4 mg norethindrone	35 mcg	$42.92
		COMBINATION: OTHER	
Seasonale	0.15 mg levonorgestrel	30 mcg	$40.19
		TRIPHASIC	
Estrostep	1.0 mg norethindrone acetate (days 1–5) 1.0 mg norethindrone acetate (days 6–12) 1.0 mg norethindrone acetate (days 13–21)	20 mcg 30 mcg 35 mcg	$38.90
Cyclessa	0.1 mg desogestrel (days 1–7) 0.125 mg desogestrel (days 8–14) 0.15 mg desogestrel (days 15–21)	25 mcg	$39.52
Ortho-Tri-Cyclen Lo	0.18 norgestimate (days 1–7) 0.21 norgestimate (days 8–14) 0.25 norgestimate (days 15–21)	25 mcg	$41.22
Triphasil Trivora Tri-Levlen	0.05 mg levonorgestrel (days 1–6) 0.075 mg levonorgestrel (days 7–11) 0.125 mg levonorgestrel (days 12–21)	30 mcg 40 mcg 30 mcg	$31.90 $27.49 $34.88
Ortho-Novum 7/7/7	0.5 mg norethindrone (days 1–7) 0.75 mg norethindrone (days 8–14) 1 mg norethindrone (days 15–21)	35 mcg	$46.13
Ortho-Tri-Cyclen	0.15 mg norgestimate (days 1–7) 0.215 mg norgestimate (days 8–14) 0.25 mg norgestimate (days 15–21)	35 mcg	$41.99

(continued)

Table 68. Commonly used low-dose oral contraceptives. (continued)

Name	Progestin	Estrogen (Ethinyl Estradiol)	Cost per Month[1]
Tri-Norinyl	0.5 mg norethindrone (days 1–7) 1 mg norethindrone (days 8–16) 0.5 mg norethindrone (days 17–21)	35 mcg	$44.08
PROGESTIN-ONLY MINIPILL			
Ortho Micronor Nor-QD	0.35 mg norethindrone to be taken continuously	(None)	$51.07 $48.80
Ovrette	0.075 mg/dL-norgestrel to be taken continuously	(None)	$35.34

[1]Average wholesale price (AWP, for AB-rated generic when available) for quantity listed. Source: *Red Book* Update, Vol. 24, No. 4, April 2005. AWP may not accurately represent the actual pharmacy cost because wide contractual variations exist among institutions.

Table 69. Contraindications to use of oral contraceptives.

Absolute contraindications
- Pregnancy
- Thrombophlebitis or thromboembolic disorders (past or present)
- Stroke or coronary artery disease (past or present)
- Cancer of the breast (known or suspected)
- Undiagnosed abnormal vaginal bleeding
- Estrogen-dependent cancer (known or suspected)
- Benign or malignant tumor of the liver (past or present)
- Uncontrolled hypertension
- Diabetes with vascular disease
- Age over 35 and smoking > 15 cigarettes daily
- Known thrombophilia
- Migraine with aura
- Active hepatitis
- Surgery or orthopedic injury requiring prolonged immobilization

Relative contraindications
- Migraine without aura
- Hypertension
- Cardiac or renal disease
- Diabetes
- Gallbladder disease
- Cholestasis during pregnancy
- Sickle cell disease (S/S or S/C type)
- Lactation

Table 70. Contraindications to IUD use.

Absolute contraindications
- Pregnancy
- Acute or subacute pelvic inflammatory disease or purulent cervicitis
- Significant anatomic abnormality of uterus
- Unexplained uterine bleeding
- Active liver disease (Mirena only)

Relative contraindications
- History of pelvic inflammatory disease since the last pregnancy
- Lack of available follow-up care
- Menorrhagia or severe dysmenorrhea (copper IUD)
- Cervical or uterine neoplasia

IUD = intrauterine device.

Table 71. Common drugs that are teratogenic or fetotoxic.[1]

- ACE inhibitors
- Alcohol
- Amantadine
- Aminopterin
- Androgens
- Anticonvulsants
  - Aminoglutethimide
  - Carbamazepine
  - Ethotoin
  - Phenytoin
  - Valproic acid
- Aspirin and other salicylates (third trimester)
- Benzodiazepines
- Carbarsone (amebicide)
- Chloramphenicol (third trimester)
- Cyclophosphamide
- Diazoxide
- Diethylstilbestrol
- Disulfiram
- Ergotamine
- Estrogens
- Griseofulvin
- Hypoglycemics, oral
- Isotretinoin
- Lithium
- Methotrexate
- Misoprostol
- NSAIDs (third trimester)
- Opioids (prolonged use)
- Progestins
- Radioiodine (antithyroid)
- Reserpine
- Ribavirin
- Sulfonamides (third trimester)
- Tetracycline (third trimester)
- Thalidomide
- Tobacco smoking
- Trimethoprim (third trimester)
- Warfarin and other coumarin anticoagulants

[1]Many other drugs are also contraindicated during pregnancy. Evaluate any drug for its need versus its potential adverse effects. Further information can be obtained from the manufacturer or from any of several teratogenic registries around the country.

ACE = angiotensin-converting enzyme; NSAIDs = nonsteroidal anti-inflammatory drugs.

Table 72. Indicators of mild to moderate versus severe preeclampsia-eclampsia.

Site	Indicator	Mild to Moderate	Severe
Central nervous system	Symptoms and signs	Hyperreflexia Headache	Seizures Blurred vision Scotomas Headache Clonus Irritability
Kidney	Proteinuria	0.3–5 g/24 h	> 5 g/24 h or catheterized urine with 4+ protein
	Uric acid	↑ > 4.5 mg/dL	↑↑ > 4.5 mg/dL
	Urinary output	> 20–30 mL/h	< 20–30 mL/h
Liver	AST, ALT, LDH	Normal	Elevated LFTs Epigastric pain Ruptured liver
Hematologic	Platelets Hemoglobin	> 100,000/mcL Normal range	< 100,000/mcL Elevated
Vascular	Blood pressure	< 160/110 mm Hg	> 160/110 mm Hg
	Retina	Arteriolar spasm	Retinal hemorrhages
Fetal-placental unit	Growth restriction Oligohydramnios Fetal distress	Absent May be present Absent	Present Present Present

AST = aspartate aminotransferase; ALT = alanine aminotransferase; LDH = lactate dehydrogenase; LFTs = liver function tests.

Table 73. Screening and diagnostic criteria for gestational diabetes mellitus.

Screening for gestational diabetes mellitus

1. 50-g oral glucose load, administered between the 24th and 28th weeks, without regard to time of day or time of last meal. Universal blood glucose screening is indicated for patients who are of Hispanic, African, Native American, South or East Asian, Pacific Island, or Indigenous Australian ancestry. Other patients who have no known diabetes in first-degree relatives, are under 25 years of age, have normal weight before pregnancy, and have no history of abnormal glucose metabolism or poor obstetric outcome do not require routine screening.
2. Venous plasma glucose measure 1 hour later.
3. Value of 130 mg/dL (7.2 mmol/L) or above in venous plasma indicates the need for a full diagnostic glucose tolerance test.

Diagnosis of gestational diabetes mellitus

1. 100-g oral glucose load, administered in the morning after overnight fast lasting at least 8 hours but not more than 14 hours, and following at least 3 days of unrestricted diet (> 150 g carbohydrate) and physical activity.
2. Venous plasma glucose is measured fasting and at 1, 2, and 3 hours. Subject should remain seated and should not smoke throughout the test.
3. Two or more of the following venous plasma concentrations must be equaled or exceeded for a diagnosis of gestational diabetes: fasting, 95 mg/dL (5.3 mmol/L); 1 hour, 180 mg/dL (10 mmol/L); 2 hours, 155 mg/dL (8.6 mmol/L); 3 hours, 140 mg/dL (7.8 mmol/L).

Table 74. Drugs and substances that require a careful assessment of risk before they are prescribed for breast-feeding women.[1]

Category	Specific Drugs or Compounds	Management Plan and Rationale
Analgesic drugs	Meperidine, oxycodone	Use alternatives to meperidine and oxycodone. Breast-fed infants whose mothers were receiving meperidine had a higher risk of neurobehavioral depression than breast-fed infants whose mothers were receiving morphine. In breast-fed infants, the level of exposure to oxycodone may reach 10% of the therapeutic dose. For potent analgesia, morphine may be given cautiously. Acetaminophen and nonsteroidal anti-inflammatory drugs are safe.
Antiarthritis drugs	Gold salts, methotrexate, high-dose aspirin	Consider alternatives to gold therapy. Although the bioavailability of elemental gold is unknown, a small amount is excreted in breast milk for a prolonged period. Therefore, the total amount of elemental gold that an infant could ingest may be substantial. No toxicity has been reported. Consider alternatives to methotrexate therapy, although low-dose methotrexate therapy for breast-feeding women with rheumatic diseases had lower risks of adverse effects in their infants than did anticancer chemotherapy. High-dose aspirin should be used with caution, since there is a case report of metabolic acidosis in a breast-fed infant whose mother was receiving high-dose therapy. Although the risk seems small, the infant's condition should be monitored clinically if the mother is receiving long-term therapy with high-dose aspirin.
Anticoagulant drugs	Phenindione[2]	Use alternatives to phenindione. Currently available vitamin K antagonists such as warfarin and acenocoumarol are considered safe, as is heparin.
Antidepressant drugs and lithium	Fluoxetine, doxepin, lithium[2]	Use fluoxetine, doxepin, and lithium with caution. Although the concentrations of these drugs in breast milk are low, colic (with fluoxetine) and sedation (with doxepin) have been reported in exposed infants. Near-therapeutic plasma concentrations of lithium were reported in an infant exposed to the drug in utero and through breast-feeding. The incidence of these adverse events is unknown.
Antiepileptic drugs	Phenobarbital, ethosuximide, primidone	In breast-fed infants, the level of exposure to phenobarbital, ethosuximide, and primidone may exceed 10% of the weight-adjusted therapeutic dose. Consider alternatives such as carbamazepine, phenytoin, and valproic acid.
Antimicrobial drugs	Chloramphenicol, tetracycline	Use alternatives to chloramphenicol and tetracycline. Idiosyncratic aplastic anemia is a possibility among breast-fed infants whose mothers are receiving chloramphenicol. Although tetracycline-induced discoloration of the teeth of breast-fed infants has not been reported, the potential risk of this event needs to be clearly communicated to lactating women.
Anticancer drugs	All (eg, cyclophosphamide,[2] methotrexate,[2] doxorubicin[2])	Because of their potent pharmacologic effects, cytotoxic drugs should not be given to breast-feeding women.
Anxiolytic drugs	Diazepam, alprazolam	Avoid long-term use of diazepam and alprazolam in breast-feeding women. Intermittent use poses little risk to their infants, but regular use may result in the accumulation of the drug and its metabolites in the infants. Lethargy and poor weight gain have been reported in an infant exposed to diazepam in breast milk, and the withdrawal syndrome was reported in a breast-fed infant after the mother discontinued alprazolam.
Cardiovascular and antihypertensive drugs	Acebutolol, amiodarone, atenolol, nadolol, sotalol	The use of acebutolol, amiodarone, atenolol, nadolol, and sotalol by breast-feeding women may cause relatively high levels of exposure among their infants, and these agents should therefore be used with caution. The two β-adrenergic antagonists propranolol and labetalol are considered safe.
Endocrine drugs and hormones	Estrogens, bromocriptine[2]	Estrogens and bromocriptine may suppress milk production. Oral contraceptives containing little or no estrogen have smaller risk than formulations with higher concentrations of estrogen. Nevertheless, caution should be exercised in their use.
Immunosuppressive drugs	Cyclosporine,[2] azathioprine	Maternal plasma concentrations of cyclosporine and azathioprine should be monitored. In nine reported cases in breast-fed infants who were exposed to azathioprine in breast milk, no obvious adverse effects were noted.
Respiratory drugs	Theophylline	Theophylline should be used with caution. When the mother's doses are high, the levels of exposure in the infant may be substantial (ie, 20% of the therapeutic dose).
Radioactive compounds	All	Breast-feeding should be stopped until the level of radioactivity in milk has returned to the background level.

(continued)

Table 74. Drugs and substances that require a careful assessment of risk before they are prescribed for breast-feeding women.[1] (continued)

Category	Specific Drugs or Compounds	Management Plan and Rationale
Drugs of abuse	All	The use of drugs of abuse precludes breast-feeding; cocaine-induced toxicity has been reported among breast-fed infants whose mothers abused cocaine. Methadone, used for the treatment of addiction, is safe for infants of breast-feeding women, at doses of up to 80 mg/d. Buprenorphine may be a safer alternative to methadone.
Nonmedicinal substances	Ethanol, caffeine, nicotine	In order to avoid exposure of the infant to ethanol, the mother should not consume alcohol or should consume no more than one drink 2 to 3 hours before breast-feeding. The ingestion of moderate amounts of caffeine should be safe. Because of the effects of second-hand smoke and the fact that nicotine is excreted in breast milk, smoking is contraindicated in breast-feeding women.
Miscellaneous compounds	Iodides and iodine, ergotamine,[2] ergonovine	Use alternatives to iodine-containing antiseptic agents. Ergotamine and ergonovine may suppress prolactin secretion in breast-feeding women. However, the use of methylergonovine to stimulate uterine involution is considered safe in breast-feeding women.

[1]Data modified from Ito S: Drug therapy for breast-feeding women. N Engl J Med 2000;343:120. Drugs for which there is no information are not included, although a careful risk assessment is necessary before such drugs are prescribed.
[2]The use of this drug or these drugs by breast-feeding women is contraindicated according to the American Academy of Pediatrics.

Table 75. Effectiveness of agents used in treatment of allergic disorders.

Drug Class	Sneezing	Pruritus	Rhinorrhea	Congestion	Inflammation	Onset of Action
Antihistamines	++++	++++	+++	+	–	Rapid
Sympathomimetics	–	–	+	++++	–	Rapid
Corticosteroids	+++	+++	+++	++++	++++	Slow (days)
Cromolyn-nedocromil sodium	++	+	+	+	++	Slow (weeks)
Anticholinergics	–	–	++++	–	–	Rapid
Immunotherapy	++++	++++	++++	++++	++++	Slow (months)

Table 76. Autoantibodies: Associations with connective tissue diseases.

Suspected Disease State	Test	Primary Disease Association (Sensitivity, Specificity)	Other Disease Associations	Comments
CREST syndrome	Anticentromere antibody	CREST (70–90%, high)	Scleroderma (10–15%), Raynaud's disease (10–30%).	Predictive value of a positive test is > 95% for scleroderma or related disease (CREST, Raynaud's). Diagnosis of CREST is made clinically.
Systemic lupus erythematosus (SLE)	Antinuclear antibody (ANA)	SLE (> 95%, low)	Rheumatoid arthritis (30–50%), discoid lupus, scleroderma (60%), drug-induced lupus (100%), Sjögren's syndrome (80%), miscellaneous inflammatory disorders.	Often used as a screening test; a negative test virtually excludes SLE; a positive test, while nonspecific, increases posttest probability of SLE. Titer does not correlate with disease activity.
	Anti-double-stranded-DNA (anti-ds-DNA)	SLE (60–70%, high)	Lupus nephritis, rarely rheumatoid arthritis, other connective tissue disease, usually in low titer.	Predictive value of a positive test is > 90% for SLE if present in high titer; a decreasing titer may correlate with worsening renal disease. Titer generally correlates with disease activity.
	Anti-Smith antibody (anti-Sm)	SLE (30–40%, high)		SLE-specific. A positive test substantially increases posttest probability of SLE. Test rarely indicated.
Mixed connective tissue disease (MCTD)	Anti-ribonucleoprotein antibody (RNP)	Scleroderma (20–30%, low), MCTD (95–100%, low)	SLE (30%), Sjögren's syndrome, rheumatoid arthritis (10%), discoid lupus (20–30%).	A negative test essentially excludes MCTD; a positive test in high titer, while nonspecific, increases posttest probability of MCTD.
Rheumatoid arthritis	Rheumatoid factor (RF)	Rheumatoid arthritis (50–90%)	Other rheumatic diseases, chronic infections, some malignancies, some healthy individuals, elderly patients.	Titer does not correlate with disease activity.
Scleroderma	Anti-Scl-70 antibody	Scleroderma (15–20%, low)		Predictive value of a positive test is > 95% for scleroderma.
Sjögren's syndrome	Anti-SS-A/Ro antibody	Sjögren's (60–70%, low)	SLE (30–40%), rheumatoid arthritis (10%), subacute cutaneous lupus, vasculitis.	Useful in counseling women of child- bearing age with known connective tissue disease, since a positive test is associated with a small but real risk of neonatal SLE and congenital heart block.
Wegener's granulomatosis	Antineutrophil cytoplasmic antibody (ANCA)	Wegener's granulomatosis (systemic necrotizing vasculitis) (56–96%, high)	Crescentic glomerulonephritis or other systemic vasculitis (eg, polyarteritis nodosa).	Ability of this assay to reflect disease activity remains unclear.

Modified, with permission, from Harvey AM et al (editors): The Principles and Practice of Medicine, 22nd ed. Appleton & Lange, 1988; White RH, Robbins DL: Clinical significance and interpretation of antinuclear antibodies. West J Med 1987;147:210; and Tan EM: Autoantibodies to nuclear antigens (ANA): their immunobiology and medicine. Adv Immunol 1982;33:167.
CREST = calcinosis, Raynaud's phenomenon, esophageal dysmotility, sclerodactyly, and telangiectasia.

Table 77. Diagnostic value of the joint pattern.

Characteristic	Status	Representative Disease
Inflammation	Present	Rheumatoid arthritis, systemic lupus erythematosus, gout
	Absent	Osteoarthritis
Number of involved joints	Monarticular	Gout, trauma, septic arthritis, Lyme disease
	Oligoarticular (2–4 joints)	Reiter's disease, psoriatic arthritis, inflammatory bowel disease
	Polyarticular (≥ 5 joints)	Rheumatoid arthritis, systemic lupus erythematosus
Site of joint involvement	Distal interphalangeal	Osteoarthritis, psoriatic arthritis (not rheumatoid arthritis)
	Metacarpophalangeal, wrists	Rheumatoid arthritis, systemic lupus erythematosus (not osteoarthritis)
	First metatarsal phalangeal	Gout, osteoarthritis

Table 79. Neurologic testing of lumbosacral nerve disorders.

Nerve Root	Motor	Reflex	Sensory Area
L4	Dorsiflexion of foot	Knee jerk	Medial calf
L5	Dorsiflexion of great toe	None	Medial forefoot
S1	Eversion of foot	Ankle jerk	Lateral foot

Table 78. Examination of joint fluid.

Measure	(Normal)	Group I (Noninflammatory)	Group II (Inflammatory)	Group III (Purulent)
Volume (mL) (knee)	< 3.5	Often > 3.5	Often > 3.5	Often > 3.5
Clarity	Transparent	Transparent	Translucent to opaque	Opaque
Color	Clear	Yellow	Yellow to opalescent	Yellow to green
WBC (per mcL)	< 200	200–300	3000–50,000	> 50,000[1]
Polymorphonuclear leukocytes	< 25%	< 25%	50% or more	75% or more[1]
Culture	Negative	Negative	Negative	Usually positive
Glucose (mg/dL)	Nearly equal to serum	Nearly equal to serum	> 25, lower than serum	< 25, much lower than serum

[1]Counts are lower with infections caused by organisms of low virulence or if antibiotic therapy has been started.

Table 80. Drugs associated with lupus erythematosus.

Definite association	
Chlorpromazine	Methyldopa
Hydralazine	Procainamide
Isoniazid	Quinidine
Possible association	
β-Blockers	Nitrofurantoin
Captopril	Penicillamine
Carbamazepine	Phenytoin
Cimetidine	Propylthiouracil
Ethosuximide	Sulfasalazine
Levodopa	Sulfonamides
Lithium	Trimethadione
Methimazole	
Unlikely association	
Allopurinol	Penicillin
Chlorthalidone	Phenylbutazone
Gold salts	Reserpine
Griseofulvin	Streptomycin
Methysergide	Tetracyclines
Oral contraceptives	

Modified and reproduced, with permission, from Hess EV, Mongey AB: Drug-related lupus. Bull Rheum Dis 1991;40:1.

Table 81. Criteria for the classification of SLE. (A patient is classified as having SLE if any 4 or more of 11 criteria are met.)

1. Malar rash
2. Discoid rash
3. Photosensitivity
4. Oral ulcers
5. Arthritis
6. Serositis
7. Renal disease
   a. > 0.5 g/d proteinuria, or—
   b. ≥ 3+ dipstick proteinuria, or—
   c. Cellular casts
8. Neurologic disease
   a. Seizures, or—
   b. Psychosis (without other cause)
9. Hematologic disorders
   a. Hemolytic anemia, or—
   b. Leukopenia (< 4000/mcL), or—
   c. Lymphopenia (< 1500/mcL), or—
   d. Thrombocytopenia (< 100,000/mcL)
10. Immunologic abnormalities
    a. Positive LE cell preparation, or—
    b. Antibody to native DNA, or—
    c. Antibody to Sm, or—
    d. False-positive serologic test for syphilis
11. Positive ANA

Modified and reproduced, with permission, from Tan EM et al: The 1982 revised criteria for the classification of systemic lupus erythematosus. Arthritis Rheum 1982;25:1271.
SLE = systemic lupus erythematosus; ANA = antinuclear antibody.

Table 82. Frequency (%) of autoantibodies in rheumatic diseases.

	ANA	Anti-Native DNA	Rheumatoid Factor	Anti-Sm	Anti-SS-A	Anti-SS-B	Anti-SCL-70	Anti-Centromere	Anti-Jo-1	ANCA
Rheumatoid arthritis	30–60	0–5	80	0	0–5	0–2	0	0	0	0
Systemic lupus erythematosus	95–100	60	20	10–25	15–20	5–20	0	0	0	0–1
Sjögren's syndrome	95	0	75	0	65	65	0	0	0	0
Diffuse scleroderma	80–95	0	30	0	0	0	33	1	0	0
Limited scleroderma (CREST syndrome)	80–95	0	30	0	0	0	20	50	0	0
Polymyositis/dermatomyositis	80–95	0	33	0	0	0	0	0	20–30	0
Wegener's granulomatosis	0–15	0	50	0	0	0	0	0	0	93–96[1]

[1]Frequency for generalized, active disease.
ANA = antinuclear antibodies; ANCA = antineutrophil cytoplasmic antibody; CREST = calcinosis cutis, Raynaud's phenomenon, esophageal motility disorder, sclerodactyly, and telangiectasia.

Table 83. Frequency of laboratory abnormalities in systemic lupus erythematosus.

Anemia	60%
Leukopenia	45%
Thrombocytopenia	30%
Biologic false-positive tests for syphilis	25%
Lupus anticoagulant	7%
Anti-cardiolipin antibody	25%
Direct Coombs-positive	30%
Proteinuria	30%
Hematuria	30%
Hypocomplementemia	60%
ANA	95–100%
Anti-native DNA	50%
Anti-Sm	20%

Modified and reproduced, with permission, from Hochberg MC et al: Systemic lupus erythematosus: a review of clinicolaboratory features and immunologic matches in 150 patients with emphasis on demographic subsets. Medicine 1985;64:285.
ANA = antinuclear antibody.

Table 84. Treatment of hyperkalemia.

EMERGENCY					
Modality	**Mechanism of Action**	**Onset**	**Duration**	**Prescription**	**K^+ Removed from Body**
Calcium	Antagonizes cardiac conduction abnormalities	0–5 minutes	1 hour	Calcium gluconate 10%, 5–30 mL intravenously; or calcium chloride 5%, 5–30 mL intravenously	0
Bicarbonate	Distributes K^+ into cells	15–30 minutes	1–2 hours	$NaHCO_3$, 44–88 mEq (1–2 ampules) intravenously	0
Insulin	Distributes K^+ into cells	15–60 minutes	4–6 hours	Regular insulin, 5–10 units intravenously, plus glucose 50%, 25 g (1 ampule) intravenously	0
Albuterol	Distributes K^+ into cells	15–30 minutes	2–4 hours	Nebulized albuterol, 10–20 mg in 4 mL normal saline, inhaled over 10 minutes	0

NONEMERGENCY				
Modality	**Mechanism of Action**	**Duration of Treatment**	**Prescription**	**K^+ Removed from Body**
Loop diuretic	↑ Renal K^+ excretion	0.5–2 hours	Furosemide, 40–160 mg intravenously or orally with or without $NaHCO_3$, 0.5–3 mEq/kg daily	Variable
Sodium polystyrene sulfonate (Kayexalate)	Ion-exchange resin binds K^+	1–3 hours	Oral: 15–30 g in 20% sorbitol (50–100 mL) Rectal: 50 g in 20% sorbitol	0.5–1 mEq/g
Hemodialysis	Extracorporeal K^+ removal	48 hours	Blood flow ≥ 200–300 mL/min Dialysate $[K^+] \sim 0$	200–300 mEq
Peritoneal dialysis	Peritoneal K^+ removal	48 hours	Fast exchange, 3–4 L/h	200–300 mEq

Modified and reproduced, with permission, from Cogan MG: *Fluid and Electrolytes: Physiology and Pathophysiology*. McGraw-Hill, 1991.

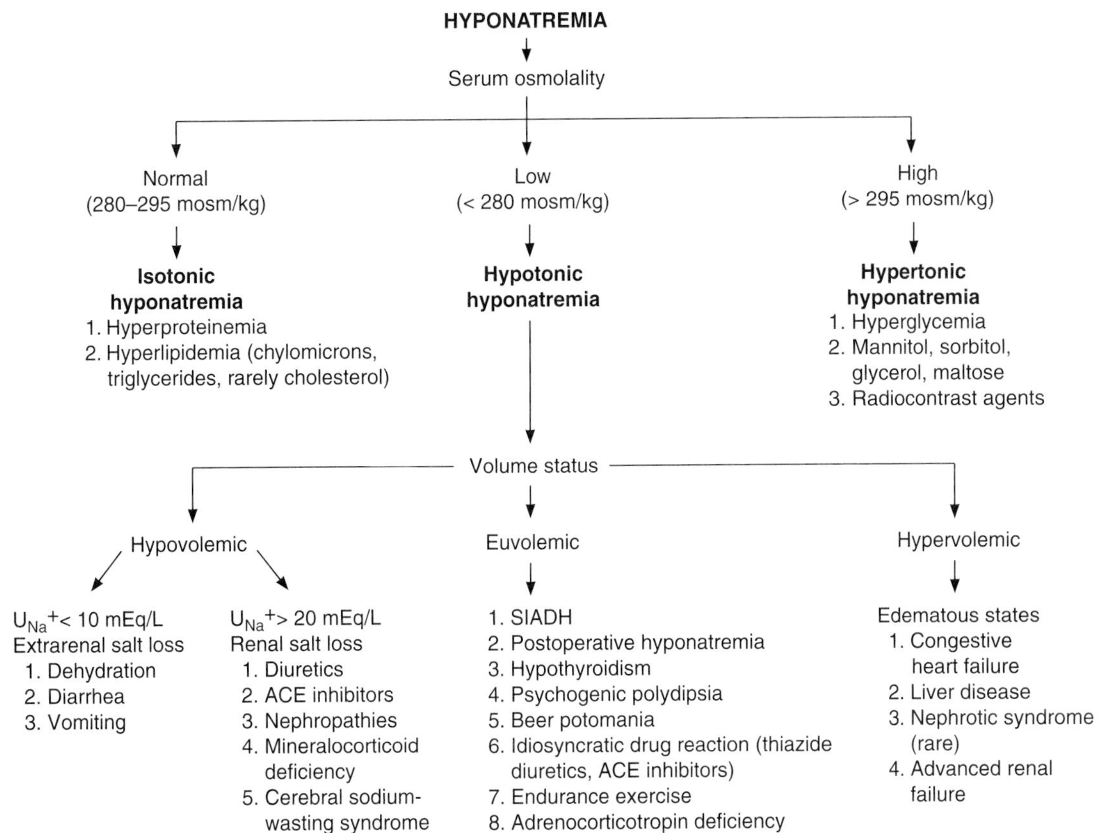

Figure 6. Evaluation of hyponatremia using serum osmolality and extracellular fluid volume status. ACE = angiotensin-converting enzyme; SIADH = syndrome of inappropriate antidiuretic hormone. (Adapted, with permission, from Narins RG et al: Diagnostic strategies in disorders of fluid, electrolyte and acid-base homeostasis. Am J Med 1982;72:496.)

Table 85. Primary acid-base disorders and expected compensation.

Disorder	Primary Defect	Compensatory Response	Magnitude of Compensation
Respiratory acidosis			
Acute	↑Pco_2	↑HCO_3^-	↑HCO_3^- 1 mEq/L per 10 mm Hg ↑Pco_2
Chronic	↑Pco_2	↑HCO_3^-	↑HCO_3^- 3.5 mEq/L per 10 mm Hg ↑Pco_2
Respiratory alkalosis			
Acute	↓Pco_2	↓HCO_3^-	↓HCO_3^- 2 mEq/L per 10 mm Hg ↓Pco_2
Chronic	↓Pco_2	↓HCO_3^-	↓HCO_3^- 5 mEq/L per 10 mm Hg ↓Pco_2
Metabolic acidosis	↓HCO_3^-	↓Pco_2	↓Pco_2 1.3 mm Hg per 1 mEq/L ↓HCO_3^-
Metabolic alkalosis	↑HCO_3^-	↑Pco_2	↑Pco_2 0.7 mm Hg per 1 mEq/L ↑HCO_3^-

Table 86. Hyperchloremic, normal anion gap metabolic acidoses.

	Renal Defect	Serum $[K^+]$	Distal H^+ Secretion: Urinary NH_4^+ Plus Minimal Urine pH	Distal H^+ Secretion: Titratable Acid	Urinary Anion Gap	Treatment
Gastrointestinal HCO_3^- loss	None	↓	< 5.5	↑↑	Negative	Na^+, K^+, and HCO_3^- as required
Renal tubular acidosis						
I. Classic distal	Distal H^+ secretion	↓	> 5.5	↓	Positive	$NaHCO_3$ (1–3 mEq/kg/d)
II. Proximal secretion	Proximal H^+	↓	< 5.5	Normal	Positive	$NaHCO_3$ or $KHCO_3$ (10–15 mEq/kg/d), thiazide
IV. Hyporeninemic hypoaldosteronism	Distal Na^+ reabsorption, K^+ secretion, and H^+ secretion	↑	< 5.5	↓	Positive	Fludrocortisone (0.1–0.5 mg/d), dietary K^+ restriction, furosemide (40–160 mg/d), $NaHCO_3$ (1–3 mEq/kg/d)

Modified and reproduced, with permission, from Cogan MG: *Fluid and Electrolytes: Physiology and Pathophysiology*. McGraw-Hill, 1991.

Table 87. Metabolic alkalosis.

Saline-Responsive (U_{Cl} < 10 mEq/d)	Saline-Unresponsive (U_{Cl} > 10 mEq/d)
Excessive body bicarbonate content	**Excessive body bicarbonate content**
Renal alkalosis	Renal alkalosis
Diuretic therapy	Normotensive
Poorly reabsorbable anion therapy: carbenicillin, penicillin, sulfate, phosphate	Bartter's syndrome (renal salt wasting and secondary hyperaldosteronism)
Posthypercapnia	Severe potassium depletion
Gastrointestinal alkalosis	Refeeding alkalosis
Loss of HCl from vomiting or nasogastric suction	Hypercalcemia and hypoparathyroidism
Intestinal alkalosis: chloride diarrhea	Hypertensive
Exogenous alkali	Endogenous mineralocorticoids
$NaHCO_3$ (baking soda)	Primary aldosteronism
Sodium citrate, lactate, gluconate, acetate	Hyperreninism
Transfusions	Adrenal enzyme deficiency: 11- and 17-hydroxylase
Antacids	Liddle's syndrome
Normal body bicarbonate content	Exogenous mineralocorticoids
"Contraction alkalosis"	Licorice

Modified and reproduced, with permission, from Narins RG et al: Diagnostic strategies in disorders of fluid, electrolyte and acid-base homeostasis. Am J Med 1982;72:496.

Table 88. Vitamin D preparations used in the treatment of hypoparathyroidism.

	Available Preparations	Daily Dose	Duration of Action
Ergocalciferol ergosterol, (vitamin D_2, calciferol)	Capsules of 50,000 international units; 8000 international units/mL oral solution	25,000–200,000 units	6–18 weeks
Dihydrotachysterol (DHT)	Tablets and capsules of 0.125, 0.2, and 0.4 mg; 0.2 mg/mL oral solution	0.2–1 mg	1–3 weeks
Calcitriol (Rocaltrol)	Capsules of 0.25 and 0.5 mcg; 1 mcg/mL oral solution; 1 mcg/mL for injection	0.25–4 mcg	½–2 weeks

Table 89. Diagnostic criteria of different types of hypercalciuria.

	Absorptive Type I	Absorptive Type II	Absorptive Type III	Resorptive	Renal
Serum					
Calcium	N	N	N	↑	N
Phosphorus	N	N	↓	↓	N
PTH	N	N	N	↑	↑
Vitamin D	N	N	↑	↑	↑
Urinary calcium					
Fasting	N	N	↑	↑	↑
Restricted	↑	N	↑	↑	↑
After calcium load	↑	↑	↑	↑	↑

PTH = parathyroid hormone; ↑ = elevated; ↓ = low; N = normal.

Table 90. American Urological Association symptom index for benign prostatic hyperplasia.[1]

Questions to Be Answered	Not at All	Less Than One Time in Five	Less Than Half the Time	About Half the Time	More Than Half the Time	Almost Always
1. Over the past month, how often have you had a sensation of not emptying your bladder completely after you finish urinating?	0	1	2	3	4	5
2. Over the past month, how often have you had to urinate again less than 2 hours after you finished urinating?	0	1	2	3	4	5
3. Over the past month, how often have you found you stopped and started again several times when you urinated?	0	1	2	3	4	5
4. Over the past month, how often have you found it difficult to post-pone urination?	0	1	2	3	4	5
5. Over the past month, how often have you had a weak urinary stream?	0	1	2	3	4	5
6. Over the past month, how often have you had to push or strain to begin urination?	0	1	2	3	4	5
7. Over the past month, how many times did you most typically get up to urinate from the time you went to bed at night until the time you got up in the morning?	0 (None)	1 (1 time)	2 (2 times)	3 (3 times)	4 (4 times)	5 (5times)

Reproduced, with permission, from Barry MJ et al: The American Urological Association symptoms index for benign prostatic hyperplasia. J Urol 1992;148:1549.
[1]Sum of seven circled numbers equals the symptom score. See text for explanation.

Table 91. Stages of chronic kidney disease: a clinical action plan.[1,2]

Stage	Description	GFR[3] (mL/min/1.73 m^2)	Action[4]
1	Kidney damage with normal or ↑ GFR	≥ 90	Diagnosis and treatment. Treatment of comorbid conditions. Slowing of progression. Cardiovascular disease risk reduction.
2	Kidney damage with mildly ↓ GFR	60–89	Estimating progression.
3	Moderately ↓ GFR	30–59	Evaluating and treating complications.
4	Severely ↓ GFR	15–29	Preparation for kidney replacement therapy.
5	Kidney failure	< 15 (or dialysis)	Replacement (if uremia is present).

[1]From National Kidney Foundation, KDOQI, chronic kidney disease guidelines.
[2]Chronic kidney disease is defined as either kidney damage or GFR < 60 mL/min/1.73 m^2 for 3 or more months. Kidney damage is defined as pathologic abnormalities or markers of damage, including abnormalities in blood or urine tests or imaging studies.
[3]GFR = glomerular filtration rate.
[4]Includes actions from preceding stages.

Table 92. Major causes of chronic renal failure.

Glomerulopathies

Primary glomerular diseases:

1. Focal and segmental glomerulosclerosis
2. Membranoproliferative glomerulonephritis
3. IgA nephropathy
4. Membranous nephropathy

Secondary glomerular diseases:

1. Diabetic nephropathy
2. Amyloidosis
3. Postinfectious glomerulonephritis
4. HIV-associated nephropathy
5. Collagen-vascular diseases
6. Sickle cell nephropathy
7. HIV-associated membranoproliferative glomerulonephritis

Tubulointerstitial nephritis

Drug hypersensitivity
Heavy metals
Analgesic nephropathy
Reflux/chronic pyelonephritis
Idiopathic

Hereditary diseases

Polycystic kidney disease
Medullary cystic disease
Alport's syndrome

Obstructive nephropathies

Prostatic disease
Nephrolithiasis
Retroperitoneal fibrosis/tumor
Congenital

Vascular diseases

Hypertensive nephrosclerosis
Renal artery stenosis

Table 93. Classification and findings in glomerulonephritis: nephrotic syndromes.

	Etiology	Histopathology	Pathogenesis
Minimal change disease (nil disease; lipoid nephrosis)	Associated with allergy, Hodgkin's disease, NSAIDs	Light: Normal (with or without mesangial proliferation) Immunofluorescence: No immunoglobulins Electron microscopy: Fusion foot processes	Unknown
Focal and segmental glomerulosclerosis	Associated with heroin abuse, HIV infection, reflux nephropathy, obesity	Light: Focal segmental sclerosis Immunofluorescence: IgM and C3 in sclerotic segments Electron microscopy: Fusion foot processes	Unknown
Membranous nephropathy	Associated with non-Hodgkin's lymphoma, carcinoma (gastrointestinal, renal, bronchogenic, thyroid), gold therapy, penicillamine, lupus erythematosus	Light: Thickened GBM and spikes Immunofluorescence: Granular IgG and C3 along capillary loops Electron microscopy: Dense deposits in subepithelial area	In situ immune complex formation
Membranoproliferative glomerulonephropathy	Type I associated with upper respiratory infection	Light: Increased mesangial cells and matrix with splitting of basement membrane Immunofluorescence: Granular C3, C1q, C4 with IgG and IgM Electron microscopy: Dense deposits in subendothelium	Unknown
	Type II	Light: Same as type I Immunofluorescence: C3 only Electron microscopy: Dense material in GBM	Unknown

NSAIDs = nonsteroidal anti-inflammatory drugs; GBM = glomerular basement membrane.

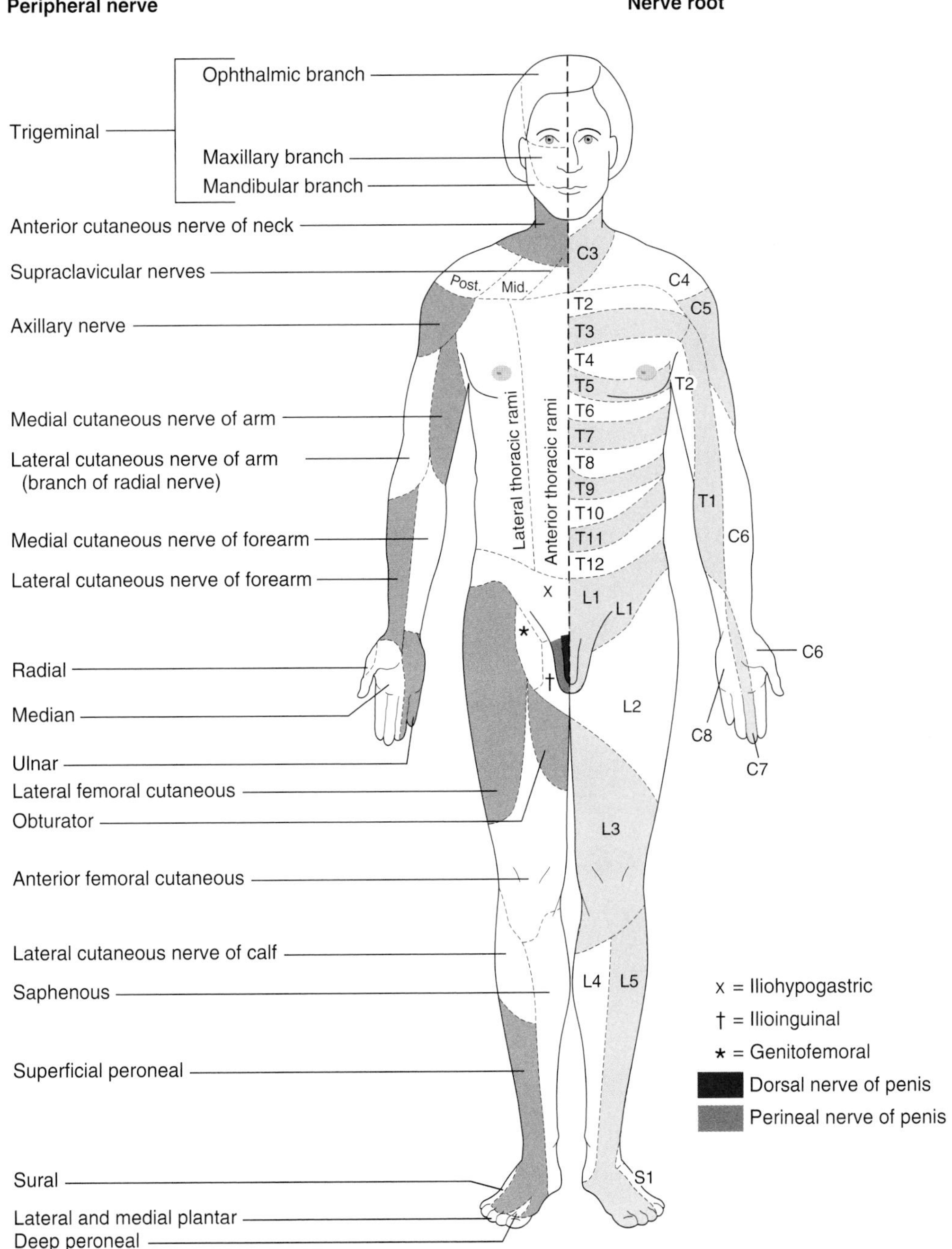

Figure 7. Cutaneous innervation. The segmental or radicular (root) distribution is shown on the left side of the body and the peripheral nerve distribution on the right side. **Above:** anterior view; **facing page:** posterior view. (Reproduced, with permission, from Simon RP, Aminoff MJ, Greenberg DA: Clinical Neurology, 4th ed. McGraw-Hill, 1999.)

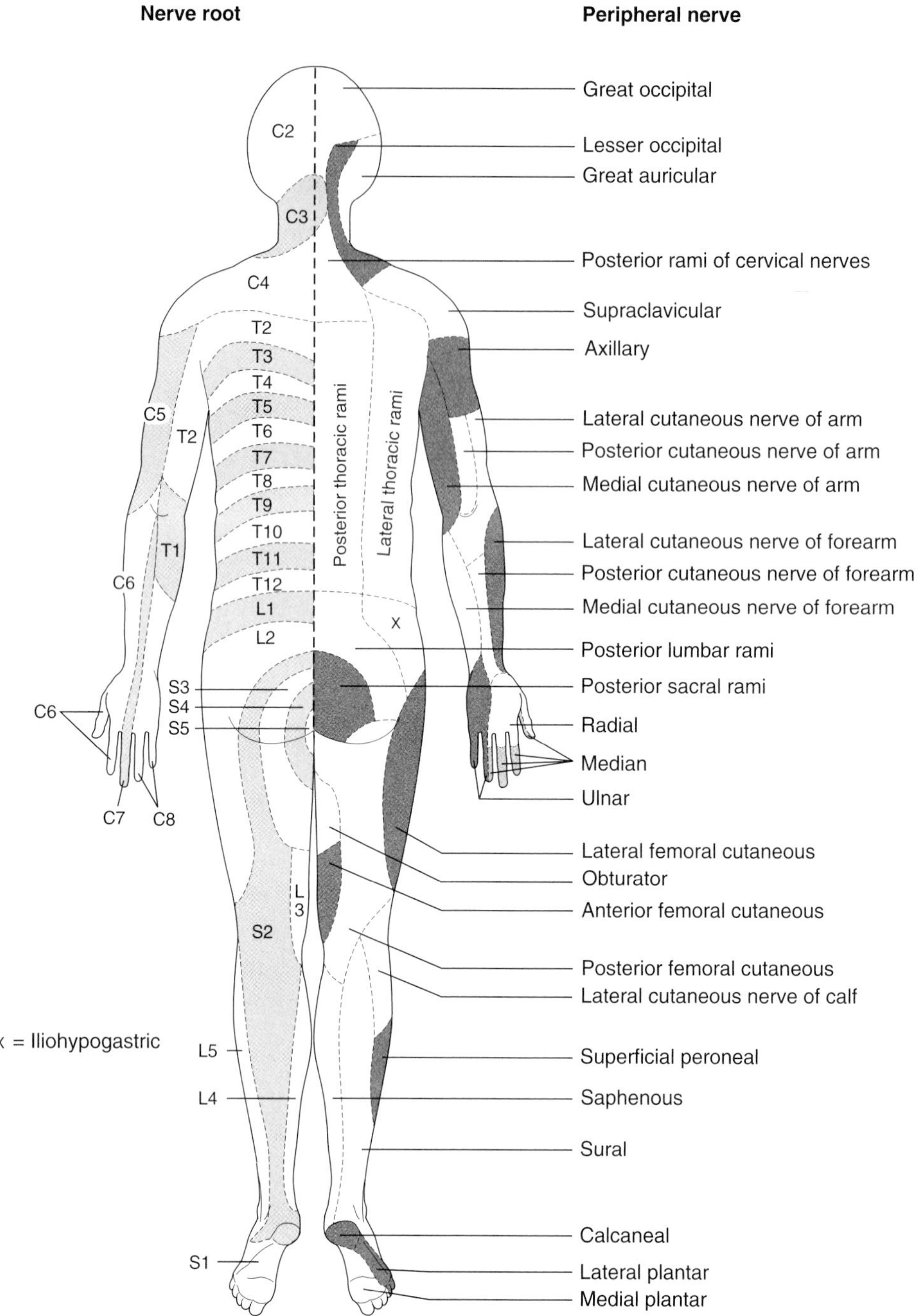
Nerve root
Peripheral nerve
C2
C3
C4
T2
T3
T4
T5
T6
T7
T8
T9
T10
T11
T12
L1
L2
C5
T2
T1
C6
S3
S4
S5
C6
C7
C8
L
3
S2
L5
L4
S1
x = Iliohypogastric
Posterior thoracic rami
Lateral thoracic rami
x
Great occipital
Lesser occipital
Great auricular
Posterior rami of cervical nerves
Supraclavicular
Axillary
Lateral cutaneous nerve of arm
Posterior cutaneous nerve of arm
Medial cutaneous nerve of arm
Lateral cutaneous nerve of forearm
Posterior cutaneous nerve of forearm
Medial cutaneous nerve of forearm
Posterior lumbar rami
Posterior sacral rami
Radial
Median
Ulnar
Lateral femoral cutaneous
Obturator
Anterior femoral cutaneous
Posterior femoral cutaneous
Lateral cutaneous nerve of calf
Superficial peroneal
Saphenous
Sural
Calcaneal
Lateral plantar
Medial plantar

Figure 7. Continued

Table 94. Clinical features associated with acute headache that warrant urgent or emergent neuroimaging.

Prior to lumbar puncture
Abnormal neurologic examination
Abnormal mental status
Abnormal funduscopic examination (papilledema; loss of venous pulsations)
Meningeal signs
Emergent (conduct prior to leaving office or emergency department)
Abnormal neurologic examination
Abnormal mental status
Thunderclap headache
Urgent (scheduled prior to leaving office or emergency department)
HIV-positive patient[1]
Age > 50 years (normal neurologic examination)

Adapted from American College of Emergency Physicians. Clinical Policy: critical issues in the evaluation and management of patients presenting to the emergency department with acute headache. Ann Emerg Med 2002;39:108.

[1]Use CT with or without contrast or MRI if HIV positive.

Table 95. Prophylactic treatment of migraine.

Drug	Usual Adult Daily Dose	Common Side Effects
Aspirin	650–1950 mg	Dyspepsia, gastrointestinal bleeding.
Propranolol[1]	80–240 mg	Fatigue, lassitude, depression, insomnia, nausea, vomiting, constipation.
Amitriptyline	10–150 mg	Sedation, dry mouth, constipation, weight gain, blurred vision, edema, hypotension, urinary retention.
Imipramine	10–150 mg	Similar to those of amitriptyline (above).
Sertraline	50–200 mg	Anxiety, insomnia, sweating, tremor, gastrointestinal disturbances.
Fluoxetine	20–60 mg	Similar to those of sertraline (above).
Ergonovine maleate	0.6–2 mg	Nausea, vomiting, abdominal pain, diarrhea.
Cyproheptadine	12–20 mg	Sedation, dry mouth, epigastric discomfort, gastrointestinal disturbances.
Clonidine	0.2–0.6 mg	Dry mouth, drowsiness, sedation, headache, constipation.
Verapamil[2]	80–160 mg	Headache, hypotension, flushing, edema, constipation. May aggravate atrioventricular nodal heart block and congestive heart failure.

[1]Other β-blockers have also been used (eg, timolol and metoprolol).

[2]Other calcium channel antagonists (eg, nimodipine, nicardipine, and diltiazem) have also been used.

Botulinum toxin type A injected locally into the scalp is effective for prophylaxis in some patients. The antiseizure agents valproic acid (500–1500 mg), gabapentin (900–2400 mg), and topiramate (50–1100 mg) are also effective and are detailed in Table 24–3. Valproic acid should be avoided during pregnancy.

Table 96. Features of the major stroke subtypes.

Stroke Type and Subtype	Clinical Features	Diagnosis	Treatment
Ischemic stroke			
Lacunar infarct	Small (< 5 mm) lesions in the basal ganglia, pons, cerebellum, or internal capsule; less often in deep cerebral white matter; prognosis generally good; clinical features depend on location, but may worsen over first 24–36 hours	CT may reveal small hypodensity but is often normal	Aspirin; long-term management is to control risk factors (hypertension and diabetes)
Carotid circulation obstruction	See text—signs vary depending on occluded vessel	Noncontrast CT to exclude hemorrhage; CT may be normal during first 6–24 hours of an ischemic stroke, whereas diffusion-weighted MRI is more sensitive; electrocardiography, blood glucose, complete blood count, and tests for hypercoagulable states, hyperlipidemia are indicated; echocardiography or Holter monitoring in selected instances	Select patients for intravenous thrombolytics (see text); aspirin (325 mg/day orally) is first-line therapy; if stroke occurs on aspirin, clopidogrel may be substituted for aspirin; anticoagulation with heparin for cardioembolic strokes, and sometimes for evolving stroke when no contraindications exist
Vertebrobasilar occlusion	See text—signs vary based on location of occluded vessel	As for carotid circulation obstruction	As for carotid circulation obstruction
Hemorrhagic stroke			
Spontaneous intracerebral hemorrhage	Commonly associated with hypertension; also with bleeding disorders, amyloid angiopathy Location: basal ganglia more common than pons, thalamus, cerebellum, or cerebral white matter	Noncontrast CT is superior to MRI for detecting bleeds of < 48 hours duration; laboratory tests to identify bleeding disorder: angiography may be indicated to exclude aneurysm or AVM. Do not perform lumbar puncture	Most managed supportively, but cerebellar bleeds or hematomas with gross mass effect benefit from urgent surgical evacuation
Subarachnoid hemorrhage	Present with sudden onset of worst headache of life, may lead rapidly to loss of consciousness; signs of meningeal irritation often present; etiology usually aneurysm or AVM, but 20% have no source identified	CT to confirm diagnosis, but may be normal in rare instances; if CT negative and suspicion high, perform lumbar puncture to look for red blood cells or xanthochromia; angiography to determine source of bleed in candidates for treatment	See sections on AVM and aneurysm
Intracranial aneurysm	Most located in the anterior circle of Willis and are typically asymptomatic until subarachnoid bleed occurs; 20% rebleed in first 2 weeks	CT indicates subarachnoid hemorrhage, and angiography then demonstrates aneurysms; angiography may not reveal aneurysm if vasospasm present	Prevent further bleeding by clipping aneurysm or coil embolization; nimodipine helps prevent vasospasm; reverse vasospasm by intravenous fluids and induced hypertension after aneurysm has been obliterated, if no other aneurysms are present; angioplasty may also reverse symptomatic vasospasm
AVMs	Focal deficit from hematoma or AVM itself	CT reveals bleed, and may reveal the AVM; may be seen by MRI. Angiography demonstrates feeding vessels and vascular anatomy	Surgery indicated if AVM has bled or to prevent further progression of neurologic deficit; other modalities to treat nonoperable AVMs are available at specialized centers

AVMs = arteriovenous malformations.

Table 97. Seizure classification.

Seizure Type	Key Features	Other Associated Features
Partial seizures	Involvement of only restricted part of brain; may become secondarily generalized	
Simple partial	Consciousness preserved	May be manifested by focal motor, sensory, or autonomic symptoms
Complex partial	Consciousness impaired	Above symptoms may precede, accompany, or follow
Generalized seizures	Diffuse involvement of brain at onset	
Absence (petit mal)	Consciousness impaired briefly; patient often unaware of attacks	May be clonic, tonic, or atonic components (ie, loss of postural tone); autonomic components (eg, enuresis); or accompanying automatisms Almost always begin in childhood and frequently cease by age 20
Atypical absences	May be more gradual onset and termination than typical absence	More marked changes in tone may occur
Myoclonic seizures	Single or multiple myoclonic jerks	
Tonic-clonic (grand mal)	Tonic phase: Sudden loss of consciousness, with rigidity and arrest of respiration, lasting < 1 minute Clonic phase: Jerking occurs, usually for < 2–3 minutes Flaccid coma: Variable duration	May be accompanied by tongue biting, incontinence, or aspiration; commonly followed by postictal confusion variable in duration
Status epilepticus	Repeated seizures without recovery between them; a fixed and enduring epileptic condition lasting 30 minutes	

Table 98. Drug treatment for seizures.

Drug	Usual Adult Daily Dose	Minimum No. of Daily Doses	Time to Steady-State Drug Levels	Optimal Drug Level	Selected Side Effects and Idiosyncratic Reactions
Generalized tonic-clonic (grand mal) or partial (focal) seizures					
Phenytoin	200–400 mg	1	5–10 days	10–20 mcg/mL	Nystagmus, ataxia, dysarthria, sedation, confusion, gingival hyperplasia, hirsutism, megaloblastic anemia, blood dyscrasias, skin rashes, fever, systemic lupus erythematosus, lymphadenopathy, peripheral neuropathy, dyskinesias.
Carbamazepine (extended-release formulation)	600–1200 mg	2–3 (2)	3–4 days	4–8 mcg/mL	Nystagmus, dysarthria, diplopia, ataxia, drowsiness, nausea, blood dyscrasias, hepatotoxicity, hyponatremia. May exacerbate myoclonic seizures.
Valproic acid	1500–2000 mg	3	2–4 days	50–100 mcg/mL	Nausea, vomiting, diarrhea, drowsiness, alopecia, weight gain, hepatotoxicity, thrombocytopenia, tremor.
Phenobarbital	100–200 mg	1	14–21 days	10–40 mcg/mL	Drowsiness, nystagmus, ataxia, skin rashes, learning difficulties, hyperactivity.
Primidone	750–1500 mg	3	4–7 days	5–15 mcg/mL	Sedation, nystagmus, ataxia, vertigo, nausea, skin rashes, megaloblastic anemia, irritability.
Felbamate[1,2]	1200–3600 mg	3	4–5 days	?	Anorexia, nausea, vomiting, headache, insomnia, weight loss, dizziness, hepatotoxicity, aplastic anemia.
Gabapentin[2]	900–1800 mg	3	1 day	?	Sedation, fatigue, ataxia, nystagmus, weight loss.
Lamotrigine	100–500 mg	2	4–5 days	?	Sedation, skin rash, visual disturbances, dyspepsia, ataxia.
Topiramate[2]	200–400 mg	2	4 days	?	Somnolence, nausea, dyspepsia, irritability, dizziness, ataxia, nystagmus, diplopia, renal calculi, weight loss, hypohidrosis, hyperthermia.
Oxcarbazepine[4]	900–1800 mg	2	2–3 days	?	As for carbamazepine.
Levetiracetam[2]	1000–3000 mg	2	2 days	?	Somnolence, ataxia, headache, behavioral changes.
Zonisamide[2]	200–600 mg	1–2	10 days	?	Somnolence, ataxia, anorexia, nausea, vomiting, rash, confusion, renal calculi. Do not use in patients with sulfonamide allergy.
Tiagabine[3]	32–56 mg	2	2 days	?	Somnolence, anxiety, dizziness, poor concentration, tremor, diarrhea.
Absence (petit mal) seizures					
Ethosuximide	100–1500 mg	2	5–10 days	40–100 mcg/mL	Nausea, vomiting, anorexia, headache, lethargy, unsteadiness, blood dyscrasias, systemic lupus erythematosus, urticaria, pruritus.
Valproic acid	1500–2000 mg	3	2–4 days	50–100 mcg/mL	See above.
Clonazepam	0.04–0.2 mg/kg	2	?	20–80 ng/mL	Drowsiness, ataxia, irritability, behavioral changes, exacerbation of tonic-clonic seizures.
Myoclonic seizures					
Valproic acid	1500–2000 mg	3	2–4 days	50–100 mcg/mL	See above.
Clonazepam	0.04–0.2 mg/kg	2	?	20–80 ng/mL	See above.

[1]Not to be used as a first-line drug; when used, blood counts should be performed regularly (every 2–4 weeks). Should be used only in selected patients because of risk of aplastic anemia and hepatic failure.
[2]Approved as adjunctive therapy for partial and secondarily generalized seizures.
[3]Approved as adjunctive therapy for partial seizures.
[4]Approved as monotherapy for partial seizures.

Table 99. Primary intracranial tumors.

Tumor	Clinical Features	Treatment and Prognosis
Glioblastoma multiforme	Presents commonly with nonspecific complaints and increased intracranial pressure. As it grows, focal deficits develop.	Course is rapidly progressive, with poor prognosis. Total surgical removal is usually not possible. Radiation therapy and chemotherapy may prolong survival.
Astrocytoma	Presentation similar to glioblastoma multiforme but course more protracted, often over several years. Cerebellar astrocytoma may have a more benign course.	Prognosis is variable. By the time of diagnosis, total excision is usually impossible; tumor often is not radiosensitive. In cerebellar astrocytoma, total surgical removal is often possible.
Medulloblastoma	Seen most frequently in children. Generally arises from roof of fourth ventricle and leads to increased intracranial pressure accompanied by brainstem and cerebellar signs. May seed subarachnoid space.	Treatment consists of surgery combined with radiation therapy and chemotherapy.
Ependymoma	Glioma arising from the ependyma of a ventricle, especially the fourth ventricle; leads to early signs of increased intracranial pressure. Arises also from central canal of cord.	Tumor is not radiosensitive and is best treated surgically if possible.
Oligodendroglioma	Slow-growing. Usually arises in cerebral hemisphere in adults. Calcification may be visible on skull x-ray.	Treatment is surgical and usually successful.
Brainstem glioma	Presents during childhood with cranial nerve palsies and then with long tract signs in the limbs. Signs of increased intracranial pressure occur late.	Tumor is inoperable; treatment is by irradiation and shunt for increased intracranial pressure.
Cerebellar hemangioblastoma	Presents with dysequilibrium, ataxia of trunk or limbs, and signs of increased intracranial pressure. Sometimes familial. May be associated with retinal and spinal vascular lesions, polycythemia, and renal cell carcinoma.	Treatment is surgical.
Pineal tumor	Presents with increased intracranial pressure, sometimes associated with impaired upward gaze (Parinaud's syndrome) and other deficits indicative of midbrain lesion.	Ventricular decompression by shunting is followed by surgical approach to tumor; irradiation is indicated if tumor is malignant. Prognosis depends on histopathologic findings and extent of tumor.
Craniopharyngioma	Originates from remnants of Rathke's pouch above the sella, depressing the optic chiasm. May present at any age but usually in childhood, with endocrine dysfunction and bitemporal field defects.	Treatment is surgical, but total removal may not be possible.
Acoustic neurinoma	Ipsilateral hearing loss is most common initial symptom. Subsequent symptoms may include tinnitus, headache, vertigo, facial weakness or numbness, and long tract signs. (May be familial and bilateral when related to neurofibromatosis.) Most sensitive screening tests are MRI and brain stem auditory evoked potential.	Treatment is excision by translabyrinthine surgery, craniectomy, or a combined approach. Outcome is usually good.
Meningioma	Originates from the dura mater or arachnoid; compresses rather than invades adjacent neural structures. Increasingly common with advancing age. Tumor size varies greatly. Symptoms vary with tumor site—eg, unilateral exophthalmos (sphenoidal ridge); anosmia and optic nerve compression (olfactory groove). Tumor is usually benign and readily detected by CT scanning; may lead to calcification and bone erosion visible on plain x-rays of skull.	Treatment is surgical. Tumor may recur if removal is incomplete.
Primary cerebral lymphoma	Associated with AIDS and other immunodeficient states. Presentation may be with focal deficits or with disturbances of cognition and consciousness. May be indistinguishable from cerebral toxoplasmosis.	Treatment is high-dose methotrexate followed by radiation therapy. Prognosis depends on CD4 count at diagnosis.

Table 100. Some anticholinergic antiparkinsonian drugs.

Drug	Usual Daily Dose
Benztropine mesylate (Cogentin)	1–6 mg
Biperiden (Akineton)	2–12 mg
Orphenadrine (Disipal, Norflex)	150–400 mg
Procyclidine (Kemadrin)	7.5–30 mg
Trihexyphenidyl (Artane)	6–20 mg

Modified, with permission, from Aminoff MJ: Pharmacologic management of parkinsonism and other movement disorders. In: *Basic & Clinical Pharmacology*, 8th ed. Katzung BG (editor). McGraw-Hill, 2001.

Table 101. Acute cerebral sequelae of head injury.

Sequelae	Clinical Features	Pathology
Concussion	Transient loss of consciousness with bradycardia, hypotension, and respiratory arrest for a few seconds followed by retrograde and posttraumatic amnesia. Occasionally followed by transient neurologic deficit.	Bruising on side of impact (coup injury) or contralaterally (contrecoup injury).
Cerebral contusion or laceration	Loss of consciousness longer than with concussion. May lead to death or severe residual neurologic deficit.	Cerebral contusion, edema, hemorrhage, and necrosis. May have subarachnoid bleeding.
Acute epidural hemorrhage	Headache, confusion, somnolence, seizures, and focal deficits occur several hours after injury and lead to coma, respiratory depression, and death unless treated by surgical evacuation.	Tear in meningeal artery, vein, or dural sinus, leading to hematoma visible on CT scan.
Acute subdural hemorrhage	Similar to epidural hemorrhage, but interval before onset of symptoms is longer. Treatment is by surgical evacuation.	Hematoma from tear in veins from cortex to superior sagittal sinus or from cerebral laceration, visible on CT scan.
Cerebral hemorrhage	Generally develops immediately after injury. Clinically resembles hypertensive hemorrhage. Surgical evacuation is sometimes helpful.	Hematoma, visible on CT scan.

Table 102. The muscular dystrophies.

Disorder	Inheritance	Age at Onset (years)	Distribution	Prognosis	Genetic Locus
Duchenne type	X-linked recessive	1–5	Pelvic, then shoulder girdle; later, limb and respiratory muscles	Rapid progression. Death within about 15 years after onset.	Xp21
Becker's	X-linked recessive	5–25	Pelvic, then shoulder girdle	Slow progression. May have normal life span.	Xp21
Limb-girdle (Erb's)	Autosomal recessive, dominant or sporadic	10–30	Pelvic or shoulder girdle initially, with later spread to the other	Variable severity and rate of progression. Possible severe disability in middle life.	Multiple
Facioscapulohumeral	Autosomal dominant	Any age	Face and shoulder girdle initially; later, pelvic girdle and legs	Slow progression. Minor disability. Usually normal life span.	4q35
Emery-Dreifuss	X-linked recessive or autosomal dominant	5–10	Humeroperoneal or scapuloperoneal	Variable.	Xq28, 1q11, 1q21.2
Distal	Autosomal dominant or recessive	40–60	Onset distally in extremities; proximal involvement later	Slow progression.	2q13, 2p13
Ocular	Autosomal dominant (may be recessive)	Any age (usually 5–30)	External ocular muscles; may also be mild weakness of face, neck, and arms		
Oculopharyngeal	Autosomal dominant	Any age	As in the ocular form but with dysphagia		14q11.2–q13

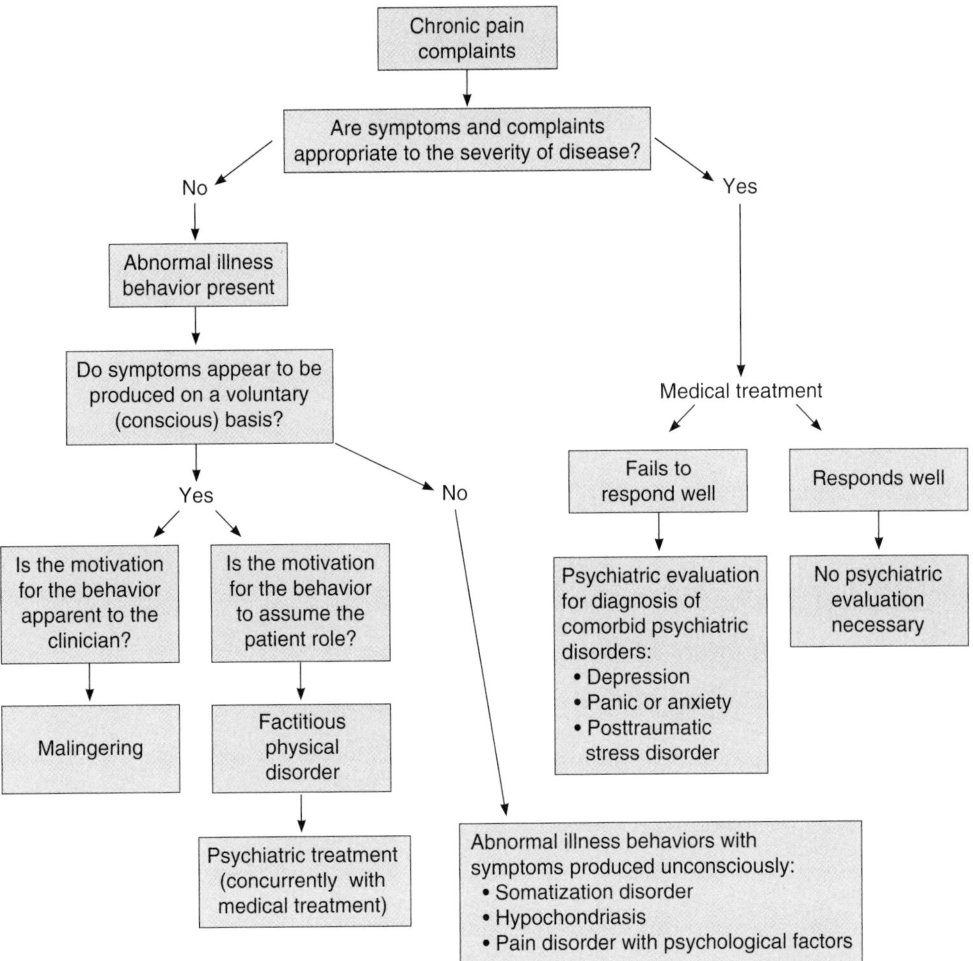

Figure 8. Algorithm for assessing psychiatric component of chronic pain. (Modified and reproduced, with permission, from Eisendrath SJ: Psychiatric aspects of chronic pain. Neurology 1995;45[Suppl 9]:S26.)

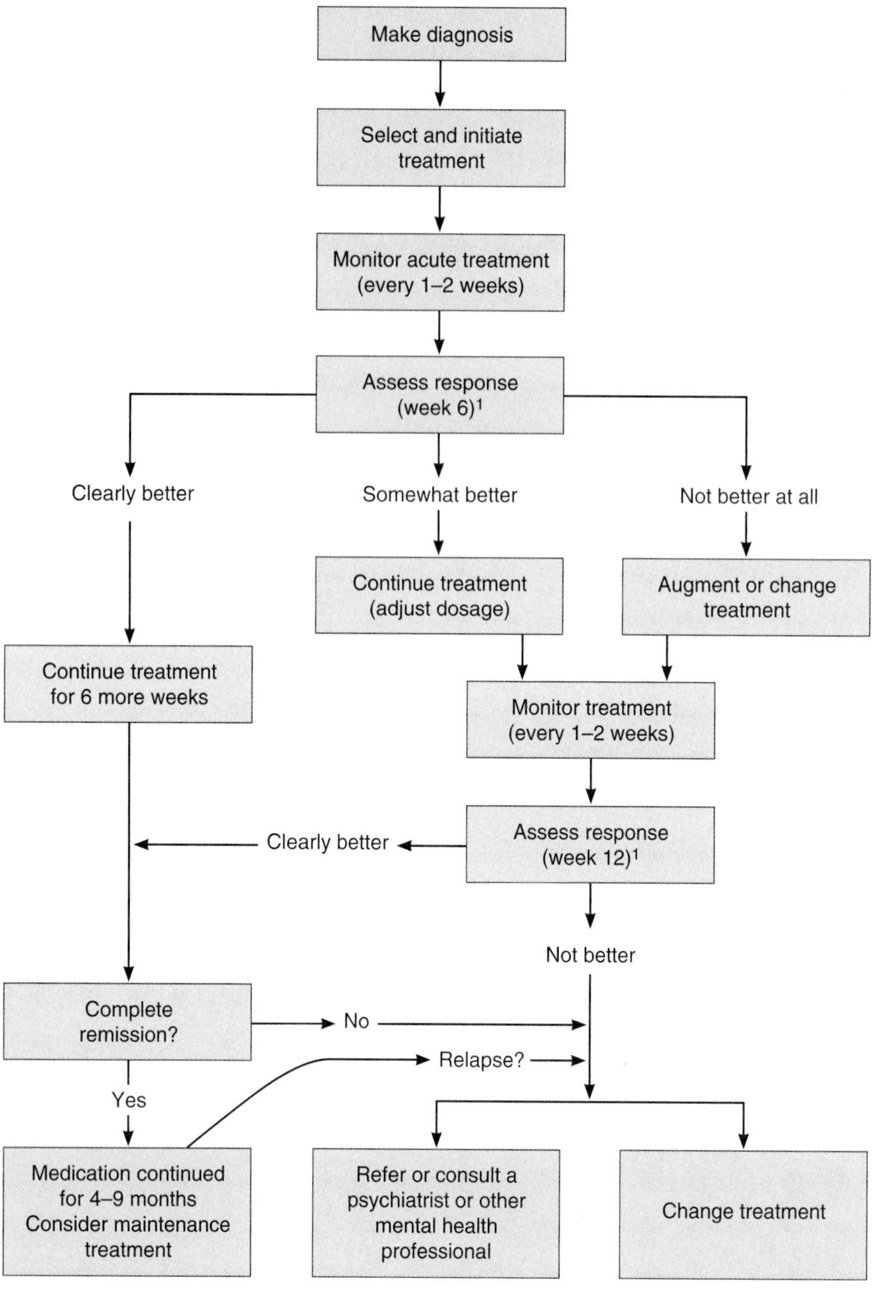

[1]Times of assessment (weeks 6 and 12) rest on very modest data. It may be necessary to revise the treatment plan earlier for patients not responding at all.

Figure 9. Overview of treatment for depression. (Reproduced, with permission, from Agency for Health Care Policy and Research: Depression in Primary Care. Vol. 2: Treatment of Major Depression. United States Department of Health and Human Services, 1993.)

Table 103. Screening for alcohol abuse.

1. CAGE screening test[1]

Have you ever felt the need to	**C**ut down on drinking?
Have you ever felt	**A**nnoyed by criticism of your drinking?
Have you ever felt	**G**uilty about your drinking?
Have you ever taken a morning	**E**ye opener?

INTERPRETATION: Two "yes" answers are considered a positive screen. One "yes" answer should arouse a suspicion of alcohol abuse.

2. The Alcohol Use Disorder Identification Test (AUDIT).[2] (Scores for response categories are given in parentheses. Scores range from 0 to 40, with a cutoff score of ≥ 5 indicating hazardous drinking, harmful drinking, or alcohol dependence.)

1. How often do you have a drink containing alcohol?	(0) Never	(1) Monthly or less	(2) Two to four times a month	(3) Two or three times a week	(4) Four or more times a week
2. How many drinks containing alcohol do you have on a typical day when you are drinking?	(0) 1 or 2	(1) 3 or 4	(2) 5 or 6	(3) 7 to 9	(4) 10 or more
3. How often do you have six or more drinks on one occasion?	(0) Never	(1) Less than monthly	(2) Monthly	(3) Weekly	(4) Daily or almost daily
4. How often during the past year have you found that you were not able to stop drinking once you had started?	(0) Never	(1) Less than monthly	(2) Monthly	(3) Weekly	(4) Daily or almost daily
5. How often during the past year have you failed to do what was normally expected of you because of drinking?	(0) Never	(1) Less than monthly	(2) Monthly	(3) Weekly	(4) Daily or almost daily
6. How often during the past year have you needed a first drink in the morning to get yourself going after a heavy drinking session?	(0) Never	(1) Less than monthly	(2) Monthly	(3) Weekly	(4) Daily or almost daily
7. How often during the past year have you had a feeling of guilt or remorse after drinking?	(0) Never	(1) Less than monthly	(2) Monthly	(3) Weekly	(4) Daily or almost daily
8. How often during the past year have you been unable to remember what happened the night before because you had been drinking?	(0) Never	(1) Less than monthly	(2) Monthly	(3) Weekly	(4) Daily or almost daily
9. Have you or has someone else been injured as a result of your drinking?	(0) No	(2) Yes, but not in the past year		(4) Yes, during the past year	
10. Has a relative or friend or a doctor or other health worker been concerned about your drinking or suggested you cut down?	(0) No	(2) Yes, but not in the past year		(4) Yes, during the past year	

[1]Modified from Mayfield D et al: The CAGE questionnaire: validation of a new alcoholism screening instrument. Am J Psychiatry 1974;131:1121.
[2]From Piccinelli M et al: Efficacy of the alcohol use disorders identification test as a screening tool for hazardous alcohol intake and related disorders in primary care: a validity study. BMJ 1997;314:420.

Table 104. Personality disorders: Classification and clinical findings.

Personality Disorder	Clinical Findings
Paranoid	Defensive, oversensitive, secretive, suspicious, hyperalert, with limited emotional response.
Schizoid	Shy, introverted, withdrawn, avoids close relationships.
Obsessive-compulsive	Perfectionist, egocentric, indecisive, with rigid thought patterns and need for control.
Histrionic (hysterical)	Dependent, immature, seductive, egocentric, vain, emotionally labile.
Schizotypal	Superstitious, socially isolated, suspicious, with limited interpersonal ability, eccentric behaviors, and odd speech.
Narcissistic	Exhibitionist, grandiose, preoccupied with power, lacks interest in others, with excessive demands for attention.
Avoidant	Fears rejection, hyperreacts to rejection and failure, with poor social endeavors and low self-esteem.
Dependent	Passive, overaccepting, unable to make decisions, lacks confidence, with poor self-esteem.
Antisocial	Selfish, callous, promiscuous, impulsive, unable to learn from experience, has legal problems.
Borderline	Impulsive; has unstable and intense interpersonal relationships; is suffused with anger, fear, and guilt; lacks self-control and self-fulfillment; has identity problems and affective instability; is suicidal (a serious problem—up to 80% of hospitalized borderline patients make an attempt at some time during treatment, and the incidence of completed suicide is as high as 5%); aggressive behavior, feelings of emptiness, and occasional psychotic decompensation. This group has a high drug abuse rate, which plays a role in symptoms. There is extensive overlap with other diagnostic categories, particularly mood disorders and posttraumatic stress disorder.

Table 105. Commonly used antianxiety and hypnotic agents.

Drug	Usual Daily Oral Dose	Usual Daily Maximum Dose	Cost for 30 Days Treatment Based on Maximum Dosage[1]
Benzodiazepines (used for anxiety)			
Alprazolam (Xanax)[2]	0.5 mg	4 mg	$117.60
Chlordiazepoxide (Librium)[3]	10–20 mg	100 mg	$40.80
Clonazepam (Klonopin)[3]	1–2 mg	10 mg	$169.50
Clorazepate (Tranxene)[3]	15–30 mg	60 mg	$260.40
Diazepam (Valium)[3]	5–15 mg	30 mg	$28.80
Lorazepam (Ativan)[2]	2–4 mg	4 mg	$76.80
Oxazepam (Serax)[2]	10–30 mg	60 mg	$94.20
Benzodiazepines (used for sleep)			
Estazolam (Prosom)[2]	1 mg	2 mg	$29.70
Flurazepam (Dalmane)[3]	15 mg	30 mg	$10.50
Midazolam (Versed IV)[4]	5 mg IV		$2.80/dose
Quazepam (Doral)[3]	7.5 mg	15 mg	$110.10
Temazepam (Restoril)[2]	15 mg	30 mg	$24.30
Triazolam (Halcion)[5]	0.125 mg	0.25 mg	$21.60
Miscellaneous (used for anxiety)			
Buspirone (Buspar)[2]	10–30 mg	60 mg	$242.40
Phenobarbital[3]	15–30 mg	90 mg	$3.15
Miscellaneous (used for sleep)			
Chloral hydrate (Noctec)[2]	500 mg	1000 mg	$8.62
Hydroxyzine (Vistaril)[2]	50 mg	100 mg	$67.20
Zolpidem (Ambien)[5]	5–10 mg	10 mg	$97.00
Zaleplon (Sonata)[6]	5–10 mg	10 mg	$84.00

[1]Average wholesale price (AWP, for AB-rated generic when available) for quantity listed. Source: *Red Book Update*, Vol. 24, No. 4, April 2005. AWP may not accurately represent the actual pharmacy cost because wide contractual variations exist among institutions.
[2]Intermediate physical half-life (10–20 hours).
[3]Long physical half-life (> 20 hours).
[4]Intravenously for procedures.
[5]Short physical half-life (1–5 hours).
[6]Short physical half-life (about 1 hour).

Table 106. Commonly used antipsychotics.

Drug	Usual Daily Oral Dose	Usual Daily Maximum Dose[1]	Cost per Unit	Cost for 30 Days Treatment Based on Maximum Dosage[2]
Phenothiazines				
Chlorpromazine (Thorazine; others)	100–400 mg	1 g	$1.05/200 mg	$157.50
Thioridazine (Mellaril)	100–400 mg	600 mg	$1.10/200 mg	$99.00
Mesoridazine (Serentil)	50–200 mg	400 mg	$1.64/100 mg	$196.80
Perphenazine (Trilafon)[3]	16–32 mg	64 mg	$1.54/16 mg	$184.80
Trifluoperazine (Stelazine)	5–15 mg	60 mg	$1.58/10 mg	$284.40
Fluphenazine (Permitil, Prolixin)[3]	2–10 mg	60 mg	$1.15/10 mg	$207.00
Thioxanthenes				
Thiothixene (Navane)[3]	5–10 mg	80 mg	$0.65/10 mg	$156.00
Dihydroindolone				
Molindone (Moban)	30–100 mg	225 mg	$3.79/50 mg	$511.65
Dibenzoxazepine				
Loxapine (Loxitane)	20–60 mg	200 mg	$2.57/50 mg	$308.40
Dibenzodiazepine				
Clozapine (Clozaril)	300–450 mg	900 mg	$3.33/100 mg	$899.10
Butyrophenone				
Haloperidol (Haldol)	2–5 mg	60 mg	$2.52/20 mg	$226.80
Benzisoxazole				
Risperidone[4] (Risperdal)	2–6 mg	10 mg	$5.87/2 mg	$731.62
Thienbenzodiazepine				
Olanzapine (Zyprexa)	5–10 mg	10 mg	$10.37/10 mg	$311.40
Dibenzothiazepine				
Quetiapine (Seroquel)	200–400 mg	800 mg	$5.89/200 mg	$706.80
Benzisothiazolyl piperazine				
Ziprasidone (Geodon)	40–160 mg	160 mg	$5.37/80 mg	$322.09
Dipiperazine				
Aripiprazole (Abilify)	10–15 mg	30 mg	$15.63/30 mg	$468.88

[1]Can be higher in some cases.

[2]Average wholesale price (AWP, for AB-rated generic when available) for quantity listed. Source: *Red Book Update*, Vol. 24, No. 4, April 2005. AWP may not accurately represent the actual pharmacy cost because wide contractual variations exist among institutions.

[3]Indicates piperazine structure.

[4]For risperidone, daily doses above 6 mg increase the risk of extrapyramidal syndrome. Risperidone 6 mg is approximately equivalent to haloperidol 20 mg.

Table 107. Relative potency and side effects of antipsychotics.

Drug	Chlorpromazine:Drug Potency Ratio	Anticholinergic Effects[1]	Extrapyramidal Effect[1]
Phenothiazines			
Chlorpromazine	1:1	4	1
Thioridazine	1:1	4	1
Mesoridazine	1:2	3	2
Perphenazine	1:10	2	3
Trifluoperazine	1:20	1	4
Fluphenazine	1:50	1	4
Thioxanthene			
Thiothixene	1:20	1	4
Dihydroindolone			
Molindone	1:10	2	3
Dibenzoxazepine			
Loxapine	1:10	2	3
Butyrophenone			
Haloperidol	1:50	1	4
Dibenzodiazepine			
Clozapine	1:1	4	—
Benzisoxazole			
Risperidone	1:50	1	1
Thienbenzodiazepine			
Olanzapine	1:20	1	1
Dibenzothiazepine			
Quetiapine	1:1	1	—
Benzisothiazolyl piperazine			
Ziprasidone	1:1	1	1
Dipiperazine			
Aripiprazole	1:20	1	0

[1]4 = strong effect; 1 = weak effect.

Table 108. Commonly used antidepressants.

Drug	Usual Daily Oral Dose (mg)	Usual Daily Maximum Dose (mg)	Sedative Effects[1]	Anticholinergic Effects[1]	Cost per Unit	Cost for 30 Days Treatment Based on Maximum Dosage[2]
SSRIs						
Fluoxetine (Prozac, Sarafem)	5–40	80	< 1	< 1	$2.67/20 mg	$320.40
Fluvoxamine (Luvox)	100–300	300	1	< 1	$2.64/100 mg	$237.60
Nefazodone (Serzone)	300–600	600	2	< 1	$1.60/200 mg	$144.00
Paroxetine (Paxil)	20–30	50	1	1	$2.64/20 mg	$158.40
Sertraline (Zoloft)	50–150	200	< 1	< 1	$2.90/100 mg	$174.00
Citalopram (Celexa)	20	40	< 1	1	$2.64/40 mg	$79.20
Escitalopram (Lexapro)	10	20	< 1	1	$2.43/20 mg	$72.90
TRICYCLIC AND CLINICALLY SIMILAR COMPOUNDS						
Amitriptyline (Elavil)	150–250	300	4	4	$1.16/150 mg	$69.60
Amoxapine (Asendin)	150–200	400	2	2	$1.67/100 mg	$200.40
Clomipramine (Anafranil)	100	250	3	3	$1.47/75 mg	$157.20
Desipramine (Norpramin)	100–250	300	1	1	$1.50/100 mg	$135.00
Doxepin (Sinequan)	150–200	300	4	3	$1.00/100 mg	$90.00
Imipramine (Tofranil)	150–200	300	3	3	$1.22/50 mg	$219.60
Maprotiline (Ludiomil)	100–200	300	4	2	$0.93/75 mg	$111.60
Nortriptyline (Aventyl, Pamelor)	100–150	150	2	2	$1.62/50 mg	$148.20
Protriptyline (Vivactil)	15–40	60	1	3	$1.58/10 mg	$248.40
MONOAMINE OXIDASE INHIBITORS						
Phenelzine (Nardil)	45–60	90	...	...	$0.57/15 mg	$102.60
Tranylcypromine (Parnate)	20–30	50	...	...	$0.80/10 mg	$120.00
OTHER COMPOUNDS						
Venlafaxine XR (Effexor)	150–225	225	1	< 1	$3.27/75 mg	$294.30
Duloxetine (Cymbalta)	40	60	2	3	$3.42/60 mg	$102.60
Mirtazapine (Remeron)	15–45	45	4	2	$2.80/30 mg	$165.46
Bupropion XL (Wellbutrin XL)	300[3]	450[3]		< 1	$3.87/300 mg	$204.20
Bupropion SR (Wellbutrin SR)	300	400[4]		< 1	$3.59/200 mg	$215.59
Trazodone (Desyrel)	100–300	400	4	< 1	$0.73/100 mg	$87.60
Trimipramine (Surmontil)	75–200	200	4	4	$2.96/100 mg	$177.60

[1]4 = strong effect; 1 = weak effect.
[2]Average wholesale price (AWP, for AB-rated generic when available) for quantity listed. Source: *Red Book Update*, Vol. 24, No. 4, April 2005. AWP may not accurately represent the actual pharmacy cost because wide contractual variations exist among institutions.
[3]Wellbutrin XL is a once-daily form of bupropion. Bupropion is still available as immediate release, and, if used, no single dose should exceed 150 mg.
[4]200 mg twice daily.
SSRIs = serotonin selective reuptake inhibitors.

Table 109. Etiology of delirium and other cognitive disorders.

Disorder	Possible Causes
Intoxication	Alcohol, sedatives, bromides, analgesics (eg, pentazocine), psychedelic drugs, stimulants, and household solvents.
Drug withdrawal	Withdrawal from alcohol, sedative-hypnotics, corticosteroids.
Long-term effects of alcohol	Wernicke-Korsakoff syndrome.
Infections	Septicemia; meningitis and encephalitis due to bacterial, viral, fungal, parasitic, or tuberculous organisms or to central nervous system syphilis; acute and chronic infections due to the entire range of microbiologic pathogens.
Endocrine disorders	Thyrotoxicosis, hypothyroidism, adrenocortical dysfunction (including Addison's disease and Cushing's syndrome), pheochromocytoma, insulinoma, hypoglycemia, hyperparathyroidism, hypoparathyroidism, panhypopituitarism, diabetic ketoacidosis.
Respiratory disorders	Hypoxia, hypercapnia.
Metabolic disturbances	Fluid and electrolyte disturbances (especially hyponatremia, hypomagnesemia, and hypercalcemia), acid-base disorders, hepatic disease (hepatic encephalopathy), renal failure, porphyria.
Nutritional deficiencies	Deficiency of vitamin B_1 (beriberi), vitamin B_{12} (pernicious anemia), folic acid, nicotinic acid (pellagra); protein-calorie malnutrition.
Trauma	Subdural hematoma, subarachnoid hemorrhage, intracerebral bleeding, concussion syndrome.
Cardiovascular disorders	Myocardial infarctions, cardiac arrhythmias, cerebrovascular spasms, hypertensive encephalopathy, hemorrhages, embolisms, and occlusions indirectly cause decreased cognitive function.
Neoplasms	Primary or metastatic lesions of the central nervous system, cancer-induced hypercalcemia.
Seizure disorders	Ictal, interictal, and postictal dysfunction.
Collagen-vascular and immunologic disorders	Autoimmune disorders, including systemic lupus erythematosus, Sjögren's syndrome, and AIDS.
Degenerative diseases	Alzheimer's disease, Pick's disease, multiple sclerosis, parkinsonism, Huntington's chorea, normal pressure hydrocephalus.
Medications	Anticholinergic drugs, antidepressants, H_2-blocking agents, digoxin, salicylates (chronic use), and a wide variety of other over-the-counter and prescribed drugs.

Table 110. Causes of hyperprolactinemia.

Physiologic Causes	Pharmacologic Causes	Pathologic Causes
Exercise	Amoxapine	Acromegaly
Idiopathic	Amphetamines	Chronic chest wall stimulation (postthoracotomy, postmastectomy, herpes zoster, breast problems, nipple rings, etc)
Macroprolactinemia ("big prolactin")	Anesthetic agents	Cirrhosis
Pregnancy	Butyrophenones	Hypothalamic disease
Puerperium	Cimetidine and ranitidine (not famotidine or nizatidine)	Hypothyroidism
Sleep (REM phase)	Estrogens	Multiple sclerosis
Stress (trauma, surgery)	Hydroxyzine	Optic neuromyelitis
Suckling	Methyldopa	Pituitary stalk section
	Metoclopramide	Prolactin-secreting tumors
	Narcotics	Pseudocyesis (false pregnancy)
	Nicotine	Renal failure (especially with zinc deficiency)
	Phenothiazines	Spinal cord lesions
	Protease inhibitors	Systemic lupus erythematosus
	Progestins	
	Reserpine	
	Risperidone	
	Selective serotonin reuptake inhibitors	
	Tricyclic antidepressants	
	Verapamil	

Table 111. The Diabetes Expert Committee criteria for evaluating the standard oral glucose tolerance test.[1]

	Normal Glucose Tolerance	Impaired Glucose Tolerance	Diabetes Mellitus[2]
Fasting plasma glucose (mg/dL)	< 100	100–125	≥ 126
Two hours after glucose load (mg/dL)	< 140	≥ 140 – 199	≥ 200

[1]Give 75 g of glucose dissolved in 300 mL of water after an overnight fast in subjects who have been receiving at least 150–200 g of carbohydrate daily for 3 days before the test.
[2]A fasting plasma glucose ≥ 126 mg/dL is diagnostic of diabetes if confirmed on a subsequent day.

Table 112. Oral antidiabetic drugs that stimulate insulin secretion.

Drug	Tablet Size	Daily Dose	Duration of Action	Cost per Unit	Cost for 30 Days Treatment Based on Maximum Dosage[1]
Sulfonylureas					
Tolbutamide (Orinase)	250 and 500 mg	0.5–2 g in 2 or 3 divided doses	6–12 hours	$0.28/500 mg	$33.60
Tolazamide (Tolinase)	100, 250, and 500 mg	0.1–1 g as single dose or in 2 divided doses	Up to 24 hours	$0.77/250 mg	$83.40
Acetohexamide (Dymelor)[2]	250 and 500 mg	0.25–1.5 g as single dose or in 2 divided doses	8–24 hours	$1.34/500 mg	$120.60
Chlorpropamide (Diabinese)[2]	100 and 250 mg	0.1–0.5 g as single dose	24–72 hours	$0.67/250 mg	$40.20
Glyburide (Diaβeta, Micronase)	1.25, 2.5, and 5 mg	1.25–20 mg as single dose or in 2 divided doses	Up to 24 hours	$0.78/5 mg	$93.60
(Glynase)	1.5, 3, and 6 mg	1.5–18 mg as single dose or in 2 divided doses	Up to 24 hours	$1.07/6 mg	$96.30
Glipizide (Glucotrol)	5 and 10 mg	2.5–40 mg as single dose or in 2 divided doses on an empty stomach	6–12 hours	$0.59/10 mg	$70.80
(Glucotrol XL)	5 and 10 mg	Up to 20 or 30 mg daily as a single dose	Up to 24 hours	$0.81/10 mg	$72.90
Gliclazide (not available in the US)	80 mg	40–80 mg as single dose; 160–320 mg as divided dose	12 hours	—	—
Glimepiride (Amaryl)	1, 2, and 4 mg	1–4 mg as single dose	Up to 24 hours	$1.31/4 mg	$39.30
Meglitinide analogs					
Repaglinide (Prandin)	0.5, 1, and 2 mg	4 mg in two divided doses given 15 minutes before breakfast and dinner	3 hours	$1.29/2 mg	$77.40
D-Phenylalanine derivative					
Nateglinide (Starlix)	60 mg and 120 mg	60 or 120 mg 3 times a day before meals	1.5 hours	$1.29/120 mg	$116.10

[1]Average wholesale price (AWP, for AB-rated generic when available) for quantity listed. Source: *Red Book* Update, Vol. 24, No. 4, April 2005. AWP may not accurately represent the actual pharmacy cost because wide contractual variations exist among institutions.
[2]There has been a decline in use of these formulations. In the case of chlorpropamide, the decline is due to its numerous side effects (see text).

Table 113. Oral antidiabetic drugs that are insulin-sparing.

Drug	Tablet Size	Daily Dose	Duration of Action	Cost per Unit	Cost for 30 Days Treatment Based on Maximum Dosage[1]
Biguanides					
Metformin (Glucophage)	500, 850, and 1000 mg	1–2.5 g; one tablet with meals 2 or 3 times daily	7–12 hours	$1.46/850 mg	$131.40
Extended-release metformin (Glucophage XR)	500 mg	500–2000 mg once a day	Up to 24 hours	$0.88/500 mg	$105.60
Thiazolidinediones					
Rosiglitazone (Avandia)	2, 4, and 8 mg	4–8 mg daily (can be divided)	Up to 24 hours	$5.59/8 mg	$167.70
Pioglitazone (Actos)	15, 30, and 45 mg	15–45 mg daily	Up to 24 hours	$6.28/45 mg	$188.42
α-Glucosidase inhibitors					
Acarbose (Precose)	50 and 100 mg	75–300 mg in 3 divided doses with first bite of food	4 hours	$0.99/100 mg	$89.10
Miglitol (Glyset)	25, 50, and 100 mg	75–300 mg in 3 divided doses with first bite of food	4 hours	$0.97/100 mg	$87.30

[1]Average wholesale price (AWP, for AB-rated generic when available) for quantity listed. Source: *Red Book* Update, Vol. 24, No. 4, April 2005. AWP may not accurately represent the actual pharmacy cost because wide contractual variations exist among institutions.

Table 114. Combination oral antidiabetic drugs.

Drug	Tablet Size	Daily Dose	Duration of Action	Cost per Unit	Cost for 30 Days Treatment Based on Maximum Dosage[1]
Glyburide/metformin (Glucovance)	1.25 mg/250 mg 2.5 mg/500 mg 5 mg/500 mg	Maximum daily dose of 20 mg glyburide/ 2000 mg metformin	See individual drugs[2]	$1.13/5/ 500 mg	$135.60
Rosiglitazone/metformin (Avandamet)	1 mg/500 mg 2 mg/500 mg 4 mg/500 mg	Maximum daily dose of 8 mg rosiglitazone/ 2000 mg metformin	See individual drugs[2]	$1.75/2/ 500 mg	$210.00

[1]Average wholesale price (AWP, for AB-rated generic when available) for quantity listed. Source: *Red Book* Update, Vol. 24, No. 4, April 2005. AWP may not accurately represent the actual pharmacy cost because wide contractual variations exist among institutions.
[2]Glyburide, Table 27–7; metformin, Table 27–8; and rosiglitazone, Table 27–8.

Table 115. Some insulin preparations available in the United States.[1]

Preparation	Species Source	Concentration	Cost[1]
Rapid-acting insulin analogs			
Insulin lispro (Humalog, Lilly)	Human analog (recombinant)	U100	$67.58
Insulin aspart (Novolog, Novo Nordisk)	Human analog (recombinant)	U100	$74.88
Insulin glulisine (Apidra, Sanofi Aventis)	Human analog (recombinant)	U100	
Short-acting regular insulins			
"Purified"[2]			
Regular Novolin (Novo Nordisk)[3]	Human	U100	$30.50
Regular Humulin (Lilly)	Human	U100, U500 20 mL	$29.28, $210.68
Regular Iletin II (Lilly)	Pork	U100	$47.98
Intermediate-acting insulins			
"Purified"[2]			
Lente Humulin (Lilly)	Human	U100	$29.28
Lente Iletin II (Lilly)	Pork	U100	$47.98
Lente Novolin (Novo Nordisk)[3]	Human	U100	$30.50
NPH Humulin (Lilly)	Human	U100	$29.28
NPH Iletin II (Lilly)	Pork	U100	$47.98
NPH Novolin (Novo Nordisk)[3]	Human	U100	$30.50
Premixed insulins			
% NPH/% regular			
Novolin 70/30 (Novo Nordisk)[3]	Human	U100	$30.50
Humulin 70/30 and 50/50 (Lilly)	Human	U100	$29.28
Other Mixes			
75% insulin lispro protamine/25% insulin lispro (Humalog Mix 75/25 [Lilly])	Human analog (recombinant)	U100 (insulin pen, prefilled syringes, 5 × 3-mL cartridges)	Pen $144.63, Vial $71.88
70% insulin aspart protamine/30% insulin aspart (Novolog Mix 70/30 [Novo Nordisk])			Pen $144.62, Vial $74.88
Long-acting insulins			
"Purified"[2]			
Ultralente Humulin (Lilly)	Human	U100	$29.28
Insulin glargine (Lantus, Aventis)	Human analog (recombinant)	U100	$66.85

[1]All of these agents (except insulin lispro and U500) are available without a prescription. Average wholesale price (AWP, for AB-rated generic when available) for 10-mL vial unless otherwise specified. Source: *Red Book* Update, Vol. 24, No. 4, April 2005. Wholesale prices for all human preparations (except insulin lispro and U500) are similar. AWP may not accurately represent the actual pharmacy cost because wide contractual variations exist among institutions.

[2]Less than 10 ppm proinsulin.

[3]Novo Nordisk human insulins are termed Novolin R, L, and N.

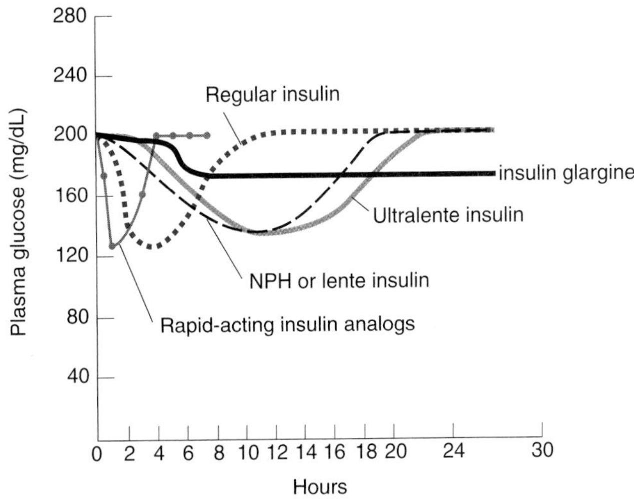

Figure 10. Extent and duration of action of various insulins (in a fasting diabetic). Duration is extended considerably when the dose of a given formulation increases above average therapeutic doses (except for insulin lispro).

Table 116. Examples of intensive insulin regimens using rapid-acting insulin analogs (insulin lispro, aspart, or glulisine) and ultralente, NPH, or insulin glargine in a 70-kg man with type 1 diabetes.[1–3]

	Pre-Breakfast	Pre-Lunch	Pre-Dinner	At Bedtime
Rapid-acting insulin analog	5 units	4 units	6 units	—
Ultralente insulin	8 units	—	8 units	—
		OR		
Rapid-acting insulin analog	5 units	4 units	6 units	—
NPH insulin	3 units	3 units	2 units	8–9 units
		OR		
Rapid-acting insulin analog	5 units	4 units	6 units	—
Insulin glargine	—	—	—	15–16 units

[1]Assumes that patient is consuming approximately 75 g carbohydrate at breakfast, 60 g at lunch, and 90 g at dinner.
[2]The dose of insulin lispro or insulin aspart can be raised by 1 or 2 units if extra carbohydrate (15–30 g) is ingested or if premeal blood glucose is > 170 mg/dL. Insulin lispro or insulin aspart can be mixed in the same syringe with ultralente or NPH insulin.
[3]Insulin glargine cannot be mixed with any of the available insulins and must be given as a separate injection.

Table 117. Secondary causes of lipid abnormalities.

Cause	Associated Lipid Abnormality
Obesity	Increased triglycerides, decreased HDL cholesterol
Sedentary lifestyle	Decreased HDL cholesterol
Diabetes mellitus	Increased triglycerides, increased total cholesterol
Alcohol use	Increased triglycerides, increased HDL cholesterol
Hypothyroidism	Increased total cholesterol
Hyperthyroidism	Decreased total cholesterol
Nephrotic syndrome	Increased total cholesterol
Chronic renal insufficiency	Increased total cholesterol, increased triglycerides
Hepatic disease (cirrhosis)	Decreased total cholesterol
Obstructive liver disease	Increased total cholesterol
Malignancy	Decreased total cholesterol
Cushing's disease (or steroid use)	Increased total cholesterol
Oral contraceptives	Increased triglycerides, increased total cholesterol
Diuretics[1]	Increased total cholesterol, increased triglycerides
β-Blockers[1,2]	Increased total cholesterol, decreased HDL

[1]Short-term effects only.
[2]β-Blockers with intrinsic sympathomimetic activity, such as pindolol and acebutolol, do not affect lipid levels.

Table 118. LDL goals and treatment cutpoints: recommendations of the NCEP Adult Treatment Panel III.

Risk Category	LDL Goal (mg/dL)	LDL Level at Which to Initiate Lifestyle Changes (mg/dL)	LDL Level at Which to Consider Drug Changes[1] (mg/dL)
High risk: CHD[2] or CHD risk equivalents[3] (10-year risk > 20%)	< 100 (optional goal: < 70 mg/dL)[4]	≥ 100[5]	≥ 100[6] (< 100: consider drug options)[1]
Moderately high risk: 2+ risk factors[7] (10-year risk 10% to 20%)[8]	< 130[9]	≥ 130[5]	≥ 130 (100–129; consider drug options)[10]
Moderate risk: 2+ risk factors[7] (10-year risk < 10%)[8]	< 130	≥ 130	≥ 160
Low risk: 0–1 risk factors[11]	< 160	≥ 160	≥ 190 (160–189: LDL-lowering drug optional)

Reproduced, with permission, from Grundy SM et al: Implications of recent clinical trials for the national cholesterol education program adult treatment panel III guidelines. Circulation 2004;110:227.
LDL = low-density lipoprotein; NCEP = National Cholesterol Education Program; CHD = coronary heart disease.
[1]When LDL-lowering drug therapy is employed, it is advised that intensity of therapy be sufficient to achieve at least a 30–40% reduction in LDL cholesterol levels.
[2]CHD includes history of myocardial infarction, unstable angina, coronary artery procedures (angioplasty or bypass surgery), or evidence of clinically significant myocardial ischemia.
[3]CHD risk equivalents include clinical manifestations of noncoronary forms of atherosclerotic disease (peripheral arterial disease, abdominal aortic aneurysm, and carotid artery disease [transient ischemic attacks or stroke of carotid origin with > 50% obstruction of a carotid artery]), diabetes mellitus, and ≥ 2 risk factors with 10-year risk for CHD > 20%.
[4]Very high risk favors the optional LDL cholesterol goal of < 70 mg/dL, or in patients with high triglycerides, non-high density lipoprotein (HDL) cholesterol < 100 mg/dL.
[5]Any person at high risk or moderately high risk who has lifestyle-related risk factors (eg, obesity, physical inactivity, elevated triglyceride, low HDL cholesterol, or metabolic syndrome) is a candidate for therapeutic lifestyle changes to modify these risk factors regardless of LDL cholesterol.
[6]If baseline LDL cholesterol is < 100 mg/dL, institution of an LDL-lowering drug is a therapeutic option on the basis of available clinical trial results. If a high-risk person has high triglycerides or low HDL cholesterol, combining a fibrate or nicotinic acid with an LDL-lowering drug can be considered.
[7]Risk factors include cigarette smoking, hypertension (blood pressure ≥ 140/90 mm Hg or on antihypertensive medication), low HDL cholesterol (< 40 mg/dL), family history of premature CHD (CHD in male first-degree relative < 55 years of age; CHD in female first-degree relative < 65 years of age), and age (men ≥ 45 years; women ≥ 55 years).
[8]Electronic 10-year risk calculators are available at www.nhlbi.nih.gov/guidelines/cholesterol.
[9]Optional LDL cholesterol goal < 100 mg/dL.
[10]For moderately high-risk persons, when the LDL cholesterol level is 100–129 mg/dL at baseline or on lifestyle therapy, initiation of an LDL-lowering drug to achieve an LDL cholesterol level < 100 mg/dL is a therapeutic option on the basis of available clinical trial results.
[11]Almost all people with zero or one risk factor have a 10-year CHD risk < 10%, and 10-year risk assessment in these people is thus not necessary.

Table 119. Effects of selected lipid-modifying drugs.

Drug	Lipid-Modifying Effects			Initial Daily Dose	Maximum Daily Dose	Cost for 30 Days Treatment with Dose Listed[1]
	LDL	HDL	Triglyceride			
Atorvastatin (Lipitor)	−25 to −40%	+5 to 10%	↓↓	10 mg once	80 mg once	$113.38 (20 mg once)
Cholestyramine (Questran, others)	−15 to −25%	+5%	±	4 g twice a day	24 g divided	$126.68 (8 g divided)
Colesevelam (WelChol)	−10 to −20%	+10%	±	625 mg, 6–7 tablets once	625 mg, 6–7 tablets once	$170.64 (6 tablets once)
Colestipol (Colestid)	−15 to −25%	+5%	±	5 g twice a day	30 g divided	$120.92 (10 g divided)
Ezetimibe (Zetia)	−20%	+5%	±	10 mg once	10 mg once	$82.04 (10 mg once)
Fluvastatin (Lescol)	−20 to −30%	+5 to 10%	↓	20 mg once	40 mg once	$63.12 (20 mg once)
Gemfibrozil (Lopid)	−10 to −15%	+15 to 20%	↓↓	600 mg once	1200 mg divided	$74.80 (600 mg twice a day)
Lovastatin (Mevacor)	−25 to −40%	+5 to 10%	↓	10 mg once	80 mg divided	$71.15 (20 mg once)
Niacin	−15 to −25%	+25 to 35%	↓↓	100 mg once	3–4.5 g divided	$7.20 (1.5 g twice a day)
Pravastatin (Pravachol)	−25 to −40%	+5 to 10%	↓	20 mg once	40 mg once	$100.53 (20 mg once)
Rosuvastatin (Crestor)	−40 to −50%	+10 to 15%	↓↓	10 mg once	40 mg once	$75.60 (20 mg once)
Simvastatin (Zocor)	−25 to −40%	+5 to 10%	↓↓	5 mg once	80 mg once	$81.94 (10 mg once)

LDL = low-density lipoprotein; HDL = high-density lipoprotein; ± = variable, if any.

[1]Average wholesale price (AWP, for AB-rated generic when available) for quantity listed. Source: *Red Book Update*, Vol. 24, No. 4, April 2005. AWP may not accurately represent the actual pharmacy cost because wide contractual variations exist among institutions.

Table 120. CDC AIDS case definition for surveillance of adults and adolescents.

Definitive AIDS diagnoses (with or without laboratory evidence of HIV infection)

1. Candidiasis of the esophagus, trachea, bronchi, or lungs.
2. Cryptococcosis, extrapulmonary.
3. Cryptosporidiosis with diarrhea persisting > 1 month.
4. Cytomegalovirus disease of an organ other than liver, spleen, or lymph nodes.
5. Herpes simplex virus infection causing a mucocutaneous ulcer that persists longer than 1 month; or bronchitis, pneumonitis, or esophagitis of any duration.
6. Kaposi's sarcoma in a patient < 60 years of age.
7. Lymphoma of the brain (primary) in a patient < 60 years of age.
8. *Mycobacterium avium* complex or *Mycobacterium kansasii* disease, disseminated (at a site other than or in addition to lungs, skin, or cervical or hilar lymph nodes).
9. *Pneumocystis jiroveci* pneumonia.
10. Progressive multifocal leukoencephalopathy.
11. Toxoplasmosis of the brain.

Definitive AIDS diagnoses (with laboratory evidence of HIV infection)

1. Coccidioidomycosis, disseminated (at a site other than or in addition to lungs or cervical or hilar lymph nodes).
2. HIV encephalopathy.
3. Histoplasmosis, disseminated (at a site other than or in addition to lungs or cervical or hilar lymph nodes).
4. Isosporiasis with diarrhea persisting > 1 month.
5. Kaposi's sarcoma at any age.
6. Lymphoma of the brain (primary) at any age.
7. Other non-Hodgkin's lymphoma of B cell or unknown immunologic phenotype.
8. Any mycobacterial disease caused by mycobacteria other than *Mycobacterium tuberculosis,* disseminated (at a site other than or in addition to lungs, skin, or cervical or hilar lymph nodes).
9. Disease caused by extrapulmonary *M tuberculosis.*
10. *Salmonella* (nontyphoid) septicemia, recurrent.
11. HIV wasting syndrome.
12. CD4 lymphocyte count below 200 cells/mcL or a CD4 lymphocyte percentage below 14%.
13. Pulmonary tuberculosis.
14. Recurrent pneumonia.
15. Invasive cervical cancer.

Presumptive AIDS diagnoses (with laboratory evidence of HIV infection)

1. Candidiasis of esophagus: (a) recent onset of retrosternal pain on swallowing; and (b) oral candidiasis.
2. Cytomegalovirus retinitis. A characteristic appearance on serial ophthalmoscopic examinations.
3. Mycobacteriosis. Specimen from stool or normally sterile body fluids or tissue from a site other than lungs, skin, or cervical or hilar lymph nodes, showing acid-fast bacilli of a species not identified by culture.
4. Kaposi's sarcoma. Erythematous or violaceous plaque-like lesion on skin or mucous membrane.
5. *Pneumocystis jiroveci* pneumonia: (a) a history of dyspnea on exertion or nonproductive cough of recent onset (within the past 3 months); and (b) chest x-ray evidence of diffuse bilateral interstitial infiltrates or gallium scan evidence of diffuse bilateral pulmonary disease; and (c) arterial blood gas analysis showing an arterial oxygen partial pressure of < 70 mm Hg or a low respiratory diffusing capacity of < 80% of predicted values or an increase in the alveolar-arterial oxygen tension gradient; and (d) no evidence of a bacterial pneumonia.
6. Toxoplasmosis of the brain: (a) recent onset of a focal neurologic abnormality consistent with intracranial disease or a reduced level of consciousness; and (b) brain imaging evidence of a lesion having a mass effect or the radiographic appearance of which is enhanced by injection of contrast medium; and (c) serum antibody to toxoplasmosis or successful response to therapy for toxoplasmosis.
7. Recurrent pneumonia: (a) more than one episode in a 1-year period; and (b) acute pneumonia (new symptoms, signs, or radiologic evidence not present earlier) diagnosed on clinical or radiologic grounds by the patient's physician.
8. Pulmonary tuberculosis: (a) apical or miliary infiltrates and (b) radiographic and clinical response to antituberculous therapy.

Table 121. Laboratory findings with HIV infection.

Test	Significance
HIV enzyme-linked immunosorbent assay (ELISA)	Screening test for HIV infection. Of ELISA tests 50% are positive within 22 days after HIV transmission; 95% are positive within 6 weeks after transmission. Sensitivity > 99.9%; to avoid false-positive results, repeatedly reactive results must be confirmed with Western blot.
Western blot	Confirmatory test for HIV. Specificity when combined with ELISA > 99.99%. Indeterminate results with early HIV infection, HIV-2 infection, autoimmune disease, pregnancy, and recent tetanus toxoid administration.
Complete blood count	Anemia, neutropenia, and thrombocytopenia common with advanced HIV infection.
Absolute CD4 lymphocyte count	Most widely used predictor of HIV progression. Risk of progression to an AIDS opportunistic infection or malignancy is high with CD4 < 200 cells/mcL.
CD4 lymphocyte percentage	Percentage may be more reliable than the CD4 count. Risk of progression to an AIDS opportunistic infection or malignancy is high with percentage < 20%.
HIV viral load tests	These tests measure the amount of actively replicating HIV virus. Correlate with disease progression and response to antiretroviral drugs. Best tests available for diagnosis of acute HIV infection (prior to serioconversion); however, caution is warrented when the test result shows low-level viremia (i.e, <500 copies) as this may represent a false-positive test.

Table 122. Health care maintenance of HIV-infected individuals.

For all HIV-infected individuals:
- CD4 counts every 3–6 months
- Viral load tests every 3–6 months and 1 month following a change in therapy
- PPD
- INH for those with positive PPD and normal chest x-ray
- RPR or VDRL
- Toxoplasma IgG serology
- CMV IgG serology
- Pneumococcal vaccine
- Influenza vaccine in season
- Hepatitis B vaccine for those who are HBsAb-negative
- *Haemophilus influenzae* type b vaccination
- Papanicolaou smears every 6 months for women
- Consider anal swabs for cytologic evaluation yearly for patients with history of receptive anal intercourse

For HIV-infected individuals with CD4 < 200 cells/mcL:
- *Pneumocystis jiroveci*[1] prophylaxis (see Table 31–6)

For HIV-infected individuals with CD4 < 75 cells/mcL:
- *Mycobacterium avium* complex prophylaxis

For HIV-infected individuals with CD4 < 50 cells/mcL:
- Consider CMV prophylaxis

PPD = purified protein derivative; INH = isonicotinic acid hydrazide (isoniazid); RPR = rapid plasma reagin; VDRL = Venereal Disease Research Laboratories; IgG = immunoglobulin G; HBsAb = antibody to the hepatitis B surface antigen; CMV = cytomegalovirus.

[1]Formerly known as *Pneumocystis carinii.*

Table 123. Treatment of AIDS-related opportunistic infections and malignancies.[1]

Infection or Malignancy	Treatment	Complications
Pneumocystis jiroveci infection[2]	Trimethoprim-sulfamethoxazole, 15 mg/kg/d (based on trimethoprim component) orally or intravenously for 14–21 days.	Nausea, neutropenia, anemia, hepatitis, drug rash, Stevens-Johnson syndrome.
	Pentamidine, 3–4 mg/kg/d IV for 14–21 days.	Hypotension, hypoglycemia, anemia, neutropenia, pancreatitis, hepatitis.
	Trimethoprim, 15 mg/kg/d orally, with dapsone, 100 mg/d orally, for 14–21 days.[3]	Nausea, rash, hemolytic anemia in G6PD[3]-deficient patients. Methemoglobinemia (weekly levels should be < 10% of total hemoglobin).
	Primaquine, 15–30 mg/d orally, and clindamycin, 600 mg every 8 hours orally, for 14–21 days.	Hemolytic anemia in G6PD-deficient patients. Methemoglobinemia, neutropenia, colitis.
	Atovaquone, 750 mg orally 3 times daily for 14–21 days.	Rash, elevated aminotransferases, anemia, neutropenia.
	Trimetrexate, 45 mg/m^2 intravenously for 21 days (given with leucovorin calcium) if intolerant of all other regimens.	Leukopenia, rash, mucositis.
Mycobacterium avium complex infection	Clarithromycin, 500 mg orally twice daily with ethambutol, 15 mg/kg/d orally (maximum, 1 g). May also add:	Clarithromycin: hepatitis, nausea, diarrhea; ethambutol: hepatitis, optic neuritis.
	Rifabutin, 300 mg orally daily.	Rash, hepatitis, uveitis.
Toxoplasmosis	Pyrimethamine, 100–200 mg orally as loading dose, followed by 50–75 mg/d, combined with sulfadiazine, 4–6 g orally daily in 4 divided doses, and folinic acid, 10 mg daily for 4–8 weeks; then pyrimethamine, 25–50 mg/d, with clindamycin, 2–2.7 g/d in 3–4 divided doses, and folinic acid, 5 mg/d, until clinical and radiographic resolution is achieved.	Leukopenia, rash.
Lymphoma	Combination chemotherapy (eg, modified CHOP,[4] M-BACOD,[4] with or without G-CSF[5] or GM-CSF[5]). Central nervous system disease: radiation treatment with dexamethasone for edema.	Nausea, vomiting, anemia, leukopenia, cardiac toxicity (with doxorubicin).
Cryptococcal meningitis	Amphotericin B, 0.6 mg/kg/d intravenously, with or without flucytosine, 100 mg/kg/d orally in 4 divided doses for 2 weeks, followed by:	Fever, anemia, hypokalemia, azotemia.
	Fluconazole, 400 mg orally daily for 6 weeks, then 200 mg orally daily.	Hepatitis.
Cytomegalovirus infection	Valganciclovir, 900 mg orally twice a day for 21 days with food (induction), followed by 900 mg daily with food (maintenance).	Neutropenia, anemia, thrombocytopenia.
	Ganciclovir, 10 mg/kg/d intravenously in 2 divided doses for 10 days, followed by 6 mg/kg 5 days a week indefinitely. (Decrease dose for renal impairment.) May use ganciclovir as maintenance therapy (1 g orally with fatty foods 3 times a day).	Neutropenia (especially when used concurrently with zidovudine), anemia, thrombocytopenia.
	Foscarnet, 60 mg/kg intravenously every 8 hours for 10–14 days (induction), followed by 90 mg/kg once daily. (Adjust for changes in renal function.)	Nausea, hypokalemia, hypocalcemia, hyperphosphatemia, azotemia.
Esophageal candidiasis or recurrent vaginal candidiasis	Fluconazole, 100–200 mg daily for 10–14 days.	Hepatitis, development of imidazole resistance.

(*continued*)

Table 123. Treatment of AIDS-related opportunistic infections and malignancies.[1] (continued)

Infection or Malignancy	Treatment	Complications
Herpes simplex infection	Acyclovir, 400 mg 3 times daily until healed; or acyclovir, 5 mg/kg intravenously every 8 hours for severe cases.	Resistant herpes simplex with chronic therapy.
	Famciclovir, 500 mg orally twice daily until healed.	Nausea.
	Valacyclovir, 500 mg orally twice daily until healed.	Nausea.
	Foscarnet, 40 mg/kg intravenously every 8 hours, for acyclovir-resistant cases. (Adjust for changes in renal function.)	See above.
Herpes zoster	Acyclovir, 800 mg orally 4 or 5 times daily for 7 days. Intravenous therapy at 10 mg/kg every 8 hours for ocular involvement, disseminated disease.	See above.
	Famciclovir, 500 mg orally 3 times daily for 7 days.	Nausea.
	Valacyclovir, 500 mg orally 3 times daily for 7 days.	Nausea.
	Foscarnet, 40 mg/kg intravenously every 8 hours for acyclovir-resistant cases. (Adjust for changes in renal function.)	See above.
Kaposi's sarcoma Limited cutaneous disease	Observation, intralesional vinblastine.	Inflammation, pain at site of injection.
Extensive or aggressive cutaneous disease	Systemic chemotherapy (eg, liposomal doxorubicin). Interferon-α (for patients with CD4 > 200 cells/mcL and no constitutional symptoms). Radiation (amelioration of edema).	Bone marrow suppression, peripheral neuritis, flu-like syndrome.
Visceral disease (eg, pulmonary)	Combination chemotherapy (eg, daunorubicin, bleomycin, vinblastine).	Bone marrow suppression, cardiac toxicity, fever.

[1]For treatment of *Mycobacterium tuberculosis* infection, see Chapter 9.
[2]For moderate to severe *P jiroveci* infection (oxygen saturation < 90%), corticosteroids should be given with specific treatment. The dose of prednisone is 40 mg twice daily for 5 days, then 40 mg daily for 5 days, and then 20 mg daily until therapy is complete.
[3]When considering use of dapsone, check glucose-6-phosphate dehydrogenase (G6PD) level in African-American patients and those of Mediterranean origin.
[4]CHOP = cyclophosphamide, doxorubicin (hydroxydaunomycin), vincristine (Oncovin), and prednisone. Modified M-BACOD = methotrexate, bleomycin, doxorubicin (Adriamycin), cyclophosphamide, vincristine (Oncovin), and dexamethasone.
[5]G-CSF = granulocyte-colony stimulating factor (filgrastim); GM-CSF = granulocyte-macrophage colony-stimulating factor (sargramostim).

Table 124. Antiretroviral therapy.

Drug	Dose	Common Side Effects	Monitoring	Cost[1]	Cost/Month
Nucleoside reverse transcriptase inhibitors					
Zidovudine (AZT) (Retrovir)	600 mg orally daily in two divided doses	Anemia, neutropenia, nausea, malaise, headache, insomnia, myopathy	Complete blood count (CBC) and differential (every 3 months once stable)	\$6.49/300 mg	\$389.36
Didanosine (ddI) (Videx)	400 mg orally daily (enteric-coated capsule) for persons ≥60 kg	Peripheral neuropathy, pancreatitis, dry mouth, hepatitis	CBC and differential, aminotransferases, K^+, amylase, triglycerides, bimonthly neurologic questionnaire for neuropathy	\$10.09/400 mg capsules	\$302.63
Zalcitabine (ddC) (Hivid)	0.375–0.75 mg orally 3 times daily	Peripheral neuropathy, aphthous ulcers, hepatitis	Monthly neurologic questionnaire for neuropathy, aminotransferases	\$2.73/0.75 mg	\$245.70
Stavudine (d4T) (Zerit)	40 mg orally twice daily for persons ≥60 kg	Peripheral neuropathy, hepatitis, pancreatitis	Monthly neurologic questionnaire for neuropathy, aminotransferases, amylase	\$6.00/40 mg	\$360.00
Lamivudine (3TC) (Epivir)	150 mg orally twice daily	Rash, peripheral neuropathy	No additional monitoring	\$5.30/150 mg	\$318.26
Emtricitabine (Emtriva)	300 mg orally once daily	Skin discoloration palms/soles (mild)	No additional monitoring	\$10.11/300 mg	\$303.40
Abacavir (Ziagen)	300 mg orally twice daily	Rash, fever—if occur, rechallenge may be fatal	No special monitoring	\$7.46/300 mg	\$447.78
Nucleotide reverse transcriptase inhibitors					
Tenofovir (Viread)	300 mg orally once daily	Gastrointestinal distress	Renal function	\$15.92/300 mg	\$477.60
Protease inhibitors					
Saquinavir hard gel (Invirase)	1000 mg twice daily with 100 mg ritonavir orally twice daily	Gastrointestinal distress	Trimonthly aminotransferases, cholesterol, triglycerides	\$5.99/500 mg	\$718.56 (plus cost of ritonavir)
Saquinavir soft gel (Fortovase)	1200 mg three times daily	Gastrointestinal distress	Trimonthly aminotransferases, cholesterol, triglycerides	\$1.34/200 mg	\$720.96
Ritonavir (Norvir)	600 mg orally twice daily or in lower doses (eg, 100 mg orally once or twice daily) for boosting other PIs	Gastrointestinal distress, peripheral paresthesias	Trimonthly aminotransferases, creatine kinase, uric acid, triglycerides	\$10.29/100 mg	\$3,704.40 (\$617.40 in lower doses)
Indinavir (Crixivan)	800 mg orally three times daily	Kidney stones	Trimonthly aminotransferases, bilirubin level, cholesterol, triglycerides	\$3.05/400 mg	\$548.12
Nelfinavir (Viracept)	750 mg orally three times daily	Diarrhea	Cholesterol, triglycerides	\$2.52/250 mg	\$680.99
Amprenavir (Agenerase)	1200 mg orally twice daily	Gastrointestinal, rash	Cholesterol, triglycerides	\$1.54/150 mg	\$740.74
Fosamprenavir (Lexiva)	1400 mg orally twice daily or 1400 mg orally once daily with ritonavir 200 mg orally once daily	Same as amprenavir	Same as amprenavir	\$10.07/700 mg	\$604.22–\$1208.44
Lopinavir/ritonavir (Kaletra)	400 mg/100 mg orally twice daily	Diarrhea	Cholesterol, triglycerides, every other month aminotransferases	\$3.91/133 mg (lopinavir)	\$703.50

Atazanavir (Reyataz)	400 mg orally once daily	Hyperbilirubinemia	Bilirubin level	$13.25/200 mg	$794.88
Nonnucleoside reverse transcriptase inhibitors (NNRTIs)					
Nevirapine (Viramune)	200 mg orally daily for 2 weeks, then 200 mg orally twice daily	Rash	No additional monitoring	$7.08/200 mg	$424.75
Delavirdine (Rescriptor)	400 mg orally three times daily	Rash	No additional monitoring	$1.76/200 mg	$316.35
Efavirenz (Sustiva)	600 mg orally daily	Neurologic disturbances	No additional monitoring	$15.53/600 mg	$465.94
Entry inhibitor					
Enfuvirtide (Fuzeon)	90 mg subcutaneously twice daily	Injection site pain and allergic reaction	No additional monitoring	$33.30/90 mg	$1999.00

[1]Average wholesale price (AWP, for AB-rated generic when available) for quantity listed. Source: *Red Book Update, Vol. 24, No.4,* April 2005. AWP may not accurately represent the actual pharmacy cost because wide contractual variations exist among institutions.

Table 125. *Pneumocystis jiroveci* prophylaxis.

Drug	Dose	Side Effects	Limitations
Trimethoprim-sulfamethoxazole	One double-strength tablet 3 times a week to one tablet daily	Rash, neutropenia, hepatitis, Stevens-Johnson syndrome	Hypersensitivity reaction is common but, if mild, it may be possible to treat through.
Dapsone	50–100 mg daily or 100 mg 2 or 3 times per week	Anemia, nausea, methemoglobinemia, hemolytic anemia	Less effective than above. Glucose-6-phosphate dehydrogenase (G6PD) level should be checked prior to therapy. Check methemoglobin level at 1 month.
Atovaquone	1500 mg daily with a meal	Rash, diarrhea, nausea	Less effective than suspension trimethoprim-sulfamethoxazole; equal efficacy to dapsone, but more expensive.
Aerosolized pentamidine	300 mg monthly	Bronchospasm (pretreat with bronchodilators); rare reports of pancreatitis	Apical *Pneumocystis jiroveci* pneumonia, extrapulmonary *P jiroveci* infections, pneumothorax.

Table 126. Diagnostic features of some acute exanthems.

Disease	Prodromal Signs and Symptoms	Nature of Eruption	Other Diagnostic Features	Laboratory Tests
Eczema herpeticum	None.	Vesiculopustular lesions in area of eczema.		Herpes simplex virus isolated in cell culture. Multinucleate giant cells in smear of lesion.
Varicella (chickenpox)	0–1 day of fever, anorexia, headache.	Rapid evolution of macules to papules, vesicles, crusts; all stages simultaneously present; lesions superficial, distribution centripetal.	Lesions on scalp and mucous membranes.	Specialized complement fixation and virus neutralization in cell culture. Fluorescent antibody test of smear of lesions.
Infectious mononucleosis (EBV)	Fever, adenopathy, sore throat.	Maculopapular rash resembling rubella, rarely papulovesicular.	Splenomegaly, tonsillar exudate.	Atypical lymphocytes in blood smears; heterophil agglutination. Monospot test.
Exanthema subitum (HHV-6, 7; roseola)	3–4 days of high fever.	As fever falls by crisis, pink maculopapules appear on chest and trunk; fade in 1–3 days.		White blood count low.
Measles (rubeola)	3–4 days of fever, coryza, conjunctivitis, and cough.	Maculopapular, brick-red; begins on head and neck; spreads downward and outward, in 5–6 days rash brownish, desquamating. See atypical measles, below.	Koplik's spots on buccal mucosa.	White blood count low. Virus isolation in cell culture. Antibody tests by hemagglutination inhibition or neutralization.
Atypical measles	Same as measles.	Maculopapular centripetal rash, becoming confluent.	History of measles vaccination.	Measles antibody present in past, with titer rise during illness.
Rubella	Little or no prodrome.	Maculopapular, pink; begins on head and neck, spreads downward, fades in 3 days. No desquamation.	Lymphadenopathy, postauricular or occipital.	White blood count normal or low. Serologic tests for immunity and definitive diagnosis (hemagglutination inhibition).
Erythema infectiosum (parvovirus B19)	None. Usually in epidemics.	Red, flushed cheeks; circumoral pallor; maculopapules on extremities.	"Slapped face" appearance.	White blood count normal.
Enterovirus infections	1–2 days of fever, malaise.	Maculopapular rash resembling rubella, rarely papulovesicular or petechial.	Aseptic meningitis.	Virus isolation from stool or cerebrospinal fluid; complement fixation titer rise.
Typhus	3–4 days of fever, chills, severe headaches.	Maculopapules, petechiae, initial distribution centrifugal (trunk to extremities).	Endemic area, lice.	Complement fixation.
Rocky Mountain spotted fever	3–4 days of fever, vomiting.	Maculopapules, petechiae, initial distribution centripetal (extremities to trunk, including palms).	History of tick bite.	Complement fixation.
Ehrlichiosis	Headache, malaise.	Rash in one-third, similiar to Rocky Mountain spotted fever.	Pancytopenia, elevated liver function tests.	Polymerase chain reaction, immunofluorescent antibody.
Scarlet fever	One-half to 2 days of malaise, sore throat, fever, vomiting.	Generalized, punctate, red; prominent on neck, in axillae, groin, skin folds; circumoral pallor; fine desquamation involves hands and feet.	Strawberry tongue, exudative tonsillitis.	Group A β-hemolytic streptococci in cultures from throat; antistreptolysin O titer rise.

(*continued*)

Table 126. Diagnostic features of some acute exanthems. (continued)

Disease	Prodromal Signs and Symptoms	Nature of Eruption	Other Diagnostic Features	Laboratory Tests
Meningococcemia	Hours of fever, vomiting.	Maculopapules, petechiae, purpura.	Meningeal signs, toxicity, shock.	Cultures of blood, cerebrospinal fluid. High white blood count.
Kawasaki disease	Fever, adenopathy, conjunctivitis.	Cracked lips, strawberry tongue, maculopapular polymorphous rash, peeling skin on fingers and toes.	Edema of extremities. Angiitis of coronary arteries.	Thrombocytosis, electrocardiographic changes.
Smallpox (based on prior experience)	Fever, malaise, prostration.	Maculopapules to vesicles to pustules to scars (lesions develop at the same pace).	Centrifugal rash; fulminant sepsis in small percentage of patients, gastrointestinal and skin hemorrhages.	Contact CDC[1] for suspicious rash; EM and gel diffusion assays.

EBV = Epstein–Barr virus; HHV = human herpesvirus.
[1]http://www.bt.cdc.gov/agent/smallpox/response-plan/.

Table 127. Drugs of choice for suspected or proved microbial pathogens, 2005.[1]

Suspected or Proved Etiologic Agent	Drug(s) of First Choice	Alternative Drug(s)
Gram-negative cocci		
Moraxella catarrhalis	TMP-SMZ,[2] a fluoroquinolone[3]	Cefuroxime, cefotaxime, ceftizoxime, ceftriaxone, cefepime, cefuroxime axetil, an erythromycin,[4] a tetracycline,[5] azithromycin, amoxicillin-clavulanic acid, clarithromycin
Neisseria gonorrhoeae (gonococcus)	Ciprofloxacin or ofloxacin	Ceftriaxone, spectinomycin, cefpodoxime proxetil
Neisseria meningitidis (meningococcus)	Penicillin[6]	Cefotaxime, ceftizoxime, ceftriaxone, ampicillin, chloramphenicol
Gram-positive cocci		
Streptococcus pneumoniae[8] (pneumococcus)	Penicillin[6]	An erythromycin,[4] a cephalosporin,[7] vancomycin, TMP-SMZ,[2] chloramphenicol, clindamycin, azithromycin, clarithromycin, a tetracycline,[5] imipenem, meropenem, quinupristin-dalfopristin, certain fluoroquinolones,[3] linezolid
Streptococcus, hemolytic, groups A, B, C, G	Penicillin[6]	An erythromycin,[4] a cephalosporin,[7] vancomycin, clindamycin, azithromycin, clarithromycin
Viridans streptococci	Penicillin[6] ± gentamicin	Cephalosporin,[7] vancomycin
Staphylococcus, methicillin-resistant	Vancomycin ± gentamicin ± rifampin	TMP-SMZ,[2] doxycycline, minocycline, a fluoroquinolone,[3] linezolid, quinupristin-dalfopristin
Staphylococcus, non-penicillinase-producing	Penicillin[6]	A cephalosporin,[8] clindamycin
Staphylococcus, penicillinase-producing	Penicillinase-resistant penicillin[9]	Vancomycin, a cephalosporin,[7] clindamycin, amoxicillin-clavulanic acid, ticarcillin-clavulanic acid, ampicillin-sulbactam, piperacillin-tazobactam, TMP-SMZ[2]
Enterococcus faecalis	Ampicillin ± gentamicin[10]	Vancomycin ± gentamicin
Enterococcus faecium	Vancomycin ± gentamicin[10]	Quinupristin-dalfopristin, linezolid
Gram-negative rods		
Acinetobacter	Imipenem or meropenem	Minocycline, doxycycline, aminoglycosides,[11] colistin
Prevotella, oropharyngeal strains	Clindamycin	Penicillin,[6] metronidazole, cefoxitin, cefotetan
Bacteroides, gastrointestinal strains	Metronidazole	Cefoxitin, clindamycin, cefotetan, ticarcillin-clavulanic acid, ampicillin-sulbactam, piperacillin-tazobactam

(continued)

Table 127. Drugs of choice for suspected or proved microbial pathogens, 2005.[1] (continued)

Suspected or Proved Etiologic Agent	Drug(s) of First Choice	Alternative Drug(s)
Gram-negative rods (continued)		
Brucella	Tetracycline + rifampin[5]	TMP-SMZ[2] ± gentamicin; chloramphenicol ± gentamicin; doxycycline + gentamicin
Campylobacter jejuni	Erythromycin[4] or azithromycin	Tetracycline,[5] a fluoroquinolone[3]
Enterobacter	TMP-SMZ,[2] imipenem, meropenem	Aminoglycoside, a fluoroquinolone,[3] cefepime
Escherichia coli (sepsis)	Cefotaxime, ceftizoxime, ceftriaxone, ceftazidime, cefepime	Imipenem or meropenem, aminoglycosides,[11] a fluoroquinolone[3]
Escherichia coli (uncomplicated urinary infection)	Fluoroquinolones,[3] nitrofurantoin	TMP-SMZ,[2] oral cephalosporin, fosfomycin
Haemophilus (meningitis and other serious infections)	Cefotaxime, ceftizoxime, ceftriaxone	Aztreonam
Haemophilus (respiratory infections, otitis)	TMP-SMZ[2]	Ampicillin, amoxicillin, doxycycline, azithromycin, clarithromycin, cefotaxime, ceftizoxime, ceftriaxone, cefuroxime, cefuroxime axetil, ampicillin-clavulanate
Helicobacter pylori	Amoxicillin + clarithromycin + proton pump inhibitor (PPI)	Bismuth subsalicylate + tetracycline + metronidazole + PPI
Klebsiella	A cephalosporin	TMP-SMZ,[2] aminoglycoside,[11] imipenem or meropenem, a fluoroquinolone,[3] piperacillin, aztreonam
Legionella species (pneumonia)	Erythromycin[4] or clarithromycin or azithromycin, or fluoroquinolones[3] ± rifampin	Doxycycline ± rifampin
Proteus mirabilis	Ampicillin	An aminoglycoside,[11] TMP-SMZ,[2] a fluoroquinolone,[3] a cephalosporin[7]
Proteus vulgaris and other species (*Morganella, Providencia*)	Cefotaxime, ceftizoxime, ceftriaxone, ceftazidime, cefepime	Aminoglycoside,[11] imipenem, TMP-SMZ,[2] a fluoroquinolone[3]
Pseudomonas aeruginosa	Aminoglycoside[11] + antipseudomonal penicillin[12]	Ceftazidime ± aminoglycoside; imipenem or meropenem ± aminoglycoside; aztreonam ± aminoglycoside; ciprofloxacin ± piperacillin; ciprofloxacin ± ceftazidime; ciprofloxacin ± cefepime
Burkholderia pseudomallei (melioidosis)	Ceftazidime	Chloramphenicol, tetracycline,[5] TMP-SMZ,[2] amoxicillin-clavulanic acid, imipenem or meropenem
Burkholderia mallei (glanders)	Streptomycin + tetracycline[5]	Chloramphenicol + streptomycin
Salmonella (bacteremia)	Ceftriaxone, a fluoroquinolone[3]	
Serratia	Cefotaxime, ceftizoxime, ceftriaxone, ceftazidime, cefepime	TMP-SMZ,[2] aminoglycosides,[11] imipenem or meropenem, a fluoroquinolone[3]
Shigella	A fluoroquinolone[3]	Ampicillin, TMP-SMZ,[2] ceftriaxone
Vibrio (cholera, sepsis)	Tetracycline[5]	TMP-SMZ,[2] a fluoroquinolone[3]
Yersinia pestis (plague, tularemia)	Streptomycin ± a tetracycline[5]	Chloramphenicol, TMP-SMZ[2]
Gram-positive rods		
Actinomyces	Penicillin[6]	Tetracycline,[5] clindamycin
Bacillus (including anthrax)	Penicillin[6] (ciprofloxacin or doxycycline for anthrax; see Table 33–2)	Erythromycin,[4] tetracycline,[5] a fluoroquinolone[3]
Clostridium (eg, gas gangrene, tetanus)	Penicillin[6]	Metronidazole, chloramphenicol, clindamycin, imipenem or meropenem
Corynebacterium diphtheriae	Erythromycin[4]	Penicillin[6]
Corynebacterium jeikeium	Vancomycin	Ciprofloxacin, penicillin + gentamicin
Listeria	Ampicillin ± aminoglycoside[11]	TMP-SMZ[2]

(continued)

Table 127. Drugs of choice for suspected or proved microbial pathogens, 2005.[1] (continued)

Suspected or Proved Etiologic Agent	Drug(s) of First Choice	Alternative Drug(s)
Acid-fast rods		
Mycobacterium tuberculosis[13]	INH + rifampin + pyrazinamide ± ethambutol (or streptomycin)	Other antituberculous drugs (see Tables 9–13 and 9–14)
Mycobacterium leprae	Dapsone + rifampin ± clofazimine	Minocycline, ofloxacin, clarithromycin
Mycobacterium kansasii	INH + rifampin ± ethambutol	Ethionamide, cycloserine
Mycobacterium avium complex	Clarithromycin or azithromycin + one or more of the following: ethambutol, rifampin or rifabutin, ciprofloxacin	Amikacin
Mycobacterium fortuitum-cheilonei	Amikacin + clarithromycin	Cefoxitin, sulfonamide, doxycycline, linezolid
Nocardia	TMP-SMZ[2]	Minocycline, imipenem or meropenem, sulfisoxazole, linezolid
Spirochetes		
Borrelia burgdorferi (Lyme disease)	Doxycycline, amoxcillin, cefuroxime axetil	Ceftriaxone, cefotaxime, penicillin, azithromycin, clarithromycin
Borrelia recurrentis (relapsing fever)	Doxycycline[5]	Penicillin[6]
Leptospira	Penicillin,[6] ceftriaxone	Doxycycline[5]
Treponema pallidum (syphilis)	Penicillin[6]	Doxycycline, ceftriaxone
Treponema pertenue (yaws)	Penicillin[6]	Doxycycline
Mycoplasmas	Erythromycin[4] or doxycycline	Clarithromycin, azithromycin, a fluoroquinolone[3]
Chlamydiae		
C psittaci	Doxycycline	Chloramphenicol
C trachomatis (urethritis or pelvic inflammatory disease)	Doxycycline or azithromycin	Ofloxacin
C pneumoniae	Doxycycline[5]	Erythromycin,[4] clarithromycin, azithromycin, a fluoroquinolone[3,14]
Rickettsiae	Doxycycline[5]	Chloramphenicol, a fluoroquinolone[3]

[1]Adapted from Med Lett Drugs Ther 2001;43:69.
[2]TMP-SMZ is a mixture of 1 part trimethoprim and 5 parts sulfamethoxazole.
[3]Fluoroquinolones include ciprofloxacin, ofloxacin, levofloxacin, moxifloxacin, gatifloxacin, and others (see text). Gatifloxacin, gemifloxacin, levofloxacin, and moxifloxacin have the best activity against gram-positive organisms, including penicillin-resistant *S pneumoniae* and methicillin-sensitive *S aureus*. Activity against enterococci and *S epidermidis* is variable.
[4]Erythromycin estolate is best absorbed orally but carries the highest risk of hepatitis; erythromycin stearate and erythromycin ethylsuccinate are also available.
[5]All tetracyclines have similar activity against most microorganisms. Minocycline and doxycycline have increased activity against *S aureus*.
[6]Penicillin G is preferred for parenteral injection; penicillin V for oral administration—to be used only in treating infections due to highly sensitive organisms.
[7]Most intravenous cephalosporins (with the exception of ceftazidime) have good activity against gram-positive cocci.
[8]Intermediate and high-level resistance to penicillin has been described. Infections caused by strains with intermediate resistance may respond to high doses of penicillin, cefotaxime, or ceftriaxone. Infections caused by highly resistant strains should be treated with vancomycin. Many strains of penicillin-resistant pneumococci are resistant to erythromycin, macrolides, and TMP-SMZ.
[9]Parenteral nafcillin or oxacillin; oral dicloxacillin, cloxacillin, or oxacillin.
[10]Addition of gentamicin indicated only for severe enterococcal infections (eg, endocarditis, meningitis).
[11]Aminoglycosides—gentamicin, tobramycin, amikacin, netilmicin—should be chosen on the basis of local patterns of susceptibility.
[12]Antipseudomonal penicillins: ticarcillin, piperacillin.
[13]Resistance may be a problem, and susceptibility testing should be done.
[14]Ciprofloxacin has inferior antichlamydial activity compared with newer fluoroquinolones.
Key: ± = alone or combined with.

Table 128. Examples of initial antimicrobial therapy for acutely ill, hospitalized adults pending identification of causative organism.

Suspected Clinical Diagnosis	Likely Etiologic Diagnosis	Drugs of Choice
(A) Meningitis, bacterial, community-acquired	Pneumococcus,[1] meningococcus	Cefotaxime,[2] 2–3 g IV every 6 hours, or ceftriaxone, 2 g IV every 12 hours plus vancomycin, 10 mg/kg every 8 hours
(B) Meningitis, bacterial, age > 50, community-acquired	Pneumococcus, meningococcus, *Listeria monocytogenes,*[3] gram-negative bacilli	Ampicillin, 2 g IV every 4 hours, plus cefotaxime or ceftriaxone and vancomycin as in (A)
(C) Meningitis, postoperative (or posttraumatic)	*S aureus,* gram-negative bacilli (pneumococcus, in posttraumatic)	Vancomycin, 10 mg/kg every 8 hours, plus ceftazidime, 3 g IV every 8 hours
(D) Brain abscess	Mixed anaerobes, pneumococci, streptococci	Penicillin G, 4 million units IV every 4 hours, + metronidazole, 500 mg PO every 8 hours, or cefotaxime or ceftriaxone as in (A) + metronidazole, 500 mg PO every 8 hours
(E) Pneumonia, acute, community-acquired, severe	Pneumococci, *M pneumoniae, Legionella, C pneumoniae*	Doxycycline, 100 mg IV or orally every 12 hours (or azithromycin), plus cefotaxime, 2 g IV every 8 hours (or ceftriaxone, 1 g IV every 24 hours); or a fluoroquinolone[5] alone
(F) Pneumonia, postoperative or nosocomial	*S aureus,* mixed anaerobes, gram-negative bacilli	Cefotaxime or ceftriaxone or cefepime, 2 g IV every 8 hours, or piperacillin-tazobactam, 4–5 g IV every 6 hours, ± tobramycin or ciprofloxacin
(G) Endocarditis, acute (including injection drug user)	*S aureus, E faecalis,* gram-negative aerobic bacteria, viridans streptococci	Vancomycin, 15 mg/kg every 12 hours, plus gentamicin, 2 mg/kg every 8 hours
(H) Septic thrombophlebitis (eg, IV tubing, IV shunts)	*S aureus,* gram-negative aerobic bacteria	Vancomycin, 15 mg/kg every 12 hours plus gentamicin,[4] 2 mg/kg every 8 hours
(I) Osteomyelitis	*S aureus*	Nafcillin, 2 g IV every 4 hours, or cefazolin, 2 g IV every 8 hours
(J) Septic arthritis	*S aureus, N gonorrhoeae*	Ceftriaxone, 1–2 g IV every 24 hours
(K) Pyelonephritis with flank pain and fever (recurrent urinary tract infection)	*E coli, Klebsiella, Enterobacter, Pseudomonas*	Ceftriaxone, 1g IV every 24 hours, or ciprofloxacin, 400 mg IV every 12 hours (500 mg PO), or levofloxacin, 500 mg once daily (IV/PO)
(L) Fever in neutropenic patient receiving cancer chemotherapy	*S aureus, Pseudomonas, Klebsiella, E coli*	Ceftazidime, 2 g IV every 8 hours, or cefepime, 2 g IV every 8 hours
(M) Intra-abdominal sepsis (eg, postoperative, peritonitis, cholecystitis)	Gram-negative bacteria, *Bacteroides,* anaerobic bacteria, streptococci, clostridia	Piperacillin-tazobactam as in (F) or ticarcillin-clavulanate, 3.1 g IV every 6 hours or ampicillin, 1–2 g every 6 hours, plus gentamicin, 2 mg/kg every 8 hours, plus metronidazole, 500 mg IV every 8 hours

[1]Some strains may be resistant to penicillin. Vancomycin can be used with or without rifampin.
[2]Cefotaxime, ceftriaxone, ceftazidime, or ceftizoxime can be used. Most studies on meningitis have been with cefotaxime or ceftriaxone (see text).
[3]TMP-SMZ can be used to treat *Listeria monocytogenes* in patients allergic to penicillin in a dosage of 15–20 mg/kg of TMP in three or four divided doses.
[4]Depending on local drug susceptibility pattern, use tobramycin, 5 mg/kg/d, or amikacin, 15 mg/kg/d, in place of gentamicin.
[5]Gatifloxacin, levofloxacin, moxifloxacin.

Table 129. Initial antimicrobial therapy for purulent meningitis of unknown cause.

Age Group	Common Microorganisms	Standard Therapy
18–50 years	*S pneumoniae,*[1] *N meningitidis*	Cefotaxime or ceftriaxone[2]
Over 50 years	*S pneumoniae,*[1] *N meningitidis, L monocytogenes,* gram-negative bacilli	Ampicillin,[3] cefotaxime, or ceftriaxone[2]
Impaired cellular immunity	*L monocytogenes,* gram-negative bacilli, *S pneumoniae*	Ampicillin[3] plus ceftazidime[4]
Postsurgical or posttraumatic	*S aureus, S pneumoniae,*[1] gram-negative bacilli	Vancomycin[5] plus ceftazidime[4]

[1]In areas where penicillin-resistant pneumococcus is prevalent, vancomycin, 10–15 mg/kg every 6 hours, should be included in the regimen.
[2]The usual dose of cefotaxime is 2 g every 6 hours and that of ceftriaxone is 2 g every 12 hours. If the organism is sensitive to penicillin, 3–4 million units IV every 4 hours is given.
[3]The dose of ampicillin is usually 2 g IV every 4 hours.
[4]Ceftazidime is given in a dose of 50–100 mg/kg every 8 hours up to 2 g every 8 hours.
[5]The dose of vancomycin is 10–15 mg/kg every 6 hours.

Table 130. Typical cerebrospinal fluid findings in various central nervous system diseases.

Diagnosis	Cells/mcL	Glucose (mg/dL)	Protein (mg/dL)	Opening Pressure
Normal	0–5 lymphocytes	45–85[1]	15–45	70–180 mm H_2O
Purulent meningitis (bacterial)[2] community-acquired	200–20,000 polymorphonuclear neutrophils	Low (< 45)	High (> 50)	Markedly elevated
Granulomatous meningitis (mycobacterial, fungal)[3]	100–1000, mostly lymphocytes[3]	Low (< 45)	High (> 50)	Moderately elevated
Spirochetal meningitis	100–1000, mostly lymphocytes[3]	Normal	Moderately high (> 50)	Normal to slightly elevated
Aseptic meningitis, viral or meningoencephalitis[4]	25–2000, mostly lymphocytes[3]	Normal or low	High (> 50)	Slightly elevated
"Neighborhood reaction"[5]	Variably increased	Normal	Normal or high	Variable

[1]Cerebrospinal fluid glucose must be considered in relation to blood glucose level. Normally, cerebrospinal fluid glucose is 20–30 mg/dL lower than blood glucose, or 50–70% of the normal value of blood glucose.
[2]Organisms in smear or culture of cerebrospinal fluid; counterimmunoelectrophoresis or latex agglutination may be diagnostic.
[3]Polymorphonuclear neutrophils may predominate early.
[4]Viral isolation from cerebrospinal fluid early; antibody titer rise in paired specimens of serum; polymerase chain reaction for herpesvirus.
[5]May occur in mastoiditis, brain abscess, epidural abscess, sinusitis, septic thrombus, brain tumor. Cerebrospinal fluid culture results usually negative.

Table 131. Acute bacterial diarrheas and "food poisoning."

Organism	Incubation Period (hours)	Vomiting	Diarrhea	Fever	Microbiology	Pathogenesis	Clinical Features and Treatment
Staphylococcus	1–8, rarely up to 18	+++	+	–	Staphylococci grow in meats, dairy, and bakery products and produce enterotoxin.	Enterotoxin acts on receptors in gut that transmit impulses to medullary centers.	Abrupt onset, intense vomiting for up to 24 hours, regular recovery in 24–48 hours. Occurs in persons eating the same food. No treatment usually necessary except to restore fluids and electrolytes.
Bacillus cereus	1–8, rarely up to 18	+++	+	–	Reheated fried rice causes vomiting or diarrhea.	Enterotoxins formed in food or in gut from growth of *B cereus*.	After 1–6 hours, mainly vomiting. After 8–16 hours, mainly diarrhea. Both self-limited to less than 1 day.
Clostridium perfringens	8–16	±	+++	–	Clostridia grow in rewarmed meat dishes and produce an enterotoxin.	Enterotoxin produced in food and in gut causes hypersecretion in small intestine.	Abrupt onset of profuse diarrhea; vomiting occasionally. Recovery usual without treatment in 1–4 days. Many clostridia in cultures of food and feces of patients.
Clostridium botulinum	24–96	±	Rare	–	Clostridia grow in anaerobic foods and produce toxin.	Toxin absorbed from gut blocks acetylcholine at neuromuscular junction.	Diplopia, dysphagia, dysphonia, respiratory embarrassment. Treatment requires clear airway, ventilation, and intravenous polyvalent antitoxin (see text). Toxin present in food and serum. Mortality rate high.
Clostridium difficile	?	–	+++	+	Associated with antimicrobial drugs, eg, clindamycin.	Enterotoxin causes epithelial necrosis in colon; pseudomembranous colitis.	Especially after abdominal surgery, abrupt bloody diarrhea and fever. Toxin in stool. Oral vancomycin or metronidazole useful in therapy.
Escherichia coli (some strains)	24–72	±	+	–	Organisms grow in gut and produce toxin. May also invade superficial epithelium.	Enterotoxin causes hypersecretion in small intestine.	Usually abrupt onset of diarrhea; vomiting rare. A serious infection in neonates. In adults, "traveler's diarrhea" is usually self-limited to 1–3 days and does respond to a fluoroquinolone.
Vibrio parahaemolyticus	6–96	+	+	±	Organisms grow in seafood and in gut and produce toxin or invade.	Hypersecretion in small intestine; stools may be bloody.	Abrupt onset of diarrhea in groups consuming the same food, especially crabs and other seafood. Recovery is usually complete in 1–3 days. Food and stool cultures are positive.
Vibrio cholerae (mild cases)	24–72	+	+++	–	Organisms grow in gut and produce toxin.	Enterotoxin causes hypersecretion in small intestine. Infective dose: 10^7–10^9 organisms.	Abrupt onset of liquid diarrhea in endemic area. Needs prompt replacement of fluids and electrolytes intravenously or orally. Tetracyclines shorten excretion of vibriones. Stool cultures positive.
Campylobacter jejuni	2–10 days	–	+++	+	Organisms grow in jejunum and ileum.	Invasion and enterotoxin production uncertain.	Fever, diarrhea; PMNs and fresh blood in stool, especially in children. Usually self-limited. Special media needed for culture at 43° C. Give a fluoroquinolone in severe cases with invasion. Recovery in 5–8 days is usual.

(continued)

Table 131. Acute bacterial diarrheas and "food poisoning." (continued)

Organism	Incubation Period (hours)	Vomiting	Diarrhea	Fever	Microbiology	Pathogenesis	Clinical Features and Treatment
Shigella species (mild cases)	24–72	±	+	+	Organisms grow in superficial gut epithelium and gut lumen and produce toxin.	Organisms invade epithelial cells; blood, mucus, and PMNs in stools. Infective dose: 10^2–10^3 organisms.	Abrupt onset of diarrhea, often with blood and pus in stools, cramps, tenesmus, and lethargy. Stool cultures are positive. Therapy depends on sensitivity testing, but the fluoroquinolones are most effective. Do not give opioids. Often mild and self-limited.
Salmonella species	8–48	±	+	+	Organisms grow in gut. Do not produce toxin.	Superficial infection of gut, little invasion. Infective dose: 10^5 organisms.	Gradual or abrupt onset of diarrhea and low-grade fever. No antimicrobials unless systemic dissemination is suspected, in which case give a fluoroquinolone. Stool cultures are positive. Prolonged carriage is common.
Yersinia enterocolitica	?	±	+	+	Fecal-oral transmission (occasionally). Foodborne. In pets.	Gastroenteritis or mesenteric adenitis. Occasional bacteremia. Enterotoxin produced.	Severe abdominal pain, diarrhea, fever. PMNs and blood in stool; polyarthritis, erythema nodosum in children. If severe, give tetracycline or gentamicin. Keep stool at 4° C before culture.

PMNs = polymorphonuclear leukocytes.

Table 132. Recommended childhood immunization schedule—United States, 2005.[1]

Range of recommended ages | Catch-up immunization | Preadolescent assessment

Vaccine ▼ / Age ▶	Birth	1 mo	2 mo	4 mo	6 mo	12 mo	15 mo	18 mo	24 mo	4–6 y	11–12 y	13–18 y
Hepatitis B[2]	HepB #1	only if mother HBsAg (-)								Hep B series		
			Hep B #2			Hep B #3						
Diphtheria,[3] Tetanus, Pertussis			DTaP	DTaP	DTaP		DTaP			DTaP	Td	Td
Haemophilus influenzae type b[4]			Hib	Hib	Hib[3]	Hib						
Inactivated Poliovirus			IPV	IPV		IPV				IPV		
Measles, Mumps, Rubella[5]						MMR #1				MMR #2	MMR #2	
Meningococcal[6]												
Varicella[7]						Varicella				Varicella		
Pneumococcal[8]			PCV	PCV	PCV	PCV			PCV	PPV		
Vaccines below this line are for selected populations												
Hepatitis A[9]										Hepatitis A series		
Influenza[10]							Influenza (yearly)					

1. Indicates the recommended ages for routine administration of currently licensed childhood vaccines, as of May 1, 2005, for children through age 18 years. Any dose not given at the recommended age should be given at any subsequent visit when indicated and feasible. Gray areas with diagonal rules indicate age groups that warrant special effort to administer those vaccines not given previously. Additional vaccines may be licensed and recommended during the year. Licensed combination vaccines may be used whenever any components of the combination are indicated and the vaccine's other components are not contraindicated. Providers should consult the manufacturers' package inserts for detailed recommendations.

2. Hepatitis B vaccine (Hep B). All infants should receive the first dose of HepB vaccine soon after birth and before hospital discharge; the first dose also may be given by age 2 months if the infant's mother is HBsAg-negative. Only monovalent HepB vaccine can be used for the birth dose. Monovalent or combination vaccine containing HepB may be used to complete the series; 4 doses of vaccine may be administered when a birth dose is given. The second dose should be given at least 4 weeks after the first dose except for combination vaccines, which cannot be administered before age 6 weeks. The third dose should be given at least 16 weeks after the first dose and at least 8 weeks after the second dose. The last dose in the vaccination series (third or fourth dose) should not be administered before age 6 months. *Infants born to HBsAg-positive mothers* should receive HepB vaccine and 0.5 mL hepatitis B immune globulin (HBIG) within 12 hours of birth at separate sites. The second dose is recommended at age 1–2 months. The last dose in the vaccination series should not be administered before age 6 months. These infants should be tested for HBsAg and anti-HBs at 9–15 months of age. *Infants born to mothers whose HBsAg status is unknown* should receive the first dose of the HepB vaccine series within 12 hours of birth. Maternal blood should be drawn as soon as possible to determine the mother's HBsAg status; if the HBsAg test is positive, the infant should receive HBIG as soon as possible (no later than age 1 week). The second dose is recommended at age 1–2 months. The last dose in the vaccination series should not be administered before age 6 months.

3. Diphtheria and tetanus toxoids and acellular pertussis vaccine (DTaP). The fourth dose of DTaP may be administered at age 12 months provided that 6 months have elapsed since the third dose and the child is unlikely to return at age 15–18 months. **Tetanus and diphtheria toxoids (Td)** are recommended at age 11–12 years if at least 5 years have elapsed since the last dose of the Td-containing vaccine. Subsequent routine Td boosters are recommended every 10 years.

4. *Haemophilus influenzae* type b (Hib) conjugate vaccine. Three Hib conjugate vaccines are licensed for infant use. If PRP-OMP (PedvaxHIB® or ComVax® [Merck]) is administered at age 2 and 4 months, a dose at age 6 months is not required. DTaP/Hib combination products should not be used for primary vaccination in infants at age 2, 4 or 6 months but can be used as boosters following any Hib vaccine.

5. Measles, mumps, and rubella vaccine (MMR). The second dose of MMR is recommended routinely at age 4–6 years but may be administered during any visit provided that at least 4 weeks have elapsed since the first dose and that both doses are administered beginning at or after age 12 months. Those who have not received the second dose previously should complete the schedule by the visit at age 11–12 years.

(continued)

Table 132. Recommended childhood immunization schedule—United States, 2005.[1] (continued)

6. Meningococcal conjugate vaccine *meningococcal (Groups A, C, Y and W-135) conjugate vaccine (MCV-4).* In February 2005, the Advisory Committee on Immunization Practices (ACIP) recommended routine vaccination of young adolescents with MCV-4 at the preadolescent visit (11- and 12-year-old). For those who have not previously received MCV-4, the ACIP recommends vaccination before high school entry (~ 15-years-old) as the most effective strategy toward reducing the incidence of meningococcal disease in adolescence and young adulthood. College freshmen who live in dormitories are at higher risk for meningococcal disease compared with other people of the same age. Because of the feasibility constraints in targeting freshmen in dormitories, colleges may elect to target their vaccination campaigns to all matriculating freshmen. The risk for meningococcal disease among non-freshmen college students is similar to that for the general population of similar age (18–24 years). However, the vaccines are safe and immunogenic and therefore can be provided to non-freshmen college students who want to reduce their risk for meningococcal disease. The vaccine is highly effective but it does not protect people against meningococcal disease caused by "type B" bacteria. The new meningococcal vaccine was licensed by the US Food and Drug Administration (FDA) in January 2005 for use in people aged 11–55 years. It is manufactured by Sanofi Pasteur and is marketed as Menactra.

7. Varicella vaccine. Varicella vaccine is recommended at any visit at or after age 12 months for susceptible children (ie, those who lack a reliable history of chickenpox). Susceptible persons aged ≥ 13 years should receive 2 doses given at least 4 weeks apart.

8. Pneumococcal vaccine. The heptavalent **pneumococcal conjugate vaccine (PCV)** is recommended for all children aged 2–23 months and for certain children aged 24–59 months. **Pneumococcal polysaccharide vaccine (PPV)** is recommended in addition to PCV for certain high-risk groups. See *MMWR* 2000;49(No. RR-9):1–37.

9. Hepatitis A vaccine. Hepatitis A vaccine is recommended for children and adolescents in selected states and regions, and for certain high-risk groups. Consult local public health authority and *MMWR* 1999;48(No. RR-12):1–37. Children and adolescents in these states, regions, and high-risk groups who have not been immunized against hepatitis A can begin the hepatitis A vaccination series during any visit. The two doses in the series should be administered at least 6 months apart.

10. Influenza vaccine. Influenza vaccine is recommended annually for children aged ≥ 6 months with certain risk factors (including but not limited to asthma, cardiac disease, sickle cell disease, HIV, and diabetes, and household members of persons in groups at high risk (see *MMWR* 2003[rr-8]:1–36), and can be administered to all others wishing to obtain immunity. In addition, healthy children age 6–23 months are encouraged to receive influenza vaccine if feasible because children in this age group are at substantially increased risk for influenza-related hospitalizations.

Additional information about vaccines, including precautions and contraindications for vaccine and vaccine shortages, is available at http://www.cdc.gov/nip or at the National Immunization hotline, 800-232-2522 (English) or 800-232-0233 (Spanish). Copies of the schedule can be obtained at http://www.cdc.gov/nip/recs/child-schedule.htm. Approved by the Advisory Committee on Immunization Practices (http://www. cdc.gov/nip/acip), the American Academy of Pediatrics (http://www.aap.org), and the American Academy of Family Physicians (http://www.aafp.org).

Table 133. Guide to tetanus prophylaxis in wound management.

History of Absorbed Tetanus Toxoid	Clean, Minor Wounds		All Other Wounds[1]	
	Td[2]	TIG[3]	Td[2]	TIG[3]
Unknown or < 3 doses	Yes	No	Yes	Yes
3 or more doses	No[4]	No	No[5]	No

From the Centers for Disease Control and Prevention. Recommended childhood immunization schedule—United States, 2002. JAMA 2002;287:707.

[1]Such as, but not limited to, wounds contaminated with dirt, feces, soil, saliva, etc; puncture wounds; avulsions; and wounds resulting from missiles, crushing, burns, and frostbite.

[2]Tetanus toxoid and diphtheria toxoid, adult form. Use only this preparation (Td-adult) in children older than 6 years.

[3]Tetanus immune globulin.

[4]Yes if more than 10 years have elapsed since last dose.

[5]Yes if more than 5 years have elapsed since last dose. (More frequent boosters are not needed and can enhance side effects.)

Table 134. Prevention regimens for infection in immunocompromised patients.

Etiology	Microorganism	Therapy	Dose/Duration
Transplant	*Pneumocystis jiroveci*	Trimethoprim-sulfamethoxazole (TMP-SMZ) In TMP-SMZ allergy: Aerosolized pentamidine Dapsone (check glucose-6 phosphate dehydrogenase levels)	One double-strength tablet three times a week or one double-strength tablet twice a day on weekends or one single-strength tablet daily for 3–6 months 300 mg once a month 50 mg daily or 100 mg three times a week
Solid organ or bone marrow herpes simplex-seropositive patients	Herpes simplex	Acyclovir or ganciclovir	200 mg orally three times daily for 4 weeks (bone marrow transplants) or for 12 weeks (other solid organ transplants)
Cytomegalovirus (CMV)-seronegative solid organ transplant patients who receive transplants from seropositive donors	CMV	Ganciclovir	2.5–5 mg/kg intravenously twice daily during hospitalization (usually about 10 days) then oral ganciclovir, 1 g three times daily, for 3 months
CMV-seropositive solid organ transplant patients	CMV; herpesvirus	Ganciclovir	2.5–5 mg/kg intravenously twice daily during hospitalization (usually about 10 days) then oral acyclovir, 800 mg four times a day or oral ganciclovir, 1 g three times daily for 3 months
Periods of rejection	CMV	Ganciclovir	2.5–5 mg/kg intravenously twice daily during rejection therapy
Bone marrow transplant[1]			
Universal prophylaxis for all seropositive patients who receive allogeneic transplants	CMV	Ganciclovir	5 mg/kg intravenously every 12 h for a week, then oral ganciclovir, 1 g three times daily to Day 100; alternatively, patients can be followed without specific therapy and have blood sampled weekly for the presence of CMV; if CMV is detected by an antigenemia assay, preemptive therapy
Preemptive therapy; less toxic than universal prophylaxis	CMV	Ganciclovir	5 mg/kg intravenously twice daily for 7–14 days, then oral ganciclovir, 1 g three times daily to Day 100
CMV-seronegative recipients			Use of CMV-negative or leukocyte-depleted blood products
Severe hypogammaglobulinemia following bone marrow transplantation		Intravenous immunoglobulin	
Neutropenia[2–4]	Fungal	Amphotericin B Liposomal preparations of amphotericin B, aerosolized amphotericin B, itraconazole (capsules and solution), voriconazole	Moderate dose (0.5 mg/kg/day) and low dose (0.1–0.25 mg/kg/day)

[1]Whether universal prophylaxis or observation with preemptive therapy is the best approach has not been determined.
[2]Routine decontamination of the gastrointestinal tract to prevent bacteremia in the neutropenic patient is not recommended.
[3]Prophylactic administration of antibiotics in the afebrile, asymptomatic neutropenic patient is controversial, though many centers have adopted this strategy.
[4]Because voriconazole appears to be more effective than amphotericin for documented aspergillus infections, one approach to prophylaxis is to use fluconazole for patients at low risk for developing fungal infections (those who receive autologous bone marrow transplants) and voriconazole for those at high risk (allogeneic transplants).

Table 135. Antimicrobial agents for treatment of or for prophylaxis against anthrax.

First-line agents and recommended doses
- Ciprofloxacin, 500 mg twice daily orally or 400 mg every 12 hours intravenously
- Doxycycline, 100 mg every 12 hours orally or intravenously

Second-line agents and recommended doses
- Amoxicillin, 500 mg three times daily orally
- Penicillin G, 2 mU every 4 hours intravenously

Alternative agents with in vitro activity and suggested doses
- Rifampin, 10 mg/kg/d orally or intravenously
- Clindamycin, 450–600 mg every 8 hours orally or intravenously
- Clarithromycin, 500 mg twice daily
- Erythromycin, 500 mg every 6 hours intravenously
- Vancomycin, 1 g every 12 hours intravenously
- Imipenem, 500 mg every 6 hours intravenously

Table 136. Endocarditis prophylaxis.[1]

	DENTAL, RESPIRATORY, OR ESOPHAGEAL PROCEDURES	
Oral	Amoxicillin	2 g 1 hour before procedure
Penicillin allergy	Clindamycin or Cephalexin or cefadroxil[2] or Azithromycin or clarithromycin	600 mg 1 hour before procedure 2 g 1 hour before procedure 500 mg 1 hour before procedure
Parenteral	Ampicillin	2 g IM or IV 30 minutes before procedure
Penicillin allergy	Clindamycin or Cefazolin[2]	600 mg IV 1 hour before procedure 1 g IM or IV 30 minutes before procedure
	GASTROINTESTINAL (EXCEPT ESOPHAGEAL) OR GENITOURINARY PROCEDURES	
High-risk patient (Table 33–3)	Ampicillin plus gentamicin	Ampicillin, 2 g IM or IV, plus gentamicin, 1.5 mg/kg (not to exceed 120 mg) 30 minutes before procedure; 6 hours later, ampicillin, 1 g IM or IV, or amoxicillin, 1 g orally
Penicillin allergy	Vancomycin plus gentamicin	Vancomycin, 1 g IV over 1–2 hours, plus gentamicin, 1.5 mg/kg (not to exceed 120 mg) IV or IM; complete infusion or injection 30 minutes before procedure
Moderate-risk patient	Amoxicillin or ampicillin	Amoxicillin, 2 g orally 1 hour before procedure, or ampicillin, 2 g IM or IV 30 minutes before starting procedure
Penicillin allergy	Vancomycin	Vancomycin, 1 g IV over 1–2 hours; complete infusion 30 minutes before procedure

Modified and reproduced, with permission, from Dajani AS et al: Prevention of bacterial endocarditis. Recommendations by the American Heart Association. JAMA 1997;277:1794.

[1]Viridans streptococci are the most common cause of endocarditis occurring after dental or upper respiratory procedures; enterococci are the most common cause after gastrointestinal or genitourinary procedures.

[2]Cephalosporins should not be used in individuals with immediate-type hypersensitivity reactions to penicillin.

Table 137. Cardiac lesions for which bacterial endocarditis prophylaxis is or is not recommended.[1]

Endocarditis prophylaxis recommended

1. High-risk category
   - Prosthetic cardiac valves, including bioprosthetic and homograft valves
   - Previous bacterial endocarditis, even in the absence of heart disease
   - Complex cyanotic congenital heart disease (eg, single ventricle states, transposition of the great arteries, tetralogy of Fallot)
   - Surgically constructed systemic pulmonary shunts or conduits
2. Moderate-risk category
   - Most congenital cardiac malformations (other than those listed above and below)
   - Rheumatic and other acquired valvular dysfunction, even after valvular surgery
   - Hypertrophic cardiomyopathy
   - Mitral valve prolapse with valvular regurgitation[2,3]

Endocarditis prophylaxis not recommended[4]

- Isolated secundum septal defect
- Surgical repair of atrial septal defect, ventricular septal defect, or patent ductus arteriosus (without residua beyond 6 months)
- Previous coronary artery bypass graft surgery
- Mitral valve prolapse without valvular regurgitation[5]
- Physiologic, functional, or innocent heart murmurs
- Previous Kawasaki disease without valvular dysfunction
- Previous rheumatic fever without valvular dysfunction
- Cardiac pacemakers (intravascular and epicardial) and implanted defibrillators

Modified and reproduced, with permission, from Dajani AS et al: Prevention of bacterial endocarditis. Recommendations by the American Heart Association. JAMA 1997;277:1794.

[1]This table lists selected conditions and is not meant to be all-inclusive.

[2]Mitral regurgitation determined by the presence of a murmur or by echo-Doppler.

[3]Men older than 45 may warrant prophylaxis even without a consistent systolic murmur.

[4]Negligible risk category—no greater than in the general population.

[5]Individuals who have a mitral valve prolapse associated with thickening or redundancy of the valve leaflets may be at increased risk for bacterial endocarditis.

Table 138. Procedures for which bacterial endocarditis prophylaxis is or is not recommended.[1]

Endocarditis prophylaxis recommended[2]	**Endocarditis prophylaxis not recommended**
1. Dental	1. Dental
Dental extractions	Restorative dentistry (filling cavities, operative and prosthodontic) with or without retraction cord[4]
Periodontal procedures	Local anesthetic injections (nonintraligamentary)
Dental implant placement or reimplantation	Intracanal endodontic treatment; post placement and buildup
Endodontic (root canal) instrumentation or surgery only beyond the apex	Placement of rubber dams, removable prosthodontic, or orthodontic appliances
Subgingival placement of antibiotic fibers or strips	Postoperative suture removal
Initial placement of orthodontic bands but not brackets	Taking of oral impression
Intraligamentary local anesthetic injections	Fluoride treatments
Prophylactic cleaning of teeth or implants where bleeding is anticipated	Orthodontic appliance adjustment
2. Respiratory tract	2. Respiratory tract
Tonsillectomy, adenoidectomy	Endotracheal intubation
Surgical operations that involve intestinal or respiratory mucosa	Bronchoscopy with a flexible bronchoscope, with or without biopsy[5]
Bronchoscopy with a rigid bronchoscope	Tympanostomy (insertion)
3. Gastrointestinal tract[3]	3. Gastrointestinal tract
Sclerotherapy for esophageal varices	Transesophageal echocardiography[5]
Esophageal stricture dilation	Endoscopy with or without gastrointestinal biopsy[5]
Endoscopic retrograde cholangiography with biliary obstruction	4. Genitourinary tract
Biliary tract surgery	Vaginal hysterectomy[5]
Surgical operations that involve intestinal mucosa	Vaginal delivery[5]
4. Genitourinary tract	Cesarean section
Prostatic surgery	In the absence of infection: urethral catheterization, uterine dilation and curettage, therapeutic abortion, sterilization procedures, insertion or removal of intrauterine devices
Cystoscopy	5. Other
Urethral dilation	Cardiac catheterization, including balloon angioplasty; implanting cardiac pacemakers or defibrillators and coronary stents; incision or biopsy of surgically scrubbed skin; circumcision

[1]This table lists selected procedures but is not meant to be all-inclusive.

[2]Recommended for individuals with high- and moderate-risk cardiac conditions (Table 33–3).

[3]Prophylaxis is recommended for high-risk patients, optional for moderate-risk patients.

[4]Clinical judgment may indicate antibiotic use in selected circumstances that may create significant bleeding.

[5]Prophylaxis is optional for high-risk patients.

Table 139. Treatment of infective endocarditis.

Condition	Standard Therapy	Remarks
Empirical regimens pending culture results	Nafcillin or oxacillin, 1.5 g intravenously every 4 h, plus penicillin, 2–3 million units every 4 h (or ampicillin, 1.5 g every 4 h), plus gentamicin, 1 mg/kg every 8 h	Should include agents active against staphylococci, streptococci, and enterococci
For penicillin allergy or if infection by methicillin-resistant staphylococci is suspected	Vancomycin, 15 mg/kg intravenously every 12 h	
Viridans streptococci		
Penicillin-susceptible viridans streptococci (ie, minimum inhibitory concentration [MIC] ≤ 0.1 μg/mL)	Penicillin G, 2–3 million units intravenously every 4 h for 4 weeks; the duration of therapy can be shortened to 2 weeks if gentamicin, 1 mg/kg every 8 h, is used with penicillin or Ceftriaxone, 2 g once daily intravenously or intramuscularly for 4 weeks	A convenient regimen for home therapy
In the penicillin-allergic patient	Vancomycin, 15 mg/kg intravenously every 12 h for 4 weeks	The 2-week regimen is not recommended for patients with symptoms of more than 3 months duration or patients with complications such as myocardial abscess or extracardiac infection; prosthetic valve endocarditis should be treated with a 6-week course of penicillin with at least 2 weeks of gentamicin
Viridans streptococci relatively resistant to penicillin (ie, MIC > 0.1 μg/mL but ≤ 0.5 μg/mL)	Penicillin G, 3 million units intravenously every 4 h for 4 weeks; combine with gentamicin, 1 mg/kg every 8 h for the first 2 weeks	
Viridans streptococci resistant to penicillin (MIC > 0.5 μg/mL)	Treat as for enterococci	
In the penicillin-allergic patient	Vancomycin, 15 mg/kg intravenously every 12 h for 4 weeks	
Enterococci	Ampicillin, 2 g intravenously every 4 h, or penicillin G, 3–4 million units every 4 h plus gentamicin, 1 mg/kg every 8 h for 4–6 weeks	The relapse rate is unacceptably high when penicillin is used alone; because aminoglycoside resistance occurs in enterococci, susceptibility should be documented; the longer duration of therapy is recommended for patients with symptoms for more than 3 months, relapse, or prosthetic valve endocarditis, though a recent retrospective study of native valve enterococcal endocarditis suggests that less than 4 weeks of an aminoglycoside may be sufficient
In the penicillin-allergic patient	Vancomycin, 15 mg/kg intravenously every 12 h, plus gentamicin, 1 mg/kg every 8 h	
Enterococci that demonstrate high-level resistance to aminoglycosides (ie, not inhibited by 500 μg/mL of gentamicin)	Ampicillin, high dose (16 g/day by continuous infusion for 8–12 weeks)	The addition of an aminoglycoside will not be beneficial. Relapse rate up to 50%. Surgery may be the only option.
Staphylococci For methicillin-susceptible *Staphylococcus aureus*	Nafcillin or oxacillin, 1.5 g intravenously every 4 h for 4–6 weeks	

(*continued*)

Table 139. Treatment of infective endocarditis. (continued)

Condition	Standard Therapy	Remarks
Staphylococci (continued)		
For methicillin-resistant strain	Vancomycin, 15 mg/kg intravenously every 12 h for 4 weeks	Aminoglycoside combination regimens may be useful in shortening the duration of bacteremia; their maximum benefit is achieved at low doses (1 mg/kg every 8 h) and in the first 3–5 days of therapy, and they should not be continued beyond the early phase of therapy; for treatment of tricuspid valve endocarditis (with or without pulmonary involvement) in the injection drug user who does not have serious extrapulmonary sites of infection, the total duration of therapy can be shortened from 4 to 2 weeks if an aminoglycoside is added to an antistaphylococcal drug for the entire 2 weeks of therapy
Coagulase-negative staphylococci	Vancomycin, 15 mg/kg intravenously for 6 weeks, plus rifampin, 300 mg orally every 8 h for 6 weeks, plus gentamicin, 1 mg/kg intravenously every 8 h for the first 2 weeks	Routinely resistant to methicillin; β-lactam antibiotics should not be used until the isolate is known to be susceptible; if the organism is sensitive to methicillin, either nafcillin or oxacillin or cefazolin can be used in combination with rifampin and gentamicin
Prosthetic valve endocarditis	Combination therapy with nafcillin or oxacillin (vancomycin for methicillin-resistant strains or patients allergic to β-lactams), rifampin, and gentamicin	
HACEK organisms (*Haemophilus aphrophilus, Haemophilus parainfluenzae, Actinobacillus actinomycetemcomitans, Cardiobacterium hominis, Eikenella corrodens,* and *Kingella kingae*)	Ceftriaxone (or some other third-generation cephalosporin), 2 g intravenously or intramuscularly once daily for 4 weeks	These organisms can produce β-lactamase; prosthetic valve endocarditis should be treated for 6 weeks
In the penicillin-allergic patient	Trimethoprim-sulfamethoxazole, quinolones, and aztreonam have in vitro activity and should be considered	

Table 140. Treatment of anaerobic intra-abdominal infections.

Oral therapy

Ciprofloxacin, 750 mg twice daily, plus metronidazole, 500 mg three times daily

Intravenous therapy

Moderate to moderately severe infections:

Ticarcillin/clavulanate, 3 g/0.1 g every 6 hours

or—

Cefotetan, 2 g every 12 hours

or—

Clindamycin, 600 mg every 8 hours, or metronidazole, 500 mg every 8 hours, plus gentamicin, 5 mg/kg/d

Severe infections:

Imipenem, 0.5 g every 6–8 hours, or ceftriaxone, 1 g every 24 hours, plus either clindamycin, 600 mg every 8 hours, or metronidazole, 500 mg every 8 hours

Table 141. Fecal leukocytes in intestinal disorders.

Infectious			Noninfectious
Present	**Variable**	**Absent**	**Present**
Shigella *Campylobacter* Enteroinvasive *E coli* (EIEC)	*Salmonella* *Yersinia* *Vibrio parahaemolytica* *Clostridium difficile* *Aeromonas*	Noroviruses Rotavirus *Giardia lamblia* *Entamoeba histolytica* *Cryptosporidium* "Food poisoning" *Staphylococcus aureus* *Bacillus cereus* *Clostridium perfringens* *Escherichia coli* Enterotoxigenic (ETEC) Enterohemorrhagic (EHEC)	Ulcerative colitis Crohn's disease Radiation colitis Ischemic colitis

Table 142. Treatment of Lyme disease.

Manifestation	Drug and Dosage
Tick bite	No treatment in most circumstances (see text); observe
Erythema migrans	Doxycycline, 100 mg twice daily, or amoxicillin, 500 mg three times daily, or cefuroxime axetil, 500 mg twice daily—all for 2–3 weeks
Neurologic disease Bell's palsy	Doxycycline, or amoxicillin as above for 2–3 weeks
Other central nervous system disease	Ceftriaxone, 2 g intravenously once daily, or penicillin G, 18–24 million units daily intravenously in 6 divided doses, or cefotaxime, 2 g intravenously every 8 hours—all for 2–4 weeks
Cardiac disease First-degree block (P-R < 0.3 seconds)	Doxycycline or amoxicillin as above for 2–3 weeks
High-degree atrioventricular block	Ceftriaxone or penicillin G as above for 30–60 days (see text)
Arthritis Oral dosage	Doxycycline or amoxicillin as above for 30–60 days (see text)
Parenteral dosage	Ceftriaxone or penicillin G as above for 2–4 weeks
Acrodermatitis chronicum atrophicans	Doxycycline or amoxicillin as above for 4 weeks
"Chronic Lyme disease" or "post-Lyme disease syndrome"	Symptomatic therapy

Table 143. Treatment of amebiasis.

Clinical Presentation	Drug(s) of Choice	Alternative Drug(s)
Asymptomatic intestinal infection	Diloxanide furoate[1,2]	Iodoquinol (diiodohydroxyquin)[3] or paromomycin[4]
Mild to moderate intestinal disease (nondysenteric colitis)	(1) Tinidazole[5] or metronidazole[5] **plus** (2) Diloxanide furoate,[1,2] iodoquinol,[3] or paromomycin[4]	(1) Diloxanide furoate[1,2] or iodoquinol[3] **plus** (2) A tetracycline[6] **followed by** (3) Chloroquine[7] **or** (1) Paromomycin[4] **followed by** (2) Chloroquine[7]
Severe intestinal disease (dysentery)	(1) Tinidazole[5] or metronidazole[5] **plus** (2) Diloxanide furoate[1,2] or iodoquinol[3] **or, if parenteral therapy is needed initially:** (1) Intravenous metronidazole[8] until oral therapy can be started; (2) Then give oral metronidazole[5] plus diloxanide furoate[1,2] or iodoquinol[3]	(1) A tetracycline[6] plus (2) Diloxanide furoate[1,2] or iodoquinol[3] **followed by** (3) Chloroquine[9] **or, if parenteral therapy is needed initially:** (1) Dehydroemetine[10] or emetine[1,10] **followed by** (2) A tetracycline[6] plus diloxanide furoate[1,2] or iodoquinol[3] **followed by** (3) Chloroquine[9]
Hepatic abscess	(1) Tinidazole[5] or metronidazole[5,8,] **plus** (2) Diloxanide furoate[1,2] or iodoquinol[3] **followed by** (3) Chloroquine[9]	(1) Dehydroemetine[11] or emetine[1,11] **followed by** (2) Chloroquine[12] **plus** (3) Diloxanide furoate[1,2] or iodoquinol[3]
Ameboma or extra-intestinal disease	As for hepatic abscess, but not including chloroquine	As for hepatic abscess, but not including chloroquine

[1]Not available in the United States.
[2]Diloxanide furoate, 500 mg three times daily with meals for 10 days.
[3]Iodoquinol (diiodohydroxyquin), 650 mg three times daily for 21 days.
[4]Paromomycin, 25–35 mg/kg (base) (maximum 3 g) in three divided doses after meals daily for 7 days.
[5]Although tinidazole and metronidazole are equally effective, tinidazole is given in a shorter course and is better tolerated. The tinidazole dosage in asymptomatic and mild intestinal infection is 2 g daily for 3 days; in severe intestinal infection and hepatic abscess, the dosage is 2 g once daily for 5 days. The metronidazole dosage is 750 mg three times daily for 10 days. The drugs should be taken with food.
[6]Tetracycline, 250 mg four times daily for 10 days; in severe dysentery, give 500 mg four times daily for the first 5 days, then 250 mg four times daily for 5 days. Tetracycline should not be used during pregnancy.
[7]Chloroquine, 500 mg (salt) daily for 7 days.
[8]An intravenous metronidazole formulation is available; change to oral medication as soon as possible. See manufacturer's recommendation for dosage and cautions.
[9]Chloroquine, 500 mg (salt) daily for 14 days.
[10]Dehydroemetine or emetine, 1 mg/kg subcutaneously (preferred) or intramuscularly daily for the least number of days necessary to control severe symptoms (usually 3–5 days) (maximum daily dose for dehydroemetine is 90 mg; for emetine, 65 mg).
[11]Use dosage recommended in footnote 10 for 8–10 days.
[12]Chloroquine, 500 mg (salt) orally twice daily for 2 days and then 500 mg orally daily for 19 days.

Table 144. Treatment of malaria in nonimmune adult populations.

<table>
<tr><th>Treatment[1] of Infection With All Species (Except Chloroquine-Resistant P falciparum or P vivax)</th><th>Treatment[1] of Infection With Chloroquine-Resistant P falciparum or P vivax Strains</th></tr>
<tr><td>
Oral treatment of uncomplicated P falciparum[2] or P malariae infection
Chloroquine phosphate, 1 g (salt)[3,4] as initial dose, then 0.5 g at 6, 24, and 48 hours.

Oral treatment of P vivax,[5] P ovale infection, or species not identified
Chloroquine[3,4] as above followed by 0.5 g on days 10 and 17 plus primaquine phosphate, 52.6 mg (salt)[3,4,5] daily for 14 days starting about day 4.

Treatment of severe attacks
Parenteral quinine dihydrochloride[6] or quinidine gluconate.[7] Start oral chloroquine therapy as soon as possible; follow with primaquine if needed.[4]

or

Parenteral artesunate,[8] artemether,[8] or chloroquine[9] until the patient can take oral chloroquine. Follow with primaquine if needed.[4]
</td><td>
Oral treatment of uncomplicated P falciparum resistant to chloroquine
Quinine sulfate, 10 mg/kg 3 times daily for 3–7 days,[10] plus one of the following: (1) doxycycline,[11] 100 mg twice daily for 7 days; (2) clindamycin,[11] 900 mg 3 times daily for 7 days; (3) tetracycline,[11] 250–500 mg 4 times daily for 7 days.

or

Malarone[11] two tablets twice daily with food for 3 days (each tablet contains atovaquone [250 mg] and proguanil [100 mg]).

or

Mefloquine,[12] 750 mg followed after 6–12 hours by 500 mg.

or

Atovaquone/doxycycline, 500 mg/100 mg, twice daily for 3 days.

or

Artesunate,[8] 4 mg/kg/d orally for 3 days plus mefloquine[12] (750 mg followed by 500 mg 12 hours later).

or

Halofantrine[13]

Oral treatment of P vivax resistant to chloroquine
Malarone or mefloquine (dosages above).

or

Quinine plus doxycycline, or tetracycline plus primaquine (dosages above).

Parenteral treatment of severe attacks[14]
Quinine dihydrochloride[6] or quinidine gluconate[7] plus intravenous doxycycline, tetracycline, or clindamycin. Start oral therapy with quinine sulfate plus the second drug as soon as possible to complete the course[10] of treatment.

or

Artemether,[8] or artesunate[8]; followed by oral mefloquine[12] (750 mg followed by 500 mg 12 hours later)
</td></tr>
</table>

[1]See text for cautions, contraindications, and side effects of each drug. For advice on management, call the Centers for Disease Control and Prevention (CDC), Atlanta, GA 770-488-7788; after business hours, 770-488-7100, or go to its website http://www.cdc.gov/malaria.

[2]In falciparum malaria, if the patient has not shown a clinical response to chloroquine (48–72 hours for mild infections, 24 hours for severe ones), parasitic resistance to chloroquine should be considered. Chloroquine should be stopped and treatment started with an oral drug used for chloroquine-resistant strains.

[3]500 mg chloroquine phosphate = 300 mg base; 52.6 mg of primaquine salt = 30 mg base.

[4]Chloroquine alone is curative for infection with sensitive strains of *P falciparum* and *P malariae*, but primaquine is needed to eradicate the persistent liver stages of *P vivax* and *P ovale*. Start primaquine after the patient has recovered from the acute illness; continue chloroquine weekly during primaquine therapy. Patients should be screened for glucose-6-phosphate dehydrogenase deficiency before use of primaquine. An alternative mode for primaquine therapy is combined primaquine, 78.9 mg (salt), and chloroquine, 0.5 g (salt), weekly for 8 weeks.

[5]Strains of *P vivax* partially resistant to primaquine have appeared in some regions (see text). This is being dealt with by an increase in the primaquine dosage to 52.6 mg (salt) daily for 14 days.

[6]Parenteral quinine dihydrochloride. As a loading dose, give 20 mg/kg (salt) in 500 mL of 5% glucose solution intravenously slowly over 4 hours; repeat using 10 mg/kg every 8 hours until oral therapy is possible (maximum, 1800 mg/d). If more than 48 hours of parenteral treatment is required, some authorities reduce the quinine dose by one-third to one-half. Total plasma concentrations of 8–15 mg/mL is effective and does not cause serious toxicity. Blood pressure and ECG should be monitored constantly to detect arrhythmias or hypotension. As severe hypoglycemia may occur, blood glucose levels should be monitored. Extreme caution is required in treating patients with quinine who previously have been taking mefloquine in prophylaxis. In the United States, quinine dihydrochloride is no longer available.

[7]When parenteral quinine is unavailable (as in the United States), quinidine gluconate can be used, administered as a continuous infusion. A loading dose of 10 mg/kg (salt) (maximum, 600 mg) is diluted in 300 mL of normal saline and administered over 1–2 hours, followed by 0.02 mg/kg/min (maximum, 10 mg/kg every 8 hours) by infusion pump until oral quinine therapy is possible. If more than 48 hours of parenteral treatment is required, some authorities reduce the quinidine dose by one-third to one-half. Total plasma concentrations of 3.5–8 mg/mL is effective and does not cause serious toxicity. Fluid status, glucose, blood pressure, and ECG should be monitored closely; widening of the QRS interval or lengthening of the QT interval requires discontinuation.

[8]Not available in the United States. Give artesunate intravenously (2.4 mg/kg on the first day, followed by 1.2 mg/kg daily) or artemether intramuscularly (3.2 mg/kg on the first day, followed by 1.6 mg/kg daily); continue the drug for a minimum of 3 days until the patient can start oral artesunate. If parenteral treatment is not available, artemisinin rectal suppositories are being evaluated (40 mg/kg loading dose, then 20 mg/kg at 24, 48, and 72 hours) followed by oral medication. With all preparations of the artemisinin drugs, as soon as oral medication can be tolerated, treat concurrently with another effective blood schizonticide (Malarone preferred).

(*continued*)

Table 144. Treatment of malaria in nonimmune adult populations. (continued)

[9]Give parenteral chloroquine (1) preferably intravenously, 10 mg base/kg in isotonic fluid by constant rate of infusion over 8 hours, followed by 15 mg/kg over the next 24 hours; or (2) intramuscularly or subcutaneously, 3.5 mg base/kg every 6 hours.
[10]Although oral quinine sulfate is usually given for 3 days, it should be continued for 7 days in patients who acquired infections in Southeast Asia and South America, where diminished responsiveness to quinine has been noted.
[11]Contraindicated in pregnant women.
[12]Serious side effects are rare. See text for cautions and contraindications. In the United States, a 250-mg tablet of mefloquine contains 228 mg of base; outside the United States, each 275-mg tablet contains 250 mg of base. Mefloquine is hazardous with quinine, quinidine, or halofantrine.
[13]The dosage is 500 mg (salt) every 6 hours for three doses and repeat in 1 week. A possible contraindication is the presence of cardiac conduction abnormalities. Do not use if mefloquine has been taken in previous 2–3 weeks or with recent use of quinine or quinidine. Not available in the United States.
[14]All of the drugs given intravenously should be administered slowly.

Table 145. Prevention of malaria in nonimmune adult travelers.[1]

TO PREVENT ATTACKS OF ALL FORMS OF MALARIA AND TO ERADICATE *P falciparum* AND *P malariae* INFECTIONS[2,3]

REGIONS WITH CHLOROQUINE-SENSITIVE *P falciparum* MALARIA: Central America west of the Panama Canal, the Caribbean, Mexico, and parts of the Middle East and China.

Chloroquine[4,5]

Dose: Chloroquine phosphate, 500 mg salt (300 mg base) weekly. Give a single dose of chloroquine weekly starting 1–2 weeks before entering the endemic area, while there, and for 4 weeks after leaving.

REGIONS WITH CHLOROQUINE-RESISTANT *P falciparum* MALARIA: All other regions of the world; the frequency and intensity of resistance vary by region.

Malarone (atovaquone [250 mg] combined with proguanil [100 mg] [preferred method])[4,6]

Dose: One tablet daily at the same time each day. Give one tablet the day before entering the endemic area, daily while there, and daily for 1 week after leaving.

Mefloquine (alternative method)[4,7]

Dose: One 250-mg tablet salt (228 mg base) weekly. Give a single dose of mefloquine weekly starting 1–3 weeks before entering the endemic area, while there, and for 4 weeks after leaving.

Doxycycline (alternative method)[4,8]

Dose: 100 mg daily. Give the daily dose for 2 days before entering the endemic area, while there, and for 4 weeks after leaving.

TO ERADICATE *P vivax* AND *P ovale* INFECTIONS[2]

Primaquine[9]

Start primaquine only after returning home, during the last 2 weeks of chemoprophylaxis. Dose: 52.6 mg salt (30 mg base) daily for 14 days. An alternative regimen in regions where chloroquine is effective in prophylaxis is chloroquine phosphate, 500 mg (salt), plus primaquine phosphate, 78.9 mg (salt), weekly for 8 weeks.

[1]See text for additional information on drug cautions, contraindications, and side effects. For additional information on prophylaxis for specific countries, see the references or call the Centers for Disease Control and Prevention, Atlanta, GA at 770-488-7788 (for fax response: 888-232-3299). The information is also available on the Internet at http://www.cdc.gov (choose the Traveler's Health category).
[2]The blood schizonticides (chloroquine, mefloquine, Malarone, and doxycycline), when taken for 4 weeks (7 days for Malarone) after leaving the endemic area, are curative for sensitive *P falciparum* and *P malariae* infections; primaquine, however, is needed to eradicate the persistent liver stages of *P vivax* and *P ovale*.
[3]See text for a standby drug for emergency self-treatment of presumptive malaria; the drug should be used only when a physician is not immediately available. It is imperative, however, that medical follow-up be sought promptly.
[4]A test dose of the selected prophylactic drug should be given before departure to allow for changing to an alternative drug in the event of significant side effects: chloroquine (once weekly for 2 weeks), Malarone (daily for 2 days), doxycycline (daily for 2 days), mefloquine (weekly for 3 weeks). Side effects from mefloquine sometimes do not appear until after the third or later doses.
[5]Chloroquine and proguanil can be used by pregnant women.
[6]Malarone is available in the United States. It eradicates falciparum infections after 1 week of postexposure treatment; its efficacy against *P malariae*, however, is undetermined. To eradicate *P vivax* and *P ovale* infections, a course of primaquine is needed, which should be started early in the final week of Malarone treatment. Malarone has not been shown to be safe in pregnancy. Malarone is more expensive than mefloquine.
[7]Because of the high frequency of resistance, mefloquine should not be used in Thailand or adjacent countries. Mefloquine is generally not recommended in the first trimester of pregnancy or under some other conditions (see text).
[8]Doxycycline is used in Thailand and adjacent countries and in other regions by persons who cannot tolerate mefloquine or Malarone. It is contraindicated in pregnant women. Take with evening meals. See text for side effects.
[9]Primaquine is indicated only for persons who have had a high probability of exposure to *P vivax* or *P ovale* (see text), and who have not taken the drug for daily prophylaxis. The drug should be taken with food and is contraindicated in pregnancy. Before use, patients must be screened for glucose-6-phosphate dehydrogenase deficiency. Note that the dosage recommended by CDC has increased.

Table 146. Currently available (prepackaged) cyanide antidotes.

Antidote	How Supplied	Dose
Amyl nitrite[1]	0.3 mL (aspirol inhalant)	Break one or two aspirols under patient's nose.
Sodium nitrite[1]	3 g/dL (300 mg in 10 mL vials)	6 mg/kg IV (0.2 mL/kg)
Sodium thiosulfate[1]	25 g/dL (12.5 g in 50 mL vials)	250 mg/kg IV (1 mL/kg)

[1]In the United States, manufactured by Taylor Pharmaceuticals.

Table 147. Clinical features of hydrocarbon poisoning.

Type	Examples	Risk of Pneumonia	Risk of Systemic Toxicity	Treatment
High-viscosity	Vaseline[1] Motor oil	Low	Low	None.
Low-viscosity, nontoxic	Furniture polish Mineral seal oil Kerosene Lighter fluid	High	Low	Observe for pneumonia. *Do not* induce emesis. *Do not* administer activated charcoal.
Low-viscosity, unknown systemic toxicity	Turpentine Pine oil	High	Variable	Observe for pneumonia. Consider activated charcoal.
Low-viscosity, known systemic toxicity	Camphor Phenol Chlorinated insecticides Aromatic hydrocarbons (benzene, toluene, etc)	High	High	Observe for pneumonia. Give activated charcoal.

[1]"Vaseline" is one of several proprietary names for petrolatum (petroleum jelly, paraffin jelly).

Table 148. Common seafood poisonings.

Type of Poisoning	Mechanism	Clinical Presentation
Ciguatera	Reef fish ingest toxic dinoflagellates, whose toxins accumulate in fish meat. Commonly implicated fish in the United States are barracuda, jack, snapper, and grouper.	1–6 hours after ingestion, victims develop abdominal pain, vomiting, and diarrhea accompanied by a variety of neurologic symptoms, including paresthesias, reversal of hot and cold sensation, vertigo, headache, and intense itching. Autonomic disturbances, including hypotension and bradycardia, may occur.
Scombroid	Improper preservation of large fish results in bacterial degradation of histidine to histamine. Commonly implicated fish include tuna, mahimahi, bonita, mackerel, and kingfish.	Allergic-like (anaphylactoid) symptoms are due to histamine, usually begin within 15–90 minutes, and include skin flushing, itching, urticaria, angioedema, bronchospasm, and hypotension as well as abdominal pain, vomiting, and diarrhea.
Paralytic shellfish poisoning	Dinoflagellates produce saxitoxin, which is concentrated by filter-feeding mussels and clams. Saxitoxin blocks sodium conductance and neuronal transmission in skeletal muscles.	Onset is usually within 30–60 minutes. Initial symptoms include perioral and intraoral paresthesias. Other symptoms include nausea and vomiting, headache, dizziness, dysphagia, dysarthria, ataxia, and rapidly progressive muscle weakness that may result in respiratory arrest.
Puffer fish poisoning	Tetrodotoxin is concentrated in liver, gonads, intestine, and skin. Toxic effects are similar to those of saxitoxin. Tetrodotoxin is also found in some North American newts and Central American frogs.	Onset is usually within 30–40 minutes but may be as short as 10 minutes. Initial perioral paresthesias are followed by headache, diaphoresis, nausea, vomiting, ataxia, and rapidly progressive muscle weakness that may result in respiratory arrest.

Table 149. Some of the "unsafe" and "probably safe" drugs used in the treatment of acute porphyrias.

Unsafe	Probably Safe
Alcohol	Acetaminophen
Alkylating agents	β-Adrenergic blockers
Barbiturates	Amitriptyline
Carbamazepine	Aspirin
Chloroquine	Atropine
Chlorpropamide	Chloral hydrate
Clonidine	Chlordiazepoxide
Dapsone	Diazepam
Ergots	Digoxin
Erythromycin	Diphenhydramine
Estrogens, synthetic	Glucocorticoids
Food additives	Guanethidine
Glutethimide	Hyoscine
Griseofulvin	Ibuprofen
Hydralazine	Imipramine
Ketamine	Insulin
Meprobamate	Lithium
Methyldopa	Naproxen
Metoclopramide	Nitrofurantoin
Nortriptyline	Opioid analgesics
Pentazocine	Penicillamine
Phenytoin	Penicillin and derivatives
Progestins	Phenothiazines
Pyrazinamide	Procaine
Rifampin	Streptomycin
Spironolactone	Succinylcholine
Succinimides	Tetracycline
Sulfonamides	Thiouracil
Theophylline	
Tolazamide	
Tolbutamide	
Valproic acid	

Table 150. Cancer screening recommendations for average-risk adults, 2003.

	Test	ACS[1]	CTF[2]	USPSTF[3]
Breast	Self-examination (BSE)	Monthly for women over age 20.	Fair evidence that BSE *should not* be used.	Insufficient evidence to recommend for or against.
	Clinical breast examination	Every 3 years age 20–40 and annually thereafter.	Every 1–2 years in women aged 40–59.	Insufficient evidence to recommend for or against.
	Mammography	Annually age 40 and older.	Every 1–2 years in women aged 40–59. Current evidence does not support the recommendation that screening mammography be included in or excluded from the periodic health examination of women aged 40–49.	Recommended every 1–2 years for women aged 40 and over (B).
Cervix	Papanicolaou test	Annually beginning within 3 years after first vaginal intercourse or no later than age 21.	Annually at age of first intercourse or by age 18; can move to every-2-year screening after two normal results.	Every 3 years beginning at onset of sexual activity.
		After age 30, women with three normal tests may be screened every 2–3 years.		
		Women may choose to stop screening after age 70 if they have had three normal (and no abnormal) results within the last 10 years.		
Colon	Stool test for occult blood*	Screening recommended, with the combination of fecal occult blood test and sigmoidoscopy preferred over stool test or sigmoidoscopy alone. Barium enema and colonoscopy also considered reasonable alternatives.	Good evidence for screening every 1–2 years over age 50.	Screening strongly recommended (A), but insufficient evidence to determine best test.
	Sigmoidoscopy		Fair evidence for screening over age 50 (insufficient evidence about combining stool test and sigmoidoscopy).	
	Double-constrast barium enema		Not addressed.	
	Colonoscopy		Insufficient evidence for or against use in screening.	
	Digital rectal exam (DRE)	Not recommended.	No recommendation.	Not recommended.
Prostate	DRE	DRE and PSA should be offered annually to men age 50 and older who have at least a 10-year life expectancy. Information should be provided to men about the benefits and risks, and they should be allowed to participate in the decision. Men without a clear preference should be screened.	Insufficient evidence for or against including in routine care.	Insufficient evidence to recommend for or against.
	Prostate-specific antigen (PSA) blood test		Fair evidence *against* including in routine care.	
Other	Cancer-related checkup	Every 3 years for men 20–40 and annually thereafter; should include counseling and perhaps oral cavity, thyroid, lymph node, or testicular examinations.	Not assessed.	Not assessed.

*Home test with three samples.

[1]American Cancer Society recommendations, available at http://www.cancer.org

[2]Canadian Task Force on Preventive Health Care recommendations available at http://www.ctfphc.org

[3]United States Preventive Services Task Force recommendations available at http://www.ahrq.gov

Recommendation A: The USPSTF strongly recommends that clinicians routinely provide the service to eligible patients. (The USPSTF found good evidence that the service improves important health outcomes and concludes that benefits substantially outweigh harms.)

Recommendation B: The USPSTF recommends that clinicians routinely provide the service to eligible patients. (The USPSTF found at least fair evidence that the service improves important health outcomes and concludes that benefits substantially outweigh harms.)

Table 151. ncidence of and mortality from the ten most common cancers in the United States in males and females (all races), 1997–2001.

Rank	Men	Incidence[1]	Mortality[1]	Women	Incidence[1]	Mortality[1]
1	Prostate	172	32	Breast	135	27
2	Lung	79	78	Lung	49	41
3	Colorectal	63	25	Colorectal	46	18
4	Bladder	36	8	Uterus[2]	33	5
5	Non-Hodgkin's lymphoma	23	11	Ovary	14	9
6	Melanoma	21	4	Non-Hodgkin's lymphoma	16	7
7	Oral cavity and pharynx[3]	16	4	Melanoma	14	2
8	Kidney	16	6	Thyroid	10	0.5
9	Leukemias[4]	16	10	Pancreas	49	2
10	Pancreas	13	12	Leukemia	9	6

Data obtained from the NCI SEER Program. Ries LAG et al (editors): *SEER Cancer Statistics Review, 1975–2001*, National Cancer Institute, 2004. http://seer.cancer.gov.csr/1975_2001/2004.

[1]Rates are per 100,000, 1996–2001, and are age adjusted to the 2000 United States population by 5-year age groups.

[2]Uterus includes the cervix and corpus uteri.

[3]Both oropharynx and larynx are included.

[4]All subtypes of leukemia are included.

Table 152. Lifetime risks for the most common cancers, 1999–2001.

Cancer	Risk of Diagnosis (%)	Risk of Death (%)
Prostate	17.8	3.0
Breast (women)	13.4	3.0
Lung		
(men)	7.6	7.43
(women)	5.7	4.8
Colorectal		
(men)	5.9	2.4
(women)	5.5	2.3
Bladder (men)	3.6	0.7
Uterus[1]	3.4	0.8
Any cancer		
(men)	45.6	23.7
(women)	38.2	20.0

Data obtained from the NCI Seer Program. Ries LAG et al (editors): *SEER Cancer Statistics Review, 1975–2001*, National Cancer Institute, 2004. http://seer.cancer.gov/csr/1975_2001/ 2004.

[1]Uterus includes the cervix and corpus uteri.

Table 153. Treatment choices for cancers responsive to systemic agents.

Diagnosis	Current Treatment of Choice	Other Valuable Agents and Procedures
Acute lymphocytic leukemia	**Induction:** combination chemotherapy. *Adults:* Vincristine, prednisone, daunorubicin, and asparaginase (DVPLasp). **Consolidation:** multiagent alternating chemotherapy. Allogeneic bone marrow transplant for young adults or high-risk disease or second remission. Central nervous system prophylaxis with intrathecal methotrexate with or without whole brain radiation. **Remission maintenance:** methotrexate, thioguanine.	Doxorubicin, cytarabine, cyclophosphamide, etoposide, teniposide, clofarabine, allopurinol[1], autologous bone marrow transplantation
Acute myelocytic and myelomonocytic leukemia	**Induction:** combination chemotherapy with cytarabine and an anthracycline (daunorubicin, idarubicin). Tretinoin with idarubicin for acute promyelocytic leukemia. **Consolidation:** high-dose cytarabine. Autologous (with or without purging) or allogeneic bone marrow transplantation for high-risk disease or second remission.	Gemtuzumab ozogamicin (Mylotarg), mitoxantrone, idarubicin, etoposide, mercaptopurine, thioguanine, azacitidine[2], amsacrine[2], methotrexate, doxorubicin, tretinoin, allopurinol[1], leukapheresis, prednisone, arsenic trioxide for acute promyelocytic leukemia
Chronic myelocytic leukemia	Imatinib mesylate (Gleevec), hydroxyurea, interferon-α. Allogeneic bone marrow transplantation for younger patients.	Busulfan, mercaptopurine, thioguanine, cytarabine, plicamycin, melphalan, autologous bone marrow transplantation[2], allopurinol[1]
Chronic lymphocytic leukemia	Fludarabine, chlorambucil, and prednisone (if treatment is indicated). Second-line therapy: alemtuzumab (Campath-1H).	Vincristine, cyclophosphamide, doxorubicin, cladribine (2-chlorodeoxyadenosine; CdA), rituximab, allogeneic bone marrow transplantation, androgens[2], allopurinol[1]
Hairy cell leukemia	Cladribine (2-chlorodeoxyadenosine; CdA).	Pentostatin (deoxycoformycin), interferon-α
Hodgkin's disease (stages III and IV)	**Combination chemotherapy:** doxorubicin (Adriamycin), bleomycin, vinblastine, dacarbazine (ABVD) or alternative combination therapy without mechlorethamine. Autologous bone marrow transplantation for high-risk patients or relapsed disease.	Mechlorethamine, vincristine, prednisone, procarbazine (MOPP); carmustine, lomustine, etoposide, thiotepa, autologous bone marrow transplantation
Non-Hodgkin's lymphoma (intermediate to high grade)	**Combination therapy:** depending on histologic classification but usually including cyclophosphamide, vincristine, doxorubicin, and prednisone (CHOP) with or without rituximab in older patients. Autologous bone marrow transplantation in high-risk first remission or first relapse.	Bleomycin, methotrexate, etoposide, chlorambucil, fludarabine, lomustine, carmustine, cytarabine, thiotepa, amsacrine, mitoxantrone, allogeneic bone marrow transplantation
Non-Hodgkin's lymphoma (low grade)	Fludarabine, rituximab, if CD20 positive; ibritumomab tiuxetan or ^{131}I tositumomab for relapsed or refractory disease.	**Combination chemotherapy:** cyclophosphamide, prednisone, doxorubicin, vincristine; chlorambucil, autologous or allogeneic transplantation
Cutaneous T cell lymphoma (mycosis fungoides)	Topical carmustine, electron beam radiotherapy, photochemotherapy, targretin, denileukin diftitox (ONTAK) for refractory disease.	Interferon, combination chemotherapy, denileukin diftitox (ONTAK), targretin
Multiple myeloma	**Combination chemotherapy:** vincristine, doxorubicin, dexamethasone; melphalan and prednisone; melphalan, cyclosphosphamide, carmustine, vincristine, doxorubicin, prednisone, thalidomide. Autologous transplantation in first complete or partial remission, miniallogeneic transplant for poor-prognosis disease. Bortezomib for relapsed or refractory disease.	Clarithromycin, etoposide, cytarabine, interferon-α, dexamethasone, autologous bone marrow transplantation

(*continued*)

Table 153. Treatment choices for cancers responsive to systemic agents. (continued)

Diagnosis	Current Treatment of Choice	Other Valuable Agents and Procedures
Waldenström's macroglobulinemia	Fludarabine **or** chlorambucil **or** cyclophosphamide, vincristine, prednisone. Allogeneic bone marrow transplantation for high-risk young patients.	Cladribine, etoposide, interferon-α, doxorubicin, dexamethasone, plasmapheresis, autologous bone marrow transplantation
Polycythemia vera, essential thrombocytosis	Hydroxyurea, phlebotomy for polycythemia. Anagrelide for thombocytosis.	Busulfan, chlorambucil, cyclophosphamide, interferon-α, radiophosphorus ^{32}P
Carcinoma of the lung Small cell	**Combination chemotherapy:** cisplatin and etoposide. Palliative radiation therapy.	Cyclophosphamide, doxorubicin, vincristine
Non-small cell[3]	**Localized disease:** cisplatin or carboplatin, docetaxel. **Advanced disease:** cisplatin or carboplatin, docetaxel, gemcitabine, gefitinib, erlotinib, etoposide, vinblastine, vinorelbine.	Doxorubicin, etoposide, pemetrexed, mitomycin, ifosfamide, paclitaxel, capecitabine, radiation therapy
Malignant pleural mesothelioma	Pemetrexed with cisplatin.	Doxorubicin, radiation, pleurectomy
Carcinoma of the head and neck[3]	**Combination chemotherapy:** cisplatin and fluorouracil, paclitaxel.	Methotrexate, bleomycin, hydroxyurea, doxorubicin, vinblastine
Carcinoma of the esophagus[3]	**Combination chemotherapy:** fluorouracil, cisplatin, mitomycin.	Methotrexate, bleomycin, doxorubicin, mitomycin
Carcinoma of the stomach and pancreas[3]	**Stomach:** etoposide, leucovorin[1], fluorouracil (ELF). **Pancreas:** fluorouracil or ELF, gemcitabine.	Carmustine, mitomycin, lomustine, doxorubicin, gemcitabine, methotrexate, cisplatin, combinations for stomach
Carcinoma of the colon and rectum[3]	**Colon:** oxaliplatin with infusional 5-fluorouracil (5-FU)/leucovorin (FOLFOX4) (adjuvant); bevacizumab with irinotecan, 5-FU/leucovorin (advanced). **Rectum:** fluorouracil with radiation therapy (adjuvant).	Cetuximab, capecitabine, methotrexate, mitomycin, carmustine, cisplatin, floxuridine
Carcinoma of the kidney[3]	Floxuridine, vinblastine, interleukin-2 (IL-2), interferon-α; consider miniallogeneic transplantation[2].	Interferon-α, progestins, infusional fluorodeoxyuridine, fluorouracil
Carcinoma of the bladder[3]	Intravesical bacillus Calmette-Guérin (BCG) or thiotepa. **Combination chemotherapy:** methotrexate, vinblastine, doxorubicin (Adriamycin), cisplatin (M-VAC) or CMV alone.	Cyclophosphamide, fluorouracil, intravesical valrubicin, gemcitabine, cisplatin
Carcinoma of the testis[3]	**Combination chemotherapy:** etoposide and cisplatin. Autologous bone marrow transplantation for high-risk or relapsed disease.	Bleomycin, vinblastine, ifosfamide, mesna[1], carmustine, carboplatin
Carcinoma of the prostate[3]	Estrogens or luteinizing hormone-releasing hormone analog (leuprolide, goserelin, or triptorelin) plus an antiandrogen (flutamide).	Ketoconazole, doxorubicin, aminoglutethimide, progestins, cyclophosphamide, cisplatin, vinblastine, etoposide, suramin[2]; PC-SPES; estramustine phosphate
Carcinoma of the uterus[3]	Progestins or tamoxifen.	Doxorubicin, cisplatin, fluorouracil, ifosfamide
Carcinoma of the ovary[3]	**Combination chemotherapy:** paclitaxel and cisplatin or carboplatin.	Docetaxel, doxorubicin, topotecan, cyclophosphamide, etoposide, liposomal doxorubicin
Carcinoma of the cervix[3]	**Combination chemotherapy:** methotrexate, doxorubicin, cisplatin, and vinblastine; or mitomycin, bleomycin, vincristine, and cisplatin with radiation therapy.	Carboplatin, ifosfamide, lomustine

(continued)

Table 153. Treatment choices for cancers responsive to systemic agents. (continued)

Diagnosis	Current Treatment of Choice	Other Valuable Agents and Procedures
Carcinoma of the breast[3]	**Combination chemotherapy:** a variety of regimens are used for adjuvant therapy. For node-positive disease—combinations including doxorubicin or epirubicin and at least one of the following additional drugs: 5-FU, cyclophosphamide, docetaxel, paclitaxel. For node-negative disease—a combination of the drugs listed above or cyclophosphamide, methotrexate, and 5-FU (CMF). For estrogen- or progesterone-positive disease, tamoxifen (premenopausal women) or anastrozole/letrozole/exemestane following or instead of tamoxifen (postmenopausal women) is given for 5 years regardless of the use of adjuvant chemotherapy.	Trastuzumab (Herceptin) with chemotherapy, paclitaxel, docetaxel, nab-paclitaxel, epirubicin, mitoxantrone, pegylated doxorubicin, capecitabine, gemcitabine, vinorelbine, thiotepa, vincristine, vinblastine, carboplatin or cisplatin, anastrozole, letrozole, exemestane, fulvestrant, toremifine, progestins
Choriocarcinoma (trophoblastic neoplasms)[3]	Methotrexate or dactinomycin (or both) plus chlorambucil.	Vinblastine, cisplatin, mercaptopurine, doxorubicin, bleomycin, etoposide
Carcinoma of the thyroid gland[3]	Radioiodine (^{131}I).	Doxorubicin, cisplatin, bleomycin, melphalan
Carcinoma of the adrenal gland[3]	Mitotane.	Doxorubicin, suramin[2]
Carcinoid[3]	Fluorouracil plus streptozocin with or without interferon-α.	Doxorubicin, cyclophosphamide, octreotide, cyproheptadine[1], methysergide[1]
Osteogenic sarcoma[3]	High-dose methotrexate, doxorubicin, vincristine.	Cyclophosphamide, ifosfamide, bleomycin, dacarbazine, cisplatin, dactinomycin
Soft tissue sarcoma[3]	Doxorubicin, dacarbazine.	Ifosfamide, cyclosphosphamide, etoposide, cisplatin, high-dose methotrexate, vincristine
Melanoma[3]	Dacarbazine, interferon-α, interleukin-2.	Carmustine, lomustine, melphalan, thiotepa, cisplatin, paclitaxel, tamoxifen, vincristine, vaccine therapy (Melacine)[2]
Kaposi's sarcoma	Doxorubicin, vincristine alternating with vinblastine or vincristine alone. Palliative radiation therapy.	Interferon-α, bleomycin, etoposide, doxorubicin
Neuroblastoma[3]	**Combination chemotherapy:** variations of cyclophosphamide, cisplatin, vincristine, doxorubicin, dacarbazine.	Melphalan, ifosfamide, autologous or allogeneic bone marrow transplantation

[1]Supportive agent; not oncolytic.
[2]Investigational agent or procedure. Treatment is available through qualified investigators and centers authorized by the National Cancer Institute and Cooperative Oncology Groups.
[3]These tumors are generally managed initially with surgery with or without radiation therapy and with or without adjuvant chemotherapy. For metastatic disease, the role of palliative radiation therapy is as important as that of chemotherapy.

Table 154. Single-agent dosage and toxicity of anticancer drugs.[1]

Drug	Dosage	Acute Toxicity	Delayed Toxicity
Alkylating agents			
Mechlorethamine	6–10 mg/m^2 intravenously every 3 weeks	Severe vesicant; severe nausea and vomiting	Moderate suppression of blood counts. Melphalan effect may be delayed 4–6 weeks. Excessive doses produce severe bone marrow suppression with leukopenia, thrombocytopenia, and bleeding. Alopecia and hemorrhagic cystitis occur with cyclophosphamide, while busulfan can cause hyperpigmentation, pulmonary fibrosis, and weakness (see text). Ifosfamide is always given with mesna to prevent cystitis. Acute leukemia may develop in 5–10% of patients receiving prolonged therapy with melphalan, mechlorethamine, or chlorambucil; all alkylators probably increase the risk of secondary malignancies with prolonged use. Most cause either temporary or permanent aspermia or amenorrhea.
Chlorambucil	0.1–0.2 mg/kg/d orally (6–12 mg/d) or 0.4 mg/kg pulse every 4 weeks	None	
Cyclophosphamide	100 mg/m^2/d orally for 14 days; 400 mg/m^2 orally for 5 days; 1–1.5 g/m^2 intravenously every 3–4 weeks	Nausea and vomiting with higher doses	
Melphalan	0.25 mg/kg/d orally for 4 days every 6 weeks	None	
Busulfan	2–8 mg/d orally; 150–250 mg/course	None	
Estramustine	14 mg/kg orally in 3 or 4 divided doses	Nausea, vomiting, diarrhea	Thrombosis, thrombocytopenia, hypertension, gynecomastia, glucose intolerance, edema.
Carmustine (BCNU)	200 mg/m^2 intravenously every 6 weeks	Local irritant	Prolonged leukopenia and thrombocytopenia. Rarely hepatitis. Acute leukemia has been observed to occur in some patients receiving nitrosoureas. Nitrosoureas can cause delayed pulmonary fibrosis with prolonged use.
Lomustine (CCNU)	100–130 mg orally every 6–8 weeks	Nausea and vomiting	
Procarbazine	100 mg/m^2/d orally for 14 days every 4 weeks	Nausea and vomiting	Bone marrow suppression, mental suppression, MAO inhibition, disulfiram-like effect.
Dacarbazine	250 mg/m^2/d intravenously for 5 days every 3 weeks; 1500 mg/m^2 intravenously as single dose	Severe nausea and vomiting; anorexia	Bone marrow suppression; flu-like syndrome.
Cisplatin	50–100 mg/m^2 intravenously every 3 weeks; 20 mg/m^2 intravenously for 5 days every 4 weeks	Severe nausea and vomiting	Nephrotoxicity, mild otic and bone marrow toxicity, neurotoxicity.
Carboplatin	360 mg/m^2 intravenously every 4 weeks	Severe nausea and vomiting	Bone marrow suppression, prolonged anemia; same as cisplatin but milder.
Oxaliplatin	85 mg/m^2 intravenously in 250–500 mL D_5W over 2 hours on day 1, with infusional 5-FU/leucovorin on days 1 and 2 every 2 weeks (FOLFOX4)	Nausea, vomiting, diarrhea, fatigue, rare anaphylactic reactions	Peripheral neuropathy, cytopenias, pulmonary toxicity (rare).
Structural analogs or antimetabolites			
Methotrexate	2.5–5 mg/d orally; 20–25 mg intramuscularly twice weekly; high-dose: 500–1000 mg/m^2 every 2–3 weeks; 12–15 mg intrathecally every week for 4–6 doses	None	Bone marrow suppression, oral and gastrointestinal ulceration, acute renal failure; hepatotoxicity, rash, increased toxicity when effusions are present. ***Note:*** Citrovorum factor (leucovorin) rescue for doses over 100 mg/m^2.
Pemetrexed (Alimta)	500 mg/m^2 intravenously every 3 weeks; given with cisplatin or alone; requires folate and vitamin B_{12} supplementation	Skin rash, cytopenias, decreased clearance of agent if given with NSAIDs, nausea, diarrhea, mucositis, hypersensitvity reactions	Cytopenias, rash, neuropathy.

(continued)

Table 154. Single-agent dosage and toxicity of anticancer drugs.[1] (continued)

Drug	Dosage	Acute Toxicity	Delayed Toxicity
Mercaptopurine	2.5 mg/kg/d orally; 100 mg/m^2/d orally for 5 days for induction	None	Well tolerated. Larger doses cause bone marrow suppression.
Thioguanine	2 mg/kg/d orally; 100 mg/m^2/d intravenously for 7 days for induction	Mild nausea, diarrhea	Well tolerated. Larger doses cause bone marrow suppression.
Fluorouracil	15 mg/kg/d intravenously for 3–5 days every 3 weeks; 15 mg/kg weekly as tolerated; 500–1000 mg/m^2 intravenously every 4 weeks	None	Nausea, diarrhea, oral and gastrointestinal ulceration, bone marrow suppression, dacrocystitis.
Capecitabine	2500 mg/m^2 orally twice daily on days 1–14 every 3 weeks	Nausea, diarrhea	Hand and foot syndrome, mucositis.
Cytarabine	100–200 mg/m^2/d for 5–10 days by continuous intravenous infusion; 2–3 g/m^2 intravenously every 12 hours for 3–7 days; 20 mg/m^2 subcutaneously daily in divided doses	High-dose: nausea, vomiting, diarrhea, anorexia	Nausea and vomiting; cystitis; severe bone marrow suppression; megaloblastosis; CNS toxicity with high-dose cytarabine.
Temozolamide	150 mg/m^2 orally for 5 days; repeat every 4 weeks	Headache, nausea, vomiting	Unknown.
Clofarabine	52 mg/m^2 intravenously daily for 5 days every 2–6 weeks	Nausea, vomiting	Bone marrow suppression, hepatobiliary and renal toxicity, capillary leak syndrome
Androgens and androgen antagonists			
Testosterone propionate	100 mg intramuscularly 3 times weekly	None	Fluid retention, masculinization, leg cramps. Cholestatic jaundice in some patients receiving fluoxymesterone.
Fluoxymesterone	20–40 mg/d orally	None	
Flutamide	250 mg 3 times a day orally	None	Gynecomastia, hot flushes, decreased libido, mild gastrointestinal side effects, hepatotoxicity.
Bicalutamide	50 mg/d orally		
Nilutamide	300 mg/d orally for 30 days, then 150 mg/d		
Ethinyl estradiol	3 mg/d orally	None	Fluid retention, feminization, uterine bleeding, exacerbation of cardiovascular disease, painful gynecomastia, thromboembolic disease.
Selective estrogen receptor modulators			
Tamoxifen	20 mg/d orally in 2 divided doses	Transient flare of bone pain; nausea, hot flushes, joint aching	Thromboembolic disease, anovulation, endometrial cancer, cataracts; vaginal bleeding, acne.
Toremifene	60 mg/d orally		
Aromatase inhibitors			
Anastrozole	1 mg orally daily	Hot flushes, joint aching	Thromboembolic disease, vaginal bleeding.
Letrozole	2.5 mg/d orally		
Exemestane	25 mg/d orally		
Pure estrogen receptor antagonist			
Fulvestrant	250 mg intramuscularly once a month	Transient injection site reactions	Nausea, vomiting, constipation, diarrhea, abdominal pain, headache, back pain, hot flushes.
Progestins			
Megestrol acetate	40 mg orally 4 times daily	Hot flushes	Fluid retention; rare thrombosis, weight gain.
Medroxyprogesterone	100–200 mg/d orally; 200–600 mg orally twice weekly	None	

(continued)

Table 154. Single-agent dosage and toxicity of anticancer drugs.[1] (continued)

Drug	Dosage	Acute Toxicity	Delayed Toxicity
GnRH analogs			
Leuprolide	7.5 mg intramuscularly (depot) once a month or 22.5 mg every 3 months as depot injection	Local irritation, transient flare of symptoms	Hot flushes, decreased libido, impotence, gynecomastia, mild gastrointestinal side effects, nausea, diarrhea, fatigue.
Goserelin acetate	3.6 mg subcutaneously monthly or 10.8 mg every 3 months as depot injection		
Triptorelin pamoate	3.75 mg intramuscularly once a month (a 3-month depot formulation also exists)		
Adrenocorticosteroids			
Prednisone	20–100 mg/d orally or 50–100 mg every other day orally with systemic chemotherapy	Alteration in mood	Fluid retention, hypertension, diabetes, increased susceptibility to infection, "moon facies," osteoporosis, electrolyte abnormalities, gastritis.
Dexamethasone	5–10 mg orally daily or twice daily		
Ketoconazole	400 mg orally 3 times daily	Acute nausea	Gynecomastia, hepatotoxicity.
Biologic response modifiers			
Interferon-α-2a Interferon-α-2b	3–5 million units subcutaneously 3 times weekly or daily	Fever, chills, fatigue, anorexia	General malaise, weight loss, confusion, hypothyroidism, retinopathy, autoimmune disease.
Aldesleukin (IL-2)	600,000 units/kg intravenously over 15 minutes every 8 hours for 14 doses, repeated after 9-day rest period. Some doses may be withheld or interrupted because of toxicity. ***Caution:*** High doses must be administered in an ICU setting by experienced personnel.	Hypotension, fever, chills, rigors, diarrhea, nausea, vomiting, pruritus; liver, kidney, and CNS toxicity; capillary leak (primarily at high doses), pruritic skin rash, infections (can be severe)	Hypoglycemia, anemia.
Peptide hormone inhibitor			
Octreotide acetate	100–600 mcg/d subcutaneously in 2 divided doses	Local irritant; nausea and vomiting	Diarrhea, abdominal pain, hypoglycemia.
Natural products and miscellaneous agents			
Vinblastine	0.1–0.2 mg/kg or 6 mg/m^2 intravenously weekly	Mild nausea and vomiting; severe vesicant	Alopecia, peripheral neuropathy, bone marrow suppression, constipation, SIADH, areflexia.
Vincristine	1.5 mg/m^2 (maximum: 2 mg weekly)	Severe vesicant	Areflexia, muscle weakness, peripheral neuropathy, paralytic ileus, alopecia (see text), SIADH.
Vinorelbine	25–30 mg/m^2 intravenously weekly	Mild nausea and vomiting, fatigue, severe vesicant	Granulocytopenia, constipation, peripheral neuropathy, alopecia.
Paclitaxel (Taxol)	175 mg/m^2 over 3 hours every 2 to 3 weeks or 80 mg/m^2 over 1 hour every week	Hypersensitivity reaction (premedicate with diphenhydramine and dexamethasone), mild nausea and vomiting	Peripheral neuropathy, bone marrow suppression, sensory neuropathy fluid retention, myalgia/arthralgias, asthenia alopecia.
Nab-paclitaxel (Abraxane)	260 mg/m^2 intravenously every 3 weeks		
Docetaxel (Taxotere)	60–100 mg/m^2 intravenously every 3 weeks		
Dactinomycin	0.04 mg/kg intravenously weekly	Nausea and vomiting; severe vesicant	Alopecia, stomatitis, diarrhea, bone marrow suppression.

(continued)

Table 154. Single-agent dosage and toxicity of anticancer drugs.[1] (continued)

Drug	Dosage	Acute Toxicity	Delayed Toxicity
Daunorubicin	30–60 mg/m^2 daily intravenously for 3 days, or 30–60 mg/m^2 intravenously weekly		Alopecia, stomatitis, bone marrow suppression, late cardiotoxicity. Risk of cardiotoxicity increases with radiation, cyclophosphamide.
Idarubicin	12 mg/m^2 daily intravenously for 3 days		
Doxorubicin	60 mg/m^2 intravenously every 3 weeks to a maximum total dose of 550 mg/m^2		
Epirubicin	60–100 mg/m^2 intravenously every 3 weeks		
Liposomal doxorubicin (Doxil)	20 mg/m^2 intravenously every 3 weeks	Mild nausea	Hand and foot syndrome; alopecia, stomatitis, and bone marrow suppression uncommon.
Liposomal daunorubicin (DaunoXome)	40 mg/m^2 intravenously every 2 weeks		
Etoposide	100 mg/m^2/d intravenously for 5 days or 50–150 mg/d orally	Nausea and vomiting; occasionally hypotension	Alopecia, bone marrow suppression, secondary leukemia.
Plicamycin (mithramycin)	25–50 mcg/kg intravenously every other day for up to 8 doses	Nausea and vomiting	Thrombocytopenia, diarrhea, hepatotoxicity, nephrotoxicity, stomatitis.
Mitomycin	10–20 mg/m^2 every 6–8 weeks	Severe vesicant; nausea	Prolonged bone marrow suppression, rare hemolytic-uremic syndrome.
Mitoxantrone	12–15 mg/m^2/d intravenously for 3 days with cytarabine; 8–12 mg/m^2 intravenously every 3 weeks	Mild nausea and vomiting	Alopecia, mild mucositis, bone marrow suppression.
Bleomycin	Up to 15 units/m^2 intramuscularly, intravenously, or subcutaneously twice weekly to a total dose of 200 units/m^2	Allergic reactions, fever, hypotension	Fever, dermatitis, pulmonary fibrosis.
Hydroxyurea	500–1500 mg/d orally	Mild nausea and vomiting	Hyperpigmentation, bone marrow suppression.
Mitotane	6–12 g/d orally	Nausea and vomiting	Dermatitis, diarrhea, mental suppression, muscle tremors.
Fludarabine	25 mg/m^2/d intravenously for 5 days every 4 weeks	Nausea and vomiting	Bone marrow suppression, diarrhea, mild hepatotoxicity, immune suppression.
Cladribine (CdA)	0.09 mg/kg/d by continuous intravenous infusion for 7 days	Mild nausea, rash, fatigue	Bone marrow suppression, fever, immune suppression.
Topotecan	1.5 mg/m^2 intravenously daily for 5 days every 3 weeks	Nausea, vomiting, diarrhea, headache, dyspnea	Alopecia, bone marrow suppression.
Gemcitabine	1000 mg/m^2 every week up to 7 weeks, then 1 week off, then weekly for 3 out of 4 weeks	Nausea, vomiting, diarrhea, fever, dyspnea	Bone marrow suppression, rash, fluid retention, mouth sores, flu-like symptoms, paresthesias.
Irinotecan	125 mg/m^2 weekly for 4 weeks, then a 2-week rest, then repeat; given with bevacizumab, 5-FU, and leucovorin	Flushing, salivation, lacrimation, bradycardia, abdominal cramps, diarrhea	Bone marrow suppression, diarrhea.

(continued)

Table 154. Single-agent dosage and toxicity of anticancer drugs.[1] (continued)

Drug	Dosage	Acute Toxicity	Delayed Toxicity
Azacitidine	75 mg/m^2 subcutaneously daily for 7 days, repeat every 4 weeks. May increase to 100 mg/m^2 after 2 cycles if no response	Nausea, fever, injection site infection	Neutropenia, thrombocytopenia, fatigue, anorexia, liver and renal toxicity (rare).
Novel therapeutic agents			
Imatinib mesylate (STI571; Gleevec)	400–600 mg/d orally	Mild nausea	Myalgias, edema, bone marrow suppression, abnormal liver function tests.
Gefitinib (Iressa)	250 mg by mouth daily	Nausea, vomiting	Diarrhea, rash, acne, dry skin, pruritus, anorexia, asthenia, interstitial lung disease (rare).
Erlotinib (Tarceva)	150 mg by mouth daily	Mild nausea	Rash, diarrhea, anorexia, fatigue, transaminitis, interstitial lung disease (rare).
Alemtuzumab (Campath-1H)	30 mg 3 times a week by subcutaneous injection for up to 12 weeks. (Use dose escalation to reduce infusion-related events.)	Severe infusion-related events, injection site irritation	Infections, short-term bone marrow suppression, autoimmune hemolytic anemia.
Gemtuzumab ozogamicin (Mylotarg)	9 mg/m^2 for 2 doses given 14 days apart	Infusion-related events	Profound bone marrow suppression.
Tretinoin	45 mg/m^2 by mouth daily until remission or for 90 days	Retinoic acid syndrome (fever, dyspnea, pleural or pericardial effusion) must be treated emergently with dexamethasone	Headache, dry skin, rash, flushing.
Arsenic trioxide	Induction: 0.15 mg/kg intravenously daily until remission; maximum 60 doses Consolidation: 0.15 mg/kg intravenously daily for 25 doses	Same as tretinoin	Nausea, vomiting, diarrhea, edema.
Trastuzumab (Herceptin)	Load: 4 mg/kg intravenously followed by 2 mg/kg weekly	Low-grade fever, chills, fatigue, constitutional symptoms with first infusion	Cardiac toxicity, especially when given with anthracyclines.
Denileukin diftitox (ONTAK)	9–10 mcg/kg/d intravenously for 5 days every 21 days	Hypersensitivity type reactions with first infusion	Vascular leak syndrome, low albumin, increased risk of infections, diarrhea, rash.
Rituximab	375 mg/m^2 intravenously weekly for 4–8 doses	Hypersensitivity type reactions with first infusion; fever, tumor lysis syndrome (can be life-threatening)	Mild cytopenias, rare red cell aplasia or aplastic anemia, severe mucocutaneous reactions.
Ibritumomab tiuxetan (Zevalin)	0.3–0.4 mCi/kg (not to exceed 32 mCi); dosing must follow rituximab	Rituximab infusion reaction symptom complex	Prolonged and severe myelosuppression, nausea, vomiting, abdominal pain, arthralgias.
Bortezomib (Velcade)	1.3 mg/m^2 by intravenous bolus twice a week for 2 weeks followed by a 10-day rest. Repeat every 3 weeks.	Low-grade nausea, diarrhea, low-grade fever, weakness	Peripheral neuropathy, thrombocytopenia, edema.

(*continued*)

Table 154. Single-agent dosage and toxicity of anticancer drugs.[1] (continued)

Drug	Dosage	Acute Toxicity	Delayed Toxicity
^{131}I Tositumomab (Bexxar)	^{131}I Tositumomab must be given with tositumomab (T). Dosimetric step: 450 mg T over 60 minutes followed by ^{131}I T containing 35 mg T with 5 mCi ^{131}I. Therapeutic step: Calculated to deliver 75 cGy total body irradiation with 35 mg T.	Hypersensitivity reactions	Prolonged and severe myelosuppression, nausea, vomiting, abdominal pains, arthralgias.
Targretin	300 mg/m^2/d orally	Nausea	Hyperlipidemia, dry mouth, dry skin, constipation, leukopenia, edema.
Bevacizumab (Avastin)	5 mg/kg intravenously every 2 weeks; given with irinotecan, 5-FU, and leucovorin (IFL)	Asthenia, hypertension, diarrhea, hypersensitivity reactions	Proteinuria, hypertension, thromboembolism, gastrointestinal perforation, wound dehiscence, hemoptysis (lung cancer).
Cetuximab (Erbitux)	400 mg/m^2 intravenous loading dose, then 250 mg/m^2 once a week; given alone or with irinotecan; requires special tubing	Rare severe infusion reactions, diarrhea, nausea, abdominal pain	Interstitial lung disease, acneiform rash, sun sensitivity.
Supportive agents			
Allopurinol	300–900 mg/d orally for prevention or relief of hyperuricemia	None	Rash, Stevens-Johnson syndrome; enhances effects and toxicity of mercaptopurine when used in combination.
Mesna	20% of ifosfamide dosage at the time of ifosfamide administration, then 4 and 8 hours after each dose of chemotherapy to prevent hemorrhagic cystitis	Nausea, vomiting, diarrhea	None.
Leucovorin	10 mg/m^2 every 6 hours intravenously or orally until serum methotrexate levels are below 5×10^{-8} mol/L with hydration and urinary alkalinization (about 72 hours)	None	Enhances toxic effects of fluorouracil.
Amifostine	910 mg/m^2 intravenously daily, 30 minutes prior to chemotherapy	Hypotension, nausea, vomiting, flushing	Decrease in serum calcium.
Dexrazoxane	10:1 ratio of anthracycline intravenously, before (within 30 minutes of) chemotherapy infusion	Pain on injection	Increased bone marrow suppression.
Palifermin	60 mcg/kg/d intravenous bolus daily for 3 days before and 3 days after myelotoxic chemotherapy (total of 6 doses separated from chemotherapy by at least 24 hours)	None	Skin rash, skin eythema, edema, pruritis, oral dysesthesias.
Pilocarpine hydrochloride	5–10 mg orally 3 times daily	Sweating, headache, flushing; nausea, chills, rhinitis, dizziness, and urinary frequency at high dosage.	

(continued)

Table 154. Single-agent dosage and toxicity of anticancer drugs.[1] (continued)

Drug	Dosage	Acute Toxicity	Delayed Toxicity
Pamidronate	90 mg intravenously every month	Symptomatic hypoglycemia (rare), flare of bone pain, local irritation	Osteonecrosis, renal insufficiency.
Zoledronic acid	4 mg intravenously every month		
Epoetin alfa (erythropoietin)	100–300 units/kg intravenously or subcutaneously 3 times a week	Skin irritation or pain at injection site	Hypertension, headache, seizures in patients on dialysis (rare).
Darbopoetin alfa	200 mcg subcutaneously every other week or 300 mcg subcutaneously every 3 weeks[2]	Injection site pain	Hypertension, thromboses, headache, diarrhea.
Filgrastim (G-CSF)	5 mcg/kg/d subcutaneously or intravenously daily until neutrophils recover	Mild to moderate bone pain, mild hypotension (rare), irritation at injection sites (rare)	Bone pain, hypoxia.
Pegfilgrastim	6 mg subcutaneously on day 2 of each 2- to 3-week chemotherapy cycle[2]	Injection site reactions	Bone pain, hypoxia.
Sargramostim (GM-CSF)	250 mcg/kg/d as a 2-hour intravenous infusion (can be given subcutaneously)	Fluid retention, dyspnea, capillary leak (rare), supraventricular tachycardia (rare), mild to moderate bone pain, irritation at injection sites	
Neumega (IL-11)	50 mcg/kg/d subcutaneously	Fluid retention, arrhythmias, headache, arthralgias, myalgias	Unknown.
Gallium nitrate	200 mg/m^2 intravenously daily by continuous infusion for 5 days	Hypocalcemia, transient hypophosphatemia	Renal insufficiency, hypocalcemia.
Samarium-153 lexidronam (Sm-153 EDTMP)	1 mCi/kg intravenously as single dose	None	Hematopoietic suppression.
Strontium-89	4 mCi every 3 months intravenously	None	Hematopoietic suppression.

[1]5-FU = 5-fluorouracil; NSAIDs = nonsteroidal anti-inflammatory drugs; MAO = monoamine oxidase; GnRH = gonadotropin-releasing hormone; CNS = central nervous system; IL = interleukin; SIADH = syndrome of inappropriate antidiuretic hormone; G-CSF = granulocyte colony-stimulating factor; GM-CSF = granulocyte-macrophage colony-stimulating factor.
[2]Off label.

Table 155. A common scheme for dose modification of cancer chemotherapeutic agents.[1]

Granulocyte Count	Platelet Count	Suggested Dosage (% of Full Dose)
> 2000/mcL	> 100,000/mcL	100%
1000–2000/mcL	75,000–100,000/mcL	50%
< 1000/mcL	< 50,000/mcL	0%

[1]In general, dose modification should be avoided to maintain therapeutic efficacy. The use of myeloid growth factors or a delay in the start of the next cycle of chemotherapy is usually effective.

Table 156. Paraneoplastic syndromes associated with common cancers.[1]

Syndromes; Hormone Excess	Small Cell Lung Cancer	Non-Small Cell Lung Cancer	Breast Cancer	Multiple Myeloma	Gastro-intestinal Cancers	Hepato-cellular Cancer	Gesta-tional Tropho-blastic Disease	Lym-phoma	Renal Cell Cancer	Carci-noid	Thymo-ma	Ovarian Cancer	Prostate Cancer	Myelo-prolifer-ative Disease	Adreno-cortical Tumors	Cerebellar Heman-gioblas-tomas
Endocrine																
Cushing's syndrome	XX	X														
SIADH[2]	XX	X														
Hypercalcemia	XX	X	X	X				X				X				
Hypoglycemia					X	X										
Gonadotropin excess	XX	X			X		X		X	X						
Hyperthyroidism							X									
Neuromuscular																
Subacute cerebellar degeneration	XX	X			X			X				X				
Sensorimotor peripheral neuropathy	XX	X														
Lambert-Eaton syndrome	XX		X		X							X				
Stiff man syndrome			X									X				
Dermatomyositis/polymyositis	XX	X	X		XX							X		X		
Skin																
Dermatomyositis	XX	X	X		XX							X		X		
Acanthosis nigricans		X	X		X					X			X	X		

Sweet's syndrome		X	X		X			XX	X			X	X	XX		
Hematologic																
Erythrocytosis						X			X			X			X	X
Pure red cell aplasia		X	X		X			X			XX					
Eosinophilia								XX								
Thrombocytosis	X	X	X	X	X	X	X	X	X	X	X	X	X	X	X	X
Coagulopathy			X					X	X				X	X		
Fever	X	X	X	X	X	X	X	X	X	X	X	X	X	X	X	X
Amyloidosis				X				X	X							

[1]XX = strong association; X = reported association.
[2]SIADH = syndrome of inappropriate antidiuretic hormone.

Index

D

G

U